Small Animal Soft Tissue Surgery

Small Animal Soft Tissue Surgery

Second Edition

Edited by

Eric Monnet, DVM, PhD, FAHA
Diplomate ACVS, ECVS
Professor, Department of Clinical Sciences
College of Veterinary Medicine and Biomedical Sciences
Colorado State University
Fort Collins, CO
USA

WILEY Blackwell

Registered Office
John Wiley & Sons, Inc., 111 River Street, Hoboken, NJ 07030, USA

For details of our global editorial offices, customer services, and more information about Wiley products visit us at www.wiley.com.

Wiley also publishes its books in a variety of electronic formats and by print-on-demand. Some content that appears in standard print versions of this book may not be available in other formats.

Library of Congress Cataloging-in-Publication Data applied for
ISBN: 9781119693680 (hardback)

Cover Design: Wiley
Cover Images: © Eric Monnet

Set in 10.5/12.5pt Minion by Straive, Pondicherry, India

Printed in Singapore
M107168_060223

Contents

List of Contributors

Pierre Amsellem
Veterinary Medical Center
University of Minnesota
St. Paul, MN, USA

Nicholas J. Bacon
AURA Veterinary
Guildford, UK

Wendy Baltzer
School of Veterinary Science
Massey University
Palmerston North, New Zealand

Yoav Bar-Am
Koret School of Veterinary Medicine
Hebrew University of Jerusalem
Jerusalem, Israel

Jamie R. Bellah
Department of Clinical Sciences
Auburn University College of Veterinary Medicine
Auburn, AL, USA

Allyson Berent
Interventional Endoscopy/Radiology
Animal Medical Center
New York, USA

Jitender Bhandal
Westbank Animal Care Hospital
West Kelowna, BC, Canada

Anthony Blikslager
College of Veterinary Medicine
North Carolina State University
Raleigh, NC, USA

Benjamin Brainard
College of Veterinary Medicine
University of Georgia
Athens, GA, USA

Ronald Bright
Retired

Floryne O. Buishand
Royal Veterinary College
University of London
London, UK

Serge Chalhoub
Faculty of Veterinary Medicine
University of Calgary
Calgary, AB, Canada

Robert Cole
Department of Clinical Sciences
Auburn University College of Veterinary Medicine
Auburn, AL, USA

William T.N. Culp
School of Veterinary Medicine
University of California–Davis
Davis, CA, USA

Daniel A. Degner
Michigan Veterinary Specialists
Auburn Hills, MI, USA

Gilles Dupré
La Garde, France

James P. Farese
Golden Gate Veterinary Specialists
San Rafael, CA, USA

Barbro Filliquist
School of Veterinary Medicine
University of California–Davis
Davis, CA, USA

Kaitlin Fiske
Department of Clinical Sciences
Auburn University College of Veterinary Medicine
Auburn, AL, USA

Erin A. Gibson
University of Pennsylvania
School of Veterinary Medicine
Philadelphia, PA, USA

Carlos Gradil
Department of Veterinary and Animal Sciences
University of Massachusetts Amherst
Amherst, MA, USA

Maureen Griffin
School of Veterinary Medicine
University of Pennsylvania
Philadelphia, PA, USA

Elizabeth M. Hardie
College of Veterinary Medicine
North Carolina State University
Raleigh, NC, USA

Robert J. Hardie
Department of Surgical Sciences
School of Veterinary Medicine
University of Wisconsin
Madison, WI, USA

John Hathcock
Department of Clinical Sciences
Auburn University College of Veterinary Medicine
Auburn, AL, USA

Tracy L. Hill
College of Veterinary Medicine
University of Minnesota
Minneapolis, MN, USA

Fiona Hollinshead
Department of Clinical Sciences
Colorado Sate University
Fort Collins, CO, USA

Naomi Hoyer
Department of Clinical Sciences
Colorado State University
Fort Collins, CO, USA

Robert Kennis
Department of Clinical Sciences
Auburn University College of Veterinary Medicine
Auburn, AL, USA

Jolle Kirpensteijn
Hill's Pet Nutrition
Topeka, KS, USA

Lisa Klopp
Department of Clinical Sciences
Colorado State University
Fort Collins, CO, USA

Dorothee Krainer
Department of Small Animal Surgery
AniCura Tierklinik
Hollabrunn, Austria

Natali Krekeler
Faculty of Veterinary Science
University of Melbourne
Melbourne, VIC, Australia

Raymond K. Kudej
Cummings School of Veterinary Medicine
Tufts University
North Grafton, MA, USA

Michelle Kutzler
College of Agricultural Sciences
Oregon State University
Corvallis, OR, USA

Cathy Langston
College of Veterinary Medicine
Ohio State University
Columbus, OH, USA

B. Duncan X. Lascelles
College of Veterinary Medicine
North Carolina State University
Raleigh, NC, USA

Julius M. Liptak
Capital City Small Animal Mobile Surgery
Ottawa, ON, Canada

Dawn Logas
Veterinary Dermatology Center
Maitland, FL, USA

Lori Ludwig
Sea Island Animal Hospital
Beaufort, SC, USA

Catriona M. MacPhail
Department of Clinical Sciences
Colorado State University
Fort Collins, CO, USA

F.A. (Tony) Mann
College of Veterinary Medicine
University of Missouri
Columbus, MO, USA

Angela J. Marolf
Department of Veterinary Clinical Sciences
Columbus, OH, USA

Kyle G. Mathews
College of Veterinary Medicine
North Caroline State University
Raleigh, NC, USA

Brad M. Matz
Department of Clinical Sciences
Auburn University College of Veterinary Medicine
Auburn, AL, USA

Marie-Pauline Maurin
School of Veterinary Medicine
University College Dublin
Dublin, Ireland

Philipp D. Mayhew
School of Veterinary Medicine
University of California—Davis
Davis, CA, USA

Elisa M. Mazzaferro
Wheat Ridge Animal Hospital
Wheat Ridge, CO, USA

Jonathan F. McAnulty
School of Veterinary Medicine
University of Wisconsin–Madison
Madison, WI, USA

Robert McCarthy
School of Veterinary Medicine
Tufts University
North Grafton, MA, USA

Janet Kovak McClaran
London Vet Specialists
London, UK

Steve J. Mehler
Hope Veterinary Specialists
Malvern, PA, USA

Carlos Henrique de Mello Souza
College of Veterinary Medicine
University of Missouri
Columbus, MO, USA

Eric Monnet
Department of Clinical Sciences
Colorado State University
Fort Collins, CO, USA

Carmel T. Mooney
School of Veterinary Medicine
University College Dublin
Dublin, Ireland

Dennis Olsen
Veterinary Clinic
College of Southern Nevada
Las Vegas, NV, USA

Ronald S. Olsen
Virginia–Maryland College of Veterinary Medicine
Blacksburg, VA, USA

E. Christopher Orton
Department of Clinical Sciences
Colorado State University
Fort Collins, CO, USA

Heidi Phillips
Department of Veterinary Clinical Medicine
University of Illinois
Urbana, IL, USA

Jennifer Prittie
Animal Medical Center
New York, NY, USA

Marije Risselada
Department of Veterinary Clinical Sciences
Purdue University
West Lafayette, IN, USA

Jeffrey J. Runge
Soft Tissue & Orthopedic Surgery
Guardian Veterinary Specialists
Brewster, NY, USA

Stewart D. Ryan
Department of Veterinary Pathology
University of Melbourne
Werribee, VIC, Australia

Nina Samuel
School of Veterinary Medicine
University of California–Davis
Davis, CA, USA

Michael Schaer
Department of Small Animal Clinical Sciences
University of Florida Veterinary Medical Center
Gainesville, FL, USA

Chad Schmiedt
Department of Small Animal Medicine and Surgery
University of Georgia
Athens, GA, USA

Bernard Séguin
Department of Surgical Oncology
Central Victoria Veterinary Hospital
Victoria, BC, Canada

Sara Shropshire
Department of Clinical Sciences
Colorado State University
Fort Collins, CO, USA

Amelia M. Simpson
Veterinary Surgical Center of Portland
Portland, OR, USA

Ramesh K. Sivacolundhu
Balcatta Vet24
Balcatta, WA, Australia

Daniel D. Smeak
College of Veterinary Medicine
Colorado State University
Fort Collins, CO, USA

Fran Smith
Smith Veterinary Hospital
Burnsville, MN, USA

Thomas J. Smith
School of Veterinary and Biomedical Sciences
James Cook University
Townsville, QLD, Australia

Jörg M. Steiner
Gastrointestinal Laboratory
Department of Veterinary Small Animal
Clinical Sciences
College of Veterinary Medicine and Biomedical
Sciences
College Station, TX, USA

Anne Sylvestre
Veterinary Referral Surgical Services
Kitchener, ON, Canada

Dawna Voelkl
Meadowlands Veterinary Hospital
Washington, PA, USA

Dietrich Volkmann
Veterinary Health Center
University of Missouri
Columbia, MO, USA

Richard Walshaw
Animal Surgical Center of Michigan
Flint, MI, USA

Kyla Walter
School of Veterinary Medicine
Veterinary Medical Teaching Hospital
University of California–Davis
Davis, CA, USA

Craig B. Webb
Department of Clinical Sciences
Colorado State University
Fort Collins, CO, USA

Chick Weisse
Animal Medical Center
New York, NY, USA

Stephen J. Withrow
Department of Clinical Sciences
Colorado State University
Fort Collins, CO, USA

Deanna R. Worley
Department of Clinical Sciences
Colorado State University
Fort Collins, CO, USA

Panagiotis G. Xenoulis
Gastrointestinal Laboratory
Department of Veterinary Small Animal
Clinical Sciences
College of Veterinary Medicine and
Biomedical Sciences
College Station, TX, USA

Kristin Zersen
Veterinary Teaching Hospital
Colorado State University
Fort Collins, CO, USA

Preface

Claude Bourgelat, Director of the Lyon Academy of Horsemanship, founded the first veterinary school in France in 1761. The main objective was to train veterinarians to protect cattle and horses against diseases. Little did he know about the amazing transformation veterinary science would go through from the time he created the first veterinary school and wrote his book *Elements of Horsemanship*. A number of specialties have evolved, including internal medicine, dermatology, ophthalmology, cardiology, neurology, oncology, radiology, dentistry, and surgery.

The limits of surgery have been extended with the development of new diagnostic tools, better understanding of pathophysiology, and new imaging techniques such as ultrasound, magnetic resonance imaging, computed tomography, and nuclear medicine. Cardiopulmonary bypass has become available to small animal surgeons. Oncologic surgery has expanded in the last 30 years because of the development of imaging technology and a better understanding of the pathophysiology of different tumors. Minimally invasive surgery and interventional radiology have emerged and have expanded exponentially in the last decade. As a consequence, veterinary surgery is becoming more specialized, with a general division between orthopedic surgery and soft tissue surgery. Thus a textbook of small animal soft tissue surgery is required.

In this second edition of this textbook, all the chapters have been revised and edited, and some new chapters have been added. This second edition of this textbook, like the first, has four goals. First, it had to be based as much as possible on evidence. Therefore, authors were selected who were known for the most recent contributions to the field. Each author was asked to perform a thorough review of the literature and to present evidence-based information. Since soft tissue surgery requires the interaction of several specialties (internal medicine, imaging, and critical care), most chapters have several authors. Each author was responsible for a specific aspect of the chapter (i.e., internal medicine, radiology, surgery, and critical care).

Second, since the textbook is strictly focused on soft tissue surgery, general chapters on surgical biology and on anesthesia and pain management are not included. Similarly, I did not include chapters on wound management or neurosurgery, since excellent textbooks on these topics are already available.

Third, I wanted the textbook to provide good documentation and illustrations. Surgery cannot be understood and performed without good illustrations. With this in mind, I selected one of the best medical illustrators, Dennis Giddings, who was the illustrator of *An Atlas of Surgical Approaches to the Bones and Joints of the Dog and Cat*, edited by Piermattei and Johnson. The illustrations went back and forth several times between the illustrator, authors, editor, and publisher to ensure the best results. Also, a website with excellent color intraoperative pictures and videos about the procedures is included with the textbook. The videos describe each surgical procedure step by step. This website is a work in progress and will be expanded with future editions.

Lastly, this textbook is intended for a wide audience, from private practitioners to specialists, including residents studying for boards. Because the most recent literature has been reviewed, the book should be of great help to residents.

The book is divided into systems, and each system subdivided into diseases or syndromes. This has allowed a thorough discussion of each important topic. The anatomy or physiology related to a certain condition is only briefly reviewed when needed. Readers are referred to specific textbooks that specialize on the topic. Knowledge of each topic is becoming so important that each chapter focuses specifically on the pathophysiology, diagnosis, and treatment of each disease or syndrome.

I would like to thank all the authors and section editors who helped me during the long process of creating the second edition of this textbook. This book will be updated as often as needed in order to stay up to date with progress in the veterinary surgery of small animals.

Eric Monnet
Professor, Small Animal Surgery,
Colorado State University

About the Companion Website

This book is accompanied by a companion website:

www.wiley.com/go/monnet/small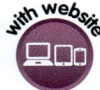

The website includes:

- Videos

Section 1

Gastrointestinal Surgery

1

Disorders of the Salivary Gland

Catriona M. MacPhail

Salivary glands can be affected by inflammation, trauma, calculus formation, and neoplasia, resulting in abscessation, rupture of the duct or gland, and formation of a salivary mucocele, obstruction, or pain on palpation or opening of the mouth. The mode of therapy is generally dictated by the type of lesion present (abscess, mucocele, neoplasia).

Anatomy

There are four paired salivary glands in the dog and cat: parotid, mandibular, sublingual, and zygomatic glands. The cat also has paired molar glands, which lie in the lower lip at the angle of the mouth. In addition, there are numerous buccal glands present in the soft palate, lips, tongue, and cheeks. The salivary glands most commonly injured or involved in pathologic processes (calculi, neoplasia, trauma) are the mandibular and sublingual salivary glands.

The mandibular salivary gland is a mixed gland (serous and mucous secretion) located in the junction of the maxillary (internal maxillary) vein and lingual facial (external maxillary) vein as they form the jugular vein. It is adherent cranially to the darker monostomatic portion of the sublingual gland, and shares a common heavy fibrous capsule with that gland. The mandibular duct leaves the medial portion of the gland near the sublingual gland and runs craniomedially, medial to the caudal sublingual gland, between the masseter muscle and mandible laterally and the digastricus muscle medially, to empty in the sublingual papilla lateral to the cranial frenulum of the tongue.

The sublingual duct originates at the caudal portion of the gland and joins the mandibular duct. The secretions of the separate lobes of the monostomatic portion of the sublingual gland drain through four to six short excretory ducts into the sublingual duct. The polystomatic portion of the sublingual gland lies under the mucosa of the tongue and secretes directly into the oral cavity rather than through the main sublingual duct.

Diseases of the parotid and zygomatic salivary glands occur infrequently in the dog and cat. The parotid gland is triangular in shape and is located at the base of the horizontal ear canal. The parotid duct runs rostrally along the lateral surface of the masseter muscle and opens into the oral cavity at the level of the second to fourth premolars. The zygomatic gland is located deep and medial to the zygomatic arch, dorsolateral to the medial pterygoid muscle. The major zygomatic duct opens into the oral cavity opposite the last upper molar.

Pathophysiology

Disorders of the salivary glands are generally uncommon in the dog and cat. Salivary gland problems most often manifest as submandibular swelling, which can either be painful or nonpainful depending on the underlying cause. Differential diagnoses for submandibular swelling include inflammation, abscess formation, lymphadenopathy, neoplasia, or salivary mucocele. Submandibular abscessation is usually secondary to bite wounds or oropharyngeal foreign body penetration. These abscesses are rarely associated with the salivary glands. Fine-needle aspiration and cytology facilitate definitive diagnosis, although diagnostic imaging may also be indicated. Both the ultrasonographic and computed tomographic appearance of sialoceles have been

Small Animal Soft Tissue Surgery, Second Edition. Edited by Eric Monnet.
© 2023 John Wiley & Sons, Inc. Published 2023 by John Wiley & Sons, Inc.
Companion website: www.wiley.com/go/monnet/small

described (Torad & Hassan 2013; Oetelaar *et al.* 2022). Removal of the affected glands is often the treatment of choice.

Specific disorders

Salivary mucocele (sialocele)

Salivary mucocele formation is the most common disease of the salivary gland in the dog and cat. The mucocele is formed from secretion of saliva from a defect in the gland or duct system. The most commonly affected glands are the mandibular and sublingual, with the sublingual gland being the most frequent source of saliva. The lining of the mucocele consists of inflammatory tissue surrounded by granulation tissue. There is no evidence of a secretory lining present in the mucocele and therefore it cannot be considered a true cyst.

There are three major types of salivary mucocele based on the location of the swelling: cervical mucocele, sublingual mucocele (ranula), and pharyngeal mucocele. Zygomatic and parotid mucoceles can also occur but are very uncommon. Nasopharyngeal sialoceles have been reported in brachycephalic breeds, thought to be a rare consequence of nonphysiologic mechanical stress on the minor salivary glands (De Lorenzi *et al.* 2018).

Cervical mucoceles are generally located on the lateral aspect of the head and neck from the level of the mandibular and sublingual salivary glands to the intermandibular space. The majority of patients present with mucoceles in the intermandibular region. Sublingual mucoceles, or ranulas, are formed from an accumulation of saliva along the base of the tongue. A less common location for salivary mucoceles is the pharynx. Pharyngeal mucoceles appear as a fluctuant, smooth, dome-shaped swelling in the lateral pharyngeal wall.

The etiology of salivary mucoceles is generally unknown, but causes such as trauma, inflammation, sialoliths, foreign bodies, and iatrogenic damage during surgery have been implicated (Figure 1.1). It is generally felt that mucoceles result from damage to the duct or gland tissue with leakage of saliva into the tissues. The monostomatic (cervical mucocele) and polystomatic (pharyngeal mucocele and ranula) portions of the sublingual salivary gland are felt to be the most commonly involved. Poodles and German shepherds are thought to be the most common breeds affected, but numerous breeds have been reported to have developed salivary mucoceles.

Cervical mucocele

The diagnosis of a cervical mucocele is based on history, physical examination, palpation, and aspiration of blood-tinged saliva. Differential diagnoses include cervical abscess, neoplasia, enlarged mandibular lymph

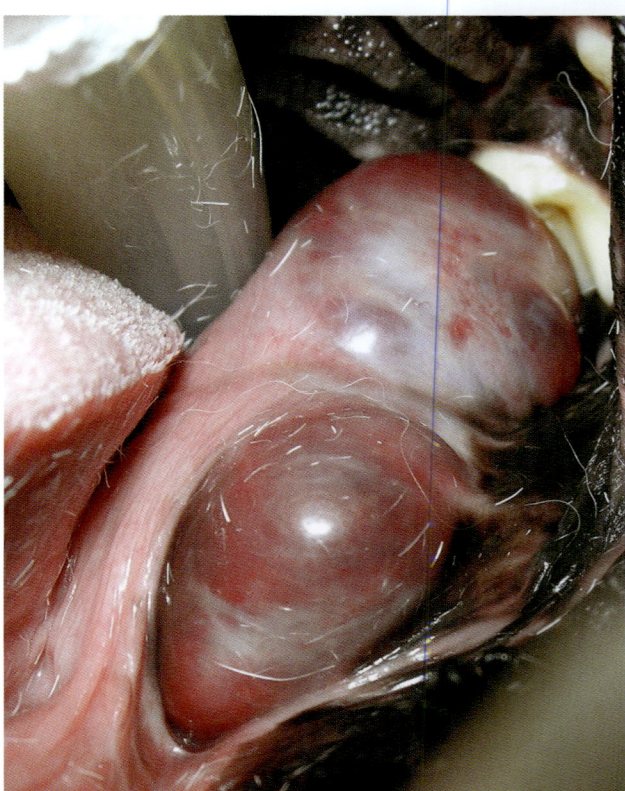

Figure 1.1 Intraoral view of an iatrogenic ranula in an 8-year-old Alaskan malamute following partial mandibulectomy.

nodes, and draining tract secondary to foreign body migration. However, the diagnosis of a mucocele is often made based on the gross appearance of the aspirated fluid. Cytology may be helpful if secondary infection is suspected. A mucus-specific stain, such as periodic acid–Schiff, will confirm that aspirated fluid is saliva, although this step is often unnecessary.

The treatment of choice for cervical mucocele is removal of the mandibular and sublingual salivary glands and associated ducts on the affected side, followed by ventral drainage of the accumulated saliva. Both the mandibular and sublingual glands are removed due to the close anatomic association between the two glands. Often, patients with cervical mucoceles will present with a midline intermandibular cervical mass, making lateralization difficult. Determination of the glands involved (right vs. left side) can be accomplished by thorough historical evaluation (which may reveal the side initially involved), careful oral examination (presence of ranula or pharyngeal mucocele), palpation of the swelling, placement of the animal in dorsal recumbency, or sialography.

Sialography is only necessary in a small percentage (5%) of cases. The technique involves injecting radiopaque contrast material retrograde into the ductal openings in the frenulum. Reflux of contrast into the swelling will determine the affected side. This procedure is time-consuming and can be technically difficult to perform.

If the affected side is unable to be determined or if the mucocele appears to be bilateral, bilateral resection of the mandibular and sublingual glands can be performed without any consequences to saliva production.

Removal of the mandibular and sublingual salivary glands is performed by first positioning the dog in lateral recumbency with the affected side facing up. The neck and jaw should be positioned slightly obliquely and towels or sandbags placed under the neck to elevate the surgical site for better visualization of the bifurcation of the jugular vein.

The incision is made from the ramus of the mandible cranially to the bifurcation of the jugular vein caudally; occlusion of the jugular vein prior to incision will facilitate visualization of landmarks. Dissection is carried into the capsule of the mandibular and sublingual salivary glands. An intracapsular dissection of the glands is performed and the ducts of the mandibular and sublingual salivary glands are followed craniomedially to the mandible. The ducts are followed as far cranially as possible and ligated or stripped out to complete the resection. Tunneling under the digastricus muscles may improve the completeness of the salivary duct excision (Marsh & Adin 2013). A small active drain can be placed in the cervical mucocele to allow drainage of the remaining saliva and accumulated fluid (Figure 1.2). The drain is typically removed 3–5 days postoperatively. If the salivary glandular tissue has an unusual appearance at the time of resection, it should be submitted for histopathologic evaluation. Closure of the incision includes apposition of muscle, subcutaneous tissues, and skin with simple interrupted or simple continuous sutures.

Alternatively, a ventral approach can be considered (Ritter *et al.* 2006). An incision is made from the level of the linguofacial vein to the rostral intermandibular space. The mandibular gland is located at the caudal aspect of this incision. An intracapsular dissection is performed as already described with dissection of the salivary chain rostrally to the level of the digastricus muscle. The digastricus muscle is then undermined from a cranial direction in order to follow the ducts as they course rostrally under the mylohyoideus muscle. This muscle is incised to gain access to residual sublingual salivary glandular tissue.

When comparing the lateral to the ventral approach, the ventral paramedian approach was associated with a lower risk of recurrence but higher rate of surgical wound complications (Cinti *et al.* 2021); long-term outcomes appear to be comparable between the two techniques (Swieton *et al.* 2022).

Complications associated with salivary gland resection are few, but may include inadvertent lymph node removal, operation on the incorrect side, incisional

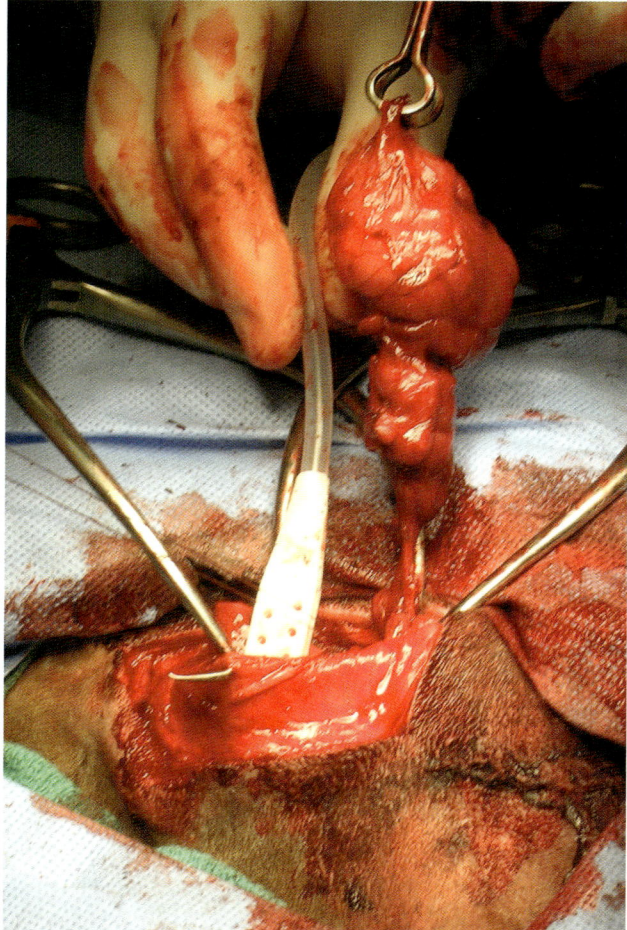

Figure 1.2 Intraoperative view of mandibular and sublingual salivary gland removal with active drain placement into the cervical mucocele.

infection, submandibular seroma, and recurrence due to incomplete removal. Prognosis following surgery is generally good to excellent, with very low recurrence rates. This is in contrast to a 42% recurrence rate associated with surgical drainage alone (Bellenger & Simpson 1992). Radiation therapy has been shown to be effective in resolving cervical sialoceles refractory to surgical management (Poirier *et al.* 2018).

Ranula

A ranula is a thin-walled linear swelling that results from ruptured sublingual or mandibular salivary ducts below the oral mucosa next to the tongue. It may also occur due to rupture of the polystomatic portion of the sublingual gland. Diagnosis is based on history, oral examination, palpation, and aspiration of the mass. Blood-tinged saliva on aspiration is diagnostic.

The treatment of choice is marsupialization of the ranula. Marsupialization is performed by incising into the swelling and resecting an elliptical segment of the overlying sublingual mucosa. The cut edges of the remaining mucosa are sutured to adjacent tissues in a simple continuous pattern with rapidly absorbable suture, thereby creating a pouch that allows saliva to drain into the oral cavity.

If there is recurrence or the ranula is associated with a cervical mucocele, the mandibular and sublingual salivary glands on the affected side should be removed.

Pharyngeal mucocele

Patients with pharyngeal mucocele may present with signs related to upper airway obstruction, since the swelling eventually becomes large enough to occlude the laryngeal orifice (Figure 1.3). Affected patients may have a history of noisy respiration progressing to intermittent dyspnea, cyanosis, and syncope in severe cases.

A presumptive diagnosis can be made by careful oral examination. The pharyngeal mucocele appears as a fluctuant, smooth, dome-shaped swelling in the lateral pharyngeal wall. Aspiration of blood-tinged saliva is diagnostic, and is generally performed when the patient is under anesthesia to avoid unnecessary stress.

Pharyngeal mucoceles are treated by marsupialization. The swelling is incised and drained by partially excising the overlying pharyngeal mucosa and suturing

the cut edges of the mucosa to the adjacent pharyngeal wall. An alternative technique is to dissect the mucocele free from the surrounding tissue and remove it en bloc. The pharyngeal wall is allowed to heal by granulation. Either procedure generally gives rewarding results. Recurrence is rare, but unilateral mandibular and sublingual salivary gland resection should be done if recurrence does occur or to avoid the potential for recurrence, due to the life-threatening clinical signs associated with this condition.

Zygomatic mucocele

Sialoceles associated with the zygomatic glands are rare. Dogs may present with a variety of clinical signs, the most common being ventral periorbital swelling. Other signs included exophthalmos, periocular pain, chemosis, and nictitating membrane protrusion. The typical location of the swelling is similar to that seen with maxillary carnassial tooth root abscesses. These conditions are differentiated by fine-needle aspiration. Advanced imaging (computed tomography [CT] or magnetic resonance imaging [MRI]) may also be beneficial in diagnosis, particularly in investigating other causes of exophthalmos. Treatment of choice is excision of the zygomatic gland, most often requiring resection of the zygomatic arch for best exposure and access. However, a ventral nonostectomy approach has been described in cadavers, allowing for complete zygomatic gland excision (Dörner *et al.* 2021). Intracanalicular injection of 10% N-acetylcysteine has also been reported with good success for resolution (Ortillés *et al.* 2020).

Parotid mucocele

Sialoceles associated with the parotid glands are also very uncommon. Dogs present with a fluctuant nonpainful swelling over the area of the parotid gland on the lateral side of the face. Advanced imaging (e.g., sialography, CT, MRI) is often required for diagnosis. Treatment is complete parotidectomy, which can be a difficult procedure due to the regional anatomy (e.g., facial nerve) and as the capsule is tightly adhered to the gland. Alternatively, the parotid duct can be ligated as close as possible to the gland to cause atrophy.

Neoplasia

Salivary gland neoplasia is a rare condition, but when it does occur it is usually adenocarcinoma of the mandibular or parotid salivary gland. Salivary gland adenocarcinoma is locally invasive and is typically associated with concurrent lymph node metastasis. Other reported salivary gland neoplasms include squamous cell carcinoma, basal cell adenocarcinoma, and mast cell tumor. Siamese cats appear to be overrepresented, although there is no

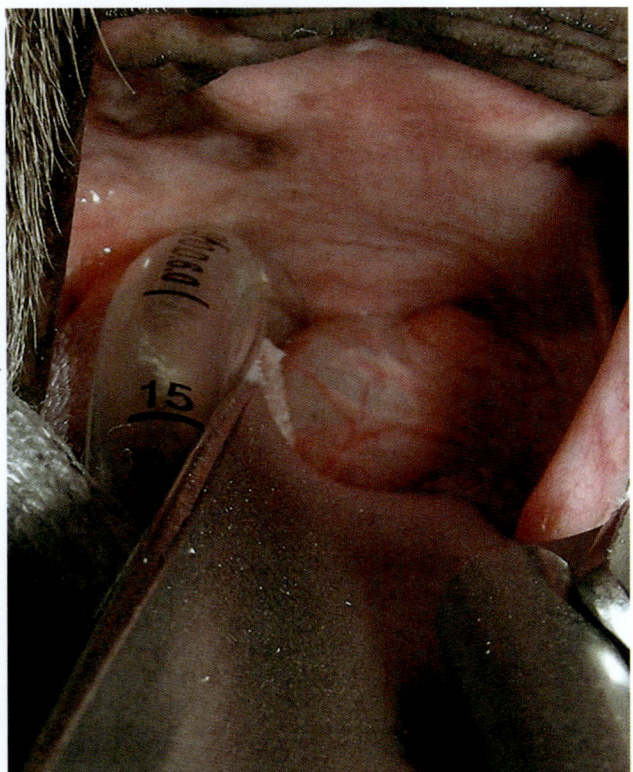

Figure 1.3 Intraoral view of a pharyngeal mucocele.

breed association in dogs. Recommended treatment is aggressive surgical resection, with or without adjunctive radiation therapy. The most recent reported median survival times for dogs and cats with salivary gland neoplasia are 550 and 516 days, respectively (Hammer *et al.* 2001).

Sialolithiasis

Salivary calculus formation is very uncommon in the dog and cat. When it does occur, salivary stones can obstruct salivary ducts, causing an acute painful swelling or rupture of the affected gland. Most stones are composed of calcium phosphate or calcium carbonate and have been reported to occur mostly in the parotid gland, although sialolithiasis associated with cervical and pharyngeal sialoceles has been reported (Han *et al.* 2016). Diagnosis is made using skull radiographs with or without sialography, although advanced imaging may also be beneficial. Surgical removal of the calculus is the treatment of choice. This is followed by cannulation and lavage of the affected salivary duct. If this is not possible due to fibrosis, inflammation, or a concurrent sialocele, surgical excision of the affected gland and duct will also be curative.

Sialoadenitis

Salivary gland inflammation (sialoadenitis) is uncommon, but has been reported in the zygomatic, mandibular, and parotid salivary glands of dogs. Causes are numerous, including blunt trauma, iatrogenic trauma, penetrating bite wounds, foreign body migration, tumor infiltration, and systemic viral infection. Severe inflammation can progress to abscess formation and require surgical intervention. Otherwise, treatment of the underlying cause may help resolve this condition.

Necrotizing Sialometaplasia

Necrotizing sialometaplasia is a benign, ischemic, and inflammatory disease of the mandibular glands, although a case involving the parotid gland has been reported (*Kim et al.* 2010). This condition is manifested by severe retropharyngeal pain, gagging, nausea, ptyalism, and dysphagia. Surgical excision of the mandibular glands tends not to resolve clinical signs, although transient administration of anticonvulsants has resulted in marked improvement (Brooks *et al.* 1995).

References

Bellenger, C. and Simpson, D.J. (1992). Canine sialoceles: 60 clinical cases. *Journal of Small Animal Practice* 33: 376–380.

Brooks, D., Hottinger, H.A., and Dunstan, R.W. (1995). Canine necrotizing sialometaplasia: a case report and review of the literature. *Journal of the American Animal Hospital Association* 31: 21–25.

Cinti, F., Rossanese, M., Buracco, P. et al. (2021). Complications between ventral and lateral approach for mandibular and sublingual sialoadenectomy in dogs with sialocele. *Veterinary Surgery* 50: 579–587.

De Lorenzi, D., Bertoncello, D., Mantovani, C., and Bottero, E. (2018). Nasopharyngeal sialoceles in 11 brachycephalic dogs. *Veterinary Surgery* 47: 431–438.

Dörner, J., Oberbacher, S., and Dupré, G. (2021). Comparison of three surgical approaches for zygomatic sialoadenectomy in canine cadavers. *Veterinary Surgery* 50: 564–570.

Hammer, A., Getzy, D., Ogilvie, G. et al. (2001). Salivary gland neoplasia in the dog and cat: survival times and prognostic factors. *Journal of the American Animal Hospital Association* 37: 478–482.

Han, H., Mann, F.A., and Park, J.Y. (2016). Canine sialolithiasis: two case reports with breed, gender, and age distribution of 29 cases (1964–2010). *Journal of the American Animal Hospital Association* 52: 22–26.

Kim, H.Y., Woo, G.H., Bae, Y.C. et al. (2010). Necrotizing sialometaplasia of the parotid gland in the dog. *Journal of Veterinary Diagnostic Investigation* 22: 975–977.

Marsh, A. and Adin, C. (2013). Tunneling under the digastricus muscle increases salivary duct exposure and completeness of excision in mandibular and sublingual sialoadenectomy in dogs. *Veterinary Surgery* 42: 238–242.

Oetelaar, G.S., Heng, H.G., Lim, C.K., and Randall, E. (2022). Computed tomographic appearance of sialoceles in 12 dogs. *Veterinary Radiology & Ultrasound* 63: 30–37.

Ortillés, Á., Leiva, M., Allgoewer, I., and Peña, M.T. (2020). Intracanalicular injection of N-acetylcysteine as adjunctive treatment for sialoceles in dogs: 25 cases (2000–2017). *Journal of the American Veterinary Medical Association* 257: 826–832.

Poirier, V.J., Mayer-Stankeová, S., Buchholz, J. et al. (2018). Efficacy of radiation therapy for the treatment of sialocele in dogs. *Journal of Veterinary Internal Medicine* 32: 107–110.

Ritter, M.J., von Pfeil, D.J., Stanley, B.J. et al. (2006). Mandibular and sublingual sialoceles in the dog: a retrospective evaluation of 41 cases, using the ventral approach for treatment. *New Zealand Veterinary Journal* 54: 333–337.

Swieton, N., Oblak, M.L., Brisson, B.A. et al. (2022). Multi-institutional study of long-term outcomes of a ventral versus lateral approach for mandibular and sublingual sialoadenectomy in dogs with a unilateral sialocele: 46 cases (1999–2019). *Journal of the American Veterinary Medical Association* 260: 634–642.

Torad, F.A. and Hassan, E.A. (2013). Clinical and ultrasonographic characteristics of salivary mucoceles in 13 dogs. *Veterinary Radiology & Ultrasound* 54: 293–298.

2

Surgical Treatment of Esophageal Disease

Eric Monnet, Jeffrey J. Runge, and William T.N. Culp

In comparison to other portions of the alimentary tract, surgery of the esophagus is associated with a greater percentage of postsurgical complications (Moore & Goldstein 1959; Bouayad *et al.* 1992). A multitude of factors have been theorized to contribute to the difficulty in achieving successful esophageal surgery. The absence of a serosal layer may prevent the formation of a quick seal as seen in other regions of the intestinal tract after a surgical incision is made (Parker & Caywood 1987; Orton 1995). Allowing tissue to rest after being incised is one of the basic requirements for wound healing; however, the esophagus is under constant motion from the head, neck, heart, diaphragm, and peristalsis and this may prevent normal wound healing (Parker & Caywood 1987; Orton 1995). Also saliva is constantly passing in the esophagus. Another concern is that the esophageal wall poorly tolerates tension, and a mortality rate as high as 33% has been reported after resection of up to one-third of the thoracic esophagus (Parker *et al.* 1989). Passage of food boluses and saliva over an anastomotic site results in delayed epithelial migration and later ultimate healing (Parker & Caywood 1987). It was once believed that the esophagus had a segmental blood supply, and that damage to these regions resulted in ischemia and poor healing; however, a rich plexus of intramural vessels exists within the submucosa, and these vessels have been shown to support segments of the esophagus that have had blood supply compromised by experimental segmental vessel ligation (Macmanus *et al.* 1950; Shamir *et al.* 1999). The mechanical problems associated with

motion from swallowing and respiration, the relatively fixed anatomic position, and the lack of a mobile omentum-like structure to help seal wounds are all factors that contribute to the susceptibility of the esophagus to various surgical complications (Orton 1995).

Prior to surgery, nutritional deficiencies associated with esophageal disease should be considered. Delaying surgery and correcting malnourishment through the use of parenteral solutions, or feeding via pharyngostomy, gastrostomy, or jejunosotomy tubes, may be indicated (Parker & Caywood 1987; Han 2004). Studies have shown that humans and animals that are nutritionally depleted have poorer recovery from surgery, decreased immune function, longer hospitalization, and increased risk of morbidity and mortality compared with well-nourished patients (Dionigi *et al.* 1977; Dempsey *et al.* 1988). The location of the esophagus allows the extension of infectious microorganisms into the mediastinum as well as other tissues within the thorax that are inherently difficult to treat (Parker & Caywood 1987). Reports have indicated that improved surgical healing is evident when infection is minimized through the prophylactic use of antibiotics in esophageal surgery (Borgstrom & Lundh 1959).

Surgical principles

The major complications associated with esophageal surgery are dehiscence, leakage, and stenosis (Parker & Caywood 1987; Flanders 1989). Many of these complications can be overcome by careful surgical technique and the selection of appropriate treatments for esophageal lesions (Flanders 1989). Because of the numerous perioperative and intraoperative factors that predispose the esophagus to complications, consideration is given to all aspects of surgical technique in order to reduce the possibility of catastrophic failure such as dehiscence. Tissue must be handled with care and attention should be paid to the numerous vital anatomic structures that are closely associated with the esophagus. To reduce confusion and to appropriately identify the adjacent anatomic structures, a stomach tube or an esophageal stethoscope should be passed (if possible) within the lumen of the esophagus to aid in the determination of esophageal location. The surgical region should be isolated and packed off with moistened laparotomy sponges to reduce spillage and to protect the surrounding structures from contamination. Stay sutures can also be placed in the esophagus to aid in the mobilization of the tissue.

In veterinary medicine some controversy exists surrounding the methods for closing esophageal incisions. Two-layer inverting esophageal suturing was first described in humans in the 1920s and was then described in the veterinary literature in 1965 (Shamir et al. 1999). More recently, incisional closures in one or two layers using various suture patterns and suture materials have been described (Renberg & Waldron 1998; Kyles 2002; Hedlund 2007). In the traditional two-layer closure, the first layer incorporates the mucosa and submucosa, with placement of the knots within the esophageal lumen; the second layer consists of an inverting suture pattern in the muscularis (Rosin 1975) or apposing the muscularis and adventitia with extramurally placed knots (Kyles 2002; Hedlund 2007). Using the single-layer technique, closure can be achieved with a simple interrupted or simple continuous suture pattern using monofilament absorbable suture. For the single-layer technique, sutures should incorporate the submucosal layer without penetrating the mucosa, and knots are tied extraluminally (Ranen et al. 2004). Various reports indicate that suturing esophageal incisions with a single-layer closure can be a rapid, safe, and effective technique (Oakes et al. 1993; Shamir et al. 1999; Ranen et al. 2004). Meticulous attention to suture placement is critical regardless of whether a one- or two-layer closure is utilized. It is generally accepted that a two-layer simple interrupted closure results in greater immediate wound strength, better tissue apposition, and improved healing after esophagotomy, but this technique takes longer to perform (Hedlund 2007). Arguments can be made to utilize a single-layer closure (Oakes et al. 1993) when prolonged anesthesia and surgery time are not possible and rapid closure is desirable.

Early reports designated the mucosa as the holding layer of the esophageal wall (Gideon 1984). In 1988, Dallman disputed these findings and reported that the submucosa is the holding layer of the esophageal wall, showing that inclusion of the mucosa in the closure did not improve the strength of the repair (Dallman 1988).

Surgical technique

Surgical approaches

Cervical esophagus

A ventral midline incision is made through the skin and subcutaneous tissue from the caudal aspect of the larynx extending to the manubrium (Figure 2.1). Using sharp dissection and limited use of electrocautery, the ventral aspect of the trachea is exposed by separating the thin raphe of the sternohyoid muscles on the midline (Hedlund 2007). The trachea is gently retracted to the right. Moistened laparotomy sponges are placed to protect the retracted trachea and surrounding neurovascular structures. Branches of the prominent thyroid vein on the ventral surface of the trachea are cauterized or ligated (Renberg & Waldron 1998). Care is taken to avoid the carotid sheath, which includes the vagosympathetic trunk, carotid artery, and internal jugular vein. An esophageal stethoscope or a stomach tube can be passed to aid in identification of the esophagus. Once the selected region is identified, additional moistened laparotomy sponges are used to pack off the region to reduce contamination during surgery. This approach can be extended through a cranial median sternotomy to expose the cranial thoracic esophagus to the level of the tracheal bifurcation.

Thoracic esophagus

The thoracic esophagus can be divided into cranial and caudal portions, and can be approached from the left or right. The patient is positioned in lateral recumbency

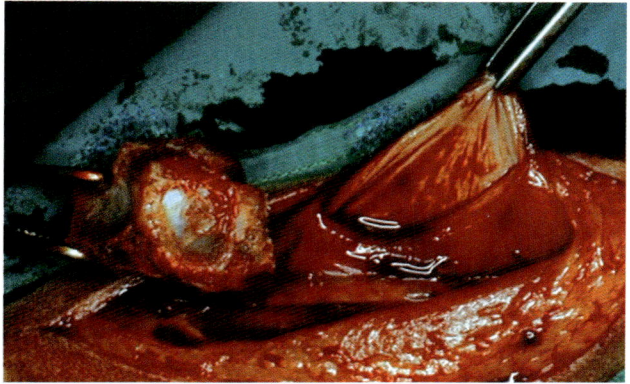

Figure 2.1 Approach to the cervical esophagus for removal of a foreign body wedged at the thoracic inlet.

and the entire hemithorax is clipped and aseptically prepared. To approach the left cranial esophagus, a left lateral thoracotomy is performed in the third or fourth intercostal space. This approach gives exposure to the esophagus at the level of the aortic arch, and improved exposure is achieved through ventral retraction of the brachiocephalic and subclavian arteries (Orton 1995). To approach the right cranial esophagus, a right lateral thoracotomy is made between the third, fourth, or fifth intercostal space. Depending on the location of the abnormality, ventral retraction of the trachea is required for proper visualization of the esophagus (Orton 1995). This can be combined with retraction or ligation of the azygous vein to increase exposure of the esophagus at the base of the heart (Kyles 2002). The caudal thoracic esophagus can be approached from either a left or right seventh, eighth, or ninth intercostal thoracotomy. The left-sided approach is generally preferred for approaching the caudal thoracic esophagus because it avoids the caudal vena cava (Orton 1995).

Abdominal esophagus

The abdominal esophagus is approached with the patient in dorsal recumbency. The hair is clipped from the ventral abdomen and caudal ventral thorax and the skin is aseptically prepared. A ventral midline skin incision is made from the xiphoid extending caudally to the umbilicus. This incision can be extended caudally if adequate exposure is not achieved. A stomach tube is placed to aid in location of the gastroesophageal junction. To expose the hiatal region of the esophagus, an incision can be made through the diaphragm to eliminate the thoracic negative pressure and thereby increase the mobility of the liver. The left lateral and left medial lobes of the liver are retracted medially to allow additional exposure. The stomach is then retracted caudally using stay sutures, and the phrenicoesophageal ligament must be incised to allow full exposure of the esophagus (Renberg & Waldron 1998). A gastrotomy can also be performed to gain access to the lumen of the caudal thoracic and abdominal esophagus.

Surgical procedures
Esophagotomy and partial esophagectomy

Indications for an esophagotomy or esophagectomy can include retrieval of foreign bodies, closure or resection of perforations and lacerations, removal or correction of diverticula, and resection of neoplasia. Esophagotomy and esophagectomy can be performed on any portion of the esophagus (Orton 1995; Ranen *et al.* 2004; Sale & Williams 2006; Doran *et al.* 2008; Leib & Sartor 2008). All the principles of esophageal surgery apply when

performing an esophagotomy and an esophagectomy, including minimal mobilization of the esophagus, atraumatic handling of tissue, and postoperative esophageal rest.

Once the surgical site is located, stay sutures are placed to aid in manipulation of the desired segment of esophagus. Remaining debris within the esophageal lumen can be manipulated cranial and caudal to the surgery site with fingers, umbilical tape, and noncrushing clamps (Kyles 2002). Esophagotomy can be performed longitudinally or transversely depending on the situation encountered (Orton 1995). The stab incision should be made in a healthy portion of the esophagus and extended as needed. If the esophageal wall appears grossly normal, the incision can be made directly over the foreign bodies; if the wall appears compromised, the incision is made just aboral to the region of interest (Hedlund 2007). For foreign body removal, gentle traction is used to remove the object from the lumen (Renberg & Waldron 1998). After foreign body removal, the remaining tissue should be palpated and inspected for devitalization; any necrotic tissue should be débrided and the site should be cultured. Perforations surrounded by healthy esophageal tissue can be débrided and closed primarily if they involve less than one-fourth of the circumference of the esophagus (Hedlund 2007).

Closure of the esophagus can be performed using a two-layer simple interrupted suture pattern, single-layer interrupted pattern, or single-layer continuous pattern. With a two-layer interrupted closure, the internal layer incorporates the mucosa and the submucosa with knots placed within the esophageal lumen; the outer layer is apposed using the adventitia and muscularis with knots placed extraluminally. The single-layer closure utilizes the submucosa as the holding layer, as shown by Dallman (1988). Single interrupted sutures are placed through the submucosa, and penetration of the mucosa is avoided; knots are tied extraluminally. Sutures should be placed 2–3 mm from the cut edge and 2 mm from each other (Rosin 1975).

A two-layer simple interrupted closure can result in greater immediate wound strength and histologically superior healing, as well as closer approximation of tissue compared with single-layer closures (Oakes *et al.* 1993). A recent report of partial esophagectomy utilizing a single-layer closure proved clinically effective, and was a simple and safe technique in esophageal closure (Ranen *et al.* 2004).

Esophageal resection and anastomosis

One of the most substantially complicating aspects of esophageal resection and anastomosis is that the esophagus has little to no redundancy and therefore autologous tissue for reconstruction is usually nonexistent. Because of the higher complications associated with esophageal healing and the excessive tension from resection of the esophagus, this method should only be considered if absolutely necessary (Renberg & Waldron 1998). However, with the use of fine nonreactive suture material, the precise apposition of tissues, and the avoidance of tension on the suture line, the esophagus can heal without complication (Flanders 1989).

Reports have shown that up to 50% of the thoracic esophagus and 20% of the cervical esophagus can be resected and anastomosed utilizing a double-layer closure without incorporating tension-relieving techniques (Saint & Mann 1929). However, tension has been reported even when 2 cm of the esophagus is removed in dogs (Renberg & Waldron 1998); in clinical patients resection of more than 3–5 cm of the esophagus increased the risk of dehiscence (Hedlund 2007). When 33% of the thoracic esophagus was resected (5 cm resection in a 20 kg dog), a positive correlation was observed between the extent of resection and the mortality associated with anastomotic breakdown; within that group of dogs a 50% success rate was reported (Muangsombut *et al.* 1974). Excessive tension at the anastomotic site is a major factor predisposing to dehiscence and stricture formation and should be avoided; various techniques have been employed to relieve tension, reinforce tissue, and bring in a new blood supply to the surgical site. If tension is excessive and all alternatives are exhausted, alternative substitution techniques are available (Kyles 2002).

Although an esophageal resection and anastomosis is an infrequent procedure in small animal surgery, it can be performed at any level of the esophagus and may be indicated for obstructions, strictures, focal necrosis, diverticula, and neoplasia. Esophageal resection requires more extensive mobilization of the esophagus than esophagotomy, but mobilization should be limited to what is necessary to control spillage and perform the surgery (Orton 1995). A number of surgical techniques for esophageal resection and anastomosis have been developed that point to the complexity of the procedure, and identification and preservation of the vagus nerve within the thoracic esophagus are crucial to maintain esophageal function postoperatively.

Approximately 2–3 cm proximal and distal to the affected esophageal region, a partial circular myotomy of the outer longitudinal muscular layer is performed to relieve anastomotic tension; avoiding a complete circular myotomy reduces injury to the submucosal vascular network (Orton 1995). The injection of saline into the muscularis aids in separation of the inner circular and outer longitudinal layers. Umbilical tape, noncrushing bowel clamps, and surgical assistant fingers are used for mobilization and control to reduce potential spillage.

Once the designated section of esophagus has been resected, stay sutures are placed to appose the anastomosis ends to avoid inappropriate torsion and properly align the esophageal segments (Figure 2.2). The ends should be sutured together using a one- or two-layer closure in a simple interrupted pattern. When utilizing a two-layer closure, appose the adventitia and muscularis on the far wall with simple interrupted sutures and extraluminal knots, then appose the submucosa and mucosa on the far wall with simple interrupted sutures with the knots intraluminal, then appose the near-side submucosa and mucosa with intraluminal knots, and lastly appose the near-side muscularis and adventitia with extraluminal knots (Figure 2.2) (Hedlund 2007). A simple continuous suture pattern is not recommended for esophageal anastomotic procedures because it resists dilation of the esophagus and may cut through the mucosa after repeated passage of food bolus (Flanders 1989). The repeated trauma from movement around the continuous suture can increase inflammation and predispose to dehiscence and stricture (Postlethwait *et al.* 1950). Stapling devices have also been used successfully for esophageal anastomosis (Pavletic 1994). An end-to-end circular stapling device may reduce operating time and contamination of the surgical field, but this technique may have greater potential for stricture formation (Hedlund 2007). Two recent reports in the human literature compared handsewn and stapled esophagogastric anastomosis for cancer resection and evaluated surgical time, site leakage, and stricture formation, with both reports concluding the techniques to be safe and efficacious; however, stricture formation was found to be significant in stapling groups (Law *et al.* 1997; Luechakiettisak & Kasetsunthorn 2008).

Patching and support techniques

Patches are used to reinforce existing esophagus ("on-lay" patch) or to provide partial circumferential replacement of the esophageal wall ("in-lay" patch) (Kyles 2002). Regions that have a risk for dehiscence due to poor perfusion or excessive tension after esophagotomy or resection and anastomosis can benefit from an on-lay patch directly over the sutured region (Fingeroth 1993). An in-lay patch serves as a viable scaffold over which the epithelium can migrate to reestablish esophageal mucosal integrity, the most common use being for esophagoplasty for relief of a longitudinal stricture (Orton 1995).

Several types of patches have been described, including muscle pedicles from the sternohyoid, sternothyroid, intercostal, and diaphragm, or epaxial muscles can be mobilized and sutured over the primary repair or esophageal defect (Figure 2.3) (Hedlund 2007). Success has also been achieved using free autogenous grafts (up to 2–3 cm

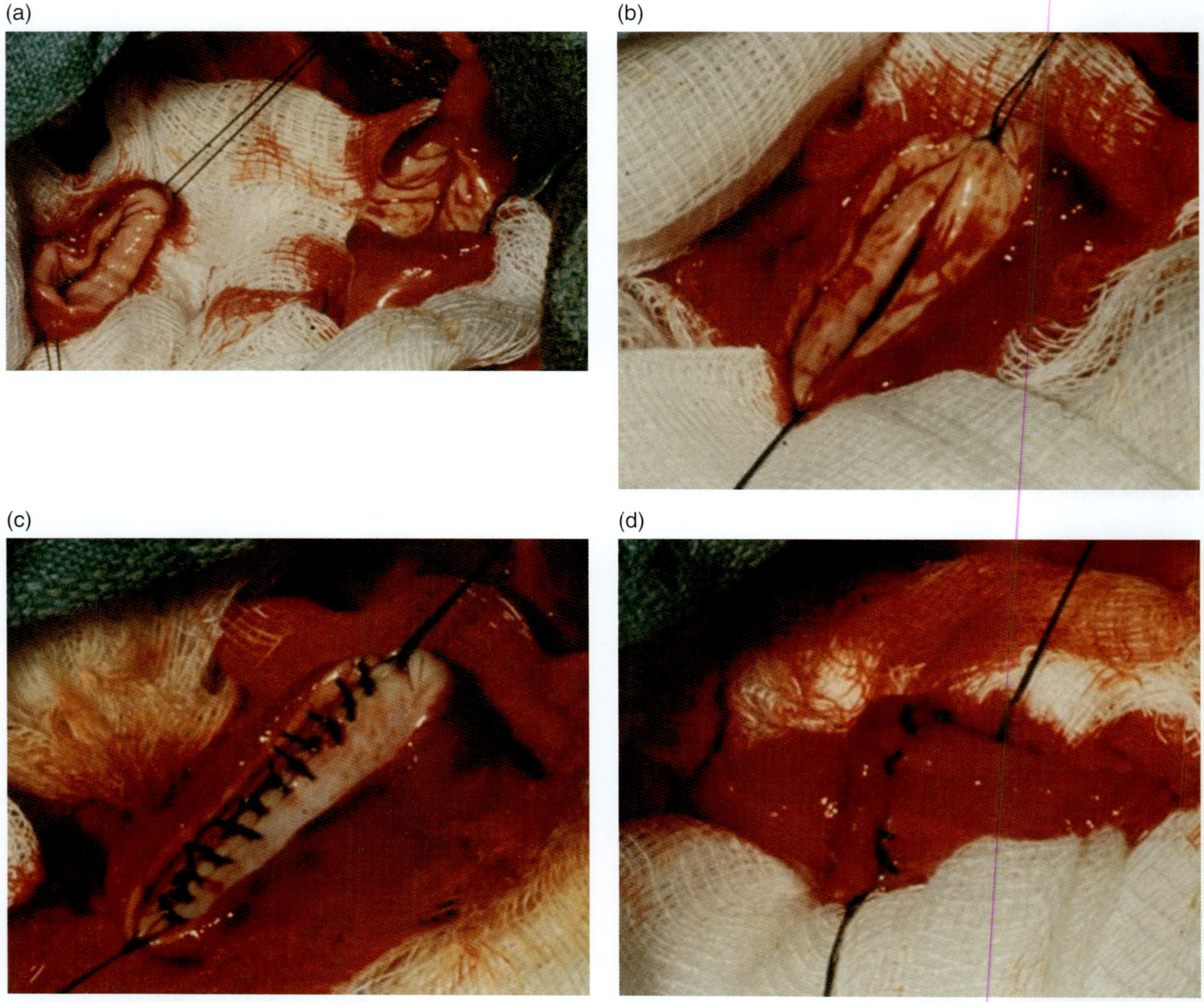

(a)

(b)

(c)

(d)

Figure 2.2 Esophagectomy in the distal thoracic esophagus. (a) Stay sutures have been placed in the cranial segment of the esophagus. (b) Two stay sutures have been placed to appose the two extremities of the esophagus. (c) The first layer of sutures has been placed in the mucosa and submucosa with knots in the lumen on the far side of the anastomosis. (d) The anastomosis is completed with a two-layer closure.

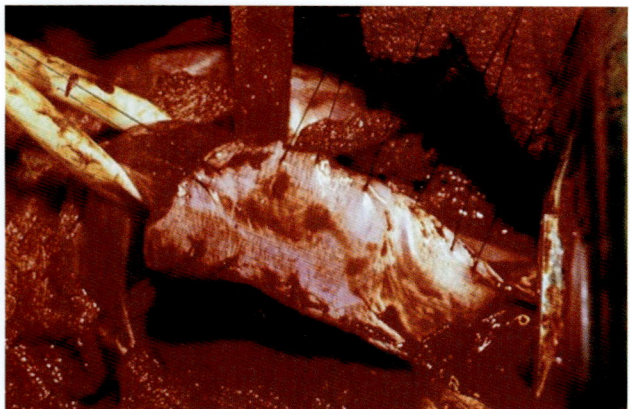

Figure 2.3 An on-lay patch of diaphragm is applied on the distal thoracic esophagus to reinforce an esophagotomy.

wide) taken from the pericardium, which significantly increases the strength of the anastomosis without increasing the risk of stricture formation (Hopper *et al.* 1963). Complete epithelialization occurs over muscle and pericardium, and normal motility is expected after healing is complete (Parker *et al.* 1989). The omentum from the greater curvature of the stomach can be detached and pulled cranially through an incision in the diaphragm and adhered to the esophageal surgical site. Saint and Mann (1929) examined the role of omentopexy in the healing of primary thoracic anastomosis and revealed that neovascularization occurred histopathologically, and that an omentopexy may improve vascularization and decrease stricture formation of the surgical site.

Esophageal substitution

Esophageal substitution is indicated for complete segmental reconstruction of the esophagus after an extensive resection. Although esophageal substitution has been performed experimentally in dogs, minimal clinical experience with these techniques in small animals has been reported. Successful two-stage reconstruction of the cervical esophagus with an inverse tubed skin graft has been reported in a dog with a severe stricture. An omocervical cutaneous island flap based on the superficial cervical branch of the omocervical artery and vein has been suggested as an alternative for one-stage reconstruction of the cervical esophagus (Pavletic 1981). Reconstruction of the distal esophagus with a jejunal or colonic pedicle has been performed experimentally in dogs, but is severely limited by the short vascular arcades of the canine gastrointestinal tract. Free jejunal segment for treatment of cervical esophageal stricture in a dog has been successful (Gregory *et al.* 1988; Bouayad *et al.* 1993). Esophageal replacement in the dog with microvascular colon transfer is associated with a high rate of complications (Kuzma *et al.* 1989). Either thrombosis of the vascular anastomosis or leakage of the colon-to-stomach anastomosis occurred in all dogs with thoracic esophageal replacement. Cervical replacement with microvascular colon transfer was more successful in three dogs (Kuzma *et al.* 1989). Use of vascular skeletal muscle graft (transverse abdominalis muscle) for esophageal reconstruction results in severe stricture of the graft (Straw *et al.* 1987). This technique is not suitable for clinical cases. Simple gastric advancement (esophagogastrostomy) to replace the distal esophagus is associated with major complications in dogs and probably should not be considered a viable alternative in small animals (Pavletic 1981). Potential complications of esophagogastrostomy are gastric dilation within the thorax and hernia of other viscera. One patient reported in the veterinary literature died of acute gastric dilatation.

Gastric tubes that incorporate the gastroepiploic vessels are probably the most feasible strategy for distal esophageal substitution in small animals, although no clinical experience with this method has been reported in small animals. Both "isoperistaltic" and "reverse" gastric tubes have been employed experimentally to replace as much as two-thirds of the thoracic esophagus in dogs (Fingeroth 1993). Reverse gastric tubes require one rather than two anastomoses and have been shown to cause minimal reflux in dogs as long as a 3–6 cm segment of the distal tube remains in the abdomen. A GIA™ surgical stapling device (Covidien USA, Minneapolis, MN, USA) greatly facilitates formation of the gastric tube. A pyloroplasty procedure to enhance gastric emptying is indicated whenever esophageal substitution is undertaken, because interruption of the vagal innervation of the stomach is usually unavoidable. Nutritional support by distal enterostomy is indicated for at least 10 days after esophageal substitution. Pedicle jejunal interposition might represent an option for replacing the distal esophagus in dogs and cats (Linder & Sugarbaker 2007).

Diagnostics

Clinical signs and physical examination findings

Diseases of the upper (cervical) and lower (thoracic) esophagus can be associated with vague signs. Taking a proper history is imperative in determining the sequence of appropriate subsequent diagnostic steps necessary to diagnose the underlying disease. Regurgitation can be singled out as a cardinal sign commonly associated with many diseases of the esophagus; an understanding of the characteristic differences between regurgitation and vomiting is crucial for a successful work-up. Regurgitation is typically a passive event and lacks the prodromal signs of restlessness, hypersalivation, lip-licking, and retching that accompany vomiting (Sellon & Willard 2003). Regurgitated food consists typically of undigested or partially digested food with copious volumes of saliva. The time between the ingestion of food and regurgitation varies, anywhere from minutes to hours (Tams 2003).

Other common clinical signs associated with esophageal disease include anorexia, decreased appetite, dysphagia, odynophagia, ptyalism, weight loss, cachexia, and pyrexia. Respiratory signs such as coughing, pulmonary crackles, dyspnea, and nasal discharge can occur with aspiration pneumonia that transpires as a sequela of esophageal disease. Physical examination findings can also prove to be unrewarding, hiding significant underlying primary esophageal disease. On occasion some abnormalities can be palpable, especially larger cervical foreign bodies.

Radiography

In normal dogs, the esophagus is not visible, except occasionally in large-breed dogs just cranial to the diaphragm in left lateral radiographs (Avner & Kirberger 2005) (Figure 2.4). The cervical esophagus silhouettes with the surrounding soft tissues, and the thoracic esophagus is surrounded by the dorsal mediastinum, fascia, and connective tissue (Watrous 2007). A small amount of gas can be observed within the lumen due to aerophagia, although if gas is observed around the esophagus one can be suspicious of a pneumothorax,

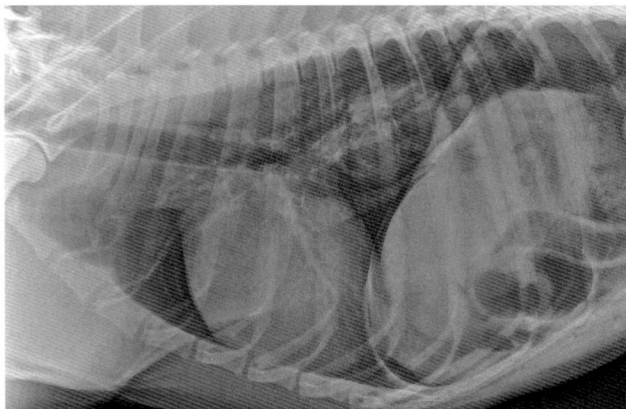

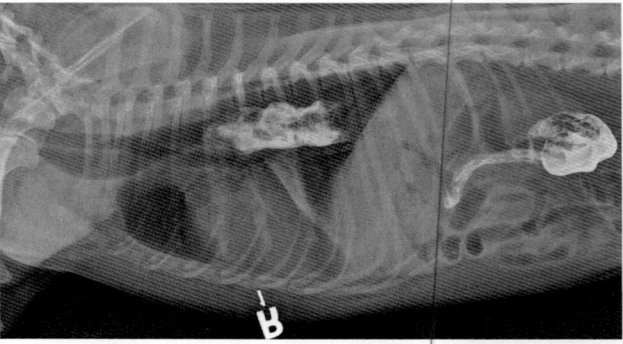

Figure 2.5 Barium esophagram in a 7-year-old male shih tzu. Esophageal foreign body with secondary multifocal aspiration pneumonia.

Figure 2.4 Survey thoracic radiograph in a 2-year-old female mixed breed taken four days after known ingestion of bone. Esophageal foreign body present in caudal thorax.

pneumomediastinum, or esophageal perforation (Owens & Biery 1999). Caudodorsal mediastinal disease, in particular that causing a mass effect, primarily involves the esophagus (Kirberger *et al.* 2009). The absence of abnormal findings on survey radiography does not preclude the presence of disease, and the treating clinician should consider further imaging.

Contrast radiography is beneficial in further characterization of underlying disease affecting the esophagus. The normal canine esophagram reveals long longitudinal parallel folds extending to the lower esophageal sphincter, while the feline esophagus shows the characteristic herringbone pattern at the caudal third due to transverse mucosal folds (Owens & Biery 1999). Contrast esophagography is indicated when esophageal pathology is suspected and survey radiographs are unremarkable, and may aid in determining the location and type of abnormality present. Liquid barium is useful for evaluating an enlarged esophagus: a food–barium mixture is helpful for distinguishing motility, while an aqueous organic iodide is used if a perforation is suspected. If a perforation is suspected, the aqueous organic iodide should be used first (Watrous 2007); if a perforation is not present, it should be followed by liquid barium.

A barium esophagram is typically used to initially evaluate the location, position, lumen, and function of the esophagus (Figure 2.5) (Owens & Biery 1999). Suspected mucosal irregularities (e.g., esophagitis, neoplastic infiltrates) can be appreciated using barium sulfate cream or paste due to its adherence to the mucosa (Watrous 2007).

Esophageal endoscopy

Esophageal endoscopy has become one of the fundamental tools in the diagnosis and treatment of esophageal disease. It is a highly reliable diagnostic method for evaluating esophageal disorders that affect the mucosa or alter the lumen of the organ (Gualtieri 2001). Thoracic radiography should be examined carefully to rule out the possibility of esophageal perforation, as insufflation of the esophagus can result in life-threatening pneumothorax (Simpson 2005). Endoscopy offers a valuable alternative to surgery and can provide direct examination of esophageal disease such as strictures, esophagitis, intraluminal masses, foreign bodies, and diverticula; it allows the procurement of biopsy samples, and can perform therapeutic options such as dilatation of esophageal strictures, retrieval of foreign bodies, and placement of feeding tubes (Figure 2.6). For diseases such as megaesophagus, diverticula, vascular ring anomalies, and hiatal disorders, contrast radiography may be more useful (Simpson 2005).

The tubular morphology of the esophagus allows for its easy evaluation during endoscopy; within the cervical region the longitudinal folds will disappear with insufflation and the mucosal surface is pale pink to gray (Gualtieri 2001). Breeds such as the chow chow and shar-pei may exhibit regions of dark pigmentation (Sherding *et al.* 1999). The normal morphology combined with the toughness of the esophageal mucosa can result in difficulty in retrieving diagnostic mucosal and submucosal biopsies with standard endoscopy equipment and specific instrumentation has been produced for this reason (Gualtieri 2001). The recent development of endoscopic ultrasonography has been a significant advance in the imaging of the gastrointestinal tract wall (Bhutani 2000; Simpson 2005). High-resolution ultrasound images of the gastrointestinal wall are achieved with the aid of an endoscope. This technique avoids the obstacles of conventional ultrasound such as loss of signal due to large penetration depths and interference with overlying gas, bones, and adipose tissue.

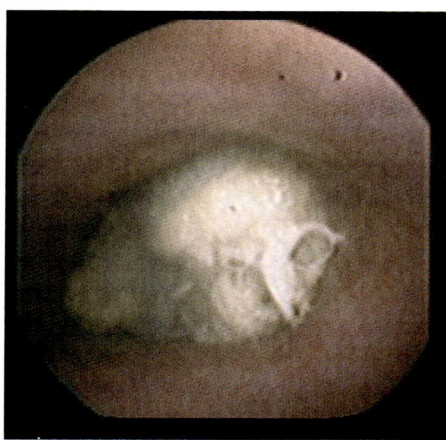

Figure 2.6 Esophagoscopy in a 7-year-old male shih tzu. Esophageal foreign body with secondary inflammation and mucosal erosions.

Computed tomography

Indications for thoracic computed tomography (CT) are the same for small animals as for humans and CT continues to play an increasing role in evaluating thoracic disease. CT and magnetic resonance imaging (MRI) are promoted as the best imaging modalities for detection and description of neoplasms, malformations, and fluid collections in the thoracic cavity (Burk 1991). CT is commonly used for disease location and surgical planning for neoplasia and parasitic *Spirocerca* infections. In recent reports CT determined the exact location, size, and shape of spirocercosis granulomatous nodules, as well as early mass mineralization indicating neoplastic transformation (Dvir *et al.* 2001).

Esophageal disease

Esophageal strictures

Esophageal stricture is an uncommon but well-documented condition in dogs and cats (Washabau 2005). Strictures can be divided into benign and malignant categories, and based on site of origin can be classified as intrinsic (intramural) or extrinsic (extramural) and further subdivided into congenital or acquired (Gualtieri 2001). Congenital strictures appear as stenotic rings or webs and have been reported in the dog and cat, but are rare (Golden *et al.* 1994).

Benign esophageal strictures are typically acquired and comprise bands of intraluminal or intramural fibrous tissue that can completely or partially obstruct the esophagus (Hedlund 2007). This form of stricture formation results from extensive damage to the esophageal lining; inflammation extends through the mucosa into the submucosa and muscularis and leads to collagen deposition and scarring (Glazer & Walters 2008). Most cases of esophageal stricture formation in dogs and cats occur from reflux esophagitis secondary to reflux of gastric acid and enzymes during general anesthesia or hiatal disease (Gualtieri 2001). Strictures have been found to be associated with anesthesia in 65% of cases, and the risk of developing a stricture after an anesthetic episode is reported as 0.7% (Melendez *et al.* 1998). Postanesthetic strictures have been reported to occur within three weeks (Harai *et al.* 1995); most strictures are single and occur at any location along the esophagus (Galatos *et al.* 1994; Hedlund 2007). The predominant clinical sign associated with esophageal strictures that occur after anesthesia is regurgitation shortly after eating, although the animal can be otherwise healthy; strictures associated with chronic or neoplastic disease can be associated with weight loss or malnutrition (Gualtieri 2001). Survey radiography is often nondiagnostic in fibrosing strictures unless the esophagus is distended with food, fluids, or air oral to the stricture (Gualtieri 2001). Definitive diagnosis of esophageal strictures requires demonstration of the esophageal abnormality by endoscopic examination or contrast esophagrams. Contrast esophagography is the best method for determining the number of strictures as well as their location and length, while esophagoscopy allows direct stricture observation and mucosal evaluation (Kyles 2002).

Treatment of esophageal strictures can either be conservative or surgical. In humans successful management of esophageal strictures requires the aggressive treatment of all pathologic processes contributing to esophageal inflammation and restricturing following dilatation (Rodriguez-Baez & Andersen 2003). Conservative treatment of esophageal strictures can be undertaken by bougienage or balloon catheter dilatation. Esophageal bougienage refers to dilation of the esophagus with mechanical dilators, also known as rigid dilators, push dilators, or bougies, and is commonly used in animals and people (Earlam & Cunha-Melo 1981; Spechler 1999). Balloon dilatation involves passing an inflatable balloon into the stricture under endoscopic or fluoroscopic guidance. The balloon is expanded with saline or a dilute contrast agent (if using fluoroscopy) to a preset diameter and pressure to gradually stretch the stricture (Glazer & Walters 2008). Dilatation with balloon catheters is thought to be safer than dilatation with traditional bougienage techniques (Leib *et al.* 2001); balloon catheters create radial stretch as a stationary force, which is considered less damaging than the longitudinal shear produced by bougienage techniques (Burk *et al.* 1987). A recent evaluation of balloon dilatation reported a successful, safe, and efficacious outcome in 88% of patients, with most animals able to eat canned, mashed, or dry food without regurgitation (Leib *et al.* 2001). Dilatation is usually required two or three times to palliate the clinical signs. In contrast, another report recently evaluated the outcome with bougienage for treatment of benign esophageal stricture in dogs and cats, with results suggesting that esophageal bougienage was a safe and effective treatment for most dogs and cats with outcomes similar to those reported for balloon dilatation (Bissett *et al.* 2009). An implantable esophageal balloon dilatation feeding tube has been used experimentally in six dogs with promising results (Weisse & Berent 2015).

Surgery is indicated for strictures that fail to respond to conservative treatment, for strictures that are too extensive to dilate, or when esophageal rupture occurs during dilatation. Surgical options include simple esophagoplasty, esophageal resection and anastomosis, patch esophagoplasty, and esophageal substitution (Orton 1995). Fortunately, the high success rate with dilatation techniques has made surgical resection for benign strictures largely unnecessary (Glazer & Walters 2008).

Esophageal diverticula

Esophageal diverticula are circumscribed sacculations in the wall of the esophagus that interfere with normal esophageal motility patterns (Washabau 2005). They are rare in small animals and are found most commonly in the proximal thoracic esophagus (middle esophageal diverticula) and distal thoracic esophagus (epiphrenic diverticula) (Gualtieri 2001). Diverticula can be single or multiple, and are divided into congenital and acquired (Kyles 2002). Congenital diverticula are rare and arise from a failure of separation between the respiratory tract and foregut (Lantz *et al.* 1976; Faulkner *et al.* 1981). Congenital diverticula have also been attributed to abnormalities in embryologic development that permit herniation of the mucosa through a defect in the muscularis (Washabau 2005).

Acquired diverticula are classified as either pulsion or traction types. Pulsion diverticula are mucosal pouches that herniate through the tunica muscularis of the esophagus, and are thought to result from high luminal pressures secondary to physiologic or mechanical (e.g., foreign body) obstruction of the esophagus (Orton 1995). Pulsion diverticula are usually globular in shape, with a well-defined neck; this allows impaction with ingested material and compromise of the adjacent esophageal lumen (Parker & Caywood 1987). Pulsion diverticula may develop as a consequence of vascular ring anomalies in the cranial thoracic esophagus, or from foreign bodies lodged in the caudal esophagus, in which case they are referred to as epiphrenic diverticula (Washabau 2005). In humans, pulsion diverticula are most frequently located in the pharyngoesophageal

region (Zenker diverticulum) or cranial to the diaphragm (epiphrenic) (Lantz *et al.* 1976).

Traction diverticula are full-thickness deviations of the esophageal wall, thought to result from outward cicatricial contraction of a resolving inflammatory process (Orton 1995). This subsequent contraction produces a distraction force that creates the diverticulum. Because of the close association of the esophagus to the trachea, bronchi, and hilar lymph nodes and the incidence of inflammation in this area, traction diverticula are usually located in the mid-thoracic region (Parker & Caywood 1987). Abscessation from grass awn migration is a common cause of traction diverticula in the western USA (Washabau 1996).

Severe complications can result from the development of a diverticulum (Lantz *et al.* 1976). Secondary chronic esophagitis and ulceration can occur and can result in stricture formation. Peridiverticulitis can cause bronchoesophageal fistulas or adhesions to adjacent lung lobes (Kyles 2002); bronchoesophageal fistulas were associated with 10 of 21 cases of esophageal diverticula in one report (Kyles 2002). Small diverticula are often asymptomatic and can be incidentally observed during radiographic and endoscopic examination. Larger diverticula have the propensity to become impacted with food and fluid (Gualtieri 2001).

A breed predilection for esophageal diverticula has been described previously in Cairn terriers. This breed predilection was noted from a series of case reports that showed an overrepresentation of the Cairn terrier breed without a specific history or signs of foreign body involvement (Thrall 1973; Caywood & Feeney 1982; Nawrocki *et al.* 2003). Miniature poodles also appear to be overrepresented in case studies, but esophageal diverticula in this breed were often due to ingested bony foreign bodies (Thrall 1973; Caywood & Feeney 1982; Nawrocki *et al.* 2003).

Plain radiographs should be evaluated for signs of aspiration pneumonia and esophageal dilatation, and for the possible presence of a soft tissue density representing the impacted diverticulum (Parker & Caywood 1987). Contrast radiography will demonstrate a focal dilated segment of esophageal lumen that fills partially or completely with contrast medium (Parker & Caywood 1987). Esophagoscopy is useful in confirming the radiographic diagnosis, although with air insufflation traction diverticula tend to disappear, whereas pulsion diverticula become more evident (Figure 2.7) (Gualtieri 2001). Esophagoscopy needs to be performed carefully since there is a risk of perforating the thin wall of the diverticulum (Figure 2.8) (Kyles 2002).

Small diverticula may be managed by feeding liquid or semi-liquid diets to minimize impaction of solid food

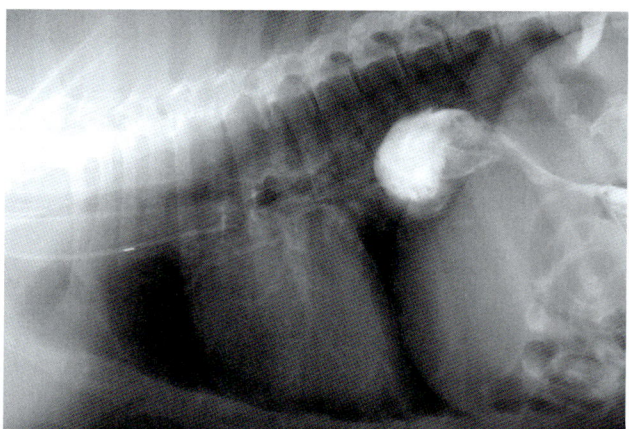

Figure 2.7 Contrast radiograph of a dog with pulsion diverticulum of the distal esophagus. A foreign body has been removed from this location three weeks before with endoscopy.

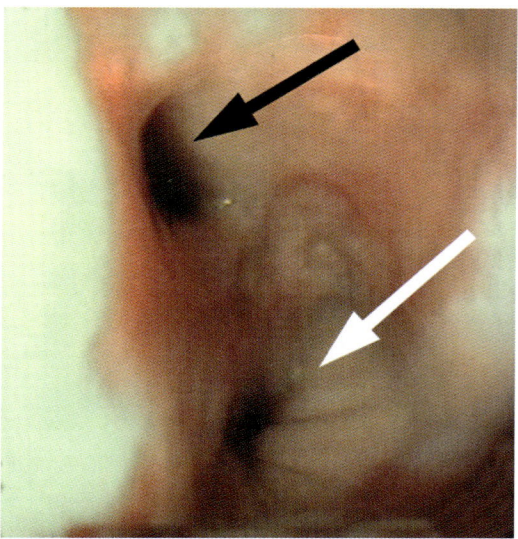

Figure 2.8 Esophagoscopy of a dog (same as in Figure 2.7) with a diverticulum (black arrow). The white arrow is pointing at the lower esophageal sphincter.

in the diverticulum (Washabau 1996). Traction diverticula rarely cause clinical signs and typically do not warrant surgical intervention (Orton 1995), whereas large diverticula generally require surgical treatment (Kyles 2002). Treatment involves surgical resection of the diverticula; epiphrenic diverticula can usually be approached at the eighth or ninth intercostal, but the space should be determined by the esophagram (Figure 2.9) (Parker & Caywood 1987). A diverticulectomy can usually be performed to excise a single diverticulum (Kyles 2002). The diverticulum is isolated from the surrounding structures and packed off with moistened laparotomy sponges. A stapling device (thoracoabdominal, TA) can be placed along the base of the

diverticulum and fired; if a stapling device is not available, noncrushing clamps can be placed at the proposed transection site. The transected edges are then apposed as for an esophagotomy utilizing either a one- or two-layer closure. Partial resection and esophaesophageal in-lay patch, complete resection and anastomosis, or esophageal substitution may be required to remove either large or multiple diverticula (Pearson *et al.* 1978; Kyles 2002). The prognosis is good if thoracic contamination is prevented and good esophageal apposition is achieved (Figure 2.10) (Hedlund 2007).

Esophageal fistula

Esophageal fistulas are an abnormal communication between the esophageal lumen and its surrounding structures (Gualtieri 2001). Esophageal fistulas can be either congenital or acquired. Congenital fistulas are rare and result from incomplete separation of the tracheobronchial tree from the digestive tract during embryologic development (Washabau 2005). Acquired fistulas of the esophagus resulting in esophagoaortic, esophagotracheal, or esophagobronchial communications are uncommon despite the intimate anatomic relationship between these structures (Parker & Caywood 1987). Acquired fistulas are more common than congenital fistulas, typically resulting from ingestion of a foreign body with pointed edges such as bones, chronic ulcerative lesions, esophageal perforation, extension of inflammation into adjacent tissue, or complications associated with esophageal surgery caused by sutures (Sherding *et al.* 1999; Washabau 2005). Bronchoesophageal fistulas are more common than tracheoesophageal fistulas in dogs (Kyles 2002). The majority of reported cases of esophagobronchial fistulas and all reported cases of esophagoaortic and esophagotracheal fistulas developed secondary to esophageal perforation by a bony foreign object (Parker *et al.* 1989).

Clinical signs are typically associated with the respiratory system. The most common clinical sign is coughing and may be associated with liquid ingestion (Parker *et al.* 1989). Other clinical signs can include regurgitation, gagging, and retching. Diagnosis can be difficult using survey radiography, which may not help to distinguish from other esophageal disease. Contrast radiography can definitively diagnose a fistula and may be more useful than esophagoscopy or bronchoscopy. A report by Nawrocki *et al.* (2003) described the fluoroscopic and endoscopic placement of a guidewire to confirm the presence and location of an esophagobronchial fistula. When utilizing contrast radiography, the choice of contrast agent varies with the site of esophageal communication (Parker *et al.* 1989). An aqueous agent is preferred if mediastinal leakage is anticipated and barium agents should be used if communication is suspected between

(a)

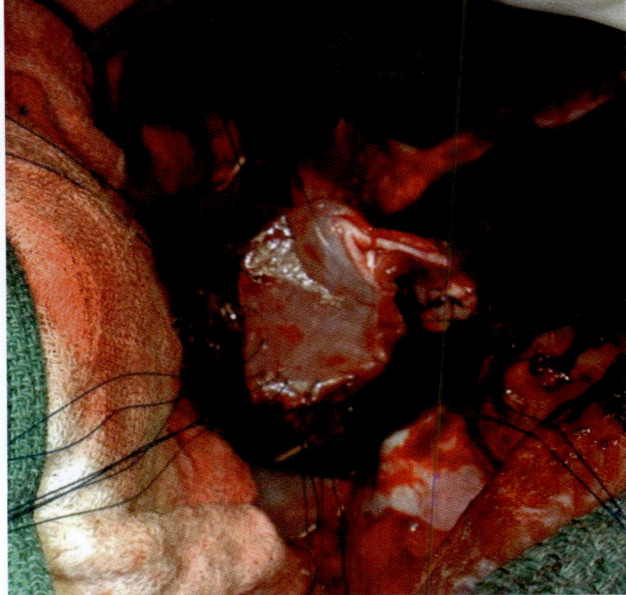

(b)

(c)

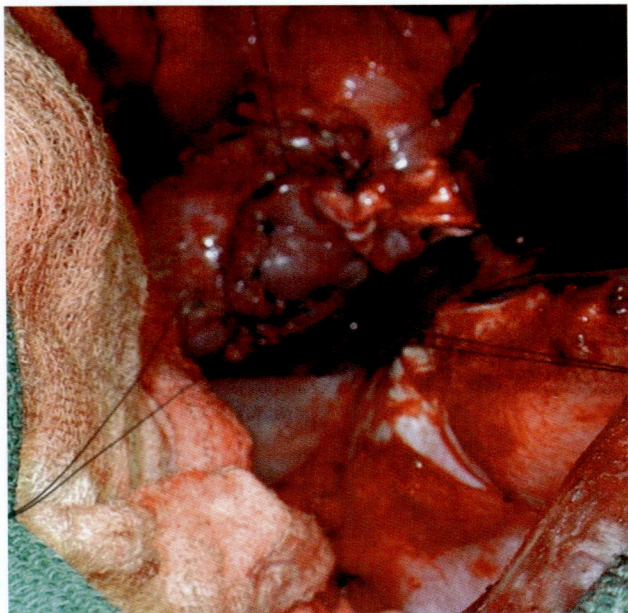

Figure 2.9 (a) Resection of a pulsion diverticulum (same dog as in Figures 2.7 and 2.8). The lumen of the esophagus is visible with a stomach tube in it. (b) An in-lay patch of diaphragm is sutured over the defect with preplaced sutures to avoid compromising the lumen of the esophagus. (c) The in-lay patch is completed. Source: Eric Monnet (author).

the esophagus and bronchus, because the hypertonicity of an iodinated agent may cause pulmonary edema (Parker *et al.* 1989).

Surgical treatment is required for the treatment of esophageal fistulas. The prognosis is guarded if secondary complications such as pneumonia, pulmonary abscess, or large quantities of pleural fluid are present (Washabau 2005). The fistulous tract is excised rather than ligated (Kyles 2002). Resection of the affected lung lobe is warranted, and a postoperative course of antibiotics should be prescribed in all cases (Washabau 2005).

Esophageal neoplasia

Esophageal neoplasia is rare in dogs, accounting for less than 0.5% of reported neoplasia (Ridgeway & Suter 1979; Withrow 2001). Most animals are older and no sex or breed predilection has been established (Withrow 2001). Esophageal neoplasia can be esophageal, periesophageal, or metastatic in origin (Washabau 2005). Esophageal neoplasia is often locally invasive, and metastasis spreads through the lymphatics to draining lymph nodes, hematogenously or both (Withrow 2001). Common reported malignant tumor types in dogs

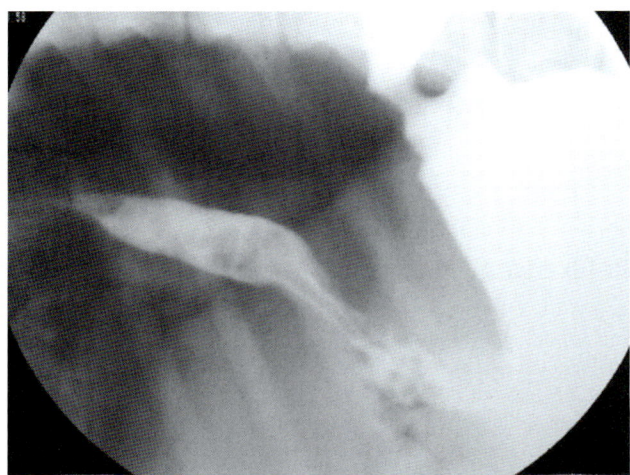

Figure 2.10 Contrast radiograph four weeks after resection of a pulsion diverticulum (same dog as in Figures 2.7–2.9). No irregularities are present in the distal esophagus.

include sarcomas secondary to *Spirocerca lupi*, squamous cell carcinoma, osteosarcoma, fibrosarcoma, and adenocarcinoma; benign tumors include leiomyosarcoma and plasmacytoma (Farese *et al.* 2008). Carcinomas can occur in any location along the esophagus, but are especially common at the thoracic inlet in the cat; in dogs, sarcomas are located in the distal third of the esophagus where the esophagus is in close contact with the aorta (Parker & Caywood 1987).

Clinical signs in affected dogs may not be present until late in the course of the disease and typically include regurgitation, inappetence, salivation, dysphagia, fetid breath, and weight loss (Jacobs & Rosen 2000). A more recent report described anorexia and vomiting with concurrent ascites and hindlimb edema due to caudal vena cava compression from a large esophageal leiomyoma (Rollois *et al.* 2003). Blood may also be noted in the regurgitated material if ulceration is present (Parker & Caywood 1987). Clinical signs develop gradually and reflect progressive esophageal obstruction or esophageal motility (Washabau 2005).

The diagnosis of esophageal neoplasia is commonly made with a combination of plain film survey and contrast radiography, endoscopy, and more recently CT (Withrow 2001). A definitive diagnosis can sometimes be made with endoscopic biopsy that involves the mucosa, but that can be unrewarding if it is submucosal in origin (Farese *et al.* 2008). Esophageal neoplasia is locally invasive, and generally advanced by the time the diagnosis is made (Orton 1995).

Chemotherapy, radiation therapy, and surgical resection are the most common treatment options for esophageal neoplasia. Chemotherapy has rarely been attempted, and radiotherapy is of limited value for intrathoracic esophageal tumors because of poor tolerance of adjacent tissues in the lung and heart (Withrow 2001). A report by Jacobs and Rosen (2000) described the use of photodynamic therapy for the treatment of esophageal squamous cell carcinoma; this therapy resulted in a partial response with a reduction in tumor size. Lymphosarcoma may be treated in some cases with chemotherapy or immunotherapy (Washabau 2005). Surgical management of esophageal neoplasia depends on the size of the primary mass and the extent of metastatic disease (Parker & Caywood 1987). A recent report evaluating esophageal leiomyosarcoma in dogs found that despite large tumor size and incomplete excision, surgical removal of a low-grade tumor can result in long-term resolution of clinical signs (Farese *et al.* 2008). In another study of esophageal sarcoma in 19 dogs that underwent surgical resection of the esophageal tumor, 10 dogs survived the surgery with an average survival time of 300 days (median survival 278 days, range 60–610 days) and an average disease-free interval of 277 days (median 260 days) (Ranen *et al.* 2004). A report evaluating partial esophagectomy described an effective, simple, and safe technique for the removal of sarcoma in the distal thoracic esophagus (Ranen *et al.* 2004). Except for the rare benign lesion or lymphosarcoma, the overall prognosis for esophageal neoplasia is poor for cure or palliation (Washabau 2005).

Esophageal foreign body

Esophageal foreign bodies are objects that do not properly pass into the stomach after being ingested. These objects can cause either a partial or full obstruction at any location along the esophagus. The most frequent type of foreign body found in dogs is ingested bone or bone fragments (Houlton *et al.* 1985). In cats, fishhooks, needles, and string foreign bodies are the most common (Kyles 2002). Foreign bodies have been shown to typically lodge in one of four regions within the esophagus based on the location of anatomic narrowing: immediately caudal to the pharynx, thoracic inlet, heart base, and distal esophagus (Sale & Williams 2006).

Clinical signs associated with esophageal foreign bodies can include lethargy, hypersalivation, regurgitation, anorexia, and distress. These signs can be present immediately or can last for several hours to weeks. A recent report characterized the presence of esophagitis in dogs after esophagoscopy for the diagnosis and treatment of esophageal foreign body and related the degree of esophageal injury to the clinical signs and outcome. This study highlighted that the degree of esophagitis is related to the duration and severity of the clinical signs of the foreign body (Rousseau *et al.* 2007).

In one study, 98.8% of foreign bodies were seen on plain film radiographs; 53% of radiographs had varying degrees of soft tissue density around the foreign body, 21% revealed air within the esophagus, and 12% had evidence of aspiration pneumonia (see Figures 2.4 and 2.5) (Houlton *et al.* 1985). In another study evaluating esophageal foreign bodies, 75.9% of foreign bodies were confirmed with plain film radiography, while the remaining 24.1% were suspicious for a foreign body (Leib & Sartor 2008). Another report indicated that lateral thoracic radiographs were diagnostic for a thoracic foreign body in 100% of cases and gave an accurate indication of the location for a thoracotomy (Sale & Williams 2006). Contrast esophagram is required if a foreign body is not visible on plain radiographs. Aqueous organic iodide should be used first in case a perforation is present. If there is no sign of perforation with aqueous organic iodide, it should be followed by barium (Parker *et al.* 1989). Esophagography was associated with a 14% false-negative rate for perforation when performed with the foreign body in place, while it was associated with a zero false-negative rate after removal of the foreign body (Parker *et al.* 1989). Therefore it has been recommended that esophagography is repeated after successful removal of a foreign body with endoscopy if a perforation is suspected. Esophageal foreign body can induce esophageal perforation, strictures, and diverticulum.

The initial treatment of esophageal foreign bodies is primarily attempted endoscopically with the use of grasping forceps, balloon catheters, or loop snares. Once the foreign body is grasped it is rotated to help free it from its position and then it is withdrawn with any sharp points facing caudally (Kyles 2002). If it cannot be successfully extracted, the foreign body can also be pushed into the stomach. After any esophageal endoscopic procedure, the region where the foreign body impacted is inspected carefully, as exploratory surgery is warranted if any significant perforation or fistula is present. A recent report evaluating esophageal obstructions from dental chews proved that these objects were difficult to remove endoscopically and resulted in moderate or severe esophageal damage, were frequently associated with stricture formation, and were associated with a high mortality rate (Leib & Sartor 2008). Esophageal penetration has an extremely guarded prognosis (Parker *et al.* 1989).

If a foreign body cannot be removed safely or pushed into the stomach, surgical intervention is indicated. Procedures such as esophagotomy (incision into the esophageal lumen) or esophagectomy (partial resection of the esophagus) can be performed on any portion of the esophagus. A recent report evaluated 14 dogs with foreign body obstruction of the esophagus that had the obstruction relieved via transthoracic esophagotomy; the clinical results of this study were considered good in 13 dogs, 2 of which had postoperative complications. The results suggest that esophagotomy is an effective surgical technique and can be performed with good outcomes (Sale & Williams 2006).

References

Avner, A. and Kirberger, R.M. (2005). Effect of various thoracic radiographic projections on the appearance of selected thoracic viscera. *Journal of Small Animal Practice* 46: 491–498.

Bhutani, M.S. (2000). Interventional endoscopic ultrasonography: state of the art at the new millenium. *Endoscopy* 32: 62–71.

Bissett, S.A., Davis, J., Subler, K., and Degernes, L.A. (2009). Risk factors and outcome of bougienage for treatment of benign esophageal strictures in dogs and cats: 28 cases (1995–2004). *Journal of the American Veterinary Medical Association* 235: 844–850.

Borgstrom, S. and Lundh, B. (1959). Healing of esophageal anastomosis: animal experiments. *Annals of Surgery* 150: 142–148.

Bouayad, H., Caywood, D.D., Alyakine, H. et al. (1992). Surgical reconstruction of partial circumferential esophageal defect in the dog. *Journal of Investigative Surgery* 5: 327–342.

Bouayad, H., Caywood, D.D., Lipowitz, A.J. et al. (1993). Replacement of the cervical and thoracic esophagus in dog using free jejunal autografts. *Journal of Investigative Surgery* 6: 157–176.

Burk, R.L. (1991). Computed tomography of thoracic diseases in dogs. *Journal of the American Veterinary Medical Association* 199: 617–621.

Burk, R.L., Zawie, D.A., and Garvey, M.S. (1987). Balloon catheter dilation of intramural esophageal strictures in the dog and cat: a description of the procedure and a report of six cases. *Seminars in Veterinary Medicine and Surgery (Small Animal)* 2: 241–247.

Caywood, D.D. and Feeney, D.A. (1982). Acquired esophagobronchial fistula in a dog. *Journal of the American Animal Hospital Association* 18: 590–594.

Dallman, M.J. (1988). Functional suture-holding layer of the esophagus in the dog. *Journal of the American Veterinary Medical Association* 192: 638–640.

Dempsey, D.T., Mullen, J.L., and Buzby, G.P. (1988). The link between nutritional status and clinical outcome: can nutritional intervention modify it? *American Journal of Clinical Nutrition* 47 (2 Suppl): 352–356.

Dionigi, R., Ariszonta, D.L., Gnes, F., and Ballabio, A. (1977). The effects of total parenteral nutrition on immunodepression due to malnutrition. *Annals of Surgery* 185: 467–474.

Doran, I.P., Wright, C.A., and Moore, A.H. (2008). Acute oropharyngeal and esophageal stick injury in forty-one dogs. *Veterinary Surgery* 37: 781–785.

Dvir, E., Kirberger, R.M., and Malleczek, D. (2001). Radiographic and computed tomographic changes and clinical presentation of spirocercosis in the dog. *Veterinary Radiology and Ultrasound* 42: 119–129.

Earlam, R. and Cunha-Melo, J.R. (1981). Benign oesophageal strictures: historical and technical aspects of dilatation. *British Journal of Surgery* 68: 829–836.

Farese, J.P., Bacon, N.J., Ehrhart, N.P. et al. (2008). Oesophageal leiomyosarcoma in dogs: surgical management and clinical outcome of four cases. *Veterinary and Comparative Oncology* 6: 31–38.

Faulkner, R.T., Caywood, D.D., Wallace, L.J., and Johnston, G.R. (1981). Epiphrenic esophageal diverticulectomy in a dog: a case report and review. *Journal of the American Animal Hospital Association* 17: 77–81.

Fingeroth, J.M. (1993). Surgical techniques for esophageal disease. In: *Textbook of Small Animal Surgery*, 3e (ed. D.H. Slatter), 549–561. Philadelphia, PA: WB Saunders.

Flanders, J.A. (1989). Problems and complications associated with esophageal surgery. *Problems in Veterinary Medicine* 1: 183–194.

Galatos, A.D., Rallis, T., and Raptopoulos, D. (1994). Post anaesthetic oesophageal stricture formation in three cats. *Journal of Small Animal Practice* 35: 638–642.

Gideon, L. (1984). Esophageal anastomosis in two foals. *Journal of the American Veterinary Medical Association* 184: 1146–1148.

Glazer, A. and Walters, P. (2008). Esophagitis and esophageal strictures. *Compendium on Continuing Education for the Practicing Veterinarian* 30: 281–292.

Golden, D.L., Henderson, R.A., and Brewer, W.G. (1994). Use of an argon laser for transendoscopic radial incision of an esophageal web in a cat. *Journal of the American Animal Hospital Association* 30: 29–32.

Gregory, C.R., Gourley, I.M., Bruyette, D.S., and Shultz, L.J. (1988). Free jejunal segment for treatment of cervical esophageal stricture in a dog. *Journal of the American Veterinary Medical Association* 193: 230–232.

Gualtieri, M. (2001). Esophagoscopy. *Veterinary Clinics of North America Small Animal Practice* 31: 605–630.

Han, E. (2004). Esophageal and gastric feeding tubes in ICU patients. *Clinical Techniques in Small Animal Practice* 19: 22–31.

Harai, B.H., Johnson, S.E., and Sherding, R.G. (1995). Endoscopically guided balloon dilatation of benign esophageal strictures in 6 cats and 7 dogs. *Journal of Veterinary Internal Medicine* 9: 332–335.

Hedlund, C.S. (2007). Surgery of the esophagus. In: *Small Animal Surgery*, 3e (ed. T.W. Fossum), 372–409. St Louis, MO: Mosby Elsevier.

Hopper, C.L., Berk, P.D., and Howes, E.L. (1963). Strength of esophageal anastomoses repaired with autogenous pericardial grafts. *Surgery, Gynecology and Obstetrics* 117: 83–86.

Houlton, J.E.F., Herrtage, M.E., Taylor, P.M., and Watkins, S.B. (1985). Thoracic oesophageal foreign bodies in the dog: a review of ninety cases. *Journal of Small Animal Practice* 26: 521–536.

Jacobs, T.M. and Rosen, G.M. (2000). Photodynamic therapy as a treatment of esophageal squamous cell carcinoma in dog. *Journal of the American Animal Hospital Association* 36: 257–261.

Kirberger, R.M., Dvir, E., and van der Merwe, L.L. (2009). The effect of positioning on the radiographic appearance of caudodorsal mediastinal masses in the dog. *Veterinary Radiology and Ultrasound* 50: 630–634.

Kuzma, A.B., Holmberg, D.L., Miller, C.W. et al. (1989). Esophageal replacement in the dog by microvascular colon transfer. *Veterinary Surgery* 18: 439–445.

Kyles, A.E. (2002). Esophagus. In: *Textbook of Small Animal Surgery*, 3e (ed. D.H. Slatter), 573–592. Philadelphia, PA: WB Saunders.

Lantz, G.C., Bojrab, M.J., and Jones, B.D. (1976). Epiphrenic esophageal diverticulectomy. *Journal of the American Animal Hospital Association* 12: 629–635.

Law, S., Fok, M., Chu, K.M., and Wong, J. (1997). Comparison of hand-sewn and stapled esophagogastric anastomosis after esophageal resection for cancer: a prospective randomized controlled trial. *Annals of Surgery* 226: 169–173.

Leib, M.S. and Sartor, L.L. (2008). Esophageal foreign body obstruction caused by a dental chew treat in 31 dogs (2000–2006). *Journal of the American Veterinary Medical Association* 232: 1021–1025.

Leib, M.S., Dinnel, H., Ward, D.L. et al. (2001). Endoscopic balloon dilation of benign esophageal strictures in dogs and cats. *Journal of Veterinary Internal Medicine* 15: 547–552.

Linder, P.A. and Sugarbaker, D.J. (2007). Surgical procedures to resect and replace the esophagus. In: *Maingot's Abdominal Operations*, 11e (ed. M. Zinner and S.W. Ashley), 305–330. McGraw-Hill: Columbus, OH.

Luechakiettisak, P. and Kasetsunthorn, S. (2008). Comparison of hand-sewn and stapled in esophagogastric anastomosis after esophageal cancer resection: a prospective randomized study. *Journal of the Medical Association of Thailand* 91: 681–685.

Macmanus, J.E., Dameron, J.T., and Paine, J.R. (1950). The extent to which one may interfere with the blood supply of the esophagus and obtain healing on antastomosis. *Surgery* 28: 11–23.

Melendez, L.D., Twedt, D.C., Weyrauch, E.A., and Willard, M.D. (1998). Conservative therapy using balloon dilatation for intramural, inflammatory esophageal strictures in dogs and cats: a retrospective study of 23 cases (1987–1997). *European Journal of Comparative Gastroenterology* 3: 31–36.

Moore, T.C. and Goldstein, J. (1959). Use of intact omentum for closure of full-thickness esophageal defects. *Surgery* 45: 899–904.

Muangsombut, J., Hankins, J.R., Mason, G.R., and McLaughlin, J.S. (1974). The use of circular myotomy to facilitate resection and end-to-end anastomosis of the esophagus. An experimental study. *Journal of Thoracic and Cardiovascular Surgery* 68: 522–529.

Nawrocki, M.A., Mackin, A.J., McLaughlin, R., and Cantwell, H.D. (2003). Fluoroscopic and endoscopic localization of an esophagobronchial fistula in a dog. *Journal of the American Animal Hospital Association* 39: 257–261.

Oakes, M.G., Hosgood, G., Snider, T.G. et al. (1993). Esophagotomy closure in the dog. A comparison of a double layer appositional and two single layer appositional techniques. *Veterinary Surgery* 22: 451–456.

Orton, E.C. (1995). Esophagus. In: *Small Animal Thoracic Surgery*, 117–132. Baltimore, MD: Lea & Febiger.

Owens, J.M. and Biery, D.N. (1999). Gastrointestinal system. In: *Radiographic Interpretation for the Small Animal Clinician*, 2e, 223–260. Baltimore, MD: Williams & Wilkins.

Parker, N.R. and Caywood, D.D. (1987). Surgical diseases of the esophagus. *Veterinary Clinics of North America Small Animal Practice* 17: 333–358.

Parker, N.R., Walter, P.A., and Gay, J. (1989). Diagnosis and surgical management of esophageal perforation. *Journal of the American Animal Hospital Association* 25: 587–594.

Pavletic, M.M. (1981). Reconstructive esophageal surgery in the dog: a literature review and case report. *Journal of the American Animal Hospital Association* 17: 435–444.

Pavletic, M.M. (1994). Stapling in esophageal surgery. *Veterinary Clinics of North America Small Animal Practice* 24: 395–412.

Pearson, H., Gibbs, C., and Kelly, D.F. (1978). Oesophageal diverticulum formation in the dog. *Journal of Small Animal Practice* 19: 341–355.

Postlethwait, R.W., Deaton, W.R. Jr., Bradshaw, H.H., and Williams, R.W. (1950). Esophageal anastomosis: types and methods of suture. *Surgery* 28: 537–542.

Ranen, E., Shamir, M.H., Shahar, R., and Johnston, D.E. (2004). Partial esophagectomy with single layer closure for treatment of esophageal sarcomas in 6 dogs. *Veterinary Surgery* 33: 428–434.

Renberg, W. and Waldron, D.R. (1998). Surgery of the esophagus. In: *Current Techniques in Small Animal Surgery*, 4e (ed. M.J. Bojrab, B. Slocum and G.W. Ellison), 187–204. Baltimore, MD: Williams and Wilkins.

Ridgeway, R.L. and Suter, P.F. (1979). Clinical and radiographic signs in primary and metastatic esophageal neoplasm in dogs. *Journal of the American Veterinary Medical Association* 174: 700–704.

Rodriguez-Baez, N. and Andersen, J.M. (2003). Management of esophageal strictures in children. *Current Treatment Options in Gastroenterology* 6: 417–425.

Rollois, M., Ruel, Y., and Besso, J.G. (2003). Passive liver congestion associated with caudal vena caval compression due to oesophageal leiomyoma. *Journal of Small Animal Practice* 44: 460–463.

Rosin, E. (1975). Surgery of the esophagus. *Veterinary Clinics of North America* 5: 557–564.

Rousseau, A., Prittie, J., Broussard, J.D. et al. (2007). Incidence and characterization of esophagitis following esophageal foreign body removal in dogs: 60 cases (1999–2003). *Journal of Veterinary Emergency and Critical Care* 17: 159–163.

Saint, J.H. and Mann, F.C. (1929). Experimental surgery of the esophagus. *Archives of Surgery* 18: 2324–2338.

Sale, C.S.H. and Williams, J.M. (2006). Results of transthoracic esophagotomy retrieval of esophageal foreign body obstructions in dogs: 14 cases (2000–2004). *Journal of the American Animal Hospital Association* 42: 450–456.

Sellon, R.K. and Willard, M.D. (2003). Esophagitis and esophageal strictures. *Veterinary Clinics of North America Small Animal Practice* 33: 945–967.

Shamir, M.H., Shahar, R., Johnston, D.E., and Mongil, C.M. (1999). Approaches to esophageal sutures. *Compendium on Continuing Education for the Practicing Veterinarian* 21: 414–421.

Sherding, R.G., Johnson, S.E., and Tams, T.R. (1999). Esophagoscopy. In: *Small Animal Endoscopy* (ed. T.R. Tams and C.A. Rawlings), 39–96. St Louis, MO: Mosby.

Simpson, J.W. (2005). Gastrointestinal endoscopy. In: *BSAVA Manual of Canine and Feline Gastroenterology*, 2 (ed. E. Hall, J.W. Simpson and D.A. Williams), 34–49. British Small Animal Veterinary Association: Gloucester.

Spechler, S.J. (1999). American Gastroenterological Association medical position statement on treatment of patients with dysphagia caused by benign disorders of the distal esophagus. *Gastroenterology* 117: 229–233.

Straw, R.C., Tomlinson, J.L., Constantinescu, G. et al. (1987). Use of a vascular skeletal muscle graft for canine esophageal reconstruction. *Veterinary Surgery* 16: 155–163.

Tams, T.R. (2003). Diseases of the esophagus. In: *Handbook of Small Animal Gastroenterology*, 151–155. Philadelphia, PA: WB Saunders.

Thrall, D.E. (1973). Esophagobronchial fistula in a dog. *Journal of the American Veterinary Radiology Society* 14: 22–26.

Washabau, R. (1996). Swallowing disorders. In: *BSAVA Manual of Canine and Feline Gastroenterology* (ed. J.E. Hall, J.W. Simpson and D.A. Williams), 67–89. Cheltenham: British Small Animal Veterinary Association.

Washabau, R. (2005). Disorders of the pharynx and oesophagus. In: *BSAVA Manual of Canine and Feline Gastroenterology*, 2e (ed. J.E. Hall, J.W. Simpson and D.A. Williams), 133–150. British Small Animal Veterinary Association: Gloucester.

Watrous, B.J. (2007). Esophagus. In: *Textbook of Veterinary Diagnostic Radiology*, 5e (ed. D.E. Thrall), 495–498. Philadelphia, PA: Saunders.

Weisse, C., Berent, A. (2015). Prospective evaluation of a one-stage esophageal balloon dilation feeding tube (EBDFT) results in 6 dogs. 2015 ACVIM Forum, Indianapolis, IN.

Withrow, S.J. (2001). Esophageal cancer. In: *Small Animal Clinical Oncology*, 3e (ed. S.J. Withrow and E.D. MacEwen), 320–321. Philadelphia, PA: Saunders.

3

Vascular Ring Anomalies

Eric Monnet

Vascular ring anomalies are a consequence of abnormal embryologic development of the aortic arches and result in abnormal vessels encircling the esophagus and trachea, causing partial obstruction of the esophagus (VanGundy 1989; Kyles 2010). During embryologic development, the six aortic arches connecting the dorsal and ventral aorta undergo remodeling with involution and reconnection that results in the definitive cardiovascular system.

The aortic arches are connected dorsally and ventrally with a dorsal and a ventral aorta. The first two aortic arches involute early during embryologic development. The ventral aorta of the first and second aortic arches forms the external carotid arteries, and the dorsal part the internal carotid arteries. The common carotid arteries are formed from the ventral aorta between the third and fourth aortic arches. The dorsal part of the aorta between the third and fourth arches involutes. The final aortic arch is formed from the left ventral aorta of the fourth aortic arch and the left aortic arch. The distal part of the dorsal aortas fuses together to create the descending aorta, while the ventral part of the right aortic arch forms the brachiocephalic trunk. The right fourth aortic arch creates the right subclavian artery. The fifth aortic arch involutes bilaterally, while the sixth aortic arch creates the pulmonary artery. The left pulmonary artery maintains a connection with the aorta to create the ductus arteriosus. The right ductus arteriosus and the right sixth dorsal aorta involute, releasing the esophagus and the trachea.

Different types of vascular ring anomalies

Seven different types of vascular ring anomaly have been described (VanGundy 1989; Kyles 2010). Persistent right aortic arch with a left ligamentum arteriosum is the most common type (type 1). When the right fourth aortic arch forms the aortic arch and a left subclavian artery originates from the right descending aorta, the left subclavian artery can result in partial compression of the esophagus (type 2). Types 1 and 2 can be combined to form type 3. Double aortic arches result from persistence of the left and right fourth aortic arches (type 4). Persistence of the right ductus arteriosus with a normal left aortic arch will result in obstruction of the esophagus (type 5). An aberrant right subclavian artery partially encircling the esophagus will induce partial obstruction of the esophagus (type 6). Combination of types 5 and 6 creates type 7.

Diagnostic

Clinical presentation

Vascular ring anomalies have been described in dogs and cats (Martin *et al.* 1983; McCandlish *et al.* 1984; Bezuidenhout 1989; Yarim *et al.* 1999; Holt *et al.* 2000; Ferrigno *et al.* 2001; White *et al.* 2003; Buchanan 2004; Vianna & Krahwinkel 2004; Du Plessis *et al.* 2006; Shojaei *et al.* 2011). No breed predisposition has been reported, but German shepherd is the breed most commonly reported to be affected. Clinical signs related to the

Small Animal Soft Tissue Surgery, Second Edition. Edited by Eric Monnet.
© 2023 John Wiley & Sons, Inc. Published 2023 by John Wiley & Sons, Inc.
Companion website: www.wiley.com/go/monnet/small

esophageal obstruction are not present until the animal is weaned and switched to solid food. Therefore most of the patients are diagnosed between 2 and 6 months of age (Shires & Liu 1981). However, older cases have been reported (Imhoff & Foster 1963; Fingeroth & Fossum 1987).

Patients suffering from a vascular ring anomaly are presented for regurgitation and slow growth. Regurgitation usually happens soon after eating. It can be associated with signs of aspiration pneumonia. It is not unusual to palpate an enlarged cervical esophagus.

Imaging techniques

Thoracic radiography reveals dilation of the cranial esophagus, which is filled with fluid, gas, and ingesta. On a ventrodorsal radiograph it might be possible to identify the right aortic arch making an indentation in the esophagus. Contrast esophagography is required to confirm the dilation of the cranial esophagus (Figure 3.1). The obstruction is localized at the base of the heart and the distal esophagus is usually normal (Buchanan 2004).

Computed tomography (CT) can be used to visualize unusual vascular ring anomalies (Figure 3.2) (Joly et al. 2008). Endoscopy is also a valuable tool for the diagnosis of a vascular ring anomaly (Townsend et al. 2016). It will identify the obstruction at the level of the heart base, and allows inspection of the esophageal mucosa. Endoscopy can also be used to decide which side to perform the thoracotomy (Figure 3.2). Most types of vascular ring anomaly can be accessed with a left-sided intercostal thoracotomy, except types 5, 6, and 7. Endoscopy can help determine if the patient has a right or left aortic arch by looking at the position of the aorta.

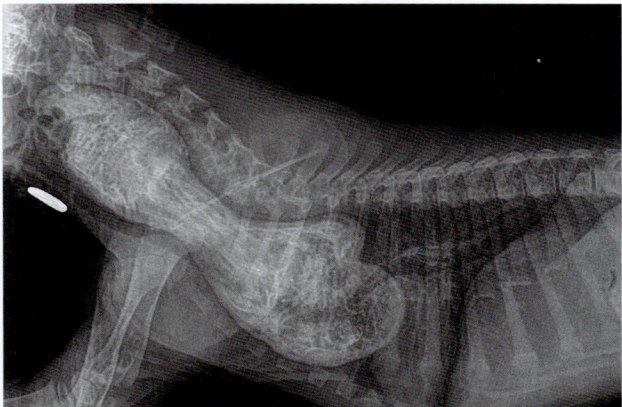

Figure 3.1 Lateral radiograph with barium of a dog with dilatation of the cranial esophagus. The esophageal dilation stops at the base of the heart.

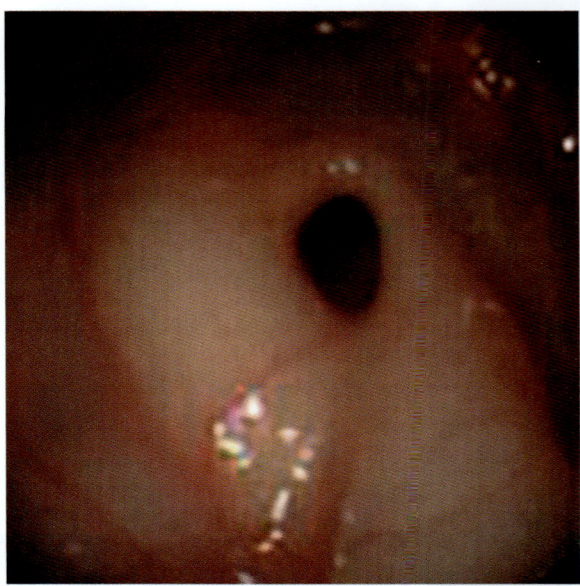

Figure 3.2 Endoscopic visualization of the ligamentum arteriosum narrowing the lumen of the esophagus. The right aortic arch is bulging on the right side of the esophagus.

Surgical treatment

Surgical treatment is indicated to relieve the obstruction. Most of the vascular ring anomalies are approached on the left side of the thoracic cavity, except types 5, 6, and 7 (Hurley et al. 1993; Muldoon et al. 1997; Holt et al. 2000; Rodrigues et al. 2007). A double aortic arch may require an angiogram or a CT scan to figure out the most important arch.

The surgery can be performed with an intercostal thoracotomy or with thoracoscopy (Muldoon et al. 1997; Holt et al. 2000; MacPhail et al. 2001; Krebs et al. 2014; Townsend et al. 2016). Thoracoscopy has been reported only for the persistence of a right aortic arch and for the ligation and division of a ligamentum arteriosum (MacPhail et al. 2001; Krebs et al. 2014; Townsend et al. 2016; Nucci et al. 2018).

Intercostal thoracotomy

A left or a right fourth intercostal thoracotomy is performed to expose the ligamentum arteriosum and/or the subclavian artery. If a patent ductus arteriosus is present, it has to be ligated at the time of surgery.

Ligamentum arteriosum

The patient is positioned in lateral recumbency. A skin incision is performed from dorsal to ventral at the level of the caudal border of the scapula. The subcutaneous tissue with the platysma muscle are incised with electrocautery to minimize bleeding. The latissimus dorsalis muscle is then exposed and incised from ventral to dorsal, preferably with electrocautery. After identifying the fourth intercostal space, the bundles of the serratus dorsalis muscles are separated at the level of the fourth intercostal space. Ventrally the scalene muscle is incised. The intercostal muscles are then incised in the fourth space. A Finochietto retractor is used to retract the ribs and expose the pleural space. The left or right cranial lung lobes are retracted caudally to expose the cranial mediastinum and the base of the heart. The ligamentum arteriosum is identified and dissected from the esophagus. The mediastinum covering the ligamentum arteriosum is incised first and then a right-angle forceps is used to dissect the ligamentum arteriosum (Figure 3.3). The vagus nerve and the laryngeal recurrent nerve should be identified before dissection and preserved. The ligamentum arteriosum is then double ligated with nonabsorbable suture and divided between the two sutures (Figure 3.3). A large Foley catheter (20 Fr) is advanced in the esophagus from the mouth beyond the area of compression. The balloon is inflated and the catheter pulled back slowly. Fibers interfering with dilatation of the esophagus should be divided. It is paramount not to damage the wall of the esophagus.

An aberrant left cranial vena cava can be present also with a vascular ring anomaly. It covers the ligamentum arteriosum. The aberrant left cranial vena cava is dissected and retracted dorsally to expose the ligamentum arteriosum. If the retraction is difficult, the aberrant cranial vena cava can be divided; usually the right cranial vena cava is present.

A thoracostomy tube is placed and the thoracotomy closed in a routine fashion.

Double aortic arch

If a double aortic is present, the dominant arch should be preserved. After performing a CT scan or magnetic resonance imaging (MRI) (Figure 3.4) to determine the major aortic arch, an intercostal thoracotomy in the fourth intercostal space in the left or right intercostal space to access the minor aortic arch. The aortic arch is exposed with caudal retraction of the left or right cranial lung lobe.

The aortic arch is dissected 360° with right-angle forceps (Figure 3.5). The dissection should be large enough to be able to place two vascular clamps across the aortic arch. A red rubber feeding tube can be used as a guide to place the vascular clamp around the aortic arch (Figure 3.6), with sufficient space between the two forceps to be able to divide the aortic arch. After application of the vascular clamp, the arterial pressure is monitored for 5 minutes to make sure it is not dropping, which would indicate that the aortic arch does not provide significant blood flow to perfuse the peripheral tissue. If the arterial pressure is decreased, the clamps are removed and applied to the other aortic arch to evaluate its contribution to the blood flow. Exposure of the contralateral aortic arch is difficult. If the arterial pressure is equally affected by clamping of either aortic arch, the ipsilateral aortic arch is clamped and divided.

After clamping the aortic arch, mattress sutures with pledgets made of Teflon are applied across the aortic arch on each side. Monofilament nonabsorbable suture size 4-0 is used. Then two simple continuous sutures with 4-0 monofilament nonabsorbable sutures are placed on each end of the aortic arch. The stitches should not be placed beyond the mattress suture to reduce the risk of bleeding. The clamps are then removed. If some bleeding is present, mattress sutures with pledgets are added. The

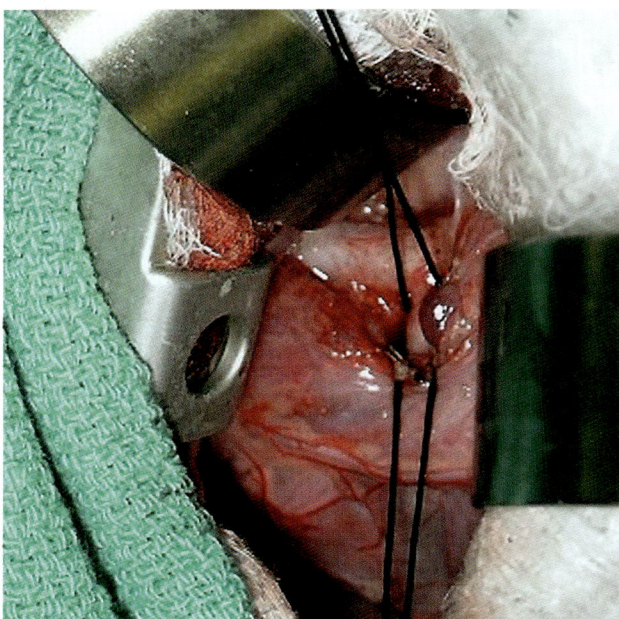

Figure 3.3 After a left intercostal thoracotomy, the ligamentum arteriosum has been dissected and mounted on two encircling sutures.

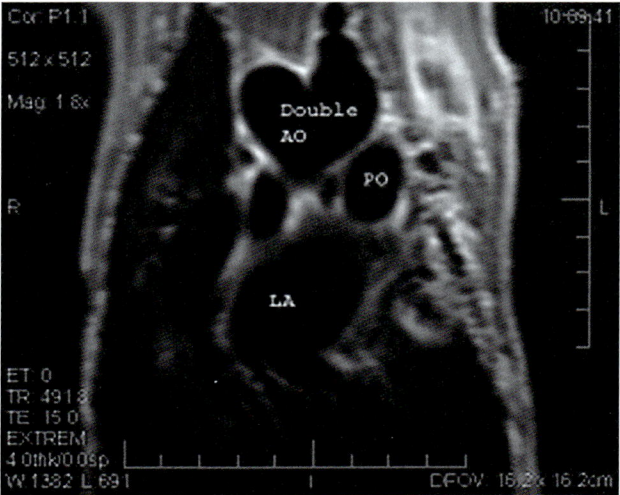

Figure 3.4 Computed tomographic scan of a dog with a double aortic arch.

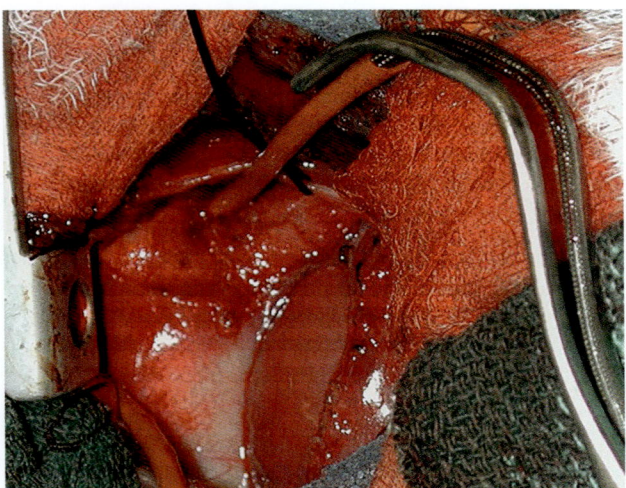

Figure 3.5 The left side of the double aortic arch has been dissected and a red rubber feeding tube has been passed around the left aortic arch to facilitate placement of vascular clamp.

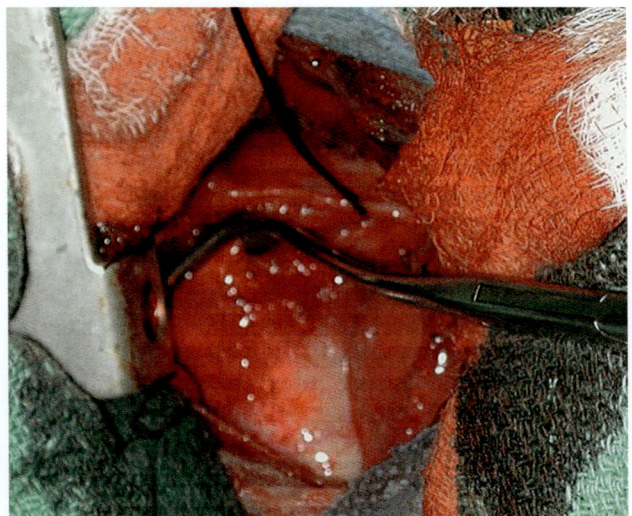

Figure 3.6 A vascular clamp has been applied to evaluate the effect of occlusion of the left aortic arch on arterial blood pressure before permanent ligation and division.

ligamentum arteriosum should be ligated and divided if the right aortic arch was preserved. If the ligamentum arteriosum is still patent it should be clamped, divided, and suture as already described for the aortic arch.

A thoracostomy tube is placed and the thoracotomy closed in a routine fashion.

Thoracoscopy

The patient is placed in right lateral recumbency. The left cranial lung lobe is excluded by placing a bronchial blocker in the left cranial bronchi. A 5 Fr endobronchial blocker is placed under bronchoscopy.

An intercostal approach with three 5 mm cannulas is performed at the eighth or ninth intercostal space on the left side. The cannulas are all placed in the same intercostal space, in the dorsal third of the intercostal space. The vagus nerve is identified. A palpation probe is used first to palpate the ligamentum arteriosum (Figure 3.7). If the ligamentum arteriosum is not identified, a stomach tube is advanced in the esophagus to visualize the area of obstruction.

A fine-teeth grasping forceps is then used to elevate the ligamentum arteriosum into the pleural space. Dissection of the mediastinum covering the ligamentum is started with electrocautery with a J hook extension to the electrocautery pencil. Then a right-angle forceps is used to complete the dissection 360° around the ligamentum arteriosum (Figure 3.8). Usually the wall of the esophagus is visible. Either clips are applied to the ligamentum arteries before transection or a vessel sealant device is used (Figure 3.9).

After transection of the ligamentum arteriosum, the esophagus is well exposed with direction of surrounding tissue and remaining fibers that could compress the esophagus.

A thoracostomy tube is then placed, the cannula removed, and each cannula site closed routinely. A local

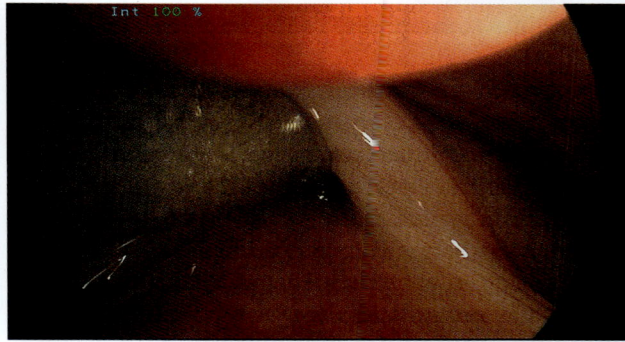

Figure 3.7 Thoracoscopic visualization of a ligamentum arteriosum.

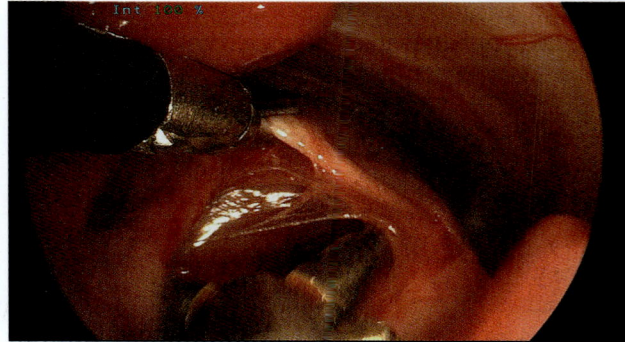

Figure 3.8 The ligamentum arteriosum has been dissected away from the esophagus.

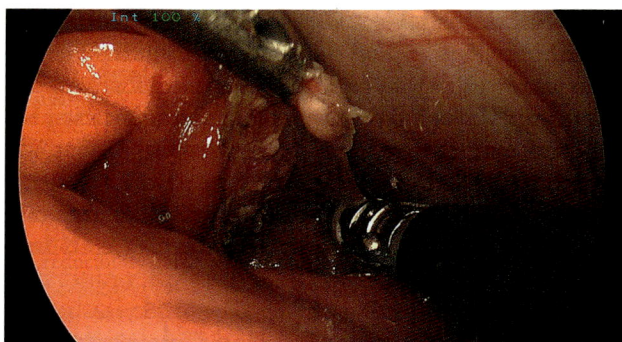

Figure 3.9 The ligamentum arteriosum is sealed and transected with a vessel sealant device.

block with a long-acting local anesthetic is performed in the intercostal space where the three cannulas were located and at the entrance of the thoracostomy tube.

Complications and aftercare

Postoperatively patients are monitored for signs of regurgitation. The thoracostomy tube is removed within 12 hours of surgery if the tube is not productive.

During surgery it is important to identify the vagus and laryngeal recurrent nerves. If the vagus nerve is damaged at the level of the ligamentum arteriosum, it induces a megaesophagus in the distal esophagus with abnormal motility. If the laryngeal recurrent nerve is damaged, it induces a unilateral laryngeal paralysis that should not be symptomatic.

After surgery dogs most likely need to be maintained in a vertical position after eating to allow the food bolus to progress to the stomach. Since dogs have a megaesophagus, they are at higher risk for regurgitation and aspiration pneumonia. It is not known if the cranial esophagus regains some function after correction of the obstruction.

Thoracoscopic treatment of a persistent aortic arch is an acceptable technique and it is not associated with higher morbidity or mortality when compared to treatment with thoracotomy (Townsend *et al.* 2016; Nucci *et al.* 2018).

The quality of life of patients is greatly improved. Owners are usually very satisfied with the improvements; however, the dogs still have to be fed in an elevated position for the rest of their life (Muldoon *et al.* 1997; Krebs *et al.* 2014; Townsend *et al.* 2016; Nucci *et al.* 2018).

References

Bezuidenhout, A.J. (1989). Anomalous origins of the right subclavian and common carotid arteries in the dog. *Journal of the South African Veterinary Association* 60: 215–218.

Buchanan, J.W. (2004). Tracheal signs and associated vascular anomalies in dogs with persistent right aortic arch. *Journal of Veterinary Internal Medicine* 18: 510–514.

Du Plessis, C.J., Keller, N., and Joubert, K.E. (2006). Symmetrical double aortic arch in a beagle puppy. *Journal of Small Animal Practice* 47: 31–34.

Ferrigno, C.R. et al. (2001). Double aortic arch in a dog (canis familiaris): aA case report. *Anatomia, Histologia, Embryologia* 30 (6): 379–381.

Fingeroth, J.M. and Fossum, T.W. (1987). Late-onset regurgitation associated with persistent right aortic arch in two dogs. *Journal of the American Veterinary Medical Association* 191: 981–983.

Holt, D., Heldmann, E., Michel, K., and Buchanan, J.W. (2000). Esophageal obstruction caused by a left aortic arch and an anomalous right patent ductus arteriosus in two German Shepherd littermates. *Veterinary Surgery* 29: 264–270.

Hurley, K., Miller, M.W., Willard, M.D., and Boothe, H.W. (1993). Left aortic arch and right ligamentum arteriosum causing esophageal obstruction in a dog. *Journal of the American Veterinary Medical Association* 203: 410–412.

Imhoff, R.K. and Foster, W.J. (1963). Persistent right aortic arch in a 10–year old dog. *Journal of the American Veterinary Medical Association* 143: 599–601.

Joly, H., D'Anjou, M.A., and Huneault, L. (2008). Imaging diagnosis: CT angiography of a rare vascular ring anomaly in a dog. *Veterinary Radiology and Ultrasound* 49: 42–46.

Krebs, I.A., Lindsley, S., Shaver, S., and Macphail, C. (2014). Short- and long-term outcome of dogs following surgical correction of a persistent right aortic arch. *Journal of the American Animal Hospital Association* 50 (3): 181–186.

Kyles, A.E. (2010). Vascular ring anomalies. In: *Mechanisms of Disease in Small Animal Surgery*, 3e (ed. M.J. Bojrab and E. Monnet), 135–137. Teton New Media: Jackson, WY.

MacPhail, C.M., Monnet, E., and Twedt, D.C. (2001). Thoracoscopic correction of persistent right aortic arch in a dog. *Journal of the American Animal Hospital Association* 37: 577–581.

Martin, D.G. et al. (1983). Double aortic arch in a dog. *Journal of the American Veterinary Medical Association* 183 (6): 697–699.

McCandlish, I.A., Nash, A.S., and Peggram, A. (1984). Unusual vascular ring in a cat: left aortic arch with right ligamentum arteriosum. *Veterinary Record* 114: 338–340.

Muldoon, M.M., Birchard, S.J., and Ellison, G.W. (1997). Long-term results of surgical correction of persistent right aortic arch in dogs: 25 cases (1980–1995). *Journal of the American Veterinary Medical Association* 210: 1761–1763.

Nucci, D.J., Hurst, K.C., and Monnet, E. (2018). Retrospective comparison of short-term outcomes following thoracoscopy versus thoracotomy for surgical correction of persistent right aortic arch in dogs. *Journal of the American Veterinary Medical Association* 253 (4): 444–451.

Rodrigues, B.A., Lamberts, M., Muccillo, M.S. et al. (2007). Successful surgical treatment of an American Staffordshire Terrier female with persistence of right aortic arch: case report. *Clinica Veterinaria* 12: 32–40.

Shires, P.K. and Liu, W. (1981). Persistent right aortic arch in dogs: a long term follow-up after surgical correction. *Journal of the American Animal Hospital Association* 17: 773–776.

Shojaei, B., Akhtardanesh, B., Kheirandish, R., and Vosough, D. (2011). Megaesophagus caused by an aberrant right subclavian artery and the brachiocephalic trunk in a cat. *Online Journal of Veterinary Research* 15: 46–52.

Townsend, S., Oblak, M.L., Singh, A. et al. (2016). Thoracoscopy with concurrent esophagoscopy for persistent right aortic arch in 9 dogs. *Veterinary Surgery* 45: O111–o118.

VanGundy, T. (1989). Vascular ring anomalies. *Compendium on Continuing Education for the Practicing Veterinarian* 11: 36–48.

Vianna, M.L. and Krahwinkel, D.J. Jr. (2004). Double aortic arch in a dog. *Journal of the American Veterinary Medical Association* 225 (1222–1224): 1196–1197.

White, R.N., Burton, C.A., and Hale, J.S.H. (2003). Vascular ring anomaly with coarctation of the aorta in a cat. *Journal of Small Animal Practice* 44: 330–334.

Yarim, M., Gültiken, M.E., Oztürk, S. et al. (1999). Double aortic arch in a Siamese cat. *Veterinary Pathology* 36: 340–341.

4

Hiatal Hernia

Eric Monnet and Ronald Bright

Hiatal hernia (HH) was first described by Gaskell *et al.* (1974). HH is a defect in the diaphragm that allows movement of the distal esophagus and a portion of the stomach into the thoracic cavity. Large hernias may also allow protrusion of other abdominal structures into the caudal thoracic cavity.

Various types of HH occur in dogs and cats. Type I is a "sliding" hernia whereby the stomach and the gastroesophageal junction (GEJ) move cranially through the defect (Figure 4.1a). The term "sliding" is applied because the proximal stomach and GEJ can move to and fro through the hiatus. This feature sometimes makes this type of hernia a diagnostic challenge. Type II herniation is when the gastric fundus and possibly other abdominal viscera are displaced cranially through the hiatus and into the chest while the GEJ remains fixed in its normal position (Figure 4.1b). This is also referred to as a paraesophageal HH. Type III features characteristics of both type I and II herniations and has rarely been reported in animals. Type IV is a type III herniation that is complicated by the herniation of abdominal viscera into the thoracic cavity, thought to be contained within a "sac" (Auger & Riley 1997; Rahal *et al.* 2003). This is also rare in the dog and cat.

Anatomy and physiology

The hiatus is a perforation of the diaphragm that allows the esophagus to course from the thoracic to the abdominal cavity. The positioning of the terminal esophagus within the abdominal cavity may act to create an intra-abdominal esophagus, thereby contributing to a reflux barrier via the law of Laplace. The esophageal wall is bound to the hiatus by the phrenicoesophageal ligament. This ligament is thought to help limit the cranial movement of the abdominal esophagus (Lecoindre & Cadore 1994).

The lower esophageal sphincter (LES) is a functional or physiologic sphincter and in the dog is composed of striated muscle and an inner layer of circular smooth muscle; in the cat it is composed only of smooth muscle (Han 2003). The circumferential striated muscle layer in the dog increases from the proximal to the distal esophagus and the maximal thickening of this muscle appears to correlate with the high-pressure zone of the GEJ. The area of increased pressure between the stomach and the esophagus (referred to as barrier pressure) helps main unidirectional flow of food and liquid and prevents reflux.

A vagally mediated relaxation of the LES begins approximately 5 seconds after swallowing. The "sphincter" mechanism at this site is thought to be augmented by various extrinsic factors. These include the diaphragmatic crural muscle, which serves as a muscular "sling" compressing the esophagus, and gastric distension, which causes the angle at which the esophagus enters the stomach to become more oblique while causing compression of the LES by the distended fundus. In addition, extrinsic factors include the acute angulation of the terminal portion of the esophagus and stomach, the gastric cardia sling fibers along the left-hand margin of the GEJ, and the short abdominal esophagus that is thought to allow a "flutter-valve" effect (Strombeck & Guilford 1983; Pratschke *et al.* 2004). The radius of the esophagus is less

(a)

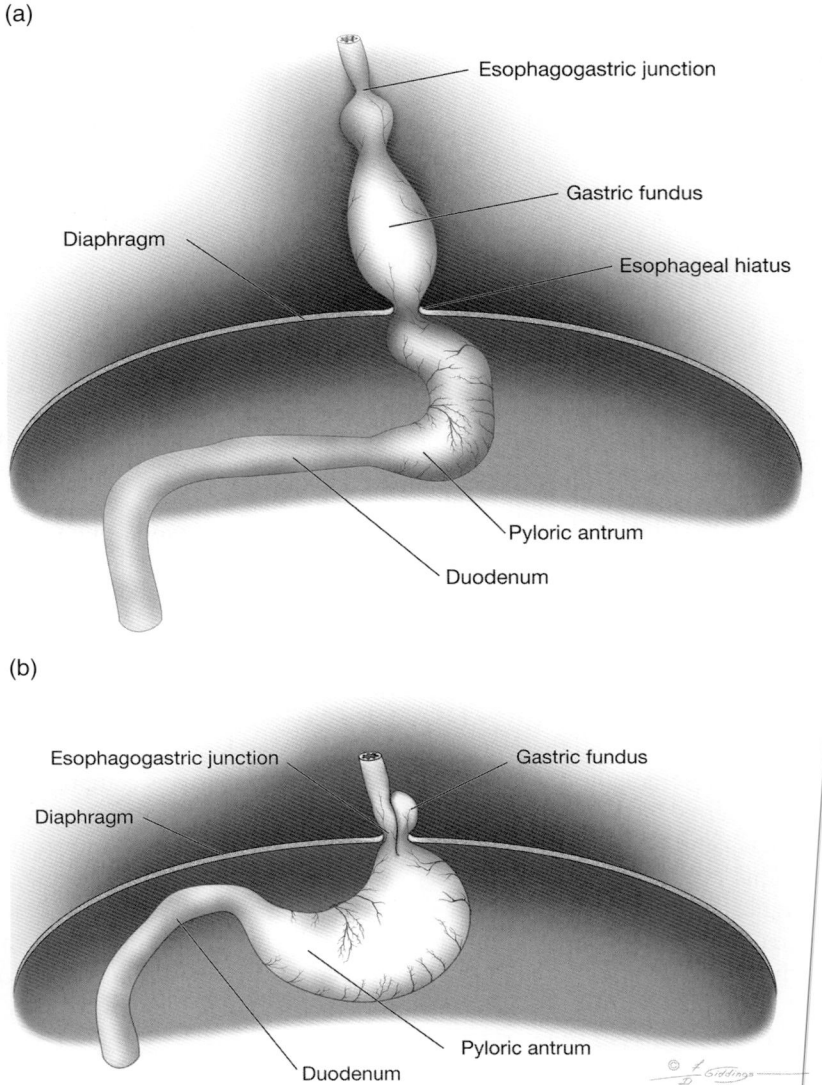

(b)

Figure 4.1 (a) Sliding hiatal hernia with the lower esophageal sphincter displaced into the thoracic cavity. (b) Paraesophageal hiatal hernia with the fundus of the stomach herniating into the thoracic cavity while the lower esophageal sphincter is still in normal position. Source: © D. Giddings.

than the gastric radius and if a short portion of the esophagus lies within the abdomen, then when both portions are exposed to the same positive intra-abdominal pressure, the pressure within the abdominal esophageal segment will always exceed that within the stomach, making it difficult for gastroesophageal reflux (GER) to occur (Van Sluijs 1993).

Pathophysiology

It is generally accepted that one of the factors involved in GER related to HH is loss of the intra-abdominal portion of the esophagus associated with cranial displacement of the gastric fundus and GEJ. This results in the absence of

a functional length of intra-abdominal esophagus (increased axial separation between the LES and hiatus), which exposes the GEJ to negative pressures, resulting in hypotonia of the sphincter, incompetence, and GER (Waldron & Lieb 1993). The contribution of the diaphragmatic crural muscle to a competent antireflux barrier has been suggested and may play an important role where the GEJ comes under increased pressure (Jackson 1922; Rådmark & Pettersson 1989). It is possible that clinical resolution of GER associated with HH may be due, at least in part, to the change in relationship between diaphragmatic crural musculature and the GEJ.

A great percentage of dogs with HH (60%) are thought to have a congenital form and mostly involve brachycephalic breeds (Guilford & Strombeck 1996; Mayhew *et al.* 2017; Reeve *et al.* 2017; Broux *et al.* 2018; Eivers *et al.* 2019; Freiche & German 2021). The cross-sectional area of the esophageal hiatus seems to be larger in brachycephalic dogs than in nonbrachycephalic dogs (Conte *et al.* 2020). The congenital form is likely due to incomplete fusion of the diaphragm during early embryonic development (Callan *et al.* 1993). The Chinese shar-pei and the English bulldog are thought to be the most commonly affected breeds. The inheritance pattern has not been established for HH type I and II in dogs. However, it has been hypothesized that the Chinese shar-pei may have a partially heritable trait, which supports the contention that it is a familial condition in these dogs (Knowles *et al.* 1990; Callan *et al.* 1993; Rahal *et al.* 2003). HH has also been described in cats (Phillips *et al.* 2019).

Reflux esophagitis due to GER is thought to be the most important cause of signs seen in type I HH (Mayhew *et al.* 2017). However, not all animals with HH and associated GER have symptomatology (Lorinson & Bright 1998). This may be due to individual variations in susceptibility of the esophagus to injury or the presence of intact factors aimed at protecting the distal esophagus from the effects of gastric contents. These include minimal exposure of material in the esophagus, normal peristalsis that provides immediate clearance of gastric contents, chemical neutralization of reflux provided by bicarbonate-rich salivary secretions, and esophageal submucosal glands secreting material that helps protect the mucosa (Han 2003). In addition, the composition and pH of the refluxed material may help determine whether esophagitis develops. Reflux often contains acid, pepsin, trypsin, bile acids, and lysolecithin, which all contribute to esophageal damage. In animals showing clinical signs, reflux esophagitis itself can cause a decrease in LES tone and diminish the antireflux barrier. Acid reflux also inhibits normal esophageal motility and the "clearing" function, thus becoming a self-perpetuating cycle (Sivacolundhu *et al.* 2002).

Because of the injury to the esophagus and subsequent negative effects on motility, megaesophagus is commonly seen with HH. Although megaesophagus is most often a secondary effect of HH, primary megaesophagus as a congenital lesion (hypomotile and redundant esophagus) has been reported in shar peis primarily, but may occur in any breed (Guiot *et al.* 2008). When megaesophagus is present, it may increase the negative effects of GER on the esophagus due to reduction of esophageal clearance. The spontaneous resolution of megaesophagus after HH surgery supports the fact that megaesophagus can be a secondary lesion rather than a primary or concurrent disease.

HH can be secondary to trauma, diaphragmatic hernia, or increased respiratory effort. Trauma is thought to cause weakening of the attachments of the esophagus at the hiatus, predisposing to HH. The HH associated with diaphragmatic hernia is usually seen within a short period of time following diaphragmatic herniorraphy (Bright *et al.* 1990; Lorinson & Bright 1998; Pratschke *et al.* 1998).

Chronic upper airway disorders such as nasal masses, brachycephalic syndrome, laryngeal paralysis, and narrowing of the intrapharyngeal opening have been associated with HH (Ellison *et al.* 1987; Pearson *et al.* 1978; Hardie *et al.* 1998; Dvir *et al.* 2003; Lecoindre & Richard 2004). The respiratory distress related to airway obstruction results in increased inspiratory effort, which causes a negative intraesophageal and intrapleural pressure that pulls the esophagus and stomach into the thorax to either cause or worsen HH. In some instances, correcting the upper airway obstruction has ameliorated signs related to HH (Dvir *et al.* 2003; Lecoindre & Richard 2004).

Dyspnea and exercise intolerance thought to be caused by HH are related to either aspiration pneumonia (more likely with type I HH) or lung compression by herniated abdominal organs, as seen with type II, III, or IV herniations (Pratschke *et al.* 1998). An experimental study in dogs revealed that the presence of gastric acid in the lower esophagus is often seen with HH, and can result in severe laryngospasm and bronchospasm that will worsen respiratory signs (Senyk *et al.* 1974). In most instances, however, dyspnea as a sole sign related to HH of any type is unusual.

There are a few reports describing HH associated with tetanus in the dog (Adamantos & Boag 2007). Many cases of HH resolved with successful treatment of the tetanus and conservative management of clinical signs related to GER.

History and clinical signs

The most common form of HH is type I, which is usually diagnosed in animals 12 months of age or less. The Chinese shar-pei and brachycephalic breeds, in particular the English bulldog, are at higher risk than most breeds. Animals with a history of trauma leading to diaphragmatic hernia will sometimes develop HH after surgical repair of the diaphragmatic hernia.

The most common signs associated with type I HH are related to GER. This includes persistent regurgitation, vomiting, ptyalism, and occasional hematemesis. Weight loss is sometimes seen. Respiratory distress due to aspiration pneumonia may be seen, but is seldom the only sign. It is important to recognize that some dogs and cats with confirmed HH have no symptomatology.

Type II (paraesophageal) HH is much less common than type I sliding HH and, unless it is combined with a sliding HH (types III and IV), is rarely associated with GER unless there is concurrent megaesophagus (Kirkby *et al.* 2005). In most instances, clinical signs likely result from the presence of the stomach and/or other organs within the thoracic cavity. This includes dyspnea, weakness, or collapse, since respiratory and cardiac compromise can result from encroachment of abdominal viscera. A type IV HH resulted in Budd–Chiari syndrome in a shar-pei dog, likely due to compression of hepatic venous outflow (Baig *et al.* 2006; Adamantos & Boag 2007).

Diagnosis

Survey radiography of the thorax may confirm HH, especially if the herniation is large and persistent (Figure 4.2). A soft tissue and gas-filled structure, usually the stomach, may be seen in the caudal dorsal aspect of the thorax. Important differential diagnoses based on plain films include esophageal epiphrenic diverticulum, gastroesophageal intussusception, neoplasia, and foreign body. Megaesophagus is often seen and aspiration pneumonia is occasionally noted.

To confirm HH, a barium esophagram with or without fluoroscopy is necessary (Figure 4.3). This helps distinguish other soft tissue densities in the caudal mediastinum from HH. This study usually demonstrates cranial displacement of the GEJ with type I, III, or IV HH. In addition, there will be retention of barium in a dilated caudal portion of the esophagus and often visualization of gastric rugal folds.

Small HH and those that are type I axial sliding forms can become a diagnostic challenge. Application of pressure on the abdomen during the esophagram may help in demonstrating the hernia. Fluoroscopy will also demonstrate GER and various degrees of to-and-fro movement of the GEJ during reflux. Hypomotility of the esophagus may also be demonstrated with fluoroscopy.

Esophagoscopy with a flexible endoscope may be necessary to confirm the presence of HH (Website Chapter 4: Gastrointestinal surgery/esophagus/hiatal hernia). An enlarged hiatal opening, mild to severe esophagitis, gastric reflux, or strictures may be seen. In some instances, gastric rugae can be seen protruding through the GEJ. Retrograde esophagoscopy is helpful in demonstrating the distortion of the hiatus and the prolapse of gastric rugae cranially through the cardia. In some dogs, minor deviation of the distal portion of the esophagus may be seen, requiring redirection of the tip of the endoscope in order to enter the stomach. Applying pressure on the abdominal wall during endoscopy might increase the chance of diagnosing a sliding HH (Broux *et al.* 2018).

Treatment

Medical treatment

Treating an underlying disorder, such as tetanus or an upper airway obstructive disease, may be sufficient to allow complete resolution of reflux esophagitis

(a)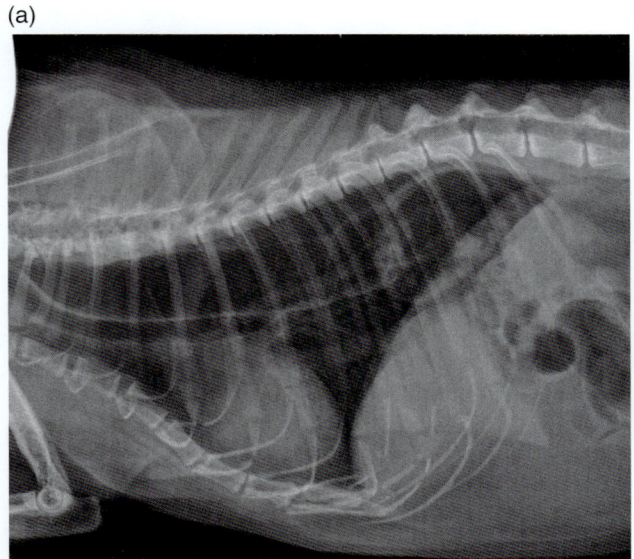

(b)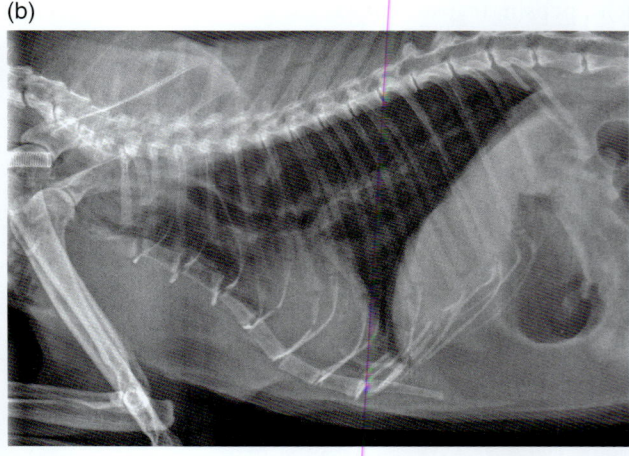

Figure 4.2 (a) Lateral radiograph of a cat with a sliding hiatal hernia with megaesophagus. This cat had a severe upper airway obstruction. (b) The hernia was not sliding after the upper airway was treated with a temporary tracheostomy.

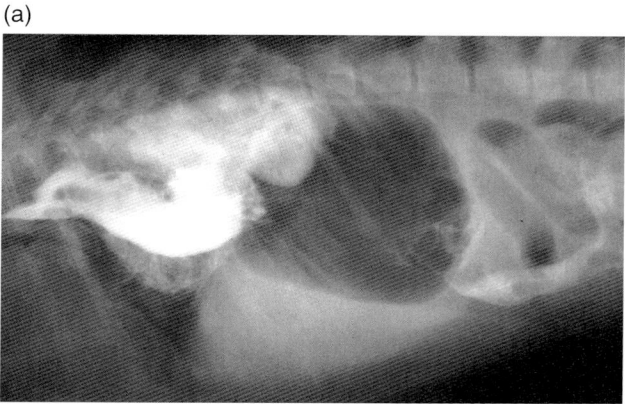

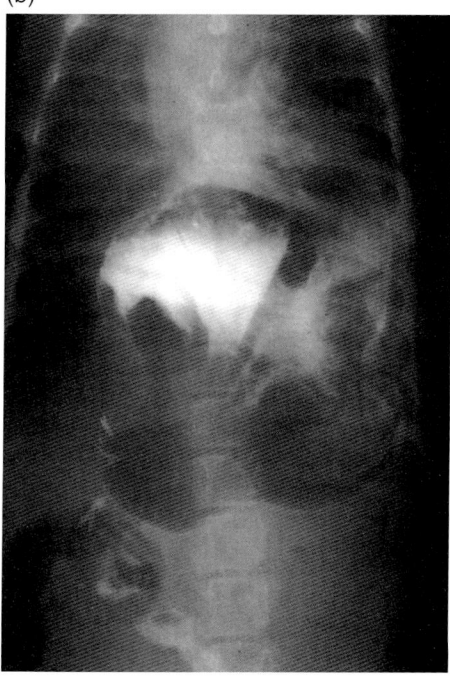

Figure 4.3 (a) Lateral view of an esophagram of a dog with a sliding hiatal hernia. (b) Ventrodorsal view of the esophagram.

secondary to GER (Dieringer & Wolf 1991; Van Ham & van Bree 1992). Feeding small portions of a low-fat softened or liquefied meal may be the only management strategy necessary for HH that has primarily GER-related signs (type I mainly). If this is unsuccessful, then medical treatment should be attempted as well. The goal of more aggressive medical therapy is to reduce signs of reflux esophagitis by helping the esophageal mucosa to heal. This is best accomplished by reducing the volume and acidity of the refluxate, increasing LES tone, improving the clearance of refluxed gastric contents, and protecting the esophageal mucosa from injury by use of a cytoprotective drug. Use of a systemic antacid, a gastric prokinetic drug that also increases LES tone, and a cytoprotective agent such as sucralfate are all recommended for a minimum of 30 days. In some instances following this period, no further therapy will be necessary with the exception of dietary management. A proton pump inhibitor is now preferred over a histamine H_2 blocker for decreasing the acid content of the refluxate.

Type II (paraesophageal) HH does not usually show signs of reflux esophagitis since the LES remains in the correct anatomic position. Instead, clinical signs likely result from the physical presence of the stomach and/or other abdominal organs in the caudal mediastinum after being displaced cranially. Type II HH is therefore unlikely to respond to any type of medical management. The only indication for medical management in type II HH would be if concurrent megaesophagus was present and thought to be responsible for GER (Kirkby *et al.* 2005).

Surgical treatment

A fundoplasty technique, Nissen fundoplication, was borrowed from human surgery and a series of cases in dogs was reported by Ellison *et al.* (1987). The goal of a fundoplasty procedure was to correct what was thought to be a primary sphincter incompetence problem associated with HH. This procedure is successful in people with HH because there is a high incidence of primary incompetence of the LES. While this procedure has been described with some success in correcting esophageal problems associated with HH in the dog and cat, a "floppy" fundoplication was described a few years later with better outcomes (Sivacolundhu *et al.* 2002). Regardless, most veterinary surgeons find the fundoplication (sphincter-enhancement technique) to be too demanding, and complication rates are higher than with techniques developed later (Lorinson & Bright 1998).

Fundoplication in animals has been shown to be associated with a "gas bloat syndrome" due to interference with eructation (Prymak *et al.* 1989). It may also prevent the animal's ability to vomit. Transient gastric tympany may be induced by the procedure (Gaskell *et al.* 1974). Fundoplication is currently thought to be reserved for those canine and feline patients that do not respond to techniques designed to correct the anatomic relationship of the stomach, diaphragm, hiatus, and stomach (Guiot *et al.* 2008).

The most successful and simplest technique is anatomic reduction and stabilization of the HH. This involves reducing the size of the esophageal hiatus (hiatal plication), securing the esophagus to the crus of the diaphragm (esophagopexy), and a left-sided gastropexy (Prymak *et al.* 1989; Mayhew *et al.* 2017; Monnet 2020, 2021). This technique is accomplished through a ventral cranial abdominal incision or with laparoscopy. The hepatogastric ligament is transected, followed by retraction of the stomach to the right and the liver medially. This allows good exposure of the distal esophagus and the hiatus. The phrenicoesophageal ligament is freed from its attachments to the esophagus, taking care to avoid the ventral branch of the vagus nerve (Figure 4.4). This allows the caudal 2–3 cm of the esophagus to be retracted into the abdomen. The left and right diaphragmatic crura are approximated with nonabsorbable suture such as polypropylene until the hiatus is reduced to approximately 1–2 cm (Figure 4.5). The circumferential esophageal rim reconstruction has been recommended (Hosgood *et al.* 2021). It requires plication of the pars lumbalis in the dorsal part of the esophageal hiatus. The esophagopexy is accomplished by placing two to three sutures between the diaphragm and the tunica muscularis of the esophagus (Figure 4.6). Lastly, the fundus of the stomach is attached to the left

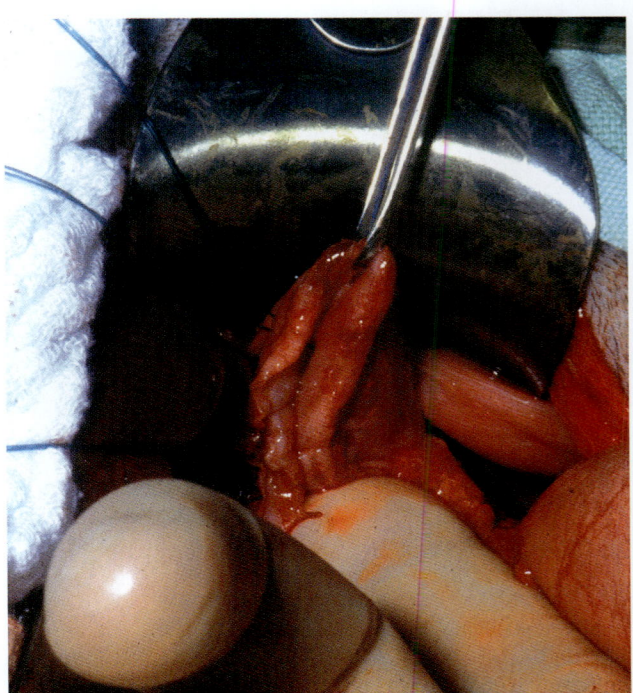

Figure 4.5 The right and left crura of the esophageal hiatus are approximated with three mattress sutures. Nonabsorbable suture has been used. The diameter is reduced to 2 cm around the finger of the surgeon.

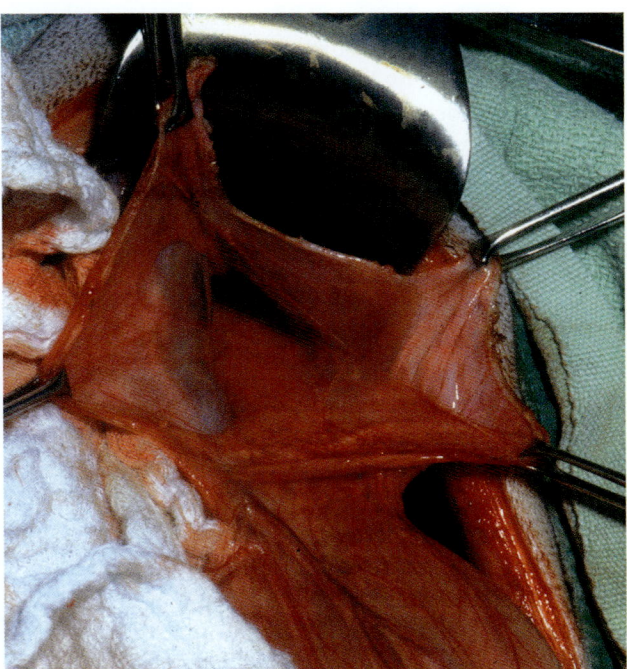

Figure 4.4 The hiatal hernia has been reduced and the phrenicoesophageal ligament is exposed.

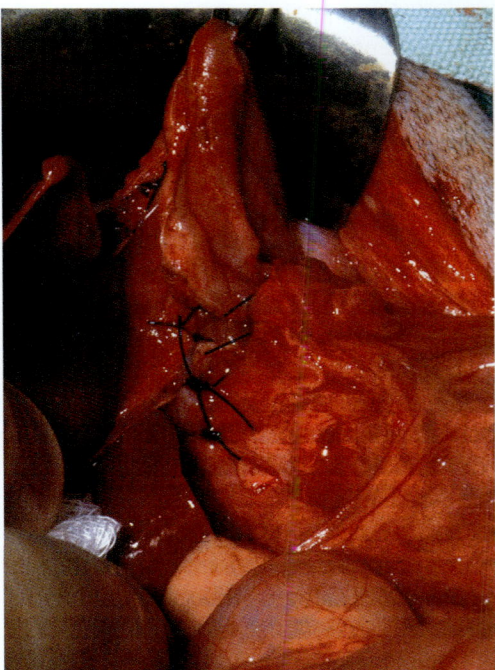

Figure 4.6 An esophagopexy is performed with three cruciate sutures between the wall of the esophagus and the crura of the esophageal hiatus.

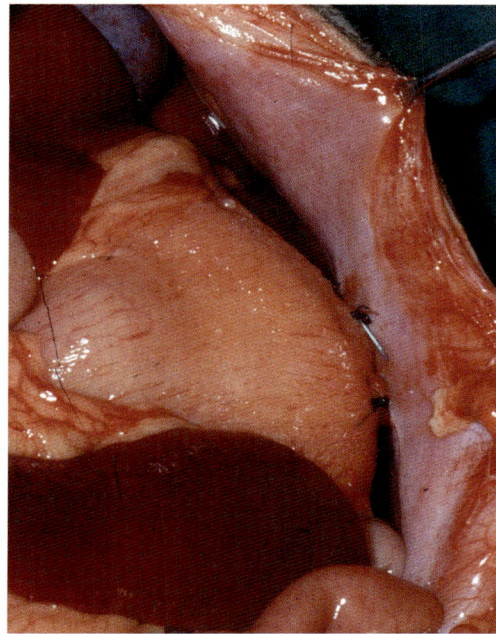

Figure 4.7 A gastropexy between the fundus of the stomach and the body wall is performed on the left side with some tension on the stomach.

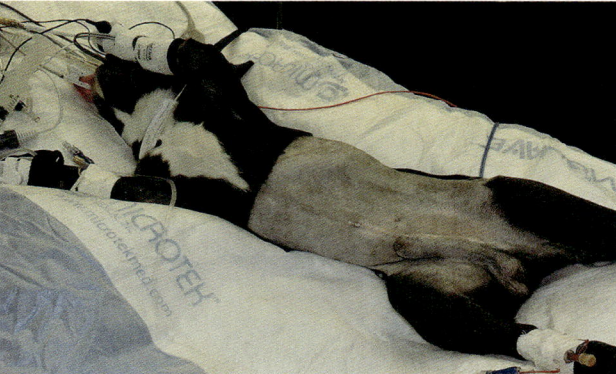

Figure 4.8 The dog has been placed in right lateral oblique recumbency to improve exposure of the esophageal hiatus.

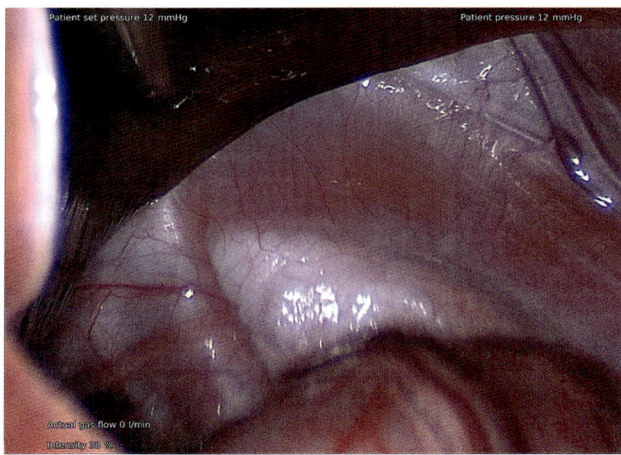

Figure 4.9 The esophageal hiatus has been exposed after transection of the triangular ligament of the left lateral liver lobe and retraction of that lobe with a palpation probe.

body wall using an incisional gastropexy (Figure 4.7). The location of the corresponding incision on the body wall is determined while applying a slight amount of caudal traction on the stomach.

Some surgeons currently believe that hernia reduction followed by gastropexy alone may be solely responsible for the good outcome (Guiot *et al.* 2008). Barrier pressure at the GEJ has been shown in the anesthetized dog to be increased following a gastropexy. The results of the increased barrier pressure at the GEJ likely explains why the risk of GER and associated reflux esophagitis decreases. This speaks to the clinical relevance of using this procedure alone (Pratschke *et al.* 2001). However, performing this procedure on immature cats and dogs may be questionable due to its possible effect on the growth of the animal. In the immature animal, therefore, it is prudent to perform an esophagopexy to prevent reherniation (Guiot *et al.* 2008). Tube gastrostomy or incisional gastropexy may be used as a primary method of gastropexy.

Correction of HH has been described with laparoscopy (Monnet 2021; Mayhew *et al.* 2021). The dog is placed in right lateral oblique recumbency (Figure 4.8) and the laparoscopic cannulas or single port are placed canal to the last rib on the left side of the abdominal cavity. After transection of the triangular ligament of the left lateral liver lobe, this lobe can be retracted with a palpation probe (Figure 4.9). With caudal traction on the body of the stomach, the hernia is reduced and the esophageal hiatus exposed. The esophageal hiatus is then plicated with unidirectional barbed sutures (Figure 4.10). The phrenicoesophageal membrane is not dissected from the esophagus to prevent induction of a pneumothorax. The esophagopexy is also performed with the same suture material (Figure 4.11). Finally, a gastropexy is performed at one of the cannula sites.

After surgery the clinical signs related to the HH are improving but do not resolve completely (Hosgood *et al.* 2021; Mayhew *et al.* 2017, 2021). GER can persist after surgery. Brachycephalic dogs with HH may be at higher risk of having esophageal motility disorders (Eivers *et al.* 2019).

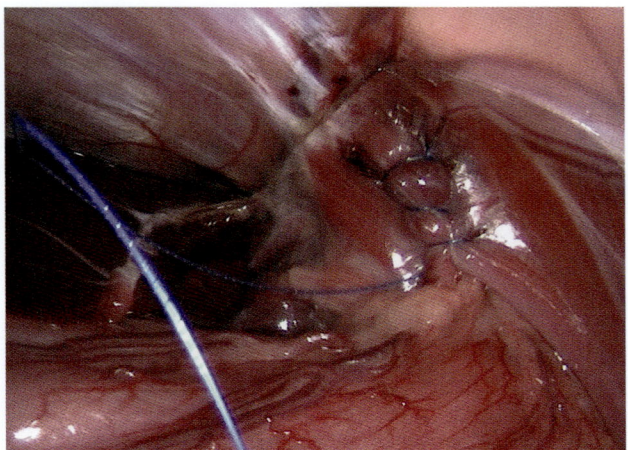

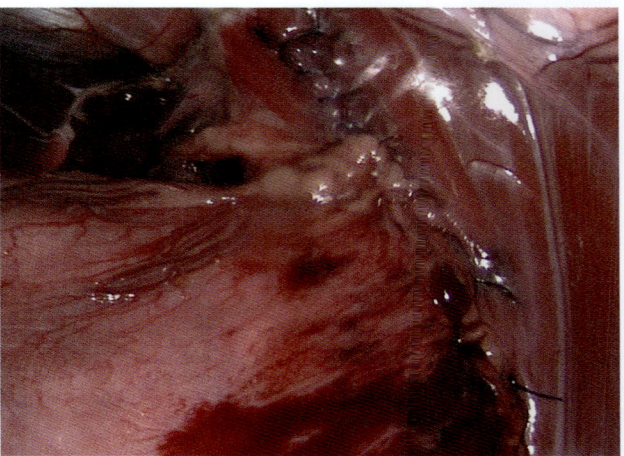

Figure 4.10 The esophageal hiatus and the phrenicoesophageal membrane have been plicated with a unidirectional barbed suture with a simple continuous pattern.

Figure 4.11 The esophagopexy has been completed on the left side of the esophagus with a unidirectional barbed suture.

References

Adamantos, S. and Boag, A. (2007). Thirteen cases of tetanus in dogs. *Veterinary Record* 161: 298–303.

Auger, J.M. and Riley, S.M. (1997). Combined hiatal and pleuroperitoneal hernia in a shar-pei. *Canadian Veterinary Journal* 38: 640–642.

Baig, M.A., Gemmill, T., Hammond, G. et al. (2006). Budd–Chiari-like syndrome caused by a congenital hiatal hernia in a shar-pei dog. *Veterinary Record* 159: 322–323.

Bright, R.M., Sackman, J.E., DeNovo, C., and Toal, C. (1990). Hiatal hernia in the dog and cat: a retrospective study of 16 cases. *Journal of Small Animal Practice* 31: 224–250.

Broux, O., Clercx, C., Etienne, A.L. et al. (2018). Effects of manipulations to detect sliding hiatal hernia in dogs with brachycephalic airway obstructive syndrome. *Veterinary Surgery* 47: 243–251.

Callan, M.B., Washabau, R.J., Saunders, H.M. et al. (1993). Congenital esophageal hiatal hernia in the Chinese shar-pei dog. *Journal of Veterinary Internal Medicine* 7: 210–215.

Conte, A., Morabito, S., Dennis, R., and Murgia, D. (2020). Computed tomographic comparison of esophageal hiatal size in brachycephalic and non-brachycephalic breed dogs. *Veterinary Surgery* 49: 1509–1516.

Dieringer, T.M. and Wolf, A.M. (1991). Esophageal hiatal hernia and megaesophagus complicating tetanus in two dogs. *Journal of the American Veterinary Medical Association* 199: 87–89.

Dvir, E., Spotswood, T.C., Lambrechts, N.E., and Lobetti, R.G. (2003). Congenital narrowing of the intrapharyngeal opening in a dog with concurrent oesophageal hiatal hernia. *Journal of Small Animal Practice* 44: 359–362.

Eivers, C., Chicon, R.R., Liuti, T., and Salavati, S.S. (2019). Retrospective analysis of esophageal imaging features in brachycephalic versus non-brachycephalic dogs based on videofluoroscopic swallowing studies. *Journal of Veterinary Internal Medicine* 33: 1740–1746.

Ellison, G.W., Lewis, D.D., Phillips, L., and Tarvin, G.B. (1987). Esophageal hiatal hernia in small animals: literature review and a modified surgical technique. *Journal of the American Animal Hospital Association* 23: 391–399.

Freiche, V. and German, A.J. (2021). Digestive diseases in brachycephalic dogs. *Veterinary Clinics of North America: Small Animal Practice* 51: 61–78.

Gaskell, C.J., Gibbs, C., and Pearson, H. (1974). Sliding hiatal hernia with reflux esophagitis in 2 dogs. *Journal of Small Animal Practice* 15: 503–510.

Guilford, W.G. and Strombeck, D.R. (1996). Diseases of swallowing. In: *Strombeck's Small Animal Gastroenterology*, 3e (ed. W.G. Guilford, S.A. Center, D.R. Strombeck, et al.), 211–238. Philadelphia, PA: WB Saunders.

Guiot, L.P., Lansdowne, J.L., Rouppert, P. and Stanley, B.J. (2008). Hiatal hernia in the dog: a clinical report of four Chinese sharpeis. *Journal of the American Animal Hospital Association* 44: 335–341.

Han, E. (2003). Diagnosis and management of reflux esophagitis. *Clinical Techniques in Small Animal Practice* 18: 231–238.

Hardie, E.M., Ramirez, O. III, Clary, E.M. et al. (1998). Abnormalities of the thoracic bellows: stress fractures of the ribs and hiatal hernia. *Journal of Veterinary Internal Medicine* 12: 279–287.

Hosgood, G.L., Appelgrein, C., and Gelmi C. (2021). Circumferential esophageal hiatal rim reconstruction for treatment of persistent regurgitation in brachycephalic dogs: 29 cases (2016–2019). *Journal of the American Veterinary Medical Association* 258: 1091–1097.

Jackson, C. (1922). The diaphragmatic pinchcock in so-called cardiospasm. *Laryngoscopy* 32: 139–145.

Kirkby, K.A., Bright, R.M., and Owen, H.D. (2005). Paraesophageal hiatal hernia and megaesophagus in a 3-week-old Alaskan malamute. *Journal of Small Animal Practice* 46: 402–405.

Knowles, K., O'Brien, D., and Amann, J. (1990). Congenital idiopathic megaesophagus in a litter of Chinese shar-peis: clinical, electrodiagnostic and pathological findings. *Journal of the American Animal Hospital Association* 26: 313–318.

Lecoindre, P. and Cadore, J.L. (1994). Disorders of the oesophagus in domestic animals. *Praktische Medizinia Chirurgia* 29: 25–43.

Lecoindre, P. and Richard, S. (2004). Digestive disorders associated with the chronic obstructive respiratory syndrome of brachycephalic dogs: 30 cases (1999–2001). *Revue de Médecine Vétérinaire* 155: 141–146.

Lorinson, D. and Bright, R.M. (1998). Long-term outcome of medical and surgical treatment of hiatal hernias in dogs and cats: 27 cases (1978–1996). *Journal of the American Veterinary Medical Association* 213: 381–385.

Mayhew, P.D., Marks, S.L., Pollard, R. et al. (2017). Prospective evaluation of surgical management of sliding hiatal hernia and gastroesophageal reflux in dogs. *Veterinary Surgery* 46: 1098–1109.

Mayhew, P.D., Balsa, I.M., Marks, S.L. et al. (2021). Clinical and videofluoroscopic outcomes of laparoscopic treatment for sliding hiatal hernia and associated gastroesophageal reflux in brachycephalic dogs. *Veterinary Surgery* 50 (Suppl 1): O67–O77.

Monnet, E. (2020). Hiatal hernia. In: *Gastrointestinal Surgical Techniques in Small Animals* (ed. E. Monnet and D. Smeak), 123–128. Hoboken, NJ: Wiley.

Monnet, E. (2021). Laparoscopic correction of sliding hiatal hernia in eight dogs: description of technique, complications, and short-term outcome. *Veterinary Surgery* 50: 230–237.

Pearson, H., Darke, P.G., Gibbs, C. et al. (1978). Reflux esophagitis and stricture formation after anesthesia: a review of seven cases in dogs and cats. *Journal of Small Animal Practice* 19: 507–519.

Phillips, H., Corrie, J., Engel, D.M. et al. (2019). Clinical findings, diagnostic test results, and treatment outcome in cats with hiatal hernia: 31 cases (1995–2018). *Journal of Veterinary Internal Medicine* 33: 1970–1976.

Pratschke, K.M., Hughes, J.M.L., Shelly, C., and Bellenger, C.R. (1998). Hiatal hernia as a complication of chronic diaphragmatic herniation. *Journal of Small Animal Practice* 39: 33–38.

Pratschke, K.M., Bellenger, C.R., McAllister, H., and Campion, D. (2001). Barrier pressure at the gastroesophageal junction in anesthetized dogs. *American Journal of Veterinary Research* 62: 1068–1072.

Pratschke, K.M., Fitzpatrick, E., Campion, D. et al. (2004). Topography of the gastroesophageal junction in the dog revisited and possible clinical implications. *Research in Veterinary Science* 76: 171–177.

Prymak, C., Saunders, H.M., and Washabau, R.J. (1989). Hiatal hernia repair by restoration and stabilization of normal anatomy in four dogs and one cat. *Veterinary Surgery* 18: 386–391.

Rådmark, T. and Pettersson, G.B. (1989). The contribution of the diaphragm as an intrinsic sphincter to the gastroesopheal reflux barrier. An experimental study in the dog. *Scandinavian Journal of Gastroenterology* 24: 85–94.

Rahal, S.C., Mamprim, M.J., Muniz, L.M., and Teixeira, C.R. (2003). Type-4 esophageal hernia in a Chinese shar-pei dog. *Veterinary Radiology and Ultrasound* 44: 646–647.

Reeve, E.J., Sutton, D., Friend, E.J., and Warren-Smith, C.M.R. (2017). Documenting the prevalence of hiatal hernia and oesophageal abnormalities in brachycephalic dogs using fluoroscopy. *Journal of Small Animal Practice* 58: 703–708.

Senyk, J., Arborelius, M. Jr., Lilja, B., and Nylander, G. (1974). Bronchogenic and angiopneumographic changes associated with esophageal hiatal hernia. An experimental study in dogs. *European Surgical Research* 6: 72–78.

Sivacolundhu, R.K., Read, R.A., and Marchevsky, A.M. (2002). Hiatal hernia controversies: a review of pathophysiology and treatment options. *Australian Veterinary Journal* 80: 48–53.

Strombeck, D. and Guilford, W.G. (1983). Pharynx and esophagus: normal structure and function. In: *Strombeck's Small Animal Gastroenterology*, 3e (ed. W.G. Guilford, S.A. Center, D.R. Strombeck, et al.), 202–209. Philadelphia, PA: WB Saunders.

Van Ham, L. and van Bree, H. (1992). Conservative treatment of tetanus associated with hiatal hernia and gastro-oesophageal reflux. *Journal of Small Animal Practice* 33: 289–294.

Van Sluijs, F. (1993). Gastroesophageal reflux disease. In: *Textbook of Small Animal Surgery*, 2e (ed. D.H. Slatter), 571–593. Philadelphia, PA: WB Saunders.

Waldron, D. and Lieb, A.S. (1993). Hiatal hernia. In: *Disease Mechanisms in Small Animal Surgery*, 2e (ed. M.J. Bojrab, D.D. Smeak and M.S. Bloomberg), 210–213. Philadelphia, PA: Lea & Febiger.

5

Pyloric Hypertrophy

Eric Monnet

Pyloric hypertrophy is probably the most common cause of gastric obstruction (Hall *et al.* 1990). It has been recognized as two different forms: congenital and acquired. The congenital form is associated with muscular hypertrophy of the pylorus, while the acquired form is presented with mucosal hypertrophy and polyps. It can be focal with one polyp, multifocal with multiple polyps or folds, or generalized with the entire pyloric astral mucosa being involved. The congenital form is more common in dogs less than 1 year old and in brachycephalic breeds (Walsh & Quigley 1966; Sikes *et al.* 1986; Prole 1989; Walter & Matthiesen 1989; Bellenger *et al.* 1990; Peeters 1991; Lecoindre & Richard 2004; Poncet *et al.* 2005). The congenital form is also referred to as pyloric stenosis, benign muscular pyloric hypertrophy, and congenital pyloric muscle hypertrophy. The acquired form, on the other hand, is more common in middle-aged male dogs in small breeds like Lhasa apso, shih tzu, Maltese, and Pekinese (Walsh & Quigley 1966; Sikes *et al.* 1986; Prole 1989; Walter & Matthiesen 1989; Bellenger *et al.* 1990; Peeters 1991; Lecoindre & Richard 2004; Poncet *et al.* 2005). A mixed form exists where muscular hypertrophy and mucosal hyperplasia are both present (Poncet *et al.* 2005).

Pathophysiology

The causes of the congenital and acquired forms are not well understood. It has been postulated that exposure to pentagastrin during pregnancy can increase the risk of developing pyloric hypertrophy. However, this hypothesis has never been proven, especially since pentagastrin cannot traverse the placenta (Dodge 1969; Dodge & Karim 1976; Janik *et al.* 1978). The acquired form may result from chronic gastritis with duodenal reflux, including bile and food stasis that stimulates cholecystokinin production (Lecoindre & Richard 2004). Histopathologic evaluation reveals hypertrophy of the mucosa with or without inflammation (Taulescu *et al.* 2014). The muscular layers can also be hypertrophied.

Clinical signs and physical examination

Dogs with pyloric hypertrophy are presented with chronic vomiting that can be projectile. At the time of presentation the owners describe an increasing frequency of vomiting over the last 3–4 months (Matthiesen & Walter 1986; Hall 2013). Usually dogs are vomiting a mixture of food and mucus. Anorexia and weight loss can be noted. The chronic vomiting can induce esophagitis and megaesophagus (Pearson *et al.* 1974). Abdominal distention is fairly common and palpation reveals a larger stomach in the cranial abdomen. Dehydration can be noted in those dogs.

Diagnostics

Bloodwork

A metabolic alkalosis is usually present with the upper gastrointestinal obstruction. Hypochloremia and hypokalemia are typically present with hypoalbuminemia (Hall 2013).

Radiographs

Plain abdominal radiographs reveal a very large stomach occupying more than half of the abdominal cavity, pushing the rest of the small intestine caudally and dorsally. The spleen is also displaced.

Contrast study with barium is required to show increased emptying time and pyloric hypertrophy. The hypertrophy is characterized by the lack of contrast material in the pyloric antrum and pylorus. The filling defect is present on serial radiographs. The "beak" appearance of the barium passing through the hypertrophied pylorus is characteristic of pyloric hypertrophy (Figure 5.1).

Usual ultrasound is not useful for the diagnosis of pyloric hypertrophy. It may show a 4 mm thick hypoechoic layer of pyloric muscle and a thickened pyloric wall. The pyloric wall can be 9 mm thick (Biller *et al.* 1994).

Endoscopy

Endoscopy of the stomach is very valuable for the diagnosis of pyloric hypertrophy. In the congenital form the mucosa should look normal, and it is difficult to impossible to advance the flexible endoscope into the duodenum. For the acquired form, flaps of mucosa and/or polyps are obstructing the pylorus (Figure 5.2). Biopsy of the mucosa is required to rule out infiltrative disease in the pylorus (Leib *et al.* 1993).

Surgical management

Pyloric hypertrophy is better treated surgically. A Billroth I procedure can be performed. Usually a Y—U pyloroplasty is recommended (Figures 5.3 and 5.4) (Bright *et al.* 1988). It is not associated with an increased risk of biliary reflux.

During the Y—U pyloroplasty it is important to resect the abnormal mucosa and appose the mucosa with a simple continuous pattern without inducing a stricture of the pylorus (Bright *et al.* 1988; Monnet 2020).

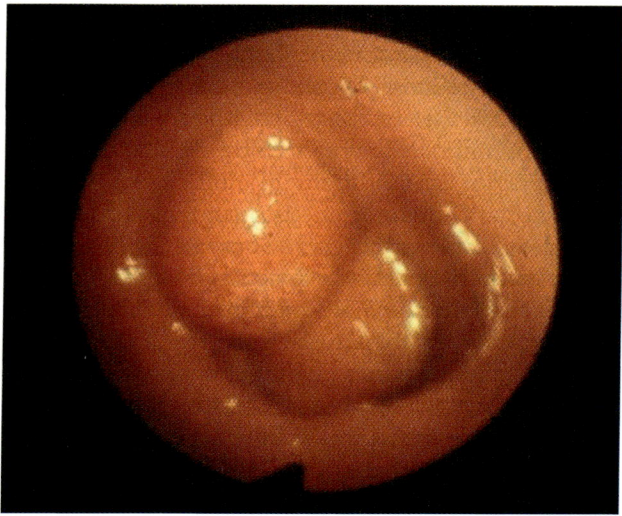

Figure 5.2 Endoscopy of polyps in the pylorus of a dog.

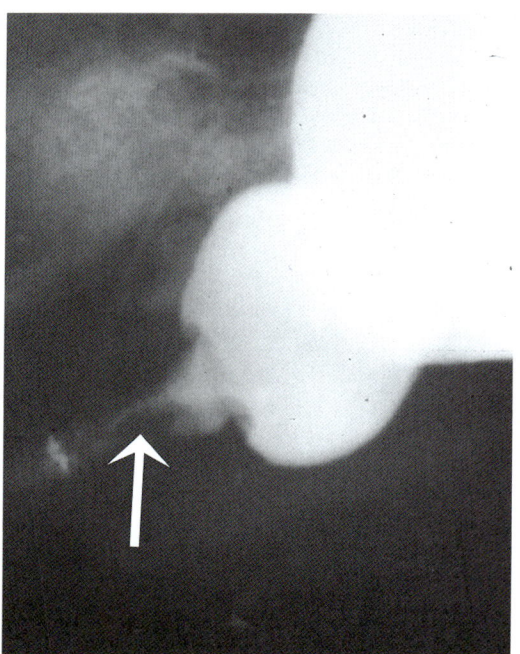

Figure 5.1 Positive contrast radiograph showing a filling defect at the level of the pylorus and a "beak" sign (white arrow).

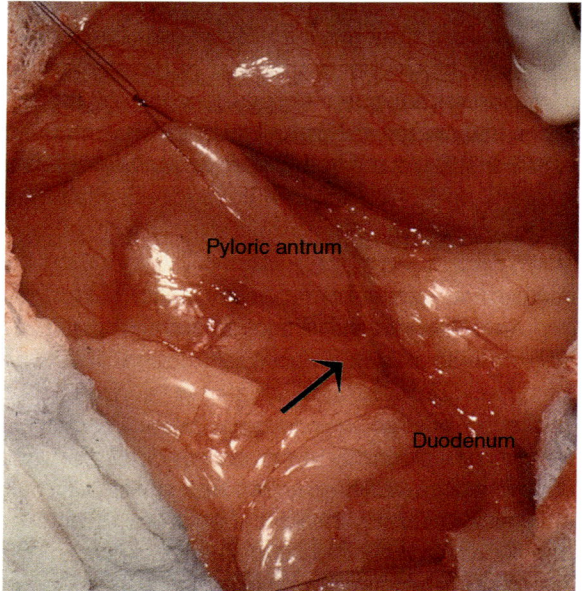

Figure 5.3 A Y incision has been marked over the pyloric antrum, the pylorus (black arrow), and the proximal duodenum.

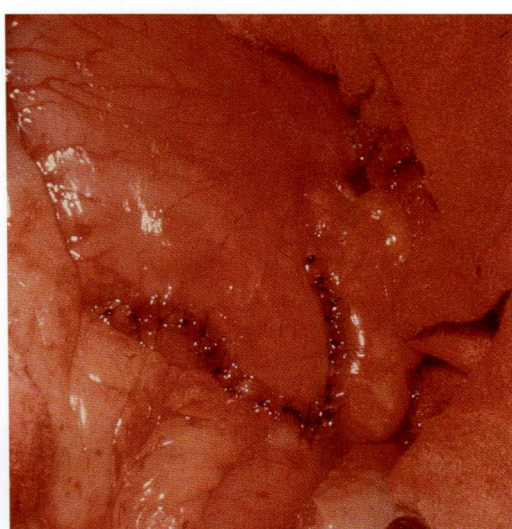

Figure 5.4 The Y incision made in Figure 5.3 has been closed with simple interrupted sutures in a U shape over the pylorus to widen the diameter of the pylorus.

The surgical treatment should be associated with medical treatment for gastritis and esophagitis. Decreased stomach motility can be present, with chronic dilatation of the stomach. Therefore cisapride might be recommended after surgery.

The prognosis is excellent since the surgery is curative.

References

Bellenger, C.R., Maddison, J.E., MacPherson, G.C., and Ilkiw, J.E. (1990). Chronic hypertrophic pyloric gastropathy in 14 dogs. *Australian Veterinary Journal* 67 (9): 317–320.

Biller, D.S., Partington, B.P., Miyabayashi, T., and Leveille, R. (1994). Ultrasonographic appearance of chronic hypertrophic pyloric gastropathy in the dog. *Veterinary Radiology & Ultrasound* 35 (1): 30–33.

Bright, R.M., Richardson, D.C., and Stanton, M.E. (1988). Y–U antral flap advancement pyloroplasty in dogs. *Compendium on Continuing Education for the Practicing Veterinarian* 10 (2): 139–144.

Dodge, J.A. (1969). Neonatal pyloric hypertrophy and duodenal ulceration produced by pentagastrin. *Gut* 10 (12): 1055–1056.

Dodge, J.A. and Karim, A.A. (1976). Induction of pyloric hypertrophy by pentagastrin. An animal model for infantile hypertrophic pyloric stenosis. *Gut* 17 (4): 280–284.

Hall, J.A. (2013). Stomach: obstruction. In: *Canine and Feline Gastroenterology* (ed. R.J. Washabau and M.J. Day), 624–650. St. Louis, Elsevier.

Hall, J.A., Twedt, D.C., and Burrows, C.F. (1990). Gastric-motility in dogs. 2. Disorders of gastric-motility. *Compendium on Continuing Education for the Practicing Veterinarian* 12 (10): 1373.

Janik, J.S., Akbar, A.M., Burrington, J.D., and Burke, G. (1978). The role of gastrin in congenital hypertrophic pyloric stenosis. *Journal of Pediatric Surgery* 13 (2): 151–154.

Lecoindre, P. and Richard, S. (2004). Digestive disorders associated with the chronic obstructive respiratory syndrome of brachycephalic dogs: 30 cases (1999–2001). *Revue de Médecine Vétérinaire* 155 (3): 141–146.

Leib, M.S., Saunders, G.K., Moon, M.L. et al. (1993). Endoscopic diagnosis of chronic hypertrophic pyloric gastropathy in dogs. *Journal of Veterinary Internal Medicine* 7 (6): 335–341.

Matthiesen, D.T. and Walter, M.C. (1986). Surgical treatment of chronic hypertrophic pyloric gastropathy in 45 dogs. *Journal of the American Animal Hospital Association* 22: 241–247.

Monnet, E. (2020). Pyloroplasty. In: *Gastrointestinal Surgical Techniques in Small Animals* (ed. E. Monnet and D.D. Smeak), 155–158. Wiley Blackwell: Hoboken, NJ.

Pearson, H., Gaskell, C.J., Gibbs, C., and Waterman, A. (1974). Pyloric and oesophageal dysfunction in the cat. *Journal of Small Animal Practice* 15 (8): 487–501.

Peeters, M.E. (1991). Pyloric stenosis in the dog: developments in its surgical treatment and retrospective study in 47 patients. *Tijdschrift voor Diergeneeskunde* 116 (3): 137–141.

Poncet, C.M., Dupre, G.P., Freiche, V.G. et al. (2005). Prevalence of gastrointestinal tract lesions in 73 brachycephalic dogs with upper respiratory syndrome. *Journal of Small Animal Practice* 46 (6): 273–279.

Prole, J.H. (1989). Acquired pyloric stenosis. *Veterinary Record* 125 (25): 630.

Sikes, R.I., Birchard, S., Patnaik, A., and Bradley, R. (1986). Chronic hypertrophicpyloric gastropathy – a review of 16 cases. *Journal of the American Animal Hospital Association* 22 (1): 99–104.

Taulescu, M.A., Valentine, B.A., Amorim, I. et al. (2014). Histopathological features of canine spontaneous non-neoplastic gastric polyps – a retrospective study of 15 cases. *Histology & Histopathology* 29 (1): 65–75.

Walsh, M.H. and Quigley, P.J. (1966). Pyloric stenosis in the dog caused by hypertrophy of the circular muscle of the pylorus. *Veterinary Record* 78 (1): 13–15.

Walter, M.C. and Matthiesen, D.T. (1989). Gastric outflow surgical problems. *Problems in Veterinary Medicine* 1 (2): 196–214.

6

Gastroduodenal Ulceration

Tracy L. Hill, B. Duncan X. Lascelles, and Anthony Blikslager

Gastroduodenal ulceration and perforation constitute an increasingly recognized cause of morbidity and mortality in dogs, although reports of prevalence of canine ulcerative disease overall or prevalence in specific canine subpopulations, such as those taking nonsteroidal anti-inflammatory drugs (NSAIDs), are lacking. With escalating use of NSAIDs for pain management, it is possible that the frequency of ulcer disease is increasing in dogs. Gastric perforation is a severe, potentially fatal, sequela of gastric ulcers that may affect up to 27% of dogs (Stanton & Bright 1989). Of dogs that suffer perforation of gastric ulcers, between 40% and 70% die or are euthanized because of their disease (Stanton & Bright 1989; Hinton *et al.* 2002; Lascelles *et al.* 2005). Reports of gastroduodenal ulceration in cats are sparse and survival rates are highly variable, ranging from 15% to 100% (Hinton *et al.* 2002; Liptak *et al.* 2002; Cariou *et al.* 2010).

Pathophysiology

The pH of a normal dog stomach is low, typically near pH 1.0 in the fed dog. Gastric pH is less than 3 for nearly 90% of the day in a normally fed dog (Bersenas *et al.* 2005). Given this prolonged exposure to high levels of acid, the gastric and duodenal mucosa have several mechanisms to prevent acid injury and rapidly repair. Awareness of these protective mechanisms helps in understanding the pathophysiology of injury. Most of the protective mechanisms have not been specifically investigated in the dog and cat, but are considered to be similar across mammalian species. The first protective mechanism is the gastric mucosal barrier, composed of primarily mucus and bicarbonate, both of which are secreted by surface epithelial cells to form a viscous layer superficial to the epithelium (Figure 6.1). Bicarbonate, secreted by surface epithelial cells, lies within the mucus layer and serves as a buffering mechanism. This helps maintain a neutral pH near the mucosal surface, neutralizing the direct effects of acid on the mucosal surface. Phospholipids, both within the mucus layer and lining the surface epithelium, add another layer of protection. Their hydrophobicity repels acid- and water-soluble toxic agents. If the mucus layer is penetrated, tight junctions between epithelial cells prevent back-diffusion of acid and other injurious agents. If epithelial cells are damaged, the resulting mucosal defect is quickly covered, usually in minutes, by epithelial restitution and later by cell proliferation. When there is penetration of acid or other damaging agents deeper than the mucosal epithelium, local mucosal blood flow quickly increases, clearing and buffering injurious agents (Laine *et al.* 2008). Duodenal surface epithelial cells also secrete bicarbonate and mucus as a protective barrier against acid (Figure 6.1); they have epithelial cell tight junctions too and can quickly increase blood flow in response to injury. In addition, bicarbonate secreted in biliary and pancreatic secretions acts to buffer acidic ingesta.

Many of these mechanisms, including mucus and bicarbonate secretion, mucosal blood flow, reduction of histamine-mediated cyclic adenosine monophosphate (AMP) to reduce proton pump activity, and epithelial restitution, are prostaglandin dependent. Prostaglandin synthesis depends on cyclooxygenase (COX) enzymes that produce prostaglandins as an end product of the arachidonic acid pathway. COX enzymes are present in two main forms that are important for gastrointestinal

Small Animal Soft Tissue Surgery, Second Edition. Edited by Eric Monnet.
© 2023 John Wiley & Sons, Inc. Published 2023 by John Wiley & Sons, Inc.
Companion website: www.wiley.com/go/monnet/small

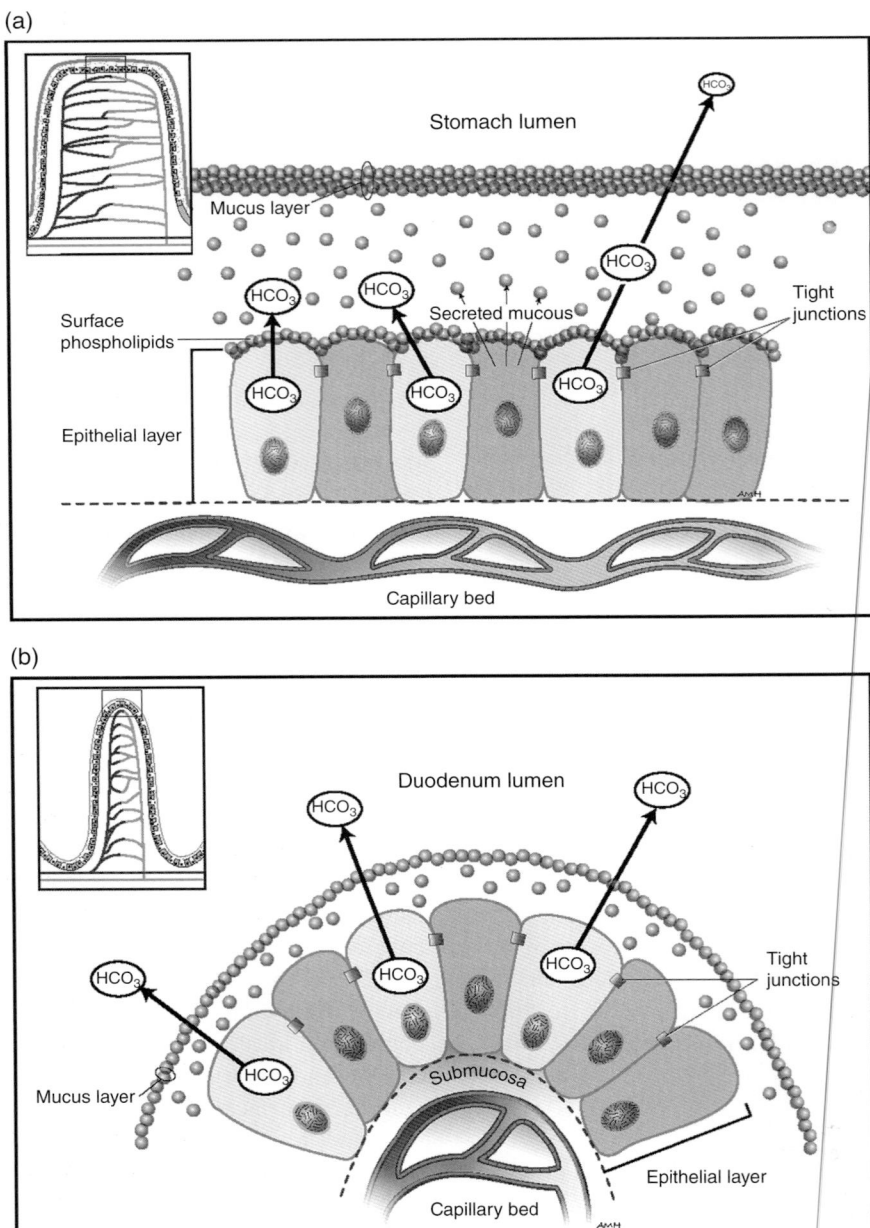

Figure 6.1 (a, b) Protective mechanisms of the gastric and duodenal mucosal epithelium. Surface epithelial cells secrete bicarbonate and mucus, while the submucosal capillary bed carries protective growth factors and carries away injurious agents. Tight junctions form a barrier against back-diffusion of acid.

health. Both forms of this enzyme convert arachidonic acid to PGH_2, which is then converted to several different prostaglandins by specific prostaglandin synthases (Figure 6.2). Traditionally, COX-1 has been considered the constitutive form, expressed in gastric and duodenal mucosa as well as other tissues, that acts to maintain gastric blood flow and perform other "housekeeping" activities, whereas COX-2 has been considered to be solely inducible, responding to inflammatory stimuli such as lipopolysaccharides, interleukin (IL)-1, and

tumor necrosis factor (TNF)-α. In many tissues and organs in the body, COX-2 is considered to be the main source of prostaglandins involved in pain and inflammation (Anderson *et al.* 1996). In the gastrointestinal tract, COX-2 expression is increased at the edges of ulcerated gastric epithelium, presumably in response to proinflammatory stimuli, and is important for ulcer healing by inducing synthesis of PGE_2. In the acute phase of injury (within the first 2 hours), PGE_2 is the primary prostaglandin synthesized at higher levels due to

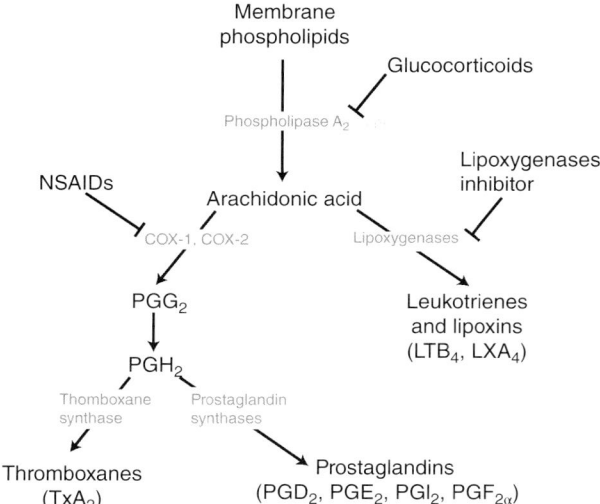

Figure 6.2 Prostanoid pathway and the role of cyclooxygenase (COX)-1 and COX-2. The site of inhibition of nonsteroidal anti-inflammatory drugs (NSIADs), lipoxygenase inhibitors, and glucocorticoids is noted.

increased COX-2 expression. At 24–48 hours of COX-2 upregulation, another PGH_2 metabolite, PGD_2, is increased, which corresponds to the resolution of inflammation and clearance of polymononuclear cells in a carrageenan rat injury model (Gilroy et al. 1999). In the early stages, NSAID treatment may inhibit healing by its inhibition of PGE_2, but in later stages it may have a proinflammatory effect through decreasing PGD_2 levels, which would also affect gastric ulcer healing. In addition to the induced expression at times of injury, COX-2 is also constitutively expressed at low levels in normal gastric and duodenal mucosa (Wilson et al. 2004; Poonam et al. 2005; Wooten et al. 2008). This background level of activity may help the gastrointestinal mucosa respond to potentially injurious events. Increased COX-2 expression exerts its protective and reparative effects by increasing PGE_2 (Poonam et al. 2005; Hatazawa et al. 2007). This important protective prostaglandin accelerates mucosal recovery and repair.

Gastroduodenal ulceration may occur when any of these protective mechanisms are disrupted. This may be due to one of several mechanisms, including altered mucosal blood flow, direct disruption of the mucosal epithelial barrier, increased acid secretion, and prostaglandin inhibition.

Pathogenesis of gastroduodenal ulcers in dogs

The most commonly identified predisposing factors for gastroduodenal ulceration in dogs include NSAID therapy, corticosteroid therapy, liver disease, shock or sepsis, and underlying neoplasia. Other less commonly reported associations include intervertebral disk disease, inflammatory bowel disease, and extreme exercise/stress in racing sled dogs (Murray et al. 1972; Stanton & Bright 1989; Neiger et al. 2000; Hinton et al. 2002; Davis et al. 2003; Lascelles et al. 2005; Cariou et al. 2009). In most retrospective studies, many of the dogs (up to 40%) showed evidence of more than one predisposing factor, supporting a multifactorial cause of ulceration in many patients (Hinton et al. 2002).

The mechanism of injury is variable depending on the associated cause. NSAIDs cause ulceration though inhibition of prostaglandin production (discussed more fully later). Likewise, corticosteroids inhibit the production of prostaglandins by inhibiting phospholipase A_2 (Figure 6.2). Phospholipase A_2 releases arachidonic acid from phospholipids in the cell membrane, which are transformed by COXs and prostaglandin synthases into various prostaglandins. Ulcerogenic doses of corticosteroids range from anti-inflammatory doses to higher shock doses (Hinton et al. 2002). The mechanisms involved with ulceration secondary to liver disease are poorly understood, but may include altered submucosal blood flow and decreased gastrin clearance (Christiansen et al. 1982). Similarly, shock and sepsis are likely associated with mucosal ulceration due to altered hemodynamics of the submucosal capillary bed (Stanton & Bright 1989). Neoplasia (such as lymphosarcoma and adenocarcinoma) may lead to ulceration by directly disrupting the mucosal epithelial layer. Additionally, neoplasia that alters acid secretion, such as gastrinomas and mast cell disease, may also lead to ulceration (Stanton & Bright 1989; Hinton et al. 2002). In dogs undergoing surgery for intervertebral disk disease, about 75% have gastric mucosal lesions. Approximately one-third of these dogs have received neither corticosteroids nor NSAIDs (Neiger et al. 2000). Potential mechanisms for ulceration associated with intervertebral disk disease include alterations in parasympathetic/sympathetic tone causing increased acid secretion and ischemic damage to the mucosa. Up to 50% of racing sled dogs may be affected with gastric erosions after strenuous activity; acute hemorrhage from ulceration is a significant cause of race-related mortality (Davis et al. 2003, 2006; Dennis et al. 2008). It is hypothesized that high-fat diets fed to these dogs may lead to delayed gastric emptying and hyperacidity. Potential contributing factors may include exercise-induced visceral ischemia, bacterial pathogens, stress, and physical trauma (foreign bodies) (Davis et al. 2003).

Helicobacter pylori is a significant cause of gastric ulceration in humans; its role in gastric ulceration in dogs has been examined. Although *H. pylori* has been reported to be associated with gastric ulcers in certain geographic regions (e.g., India), there has not been a confirmed report of gastric ulceration due to *Helicobacter* species in the USA and up to 100% of unaffected healthy dogs may be positive for various *Helicobacter* species (Simpson *et al.* 2000; Kavitha *et al.* 2007; Jergens *et al.* 2009). As opposed to *Helicobacter* infection in humans, natural infection with *Helicobacter* in dogs does not significantly increase gastrin levels (Simpson *et al.* 1999). Although *Helicobacter* has been associated with gastritis and duodenitis, it has not yet shown a significant association with ulcer disease (Leib *et al.* 2007; Jergens *et al.* 2009).

The most common locations for gastroduodenal ulceration, regardless of cause, are the antrum, pylorus, and proximal duodenum. In normal dogs, PGE_2 levels are highest in the pylorus and proximal duodenum (Wilson *et al.* 2004; Punke *et al.* 2008; Wooten *et al.* 2008). These locations may be the most predisposed to ulceration because they can be exposed to high levels of acid and ingesta that damage epithelium, through either chemical or mechanical trauma. In addition, bile salts and bile acids may contribute to injury in the pyloric antrum, via biliary reflux into the stomach. Biliary contents can damage mucosa by dissolution of mucosal lipids as well as mucosal absorption of toxic bile acids (Duane & Wiegand 1980; Duane *et al.* 1982).

Nonsteroidal anti-inflammatory drugs and gastroduodenal ulcers

In humans, chronic NSAID therapy is a common cause of gastric and duodenal lesions, affecting up to 9% of patients within the first 2 weeks of treatment with NSAID or aspirin therapy. Importantly, up to 40% of these patients can be asymptomatic (Schoenfeld *et al.* 1999). There are no similar studies in dogs and cats receiving chronic NSAID therapy, but if veterinary patients are at all similar to their human counterparts in the prevalence of subclinical disease, then NSAID-induced gastroduodenal irritation is likely to be an underrecognized disease in patients receiving NSAID therapy. However, it is the most well-examined, and most commonly reported, cause of gastric ulcers in dogs. NSAID-associated ulcers are reported with both acute (one to two doses) and chronic (months to years) therapy using these drugs (Hinton *et al.* 2002). Ulcers have been associated with most NSAIDs, including nonselective COX inhibitors such as aspirin, phenylbutazone, ketoprofen, flunixin, piroxicam, ibuprofen, and naproxen, as well as with the preferential COX-2 inhibitors carprofen and meloxicam, and selective COX-2 inhibitors (coxibs) (Wallace *et al.* 1990; Gfeller & Sandors 1991; Godshalk *et al.* 1992; Knapp *et al.* 1992; Vonderhaar &

Salisbury 1993; Forsyth *et al.* 1998; Reed 2002; Lascelles *et al.* 2005). Administration at higher than approved doses, or close association temporally of two different NSAIDs or an NSAID and a corticosteroid, increases the risk of ulceration, though there are reports of ulceration in dogs treated with NSAIDs at prescribed doses (Lascelles *et al.* 2005; Cariou *et al.* 2009).

NSAIDs can induce gastric injury leading to ulcers via a variety of mechanisms. First, aspirin in particular is a weak acid that becomes nonionized in contact with gastric acid. In its nonionized form, aspirin more readily diffuses across membranes into epithelial cells. Within the neutral pH of the epithelial cell, aspirin then becomes ionized, releasing hydrogen ions that disrupt cell function. This mechanism does not seem to be a significant cause of injury in other clinically utilized NSAIDs.

For most NSAIDs, the primary mechanism of injury leading to gastroduodenal ulceration is thought to be via COX inhibition, depressing prostaglandin synthesis. Because of the presumed role of COX-1 as the constitutively expressed COX enzyme in the gastrointestinal tract, COX-2 selective inhibitors were developed in an attempt to decrease adverse gastrointestinal events such as ulceration and perforation. Though many of these COX-2 selective inhibitors (meloxicam, carprofen, deracoxib, firocoxib) do show COX-2 selectivity in whole blood assays, evidence of the selectivity of these drugs at the gastrointestinal mucosa is conflicting; selectivity of NSAIDs in whole blood (Jones *et al.* 2002) may be lost at the tissue level (Jones & Budsberg 2000). Several studies show maintenance of normal prostaglandin levels in mucosal tissue with COX-2 selective NSAIDs, supportive of COX-2 selectivity, while others show some suppression of baseline prostaglandin levels (Poortinga & Hungerford 1998; Jones & Budsberg 2000; Jones *et al.* 2002; Agnello *et al.* 2005; Sessions *et al.* 2005; Punke *et al.* 2008; Wooten *et al.* 2009). When gastric mucosa is examined endoscopically after administration of various NSAIDs, reports are somewhat contradictory as to which NSAIDs produce the most severe lesions, although the nonselective COX inhibitors tend to induce lesions more reliably than COX-2 selective drugs (Reimer *et al.* 1999; Sessions *et al.* 2005; Sennello & Leib 2006; Wooten *et al.* 2009). As stated previously, COX-2 is upregulated with gastrointestinal injury associated with the reparative process. The administration of a COX-2 inhibitor concurrent with another cause of gastrointestinal injury (liver disease, ischemic/hypovolemic injury, etc.) may exacerbate injury. In humans, the presence of concurrent diseases, such as sepsis and liver cirrhosis, has been associated with a poorer outcome in patients with peptic ulcers (Kitano & Dolgor 2000; Møller *et al.* 2009).

Another mechanism by which many NSAIDs can induce epithelial injury is via increased leukotriene synthesis and neutrophil-mediated damage. Suppression of COX enzymes may increase leukotriene synthesis by shuttling arachidonic acid conversion to leukotrienes, such as LTB_4, via lipoxygenases (LOX). However, whether this occurs in tissues in response to NSAIDs has been debated. Nonetheless, increased LTB_4 would lead to neutrophil recruitment to the gastrointestinal mucosa, causing further mucosal damage (Tomlinson & Blikslager 2003). Dual COX/LOX inhibitors (tepoxalin) have been developed in an attempt to reduce gastric injury with this potential mechanism as a consideration. When compared with a highly selective COX-2 inhibitor (firo-coxib), the dual COX/LOX inhibitor tepoxalin did inhibit healing after endoscopic biopsy of the duodenal mucosa less than the COX-2 selective inhibitor firocoxib (Goodman *et al.* 2009).

Much is yet to be understood regarding the role of various NSAIDs in gastrointestinal ulceration. It is important to recognize that any NSAID, regardless of selectivity, may cause gastroduodenal ulceration and perforation, especially in dogs with a predisposing cause. However, there is support that more COX-2 selective inhibitors, such as firocoxib and deracoxib, reduce gastrointestinal side effects in research animals (Ryan *et al.* 2006, 2007; Sennello & Leib 2006; Roberts *et al.* 2009). Caution should be taken any time an NSAID, even a COX-2 selective inhibitor, is administered and owners should be warned to watch for and report signs suggestive of potential ulceration. Additionally, switching therapy between NSAIDs or between a corticosteroid and an NSAID should only be undertaken after a sufficient washout period. The appropriate length of this washout period is unknown, but is likely anywhere from a few days up to one week or more, depending on the duration of therapy and drug. It must be noted that this is our recommendation and is not supported (or refuted) by current evidence.

Pathogenesis of gastroduodenal ulceration in cats

Gastroduodenal ulceration and perforation are less frequently recognized in cats. Most commonly, ulceration is described secondary to neoplasia, including systemic mastocytosis, gastric lymphosarcoma and adenocarcinoma, and gastrinoma (Liptak *et al.* 2002). Additional diseases that have been described and associated with ulceration include inflammatory bowel disease, hypovolemia, renal disease, toxic ingestion, and infectious causes (endoparasites, bacterial granuloma) (Hinton *et al.* 2002; Liptak *et al.* 2002). There are reports of cats

developing gastroduodenal ulceration secondary to anti-inflammatory therapy with carprofen, meloxicam, and prednisolone (Cariou *et al.* 2010; Runk *et al.* 1999). It is unclear whether cats are more resistant to adverse gastrointestinal side effects of NSAID therapy or if the paucity of reports on NSAID-associated ulceration in cats is because these drugs are less commonly prescribed for use in cats than in dogs (Lascelles *et al.* 2007).

Clinical presentation of dogs and cats with gastroduodenal ulceration

Dogs presenting for spontaneous gastroduodenal ulceration or perforation are most often large-breed dogs (average 35 kg) that are middle-aged (5–7 years). The most common breeds reported include larger-breed dogs such as Labrador retrievers, Doberman pinschers, German shepherd dogs, and Rottweilers (Stanton & Bright 1989; Wallace *et al.* 1990; Hinton *et al.* 2002; Lascelles *et al.* 2005). In one report, affected Rottweilers were younger at age of presentation (3.5 years on average) (Hinton *et al.* 2002). It is not known if there is something inherent in these dogs that predisposes them to gastroduodenal ulceration, or if other factors (such as that these are the breeds most likely to be administered NSAIDs) skew reports of ulceration. Reported duration of clinical signs prior to presentation ranges from less than 24 hours to several months (Stanton & Bright 1989; Wallace *et al.* 1990; Hinton *et al.* 2002; Lascelles *et al.* 2005; Cariou *et al.* 2009). Most commonly, owners report nonspecific signs such as lethargy, vomiting, inappetence, and weakness (Table 6.1). Fewer dogs present with more obvious signs such as hematemesis or melena, although melena is more common than hematemesis. Described physical examination findings in dogs with spontaneous gastroduodenal perforation include dehydration, compensated or decompensated shock, abdominal pain, and abdominal distension (Stanton & Bright 1989; Wallace *et al.* 1990; Hinton *et al.* 2002; Lascelles *et al.* 2005; Cariou *et al.* 2009).

Although reports of gastroduodenal ulceration in cats are less common, affected cats also have nonspecific presenting signs including lethargy, weight loss, vomiting, and inappetence (Hinton *et al.* 2002; Liptak *et al.* 2002; Cariou *et al.* 2010). Hematemesis and melena seem to be even less common in cats. Cats are older on presentation, on average 10 years, and are mostly domestic shorthair and domestic longhair (Hinton *et al.* 2002). In cats with ulceration-associated tumors, duration of clinical signs is longer than in cats with nonneoplastic disease (4–5 months vs. about 1 month for nonneoplastic disease) (Liptak *et al.* 2002). Cats with gastroduodenal perforation present similarly to dogs, with dehydration,

Table 6.1 Common clinical signs of gastroduodenal ulceration.

Clinical sign	Frequency in dogs (%)	Frequency in cats (%)
Lethargy	95*	100*
Vomiting	81*	87*
Inappetence/anorexia	52*	73
Melena	40	20
Diarrhea	29	50
Hematemesis	29	23
Abdominal pain	22	31
Weight loss	11	80*
Weakness	6	0
Polyuria/polydipsia	5	33

Most common clinical signs with gastroduodenal ulceration and/or perforation in dogs and cats. The three most common signs for each species are marked with an asterisk.
Source: Data from Cariou *et al.* (2009), Wallace *et al.* (1990), Hinton *et al.* (2002), and Liptak *et al.* (2002).

shock, and abdominal pain and distension being the most common findings (Hinton *et al.* 2002; Liptak *et al.* 2002; Cariou *et al.* 2010).

Diagnosis of gastroduodenal ulceration

The most common hematologic abnormalities in dogs include a leukocytosis characterized by neutrophilia with a left shift and lymphopenia, and less consistently anemia. Anemia is commonly normocytic normochromic, but may be microcytic hypochromic depending on duration of ulceration and significance of gastrointestinal hemorrhage. Clinical pathologic analyses of ulcerated dogs most commonly show hypoproteinemia and hypoalbuminemia. Other frequent findings include hyponatremia and hypocalcemia. If a concurrent disease is present, supportive abnormalities of that condition may also be seen, such as elevation in liver enzymes (Stanton & Bright 1989; Wallace *et al.* 1990; Hinton *et al.* 2002; Cariou *et al.* 2009).

In cats, neutrophilia with a left shift, lymphopenia, and anemia are most commonly detected. Cats likewise demonstrate hypoproteinemia and hypoalbuminemia as well as hyponatremia and hypocalcemia. In addition, clinical pathologic biochemical abnormalities in cats may include azotemia and elevation in creatine kinase (Hinton *et al.* 2002; Liptak *et al.* 2002). It is unclear whether these biochemical changes (azotemia, elevated creatine kinase) are directly related to gastrointestinal ulceration in cats or are due to concurrent diseases.

Orthogonal abdominal radiographs often show evidence of gastroduodenal perforation more consistently than in patients without perforation (Figure 6.3). Dogs and cats with perforation have decreased abdominal detail in about 75% of cases (Hinton *et al.* 2002; Cariou *et al.* 2009). Cats with gastroduodenal perforation frequently have pneumoperitoneum, whereas fewer canine cases present with pneumoperitoneum (approximately 50%) (Hinton *et al.* 2002; Liptak *et al.* 2002; Cariou *et al.* 2010). Abdominal radiographs are often normal in patients with gastroduodenal ulceration without perforation, although they may demonstrate a mass effect if there is underlying gastrointestinal neoplasia (Barber 1982; Wallace *et al.* 1990). Contrast radiography has a higher sensitivity for gastroduodenal ulceration than plain radiography, although only approximately 25% of gastroduodenal ulcers are detected, and this technique has a higher complication rate than either plain radiography or ultrasound (Stanton & Bright 1989). Contrast radiography may show a filling defect representative of the ulcer and/or delayed gastric emptying (Vonderhaar & Salisbury 1993; Hinton *et al.* 2002). In patients where perforation is known or suspected, contrast radiography should not be performed due to the risk of barium peritonitis. Abdominal ultrasound is generally considered a better modality to diagnose perforation and often ulceration as well. With perforation, dogs and cats commonly (80–100%) have free peritoneal effusion. Additional findings include "bright" (highly echogenic) mesenteric fat, gastric or duodenal mucosal thickening, and pneumoperitoneum (Hinton *et al.* 2002; Boysen *et al.* 2003; Cariou *et al.* 2009). Ultrasonographic changes with ulceration include thickening of the gastric or duodenal wall, loss of normal layering, presence of a crater with accumulation of microbubbles (a collection of small dense echoes associated with strong acoustic shadowing), and decreased gastric motility (Figures 6.4 and 6.5). If there is underlying gastrointestinal neoplasia, it is often also visualized by ultrasonography (Penninck *et al.* 1997; Liptak *et al.* 2002). This modality is also useful for detecting nongastrointestinal neoplasias that can cause ulcers, such as gastrinomas and mast cell disease. Abdominal cytology may be performed if free fluid is present. About 50% of dogs and cats with perforation of the gastric or duodenal mucosa secondary to ulceration have septic suppurative inflammation; nonseptic suppurative inflammation is seen in the remainder of cases. Likewise, culture of abdominal fluid is positive for growth in about half of dogs and cats, though the likelihood of a positive culture was not associated with the presence of bacteria, cytologic neutrophil count, or morphology (Hinton *et al.* 2002; Cariou *et al.* 2009).

(a)

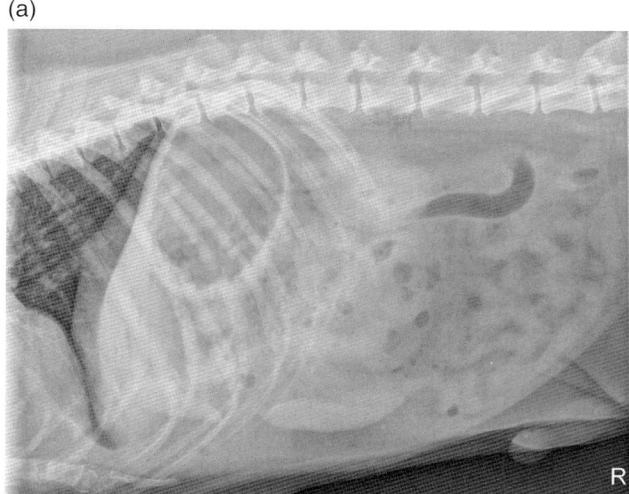

(b)

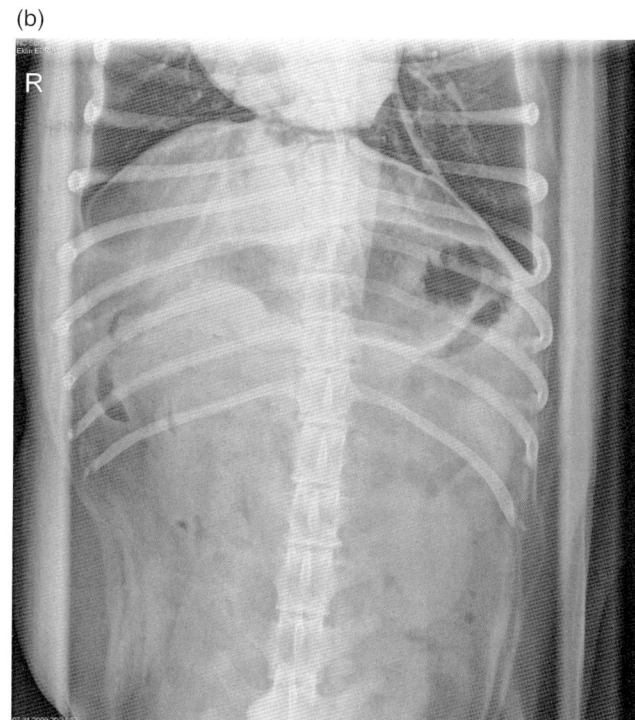

Figure 6.3 (a, b) Abdominal radiographs of a dog. There is peritoneal fluid and pneumoperitoneum, consistent with intestinal perforation. The pylorus appears thickened, consistent with a gastric ulcer.

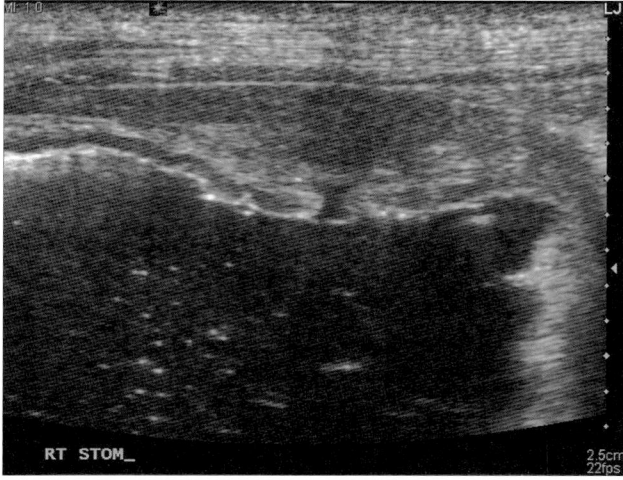

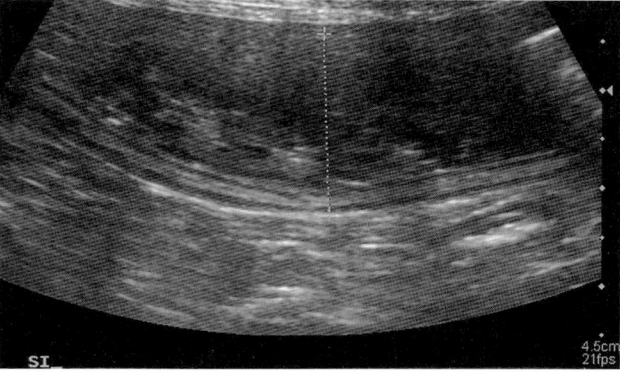

Figure 6.5 Ultrasonographic image of a duodenal ulcer, showing duodenal wall thickening and bright surrounding mesentery.

Figure 6.4 Ultrasonographic image of a gastric ulcer, showing gastric wall thickening.

Endoscopy is commonly cited as the most reliable test for gastroduodenal ulceration, detecting up to 100% of ulcers (Stanton & Bright 1989; Wallace *et al.* 1990). Endoscopy offers the advantage that in addition to visualization of the ulcer and assessment for gastrointestinal masses not detected with other modalities, it may allow biopsy of surrounding mucosal tissue for diagnostic purposes. Though it may be impossible to determine the depth of injury, and therefore whether the defect is truly an ulcer or superficial erosion, the severity of lesions can be judged subjectively, which can help make the determination of whether surgical intervention is required or if medical management is appropriate (Figure 6.6). Hemorrhage from the ulcer or gastric contents may obscure visualization and make diagnosis difficult (Hinton *et al.* 2002). If a perforation is present or the ulcer is very deep, insufflation of the stomach and duodenum with air may potentially worsen the defect or cause perforation. Endoscopy, though a valuable tool for

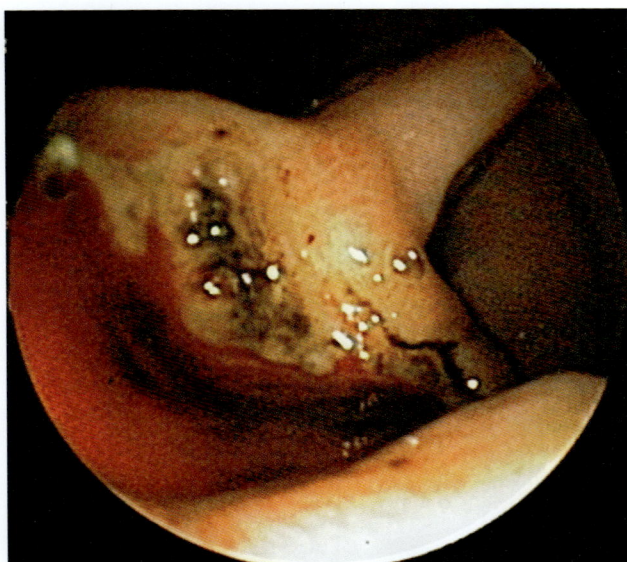

Figure 6.6 Endoscopic image of a gastric ulcer showing evidence of necrosis and active hemorrhage.

detection of ulceration, should not be performed without preparation to move to exploratory surgery if a perforation is observed or hemorrhage is severe.

Exploratory celiotomy is the gold standard for gastroduodenal ulceration. Examination of the gastric and duodenal mucosa allows the assessment of both depth and severity of ulceration, and provides a means of treatment via resection of the ulceration or perforation. The surgeon should ensure that all surfaces of the stomach and duodenum are inspected, including the difficult to access dorsal surface of the stomach and the cardia area.

Treatment of gastroduodenal ulceration

Effective treatment begins by addressing the underlying causes of ulceration when applicable. NSAID therapy should be discontinued immediately upon suspicion of ulceration. Any underlying hemodynamic abnormalities and dehydration should be corrected. If possible, concurrent diseases should be treated appropriately (liver disease, renal disease, neoplasia). Minimizing the cause of gastroduodenal ulceration is the first step in treatment. In addition, two important arms of treatment specific for ulceration and perforation are medical management and surgical therapy. Less severely affected animals may often be successfully managed with medical therapy alone. There are many available drug therapies aimed at decreasing or neutralizing acid secretion or directed at cytoprotection. Usually, a combination of acid-suppressing treatments and cytoprotective agents is used. Commonly prescribed medications include histamine

H_2-receptor antagonists, proton pump inhibitors (PPIs), prostaglandin analogs, sucralfate, and antacids (Table 6.2).

Acid suppression therapy

Although the minimum level or time of total acid suppression that is required in dogs and cats to best facilitate ulcer healing is unknown, examination of human data suggests that for optimal healing gastric pH should be maintained above 3 for at least 75% of the day (Green *et al.* 1978). If active hemorrhage is present, a pH above 6 is required to allow platelet aggregation and hemostasis (Green *et al.* 1978). Effective acid suppression may be attempted with one of two main classes of drugs: H_2-receptor antagonists and PPIs.

H_2-receptor antagonists exert their activity by reversibly binding the histamine receptor on the gastric parietal cell. Of the most commonly used H_2-receptor antagonists, famotidine, cimetidine, and ranitidine, famotidine achieves the most effective acid suppression, reducing maximal acid output by 50–70% (Katz *et al.* 1987; Bersenas *et al.* 2005). Famotidine also prevents NSAID-induced decrease in mucosal blood flow by an unknown mechanism (Hata *et al.* 2005). In this way, famotidine may serve in the prevention of gastric ulcers, as well as for treatment. Famotidine, administered daily at 1 mg/kg, tended to decrease gastric lesion score following an exercise trial in Alaskan racing sled dogs (Williamson *et al.* 2007).

PPIs, by binding irreversibly to H^+/K^+-ATPase, can achieve more effective acid suppression than H_2-receptor antagonists (Abelö *et al.* 2002). PPIs are weak bases that diffuse into cells in a nonprotonated form. For activation, PPIs need to be exposed to the acidity of the canaliculi within the parietal cell, where they become activated to bind to the proton pump. In clinical patients, time to effective acid suppression is approximately 2–6 days. Omeprazole at 1–2.5 mg/kg once a day is more effective than famotidine for acid suppression. Twice-daily treatment may increase the efficacy of acid suppression (Bersenas *et al.* 2005; Tolbert *et al.* 2010). PPIs may have additional beneficial effects besides acid suppression. In human neutrophils, omeprazole treatment *in vitro* decreased the production of free radicals produced with NSAID-induced injury (Suzuki *et al.* 1996). For patients unable to tolerate oral medication due to vomiting, PPIs are available in intravenous injectable form, such as pantoprazole, that also effectively increases gastric pH in dogs (Postius *et al.* 1991). When administered intravenously (1 mg/kg once daily), pantoprazole suppressed acid secretion similarly to, though slightly less than, oral omeprazole at 1 mg/kg once daily (Bersenas *et al.* 2005). The time to onset of acid suppression was also similar between the injected and oral PPI.

Table 6.2 Frequently prescribed medications for management of gastroduodenal ulceration.

Drug	Use	Dose	Route	Frequency
Famotidine	Acid suppressant	0.5–1 mg/kg	i.v., s.c., p.o.	q12–24 h
Omeprazole	Acid suppressant	0.5–1 mg/kg	p.o.	q12–24 h
Pantoprazole	Acid suppressant	0.5–1 mg/kg	i.v.	q12 h on day 1, then q24 h
Misoprostol	Prostaglandin analog	Dog: 2–5 µg/kg Cat: no known dose	p.o.	q12 h
Sucralfate	Cytoprotectant	Dog: 0.5–1 g/dog Cat: 0.25 g/cat	p.o. as slurry in water	q8–12 h
Buprenorphine	Pain management	0.01–0.02 mg/kg	i.v., i.m., p.o. in cats	q6–12 h
Ondansetron	Antiemetic	0.25–1 mg/kg	i.v., p.o.	q6–12 h
Dolasetron	Antiemetic	0.5–1 mg/kg	i.v., p.o.	q24 h
Aprepitant	Antiemetic	1–2 mg/kg	p.o.	q24 h
Maropitant	Antiemetic	s.c. 1 mg/kg p.o. 2 mg/kg		q24 h for 5 d
Metoclopramide	Antiemetic, promotility	0.2–0.5 mg/kg 1–2 mg/kg daily	i.v., i.m., p.o. i.v.	q6–8 h Constant-rate infusion
Magnesium hydroxide	Antacid	5–10 mL/animal		q4–6 h

i.m., intramuscularly; i.v., intravenously; p.o., orally; q, every; s.c., subcutaneously.

Because this class of drugs is dependent on acid for activation, it is generally not recommended that they be coadministered with H_2-receptor antagonists, which may inhibit activation of the proton pump and thereby decrease PPI activity. In humans, it is recommended that PPIs be administered approximately 15 minutes prior to eating (Thomson *et al.* 1997; Vaz-da-Silva *et al.* 2005).

Cytoprotection

Misoprostol is a PGE_1 analog that acts similarly to endogenous prostaglandins by increasing gastric mucosal blood flow, stimulating bicarbonate and mucus secretion, and increasing epithelial turnover (Goodlad *et al.* 1990; Larsen *et al.* 1992). It has been shown to decrease gastric erosions associated with aspirin treatment in dogs, suggesting its utility in prevention of NSAID-induced ulcers (Johnston *et al.* 1995). The use of misoprostol for treatment of preexisting ulcers has not been examined in dogs, but its ability to promote and support protective mechanisms implies that it may serve a role in gastric ulcer treatment as well as prevention. Additional studies examining the efficacy of different dosing intervals of misoprostol (every 8, 12, or 24 hours) showed that misoprostol twice daily prevented the development of gastric lesions associated with aspirin treatment just as well as three times a day treatment

(Ward *et al.* 2003). Misoprostol, as a prostaglandin analog, is probably most effectively used in the prevention of NSAID- and corticosteroid-induced ulcers.

Sucralfate is a mucosal cytoprotective drug that dissociates in the acid contents of the stomach to aluminum hydroxide and sucrose octosulfate. It then electrostatically binds to positively charged proteins exposed at the base of the ulcer, forming a barrier against further diffusion of acid into the mucosa (Steiner *et al.* 1982). As such, sucralfate is only useful as an ulcer treatment and not as protective therapy against ulceration. Binding to ulcerated gastric mucosa is not adversely affected by concurrent administration with acid suppressants or antacids (Steiner *et al.* 1982). In addition, sucralfate stimulates PGE_2 production, thereby promoting prostaglandin-mediated cytoprotective mechanisms (increased mucosal blood flow, decreased acid secretion, increased mucus and bicarbonate secretion) as well as increasing expression of epidermal growth factor (Slomiany *et al.* 1991, 1992).

Antacids, such as magnesium hydroxide and aluminum hydroxide, act in cytoprotection of the gastric mucosa by neutralizing acid and inactivating pepsin. In addition, they can also induce local PGE_2 synthesis (Dowling 1995). The disadvantage of these treatments is that to maintain efficacy they must be given very frequently, up to every 2–3 hours, to prevent rebound hyperacidity between dosing. Given at these high frequencies and therefore relatively high total dose, acid–base derangements, phosphate depletion, and diarrhea can occur, which limits their clinical utility in most patients.

Adjunctive treatments

In addition to the targeted therapies for ulceration already discussed, additional therapy may be warranted based on individual assessment of the patient. This may include pain management with opioids such as buprenorphine to manage acute pain associated with ulceration. Buprenorphine has less effect on gastrointestinal motility than a more potent μ-agonist such as morphine or hydromorphone, but can still be administered intravenously. Vomiting is a common sign in patients with gastroduodenal ulceration and may be due to either locally mediated effects (stimulation of vagal afferents due to ulceration) or centrally acting effects with concurrent diseases (stimulation of the chemoreceptor trigger zone, i.e., liver disease, renal disease, neoplasia). If vomiting is present, antiemetics should be prescribed. Many highly effective intravenous antiemetics are available and relatively inexpensive, including serotonin receptor antagonists (ondansetron and dolasetron), NK-1 receptor antagonists (aprepitant and maropitant), and more conventional antiemetics such as metoclopramide and chlorpromazine. Serotonin receptor antagonists are effective peripherally acting antiemetics and are therefore appropriate for treatment of ulcerogenic vomiting. NK-1 receptor antagonists act both locally and centrally to protect against emetogens. Metoclopramide, as a dopaminergic antagonist, works primarily in the chemoreceptor trigger zone, so may be less effective in treating visceral afferent-mediated vomiting as is often present with ulceration. Chlorpromazine, because of its potential hemodynamic and anticholinergic effects, is not recommended for most patients with ulceration. Many of the recommended antiemetic therapies have relatively wide effective therapeutic dosing ranges, so dosing may be tailored to each individual patient based on the frequency and severity of emesis.

Surgical treatment

For patients with gastroduodenal perforation, severe ulceration with hemorrhage, or failure to respond to medical therapy, surgery is typically warranted. In critically ill patients, appropriate stabilization measures should be taken prior to surgery and may include fluid resuscitation and/or blood transfusions if anemia is severe. At surgery, the ulcerated mucosa is resected. Occasionally Billroth procedures are required for more severely affected animals or in patients with gastrointestinal tumors where the lesions are located in or near the pylorus (Liptak et al. 2002). Often, dogs and cats with gastroduodenal perforations will have local or generalized peritonitis that will need to be managed appropriately with lavage and placement of drains as necessary (Hinton et al. 2002; Cariou et al. 2010). If ulcerations or perforations are difficult to identify, intraoperative endoscopy or ultrasonography may aid in localization of disease. Subsequent to surgery, appropriate medical therapy should also be employed, including antibiotic therapy, acid suppression therapy, and nutritional management.

Outcome

There are few reports in the literature describing short- and long-term survival of dogs and cats with gastroduodenal ulceration, though reported survival rates following medical or surgical management are quite variable. In dogs with perforations, survival to discharge rates have ranged from 30% to 60% (Hinton et al. 2002; Lascelles et al. 2005; Cariou et al. 2009). In cases where perforation is not present and treatment consists of aggressive medical management, survival is reportedly as good as 100% (Wallace et al. 1990). Survival rates in cats following spontaneous perforation appear to be higher following surgical management, often reaching 100%. In the few reports of cats with ulceration without perforation, survival rates range from 14% to 100% (Liptak et al. 2002; Cariou et al. 2010). Early recognition of potential ulceration and prompt treatment are the optimal approach for achieving the best outcome. In addition, as effective acid suppression drugs such as PPIs become more common, successful treatment with medical management of ulceration in dogs and cats will likely improve.

References

Abelö, A., Holstein, B., Eriksson, U.G. et al. (2002). Gastric acid secretion in the dog: a mechanism-based pharmacodynamic model for histamine stimulation and irreversible inhibition by omeprazole. *Journal of Pharmacokinetics and Pharmacodynamics* 29: 365–382.

Agnello, K.A., Reynolds, L.R., and Budsberg, S.C. (2005). in vivo effects of tepoxalin, an inhibitor of cyclooxygenase and lipoxygenase, on prostanoid and leukotriene production in dogs with chronic osteoarthritis. *American Journal of Veterinary Research* 66: 966–972.

Anderson, G.D., Hauser, S.D., McGarity, K.L. et al. (1996). Selective inhibition of cyclooxygenase (COX)-2 reverses inflammation and expression of COX-2 and interleukin 6 in rat adjuvant arthritis. *Journal of Clinical Investigation* 97: 2672–2679.

Barber, D.L. (1982). Radiographic aspects of gastric ulcers in dogs: a comparative review and report of 5 case histories. *Veterinary Radiology* 23: 109–116.

Bersenas, A.M., Mathews, K.A., Allen, D.G., and Conlon, P.D. (2005). Effects of ranitidine, famotidine, pantoprazole, and omeprazole on intragastric pH in dogs. *American Journal of Veterinary Research* 66: 425–431.

Boysen, S.R., Tidwell, A.S., and Penninck, D.G. (2003). Ultrasonographic findings in dogs and cats with gastrointestinal perforation. *Veterinary Radiology and Ultrasound* 44: 556–564.

Cariou, M., Lipscomb, V.J., Brockman, D.J. et al. (2009). Spontaneous gastroduodenal perforations in dogs: a retrospective study of 15 cases. *Veterinary Record* 165: 436–441.

Cariou, M.P., Halfacree, Z.J., Lee, K.C., and Baines, S.J. (2010). Successful surgical management of spontaneous gastric perforations in three cats. *Journal of Feline Medicine and Surgery* 12: 36–41.

Christiansen, L.A., Keiding, S., and Winkler, K. (1982). Hepatic elimination of endogenous gastrin in pigs. *Scandinavian Journal of Gastroenterology* 17: 113–120.

Davis, M.S., Willard, M.D., Nelson, S.L. et al. (2003). Prevalence of gastric lesions in racing Alaskan sled dogs. *Journal of Veterinary Internal Medicine* 17: 311–314.

Davis, M.S., Willard, M., Williamson, K. et al. (2006). Temporal relationship between gastrointestinal protein loss, gastric ulceration or erosion, and strenuous exercise in racing Alaskan sled dogs. *Journal of Veterinary Internal Medicine* 20: 835–839.

Dennis, M.M., Nelson, S.N., Cantor, G.H. et al. (2008). Assessment of necropsy findings in sled dogs that died during Iditarod Trail sled dog races: 23 cases (1994–2006). *Journal of the American Veterinary Medical Association* 232: 564–573.

Dowling, P.M. (1995). Therapy of gastrointestinal ulcers. *Canadian Veterinary Journal* 36: 276–277.

Duane, W.C. and Wiegand, D.M. (1980). Mechanism by which bile salt disrupts the gastric mucosal barrier in the dog. *Journal of Clinical Investigation* 66: 1044–1049.

Duane, W.C., Wiegand, D.M., and Sievert, C.E. (1982). Bile acid and bile salt disrupt gastric mucosal barrier in the dog by different mechanisms. *American Journal of Physiology* 242: G95–G99.

Forsyth, S.F., Guilford, W.G., Haslett, S.J., and Godfrey, J. (1998). Endoscopy of the gastroduodenal mucosa after carprofen, meloxicam and ketoprofen administration in dogs. *Journal of Small Animal Practice* 39: 421–424.

Gfeller, R.W. and Sandors, A.D. (1991). Naproxen-associated duodenal ulcer complicated by perforation and bacteria- and barium sulfate-induced peritonitis in a dog. *Journal of the American Veterinary Medical Association* 198: 644–646.

Gilroy, D.W., Colville-Nash, P.R., Willis, D. et al. (1999). Inducible cyclooxygenase may have anti-inflammatory properties. *Nature Medicine* 5: 698–701.

Godshalk, C.P., Roush, J.K., Fingland, R.B. et al. (1992). Gastric perforation associated with administration of ibuprofen in a dog. *Journal of the American Veterinary Medical Association* 201: 1734–1736.

Goodlad, R.A., Madgwick, A.J., Moffatt, M.R. et al. (1990). The effects of the prostaglandin analog, misoprostol, on cell proliferation and cell migration in the canine stomach. *Digestion* 46 (Suppl 2): 182–187.

Goodman, L., Torres, B., Punke, J. et al. (2009). Effects of firocoxib and tepoxalin on healing in a canine gastric mucosal injury model. *Journal of Veterinary Internal Medicine* 23: 56–62.

Green, F.W. Jr., Kaplan, M.M., Curtis, L.E., and Levine, P.H. (1978). Effect of acid and pepsin on blood coagulation and platelet aggregation. A possible contributor prolonged gastroduodenal mucosal hemorrhage. *Gastroenterology* 74: 38–43.

Hata, J., Kamada, T., Manabe, N. et al. (2005). Famotidine prevents canine gastric blood flow reduction by NSAIDs. *Alimentary Pharmacology and Therapeutics* 21 (Suppl 2): 55–59.

Hatazawa, R., Tanaka, A., Tanigami, M. et al. (2007). Cyclooxygenase-2/prostaglandin E-2 accelerates the healing of gastric ulcers via EP4 receptors. *American Journal of Physiology* 293: G788–G797.

Hinton, L.E., McLoughlin, M.A., Johnson, S.E., and Weisbrode, S.E. (2002). Spontaneous gastroduodenal perforation in 16 dogs and seven cats (1982–1999). *Journal of the American Animal Hospital Association* 38: 176–187.

Jergens, A.E., Pressel, M., Crandell, J. et al. (2009). Fluorescence in situ hybridization confirms clearance of visible *Helicobacter* spp. associated with gastritis in dogs and cats. *Journal of Veterinary Internal Medicine* 23: 16–23.

Johnston, S.A., Leib, M.S., Forrester, S.D., and Marini, M. (1995). The effect of misoprostol on aspirin-induced gastroduodenal lesions in dogs. *Journal of Veterinary Internal Medicine* 9: 32–38.

Jones, C.J. and Budsberg, S.C. (2000). Physiologic characteristics and clinical importance of the cyclooxygenase isoforms in dogs and cats. *Journal of the American Veterinary Medical Association* 217: 721–729.

Jones, C.J., Streppa, H.K., Harmon, B.G., and Budsberg, S.C. (2002). in vivo effects of meloxicam and aspirin on blood, gastric mucosal, and synovial fluid prostanoid synthesis in dogs. *American Journal of Veterinary Research* 63: 1527–1531.

Katz, L.B., Tobia, A.J., and Shriver, D.A. (1987). Effects of ORF 17583, other histamine H-2-receptor antagonists and omeprazole on gastric acid secretory states in rats and dogs. *Journal of Pharmacology and Experimental Therapeutics* 242: 437–442.

Kavitha, S., Prathaban, S., Vasu, K., and Dhanapalan, P. (2007). Endoscopic isolation of *Helicobacter pylori* from gastric ulcer dogs. *Indian Journal of Veterinary Medicine* 27: 1–4.

Kitano, S. and Dolgor, B. (2000). Does portal hypertension contribute to the pathogenesis of gastric ulcer associated with liver cirrhosis? *Journal of Gastroenterology* 35: 79–86.

Knapp, D.W., Richardson, R.C., Bottoms, G.D. et al. (1992). Phase I trial of piroxicam in 62 dogs bearing naturally occurring tumors. *Cancer Chemotherapy and Pharmacology* 29: 214–218.

Laine, L., Takeuchi, K., and Tarnawski, A. (2008). Gastric mucosal defense and cytoprotection: bench to bedside. *Gastroenterology* 135: 41–60.

Larsen, K.R., Dajani, E.Z., and Ives, M.M. (1992). Antiulcer drugs and gastric mucosal integrity. Effects of misoprostol, 16,16-dimethyl PGE2, and cimetidine on hemodynamics and metabolic rate in canine gastric mucosa. *Digestive Diseases and Sciences* 37: 1029–1038.

Lascelles, B.D., Blikslager, A.T., Fox, S.M., and Reece, D. (2005). Gastrointestinal tract perforation in dogs treated with a selective cyclooxygenase-2 inhibitor: 29 cases (2002–2003). *Journal of the American Veterinary Medical Association* 227: 1112–1117.

Lascelles, B.D., Court, M.H., Hardie, E.M., and Robertson, S.A. (2007). Nonsteroidal anti-inflammatory drugs in cats: a review. *Veterinary Anaesthesia and Analgesia* 34: 228–250.

Leib, M.S., Duncan, R.B., and Ward, D.L. (2007). Triple antimicrobial therapy and acid suppression in dogs with chronic vomiting and gastric *Helicobacter* spp. *Journal of Veterinary Internal Medicine* 21: 1185–1192.

Liptak, J.M., Hunt, G.B., Barrs, V.R. et al. (2002). Gastroduodenal ulceration in cats: eight cases and a review of the literature. *Journal of Feline Medicine and Surgery* 4: 27–42.

Møller, M.H., Adamsen, S., Wøjdemann, M., and Møller, A.M. (2009). Perforated peptic ulcer: how to improve outcome? *Scandinavian Journal of Gastroenterology* 44: 15–22.

Murray, M., Robinson, P.B., McKeating, F.J. et al. (1972). Peptic ulceration in the dog: a clinico-pathological study. *Veterinary Record* 91: 441–447.

Neiger, R., Gaschen, F., and Jaggy, A. (2000). Gastric mucosal lesions in dogs with acute intervertebral disc disease: characterization and effects of omeprazole or misoprostol. *Journal of Veterinary Internal Medicine* 14: 33–36.

Penninck, D., Matz, M., and Tidwell, A. (1997). Ultrasonography of gastric ulceration in the dog. *Veterinary Radiology and Ultrasound* 38: 308–312.

Poonam, D., Vinay, C.S., and Gautam, P. (2005). Cyclo-oxygenase-2 expression and prostaglandin E-2 production in experimental chronic gastric ulcer healing. *European Journal of Pharmacology* 519: 277–284.

Poortinga, E.W. and Hungerford, L.L. (1998). A case–control study of acute ibuprofen toxicity in dogs. *Preventive Veterinary Medicine* 35: 115–124.

Postius, S., Bräuer, U., and Kromer, W. (1991). The novel proton pump inhibitor pantoprazole elevates intragastric pH for a prolonged period when administered under conditions of stimulated gastric acid secretion in the gastric fistula dog. *Life Sciences* 49: 1047–1052.

Punke, J.P., Speas, A.L., Reynolds, L.R., and Budsberg, S.C. (2008). Effects of firocoxib, meloxicam, and tepoxalin on prostanoid and leuko triene production by duodenal mucosa and other tissues of osteoarthritic dogs. *American Journal of Veterinary Research* 69: 1203–1209.

Reed, S. (2002). Nonsteroidal anti-inflammatory drug-induced duodenal ulceration and perforation in a mature rottweiler. *Canadian Veterinary Journal* 43: 971–972.

Reimer, M.E., Johnston, S.A., Leib, M.S. et al. (1999). The gastroduodenal effects of buffered aspirin, carprofen, and etodolac in healthy dogs. *Journal of Veterinary Internal Medicine* 13: 472–477.

Roberts, E.S., Van Lare, K.A., Marable, B.R., and Salminen, W.F. (2009). Safety and tolerability of 3-week and 6-month dosing of Deramaxx (deracoxib) chewable tablets in dogs. *Journal of Veterinary Pharmacology and Therapeutics* 32: 329–337.

Runk, A., Kyles, A.E., and Downs, M.O. (1999). Duodenal perforation in a cat following the administration of nonsteroidal anti-inflammatory medication. *Journal of the American Animal Hospital Association* 35: 52–55.

Ryan, W.G., Moldave, K., and Carithers, D. (2006). Clinical effectiveness and safety of a new NSAID, firocoxib: a 1,000 dog study. *Veterinary Therapeutics* 7: 119–126.

Ryan, W.G., Moldave, K., and Carithers, D. (2007). Switching NSAIDs in practice: insights from the Previcox (firocoxib) experience trial. *Veterinary Therapeutics* 8: 263–271.

Schoenfeld, P., Kimmey, M.B., Scheiman, J. et al. (1999). Review article: Nonsteroidal anti-inflammatory drug-associated gastrointestinal complications: guidelines for prevention and treatment. *Alimentary Pharmacology and Therapeutics* 13: 1273–1285.

Sennello, K.A. and Leib, M.S. (2006). Effects of deracoxib or buffered aspirin on the gastric mucosa of healthy dogs. *Journal of Veterinary Internal Medicine* 20: 1291–1296.

Sessions, J.K., Reynolds, L.R., and Budsberg, S.C. (2005). in vivo effects of carprofen, deracoxib, and etodolac on prostanoid production in blood, gastric mucosa, and synovial fluid in dogs with chronic osteoarthritis. *American Journal of Veterinary Research* 66: 812–817.

Simpson, K.W., Strauss-Ayali, D., McDonough, P.L. et al. (1999). Gastric function in dogs with naturally acquired gastric *Helicobacter* spp. infection. *Journal of Veterinary Internal Medicine* 13: 507–515.

Simpson, K., Neiger, R., DeNovo, R., and Sherding, R. (2000). The relationship of *Helicobacter* spp. infection to gastric disease in dogs and cats. *Journal of Veterinary Internal Medicine* 14: 223–227.

Slomiany, B.L., Piotrowski, J., Tamura, S., and Slomiany, A. (1991). Enhancement of the protective qualities of gastric mucus by sucralfate: role of phosphoinositides. *American Journal of Medicine* 91 (2A): 30S–36S.

Slomiany, B.L., Liu, J., Keogh, J.P. et al. (1992). Enhancement of gastric mucosal epidermal growth factor and platelet-derived growth factor receptor expression by sucralfate. *General Pharmacology* 23: 715–718.

Stanton, M.E. and Bright, R.M. (1989). Gastroduodenal ulceration in dogs. Retrospective study of 43 cases and literature review. *Journal of Veterinary Internal Medicine* 3: 23 –244.

Steiner, K., Bühring, K.U., Faro, H.P. et al. (1982). Sucralfate: pharmacokinetics, metabolism and selective binding to experimental gastric and duodenal ulcers in animals. *Arzneimittel-Forschung* 32: 512–518.

Suzuki, M., Mori, M., Miura, S. et al. (1996). Omeprazole attenuates oxygen-derived free radical production from human neutrophils. *Free Radical Biology and Medicine* 21: 727–731.

Thomson, A.B., Sinclair, P., Matisko, A. et al. (1997). Influence of food on the bioavailability of an enteric-coated tablet formulation of omeprazole 20 mg under repeated dose conditions. *Canadian Journal of Gastroenterology* 11: 663–667.

Tolbert, K., Bissett, S., King, A. et al. (2010). Efficacy of oral famotidine and two omeprazole formulations for the control of intragastric pH in dogs. *Journal of Veterinary Internal Medicine* 25: 47–54.

Tomlinson, J. and Blikslager, A. (2003). Role of nonsteroidal anti-inflammatory drugs in gastrointestinal tract injury and repair. *Journal of the American Veterinary Medical Association* 222: 946–951.

Vaz-da-Silva, M., Loureiro, A.I., Nunes, T. et al. (2005). Bioavailability and bioequivalence of two enteric-coated formulations of omeprazole in fasting and fed conditions. *Clinical Drug Investigation* 25: 391–399.

Vonderhaar, M.A. and Salisbury, S.K. (1993). Gastroduodenal ulceration associated with flunixin meglumine administration in three dogs. *Journal of the American Veterinary Medical Association* 203: 92–95.

Wallace, M.S., Zawie, D.A., and Garvey, M.S. (1990). Gastric ulceration in the dog secondary to the use of nonsteroidal antiinflammatory drugs. *Journal of the American Animal Hospital Association* 26: 467–472.

Ward, D.M., Leib, M.S., Johnston, S.A., and Marini, M. (2003). The effect of dosing interval on the efficacy of misoprostol in the prevention of aspirin-induced gastric injury. *Journal of Veterinary Internal Medicine* 17: 282–290.

Williamson, K.K., Willard, M.D., McKenzie, E.C. et al. (2007). Efficacy of famotidine for the prevention of exercise-induced gastritis in racing Alaskan sled dogs. *Journal of Veterinary Internal Medicine* 21: 924–927.

Wilson, J.E., Chandrasekharan, N.V., Westover, K.D. et al. (2004). Determination of expression of cyclooxygenase-1 and -2 isozymes in canine tissues and their differential sensitivity to nonsteroidal anti-inflammatory drugs. *American Journal of Veterinary Research* 65: 810–818.

Wooten, J.G., Blikslager, A.T., Ryan, K.A. et al. (2008). Cyclooxygenase expression and prostanoid production in pyloric and duodenal mucosae in dogs after administration of nonsteroidal anti-inflammatory drugs. *American Journal of Veterinary Research* 69: 457–464.

Wooten, J.G., Blikslager, A.T., Marks, S.L. et al. (2009). Effect of nonsteroidal anti-inflammatory drugs with varied cyclooxygenase-2 selectivity on cyclooxygenase protein and prostanoid concentrations in pyloric and duodenal mucosa of dogs. *American Journal of Veterinary Research* 70: 1243–1249.

7

Gastric Dilatation Volvulus

Elisa M. Mazzaferro and Eric Monnet

Gastric dilatation volvulus (GDV) syndrome is characterized by accumulation of air within the stomach with a rapid rise in intraluminal pressure, gastric malpositioning, compression of the diaphragm and caudal vena cava, and impaired respiratory and cardiovascular function (Passi *et al.* 1969; Matthiesen 1993; Brockman *et al.* 2000; Evans & Adams 2010). A variety of intrinsic and extrinsic risk factors for the development of GDV have been investigated. To date, no one causative factor has been found, and the etiology and even pathophysiology are not fully understood (Brockman *et al.* 2000). While GDV is most commonly seen in large or giant deep-chested dogs, it has also been documented in guinea pigs (Nogradi *et al.* 2017), cats (Leary & Sinnott-Stutzman 2018), and small dogs (Brockman *et al.* 1995; Glickman *et al.* 2000a; Formaggini *et al.* 2008; Mitchell *et al.* 2010). In large-breed dogs, GDV is reported to be the second leading cause of death (Glickman *et al.* 1994, 2000a).

Etiology

Intrinsic risk factors

Body size, thoracoabdominal dimensions, and genetics

Dogs with higher thoracic depth to width ratios on radiographs and external thoracic measurements have a significantly increased risk of developing GDV during their lifetime, particularly if a family member or parent has also had GDV (Glickman *et al.* 1996, 2000a; Schaible *et al.* 1997; Schellenberg *et al.* 1998; Raghavan *et al.* 2004). Dogs with leaner body condition are also at higher risk compared with overweight dogs (Schaible *et al.* 1997).

The Great Dane (odds ratio [OR] 10), Weimaraner (OR 4.6), St Bernard (OR 4.2), and Irish setter (OR 3.5) have been shown to be at greater risk for developing GDV (Glickman *et al.* 1994). The Irish wolfhound, borzoi, mastiff, Akita, bull mastiff, pointers, bloodhound, Grand Bleu de Gascogne, and standard poodle also have an increased risk for developing GDV because of their conformation (Glickman *et al.* 1994, 2000b; Schaible *et al.* 1997; Elwood 1998; Evans & Adams 2010). Large- and giant-breed dogs appear to have a 7% risk of death from GDV throughout their lifetime (Glickman *et al.* 2000a,b). Great Danes have a 42.4% chance of developing GDV (Glickman *et al.* 2000a,b). Recent studies in Great Danes have documented that dogs with specific alleles of the canine immune genes (Harkey *et al.* 2018) along with a more diverse gut microbiome (Hullar *et al.* 2018) have an increased risk of GDV, further supporting a role of genetic and other intrinsic risk factors.

Serum gastrin concentration

Serum gastrin concentrations have been investigated as a potential cause of GDV, with the presumption that hypergastrinemia would cause pyloric hypertrophy, resulting in partial pyloric outflow obstruction and delayed gastric emptying (Hosgood 1994). While one study showed elevated serum gastrin concentrations in dogs with GDV, a second study failed to replicate these same results (Leib *et al.* 1984; Hall *et al.* 1989). Further, it remained unclear whether hypergastrinemia was the primary cause of GDV, or rather was a consequence of GDV, hypoperfusion, and impaired renal clearance

Small Animal Soft Tissue Surgery, Second Edition. Edited by Eric Monnet.
© 2023 John Wiley & Sons, Inc. Published 2023 by John Wiley & Sons, Inc.
Companion website: www.wiley.com/go/monnet/small

(Leib *et al.* 1984; Hosgood 1994). Postprandial gastrin concentrations have been found to be elevated in dogs fed once daily compared with dogs fed more than once daily (Hall *et al.* 1989). It has been shown that pyloric hypertrophy is not associated with GDV in dogs (Greenfield *et al.* 1989).

Gastric myoelectric function

Gastric myoelectric function has also been investigated as a putative/potential cause of GDV, with the hypothesis that impaired gastric contractility could result in delayed gastric emptying (Stampley *et al.* 1992). Researchers found that gastric myoelectric function was impaired in animals with experimentally induced GDV for up to 48–72 hours postoperatively, but similar results were also found in animals who had gastrotomy alone without GDV, and without an intraoperative gastropexy. Stampley *et al.* (1992) documented normal gastric emptying in dogs 3 months after GDV.

Impaired esophageal motility and aerophagia

Impaired esophageal motility with aerophagia has also been implicated as a potential cause of GDV (Caywood *et al.* 1977; van Sluijs & van den Brom 1989). Aerophagia secondary to reverse sneezing has been implicated as a putative risk factor for GDV development, as one study reported a higher incidence of nasal mites in dogs with GDV (Bredal 1998). Stomach gas analysis of dogs with GDV documented concentrations of hydrogen (29%) and carbon dioxide (13–20%) that are higher than those of room air, suggesting that fermentation of food with gastric acid more likely plays some role in the development of GDV (Van Kruiningen *et al.* 2013). Additionally, 12% of dogs with GDV have a prior history of gastrointestinal-related illness, and 61% of dogs with GDV were found to have inflammatory bowel disease (Braun *et al.* 1996; Glickman *et al.* 2000b).

Age

GDV has been reported in animals whose ages ranged from less than 1 year to greater than 14 years. In a number of studies, the risk of GDV occurrence increases with advancing age, although the cutoff age range differs among large- and giant-breed dogs (Theyse *et al.* 1998; Glickman *et al.* 2000a,b). In large-breed dogs, the risk of GDV increases after 3 years of age, while giant breeds have a greater risk before 3 years of age (Glickman *et al.* 2000a,b).

Extrinsic risk factors

Diet and eating

One study documented an increased risk of GDV when dogs were fed dry food (Elwood 1998; Pipan *et al.* 2012).

In another study, feeding food whose particles were greater than 30 mm in size decreased the risk of GDV fourfold. Feeding table scraps, particularly fish or eggs, with dog food was shown to decrease the risk of GDV by 28% (Glickman *et al.* 1997; Pipan *et al.* 2012). Irish setters have been shown to be three times more likely to develop GDV if fed one food type, rather than a mixture of food types (Elwood 1998).

The use of raised feeding bowls was documented to actually increase the risk of GDV in one study (Glickman *et al.* 1997). Faster, more rapid eating has been shown to increase the risk of GDV (Elwood 1998; Glickman *et al.* 2000a). In addition, feeding just once daily rather than more than once daily has also been implicated as increasing the risk of GDV (Glickman *et al.* 1997). In another study, there was increased risk with feeding larger volumes of food, irrespective of whether feeding was scheduled once or more than once daily (Raghavan *et al.* 2004). Gastric foreign material also has been documented to increase the risk of GDV in large- and giant-breed dogs (de Battisti *et al.* 2012).

Stress

Stress has been documented to be a risk factor for the development of GDV. In one study, dogs that presented with GDV had a higher incidence of kenneling or transport/car ride within 24 hours preceding GDV (Elwood 1998). Fearful and anxious dogs have been shown to have an increased risk of GDV, while happier dogs appear to have a decreased risk (Glickman *et al.* 1997, 2000b; Elwood 1998; Pipan *et al.* 2012).

Climatic factors

There appears to be a seasonal increase in the incidence of GDV in some studies, although climatic change appears to vary according to location. In one study, the incidence of GDV increased during the summer (June, July, August, and September), while in another study of military working dogs, a seasonal increase occurred in the winter months (November, December, and January) (Herbold *et al.* 2002; Dennler *et al.* 2005). The effects of ambient temperature, humidity, and barometric pressure were variable, although the incidence of GDV did appear to increase with falling barometric pressure (Herbold *et al.* 2002; Dennler *et al.* 2005).

Previous splenectomy

Splenectomy has been researched as a potential risk factor for subsequent development of GDV in dogs in multiple retrospective studies (Goldhammer *et al.* 2010; Grange *et al.* 2012; Sartor *et al.* 2013) with equivocal results. GDV has been documented in two dogs following splenectomy for splenic torsion and removal of a large splenic mass, respectively (Millis *et al.* 1995; Marconato 2006). The largest case–control study evaluated 453 cases of splenectomized dogs and determined that previous splenectomy increased the relative risk of GDV by 5.3 times (Sartor *et al.* 2013). Smaller studies that evaluated 219 splenectomized dogs compared with 47 dogs undergoing enterotomy (Grange *et al.* 2012) and 37 splenectomized dogs with 43 dogs undergoing other abdominal surgery (Goldhammer *et al.* 2010) showed no significant association with splenectomy and the development of GDV. In dogs with other predisposing factors for GDV, prophylactic gastropexy can be considered following splenectomy or other abdominal surgery, provided that the patient is stable and the procedure will not significantly increase surgical or anesthesia time.

Pathophysiology

It is unknown if volvulus of the stomach occurs prior to dilatation or vice versa. Malposition of the stomach will result in occlusion of the lower esophageal sphincter and the pylorus. Therefore, fermentation of gastric contents will induce dilation of the stomach (Passi *et al.* 1969; Wingfield *et al.* 1974; Brockman *et al.* 2000). Volvulus has been documented in some patients without gastric dilatation (Boothe & Ackerman 1976; Frendin *et al.* 1988). Hepatogastric ligaments were measured in dogs with and without GDV and were found to be significantly longer in dogs with GDV (Hall *et al.* 1995). With elongation or stretching of the hepatogastric ligaments, the stomach can twist. Histologically, the ligaments from GDV and control dogs appeared similar (Hall *et al.* 1995). Gastric dilatation can occur without malposition of the stomach, and often occurs secondary to aerophagia. Computed tomography has been used to document chronic gastric instability in a Great Dane that then progressed to GDV (Czajkowski & Hallman 2018). Gastric dilatation has been diagnosed in dogs without volvulus, and in dogs with gastropexy (Ende 1980; Leib *et al.* 1985; Woolfson & Kostolich 1986; Eggertsdottir *et al.* 2008). Once intragastric pressures exceed a cutoff point, increased pressure on the lower esophageal sphincter exceeds the sphincter's ability to open and allow eructation. An acute gastric angle accompanied by the presence of intragastric bacteria and bacterial fermentation results in further gastric distension, and finally rotation. The stomach rotates in a clockwise direction in more than 90% of cases. The pyloric antrum moves from a right-sided position ventrally across the abdomen to a dorsal position in the left side of the abdomen. Most often the rotation is 270°, but rotations of more than 360° have been reported. In 10%

of cases the stomach is in a normal position at the time of surgery. This most likely occurs because the stomach derotates on its own after decompression.

GDV is associated with severe changes in cardiovascular, respiratory, renal, and gastrointestinal physiology (Passi *et al.* 1969; Wingfield *et al.* 1974; Orton & Muir 1983a; Matthiesen 1993; Sharp & Rozanski 2014). If not treated correctly, these changes lead to the development of shock and the death of the patient.

Elevation of the pressure in the abdominal cavity compresses the portal vein and the vena cava. It reduces venous return to the heart, cardiac output, and arterial pressure (Passi *et al.* 1969; Orton & Muir 1983a; Brockman *et al.* 2000). It has been shown in a model of acute gastric dilatation that flow in the caudal vena cava dropped from 51 to 0.9 mL/kg per min (Passi *et al.* 1969). Blood flow in the cranial vena cava was also decreased (Passi *et al.* 1969). Acute gastric dilatation resulted in a significant reduction in mean arterial pressure that responded to intravenous fluid administration (Passi *et al.* 1969). Orton and Muir (1983a,b) further demonstrated that acute gastric dilatation is associated with a reduction in cardiac output and contractility. Wingfield *et al.* (1975b) showed with an angiographic study that acute gastric dilatation induces obstruction of the caudal vena cava. Barnes *et al.* (1985) demonstrated that increasing intra-abdominal pressure by 40 mmHg induces occlusion of the caudal vena cava. Compression of the portal vein induces edema and congestion of the gastrointestinal system and a reduction in vascular volume. Elevated portal pressure compromises microcirculation in the viscera and reduces oxygen delivery to the gastrointestinal tract. Under ischemic conditions the pancreas produces a "myocardial depressant factor" (Orton & Muir 1983b). Ischemia, acidosis, liberation of myocardial depressant factor by the pancreas, and the production of free oxygen radicals induces myocardial ischemia and reduces cardiac contractility (Orton & Muir 1983b; Horne *et al.* 1985).

The reduction in cardiac output has not always been documented in clinical cases (Wagner *et al.* 1999). Horne *et al.* (1985) documented a reduction in myocardial blood flow and an increase in myocardial oxygen consumption resulting in myocardial necrosis. MacPhail *et al.* (2006) demonstrated a reduction in cardiac efficiency after induction of portal hypertension and ischemia of the stomach wall. Reduction in perfusion triggers the release of catecholamines that induces an intense vasoconstriction and redirects blood flow to the essential organs (brain and kidney), to the detriment of other organs (Davidson *et al.* 1992). Subendocardial ischemia and necrosis combined with tachycardia and acid–base imbalance induce dysrhythmias (most frequently ventricular tachycardia)

(Wingfield *et al.* 1974, 1982; Muir 1982a,b; Miller *et al.* 2000). Atrial fibrillation and supraventricular tachycardia have been also documented during GDV in dogs (Muir 1982b).

Distension of the stomach limits motion of the diaphragm during inspiration, and reduces the tidal volume (Wingfield *et al.* 1974, 1975a; Merkley *et al.* 1976a; Wingfield 1981). This results in reduction of ventilation with a rise in partial pressure of arterial carbon dioxide (PaCO$_2$) (Wingfield *et al.* 1982). As the severity of the condition increases, atelectasis of the lungs develops, resulting in a reduction of arterial oxygen saturation (Wingfield *et al.* 1982). Reduction in oxygen saturation further reduces arterial oxygen content and oxygen delivery.

Increased intragastric pressure collapses the capillaries in the wall of the stomach, resulting in ischemia and necrosis of the gastric mucosa (Lantz *et al.* 1984). If the intragastric pressure continues rising, perfusion of the muscularis and serosa becomes compromised (Monnet *et al.* 2006). This results in full-thickness ischemia and necrosis of the stomach. Reduction in cardiac output contributes to the development of ischemia of the stomach wall and other organs in the abdomen (Komtebedde *et al.* 1991). The short gastric arteries are commonly avulsed during rotation of the stomach, which reduces perfusion of the body of the stomach along the greater curvature (Lantz *et al.* 1984). Breakdown of the gastrointestinal mucosa allows bacterial translocation and endotoxemia (Davidson *et al.* 1992; Winkler *et al.* 2003; Peycke *et al.* 2005; Walker *et al.* 2007). The local immune system that controls bacterial translocation is altered by ischemia. When circulation is restored, bacteria and endotoxins are liberated into the circulation. Endotoxins induce damage to cellular membranes, activate the complement and the coagulation cascade, activate platelets, increase vascular permeability, induce renal and hepatic damage, and cause fever. Dogs shift from hypovolemic shock to septic shock.

Reduction of peripheral perfusion overwhelms the inherent renal mechanisms and reduction in kidney function occurs. The decrease in glomerular filtration rate is manifested as prerenal oliguria and finally anuria. Poor perfusion of the peripheral tissue results in severe cellular hypoxemia and cell death. Lactic acid production is increased due to anaerobic metabolism and endotoxin. Finally, multiple organ failure occurs, with death of the patient.

Clinical signs

Clinical signs of GDV can be variable, depending on the body conformation of the dog, and the degree of rotation and dilatation of the stomach. The most common presenting complaint and clinical signs include gastric distension, nonproductive retching, ptyalism or hypersalivation, restlessness, anxiousness, and stretching or adopting a "prayer position" (Brockman *et al.* 1995; Brourman *et al.* 1996; Broome & Walsh 2003; Bhatia *et al.* 2010; Mackenzie *et al.* 2010; Zacher *et al.* 2010). In some instances, gastric distension may not be obvious in extremely deep-chested dogs. Additionally, depending on the degree of gastric distension and duration of clinical signs, affected animals can present with varying degrees of hypovolemic or distributive shock.

In early compensatory shock, the affected animal may demonstrate signs of tachycardia, rapid capillary refill time, and bounding femoral pulses. As shock progresses and the patient is no longer able to compensate, pulse quality, blood pressure, and body temperature decrease, and hypoperfusion ensues and leads to transition from aerobic to anaerobic metabolism and the development of metabolic acidosis. A body temperature of less than 38 °C (100.4 °F) has been associated with increased mortality (Buber *et al.* 2007). Finally, worsening of cardiac output and decompensatory shock impair the ability to ambulate, decrease mentation, and in the end stages of shock lead to coma and death. It has been shown that recumbent patients have a 4.4 times greater probability of dying than dogs that are ambulatory. If the patient is comatose it has a 36 times greater probability of dying. Dogs that appear depressed on presentation have a 3 times greater probability of dying (Glickman *et al.* 1998). Time is of the essence when making a diagnosis and treating a patient with GDV. The risk of comorbidity and mortality significantly increases if treatment lags behind the onset of clinical signs by more than 5 hours (Glickman *et al.* 1998; Beck *et al.* 2006; Buber *et al.* 2007).

Bloodwork

Serum biochemical and hemostatic abnormalities have been documented in animals with GDV. Early on, the complete blood count often reveals a stress leukogram with neutrophilic leukocytosis and lymphopenia (Merkley *et al.* 1976b; Leib & Martin 1987; Brockman *et al.* 1995; Brockman & Holt 2000; Monnet 2003). As GDV syndrome progresses, leukopenia may be present (Glickman *et al.* 1998). Thrombocytopenia and hemoconcentration also may be present (Merkley *et al.* 1976b; Glickman *et al.* 1998). Biochemical evidence of hepatocellular damage and cholestasis, with elevations in alanine aminotransferase (ALT) and total bilirubin, azotemia with elevations in blood urea nitrogen (BUN) and creatinine, and hypokalemia may also be present (Wingfield *et al.* 1975c; Merkley *et al.* 1976b). Canine pancreatic lipase immunoreactivity (cPLI) and lipase are frequently increased in dogs with GDV;

however, they cannot be used to prognosticate the outcome at this time (Spinella *et al.* 2018).

Abnormalities of coagulation with either prolonged or rapid prothrombin time (PT), partial thromboplastin time (PTT), and activated clotting time (ACT) may be present, depending on whether the patient is hypocoagulable or hypercoagulable (Millis *et al.* 1993; Sharp & Rozanski 2014). That, along with increased fibrin degradation products, decreased antithrombin, elevated D-dimers, and thrombocytopenia, may be used to determine the presence of disseminated intravascular coagulation (DIC) (Millis *et al.* 1993). One study documented abnormal hemostasis and coagulation abnormalities consistent in 40% of dogs with GDV (Millis *et al.* 1993). A multiple regression analysis based on fibrin degradation product concentration, activated (A)PTT, and antithrombin III activity was predictive of gastric necrosis (86% sensitivity, 100% specificity) (Millis *et al.* 1993). In another study, prolongation of PT within 12 hours of admission for GDV was associated with a significantly increased risk of death (Buber *et al.* 2007).

Prognostic tests

Myoglobin

Myoglobin at time of presentation was significantly higher in nonsurvivors than in survivors, although the authors concluded that myoglobin alone is not a sensitive or specific indicator to predict death in naturally occurring cases of GDV. Myoglobin may instead be more useful at predicting inadequate resuscitation, or ongoing cell damage if levels continue to rise in the postoperative period (Adamik *et al.* 2009).

Cardiac biomarkers and echocardiography

Elevations in serum concentrations of cardiac troponins I and T, markers of myocardial cell damage, have been documented in dogs with GDV (Schober *et al.* 2002). Elevations in cardiac troponin values have been positively correlated with an increased risk of ventricular dysrhythmias and death (Schober *et al.* 2002; Aona *et al.* 2017). Dogs who have echocardiographic measurements consistent with decreased ventricular preload and who do not receive adequate intravascular fluid resuscitation have a significantly increased relative risk of death from GDV (Aona *et al.* 2017).

Serum lactate

Cardiovascular instability and decreased organ perfusion are among the causative factors of the complications associated with GDV syndrome. A switch from aerobic to anaerobic metabolism ensues, as oxygen utilization becomes dependent on what is supplied. Lactate is produced as a byproduct of anaerobic metabolism and has been shown to be elevated in animals with GDV (de Papp *et al.* 1999; Zacher *et al.* 2010; Green *et al.* 2011; Beer *et al.* 2013; Verschoof *et al.* 2015; Oron *et al.* 2018; Sharp *et al.* 2020). While an initial study suggested that a cutoff of greater than 6.6 mmol/L at the time of presentation was associated with a greater risk for gastric necrosis and death, more recent studies refuted this value and found instead that initial serum lactate concentrations at the time of presentation were not significantly different among survivors of GDV and nonsurvivors (de Papp *et al.* 1999; Zacher *et al.* 2010). Following resuscitation, a lactate value of less than 6.4 mmol/L, a decrease of 4 mmol/L or more, or a percentage change (decrease) in lactate by more than 42.5% of the original value was associated more closely with survival (Zacher *et al.* 2010; Green *et al.* 2011).

Inflammatory biomarkers C-reactive protein, high-mobility group box 1, and procalcitonin

In dogs with GDV, relative hypovolemia, hypoperfusion, and tissue necrosis predispose patients to the development of systemic inflammatory response syndrome (SIRS). C-reactive protein (CRP), high-mobility group box 1 (HMGB1), and procalcitonin are biomarkers of inflammation that have been shown to be elevated in dogs with GDV (Uhrikova *et al.* 2015; Israeli *et al.* 2012; Troia *et al.* 2018). In one study procalcitonin levels were significantly higher in nonsurvivors and were prognostic for survival (Troia *et al.* 2018), and in another study HMGB1 was significantly different in survivors versus nonsurvivors (Uhrikova *et al.* 2015). More research is required to determine the sensitivity and specificity of these biomarkers when considering prognosis in dogs with GDV.

Immediate diagnostics and treatment/ stabilization

Because of the urgency of stabilization and surgical intervention, diagnostics and immediate treatment should occur simultaneously. Diagnosis is mostly based on signalment and clinical signs on presentation. Abdominal radiographs might be required if the diagnosis is not obvious or if a mesenteric volvulus is suspected. Treatment is directed at restoring perfusion and blood pressure and providing analgesia for the patient. Identifying complications that could make an animal a higher anesthetic and surgical risk is also paramount, as interventions can be started.

Intravenous fluid therapy

The use of isotonic crystalloid fluids (0.9% NaCl, lactated Ringer solution, Normosol-R, Plasmalyte-A) is administered preferably through one or two large-bore catheters placed in the cephalic veins. Lateral saphenous veins can also be used, since fluid instilled into the lateral saphenous vein enters circulation through the paravertebral sinuses (Wingfield et al. 1975b). Incremental boluses of one-fourth of a shock volume of fluid should be administered as quickly as possible during intravenous fluid resuscitation. The shock volume of fluid in the dog is 90 mL/kg. Once one-fourth of the shock volume has been administered, blood pressure, mucous membrane color, capillary refill time, and urine output should be assessed. If the patient is still hypotensive, an additional one-fourth shock bolus of fluid should be administered as rapidly as possible, then perfusion parameters are once again reassessed.

If more than 90 mL/kg of crystalloid fluid has been administered and the patient is still hypotensive or not responding to crystalloid fluid alone, a colloid such as hydroxyethyl starch can be administered in incremental boluses of 5 mL/kg to augment blood pressure and perfusion. Hydroxyethyl starch is a polymer of amylopectin and will cause prolongations of APTT and ACT, although it has not been associated with clinical bleeding in animals, except those with von Willebrand disease or in von Willebrand carriers. Hydroxyethyl starch will bind von Willebrand factor and can worsen clinical bleeding in affected animals, so should be avoided in von Willebrand patients. The use of a colloid in combination with a crystalloid will help maintain the crystalloid volume infused for a longer period of time than if the crystalloid fluid was infused alone.

Hypertonic saline with dextran-70 (7% hypertonic saline with dextran 5 mL/kg over 15 minutes) has been shown to provide more rapid resuscitation and a longer duration of action than resuscitation of GDV dogs with 0.9% saline alone (Allen et al. 1991; Schertel et al. 1997).

When available, hemoglobin-based oxygen carriers (HBOC) can be used as a potent colloid and oxygen carrier past sites of impaired perfusion. Comparison of an HBOC with 6% hetastarch as an initial resuscitative fluid showed that the HBOC was superior to the starch product at reaching end-point goals of fluid resuscitation in less time and with a smaller mL/kg volume (Haak et al. 2012). Although HBOC are not currently available at the time of this writing, they should be considered if the products resurface on the veterinary market.

Positive inotropes and vasopressors

If fluid therapy, analgesia, and antiarrhythmic drugs alone are unsuccessful at augmenting and normalizing blood pressure, positive inotropic and vasopressor drugs should be considered. Dobutamine (5–15 µg/kg per min intravenously [i.v.] by continuous-rate infusion) and/or dopamine (3–10 µg/kg per min i.v. by continuous-rate infusion) can be administered to improve inotropy. Intraoperatively, ephedrine (0.1–0.2 mg/kg i.v.) or phenylephrine (0.1 mg i.v., then as a continuous-rate infusion 3–5 µg/kg per min) can be used. Vasopressors such as epinephrine (0.05–0.4 µg/kg per min i.v. by continuous-rate infusion) or norepinephrine (0.05–0.4 µg/kg per min i.v. by continuous-rate infusion) can be considered. The use of vasopressors will result in vasoconstriction to improve blood pressure. Blood pressure, particularly when vascular beds are constricted from α-adrenergic stimulation, may increase at the expense of perfusion. Therefore, the use of vasopressor drugs should be limited to a last effort to stabilize cardiovascular status before and during general anesthesia for surgical correction of GDV.

Antiarrhythmic drugs

Cardiac dysrhythmias have been documented in up to 10–42% of dogs with GDV preoperatively (Muir & Lipowitz 1978; Brourman et al. 1996). A variety of supraventricular and ventricular dysrhythmias have been documented in dogs with GDV, with ventricular tachycardia being the most common (Muir & Lipowitz 1978; Muir 1982b; Muir & Bonagura 1984; Brourman et al. 1996). It is advisable to treat ventricular dysrhythmias before the onset of general anesthesia whenever possible. Common treatments include lidocaine (1–2 mg/kg i.v., followed by a constant-rate infusion of 50–100 µg/kg per min) or procainamide (10–15 mg/kg i.v. slowly over 10 min, then 25–50 µg/kg per min i.v. by constant-rate infusion) (Muir & Bonagura 1984; Chandler et al. 2006). As the irritated myocardium is sensitive to the effects of catecholamines, decreasing anxiety, stress, and discomfort with opioid analgesia is also recommended. In the preoperative and postoperative periods, ventricular dysrhythmias should be treated with antiarrhythmic drugs if the ectopic beats/premature ventricular contractions are more than 160 beats per minute (bpm) (Figure 7.1), are multifocal in nature (indicating more than one irritable location within the ventricles), or exhibit R-on-T phenomena in which the repolarization of one beat is superimposed on the depolarization of the previous beat (Figure 7.2). Ventricular dysrhythmias, even if they do not meet the criteria listed, should also be treated when they are associated with hypotension. In one study, the administration of lidocaine (2 mg/kg i.v. bolus, then 50 µg/kg per min) was not shown to prevent cardiac dysrhythmias or other complications assumed to be secondary to reperfusion injury (Buber et al. 2007);

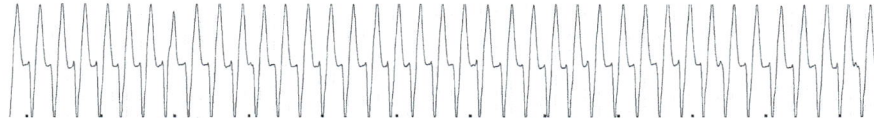

Figure 7.1 Sustained ventricular tachycardia with more than 160 beats per minute.

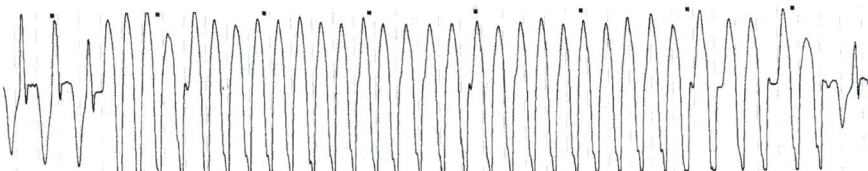

Figure 7.2 R-on-T phenomenon, where the T wave of repolarization is superimposed on the previous QRS complex. This is a prefibrillatory rhythm and must be treated with antiarrhythmic drugs.

however, a more recent study showed that pretreatment with lidocaine to dogs with GDV as a bolus (2 mg/kg i.v.) followed by a continuous-rate infusion of lidocaine (50 μg/kg per min i.v.) for a minimum of 24 hours after surgery was found to decrease the incidence of cardiac dysrhythmias, acute kidney injury, and hospitalization time compared with nontreated control dogs (Bruchim *et al*. 2012). In many cases, hypokalemia and hypomagnesemia can also predispose a patient to ventricular dysrhythmias. Maintenance of normokalemia with potassium supplementation, and supplementation with magnesium chloride (0.75 mEq/kg daily), should be considered in cases with refractory ventricular dysrhythmias.

Antibiotics

During GDV, decreased oxygen delivery to the small and large intestine and cellular membrane dysfunction has been associated with bacterial translocation (Winkler *et al*. 2003). One study documented bacteremia in 43% of dogs with GDV, but also documented bacteremia in 40% of control dogs. The presence of bacteremia did not appear to be associated with, or predictive of, survival in dogs with GDV (Winkler *et al*. 2003). While bacterial translocation from the stomach was not documented, the stomach normally has a lower population of bacteria than the small and large intestines. Elevated portal pressures and cellular membrane damage in the jejunum have been documented in experimentally induced GDV. Broad-spectrum antibiotics in the immediate perioperative period (cefazolin 22 mg/kg i.v.) is still advised.

Adjunct therapies

Impaired perfusion and impaired oxygen delivery can result in a switch from aerobic to anaerobic metabolism, production of lactic acid, and metabolic acidosis. Myocardial and cellular acidosis can be impaired and

result in further complications of cardiac dysrhythmias and decreased oxygen extraction or utilization. In addition, once perfusion is reestablished, using either gastric decompression or decompression and derotation, with the addition of intravenous fluid therapy, reperfusion is often characterized by the release of oxygen-derived free radical species and by cellular damage secondary to the activation of arachidonic acid and the inflammatory cascade. Urinary thromboxane derivatives – markers of arachidonic acid activation and inflammation – were found to be significantly higher in dogs with GDV at the time of admission and one hour postoperatively (Baltzer *et al*. 2006). The elevation was positively correlated with a significant increase in the incidence of postoperative complications, including gastric necrosis, cardiac dysrhythmias, and death (Winkler *et al*. 2003). That, along with vascular endothelial damage and sluggish blood flow, can activate DIC and multiple organ damage. DIC has been documented in 8 of 20 dogs with GDV, with the affected animals exhibiting thrombocytopenia, prolonged PT and APTT, decreased antithrombin, increased fibrin degradation products, and hypofibrinogenemia (Millis *et al*. 1993). DIC is associated with a poor prognosis (Beck *et al*. 2006). For these reasons, interventions have been evaluated to help decrease the effect of reperfusion injury.

In dogs with experimental GDV, the use of lipid peroxidation inhibitors was found to inhibit lipid peroxidation in the small and large intestine, liver, and pancreas if given before GDV was established, while the use of allopurinol failed to inhibit lipid peroxidation experimentally (Guilford *et al*. 1989; Badylak *et al*. 1990; Davidson *et al*. 1992; Lantz *et al*. 1992; Costa *et al*. 2004; Buber *et al*. 2007). Bacterial endotoxin and prostaglandin concentrations have also been found to be elevated in dogs with experimentally induced GDV. Flunixin meglumine, a prostaglandin synthesis inhibitor, administered at the time of gastric derotation, was not found to be useful in improving hemodynamics in the perioperative period (Davidson *et al.* 1992). However, administration of intra-operative flunixin meglumine may have helped blunt or attenuate the effects of bacterial endotoxin. Because of the inherent risks of administration of a prostaglandin synthesis inhibitor to a patient with impaired gastric and intestinal mucosal blood flow and portal hypertension, the risks associated with its administration greatly outweigh the potential but unproven benefits of its use, so the use of flunixin meglumine, glucocorticosteroids, and nonsteroidal anti-inflammatory drugs in patients with GDV is considered contraindicated at this time (Hosgood 1994).

Gastric decompression techniques

Percutaneous decompression

Percutaneous decompression of the stomach is one of the easiest techniques to perform, particularly if there is a limited number of personnel available to restrain the dog. To perform percutaneous gastric decompression, the abdomen should be auscultated and percussed to find the area with a sharp pinging sound (Walshaw & Johnston 1976; Brockman *et al.* 1995; Eggertsdottir & Moe 1995; Mackenzie *et al.* 2010) (Figure 7.3). A dull

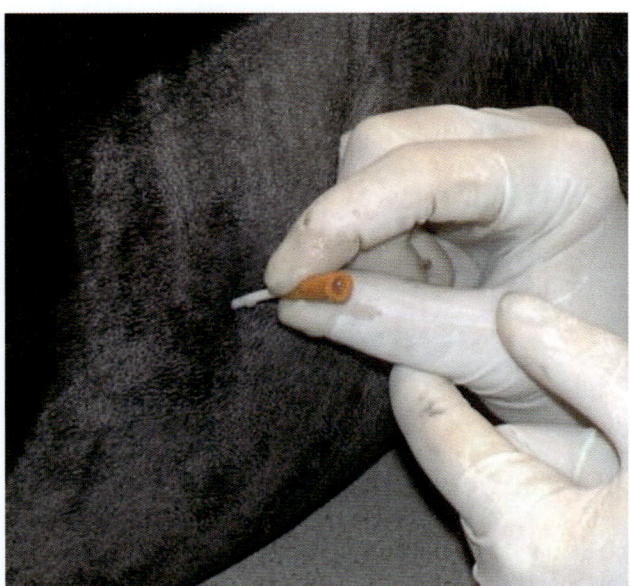

Figure 7.3 Percutaneous decompression of the stomach with a large over-the-needle catheter. Flicking the lateral abdomen with the thumb and forefinger while simultaneously auscultating the abdomen with a stethoscope can allow the operator to determine the area of gas distension and make sure the spleen is not present. After clipping and aseptically scrubbing the lateral abdominal wall, a large-bore catheter is inserted through the skin into the dilated stomach, to relieve the gas and lower intragastric pressure.

"thud" is often associated with the presence of the spleen entrapped between the stomach and the abdominal wall and should be avoided. Clip and aseptically scrub over the area of greatest gastric tympany, then insert a large-bore catheter (14–18 gauge) or needle through the skin briskly into the gastric lumen (Figure 7.3). Risks associated with percutaneous gastric decompression are iatrogenic laceration or puncture of the spleen with subsequent hemorrhage, and perforation of necrotic stomach with leakage of gastric contents into the abdominal cavity. The spleen and stomach will be exteriorized and evaluated at the time of surgery, and any complications associated with percutaneous decompression can be dealt with at that time.

Orogastric intubation

Orogastric intubation can be performed in some cases, where a number of personnel are available to restrain the dog and the dog is cooperative. Because many dogs with GDV are large and giant breeds, orogastric intubation for gastric decompression can be challenging. To perform orogastric intubation, two large buckets (one filled with tepid water), a large-bore orogastric tube, and a gavage pump are needed. The stiff orogastric tube should be measured from the tip of the nose to the last rib, so that the tube will enter the stomach through the lower esophageal sphincter (Figure 7.4). Mark the tube at the tip of the nose to prevent inserting the tube too far. Next, use a roll of 5 cm white surgical tape and place it behind the incisors (Figure 7.5). Tape the mouth closed over the roll of tape, then insert the lubricated tube through the roll of tape, simultaneously pushing slowly and twisting as the tube approaches the lower esophageal sphincter. Once the tube enters the stomach, air is expressed through the tube opening, often with the characteristic odor of fermented gastric contents. In some cases, a large amount of resistance will be felt at the lower esophageal sphincter due to high intragastric pressures. Placing the forelimbs of the dog on the table and hindlimbs on the ground can sometimes help decrease

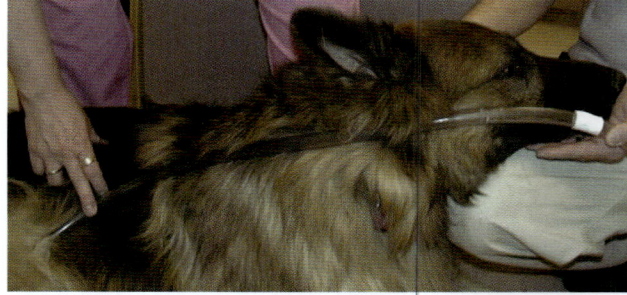

Figure 7.4 Orogastric decompression: an orogastric tube is measured from the tip of the patient's nose to the level of the last rib.

(a)

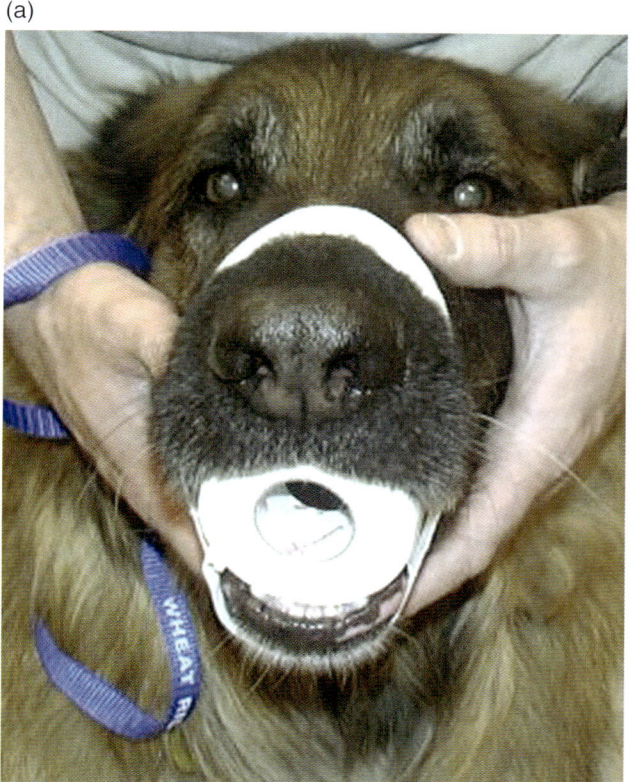

(b)

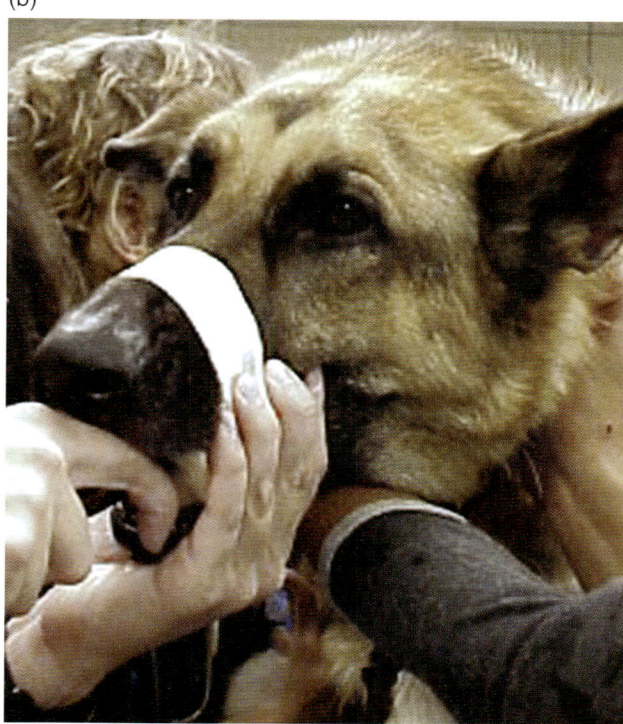

Figure 7.5 Orogastric decompression: (a) a 5 cm roll of tape is inserted in the mouth of the patient, behind the incisors, and tape is placed around the muzzle; (b) the orogastric tube can then be inserted through the hole in the middle of the roll of tape.

pressure from within the stomach on the lower esophageal sphincter and diaphragm to allow successful passing of the tube. Once the orogastric tube is passed, the stomach is lavaged with warm water in boluses of 5–10 mL/kg until the efflux runs clear (Walshaw & Johnston 1976; Wingfield 1981; Matthiesen 1983; Brockman & Holt 2000). The presence of red or black gastric mucosa is an indicator of gastric necrosis (Figure 7.6). In the event that fluid infused into the stomach is not returned, gastric perforation should be suspected.

Temporary gastrostomy and gastrostomy catheter placement

Temporary gastrostomy or placement of a temporary gastrostomy catheter can be performed to maintain gastric decompression if surgery is to be delayed for a period of time, for example if the patient must be transported to another facility and continues to bloat as soon as the gastrostomy tube is removed. The techniques are attempted only if other techniques to keep the stomach decompressed have failed. Both procedures are performed with only a local block (Pass & Johnston 1973; Walshaw & Johnston 1976; Fox-Alvarez *et al.* 2019). To place a

temporary gastrostomy catheter, put the patient in left lateral recumbency, then clip the fur over the dorsolateral right 13th rib, extending caudally at least 4 cm. Use an ultrasound probe and auscultation to confirm an area of gastric tympany in the clipped area. Next, aseptically scrub the area, and insert three T-fasteners percutaneously into the gastric lumen, 1.5 cm apart in a triangular pattern to perform a temporary gastropexy (Fox-Alvarez *et al.* 2019). Syringes filled with 6 mL of saline can be attached to each T-fastener to examine for air bubbles to confirm placement into the gastric lumen. In the center of the triangle/gastropexy site created by the T-fasteners, a 5 Fr over-the-wire pigtail catheter is inserted, then left in place to maintain gastric decompression (Fox-Alvarez *et al.* 2019).

To perform a temporary gastrostomy, place the patient in left lateral recumbency and clip and aseptically scrub the right lateral abdominal wall. After parenteral analgesia, a local block in the skin and abdominal wall 2 cm caudal to the last rib in the right paracostal area is performed with 2% lidocaine (1 mg/kg, diluted with sterile saline). A 2 cm incision is made through the skin. After blunt dissection through the abdominal muscles into the peritoneal cavity, the stomach is pulled through and

(a)

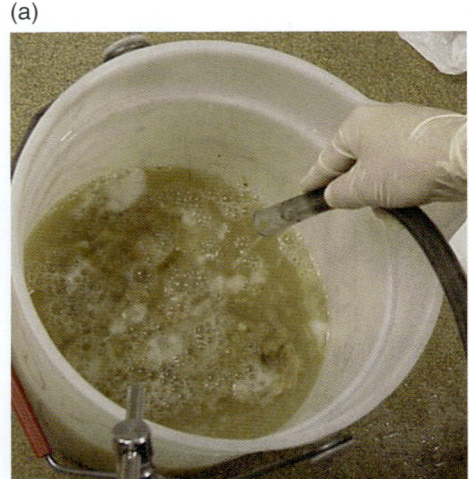

(b)

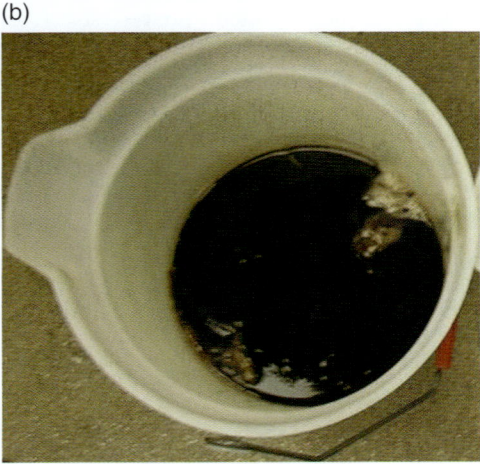

Figure 7.6 Fluid retrieval during stomach lavage: (a) stomach content retrieved from a dog that did not have necrosis of its stomach; (b) hemorrhagic fluid retrieved from a stomach that required resection.

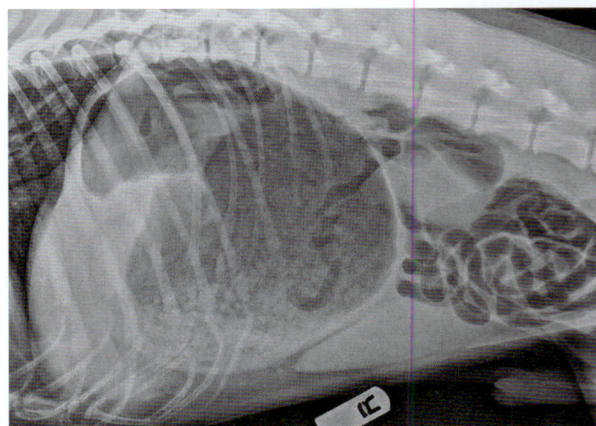

Figure 7.7 Right lateral abdominal radiograph of a dog with gastric dilatation volvulus. Note the line of demarcation between the gastric fundus and pylorus, and cranial displacement of the pylorus.

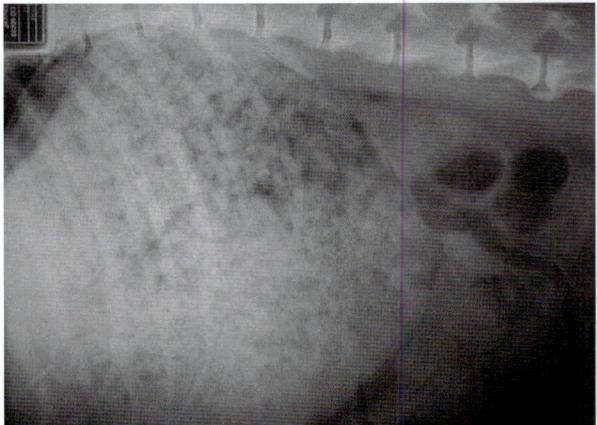

Figure 7.8 Lateral abdominal radiograph of a dog with a stomach engorged with ingesta (also known as "food bloat").

sutured to the abdominal incision with a continuous suture pattern. The stomach is then opened and the edges of the stomach are sutured to the skin to prevent iatrogenic contamination of the peritoneal cavity. The animal can then be transported and have surgery immediately upon arrival following transport.

Diagnostic imaging

If a radiograph is required for the diagnosis of GDV, a right lateral abdominal radiograph is the view of choice to make a diagnosis (Hathcock 1984). Most commonly, there is gas distension of the body of the stomach, with dorsocranial displacement of the gas-filled pyloric antrum (Figure 7.7). If gastric distension is present on the radiographs, it can be due to GDV that derotated on its own, or it can be secondary to food engorgement (Figure 7.8). If the stomach is full of fluid and food

without any gas, the double bubble might be difficult to visualize on radiographs (Figure 7.9). If only food engorgement is present, a preventive gastropexy might be recommended. If gastric dilatation is present without signs of food engorgement, an abdominal exploration is recommended to evaluate the integrity of the stomach wall and spleen, as well as to perform a gastropexy. The presence of gas within the stomach wall (gastric pneumatosis) has been shown to be relatively sensitive in diagnosing the presence of gastric necrosis (Figure 7.10) (Fischetti *et al.* 2004). However, the absence of gastric pneumatosis is relatively insensitive at ruling out gastric necrosis (Fischetti *et al.* 2004). For this reason, if pneumatosis is present, the client should be alerted to the probable need for partial gastric resection, and a potential increase in postoperative morbidity. Radiographic findings on preoperative thoracic radiographs in dogs

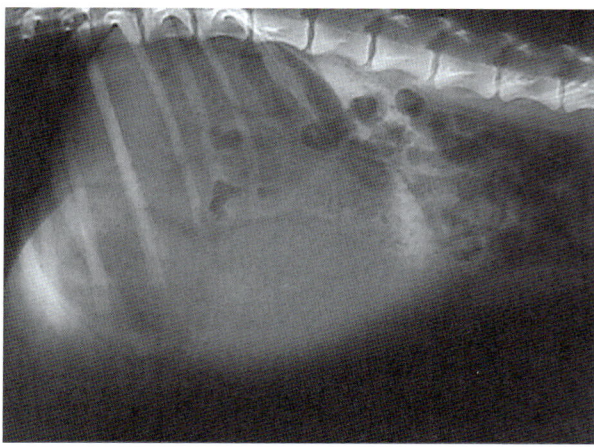

Figure 7.9 Right lateral abdominal radiograph of a dog with gastric dilatation volvulus. Note that the stomach is distended with fluid, not air, making a diagnosis more challenging, as the classic "Popeye" arm is not readily visible.

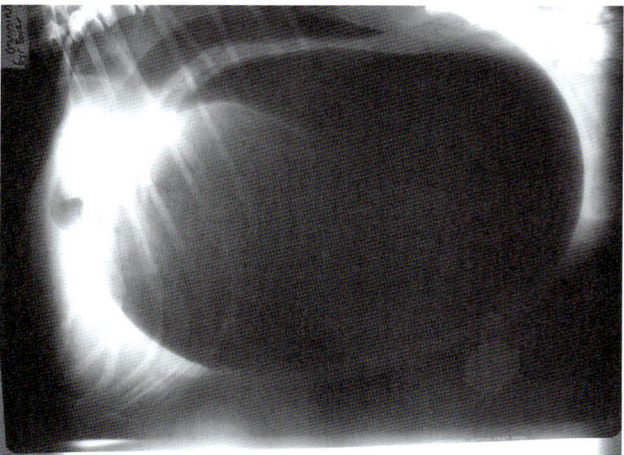

Figure 7.10 Gastric dilatation volvulus with pneumatosis. Small dark gas bubbles are present between the fundus and the pylorus.

with GDV have shown evidence of hypovolemia (microcardia, small caudal vena cava), aspiration pneumonia, pulmonary nodules, cardiomegaly, and pulmonary edema (Green *et al.* 2012). Preoperative radiographs should be recommended to document comorbidities that may influence ongoing therapy and the client's decision on whether to proceed with surgery.

Exploratory laparotomy

Dogs with GDV should be directed toward surgery as soon as they are stabilized. The goals of the surgery are to reposition the stomach in a normal anatomic position, inspect the wall of the stomach for viability, perform a gastrectomy if needed, and finally fix the stomach to the abdominal wall (Matthiesen 1983; Brockman

et al. 1995; Buber *et al.* 2007). Following routine preparation of the ventral abdomen, a ventral midline incision should be made through the skin and linea from xiphoid to pubis, to allow maximal visualization of the stomach and other abdominal organs. If the stomach is in an abnormal position, the omentum will be visualized over the stomach (on the ventral surface) as the peritoneal cavity is opened. Abdominal hemorrhage may be present from rupture of the short gastric vessels or vessels along the splenic hilus. The stomach is repositioned into its normal anatomic location as rapidly as possible. The stomach can rotate in a clockwise direction (up to 360°) (Website Chapter 7: Gastrointestinal surgery/stomach/GDV derotation and viability). Most frequently, the stomach is rotated 180–270° in a clockwise direction. With the surgeon standing on the right side of the dog, the stomach can be repositioned by pulling up on the pylorus/pyloric antrum with the right hand and pushing the body of the stomach into the abdominal cavity with the left hand. If severe gastric dilatation prevents derotation, an orogastric tube can be passed into the stomach by an assistant, with the surgeon directing the tip of the orogastric tube through the lower esophageal sphincter into the gastric lumen. A needle can be used to pierce the gastric wall and suction air from the stomach to aid in decompression and derotation.

Once the stomach is derotated, it should be inspected initially for viability; the rest of the abdominal cavity is routinely explored while the stomach is reperfused (Website Chapter 7: Gastrointestinal surgery/stomach/ GDV derotation and viability). Only after reperfusion can adequate subjective assessment of gastric wall viability be performed (Matthiesen 1983, 1985, 1987).

The liver, gallbladder, duodenum, pancreas, jejunum, ileum, and colon should be assessed. The spleen should be exteriorized from the abdominal cavity and palpated carefully for perfusion along the splenic hilus. If there are no palpable pulses or if splenic viability is questioned, a complete splenectomy should be performed. If the spleen is rotated along with the stomach, the spleen should be removed without untwisting the pedicle, to prevent recirculation of proinflammatory cytokines. Very often the spleen appears congested because of mild portal hypertension. This congestion will correct itself very quickly and should not warrant a splenectomy. Avulsion of the short gastric artery between the spleen and the fundus of the stomach is very common and usually without any consequences unless there is active bleeding (Lantz *et al.* 1984). The kidneys, adrenal glands, and urinary bladder should also be assessed for normalcy. Following routine exploration, gastric viability can be evaluated.

(a)

(b)

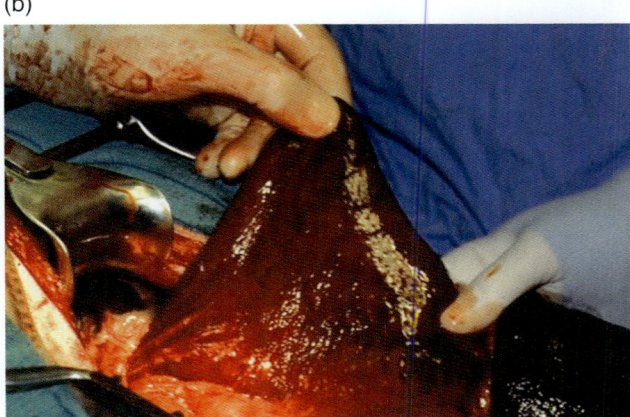

Figure 7.11 Necrosis along the greater curvature in the body of the stomach. (a) The color (black) of the serosa is an indicator of ischemia. More than 60% of the stomach is necrotic in this case. (b) Pinching the wall of the stomach also gives an indication of the viability of the stomach wall. If the serosa and muscularis are not slipping between the fingers, it means that the stomach wall is necrotic.

Assessment of gastric wall viability

Gastric necrosis has been reported in 10–25% of patients with GDV. The greater curvature and gastric fundus along the dorsal aspect of the stomach near the esophageal hiatus are most commonly affected by necrosis (Figure 7.11). It is important to exteriorize the stomach and visually and digitally inspect all areas for viability. Normal tissue appears pink to red in color, and feels thick. Subjectively, necrotic sections of stomach will appear gray to black in color, and have decreased thickness (Matthiesen 1983, 1985). The separate wall layers may palpably slide over one another when pinched between the fingers. If the layers are not slipping between the fingers, more likely the mucosa and submucosa are necrotic. The tissue may feel friable, or perforate in the most extreme cases. In one study, subjective evaluation of gastric viability was accurate in only 60% of clinical cases (Matthiesen 1983). For this reason, more objective parameters for assessing gastric viability have been investigated.

Bleeding from the cut surface is associated with perfusion to that area of serosa, but is not 100% sensitive at predicting whether gastric necrosis will occur postoperatively (Matthiesen 1983). Experimentally, intravenous fluorescein dye has not been shown to be sensitive at determining gastric wall viability (Wheaton et al. 1986). Nuclear scintigraphy with technetium pertechnetate administered postoperatively has been shown to be more accurate at predicting ischemic areas of the stomach postoperatively, but is not routinely available at all hospitals and requires postoperative isolation until radioactivity has decayed to a safe level for personnel (Berardi et al. 1991, 1993). Also, the scintigraphy does not provide landmarks for the surgeon on where to perform the gastrectomy. Laser Doppler flowmetry was used to document capillary blood flow in the stomach of experimental dogs with portal hypertension and gastric ischemia, and in clinical dogs with GDV (Monnet et al. 2006). Laser Doppler flowmetry accurately measured reduction of blood flow within the wall of the stomach during ischemia. Capillary blood flow was found to be significantly lower in dogs that required partial gastric resection compared with those that did not require gastric resection, and may be superior to subjective methods of evaluating gastric wall viability (Monnet et al. 2006).

Partial gastrectomy

If gastric viability is compromised or questionable, gastric resection with partial gastrectomy is necessary; 60% of the stomach can be removed without compromising the quality of life of the dog. If the area of necrosis is affecting the cardia, the prognosis is more guarded because of the risk of reflux esophagitis (Beck et al. 2006). Invagination techniques have been described (MacCoy et al. 1986). The area of necrosis is invaginated by placing a continuous line of absorbable (3-0) suture in a healthy portion of stomach adjacent to the area of necrosis and inverting the area with a continuous pattern of inverting sutures (MacCoy et al. 1986). When left in place, the area will eventually autodigest by gastric acid within the gastric lumen. Severe hemorrhage and gastric ulceration, with need for subsequent surgery and multiple transfusions, have been reported following invagination of necrotic areas of stomach during surgical correction of GDV (Parton et al. 2006). This technique is not recommended for the treatment of gastric necrosis, since stapling equipment is readily available in

(a)

(b)

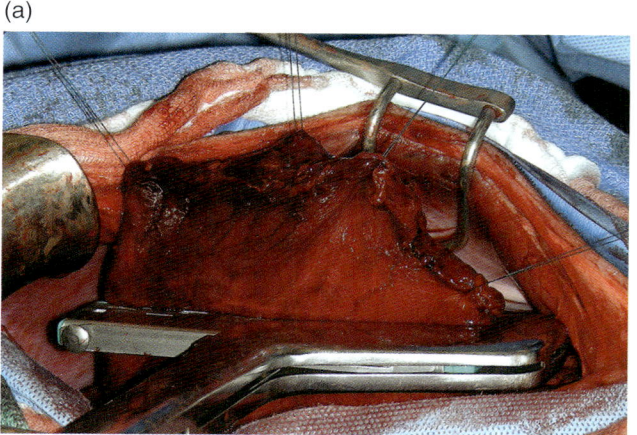
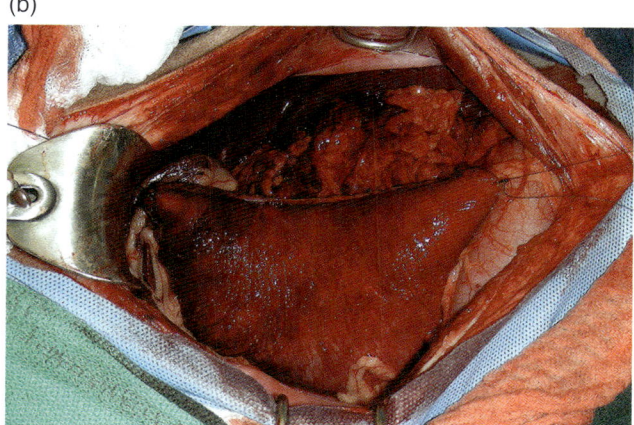

Figure 7.12 (a) Partial gastrectomy is performed with automatic stapling equipment. (b) The staple line can be oversewn with an inverting suture pattern.

the veterinary surgery and has been shown to provide a safe gastrectomy (Clark & Pavletic 1991).

Partial gastrectomy is the technique of choice for treating stomach necrosis (Figure 7.12). The stomach is exteriorized as much as possible and packed off from the rest of the abdominal cavity with laparotomy towels. Stay sutures are placed in areas of healthy tissue to assist in gastric exteriorization. It is preferable to use automatic stapling devices, placed across an area of healthy tissue adjacent to the area of gastric necrosis (Website Chapter 7: Gastrointestinal surgery/stomach/GDV gastrectomy). Once the automatic stapling device has been employed and staples are in place, the area of necrosis is removed with a scalpel blade or scissors and the area oversewn with an inverting suture pattern (Clark & Pavletic 1991). If automatic stapling equipment is not available, the area of gastric necrosis is surgically removed with a scalpel blade, making sure that bleeding occurs on all cut edges. The stomach is then closed with a two-layer closure, the second layer being an inverting layer. Partial gastrectomy using stapling devices is thought to be superior to hand sutures and has been associated with a lower incidence of postoperative mortality (Matthiesen 1983, 1985, 1987; Clark & Pavletic 1991).

Gastropexy techniques

The goal of surgical gastropexy is to create a permanent adhesion of the pyloric antrum to the right-side body wall to prevent recurrence of gastric volvulus. Recurrence rates of GDV can approach 80% if surgical gastropexy is not performed at the time of gastric derotation (Dann 1976; Ellison 1993; Eggertsdottir & Moe 1995; Glickman et al. 1998). Several techniques of permanent gastropexy have been described in the literature: balloon

gastropexy, incisional gastropexy, circumcostal gastropexy, and belt loop gastropexy (Parks & Greene 1976; Fallah et al. 1982; Johnson et al. 1984; Fox et al. 1985, 1988; Leib et al. 1985; Woolfson & Kostolich 1986; Whitney et al. 1989; Waschak et al. 1997; Eggertsdottir et al. 2001; Allen & Paul 2014; Smeak 2020). All these techniques have been associated with a GDV recurrence rate of less than 7% (Johnson et al. 1984; Woolfson & Kostolich 1986; Eggertsdottir et al. 2008). Dilatation can still occur after gastropexy, but the pyloric antrum cannot move to an abnormal position (Przywara et al. 2014). Modifications of each of these techniques have been described (Pope & Jones 1999; Degna et al. 2001). A gastrocolopexy has been evaluated in dogs and has been associated with a GDV recurrence rate of 20% (Eggertsdottir et al. 2001). Biomechanical testing has shown that circumcostal gastropexy is the strongest technique, while balloon and incisional gastropexies are the weakest (Levine & Caywood 1983; Fox et al. 1985, 1988). However, it is not known how strong the gastropexy has to be in a clinical situation to prevent a volvulus. It is likely that each technique is strong enough to prevent a volvulus in a clinical situation. Therefore, any gastropexy technique is appropriate except the incorporating gastropexy. The tube gastropexy has been shown to affect the myoelectrical function of the stomach (Stampley et al. 1992). The incorporating gastropexy is performed by incorporating the wall of the body of the stomach in the linea alba closure (Meyer-Lindenberg et al. 1993). This technique is inappropriate, since it does not stabilize the pyloric antrum on the right side of the abdominal cavity.

Incisional gastropexy

Incisional gastropexy involves making a 4–6 cm incision in the gastric serosa, between the greater and lesser

(a)
(b)
(c)

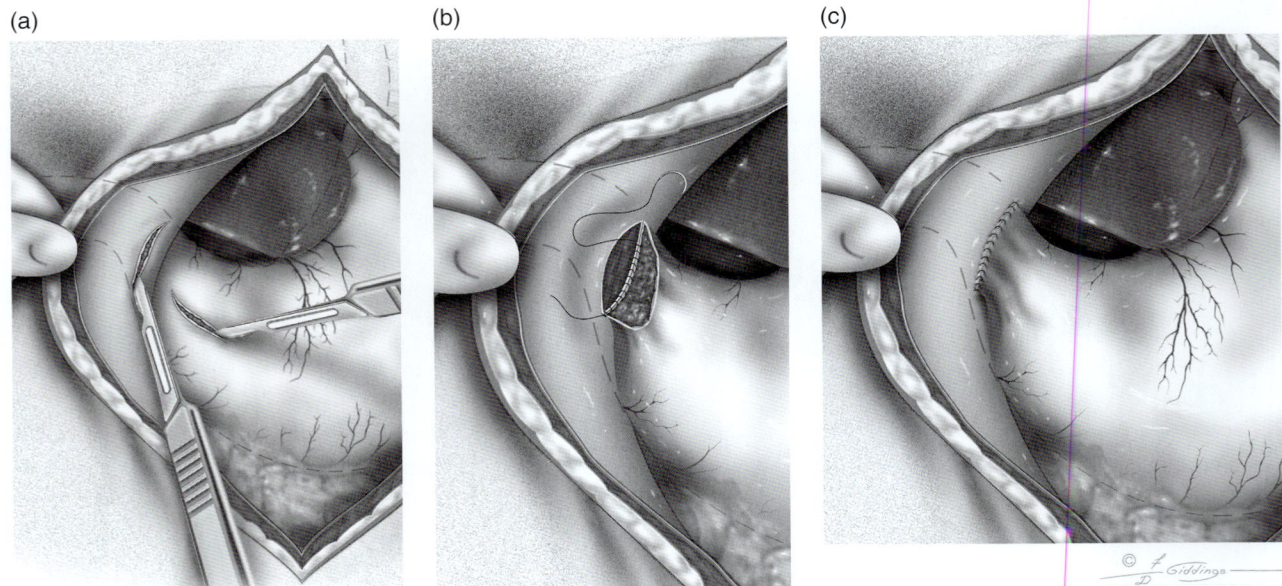

Figure 7.13 Incisional gastropexy. (a) A seromuscular incision is made over the pyloric antrum. A second incision is made in the transversus abdominalis muscle in the right lateral body wall caudal to the last rib. (b, c) The two incisions are apposed with two simple continuous suture patterns. Source: © D. Giddings.

curvatures of the pyloric antrum, through the seromuscular layers (Figure 7.13). A similar-sized incision is created in the peritoneum and transversus abdominis muscles caudal to the last rib in the right paracostal area of the ventrolateral abdominal wall. The two incisions are then apposed with a continuous pattern using 2-0 or 0 absorbable or nonabsorbable suture, starting at the most cranial margin, then caudal margin, working dorsally to ventrally. With this technique, two parallel incisions create a seal between the seromuscular layer of the stomach at the pylorus and the abdominal wall (MacCoy *et al.* 1982). More recently, the use of automated stapling equipment has also been described to secure the stomach to the body wall (Belandria *et al.* 2009). This type of gastropexy has been shown to have a recurrence rate of 0–4% (MacCoy *et al.* 1982; Hammel & Novo 2006).

Belt loop gastropexy

A seromuscular flap is created in the pyloric antrum with its base along the greater curvature of the stomach. The flap should incorporate two or three perforating branches from the right gastroepiploic artery. Two transverse 4 cm incisions are made approximately 3–4 cm apart in the right ventrolateral abdominal wall, through the peritoneum and transversus abdominis muscles (Figure 7.14) (Website Chapter 7: Gastrointestinal surgery/stomach/GDV belt loop gastropexy). A tunnel is created between the two incisions, under the abdominal musculature. The seromuscular flap from the stomach is pulled through the tunnel (Whitney *et al.* 1989). The

seromuscular flap is then replaced and secured onto its original location on the pyloric antrum with 3-0 absorbable suture. The flap can be secured either with sutures or with standard skin staples (Whitney *et al.* 1989; Coolman *et al.* 1999). A modification of the standard belt loop gastropexy has been described in which a fold of seromuscular tissue rather than a flap is created in the gastric antrum (Formaggini & Tommasini Degna 2018). The fold of tissue is passed through the belt loop in the transversus abdominus, then is sutured to the gastric serosa and cut edge of the abdominal wall. This modification could potentially decrease surgical time, is associated with few complications, and is successful at preventing the recurrence of GDV.

Circumcostal gastropexy

For circumcostal gastropexy, a seromuscular flap is created in the pyloric antrum similar to that described for belt loop gastropexy, but is placed around the last rib (Fallah *et al.* 1982). Stay sutures are placed in the seromuscular flap, allowing them to be pulled through the tunnel and around the rib. The seromuscular flap is then sutured back to its original position on the stomach using 3-0 absorbable suture. While technically more difficult, the circumcostal gastropexy is stronger than tube or incisional gastropexy techniques. Potential complications of circumcostal gastropexy include iatrogenic pneumothorax and rib fracture (Leib *et al.* 1985; Woolfson & Kostolich 1986; Eggertsdottir *et al.* 2008).

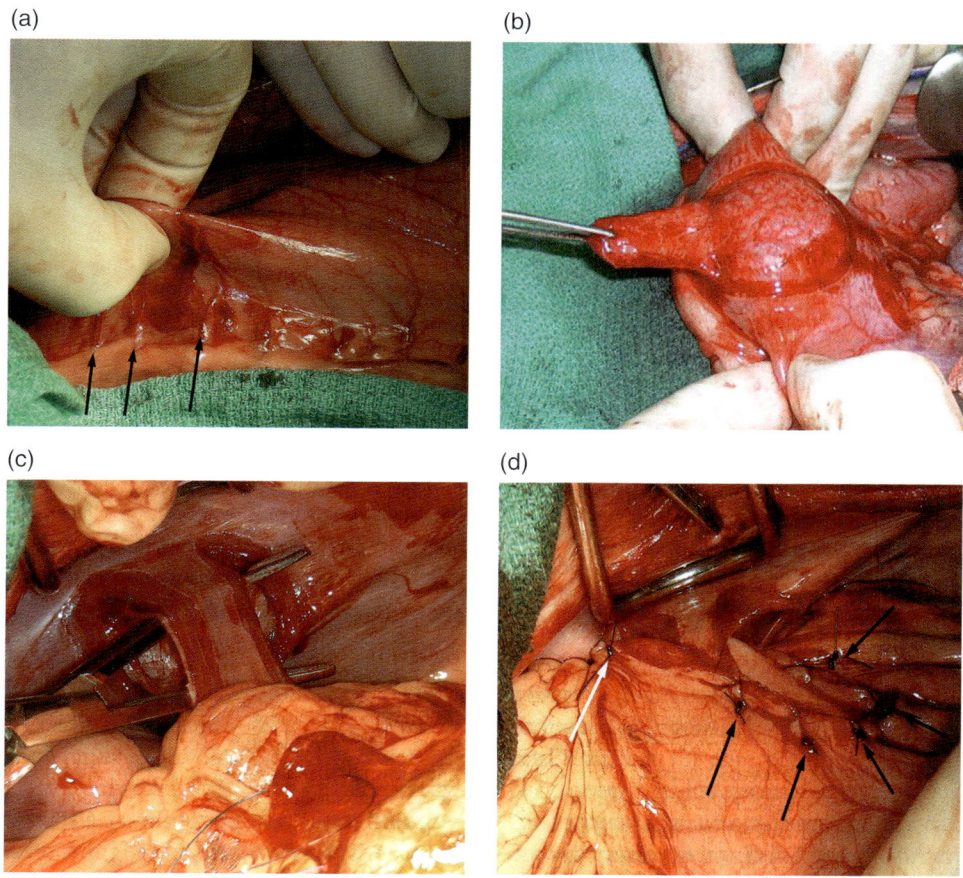

Figure 7.14 Belt loop gastropexy. (a) A seromuscular flap based on the greater curvature is dissected on the pyloric antrum. Two or three branches (black arrows) of the gastroepiploic artery are incorporated in the base of the seromuscular flap. (b) The seromuscular flap has been completely dissected. (c) A flap is created in the transversus abdominalis muscle in the right side behind the last rib. (d) The flap from the pyloric antrum is introduced in a caudocranial direction around the flap in the transversus abdominalis muscle. The flap from the pyloric antrum is sutured back in its original position with 3-0 absorbable suture (black arrows). A stay suture can be placed between the abdominal wall and the pyloric antrum (white arrow).

Laparoscopic-assisted derotation and gastropexy

Laparoscopic-assisted derotation and gastropexy have been described for treatment of GDV in two clinical cases with good outcomes (Rawlings *et al.* 2001, 2002). In this technique, grasping instruments are used to derotate the stomach into its normal anatomic position with laparoscopic visualization. After inspection of the wall of the stomach for viability, a laparoscopic-assisted incisional gastropexy is performed (Rawlings *et al.* 2001). This technique does not allow good evaluation of stomach viability and splenic perfusion. If gastric resection or splenectomy is required, the technique would need to be transitioned to a full routine exploratory surgery.

Prophylactic gastropexy

Prophylactic gastropexy has been recommended to prevent GDV in dogs at high risk of GDV (Irish Wolfhound, borzoi, mastiff, Akita, bull mastiff, setter, Weimaraner, Great Dane, and standard poodle) (Glickman *et al.* 1994; Schaible *et al.* 1997; Elwood 1998; Glickman *et al.* 2000b; Evans & Adams 2010). Large- and giant-breed dogs appear to have a 7% risk of death from GDV throughout their lifetime (Glickman *et al.* 2000b). Great Danes, however, have a 42.4% chance of developing GDV, and a 12.6% chance of dying from GDV in their lifetime (Glickman *et al.* 2000a,b). Preventive gastropexy can be performed with an open abdomen during an ovariohysterectomy or an abdominal surgery, a grid approach, laparoscopy to minimize soft tissue trauma, or with endoscopy (Rawlings *et al.* 2001; Dujowich & Reimer 2008; Mayhew & Brown 2009; Runge *et al.* 2009; Dujowich *et al.* 2010; Rivier *et al.* 2011; Loy Son *et al.* 2016; Tavakoli *et al.* 2016). Several techniques of laparoscopic gastropexy have been described using intracorporeal knot tying, staples, laparoscopically assisted, or with laparoscopy and intracorporeal suturing (Hardie *et al.* 1996; Rawlings *et al.* 2001; Mayhew & Brown 2009; Runge *et al.* 2009; Coleman *et al.* 2016; Coleman & Monnet 2017). The laparoscopically assisted incisional gastropexy seems to be the easiest procedure to perform and provides strong adhesions (Rawlings *et al.* 2002; Loy Son *et al.* 2016), decreases surgical time (Haraguchi *et al.* 2017), and does not appear to adversely impact gastrointestinal transit time (Balsa *et al.* 2017). Laparoscopic-assisted gastropexy is associated with a complication rate of 19% (Baron *et al.* 2020). The most common complication was seroma in 12% of cases. Laparoscopic gastropexy is now more commonly performed and eliminates the risk of surgical site complication related to the laparoscopic-assisted gastropexy (Coleman *et al.* 2016; Coleman & Monnet 2017; Takacs *et al.* 2017). It is usually performed with unidirectional barbed suture with needle holders and endoscopic suturing devices (Spah *et al.* 2013; Coleman *et al.* 2016; Coleman & Monnet 2017; Takacs *et al.* 2017).

Postoperative management

Postoperative management of the GDV patient involves maintaining fluid balance and blood pressure, and administration of gastroprotectant drugs, promotility agents, analgesia, and antiarrhythmic agents as warranted (Bruchim & Kelmer 2014). In the most critical animals, positive inotropes and vasopressor drugs may also be necessary to maintain myocardial contractility, cardiac output, and blood pressure.

In many cases, intravenous crystalloid fluids are continued until the patient is eating and drinking. If hypoproteinemia exists, a synthetic colloid such as hydroxyethyl starch can also be administered at a daily rate of 20–30 mL/kg i.v. as a continuous-rate infusion. Gastroprotectant drugs such as histamine-receptor blockers, sucralfate, or proton pump inhibitors may be necessary if gastric mucosal integrity has been severely compromised, and especially if gastrectomy was performed. Cardiac dysrhythmias should be treated with intravenous or oral antiarrhythmic drugs, and care should be exercised in monitoring and maintaining normal serum acid–base and electrolyte status. When necessary, supplementation with potassium chloride and magnesium chloride may be necessary to maintain normokalemia and aid in the treatment of ventricular dysrhythmias.

A continuous electrocardiogram (ECG) should be performed to evaluate for the presence of dysrhythmias. Blood pressure should be monitored, and interventions implemented when mean arterial blood pressure is less than 60 mmHg or if diastolic blood pressure is less than 40 mmHg at any time. Packed cell volume, total solids,

and postoperative lactate should be performed within the first 6–12 hours postoperatively and be monitored twice daily. Glucose, acid–base, and electrolyte status should be monitored at least twice daily in the most critical patients. If hypotension has occurred, the potential for renal insufficiency or failure exists, and BUN, creatinine, and urine output should be carefully monitored. Nutrition should be administered in the form of enteral nutrition whenever possible, ideally within the first 12–24 hours postoperatively. If enteral nutrition is discouraged, then parenteral nutrition should be considered. Coagulation status should be monitored at least once daily, as DIC is a major complication in the immediate postoperative period. If there are signs of coagulopathies (thrombocytopenia; prolonged PT, APTT, or ACT; elevated D-dimers; decreased antithrombin; petechiation or ecchymosis), fresh frozen plasma should be administered (15–20 mL/kg) to help replenish antithrombin and clotting factors.

Prognosis

Postoperative complication rates have been reported to be up to 90% in dogs with GDV and gastropexy (Matthiesen 1983, 1985). The short-term mortality rate after GDV is 10–60% (Matthiesen 1985; Clark & Pavletic 1991; Glickman *et al.* 1994, 1998; Brourman *et al.* 1996; Beck *et al.* 2006; Buber *et al.* 2007; Mackenzie *et al.* 2010). In one retrospective study that evaluated risk factors for mortality, the majority of dogs with GDV that were euthanized were euthanized prior to surgery due to financial constraints, age, and the presence of other comorbidities, and not due to intra- or postoperative findings or complications (Sharp *et al.* 2020).

Gastrectomy has been associated with poor outcomes in several studies (Matthiesen 1985; Glickman *et al.* 1994; Brourman *et al.* 1996; Buber *et al.* 2007). Matthiesen (1985) reported a mortality rate up to 60% after gastrectomy with hand suture. With the development of stapling equipment, and better understanding of the pathophysiology resulting in better critical care management of cases, gastrectomy is no longer associated with such a high mortality rate (Clark & Pavletic 1991; Glickman *et al.* 1994, 1998; Brourman *et al.* 1996; Buber *et al.* 2007; Mackenzie *et al.* 2010). Glickman *et al.* (1998) showed that gastrectomy was associated with an OR of 11. Beck *et al.* (2006) showed that gastrectomy alone was not associated with an increased mortality rate (OR 2.28, $P = 0.76$), but that a combination of gastrectomy and splenectomy was associated with a worse outcome (OR 3.15, $P = 0.025$). Mackenzie *et al.* (2010) also showed that gastrectomy was not associated with an increased mortality rate (OR 0.31, $P = 0.496$), while splenectomy was associated with an increased mortality rate

(OR 247.67, $P = 0.008$). The combination of splenectomy and gastrectomy was not associated with an increased mortality rate in that study. Brourman *et al.* (1996) showed that mortality was significantly increased if a splenectomy had to be performed at the same time as a gastrectomy. Gastrectomy has been associated with increased morbidity (Beck *et al.* 2006). After a gastrectomy, dogs were more at risk of developing peritonitis (OR 7.33, $P = 0.009$), DIC (OR 7.75, $P < 0.001$), arrhythmias (OR 5.0, $P = 0.001$), and sepsis (OR 12.58, $P = 0.31$). Each of these complications was associated with an increased mortality rate. Other risk factors associated with short-term survival are clinical signs for more than 6 hours (OR 3.25, $P = 0.01$), hypotension (OR 6.5, $P = 0.001$), need for a blood transfusion (OR 5.4, $P = 0.001$), sepsis (OR 17.25, $P = 0.015$), peritonitis (OR 10.8, $P = 0.002$), and DIC (OR 5.38, $P = 0.005$) (Beck *et al.* 2006). Presence of clinical signs for more than 6 hours was associated with a higher rate of gastrectomy (OR 2.6, $P = 0.024$), arrhythmias (OR 3.6, $P = 0.001$), and splenectomy (OR 2.9, $P = 0.023$) (Beck *et al.* 2006). Preoperative arrhythmias were associated with a higher mortality rate (Brourman *et al.* 1996; Mackenzie *et al.* 2010). Elevations in cardiac troponin values have been positively correlated with an increased risk of ventricular dysrhythmias and death (Schober *et al.* 2002). In another study, the presence of dysrhythmias was common, but did not appear to be positively correlated with an increased risk of death (Buber *et al.* 2007). In one study that investigated intracellular magnesium concentration in dogs with GDV, there was no significant difference in intracellular magnesium concentration in dogs that developed cardiac dysrhythmias and GDV compared with GDV dogs without dysrhythmias (Bebchuk *et al.* 2000).

Gastric dilatation can still occur after gastropexy; however, if the gastropexy has been performed correctly, the stomach should not be able to rotate (Matthiesen 1983; Flanders & Harvey 1984; Johnson *et al.* 1984; Jennings *et al.* 1992; Ellison 1993; Eggertsdottir *et al.* 2008).

References

Adamik, K.N., Burgener, I.A., Kovacevic, A. et al. (2009). Myoglobin as a prognostic indicator for outcome in dogs with gastric dilatation-volvulus. *Journal of Veterinary Emergency and Critical Care* 19: 247–253.

Allen, P. and Paul, A. (2014). Gastropexy for prevention of gastric dilatation-volvulus in dogs: history and techniques. *Topics in Companion Animal Medicine* 29: 77–80.

Allen, D.A., Schertel, E.R., Muir, W.W., and Valentine, A.K. (1991). Hypertonic saline/dextran resuscitation of dogs with experimentally induced gastric dilatation-volvulus shock. *American Journal of Veterinary Research* 52: 92–96.

Aona, B.D., Rush, J.E., Rozanski, E.A. et al. (2017). Evaluation of echocardiography and cardiac biomarker concentrations in dogs with gastric dilatation volvulus. *Journal of Veterinary Emergency and Critical Care* 27: 631–637.

Badylak, S.F., Lantz, G.C., and Jeffries, M. (1990). Prevention of reperfusion injury in surgically induced gastric dilatation-volvulus in dogs. *American Journal of Veterinary Research* 51: 294–299.

Balsa, I.M., Culp, W.T.N., Drobatz, K.J. et al. (2017). Effect of laparoscopic-assisted gastropexy on gastrointestinal transit time in dogs. *Journal of Veterinary Internal Medicine* 31: 1680–1685.

Baltzer, W.I., McMichael, M.A., Ruaux, C.G. et al. (2006). Measurement of urinary 11-dehydro-thromboxane B2 excretion in dogs with gastric dilatation-volvulus. *American Journal of Veterinary Research* 67: 78–83.

Barnes, G.E., Laine, G.A., Giam, P.Y. et al. (1985). Cardiovascular responses to elevation of intra-abdominal hydrostatic pressure. *American Journal of Physiology* 248: R208–R213.

Baron, J.K., Casale, S.A., Monnet, E. et al. (2020). Paramedian incisional complications after prophylactic laparoscopy-assisted gastropexy in 411 dogs. *Veterinary Surgery* 49 (S1): O148–O155.

de Battisti, A., Toscano, M.J., and Formaggini, L. (2012). Gastric foreign material as a risk factor for gastric dilatation and volvulus in dogs. *Journal of the American Veterinary Medical Association* 241: 1190–1193.

Bebchuk, T.N., Hauptman, J.G., Braselton, W.E., and Walshaw, R. (2000). Intracellular magnesium concentrations in dogs with gastric dilatation-volvulus. *American Journal of Veterinary Research* 61: 1415–1417.

Beck, J.J., Staatz, A.J., Pelsue, D.H. et al. (2006). Risk factors associated with short-term outcome and development of perioperative complications in dogs undergoing surgery because of gastric dilatation-volvulus: 166 cases (1992–2003). *Journal of the American Veterinary Medical Association* 229: 1934–1939.

Beer, K.A., Syring, E.S., and Drobatz, K.J. (2013). Evaluation of plasma lactate concentration and base excess at the time of hospital admission as predictors of gastric necrosis and outcome and correlation between those variables in dogs with gastric dilatation-volvulus: 78 cases (2004–2009). *Journal of the American Veterinary Medical Association* 242: 54–58.

Belandria, G.A., Pavletic, M.M., Boulay, J.P. et al. (2009). Gastropexy with an automatic stapling instrument for the treatment of gastric dilatation and volvulus in 20 dogs. *Canadian Veterinary Journal* 50: 733–740.

Berardi, C., Wheaton, L.G., Twardock, A.R., and Schaeffer, D.J. (1991). Use of a nuclear imaging technique to detect gastric wall ischemia. *American Journal of Veterinary Research* 52: 1089–1096.

Berardi, C., Wheaton, L.G., Twardock, A.R., and Barbee, D.D. (1993). Nuclear imaging to evaluate gastric mucosal viability following surgical correction of gastric dilatation/volvulus. *Journal of the American Animal Hospital Association* 29: 239–246.

Bhatia, A.S., Tank, P.H., Karle, A.S. et al. (2010). Gastric dilation and volvulus syndrome in dog. *Veterinary World* 3: 554–557.

Boothe, H.W. and Ackerman, N. (1976). Partial gastric torsion in two dogs. *Journal of the American Animal Hospital Association* 12: 27–30.

Braun, L., Lester, S., Kuzma, A.B., and Hosie, S.C. (1996). Gastric dilatation volvulus in the dog with histological evidence of preexisting inflammatory bowel disease: a retrospective study of 23 cases. *Journal of the American Animal Hospital Association* 32: 287–290.

Bredal, W.P. (1998). *Pneumonyssoides caninum* infection: a risk factor for gastric dilatation-volvulus in dogs. *Veterinary Research Communications* 22: 225–231.

Brockman, D.J. and Holt, D.E. (2000). Management protocol for acute gastric dilatation-volvulus syndrome in dogs. *Compendium on Continuing Education for the Practicing Veterinarian* 22: 1025–1034.

Brockman, D.J., Washabau, R.J., and Drobatz, K.J. (1995). Canine gastric dilatation/volvulus syndrome in a veterinary critical care unit: 295 cases (1986–1992). *Journal of the American Veterinary Medical Association* 207: 460–464.

Brockman, D.J., Holt, D.E., and Washabau, R.J. (2000). Pathogenesis of acute canine gastric dilatation-volvulus syndrome: is there a unifying hypothesis? *Compendium on Continuing Education for the Practicing Veterinarian* 22: 1108–1113.

Broome, C.J. and Walsh, V.P. (2003). Gastric dilatation volvulus in dogs. *New Zealand Veterinary Journal* 51: 275–283.

Brourman, J.D., Schertel, E.R., Allen, D.A. et al. (1996). Factors associated with perioperative mortality in dogs with surgically managed gastric dilatation-volvulus: 137 cases (1988–1993). *Journal of the American Veterinary Medical Association* 208: 1855–1858.

Bruchim, Y. and Kelmer, E. (2014). Post-operative management of dogs with gastric dilatation and volvulus. *Topics in Companion Animal Medicine* 29: 81–85.

Bruchim, Y., Itay, S., Shira, B.H. et al. (2012). Evaluation of lidocaine treatment on frequency of cardiac arrhythmias, acute kidney injury, and hospitalization time in dogs with gastric dilatation volvulus. *Journal of Veterinary Emergency and Critical Care* 22: 419–427.

Buber, T., Saragusty, J., Ranen, E. et al. (2007). Evaluation of lidocaine treatment and risk factors for death associated with gastric dilatation and volvulus in dogs: 112 cases (1997–2005). *Journal of the American Veterinary Medical Association* 230: 1334–1339.

Caywood, D.D., Teague, H.D., Jackson, D.A. et al. (1977). Gastric gas analysis in the canine gastric dilation-volvulus syndrome. *Journal of the American Animal Hospital Association* 13: 459–462.

Chandler, J.C., Monnet, E., and Staatz, A.J. (2006). Comparison of acute hemodynamic effects of lidocaine and procainamide for postoperative ventricular arrhythmias in dogs. *Journal of the American Animal Hospital Association* 42: 262–268.

Clark, G.N. and Pavletic, M.M. (1991). Partial gastrectomy with an automatic stapling instrument for treatment of gastric necrosis secondary to gastric dilatation-volvulus. *Veterinary Surgery* 20: 61–68.

Coleman, K.A. and Monnet, E. (2017). Comparison of laparoscopic gastropexy performed via intracorporeal suturing with knotless unidirectional barbed suture using a needle driver versus a roticulated endoscopic suturing device: 30 cases. *Veterinary Surgery* 46 (7): 1002–1007.

Coleman, K.A., Adams, S., Smeak, D.D., and Monnet, E. (2016). Laparoscopic gastropexy using knotless unidirectional suture and an articulated endoscopic suturing device: seven cases. *Veterinary Surgery* 45 (S1): O95–O101.

Coolman, B.R., Manfra Marretta, S., Pijanowski, G.J., and Coolman, S.L. (1999). Evaluation of a skin stapler for belt-loop gastropexy in dogs. *Journal of the American Animal Hospital Association* 35: 440–444.

Costa, P.R.d.S., Carlo, R.J., Viana, J.A. et al. (2004). Deferoxamine for treatment in dogs with experimentally induced gastric dilatation-volvulus. *Veterinária Notícias* 10: 55–61.

Czajkowski, P.S. and Hallman, R.M. (2018). Diagnosis of chronic gastric instability using computed tomography in a great Dane that progressed to gastric dilatation and volvulus: a literature review and a case report. *Open Veterinary Journal* 8: 219–223.

Dann, J.R. (1976). Medical and surgical treatment of canine acute gastric dilatation. *Journal of the American Animal Hospital Association* 12: 17–22.

Davidson, J.R., Lantz, G.C., Salisbury, S.K. et al. (1992). Effects of flunixin meglumine on dogs with experimental gastric dilatation-volvulus. *Veterinary Surgery* 21: 113–120.

Degna, M.T., Formaggini, L., Fondati, A., and Assin, R. (2001). Using a modified gastropexy technique to prevent recurrence of gastric dilatation volvulus in dogs. *Veterinary Medicine* 96: 39–50.

Dennler, R., Koch, D., Hassig, M. et al. (2005). Climatic conditions as a risk factor in canine gastric dilatation volvulus. *Veterinary Journal (London)* 169: 97–101.

Dujowich, M. and Reimer, S.B. (2008). Evaluation of an endoscopically assisted gastropexy technique in dogs. *American Journal of Veterinary Research* 69: 537–541.

Dujowich, M., Keller, M.E., and Reimer, S.B. (2010). Evaluation of short- and long-term complications after endoscopically assisted gastropexy in dogs. *Journal of the American Veterinary Medical Association* 236: 177–182.

Eggertsdottir, A.V. and Moe, L. (1995). A retrospective study of conservative treatment of gastric dilatation-volvulus in the dog. *Acta Veterinaria Scandinavica* 36: 175–184.

Eggertsdottir, A.V., Stigen, Ø., Lønaas, L. et al. (2001). Comparison of the recurrence rate of gastric dilatation with or without volvulus in dogs after circumcostal gastropexy versus gastrocolopexy. *Veterinary Surgery* 30: 546–551.

Eggertsdottir, A.V., Langeland, M., Fuglem, B. et al. (2008). Long-term outcome in dogs after circumcostal gastropexy or gastrocolopexy for gastric dilatation with or without volvulus. *Veterinary Surgery* 37: 809–810.

Ellison, G.W. (1993). Gastric dilatation volvulus. Surgical prevention. *Veterinary Clinics of North America Small Animal Practice* 23: 513–530.

Elwood, C.M. (1998). Risk factors for gastric dilatation in Irish setter dogs. *Journal of Small Animal Practice* 39: 185–190.

Ende, C.W. (1980). Recurrent canine gastric dilation corrected by gastropexy and pyloroplasty. *Canadian Veterinary Journal* 21: 60.

Evans, K.M. and Adams, V.J. (2010). Mortality and morbidity due to gastric dilatation-volvulus syndrome in pedigree dogs in the UK. *Journal of Small Animal Practice* 51: 376–381.

Fallah, A.M., Lumb, W.V., Nelson, A.W. et al. (1982). Circumcostal gastropexy in the dog: a preliminary study. *Veterinary Surgery* 11: 9–12.

Fischetti, A.J., Saunders, H.M., and Drobatz, K.J. (2004). Pneumatosis in canine gastric dilatation volvulus syndrome. *Veterinary Radiology and Ultrasound* 45: 205–209.

de Papp, E., Drobatz, K.J., and Hughes, D. (1999). Plasma lactate concentration as a predictor of gastric necrosis and survival among dogs with gastric dilatation-volvulus: 102 cases (1995–1998). *Journal of the American Veterinary Medical Association* 215: 49–52.

Flanders, J.A. and Harvey, H.J. (1984). Results of tube gastrostomy as treatment for gastric volvulus in the dog. *Journal of the American Veterinary Medical Association* 185: 74–77.

Formaggini, L., Schmidt, K., and De Lorenzi, D. (2008). Gastric dilatation volvulus associated with diaphragmatic hernia in three cats: clinical presentation, surgical treatment and presumptive aetiology. *Journal of Feline Medicine and Surgery* 10: 198–201.

Formaggini, L. and Tommasini Degna, M. (2018). A prospective evaluation of a modified belt-loop gastropexy in 100 dogs with gastric dilatation-volvulus. *Journal of the American Animal Hospital Association* 54: 239–245.

Fox, S.M., Ellison, G.W., Miller, G.J., and Howells, D. (1985). Observations on the mechanical failure of three gastropexy techniques. *Journal of the American Animal Hospital Association* 21: 729–734.

Fox, S.M., McCoy, C.P., Cooper, R.C., and Baine, J.C. (1988). Circumcostal gastropexy versus tube gastrostomy: histological comparison of gastropexy adhesions. *Journal of the American Animal Hospital Association* 24: 273–279.

Fox-Alvarez, W.A., Case, J.B., Lewis, D.D. et al. (2019). Evaluation of a novel technique involving ultrasound-guided, temporary, percutaneous gastropexy and gastrostomy catheter placement for providing sustained gastric decompression in dogs with gastric dilatation-volvulus. *Journal of the American Veterinary Medical Association* 255: 1027–1034.

Frendin, J., Funkquist, B., and Stavenborn, M. (1988). Gastric displacement in dogs without clinical signs of acute dilatation. *Journal of Small Animal Practice* 29: 775–779.

Glickman, L.T., Emerick, T., Glickman, N.W. et al. (1996). Radiological assessment of the relationship between thoracic conformation and the risk of gastric dilatation-volvulus in dogs. *Veterinary Radiology and Ultrasound* 37: 174–180.

Glickman, L.T., Glickman, N.W., Perez, C.M. et al. (1994). Analysis of risk factors for gastric dilatation and dilatation volvulus in dogs. *Journal of the American Veterinary Medical Association* 204: 1465–1471.

Glickman, L.T., Glickman, N.W., Schellenberg, D.B. et al. (2000a). Incidence of and breed-related risk factors for gastric dilatation-volvulus in dogs. *Journal of the American Veterinary Medical Association* 216: 40–45.

Glickman, L.T., Glickman, N.W., Schellenberg, D.B. et al. (2000b). Non-dietary risk factors for gastric dilatation-volvulus in large and giant breed dogs. *Journal of the American Veterinary Medical Association* 217: 1492–1499.

Glickman, L.T., Glickman, N.W., Schellenberg, D.B. et al. (1997). Multiple risk factors for the gastric dilatation-volvulus syndrome in dogs: a practitioner/owner case–control study. *Journal of the American Animal Hospital Association* 33: 197–204.

Glickman, L.T., Lantz, G.C., Schellenberg, D.B., and Glickman, N.W. (1998). A prospective study of survival and recurrence following the acute gastric dilatation-volvulus syndrome in 136 dogs. *Journal of the American Animal Hospital Association* 34: 253–259.

Goldhammer, M.A., Haining, H., Milne, E.M. et al. (2010). Assessment of the incidence of GDV following splenectomy in dogs. *Journal of Small Animal Practice* 51: 23–28.

Grange, A.M., Cough, W., and Casale, S.A. (2012). Evaluation of splenectomy as a risk factor for gastric dilatation-volvulus. *Journal of the American Veterinary Medical Association* 241: 461–466.

Green, J.L., Cimino Brown, D., and Agnello, K.A. (2012). Preoperative thoracic radiographic findings in dogs presenting for gastric dilatation-volvulus (2000–2010):101 cases. *Journal of Veterinary Emergency and Critical Care* 22: 595–600.

Green, T.I., Tonozzi, C.C., Kirby, R., and Rudloff, E. (2011). Evaluation of initial plasma lactate values as predictor of gastric necrosis and initial and subsequent plasma lactate values as predictor of survival in dogs with gastric dilatation-volvulus: 84 dogs (2003–2007). *Journal of Veterinary Emergency and Critical Care* 21: 36–44.

Greenfield, C.L., Walshaw, R., and Thomas, M.W. (1989). Significance of Heineke–Mikulicz pyloroplasty in the treatment of gastric dilatation-volvulus: a prospective clinical study. *Veterinary Surgery* 18: 22–26.

Guilford, W.G., Komtebedde, J., Haskins, S.C. et al. (1989). Effect of allopurinol (APL) on experimental gastric dilation-volvulus (GDV) [abstract]. *Journal of Veterinary Internal Medicine* 3: 133.

Haak, C.E., Rudloff, E., and Kirby, R. (2012). Comparison of Hb-200 and 6% hetastarch 450/0.7 during initial fluid resuscitation of 20 dogs with gastric dilatation-volvulus. *Journal of Veterinary Emergency and Critical Care* 22: 201–210.

Hall, J.A., Twedt, D.C., and Curtis, C.R. (1989). Relationship of plasma gastrin immunoreactivity and gastroesophageal sphincter pressure in clinically normal dogs and in dogs with previous gastric dilatation volvulus. *American Journal of Veterinary Research* 50: 1228–1232.

Hall, J.A., Willer, R.L., Seim, H.B., and Powers, P.E. (1995). Gross and histologic evaluation of hepatogastric ligaments in clinically normal dogs and dogs with gastric dilatation-volvulus. *American Journal of Veterinary Research* 56: 1611–1614.

Hammel, S.P. and Novo, R.E. (2006). Recurrence of gastric dilatation-volvulus after incisional gastropexy in a rottweiler. *Journal of the American Animal Hospital Association* 42: 147–150.

Haraguchi, T., Kimura, S., Itoh, H. et al. (2017). Comparison of postoperative pain and inflammation reaction in dogs undergoing preventional laparoscopic-assisted and incisional gastropexy. *Journal of Veterinary Medical Science* 79: 1524–1531.

Hardie, R.J., Flanders, J.A., Schmidt, P. et al. (1996). Biomechanical and histological evaluation of a laparoscopic stapled gastropexy technique in dogs. *Veterinary Surgery* 25: 127–133.

Harkey, M.A., Villagran, A.M., Venkataraman, G.M. et al. (2018). Associations between gastric dilatation-volvulus in great Danes and specific alleles of the canine immune-system genes DLA88, DRBI and TLR5. *American Journal of Veterinary Research* 78: 934–945.

Hathcock, J.T. (1984). Radiographic view of choice for the diagnosis of gastric volvulus: the right lateral recumbent view. *Journal of the American Animal Hospital Association* 20: 967–969.

Herbold, J.R., Moore, G.E., Gosch, T.L., and Bell, B.S. (2002). Relationship between incidence of gastric dilatation-volvulus and biometeorologic events in a population of military working dogs. *American Journal of Veterinary Research* 63: 47–52.

Horne, W.A., Gilmore, D.R., Dietze, A.E. et al. (1985). Effects of gastric distention-volvulus on coronary blood flow and myocardial oxygen consumption in the dog. *American Journal of Veterinary Research* 46: 98–104.

Hosgood, G. (1994). Gastric dilatation-volvulus in dogs. *Journal of the American Veterinary Medical Association* 204: 1742–1747.

Hullar, M.A.J., Lampe, J.W., Torok-Storb, B.J., and Harkey, M.A. (2018). The canine gut microbiome is associated with higher risk of gastric dilatation-volvulus and high risk genetic variants of the immune system. *PLoS One* 13: e0197686.

Israeli, I., Steiner, J., Segev, G. et al. (2012). Serum pepsinogen-A, canine pancreatic lipase immunoreactivity, and C-reactive protein as prognostic markers in dogs with gastric dilatation-volvulus. *Journal of Veterinary Internal Medicine* 26: 920–928.

Jennings, P.B. Jr., Mathey, W.S., and Ehler, W.J. (1992). Intermittent gastric dilatation after gastropexy in a dog. *Journal of the American Veterinary Medical Association* 200: 1707–1708.

Johnson, R.G., Barrus, J., and Greene, R.W. (1984). Gastric dilatation-volvulus: recurrence rate following tube gastrostomy. *Journal of the American Animal Hospital Association* 20: 33–37.

Komtebedde, J., Gullford, W.G., Haskins, S.C., and Snyder, J.R. (1991). Evaluation of systemic and splanchnic visceral oxygen variables in dogs with surgically induced gastric dilatation-volvulus. *Journal of Veterinary Emergency and Critical Care* 1: 5–13.

Lantz, G.C., Badylak, S.F., Hiles, M.C., and Arkin, T.E. (1992). Treatment of reperfusion injury in dogs with experimentally induced gastric dilatation-volvulus. *American Journal of Veterinary Research* 53: 1594–1598.

Lantz, G.C., Bottoms, G.D., Carlton, W.W. et al. (1984). The effects of 360° gastric volvulus on the blood supply of the nondistended normal dog stomach. *Veterinary Surgery* 13: 189–196.

Leary, M.L. and Sinnott-Stutzman, V. (2018). Spontaneous gastric dilatation-volvulus in two cats. *Journal of Veterinary Emergency and Critical Care* 28: 346–355.

Leib, M.S., Konde, L.J., Wingfield, W.E., and Twedt, D.C. (1985). Circumcostal gastropexy for preventing recurrence of gastric dilatation-volvulus in the dog: an evaluation of 30 cases. *Journal of the American Veterinary Medical Association* 187: 245–248.

Leib, M.S. and Martin, R.A. (1987). Therapy of gastric dilatation-volvulus in dogs. *Compendium on Continuing Education for the Practicing Veterinarian* 9: 1155–1163.

Leib, M.S., Wingfield, W.E., Twedt, D.C., and Bottoms, G.D. (1984). Plasma gastrin immunoreactivity in dogs with acute gastric dilatation volvulus. *Journal of the American Veterinary Medical Association* 185: 205–208.

Levine, S.H. and Caywood, D.D. (1983). Biomechanical evaluation of gastropexy techniques in the dog. *Veterinary Surgery* 12: 166–169.

Loy Son, N.K., Singh, A., Amsellem, P. et al. (2016). Long-term outcome and complications following laparoscopic-assisted gastropexy in dogs. *Veterinary Surgery* 45: 077–083.

MacCoy, D.M., Kneller, S.K., Sundberg, J.P., and Harari, J. (1986). Partial invagination of the canine stomach for treatment of infarction of the gastric wall. *Veterinary Surgery* 15: 237–245.

MacCoy, D.M., Sykes, G.P., Hoffer, R.E., and Harvey, H.J. (1982). A gastropexy technique for the permanent fixation of the pyloric antrum. *Journal of the American Animal Hospital Association* 18: 763–768.

Mackenzie, G., Barnhart, M., Kennedy, S. et al. (2010). A retrospective study of factors influencing survival following surgery for gastric dilatation-volvulus syndrome in 306 dogs. *Journal of the American Animal Hospital Association* 46: 97–102.

MacPhail, C.M., Monnet, E., Pelsue, D.H., and Gaynor, J.S. (2006). Evaluation of cardiac performance of the dog after induction of portal hypertension and gastric ischemia. *Journal of Veterinary Emergency and Critical Care* 16: 192–198.

Marconato, L. (2006). Gastric dilatation-volvulus as complication after surgical removal of a splenic haemangiosarcoma in a dog. *Journal of Veterinary Medicine. A, Physiology, Pathology, Clinical Medicine* 53: 371–374.

Matthiesen, D.T. (1983). The gastric dilatation-volvulus complex: medical and surgical considerations. *Journal of the American Animal Hospital Association* 19: 925–932.

Matthiesen, D.T. (1985). Partial gastrectomy as treatment of gastric volvulus: results in 30 dogs. *Veterinary Surgery* 14: 185–193.

Matthiesen, D.T. (1987). Indications and techniques of partial gastrectomy in the dog. *Seminars in Veterinary Medicine and Surgery (Small Animal)* 2: 248–256.

Matthiesen, D.T. (1993). Pathophysiology of gastric dilatation volvulus. In: *Disease Mechanisms in Small Animal Surgery*, 2e (ed. M.J. Bojrab, D.D. Smeak and M.S. Bloomberg), 220–231. Philadelphia, PA: Lea & Febiger.

Mayhew, P.D. and Brown, D.C. (2009). Prospective evaluation of two intracorporeally sutured prophylactic laparoscopic gastropexy techniques compared with laparoscopic-assisted gastropexy in dogs. *Veterinary Surgery* 38: 738–746.

Merkley, D.F., Howard, D.R., Eyster, G.E. et al. (1976a). Experimentally induced acute gastric dilation in the dog: cardiopulmonary effects. *Journal of the American Animal Hospital Association* 12: 143–148.

Merkley, D.F., Howard, D.R., Krehbiel, J.D. et al. (1976b). Experimentally induced acute gastric dilatation in the dog: clinico-pathologic findings. *Journal of the American Animal Hospital Association* 12: 149–153.

Meyer-Lindenberg, A., Harder, A., Fehr, M. et al. (1993). Treatment of gastric dilatation-volvulus and a rapid method for prevention of relapse in dogs: 134 cases (1988–1991). *Journal of the American Veterinary Medical Association* 203: 1303–1307.

Miller, T.L., Schwartz, D.S., Nakayama, T., and Hamlin, R.L. (2000). Effects of acute gastric distention and recovery on tendency for ventricular arrhythmia in dogs. *Journal of Veterinary Internal Medicine* 14: 436–444.

Millis, D.L., Hauptman, J.G., and Fulton, R.B. (1993). Abnormal hemostatic profiles and gastric necrosis in canine gastric dilatation-volvulus. *Veterinary Surgery* 22: 93–97.

Millis, D.L., Nemzek, J., Riggs, C., and Walshaw, R. (1995). Gastric dilatation volvulus after splenic torsion in two dogs. *Journal of the American Veterinary Medical Association* 207: 314–315.

Mitchell, E.B., Hawkins, M.G., Gaffney, P.M., and Macleod, A.G. (2010). Gastric dilatation-volvulus in a guinea pig (*Cavia porcellus*). *Journal of the American Animal Hospital Association* 46: 174–180.

Monnet, E. (2003). Gastric dilatation-volvulus syndrome in dogs. *Veterinary Clinics of North America. Small Animal Practice* 33: 987–1005.

Monnet, E., Pelsue, D., and MacPhail, C. (2006). Evaluation of laser Doppler flowmetry for measurement of capillary blood flow in the stomach wall of dogs during gastric dilatation-volvulus. *Veterinary Surgery* 35: 198–205.

Muir, W.W. (1982a). Acid–base and electrolyte disturbances in dogs with gastric dilatation-volvulus. *Journal of the American Veterinary Medical Association* 181: 229–231.

Muir, W.W. (1982b). Gastric dilatation-volvulus in the dog, with emphasis on cardiac arrhythmias. *Journal of the American Veterinary Medical Association* 180: 739–742.

Muir, W.W. and Bonagura, J.D. (1984). Treatment of cardiac arrhythmias in dogs with gastric distention-volvulus. *Journal of the American Veterinary Medical Association* 184: 1366–1371.

Muir, W.W. and Lipowitz, A.J. (1978). Cardiac dysrhythmias associated with gastric dilatation-volvulus in the dog. *Journal of the American Veterinary Medical Association* 172: 683–689.

Nogradi, A.L., Cope, I., Balogh, M., and Gal, J. (2017). Review of gastric torsion in eight guinea pigs (*Cavia porcellus*). *Acta Veterinaria Hungarica* 65: 487–499.

Oron, L.D., Klainbart, S., Bruchim, Y. et al. (2018). Comparison of saphenous and cephalic blood lactate concentrations in dogs with gastric dilatation and volvulus: 45 cases. *Canadian Journal of Veterinary Research* 82: 271–277.

Orton, E.C. and Muir, W.W. (1983a). Hemodynamics during experimental gastric dilatation-volvulus in dogs. *American Journal of Veterinary Research* 44: 1512–1515.

Orton, E.C. and Muir, W.W. (1983b). Isovolumetric indices and humoral cardioactive substance bioassay during clinical and experimentally induced gastric dilatation-volvulus in dogs. *American Journal of Veterinary Research* 44: 1516–1520.

Parks, J.L. and Greene, R.W. (1976). Tube gastrostomy for the treatment of gastric volvulus. *Journal of the American Animal Hospital Association* 12: 168–172.

Parton, A.T., Volk, S.W., and Weisse, C. (2006). Gastric ulceration subsequent to partial invagination of the stomach in a dog with gastric dilatation-volvulus. *Journal of the American Veterinary Medical Association* 228: 1895–1900.

Pass, M.A. and Johnston, D.E. (1973). Treatment of gastric dilation and torsion in the dog. Gastric decompression by gastrostomy under local analgesia. *Journal of Small Animal Practice* 14: 131–142.

Passi, R.B., Kraft, A.R., and Vasko, J.S. (1969). Pathophysiologic mechanisms of shock in acute gastric dilatation. *Surgery* 65: 298–303.

Peycke, L.E., Hosgood, G., Davidson, J.R. et al. (2005). The effect of experimental gastric dilatation-volvulus on adenosine triphosphate content and conductance of the canine gastric and jejunal mucosa. *Canadian Journal of Veterinary Research* 69: 170–179.

Pipan, M., Brown, D.C., Battaglia, C.L., and Otto, C.M. (2012). An internet-based survey of risk factors for surgical gastric dilatation-volvulus in dogs. *Journal of the American Veterinary Medical Association* 240: 1456–1462.

Pope, E.R. and Jones, B.D. (1999). Clinical evaluation of a modified circumcostal gastropexy in dogs. *Journal of the American Veterinary Medical Association* 215: 952–955.

Przywara, J.F., Abel, S.B., Peacock, J.T., and Shott, S. (2014). Occurrence and recurrence of gastric dilatation with or without volvulus after incisional gastropexy. *Canadian Veterinary Journal* 55: 981–984.

Raghavan, M., Glickman, N.W., McCabe, G. et al. (2004). Diet-related risk factors for gastric dilatation-volvulus in dogs of high-risk breeds. *Journal of the American Animal Hospital Association* 40: 192–203.

Rawlings, C.A., Foutz, T.L., Mahaffey, M.B. et al. (2001). A rapid and strong laparoscopic-assisted gastropexy in dogs. *American Journal of Veterinary Research* 62: 871–875.

Rawlings, C.A., Mahaffey, M.B., Bement, S., and Canalis, C. (2002). Prospective evaluation of laparoscopic-assisted gastropexy in dogs susceptible to gastric dilatation. *Journal of the American Veterinary Medical Association* 221: 1576–1581.

Rivier, P., Furneaux, R., and Viguier, E. (2011). Combined laparoscopic ovariectomy and laparoscopic-assisted gastropexy in dogs susceptible to gastric dilatation-volvulus. *Canadian Veterinary Journal* 52: 62–66.

Runge, J.J., Mayhew, P., and Rawlings, C.A. (2009). Surgical views: laparoscopic assisted and laparoscopic prophylactic gastropexy: indications and techniques. *Compendium on Continuing Education for the Practicing Veterinarian* 31: 58–65.

Sartor, A.J., Bentley, A.M., and Brown, D.C. (2013). Association between previous splenectomy and gastric dilatation-volvulus in dogs: 453 cases (2004–2009). *Journal of the American Veterinary Medical Association* 242: 1381–1384.

Schaible, R.H., Ziech, J., Glickman, N.W. et al. (1997). Predisposition to gastric dilatation-volvulus in relation to genetics of thoracic conformation in Irish setters. *Journal of the American Animal Hospital Association* 33: 379–383.

Schellenberg, D., Yi, Q., Glickman, N.W., and Glickman, L.T. (1998). Influence of thoracic conformation and genetics on the risk of gastric dilatation-volvulus in Irish setters. *Journal of the American Animal Hospital Association* 34: 64–73.

Schertel, E.R., Allen, D.A., Muir, W.W. et al. (1997). Evaluation of a hypertonic saline-dextran solution for treatment of dogs with shock induced by gastric dilatation-volvulus. *Journal of the American Veterinary Medical Association* 210: 226–230.

Schober, K.E., Cornand, C., Kirbach, B. et al. (2002). Serum cardiac troponin I and cardiac troponin T concentrations in dogs with gastric dilatation-volvulus. *Journal of the American Veterinary Medical Association* 221: 381–388.

Sharp, C.R. and Rozanski, E.A. (2014). Cardiovascular and systemic effects of gastric dilatation and volvulus in dogs. *Topics in Companion Animal Medicine* 29: 67–70.

Sharp, C.R., Rozanski, E.A., Finn, E., and Borrego, E.J. (2020). The pattern of mortality in dogs with gastric dilatation volvulus. *Journal of Veterinary Emergency and Critical Care* 30: 232–238.

Smeak, D.D. (2020). Gastropexy. In: *Gastro-Intestinal Surgical Techniques in Small Animals* (ed. E. Monnet and D.D. Smeak), 165–178. Hoboken, NJ: Wiley Blackwell.

Spah, C.E., Elkins, A.D., Wehrenberg, A. et al. (2013). Evaluation of two novel self-anchoring barbed sutures in a prophylactic laparoscopic gastropexy compared with intracorporeal tied knots. *Veterinary Surgery* 42 (8): 932–942.

Spinella, G., Dondi, F., Grassato, L. et al. (2018). Prognostic value of canine pancreatic lipase immunoreactivity and lipase activity in dogs with gastric dilatation-volvulus. *PLoS One* 13: e0204216.

Stampley, A.R., Burrows, C.F., Ellison, G.W., and Tooker, J. (1992). Gastric myoelectric activity after experimental gastric dilatation-volvulus and tube gastrostomy in dogs. *Veterinary Surgery* 21: 10–14.

Takacs, J.D., Singh, A., Case, J.B. et al. (2017). Total laparoscopic gastropexy using 1 simple continuous barbed suture line in 63 dogs. *Veterinary Surgery* 46 (2): 233–241.

Tavakoli, A., Mahmoodifard, M., and Razavifard, A.H. (2016). The superiority of paracostal endoscopic-assisted gastropexy over open incisional and belt-loop gastropexy in dogs: a comparison of three prophylactic techniques. *Iranian Journal of Veterinary Research* 17: 118–123.

Theyse, L.F., van den Brom, W.E., and van Sluijs, F.J. (1998). Small size of food particles and age as risk factors for gastric dilatation volvulus in great Danes. *Veterinary Record* 143: 48–50.

Troia, R., Giunti, M., Calipa, S., and Goggs, R. (2018). Cell-free DNA, high-mobility group box-1 and procalcitonin concentrations in dogs with gastric dilatation-volvulus syndrome. *Frontiers in Veterinary Science* 5: –67.

Uhrikova, I., Rauserova-Lexmaulova, L., Rehakova, K. et al. (2015). C-reactive protein and high mobility group box-1 in dogs with gastric dilatation and volvulus. *Journal of Veterinary Emergency and Critical Care* 25: 488–494.

Van Kruiningen, H.J., Gargamelli, C., Havier, J. et al. (2013). Stomach gas analyses in canine acute gastric dilatation with volvulus. *Journal of Veterinary Internal Medicine* 27: 1260–1261.

van Sluijs, F.J. and van den Brom, W.E. (1989). Gastric emptying of a radionuclide-labeled test meal after surgical correction of gastric dilatation-volvulus in dogs. *American Journal of Veterinary Research* 50: 433–435.

Verschoof, J., Moritz, A., Kramer, M., and Bauer, N. (2015). Hemostatic variables, plasma lactate concentration and inflammatory biomarkers in dogs with gastric dilatation-volvulus. *Tierärztliche Praxis Ausgabe K Kleintiere Heimtiere* 43: 389–398.

Wagner, A.E., Dunlop, C.I., and Chapman, P.L. (1999). Cardiopulmonary measurements in dogs undergoing gastropexy without gastrectomy for correction of gastric dilatation-volvulus. *Journal of the American Veterinary Medical Association* 215: 484–488.

Walker, T.G., Chan, D.L., Freeman, L.M. et al. (2007). Serial determination of biomarkers of oxidative stress and antioxidant status in dogs with naturally occurring gastric dilatation volvulus. *Journal of Veterinary Emergency and Critical Care* 17: 250–256.

Walshaw, R. and Johnston, D.E. (1976). Treatment of gastric dilatation volvulus by gastric decompression and patient stabilization before major surgery. *Journal of the American Animal Hospital Association* 12: 162–167.

Waschak, M.J., Payne, J.T., Pope, E.R. et al. (1997). Evaluation of percutaneous gastrostomy as a technique for permanent gastropexy. *Veterinary Surgery* 26: 235–241.

Wheaton, L.G., Thacker, H.L., and Caldwell, S. (1986). Intravenous fluorescein as an indicator of gastric viability in gastric dilation-volvulus. *Journal of the American Animal Hospital Association* 22: 197–204.

Whitney, W.O., Scavelli, T.D., Matthiesen, D.T., and Burk, R.I. (1989). Belt-loop gastropexy: technique and surgical results in 20 dogs. *Journal of the American Animal Hospital Association* 25: 75–83.

Wingfield, W.E. (1981). Acute gastric dilatation-volvulus. *Veterinary Clinics of North America Small Animal Practice* 11: 147–155.

Wingfield, W.E., Betts, C.W., and Greene, R.W. (1975a). Operative techniques and recurrence rates associated with gastric volvulus in the dog. *Journal of Small Animal Practice* 16: 427–432.

Wingfield, W.E., Cornelius, L.M., Ackerman, N., and DeYoung, D.W. (1975b). Experimental acute gastric dilatation and torsion in the dog. 2. Venous angiographic alterations seen in gastric dilation. *Journal of Small Animal Practice* 16: 55–60.

Wingfield, W.E., Cornelius, L.M., and DeYoung, D.W. (1974). Pathophysiology of the gastric dilation-torsion complex in the dog. *Journal of Small Animal Practice* 15: 735–739.

Wingfield, W.E., Cornelius, L.M., and DeYoung, D.W. (1975c). Experimental acute gastric dilation and torsion in the dog. 1. Changes in biochemical and acid–base parameters. *Journal of Small Animal Practice* 16: 41–53.

Wingfield, W.E., Twedt, D.C., Moore, R.W. et al. (1982). Acid–base and electrolyte values in dogs with acute gastric dilatation-volvulus. *Journal of the American Veterinary Medical Association* 180: 1070–1072.

Winkler, K.P., Greenfield, C.L., and Schaeffer, D.J. (2003). Bacteremia and bacterial translocation in the naturally occurring canine gastric dilatation-volvulus patient. *Journal of the American Animal Hospital Association* 39: 361–368.

Woolfson, J.M. and Kostolich, M. (1986). Circumcostal gastropexy: clinical use of the technique in 34 dogs with gastric dilation-volvulus. *Journal of the American Animal Hospital Association* 22: 825–830.

Zacher, L.A., Berg, J., Shaw, S.P., and Kudej, R.K. (2010). Association between outcome and changes in plasma lactate concentration during presurgical treatment in dogs with gastric dilatation-volvulus: 64 cases (2002–2008). *Journal of the American Veterinary Medical Association* 236: 892–897.

8

Focal and Linear Gastrointestinal Obstructions

Nina Samuel, Barbro Filliquist, and William T.N. Culp

Focal and linear gastrointestinal obstructions in dogs and cats are commonly seen and often require emergency surgical intervention in conjunction with attentive medical management. Reported causes of gastrointestinal obstruction include foreign bodies, intussusception, neoplasia, abscessation, granulomas, and stricture formation. Clinical signs, physical examination findings, and diagnostic results vary depending on the underlying cause and location of the obstruction. This chapter focuses on focal and linear gastrointestinal obstruction due to foreign body ingestion as well as intussusception.

The most commonly reported foreign bodies in dogs include latex, rubber, or plastic objects, stones, balls, underwear, pantyhose, towel or fabric, carpet, and corn cobs (Evans *et al.* 1994; Hayes 2009). Cats are more likely to ingest linear foreign material, such as string or thread with or without needle attached, but focal obstructions have been reported (Basher & Fowler 1987; Bebchuk 2002; Hayes 2009). Trichobezoars are also a reported cause of obstruction in cats (Barrs *et al.* 1999).

Pathophysiology

Gastrointestinal obstruction causes many local and systemic abnormalities that contribute to the development of the clinical signs observed. An atropine-mediated increase in intestinal motor activity occurs proximal to the obstruction, while a decrease in motor activity occurs distal to the obstruction (Prihoda *et al.* 1984). The decrease in motor activity is due to reduced intestinal content as well as inhibition of motor activity. With sustained obstruction, the overall motor activity orad to

the obstruction will decrease as periods of increased myoelectric spike activity are interspersed with long periods of absent motor activity (Summers *et al.* 1983). These factors result in a generalized ileus.

The development of ileus leads to subsequent increase in intraluminal pressure, dilatation of the intestines, and tissue ischemia. Intestinal dilatation is thought to be mediated by nitric oxide, which is released in the intestinal muscle secondary to the inflammation, resulting in inhibition of smooth muscle tone. Systemic sequelae of ileus include gastroduodenal reflux leading to an increased risk of aspiration pneumonia, hypovolemia due to fluid imbalances, bacterial overgrowth and translocation, and, more seriously, intra-abdominal hypertension, systemic inflammation, and multiorgan dysfunction syndrome (MODS) (Madl & Druml 2003). MODS is characterized by systemic organ failure, including acute renal failure, acute respiratory distress syndrome, and disseminated intravascular coagulation, and has a poor prognosis (Osterbur *et al.* 2014).

Obstruction of the gastrointestinal tract has been shown experimentally to alter mesenteric blood flow by significantly increasing blood flow oral to the obstructed section and decreasing mesenteric blood flow aboral to that section (Papanicolaou *et al.* 1985). Intestinal fluid accumulation occurs as a result of increased secretion from the gastrointestinal tract, pancreas, and biliary system, along with retention of ingested fluids (Papazoglou *et al.* 2003). Intestinal fluid accumulation increases as the duration of a proximal obstruction progresses (Mishra *et al.* 1974). Direct distension of the intestinal wall by the foreign body can lead to venous stasis and edema, followed by more significant vascular compromise and necrosis.

Gastrointestinal obstruction results in electrolyte disturbances and acid–base abnormalities as the normal state of secretion and resorption is altered (Papazoglou *et al.* 2003). Vomiting and diarrhea associated with intestinal obstruction will also alter electrolyte levels along with acid–base status as hypovolemia and hemoconcentration develop. The most common electrolyte disturbances include hypochloremia, hyperlactatemia, hypokalemia, and hyponatremia, and patients commonly develop metabolic alkalosis (Boag *et al.* 2005). These changes do not appear to be linked to a specific site of obstruction.

Aborally directed peristaltic movement of the intestines over a linear structure fixed under the tongue or in the pylorus leads to pleating of the intestine with subsequent partial or complete obstruction. Secondary to this phenomenon, linear foreign body obstructions are commonly associated with mucosal injury and perforation on the mesenteric aspect (Bebchuk 2002; MacPhail 2002). Plication of the small intestines has also been reported in a cat infected with tapeworms (Papazoglou *et al.* 2006).

Bacterial sepsis caused by gastrointestinal obstruction and perforation leads to systemic illness as a result of the release of proinflammatory mediators, activation of the cytokine cascade, and liberation of other inflammatory factors, including histamine, serotonin, and arachidonic acid metabolites (Swann & Hughes 2000). The overall effect of these factors leads to a systemic inflammatory response syndrome with detrimental global effects on the patient. MODS can occur as well.

Intussusception typically affects young dogs and cats, although intussusception secondary to intestinal neoplasia is seen in older animals (Figure 8.1). Reported causes

for intussusception include viral enteritis, intestinal parasitism, gastrointestinal foreign bodies, recent gastrointestinal surgery, intestinal masses, and gastroenteritis. Cecal inversion has also been reported in conjunction with intussusception (Bhandal *et al.* 2008). Most cases of intussusception in dogs and cats have an idiopathic etiology (Levitt & Bauer 1992; Oakes *et al.* 1994; Burkitt *et al.* 2009); however, an abnormality in an intestinal segment with a sudden change in intestinal diameter or motility has been suggested as a cause (Klinger *et al.* 1990; Levitt & Bauer 1992; Oakes *et al.* 1994; Burkitt *et al.* 2009). The intussusceptum becomes invaginated into the intussuscipiens, causing an obstruction. Arterial and venous blood flow becomes occluded and intestinal ischemia leads to necrosis and ulceration. The most commonly reported locations for intussusception in the dog and cat are enterocolic and enteroenteric, while gastroesophageal, pylorogastric, and colorectal intussusceptions have been reported as well (Wilson & Burt 1974; Levitt & Bauer 1992; Applewhite *et al.* 2001a; Patsikas *et al.* 2003; Burkitt *et al.* 2009).

Clinical signs and physical examination

The mean reported age of dogs with gastrointestinal foreign bodies ranges from 2.5 to 4.5 years (Evans *et al.* 1994; Hayes 2009). Cats also tend to be young at the time of evaluation, with a mean reported age ranging from 1.8 to 2.7 years (Felts *et al.* 1984; Hayes 2009). The most common clinical signs associated with gastrointestinal obstructions secondary to foreign bodies and intussusception include vomiting, anorexia, lethargy, abdominal pain, and diarrhea (Anderson *et al.* 2021). Physical examination findings include abdominal pain, dehydration, and palpation of an abdominal mass lesion. One study reported a palpable abdominal mass in 53% of animals with intussusception (Levitt & Bauer 1992). In cats, linear foreign material, including string or thread, commonly becomes lodged around the base of the tongue and will be noted on careful physical examination.

The presence of abdominal effusion is suggestive of septic peritonitis, and abnormal mentation, bright red mucous membranes, hypotension, hyperthermia or hypothermia, altered cardiac output, and abdominal pain can also be detected in the septic patient (King 1994; Hauptman *et al.* 1997). Cats with septic peritonitis have been reported to have a relative bradycardia (Costello *et al.* 2004).

Diagnostics

Bloodwork

Bloodwork abnormalities in animals with gastrointestinal obstruction are often nonspecific: the most

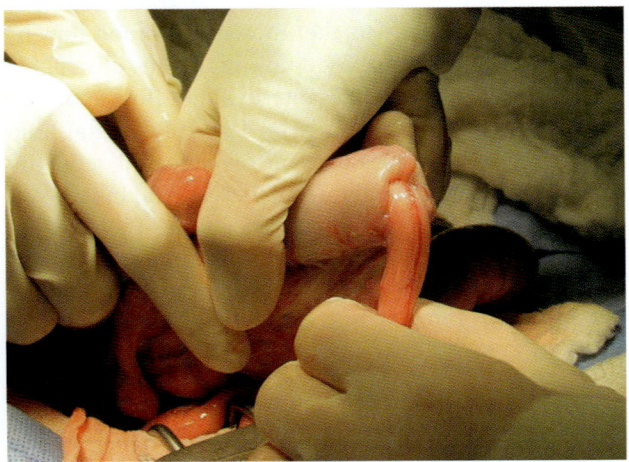

Figure 8.1 Intussusception involving the jejunum and ileum in a dog.

commonly reported biochemical abnormality is azotemia (Felts *et al.* 1984; Evans *et al.* 1994). Hypochloremia, hyponatremia, and hypokalemia are associated with vomiting and sequestration within the gastrointestinal tract (Boag *et al.* 2005). Metabolic alkalosis is the most common acid–base abnormality, but a metabolic acidosis can be seen secondary to hypovolemia and hyperlactatemia (Papazoglou *et al.* 2003; Boag *et al.* 2005). In cats with septic peritonitis, mean blood glucose at time of presentation has been shown to be significantly higher in nonsurvivors versus survivors (Scotti *et al.* 2019). A leukocytosis due to neutrophilia with or without a left shift can be noted preoperatively. One study reported that the probability of survival following small intestinal surgery was not affected by the preoperative neutrophil count or the presence of preoperative bands (Wylie & Hosgood 1994). Decreased protein C and antithrombin has been shown to be associated with increased mortality (Bentley *et al.* 2013).

Fluid analysis

Peritoneal effusion should be collected if present. Fluid should be evaluated to determine type of fluid, nucleated cell count, and glucose and lactate concentrations. A septic effusion is suspected if degenerative neutrophils are present. A total nucleated cell count in excess of $13 \times 10^9/L$ is 86% sensitive and 100% specific for septic effusion in the dog and 100% sensitive and specific in the cat (Bonczynski *et al.* 2003). Intracellular bacteria confirms the diagnosis and a cytologic evaluation of a septic effusion is 57–100% accurate in diagnosing a septic peritonitis (Mueller *et al.* 2001; Bonczynski *et al.* 2003; Levin *et al.* 2004). Culture and sensitivity should always be performed on the fluid. The most commonly isolated organisms associated with foreign body obstruction in dogs include *Escherichia coli*, *Enterococcus* spp., *Enterobacter* spp., *Klebsiella* spp., and *Pseudomonas* spp. (Evans *et al.* 1994). Septic peritonitis in cats is typically associated with *E. coli*, *Enterococcus* spp., *Clostridium* spp., and *Pseudomonas* spp. (Costello *et al.* 2004).

Patients with septic peritonitis have a peritoneal fluid lactate concentration greater than patients with nonseptic effusion, and a fluid lactate concentration above 2.5 mmol/L has been found to be 100% sensitive and 91% specific for septic peritonitis in the dog (Levin *et al.* 2004). This same study found that a fluid lactate concentration above 2.5 mmol/L in cats is only 67% sensitive and specific for the diagnosis of a septic peritonitis. A blood to peritoneal fluid lactate difference of less than −2.0 mmol/L is 63–100% sensitive and 100% specific for a septic effusion in the dog. Fluid lactate concentration and blood to fluid lactate difference are not consistent markers of septic effusion in the cat, despite

being statistically significant. Comparing blood with peritoneal fluid glucose, a difference of more than 20 mg/dL is 100% sensitive and specific for septic peritonitis in the dog and 86% sensitive and 100% specific in the cat (Bonczynski *et al.* 2003). These parameters are not utilized postoperatively as an indicator of septic peritonitis in patients in which a closed-suction drain has been placed (Szabo *et al.* 2011; Mouat *et al.* 2014).

Radiography

Abdominal radiography is frequently used to assess the abdomen in vomiting patients. Radiographic findings associated with a focal foreign body obstruction include intestinal dilatation, presence of ingesta oral to the obstruction, and detection of foreign material within the intestinal tract (Graham *et al.* 1998; Tyrell & Beck 2006). Comparing the maximum small intestinal diameter to the height of L5 on a lateral abdominal radiograph has been evaluated as a diagnostic tool for determining the presence of an intestinal foreign body in dogs (Graham *et al.* 1998). A ratio of 1.6 is the upper range of normal and animals with a value greater than 2.07 have a 90% probability of having an obstruction. However, this study was done by a single examiner and when this method was used by examiners with different levels of experience, the specificity and sensitivity were both only 66% and use of the ratio did not correlate with an increase in diagnostic accuracy (Ciasca *et al.* 2013). Using three small intestinal diameter ratios has also been proposed as another means of assessing for mechanical obstruction, where patients with maximum small intestinal diameter : L5 $\geq$2.4, small intestinal maximum diameter : small intestinal minimum diameter $\geq$3.4, and small intestinal maximum diameter : small intestinal average diameter $\geq$1.9 were considered likely to be obstructed (Finck *et al.* 2014). Comparing the maximum small intestinal diameter to the height of the cranial endplate of L2 has been used to assess for mechanical obstruction in cats. In those patients with a ratio $\geq$3.0, there was a >70% probability of mechanical obstruction in one study (Adams *et al.* 2010).

Linear foreign bodies are suspected when there is plication of the intestines and gathering of the small intestines to the right side of the abdomen. In one report, the presence of luminal gas bubbles that were tapered at one or both ends was suggestive of a linear foreign body and the presence of three or more of these bubbles was always associated with a linear foreign body (Figure 8.2) (Felts *et al.* 1984). Another study found that the probability of intestinal plication was highest with a combination of a linear and comma-shaped gas pattern together or linear, bubble, and comma patterns combined. In the same study, 8 of 10 cats had comma-shaped gas patterns with the presence of plication (Adams *et al.* 2010).

The presence of a pneumoperitoneum is consistent with perforation due to a foreign body. The presence of free gas on preoperative radiographs was associated with 100% mortality in one study (Evans *et al.* 1994). Another report looking at outcome and prognosis in dogs and cats with nontraumatic pneumoperitoneum reported a survival rate of 44% (Smelstoys *et al.* 2004). Decreased serosal detail is a nonspecific finding and can be caused by decreased intra-abdominal fat or peritoneal effusion (Tyrell & Beck 2006).

Radiographic findings without the presence of radiopaque material are often nonspecific, and in one study a radiographic diagnosis of gastrointestinal foreign bodies was only achieved in 56% of the animals (Tyrell & Beck 2006). Another study found no radiographic abnormalities in 14% of cats with linear foreign bodies (Felts *et al.* 1984). To aid with the diagnosis, the opposite lateral view may help identify a foreign body, as gas distribution will change within the gastrointestinal tract. For example, a left lateral radiograph will shift gas from the fundus to the pylorus and can outline pyloric foreign bodies (Armbrust *et al.* 2000). Animals with an intussusception can have radiographic evidence of an intestinal mass effect in addition to intestinal distension; however, diagnosis of intussusception is not made consistently with plain film radiography (Levitt & Bauer 1992; Burkitt *et al.* 2009).

Contrast radiography can aid in a radiographic diagnosis of an intestinal obstruction when plain film radiography does not lead to a diagnosis (Figure 8.3). The upper gastrointestinal series using barium is the standard for evaluation of the stomach and small intestine using contrast radiography; however, barium should be used with caution if perforation is suspected or when surgery is inevitable, as it is very irritating to the peritoneum (Brawner & Bartels 1983) and can result in the progression of extracellular fluid and albumin exudate as well as the formation of severe adhesions (Ko & Mann 2014). In cases of gastrointestinal obstructions or perforations, it is advisable to use a nonionic iodinated contrast agent with low osmolality such as iohexol to achieve radiographic diagnosis (Williams *et al.* 1993) or to avoid contrast studies if possible.

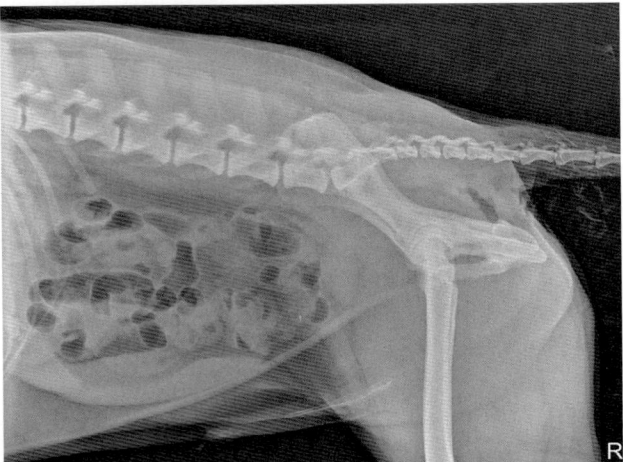

Figure 8.2 Lateral abdominal radiograph of a dog with a linear foreign body demonstrating multiple comma-shaped to rounded gas opacities throughout the small intestines, consistent with plication.

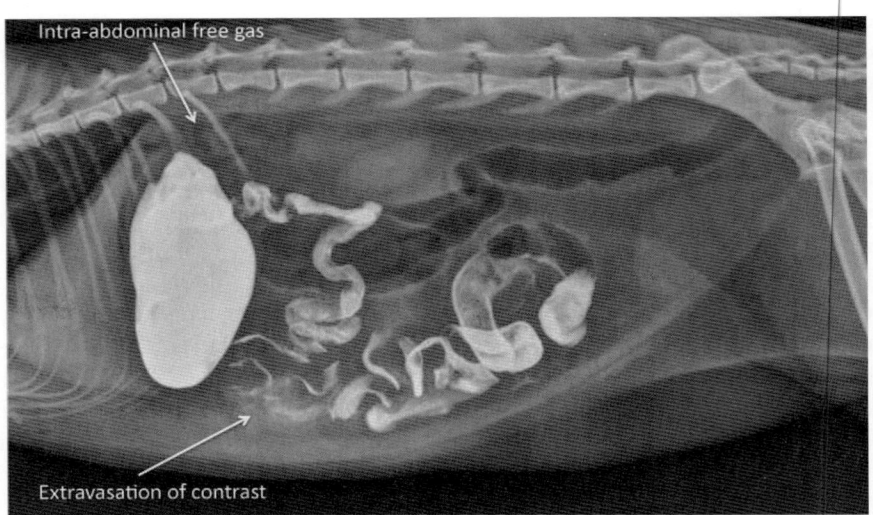

Figure 8.3 Lateral radiograph of a cat that presented with clinical signs of anorexia and vomiting. An upper gastrointestinal contrast study was performed. Note the presence of free gas and extravasation of barium into the peritoneal cavity consistent with perforation. Plication of the small intestine is consistent with a linear foreign body.

Barium sulfate enema can be used in patients suspected of having ileocolic or cecocolic intussusceptions. Radiographs will show distension of the intussuscipiens while the intussusceptum will appear lucent, and there is often an abrupt end to the involved intestinal loop (Wilson & Burt 1974).

In patients in which radiography is equivocal for mechanical obstruction, a repeated acquisition of radiographs is sometimes recommended. However, in one study there was no increase in accuracy of diagnosis when radiographs were repeated within 7–28 hours. Therefore, alternative imaging methods, such as ultrasonography, may be recommended in cases where radiographs are not definitive for a diagnosis (Elser et al. 2020).

Ultrasound

Ultrasonography is readily available in veterinary medicine and is useful for the diagnosis of intestinal obstructions. Ultrasonographic findings in animals with intestinal obstruction include gastrointestinal distension, fluid-filled intestinal loops, intestinal hypermotility and hypomotility, identification of a foreign body, and hyperechoic mesentery (Tidwell & Penninck 1992; Tyrell & Beck 2006). In a study comparing plain film radiography with ultrasonography, a foreign body was identified in 100% of the cases using ultrasound (Tyrell & Beck 2006). In this study, ultrasonography also allowed evaluation of intestinal wall integrity and was more sensitive in detecting intestinal perforation compared with radiographic evaluation. In another study, ultrasonography definitively determined whether a patient was obstructed 97% of the time, whereas radiography was only 70% accurate (Sharma et al. 2011). Ultrasonographic findings in dogs and cats with gastrointestinal perforation secondary to intestinal foreign body obstruction or intussusception include hyperechoic mesentery, effusion, pneumoperitoneum, loss of normal gastrointestinal wall layer, and lymphadenopathy (Boysen et al. 2003).

The ultrasonographic diagnosis of an intussusception in dogs and cats is based on the presence of a target-like mass with multiple hyperechoic and hypoechoic rings around a hyperechoic center in the transverse view. The hyperechoic center represents mesenteric fat associated with the intussusceptum. Consequently, in longitudinal sections, hyperechoic and hypoechoic parallel lines are apparent. One study found Doppler ultrasonography helpful for identifying mesenteric blood flow within the intussuscepted intestine, and 75% of the cases where blood flow was identified could be reduced at the time of surgery (Patsikas et al. 2005). Dogs in which Doppler ultrasonography failed to identify mesenteric blood flow were diagnosed with an irreducible intussusception during surgery. Normal and abnormal findings can mimic the ultrasonographic appearance of an intussusception; it is important to use a multiplane imaging technique and to look for complete rings at the periphery of the target-like mass (Patsikas et al. 2004).

Endoscopy

Endoscopy is commonly used for foreign body removal in the esophagus and the stomach, but little is published in veterinary and human literature on the use of endoscopy with small intestinal obstruction. Endoscopic removal of foreign bodies in the stomach is attractive due to lower cost and the decreased invasiveness compared with surgical removal. One study found an association between complications and bone foreign bodies, body weight below 10 kg, and time of foreign body presence; however, in this report the bone was located in the esophagus in the cases that died (Gianella et al. 2009). Endoscopic evaluation of the esophagus and stomach may be useful in obstructed animals that exhibit signs consistent with esophageal disease. It may also be advantageous to use endoscopy for evaluation of the esophagus and stomach in cats with a linear foreign body anchored to the tongue and in cases of ingestion of sharp objects, such as sewing needles, to prevent future perforation of the gastrointestinal tract (Pratt et al. 2014).

Computed tomography

Computed tomography (CT) is not commonly used for the diagnosis of gastrointestinal foreign body obstruction and intussusception in dogs and cats. In human medicine, CT is used frequently to diagnose abdominal disease, although obstruction due to an intestinal foreign body is rare. When comparing the role of plain film radiography and CT for the diagnosis of small intestinal obstruction, a study reported similar overall accuracies in revealing the obstruction (Maglinte et al. 1996). CT was often able to reveal the cause of obstruction and remains an important diagnostic tool when managing cases; however, the consensus was that plain film radiography should be part of the initial diagnosis. An earlier report found plain film radiography insensitive, with a diagnosis of complete obstruction in only 46% of cases, whereas the use of CT confirmed obstruction in all cases (Frager et al. 1994). Reported CT findings of small intestinal perforations secondary to foreign body ingestion in humans include localized pneumoperitoneum, infiltrative fat near a thickened intestinal loop, and evidence of obstruction (Coulier et al. 2004; Zissin et al. 2009). In veterinary medicine, recent studies have shown 100% accuracy in diagnosing mechanical obstructions with the use of CT scans (Winter et al. 2017; Miniter et al. 2019). Although CT has the benefit of taking significantly less time for acquiring images as compared to ultrasonography (Winter *et al.* 2017), the cost and requirement for profound sedation or anesthesia are a major limitation for using CT in small animal medicine.

Magnetic resonance imaging

Magnetic resonance imaging (MRI) has several limitations regarding abdominal imaging, including excessive motion artifact due to long acquisition time, peristalsis, and respiration, in addition to low signal-to-noise ratio and lack of suitable oral contrast agents (Paley & Ros 1997). The usefulness of MRI for detecting gastrointestinal disease in humans is still being investigated. HASTE (half-Fourier acquisition single-shot turbo spin-echo) is a high-speed MRI technique that allows great sensitivity of fluid detection and good images of the abdominal cavity, and can be considered an alternative diagnostic tool for gastrointestinal obstruction and masses in human medicine (Kim *et al.* 2000). According to this study, MRI provided the correct diagnosis in 73% of the cases compared with CT (60%).

As radiography, ultrasound, and surgical exploration commonly provide the veterinarian with a diagnosis, it is difficult to justify the high cost of MRI; however, as technology improves and the cost of new imaging techniques decreases, this technique may become more viable.

Surgical management

Surgical considerations

The type of surgery performed is dependent on the extent of injury to the intestine. A careful and thorough inspection of the entire gastrointestinal tract should be performed. A review of gastrointestinal foreign bodies in 208 dogs and cats found that gastric foreign bodies represented 24% of the feline cases and 16% of the canine cases (Hayes 2009). In a separate report, 50% of the canine foreign bodies were located in the stomach (Boag *et al.* 2005). Of the feline obstructions, 47% occurred in the jejunum, 24% in the duodenum, and 6% in the ileum. In dogs, 62% of the obstructions occurred in the jejunum, 14% in the duodenum, and 3% in the ileum (Figure 8.4) (Hayes 2009).

Linear foreign bodies are more commonly seen in cats than in dogs and represent 33% of feline gastrointestinal obstructions (Hayes 2009). The foreign material typically becomes lodged at the base of the tongue or the pylorus. One study compared medical management with surgical management of gastrointestinal linear foreign bodies in the cat and found conservative management successful in 9 of 24 cases (Basher & Fowler 1987).

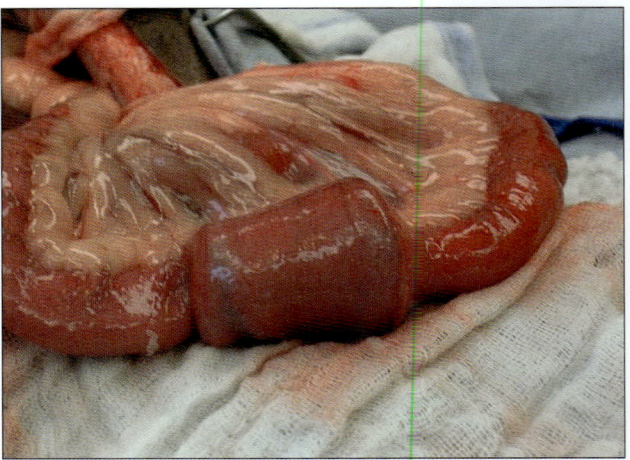

Figure 8.4 Intraoperative image of focal jejunal foreign body. Note the erythema associated with the oral aspect of the intestine and the normal appearance of the intestine aboral to the foreign body.

In the same study, an additional 10 cases failed conservative management, and on surgical exploration 3 of these cats were found to have intestinal perforations. A review of 64 feline cases of thread and needle linear foreign bodies found that 10 of 63 surgical cases had evidence of perforation secondary to the thread (Felts *et al.* 1984). An overall success rate of 84% was reported, but only 50% of the cases with perforations recovered. Because of the poor survival rate in cats with perforation, conservative management of linear foreign bodies cannot be recommended.

Linear foreign body obstruction in the dog reportedly occurs in approximately 16% of canine gastrointestinal obstructions (Hayes 2009). A study evaluating gastrointestinal foreign bodies in the dog found the linear foreign material to be anchored in the pylorus in 87% of the cases and under the tongue in only 6% of dogs (Evans *et al.* 1994). Perforations were found in 31% of the dogs, while intussusceptions were present in 25% of the dogs suffering from linear foreign bodies (Figures 8.5 and 8.6). The presence of a linear foreign body has been associated with an increased mortality rate compared with a discrete obstruction in one study (Hayes 2009). However, a subsequent study found no difference in outcome between dogs with linear versus nonlinear foreign bodies, with 96% of each patient population surviving to discharge (Hobday *et al.* 2014).

Intussusception often requires enterectomy followed by anastomosis due to compromised blood flow and necrosis or inability to reduce secondary to adhesions. Manual reduction is typically attempted first, but variable success has been reported (Wilson & Burt 1974; Levitt & Bauer 1992; Burkitt *et al.* 2009). Spontaneous

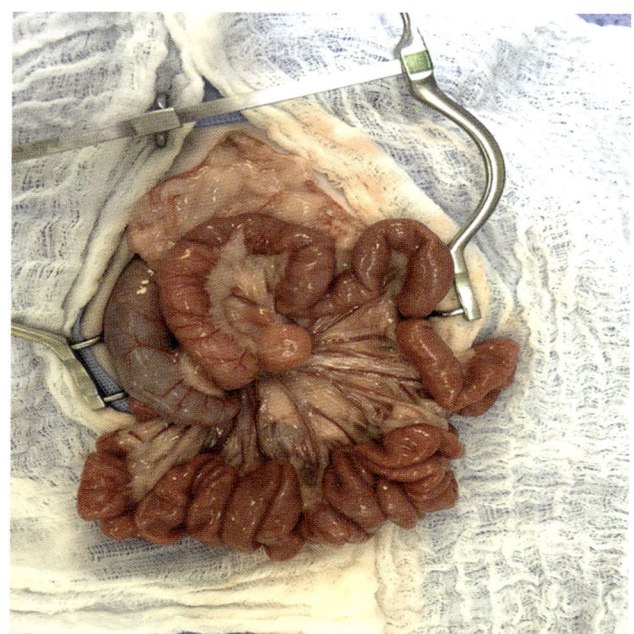

Figure 8.5 Plication of the jejunum because of a linear foreign body. Source: Courtesy of Dr. Philipp Mayhew.

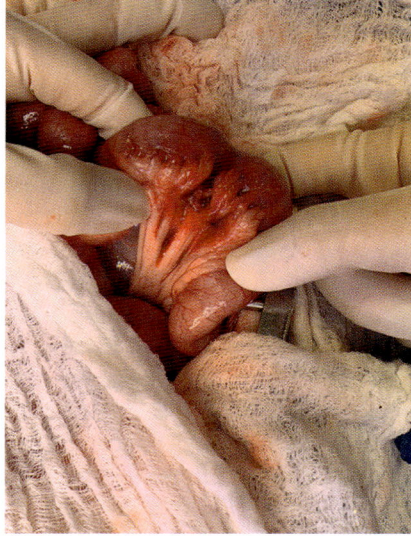

Figure 8.6 A linear foreign body has perforated the wall of the jejunum along the mesenteric border. Source: Courtesy of Dr. Karen Park.

reduction of intestinal intussusception has been reported in dogs (Patsikas *et al.* 2008), where the diagnosis was made based on clinical signs and ultrasonographic findings but surgical findings were normal. One dog developed clinical signs again within 48 hours and a second surgical exploration revealed an enteroenteric intussusception.

Reported recurrence rates for intussusception in dogs range from 18.5% to 27% (Levitt & Bauer 1992; Oakes *et al.* 1994), though more recently recurrence rates as low as 3% have been reported (Larose *et al.* 2020). Enteroplication following resolution of the intussusception has been proposed to minimize the risk of recurrence. Due to small numbers of cases, statistical difference in cases undergoing enteropexy or enteroplication versus cases without the additional procedure has not been established, and the decision to perform enteroplication is surgeon dependent (Levitt & Bauer 1992; Applewhite *et al.* 2001a,b; Burkitt *et al.* 2009, Larose *et al.* 2020). The use of butorphanol and morphine as part of the preoperative and intraoperative protocol for prevention of intussusception in canine renal transplant patients is reportedly effective (McAnulty *et al.* 1989; Klinger *et al.* 1990).

Animals with evidence of septic peritonitis at the time of surgery should be lavaged with large amounts of a warm balanced electrolyte solution. It is important to remove as much of the lavage as possible, as bacterial clearance can be reduced with the presence of fluid (Ahrenholz 1979). Following lavage of the peritoneum, a multidrug-resistant bacteria is less likely to be cultured (Marshall *et al.* 2019). Serosal patching has been proposed to reinforce intestinal closures, which may be useful in patients with septic peritonitis; however, in one study the use of a serosal patch did not result in protection from postoperative septic peritonitis or death (Grimes *et al.* 2013). Open peritoneal drainage has been used in both humans and animals with gross abdominal contamination. One study comparing open peritoneal drainage with primary closure in dogs and cats found no difference in mortality rate between the two groups, with an overall mortality rate of 29% (Staatz *et al.* 2002). Open peritoneal drainage requires at least one additional surgical procedure. The use of closed-suction drains has been evaluated for the management of peritonitis in dogs and cats (Mueller *et al.* 2001). Except for minor trauma to the drainage bulb, there were no complications associated with management of septic peritonitis using closed-suction drains and the mortality rate in this study was 30%. In a subsequent study that employed closed-suction drainage for postoperative management, 85% of dogs survived to discharge (Adams *et al.* 2014). Vacuum-assisted peritoneal drainage has been evaluated as an alternative to other drainage methods for postoperative management of septic peritonitis, and has been found to have similar issues, including nosocomial infections and hypoproteinemia (Cioffi *et al.* 2012; Buote & Havig 2012; Spillebeen *et al.* 2017). A case report of management of a dehisced resection and anastomosis site with extra-abdominal exteriorization and bandaging of the affected segment following repeat resection and anastomosis has also been described (Tzimtzimis *et al.* 2016).

Surgical techniques

Gastrotomy

Gastric foreign bodies are removed through a longitudinal gastrotomy incision on the ventral surface of the stomach. Stay sutures are placed on either end of the proposed incision (Website Chapter 8: Gastrointestinal surgery/stomach/gastrotomy foreign body). The body of the stomach is opened with a stab incision into the lumen in a relatively avascular area between the greater and lesser curvatures and the incision is continued with Metzenbaum scissors (Figure 8.7). The length of the incision is based on the anticipated size of the foreign material to be removed. Several techniques have been described for closure of the stomach, including inverting, appositional, single-layer, and double-layer patterns. The standard technique described is a two-layer closure, with the first layer incorporating the mucosa and submucosa in a simple continuous pattern using 3-0 or 4-0 absorbable monofilament suture. The second layer may be a simple continuous or inverting pattern, such as Connell or Cushing, using 3-0 or 4-0 absorbable monofilament suture spaced 3–4 mm apart and 3–4 mm from the edges (Figure 8.8).

Enterotomy

A focal obstruction with no evidence of perforation or intestinal wall compromise is removed via a single enterotomy just aboral to the foreign body along the antimesenteric border. To perform the enterotomy, the affected area of intestine is first isolated from surrounding organs

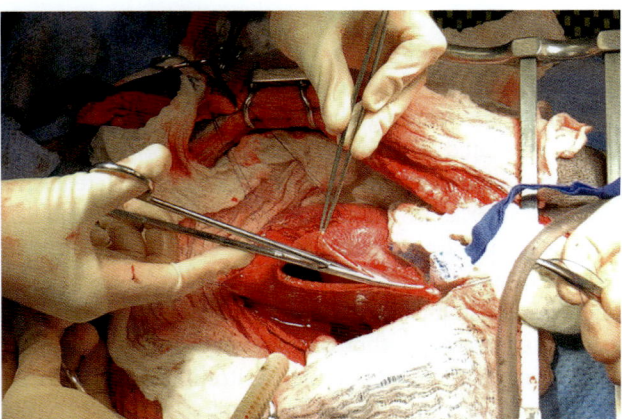

Figure 8.7 A gastrotomy is performed with an incision between the greater and lesser curvature of the stomach. Stay sutures are placed to help prevent contamination. The stomach is also packed off from the rest of the abdominal cavity with laparotomy sponges.

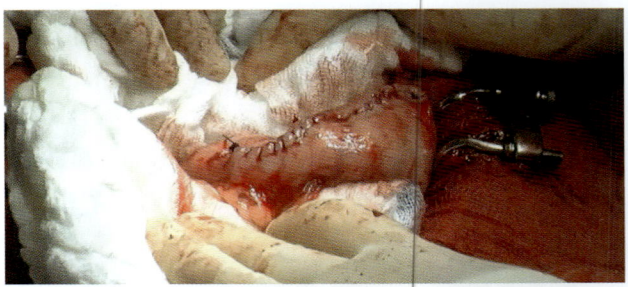

Figure 8.8 The gastrotomy has been closed with 4-0 monofilament suture in a simple continuous pattern. The suture was started and ended past the incision to provide a better seal.

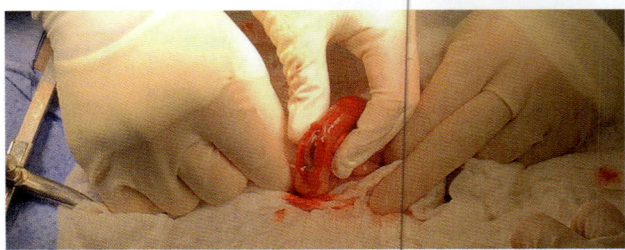

Figure 8.9 An enterotomy has been performed to remove a single foreign body in the jejunum. The fingers of an assistant are holding the loop of jejunum to prevent contamination from intestinal content.

by several moistened, sterile laparotomy sponges. Intestinal contents are milked orally and aborally away from the proposed enteric incision. The finger of an assistant or Doyen clamps are used to prevent the intestinal contents from leaking into the surgical field (Figure 8.9). A linear incision is made into the intestine of sufficient size to allow the foreign material to be removed. Suction should be available to assist in the removal of any intestinal contents that spill from the intestine. Several closure techniques have been described in the veterinary literature. The standard technique described is a full-thickness simple interrupted or continuous closure using 3-0 or 4-0 synthetic absorbable monofilament sutures spaced 3–4 mm apart (Figure 8.10) (Weisman *et al.* 1999). The use of nonabsorbable suture in enteric closure has been associated with foreign body attachment and subsequent obstruction (Milovancev *et al.* 2004).

A study comparing a modified continuous suture pattern to a simple interrupted pattern found the continuous pattern comparable to an interrupted pattern (Weisman *et al.* 1999). A technique has also been described using skin staples in the rapid closure of cases needing multiple enterotomies (Coolman *et al.* 2000a,b). With this technique, a stay suture using a monofilament absorbable suture is placed at each end of the enterotomy to provide tension. As the incisional

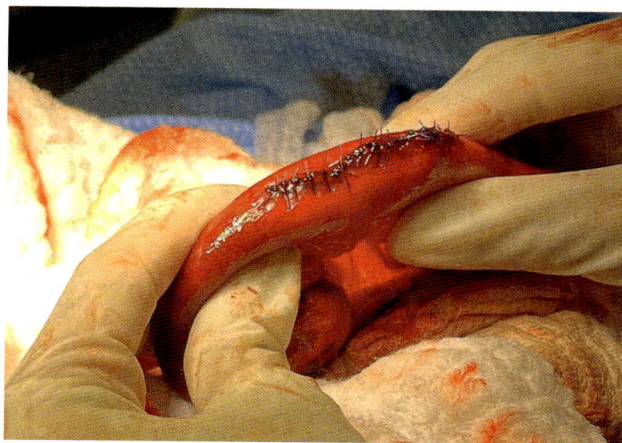

Figure 8.10 The enterotomy has been closed with 3-0 monofilament absorbable suture with a simple interrupted pattern.

edges are opposed with tension, regular dimension skin staples are placed approximately 2–3 mm apart to close the enterotomy.

Animals with linear foreign bodies are frequently treated with multiple enterotomies in order to minimize continued mucosal injury and iatrogenic perforation. The pyloric anchor is first released with a gastrotomy. There is evidence that animals undergoing multiple enterotomies have a higher mortality rate compared with animals with a single enterotomy (Wylie & Hosgood 1994; Hayes 2009).

A surgical report describing a single enterotomy technique in cats for removal of gastrointestinal linear foreign bodies has been published (Anderson *et al.* 1992). Using this technique, an incision is made on the antimesenteric surface at the most oral extent of the intestinal plication. A red rubber catheter is sewn to the foreign material using suture and the enterotomy is closed once the catheter has been fed into the intestinal tract. The catheter is then passed aborally through the intestinal tract by milking the intestine until the intestinal plication is relieved and the catheter with the foreign material is passed out through the anus. This technique can be used in animals with a pyloric anchor by performing a gastrotomy and attaching the catheter to the material as described. Patient selection is important and this technique should only be used in animals with no evidence of necrosis or perforation.

Intestinal resection and anastomosis

Animals with evidence of perforation or significant intestinal injury and necrosis should be treated with resection and anastomosis that allows removal of the compromised section of intestine (Figures 8.11–8.13) (Website Chapter 8: Gastrointestinal surgery/small

intestine/enterectomy). The affected intestinal segment is isolated as already described. The segment to be removed is identified including a margin of grossly normal tissue. The blood supply to the segment being removed is identified and ligation commences with the placement of ligatures or use of a vessel-sealing device around the vasa recta blood supply along the mesenteric border of the intestine. Sufficient mesenteric tissue should be maintained for closure of the subsequent mesenteric defect. If intestinal contents can be milked away from the surgical site, this should be performed, and Carmalt clamps can be placed on the section of bowel to be removed to prevent spillage of intestinal contents after transection. Noncrushing Doyen forceps can be placed on the intestinal segments that will be anastomosed to prevent spillage of intestinal contents; alternatively, an assistant's fingers can be used to hold the segments (Figures 8.11 and 8.12). The damaged intestine is sharply transected using a scalpel blade.

The traditional full-thickness closure consists of opposing the intestinal ends followed by anastomosis using a simple interrupted pattern and absorbable sutures (Coolman *et al.* 2000a,b). A simple continuous suture pattern for enterectomy and anastomosis has also been described (Weisman *et al.* 1999). Using this technique, two separate sutures are placed at the mesenteric and the antimesenteric borders and the ends left as stay sutures, keeping the needle and strand intact (Figure 8.12). Tension is applied as the continuous pattern is advanced from one border to the opposite side, where it is ligated to the tagged suture of the opposite border. The bites are taken approximately 3–4 mm from the cut edge and 3 mm apart (Figure 8.13).

Several surgical stapling devices can be used for anastomosis following enterectomy. The gastrointestinal anastomosis or intestinal linear anastomosis stapler creates a side-to-side or functional end-to-end anastomosis and the remaining open edge is then sealed using a thoracoabdominal stapler (Figure 8.14) (Tobias 2007). The use of skin staples has also been described for anastomosis of the small intestine in dogs (Coolman *et al.* 2000a,b). Because of the limited intestinal diameter, surgical stapling devices are typically not used in cats except for colonic surgery. Trichobezoar obstruction has been reported in a Labrador retriever at the site of a jejunal enterectomy and stapled anastomosis (Carobbi *et al.* 2009).

Use of the gastrointestinal anastomosis stapler has been shown to be safe and fast when performed by nonexpert, trained surgeons (end of internship or first-year surgery residents) (Jardel *et al.* 2011). In addition, studies have shown that in patients with preoperative septic peritonitis, dehiscence is less likely with stapled

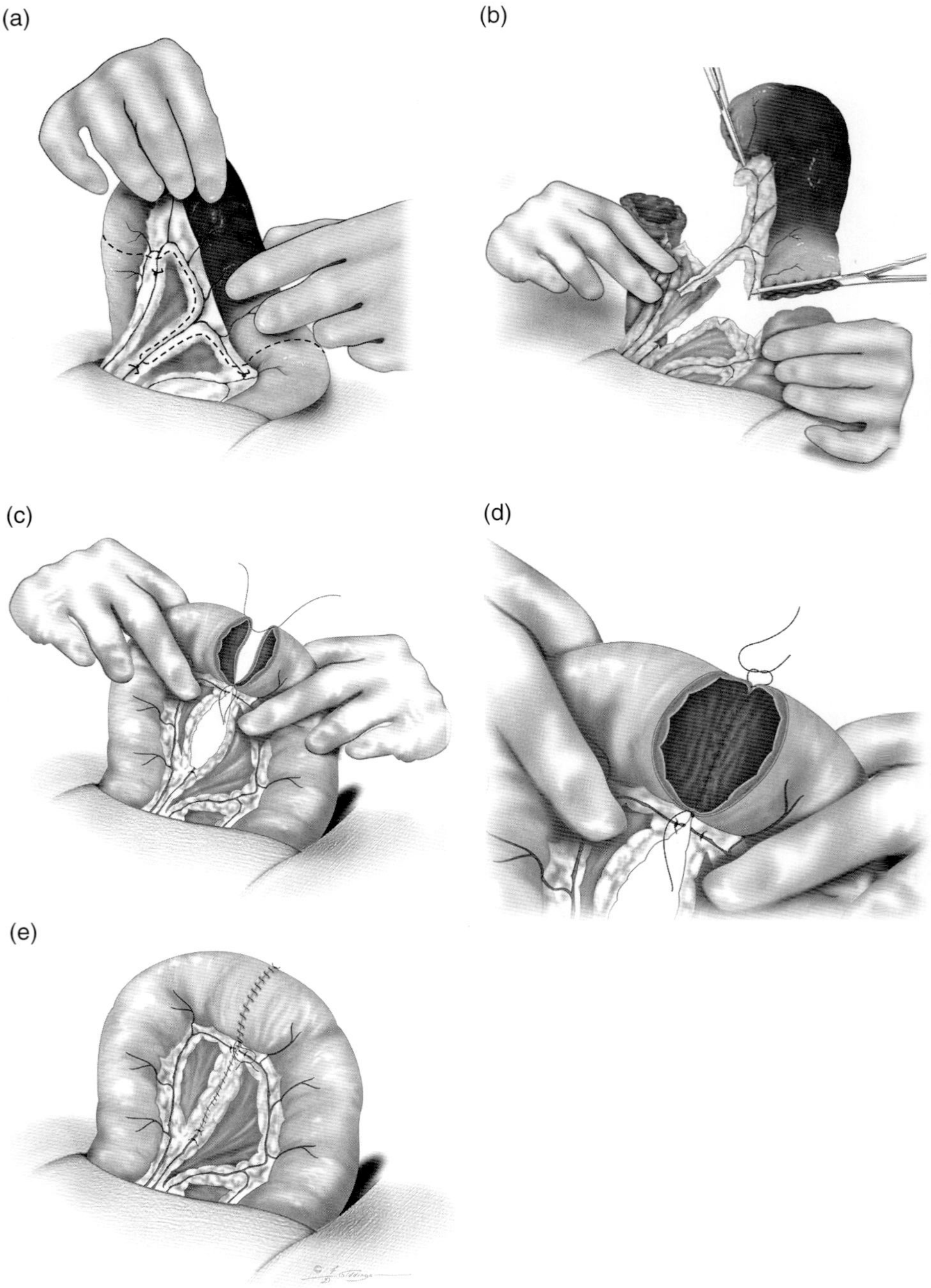

(a)

(b)

(c)

(d)

(e)

Figure 8.11 Enterectomy. (a) The mesenteric artery and vein have been ligated at the root of the mesentery and also along the mesenteric side. The content of the intestine is milked away. (b) The fingers of an assistant are holding the loop of intestine and prevent contamination of the surgical field. Crushing clamps have been placed on the loop of intestine that is resected to prevent contamination. (c) Stay sutures are preplaced at the mesenteric and antimesenteric borders. (d, e) The anastomosis has been completed with two simple continuous pattern sutures using 4-0 monofilament absorbable material. One simple continuous suture goes from the mesenteric to the antimesenteric side and the other from the antimesenteric to the mesenteric side.

anastomoses versus handsewn anastomoses (Davis *et al.* 2018). It is recommended to oversew the transverse staple line with the functional end-to-end anastomosis technique, as this has been associated with a decreased incidence of postoperative dehiscence (Sumner *et al.* 2019).

Minimally invasive techniques

As minimally invasive techniques have become commonplace in human medicine, these methods have been explored in veterinary patients in order to reduce morbidity. For intestinal surgery, laparoscopic-assisted

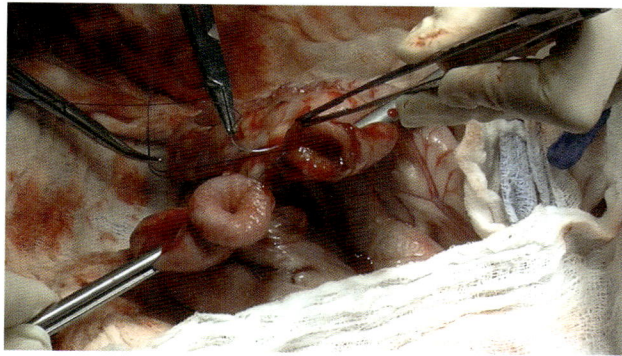

Figure 8.12 Stay sutures are preplaced at the mesenteric and antimesenteric borders.

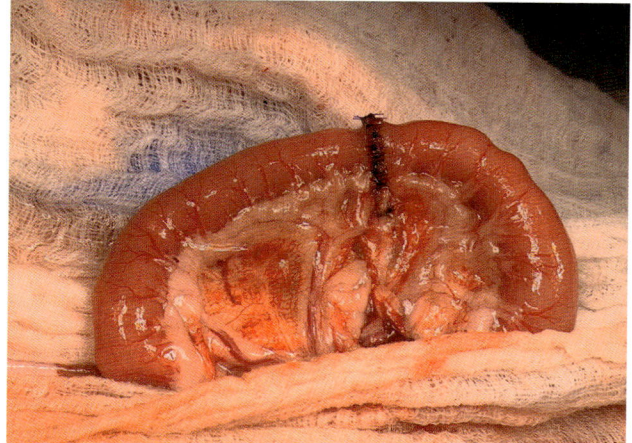

Figure 8.13 The anastomosis has been completed with a simple interrupted suture pattern. Source: Courtesy of Dr. Andrea Castilla.

techniques have been shown to allow for adequate exploration of the abdomen and completion of basic intestinal procedures, including enterotomy, resection and anastomosis, and biopsy. Patient selection is important, though conversion to an open laparotomy may still be necessary (Gower & Mayhew 2011; Case & Ellison 2013; Barry *et al.* 2017). One study showed that there was no difference in surgical time, length of hospitalization, or length of recovery in patients that underwent open laparotomy for foreign body removal versus those that underwent single-incision laparoscopic-assisted intestinal surgery (Otomo *et al.* 2019). Additionally, a laparoscopic-assisted gastrotomy technique for foreign body has been described in dogs (Gibson *et al.* 2020).

Biopsies

Surgical biopsies should be obtained if there is evidence of focal or diffuse intestinal abnormalities. Sharp excision of a small sample from the antimesenteric aspect of the intestine is commonly used. A stab incision is made with a scalpel blade and the intestinal biopsy is excised using scissors; the mucosa should always be included in the biopsy sample (Figure 8.15). The intestinal defect is then closed as a standard enterotomy using an interrupted suture technique; however, a simple continuous closure can also be used (Keats *et al.* 2004).

A different technique using the Keyes skin biopsy punch has been evaluated for intestinal biopsy collection (Keats *et al.* 2004). A full-thickness biopsy was collected using a no. 6 Keyes biopsy punch from the

(a) (b) (c)

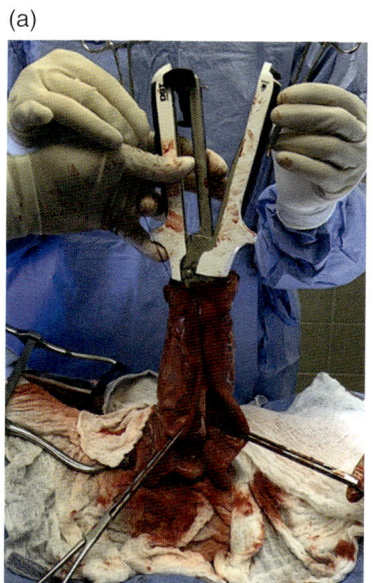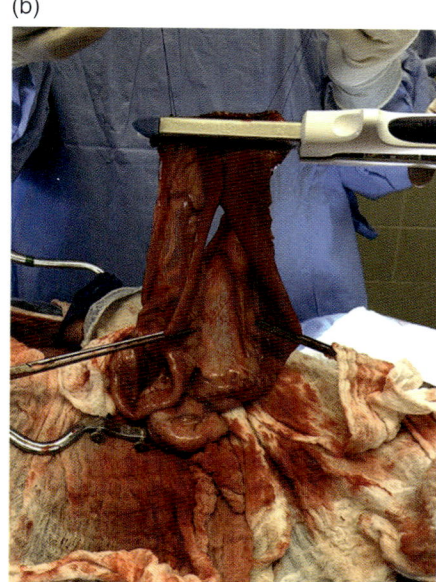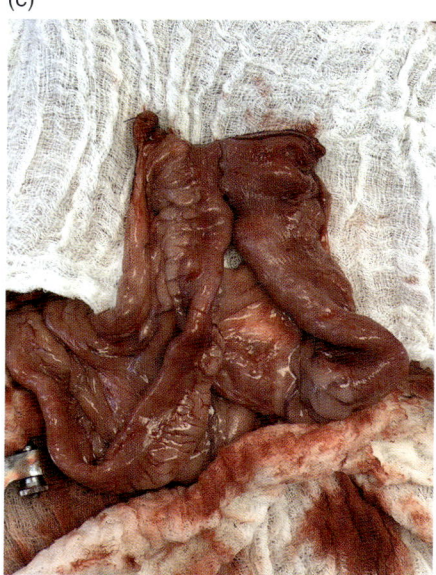

Figure 8.14 Enterectomy performed with staples. (a) A gastrointestinal stapler is introduced in both sides of the anastomosis to create a side-to-side anastomosis. (b) A thoracoabdominal stapler is used to close the enterectomy. The excess tissue is trimmed with a surgical blade. (c) The enterectomy is completed. It is recommended to add a simple interrupted suture at the distal end of the anastomosis for safety. Source: Courtesy of Dr. Philipp Mayhew.

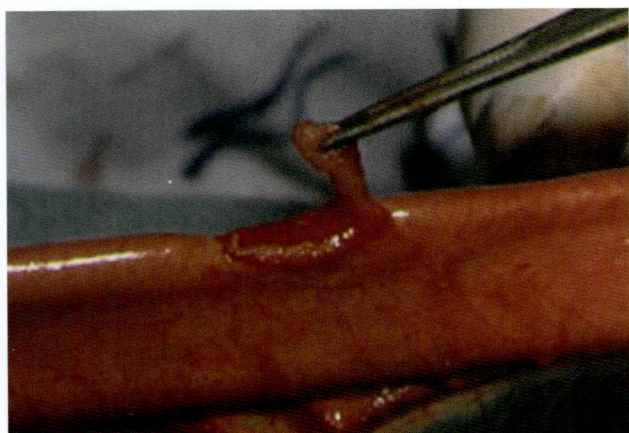

Figure 8.15 Jejunal biopsy taken from the antimesenteric border of the jejunum.

antimesenteric border and this was compared with sharp excision using a blade and Metzenbaum scissors. Both sites were closed using an appositional simple interrupted technique. The same clinical diagnosis was achieved in the two groups and although not statistically significant, use of the biopsy punch was generally faster. It has been suggested that closure of the biopsy site in a transverse orientation instead of a longitudinal orientation may result in less decrease in intestinal luminal diameter (Matz *et al.* 2014).

A minimally invasive technique for intestinal exploration and targeted biopsies using a wound retraction device has also been described as an effective way to obtain samples (Shamir *et al.* 2019). In a study that compared different access incisions along the linea alba for minimally invasive biopsy of various organs in cats, the optimal access location was found to be halfway between the umbilicus and caudal aspect of the xiphoid (Mayhew *et al.* 2014).

Leak testing

Leak testing of the enterotomy, biopsy, or resection and anastomosis suture line is commonly performed following the procedure to assess for any leakage of contents. This can be performed by milking intestinal contents away from the surgical site or isolating the intestinal segment and introducing a volume of sterile saline to distend the lumen. One study demonstrated that saline volumes of 16–19 mL with digital occlusion and 12–15 mL with Doyen occlusion were required to achieve a normal peristaltic pressure of approximately 34 cm of water (Saile *et al.* 2010). Although commonly performed, leak testing was not shown to be associated with a reduction in postoperative intestinal suture line

dehiscence with either handsewn or stapled anastomosis techniques in a 2021 study (Mullen *et al.* 2021).

Enteroplication

Enteroplication is performed by suturing adjacent loops of intestine to each other using absorbable or nonabsorbable suture midway between the mesenteric and antimesenteric surface and penetrating the submucosa (Figure 8.16). Enteroplication has been used in animals to reduce the recurrence of intussusception; however, statistically significant differences in outcome in patients that have enteroplication performed versus those that do not have not been demonstrated in the veterinary literature (Larose *et al.* 2020).

Postoperative care

Supportive care during the postoperative period is highly critical to a successful outcome. Dehydration and electrolyte and acid–base abnormalities are treated with intravenous crystalloid administration and the choice of fluid is based on the abnormalities present (Papazoglou *et al.* 2003). Colloids can be used in patients with a low colloid oncotic pressure. The plasma oncotic pressure is affected by albumin levels and the sequelae of a low plasma oncotic pressure may include fluid loss from the intravascular space, peripheral edema, and pleural effusion (Smiley & Garvey 1994). Colloids are effective in increasing plasma oncotic pressure and can be used for supportive treatment of patients with gastrointestinal foreign bodies (Smiley & Garvey 1994). Care should be taken, as coagulopathies can reportedly develop at higher doses (Smiley & Garvey 1994).

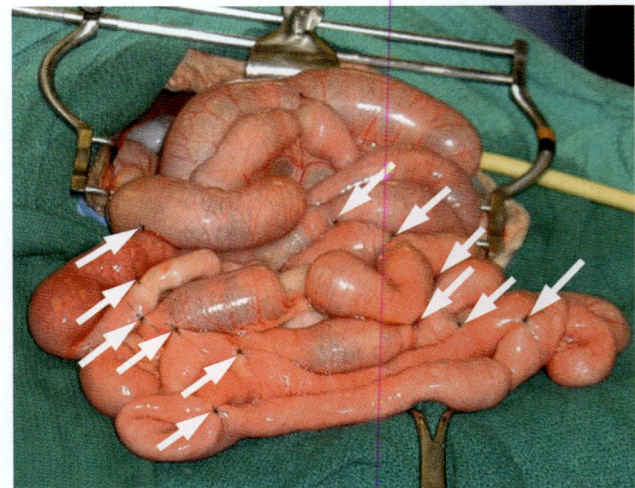

Figure 8.16 Enteroplication in a cat with an intussusception. Adjacent loops of intestine have been sutured to each other with simple interrupted sutures (white arrow) without penetrating the lumen.

Preoperative factors that have been shown to be associated with development of postoperative septic peritonitis following gastrointestinal surgery include preoperative hypoalbuminemia or hypoproteinemia, preoperative septic peritonitis, and intraoperative hypotension (Grimes *et al.* 2013). In patients with septic peritonitis, broad-spectrum intravenous antibiotic administration should be instituted empirically and should be targeted toward Gram-positive, Gram-negative, and anaerobic bacteria (Swann & Hughes 2000); culture results of the peritoneal effusion will ultimately guide the antibiotic choice. Appropriateness of initial antimicrobial choice has not been associated with treatment outcome in dogs in one study (Dickinson *et al.* 2015); however, a study in cats demonstrated that appropriate empirical antimicrobial choice improved survival (Scotti *et al.* 2019). Animals with septic peritonitis consistently develop hypoalbuminemia, but it was not found to affect survival in one study (King 1994), while others have demonstrated an association between hypoalbuminemia and failure to survive (Grimes *et al.* 2013). Canine-specific albumin may be a useful tool to combat severe hypoalbuminemia postoperatively, as it has been shown to improve serum albumin concentration, colloid osmotic pressure, and Doppler blood pressure postoperatively in patients that underwent surgery for septic peritonitis (Craft & Powell 2012). Additionally, management of septic peritonitis with open peritoneal drainage reportedly leads to hypoalbuminemia (Staatz *et al.* 2002). Refractory hypotension associated with septic peritonitis carries a poor prognosis (King 1994).

Nutrition is an important component of the postoperative recovery in dogs and cats with gastrointestinal obstruction. Enteral feeding should be instituted within 24 hours as long as the patient is not vomiting (Papazoglou *et al.* 2003). The benefits of enteral feeding in humans and animals include stimulation of mucosal growth, maintenance of gastrointestinal mucosal integrity, and decreased risk of bacterial translocation across the intestinal wall (Tara & Jacobs 1998; Swann & Hughes 2000). In addition, patients that receive early nutrition have been shown to have significantly shorter hospital stays. The same study did not find an association between hospitalization length and route of the nutrition provided, whether enteral or central parenteral nutrition (Liu *et al.* 2012).

In critically ill patients, a gastrojejunostomy feeding tube can be placed during surgery to provide enteral nutrition in the postoperative period (Cavanaugh *et al.* 2008). The reported complication rate is high, but most complications are minor and include erythema, cellulitis, and discharge at the stoma site, while mechanical tube complications are seen in 46% of cases (Cavanaugh *et al.* 2008).

Parenteral intravenous feeding via either total parenteral nutrition (TPN) or peripheral parenteral nutrition can be provided to critically ill patients that are anorexic or in patients with vomiting or regurgitation postoperatively (Reuter *et al.* 1998; Chandler & Payne-James 2006). Complications associated with TPN feeding include electrolyte abnormalities, hyperglycemia, and catheter-related sepsis (Reuter *et al.* 1998).

Expected postoperative ultrasonographic changes seen in dogs with uncomplicated enterotomy or enterectomy have been described (Matthews *et al.* 2008). Absent wall layering, improving generalized abdominal effusion, resolving pneumoperitoneum, and hyperechoic omental and mesenteric fat localized to the surgical site are normal changes associated with intestinal surgery (Matthews *et al.* 2008).

Surgical complications and outcome

Complications associated with gastrointestinal obstructions such as malabsorption, perforation and septic peritonitis, and postoperative dehiscence of the surgical site affect the prognosis and alter the postoperative course of patients undergoing surgery. Extensive resection can cause short bowel syndrome, with clinical signs including diarrhea, malabsorption, weight loss, and fluid and electrolyte abnormalities (Gorman *et al.* 2006). In one study, most dogs and cats tolerated a resection of 50% or more of the small intestine; 8 of 10 dogs and 4 of 5 cats were reported to have a good outcome. Clinical signs in dogs and cats associated with a poor outcome included weight loss and diarrhea (Gorman *et al.* 2006).

Septic peritonitis is diagnosed in 41% of dogs treated for a linear foreign body at the time of surgery, and this is associated with a significantly higher probability of death compared with dogs without peritonitis (Evans *et al.* 1994). Septic peritonitis was present in 16% of feline cases of linear foreign bodies (Felts *et al.* 1984). A mortality rate of 31% has been reported in animals with peritonitis associated with small and large intestinal surgery (Wylie & Hosgood 1994). Plasma lactate concentration and serial evaluation of plasma lactate have been studied as prognostic indicators in patients with septic peritonitis. One study demonstrated that an admission plasma lactate concentration >2.5 mmol/L was correlated with mortality. Additionally, inability to correct hyperlactatemia within 6 hours of presentation resulted in a sensitivity of 76% and specificity of 100% for mortality (Cortellini *et al.* 2015).

Reported dehiscence rates following surgery for gastrointestinal foreign body obstruction have been reported to range from 2% to 27.7% (Allen *et al.* 1992;

Weisman *et al.* 1999; Ralphs *et al.* 2003; Boag *et al.* 2005; Strelchik *et al.* 2019). The presence of an intestinal foreign body, septic peritonitis, and hypoalbuminemia of 2.5 g/dL or less have been identified as risk factors for anastomotic dehiscence (Ralphs *et al.* 2003). In a separate study, dogs that developed intestinal dehiscence had a much higher band neutrophil count postoperatively compared with dogs without dehiscence, and albumin levels were consistently lower in the dehiscence group compared with the nondehiscence group (Allen *et al.* 1992). Inflammatory bowel disease has also been associated with anastomotic dehiscence (Snowdon *et al.* 2016). Dogs with dehiscence of the surgical site have a reported mortality rate of 74–80% (Allen *et al.* 1992; Wylie & Hosgood 1994).

A study looking at complications following full-thickness small intestinal biopsy collection in dogs reported a dehiscence rate of 11% and there were no predictors for dehiscence identified (Shales *et al.* 2005). Another study looking specifically at complications in hypoalbuminemic dogs that underwent full-thickness gastrointestinal biopsy found no difference in complication rate in hypoalbuminemic dogs compared with dogs with a normal plasma albumin level (Harvey 1990). Dehiscence following full-thickness gastrointestinal surgery in cats with gastrointestinal lymphoma has been evaluated, with one study demonstrating no increased risk (Smith *et al.* 2011).

Reported complications following surgical correction of intussusception include recurrence, ileus, intestinal obstruction, intestinal strangulation, diarrhea, regurgitation, and peritonitis (Levitt & Bauer 1992; Applewhite *et al.* 2001a,b; Burkitt *et al.* 2009, Larose *et al.* 2020). The overall recurrence rate for dogs with intussusception ranges from 3% to 19% (Levitt & Bauer 1992; Oakes *et al.* 1994; Applewhite *et al.* 2001a; Larose *et al.* 2020). Intestinal obstruction secondary to enteroplication was observed in two dogs and the obstruction was located at the bend of the intestinal loop (Applewhite *et al.* 2001a). Severe ileus and subsequent death were reported in two of three cats that underwent enteroplication, but due to the overall low number of cats that underwent this procedure, conclusions cannot be drawn from these data (Burkitt *et al.* 2009). The reported short-term survival rate for cats with surgical treatment for intussusception ranges from 74% to 80% (Levitt & Bauer 1992; Burkitt *et al.* 2009).

The overall survival rate in one study of dogs and cats with focal gastrointestinal foreign body removal was 92% and 88%, respectively; a survival rate of 99% was reported for dogs in a separate study (Boag *et al.* 2005; Hayes 2009). Cats with linear foreign body obstruction have a reported survival rate between 63% and 100% (Felts *et al.* 1984; Basher & Fowler 1987; Hayes 2009) and the reported survival rate for dogs with linear foreign body obstruction is approximately 80% (Evans *et al.* 1994; Hayes 2009).

Conclusion

Dogs and cats with gastrointestinal focal and linear obstructions due to foreign body ingestion and intussusception represent challenging but common cases for veterinary surgeons. A thorough diagnostic work-up is important to maximize the treating clinician's ability to provide appropriate care. Prompt surgical intervention is warranted to minimize continued intestinal damage and compromise. Attentive postoperative management and monitoring for complications such as surgical dehiscence are critical for achieving clinical success.

References

Adams, W.M., Sisterman, L.A., Klauer, J.M. et al. (2010). Association of intestinal disorders in cats with findings of abdominal radiography. *Journal of the American Veterinary Medical Association* 236 (8): 880–886.

Adams, R.J., Doyle, R.S., Bray, J.P., and Burton, C.A. (2014). Closed suction drainage for treatment of septic peritonitis of confirmed gastrointestinal origin in 20 dogs. *Veterinary Surgery* 43 (7): 843–851.

Ahrenholz, D.H. (1979). Effect of intraperitoneal fluid on mortality of *Escherichia coli* peritonitis. *Surgical Forum* 30: 483–484.

Allen, D.A., Smeak, D.D., and Schertel, E.R. (1992). Prevalence of small intestinal dehiscence and associated clinical factors: a retrospective study of 121 dogs. *Journal of the American Animal Hospital Association* 28: 70–76.

Anderson, S., Lippincott, C.L., and Gill, P.J. (1992). Single enterotomy removal of gastrointestinal linear foreign bodies. *Journal of the American Animal Hospital Association* 28: 487–490.

Anderson, T., Beever, L., Hall, J. et al. (2021). Outcome following surgery to treat septic peritonitis in 95 cats in the United Kingdom. *Journal of Small Animal Practice* 62 (9): 744–749.

Applewhite, A.A., Cornell, K.K., and Selcer, B.A. (2001a). Pylorogastric intussusception in the dog: a case report and literature review. *Journal of the American Animal Hospital Association* 37: 238–243.

Applewhite, A.A., Hawthorne, J.C., and Cornell, K.K. (2001b). Complications of enteroplication for the prevention of intussusception recurrence in dogs: 35 cases (1989–1999). *Journal of the American Veterinary Medical Association* 219: 1415–1418.

Armbrust, L.J., Biller, D.S., and Hoskinson, J.J. (2000). Case examples demonstrating the clinical utility of obtaining both right and left lateral abdominal radiographs in small animals. *Journal of the American Animal Hospital Association* 36: 531–536.

Barrs, V.R., Beatty, J.A., Tisdall, P.L. et al. (1999). Intestinal obstruction of trichobezoars in five cats. *Journal of Feline Medicine and Surgery* 1: 199–207.

Barry, K.S., Case, J.B., Winter, M.D. et al. (2017). Diagnostic usefulness of laparoscopy versus exploratory laparotomy for dogs with suspected gastrointestinal obstruction. *Journal of the American Veterinary Medical Association* 251 (3): 307–314.

Basher, A.W.P. and Fowler, J.D. (1987). Conservative versus surgical management of gastrointestinal linear foreign bodies in the cat. *Veterinary Surgery* 16: 135–138.

Bebchuk, T.N. (2002). Feline gastrointestinal foreign bodies. *Veterinary Clinics of North America Small Animal Practice* 32: 861–880.

Bentley, A.M., Mayhew, P.D., Culp, W.T.N., and Otto, C.M. (2013). Alterations in the hemostatic profiles of dogs with naturally occurring septic peritonitis. *Journal of Veterinary Emergency and Critical Care* 23 (1): 14–22.

Bhandal, J., Kuzma, A., and Head, L. (2008). Cecal inversion followed by ileocolic intussusception in a cat. *Canadian Veterinary Journal* 49 (5): 483–484.

Boag, A.K., Coe, R.J., Martinez, T.A., and Hughes, D. (2005). Acid–base and electrolyte abnormalities in dogs with gastrointestinal foreign bodies. *Journal of Veterinary Internal Medicine* 19: 816–821.

Bonczynski, J.J., Ludwig, L.L., Barton, L.J. et al. (2003). Comparison of peritoneal fluid and peripheral blood pH, bicarbonate, glucose, and lactate concentration as a diagnostic tool for septic peritonitis in dogs and cats. *Veterinary Surgery* 32: 161–166.

Boysen, S.R., Tidwell, A.S., and Penninck, D.G. (2003). Ultrasonographic findings in dogs and cats with gastrointestinal perforation. *Veterinary Radiology and Ultrasound* 44: 556–564.

Brawner, W.R. Jr. and Bartels, J.E. (1983). Contrast radiography of the digestive tract. *Veterinary Clinics of North America Small Animal Practice* 13: 599–626.

Buote, N.J. and Havig, M.E. (2012). The use of vacuum-assisted closure in the management of septic peritonitis in six dogs. *Journal of the American Animal Hospital Association* 48 (3): 164–171.

Burkitt, J.M., Drobatz, K.J., Saunders, H.M., and Washabau, R.J. (2009). Signalment, history, and outcome of cats with gastrointestinal tract intussusception: 20 cases (1986–2000). *Journal of the American Veterinary Medical Association* 234: 771–776.

Carobbi, B., Foale, R.D., and White, R.A. (2009). Trichobezoar obstruction after stapled jejunal anastomosis in a dog. *Veterinary Surgery* 38: 417–420.

Case, J.B. and Ellison, G. (2013). Single incision laparoscopic-assisted intestinal surgery (SILAIS) in 7 dogs and 1 cat. *Veterinary Surgery* 42 (5): 629–634.

Cavanaugh, R.P., Kovak, J.R., Fischetti, A.J. et al. (2008). Evaluation of surgically placed gastrojejunostomy feeding tubes in critically ill dogs. *Journal of the American Veterinary Medical Association* 232: 380–388.

Chandler, M.L. and Payne-James, J.J. (2006). Prospective evaluation of a peripherally administered three-in-one parenteral nutrition product in dogs. *Journal of Small Animal Practice* 47: 518–523.

Ciasca, T.C., David, F.H., and Lamb, C.R. (2013). Does measurement of small intestinal diameter increase diagnostic accuracy of radiography in dogs with suspected intenstial obstruction? *Veterinary Radiology & Ultrasound* 54 (3): 207–211.

Cioffi, K.M., Schmiedt, C.W., Cornell, K.K., and Radlinsky, M.G. (2012). Retrospective evaluation of vacuum-assisted peritoneal drainage for the treatment of septic peritonitis in dogs and cats: 8 cases (2003–2010). *Journal of Veterinary Emergency and Critical Care* 22 (5): 601–609.

Coolman, B.R., Ehrhart, N., and Marretta, S.M. (2000a). Use of skin staples for rapid closure of gastrointestinal incisions in the treatment of canine linear foreign bodies. *Journal of the American Animal Hospital Association* 36: 542–547.

Coolman, B.R., Ehrhart, N., Pijanowski, G. et al. (2000b). Comparison of skin staples with sutures for anastomosis of the small intestine in dogs. *Veterinary Surgery* 29: 293–302.

Cortellini, S., Seth, M., and Kellett-Gregory, L.M. (2015). Plasma lactate concentrations in septic peritonitis: a retrospective study of 83 dogs (2007–2012). *Journal of Veterinary Emergency and Critical Care* 25 (3): 388–395.

Costello, M.F., Drobatz, K.J., Aronson, L.R., and King, L.G. (2004). Underlying cause, pathophysiologic abnormalities and response to treatment in cats with septic peritonitis: 51 cases (1990–2001). *Journal of the American Veterinary Medical Association* 225: 897–902.

Coulier, B., Tancredi, M.H., and Ramboux, A. (2004). Spiral CT and multidetector-row CT diagnosis of perforation of the small intestine caused by ingested foreign bodies. *European Radiology* 14: 1918–1925.

Craft, E.M. and Powell, L.L. (2012). The use of canine-specific albumin in dogs with septic peritonitis. *Journal of Veterinary Emergency and Critical Care* 22 (6): 631–639.

Davis, D.J., Demianiuk, R.M., Musser, J. et al. (2018). Influence of pre-operative septic peritonitis and anastomotic technique on the dehiscence of enterectomy sites in dogs: a retrospective review of 210 anastomoses. *Veterinary Surgery* 47 (1): 125–129.

Dickinson, A.E., Summers, J.F., Wignal, J. et al. (2015). Impact of appropriate empirical antimicrobial therapy on outcome of dogs with septic peritonitis. *Journal of Veterinary Emergency and Critical Care* 25 (1): 152–159.

Elser, E.B., Mai, W., Reetz, J.A. et al. (2020). Serial abdominal radiographs do not significantly increase accuracy of diagnosis of gastrointestinal mechanical obstruction due to occult foreign bodies in dogs and cats. *Veterinary Radiology & Ultrasound* 61 (4): 399–408.

Evans, K.L., Smeak, D.D., and Biller, D.S. (1994). Gastrointestinal linear foreign bodies in 32 dogs: a retrospective evaluation and feline comparison. *Journal of the American Animal Hospital Association* 30: 445–450.

Felts, J.F., Fox, P.R., and Burk, R.L. (1984). Thread and sewing needles as gastrointestinal foreign bodies in the cat: a review of 64 cases. *Journal of the American Veterinary Medical Association* 184: 56–59.

Finck, C., D'anjou, M.-A., Alexander, K. et al. (2014). Radiographic diagnosis of mechanical obstruction in dogs based on relative small intestinal external diameters. *Veterinary Radiology and Ultrasound* 55 (5): 472–479.

Frager, D., Medwid, S.W., Baer, J.W. et al. (1994). CT of small-bowel obstruction: value in establishing the diagnosis and determining the degree and cause. *American Journal of Roentgenology* 162: 37–41.

Gianella, P., Pfammatter, N.S., and Burgener, I.A. (2009). Oesophageal and gastric endoscopic foreign body removal: complications and follow-up of 102 dogs. *Journal of Small Animal Practice* 50: 649–654.

Gibson, E.A., Culp, W., Mayhew, P. et al. (2020). Laparoscopic-assisted gastrotomy for foreign body retrieval in four dogs. *Veterinary Record Case Reports* 8: e000966.

Gorman, S.C., Freeman, L.M., Mitchell, S.L., and Chan, D.L. (2006). Extensive small bowel resection in dogs and cats: 20 cases (1998–2004). *Journal of the American Veterinary Medical Association* 228: 403–407.

Gower, S.B. and Mayhew, P.D. (2011). A wound retraction device for laparoscopic-assisted intestinal surgery in dogs and cats. *Veterinary Surgery* 40 (4): 485–488.

Graham, J.P., Lord, P.F., and Harrison, J.M. (1998). Quantitative estimation of intestinal dilation as a predictor of obstruction in the dog. *Journal of Small Animal Practice* 39: 521–524.

Grimes, J., Schmiedt, C., Milovancev, M. et al. (2013). Efficacy of serosal patching in dogs with septic peritonitis. *Journal of the American Animal Hospital Association* 49 (4): 246–249.

Harvey, H.J. (1990). Complications of small intestinal biopsy in hypo-albuminemic dogs. *Veterinary Surgery* 19: 289–292.

Hauptman, J.G., Walshaw, R., and Olivier, N.B. (1997). Evaluation of the sensitivity and specificity of diagnostic criteria for sepsis in dogs. *Veterinary Surgery* 26: 393–397.

Hayes, G. (2009). Gastrointestinal foreign bodies in dogs and cats: a retrospective study of 208 cases. *Journal of Small Animal Practice* 50: 576–583.

Hobday, M.M., Pachtinger, G.E., Drobatz, K.J., and Syring, R.S. (2014). Linear versus non-linear gastrointestinal foreign bodies in 499 dogs: clinical presentation, management and short-term outcome. *Journal of Small Animal Practice* 55 (11): 560–565.

Jardel, N., Hidalgo, A., Leperlier, D. et al. (2011). One stage functional end-to-end stapled intestinal anastomosis and resection performed by nonexpert surgeons for the treatment of small intestinal obstruction in 30 dogs. *Veterinary Surgery* 40 (2): 216–222.

Keats, M.M., Weeren, R., Greenlee, P. et al. (2004). Investigation of Keyes skin biopsy instrument for intestinal biopsy versus a standard biopsy technique. *Journal of the American Animal Hospital Association* 40: 405–410.

Kim, J.H., Ha, H.K., Sohn, M.J. et al. (2000). Usefulness of MR imaging for diseases of the small intestine: comparison with CT. *Korean Journal of Radiology* 1: 43–50.

King, L.G. (1994). Postoperative complications and prognostic indicators in dogs and cats with septic peritonitis: 23 cases (1989–1992). *Journal of the American Veterinary Medical Association* 204: 407–414.

Klinger, M., Cooper, J., and McCabe, R. (1990). The use of butorphanol tartrate for the prevention of canine intussusception following renal transplantation. *Journal of Investigative Surgery* 3: 229–233.

Ko, J.J. and Mann, F.A. (2014). Barium peritonitis in small animals. *Journal of Veterinary Medical Science* 76 (5): 621–628.

Larose, P.C., Singh, A., Giuffrida, M.A. et al. (2020). Clinical findings and outcomes of 153 dogs surgically treated for intestinal intussusceptions. *Veterinary Surgery* 49 (5): 870–878.

Levin, G.M., Bonczynski, J.J., Ludwig, L.L. et al. (2004). Lactate as a diagnostic test for septic peritoneal effusions in dogs and cats. *Journal of the American Animal Hospital Association* 40: 364–371.

Levitt, L. and Bauer, M.S. (1992). Intussusception in dogs and cats: a review of thirty-six cases. *Canadian Veterinary Journal* 33: 660–664.

Liu, D.T., Brown, D.C., and Silverstein, D.C. (2012). Early nutritional support is associated with decreased length of hospitalization in dogs with septic peritonitis: a retrospective study of 45 cases (2000–2009). *Journal of Veterinary Emergency and Critical Care* 22 (4): 453–459.

MacPhail, C. (2002). Gastrointestinal obstruction. *Clinical Techniques in Small Animal Practice* 17: 178–183.

Madl, C. and Druml, W. (2003). Systemic consequences of ileus. *Best Practice and Research in Clinical Gastroenterology* 17 (3): 445–456.

Maglinte, D.D., Reyes, B.L., Harmon, B.H. et al. (1996). Reliability and role of plain film radiography and CT in the diagnosis of small-bowel obstruction. *American Journal of Roentgenology* 167: 1451–1455.

Marshall, H., Sinnott-Stutzman, V., Ewing, P. et al. (2019). Effect of peritoneal lavage on bacterial isolates in 40 dogs with confirmed septic peritonitis. *Journal of Veterinary Emergency and Critical Care* 29 (6): 635–642.

Matthews, A.R., Penninck, D.G., and Webster, C.R.L. (2008). Postoperative ultrasonographic appearance of uncomplicated enterotomy or enterectomy sites in dogs. *Veterinary Radiology and Ultrasound* 49: 477–483.

Matz, B.M., Boothe, H.W., Wright, J.C., and Boothe, D.M. (2014). Effect of enteric biopsy closure orientation on enteric circumference and volume of saline needed for leak testing. *Canadian Veterinary Journal* 55 (1): 1255–1257.

Mayhew, P.D., Mayhew, K.N., Shilo-Benjamini, Y. et al. (2014). Prospective evaluation of access incision position for minimally invasive surgical organ exposure in cats. *Journal of the American Veterinary Medical Association* 245 (10): 1129–1134.

McAnulty, J.F., Southard, J.H., and Belzer, F.O. (1989). Prevention of postoperative intestinal intussusception by prophylactic morphine administration in dogs used for organ transplantation. *Surgery* 105: 494–495.

Milovancev, M., Weisman, D.L., and Palmisano, M.P. (2004). Foreign body attachment to polypropylene suture material extruded into the small intestinal lumen after enteric closure in three dogs. *Journal of the American Veterinary Medical Association* 225: 1713–1715.

Miniter, B.M., Arruda, A.G., Zuckerman, J. et al. (2019). Use of computed tomography (CT) for the diagnosis of mechanical gastrointestinal obstruction in canines and felines. *PLOS ONE* 14 (8): e0219748.

Mishra, N.K., Appert, H.E., and Howard, J.M. (1974). The effects of distention and obstruction on the accumulation of fluid in the lumen of small bowel of dogs. *Annals of Surgery* 180: 791–795.

Mouat, E.E., Davis, G.J., Drobatz, K.J., and Wallace, K.A. (2014). Evaluation of data from 35 dogs pertaining to dehiscence following intestinal resection and anastomosis. *Journal of the American Animal Hospital Association* 50 (4): 254–263.

Mueller, M.G., Ludwig, L.L., and Barton, L.J. (2001). Use of closed-suction drains to treat generalized peritonitis in dogs and cats: 40 cases (1997–1999). *Journal of the American Veterinary Medical Association* 219: 789–794.

Mullen, K.M., Regier, P.J., Fox-Alvarez, W.A. et al. (2021). Evaluation of intraoperative leak testing of small intestinal anastomoses performed by hand-sewn and stapled techniques in dogs: 131 cases (2008–2019). *Journal of the American Veterinary Medical Association* 258 (9): 991–998.

Oakes, M.G., Lewis, D.D., Hosgood, G., and Beale, B.S. (1994). Enteroplication for the prevention of intussusception recurrence in dogs: 31 cases (1978–1992). *Journal of the American Veterinary Medical Association* 205: 72–75.

Osterbur, K., Mann, F.A., Kuroki, K., and Declue, A. (2014). Multiple organ dysfunction syndrome in humans and animals. *Journal of Veterinary Internal Medicine* 28 (4): 1141–1151.

Otomo, A., Singh, A., Valverde, A. et al. (2019). Comparison of outcome in dogs undergoing single-incision laparoscopic-assisted intestinal surgery and open laparotomy for simple small intestinal foreign body removal. *Veterinary Surgery* 48 (S1): O83–O90.

Paley, M.R. and Ros, P.R. (1997). MRI of the gastrointestinal tract. *European Radiology* 7: 1387–1397.

Papanicolaou, G., Nikas, D., Ahn, Y. et al. (1985). Regional blood flow and water content of the obstructed small intestine. *Archives of Surgery* 120: 926–932.

Papazoglou, L.G., Patsikas, M.N., and Rallis, T. (2003). Intestinal foreign bodies in dogs and cats. *Compendium on Continuing Education for the Practicing Veterinarian* 25: 830–843.

Papazoglou, L.G., Diakou, A., Patsikas, M.N. et al. (2006). Intestinal pleating associated with Joyeuxiella pasqualei infection in a cat. *Veterinary Record* 159 (19): 634–635.

Patsikas, M.N., Papazoglou, L.G., Papaioannou, N.G. et al. (2003). Ultrasonographic findings of intestinal intussusception in seven cats. *Journal of Feline Medicine and Surgery* 5: 335–343.

Patsikas, M.N., Papazoglou, L.G., Papaioannou, N.G., and Dessiris, A.K. (2004). Normal and abnormal ultrasonographic findings that mimic small intestinal intussusception in the dog. *Journal of the American Animal Hospital Association* 40: 147–151.

Patsikas, M.N., Papazoglou, L.G., Jakovljevic, S., and Dessiris, A.K. (2005). Color Doppler ultrasonography in prediction of the reducibility of intussuscepted bowel in 15 young dogs. *Veterinary Radiology and Ultrasound* 46: 313–316.

Patsikas, M.N., Papazoglou, L.G., and Adamama-Moraitou, K.K. (2008). Spontaneous reduction of intestinal intussusception in five young dogs. *Journal of the American Animal Hospital Association* 44: 41–47.

Pratt, C.L., Reineke, E.L., and Drobatz, K.J. (2014). Sewing needle foreign body ingestion in dogs and cats: 65 cases (2000–2012). *Journal of the American Veterinary Medical Association* 245 (3): 302–308.

Prihoda, M., Flatt, A., and Summers, R.W. (1984). Mechanisms of motility changes during acute intestinal obstruction in the dog. *American Journal of Physiology* 247: G37–G42.

Ralphs, S.C., Jessen, C.R., and Lipowitz, A.J. (2003). Risk factors for leakage following intestinal anastomosis in dogs and cats: 115 cases (1991–2000). *Journal of the American Veterinary Medical Association* 223: 73–77.

Reuter, J.D., Marks, S.L., Rogers, Q.R., and Farver, T.B. (1998). Use of total parenteral nutrition in dogs: 209 cases (1988–1995). *Journal of Veterinary Emergency and Critical Care* 8: 201–213.

Saile, K., Boothe, H.W., and Boothe, D.M. (2010). Saline volume necessary to achieve predetermined intraluminal pressures during leak testing of small intestinal biopsy sites in the dog. *Veterinary Surgery* 39 (7): 900–903.

Scotti, K.M., Koenigshof, A., Sri-Jayantha, L.S.H. et al. (2019). Prognostic indicators in cats with septic peritonitis (2002–2015): 83 cases. *Journal of Veterinary Emergency and Critical Care* 29 (6): 647–652.

Shales, C.J., Warren, J., Anderson, D.M. et al. (2005). Complications following full-thickness small intestinal biopsy in 66 dogs: a retrospective study. *Journal of Small Animal Practice* 46: 317–321.

Shamir, S.K., Singh, A., Mayhew, P.D. et al. (2019). Evaluation of minimally invasive small intestinal exploration and targeted abdominal organ biopsy with use of a wound retraction device in dogs: 27 cases (2010–2017). *Journal of the American Veterinary Medical Association* 255 (1): 78–84.

Sharma, A., Thompson, M.S., Scrivani, P.V. et al. (2011). Comparison of radiography and ultrasonography for diagnosing small-intestinal mechanical obstruction in vomiting dogs. *Veterinary Radiology & Ultrasound* 52 (3): 248–255.

Smelstoys, J.A., Davis, G.J., Learn, A.E. et al. (2004). Outcome of and prognostic indicators for dogs and cats with pneumoperitoneum and no history of penetrating trauma: 54 cases (1988–2002). *Journal of the American Veterinary Medical Association* 225: 251–255.

Smiley, L.E. and Garvey, M.S. (1994). The use of hetastarch as adjunct therapy in 26 dogs with hypoalbuminemia: a phase two clinical trial. *Journal of Veterinary Internal Medicine* 8: 195–202.

Smith, A.L., Wilson, A.P., Hardie, R.J. et al. (2011). Perioperative complications after full-thickness gastrointestinal surgery in cats with alimentary lymphoma. *Veterinary Surgery* 40: 849–852.

Snowdon, K.A., Smeak, D.D., and Chiang, S. (2016). Risk factors for dehiscence of stapled functional end-to-end intestinal anastomoses in dogs: 53 cases (2001–2012). *Veterinary Surgery* 45: 91–99.

Spillebeen, A.L., Robben, J.H., Thomas, R. et al. (2017). Negative pressure therapy versus passive open abdominal drainage for the treatment of septic peritonitis in dogs: a randomized, prospective study. *Veterinary Surgery* 46 (8): 1086–1097.

Staatz, A.J., Monnet, E., and Seim, H.B. (2002). Open peritoneal drainage versus primary closure for the treatment of septic peritonitis in dogs and cats: 42 cases (1993–1999). *Veterinary Surgery* 31: 174–180.

Strelchik, A., Coleman, M.C., Scharf, V.F. et al. (2019). Intestinal incisional dehiscence rate following enterotomy for foreign body removal in 247 dogs. *Journal of the American Veterinary Medical Association* 255 (6): 695–699.

Summers, R.W., Yanda, R., Prihoda, M., and Flatt, A. (1983). Acute intestinal obstruction: an electromyographic study in dogs. *Gastroenterology* 85: 1301–1306.

Sumner, S.M., Regier, P.J., Case, J.B., and Ellison, G.W. (2019). Evaluation of suture reinforcement for stapled intestinal anastomoses: 77 dogs (2008–2018). *Veterinary Surgery* 48 (7): 1188–1193.

Swann, A. and Hughes, D. (2000). Diagnosis and management of peritonitis. *Veterinary Clinics of North America Small Animal Practice* 30: 603–615.

Szabo, S.D., Jermyn, K., Neel, J., and Mathews, K.G. (2011). Evaluation of postceliotomy peritoneal drain fluid volume, cytology, and blood-to-peritoneal fluid lactate and glucose differences in normal dogs. *Veterinary Surgery* 40 (4): 444–449.

Tara, T.M. and Jacobs, D.O. (1998). Effect of critical illness and nutritional support on mucosal mass and function. *Clinical Nutrition* 17: 99–105.

Tidwell, A.S. and Penninck, D.G. (1992). Ultrasonography of gastrointestinal foreign bodies. *Veterinary Radiology and Ultrasound* 33: 160–169.

Tobias, K.M. (2007). Surgical stapling devices in veterinary medicine: a review. *Veterinary Surgery* 36: 341–349.

Tyrell, D. and Beck, C. (2006). Survey of the use of radiography vs. ultrasonography in the investigation of gastrointestinal foreign bodies in small animals. *Veterinary Radiology and Ultrasound* 47: 404–408.

Tzimtzimis, E., Kouki, M., Rampidi, S. et al. (2016). Successful management of jejunojejunal anastomosis dehiscence by extra-abdominal exteriorization and bandaging in a cat with septic peritonitis. *Canadian Veterinary Journal* 57 (5): 507–510.

Weisman, D.L., Smeak, D.D., Birchard, S.J., and Zweigart, S.L. (1999). Comparison of a continuous suture pattern with a simple interrupted pattern for enteric closure in dogs and cats: 83 cases (1991–1997). *Journal of the American Veterinary Medical Association* 214: 1507–1510.

Williams, J., Biller, D.S., Myer, C.W. et al. (1993). Use of iohexol as a gastrointestinal contrast agent in three dogs, five cats and one bird. *Journal of the American Veterinary Medical Association* 202: 624–627.

Wilson, G.P. and Burt, J.K. (1974). Intussusception in the dog and cat: a review of 45 cases. *Journal of the American Veterinary Medical Association* 164: 515–518.

Winter, M.D., Barry, K.S., Johnson, M.D. et al. (2017). Ultrasonographic and computed tomographic characterization and localization of suspected mechanical gastrointestinal obstruction in dogs. *Journal of the American Veterinary Medical Association* 251 (3): 315–321.

Wylie, K.B. and Hosgood, G. (1994). Mortality and morbidity of small and large intestinal surgery in dogs and cats: 74 cases (1980–1992). *Journal of the American Animal Hospital Association* 30: 469–474.

Zissin, R., Osadchy, A., and Gayer, G. (2009). Abdominal CT findings in small bowel perforation. *British Journal of Radiology* 82: 162–171.

9

Mesenteric Volvulus and Colonic Torsion

Catriona M. MacPhail

Mesenteric volvulus is a rare but often fatal condition in dogs. It occurs when the small intestine twists around the mesenteric axis, resulting in a strangulating obstruction. This is in contrast to when the small intestine twists along the long axis, resulting in an intestinal torsion. There are only isolated case reports of mesenteric volvulus in cats (Knell *et al*. 2010). Volvulus and torsion of the colon are even less common conditions.

Mesenteric volvulus

Pathophysiology

Mesenteric volvulus is thought to be an uncommon condition in small animals due to short mesenteric attachments. When there is abnormal twisting of the intestine around the root, a series of significant consequences occurs. The volvulus may be partial (incomplete) or complete. When the volvulus is complete, venous obstruction occurs first and results in edema and vascular congestion of the intestinal wall, disruption of peristalsis, and tissue anoxia. Fluid and gas begin to accumulate within the lumen, resulting in rapid intestinal distension. Sloughing of the mucosal epithelium follows and blood begins accumulating in the intestinal lumen and may extravasate into the peritoneal cavity. Within several hours, the intestine reaches maximal distension and full-thickness disintegration of the intestinal wall occurs (Figure 9.1). With complete arterial occlusion, branches of the cranial mesenteric artery are affected, causing ischemic necrosis of the distal duodenum, jejunum, ileum, cecum, ascending colon, transverse colon, and proximal descending colon. Significant bacterial proliferation with endotoxin and exotoxin production also occurs, contributing to hypovolemic shock and sepsis and ultimately resulting in death.

Etiology

No identifiable cause of mesenteric volvulus has been recognized in dogs, although there is often an association with other gastrointestinal conditions. Such conditions include, but are not limited to, exocrine pancreatic insufficiency, inflammatory bowel disease, gastrointestinal foreign bodies, recent gastrointestinal surgery, ileocolic carcinoma, blunt abdominal trauma, and gastric dilatation-volvulus syndrome. In military working dogs, identified risk factors for mesenteric volvulus include German shepherd dog breed, increasing age, and history of gastrointestinal disease, prophylactic gastropexy, or abdominal surgery (Andrews *et al*. 2018).

Intestinal volvulus in humans is uncommon and is mostly associated with infants (midgut volvulus) due to congenital intestinal malrotation. Intestinal volvulus in adults may be primary (associated with a normal abdominal cavity) or secondary due to adhesions, tumors, or diverticula (Huang *et al*. 2005).

Diagnosis

Mesenteric volvulus most commonly occurs in young male large-breed dogs. German shepherd dogs are overly represented, but other sporting or working breeds have been reported (e.g., English pointers). Dogs with mesenteric volvulus typically present with peracute abdominal pain, retching, vomiting, hematochezia, weakness, and/or recumbency. Chronic partial mesenteric volvulus associated with intermittent vomiting and diarrhea has been reported in one dog (Spevakow *et al*. 2010).

Small Animal Soft Tissue Surgery, Second Edition. Edited by Eric Monnet.
© 2023 John Wiley & Sons, Inc. Published 2023 by John Wiley & Sons, Inc.
Companion website: www.wiley.com/go/monnet/small

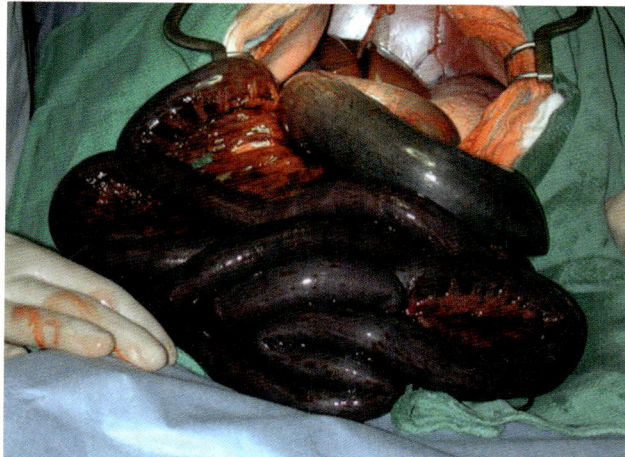

Figure 9.1 Mesenteric volvulus with severe ischemia of the entire jejunum in a 6-year-old German shepherd dog.

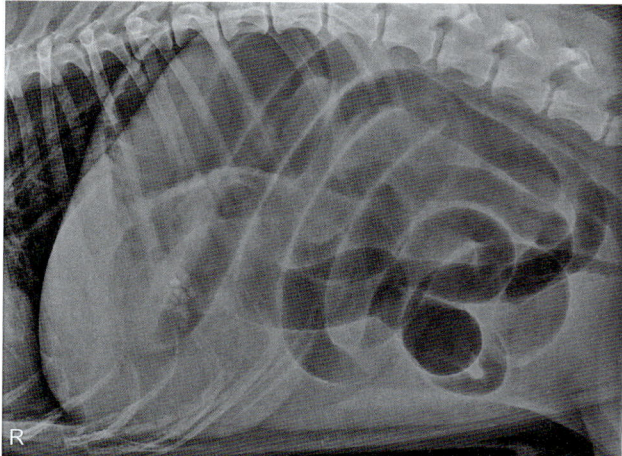

Figure 9.2 Lateral abdominal radiograph of a dog with mesenteric volvulus. Multiple loops of intestine are severely dilated.

Physical examination reveals evidence of shock (tachycardia, weak peripheral pulses, slow capillary refill time, and pale or injected mucous membranes) and sharp pain on abdominal palpation. Dogs may have varying degrees of abdominal distension that is not relieved by orogastric intubation.

Plain abdominal radiographs are often diagnostic as there is extensive uniform distension of the intestinal tract (Figure 9.2). The stomach and colon are typically in a normal position and not distended with gas. Generalized loss of serosal detail due to free abdominal fluid may also be present.

Laboratory findings are fairly nonspecific, but may include leukocytosis, hypoalbuminemia, and hypokalemia. Retrieval of free abdominal fluid may reveal a transudate associated with venous and lymphatic congestion, a serosanguineous modified transudate due to

acute vascular insult, or a septic suppurative exudate due to disruption of the mucosal barrier and translocation of bacteria.

Treatment

Mesenteric volvulus is a surgical emergency. Immediate recognition and diagnosis are critical for survival and surgery should not be delayed. In preparation of the animal for surgery, aggressive therapy of hypovolemic shock and electrolyte and acid–base abnormalities should be instituted. A central venous catheter is placed in a jugular vein and crystalloid and/or colloid fluids are administered rapidly. Central venous pressure can be monitored to avoid volume overload. Broad-spectrum antimicrobials (e.g., ampicillin plus enrofloxacin) should also be administered.

The goal of surgery is to confirm the diagnosis and quickly identify the direction of the mesenteric twist. The intestines are derotated and given time to reperfuse. A complete abdominal exploratory is then performed, evaluating for intestinal viability. Subjective criteria of intestinal viability include intestinal color, intestinal wall texture, arterial pulsations, and peristalsis. Assessment of viability may be difficult, particularly when the entire small intestine is affected, as with mesenteric volvulus. Objective means of viability assessment are available, but are not often used clinically. When resection is performed, it is typically extensive and short bowel syndrome is a possible postoperative complication.

Prognosis

The prognosis for dogs with mesenteric volvulus is uniformly poor. Early studies report close to 100% mortality (Westermarck & Rimaila-Pärnänen 1989; Nemzek et al. 1993; Cairó et al. 1999). More recent studies report improved outcomes, with a 42% survival rate (Junius et al. 2004). Reasons for reduced mortality are thought to be early surgical intervention, cases of partial torsion, and breed variety. Nearly all reported cases of mesenteric volvulus in German shepherd dogs have resulted in death.

Colonic torsion/volvulus

The terms volvulus and torsion are often used interchangeably or in combination when describing twisting of the large intestine. By definition, volvulus is rotation of viscera around its mesenteric attachment (e.g., gastric dilatation-volvulus syndrome), while torsion is rotation of viscera around its long axis (e.g., splenic torsion).

Pathophysiology

The most typical colonic displacement involves the descending colon shifting to the right, with focal narrowing at the distal descending colon (Figure 9.3).

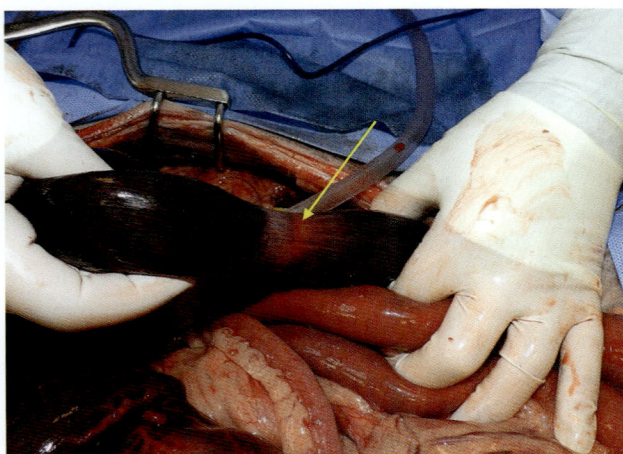

Figure 9.3 Intraoperative photograph of an 8-year-old male Alaskan malamute with a colonic torsion following derotation, showing site of counterclockwise twist in the descending colon (arrow).

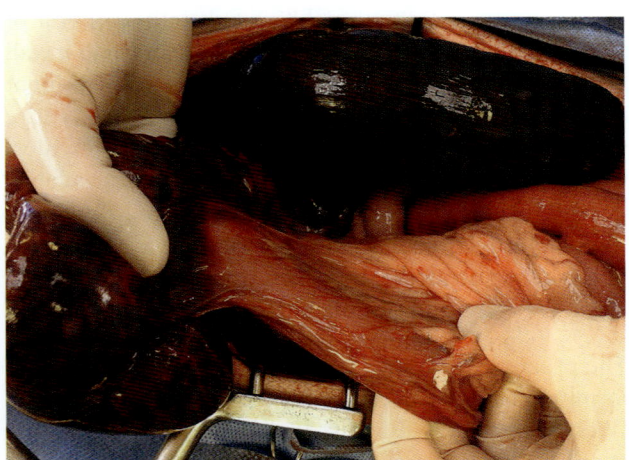

Figure 9.4 Intraoperative photograph of the same dog as in Figure 9.3 demonstrating complete devitalization of the cecum and the ascending, transverse, and descending colon, with blood supply to the small intestine preserved.

The cecum is displaced to the left. The degree of rotation can be 180° to 360° with or without involvement of the ileocecal segment (Figure 9.4) (Plavec *et al.* 2017).

Etiology

There is no known etiology of colonic torsion. Like mesenteric volvulus, cases of colonic torsion have been reported in dogs with concurrent gastrointestinal disease or previous history of a therapeutic or elective gastropexy.

Diagnosis

Like dogs with mesenteric volvulus, dogs with colonic torsion tend to be male, large-breed dogs, but approaching

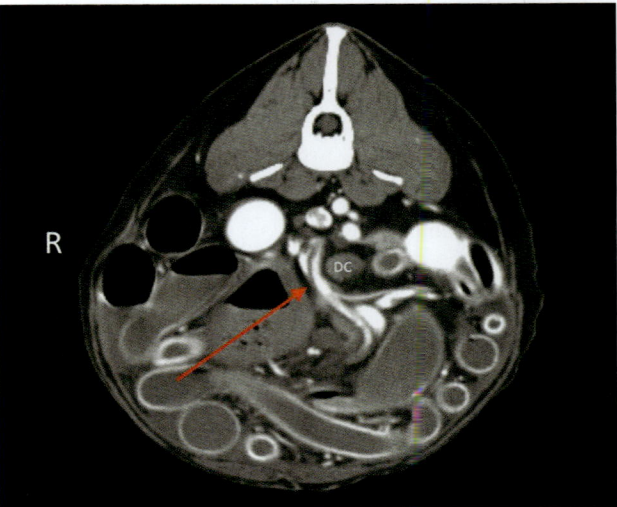

Figure 9.5 Computed tomographic transverse section of a dog with colonic volvulus demonstrating the whirl sign (arrow). DC, descending colon.

middle age (~6–7 years old). Clinical signs include vomiting, lethargy, tenesmus, diarrhea, and hematochezia.

Abdominal radiographs demonstrate severe segmental distension and malpositioning of the descending colon from left to right. Barium enemas may show helical striations in the distal descending colon, known as the "torsion" sign (Gremillion *et al.* 2018). Computed tomographic findings not seen on radiographs include distension of mesenteric vasculature and the "whirl" sign, spiral path of the rotated viscera, and blood supply (Figure 9.5) (Barge *et al.* 2020). In colonic torsion, this occurs in the distal descending colon in a counterclockwise direction.

Treatment

Immediate surgical intervention is indicated when colonic displacement is recognized. The large intestine is rotated clockwise from the right to left side of the abdomen. If the bowel is or becomes viable, a left-sided colopexy of the descending colon is performed. Matching longitudinal incisions are made in the seromuscular layer of the left lateral wall of the colon and in through the peritoneum and into the transversus abdominus of the left abdominal wall. The incisions are sutured together using a 2-0 or 3-0 standard absorbable monofilament suture (e.g., PDS®, Ethicon, Raritan, NJ, USA) without entering the lumen of the colon. If the large intestine is not viable, ileorectal resection and anastomosis can be considered.

Prognosis

Short-term survival was reported in 10 of 13 dogs (77%) with either colonic or ileocecocolic volvulus (Plavec *et al.* 2017).

References

Andrews, S.J., Thomas, T.M., Hauptman, J.G., and Stanley, B.J. (2018). Investigation of potential risk factors for mesenteric volvulus in military working dogs. *Journal of the American Veterinary Medical Association* 253: 877–885.

Barge, P., Fina, C.J., Mortier, J.R., and Jones, I.D. (2020). CT findings in five dogs with surgically confirmed colonic torsion. *Veterinary Radiology & Ultrasound* 61: 190–196.

Cairó, J., Font, J., Gorraiz, J. et al. (1999). Intestinal volvulus in dogs: a study of four clinical cases. *Journal of Small Animal Practice* 40: 136–140.

Gremillion, C.L., Savage, M., and Cohen, E.B. (2018). Radiographic findings and clinical factors in dogs with surgically confirmed or presumed colonic torsion. *Veterinary Radiology & Ultrasound* 59: 272–278.

Huang, J.C., Shin, J.S., Huang, Y.T. et al. (2005). Small bowel volvulus among adults. *Journal of Gastroenterology and Hepatology* 20: 1906–1912.

Junius, G., Appeldoorn, A.M., and Schrauwen, E. (2004). Mesenteric volvulus in the dog: a retrospective study of 12 cases. *Journal of Small Animal Practice* 45: 104–107.

Knell, S.C., Andreoni, A.A., Dennler, M., and Venzin, C.M. (2010). Successful treatment of small intestinal volvulus in two cats. *Journal of Feline Medicine and Surgery* 12: 874–877.

Nemzek, J.A., Walshaw, R., and Hauptman, J.G. (1993). Mesenteric volvulus in the dog: a retrospective study. *Journal of the American Animal Hospital Association* 29: 357–362.

Plavec, T., Rupp, S., and Kessler, M. (2017). Colonic or ileocecocolic volvulus in 13 dogs (2005–2016). *Veterinary Surgery* 46: 851–859.

Spevakow, A.B., Nibblett, B.M., Carr, A.P., and Linn, K.A. (2010). Chronic mesenteric volvulus in a dog. *Canadian Veterinary Journal* 51: 85–88.

Westermarck, E. and Rimaila-Pärnänen, E. (1989). Mesenteric torsion in dogs with exocrine pancreatic insufficiency: 21 cases (1978–1987). *Journal of the American Veterinary Medical Association* 195: 1404–1494.

10

Gastrointestinal Neoplasia

Deanna R. Worley

One of the challenges of veterinary oncology is determining optimal treatment recommendations and prognosis for an affected patient despite the limited numbers of robust clinical trials and plethora of small case reports. The goal of this chapter is to provide a synopsis of insights from the recent literature with particular focus on more commonly occurring tumor types. Attention will focus on neoplasia of the stomach, small intestine, large intestine, and exocrine pancreas. Primary neoplasia affecting the alimentary tract cranial to the stomach and the liver is addressed in other sections.

Tumors of the stomach, small intestine, colon, and rectum

In general, gastrointestinal neoplasia occurs rarely in the dog and cat. Adenocarcinoma is the more commonly occurring tumor in the dog stomach (Swann & Holt 2002; Eisele *et al.* 2010), while lymphoma is the more common feline gastric neoplasia. Other tumors commonly affecting the stomach include leiomyoma, leiomyosarcoma, mast cell tumor, extramedullary plasmacytoma, fibrosarcoma, and gastrointestinal stromal tumor (GIST), though this is not an exclusive list. Lymphoma is also the more commonly occurring feline intestinal neoplasia, with lymphoma or adenocarcinoma being the more commonly occurring canine intestinal tumor (Rissetto *et al.* 2011). In the intestines, leiomyosarcoma, GIST, mast cell tumor, carcinoids (arising from the diffuse endocrine system), and others are tumor types that can also occur. The various tumor histotypes that can affect the gastrointestinal tract arise from any of the multiple diverse normally occurring cells.

Pathology

Feline

Lymphoma is the most commonly occurring neoplasia in cats, the gastrointestinal tract being a common site of feline lymphoma (Grover 2005). It typically occurs in older cats, with a median age of diagnosis of 9–13 years. The cecum and colon are rarely affected. Surgery is indicated for obtaining a diagnosis or when obstruction or perforation is present. There is low risk of postoperative dehiscence following full-thickness gastrointestinal biopsies in cats having gastrointestinal lymphoma, even with concurrent hypoalbuminemia (Smith *et al.* 2011). Following surgery, initiation of chemotherapy is typically delayed by 10–14 days. For cats experiencing a poor appetite, parenteral nutrition is important and can be delivered by esophagostomy, gastrostomy, or jejunostomy tube.

The most significant prognostic indicator is the initial response to chemotherapy, as cats experiencing complete remission have longer survival times. There is a poorer prognosis and shorter survival with high-grade lymphoma, and the response rate and remission duration are better for low-grade lymphoma. In feline lymphoma patients, those with lymphoma substage a (no clinical signs) have a better response to treatment and longer survival than do those with substage b; however, all cats with extranodal gastrointestinal lymphoma are either ill or presenting with clinical signs at the time of

Small Animal Soft Tissue Surgery, Second Edition. Edited by Eric Monnet.
© 2023 John Wiley & Sons, Inc. Published 2023 by John Wiley & Sons, Inc.
Companion website: www.wiley.com/go/monnet/small

diagnosis. Furthermore, B-cell or T-cell immunophenotype does not correlate with treatment response or survival in cats (Grover 2005). It has been reported that cats receiving chemotherapy for discrete intestinal lymphoma have a median survival time of 75–270 days (Simon *et al.* 2008; Teske *et al.* 2002; Limmer *et al.* 2016), whereas cats receiving both chemotherapy and surgery had a median survival time of 417 days (Gouldin *et al.* 2017). Another study of 40 cats receiving surgery for discrete gastrointestinal lymphoma reported a median survival time of 96 days, and survival improved when assessing cats that survived to suture removal, who had a median survival time of 185 days (Tidd *et al.* 2019). Also in that study, the presence of septic peritonitis at the time of surgery was not associated with patient outcome (Tidd *et al.* 2019). Cats with small cell, T-cell, intestinal lymphoma have a better prognosis, with median survival times exceeding 600 days with chemotherapy. One pilot study investigated the incidence of postchemotherapy perforation in cats with intermediate- or large-cell gastrointestinal lymphoma and found it to occur in 4 out of 23 cats, with a median time of 57.5 days after induction, and in cats that might have had greater than 5% weight loss following induction (Crouse *et al.* 2018).

A recent survey of the Veterinary Medical Database from 1964 to 2004 reviewed the prevalence of feline intestinal neoplasia from 1129 cases (Rissetto *et al.* 2011), in which lymphoma represented 47% of all feline intestinal tumors, which compares with a historical range of 44–63%. Lymphoma represents 59% of feline small intestinal tumors and 18% of large intestinal tumors, which differs from the historical values of 50% for small intestinal tumors and 40% for large intestinal tumors. Of all intestinal lymphoma cases, 79% occurred in the small intestine and 22% in the large intestine, similar to the historical distribution. It is also interesting to note that cases of feline intestinal lymphoma were typically in feline leukemia virus-negative cats.

Adenocarcinoma comprised 0.4–3% of all feline tumors, and 7–27% of alimentary tumors. Differing from the historical trend that showed a greater prevalence in the small intestine, 69% of intestinal adenocarcinomas occurred in the large intestine. Adenocarcinoma accounted for 45% of all feline large intestinal tumors, similar to the historical values of 46–100%. The large intestine is the more common location for adenocarcinoma, and adenocarcinomas are the most commonly occurring neoplasia in the large intestine.

Mast cell tumors were reported in 4% of intestinal tumor cases, similar to the historical value of 5%. Intestinal leiomyosarcomas comprised 1.1% of all intestinal tumors, with equal distribution by location, which differs from historical accounts where it is mostly a small intestinal tumor. From the same survey, it was found that there was an increased risk of intestinal neoplasia with increasing age after age 7 years, and that the Siamese breed has an increased risk for developing intestinal neoplasia (Rissetto *et al.* 2011). There was also a possible decreased risk of developing intestinal neoplasia in intact males and female cats, but this may be skewed as intact individuals are commonly younger cats (Rissetto *et al.* 2011). A limitation of the study is that the data represent prevalence or the number of newly reported cases, not incidence or all currently affected individuals in an entire population.

Canine

Gastric carcinomas occur rarely in dogs (Seim-Wikse *et al.* 2013). As reported in one case series of 19 dogs with gastric adenocarcinoma, 74% had metastasis at the time of diagnosis, including to regional lymph nodes, omentum, duodenum, liver, pancreas, spleen, esophagus, adrenal glands, and lungs (Swann & Holt 2002). Two dogs with gastric leiomyosarcomas in the same case series had metastatic disease to liver and duodenum discovered at diagnosis (Swann & Holt 2002). Clinical signs included vomiting, anorexia, weight loss, melena, lethargy, abdominal pain, and ptyalism. Palliative Billroth I or gastrojejunostomy provided immediate relief from obstruction, with clinical signs recurring anywhere from 3 days to 10 months after surgery. The role of chemotherapy is not clear for gastric adenocarcinoma. Gastric neoplasia can affect dogs of any age range, though it more commonly affects older dogs. In the cited case series there was a poor prognosis, as survival ranged from time of diagnosis to 10 months post, with euthanasia elected for in all cases (Swann & Holt 2002). Linitis plastica (or "leather bottle" stomach) is a popular descriptive term for carcinoma infiltration of the stomach, rendering it thickened, difficult to distend, and very rigid. Hereditary breed predisposition for gastric carcinoma has been found in Tervueren, bouvier des Flandres, Groenendael, collie, standard poodle, and Norwegian elkhound dogs following studies of the Norwegian Canine Cancer Register (Seim-Wikse *et al.* 2013). There is a rare condition of hypertrophic gastropathy due to epithelial hyperplasia or Ménétrier disease that might have an association with gastric carcinoma, as reported in one West Highland white terrier and in three Cairn terrier littermates (Lecoindre *et al.* 2012; Munday *et al.* 2012).

Limited case series exist for canine intestinal adenocarcinoma (Figure 10.1). In one study of 23 dogs from seven institutions who received primary resection, all survived the immediate postoperative period

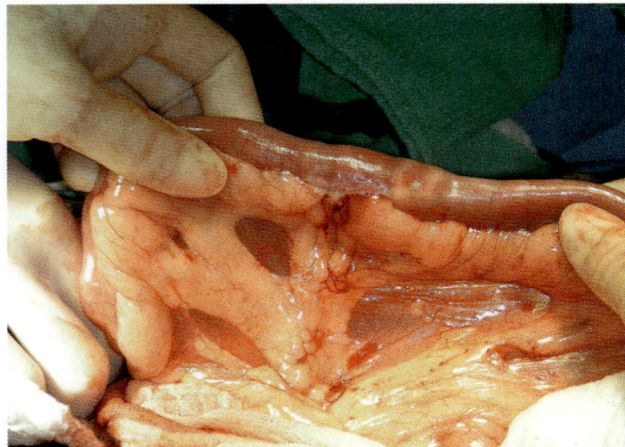

Figure 10.1 Jejunal adenocarcinoma with metastasis extending along the mesentery in a dog.

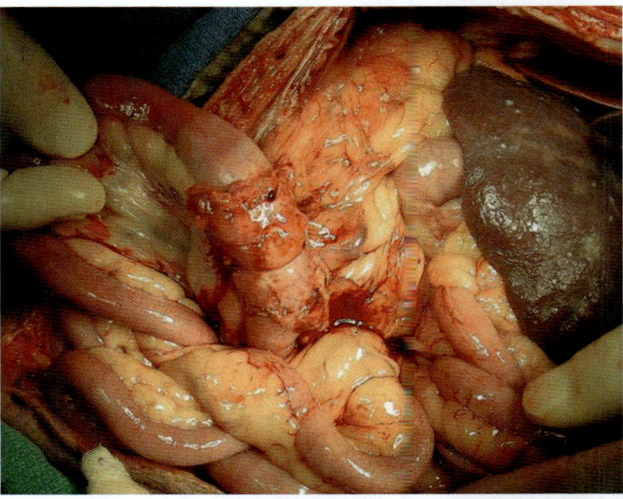

Figure 10.2 Gastrointestinal lymphoma with disease present within the jejunum, omentum, and liver. Grossly these lesions could be associated with many different types of gastrointestinal neoplasia. Histopathology is necessary for diagnosis and prognosis, despite how these lesions might appear.

(Crawshaw *et al.* 1998). Of the 23 dogs, 12 received intraoperative lymph node staging, with metastasis detected in 7 and presumed intra-abdominal extranodal metastasis in another 4. Histopathology confirmed metastasis in 43.5% of cases. Of dogs with metastasis, the median survival time was 3 months; for dogs staging free of metastasis, the median survival time was 15 months (Crawshaw *et al.* 1998). Malignant transformation of adenomatous polyps and carcinoma in situ to invasive carcinoma has been documented in the canine colon and rectum (Valerius *et al.* 1997). In a case series of 11 dogs with colorectal carcinoma, the local recurrence rate was 18% and the metastatic rate 0%; the median disease-free interval and the median survival times were not reached. The lower end of the 95% confidence intervals was 4.5 months for median disease-free interval and 6 months for median survival time (Morello *et al.* 2008). The survival time of the 11 dogs ranged from 0 to 72 months. Historical metastatic rates range from 0% to 80%.

In humans, altered intestinal microbiota has been linked with colorectal tumorigenesis. A recent study observed significantly different fecal microbiota profiles in dogs with colorectal epithelial tumors, both polyps, adenomas, and carcinomas, when compared to the fecal microbiota of control dogs (Herstad *et al.* 2018).

There is a condition occurring in miniature dachshunds, recognized in Japan as inflammatory polyp of miniature dachshunds (IPMD) (Saito *et al.* 2018). IPMD consists of nonneoplastic inflammatory polyps localized to the colorectum. In one study of sequential colorectal biopsies occurring over time in dachshunds with IPMD, interestingly half of the dogs were found to develop adenomas and or adenocarcinomas (Itoh *et al.* 2021).

Gastrointestinal lymphoma is the most common extranodal form of canine lymphoma (Figure 10.2). Clinical signs include anorexia, lethargy, vomiting, and hemorrhagic diarrhea. Diagnosis of concurrent hypoalbuminemia is not uncommon (Frank *et al.* 2007). Indications for surgical treatment in dogs with intestinal lymphoma include perforation, obstruction, peritonitis, or diagnosis (Sogame *et al.* 2018). In a series of 30 dogs, surgery was either for diagnostic purposes or for correction of perforation. Reported median survival times for canine gastrointestinal lymphoma range from 6 to 12 months, with complete remission occurring in 60–90% of cases. This series of 30 dogs exhibited short median survival times and poor response to variable treatments. Most gastrointestinal lymphoma is of T-cell origin (Frank *et al.* 2007). A study comparing either surgical resection (median overall survival 120 days) or chemotherapy (median survival 98 days) for primary high-grade small intestinal lymphoma in dogs revealed no significant difference in overall survival between the therapies (Yamazaki *et al.* 2021). Similar findings were reported in another study of primary canine intestinal lymphoma, whereby the median survival time for dogs receiving surgery was 125 days versus 129 days for dogs not receiving surgery, with most having received chemotherapy (Sogame *et al.* 2018). In that study a 10% postoperative complication rate was reported for 3 of the 31 dogs receiving intestinal surgery (Sogame *et al.* 2018). Dogs with small cell, T-cell, intestinal lymphoma receiving mostly nonsurgical therapies have a reported median survival time of 628 days; this may be a distinct clinical entity and is also echoed in another study of canine low-grade intestinal lymphoma with a median survival time of 424 days (Couto *et al.* 2018; Lane *et al.* 2018). Primary colorectal lymphoma described in 31 dogs had a reported progression-free interval of 1318 days and a median survival time of 1845 days (Desmas *et al.* 2017).

Leiomyosarcomas are the most common sarcoma of the canine intestinal tract and arise from smooth muscle (Figure 10.3). GIST are derived from interstitial cells of Cajal (pacemaker cells of the gastrointestinal tract) and not from smooth muscle, but the interstitial cells of Cajal are commonly within smooth muscle. Immunohistochemical staining for expression of c-KIT (CD117) is necessary to distinguish between the two histotypes, as leiomyosarcomas do not express c-KIT protein. GIST develop most commonly in the cecum and large intestine, and less commonly in the stomach or small intestine. Leiomyosarcomas are more commonly found in the stomach and small intestine and less commonly in the large intestine. Only GIST have been diagnosed with perforation of the gastrointestinal wall subsequent to tumor invasion and only within the cecum (Russell *et al.* 2007). Surgical therapy alone for GIST in the same study had a median survival time of 11.6 months, not significantly different from the median survival time for leiomyosarcomas (7.8 months) (Russell *et al.* 2007).

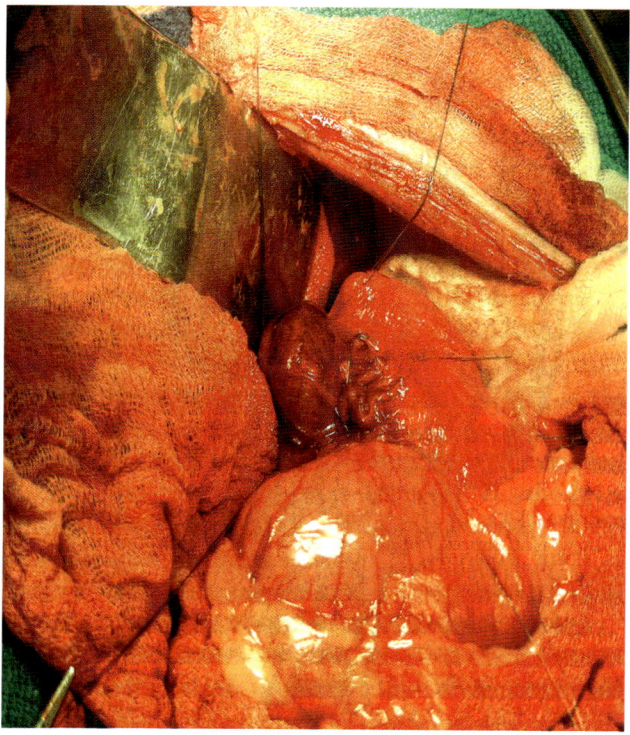

Figure 10.3 Well-differentiated pyloric leiomyosarcoma in a dog. Source: Eric Monnet (Author).

Another study evaluating reclassified leiomyosarcomas found that regardless of classification or immunohistochemistry, there were no prognostic differences following surgical excision (Maas *et al.* 2007). Dogs that were neutered or spayed had better survival than intact dogs, speculated to be due to lack of sex hormones stimulating activation of epidermal growth factor receptor by transforming growth factor (TGF)-α (Maas *et al.* 2007). Humans with c-KIT expressing gastrointestinal tumors experience a positive therapeutic response to the tyrosine kinase inhibitor imatinib mesilate (Gleevec®, Novartis, Basel, Switzerland). The role of tyrosine kinase inhibitors is currently unproven for canine GIST using drugs such as Gleevec or even toceranib phosphate (Palladia®, Zoetis, Parsippany, NJ, USA), another tyrosine kinase inhibitor. One-year and two-year survival times for small intestinal tumors in the cited series were 62.6% and 52.3% in 42 dogs treated with surgery and 84.2% and 66% for the 19 cecal tumors treated with surgery (Maas *et al.* 2007). Weight loss, a painful abdomen, and tumor diameter were associated with a poorer prognosis, whereas neutering status was associated with a more favorable prognosis (Maas *et al.* 2007).

In a recent retrospective case series of 14 dogs with leiomyosarcoma, the tumor was typically seen in older dogs, commonly involving the cecum and jejunum, and with a median age of onset of 10.5 years (Cohen *et al.* 2003). The most common clinical signs reported were anorexia, lethargy, vomiting, weight loss, abdominal distension, and diarrhea, and symptoms were typically acute to subacute. Additional reported findings on evaluation were intestinal obstruction, anemia, bowel perforation, and peritonitis. In the same study half of the dogs had histologic confirmation of metastasis (to mesenteric lymph nodes, peritoneum, and liver) (Cohen *et al.* 2003). Historical rates of metastasis diagnosed at the time of surgery are low, ranging from 16% to 37.5% and more commonly occurring within the liver. In this same population of 14 dogs, the mesentery was the most common site of metastasis (Cohen *et al.* 2003). Most dogs survived the immediate postoperative period, and evidence of perforation was present in 50% of cases. Of dogs with bowel perforation who survived the immediate postoperative period, the long-term survival ranged from 36.3 to 72.7 months (Cohen *et al.* 2003). Hypoglycemia as a paraneoplastic syndrome was seen in this case series in 43% of dogs; this may be falsely high due to peritonitis in four of the dogs. Polyuria/polydipsia was also documented, perhaps caused by tumor-associated nephrogenic diabetes insipidus. Median survival for dogs surviving the immediate postoperative period was 21.3 months. The one-year, two-year, and three-year survival rates were 75%, 66%, and 60%, respectively. Of the seven dogs with perforation, three died in the immediate postoperative period. Of dogs with metastasis, the median survival was 21.7 months, with one dog dying in the immediate postoperative period. The role of chemotherapy could not be discerned in this series as only two dogs received adjuvant therapy (Cohen *et al.* 2003).

Extramedullary solitary colorectal plasmacytomas occur rarely. It is important to rule out systemic involvement. The preferred treatment is local excision, but plasmacytomas will recur if not completely excised. The role for adjuvant chemotherapy is currently unknown (Kupanoff *et al.* 2006). Extramedullary plasmacytomas are not aggressive tumors. The median survival time was 15 months in one case series (Kupanoff *et al.* 2006).

Gastric neuroendocrine carcinoma may be associated with chronic atrophic gastritis in the Norwegian lundehund due to possible hypergastrinemia, secondary to fundic atrophy (Qvigstad *et al.* 2008). Proposed pathogenesis in a small group of Norwegian lundehunds includes chronic inflammation of fundic mucosa leading to mucosal atrophy, a hypoacidic local environment that progresses to carcinoma, and a probable neuroendocrine origin (Qvigstad *et al.* 2008). Other rare canine neuroendocrine gastrointestinal tumors occur and are commonly referred to as carcinoids, which are slow growing and tend to metastasize (Sako *et al.* 2003; Tappin *et al.* 2008).

Clinical signs

Stomach and intestinal neoplasia frequently present with vague nonspecific clinical signs, in varying prevalence, of weight loss, lethargy, and inappetence (Abrams *et al.* 2019). In the early stages of disease clinical signs may be mild, if present at all, and this is a possible reason why patients present with advanced-stage disease such as with gastric carcinoma (Hugen *et al.* 2017). Surprisingly, symptoms of nausea and vomiting may be seen of a more chronic and intermittent nature. Other clinical signs include melena, hematemesis, ptyalism, and hematochezia, depending on tumor location (Abrams *et al.* 2019). One prospective study comparing dogs with gastric carcinoma versus those with chronic gastritis found that dogs with gastric carcinoma were older and had poorer body condition scores (Seim-Wikse *et al.* 2019). Serum C-reactive protein concentration was elevated in some of the dogs with gastric carcinoma and some of those dogs had abnormally low serum folate concentrations (Seim-Wikse *et al.* 2019). Sometimes a mass may be palpable on examination. Hypoglycemia and/or polyuria/polydipsia as a paraneoplastic syndrome in some dogs with gastrointestinal

leiomyosarcomas can present as an emergency (Cohen *et al.* 2003). Removal of the tumor can resolve these symptoms.

Though not reported in the dog, carcinoid syndrome affects humans and produces a range of symptoms, including diarrhea, episodic flushing, bronchospasm, cyanosis, telangiectasia, skin lesions, and endocardial plaque formation (Sako *et al.* 2003; Tappin *et al.* 2008). There is a single veterinary report suggesting the presence of paraneoplastic paroxysmal ventricular tachycardia and melena that resolved following resection of an ileocecal carcinoid (Tappin *et al.* 2008).

Hypergastrinemia has been reported in a single dog secondary to gastric carcinoma and carcinomatosis, which is unusual and more commonly associated with gastrinoma arising from the pancreas (de Brito Galvao *et al.* 2009).

For older animals presenting with intestinal intussusception, a gastrointestinal tumor needs to be considered as an inciting cause (Levien & Baines 2011).

Clinical signs associated with colorectal tumors often include hematochezia, tenesmus, constipation, diarrhea, rectal prolapse, and/or excessive licking (Nucci *et al.* 2014).

Diagnosis

Cytology and endoscopic biopsy

Noninvasive diagnosis of stomach and intestinal tumors can be challenging. Tools available include transcutaneous fine-needle aspiration, transcutaneous needle-core biopsies for solid masses, and endoscopic biopsies. Cytologic analysis of fine-needle aspirates showed complete or partial agreement when compared with histologic analysis in 72% of cases in one series (Bonfanti *et al.* 2006). Often for canine gastric tumors, cytology samples are frequently either nondiagnostic or inconclusive (Abrams *et al.* 2019). Interestingly, intraoperative impression smears showed 96% agreement with histopathologic diagnosis (Bonfanti *et al.* 2006). Endoscopic biopsies did not match with surgical histopathology when gastrointestinal neoplasia was present (Desmas *et al.* 2010), but a more recent study of canine gastric carcinoma revealed concordance of endoscopic biopsies with surgical biopsies in 16 of 24 dogs (Abrams *et al.* 2019). Even though agreement of presurgical endoscopic biopsies with full-thickness surgical biopsies is better in the stomach, it is not common for an endoscopic mucosal biopsy of the proximal small intestine to yield a diagnosis of inflammatory bowel disease when in fact lymphoma may be present, as confirmed with full-thickness biopsies (Evans *et al.* 2006; Kleinschmidt *et al.* 2010). If lymphoma is suspected and endoscopic canine alimentary tract mucosal biopsies are planned, polymerase chain reaction for antigen receptor gene rearrangement analysis may be a useful tool and a sensitive adjunct in detecting lymphoma (Kaneko *et al.* 2009). Leiomyosarcomas will appear identical to GIST on routine hematoxylin and eosin staining, but can be differentiated by CD117 immunohistochemistry for the presence of c-KIT activity. Both of these tumors are more common in the small intestine and cecum, with GIST more common in the cecum and more likely to be associated with septic peritonitis following perforation as compared with leiomyosarcoma. Thus clinical suspicion for a neoplastic mass should trump less invasive diagnostics that have not confirmed the presence of neoplasia.

Imaging

Abdominal ultrasound may be the more commonly utilized imaging when working up gastrointestinal disease, though one should recognize the diagnostic limitations of ultrasound when evaluating the stomach for neoplastic disease (Marolf *et al.* 2015). Abdominal computed tomography (CT) with contrast is an important staging tool for human gastric tumors and is well described for the dog (Tanaka *et al.* 2019). For many gastric tumors, utilizing both an abdominal CT study with an endoscopic study and transabdominal needle aspirates (via ultrasound or CT guidance) and/or intraluminal endoscopic biopsies will maximize diagnostic understanding of a suspected gastric tumor prior to an abdominal exploratory, and also optimize patient staging with regional lymph node assessment and evaluation of distant organs for metastatic spread. Additional diagnostic tools can include abdominal radiography, positive-contrast gastrogram, abdominal ultrasound, and exploratory surgery. Functional changes suggestive of gastric neoplasia can include gastric ulceration, delayed gastric emptying, poor motility, and delayed adherence of contrast material to an ulcerated tumor.

Regarding canine colorectal lesions, intraluminal imaging options classically include colonoscopy as well as proctoscopy (performed without insufflation) and transanal laparoscopic single-port evaluation (Adamovich-Rippe *et al.* 2017). A retrospective multi-institutional study of canine rectal masses visualized with colonoscopy found multiple rectal masses in 6 of 82 dogs and no lesions visualized orad to the colorectal junction (Adamovich-Rippe *et al.* 2017). Other studies evaluating canine rectal tumors reported concurrent lesions occurring in both colon and rectum in some dogs (Valerius *et al.* 1997). A colonoscopy procedure is considered safe, with minor complications noted in only 3 out of 82 dogs being evaluated (Adamovich-Rippe *et al.* 2017).

In cats, when the ultrasound appearance of the muscularis propria layer was thickened, it was more commonly associated with lymphoma as opposed to inflammatory bowel disease or normal bowel (Zwingenberger *et al.* 2010). However, this should not be seen as a reason to avoid pursuing cytologic or histologic diagnosis. Also noteworthy is that lymphomatous involvement of the mesentery in the cat may appear ultrasonographically as carcinomatosis, and also that peritoneal lymphomatosis appears identically to carcinomatosis (Oetelaar *et al.* 2020; Morgan *et al.* 2018).

Surgical treatment

The extent of surgery is dependent on surgical goals. When performing a diagnostic exploratory with unknown histopathology, incisional biopsies or even intraoperative frozen histopathologic sections can be obtained before embarking on extensive tumor resection. Extreme caution is merited before recommending euthanasia intraoperatively, for example because diffuse lymphoma can mirror the appearance of carcinomatosis and the extent of any malignant disease may appear worse than what the patient is truly experiencing clinically. For hospitals not equipped to evaluate intraoperative frozen histopathologic samples, intraoperative impression smears can be the next best alternative.

The decision to pursue extensive surgical procedures such as Billroth I or Billroth II can be controversial without a prior histologic diagnosis, unless the presenting clinical signs are due to obstruction, as the morbidity associated particularly with a Billroth II has been reported to be significant (Ahmadu-Suka *et al.* 1988). In one case series, it was concluded that a Billroth I procedure was reasonable when obtaining a histopathologic diagnosis and to increase gastric outflow regardless of whether the obstruction was due to neoplastic or nonneoplastic disease, as more than 75% of dogs in the series survived the short-term period of more than 14 days (Desmas *et al.* 2010). In a retrospective study of 40 dogs receiving surgical resections for gastric carcinoma, 9 dogs had Billroth I performed, with 2 of those dogs requiring cholecystoduodenostomies (Abrams *et al.* 2019). One of these 9 dogs having a Billroth I procedure experienced major hemorrhage intraoperatively and 3 dogs experienced postoperative pancreatitis, with 1 also having ascending cholangiohepatitis (Abrams *et al.* 2019). Of the other 40 dogs in the study, partial gastrectomy was done in 28, subtotal gastrectomy in 2, and a submucosal resection in 1 (Abrams *et al.* 2019). In that study 3 dogs experienced major intraoperative complications and all 3 also developed septic peritonitis, with 2 being euthanized. In addition to the 5 dogs experiencing postoperative complications following Billroth

I, 9 other dogs having varying other levels of gastrectomy also experienced postoperative complications, including septic peritonitis in 4, cardiopulmonary arrest in 2, and protracted pancreatitis and/or ileus in 2 dogs resulting in euthanasia. In almost half of the dogs metastatic disease was identified histologically at the time of surgery, with metastasis in regional lymph nodes in 14 dogs, the mesentery in 3, and in 1 also in the liver and nodes (Abrams *et al.* 2019). This highlights the value of regional lymph node assessment with gastric tumors.

Wide excision of any alimentary neoplasia is recommended; reported margins range from 4 to 10 cm in the intestine, though 5 cm is most commonly attempted for small intestinal tumors and at least 1 cm wide (or 2 cm) in the stomach (Hugen *et al.* 2017) and rectum (Figure 10.4). Wider margins in the stomach and rectum may be anatomically limited (Morello *et al.* 2008). In a prospective *ex vivo* study of nonlymphoma canine small intestinal specimens, orad and aborad surgical margins of 3 cm from the palpable edge of a tumor resulted in tumor-free margins for all of the 10 carcinoma and 11 sarcoma small intestinal tumor samples, 95% tumor-free margins following 2 cm resection margins, and 76% tumor-free margins following 1 cm margins (Morrice *et al.* 2019a). A similar study was conducted with a variety of solitary feline intestinal tumors, which concluded that the aim was to achieve at least 4 cm orad and aborad surgical

margins for most discrete small intestinal tumors, but that marginal resection was sufficient for lymphoma lesions (Morrice *et al.* 2019b). For masses such as leiomyomas or even grade 1 leiomyosarcomas, marginal resection may be sufficient. Hypoalbuminemia is a risk factor for intestinal resection and anastomotic dehiscence, as is the presence of a tumor, but hypoalbuminemia has not been proven a risk factor for Billroth I (Desmas *et al.* 2010).

It is essential to perform a full abdominal exploration, especially as many metastatic lesions can be hidden within the liver and regional lymph nodes (Figure 10.5). A consistent staging system for evaluating draining lymph nodes in the dog and cat is lacking, with anecdotal reports of sentinel lymph node mapping techniques utilizing methylene blue and filtered technetium sulfur colloid being feasible and well tolerated.

There are many opinions regarding the tolerability of pylorectomy and gastrojejunostomy (Billroth II) for resection of extensive gastric and duodenal neoplastic lesions. The most notable considerations include the poor long-term survival of a patient if an adenocarcinoma is present and postoperative dumping syndrome. Gastrojejunostomy alone could be another palliative option for relieving a neoplastic gastric obstruction. Jejunocolonic anastomosis has been reported to be tolerated in dogs (Crawshaw *et al.* 1998).

With large intestinal tumors requiring colorectal anastomosis, there is a case report that the caudal mesenteric artery can be ligated in the dog without resulting in ischemic necrosis of the anastomotic region (Sarathchandra *et al.* 2009). For tumors located in the distal colon or mid-cranial rectum, a combined caudal celiotomy and transanal pull-through technique has been described as an alternative to pelvic osteotomy

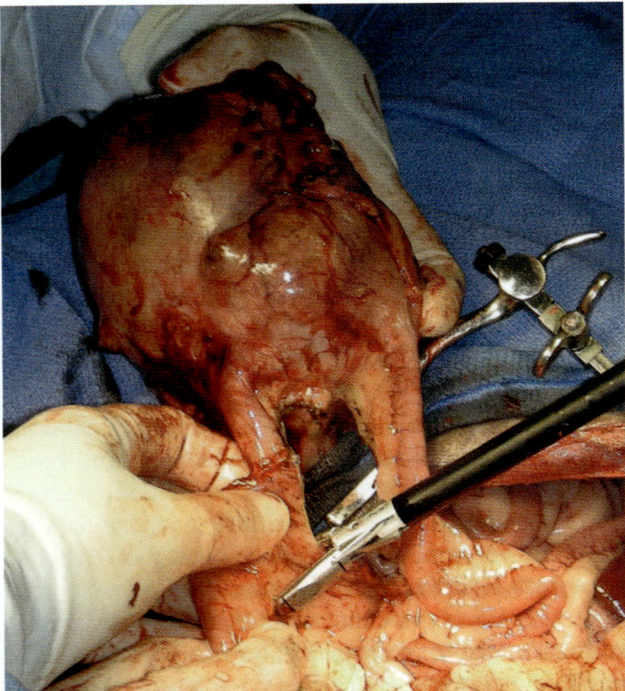

Figure 10.4 Canine patient receiving a palliative intestinal resection with wide margin and anastomosis for metastatic and obstructive leiomyosarcoma.

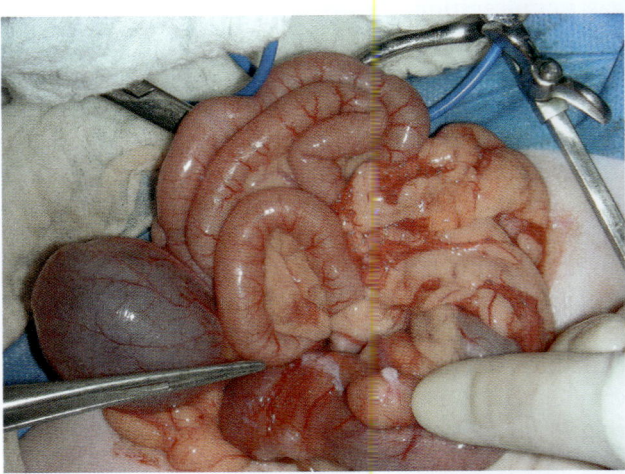

Figure 10.5 Colonic adenocarcinoma in a cat with mesenteric metastasis.

(Morello *et al.* 2008). There is conflicting and limited information in the dog regarding maintenance of fecal continence if the cranial rectal peritoneal reflection (which carries the neurovascular supply to the rectum and sphincter) is surgically disturbed, such as with pelvic osteotomy. The case series of two dogs with caudal mesenteric artery ligations did not experience long-term incontinence (Sarathchandra *et al.* 2009), nor was permanent fecal incontinence encountered with wide rectal resections, though transient incontinence persisted for months (Morello *et al.* 2008). Sparing of the distal 1–1.5 cm of rectum has been recommended for preserving fecal continence and external anal sphincter function.

Transanal rectal pull-through surgical procedures were retrospectively assessed in 74 dogs (Nucci *et al.* 2014). The length of the resected rectum ranged from 0.5 cm to 14 cm, with a mean of 6.3 cm in the study (Nucci *et al.* 2014). In half of the dogs in the study the anocutaneous junction was resected, and in dogs where a cuff of the distal rectum was preserved the mean length was 1.8 cm (Nucci *et al.* 2014). Of the 74 dogs, 58 (78.4%) developed postoperative complications. Fecal incontinence was seen in 42 (56.8%) of the dogs, with half of these being permanent incontinence, and this was not associated with the length of resected rectum. The median duration for transient fecal incontinence was 14 days (range 3–180 days). Other complications included diarrhea in half of the dogs, which was dependent on the length of resected rectum (and permanent in eight dogs), tenesmus in 40% (and permanent in five dogs), stricture formation in just over a quarter of the dogs, rectal bleeding, constipation, dehiscence in 10% (with resulting septic peritonitis and euthanasia in one dog and pararectal abscesses in three), and infection (Nucci *et al.* 2014). The hazard of death was greater for dogs with incompletely excised rectal masses (Nucci *et al.* 2014). For rectal lesions in the proximal rectum, complete tumor resection may require a combined abdominal transanal pull-through colorectal amputation, whereby a laparotomy is necessary for performing the colonic transection and then with patient repositioning to a perineal position to complete the transanal portion for delivery and removal of the colorectal segment, and colorectal anastomosis of the normal colon to the distal rectum (Figure 10.6).

A minimally invasive endoscopic mucosal resection of a colorectal polypoid adenoma has been reported in a dog (Coleman *et al.* 2014). Canine cadaveric studies have been done via transanal minimally invasive surgery used in humans to assess submucosal rectal resections, as an alternative to rectal pull-through procedures in dogs (Mayhew *et al.* 2020). Challenges to reconcile prior

to clinical use in dogs include the thinner rectal walls compared to humans, along with additional anatomic differences such as a more caudally located peritoneal reflection in dogs, and the need to establish surgical criteria for safe transanal minimally invasive submucosal tumor resections in dogs (Mayhew *et al.* 2020).

Marking of the *ex vivo* resection specimen is critical, whether with ink, suture, or other commercially available tissue tags, to orient the histopathology team when evaluating the surgical margins for completeness of excision. When a histopathologic diagnosis of leiomyosarcoma is obtained, it is important to request immunohistochemical special stains for CD117, which is the sole means of distinguishing leiomyosarcoma from GIST. In humans this is particularly important, as adjuvant chemotherapy for GIST using imatinib mesilate (Gleevec) has dramatically improved long-term survival (Russell *et al.* 2007; Maas *et al.* 2007).

Many canine and feline patients presenting to the operating room for laparotomy for alimentary neoplasia have a clinical history of inappetence and weight loss, such that consideration needs to be given to parenteral nutrition and placement of a percutaneous feeding tube for support in qualifying patients. Nielsen and Anderson (2005) reported probable local tumor progression and spread from tumor seeding in a gastrostomy stoma in a patient with an incompletely excised gastric adenocarcinoma via Billroth I. However, this should not discourage the placement of enteral feeding tubes for nutritional support in patients receiving therapy for gastrointestinal neoplasia.

Use of second-look laparotomy for staging and assessment of treatment response has been described for intestinal and gastric adenocarcinomas, but its practical incorporation is still undetermined (Stanclift & Gilson 2004). Interestingly, two dogs in that case report with metastatic intestinal adenocarcinoma had survival times of 17 and 35 months following treatment with cisplatin and 5-fluorouracil (Stanclift & Gilson 2004). The single dog with gastric adenocarcinoma had a survival time of 4 months, which does not differ from the expected survival data of less than 6 months, and had no apparent response to cisplatin and 5-fluorouracil (Stanclift & Gilson 2004).

Palliative treatments: stenting/rerouting/bypass

In dogs receiving a Billroth I procedure, overall median survival times in dogs undergoing incomplete resection were not significantly different from those in dogs undergoing complete tumor resection (Desmas *et al.* 2010). Dogs receiving Billroth I for malignant neoplasia had an overall median survival time of 33 days,

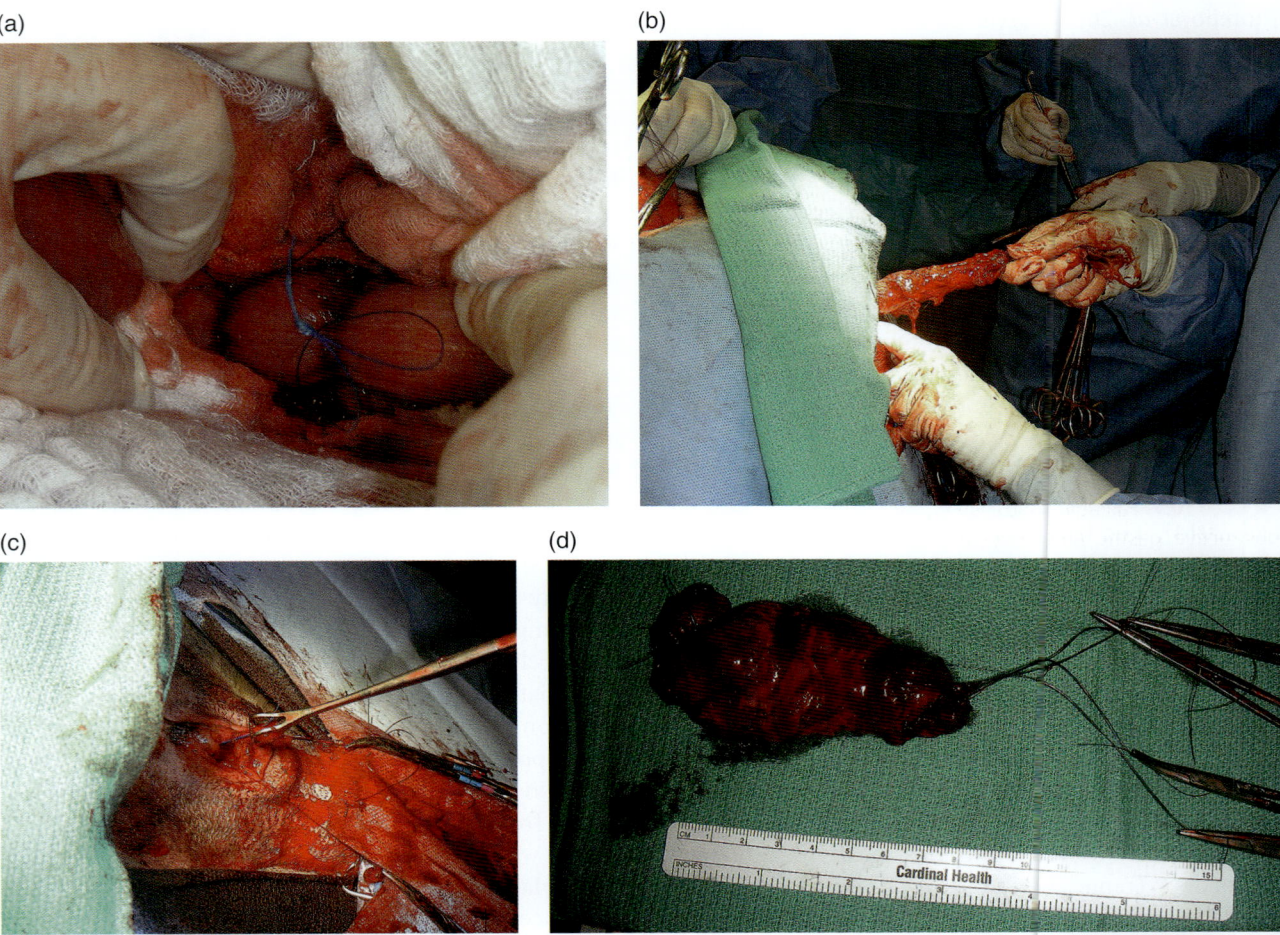

Figure 10.6 Collection of four pictures illustrating combined abdominal transanal pull-through colorectal amputation of a proximal rectal carcinoma in a dog. (a) Within the abdomen the descending normal colon and the planned colonic surgical resection margin for the rectal carcinoma have been secured using a Furness purse-string clamp. (b) From a transanal approach with the dog in dorsal recumbency, the distal rectum has been incised full thickness and the proximal rectum is being delivered. Note that a second surgeon assisted in mobilizing the colon via open celiotomy during transanal delivery. (c) Close-up view of the stay sutures that were attached to the delivered colorectal segment and to the stump of normal colon being exteriorized for eventual anal anastomosis. (d) *ex vivo* amputated colorectal segment for wide excision of rectal carcinoma.

and this was significantly different from dogs receiving an identical procedure for benign diseases in the same case series (Desmas *et al.* 2010). It is important to note that if a mass is not amenable to perceived wide complete excision, a marginal or intralesional cytoreductive procedure should not be attempted, as the risk of anastomotic leakage would be great and typical survival expectations for septic peritonitis approach 50%.

Gastrojejunostomy alone could be another palliative option for relieving a neoplastic gastric obstruction. Jejunocolonic anastomosis has also been reported to be tolerated in dogs. Other palliative bypass procedures for the alimentary tract include Roux-en-Y type anastomoses (Figure 10.7).

In cats with tenesmus due to extraluminal colonic obstruction secondary to adenocarcinoma infiltration, colonic stenting with a metallic self-expanding stent has been successful in palliating the obstruction and improving the tenesmus, even in the face of metastatic disease. This procedure was performed in under 40 minutes by the authors of this report (Hume *et al.* 2006). It is reasonable to consider such an option for similarly affected dogs.

There are isolated reports of varying temporary and permanent colostomy procedures being done to dogs and cat for fecal diversion. A practical challenge with this procedure is managing fecal incontinence, as human fecal collection bags and adhesive flange products do not substantively adhere to the skin (Cinti & Pisani 2019). Patients experience significant dermatitis from the fecal incontinence. As fecal continence is a commonly accepted and reliable indicator of quality of life, the

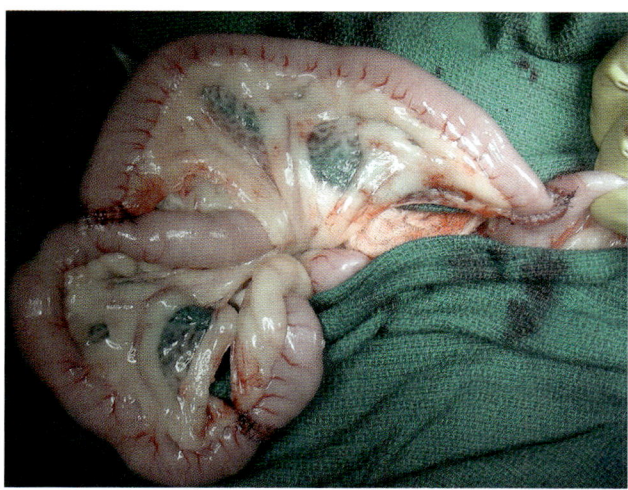

Figure 10.7 Palliative Roux-en-Y procedure in a cat with an obstructive gastric and proximal duodenal mass. Source: Eric Monnet (Author).

decision to perform a permanent colostomy for palliation of certain alimentary tumors is highly controversial and raises ethical questions.

Intracavitary chemotherapy is well tolerated, can improve symptoms relating to effusive carcinomatosis, and may temporarily resolve the effusion (Charney *et al.* 2005). Suitable chemotherapy drugs for intraperitoneal instillation include carboplatin and mitoxantrone (Charney *et al.* 2005; Spugnini *et al.* 2008).

Adjuvant therapy

Chemotherapy

In one study, 19 of 40 dogs received varying adjuvant chemotherapy protocols following gastric carcinoma resections and multivariant analysis results demonstrated correlation of improved survival for those dogs receiving chemotherapy, with inability to identify an ideal chemotherapy protocol (Abrams *et al.* 2019).

Limited retrospective case series address the efficacy of adjuvant chemotherapy for intestinal tumors, and there is limited information in general on the role of adjuvant chemotherapy for intestinal adenocarcinoma in the dog and cat (Smith *et al.* 2019). Systemic chemotherapeutic agents for metastatic carcinomas include doxorubicin and carboplatin-based regimens. Toceranib was found to increase the time to tumor progress in dogs with a variety of surgically resected adenocarcinomas, including intestinal (Yamazaki *et al.* 2020). Adjuvant nonsteroidal anti-inflammatory drugs may have a role in colorectal carcinomas. Humans with c-KIT-expressing gastrointestinal tumors experience a positive therapeutic response with the tyrosine kinase inhibitor imatinib mesilate (Gleevec). Toceranib, another tyrosine kinase

inhibitor, has demonstrated clinical benefit for gross canine GIST lesions, but the clinical benefit as adjuvant therapy following surgical resection of canine GIST lesions is unknown (Berger *et al.* 2018). Multiple varying protocols have been published for the treatment of gastrointestinal lymphoma.

Radiation therapy

Curative-intent or definitive radiation therapy of the abdomen is limited to the tolerance of normal tissues in the area, particularly the small intestine, colon, rectum, urethra, and spinal cord. Because of the sensitivity of these tissues to radiation, definitive radiation and adjuvant radiation of the gastrointestinal tract are typically not performed. Side effects of radiation therapy are grouped into two categories: acute, which occur within 10–14 days following radiation; and late, occurring 6 months or longer following radiation therapy. Acute side effects can include mucositis and moist and/or dry epithelial desquamation. Late side effects to the abdomen include strictures (rectal, vaginal, urethral), chronic colitis, necrotic tissue, persistent ulceration, rectal perforation, bladder wall thickening, osteopenia, pain, and edema. These late side effects occurred in 39% of a cohort of 51 dogs following pelvic radiation (Arthur *et al.* 2008). In the case series, it was concluded that a smaller dose of radiation per fraction (with an increased number of fractions) of the planned total dose to be delivered would decrease the occurrence of late complications (Arthur *et al.* 2008).

Prognosis

Following curative-intent therapy of gastrointestinal neoplasia, additional monitoring is recommended. Generically this would include reexamination every 3 months for the first year, then every 6 months thereafter. Each reexamination should also include serial staging to include three-view thoracic radiography, abdominal ultrasound, bloodwork, and/or other monitoring to detect either local recurrence of disease or metastasis. Of interest is that in a case series of 40 dogs receiving surgical resection of gastric carcinoma, sites of metastatic progression included regional lymph nodes, mesentery, abdominal wall, spleen, ureter, bladder, and ulna, and local recurrence was confirmed or suspected in 12 dogs (Abrams *et al.* 2019). This suggests consideration of additional endoscopy and/or CT abdominal imaging for staging of gastric tumors in dogs.

In general, positive prognostic factors for gastrointestinal tumors include a solitary mass, surgical margins complete and free of any tumor cells, and (for cats) response to chemotherapy for gastrointestinal lymphoma. Negative prognostic factors include the presence of metastasis to regional lymph nodes, lung, or peritoneum. For colorectal tumors, pedunculated or polypoid lesions have a better postsurgical prognosis than annular colorectal adenocarcinoma historically, with mean survival times for postoperative colorectal carcinomas ranging from 6 to 22 months. The survival time for dogs with nonlymphoma small intestinal masses without evidence of metastasis is described to be 15 months, as opposed to 3 months for dogs with concurrent metastasis (Crawshaw *et al.* 1998). A median survival time of 544 days was reported in a retrospective study of 29 dogs following resections for small intestinal adenocarcinomas (Smith *et al.* 2019). In dogs with either a leiomyosarcoma or GIST, a history of weight loss, a painful abdomen, and tumor diameter were associated with a poorer prognosis, whereas neutering status was associated with a more favorable prognosis (Maas *et al.* 2007). Cats with lymphoma localized to the small intestine might do better than those with lymphoma localized to the large intestine. Surgical resection of small intestinal adenocarcinoma improves long-term survival, with a median survival time of 365 days versus 22 days for cats that did not receive surgery (Green *et al.* 2011). A median survival time of 269 days was found in 18 cats with colonic adenocarcinoma that was treated with subtotal colectomy and adjuvant carboplatin (Arteaga *et al.* 2012). Overall median survival time for 31 cats with gastrointestinal mast cell tumors was 531 days and was not impacted by treatment type, including surgery (Barrett *et al.* 2018). For dogs receiving a Billroth I procedure for a primary neoplastic obstruction, median survival time was 33 days for dogs with metastasis. Preoperative weight loss and presence of malignant neoplasia were the only factors associated with decreased overall survival following a Billroth I (Desmas *et al.* 2010). Dogs receiving varying levels of surgical resections for gastric carcinoma have reported median survival times of 6 months (178 days) (Abrams *et al.* 2019). For dogs not receiving treatment for gastric carcinoma, anticipated survival times are less than 3 months following the development of clinical signs (Swann & Holt 2002). Of 31 dogs receiving transanal rectal pull-through procedures for rectal carcinoma, 7 dogs had metastatic disease discovered prior to surgery, and 4 dogs developed metastasis, with the median time to metastasis being about a year. The median survival time for 31 dogs was 696 days and 1006 days for renal carcinoma in situ (Nucci *et al.* 2014).

Exocrine pancreatic tumors

Feline pancreatic tumors are rare. In two case series of feline exocrine pancreatic neoplasia, there was no clear breed or age predisposition (Seaman 2004; Linderman *et al.* 2013). Cats with adenocarcinoma presented with clinical signs relating to acute pancreatitis (anorexia, vomiting, abdominal pain, and/or jaundice), while cats with pancreatic adenomas did not demonstrate any clinical signs (Seaman 2004). In two case series, there was a possible association between concurrent diabetes mellitus and exocrine pancreatic neoplasia (Linderman *et al.* 2013; Seaman 2004). Thoracic radiographs performed in 23 of 34 cats revealed pulmonary masses in 3 (with 2 being of diffuse nodules), sternal lymphadenopathy in 2, and pleural effusions in 2 (Linderman *et al.* 2013). Many pancreatic adenocarcinomas have metastasized by the time of diagnosis (Seaman 2004; Linderman *et al.* 2013).

Canine exocrine pancreatic tumors are similarly rare (Bennett *et al.* 2001; Pinard *et al.* 2021). Of 8 dogs in one case series, ages ranged from 5 to 13 years, 5 of the dogs had necropsy performed and all had metastatic disease (Bennett *et al.* 2001). In another case series of 23 dogs with exocrine pancreatic carcinomas, the median age was 11 years and pancreatic tumors were either diffuse or localized (Pinard *et al.* 2021). Of the 23 dogs, 18 (78%) had evidence of metastasis at the time of diagnosis (Pinard *et al.* 2021).

Clinical signs

Clinical signs relating to pancreatic neoplasia are vague and nonspecific or similar to those associated with pancreatitis. The most common clinical signs in cats with exocrine pancreatic tumors are weight loss, decreased appetite, vomiting, palpable abdominal mass, and diarrhea (Seaman 2004; Linderman *et al.* 2013). The physical presence of a pancreatic tumor can obstruct the common bile duct, leading to clinical signs of extrahepatic biliary duct obstruction (Vergine *et al.* 2005). Described clinical signs associated with gastrinomas include severe vomiting, melena, anorexia, depression, weight loss, iron-deficiency anemia from upper gastrointestinal tract bleeding, and risk of perforation (Fukushima *et al.* 2004a,b).

Dogs with exocrine pancreatic carcinoma are reported to present similarly with anorexia, lethargy, vomiting, and abdominal pain (Pinard *et al.* 2021).

Two different paraneoplastic conditions have been described for cats with pancreatic exocrine tumors. There is a paraneoplastic dermatologic condition consisting of nonpruritic symmetric alopecia on the face, ventral body, and medial aspect of limbs, with glistening nonfragile skin and crusting present on the foot pad. This paraneoplastic condition can also be seen with bile duct carcinomas (Seaman 2004). The other described paraneoplastic condition is necrotizing panniculitis and steatitis (or steatonecrosis and lipodystrophy), which occurred in a cat with a pancreatic adenocarcinoma, possibly due to systemic pancreatic lipolytic enzyme release (Fabbrini *et al.* 2005).

In the dog, canine superficial necrolytic dermatitis has been reported in association with a glucagonoma, but is more commonly associated with hepatic disease (Gross *et al.* 1990; Torres *et al.* 1997; Turek 2003; Mizuno *et al.* 2009; Oberkirchner *et al.* 2010).

Diagnosis

Measurement of blood gastrin levels can be helpful in diagnosing canine gastrinoma. If blood gastrin concentrations are only mildly elevated, a secretin challenge test may help as well as a calcium gluconate challenge test (Fukushima *et al.* 2004b).

If a pancreatic mass is seen with ultrasound, it can be aspirated for a diagnosis or an ultrasound-guided biopsy can be performed (Bennett *et al.* 2001). Of 34 cats with exocrine pancreatic tumors, 33 received abdominal ultrasounds, of which localizing a lesion in the pancreas was not possible or diffuse in 17 cats, focal pancreatic lesions were seen in 13 cats, abdominal effusion was seen in 16 cats, abdominal lymphadenopathy in 11, and in 2 cats bile and pancreatic duct dilatation was found (Linderman *et al.* 2013). In cats, radiography and ultrasound may be helpful in identifying a pancreatic tumor, but suspicion should not trump cytologic or histologic diagnosis, as nodular hyperplasia can appear similar to malignant pancreatic tumors (Hecht *et al.* 2007). Accuracy of ultrasound is also reliant upon the experience of the ultrasonographer.

In a study evaluating the effectiveness of ultrasound, CT, and single-photon emission CT in evaluation of the canine pancreas, it was found that CT could identify more lesions, but that single-photon emission CT was as effective as either CT or ultrasound (Robben *et al.* 2005). However, surgery was the ultimate diagnostic test and more sensitive than any of these imaging modalities (Robben *et al.* 2005).

Surgical treatment

Surgery is the treatment of choice for pancreatic tumors in general, as it is in humans, whether for obtaining a diagnosis, staging extent of disease, treatment, or palliation. For three cats in which only incisional biopsies were possible and not excision of exocrine pancreatic tumor, the reported survival times were 48, 135, and 570 days (Linderman *et al.* 2013).

Chemotherapy

Published reports investigating adjuvant chemotherapy for exocrine pancreatic tumors are lacking. The overall median survival time of 33 cats receiving varying chemotherapy protocols or varying adjuvant chemotherapy following resection of exocrine pancreatic tumors was 165 days (Linderman *et al.* 2013). Toceranib has been found to have clinical benefit in dogs with exocrine pancreatic adenocarcinoma. It was used in six dogs for treatment of gross disease and in two dogs for microscopic disease following surgical resection, with an overall clinical benefit rate of 75% (Musser & Johannes 2021).

Radiation therapy

One 16-year-old cat received three every-other-day fractions of stereotactic radiation therapy for an exocrine pancreatic carcinoma, with documented partial tumor response (Gaitan-Cobo *et al.* 2021). Carcinomatosis and abdominal effusion were noted 15 months later, which resolved following carboplatin chemotherapy. The cat was euthanized 589 days after initiation of radiation therapy (Gaitan-Cobo *et al.* 2021).

One dog with exocrine pancreatic carcinoma was treated with a single fraction of stereotactic radiation therapy for a lesion discovered to be inoperable during an abdominal surgery. This patient had stable disease for one month until it was lost to follow-up (Pinard *et al.* 2021).

Prognosis

Most feline pancreatic adenocarcinomas have evidence of metastasis at the time of diagnosis. One report describes cats as either euthanized or dying within 7 days of diagnosis (Seaman 2004). The median survival time of nine cats not receiving surgery or chemotherapy in another study was 6 days (Linderman *et al.* 2013). The median survival time for cats with abdominal effusion was 30 days when compared to cats with no effusion (Linderman *et al.* 2013). The median survival time for cats having resection of exocrine pancreatic tumors was 165 days when compared to 30 days for cats not receiving surgery (Linderman *et al.* 2013).

The reported median survival time for 20 dogs diagnosed with exocrine pancreatic carcinoma prior to necropsy was 1 day, with a mean overall survival time of 8 days for all 23 dogs (Pinard *et al.* 2021). Another study of eight dogs receiving toceranib either for treatment of gross exocrine pancreatic adenocarcinoma disease or for microscopic disease following surgery had an overall median survival time of 89.5 days (range 14–506 days) (Musser & Johannes 2021).

References

Abrams, B., Wavreille, V.A., Husbands, B.D. et al. (2019). Perioperative complications and outcome after surgery for treatment of gastric carcinoma in dogs: a Veterinary Society of Surgical Oncology retrospective study of 40 cases (2004–2018). *Veterinary Surgery* 48: 923–932.

Adamovich-Rippe, K.N., Mayhew, P.D., Marks, S.L. et al. (2017). Colonoscopic and histologic features of rectal masses in dogs: 82 cases (1995–2012). *Journal of the American Veterinary Medical Association* 250: 424–430.

Ahmadu-Suka, F., Withrow, S.J., Nelson, A.W. et al. (1988). Billroth II gastrojejunostomy in dogs. Stapling technique and postoperative complications. *Veterinary Surgery* 17: 211–219.

Arteaga, T.A., McKnight, J., and Bergman, P.J. (2012). A review of 18 cases of feline colonic adenocarcinoma treated with subtotal colectomies and adjuvant carboplatin. *Journal of the American Animal Hospital Association* 48: 399–404.

Arthur, J.J., Kleiter, M.M., Thrall, D.E., and Pruitt, A.F. (2008). Characterization of normal tissue complications in 51 dogs undergoing definitive pelvic region irradiation. *Veterinary Radiology and Ultrasound* 49: 85–89.

Barrett, L.E., Skorupski, K., Brown, D.C. et al. (2018). Outcome following treatment of feline gastrointestinal mast cell tumours. *Veterinary and Comparative Oncology* 16: 188–193.

Bennett, P.F., Hahn, K.A., Toal, R.L., and Legendre, A.M. (2001). Ultrasonographic and cytopathological diagnosis of exocrine pancreatic carcinoma in the dog and cat. *Journal of the American Animal Hospital Association* 37: 466–473.

Berger, E.P., Johannes, C.M., Jergens, A.E. et al. (2018). Retrospective evaluation of toceranib phosphate (Palladia®) use in the treatment of gastrointestinal stromal tumors of dogs. *Journal of Veterinary Internal Medicine* 32: 2045–2053.

Bonfanti, U., Bertazzolo, W., Bottero, E. et al. (2006). Diagnostic value of cytologic examination of gastrointestinal tract tumors in dogs and cats: 83 cases (2001–2004). *Journal of the American Veterinary Medical Association* 229: 1130–1133.

de Brito Galvao, J.F., Pressler, B.M., Freeman, L.J. et al. (2009). Mucinous gastric carcinoma with abdominal carcinomatosis and hypergastrinemia in a dog. *Journal of the American Animal Hospital Association* 45: 197–202.

Charney, S.C., Bergman, P.J., McKnight, J.A. et al. (2005). Evaluation of intracavitary mitoxantrone and carboplatin for treatment of carcinomatosis, sarcomatosis and mesothelioma, with or without malignant effusions: a retrospective analysis of 12 cases (1997–2002). *Veterinary and Comparative Oncology* 3: 171–181.

Cinti, F. and Pisani, G. (2019). Temporary end-on colostomy as a treatment for anastomotic dehiscence after a transanal rectal pull-through procedure in a dog. *Veterinary Surgery* 48: 897–901.

Cohen, M., Post, G.S., and Wright, J.C. (2003). Gastrointestinal leiomyosarcoma in 14 dogs. *Journal of Veterinary Internal Medicine* 17: 107–110.

Coleman, K.A., Berent, A.C., and Weisse, C.W. (2014). Endoscopic mucosal resection and snare polypectomy for treatment of a colorectal polypoid adenoma in a dog. *Journal of the American Veterinary Medical Association* 244: 1435–1440.

Couto, K.M., Moore, P.F., Zwingenberger, A.L. et al. (2018). Clinical characteristics and outcome in dogs with small cell T-cell intestinal lymphoma. *Veterinary and Comparative Oncology* 16: 337–343.

Crawshaw, J., Berg, J., Sardinas, J.C. et al. (1998). Prognosis for dogs with nonlymphomatous, small intestinal tumors treated by surgical excision. *Journal of the American Animal Hospital Association* 34: 451–456.

Crouse, Z., Phillips, B., Flory, A. et al. (2018). Post-chemotherapy perforation in cats with discrete intermediate- or large-cell gastrointestinal lymphoma. *Journal of Feline Medicine and Surgery* 20: 696–703.

Desmas, I., Burton, J.H., Post, G. et al. (2017). Clinical presentation, treatment and outcome in 31 dogs with presumed primary colorectal lymphoma (2001–2013). *Veterinary and Comparative Oncology* 15: 504–517.

Eisele, J., McClaran, J.K., Runge, J.J. et al. (2010). Evaluation of risk factors for morbidity and mortality after pylorectomy and gastroduodenostomy in dogs. *Veterinary Surgery* 39: 261–267.

Evans, S.E., Bonczynski, J.J., Broussard, J.D. et al. (2006). Comparison of endoscopic and full-thickness biopsy specimens for diagnosis of inflammatory bowel disease and alimentary tract lymphoma in cats. *Journal of the American Veterinary Medical Association* 229: 1447–1450.

Fabbrini, F., Anfray, P., Viacava, P. et al. (2005). Feline cutaneous and visceral necrotizing panniculitis and steatitis associated with a pancreatic tumour. *Veterinary Dermatology* 16: 413–419.

Frank, J.D., Reimer, S.B., Kass, P.H., and Kiupel, M. (2007). Clinical outcomes of 30 cases (1997–2004) of canine gastrointestinal lymphoma. *Journal of the American Animal Hospital Association* 43: 313–321.

Fukushima, R., Ichikawa, K., Hirabayashi, M. et al. (2004a). A case of canine gastrinoma. *Journal of Veterinary Medical Science* 66: 993–995.

Fukushima, U., Sato, M., Okano, S. et al. (2004b). A case of gastrinoma in a Shih-Tzu dog. *Journal of Veterinary Medical Science* 66: 311–313.

Gaitan-Cobo, A.L., Griffin, L.R., and Kruckman-Gatesy, C.R. (2021). Use of stereotactic body radiation therapy for treatment of a pancreatic tumor in a cat. *Journal of the American Veterinary Medical Association* 259: 184–189.

Gouldin, E.D., Mullin, C., Morges, M. et al. (2017). Feline discrete high-grade gastrointestinal lymphoma treated with surgical resection and adjuvant CHOP-based chemotherapy: retrospective study of 20 cases. *Veterinary and Comparative Oncology* 15: 328–335.

Green, M.L., Smith, J.D., and Kass, P.H. (2011). Surgical versus nonsurgical treatment of feline small intestinal adenocarcinoma and the influence of metastasis on long-term survival in 18 cats (2000–2007). *Canadian Veterinary Journal* 52: 1101–1105.

Gross, T.L., O'Brien, T.D., Davies, A.P., and Long, R.E. (1990). Glucagon-producing pancreatic endocrine tumors in two dogs with superficial necrolytic dermatitis. *Journal of the American Veterinary Medical Association* 197: 1619–1622.

Grover, S. (2005). Gastrointestinal lymphoma in cats. *Compendium: Continuing Education for Veterinarians* 27: 741–751.

Hecht, S., Penninck, D.G., and Keating, J.H. (2007). Imaging findings in pancreatic neoplasia and nodular hyperplasia in 19 cats. *Veterinary Radiology and Ultrasound* 48: 45–50.

Herstad, K.M.V., Moen, A.E.F., Gaby, J.C. et al. (2018). Characterization of the fecal and mucosa-associated microbiota in dogs with colorectal epithelial tumors. *PLOS ONE* 13: e0198342.

Hugen, S., Thomas, R.E., German, A.J. et al. (2017). Gastric carcinoma in canines and humans, a review. *Veterinary and Comparative Oncology* 15: 692–705.

Hume, D.Z., Solomon, J.A., and Weisse, C.W. (2006). Palliative use of a stent for colonic obstruction caused by adenocarcinoma in two cats. *Journal of the American Veterinary Medical Association* 228: 392–396.

Itoh, T., Kojimoto, A., Uchida, K. et al. (2021). Long-term postsurgical outcomes of mast cell tumors resected with a margin proportional to the tumor diameter in 23 dogs. *Journal of Veterinary Medical Science* 83: 230–233.

Kaneko, N., Yamamoto, Y., Wada, Y. et al. (2009). Application of polymerase chain reaction to analysis of antigen receptor rearrangements to support endoscopic diagnosis of canine alimentary lymphoma. *Journal of Veterinary Medical Science* 71: 555–559.

Kleinschmidt, S., Harder, J., Nolte, I. et al. (2010). Chronic inflammatory and non-inflammatory diseases of the gastrointestinal tract in cats: diagnostic advantages of full-thickness intestinal and extraintestinal biopsies. *Journal of Feline Medicine and Surgery* 12: 97–103.

Kupanoff, P.A., Popovitch, C.A., and Goldschmidt, M.H. (2006). Colorectal plasmacytomas: a retrospective study of nine dogs. *Journal of the American Animal Hospital Association* 42: 37–43.

Lane, J., Price, J., Moore, A. et al. (2018). Low-grade gastrointestinal lymphoma in dogs: 20 cases (2010 to 2016). *Journal of Small Animal Practice* 59: 147–153.

Lecoindre, P., Bystricka, M., Chevallier, M., and Peyron, C. (2012). Gastric carcinoma associated with Menetrier's-like disease in a West Highland white terrier. *Journal of Small Animal Practice* 53: 714–718.

Levien, A.S. and Baines, S.J. (2011). Histological examination of the intestine from dogs and cats with intussusception. *Journal of Small Animal Practice* 52: 599–606.

Limmer, S., Eberle, N., Nerschbach, V. et al. (2016). Treatment of feline lymphoma using a 12-week, maintenance-free combination chemotherapy protocol in 26 cats. *Veterinary and Comparative Oncology* 14 (Suppl 1): 21–31.

Linderman, M.J., Brodsky, E.M., de Lorimier, L.P. et al. (2013). Feline exocrine pancreatic carcinoma: a retrospective study of 34 cases. *Veterinary and Comparative Oncology* 11: 208–218.

Maas, C.P., ter Haar, G., van der Gaag, I., and Kirpensteijn, J. (2007). Reclassification of small intestinal and cecal smooth muscle tumors in 72 dogs: clinical, histologic, and immunohistochemical evaluation. *Veterinary Surgery* 36: 302–313.

Marolf, A.J., Bachand, A.M., Sharber, J., and Twedt, D.C. (2015). Comparison of endoscopy and sonography findings in dogs and cats with histologically confirmed gastric neoplasia. *Journal of Small Animal Practice* 56: 339–344.

Mayhew, P.D., Balsa, I.M., Guerzon, C.N. et al. (2020). Evaluation of transanal minimally invasive surgery for submucosal rectal resection in cadaveric canine specimens. *Veterinary Surgery* 49: 1378–1387.

Mizuno, T., Hiraoka, H., Yoshioka, C. et al. (2009). Superficial necrolytic dermatitis associated with extrapancreatic glucagonoma in a dog. *Veterinary Dermatology* 20: 72–79.

Morello, E., Martano, M., Squassino, C. et al. (2008). Transanal pull-through rectal amputation for treatment of colorectal carcinoma in 11 dogs. *Veterinary Surgery* 37: 420–426.

Morgan, K.R.S., North, C.E., and Thompson, D.J. (2018). Sonographic features of peritoneal lymphomatosis in 4 cats. *Journal of Veterinary Internal Medicine* 32: 1178–1184.

Morrice, M., Polton, G., and Beck, S. (2019a). Evaluation of the extent of neoplastic infiltration in small intestinal tumours in dogs. *Veterinary Medicine and Science* 5: 189–198.

Morrice, M., Polton, G., and Beck, S. (2019b). Evaluation of the histopathological extent of neoplastic infiltration in intestinal tumours in cats. *Veterinary Medicine and Science* 5: 307–316.

Munday, J.S., Aberdein, D., Cullen, G.D., and French, A.F. (2012). Menetrier disease and gastric adenocarcinoma in 3 Cairn terrier littermates. *Veterinary Pathology* 49: 1028–1031.

Musser, M.L. and Johannes, C.M. (2021). Toceranib phosphate (Palladia) for the treatment of canine exocrine pancreatic adenocarcinoma. *BMC Veterinary Research* 17: 269.

Nielsen, C. and Anderson, G.M. (2005). Metastasis of gastric adenocarcinoma to the abdominal wall following placement of a gastrostomy tube in a dog. *Canadian Veterinary Journal* 46: 641–643.

Nucci, D.J., Liptak, J.M., Selmic, L.E. et al. (2014). Complications and outcomes following rectal pull-through surgery in dogs with rectal masses: 74 cases (2000–2013). *Journal of the American Veterinary Medical Association* 245: 684–695.

Oberkirchner, U., Linder, K.E., Zadrozny, L., and Olivry, T. (2010). Successful treatment of canine necrolytic migratory erythema (superficial necrolytic dermatitis) due to metastatic glucagonoma with octreotide. *Veterinary Dermatology* 21: 510–516.

Oetelaar, G.S., Lim, C.K., Heng, H.G. et al. (2020). Ultrasonographic features of colonic B-cell lymphoma with mesenteric lymphomatosis in a cat. *Veterinary Radiology and Ultrasound* 61: E60–E63.

Pinard, C.J., Hocker, S.E., and Weishaar, K.M. (2021). Clinical outcome in 23 dogs with exocrine pancreatic carcinoma. *Veterinary and Comparative Oncology* 19: 109–114.

Qvigstad, G., Kolbjornsen, O., Skancke, E., and Waldum, H.L. (2008). Gastric neuroendocrine carcinoma associated with atrophic gastritis in the Norwegian Lundehund. *Journal of Comparative Pathology* 139: 194–201.

Rissetto, K., Villamil, J.A., Selting, K.A. et al. (2011). Recent trends in feline intestinal neoplasia: an epidemiologic study of 1,129 cases in the veterinary medical database from 1964 to 2004. *Journal of the American Animal Hospital Association* 47: 28–36.

Robben, J.H., Pollak, Y.W., Kirpensteijn, J. et al. (2005). Comparison of ultrasonography, computed tomography, and single-photon emission computed tomography for the detection and localization of canine insulinoma. *Journal of Veterinary Internal Medicine* 19: 15–22.

Russell, K.N., Mehler, S.J., Skorupski, K.A. et al. (2007). Clinical and immunohistochemical differentiation of gastrointestinal stromal tumors from leiomyosarcomas in dogs: 42 cases (1990–2003). *Journal of the American Veterinary Medical Association* 230: 1329–1333.

Saito, T., Chambers, J.K., Nakashima, K. et al. (2018). Histopathologic features of colorectal adenoma and adenocarcinoma developing within inflammatory polyps in miniature dachshunds. *Veterinary Pathology* 55: 654–662.

Sako, T., Uchida, E., Okamoto, M. et al. (2003). Immunohistochemical evaluation of a malignant intestinal carcinoid in a dog. *Veterinary Pathology* 40: 212–215.

Sarathchandra, S.K., Lunn, J.A., and Hunt, G.B. (2009). Ligation of the caudal mesenteric artery during resection and anastomosis of the colorectal junction for annular adenocarcinoma in two dogs. *Australian Veterinary Journal* 87: 356–359.

Seaman, R.L. (2004). Exocrine pancreatic neoplasia in the cat: a case series. *Journal of the American Animal Hospital Association* 40: 238–245.

Seim-Wikse, T., Jorundsson, E., Nodtvedt, A. et al. (2013). Breed predisposition to canine gastric carcinoma – a study based on the Norwegian canine cancer register. *Acta Veterinaria Scandinavica* 55: 25.

Seim-Wikse, T., Skancke, E., Nødtvedt, A. et al. (2019). Comparison of body condition score and other minimally invasive biomarkers between dogs with gastric carcinoma and dogs with chronic gastritis. *Journal of the American Veterinary Medical Association* 254: 226–235.

Simon, D., Eberle, N., Laacke-Singer, L., and Nolte, I. (2008). Combination chemotherapy in feline lymphoma: treatment outcome, tolerability, and duration in 23 cats. *Journal of Veterinary Internal Medicine* 22: 394–400.

Smith, A.L., Wilson, A.P., Hardie, R.J. et al. (2011). Perioperative complications after full-thickness gastrointestinal surgery in cats with alimentary lymphoma. *Veterinary Surgery* 40: 849–852.

Smith, A.A., Frimberger, A.E., and Moore, A.S. (2019). Retrospective study of survival time and prognostic factors for dogs with small intestinal adenocarcinoma treated by tumor excision with or without adjuvant chemotherapy. *Journal of the American Veterinary Medical Association* 254: 243–250.

Sogame, N., Risbon, R., and Burgess, K.E. (2018). Intestinal lymphoma in dogs: 84 cases (1997–2012). *Journal of the American Veterinary Medical Association* 252: 440–447.

Spugnini, E.P., Crispi, S., Scarabello, A. et al. (2008). Piroxicam and intracavitary platinum-based chemotherapy for the treatment of advanced mesothelioma in pets: preliminary observations. *Journal of Experimental and Clinical Cancer Research* 27: 6.

Stanclift, R.M. and Gilson, S.D. (2004). Use of cisplatin, 5-fluorouracil, and second-look laparotomy for the management of gastrointestinal adenocarcinoma in three dogs. *Journal of the American Veterinary Medical Association* 225 (1412–7): 393.

Swann, H.M. and Holt, D.E. (2002). Canine gastric adenocarcinoma and leiomyosarcoma: a retrospective study of 21 cases (1986–1999) and literature review. *Journal of the American Animal Hospital Association* 38: 157–164.

Tanaka, T., Akiyoshi, H., Mie, K. et al. (2019). Contrast-enhanced computed tomography may be helpful for characterizing and staging canine gastric tumors. *Veterinary Radiology and Ultrasound* 60: 7–18.

Tappin, S., Brown, P., and Ferasin, L. (2008). An intestinal neuroendocrine tumour associated with paroxysmal ventricular tachycardia and melaena in a 10-year-old boxer. *Journal of Small Animal Practice* 49: 33–37.

Teske, E., van Straten, G., van Noort, R., and Rutteman, G.R. (2002). Chemotherapy with cyclophosphamide, vincristine, and prednisolone (COP) in cats with malignant lymphoma: new results with an old protocol. *Journal of Veterinary Internal Medicine* 16: 179–186.

Tidd, K.S., Durham, A.C., Brown, D.C. et al. (2019). Outcomes in 40 cats with discrete intermediate- or large-cell gastrointestinal lymphoma masses treated with surgical mass resection (2005–2015). *Veterinary Surgery* 48: 1218–1228.

Torres, S.M., Caywood, D.D., O'Brien, T.D. et al. (1997). Resolution of superficial necrolytic dermatitis following excision of a glucagon-secreting pancreatic neoplasm in a dog. *Journal of the American Animal Hospital Association* 33: 313–319.

Turek, M.M. (2003). Cutaneous paraneoplastic syndromes in dogs and cats: a review of the literature. *Veterinary Dermatology* 14: 279–296.

Valerius, K.D., Powers, B.E., McPherron, M.A. et al. (1997). Adenomatous polyps and carcinoma in situ of the canine colon and rectum: 34 cases (1982–1994). *Journal of the American Animal Hospital Association* 33: 156–160.

Vergine, M., Pozzo, S., Pogliani, E. et al. (2005). Common bile duct obstruction due to a duodenal gastrinoma in a dog. *Veterinary Journal* 170: 141–143.

Yamazaki, H., Tanaka, T., Mie, K. et al. (2020). Assessment of postoperative adjuvant treatment using toceranib phosphate against adenocarcinoma in dogs. *Journal of Veterinary Internal Medicine* 34: 1272–1281.

Yamazaki, H., Sasai, H., Tanaka, M. et al. (2021). Assessment of biomarkers influencing treatment success on small intestinal lymphoma in dogs. *Veterinary and Comparative Oncology* 19: 123–131.

Zwingenberger, A.L., Marks, S.L., Baker, T.W., and Moore, P.F. (2010). Ultrasonographic evaluation of the muscularis propria in cats with diffuse small intestinal lymphoma or inflammatory bowel disease. *Journal of Veterinary Internal Medicine* 24: 289–292.

11

Megacolon

Stewart D. Ryan

Megacolon is a disorder of both colonic structure and function, in which gross dilatation of the large intestine and inability to evacuate fecal material result in severe chronic constipation or obstipation. Megacolon describes a clinical condition with many possible etiologies, rather than a distinct disease entity.

Megacolon can be classified in a number of ways (primary or secondary, congenital or acquired, functional or mechanical) that provide some indication of the underlying pathophysiology. Functionally, causes of megacolon can be divided into colonic inertia or outlet obstruction, which is useful in selecting appropriate therapeutic options (Bertoy 2002; Zalcman & Bright 2010).

The most common presentation of primary megacolon is idiopathic megacolon in cats. The underlying pathophysiology in feline idiopathic megacolon is dysfunction of smooth muscle in the colon. The diagnosis of idiopathic megacolon is made after mechanical, neurologic, or endocrine causes cannot be identified. Secondary megacolon can occur as a sequela to any lesion that prevents defecation for a prolonged period of time. Common causes of secondary megacolon include outflow obstruction of the pelvic canal, such as pelvic fracture malunion, neoplasia (colonic, rectoanal tumors, intrapelvic extraluminal tumors), anal or rectal stricture, anal atresia, and neurologic conditions (spinal cord or pelvic nerve injury, feline dysautonomia). Other less common causes of secondary megacolon include colonic inflammatory conditions, metabolic and endocrine disease, and pharmacologic, environmental, and behavioral causes.

Pathophysiology

The underlying pathophysiology of megacolon can be divided functionally into colonic inertia or outlet obstruction (Bertoy 2002). Regardless of the cause, chronic obstipation with colonic distension eventually renders the colonic muscle nonfunctional, leading to irreversible changes in colonic smooth muscle and nerves, and subsequently causing inertia. Feces retained in the colon for prolonged periods will dehydrate and solidify, forming concretions that are difficult to eliminate. Absorption of bacterial toxins from the retained feces may cause depression, anorexia, and weakness. Prolonged colonic distension eventually causes irreversible damage to the colonic smooth muscle and nerves. Vomiting may be observed secondary to obstruction, absorbed toxins, or vagal stimulation.

Congenital megacolon (Hirschsprung disease)

Congenital megacolon is a well-recognized condition in human pediatric gastroenterology. The underlying pathophysiology in Hirschsprung disease is congenital absence of intramural myenteric ganglion cells in the submucosal plexus (part of the parasympathetic nervous system) that leads to loss of peristaltic activity (segmental aganglionic megacolon). Congenital segmental aganglionosis is extremely rare in dogs and cats. A single case diagnosed on post-mortem histopathology was recently reported in a kitten (Roe *et al.* 2010).

Small Animal Soft Tissue Surgery, Second Edition. Edited by Eric Monnet.
© 2023 John Wiley & Sons, Inc. Published 2023 by John Wiley & Sons, Inc.
Companion website: www.wiley.com/go/monnet/small

Idiopathic megacolon

Idiopathic megacolon is the most common type of megacolon observed in the cat. The exact underlying etiology is unknown. The pathophysiology of idiopathic megacolon is thought to be a primary acquired disorder resulting from generalized dysfunction of the smooth muscle of the colon, rather than dysfunction of nerves supplying the colon. Contraction of feline colonic smooth muscle is mediated by serotonin (5-hydroxytryptamine, 5-HT). In a series of *in vitro* experiments by Washabau and Zhukovskaya (1994) and Washabau and Stalis (1996), isolated colonic smooth muscle samples from feline normal colons and colons affected with idiopathic megacolon were subjected to isometric stress under the influence of various neurotransmitters, membrane depolarization, and electrical field stimulation. The smooth muscle from the idiopathic megacolon samples developed less isometric stress compared with normal colon. No histologic abnormalities of the myenteric neurons or smooth muscle of these colon samples were observed.

Functional outlet obstruction

Functional outlet obstruction can be due to mechanical outlet obstruction such as pelvic fractures; neoplasia of the colon, rectum, or anus; intrapelvic extraluminal tumors; rectal strictures; intraluminal foreign bodies of the rectum or distal colon; or anal or rectal atresia. Pelvic fracture malunion is the most common cause of outlet obstruction megacolon in the dog and cat. Chronic outflow obstruction leads to colonic distension, irreversible changes in colonic motility, and eventual colonic inertia. Other nonmechanical causes of functional obstruction include distal spinal cord pathology, dysautonomia, and chronic colonic inflammation. Some reports note that Manx cats may have an increased incidence of megacolon (De Haan *et al.* 1992). The pathophysiology of megacolon in these cases is related to the premature ending of the spinal cord in these animals, with absence of spinal cord nerves from the sacral cord segments that supply innervation to the colon and bladder, hindlimbs, and perineal region (Deforest & Basrur 1979).

Clinical presentation

Feline megacolon

Primary idiopathic megacolon can be diagnosed in cats of any age, although it is most commonly diagnosed in middle-aged to older cats, with a mean age at diagnosis of 5.8 years (Greenfield 1991; Holt & Johnston 1991; Salisbury 1991; Washabau & Holt 1999; Bertoy 2002; Byers *et al.* 2006; Dimski 2008). Males are reported to be more commonly affected than females. Affected animals typically present for recurrent progressive episodes of constipation or obstipation, often with a history over months to years. Affected animals are typically anorectic, dehydrated, and lethargic, and may have experienced significant weight loss. They can be anemic and may exhibit vomiting and ptyalism. Some animals will have tenesmus and may pass mucoid liquid feces. Hypokalemia can result secondary to vomiting and anorexia.

Canine megacolon

Canine megacolon is diagnosed much less frequently than feline megacolon. Dogs with megacolon commonly have a history of a bony diet, low exercise levels, and chronic constipation with dyschezia and tenesmus (Nemeth *et al.* 2008; Prokić *et al.* 2010) There is a male sex and large-breed predisposition. Histopathology shows thickening of the colon wall with hypertrophy of the smooth muscle cells.

Diagnosis

The diagnosis of idiopathic megacolon is made based on characteristic clinical presentation and diagnostic imaging and after ruling out all other causes of constipation. The diagnosis is confirmed after exploratory surgery, colectomy, and histopathology.

The clinical history and physical examination findings are highly suggestive of a diagnosis of megacolon. Digital rectal examination may demonstrate scant feces in the rectum, pelvic outlet obstruction, and ability to palpate a firm fecalith. Abdominal palpation will generally reveal firm feces within the colon. Normal fecal material within the colon should be able to be deformed with abdominal palpation, whereas neoplastic mass lesions will not. Neurologic examination, especially assessment of lower motor neuron function, is important for establishing whether an underlying neurologic cause is present.

Abdominal and pelvic radiographs confirm the presence of a large, distended colon filled with fecal material (Figure 11.1). Radiography can also identify underlying causes for megacolon such as pelvic fracture malunion, sacrocaudal spinal trauma or deformity, and rectoanal obstructive lesions.

Concurrent conditions

Perineal hernia

Perineal hernia may develop secondary to chronic tenesmus and constipation associated with megacolon (Welches *et al.* 1992). Perineal hernia in cats is most frequently bilateral. If perineal hernia is secondary to megacolon, subtotal colectomy alone will often resolve the clinical signs and perineal herniorrhaphy may not be required.

(a)

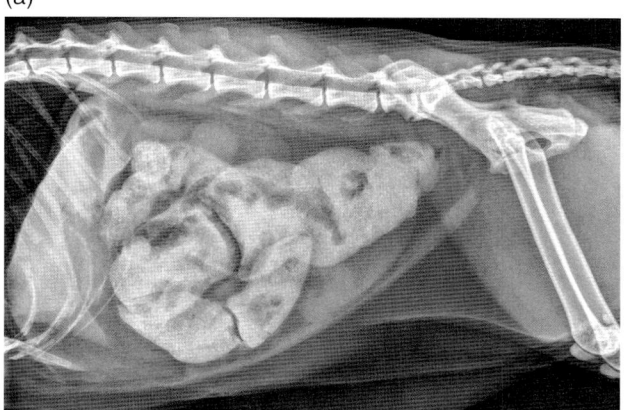

(b)

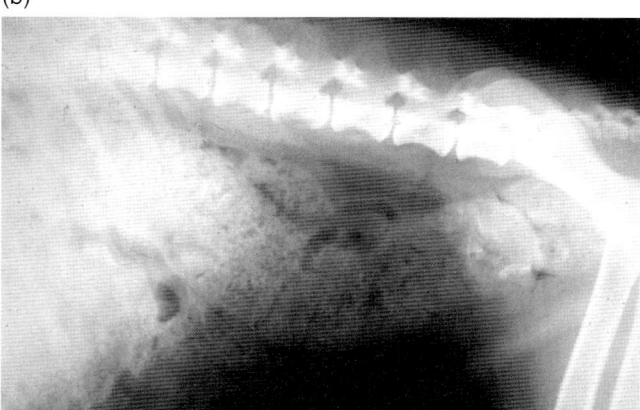

Figure 11.1 (a) Lateral abdominal radiograph of a cat with megacolon. The colon is dilated and full of feces. (b) Lateral abdominal radiograph of a dog with megacolon.

Inflammatory bowel disease

Inflammatory bowel disease (IBD) may be present concurrently with megacolon. Occult IBD may be a cause of persistent gastrointestinal clinical signs after surgical therapy for megacolon. If this is suspected, full-thickness intestinal biopsies of the small intestine and appropriate medical and dietary therapy are indicated (Krecic 2001; Trepanier 2009).

Medical treatment

Medical therapy is indicated prior to surgical intervention in mild cases of megacolon. However, most cases of idiopathic megacolon are progressive and surgical intervention is ultimately required for a successful outcome. Correction of fluid, acid–base, and electrolyte abnormalities (hypokalemia) are very important for successful case management and are essential prior to general anesthesia.

Laxatives that act by bulk forming (e.g., psyllium, bran, or canned pumpkin) or osmotic gradient (e.g., lactulose) or as emollients (e.g., dioctyl sodium sulfosuccinate) can be used in combination with low-residue dietary modification to reduce the amount of fecal material and produce a softer fecal consistency. Lactulose increases the osmotic pressure gradient across the colonic wall to draw water into the bowel lumen. It is well tolerated in the cat at doses of 1 mL per 4.5 kg orally three times daily.

Colonic motility modification using a serotonin (5-HT) agonist such as cisapride (0.5–1.0 mg/kg three times daily or 1.5 mg/kg twice daily) may be beneficial in mild to moderate cases of idiopathic megacolon that have some remaining colonic smooth muscle function. Cisapride mediates contraction of feline colonic smooth muscle by increasing longitudinal smooth muscle

contraction (Hasler & Washabau 1997). The dose of cisapride should be decreased in older cats with hepatic disease (FitzSimons 1999). Histamine H_2-receptor antagonists (e.g., ranitidine, nizatidine) may be used to stimulate colonic contraction through a cholinergic mechanism by the inhibition of synaptic anticholinesterase.

Mechanical removal of retained fecal material can be achieved with enemas of warm water or lubricating enemas under general anesthesia. Enemas should be administered under gravity flow and any manual manipulation of the colon should be gentle to minimize the risk of colonic mucosal damage and bacterial translocation. Enemas containing phosphate should be steered clear of in cats to avoid risk of hypocalcemia, hyperphosphatemia, and death (Bright 1990; Holt & Johnston 1991; Salisbury 1991; Byers *et al.* 2006; Dimski 2008).

Surgical treatment

The decision to proceed to surgical therapy is based on worsening clinical signs (constipation or obstipation) that are refractory to appropriate medical therapy with dietary modification, laxatives, prokinetic therapy, and enemas. Without surgery, many owners elect euthanasia for their pet rather than chronic ineffective medical management. The main goal of the surgery is to improve the quality of life of the patient.

Subtotal colectomy, with or without preservation of the ileocolic valve, is the surgical procedure of choice for treatment of idiopathic megacolon. Careful evaluation for concurrent diseases such as perineal hernia, neurologic dysfunction that may cause decreased anal sphincter tone, or IBD is recommended before surgery.

Patients that are dehydrated should have their fluid deficits and electrolyte and acid–base imbalances corrected before surgery. Preoperative enemas are not recommended prior to surgery. Preoperative enemas are generally ineffective in relieving colonic obstruction in idiopathic megacolon, and can cause liquefaction of colonic contents and be associated with an increased risk of contamination during surgery (Pavletic & Berg 1996).

The risk of infection after colorectal surgery is high due to the high concentration (up to 10^{10}–10^{11} bacteria per gram of feces) of normal resident bacterial flora in the colon. Anaerobic bacteria predominate over aerobic bacteria. Anastomotic leakage or dehiscence can result in septic peritonitis and death. The number of colonic bacteria can be reduced by withholding food for 24 hours before surgery, as well as using oral antimicrobials such as a combination of neomycin and erythromycin or metronidazole combined with first-generation cephalosporins, aminoglycosides, or trimethoprim sulfa. Perioperative antimicrobial prophylaxis is recommended during surgical therapy for megacolon (Ly 1977; Bright *et al.* 1986; Bertoy & MacCoy 1988; Rosin *et al.* 1988a; Kudisch & Pavletic 1993; Pavletic & Berg 1996) The antimicrobial(s) selected should be effective against anaerobic and Gram-negative aerobic bacteria. Second-generation cephalosporins such as cefoxitin (20–30 mg/kg), cefmetazole, or cefotetan are appropriate choices. Metronidazole has been used very frequently as well (Bright 1990, 1991; Greenfield 1991; Pavletic & Berg 1996). The antimicrobial should be administered intravenously 20–30 minutes prior to surgery and repeated every 90 minutes during surgery. Antimicrobial therapy should not be continued in the postoperative period after uncomplicated subtotal colectomy.

A midline ventral laparotomy approach is used for colotomy and colectomy surgical procedures. The colon should be exteriorized from the abdominal cavity and packed off with moistened laparotomy sponges (Figure 11.2). General surgical principles of atraumatic tissue handling, accurate mucosal apposition, tension-free closure, and preservation of blood supply are important for a successful outcome in any colonic surgery.

Gloves and instruments should be changed after closure of the colon. The peritoneal cavity should be lavaged with 0.9% saline prior to abdominal closure. Any resected colon or other tissues should be submitted for histopathology.

The healing of the large intestine is delayed compared with the small intestine due to the action of collagenases (van der Stappen *et al.* 1992). The risk of dehiscence is highest in the first 3–5 days after surgery due to the extended lag phase of healing.

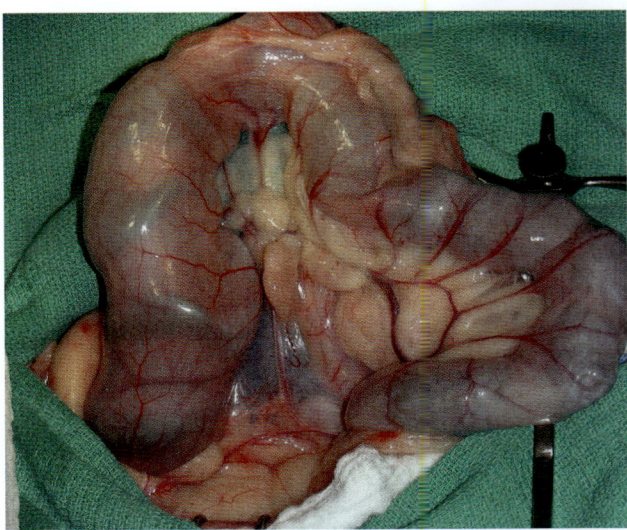

Figure 11.2 Megacolon in a cat. The colon has been exteriorized and isolated with laparotomy sponges and towels to limit contamination during the procedure.

Colotomy

Colotomy involves a linear incision into the antimesenteric colon wall to remove colonic content such as a foreign body or impacted fecal material. The incision is closed with simple interrupted appositional sutures. Colotomy is rarely indicated for the treatment of megacolon, as the underlying pathology is not addressed and constipation or obstipation usually recurs. Colotomy, in combination with intensive postoperative medical therapy, was recently described as a successful therapy for canine acquired hypertrophic megacolon in 26 cases (Prokić *et al.* 2010). The colon was exteriorized, packed off with abdominal sponges, and a longitudinal incision made in the colon wall, followed by manual extraction of the large intestinal contents. Dietary therapy and colonic motility modifiers were used postoperatively.

Subtotal colectomy

Subtotal colectomy, with or without preservation of the ileocolic valve, is the surgical procedure of choice for treatment of idiopathic megacolon (Figure 11.3). Subtotal colectomy will remove 90–95% of the colon. It is important to remove this amount of colon, regardless of how much colon appears to be involved grossly at the time of surgery, as recurrent constipation can be observed if an insufficient length of colon is removed. Partial colectomy, removing only the grossly affected colon, has been described, but is not recommended due to the high rate of recurrent constipation and histologic evidence that the entire colon is affected in cases of idiopathic megacolon (Fellenbaum 1978). The level of proximal resection will be determined by whether the

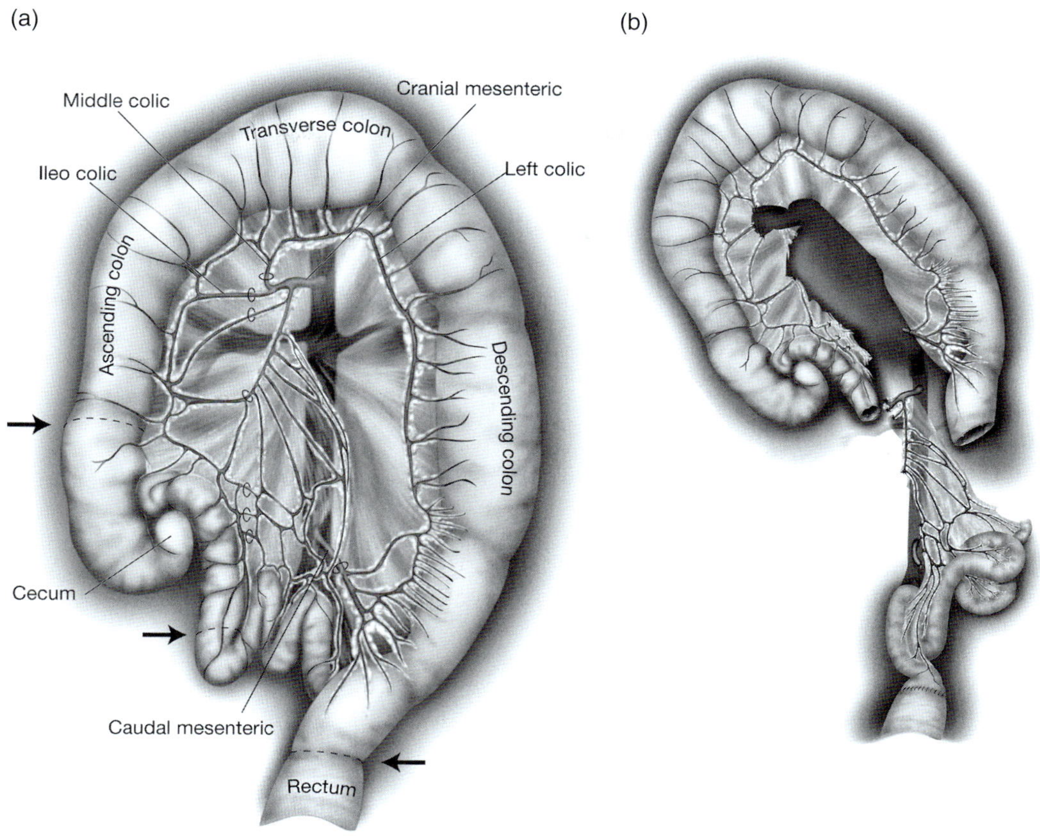

(a)

Middle colic

Cranial mesenteric

Transverse colon

Ileo colic

Left colic

Ascending colon

Descending colon

Cecum

Caudal mesenteric

Rectum

(b)

(c)

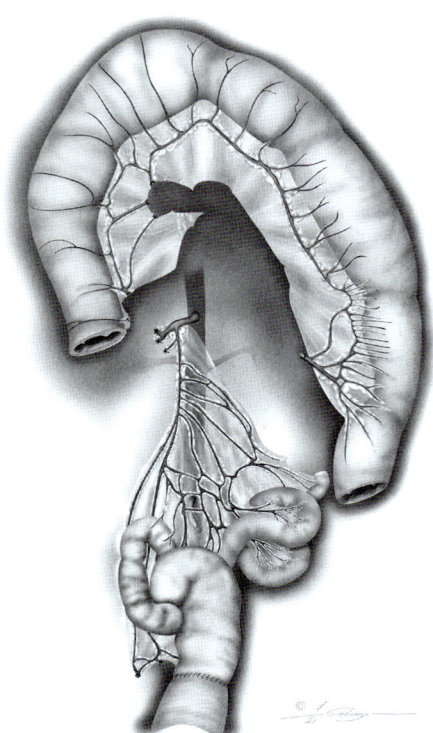

Figure 11.3 Anatomy of the colon in a cat: (a) the different levels of resection are identified; (b) resection of the ileocolic valve with ileocolic anastomosis; (c) preservation of the ileo-colic valve and colocolic anastomosis. © D. Giddings.

ileocolic valve is retained or not. If the ileocolic valve is removed, an ileocolic anastomosis is done and there will be luminal disparity between the ends of the anastomosis. If the ileocolic valve is preserved, 2–3 cm of the ascending colon should be retained and a colocolic anastomosis performed. The descending colon is transected approximately 2–4 cm cranial to the pubis to facilitate anastomosis in both cases. The ileocolic valve should be preserved if possible (Bright 1991; *Sweet et al.* 1994). Preservation of the ileocolic valve is strongly recommended in cases of canine acquired hypertrophic megacolon (Nemeth *et al.* 2008). Tension at the anastomosis site is more likely with preservation of the ileocolic valve due to the short mesocolon. If tension at the anastomosis is likely, then removal of the ileocolic valve and ileocolic anastomosis is indicated for a tension-free anastomosis.

Prior to making the intestinal incisions, the terminal ileum and colon are exteriorized from the abdominal cavity and packed off with laparotomy sponges. The colonic luminal contents should be gently milked away from the proposed incision sites. Atraumatic intestinal clamps (e.g., Doyen intestinal forceps) or surgical assistant's fingers can be used to keep intestinal contents from the incision site.

The vasa recta vessels supplying the colonic segments to be removed should be ligated according to the level of resection. If the ileocecal valve is preserved, the right colic, middle colic, and left colic vessels will be ligated. If the ileocecal valve is removed, the ileocolic and mesenteric and antimesenteric branches of the ileal artery (terminal arcade of jejunal vessels) need to be ligated in addition to the vessels already described. Care must be taken not to damage the cranial or caudal mesenteric arteries.

Methods of anastomosis

There are several anastomotic methods available to reestablish continuity of the gastrointestinal tract after subtotal colectomy (White 2002). The most appropriate method will depend on the amount of colon removed (i.e., whether the anastomosis is an ileocolic or colocolic anastomosis) as well as surgeon experience, preference, and equipment availability. It is important to ensure that the anastomosis is not under tension regardless of technique used. The anastomosis configuration can be an end-to-end, end-to-side, or side-to-side anastomosis and can be achieved with sutures, surgical stapling devices, or a biofragmentable anastomotic ring (BAR).

An ileocolic or colocolic anastomosis can be performed as an end-to-end anastomosis (EEA) (White 2002). If the ileocolic valve is removed, there will be significant luminal disparity between the ileal and

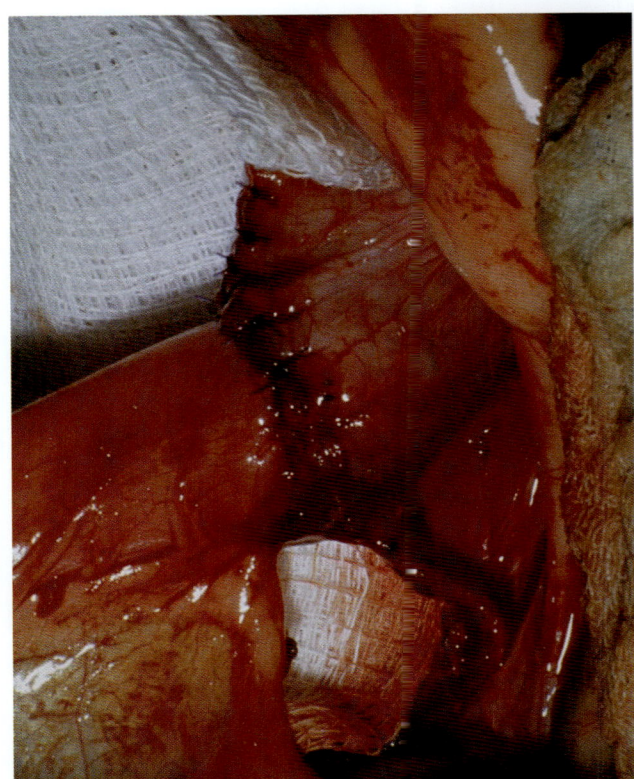

Figure 11.4 End-to-end ileocolic anastomosis. The lumen disparity has been corrected by partially closing the colon.

colonic ends of the anastomosis (Figure 11.4). To address this luminal disparity, the diameter of the colonic lumen is reduced to match that of the ileal lumen by suturing the antimesenteric margin of the colon with simple interrupted or continuous appositional sutures until the lumens are a similar size (Figure 11.4). If the luminal disparity is only mild, then the terminal ileal segment can be spatulated by incising the antimesenteric border to match the lumen diameters.

If an end-to-side anastomosis is used, the entire length of the distal colonic segment is oversewn with a double-layer inverting pattern. The ileal segment or the ascending colon is then anastomosed to an ostomy incision made in the lateral aspect of the distal colonic segment (Bright *et al.* 1986). The anastomosis should not be located too far from the oversewn end to avoid a diverticulum that could accumulate feces. A side-to-side, functional EEA can be achieved with a gastrointestinal anastomosis (GIA) stapler and a thoracoabdominal (TA) stapler (Ullman *et al.* 1991).

Anastomosis after subtotal colectomy can be achieved using sutures, surgical stapling devices, or a BAR. For suture anastomosis, monofilament absorbable or nonabsorbable sutures (e.g., polydioxanone, polyglyconate, polyglactin 910) of 3/0 or 4/0 size with a taper swaged on a curved needle are appropriate after subtotal colectomy. An appositional technique is preferred over inverting or everting techniques and single-layer closure is preferred over a two-layer closure (Richardson *et al.* 1982). Simple interrupted sutures should be placed at the mesenteric and antimesenteric margins to facilitate alignment of the anastomosis. If the ends of these sutures are left long, they can be used as stay sutures to facilitate retraction and movement of the anastomosis, reducing the need to directly handle the colonic tissue. Sutures can be placed in either a simple interrupted or modified continuous appositional suture pattern. If a continuous suture pattern is used, a maximum of 180° of the anastomosis should be done before tying the suture off to avoid a purse-string effect. Each suture throw should be placed approximately 5 mm from the anastomosis margin and sutures should be spaced 3–5 mm apart (Figure 11.5). Care should be taken to ensure that the submucosal layer is incorporated in the sutures, as this is the primary holding layer of the colon. The easiest way to do this is to use full-thickness suture bites incorporating all four histologic layers.

An EEA circular stapling instrument has been described for successful colocolic anastomosis in cats with idiopathic megacolon (Kudisch & Pavletic 1993). The EEA stapler creates an inverting anastomosis. A Furness clamp is very useful to create the purse-string sutures required for positioning the anvil of the EEA stapling device within the lumen (Figure 11.6). In cats, the disposable 21 mm or 25 mm diameter EEA stapling device is introduced through a transcecal access site into the bowel, as the transanal retrograde approach is very difficult in cats due to their narrow pelvic canal. Also it can result in significant contamination of the surgical site (Figures 11.7 and 11.8). Passage of the EEA stapler

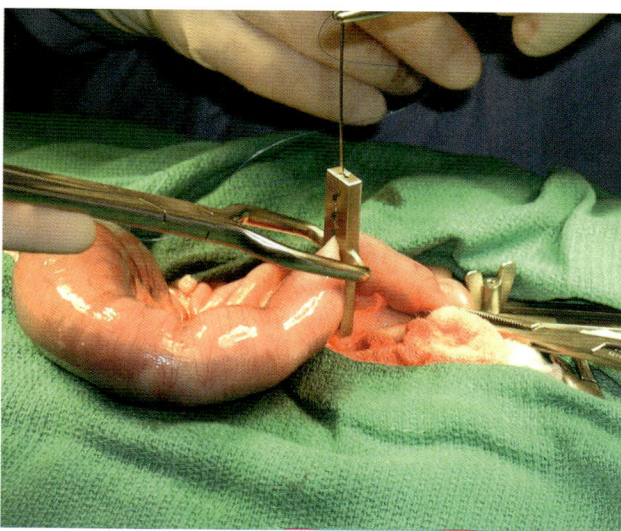

Figure 11.6 A Furness clamp is used to place purse-string sutures on both ends of the colonectomy. A 2-0 monofilament suture is used.

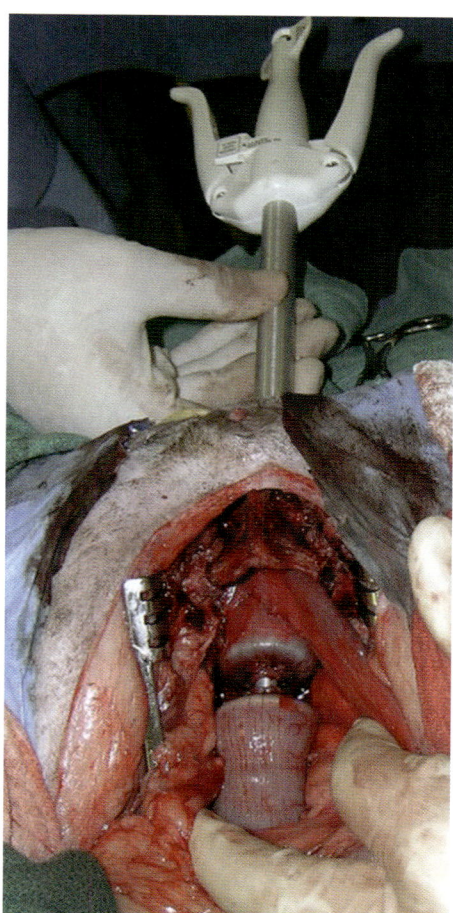

Figure 11.7 Retrograde placement of an end-to-end anastomosis (EEA) stapling device. This procedure can result in significant contamination of the abdominal cavity. It is not always possible in cats because of the diameter of the EEA apparatus.

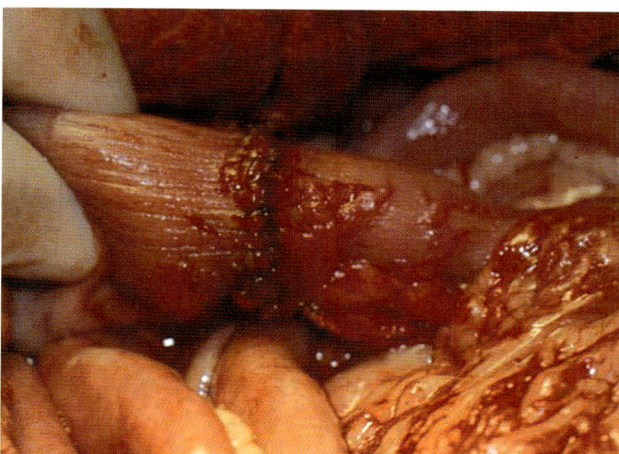

Figure 11.5 Colocolic anastomosis performed with 4-0 monofilament absorbable suture.

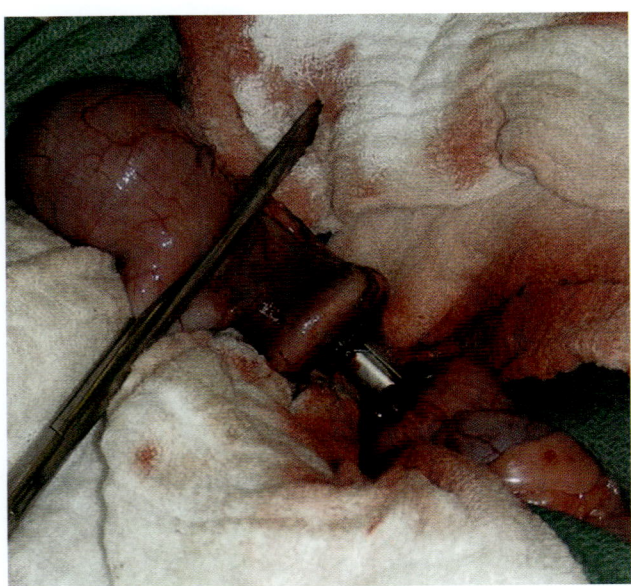

Figure 11.8 The colocolic anastomosis is ready to be completed. Both ends of the colon have been loaded on the end-to-end anastomosis apparatus and the purse-string sutures tightened.

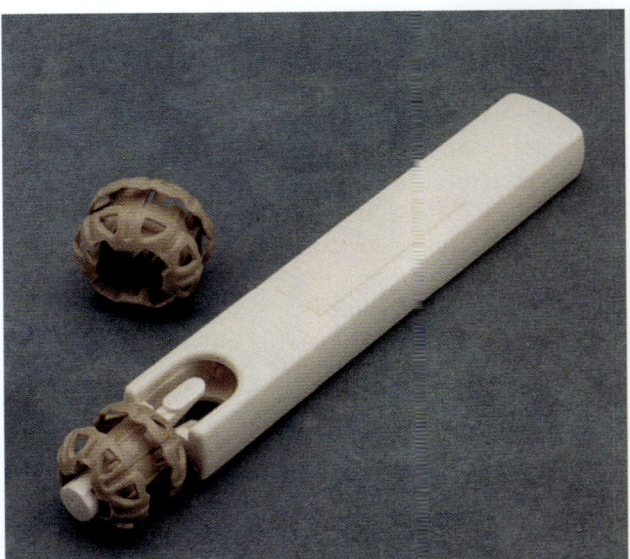

Figure 11.9 Biofragmentable anastomosis ring. This device has a handle to facilitate manipulation during its insertion in the first side of the colon.

through the cecal access site may require dilatation with a series of ovoid sizes. The cecal access site is closed with a TA stapler. The main complication observed with this technique was postoperative bleeding that required treatment with a blood transfusion in 2 of 15 cats. Long-term outcome results in this study were excellent. A transrectal approach for introduction of the EEA stapling device has been described for colonic anastomosis in dogs (Banz et al. 2008). Stapled colonic anastomoses in dogs are reported to have less tissue reaction and a higher tensile strength than inverting or crushing suture methods (Stoloff et al. 1984).

A side-to-side, functional EEA can be achieved with a combination of the GIA and TA staplers (Ullman et al. 1991). If this method is used, an appropriate length of colon, which is not indicated for the treatment of megacolon, should be retained to facilitate the anastomosis. Stapled anastomoses offer the advantage of reliable bursting pressure and tensile wound strength during the lag phase of healing when anastomotic strength is weakest (Stoloff et al. 1984). Stapled anastomoses heal by primary intention with minimal inflammatory response. Stapled anastomoses are quick to perform. As an inverting anastomosis is produced, there is a risk of stricture at the anastomosis site.

The BAR was developed to create a sutureless inverted colonic anastomosis for enterectomy and colonectomy in human patients (Figure 11.9) (Hardy et al. 1985, 1987). The BAR is composed of 87.5% polyglycolic acid and 12.5% barium sulfate and is available in a range of

external diameters and gap sizes. The barium sulfate makes the device radiopaque, so fragmentation and elimination can be monitored radiographically. Potential advantages of the BAR are that it can be placed at the surgical site without an additional incision in the gastrointestinal tract and without retrograde introduction through the anus (Figure 11.10). The inverted tissue will go under necrosis because of the pressure applied by the BAR device (Figure 11.11). After the BAR has fragmented and been eliminated, there is no foreign material remaining at the anastomosis site. The use of a Furness clamp to facilitate purse-string suture placement before colonic resection is recommended to avoid retraction of the colon edges (Figure 11.6) (Huss et al. 1994).

The BAR device has been evaluated for anastomosis after subtotal colectomy in a population of normal cats (Huss et al. 1994). The BAR fragmented in a predictable manner 10–12 days after implantation and was passed in the stool 2–5 days after fragmentation without clinical signs. A 25 mm external diameter BAR with a 1.5 mm gap size was used in a retrospective study comparing the BAR with sutured anastomoses in cats affected by idiopathic megacolon (Figure 11.11) (Ryan et al. 2006). The 25 mm BAR is the smallest diameter commercially available. Reported intraoperative complications with the BAR include narrow luminal diameter causing difficulty in insertion of the smallest diameter device, and serosal splitting after placement of the device (Corman et al. 1989; Huss et al. 1994; Ryan et al. 2006). Warm saline irrigation and intravenous glucagon have been recommended in human patients to allow the bowel to

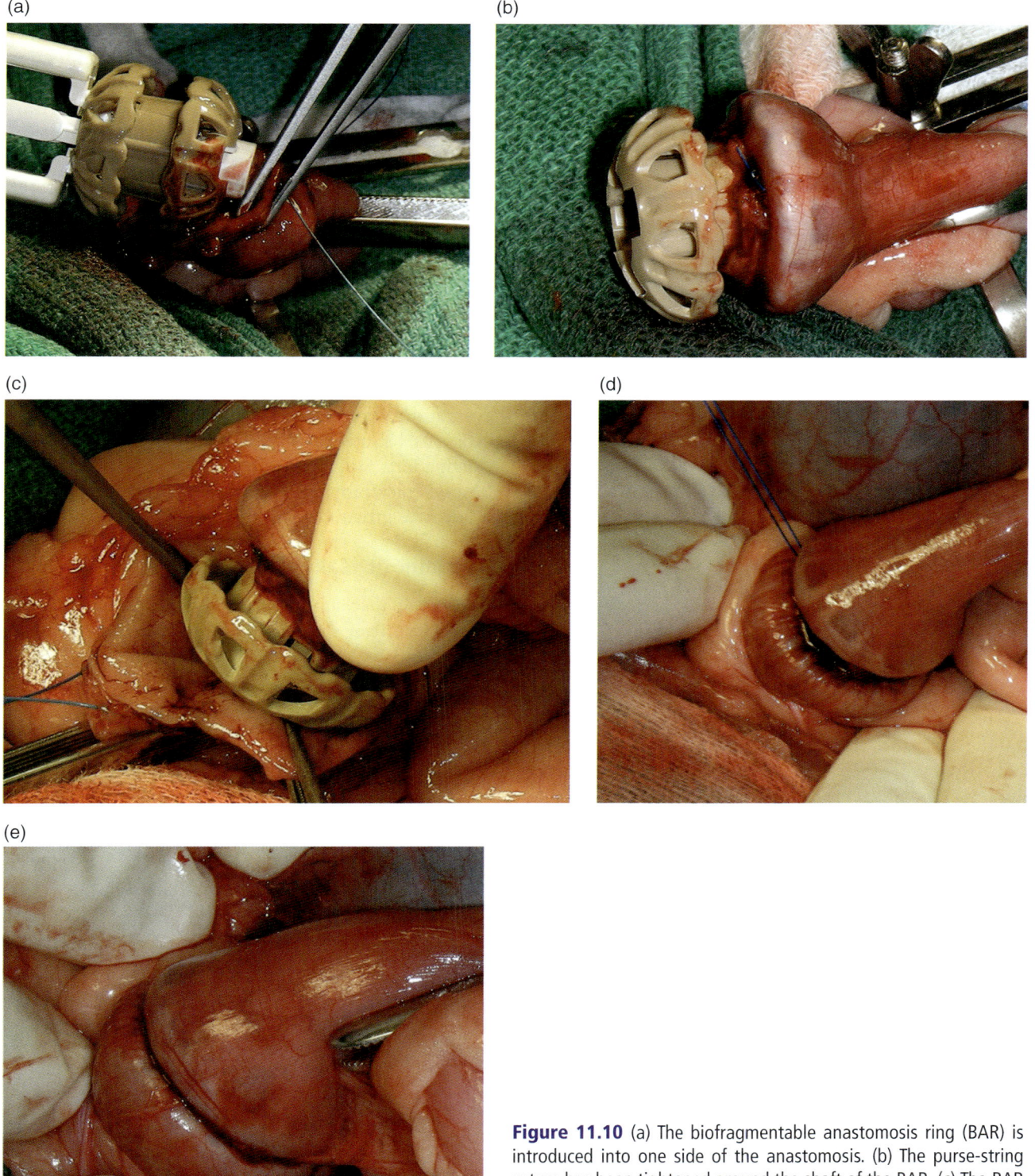

Figure 11.10 (a) The biofragmentable anastomosis ring (BAR) is introduced into one side of the anastomosis. (b) The purse-string suture has been tightened around the shaft of the BAR. (c) The BAR is introduced into the other segment of the colonectomy. (d) The second purse-string suture has been tightened. (e) The BAR is closed with finger pressure. No serosal-to-serosal suture is required.

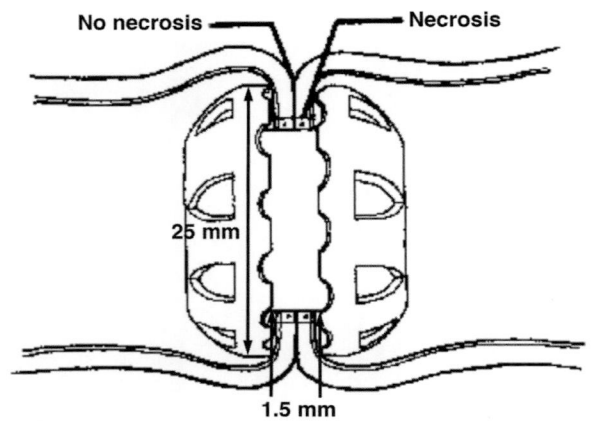

Figure 11.11 The biofragmentable anastomosis ring device used in cats clamps down to 1.5 mm and is 25 mm in diameter.

maximally dilate and facilitate BAR placement. If required, we have used papaverine topically, instead of glucagon, to relax the smooth muscle in the wall of the colon.

Pelvic canal osteotomy

Obstructive megacolon can develop secondary to pelvic canal obstruction, and the most common cause is pelvic fracture malunion. In cases of megacolon secondary to pelvic canal obstruction that have been present for less than six months, pelvic osteotomy or pelvic canal widening procedures are indicated, because the megacolon and the damage to the colonic smooth muscle are potentially reversible (Schrader 1992). Subtotal colectomy alone or in addition to pelvic canal reconstruction may be required if colonic changes are irreversible (Matthiesen et al. 1991). Removal of the ileocolic valve may be indicated in cats affected by megacolon secondary to pelvic outlet obstruction to produce softer stool consistency.

With the patient in dorsal recumbency, a midline approach to the pubic symphysis is made. An osteotomy along the pubic symphysis is made with a saw or osteotome and the pubic bones are retracted laterally. A spacer (allograft or autograft bone, methyl methacrylate spacer, spiral wire, syringe case) is interposed between the pubic bones to increase the pelvic canal diameter (Webb 1985; McKee & Wong 1994; Prassinos et al. 2007).

Postoperative management and outcome

Intravenous fluid therapy should be continued in the postoperative period for 1–3 days to prevent or correct dehydration and electrolyte and acid–base abnormalities. Postoperative analgesics should be administered for 3–5 days. Oral water should be offered 8–12 hours after surgery and a bland low-fat diet offered within 12–24 hours after surgery. Early enteral nutrition helps to promote healing of colonic anastomoses.

Anorexia can be persistent after surgery and appetite stimulants (cyproheptadine/mirtazapine) may be required. Animals may have 10–15% weight loss during the first 2–3 weeks after surgery and then regain body weight within 3–7 weeks. Fecal passage may be more frequent and blood or tenesmus can be common, so regular litterbox changes are important. Fecal continence is usually retained after subtotal colectomy.

Complications

More than 90% of cats have an uncomplicated recovery after subtotal colectomy for treatment of megacolon. Possible short-term postoperative complications include anastomosis dehiscence, peritonitis, anorexia, anemia, fever, and gastrointestinal bleeding. Longer-term complications include anastomotic stricture and recurrent constipation. Soft stool consistency is expected after subtotal colectomy while the terminal ileum undergoes an adaptive process.

Anastomotic leakage/dehiscence

Dehiscence after subtotal colectomy has been reported, but is a relatively rare complication. Patients should be monitored very closely in the immediate postoperative period for evidence of peritonitis. The risk of dehiscence is greatest in the first 3–7 days after surgery due to the lag phase of healing, when collagen lysis exceeds collagen synthesis with a resultant decrease in tensile wound strength. High intraluminal pressures can develop during the passage of fecal material that place mechanical stress on the anastomosis.

Post-colectomy intestinal adaptation

Watery to mucoid stools are expected during the first 3–7 weeks, followed by mucoid to semi-solid to formed stools by 3–6 months (Sweet et al. 1994). In a study of normal cats that underwent colectomy, histology of the ileum showed increases in villus and enterocyte height, which led to adaptive changes in intestinal physiology whereby water resorption and storage capabilities increased, thus normalizing bowel function after subtotal colectomy (Bertoy et al. 1989). In another study, enteric function after subtotal colectomy was compared in cats affected by idiopathic megacolon and in normal cats, and no differences in enteric function were reported (Gregory et al. 1990).

Increased frequency of defecation is noted in 30–50% of cases after subtotal colectomy due to the decreased storage capacity for fecal material. Fecal consistency is looser if the ileocecal junction is excised, so preservation of the ileocolic valve is recommended when possible (Sweet *et al.* 1994). In dogs, normal defecation and fecal consistency occurred at a mean of seven weeks after surgery (Nemeth *et al.* 2008).

Stricture

Stricture at the anastomotic site is a reported complication after subtotal colectomy in dogs and cats (Rosin *et al.* 1988b). One dog and one cat out of ten animals treated with a circular EEA stapler developed postoperative stricture (Banz *et al.* 2008). Colonic anastomosis stricture can be treated with balloon dilatation and triamcinolone injections (Webb *et al.* 2007).

Recurrent constipation

The recurrence rate for constipation was 45% in one study, with recurrence rates the same whether the ileocolic junction was preserved or excised (Sweet *et al.* 1994). It is important to remove the entire colon regardless of gross appearance, so as to decrease the risk of postoperative recurrent constipation as a complication.

Fecal incontinence

Fecal continence is usually preserved after subtotal colectomy. If clinical signs of tenesmus and increased defecation frequency persist after the anticipated adaptation period, further diagnostic investigation is indicated to rule out concurrent IBD.

Prognosis

The long-term prognosis after surgical treatment of megacolon with subtotal colectomy in both cats and dogs is excellent regardless of the anastomotic technique used (Kudisch & Pavletic 1993; Rosin 1993; Ryan *et al.* 2006). The four-year survival rate has been reported as 90–100% in cats, depending on the surgical technique used (Ryan *et al.* 2006).

References

Banz, W.J., Jackson, J., Richter, K., and Launer, D.P. (2008). Transrectal stapling for colonic resection and anastomosis (10 cases). *Journal of the American Animal Hospital Association* 44: 198–204.

Bertoy, R.W. (2002). Megacolon in the cat. *Veterinary Clinics of North America Small Animal Practice* 32: 901–915.

Bertoy, R.W. and MacCoy, D.M. (1988). Total colectomy with ileorectal anastomosis in the cat [abstract]. *Veterinary Surgery* 17: 28.

Bertoy, E.W., MacCoy, D.M., Wheaton, L.G., and Gelberg, H.B. (1989). Total colectomy with ileorectal anastomosis in the cat. *Veterinary Surgery* 18: 204–210.

Bright, R.M. (1990). Treatment of feline colonic obstruction (megacolon). In: *Current Techniques in Small Animal Surgery* (ed. M.J. Bojrab), 263–265. Philadelphia, PA: Lea & Febiger.

Bright, R.M. (1991). Idiopathic megacolon in the cat. Subtotal colectomy with preservation of the ileocolic valve. *Veterinary Medicine Report* 3: 183–187.

Bright, R.M., Burrows, C.F., Goring, R. et al. (1986). Subtotal colectomy for treatment of acquired megacolon in the dog and cat. *Journal of the American Veterinary Medical Association* 188: 1412–1416.

Byers, C.G., Leasure, C.S., and Sanders, N.A. (2006). Feline idiopathic megacolon. *Compendium on Continuing Education for the Practicing Veterinarian* 28: 658–665.

Corman, M.L., Prager, E.D., Hardy, T.G. Jr., and Bubrick, M.P. (1989). Comparison of the Valtrac biofragmentable anastomosis ring with conventional suture and stapled anastomosis in colon surgery. Results of a prospective, randomized clinical trial. *Diseases of the Colon and Rectum* 32: 183–187.

De Haan, J.J., Ellison, G.W., and Bellah, J.R. (1992). Surgical correction of idiopathic megacolon in cats. *Feline Practice* 20: 6–11.

Deforest, M.E. and Basrur, P.K. (1979). Malformations and the Manx syndrome in cats. *Canadian Veterinary Journal* 20: 304–314.

Dimski, D.S. (2008). Feline megacolon. In: *Proceedings of the North American Veterinary Conference, Small Animals and Exotics*, vol. 22, 527. Gainesville, FL: North American Veterinary Conference.

Fellenbaum, S. (1978). Partial colectomy in the treatment of recurrent obstipation/megacolon in the cat. *Veterinary Medicine/Small Animal Clinician* 73: 737–742.

FitzSimons, H. (1999). Cisapride. *Compendium on Continuing Education for the Practicing Veterinarian* 21: 324–326.

Greenfield, C.L. (1991). Idiopathic megacolon in the cat. Subtotal colectomy with removal of the ileocolic valve. *Veterinary Medicine Report* 3: 182–185.

Gregory, C.R., Guilford, W.G., Berry, C.R. et al. (1990). Enteric function in cats after subtotal colectomy for treatment of megacolon. *Veterinary Surgery* 19: 216–220.

Hardy, T.G. Jr., Pace, W.G., Maney, J.W. et al. (1985). A biofragmentable ring for sutureless bowel anastomosis. An experimental study. *Diseases of the Colon and Rectum* 28: 484–490.

Hardy, T.G. Jr., Aguilar, P.S., Stewart, W.R. et al. (1987). Initial clinical experience with a biofragmentable ring for sutureless bowel anastomosis. *Diseases of the Colon and Rectum* 30: 55–61.

Hasler, A.H. and Washabau, R.J. (1997). Cisapride stimulates contraction of idiopathic megacolonic smooth muscle in cats. *Journal of Veterinary Internal Medicine* 11: 313–318.

Holt, D. and Johnston, D.E. (1991). Idiopathic megacolon in cats. *Compendium on Continuing Education for the Practicing Veterinarian* 13: 1411–1416.

Huss, B.T., Payne, J.T., Johnson, G.C., and Wagner-Mann, C.C. (1994). Comparison of a biofragmentable intestinal anastomosis ring with appositional suturing for subtotal colectomy in normal cats. *Veterinary Surgery* 23: 466–474.

Krecic, M.R. (2001). Feline inflammatory bowel disease: treatment, prognosis, and new developments. *Compendium on Continuing Education for the Practicing Veterinarian* 23: 964–973.

Kudisch, M. and Pavletic, M.M. (1993). Subtotal colectomy with surgical stapling instruments via a trans-cecal approach for treatment of acquired megacolon in cats. *Veterinary Surgery* 22: 457–463.

Ly, J.T. (1977). Surgical correction of megacolon in a cat. *Australian Veterinary Practitioner* 7: 210–212.

Matthiesen, D.T., Scavelli, T.D., and Whitney, W.O. (1991). Subtotal colectomy for the treatment of obstipation secondary to pelvic fracture malunion in cats. *Veterinary Surgery* 20: 113–117.

McKee, W.M. and Wong, W.T. (1994). Symphyseal distraction-osteotomy using an ulnar autograft for the treatment of pelvic canal stenosis in three cats. *Veterinary Record* 134: 132–135.

Nemeth, T., Solymosi, N., and Balka, G. (2008). Long-term results of subtotal colectomy for acquired hypertrophic megacolon in eight dogs. *Journal of Small Animal Practice* 49: 618–624.

Pavletic, M.M. and Berg, J. (1996). Gastrointestinal surgery. In: *Complications in Small Animal Surgery* (ed. A.J. Lipowitz, D.D. Caywood, C. Newton, et al.), 365–398. Philadelphia, PA: Lippincott Williams & Wilkins.

Prassinos, N.N., Adamama-Moraitou, K.K., Gouletsou, P.G., and Rallis, T.S. (2007). Symphyseal distraction-osteotomy using a novel spacer of spirally fashioned orthopaedic wire for the management of obstipation. *Journal of Feline Medicine and Surgery* 9: 23–28.

Prokić, B., Todorović, V., Mitrović, O. et al. (2010). Ethiopathogenesis, diagnosis and therapy of acquired megacolon in dogs. *Acta Veterinaria (Beograd)* 60: 273–284.

Richardson, D.C., Duckett, K.E., Krahwinkel, D.J., and Shipman, L.W. (1982). Colonic anastomosis: evaluation of an end-to-end crushing and inverting technique. *American Journal of Veterinary Research* 43: 436–442.

Roe, K.A., Syme, H.M., and Brooks, H.W. (2010). Congenital large intestinal hypoganglionosis in a domestic shorthair kitten. *Journal of Feline Medicine and Surgery* 12: 418–420.

Rosin, E. (1993). Megacolon in cats. The role of colectomy. *Veterinary Clinics of North America Small Animal Practice* 23: 587–608.

Rosin, E., Walshaw, R., Mehlhaff, C. et al. (1988a). Subtotal colectomy for treatment of chronic constipation associated with idiopathic megacolon in cats: 38 cases (1979–1985). *Journal of the American Veterinary Medical Association* 193: 850–893.

Rosin, E., Walshaw, R., Mehlhaff, C. et al. (1988b). Subtotal colectomy for treatment of chronic constipation associated with idiopathic megacolon in 38 cats. *Veterinary Surgery* 17: 39–39.

Ryan, S., Seim, H. III, MacPhail, C. et al. (2006). Comparison of biofragmentable anastomosis ring and sutured anastomoses for subtotal colectomy in cats with idiopathic megacolon. *Veterinary Surgery* 35: 740–748.

Salisbury, S.K. (1991). Feline megacolon. *Veterinary Medicine Report* 3: 131–138.

Schrader, S.C. (1992). Pelvic osteotomy as a treatment for obstipation in cats with acquired stenosis of the pelvic canal: six cases (1978–1989). *Journal of the American Veterinary Medical Association* 200: 208–213.

van der Stappen, J.W., Hendriks, T., de Boer, H.H. et al. (1992). Collagenolytic activity in experimental intestinal anastomoses. Differences between small and large bowel and evidence for the presence of collagenase. *Internationa Journal of Colorectal Disease* 7: 95–101.

Stoloff, D., Snider, T.G. III, Crawford, M.P. et al. (1984). End-to-end colonic anastomosis: a comparison of techniques in normal dogs. *Veterinary Surgery* 13: 76–82.

Sweet, D.C., Hardie, E.M., and Stone, E.A. (1994). Preservation versus excision of the ileocolic junction during colectomy for megacolon: a study of 22 cats. *Journal of Small Animal Practice* 35: 358–363.

Trepanier, L. (2009). Idiopathic inflammatory bowel disease in cats. Rational treatment selection. *Journal of Feline Medicine and Surgery* 11: 32–38.

Ullman, S.L., Pavletic, M.M., and Clark, G.J. (1991). Open intestinal anastomosis with surgical stapling equipment in 24 dogs and cats. *Veterinary Surgery* 20: 385–391.

Washabau, R.J. and Holt, D. (1999). Pathogenesis, diagnosis, and therapy of feline idiopathic megacolon. *Veterinary Clinics of North America Small Animal Practice* 29: 589–603.

Washabau, R.J. and Stalis, I.H. (1996). Alterations in colonic smooth muscle function in cats with idiopathic megacolon. *American Journal of Veterinary Research* 57: 580–587.

Washabau, R.J. and Zhukovskaya (1994). Alterations in colonic smooth muscle function in cats affected with idiopathic megacolon [abstract]. *Veterinary Surgery* 23: 20.

Webb, S.M. (1985). Surgical management of acquired megacolon in the cat. *Journal of Small Animal Practice* 26: 399–405.

Webb, C.B., McCord, K.W., and Twedt, D.C. (2007). Rectal strictures in 19 dogs: 1997–2005. *Journal of the American Animal Hospital Association* 43: 332–336.

Welches, C.D., Scavelli, T.D., Aronsohn, M.G., and Matthiesen, D.T. (1992). Perineal hernia in the cat: a retrospective study of 40 cases. *Journal of the American Animal Hospital Association* 28: 431–438.

White, R.N. (2002). Surgical management of constipation. *Journal of Feline Medicine and Surgery* 4: 129–138.

Zalcman, A. and Bright, R.M. (2010). Megacolon. In: *Mechanism of Disease in Small Animal Surgery*, 3e (ed. M.J. Bojrab), 200–203. Teton NewMedia: Jackson, WY.

12

Anal Sac Disease

Maureen Griffin and William T.N. Culp

Anatomy

The anal sacs are paired organs found ventrolateral and cranial to the anal orifice. The anal sacs are located between the external and internal anal sphincters and can be palpated externally or from within the rectum (Baker 1962; Dyce *et al.* 1996). Anal sacs in normal dogs tend to be empty or soft when palpated (Robson *et al.* 2003). Each anal sac has a duct that extends to the anal orifice and from which a secretion produced by the glands of the anal sac can be discharged near the anocutaneous junction (Baker 1962; Marretta 1998). As opposed to dogs, the orifice of the anal sac duct in cats opens on a pyramidal prominence 0.25 cm lateral to the anus (Marretta 1998).

The anal sac is a pouch consisting of a fundus and neck that are lined by thin stratified squamous epithelium (Montagna & Parks 1948; Al-Bagdadi 1993). Sebaceous glands line the neck of the anal sac, while apocrine glands line the fundus of the anal sac. Together these glands form the secretion that is discharged from the anal sac duct onto the anal orifice surface. This secretion is utilized for scenting, and individual olfactory signals are generated by an animal's secretion (Meyer *et al.* 2001). The secretion is 88% water and 12% dry matter.

Several studies have characterized the contents of the anal sacs in dogs (Pappalardo *et al.* 2002; Robson *et al.* 2003; Lake *et al.* 2004). The majority of anal sacs contain keratinocytes as well as leukocytes. Over 75% of the leukocytes are degenerate and bacteria are rarely found intracellularly. The number of bacilli and cocci are variable in the normal anal sac, and it is unlikely that quantitative bacterial counts will be useful in the diagnosis of anal sac disease. In one study, Gram-positive cocci were found in higher numbers in 86% of anal sac secretion samples, while Gram-positive rods predominated in only 14% of samples (Lake *et al.* 2004). The total number of yeasts in anal sac secretions is generally low, although some dogs have a large quantity and 63% of dogs will have at least one yeast per high-power field. Erythrocytes are very uncommon in canine anal sac secretions. The left and right anal sacs in dogs without anal sac disease may differ in gross characteristics but tend to have similar microscopic characteristics.

The normal anal sac contents of cats have also been described and are similar to what is seen in dogs (Lake *et al.* 2004; Frankel *et al.* 2008). Cats less than 1 year old are significantly more likely to have watery secretions as opposed to older cats. Gross characteristics such as color and consistency are variable among different cats. Epithelial cells are found commonly in feline anal sac secretions, and 63% of samples will contain neutrophils. Erythrocytes and intracellular bacteria are not normally part of the anal sac secretion. Similar to dogs, the majority of feline anal sac secretions are dominated by Gram-positive cocci (63%).

Important arterial branches are found in the region of the anal sacs and include the caudal rectal and perianal arteries, as well as the caudal gluteal artery, which is a branch of the internal iliac artery. The perineal nerve provides the nervous supply to the anal sacs.

Small Animal Soft Tissue Surgery, Second Edition. Edited by Eric Monnet.
© 2023 John Wiley & Sons, Inc. Published 2023 by John Wiley & Sons, Inc.
Companion website: www.wiley.com/go/monnet/small

Anal sac diseases

Neoplasia

Historically, female dogs were found to be more likely to develop anal sac adenocarcinoma compared with male dogs (Goldschmidt & Zoltowski 1981; Meuten *et al.* 1981). Other studies have called this into question, as females have accounted for 42–54% of cases in these cohorts (Bennett *et al.* 2002; Williams *et al.* 2003; Polton *et al.* 2006; Polton & Brearley 2007). Most dogs diagnosed with anal sac adenocarcinoma are geriatric, with a median age between 10 and 11 years at the time of diagnosis. Many studies note that mixed-breed dogs are most commonly affected with anal sac adenocarcinoma; however, in a study of British dogs, English cocker spaniels were estimated to have a mean relative risk of 7.3 (Polton *et al.* 2006).

Dogs diagnosed with anal sac adenocarcinoma are presented for evaluation of a myriad of clinical signs, the most common historical complaints including perianal swelling/rectal mass and tenesmus. Other common signs associated with anal sac neoplasia include anorexia/inappetence, polyuria/polydipsia, lethargy, weight loss, urinary incontinence, constipation, and posterior weakness. At the time of referral, 39% of dogs will have more than one clinical sign (Bennett *et al.* 2002).

Between 7% and 34% of anal sac adenocarcinomas are diagnosed incidentally during routine rectal examination (Bennett *et al.* 2002). Several aspects of the rectal examination are essential in the staging of anal masses. First, the anal sac mass should be palpated for size and adherence to underlying tissues, in particular the rectum. Second, palpation of the vertebral bodies and pelvis is important in order to discover evidence of pain, which may suggest metastatic bone disease. Lastly, palpation of the sublumbar lymph nodes should be attempted, as metastatic disease may be palpable due to lymphadenopathy. The majority of anal sac adenocarcinomas are unilateral, but bilateral cases have been reported (Meuten *et al.* 1981).

Tumor size has been shown to affect outcome in several studies (Williams *et al.* 2003; Polton & Brearley 2007; Simeonov & Simeonova 2008; Schlag *et al.* 2020). Dogs with tumors larger than 2.5 cm have been reported to have a worse prognosis and are more likely to present with metastatic disease (Polton & Brearley 2007; Schlag *et al.* 2020). In a separate study, dogs with tumors of 10 cm² or more had a median survival time of 292 days compared with dogs with tumors of less than 10 cm², which had a median survival time of 584 days (Williams *et al.* 2003). Approximately 86% of cases with tumor diameter above 5 cm will have metastases in the regional lymph nodes at the time of diagnosis (Simeonov & Simeonova 2008).

Bloodwork (complete blood count, serum chemistry panel) must be performed in all dogs diagnosed with an anal sac mass. Hypercalcemia has been documented in 25–90% of dogs diagnosed with anal sac adenocarcinoma (Meuten *et al.* 1981; Bennett *et al.* 2002; Williams *et al.* 2003). Many of the clinical signs (polyuria/polydipsia, lethargy, weakness, vomiting) regularly noted can be attributed to hypercalcemia (Meuten *et al.* 1981; Elliott *et al.* 1991). Anal sac adenocarcinomas are the second most likely neoplastic disease after lymphoma to cause hypercalcemia (Messinger *et al.* 2009). Additionally, dogs with anal sac adenocarcinoma have statistically higher concentrations of ionized serum calcium compared with dogs with renal failure, carcinoma, hypoadrenocorticism, and noncarcinomatous neoplasia, as well as statistically higher total serum calcium compared with dogs with renal failure, nonmalignant neoplasia, granulomas, carcinoma, and noncarcinomatous neoplasia.

Dogs with anal sac adenocarcinomas that develop hypercalcemia typically also have low or undetectable serum parathyroid hormone and increased urinary excretion of calcium, hydroxyproline, and cyclic adenosine monophosphate (AMP); these findings occur in concordance with increased levels of parathyroid hormone-related protein (PTHrp) (Rosol *et al.* 1986, 1992). Canine anal sac adenocarcinomas express mRNA for PTHrp and also produce a PTHrp that is homologous to human PTHrp (Meuten *et al.* 1982; Weir *et al.* 1988; Rosol *et al.* 1990). PTHrp is secreted by tumor cells and has the capacity to bind to parathyroid hormone receptors, thereby causing stimulation of osteoclastic bone resorption and increased reabsorption of calcium in the kidneys (Rosol *et al.* 1990; Rosol & Capen 1996; Gröne *et al.* 1998). In dogs with hypercalcemia and increased concentrations of PTHrp (1.5 pmol/L), the positive predictive value for a malignant disorder (anal sac adenocarcinoma, lymphoma, parathyroid carcinoma) is 100%, and the sensitivity with similar parameters is 86% (Mellanby *et al.* 2006).

The total serum calcium in hypercalcemic dogs with anal sac adenocarcinoma has a significant linear correlation with the concentration of PTHrp (Rosol *et al.* 1992). Serum calcium levels will often return to normal after removal of the anal sac adenocarcinoma, likely due to alteration in PTHrp concentrations. However, if recurrence occurs or metastatic disease is noted, hypercalcemia may return. The presence of hypercalcemia negatively affects survival times (Ross *et al.* 1991; Williams *et al.* 2003).

In addition to these biochemical profile abnormalities, many dogs will demonstrate hypophosphatemia. Up to 71% of cases of canine anal sac adenocarcinomas have been documented to have hypophosphatemia. Similar to calcium concentrations, hypophosphatemia will often resolve when the anal sac adenocarcinoma has been removed.

Nuclear morphometric analysis has been utilized to evaluate anal sac adenomas and adenocarcinomas (Simeonov & Simeonova 2008). Certain nuclear parameters (mean nuclear area, mean nuclear perimeter, mean nuclear diameter, nuclear roundness) differ significantly between canine anal sac adenoma and adenocarcinoma. Additionally, in cases with anal sac adenocarcinoma, mean nuclear area, mean nuclear perimeter, and mean nuclear diameter are significantly higher in cases that metastasize compared with those that do not. Additional histopathologic findings associated with a worse prognosis in dogs with anal sac adenocarcinoma include tumor necrosis, solid pattern, and vascular invasion (Wong *et al.* 2021). One study showed no prognostic significance of Ki67 index in dogs with anal sac adenocarcinoma (Morello *et al.* 2021).

Fine-needle aspiration of anal sac masses can be performed prior to surgical removal. Fine-needle aspiration of these masses is not well described in the veterinary literature, but cytology can be used to confirm a diagnosis of anal sac adenocarcinoma, as these cells exfoliate well and diagnostic samples can often be obtained. Incisional biopsies are generally not recommended. When possible, excisional biopsies should be performed and the entire mass should be submitted. Anal sac adenocarcinomas have a unique and characteristic histologic appearance, as these tumors are derived from the apocrine glands of the anal sac and therefore have distinct tubular structures noted on histopathologic evaluation. The glands of the anal sac merge directly with the tumor, adding another distinguishing feature to this malignant neoplasm. Other authors have characterized three distinct histologic patterns: a solid pattern, a tubular pattern, and a rosette pattern (Goldschmidt & Zoltowski 1981).

Metastasis is common with canine anal sac adenocarcinomas, and lymph node and pulmonary metastases have been shown to be negative prognostic indicators (Williams *et al.* 2003; Polton & Brearley 2007). Up to 96% of cases will have metastatic disease at the time of diagnosis (Ross *et al.* 1991). As such, thoracic radiography is always indicated when evaluating patients with anal sac masses. Three-view thoracic radiography should be performed and should be assessed for the presence of metastatic disease; the cardiopulmonary structures should also be evaluated to ensure that there are no obvious contraindications to anesthesia. Pulmonary metastases are noted in 8–22% of cases with confirmed anal sac adenocarcinoma (Goldschmidt & Zoltowski 1981;

Meuten *et al.* 1981; Ross *et al.* 1991; Bennett *et al.* 2002; Williams *et al.* 2003; Sutton *et al.* 2022). Dogs with anal sac adenocarcinoma and distant pulmonary metastasis generally also have concurrent locoregional lymphadenopathy, and staging of the abdomen is very important in these dogs (Sutton *et al.* 2022).

In addition to thoracic imaging, abdominal radiography, ultrasound, and/or computed tomography (CT) should be performed in all patients with anal sac adenocarcinoma. Importantly, no association between anal sac mass size and presence or absence of sublumbar lymph node metastasis has been detected, such that abdominal staging is indicated in all cases of anal sac tumors (Sutton *et al.* 2022). Sublumbar lymphadenopathy can occur secondary to metastatic disease and can occasionally be visible on abdominal radiographs. Metastatic disease to the sublumbar lymph nodes occurs frequently (47–96%) (Goldschmidt & Zoltowski 1981; Meuten *et al.* 1981; Ross *et al.* 1991; Bennett *et al.* 2002; Williams *et al.* 2003; Emms 2005; Polton & Brearley 2007; Sutton *et al.* 2022). The abdominal radiographs may also reveal metastatic lesions to the lumbar vertebrae or pelvis. Other metastatic sites may include liver, spleen, femur, inguinal lymph node, pancreas, heart, and mediastinum. Ultrasound or CT examination of the abdomen should be performed prior to definitive therapy to evaluate dogs for signs of intra-abdominal disease. When comparing the efficacy of abdominal ultrasound and CT for staging of dogs with anal sac adenocarcinoma, one study showed that although abdominal ultrasound identified at least one enlarged lymph node in all dogs with enlarged lymph nodes on CT, ultrasound correctly identified all enlarged lymph nodes in only 31% of dogs (Palladino *et al.* 2016). The most common site to have visible metastatic disease is the sublumbar lymph nodes (Goldschmidt & Zoltowski 1981; Meuten *et al.* 1981; Ross *et al.* 1991; Bennett *et al.* 2002; Williams *et al.* 2003; Emms 2005; Hobson *et al.* 2006; Polton & Brearley 2007). Sentinel lymph node mapping via indirect CT lymphography and lymphoscintigraphy has been reported in dogs with and without anal sac adenocarcinoma, demonstrating a widely variable pattern of lymphatic drainage (Majeski *et al.* 2017; Linden *et al.* 2019). For dogs with anal sac adenocarcinoma, sentinel lymph nodes were ipsilateral to the tumor in 8/12 and contralateral to the tumor in 4/12 cases, and sentinel lymph nodes included sacral, internal iliac, and medial iliac lymph nodes (Majeski *et al.* 2017). Fine-needle aspiration and cytologic examination can confirm the diagnosis of metastatic disease and may direct the surgeon removing the primary tumor to also perform an abdominal exploration. Dogs with metastatic disease from a primary anal sac adenocarcinoma to the medial iliac lymph nodes have more lymph nodes identified by ultrasound as well as more heterogeneous lymph nodes than dogs without metastatic disease (Llabrés-Díaz 2004).

Surgery is generally considered the first-line therapy for the treatment of primary anal sac adenocarcinomas. There are several documented postoperative complications that may occur after the removal of anal sac adenocarcinoma. Recurrence (both locally and to sublumbar lymph nodes) is most common. Local recurrence rates of 12–45% have been reported (Ross *et al.* 1991; Bennett *et al.* 2002; Barnes & Demetriou 2017; Sterman *et al.* 2021). The only risk factor significantly associated with local recurrence in one study was the presence of vascular or lymphatic invasion (Sterman *et al.* 2021). Incomplete or narrow excision of the anal sac tumor (with residual microscopic disease) has not been demonstrated to have an association with local disease recurrence. Postoperative development or recurrence of lymph node metastasis has been reported in 42% of dogs (Barnes & Demetriou 2017). In addition, one study reported anorectal wall perforation as the most common intraoperative complication, and local infection rates as high as 12% have been reported (Sterman *et al.* 2021). In another study, 5 of 27 dogs developed incontinence postoperatively (two cases resolved). In a large case series involving 81 dogs that underwent surgery as part of the treatment regimen, surgical complications included infection (2 dogs), fecal incontinence (2 dogs), hypocalcemia (1 dog), sudden death (1 dog), tenesmus (1 dog), and perianal fistula (1 dog) (Williams *et al.* 2003). Clinical hypocalcemia following anal sacculectomy for adenocarcinoma in dogs with preoperative hypercalcemia has been reported in several cases (Olsen & Sumner 2019).

Historically, dogs undergoing surgery alone have had median survival times between 7.9 and 16.4 months (Bennett *et al.* 2002; Williams *et al.* 2003). However, for dogs with early stage (<3.2 cm diameter, nonmetastatic) anal sac adenocarcinoma, median survival time as high as 1237 days has been reported with surgical treatment alone (Skorupski *et al.* 2018). In one study, dogs undergoing any type of surgery as part of their treatment had significantly improved median survival times (548 vs. 402 days) (Williams *et al.* 2003).

Sublumbar lymphadenectomy has been performed successfully in several studies, and the results for long-term outcome are encouraging. In one study of five dogs, no intraoperative or immediately postoperative complications were noted in dogs undergoing lymph node removal (Hobson *et al.* 2006). Of three dogs that were euthanized in this study, the median survival time was 20.6 months. Another case in this study underwent five surgeries for removal of metastatic disease to the lymph nodes and was still alive 54 months after the initial surgery. In a separate study evaluating resection of metastatic disease from anal sac adenocarcinomas, the mean survival time for two dogs undergoing surgery was 3 years (Jeffery *et al.* 2000). An additional study on dogs with anal sac adenocarcinoma with nodal metastasis that were treated with anal sacculectomy and lymph node extirpation revealed a median disease-specific survival of 340 days, and the number, but not size, of metastatic lymph nodes was negatively associated with outcome (Tanis *et al.* 2022). Extirpation of sublumbar lymph nodes in dogs without distant metastasis significantly improves survival times (Polton & Brearley 2007). Subsequent surgical treatment for local disease recurrence and/or metastatic disease has resulted in median additional survival of 283 days, supporting a role for subsequent surgical procedures in these patients with progressive disease (Barnes & Demetriou 2017).

Because of the highly metastatic nature of anal sac adenocarcinomas, many clinicians recommend chemotherapy as part of the treatment protocol. For dogs with documented nodal metastasis, one study showed no association between chemotherapy administration and outcome (Tanis *et al.* 2022). Of 61 dogs receiving chemotherapy in another study, adjuvant chemotherapy and solo chemotherapy were used in 50 and 11 cases, respectively (Williams *et al.* 2003). No specific chemotherapy protocol was found to be more effective than another in this study; however, dogs with iliac lymphadenopathy were significantly more likely to receive chemotherapy.

In a series of dogs, 46 of 80 with anal sac adenocarcinomas received carboplatin (Polton & Brearley 2007). Chemotherapy did not impact survival times in the entire cohort of this study, but cases with unresectable lymph node metastases and without distant metastases did have significantly improved survival times with chemotherapy administration. The administration of carboplatin allowed surgery to be pursued in 2 of 4 dogs with previously deemed unresectable primary tumors and improved the clinical signs in 12 of 40 dogs with fecal obstruction secondary to unresectable lymph nodes. Another study on adjuvant carboplatin chemotherapy for dogs with surgically excised anal sac adenocarcinomas showed no significant difference in outcome associated with carboplatin administration (Wouda *et al.* 2016).

The response of anal sac adenocarcinomas to various chemotherapeutic regimens in 20 dogs has been evaluated (Bennett *et al.* 2002). No dogs achieved a complete response, five achieved a partial remission, and five were noted to have stable disease. Of the dogs in this study, 25% developed mild gastrointestinal side effects. Six dogs that received platinum chemotherapy developed azotemia, although it was deemed clinically nonevident.

Other chemotherapeutic protocols that have been reported in the treatment of anal sac adenocarcinomas include doxorubicin, mitoxantrone, melphalan, actinomycin D, piroxicam, epirubicin, chlorambucil, prednisolone, vincristine, l-asparaginase, cyclophosphamide, and toceranib (Goldschmidt & Zoltowski 1981; Ross et al. 1991; Williams et al. 2003; Emms 2005; Heaton et al. 2020). Melphalan administration after cytoreductive surgery has been described in dogs with and without lymph node metastases (Emms 2005). In dogs with sublumbar lymph node metastases the median survival time was 20 months, and in dogs without sublumbar metastases the median survival time was 29.3 months; 86% of dogs with and without lymph node metastasis were alive at one year. One study showed a clinical benefit in 69% of dogs with anal sac adenocarcinoma treated with toceranib alone or in combination with other therapies (Heaton et al. 2020).

Radiotherapy has also been used as both primary and adjuvant therapy in the treatment of anal sac adenocarcinomas. In 10 dogs undergoing radiotherapy alone for the treatment of anal sac adenocarcinoma, a median survival time of 657 days was achieved (Williams et al. 2003). Promising findings in another study combining postoperative radiotherapy with mitoxantrone have also been reported (Turek et al. 2003). Median event-free survival in this group of dogs was 287 days and median overall survival was 956 days. At one year, 87% of dogs were still alive; at two years, 66% of dogs were still alive. Another study showed that hypofractionated radiation therapy for treatment of gross anal sac adenocarcinoma (primary or metastatic disease) in 77 dogs resulted in a partial response in 38% of cases, median overall survival of 329 days, and only mild and infrequent radiation toxicities (McQuown et al. 2017). In addition, one study reported the use of a definitive-intent, moderately hypofractionated radiation therapy protocol with image-guided intensity modulation in dogs with or without prior surgery for anal sac adenocarcinoma; this study demonstrated a median progression-free survival of 908 days with acute grade 2 toxicities in 73% and grade 1 toxicities in 36% of dogs, all of which resolved, and no documented late toxicities (Körner et al. 2022).

Feline anal sac adenocarcinomas occur rarely and are poorly described in comparison to their canine counterparts; however, there are multiple case series and case reports (Mellanby et al. 2002; Parry 2006; Cavanaugh et al. 2008; Amsellem et al. 2019). Feline anal sac adenocarcinomas were considered skin neoplasms in one study and accounted for 0.5% of all skin neoplasm submissions (Shoieb & Hanshaw 2009). Domestic shorthair cats account for 52–81% of all cases of feline anal sac

adenocarcinomas, and the female to male ratio is 1.56. The most common clinical signs in cats include rectal bleeding, perianal ulceration, dyschezia, tenesmus, and change in volume or character of feces. Of the 30 cats with available biochemistry results at the time of diagnosis of anal sac adenocarcinoma, only one had hypercalcemia; this case exhibited marginal hypercalcemia with an ionized calcium concentration of 2.6 mmol/L (laboratory reference range 1.6–2.5 mmol/L). Local recurrence after surgical excision appears to be a common complication in cats, occurring in 35–41% of cases; however, presumed or confirmed metastasis occurs less frequently (13–15%). In one study, 85% of cats were euthanized or died for reasons directly related to the primary tumor or presumptive metastatic disease (Shoieb & Hanshaw 2009). Median survival time in this study was three months. In a separate study, median survival time was approximately one year (Cavanaugh et al. 2008). One study on 30 cats with anal sac adenocarcinoma that underwent anal sacculectomy reported a local recurrence rate of 37% at a median of 96 days postoperatively, negative prognostic indicators including development of local recurrence and a high nuclear pleomorphic score, and overall median survival time of 260 days (Amsellem et al. 2019).

Other tumors that have been described as affecting the canine anal sacs include adenomas, squamous cell carcinomas, and malignant melanomas, each of which is very rare. Among seven dogs diagnosed with anal sac adenoma, five were female, and the mean age at the time of diagnosis was 6.3 years (Simeonov & Simeonova 2008). In a case series of five dogs with squamous cell carcinoma of the anal sac, metastasis was not noted, but four of five dogs were euthanized due to the severity of local disease (Esplin et al. 2003). The fifth case was still alive at seven months after tumor removal, with no signs of local recurrence. Squamous cell carcinoma of the anal sac has also been reported in cats (Kopke et al. 2021). A case series on 11 dogs with malignant anal sac melanoma demonstrated a poor prognosis (median survival time 107 days) regardless of treatment pursued, including surgery (8/11), melanoma vaccine administration (4/11), palliative treatment with analgesics and stool softeners (2/11), and chemotherapy (1/11) (Vinayak et al. 2017).

Anal sacculitis/impaction/abscessation

Inflammation of the anal sacs occurs commonly in dogs. Incidence rates as high as 12.5% have been recorded (Halnan 1976a,b). Clinical signs that may be seen include licking or biting at the perineum, rubbing the anus along the floor, tenesmus, and changes in temperament. When anal sacs become infected or develop an abscess, the anal sac and surrounding region often become inflamed, swollen, and painful. A fistulous tract can develop that may be noted on the perineum, and discharge with blood contamination may also occur. When impacted anal sacs are encountered, a thick, difficult-to-express secretion is noted within the anal sac. Dogs with chronic anal sac disease may also show signs of a more generalized dermatitis (Walshaw 1983; Marretta & Matthiesen 1989).

During physical examination of a patient with suspected anal sac disease, a rectal examination and careful palpation of the anal sacs are essential. Impacted anal sacs will often feel firm and enlarged, but can usually be expressed with gentle forcefulness. When an anal sac develops an abscess, the anal sac itself and the surrounding region are very painful, and the patient will resent any palpation in that area. Sedation may be necessary to fully examine a patient with suspected anal sac abscessation. Pyrexia is often noted in these cases, although it can be difficult to obtain a rectal temperature, as affected patients often do not tolerate the use of a rectal thermometer. Aspiration and cytologic evaluation of an anal sac that is inflamed are usually unrewarding, as the flora of diseased anal sacs is similar to what is cultured from normal anal sacs (Frankel *et al.* 2008). One study showed no statistically significant cytologic differences between normal dogs and dogs with nonneoplastic anal sac disease, such that cytology appears to be an ineffective method for diagnosing anal sac disease (James *et al.* 2011).

Anal sacculitis and impaction can often be treated without surgical intervention by a combination of emptying of the anal sacs, drainage, warm packing, anti-inflammatory medications, and systemic antibiotics. Additionally, skin disease and diarrhea should be treated, as these conditions may be contributing to anal sac disease. When these techniques are unsuccessful in cases of abscessation, an incision can be made over the anal sac region to allow for open drainage. Flushing of the anal sacs can be performed by introducing a sterile catheter or tube into the anal sac duct and flushing with a mild antiseptic solution or 10% povidone-iodine solution (Marretta & Matthiesen 1989).

In cases where these treatments are unsuccessful or in patients with recurrent disease, anal sacculectomy should be considered. An anal sacculectomy is indicated if the patient has become refractory to medical management, if an abscess has developed that does not resolve with open drainage, or when severe fistulous tracts have developed. Anal sacculectomies are also recommended in many dogs with perianal fistula development (Walshaw 1983; Marretta 1998).

Techniques used for anal sacculectomy are described in the following sections. Complications that may be encountered intraoperatively include bleeding, nerve damage from excessive or uncontrolled dissection, and laceration of the rectum. Complications encountered postoperatively include fecal incontinence, draining tracts, tenesmus, dehiscence, and dyschezia. Incontinence is generally not seen when unilateral anal sacculectomy is performed; however, incontinence lasting longer than 3–4 months is unlikely to resolve (Marretta & Matthiesen 1989). One study reported on bilateral closed anal sacculectomy for treatment of non-neoplastic anal sac disease in 62 dogs (Charlesworth 2014). In this study, 32% of dogs developed mild and self-limiting complications, with no dog developing permanent fecal incontinence, small dogs (<15 kg) were more likely to develop complications, and instillation of gel to distend the anal sac was associated with a higher rate of complications. For cats that undergo anal sacculectomy for nonneoplastic disease, minor and self-limiting complications have been reported in 50% of cases, with no permanent fecal incontinence documented (Jimeno Sandoval *et al.* 2022).

Comparisons have been made between open and closed techniques for anal sacculectomy for the treatment of anal sacculitis/impaction/abscessation (Hill & Smeak 2002). In 95 dogs, only 3 developed short-term complications (excessive drainage, seroma, scooting/inflammation); 14 dogs developed long-term complications and, of these, 11 had undergone open sacculectomy. The long-term complications in the open sacculectomy group included continued licking (3 dogs), fistulation (3 dogs), anal stricture (3 dogs), and fecal incontinence (2 dogs). Fistulation was the only long-term complication in the closed sacculectomy group.

Surgery of the anal sacs

Open anal sacculectomy

Open anal sacculectomy should not be utilized in cases of anal sac neoplasia. When not performing abdominal exploratory surgery or sublumbar lymphadenectomy, the patient should be positioned in ventral recumbency, preferably in a perineal stand. The perineum should be clipped free from fur, and the tail should be secured cranially to prevent it from contaminating the surgical field. The surgical site should be prepared with aseptic technique and draped.

The open procedure can be performed using a scalpel blade or sharp scissors. If a scalpel blade is selected, a blunt probe is first inserted into the orifice of the anal duct at the anal orifice and directed into the anal sac. The blade is then pressed down onto the blunt probe to incise through the skin, anal duct, and anal sac. If scissors are selected, the tips are pointed up to prevent

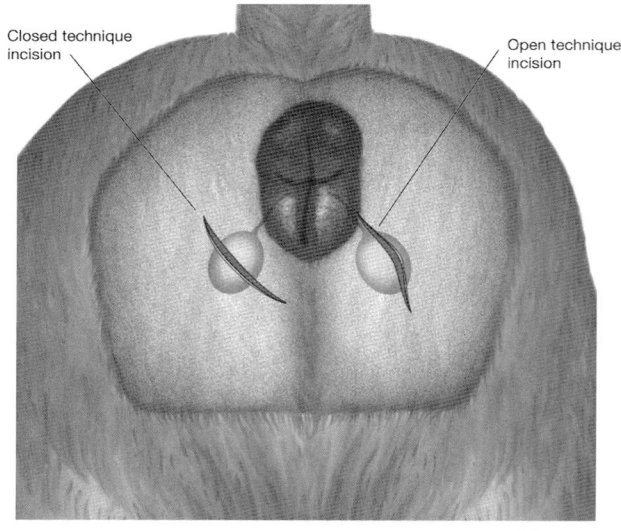

Closed technique incision

Open technique incision

Figure 12.1 Incision for a closed and an open anal sacculectomy.

accidental incision of the external sphincter muscle (Figure 12.1). The anal sac duct is gently incised open, starting at the terminal end of the duct (at the anal orifice) and extending toward the anal sac. During this procedure, the skin overlying the anal sac as well as the anal sac and anal duct are all incised open.

After an incision has been made, blunt and sharp dissection is used to separate the surrounding connective tissue and external sphincter muscle from the anal sac and duct, and the boundaries of these organs are determined. A tissue forceps can be placed on the most ventral and lateral aspect of the anal sac when it has been exposed, but manipulation should be performed gently, as tearing of the sac and release of the contents into the surgical site are contraindicated. Additionally, the surgeon should avoid damaging the caudal rectal branch of the pudendal nerve, as this may result in fecal incontinence. When the entire sac and duct have been completely freed from the surrounding tissue, two ligatures (2-0 to 3-0 monofilament absorbable suture) can be placed around the most terminal aspect of the duct, and a scalpel blade can be used to remove the duct; alternatively, the duct can be excised at the level of the anocutaneous junction, with subsequent closure of the remaining defect with a cruciate or mattress suture pattern (2-0 to 3-0 monofilament absorbable suture) from within the surgical site. The entire anal sac and duct should be removed to ensure that no secretory epithelium remains in the patient. When the anal sac and duct have been removed, the surgical site should be copiously lavaged. The muscles and subcutaneous tissue are closed with 3-0 monofilament absorbable suture and the skin is closed with 3-0 nylon or 3-0 monofilament absorbable suture placed intradermally.

Closed anal sacculectomy

Some surgeons prefer filling or packing the anal sacs prior to resection to improve delineation of the organ. Products that have been described for this use include string, yarn, plaster of Paris, agar base gel, dental molds, hydrocolloid, and silicone sealant (MacPhail 2008). In general, these products are injected into the anal sac to fill and outline the sac for dissection. When anal sac neoplasia is suspected or has been diagnosed preoperatively, no material should be injected into the anal sac duct.

Another technique that has been described to delineate the anal sac includes the use of a Foley (balloon-tipped) catheter (Downs & Stampley 1998). For this procedure, a Foley catheter is placed within the anal sac, the entire balloon being seated within the sac. The balloon is then distended with sterile saline to firmly delineate the perimeter of the anal sac. When a medium has been injected to fill the sac or the Foley catheter technique has been used, a closed anal sacculectomy technique is then performed, as described shortly. Alternatively, the duct can be ligated and transected prior to Foley catheter placement and subsequent closed anal sac dissection and excision (Diaz *et al.* 2019).

Patient positioning and preparation are the same for closed anal sacculectomy as for open sacculectomy. Some surgeons recommend placing a hemostat or probe into the anal sac duct to orient oneself to the location of the anal sac. A skin incision is made over the anal sac in the perineum 1–2 cm lateral to the anal orifice and is curved so that the concave side is pointed toward the anus (Figure 12.1) (Website Chapter 12: Gastrointestinal tract/ anal sac). The subcutaneous tissues are bluntly and sharply dissected to expose the perimeter of the anal sac and anal duct. If a tumor is suspected, a connective tissue layer immediately surrounding the anal sac and duct can be included in the removed portion in order to possibly decrease the chance of local recurrence. However, care should be taken to avoid the caudal rectal artery and caudal rectal branch of the pudendal nerve during the surgery. If bleeding is encountered, it may be excessive and can obstruct visualization. If tissue forceps are utilized to grasp the anal sac, care should be taken to prevent tearing of the organ and potential seeding of the surgical site. As with open anal sacculectomy, the terminal part of the anal sac duct should be ligated as close to the rectum as possible once the anal sac and anal sac duct have been completely freed from the surrounding tissue. When the anal sac and duct have been removed, the surgical site should be copiously lavaged. The subcutaneous tissue is closed with 3-0 monofilament absorbable suture and the skin is closed with 3-0 nylon or 3-0 monofilament absorbable suture placed intradermally.

Anal sac tumors may be locally extensive and resection of part of the rectum may be necessary. When the anal sac tumor and duct have been freed as extensively as possible, an incision is made into the rectum, providing a narrow margin of grossly normal tissue around the tumor when possible. The rectum is then closed in one to two layers in a simple interrupted or simple continuous pattern (3-0 or 4-0 monofilament absorbable suture). Closure of the subcutaneous tissue and skin continues as earlier described.

References

Al-Bagdadi, F. (1993). The integument. In: *Miller's Anatomy of the Dog*, 3e (ed. H.E. Evans), 115–116. Philadelphia, PA: WB Saunders.

Amsellem, P.M., Cavanaugh, R.P., Chou, P.Y. et al. (2019). Apocrine gland anal sac adenocarcinoma in cats: 30 cases (1994–2015). *Journal of the American Veterinary Medical Association* 254 (6): 716–722.

Baker, E. (1962). Diseases and therapy of the anal sacs. *Journal of the American Veterinary Medical Association* 141: 1347–1350.

Barnes, D.C. and Demetriou, J.L. (2017). Surgical management of primary, metastatic and recurrent anal sac adenocarcinoma in the dog: 52 cases. *Journal of Small Animal Practice* 58 (5): 263–268.

Bennett, P.F., DeNicola, D.B., Bonney, P. et al. (2002). Canine anal sac adenocarcinoma: clinical presentation and response to therapy. *Journal of Veterinary Internal Medicine* 16: 100–104.

Cavanaugh, R., Bacon, N.J., Schallberger, S. et al. (2008). Biologic behavior and clinical outcome of cats with anal sac adenocarcinoma: a Veterinary Society of Surgical Oncology retrospective study of 23 cats [Abstract]. Presented at Veterinary Cancer Society Meeting, Seattle, WA, October.

Charlesworth, T.M. (2014). Risk factors for postoperative complications following bilateral closed anal sacculectomy in the dog. *Journal of Small Animal Practice* 55 (7): 350–354.

Diaz, D., Boston, S., Ogilvie, A. et al. (2019). Modified balloon-catheter-assisted closed anal sacculectomy in the dog: description of surgical technique. *Canadian Veterinary Journal* 60 (6): 601.

Downs, M.O. and Stampley, A.R. (1998). Use of a Foley catheter to facilitate anal sac removal in the dog. *Journal of the American Animal Hospital Association* 34: 395–397.

Dyce, K., Sack, W.O., and Wensing, C.J.G. (1996). The pelvis and reproductive organs of the carnivores. In: *Textbook of Veterinary Anatomy*, 2e, 438. Philadelphia, PA: WB Saunders.

Elliott, J., Dobson, J.M., Dunn, J.K. et al. (1991). Hypercalcemia in the dog: a study of 40 cases. *Journal of Small Animal Practice* 32: 564–571.

Emms, S.G. (2005). Anal sac tumours of the dog and their response to cytoreductive surgery and chemotherapy. *Australian Veterinary Journal* 83: 340–343.

Esplin, D.G., Wilson, S.R., and Hullinger, G.A. (2003). Squamous cell carcinoma of the anal sac in five dogs. *Veterinary Pathology* 40: 332–334.

Frankel, J.L., Scott, D.W., and Erb, H.N. (2008). Gross and cytological characteristics of normal feline anal-sac secretions. *Journal of Feline Medicine and Surgery* 10: 319–323.

Goldschmidt, M.H. and Zoltowski, C. (1981). Anal sac gland adenocarcinoma in the dog: 14 cases. *Journal of Small Animal Practice* 22: 119–128.

Gröne, A., Weckmann, M.T., Blomme, E.A. et al. (1998). Dependence of humoral hypercalcemia of malignancy on parathyroid hormone-related protein expression in the canine anal sac apocrine gland adenocarcinoma (CAC-8) nude mouse model. *Veterinary Pathology* 35: 344–351.

Halnan, C.R.E. (1976a). The diagnosis of anal sacculitis in the dog. *Journal of Small Animal Practice* 17: 527–535.

Halnan, C.R.E. (1976b). Therapy of anal sacculitis in the dog. *Journal of Small Animal Practice* 17: 685–691.

Heaton, C.M., Fernandes, A.F., Jark, P.C., and Pan, X. (2020). Evaluation of toceranib for treatment of apocrine gland anal sac adenocarcinoma in dogs. *Journal of Veterinary Internal Medicine* 34 (2): 873–881.

Hill, L.N. and Smeak, D.D. (2002). Open versus closed bilateral anal sacculectomy for treatment of non-neoplastic anal sac disease in dogs: 95 cases (1969–1994). *Journal of the American Veterinary Medical Association* 221: 662–665.

Hobson, H.P., Brown, M.R., and Rogers, K.S. (2006). Surgery of metastatic anal sac adenocarcinoma in five dogs. *Veterinary Surgery* 35: 267–270.

James, D.J., Griffin, C.E., Polissar, N.L., and Neradilek, M.B. (2011). Comparison of anal sac cytological findings and behaviour in clinically normal dogs and those affected with anal sac disease. *Veterinary Dermatology* 22 (1): 80–87.

Jeffery, N., Phillips, S.M., and Brearly, M.J. (2000). Surgical management of metastases from anal sac apocrine gland adenocarcinoma of dogs. *Journal of Small Animal Practice* 41: 390.

Jimeno Sandoval, J.C., Charlesworth, T., and Anderson, D. (2022). Outcomes and complications of anal sacculectomy for non-neoplastic anal sac disease in cats: 8 cases (2006–2019). *Journal of Small Animal Practice* 63 (1): 56–61.

Kopke, M.A., Gal, A., Piripi, S.A., and Poirier, V.J. (2021). Squamous cell carcinoma of the anal sac in two cats. *Journal of Small Animal Practice* 62 (8): 704–708.

Körner, M., Staudinger, C., Meier, V., and Rohrer Bley, C. (2022). Retrospective assessment of radiation toxicity from a definitive-intent, moderately hypofractionated image-guided intensity-modulated protocol for anal sac adenocarcinoma in dogs. *Veterinary and Comparative Oncology* 20 (1): 8–19.

Lake, A.M., Scott, D.W., Miller, W.H. Jr., and Erb, H.N. (2004). Gross and cytological characteristics of normal canine anal-sac secretions. *Journal of Veterinary Medicine A Physiology, Pathology, Clinical Medicine* 51: 249–253.

Linden, D.S., Cole, R., Tillson, D.M. et al. (2019). Sentinel lymph node mapping of the canine anal sac using lymphoscintigraphy: a pilot study. *Veterinary Radiology & Ultrasound* 60 (3): 346–350.

Llabrés-Díaz, F.J. (2004). Ultrasonography of the medial iliac lymph nodes in the dog. *Veterinary Radiology and Ultrasound* 45: 156–165.

MacPhail, C. (2008). Surgical views: anal sacculectomy. *Compendium on Continuing Education for Practicing Veterinarians* 30: 530–535.

Majeski, S.A., Steffey, M.A., Fuller, M. et al. (2017). Indirect computed tomographic lymphography for iliosacral lymphatic mapping in a cohort of dogs with anal sac gland adenocarcinoma: technique description. *Veterinary Radiology & Ultrasound* 58 (3): 295–303.

Marretta, S. (1998). Anal sac disease and removal. In: *Current Techniques in Small Animal Surgery*, 2e (ed. M.J. Bojrab), 283–286. Philadelphia, PA: WB Saunders.

Marretta, S.M. and Matthiesen, D.T. (1989). Problems associated with the surgical treatment of diseases involving the perineal region. *Problems in Veterinary Medicine* 1: 215–242.

McQuown, B., Keyerleber, M.A., Rosen, K. et al. (2017). Treatment of advanced canine anal sac adenocarcinoma with hypofractionated radiation therapy: 77 cases (1999–2013). *Veterinary and Comparative Oncology* 15 (3): 840–851.

Mellanby, R.J., Craig, R., Evans, H., and Herrtage, M.E. (2006). Plasma concentrations of parathyroid hormone-related protein in dogs with potential disorders of calcium metabolism. *Veterinary Record* 159: 833–838.

Mellanby, R.J., Foale, R., Friend, E. et al. (2002). Anal sac adenocarcinoma in a Siamese cat. *Journal of Feline Medicine and Surgery* 4: 205–207.

Messinger, J.S., Windham, W.R., and Ward, C.R. (2009). Ionized hypercalcemia in dogs: a retrospective study of 109 cases (1998–2003). *Journal of Veterinary Internal Medicine* 23: 514–519.

Meuten, D.J., Capen, C.C., Kociba, G.J. et al. (1982). Ultrastructural evaluation of adenocarcinomas derived from apocrine glands of the anal sac associated with hypercalcemia in dogs. *American Journal of Pathology* 107: 167–175.

Meuten, D.J., Cooper, B.J., Capen, C.C. et al. (1981). Hypercalcemia associated with an adenocarcinoma derived from the apocrine glands of the anal sac. *Veterinary Pathology* 18: 454–471.

Meyer, W., Tsukise, A., Neurand, K., and Hirabayashi, Y. (2001). Cytological and lectin histochemical characterization of secretion production and secretion composition in the tubular glands of the canine anal sacs. *Cells Tissues Organs* 168: 203–219.

Montagna, W. and Parks, H.F. (1948). A histochemical study of the glands of the anal sac of the dog. *Anatomical Record* 100: 297–317.

Morello, E.M., Cino, M., Giacobino, D. et al. (2021). Prognostic value of Ki67 and other clinical and histopathological factors in canine apocrine gland anal sac adenocarcinoma. *Animals* 11 (6): 1649.

Olsen, J.A. and Sumner, J.P. (2019). Clinical hypocalcemia following surgical resection of apocrine gland anal-sac adenocarcinomas in 3 dogs. *Canadian Veterinary Journal* 60 (6): 591.

Palladino, S., Keyerleber, M.A., King, R.G., and Burgess, K.E. (2016). Utility of computed tomography versus abdominal ultrasound examination to identify iliosacral lymphadenomegaly in dogs with apocrine gland adenocarcinoma of the anal sac. *Journal of Veterinary Internal Medicine* 30 (6): 1858–1863.

Pappalardo, E., Martino, P.A., and Noli, C. (2002). Macroscopic, cytological and bacteriological evaluation of anal sac content in normal dogs and in dogs with selected dermatological diseases. *Veterinary Dermatology* 13: 315–322.

Parry, N.M. (2006). Anal sac gland carcinoma in a cat. *Veterinary Pathology* 43: 1008–1009.

Polton, G.A. and Brearley, M.J. (2007). Clinical stage, therapy, and prognosis in canine anal sac gland carcinoma. *Journal of Veterinary Internal Medicine* 21: 274–280.

Polton, G.A., Mowat, V., Lee, H.C. et al. (2006). Breed, gender and neutering status of British dogs with anal sac carcinoma. *Veterinary and Comparative Oncology* 4: 125–131.

Robson, D.C., Burton, G.G., and Lorimer, M.F. (2003). Cytological examination and physical characteristics of the anal sacs in 17 clinically normal dogs. *Australian Veterinary Journal* 81: 36–41.

Rosol, T.J. and Capen, C.C. (1996). Pathophysiology of calcium, phosphorus, and magnesium metabolism in animals. *Veterinary Clinics of North America Small Animal Practice* 26: 1155–1175.

Rosol, T.J., Capen, C.C., Danks, J.A. et al. (1990). Identification of parathyroid hormone-related protein in canine apocrine adenocarcinoma of the anal sac. *Veterinary Pathology* 27: 89–95.

Rosol, T.J., Capen, C.C., Weisbrode, S.E., and Horst, R.L. (1986). Humoral hypercalcemia of malignancy in nude mouse model of a canine adenocarcinoma derived from apocrine glands of the anal sac. Biochemical, histomorphometric, and ultrastructural studies. *Laboratory Investigation* 54: 679–688.

Rosol, T.J., Nagode, L.A., Couto, C.G. et al. (1992). Parathyroid hormone (PTH)-related protein, PTH, and 1,25-dihydroxyvitamin D in dogs with cancer-associated hypercalcemia. *Endocrinology* 131: 1157–1164.

Ross, J.T., Scavelli, T.D., Mathiesen, D.T., and Patnaik, A.K. (1991). Adenocarcinoma of the apocrine glands of the anal sac in dogs: a review of 32 cases. *Journal of the American Animal Hospital Association* 27: 349–355.

Schlag, A.N., Johnson, T., Vinayak, A. et al. (2020). Comparison of methods to determine primary tumour size in canine apocrine gland anal sac adenocarcinoma. *Journal of Small Animal Practice* 61 (3): 185–189.

Shoieb, A.M. and Hanshaw, D.M. (2009). Anal sac gland carcinoma in 64 cats in the United Kingdom (1995–2007). *Veterinary Pathology* 46: 677–683.

Simeonov, R. and Simeonova, G. (2008). Quantitative analysis in spontaneous canine anal sac gland adenomas and carcinomas. *Research in Veterinary Science* 85: 559–562.

Skorupski, K.A., Alarcón, C.N., De Lorimier, L.P. et al. (2018). Outcome and clinical, pathological, and immunohistochemical factors associated with prognosis for dogs with early-stage anal sac adenocarcinoma treated with surgery alone: 34 cases (2002–2013). *Journal of the American Veterinary Medical Association* 253 (1): 84–91.

Sterman, A., Butler, J.R., Chambers, A. et al. (2021). Post-operative complications following apocrine gland anal sac adenocarcinoma resection in dogs. *Veterinary and Comparative Oncology* 19 (4): 743–749.

Sutton, D.R., Hernon, T., Hezzell, M.J. et al. (2022). Computed tomographic staging of dogs with anal sac adenocarcinoma. *Journal of Small Animal Practice* 63 (1): 27–33.

Tanis, J.B., Simlett-Moss, A.B., Ossowksa, M. et al. (2022). Canine anal sac gland carcinoma with regional lymph node metastases treated with sacculectomy and lymphadenectomy: outcome and possible prognostic factors. *Veterinary and Comparative Oncology* 20 (1): 276–292.

Turek, M.M., Forrest, L.J., Adams, W.M. et al. (2003). Postoperative radiotherapy and mitoxantrone for anal sac adenocarcinomas in the dog: 15 cases (1991–2001). *Veterinary and Comparative Oncology* 1: 94–104.

Vinayak, A., Frank, C.B., Gardiner, D.W. et al. (2017). Malignant anal sac melanoma in dogs: eleven cases (2000 to 2015). *Journal of Small Animal Practice* 58 (4): 231–237.

Walshaw, R. (1983). Anal sac disease. In: *Current Techniques in Small Animal Surgery*, 2e (ed. M.J. Bojrab), 196–201. Philadelphia, PA: WB Saunders.

Weir, E.C., Burtis, W.J., Morris, C.A. et al. (1988). Isolation of 16,000–Dalton parathyroid hormone-like proteins from two animal tumors causing humoral hypercalcemia of malignancy. *Endocrinology* 123: 2744–2751.

Williams, L.E., Gliatto, J.M., Dodge, R.K. et al. (2003). Carcinoma of the apocrine glands of the anal sac in dogs: 113 cases (1983–1995). *Journal of the American Veterinary Medical Association* 223: 825–831.

Wong, H., Byrne, S., Rasotto, R. et al. (2021). A retrospective study of clinical and histopathological features of 81 cases of canine apocrine gland adenocarcinoma of the anal sac: independent clinical and histopathological risk factors associated with outcome. *Animals* 11 (11): 3327.

Wouda, R.M., Borrego, J., Keuler, N.S., and Stein, T. (2016). Evaluation of adjuvant carboplatin chemotherapy in the management of surgically excised anal sac apocrine gland adenocarcinoma in dogs. *Veterinary and Comparative Oncology* 14 (1): 67–80.

Section 2

Liver, Gallbladder, and Pancreas

13

Portosystemic Shunts

Lisa Klopp, Angela J. Marolf, Eric Monnet, and Craig B. Webb

The classification and grouping of circulatory disorders of the liver were standardized by the World Small Animal Veterinary Association, Liver Standardization Group (Table 13.1) (Rothuizen *et al.* 2006). A clear understanding of the pathophysiology behind this terminology is essential for interpreting diagnostic test results, as well as determining whether a particular portosystemic vascular anomaly (PSVA) is a surgical condition.

The most common PSVA is a congenital portosystemic shunt (CPSS). This is a single and direct vascular connection between the portal and systemic circulation that may be located either within the hepatic parenchyma (intrahepatic) or outside the liver (extrahepatic) (Table 13.2). CPSS results from abnormal development of the umbilical vein, vitelline vein, and caudal cardinal vein (Payne *et al.* 1990). The origin, insertion, and caliber of the abnormal vasculature may impact the fraction of the liver that is hypoperfused, the severity of the histopathologic changes, and the severity and progression of the clinical signs (Windsor & Olby 2007). Whereas surgery is the preferred treatment for a CPSS, all the listed variables may impact the surgical accessibility, the likelihood of postsurgical complications, and the long-term prognosis for surgical treatment compared with medical management of the condition. The tendency is to assume that the diagnosis of a portosystemic shunt (PSS) in an older dog represents an acquired condition with a poor prognosis. However, it appears that some of these dogs may have a congenital shunt that initially manifests with minimal or mild clinical signs and is slowly progressive. There are a number of nonsurgical PSVAs, both acquired shunts and congenital conditions other than single-vessel CPSS (Table 13.2).

The nomenclature can be particularly confusing, as it is still unclear whether these vascular abnormalities have distinct and separate etiologies or belong on a continuum with a shared underlying cause.

Regardless of the underlying disease process, the majority of pets with PSVAs demonstrate similar clinical signs, biochemical changes, and histopathologic markers. In some cases, there are only subtle differences with even more specialized testing.

Hepatic encephalopathy

Hepatic encephalopathy (HE) is a metabolic syndrome associated with significant liver dysfunction and is characterized by diffuse cerebral and neuropsychiatric dysfunction (Zieve 1979a; Tarter *et al.* 1984). The syndrome is well described and contributing factors have been established, but the precise mechanisms are not truly known (Pilbeam *et al.* 1983a, b; Jensen 1986; Hardy 1990; Basile *et al.* 1991; Binesh *et al.* 2006). Accordingly, studies evaluating biochemical contributors are often contradictory and confusing. It is accepted that HE is related to alterations stemming from a gastrointestinal–hepatic–central nervous system (CNS) axis. When portal blood bypasses the liver or the liver is unable to metabolize endogenous toxins and those derived from gastrointestinal bacterial metabolism, clinical signs may occur. The concept of this axis is supported by improvement in clinical signs when treatment is aimed at managing the bacterial microbiota and decreasing gastrointestinal absorption of bacterial metabolic byproducts.

The putative cause(s) of HE should have the following attributes: (i) there should be elevated concentrations in

Small Animal Soft Tissue Surgery, Second Edition. Edited by Eric Monnet.
© 2023 John Wiley & Sons, Inc. Published 2023 by John Wiley & Sons, Inc.
Companion website: www.wiley.com/go/monnet/small

Table 13.1 Classification of circulatory disorders of the liver.

Name	Anatomy	Location	Pressure changes	Preferred treatment
Congenital portosystemic shunt	Single vessel	Intrahepatic (large breed, feline) Extrahepatic (small breed, feline)	No portal hypertension	Surgical
Outflow disturbance	Impaired venous outflow	Cardiac failure, caudal vena cava obstruction or compression, intrahepatic outflow obstruction[a]	Passive congestion	Medical
Portal vein obstruction	Thrombosis, inflammation, neoplasia, *Heterobilharzia americana*	Intraluminal, extraluminal	Portal hypertension	Medical
Primary hypoplasia of the portal vein[b]	Congenital malformation	Intrahepatic	Portal hypertension	Medical
Intrahepatic arteriovenous fistulas	One or more liver lobes	Hepatic artery and portal venous radicles	Aneurysmal distension of portal veins; portal hypertension	± Surgical
Primary (intrinsic) hepatic disease	Cirrhosis, fibrosis, cholestasis	Multiple liver lobes	Portal hypertension	Medical

[a] The terms "Budd–Chiari syndrome" or "Budd–Chiari-like syndrome" are no longer used to describe venous outflow obstructions in dogs or cats.
[b] Formerly known as noncirrhotic portal hypertension and/or microvascular dysplasia (MVD).
Source: Rothuizen J, Bunch BL, Charles JA et al. (2006) / with permission of Elsevier.

Table 13.2 Classification and acronyms for portosystemic vascular anomalies.

Portosystemic shunt (PSS)
Congenital (CPSS)
    Single extrahepatic (single EHPSS)
    Single intrahepatic (single IHPSS)
        Left divisional
        Right divisional
        Central divisional
    Portal vein atresia
Acquired (acquired EHPSS)
    Multiple extrahepatic (multiple EHPSS) (synonym: acquired portosystemic collaterals, APSC)
Primary hypoplasia of the portal vein (PHPV); formerly microvascular dysplasia (MVD)
    (synonym: portal venous hypoplasia, PVH)
Noncirrhotic portal hypertension (NCPH)
(Intra)hepatic arteriovenous fistulas (HAVF)
    (synonym: hepatic arteriovenous malformation, HAVM)

the brain or serum of HE patients when clinical signs are observed; (ii) clinical signs should be induced when the factor is administered experimentally; and (iii) clinical signs should resolve when the substance is removed from the circulation (or brain). Many factors have been studied and none has unequivocally been shown to be the single cause. Therefore, HE should be considered a multifactorial metabolic disease (Butterworth 2008). The contribution of any single factor may differ in the type of liver disease (e.g., fulminant hepatic failure vs. portosystemic encephalopathy vs. chronic liver failure) and even between individual patients with the same disease.

Pathogenic factors implicated in hepatic encephalopathy

Hyperammonemia

Ammonia is an essential precursor for nitrogenous compounds (amino acids, proteins, nucleic acids, and coenzymes) (Swart & Van den Berg 1991). About 40% of ammonia is produced in the gastrointestinal tract as a byproduct of bacterial metabolism of nitrogenous compounds (dietary protein, bacterial degradation, and epithelial debris) (Lockwood *et al.* 1979; van Leeuwen *et al.* 1984; Swart & Van den Berg 1991; Maddison 1992). Ammonia enters the systemic circulation by diffusion into the portal circulation. In addition, there are other endogenous sources of ammonia production (Wolpert *et al.* 1971; Lowenstein 1972; Maddison 1991, 1992; Dimski 1994). Blood urea nitrogen (BUN) produced by liver metabolism of ammonia diffuses into the colon and is recycled to ammonia by the microbiota. In the small intestine, mucosal cells use glutamine as a primary nutritional source. As a consequence, intestinal metabolism of glutamine by deamination and transamination liberates ammonia (Lowenstein 1972; van Leeuwen *et al.* 1984). Additionally, skeletal muscle and kidneys contribute to ammonia production (Duda & Handler 1958; Lowenstein 1972; Onstad & Zieve 1979).

The liver is the major organ responsible for ammonia metabolism. Gastrointestinal-derived ammonia is presented to the liver via the portal circulation (Dimski 1994). Ammonia metabolism occurs primarily (81–87%) via the urea cycle (Cooper *et al.* 1987; Bachmann 2002). The urea cycle prevents accumulation of excess nitrogen that is not used for biosynthesis by incorporating it into urea. A secondary system for ammonia metabolism involves glutaminase, and is found primarily in the centrilobular area. Glutaminase plays a role in metabolizing ammonia that has not passed through the urea cycle (Duda & Handler 1958; Onstad & Zieve 1979; Cooper *et al.* 1987). The genesis of hyperammonemia in animals with HE may be due to shunting of portal blood around the liver or a proportional functional reduction of ammonia in the urea cycle secondary to a decrease in functional hepatic mass (Hardy 1990; Swart & Van den Berg 1991). Because of the functional reserve of the liver, hyperammonemia usually develops only when there is a 70% reduction in liver function.

Ammonia passively diffuses into the brain along a concentration gradient and is captured in the parenchyma due to a difference between systemic and brain pH values. Normal systemic pH is 7.4, but the pH of the brain is reported to be somewhat lower (range of 6.5–8.0, depending on the region of the brain tested) (Lockwood *et al.* 1980; Brooks *et al.* 1984; Zauner *et al.* 1995; Barker *et al.* 1999; Chung *et al.* 1999). Ammonia will diffuse toward a lower concentration gradient, and because the pH in the brain is lower, the ammonia will be converted to the ammonium ion. Entrapment of ammonia within the CNS occurs because the ammonium ion is not readily diffusible across membranes.

While most studies have supported hyperammonemia as a contributing factor in HE, there are conflicting data (Walker & Schenker 1970; Record *et al.* 1976; Zieve 1981; Theoret & Bossu 1985). The role of ammonia in HE is supported by data derived from experimental and naturally occurring liver disease. Increased arterial and cerebrospinal fluid (CSF) ammonia levels are observed in HE patients (Neary *et al.* 1987; Albrecht & Faff 1994; de Knegt *et al.* 1994; Bachmann 2002; Brusilow 2002; Zwingmann & Butterworth 2005; Devriendt *et al.* 2017). Signs of HE have been observed in children and animals with healthy livers and genetic abnormalities of urea cycle enzymes (arginosuccinate synthetase deficiency) (Shih 1976; Morris & Rogers 1978; Flannery *et al.* 1982; Zieve 1986). Similarly, arginine deficiency in the cat results in signs of HE, as cats require arginine to synthesize the urea cycle intermediate ornithine (Morris & Rogers 1978; Stewart *et al.* 1981; Zieve 1986).

Clinical signs in affected patients are precipitated by high-protein meals or gastrointestinal bleeding (Kromhout *et al.* 1980; Jensen 1986; Maqsood *et al.* 2006). These clinical signs are improved by decreasing production/absorption of ammonia in the gastrointestinal tract (Conn *et al.* 1977; Huchzermeyer & Schumann 1997; Bajaj *et al.* 2010; Phongsamran *et al.* 2010; Sharma *et al.* 2010). It has been shown that patients with HE have an increased blood–brain barrier permeability to ammonia (Knudsen *et al.* 1993; Albrecht & Faff 1994) and uptake and metabolism of ammonia in the brain (positron emission tomography scan with ^{13}N isotope). This has been shown to be associated with changes to astrocytes (Blei 2005; Norenberg *et al.* 2007; Sorensen & Keiding 2007; Jayakumar & Norenberg 2010; Keiding *et al.* 2010). The exact mechanisms behind ammonia-induced neurotoxicity are not known, but have been proposed to include depressed ATP synthesis, decreased Na^+/K^+-ATPase pump activity, perturbed cerebral blood flow and oxygen utilization, alterations in neurotransmission, and inhibition of neuronal chloride transport (Lux & Loracher 1970; Cooper & Plum 1987; Inagaki *et al.* 1987; Hawkins & Mans 1989).

Ammonia has both direct and indirect neurotoxic effects. It has been implicated in injury to astrocytes – highly metabolic cells that comprise about one-third of the entire brain volume (Butterworth 1993, 2002; Dombro *et al.* 1993; Albrecht & Faff 1994; Albrecht *et al.* 1997; Rao & Norenberg 2001; Bachmann 2002; Blei 2005; Ott *et al.* 2005; Rao *et al.* 2005; Albrecht & Norenberg 2006; Lemberg & Fernandez 2009). The astrocyte contributes to the formation of the blood–brain barrier, the physiologic barrier that segregates neurons from the systemic environment. In addition, the astrocyte is integral in the detoxification of ammonia in the CNS, a process that occurs via the glutamine synthetase reaction using glutamate (Maddison 1992).

Excess CNS glutamine has been implicated in the pathogenesis of HE (Schenker *et al.* 1967; Norenberg *et al.* 1997, 2007; Suarez *et al.* 2002; Binesh *et al.* 2006; Lemberg & Fernandez 2009; Albrecht *et al.* 2010). Specifically, the concentration of CNS glutamine has been correlated with the degree of HE and has been found in concentrations 5–10 times normal levels in HE patients. Glutamate is derived from α-ketoglutarate, an intermediate in the tricarboxylic acid (TCA) cycle. High levels of ammonia result in diversion of α-ketoglutarate away from this cycle while simultaneously inhibiting Na$^+$/K$^+$-ATPase pumps. These both contribute to decreased ATP production and brain energy depletion in the late stages of HE.

Aberrations in key astrocytic protein production secondary to hyperammonemia are observed and result in impairment of astrocyte function (Butterworth 1993, 2000, 2008; Rama Rao *et al.* 2003; Ott *et al.* 2005; Rama Rao & Norenberg 2007; Lemberg & Fernandez 2009). Extracellular-regulated protein kinases, glial fibrillary acid protein (a structural protein), and glutamine synthetase and glutamate transporter protein (GLT-1) have all been shown to be decreased. Conversely, peripheral-type benzodiazepine receptors (BDZ-Rs), intracellular calcium, and aquaporin IV (water channel proteins) have been shown to be increased in hyperammonemia.

In addition to astrocyte injury, hyperammonemia affects postsynaptic inhibition and may inhibit excitatory neurotransmission in the cerebral cortex, brainstem, and spinal cord (Lux & Loracher 1970; Inagaki *et al.* 1987). Excess cerebral ammonia may impair the chloride pump, rendering the neuron hyperpolarized and unable to generate postsynaptic potentials, which are generally inhibitory (Raabe & Gumnit 1975). This may explain some conflicting findings of hyperkinetic and excitatory neuronal function rather than cerebral depression with high CNS ammonia concentrations (Theoret & Bossu 1985). Eventually, excitatory postsynaptic potentials are depressed as well, resulting in conduction block and diffuse neuronal inhibition. Postsynaptic potentials have been studied in cats with portosystemic encephalopathy (Raabe 1981, 1987; Raabe & Gumnit 1975; Raabe & Lin 1983; Raabe & Onstad 1985). These animals appeared to have normal postsynaptic inhibitory potentials, but did not tolerate additional acute metabolic and toxic insults. This suggests that hyperammonemia may sensitize the CNS.

Both the kidneys and skeletal muscle can help buffer hyperammonemia, the kidneys through excretion and skeletal muscle through conversion to glutamine.

Despite its role in the pathogenesis of HE and the correlation between ammonia and grade of HE in populations, ammonia concentration is a poor predictor of HE in any one individual dog (Gow 2017; Tivers *et al.* 2014).

Brain edema

For the most part HE is considered a biochemical disease. However, edema is sometimes a structural factor seen in fulminant hepatic failure. Brain edema is both cytotoxic (glutamine osmosis in astrocytes and inhibition of Na$^+$/K$^+$-ATPase pumps) and vasogenic (increased blood–brain barrier permeability) in nature (Ede & Williams 1986; Vaquero *et al.* 2003; Blei 2005).

Glutamate, gamma-aminobutyric acid and benzodiazepine receptors

In the last 20 years, more focus has been given to the role of glutamate, γ-aminobutyric acid (GABA), and the benzodiazepine portion of the GABA receptor in HE (Zieve 1979a; Basile *et al.* 1991; Maddison 1992; Basile & Jones 1994, 1997). Glutamate is one of the most important excitatory neurotransmitters in the CNS. Metabolism of glutamate is intimately associated with GABA and glutamine via astrocyte–neuron trafficking (Bradford & Ward 1976; Bradford *et al.* 1978; Norenberg *et al.* 1997; Monfort *et al.* 2002; Chan & Butterworth 2003; Lemberg & Fernandez 2009). Fluctuation in the level of one component is associated with an opposite change in the others. Glutamate is synthesized in nerve terminals from many substrates, but glutamine may be the most important. Glutaminase converts glutamine to glutamate, effectively recycling glutamine. Glutamate also plays roles other than that of a neurotransmitter, including synthesis of GABA, glutathione, proteins, and ammonia. In addition, it has a role in energy metabolism.

It has been proposed that excitatory neurotransmission is depressed in animal models and human patients with HE (Watanabe *et al.* 1984; Chan & Butterworth 1999; Rose 2002; Rose *et al.* 2005; Kelly *et al.* 2009; Lemberg & Fernandez 2009). When cerebral ammonia concentrations are elevated, glutamate is converted to glutamine, thus depleting the glutamate supply that would otherwise be used for neurotransmitter production.

GABA is an important inhibitory neurotransmitter in the CNS. Interest in GABA and its receptor (GABA-R) arose from observations that HE patients were very sensitive to barbiturates and benzodiazepine medications, both of which act on this receptor (Maddison 1992). The GABA-R is a hetero-oligomeric complex composed of α, β, and γ subunits (Basile *et al.* 1991). The receptor is classified into GABA-RA and GABA-RB. The GABA-RA is pharmacologically divided into the GABA-R, the BDZ-R, and the chloride ionophore, but they are coupled both physically and pharmacologically. The receptor forms an ion-gated channel that facilitates entry of chloride into the postsynaptic neuron, resulting in hyperpolarization.

The BDZ-R portion of the receptor modulates receptor affinity for GABA (and other agonists) and therefore increases duration of chloride channel opening (Basile et al. 1991). The barbiturate portion of the receptor is associated with the ion channel and binding of barbiturate is associated with GABA-mediated chloride entry into the neuron. In addition, the ion channel can also be influenced by ammonia and astrocyte-derived neurosteroids, which increase the affinity of the GABA-R for GABA and enhance benzodiazepine binding to the BDZ-R complex (Basile & Jones 1994, 1997; Desjardins & Butterworth 2002; Ahboucha 2011). Therefore, ammonia enhances neuroinhibitory effects by modulating these receptor binding sites. Ammonia is also associated with upregulation of peripheral-type BDZ-Rs located on the outer mitochondrial membrane of astrocytes.

While studies evaluating agonists and antagonists of the GABA-R support increase in "GABAergic tone" in HE patients, it is not known how this physiologic phenomenon originated. Proposed theories include alterations in the density or affinity of GABA-R and the presence of endogenous ligands (Basile et al. 1991; Basile & Jones 1994). A more popular theory arose suggesting that HE patients had increases in naturally occurring benzodiazepine-like receptor agonists (Asano & Spector 1979; Möhler et al. 1979; Sangameswaran et al. 1986; Wildmann et al. 1986, 1987; Medina et al. 1989; Unseld et al. 1989; Basile et al. 1990). Various compounds have been shown to have affinity for the BDZ-R. These include purines, 1,4-benzodiazepines (diazepam, N-desmethyldiazepam, oxazepam, lorazepam, and deschlorodiazepam), and nicotinamide. It is proposed that benzodiazepine- and GABA-like molecules may be a product of bacterial metabolism or synthesized by the gastrointestinal mucosa. Additionally, certain foods (wheat, potatoes, soybean, rice, and mushrooms) have been shown to possess 1,4-benzodiazepine activity (Asano & Spector 1979; Möhler et al. 1979; Sangameswaran et al. 1986; Wildmann et al. 1986, 1987; Medina et al. 1989; Unseld et al. 1989; Basile et al. 1990). Similar to ammonia, these compounds would normally be extracted and metabolized by the liver. However, they would not be efficiently removed in severe liver disease or PSS.

Benzodiazepine-like agonists are believed to contribute to the pathogenesis of HE by an inherent ability to stimulate GABA-R (Asano & Spector 1979; Möhler et al. 1979; Sangameswaran et al. 1986; Wildmann et al. 1986, 1987; Medina et al. 1989; Unseld et al. 1989; Basile et al. 1990). Studies have shown that the ligand is reversibly bound to 20–40% of BDZ-Rs (Basile et al. 1990). Concentrations of the benzodiazepine-like compounds are less than those required to induce encephalopathy with diazepam; however, they may be present in concentrations that mediate clinical signs in combination with other derangements (Bassett et al. 1987; Basile & Gammal 1988).

Alteration of amino acid metabolism

Changes in the concentration and nature of plasma and brain amino acids are reported in both acute and chronic liver disease, as well as in cases of portosystemic encephalopathy (Iber et al. 1957; Ansley et al. 1978; Cascino et al. 1978, 1982; James et al. 1979; Nagasue et al. 1981). These alterations are proposed to be either directly or indirectly related to hyperammonemia. Hyperammonemia is associated with changes in metabolic hormones (glucagon and insulin) (Soeters & Fischer 1976; Marchesini et al. 1979). Hyperammonemia induces glucagon-mediated gluconeogenesis from nitrogenous sources (amino acids). Enhanced gluconeogenesis results in hyperinsulinism, which initiates catabolism and release of muscle stores of branched-chain amino acids (BCAAs). In addition, malnutrition, which is common with chronic hepatic diseases, promotes muscle catabolism. Alteration in the ratio of BCAAs to aromatic amino acids (AAAs) has been shown to occur (Record et al. 1976; Zieve 1979b; Schäfer et al. 1985; Maddison et al. 1986; Knudsen et al. 1993). The BCAAs are valine, leucine, and isoleucine. These amino acids are used by skeletal muscle for metabolism. The AAAs are tyrosine, tryptophan, and phenylalanine. The normal ratio of BCAA to AAA is 3.03 : 1, but changes to 1.5 : 1 in liver failure. BCAAs and AAAs compete for the same receptor transporting into and out of the CNS (Fischer 1975; Ansley et al. 1978). BCAAs are usually more abundant and are preferentially transported across the blood–brain barrier. Glutamine and AAAs compete for the same receptor to exit the brain (Cangiano et al. 1983; Mans et al. 1983, 1984; Cardelli-Cangiano et al. 1984). When there is excess glutamine (e.g., as observed with hyperammonemia), AAAs will tend to remain in higher than usual concentrations in the brain.

BCAAs are used in the brain to synthesize the excitatory amino acids dopamine (DA) and norepinephrine (NE) (Hardy 1990). It is believed that relative elevation in concentrations of AAAs results in generation of "false neurotransmitters" by impairing catecholamine synthesis (Fischer 1975; Faraj et al. 1981; Jensen 1986; Maddison 1992; Saleem et al. 2008). Tyrosine is believed to be converted to tyramine and octopamine and phenylalanine to phenylethylamine. False neurotransmitters may alter cerebral function in several ways. Octopamine is stored and released at nerve terminals and may displace the true neurotransmitters (DA and NE) from synaptic vesicles, allowing rapid cytosolic degradation. Octopamine and phenylethylamine only serve as weak neurotransmitters, acting as catecholamine receptor agonists by competing with true neurotransmitters for receptor binding. In addition, false neurotransmitters may also compete for enzymes involved in true neurotransmitter synthesis (tyrosine hydroxylase and dopamine 6-hydroxylase). Studies have both supported and refuted the role of false neurotransmitters in the pathogenesis of HE (Dodsworth *et al.* 1974; Boulton *et al.* 1975; Zieve & Olsen 1977; Cuilleret *et al.* 1980; Hauger *et al.* 1982).

In addition to the generation of false neurotransmitters, tryptophan can be neurotoxic in high concentrations and has been shown to induce neurologic disturbances in humans (Smith & Prockop 1962; Hirayama 1971; Ono *et al.* 1978; Rossi-Fanelli *et al.* 1982; Holt *et al.* 2002). In some animal models of HE, elevated brain and CSF concentrations of serotonin and its metabolite, 5-hydroxyindoleacetic acid, were observed (Cummings *et al.* 1976; Koyuncuoğlu *et al.* 1978; Simert *et al.* 1978; Bengtsson *et al.* 1989a, b, 1991; Basile *et al.* 1991). Elevation of 5-hydroxyindoleacetic acid was also reported in human patients with HE and fulminant hepatic failure (Knell *et al.* 1974; Bergeron *et al.* 1995). However, evidence for an important role in the pathogenesis of HE is lacking (Walker & Schenker 1970; Knell *et al.* 1974; Bergeron *et al.* 1995).

Mercaptans

Gastrointestinal metabolism of methionine, a sulfur-containing amino acid, is believed to generate various toxic metabolites known as mercaptans (methanethiol, ethanethiol, and dimethylsulfoxide) (Phear *et al.* 1956; Hardy 1990). In addition, the liver itself may be involved in the production of these compounds (Blom *et al.* 1990). Mercaptans have been shown to have both anesthetic and antiepileptic properties (Pappas *et al.* 1984). They have been demonstrated to precipitate hepatic coma in patients with a cirrhotic liver, and can cause reversible coma in animal models of HE (Challenger & Walshe 1955; Foster *et al.* 1974; Windus-Podehl *et al.* 1983). Biochemically, mercaptans have been shown to alter the function of Na^+/K^+-ATPase pumps, inhibit hepatic urea synthesis, and potentiate the neurotoxicity of ammonia (Foster *et al.* 1974; Zieve *et al.* 1974b; Windus-Podehl *et al.* 1983).

Short-chain fatty acids

Short-chain fatty acids (5, 6, and 8 carbons) are produced from bacterial metabolism of carbohydrates and amino acids in the gastrointestinal tract and from incomplete β-oxidation of long-chain fatty acids in hepatic mitochondria (Rabinowitz *et al.* 1983, 1991). Short-chain fatty acids have been shown to uncouple oxidative phosphorylation and depress Na^+/K^+-ATPase pump activity (Hird & Weidemann 1966). They may also be synergistic with ammonia and mercaptans in creating clinical signs (Zieve 1981). Short-chain fatty acids have been shown to induce coma in a chain length-dependent manner (Zieve *et al.* 1974a, b; Baraldi *et al.* 1984).

Phenols

Metabolism of the aliphatic amino acids tyrosine and phenylalanine results in the production of phenols (Maddison 1992). Plasma and CSF concentrations have been shown to be elevated in patients with acute and chronic liver disease (Crossley *et al.* 1983; Windus-Podehl *et al.* 1983). Phenols are both neurotoxic and hepatotoxic, and have been reported to induce coma and to act synergistically with other toxins in HE (Crossley *et al.* 1983; Windus-Podehl *et al.* 1983). Experimental models report that much higher concentrations of phenols are required to induce coma compared with levels found in patients with hepatic coma (Windus-Podehl *et al.* 1983). Because of a paucity of studies, the role of phenols in the pathogenesis of HE is poorly understood.

Other identified factors

Manganese, a neurotoxic paramagnetic metal, has been implicated in HE (Hazell & Norenberg 1997; Chetri & Choudhuri 2003; Rao & Norenberg 2004; Rama Rao & Norenberg 2007; Rama Rao *et al.* 2007; Rovira *et al.* 2008). Manganese has been shown to accumulate in the brain of patients with cirrhotic livers and is believed to contribute to the Alzheimer type II astrocytic changes by acting synergistically with ammonia. On magnetic resonance images of patients with HE, accumulation of manganese in the basal ganglia is observed as hyperintensity on T2-weighted images. At necropsy, the brain concentrations of manganese in HE patients were 2–7 times greater than concentrations in patients with normal brains.

Low plasma levels of zinc have been identified in patients with cirrhosis and PSS (Marchesini *et al.* 1996; Chetri & Choudhuri 2003; Katayama 2004; Schliess *et al.* 2009; Coughlan *et al.* 2010; Takuma *et al.* 2010). Zinc is a cofactor for two of five enzymes in the urea cycle and experimental deficiency in rats results in altered nitrogen metabolism. Histamine H_1 receptors have been shown to be upregulated in naturally occurring liver disease and experimentally induced PSS in rats (Lozeva *et al.* 2001, 2003). Histamine in the nervous system plays a role in arousal and the circadian rhythm. Blockade of H_1 receptors was shown to improve locomotor activity and circadian cycles in rats with HE. Taurine acts as an agonist on GABA receptors (Rao *et al.* 1995; Butterworth 1996; Hilgier *et al.* 1996, 2000; Chepkova *et al.* 2006). Massive release of taurine in the brain has been demonstrated after ammonia administration. Taurine is also believed to play a role in the perturbed astrocyte osmoregulation and cerebral edema observed with hyperammonemia. An aberration in endogenous opioid biochemistry has also been identified (Yurdaydin *et al.* 1995, 1998; Bergasa *et al.* 2002; Davis 2007; Kamel *et al.* 2007). Arginine deficiency impacts the urea cycle in cats with hepatic lipidosis and precipitates HE. C-reactive protein is increased in dogs with CPSS and clinical HE and reduced following treatment, consistent with inflammation acting as a potentiating factor for HE in humans (Center *et al.* 1993; Gow *et al.* 2012; Kilpatrick *et al.* 2014; Tivers *et al.* 2015). Neurosteroids accumulate in the brain of people with HE, modulate GABA receptors, and may contribute to astrocyte swelling (Ahboucha *et al.* 2005).

Signalment, clinical signs, and physical examination

The majority (75%) of CPSS are identified in dogs less than 2 years of age, but they have been diagnosed in dogs 10 years of age and older (Tobias & Rohrbach 2003; Windsor & Olby 2007). CPSS are common in a variety of breeds, including the Yorkshire terrier, Maltese, Cairn terrier, Dandie Dinmont terrier, pug, miniature schnauzer, shih tzu, Lhasa apso, chihuahua, dachshunds, Australian cattle dog, Irish wolfhounds, bichon frisé, Tibetan spaniel, and Havanese (Table 13.3) (Johnson *et al.* 1987; Tisdall *et al.* 1994; Tobias & Rohrbach 2003; Hunt 2004; van Steenbeek *et al.* 2009).

Clinical signs consistent with CPSS revolve around the neurologic, gastrointestinal, and urologic systems, and are often intermittent (Table 13.4). Signs of HE occur in 95% of dogs with a CPSS, but can also appear as a result of severe hepatocellular disease or, rarely, a congenital urea cycle enzyme disorder. Clinical signs of HE can be as striking as a partial or grand mal seizure, blindness, or coma. However, usually the signs are more subtle and include changes in behavior or activity, weakness, trembling or shaking, aimless pacing or circling, vocalization, staring into space or head pressing, blindness, drooling, or ptyalism (especially in cats). The neurologic signs are usually exacerbated two hours after a high-protein meal.

Table 13.3 Defining characteristics and breed predispositions for portosystemic vascular anomalies.

Portosystemic shunt	
Congenital	Young dogs > older dogs
Single extrahepatic	Small/toy breeds (Yorkshire terrier, schnauzer, poodle, Maltese, shih tzu, dachshund, pug, Havanese, Dinmont, bichon frisé, Tibetan spaniel), cats (Persian, Siamese, Himalayan, Burmese)
Single intrahepatic	Large breed (golden and Labrador retrievers, Bernese mountain dog, Old English sheepdog, Samoyed, Australian shepherd), cats
Left divisional	Irish wolfhound
Right divisional	Australian cattle dogs
Central divisional	
Portal vein atresia	Multiple portocaval anastomoses
Acquired	Older dogs > younger dogs
Multiple extrahepatic	Ascites secondary to portal hypertension or hypoalbuminemia, German shepherd dog
Primary hypoplasia of the portal vein	
Noncirrhotic portal hypertension	Idiopathic, <4 years old and >10 kg, no macrovascular shunt, portal hypertension and ascites, may develop multiple extrahepatic portosystemic shunts (EHPSS), Doberman pinscher
Microvascular dysplasia	No macrovascular shunt, no portal hypertension, Cairn and Yorkshire terriers, Maltese, cocker spaniel, poodle
Arteriovenous fistulas	Ascites, multiple acquired EHPSS, portal vein dilatation, portal hypertension, hepatofugal flow

Table 13.4 Clinicopathologic characteristics of portosystemic vascular anomalies.

	Neurologic	Gastrointestinal	Urinary	Other
History	Dull mentation, abnormal behavior, delayed recovery from anesthesia	Vomiting, pica, anorexia, diarrhea	Hematuria, stranguria, PU/PD, uroliths	Small stature, poor growth, lethargy, weight loss
Clinical signs	Head pressing, vocalization, staring, intermittent blindness, ataxia, seizures	Nausea, diarrhea, gastrointestinal ulceration, melena, hematemesis	Ammonium urate stones, secondary bacterial infections	Ptyalism or copper-colored irises in cats
Ascites	Not seen in CPSS or MVD unless secondary to hepatic failure or hypoalbuminemia Possible in HAVM, NCPH, acquired EHPSS secondary to hepatic cirrhosis			
Biochemistry	Hypoalbuminemia (dogs), low BUN, hypocholesterolemia, hypoglycemia, elevated liver enzyme activity (bone growth)			
Complete blood count	Microcytosis, hypochromasia, anemia, leukocytosis, low mean corpuscular hemoglobin (MCH), target cells (D), poikilocytes (C)			
Urinalysis	Low urine specific gravity, ammonium (bi)urate crystalluria, uroliths (with secondary cystitis and an active sediment or proteinuria)			
Coagulation	Normal to prolonged (although not usually clinical)			
Bile acids test	**1** Fasted preprandial serum sample: normal or elevated **2** Feed tablespoon(s) of food (high fat), insure ingestion **3** 2 h postprandial serum sample: elevated			
Basal ammonia	Fasted plasma sample: elevated (may be normal with prolonged fast)			
Ammonia tolerance test	**1** Fasted (heparinized) plasma sample **2** Ammonium chloride (2 mL/kg of 5% solution in water) administered rectally (deep) with catheter **3** 30 min post administration of plasma sample (samples on ice, process within 20 min of collection) or calibrated in-house auto-analyzer			
Postprandial ammonia tolerance test	Heparinized plasma 6 h postprandial (12 h fast, then 33 kcal/kg)			
Protein C	PSVA < MVD			

BUN, blood urea nitrogen; CPSS, congenital portosystemic shunt; EHPSS, extrahepatic portosystemic shunt; HAVM, hepatic arteriovenous malformation; MVD, microvascular dysplasia; NCPH, noncirrhotic portal hypertension; PSVA, portosystemic vascular anomaly; PU/PD, polyuria/polydipsia.

The polydipsia with secondary polyuria seen in dogs with shunts may be a sign of HE. In older dogs the neurologic signs of a PSS may be more severe, reflect brainstem and cerebellar abnormalities, and appear asymmetric (Windsor & Olby 2007).

Diarrhea (with or without melena), inappetence, and occasionally vomiting are gastrointestinal signs seen in dogs with a CPSS, but obviously are very nonspecific. Although there may be some variation in the breed, age of onset, and severity of clinical signs, the majority of PSVAs, congenital or acquired, present with a clinical picture similar to, or even indistinguishable from, those dogs with classic CPSS.

The physical examination may be normal or may reveal a dog that is abnormally small in size or stature for the age and breed. An abnormal mentation may be appreciated or may require historical confirmation. Even with an owner reporting neurologic signs, the neurologic examination may fail to reveal any abnormalities. Alternatively, marked deficits in conscious proprioception, hopping, and placing may be present. Lateralizing signs may be revealed, such as a head tilt, anisocoria, or nystagmus. Dogs suspected of having a CPSS should not have evidence of ascites. For example, in a young Yorkshire terrier with biochemical changes consistent with abnormal liver function (i.e., hypoalbuminemia and hypocholesterolemia) and a "big belly" (i.e., ascites), lymphangiectasia is the differential that should be pursued, not a CPSS.

Acquired extrahepatic portosystemic shunts (EHPSS) are most often diagnosed in older dogs and do not represent a surgical condition. The most common causes of

EHPSS are severe chronic hepatic disease leading to cirrhosis, or PSVA including primary hypoplasia of the portal vein (PHPV, also known as noncirrhotic portal hypertension), or intrahepatic arteriovenous fistulas.

Biochemical profile, hematology, and urinalysis

Commonly reported biochemical abnormalities in dogs with PSVA include hypoalbuminemia, hypoglycemia, hypocholesterolemia, low BUN, and mildly elevated liver enzymes (Table 13.4). Microcytosis and hypochromasia may be seen on a complete blood count. Ammonium (bi)urate crystals and a low urine specific gravity secondary to polydipsia may appear in the urinalysis (Winkler *et al.* 2003; Broome *et al.* 2004; Caporali *et al.* 2015). Total bilirubin concentration is normal in dogs with vascular anomalies. A mildly prolonged partial thromboplastin time has been reported in dogs with CPSS, but none of these abnormalities will distinguish between a surgical and nonsurgical problem in patients with hepatic disease or vascular abnormalities (Niles *et al.* 2001).

Special blood tests

Measurement of fasted and two-hour postprandial total serum bile acid concentration is a test of liver function and frequently performed early in the diagnostic work-up of a suspect PSVA case (Table 13.4). However, this "bile acids test" is not specific for a PSS, and the test certainly does not distinguish a surgical from a nonsurgical condition. Differentials for an elevation in postprandial serum bile acids include chronic hepatitis, extrahepatic bile duct obstruction, hepatic cirrhosis and necrosis, congenital and acquired PSVA, microvascular dysplasia (MVD, now considered a variation of PHPV), intrahepatic cholestasis, steroid or vacuolar hepatopathy, neoplasia, hepatotoxins, hepatic failure secondary to infections (such as leptospirosis), and hepatocutaneous syndrome. Although the fasted serum bile acid concentration (preprandial bile acids) is often significantly elevated in dogs with a PSVA, it may be within normal limits. Studies suggest that if the fasted serum bile acid concentration is greater than 20, 30, or 50 μmol/L, the specificity for liver disease approaches 100% and the additional effort and expense of obtaining a postprandial serum bile acids are unnecessary. However, the greatest sensitivity for liver disease remains a combination of preprandial and postprandial values (Center *et al.* 1985a, b, 1991, 1995). Similar results are found for the sensitivity and specificity of serum bile acids in cats suspected of having hepatobiliary disease (Center *et al.* 1995).

Fasted serum ammonium levels and the ammonium tolerance test (ATT) require special sample handling and processing that make them technically more demanding than the serum bile acids test, although this is changing with improved technology (i.e., in-house auto-analyzers for ammonia concentrations). The specificity of a fasted plasma ammonia level is significantly greater than the fasted serum bile acids for detection of a PSVA, again emphasizing the intent of the bile acids test as a determinant of liver function (Gerritzen-Bruning *et al.* 2006). One publication describes a protocol for a postprandial ATT that was designed to circumvent some of the problems with the rectal administration of ammonia in the ATT (Walker *et al.* 2001). The test appeared to be sensitive for the detection of PSVAs, but not other hepatocellular diseases. The protocol also requires that each laboratory or analyzer establish a normal reference range. Multiple parameters, including positive predictive value and negative predictive value (PPV and NPV), were determined for the diagnosis of PSS using fasting bile acids (FBA), fasting ammonia concentration (FA), and the ATT (rectal application). No single test was sufficient for both detecting and excluding PSS. The ATT and FBA are more sensitive than FA for detection, but FA was more specific. The sensitivity and NPV of the ATT (at the 40-minute collection point) for detection of a PSS were 100%. Serial testing using FBA and either FA or ATT increased specificity and PPV in a symptomatic population, and an increase in both FBA and FA was sufficient for making the diagnosis (van Straten *et al.* 2015).

It is important to note that a number of Maltese dogs have been found to have elevated postprandial serum bile acids with a normal ATT and no significant hepatic disease or dysfunction. In one Maltese there were histopathologic changes consistent with microscopic portosystemic connections, a hepatic vascular anomaly that is not surgically correctable (Tisdall *et al.* 1995). Elevations in postprandial bile acids have also been found in dogs with tracheal collapse, although the clinical relevance of this finding is unclear (Bauer *et al.* 2006).

Plasma protein C activity (vitamin K-dependent anticoagulant) has been used to help distinguish between cases of PSS and hepatic failure. Dogs with hepatobiliary disease had a significantly lower protein C activity than clinically ill dogs without hepatobiliary disease, and dogs with PSVA had significantly lower protein C activity than dogs with MVD, a nonsurgical condition. However, there is no significant difference in protein C activity between dogs with congenital PSVA, acquired PSS, or hepatic failure, the latter two being nonsurgical conditions. Using specific cutoff values and combining protein C activity with cholesterol concentration and red cell microcytosis may help discriminate between macroscopic PSVA and MVD (Toulza *et al.* 2006).

Imaging

Multiple imaging modalities can be utilized in the diagnosis of shunting conditions. However, computed tomography angiography (CTA), with its ability to capture timed vascular phases, has emerged as the optimal imaging modality for diagnosing a variety of shunting lesions. Ultrasound continues to be utilized frequently due to its ubiquity and ability to perform in awake patients. Nuclear medicine and magnetic resonance imaging (MRI) are less commonly used to diagnose PSS anomalies.

Radiography

Digital radiography is a front-line imaging choice for many patients presenting with abdominal disease. Radiographic findings for dogs with shunting conditions are usually nonspecific and may reveal microhepatica or renomegaly in dogs with various portal vein vascular anomalies. Decreased serosal detail consistent with ascites may be present in cases of portal hypertension and acquired shunts.

Ultrasound

Ultrasound imaging has been well established in diagnosing PSS and assessing the liver parenchyma, kidneys, and urinary bladder prior to surgical intervention. CPSS

can be characterized as intrahepatic or extrahepatic (Lamb *et al.* 1996; Lamb & White 1998; d'Anjou *et al.* 2004). Intrahepatic shunts tend to be easier to identify due to their large size and location within the liver (Figure 13.1). Extrahepatic shunts are more challenging to find, as they are often small and tortuous and may be masked by overlying gastric and intestinal gas (Figure 13.2). Sonographic changes consistent with a portosystemic shunt include observation of an anomalous vessel connecting to the portal vein, evidence of turbulent flow within the caudal vena cava, comparison of cross-sectional diameters of the portal vein relative to the aorta or caudal vena cava, small liver size, and presence of nephroliths and/or cystoliths (d'Anjou *et al.* 2004). The origin and insertion of the shunting vessel are occasionally found. Ultrasound is an accurate imaging modality for diagnosis of portosystemic shunts, with 92% sensitivity and 98% specificity (d'Anjou *et al.* 2004). In patients with portal hypertension, acquired portosystemic shunts may be more difficult to identify sonographically. These small and numerous vessels may be found in many parts of the abdomen, but can often be identified caudal to the left kidney. (Figure 13.3). Other sonographic findings include splenomegaly and anechoic free fluid. Ultrasound evaluation of patients with shunting lesions is operator dependent, with more experienced sonographers more likely to identify shunts accurately. There is the potential to miss small or complicated congenital and acquired shunts with ultrasound imaging.

(a) (b)

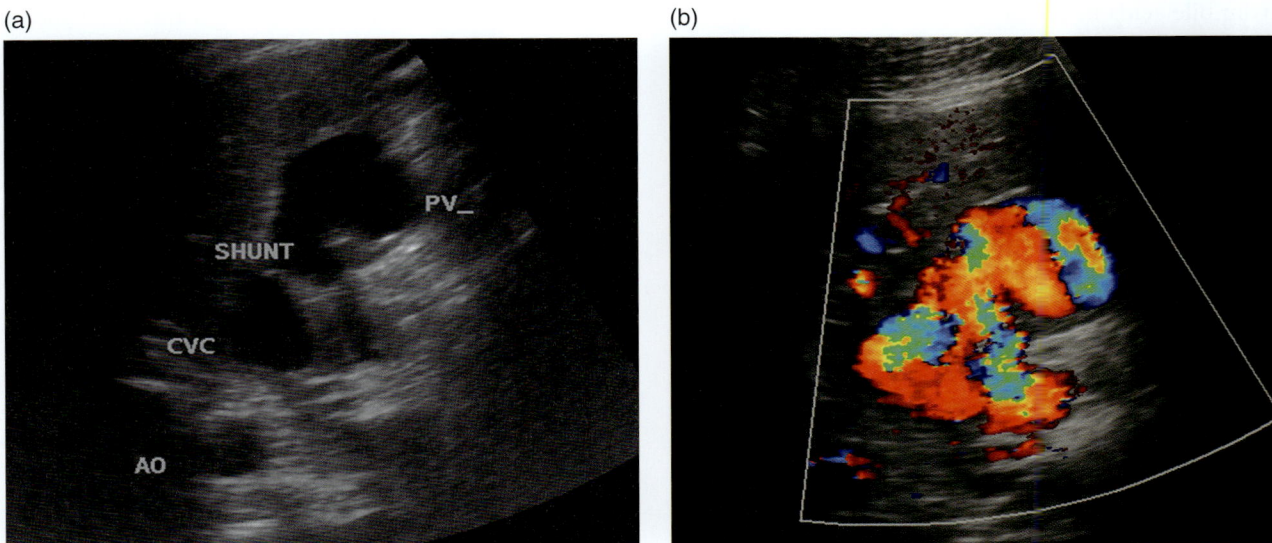

Figure 13.1 (a) Transverse plane image of the liver with a large intrahepatic portosystemic shunt. Note the large portal vein (PV) with anomalous shunting vessel (SHUNT) connecting to the caudal vena cava (CVC). The aorta (AO) is identified dorsal to the portal vein and caudal vena cava. (b) Transverse plane color Doppler image of the same intrahepatic shunt. The mosaic of colors within the shunting vessel, portal vein, and caudal vena cava indicates turbulent flow associated with the shunt.

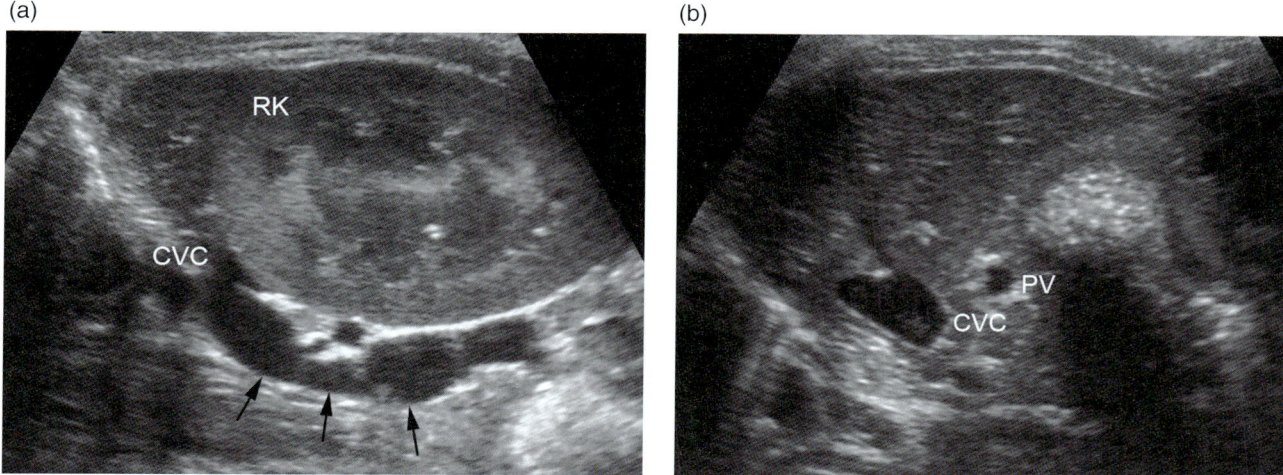

Figure 13.2 (a) Dorsal plane image of the medial aspect of the right kidney (RK) with an adjacent extrahepatic portocaval shunt. A tortuous vessel (arrows) is entering the caudal vena cava (CVC). (b) Transverse plane image of the porta hepatis of the same patient. The CVC is enlarged compared with the small portal vein (PV). The PV is small at this level due to shunting of blood from the upstream extrahepatic portocaval shunt.

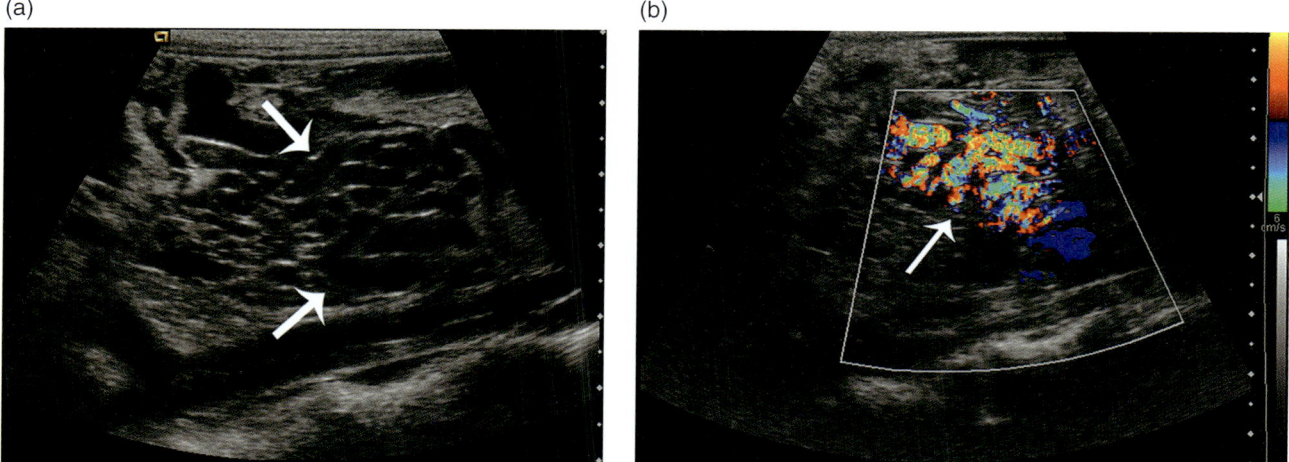

Figure 13.3 (a) Ultrasound sagittal plane B mode image medial to the left kidney. Note the large number of anechoic tubular structures in this region (arrows). (b) Ultrasound sagittal plane color Doppler image of the same region. Note the turbulent blood flow (mosaic of colors) within these vessels consistent with acquired shunts (arrow). This dog had portal hypertension secondary to an arterioportal fistula.

Computed tomography

CTA utilizes intravenous positive iodinated contrast media and is a fast and accurate means for diagnosing shunting lesions (Frank *et al.* 2003; Zwingenberger *et al.* 2005b; Bertolini *et al.* 2006). Contrast bolus tracking and time to peak enhancement in the arterial and portal phases are essential for recognizing arterial, portal, and venous vasculature (Zwingenberger *et al.* 2005b; Bertolini *et al.* 2006; Zwingenberger & Shofer 2007; Zwingenberger 2009). Excellent anatomic detail allows identification of the origin and insertion of congenital and acquired portosystemic shunts when using CTA, which has 100% sensitivity and 100% specificity (Bertolini *et al.* 2006). This excellent anatomic detail can be valuable for presurgical planning. CTA allows for optimal identification of extrahepatic, intrahepatic, and acquired portosystemic shunts. Extrahepatic portosystemic shunts have a variety of courses due to different origins and insertions (Figure 13.4). With CTA evaluation, six general shunt types have been identified: splenocaval, splenoazygous, splenophrenic, right gastric-caval, right gastric-caval with a caudal shunt

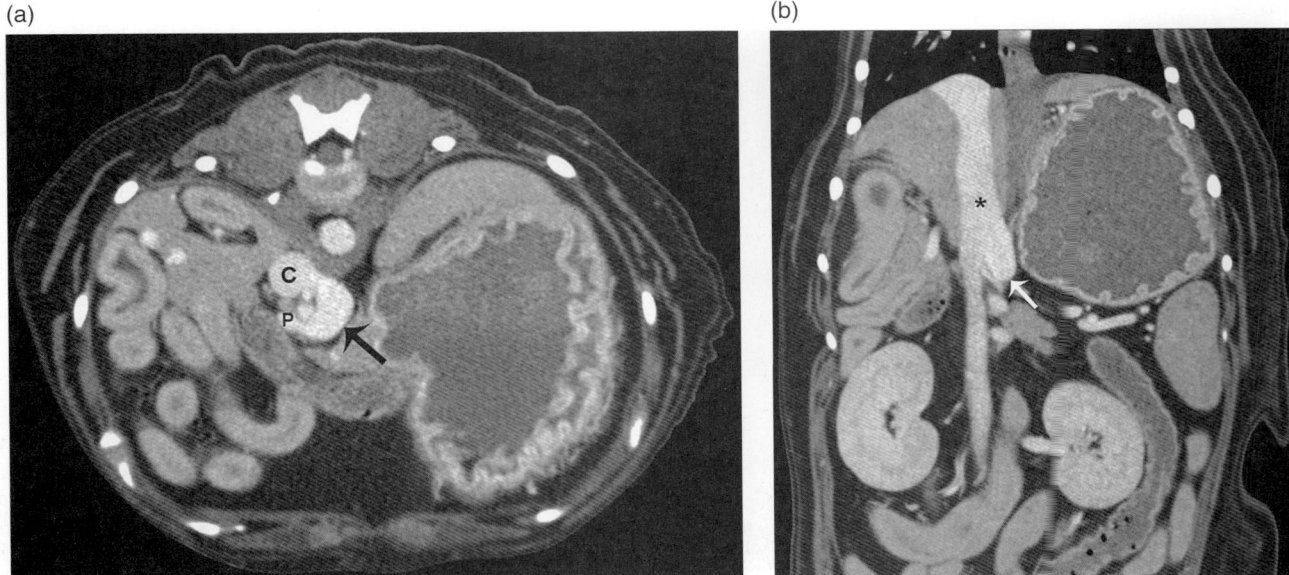

Figure 13.4 (a) Computed tomography angiography (CTA) venous phase transverse plane image of dog with an extrahepatic portocaval shunt. Note the curved anomalous vessel (arrow) connecting the portal vein (P; origin) with the caudal vena cava (C; insertion). (b) CTA venous phase dorsal multiplanar reconstruction (MPR) image of the cranial abdomen in the same patient. Note the insertion of the shunting vessel into the caudal vena cava (arrow). The caudal vena cava is distended cranial to the insertion of the shunt (asterisk).

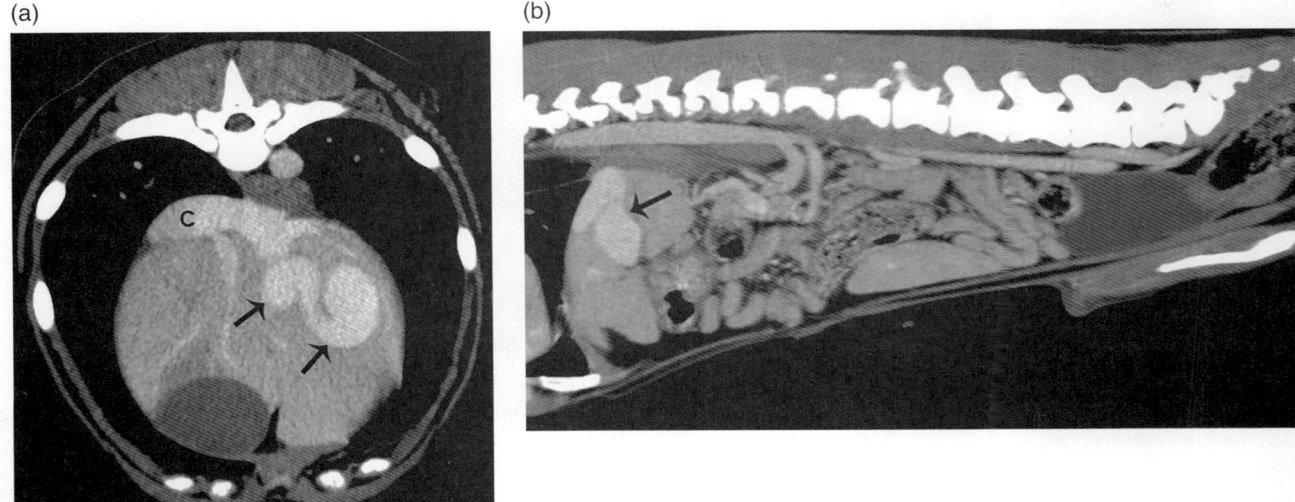

Figure 13.5 (a) Computed tomography angiography (CTA) venous phase transverse plane image of a dog with an intrahepatic shunt. Note the large, tortuous shunting vessel in the left aspect of the liver (arrows). The caudal vena cava is distended (C). (b) CTA venous phase sagittal multiplanar reconstruction (MPR) of the same shunt. Note the large shunt in the dorsal aspect of the liver (arrow). The liver is also decreased in size

loop, and right gastric-azygous with a caudal shunt loop (Nelson & Nelson 2011). Many of these complex shunts will be difficult to characterize fully with ultrasound. CTA diagnosis of intrahepatic shunts can determine if a shunt is left, right, or central divisional (Figure 13.5). CTA studies can allow for measurement of the shunt and

caval diameters if intravascular interventional procedures, such as stents, are performed (Zwingenberger 2009).

In the diagnosis of portal hypertension, identification of acquired shunting vessels noninvasively is advantageous. With CTA imaging, these small, tortuous vessels are readily identified and can be located anywhere in the

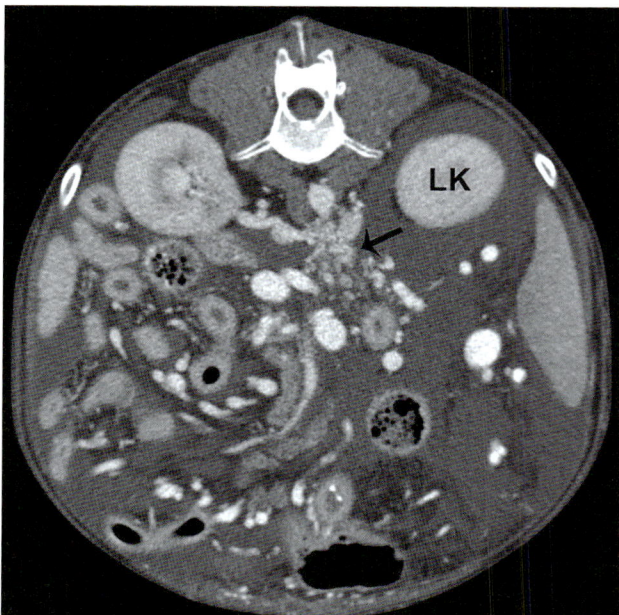

Figure 13.6 Computed tomography angiography (CTA) venous phase transverse plane image of a dog with acquired shunts. Note the small, tortuous vessels at the level of the portal vein (arrow). The left kidney (LK) is lateral to these acquired vessels. There is a large amount of hypoattenuating free fluid throughout the abdomen.

abdomen, although they often form between the portal vein and left renal vein (Zwingenberger 2009) (Figure 13.6). It is possible to identify even smaller acquired portal varices with CTA imaging. Varix formation can occur around the gallbladder and choledochal, omental, duodenal, and phrenicoabdominal locations (Bertolini 2010). Detection of these varices is important prior to interventional procedures or surgery to avoid serious hemorrhage (Bertolini 2010) (Figure 13.7). A less common cause of portal hypertension is congenital arterioportal fistulas/malformations. This condition causes ascites and acquired shunts. With CTA imaging, arterioportal fistulas/malformations are recognized when intravenous contrast is noted immediately in the hepatic portal veins during the arterial phase of the CTA study. The fistula is identified around the aneurysmal dilation of the portal veins (Specchi *et al.* 2018; Zwingenberger *et al.* 2005a; Zwingenberger 2009) (Figure 13.8). Causes of portal hypertension, such as portal vein thrombosis, are readily identified with CTA imaging as large intraluminal filling defects in any portion of the portal system (Figure 13.7).

CTA is highly advantageous due to its sequential images that assist in anatomic orientation and identification of shunts, decreased reliance on operator dependence, and swift diagnostic results from fast scan times

when using multislice CT scanners (Zwingenberger *et al.* 2005a, b; Bertolini *et al.* 2006; Zwingenberger & Shofer 2007).

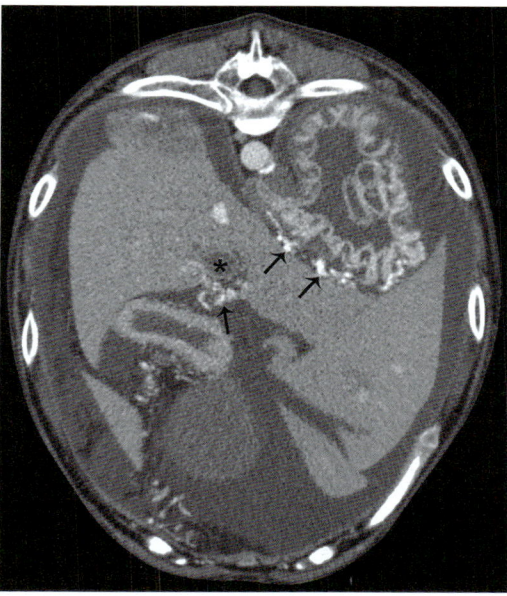

Figure 13.7 Computed tomography angiography (CTA) venous phase transverse plane image of a dog with portal hypertension. Note the varices along the liver and stomach and around the portal vein (arrows). A large thrombus occludes the portal vein (asterisk). There is a large amount of free fluid surrounding the liver.

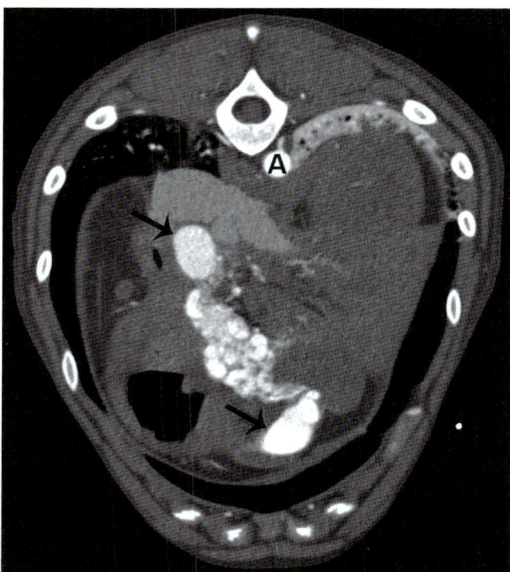

Figure 13.8 Computed tomography angiography (CTA) arterial phase transverse plane image of a dog with an arterioportal malformation. Note contrast within the aorta (A) and simultaneous contrast within the distended portal vasculature (arrows). Numerous tortuous vessels within the malformation are present surrounding the portal vasculature.

Nuclear medicine

Nuclear medicine imaging is less commonly performed due to limited availability and lack of specificity compared to other imaging modalities. Scintigraphic examination of PSS is divided into two categories: per-rectal portal and trans-splenic portal scintigraphic techniques (Daniel *et al.* 1990, 1991; Cole *et al.* 2005; Morandi *et al.* 2005). The per-rectal procedure involves injecting radiopharmaceutical via a catheter into the rectum, while the trans-splenic procedure uses ultrasound guidance to inject radiopharmaceutical into the splenic parenchyma. Both methods acquire dynamic images with the patient lying on a gamma camera to evaluate radiopharmaceutical uptake in the liver and heart (Cole *et al.* 2005). Radiopharmaceutical uptake in the heart prior to the liver indicates portosystemic shunting. The trans-splenic technique utilizes a much smaller dose (less than half) than the per-rectal technique, allowing patients to be discharged sooner or released earlier for surgical intervention (Cole *et al.* 2005; Morandi *et al.* 2005). Unlike per-rectal portal scintigraphy, the trans-splenic method can classify the type of portosystemic shunt present, including portoazygous, portocaval, and acquired shunts. However, the technique cannot differentiate intrahepatic from extrahepatic shunts (Morandi *et al.* 2005, 2010; Sura *et al.* 2007). Both methods have 100% sensitivity, and the trans-splenic technique is 100% specific for categorizing portosystemic shunts (Morandi *et al.* 2010). Both procedures can be performed on sedated patients, so general anesthesia is not required. The need for a gamma camera, radionuclide supplier, and radiation safety requirements are limitations of performing scintigraphic studies. Neither scintigraphic method has the anatomic detail inherent in the cross-sectional imaging modalities of CTA and MRI.

Magnetic resonance imaging

Multiple MRI methods have been developed to diagnose portosystemic shunts. Contrast-enhanced magnetic resonance angiography (MRA), which uses intravenous paramagnetic contrast media, is preferred to noncontrast protocols such as time-of-flight and phase-contrast sequences (Seguin *et al.* 1999; Mai 2009; Bruehschwein *et al.* 2010; Mai & Weisse 2011). Utilizing positive-pressure ventilation and breath-hold techniques, contrast-enhanced MRA sequences can be obtained quickly and free from motion artifacts (Bruehschwein *et al.* 2010; Mai & Weisse 2011). Good anatomic detail can be achieved with contrast-enhanced MRA and can be useful for presurgical planning. The accurate characterization of PSS, including the origin and insertion, can be identified with nearly 100% sensitivity and 100% specificity (Bruehschwein *et al.* 2010; Mai & Weisse 2011). With contrast-enhanced MRA, there is no need for bolus tracking of the contrast. Consequently, MRA does not require the exact timing necessary with CTA. MRI studies require longer acquisition times than CTA, and are more limited in availability.

Nonsurgical differentials

For dogs and cats with a surgically correctable CPSS, the signalment, presenting complaint, biochemical, hematologic, and urinary abnormalities, as well as abnormal preprandial and/or postprandial bile acid concentrations, can look very much the same as a dog or cat with a nonsurgical vascular anomaly. Patients with PHPV or multiple EHPSS secondary to hepatic cirrhosis can produce many of the same diagnostic test results as those pets that would benefit from surgical intervention.

One clear demarcation is the presence of ascites. A large single CPSS is flowing through the vascular route of least resistance and does not result in an increase in portal pressures. Ascites commonly develops in response to a low oncotic pressure because of significant hypoalbuminemia, usually the result of protein-losing nephropathy, protein-losing enteropathy, or liver failure. Ascites in the absence of hypoalbuminemia is due to presinusoidal portal hypertension and may be seen in heart failure, blockage of the caudal vena cava, intrahepatic arteriovenous fistulas, and severe hepatic fibrosis or chronic hepatitis. Like portal vein atresia and segmental caudal vena cava aplasia, PHPV has been reported as likely being a congenital cause of portal hypertension in a number of young dogs (Harder *et al.* 2002; Schwarz *et al.* 2009). The predominant clinical signs are stunted growth, lethargy, diarrhea and vomiting, polydipsia, anorexia, abdominal distension, and HE. Hypoalbuminemia and elevation of bile acids were similar to those seen in dogs with a single congenital shunt, but PHPV is another example of a congenital PSVA that is nonsurgical (van den Ingh *et al.* 1995). Also classified as a form of PHPV, idiopathic or noncirrhotic portal hypertension is a further nonsurgical PSVA found in a small number of dogs that results in ascites (DeMarco *et al.* 1998; Bunch *et al.* 2001). This vascular anomaly has been found in a number of breeds, although Doberman pinschers maybe overrepresented, and it can only be distinguished from hepatic cirrhosis with histopathology. In one rare example, a young wheaten terrier was presented for ascites and segmental aplasia of the caudal vena cava with azygos continuation was revealed; surgery was performed to remove thrombi that had formed and to increase shunting of blood through the azygos vein (as opposed to surgical repair of a shunting vessel) (Harder *et al.* 2002).

Abdominal ultrasound performed by an experienced ultrasonographer will frequently resolve the diagnostic dilemma. Because sonographic images are best for the vasculature surrounded by tissue, ultrasonography is most sensitive for single intrahepatic shunts. Congenital extrahepatic shunts can be a more challenging diagnostic endpoint for an ultrasonographer. The appearance of a cirrhotic liver is usually quite distinct, and multiple acquired extrahepatic shunting vessels may then be identified, frequently in the vicinity of the left kidney. There may be bilateral renomegaly as the kidneys become hyperperfused in such cases. There is now a variety of more advanced imaging modalities that can be used to further delineate the nature of the shunting vasculature and discriminate between surgical and nonsurgical cases.

Perhaps the most challenging diagnostic dilemma is the patient that presents with all the clinical signs, biochemical changes, and bile acids test results indicative of a surgically correctable CPSS, and yet the ultrasound study appears sonographically normal. It may be that ultrasound was not sensitive enough to detect an extrahepatic shunt, and yet rectal scintigraphy reveals a significant shunt fraction. This case is very likely one that is amenable to surgery. On the other hand, if rectal scintigraphy fails to reveal a significant shunt fraction in a dog that by all other measures should have a PSVA, that anomaly is likely a version of PHPV formerly referred to as MVD. In a group of Cairn terriers with MVD, the history, physical examination findings, clinicopathologic abnormalities, and abdominal imaging, including radiographs, ultrasound, and transcolonic scintigraphy, were indistinguishable from those of dogs that had a portosystemic shunt (Schermerhorn *et al.* 1996). Contrast portography revealed abnormalities of terminal twigs of the portal vasculature without large intrahepatic or extrahepatic shunting vessels, but this is rarely performed. Dogs with MVD were found to be older, with less marked biochemical abnormalities than dogs with both MVD and CPSS (Allen *et al.* 1999). Laparoscopy is a minimally invasive means of obtaining liver biopsies for histopathologic confirmation of MVD in dogs where diagnostic test results are consistent with a PSS but ultrasonographic and transcolonic scintigraphy results appear normal.

Medical treatment of dogs with portosystemic shunt

If possible, surgical correction of a CPSS has been shown to result in a significantly improved survival rate and lower frequency of clinical signs compared to medical management (Greenhalgh *et al.* 2014), but for a variety of reasons a number of cases will be managed medically.

The primary goals of treatment include addressing and/or reversing the underlying liver disease if possible and managing clinical signs of HE. Treatment of HE can be separated into methods that decrease the systemic concentration of ammonia and other neurotoxins, prevent/control precipitating factors, dietary management, and treatment of increased GABAergic tone.

Decreased production and absorption of ammonia and other neurotoxins

Therapies used to decrease the concentration of circulating ammonia and other neurotoxins can be divided into three categories: (i) those that decrease absorption of ammonia from the gastrointestinal tract; (ii) those that improve ammonia conversion through the urea cycle; and (iii) those that increase removal of ammonia from the systemic circulation.

Lactulose

The main therapy for decreasing absorption of ammonia and other neurotoxins has been lactulose (Conn 1972; Conn *et al.* 1977; van Leeuwen *et al.* 1984; Huchzermeyer & Schumann 1997; Bajaj *et al.* 2010; Sharma *et al.* 2010; Favier *et al.* 2020). (Lactitol and kristalose, powder forms, may be better tolerated in cats, with mechanism of action and dosing to effect being the same as with lactulose.) Lactulose is a nonmetabolized, nonabsorbable disaccharide that is administered orally or rectally. Lactulose, despite the simplicity of the concept behind its use, is quite effective. The mechanism of action of lactulose in preventing absorption of ammonia is multifold. Lactulose is used by colonic bacteria as a carbohydrate source and in the process is metabolized to organic acids (propionic, acetic, formic, and lactic). The presence of the organic acids in the colon reduces colonic pH. Decreasing pH results in increased ammonia removal through the feces by decreasing fecal pH. This occurs via conversion of the reabsorbable ammonia to the ammonium ion, which does not readily diffuse through the colonic mucosa, creating a passive concentration gradient for ammonia to diffuse into the colon from the blood due to a higher pH on the systemic side. This in turn induces catharsis, thereby shortening fecal retention times of ammonia. Lactulose can also be used as a 20% solution in a retention enema. The goals of lactulose therapy include 2–4 soft stools per day and a fecal pH below 6. Because of its mechanisms of action, adverse effects include bloating, flatulence, and diarrhea.

Antibiotics

Antibiotics are used to change or decrease the colonic concentration of urease-producing bacteria in the colon

(Conn 1972; Conn *et al.* 1977; van Leeuwen *et al.* 1984; Phongsamran *et al.* 2010). Ideal antibiotics are poorly absorbed so that their actions are maintained in the intestinal tract. Most commonly used are neomycin, metronidazole, and ampicillin. Neomycin is 97% nonabsorbable and may be synergistic with lactulose, but because 3% of the medication is absorbed and neomycin is nephrotoxic and ototoxic, it is no longer recommended as a treatment for human or veterinary patients. Metronidazole is commonly used to treat HE. Recommended dosage is 7.5 mg/kg 2–3 times daily. Metronidazole is metabolized by the liver. This antibiotic should be used judiciously because, while uncommon, metronidazole toxicity has been observed in portosystemic shunt patients. Ampicillin is also a drug that can be used very safely in cases of HE. It is only about 30% absorbed when administered orally and is associated with minimal side effects. Rifaximin, a rifamycin derivative, has been approved for the treatment of HE in human patients (Phongsamran *et al.* 2010). Less than 1% is absorbed.

Retention enema

Under conditions where emergency treatment is required and the patient is too moribund to administer oral medications, retention enemas can be used to obtain similar results of decreasing ammonia absorption. This can be achieved by administering 15–60 mL (weight dependent) of 20% lactulose and using a tampon to prevent evacuation. The enema should be retained for about 20 minutes if possible. Povidone iodine in a 1 in 10 solution or a 1% neomycin solution can also be used.

Probiotics and fecal transplantation

Administration of probiotic bacterial cultures (e.g., *Lactobacillus*) is one of the more recent treatments for HE in human medicine (Bajaj *et al.* 2008; Sharma *et al.* 2008; Sheth & Garcia-Tsao 2008; Foster *et al.* 2010; Malaguarnera *et al.* 2010; Pereg *et al.* 2011). The growth of probiotic bacteria results in a shift in the colonic environment to non-urease-producing bacteria. It appears that the beneficial effect of lactulose may be due, in part, to its impact on the microbiota (Ferreira *et al.* 2019). Recent systematic reviews concluded that although the data was of "low quality," probiotics seem to improve recovery, development of overt HE, quality of life, and plasma ammonia concentrations (Dalal *et al.* 2017; Hörner *et al.* 2017). There may even be a place for fecal microbiota transplantation in the treatment of HE (Hassouneh & Bajah 2021; Bloom *et al.* 2021).

Acarbose

Acarbose is a therapy reported for the treatment of HE in human patients (Gentile *et al.* 2005; Mullen & Howard 2005; Stewart & Vella 2005). Acarbose is a hypoglycemic agent used for type 2 diabetes mellitus. It acts through the inhibition of glucose absorption in the gut and promotion of intestinal saccharolytic bacterial flora at the expense of proteolytic flora. A randomized controlled crossover clinical trial of 107 human cirrhosis patients showed significant decrease in levels of ammonia and improvement in HE symptoms versus placebo-treated patients. However, it is recommended by the manufacturer that this medication is contraindicated in hepatic cirrhosis.

L-ornithine-L-aspartate

Ornithine is an intermediate in the urea cycle. Providing L-ornithine-L-aspartate is believed to improve and upregulate the urea cycle conversion of ammonia to urea. It has been administered both orally and parenterally at 5–10 g/day in human patients (Kircheis *et al.* 1997; Poo *et al.* 2006; Ahmad *et al.* 2008; Acharya *et al.* 2009; Jiang *et al.* 2009; Soarez *et al.* 2009; Schmid *et al.* 2010). Dogs with hyperammonemia as a result of liver disease responded to L-ornithine-L-aspartate treatment with a decrease in blood ammonia levels and improved clinical signs of HE compared to controls (Ahn *et al.* 2016). Randomized clinical trials show that L-ornithine-L-aspartate is comparable (or superior) in efficacy to nonabsorbable disaccharides or probiotics in lowering blood ammonia levels (Butterworth & McPhail 2019).

Dietary management

For many years, protein restriction was considered a necessary component of dietary management in HE. Now restriction or abstinence from protein in the diet is no longer recommended (Thompson *et al.* 1986; Meyer & Rothuizen 1992; Laflamme *et al.* 1993, 1994; Michel 1995; Center 1998; Proot *et al.* 2009). Protein restriction results in further muscle catabolism of muscle protein, which enhances cachexia. The muscle tissue is rendered less able to metabolize ammonia and a negative nitrogen balance is associated with an alteration in the ratio of BCAAs to AAAs. A positive nitrogen balance is suggested and the recommended daily protein requirement is a minimum of 2.1 g/kg. While BCAA therapy is controversial, the protein source should favor these amino acids. One study revealed that dogs on moderate protein restriction (vs. severe protein restriction) were improved clinically and that dietary provision of BCAAs was neurologically protective (Laflamme *et al.* 1993). In people, it has been shown that vegetable protein both improves nitrogen balance and provides soluble fiber that promotes colonic fermentation and ammonia excretion. Cats should be provided with adequate taurine and arginine sources (Meyer & Rothuizen 1992; Michel 1995; Center 1998). Small, frequent meals with adequate calories are recommended. Restriction or abstinence from protein should only be undertaken on a short-term basis in acute or chronic disease or long term in refractory cases only. In long-term protein restriction, BCAAs should be supplemented.

Adequate amounts of L-carnitine are also recommended in the dietary management of HE (O'Connor & Costell 1990; Therrien *et al.* 1997; Malaguarnera *et al.* 2005, 2009; Siciliano *et al.* 2006; Shores & Keeffe 2008; Foster *et al.* 2010). Carnitine helps shuttle long-chain fatty acids across the mitochondrial membrane, which allows complete oxidation of these substances.

Addition of soluble fiber to the diet of patients with HE is highly recommended (Weber *et al.* 1985; Liu *et al.* 2004; Swennen *et al.* 2006). In essence, the benefit of soluble fiber is similar to that attained by the use of lactulose and probiotic therapies.

A number of commercially available diets have been specifically formulated to address all the dietary recommendations for dogs and cats with HE. They have a moderate protein content of high biological value (egg and soy source) and provide high BCAA levels, soluble fiber, high buffering capacity, high potassium/sodium ratio, and high concentrations of antioxidants (e.g., vitamins E and C, β-carotene, and selenium).

Controlling precipitating factors

Precipitating factors are often associated with increased systemic ammonia concentrations. Table 13.5 indicates the precipitating factor, the ultimate interaction with clinical signs, and the recommended therapy (Jensen 1986; Katayama 2004; Maqsood *et al.* 2006; Bajaj *et al.* 2010; Mumtaz *et al.* 2010; Lidbury *et al.* 2015, 2016).

Table 13.5 Risk factors for the development of hepatic encephalopathy (HE).

Precipitating factor	Mode of action increasing clinical signs of HE	Recommended therapy
Gastrointestinal hemorrhage	Endogenous protein source (15–20 g/dL blood) Increases ammonia in the colon Hypovolemia Prerenal azotemia	Treat gastrointestinal hemorrhage with H_2 blockers, proton pump inhibitors Volume expansion, blood and/or plasma if indicated Lactulose
High dietary protein	Increased dietary protein converted to ammonia	Dietary management Lactulose
Azotemia	Increased amount of urea in colon metabolized to ammonia	Discontinue diuretics Volume expansion Albumin
Infection/endotoxemia	Increased peripheral ammonia from decreased liver metabolism and increased muscle breakdown	Antibiotics Lactulose
Constipation	Increased retention of nitrogen and proteins in colon converted to ammonia Improved efficiency of formation of ammonia by bacteria	Lactulose Fiber
Metabolic alkalosis	Increased diffusion of ammonia across the blood–brain barrier	Addition of potassium
Metabolic acidosis	Impairment of hepatic urea synthesis	Fluid therapy Treatment of infection Sodium bicarbonate
Sedation/anesthesia	Increased sedation in depressed animal Decreased liver metabolism of drugs Interaction at GABA/BDZ receptors	Judicious use of sedatives and anesthetics

BDZ, benzodiazepine; GABA, γ-aminobutyric acid.

Benzodiazepine receptor modulators

As previously discussed, the presence or nature of endogenous BDZ-R ligands has not been well established. BDZ-R modulators can be categorized as agonists, antagonists, and inverse agonists. Agonists function by increasing postsynaptic GABA effects and the affinity of GABA for the receptor (benzodiazepine derivatives). Antagonists (i.e., flumazenil) directly bind to the BDZ-R. These medications, dependent on their intrinsic activity, may also have partial agonist and inverse agonist effects at high dosages. This may be one reason that both human and animal clinical studies on flumazenil have, for the most part, been conflicting and disappointing (Bassett *et al.* 1987; Butterworth 1990; Jones *et al.* 1990; Meier & Bansky 1990; Laccetti *et al.* 2000; Foster *et al.* 2010). Inverse agonists have directly opposite effects to agonists. Sarmazenil is both an antagonist and an inverse agonist. In rat studies, results for use in the treatment of HE were better than those for flumazenil. In one study, the benefits and effects of sarmazenil and flumazenil in dogs with surgically induced portocaval shunts and partial hepatectomy were evaluated (Meyer *et al.* 1998). These dogs were found to have similar plasma and CSF concentrations of ammonia to those of human patients with chronic HE. No significant improvement was identified with flumazenil, but a positive response was observed with sarmazenil. Recommended dosages for dogs are 3–8 mg/kg intravenously (i.v.). The reason for an improved response is not entirely known, but it is postulated that sarmazenil may work at regions of the GABA-R not involved with the BDZ-R (ion channel) and may modulate presynaptic release of GABA.

Surgical treatment

The main goal for surgical treatment of patients with macrovascular PSS is to redirect portal blood flow into the liver parenchyma to improve liver function. Successful attenuation of PSS with several surgical modalities results in increased development of portal vasculature in the liver parenchyma and also an increase in liver volume (Lee *et al.* 2006; Lipscomb *et al.* 2009; Kummeling *et al.* 2010). PSS have been treated surgically with open laparotomy; however, laparoscopy is possible for extrahepatic shunts (Poggi *et al.* 2022). Extrahepatic shunts in the epiploic foramen seem to be easier to approach with laparoscopy than any other extrahepatic shunts. Three to four cannulas are required with a lateral approach. The lateral approach is on the right side for shunts in the epiploic foramen versus being on the left side for portoazygous shunts or shunts connected to the phonic vein. Therefore, an ultrasound evaluation or a CT scan is required to have a better idea of the location of the shunt and to plan the approach appropriately. The laparoscopic approach was associated with a 25% conversion rate (Poggi *et al.* 2022).

Identification of a portosystemic shunt in surgery

Once a single macrovascular shunt has been identified with imaging, the first step in surgical treatment is to accurately identify the shunt within the abdomen. A thorough abdominal exploration through a generous midline laparotomy is required to achieve this goal.

Following complete abdominal exploration, the caudal vena cava is inspected on the right side of the dorsal abdominal cavity after retraction of the descending duodenum to the left. Between the right renal vein and the hilus of the liver there should be no vessel entering the caudal vena cava, with the exception of the phrenicoabdominal vein. The right phrenicoabdominal vein is identified as it courses over the adrenal gland. Therefore any other vessel entering the caudal vena cava in this area is suspect for a PSS. Turbulent flow can often be observed in the vena cava cranial to the abnormal vessel because flow from the shunt disrupts the caval laminar flow. Most extrahepatic shunts are found in the region of the epiploic foramen (Figure 13.2). They are exposed by retracting ventrally the hepatic artery and portal vein just caudal to the liver. If the shunt is not visualized with this maneuver, open into the omental bursa by digitally breaking down an avascular area of the greater omentum. Once the omental bursa is opened, inspect the portal vein and its branches. Any large venous structures not supplying the portal vein are suspect for a PSS. Most extrahepatic shunts originate from either the splenic vein, the left gastroepiploic vein, or the left gastric vein. The suspected shunt should be traced until it branches into the vena cava, thus confirming the diagnosis. The shunt can connect to the caudal vena cava anywhere in the abdomen, or it may course in front of the liver, and even through the diaphragm. It is not unusual to see a shunt traveling dorsal to the stomach around the distal esophagus and passing cranial to the liver to finally empty into the caudal vena cava just caudal to the diaphragm. A PSS can also connect with the azygos vein instead of the caudal vena cava. Since the azygos vein resides in the left side of the abdominal cavity next to the aorta, retract the fundus of the stomach to the right to expose the aortic hiatus of the diaphragm. The portoazygous shunt is visualized traveling along the dorsal stomach region and distal esophagus before traversing the aortic hiatus.

If a shunt cannot be identified at this point, begin to search for an intrahepatic shunt. Intrahepatic shunts have been described in all divisions of the terminal portal vein. First, search for an intrahepatic shunt entering the caudal vena cava between the diaphragm and the liver. Observe the hepatic veins closely: the hepatic vein draining the PSS is usually enlarged with obvious turbulent flow. Plested *et al.* (2020) showed that 92% of intrahepatic shunts inserted in a hepatic vein, therefore evaluation of hepatic veins for signs of dilatation and turbulence is very important to identify the vein that is draining the shunt. Single right divisional shunts (44%) inserted in the caudal vena cava via the right lateral hepatic vein or the caudate hepatic vein. Left divisional IHPSS (33%) inserted into the left hepatic vein or left phrenic vein. Central divisional IHPSS (13%) inserted into the quadrate hepatic vein, central hepatic vein, dorsal right medial hepatic vein, or directly into the ventral aspect of the intrahepatic caudal vena cava (Plested *et al.* 2020).

The hepatic veins from the right medial and lateral liver lobes are more difficult to visualize and retraction of those liver lobes medially is required to find these veins. The hepatic vein of the quadrate lobe usually has a broad insertion to the vena cava. Branches of the portal vein entering the liver lobes should also be inspected. The branch of the portal vein feeding the shunt is often obviously enlarged. Also, inspection and palpation of the liver lobes can reveal an aneurysmal dilatation or a collapsible area (soft spot) within a liver lobe due to the presence of the shunt. If a shunt is still not found, place a catheter in a jejunal vein to measure portal pressure. Baseline portal pressure is recorded and then the hepatic veins are occluded one by one until the portal pressure rises. This allows identification of the hepatic vein draining the intrahepatic shunt. Alternately, a long catheter can also be introduced from the splenic vein and advanced into the portal vein. The catheter should follow the path of least resistance and travel through the shunt into the caudal vena cava. Palpation of the catheter within the affected hepatic vein should help identify which vein is draining the shunt (Tobias & Rawlings 1996). Intraoperative ultrasound or a portovenogram has also been used to help localize the shunt (Wrigley *et al.* 1983; Tobias *et al.* 1996). Other imaging modalities have been used before surgery to help determine the location of an intrahepatic shunt (Wrigley *et al.* 1987; Seguin *et al.* 1999; d'Anjou *et al.* 2004; d'Anjou & Huneault 2008; Bruehschwein *et al.* 2010). Contrast three-dimensional reconstructions of the liver vasculature may provide valuable information about the shunt location preoperatively to better prepare for the dissection.

The most difficult aspect of the surgery for intrahepatic shunt attenuation is not in the localization, but in the dissection. Many intrahepatic shunts are at least partially encircled with vascular hepatic tissue, so complete shunt dissection is difficult. Subtraction angiography and an ultrasonic aspirator have been used to improve visualization and isolation of intrahepatic shunts (Tobias *et al.* 1996). In our opinion, since intrahepatic shunt location is generally not difficult during surgery and shunt location is not a prognostic indicator, there is not much value in routinely performing advanced imaging before surgery (Papazoglou *et al.* 2002).

Where to attenuate a shunt

Along their course, PSS may have several contributing venous tributaries before they anastomose with the systemic circulation. Therefore, although it is important to identify the shunt throughout its length, dissection should be directed at the point where the shunt connects with the caudal vena cava or the azygos vein. If the shunt is attenuated too far from its connection with the systemic circulation and a tributary is still perfusing the shunt distal to the attenuation site, continuation of shunting is expected and the patient may not improve after surgery.

After identification of an intrahepatic shunt, it is more logical to attenuate the hepatic vein draining the shunt cranial to the liver, rather than to attenuate the branch of the portal vein feeding into the shunt (Breznock *et al.* 1983). Attenuation or complete occlusion of the hepatic vein draining the left liver lobes did not induce any significant changes in the biochemistry and liver histology of normal dogs (Payne *et al.* 1991). However, occlusion of a branch of the portal vein will induce atrophy of the respective liver lobe, because the lobe is deprived of its important hepatotropic factors coming from the splanchnic circulation (Rozga *et al.* 1986a, b; Rozga 2001). Since dogs or cats with a PSS already have a small liver, induction of additional liver atrophy is less desirable. Successful ligation of the terminal branches of the portal vein have been described, but this should be used as the last option to correct intrahepatic shunts (Hunt *et al.* 1996; Tobias *et al.* 2004).

Attenuation of the shunt

It has been shown that complete occlusion of the shunt is the most desirable goal of surgery in order to achieve the best long-term outcome (Hottinger *et al.* 1995). Dogs with complete occlusion did not have any clinical signs one year after surgery, while only 11% of dogs with partial occlusion eventually became asymptomatic (Hottinger *et al.* 1995). In another study of 64 cases, partial occlusion of the shunt was associated with a 42%

complication rate, while complete occlusion had a 9% complication rate (Winkler *et al.* 2003). Hunt and Hughes (1999) showed that 92% of dogs with complete shunt occlusion recovered normal liver function compared with only 70% of dogs with partial occlusion. The ability to completely close a portosystemic shunt in surgery depends on whether signs of acute portal hypertension develop during temporary ligation (Swalec & Smeak 1990). Since occlusion of the shunt results in increased portal blood flow toward the liver, it may induce acute portal hypertension if the portal vasculature is not well developed. Between 15% and 50% of shunts can be completely occluded safely at the time of the first attenuation attempt (Breznock *et al.* 1983; Swalec & Smeak 1990; Komtebedde *et al.* 1991, 1995; Smith *et al.* 1995; Hunt *et al.* 1996; White *et al.* 1998; Hunt & Hughes 1999; Kyles *et al.* 2001). Techniques that produce sudden and complete attenuation of shunts, such as ligation, are less desirable since they may lead to acute portal hypertension and death, or chronic portal hypertension and the development of acquired multiple shunts. It has been shown that portal vasculature improves with time even after partial attenuation of a shunt (Lee *et al.* 2006; Lipscomb *et al.* 2009). Therefore, techniques of progressive occlusion are now favored since they reduce the risk of acute portal hypertension, and may help reduce the development of multiple shunts. These progressive occlusion techniques may eventually achieve complete occlusion and, since the diversion of blood flow is progressive, may allow slow adaptation of the portal vasculature. This is desirable, because this adaptation may help the liver accept more blood flow and reduce the risk of chronic portal hypertension and the development of acquired shunts.

Attenuation of PSS can be accomplished by ligature, ameroid ring, cellophane banding, hydraulic occluder, and intravascular stent with coils (Murphy *et al.* 2001; Havig & Tobias 2002; Kyles *et al.* 2002; Winkler *et al.* 2003; Mehl *et al.* 2005; Adin *et al.* 2006; Bright *et al.* 2006; Lee *et al.* 2006; Lipscomb *et al.* 2007, 2009; Mehl *et al.* 2007; Worley & Holt 2008). Note that not all of the following attenuation techniques provide progressive closure of the shunt.

Ligature

In the traditional ligature technique, either a silk or a polypropylene suture is placed around the shunt. The suture is tightened as much as possible without inducing acute portal hypertension. Measurement of portal pressure with a catheter in a branch of the portal vein and a water manometer is required to help determine optimal ligature tightness (Swalec & Smeak 1990; Meyer

et al. 1999; Winkler *et al.* 2003; Kummeling *et al.* 2004, 2010; Lee *et al.* 2006; Lipscomb *et al.* 2007, 2009). Baseline portal pressure should not be increased by more than 9–10 cmH$_2$O and the final portal pressure should not be greater than 17 cmH$_2$O (Swalec & Smeak 1990). In addition, central venous pressure measured soon after temporary shunt occlusion should not decrease by more than 1 cmH$_2$O. Other surgeons have used a calibrated set of stainless steel rods to gauge the amount of shunt attenuation, and/or observations of the intestine and pancreas intraoperatively to determine the degree of attenuation possible (Meyer *et al.* 1999; Wolschrijn *et al.* 2000; Szatmari *et al.* 2004). During temporary shunt occlusion, signs of increased intestinal motility and spasming and cyanosis of the pancreas suggest that portal hypertension is imminent. This visceral observation technique to predict portal hypertension is associated with a mortality rate of 29% (Wolschrijn *et al.* 2000).

Occlusion with a suture does not provide consistent slow, progressive, and complete occlusion of the shunt over time, and a second surgery is usually required to attain complete occlusion (Hottinger *et al.* 1995; Lee *et al.* 2006; Lipscomb *et al.* 2007). Silk may trigger enough inflammatory reaction around the shunt to induce complete occlusion in 20–74% of cases after partial attenuation (Van Vechten *et al.* 1994; White *et al.* 1998; Hunt & Hughes 1999; Meyer *et al.* 1999; Burton & White 2001). However, this observation was not reproduced using silk to partially ligate the femoral vein in a research model (Youmans & Hunt 1999). Silk acts as a foreign body, so the amount of reaction and fibrosis would likely be a function of the amount of silk implanted at the time of surgery. Nevertheless, it has been shown that the size of silk used for vasculature attenuation does not make a difference in the amount of occlusion achieved in the long term (Hunt & Hughes 1999). Simply the surgical trauma involved in passing silk suture around the shunt can also induce temporary vascular spasm and induce acute thrombosis of the vessel (Van Vechten *et al.* 1994).

Ameroid ring

The ameroid ring was the first occlusive device used on clinical animals to slowly attenuate shunts (Vogt *et al.* 1996). An ameroid ring has been used in the past as a research tool to induce chronic myocardial infarction in research settings (Elzinga 1969; Bredée *et al.* 1975; Firoozan *et al.* 1999). It induced complete occlusion of the coronary artery by triggering an inflammatory reaction and fibrosis. The device was then examined to see how completely and how quickly it could occlude veins in dogs (Vogt *et al.* 1996). In the first experiment, the ameroid ring was placed around the splenic vein of three dogs and it resulted in the occlusion of the vein in 4–5 weeks. These results appeared promising for ameroid use in clinically affected dogs with PSS.

The ameroid occluder is an incomplete stainless steel cylinder with hydrophilic casein inside (Figure 13.4). Ameroid rings are available in the following internal diameters: 3.5, 5.0, and 6.5 mm. The ring should be placed close to the vena cava with minimal dissection around the shunt. The surrounding tissue stabilizes the ameroid ring and this helps prevent acute occlusion associated with kinking of the shunt by the device. The inside diameter of the ring is chosen to create minimal initial occlusion of the shunt vessel (Vogt et al. 1996). The ring is placed around the vessel and the open slot is closed with a small casein key.

The ameroid ring was first placed around an extrahepatic shunt in 12 dogs and 2 cats. Two dogs died of acute portal hypertension after surgery and one dog and one cat developed multiple acquired shunts. In the remaining animals, scintigraphy showed complete occlusion of the shunts between 30 and 210 days in 10 patients, with reduction of the shunt fraction at days 30 and 60 after surgery. Serum bile acids significantly decreased at days 30 and 60 after surgery (Vogt et al. 1996).

Outcome after the use of ameroid constrictors in series of dogs and cats with extrahepatic and intrahepatic shunts has been reported (Vogt et al. 1996; Kyles et al. 2001, 2002; Murphy et al. 2001; Winkler et al. 2003; Mehl et al. 2005, 2007; Lipscomb et al. 2007; Worley & Holt 2008; Otomo et al. 2020; Matiasovic et al. 2020). Ameroid rings have been associated with shorter surgical time and fewer complications than suture ligations (Murphy et al. 2001). In that study of 10 dogs treated with an ameroid ring, per-rectal scintigraphy showed residual shunting (shunt fraction >55%) in 3 of 5 dogs 2.5–4 months after surgery. In a study of 168 dogs with extrahepatic shunts, Mehl et al. (2005) reported an excellent clinical outcome in 80% of cases with a median follow-up of three years. Postoperative complications included seizures, abdominal distension, and hemoperitoneum. The postoperative mortality rate was 7.1%. Residual shunting was present on scintigraphy 6–10 weeks after surgery in 21% (21 of 99) of the cases. Within those dogs with residual shunting, 50% had an excellent clinical outcome. Low plasma albumin concentration and high portal pressure with temporary complete occlusion of the shunt were risk factors for residual shunting on scintigraphy. When placed on the left hepatic vein to treat a patent ductus venosus, ameroid rings were associated with excellent outcome in 20% of cases, while partial ligation with suture was associated with 92% excellent outcomes (Mehl et al. 2007). However, per-rectal scintigraphy showed residual shunting in 7 of 8 dogs with partial

ligation and in 3 of 7 with the ameroid ring. In cats, the outcome of portosystemic shunt occlusion with ameroid rings ranged from poor in one study (Havig & Tobias 2002) to excellent in 75% of cases in another (Kyles et al. 2002). Postoperative complications were present in 77% of cases and included blindness, generalized seizures, abnormal behavior, and hyperthermia (Kyles et al. 2002). Per-rectal scintigraphy revealed 57% residual shunting in cats even with normal clinical signs. In the study by Havig and Tobias (2002), long-term follow-up on nine cats showed that four cats were euthanized because of progressive neurologic disease. Four of the seven cats with abnormal neurologic activity either did not exhibit residual shunting on scintigraphy or had normal liver function (Havig & Tobias 2002). Therefore, neurologic signs developing after surgery in cats treated with ameroid constrictors should not necessarily be blamed on incomplete shunt occlusion. Outcome results after ameroid constrictor treatment of shunts appears to be good in dogs and variable in cats. While the rate of shunt occlusion is variable and eventual shunt occlusion is not guaranteed with ameroid constrictors, clinical outcomes are comparable with other progressive occlusive devices.

Because of the inconsistent attenuation documented in case studies, research was conducted to determine factors that might influence the fluid content within the casein core. Casein present in the ameroid ring is hydrophilic and absorbs water in the early postoperative period. It has been shown that protein content in the fluid around the ameroid ring does not have an effect on the rate of closure of the ameroid ring in vitro (Monnet & Rosenberg 2005). In the in vitro model, closure of the ameroid ring was never complete (Monnet & Rosenberg 2005). Therefore another mechanism, such as inflammation and fibrosis, likely contributes to complete closure of the shunt. Ameroid rings can induce complete occlusion of shunts by as soon as 7–10 days (Youmans & Hunt 1999; Besancon et al. 2004). This rapid occlusion is probably due to inflammation and vasculitis, which can induce thrombus and premature closure of the shunt. The rapid occlusion is thought to have contributed to the development of acquired shunts in 17% of cases in two different studies using the ameroid constrictor (Vogt et al. 1996; Mehl et al. 2005). Application of petrolatum to the ameroid ring has been attempted to reduce the inflammatory reaction and slow down the rate of closure, without success (Adin et al. 2004).

Silicone-polyacrylic acid gradual venous occlusion device

A silicone-polyacrylic acid gradual venous occlusion device has been developed to achieve gradual and complete occlusion of a shunt in 6–8 weeks (Wallace *et al.* 2016, 2018a, b). This device should not induce thrombosis of the shunt, which can induce a very premature closure of the shunt with mid-portal hypertension.

Cellophane or thin film banding

Like ameroid rings, cellophane banding was originally used to induce slow progressive occlusion of blood vessels in experimental situations (Wiles *et al.* 1952). Cellophane banding as originally described for portosystemic shunt treatment consists of placing a three-layer 3 mm wide band of cellophane around the shunt (Harari *et al.* 1990; Youmans & Hunt 1998). Since no medical-grade cellophane is available, cellophane is collected from different sources and aseptically prepared with cold sterilization. Diacetyl phosphate present in cellophane induces an inflammatory reaction, resulting in fibrosis and progressive closure of the vessel (Wiles *et al.* 1952). Cellophane banding has been used for the treatment of PSS in dogs and cats since 1998 (Youmans & Hunt 1998; Hunt *et al.* 2004; Frankel *et al.* 2006; Landon *et al.* 2008; Cabassu *et al.* 2011; Serrano *et al.* 2019; Otomo *et al.* 2020; Matiasovic *et al.* 2020). Cellophane banding has also been called thin film banding.

These bands are placed around the shunt similar to a ligature (Youmans & Hunt 1998). The tape is pliable and thin, and requires minimal dissection. These characteristics are highly desirable for use particularly around intrahepatic shunts in tight confines (Hunt *et al.* 2004). The cellophane band is secured around the shunt with vascular clips (Website Chapter 13: Liver and gall bladder/PSS cellophane) (Figure 13.5). Several clips placed in opposing directions are required to hold the original intrinsic tension of the cellophane band (McAlinden *et al.* 2010).

Cellophane banding has been used to close shunts of different sizes. It was originally recommended to place the band while monitoring heart rate, arterial pressure, and color of the intestine, or while measuring portal pressure. This was done to help safely attenuate the shunt at the time of the original surgery (Youmans & Hunt 1998; Hunt *et al.* 2004). The goal was to reduce the diameter of the shunt to less than 3 mm (Youmans & Hunt 1998). However, Frankel *et al.* (2006) showed in a clinical study that dogs with portosystemic shunts larger than 3 mm had normal liver function tests within six months after surgery when they were not attenuated during the initial cellophane banding. Partial attenuation of the larger shunts to a diameter of less than 3 mm seemed detrimental. Animals with larger shunts that were partially attenuated had normal liver function within 2–3 months after surgery, but they experienced an elevation of their postprandial bile acids 4–6 months after surgery. These animals likely developed acquired shunts due to chronic portal hypertension (Frankel *et al.* 2006).

In a study of 106 dogs and 5 cats with PSS, Hunt *et al.* (2004) reported that 85% of the dogs and 60% of the cats had normal bloodwork eight weeks after cellophane banding. These patients were either clinically improved or were asymptomatic according to the owners. The postoperative mortality rate in this study was low (5.5%), and deaths were due to either portal hypertension or seizures. Of the dogs with an intrahepatic shunt that survived the surgery, 71% eventually had normal hepatic function tests, while 87% of the patients with extrahepatic shunts had normal hepatic function tests. Half of the cases with intrahepatic shunts survived without clinical signs compared with 84% of the cases with extrahepatic shunts. Resolution of clinical signs was observed in 66% of the cats. Cabassu *et al.* (2011) reported the results of PSS attenuation with cellophane banding in nine cats. The three-year survival rate was 66%, and five cats had normal liver function tests in the long term. Generally, dogs with extrahepatic shunts have a more favorable outcome compared to dogs with intrahepatic shunts or cats when treated with cellophane or ameroid constrictors.

In a study including 123 dogs with extrahepatic portosystemic shunts treated with thin film banding (85 cases) or ameroid constrictor (38 cases) with an ameroid ring, the short- and long-term outcomes were similar between the two treatment modalities (Otomo *et al.* 2020). However, in another study with 53 cases treated with thin film banding and 23 with an ameroid constrictor, thin film banding seemed to be associated with a higher rate of residual shunting and required a second intervention (Matiasovic *et al.* 2020). In a meta-analysis ameroid constrictors may be superior to cellophane banding to induce complete occlusion of PSS in the long term; however, evidence is very weak and a randomized clinical trial is lacking (Serrano *et al.* 2019).

Hydraulic occluder

Hydraulic occluders are inflatable silicon cuffs imbedded with polyester for support. They exist in three different internal diameters: 2, 5, and 20 mm. The occluder is placed around a blood vessel similar to an ameroid constrictor, but is maintained in position with a suture placed through holes at the apex of the cuff, rather than a key (Figure 13.6). A tube connects the occluder to a port placed under the skin. Percutaneous inflation of the cuff and occlusion of the encircled shunt are controlled by injecting or removing sterile saline from the port. Injection of sterile saline or sodium hyaluronate solutions will maintain insufflation of the cuff for at least 90–99% of its original volume at 133 days (Sereda *et al.* 2006). Hydraulic occluders have been used to experimentally decrease blood flow in the vena cava in rats and dogs (Bache *et al.* 1974; Park *et al.* 1985; Peacock *et al.* 2003). It has been shown that the hydraulic occluder can decrease blood flow in the vena cava in rats and dogs (Peacock *et al.* 2003; Sereda *et al.* 2005). Blood flow in the caudal vena cava was decreased from 40.7 to 4.7 mL/min/kg in the rat after eight weeks of gradual occlusion. The presence of occluders by themselves does not influence blood flow in the caudal vena cava, since application of the hydraulic occluder without inflation of the cuff did not change blood flow over eight weeks (Sereda *et al.* 2005).

In a clinical study of 10 dogs with intrahepatic shunts, serum biochemical values and clinical signs improved in all dogs after occluder treatment. The hydraulic occluders were inflated by 25% increments at 2, 4, 6, and 8 weeks after surgery. Dogs were monitored for signs of acute portal hypertension after inflation. Of the 10 dogs, 6 had normal postprandial bile acids two weeks after complete occlusion of the shunt. Three dogs experienced a deflation of the hydraulic occluder and showed elevation of postprandial bile acids. This confirmed the impression that the occluder cannot, by itself, induce closure of the shunt and will more likely not maintain complete occlusion of the shunt in the long term (Adin *et al.* 2006). Two dogs developed ascites after surgery that resolved in one or two weeks. Inflation of the cuff was delayed in those two cases. It is likely that these shunts undergo thrombosis when blood flow is completely interrupted, which should help maintain complete occlusion in the long term even if the cuff deflates. This is supported by the observation that at least one year after occluder implantation postprandial bile acids were within reference range in 8 of 10 dogs. One dog required another injection of saline in the subcutaneous port eight months after surgery to finally achieve normal postprandial bile acids (Adin *et al.* 2006).

Hydraulic occluders are bulky and more difficult to place around an intrahepatic shunt than silk or cellophane. Because of the technical difficulty in placement, in one study hydraulic occluders were not placed around the hepatic vein draining the shunt, but rather were secured around the branch of the portal vein feeding the shunt (Adin *et al.* 2006). This approach will completely interrupt portal blood flow in the liver lobe and should result in liver lobe atrophy in the long term, which might not be desirable in dogs with PSS and microhepatica (Rozga *et al.* 1986a, b; Rozga 2001). The advantage of the hydraulic occluder is that it allows complete and progressive occlusion of the shunt that can be titrated to each patient's needs according to clinical signs and serum biochemistry values (Adin *et al.* 2006).

Embolization with stent and coils

Embolization of intrahepatic and extrahepatic shunts using fluoroscopic guidance has been successfully performed in dogs and cats (Gonzalo-Orden *et al.* 2000; Weisse *et al.* 2002, 2005, 2006; Asano *et al.* 2003; Leveille *et al.* 2003; Bussadori *et al.* 2008; Case *et al.* 2018; Culp *et al.* 2018). To prevent migration of the coils, a stent is first placed in the caudal vena cava at the level of the shunt entrance site. Following similar guidelines used with ligatures, coils are delivered in the PSS while portal pressure is monitored. In order to attenuate blood flow into the shunt, 1–9 coils have been needed in previous reports (Weisse *et al.* 2006; Bussadori *et al.* 2008). Bussadori *et al.* (2008) placed enough coils to fill about 75% of the diameter of the shunt as measured on radiographs. At 1–2 months after coil placement, the shunts were closed in five of six dogs based on liver function tests and ultrasonography. One dog was euthanized six months after coil placement because of persistence of clinical signs (Bussadori *et al.* 2008). Weisse *et al.* (2006) measured portal pressures to decide how many coils to place in their patients with PSS. The perioperative mortality rate in this study was 8% and death was due to portal hypertension, seizure, aspiration pneumonia, and gastrointestinal ulceration. In the long term, the mortality rate was 31%, and 47% of the dogs did not show clinical signs. The coil occlusion technique is the least invasive method for attenuation of shunts, but requires expensive imaging modalities and operator experience. Bloodwork values improved by at least 50% of their initial value by three months after percutaneous transvenous coil embolization in 25 dogs (Culp *et al.* 2018). At three months 24 of 25 dogs were available for reevaluation, and all abnormal clinical signs had resolved in 22 of those 24 dogs.

In a study including 31 dogs with intrahepatic shunts treated with cellophane banding and 27 treated with percutaneous transvenous coil embolization, the long-term survival was not different between the two treatment modalities (Case *et al.* 2018). The one-year and two-year survival rates were 89% for the cellophane banding group and 87% and 80% for the percutaneous transvenous coil embolization group, respectively. The proportion surviving at five years was 75% and 80% for the cellophane banding group and percutaneous transvenous coil embolization group, respectively.

Other techniques for intrahepatic shunts

Some intrahepatic shunts, particularly right-sided ones, are difficult to dissect and expose. Placement of even a suture around the shunt may be dangerous to the patient. Several possibilities exist to partially attenuate the shunts in these cases. First, if the shunt is partially exposed, a mattress suture with pledgets can be placed across a portion of the shunt. The suture is progressively tightened while portal pressures are monitored. As a second option, an extrahepatic shunt can be created with a vascular graft (Kyles et al. 2001, 2004). The jugular vein can be harvested and then sutured between the portal vein and the caudal vena cava in the right side to create an extrahepatic portosystemic conduit. This is similar in theory to an Eck fistula. An ameroid constrictor, a cellophane band, or a hydraulic occluder can be placed around the conduit while the intrahepatic shunt is completely ligated or the liver lobe containing the intrahepatic shunt is resected. The extrahepatic shunt should prevent the development of acute portal hypertension. However, in two different studies this technique did not seem to be sufficient to prevent the development of portal hypertension, even without progressive occlusion of the conduit (Kyles et al. 2004). Creation of a conduit larger than the jugular vein might prove necessary for this complicated method to be successful.

Intravascular procedures for shunt attenuation during inflow occlusion of blood flow to the liver have been reported (Breznock et al. 1983; Hunt et al. 1996). Under venous inflow occlusion, a venotomy is performed in either the caudal vena cava at a level cranial to the liver or the portal vein at the level of the porta hepatis. The shunt is then identified inside the lumen of the vein, because its borders are more irregular than the normal branches of the portal vein or the hepatic veins. A mattress suture is placed across the abnormal vessel under visualization within the portal vein or the vena cava. The free ends of the suture are left loose outside the portal vein or the vena cava. After closure of the venotomy and release of the inflow occlusion, the shunt can then be progressively closed by tying the mattress suture while monitoring portal pressure.

Prognostic indicators

Preoperative prognostic indicators for long-term outcome have been difficult to identify in dogs and cats with PSS. Low body weight (hazard ratio [HR] 0.89, $P = 0.0320$), low total protein (HR 0.397, $P = 0.02$), low albumin (HR 0.35, $P = 0.03$), and low BUN (HR 1.127, $P = 0.023$) were identified as negative short-term prognostic indicators for dogs with intrahepatic shunts (Papazoglou et al. 2002). Low total protein (HR 0.432, $P = 0.019$) and low packed cell volume (HR 0.933, $P = 0.0390$) were risk factors for negative long-term outcome (Papazoglou et al. 2002). High white blood cell counts before surgery appear to be a negative long-term prognostic indicator for extrahepatic shunts (Mehl et al. 2005). Elevated portal pressure during temporary complete occlusion of the shunt is a prognostic indicator for residual shunting postoperatively and a long-term negative outcome for patients with extrahepatic shunts (odds ratio [OR] 1.07–1.09) (Mehl et al. 2005). The presence of abdominal distension has been recognized as a negative prognostic indicator for short-term outcome after extrahepatic shunt surgery (OR 19.7) (Mehl et al. 2005). Presence of residual shunting on portal scintigraphy eight weeks after surgery with an ameroid ring has been identified as a negative long-term prognostic indicator (Mehl et al. 2005). Parker et al. (2008) evaluated histopathologic features of the liver of dogs with portosystemic shunts and could not identify any prognostic indicator. Presence of seizures after surgery is a negative prognostic indicator for short-term (OR 27.9) and long-term (OR 16.4) outcomes (Mehl et al. 2005). Opacification of portal vasculature branching during portovenography was associated with a higher likelihood of safe complete ligation of the shunt at surgery in dogs but not cats (Lee et al. 2006; Lipscomb et al. 2009). The amount of opacification of the intrahepatic portal vasculature was not different between intrahepatic and extrahepatic shunts in a series of dogs and cats (Lee et al. 2006; Lipscomb et al. 2009). The amount of opacification of the portal vasculature seems to have a very weak correlation with the degree of safe occlusion of the shunt for extrahepatic shunts ($r = 0.45$, $P = 0.001$) and intrahepatic shunts ($r = 0.52$, $P = 0.011$) (Kummeling et al. 2004). The degree of occlusion of the shunt at the time of surgery is not different between intrahepatic and extrahepatic shunts in dogs (Lee et al. 2006). The amount of improvement in clinical signs seen after surgery does not correlate with the amount of opacification of the portal vasculature during portovenography (Lee et al. 2006; Lipscomb et al. 2009). Improvement of bile acids and the number of body systems affected after surgery were very weakly correlated to the improved branching of the portal vasculature after shunt surgery ($r = -0.42$, $P = 0.012$ and $r = -0.479$, $P = 0.006$, respectively) (Lee et al. 2006). Redirection of portal blood flow toward the liver improves the development of the portal vasculature and augments liver volume (Lee et al. 2006; Lipscomb et al. 2009; Kummeling et al. 2010). Augmentation of liver volume is mostly present in the first eight days after surgery, then reaches a plateau during the following two months. Development of acquired shunts has been described with any techniques used to attenuate an extrahepatic or an intrahepatic shunt (Vogt et al. 1996; Heldmann et al. 1999; Hunt & Hughes 1999; Tisdall et al. 2000; Hunt et al. 2004; Mehl et al. 2005;

Worley & Holt 2008; Cabassu *et al.* 2011; Wallace *et al.* 2018a, b; Otomo *et al.* 2020; Mullins *et al.* 2020, 2022; Escribano *et al.* 2021). The acquired shunt results from the progression of liver dysfunction (Anglin *et al.* 2021).

Neurologic complications including ataxia, blindness, and seizures have been reported in 3.6–17% after shunt surgery (Hardie *et al.* 1990; Matushek *et al.* 1990; Heldmann *et al.* 1999; Hunt & Hughes 1999; Tisdall *et al.* 2000; Hunt *et al.* 2004; Mehl *et al.* 2005; Worley & Holt 2008; Cabassu *et al.* 2011; Wallace *et al.* 2018a, b; Otomo *et al.* 2020; Mullins *et al.* 2020, 2022; Escribano *et al.* 2021). Short- and long-term prognosis for patients developing seizures after surgery is poor (OR 27.9) (Mehl *et al.* 2005). Dogs that develop postattenuation neurologic signs without seizures can have a survival time above six months and a good quality of life if they survive the first 30 days after surgery (Escribano *et al.* 2021). Hunt *et al.* (2004) reported 11 cases developing neurologic deficits severe enough to require treatment after surgery. Seven cases made a full recovery with a combination of phenobarbital, propofol, midazolam, and acepromazine. Tisdall *et al.* (2000) reported 11 dogs with neurologic complications after PSS attenuation with either silk or cellophane. Three dogs developed seizures and only one had a partial recovery. Heldmann *et al.* (1999) reported the use of propofol to treat seizures after PSS ligation with a favorable outcome in two of five cases. Levetiracetam and α2 antagonist have also been used for the treatment of postattenuation neurologic syndrome and seizures (Escribano *et al.* 2021).

Risk factors for the development of seizures have not been identified. Pretreatment with phenobarbital is not warranted since it does not seem to affect the risk of seizures after surgery (Tisdall *et al.* 2000). Levetiracetam has been advocated to prevent postattenuation seizures; however, the effect is not consistent (Fryer *et al.* 2011; Mullins *et al.* 2019, 2020). The frequency of seizure development after shunt surgery appears to be similar among dogs with extrahepatic and intrahepatic shunts (Hunt & Hughes 1999; Hunt *et al.* 2004; Mullins *et al.* 2020, 2022; Escribano *et al.* 2021). Older patients may be more at risk than younger dogs or cats (Hardie *et al.* 1990; Matushek *et al.* 1990). Worley and Holt (2008) reported neurologic complications in 17% of cases older than 5 years. However, Hunt *et al.* (2004) did not report a significant age difference among patients that developed postoperative neurologic complications. The degree of attenuation of the shunt at the time of surgery might be a factor in the development of neurologic complications. Pugs might be at increased risk of seizures after surgery for a PSS (Wallace *et al.* 2018a, b). Cats with better development of portal vasculature may have a lower risk of neurologic complications after

surgery (Lipscomb *et al.* 2009), and the presence of seizures before surgery does not seem to be a risk factor for the development of refractory seizures after surgery (Cabassu *et al.* 2011).

Continued evidence of abnormal liver function or residual shunting in patients with no associated clinical signs or significantly improved clinical signs after PSS surgery is common in dogs and cats (Hunt *et al.* 2004; Mehl *et al.* 2005; Bristow *et al.* 2017). Mehl *et al.* (2005) documented abnormal scintigraphy results in 21% of the dogs 10 weeks after ameroid ring application. Those dogs experienced an excellent outcome after surgery according to the owners. Three dogs were still showing evidence of shunting 16 weeks after surgery due to the development of acquired shunts in one dog and continued portoazygous shunting in another. Hunt *et al.* (2004) examined 12 dogs and 2 cats with abnormal liver function based on ATT or bile acids at eight weeks following PSS surgery. The owners of those dogs reported an absence or significant improvement of clinical signs. Multiple acquired shunts were present in two cases and one dog developed ascites 10 days after surgery, suggesting the abnormal liver function tests were the result of chronic portal hypertension. Cellophane bands were applied with some occlusion of the shunt in this case series. Frankel *et al.* (2006) showed that partial occlusion of the shunt at the time of cellophane banding to a diameter of less than 3 mm is not desirable. Dogs that had no attenuation at the time of cellophane implantation had normal bile acids more than six months after surgery. This suggests that surgeons should strive to place cellophane with the goal of minimally attenuating the shunt. It has been shown in a study of 51 dogs with complete occlusion of the shunt at the time of surgery that mild increases in serum bile acids are not clinically relevant if there are no physical examination abnormalities, a normal body condition score, and no relapse in clinical signs (Bristow *et al.* 2017).

A lidocaine/monoethylglycylxylidide (MEGX) test has been advocated to evaluate closure of PSS (Devriendt *et al.* 2021). Monoethylglycylxylidide is higher 15 minutes after injection of lidocaine in cases with the shunt completely closed. The sensitivity of the test was 96.2% and specificity 82.8% to determine shunt closure. Dogs with PSS have an altered blood amino acid profile, with an abnormal BCAA to AAA ratio being the most common abnormality. The ratio has been shown not to improve with medical treatment but to significantly improve after surgery. However, it remains abnormal, indicating moderate to severe hepatic dysfunction (Devriendt *et al.* 2021).

Overall median survival time of dogs treated for PSS is between four and five years (Papazoglou *et al.* 2002;

Parker *et al.* 2008; Worley & Holt 2008). In these studies, most shunts were ligated with suture and were not attenuated with an ameroid ring or cellophane. In a study of nine cats treated with cellophane, 65% were still alive five years after surgery (Cabassu *et al.* 2011). In the study by Greenhalgh *et al.* (2010), median survival time was not reached, as 90% of the dogs were still alive five years after surgery. These shunts were either ligated with suture or attenuated with ameroid rings or cellophane. In that same study, 60% of dogs treated with medical therapy alone were still alive at five years. The difference in median survival was no different between medical and surgical treatment in that study; however, Cox analysis showed that surgical treatment was associated with a longer survival time (HR 2.9). In a case series of 27 dogs that were medically treated for PSS, 14 dogs were euthanized 10 months after diagnosis at owner request because of neurologic signs and unrewarding medical therapy; however, 9 dogs (33%) were still alive five years later (Watson & Herrtage 1998). Most of these cases were treated medically because the owners could not afford surgery, which may have instilled a bias into the data. Age above 2–5 years at the time of diagnosis has been shown to be associated with a higher risk of posttenuation neurologic syndrome, although it has been shown that dogs above 5 years old still benefit from medical treatment (Mullins *et al.* 2022; Wallace *et al.* 2022). At present, there is no randomized clinical trial that allows a valid comparison of medical and surgical treatment of PSS in dogs and cats. It appears, though, that up to 50% of dogs with PSS may thrive for many years with medical therapy alone.

References

Acharya, S.K., Bhatia, V., Sreenivas, V. et al. (2009). Efficacy of l-ornithine l-aspartate in acute liver failure: a double-blind, randomized, placebo-controlled study. *Gastroenterology* 136: 2159–2168.

Adin, C.A., Gregory, C.R., Kyles, A.E. et al. (2004). Effect of petrolatum coating on the rate of occlusion of ameroid constrictors in the peritoneal cavity. *Veterinary Surgery* 33: 11–16.

Adin, C.A., Sereda, C.W., Thompson, M.S. et al. (2006). Outcome associated with use of a percutaneously controlled hydraulic occluder for treatment of dogs with intrahepatic portosystemic shunts. *Journal of the American Veterinary Medical Association* 229: 1749–1755.

Ahboucha, S. (2011). Neurosteroids and hepatic encephalopathy: an update on possible pathophysiologic mechanisms. *Current Molecular Pharmacology* 4: 1–13.

Ahboucha, S., Layrargues, G.P., Mamer, O. et al. (2005). Increased brain concentrations of neurohinhibitory steroid in human hepatic encephalopathy. *Annals of Neurology* 58: 169–170.

Ahmad, I., Khan, A.A., Alam, A. et al. (2008). l-Ornithine-l-aspartate infusion efficacy in hepatic encephalopathy. *Journal of the College of Physicians and Surgeons Pakistan* 18: 684–687.

Ahn, J.O., Li, Q., Lee, Y.H. et al. (2016). Hyperammonemic hepatic encephalopathy management through L-ornithin-L-aspartate administration in dogs. *Journal of Veterinary Science* 17: 431–433.

Albrecht, J. and Faff, L. (1994). Astrocyte-neuron interactions in hyperammonemia and hepatic encephalopathy. *Advances in Experimental Medicine and Biology* 368: 45–54.

Albrecht, J. and Norenberg, M.D. (2006). Glutamine: a Trojan horse in ammonia neurotoxicity. *Hepatology* 44: 788–794.

Albrecht, J., Waskiewicz, J., Dolinska, M., and Rafalowska, U. (1997). Synaptosomal uptake of alpha-ketoglutarate and glutamine in thioacetamide-induced hepatic encephalopathy in rats. *Metabolic Brain Disease* 12: 281–286.

Albrecht, J., Zielinska, M., and Norenberg, M.D. (2010). Glutamine as a mediator of ammonia neurotoxicity: a critical appraisal. *Biochemical Pharmacology* 80: 1303–1308.

Allen, L., Stobie, D., Mauldin, G.N., and Baer, K.E. (1999). Clinicopathologic features of dogs with hepatic microvascular dysplasia with and without portosystemic shunts: 42 cases (1991–1996). *Journal of the American Veterinary Medical Association* 214: 218–220.

Anglin, E.V., Lux, C.N., Sun, X. et al. (2021). Clinical characteristics of, prognostic factors for, and long-term outcome of dogs with multiple acquired portosystemic shunts: 72 cases (2000–2018). *Journal of the American Veterinary Medical Association* 260: S30–S39.

Ansley, J.D., Isaacs, J.W., Rikkers, L.F. et al. (1978). Quantitative tests of nitrogen metabolism in cirrhosis: relation to other manifestations of liver disease. *Gastroenterology* 75: 570–579.

Asano, T. and Spector, S. (1979). Identification of inosine and hypoxanthine as endogenous ligands for the brain benzodiazepine-binding sites. *Proceedings of the National Academy of Sciences USA* 76: 977–981.

Asano, K., Watari, T., Kuwabara, M. et al. (2003). Successful treatment by percutaneous transvenous coil embolization in a small-breed dog with intrahepatic portosystemic shunt. *Journal of Veterinary Medical Science* 65: 1269–1272.

Bache, R.J., Cobb, F.R., and Greenfield, J.C. Jr. (1974). Myocardial blood flow distribution during ischemia-induced coronary vasodilation in the unanesthetized dog. *Journal of Clinical Investigation* 54: 1462–1472.

Bachmann, C. (2002). Mechanisms of hyperammonemia. *Clinical Chemistry and Laboratory Medicine* 40: 653–662.

Bajaj, J.S., Saeian, K., Christensen, K.M. et al. (2008). Probiotic yogurt for the treatment of minimal hepatic encephalopathy. *American Journal of Gastroenterology* 103: 1707–1715.

Bajaj, J.S., Sanyal, A.J., Bell, D. et al. (2010). Predictors of the recurrence of hepatic encephalopathy in lactulose-treated patients. *Alimentary Pharmacology and Therapeutics* 31: 1012–1017.

Baraldi, M., Pinelli, G., Ricci, P., and Zeneroli, M.L. (1984). Toxins in hepatic encephalopathy: the role of the synergistic effect of ammonia, mercaptans and short chain fatty acids. *Archives of Toxicology Supplement* 7: 103–105.

Barker, P.B., Butterworth, E.J., Boska, M.D. et al. (1999). Magnesium and pH imaging of the human brain at 3.0 Tesla. *Magnetic Resonance in Medicine* 41: 400–406.

Basile, A.S. and Gammal, S.H. (1988). Evidence for the involvement of the benzodiazepine receptor complex in hepatic encephalopathy. Implications for treatment with benzodiazepine receptor antagonists. *Clinical Neuropharmacology* 11: 401–422.

Basile, A.S. and Jones, E.A. (1994). The involvement of benzodiazepine receptor ligands in hepatic encephalopathy. *Hepatology* 20: 541–543.

Basile, A.S. and Jones, E.A. (1997). Ammonia and GABA-ergic neurotransmission: interrelated factors in the pathogenesis of hepatic encephalopathy. *Hepatology* 25: 1303–1305.

Basile, A.S., Ostrowski, N.L., Gammal, S.H. et al. (1990). The GABAA receptor complex in hepatic encephalopathy. Autoradiographic evidence for the presence of elevated levels of a benzodiazepine receptor ligand. *Neuropsychopharmacology* 3: 61–71.

Basile, A.S., Jones, E.A., and Skolnick, P. (1991). The pathogenesis and treatment of hepatic encephalopathy: evidence for the involvement of benzodiazepine receptor ligands. *Pharmacological Reviews* 43: 27–71.

Bassett, M.L., Mullen, K.D., Skolnick, P., and Jones, E.A. (1987). Amelioration of hepatic encephalopathy by pharmacologic antagonism of the GABAA–benzodiazepine receptor complex in a rabbit model of fulminant hepatic failure. *Gastroenterology* 93: 1069–1077.

Bauer, N.B., Schneider, M.A., Neiger, R., and Moritz, A. (2006). Liver disease in dogs with tracheal collapse. *Journal of Veterinary Internal Medicine* 20: 845–849.

Bengtsson, F., Bugge, M., Hall, H., and Nobin, A. (1989a). Brain 5-Ht1 and 5-Ht2 binding sites following portacaval shunt in the rat. *Research in Experimental Medicine* 189: 249–256.

Bengtsson, F., Bugge, M., Herlin, P. et al. (1989b). Serotonin metabolism in the central nervous system in portacaval shunted rats infused with fat emulsion. *Journal of Parenteral and Enteral Nutrition* 13: 65–70.

Bengtsson, F., Bugge, M., Johansen, K.H., and Butterworth, R.F. (1991). Brain tryptophan hydroxylation in the portacaval shunted rat: a hypothesis for the regulation of serotonin turnover in vivo. *Journal of Neurochemistry* 56: 1069–1074.

Bergasa, N.V., Rothman, R.B., Mukerjee, E. et al. (2002). Up-regulation of central mu-opioid receptors in a model of hepatic encephalopathy: a potential mechanism for increased sensitivity to morphine in liver failure. *Life Sciences* 70: 1701–1708.

Bergeron, M., Swain, M.S., Reader, T.A., and Butterworth, R.F. (1995). Regional alterations of dopamine and its metabolites in rat brain following portacaval anastomosis. *Neurochemical Research* 20: 79–86.

Bertolini, G. (2010). Acquired portal collateral circulation in the dog and cat. *Veterinary Radiology and Ultrasound* 51: 25–33.

Bertolini, G., Rolla, E.C., Zotti, A., and Caldin, M. (2006). Three-dimensional multislice helical computed tomography techniques for canine extra-hepatic portosystemic shunt assessment. *Veterinary Radiology and Ultrasound* 47: 439–443.

Besancon, M.F., Kyles, A.E., Griffey, S.M., and Gregory, C.R. (2004). Evaluation of the characteristics of venous occlusion after placement of an ameroid constrictor in dogs. *Veterinary Surgery* 33: 597–605.

Binesh, N., Huda, A., Thomas, M.A. et al. (2006). Hepatic encephalopathy: a neurochemical, neuroanatomical, and neuropsychological study. *Journal of Applied Clinical Medical Physics* 7: 86–96.

Blei, A.T. (2005). The pathophysiology of brain edema in acute liver failure. *Neurochemistry International* 47: 71–77.

Blom, H.J., Chamuleau, R.A., Rothuizen, J. et al. (1990). Methanethiol metabolism and its role in the pathogenesis of hepatic encephalopathy in rats and dogs. *Hepatology* 11: 682–689.

Bloom, P.P., Tapper, E.B., Young, V.B. et al. (2021). Microbiome therapeutics for hepatic encephalopathy. *Journal of Hepatology* 75: 1452–1464.

Boulton, A.A., Juorio, A.V., Philips, S.R., and Wu, P.H. (1975). Some arylalkylamines in rabbit brain. *Brain Research* 96: 212–216.

Bradford, H.F. and Ward, H.K. (1976). On glutaminase activity in mammalian synaptosomes. *Brain Research* 110: 115–125.

Bradford, H.F., Ward, H.K., and Thomas, A.J. (1978). Glutamine: a major substrate for nerve endings. *Journal of Neurochemistry* 30: 1453–1459.

Bredée, J.J., Blickman, J.R., Holman van der Heide, J.N. et al. (1975). Standardized induction of myocardial ischaemia in the dog. *European Surgical Research* 7: 269–286.

Breznock, E.M., Berger, B., Pendray, D. et al. (1983). Surgical manipulation of intrahepatic portocaval shunts in dogs. *Journal of the American Veterinary Medical Association* 182: 798–804.

Bright, S.R., Williams, J.M., and Niles, J.D. (2006). Outcomes of intrahepatic portosystemic shunts occluded with ameroid constrictors in nine dogs and one cat. *Veterinary Surgery* 35: 300–309.

Bristow, P., Tivers, M., Packer, R. et al. (2017). Long-term serum bile acid concentrations in 51 dogs after complete extrahepatic congenital portosystemic shunt ligation. *Journal of Small Animal Practice* 58: 454–460.

Brooks, D.J., Lammertsma, A.A., Beaney, R.P. et al. (1984). Measurement of regional cerebral pH in human subjects using continuous inhalation of $^{11}CO_2$ and positron emission tomography. *Journal of Cerebral Blood Flow and Metabolism* 4: 458–465.

Broome, C.J., Walsh, V.P., and Braddock, J.A. (2004). Congenital portosystemic shunts in dogs and cats. *New Zealand Veterinary Journal* 52: 154–162.

Brueschwein, A., Foltin, I., Flatz, K. et al. (2010). Contrast-enhanced magnetic resonance angiography for diagnosis of portosystemic shunts in 10 dogs. *Veterinary Radiology and Ultrasound* 51: 116–121.

Brusilow, S.W. (2002). Hyperammonemic encephalopathy. *Medicine* 81: 240–249.

Bunch, S.E., Johnson, S.E., and Cullen, J.M. (2001). Idiopathic noncirrhotic portal hypertension in dogs: 33 cases (1982–1998). *Journal of the American Veterinary Medical Association* 218: 392–399.

Burton, C.A. and White, R.N. (2001). Portovenogram findings in cases of elevated bile acid concentrations following correction of portosystemic shunts. *Journal of Small Animal Practice* 42: 536–540.

Bussadori, R., Bussadori, C., Millán, L. et al. (2008). Transvenous coil embolisation for the treatment of single congenital portosystemic shunts in six dogs. *Veterinary Journal (London)* 176: 221–226.

Butterworth, R.F. (1990). Brain GABA and benzodiazepine receptors in hepatic encephalopathy. *Revista de Investigacion Clinica* 42 (Suppl): 137–140.

Butterworth, R.F. (1993). Portal–systemic encephalopathy: a disorder of neuron–astrocytic metabolic trafficking. *Developmental Neuroscience* 15: 313–319.

Butterworth, R.F. (1996). Taurine in hepatic encephalopathy. *Advances in Experimental Medicine and Biology* 403: 601–606.

Butterworth, R.F. (2000). The astrocytic ("peripheral-type") benzodiazepine receptor: role in the pathogenesis of portal–systemic encephalopathy. *Neurochemistry International* 36: 411–416.

Butterworth, R.F. (2002). Pathophysiology of hepatic encephalopathy: a new look at ammonia. *Metabolic Brain Disease* 17: 221–227.

Butterworth, R.F. (2008). Pathophysiology of hepatic encephalopathy: the concept of synergism. *Hepatology Research* 38 (Suppl 1): S116–S121.

Butterworth, R.F. and McPhail, M.J.W. (2019). L-Ornithine L-Aspartate (LOLA) for hepatic encephalopathy in cirrhosis: results of randomized controlled trials and meta-analysis. *Drugs* 79: S31–S37.

Cabassu, J., Seim, H.B. III, MacPhail, C.M., and Monnet, E. (2011). Outcomes of cats undergoing surgical attenuation of congenital extrahepatic portosystemic shunts through cellophane banding:

9 cases (2000–2007). *Journal of the American Veterinary Medical Association* 238: 89–93.

Cangiano, C., Cardelli-Cangiano, P., James, J.H. et al. (1983). Brain microvessels take up large neutral amino acids in exchange for glutamine. Cooperative role of Na+-dependent and Na+-independent systems. *Journal of Biological Chemistry* 258: 8949–8954.

Caporali, E.H., Philips, H., Underwood, L. et al. (2015). Risk factors for urolithiasis in dogs with congenital extrahepatic portosystemic shunts: 95 cases (1999–2013). *Journal of the American Medical Association* 246: 530–536.

Cardelli-Cangiano, P., Cangiano, C., James, J.H. et al. (1984). Effect of ammonia on amino acid uptake by brain microvessels. *Journal of Biological Chemistry* 259: 5295–5300.

Cascino, A., Cangiano, C., Calcaterra, V. et al. (1978). Plasma amino acids imbalance in patients with liver disease. *American Journal of Digestive Diseases* 23: 591–598.

Cascino, A., Cangiano, C., Fiaccadori, F. et al. (1982). Plasma and cerebrospinal fluid amino acid patterns in hepatic encephalopathy. *Digestive Diseases and Sciences* 27: 828–832.

Case, J.B., Marvel, S.J., Stiles, M.C. et al. (2018). Outcomes of cellophane banding or percutaneous transvenous coil embolization of canine intrahepatic portosystemic shunts. *Veterinary Surgery* 47: O59–O66.

Center, S.A. (1998). Nutritional support for dogs and cats with hepatobiliary disease. *Journal of Nutrition* 128 (12 Suppl): 2733S–2746S.

Center, S.A., Baldwin, B.H., Erb, H.N., and Tennant, B.C. (1985a). Bile acid concentrations in the diagnosis of hepatobiliary disease in the dog. *Journal of the American Veterinary Medical Association* 187: 935–940.

Center, S.A., Baldwin, B.H., de Lahunta, A. et al. (1985b). Evaluation of serum bile acid concentrations for the diagnosis of portosystemic venous anomalies in the dog and cat. *Journal of the American Veterinary Medical Association* 186: 1090–1094.

Center, S.A., ManWarren, T., Slater, M.R., and Wilentz, E. (1991). Evaluation of twelve hour preprandial and two hours postprandial serum bile acids concentrations for diagnosis of hepatobiliary disease in dogs. *Journal of the American Veterinary Medical Association* 199: 217–226.

Center, S.A., Crawford, M.A., Guida, L. et al. (1993). A retrospective study of 77 cats with severe hepatic lipidosis: 1975–1990. *Journal of Veterinary Internal Medicine* 7: 349–359.

Center, S.A., Erb, H.N., and Joseph, S.A. (1995). Measurement of serum bile acids concentrations for diagnosis of hepatobiliary disease in cats. *Journal of the American Veterinary Medical Association* 207: 1048–1054.

Challenger, R.F. and Walshe, J.M. (1955). Methyl mercaptan in relation to foetor hepaticus. *Biochemical Journal* 59: 372–375.

Chan, H. and Butterworth, R.F. (1999). Evidence for an astrocytic glutamate transporter deficit in hepatic encephalopathy. *Neurochemistry Research* 24: 1397–1401.

Chan, H. and Butterworth, R.F. (2003). Cell-selective effects of ammonia on glutamate transporter and receptor function in the mammalian brain. *Neurochemistry International* 43: 525–532.

Chepkova, A.N., Sergeeva, O.A., and Haas, H.L. (2006). Taurine rescues hippocampal long-term potentiation from ammonia-induced impairment. *Neurobiology of Disease* 23: 512–521.

Chetri, K. and Choudhuri, G. (2003). Role of trace elements in hepatic encephalopathy: zinc and manganese. *Indian Journal of Gastroenterology* 22 (Suppl 2): S28–S30.

Chung, Y.L., Williams, S.C., Hope, J., and Bell, J.D. (1999). Brain bioenergetics in murine models of scrapie using in vivo ^{31}P magnetic resonance spectroscopy. *Neuroreport* 10: 1899–1901.

Cole, R.C., Morandi, F., Avenell, J., and Daniel, G.B. (2005). Transsplenic portal scintigraphy in normal dogs. *Veterinary Radiology and Ultrasound* 46: 146–152.

Conn, H.O. (1972). Interactions of lactulose and neomycin. *Drugs* 4: 4–6.

Conn, H.O., Leevy, C.M., Vlahcevic, Z.R. et al. (1977). Comparison of lactulose and neomycin in the treatment of chronic portal-systemic encephalopathy. A double blind controlled trial. *Gastroenterology* 72: 573–583.

Cooper, A.J. and Plum, F. (1987). Biochemistry and physiology of brain ammonia. *Physiological Reviews* 67: 440–519.

Cooper, A.J., Nieves, E., Coleman, A.E. et al. (1987). Short-term metabolic fate of [^{13}N]ammonia in rat liver in vivo. *Journal of Biological Chemistry* 262: 1073–1080.

Coughlan, J., Hamlin, P.J., and Ford, A.C. (2010). Effect of oral zinc in hepatic encephalopathy remains unclear. *Alimentary Pharmacology and Therapeutics* 32: 1405–1406.

Crossley, I.R., Wardle, E.N., and Williams, R. (1983). Biochemical mechanisms of hepatic encephalopathy. *Clinical Science* 64: 247–252.

Cuilleret, G., Pomier-Layrargues, G., Pons, F. et al. (1980). Changes in brain catecholamine levels in human cirrhotic hepatic encephalopathy. *Gut* 21: 565–569.

Culp, W.T.N., Zwingenberger, A.L., Giuffrida, M.A. et al. (2018). Prospective evaluation of outcome of dogs with intrahepatic portosystemic shunts treated via percutaneous transvenous coil embolization. *Veterinary Surgery* 47: 74–85.

Cummings, M.G., Soeters, P.B., James, J.H. et al. (1976). Regional brain indoleamine metabolism following chronic portacaval anastomosis in the rat. *Journal of Neurochemistry* 27: 501–509.

Dalal, R., McGee, R.G., Riordan, S.M. et al. (2017). Probiotics for people with hepatic encephalopathy. *Cochrane Database of Systematic Reviews* 2: CD008716. https://doi.org/10.1002/14651858.CD008716.

Daniel, G.B., Bright, R., Monnet, E. et al (1990). Comparison of per rectal portal scintigraphy using 99 m technetium pertechnate to mesenteric injection of radioactive microspheres for quantification of portosystemic shunts in an experimental dog model. *Veterinary Radiology* 31: 175–181.

Daniel, G.B., Bright, R., Ollis, P., and Shull, R. (1991). Per rectal portal scintigraphy using 99 m-technetium pertechnetate to diagnose portosystemic shunts in dogs and cats. *Journal of Veterinary Internal Medicine* 5: 23–27.

d'Anjou, M.A. and Huneault, L. (2008). Imaging diagnosis: complex intrahepatic portosystemic shunt in a dog. *Veterinary Radiology and Ultrasound* 49: 51–55.

d'Anjou, M.A., Penninck, D., Cornejo, L., and Pibarot, P. (2004). Ultrasonographic diagnosis of portosystemic shunting in dogs and cats. *Veterinary Radiology and Ultrasound* 45: 424–437.

Davis, M. (2007). Cholestasis and endogenous opioids: liver disease and exogenous opioid pharmacokinetics. *Clinical Pharmacokinetics* 46: 825–850.

DeMarco, J., Center, S.A., Dykes, N. et al. (1998). A syndrome resembling idiopathic noncirrhotic portal hypertension in 4 young Doberman pinschers. *Journal of Veterinary Internal Medicine* 12: 147–156.

Desjardins, P. and Butterworth, R.F. (2002). The "peripheral-type" benzodiazepine (omega 3) receptor in hyperammonemic disorders. *Neurochemistry International* 41: 109–114.

Devriendt, N., Kitshoff, A.M., Peremans, K. et al. (2017). Ammonia concentrations in arterial blood, venous blood, and cerebrospinal fluid of dogs with and without congenital extrahepatic portosystemic shunts. *American Journal of Veterinary Research* 78: 1313–1318.

Devriendt, N., Paepe, D., Serrano, G. et al. (2021). Plasma amino acid profiles in dogs with closed extrahepatic portosystemic shunts are only partially improved 3 months after successful gradual attenuation. *Journal of Veterinary Internal Medicine* 35: 1347–1354.

Dimski, D.S. (1994). Ammonia metabolism and the urea cycle: function and clinical implications. *Journal of Veterinary Internal Medicine* 8: 73–78.

Dodsworth, J.M., James, J.H., Cummings, M.C., and Fischer, J.F. (1974). Depletion of brain norepinephrine in acute hepatic coma. *Surgery* 75: 811–820.

Dombro, R.S., Hutson, D.G., and Norenberg, M.D. (1993). The action of ammonia on astrocyte glycogen and glycogenolysis. *Molecular and Chemical Neuropathology* 19: 259–268.

Duda, G.G. and Handler, P. (1958). Kinetics of ammonia metabolism in vivo. *Journal of Biological Chemistry* 232: 303–314.

Ede, R.J. and Williams, R.W. (1986). Hepatic encephalopathy and cerebral edema. *Seminars in Liver Disease* 6: 107–118.

Elzinga, W.E. (1969). Ameroid constrictor: uniform closure rates and a calibration procedure. *Journal of Applied Physiology* 27: 419–421.

Escribano, C.A., Morrissey, A.M., Lipscomb, V.J. et al. (2021). Long-term outcome and quality of life of dogs that developed neurologic signs after surgical treatment of a congenital portosystemic shunt: 50 cases (2005–2020). *Journal of the American Veterinary Medical Association* 260: 326–334.

Faraj, B.A., Camp, V.M., Ansley, J.D. et al. (1981). Evidence for central hypertyraminemia in hepatic encephalopathy. *Journal of Clinical Investigation* 67: 395–402.

Favier, R.P., de Graaf, E., Corbee, R.J. et al. (2020). Outcome of non-surgical dietary treatment with or without lactulose in dogs with congenital portosystemic shunts. *Veterinary Quarterly* 40: 108–114.

Ferreira, M.F., Schmitz, S.S., Schoenbeck, J.J. et al. (2019). Lactulose drives a reversible reduction and qualitative modulation of the faecal microbiota diversity in healthy dogs. *Scientific Reports* 9: 13350.

Firoozan, S., Wei, K., Linka, A. et al. (1999). A canine model of chronic ischemic cardiomyopathy: characterization of regional flow-function relations. *American Journal of Physiology* 276: H446–H455.

Fischer, J.E. (1975). On the occurrence of false neurochemical transmitter. In: *Artificial Liver Support* (ed. R. Williams and I. Murray-Lyons), 31–48. Tunbridge Wells: Pitman Medical.

Flannery, D.B., Hsia, Y.E., and Wolf, B. (1982). Current status of hyperammonemic syndromes. *Hepatology* 2: 495–506.

Foster, D., Ahmed, K., and Zieve, L. (1974). Action of methanethiol on Na^+, K^+ATPase: implications for hepatic coma. *Annals of the New York Academy of Sciences* 242: 573–576.

Foster, K.J., Lin, S., and Turck, C.J. (2010). Current and emerging strategies for treating hepatic encephalopathy. *Critical Care Nursing Clinics of North America* 22: 341–350.

Frank, P., Mahaffey, M., Egger, C., and Cornell, K.K. (2003). Helical computed tomographic portography in ten normal dogs and ten dogs with a portosystemic shunt. *Veterinary Radiology and Ultrasound* 44: 392–400.

Frankel, D., Seim, H., MacPhail, C., and Monnet, E. (2006). Evaluation of cellophane banding with and without intraoperative attenuation for treatment of congenital extrahepatic portosystemic shunts in dogs. *Journal of the American Veterinary Medical Association* 228: 1355–1360.

Fryer, K.J., Levine, J.M., Peycke, L.E. et al. (2011). Incidence of postoperative seizures with and without levetiracetam pretreatment in dogs undergoing portosystemic shunt attenuation. *Journal of Veterinary Internal Medicine* 25: 1379–1384.

Gentile, S., Guarino, G., Romano, M. et al. (2005). A randomized controlled trial of acarbose in hepatic encephalopathy. *Clinical Gastroenterology and Hepatology* 3: 184–191.

Gerritzen-Bruning, M.J., van den Ingh, T.S., and Rothuizen, J. (2006). Diagnostic value of fasting plasma ammonia and bile acid concentrations in the identification of portosystemic shunting in dogs. *Journal of Veterinary Internal Medicine* 20: 13–19.

Gonzalo-Orden, J.M., Altonaga, J.R., Costilla, S. et al. (2000). Transvenous coil embolization of an intrahepatic portosystemic shunt in a dog. *Veterinary Radiology and Ultrasound* 41: 516–518.

Gow, A.G. (2017). Hepatic encephalopathy. *Veterinary Clinics of North America. Small Animal Practice* 47: 585–599.

Gow, A.G., Marques, A.I., Yool, D.A. et al. (2012). Dogs with congenital porto-systemic shunting (cPSS) and hepatic encephalopathy have higher serum concentrations of C-reactive protein than asymptomatic dogs with cPSS. *Metabolism and Brain Disease* 27: 227–229.

Greenhalgh, S.N., Dunning, M.D., McKinley, T.J. et al. (2010). Comparison of survival after surgical or medical treatment in dogs with a congenital portosystemic shunt. *Journal of the American Veterinary Medical Association* 236: 1215–1220.

Greenhalgh, S.N., Reeve, J.A., Johnstone, T. et al. (2014). Long-term survival and quality of life in dogs with clinical signs associated with a congenital portosystemic shunt after surgical or medical treatment. *Journal of the American Medical Association* 245: 527–533.

Harari, J., Lincoln, J., Alexander, J., and Miller, J. (1990). Lateral thoracotomy and cellophane banding of a congenital portoazygous shunt in a dog. *Journal of Small Animal Practice* 31: 571–573.

Harder, M.A., Fowler, D., Pharr, J.W. et al. (2002). Segmental aplasia of the caudal vena cava in a dog. *Canadian Veterinary Journal* 43: 365–368.

Hardie, E.M., Kornegay, J.N., and Cullen, J.M. (1990). Status epilepticus after ligation of portosystemic shunts. *Veterinary Surgery* 19: 412–417.

Hardy, R.M. (1990). Pathophysiology of hepatic encephalopathy. *Seminars in Veterinary Medicine and Surgery (Small Animal)* 5: 100–106.

Hassouneh, R. and Bajaj, J.S. (2021). Gut microbiota modulation and fecal transplantation: An overview on innovative strategies for hepatic encephalopathy treatment. *Journal of Clinical Medicine* 10: 330.

Hauger, R.L., Skolnick, P., and Paul, S.M. (1982). Specific [³H] beta-phenylethylamine binding sites in rat brain. *European Journal of Pharmacology* 83: 147–148.

Havig, M. and Tobias, K.M. (2002). Outcome of ameroid constrictor occlusion of single congenital extrahepatic portosystemic shunts in cats: 12 cases (1993–2000). *Journal of the American Veterinary Medical Association* 220: 337–341.

Hawkins, R.A. and Mans, A.M. (1989). Brain energy metabolism in hepatic encephalopathy. In: *Hepatic Encephalopathy* (ed. R.F. Butterworth and G. Pomier Layrargues), 159–176. Clifton, NJ: Humana Press.

Hazell, A.S. and Norenberg, M.D. (1997). Manganese decreases glutamate uptake in cultured astrocytes. *Neurochemical Research* 22: 1443–1447.

Heldmann, E., Holt, D.E., Brockman, D.J. et al. (1999). Use of propofol to manage seizure activity after surgical treatment of portosystemic shunts. *Journal of Small Animal Practice* 40: 590–594.

Hilgier, W., Olson, J.E., and Albrecht, J. (1996). Relation of taurine transport and brain edema in rats with simple hyperammonemia or liver failure. *Journal of Neuroscience Research* 45: 69–74.

Hilgier, W., Law, R.O., Zielińska, M., and Albrecht, J. (2000). Taurine, glutamine, glutamate, and aspartate content and efflux, and cell volume of cerebrocortical minislices of rats with hepatic encephalopathy: influence of ammonia. *Advances in Experimental Medicine and Biology* 483: 305–312.

Hirayama, C. (1971). Tryptophan metabolism in liver disease. *Clinica Chimica Acta* 32: 191–197.

Hird, F.J. and Weidemann, M.J. (1966). Oxidative phosphorylation accompanying oxidation of short-chain fatty acids by rat-liver mitochondria. *Biochemical Journal* 98: 378–388.

Holt, D.E., Washabau, R.J., Djali, S. et al. (2002). Cerebrospinal fluid glutamine, tryptophan, and tryptophan metabolite concentrations in dogs with portosystemic shunts. *American Journal of Veterinary Research* 63: 1167–1171.

de Knegt, R.J., Groeneweg, M., Schalm, S.W., and Hekking-Weijma, I. (1994). Encephalopathy from acute liver failure and from acute hyperammonemia in the rabbit. A clinical and biochemical study. *Liver* 14: 25–31.

Hörner, D.V., Avery, A., and Stow, R. (2017). The effects of probiotics and symbiotics on risk factors for hepatic encephalopathy. *Journal of Clinical Gastroenterology* 51: 312–323.

Hottinger, H.A., Walshaw, R., and Hauptman, J.G. (1995). Long-term results of complete and partial ligation of congenital portosystemic shunts in dogs. *Veterinary Surgery* 24: 331–336.

Huchzermeyer, H. and Schumann, C. (1997). Lactulose: a multifaceted substance. *Zeitschrift fur Gastroenterologie* 35: 945–955.

Hunt, G.B. (2004). Effect of breed on anatomy of portosystemic shunts resulting from congenital diseases in dogs and cats: a review of 242 cases. *Australian Veterinary Journal* 82: 746–749.

Hunt, G.B., Bellenger, C.R., and Pearson, M.R. (1996). Transportal approach for attenuating intrahepatic portosystemic shunts in dogs. *Veterinary Surgery* 25: 300–308.

Hunt, G.B. and Hughes, J. (1999). Outcomes after extrahepatic portosystemic shunt ligation in 49 dogs. *Australian Veterinary Journal* 77: 303–307.

Hunt, G.B., Kummeling, A., Tisdall, P.L. et al. (2004). Outcomes of cellophane banding for congenital portosystemic shunts in 106 dogs and 5 cats. *Veterinary Surgery* 33: 25–31.

Iber, F.L., Rosen, H., Levenson, S.M., and Chalmers, T.C. (1957). The plasma amino acids in patients with liver failure. *Journal of Laboratory and Clinical Medicine* 50: 417–425.

Inagaki, C., Oda, W., Kondo, K., and Kusumi, M. (1987). Histochemical demonstration of Cl(−)-ATPase in rat spinal motoneurons. *Brain Research* 419: 375–378.

James, J.H., Ziparo, V., Jeppsson, B., and Fischer, J.E. (1979). Hyperammonaemia, plasma aminoacid imbalance, and blood–brain aminoacid transport: a unified theory of portal–systemic encephalopathy. *Lancet* ii: 772–775.

Jayakumar, A.R. and Norenberg, M.D. (2010). The Na–K–Cl co-transporter in astrocyte swelling. *Metabolic Brain Disease* 25: 31–38.

Jensen, D.M. (1986). Portal–systemic encephalopathy and hepatic coma. *Medical Clinics of North America* 70: 1081–1092.

Jiang, Q., Jiang, X.H., Zheng, M.H., and Chen, Y.P. (2009). l-Ornithine-l-aspartate in the management of hepatic encephalopathy: a metaanalysis. *Journal of Gastroenterology and Hepatology* 24: 9–14.

Johnson, C.A., Armstrong, P.J., and Hauptman, J.G. (1987). Congenital portosystemic shunts in dogs: 46 cases (1979–1986). *Journal of the American Veterinary Medical Association* 191: 1478–1483.

Jones, E.A., Basile, A.S., Mullen, K.D., and Gammal, S.H. (1990). Flumazenil: potential implications for hepatic encephalopathy. *Pharmacology and Therapeutics* 45: 331–343.

Kamel, L., Saleh, A., Morsy, A. et al. (2007). Plasma met-enkephalin, beta-endorphin and leu-enkephalin levels in human hepatic encephalopathy. *East Mediterranean Health Journal* 13: 257–265.

Katayama, K. (2004). Ammonia metabolism and hepatic encephalopathy. *Hepatology Research* 30 S: 73–80.

Keiding, S., Sorensen, M., Munk, O.L., and Bender, D. (2010). Human (13) N-ammonia pet studies: the importance of measuring (13) N-ammonia metabolites in blood. *Metabolic Brain Disease* 25: 49–56.

Kelly, T., Kafitz, K.W., Roderigo, C., and Rose, C.R. (2009). Ammonium-evoked alterations in intracellular sodium and pH reduce glial glutamate transport activity. *Glia* 57: 921–934.

Kilpatrick, S., Gow, A.G., Foale, R.D. et al. (2014). Plasma cytokine concentrations in dogs with congenital portosystemic shunt. *Veterinary Journal* 200: 197–199.

Kircheis, G., Nilius, R., Held, C. et al. (1997). Therapeutic efficacy of l-ornithine-l-aspartate infusions in patients with cirrhosis and hepatic encephalopathy: results of a placebo-controlled, double-blind study. *Hepatology* 25: 1351–1360.

Knell, A.J., Davidson, A.R., Williams, R. et al. (1974). Dopamine and serotonin metabolism in hepatic encephalopathy. *British Medical Journal* 1: 549–551.

Knudsen, G.M., Schmidt, J., Almdal, T. et al. (1993). Passage of amino acids and glucose across the blood–brain barrier in patients with hepatic encephalopathy. *Hepatology* 17: 987–992.

Komtebedde, J., Forsyth, S.F., Breznock, E.M., and Koblik, P.D. (1991). Intrahepatic portosystemic venous anomaly in the dog. Perioperative management and complications. *Veterinary Surgery* 20: 37–42.

Komtebedde, J., Koblik, P.D., Breznock, E.M. et al. (1995). Long-term clinical outcome after partial ligation of single extrahepatic vascular anomalies in 20 dogs. *Veterinary Surgery* 24: 379–383.

Koyuncuoğlu, H., Keyer, M., Simşek, S., and Sağduyu, H. (1978). Ammonia intoxication: changes of brain levels of putative neurotransmitters and related compounds and its relevance to hepatic coma. *Pharmacological Research Communications* 10: 787–807.

Kromhout, J., McClain, C.J., Zieve, L. et al. (1980). Blood mercaptan and ammonia concentrations in cirrhotics after a protein load. *American Journal of Gastroenterology* 74: 507–511.

Kummeling, A., Van Sluijs, F.J., and Rothuizen, J. (2004). Prognostic implications of the degree of shunt narrowing and of the portal vein diameter in dogs with congenital portosystemic shunts. *Veterinary Surgery* 33: 17–24.

Kummeling, A., Vrakking, D.J., Rothuizen, J. et al. (2010). Hepatic volume measurements in dogs with extrahepatic congenital portosystemic shunts before and after surgical attenuation. *Journal of Veterinary Internal Medicine* 24: 114–119.

Kyles, A.E., Gregory, C.R., and Adin, C.A. (2004). Re-evaluation of a portocaval venograft without an ameroid constrictor as a method for controlling portal hypertension after occlusion of intrahepatic portocaval shunts in dogs. *Veterinary Surgery* 33: 691–698.

Kyles, A.E., Gregory, C.R., Jackson, J. et al. (2001). Evaluation of a portocaval venograft and ameroid ring for the occlusion of intrahepatic portocaval shunts in dogs. *Veterinary Surgery* 30: 161–169.

Kyles, A.E., Hardie, E.M., Mehl, M., and Gregory, C.R. (2002). Evaluation of ameroid ring constrictors for the management of single extrahepatic portosystemic shunts in cats: 23 cases (1996–2001). *Journal of the American Veterinary Medical Association* 220: 1341–1347.

Laccetti, M., Manes, G., Uomo, G. et al. (2000). Flumazenil in the treatment of acute hepatic encephalopathy in cirrhotic patients: a double blind randomized placebo controlled study. *Digestive and Liver Disease* 32: 335–338.

Laflamme, D.P., Allen, S.W., and Huber, T.L. (1993). Apparent dietary protein requirement of dogs with portosystemic shunt. *American Journal of Veterinary Research* 54: 719–723.

Laflamme, D.P., Allen, S.A., and Huber, T.L. (1994). Recent advances in dietary management of hepatic diseases. *Veterinary Quarterly* 16 (Suppl 1): 34 S–35 S.

Lamb, C.R., Forster van Hijfte, M.A., White, R.N. et al. (1996). Ultrasonographic diagnosis of congenital portosystemic shunt in 14 cats. *Journal of Small Animal Practice* 37: 205–209.

Lamb, C.R. and White, R.N. (1998). Morphology of congenital intra-hepatic portacaval shunts in dogs and cats. *Veterinary Record* 142: 55–60.

Landon, B.P., Abraham, L.A., and Charles, J.A. (2008). Use of transcolonic portal scintigraphy to evaluate efficacy of cellophane banding of congenital extrahepatic portosystemic shunts in 16 dogs. *Australian Veterinary Journal* 86: 169–179.

Lee, K.C., Lipscomb, V.J., Lamb, C.R. et al. (2006). Association of portovenographic findings with outcome in dogs receiving surgical treatment for single congenital portosystemic shunts: 45 cases (2000–2004). *Journal of the American Veterinary Medical Association* 229: 1122–1129.

Lemberg, A. and Fernandez, M.A. (2009). Hepatic encephalopathy, ammonia, glutamate, glutamine and oxidative stress. *Annals of Hepatology* 8: 95–102.

Leveille, R., Johnson, S.E., and Birchard, S.J. (2003). Transvenous coil embolization of portosystemic shunt in dogs. *Veterinary Radiology and Ultrasound* 44: 32–36.

Lidbury, J.A., Cook, A.K., and Steiner, J.M. (2016). Hepatic encephalopathy in dogs and cats. *Journal of Veterinary Emergency and Critical Care* 26: 471–487.

Lidbury, J.A., Ivanek, R., Suchodolski, J.S. et al. (2015). Putative precipitating factors for hepatic encephalopathy in dogs: 118 cases (1991–2014). *Journal of the American Veterinary Medical Association* 247: 176–183.

Lipscomb, V.J., Jones, H.J., and Brockman, D.J. (2007). Complications and long-term outcomes of the ligation of congenital portosystemic shunts in 49 cats. *Veterinary Record* 160: 465–470.

Lipscomb, V.J., Lee, K.C., Lamb, C.R., and Brockman, D.J. (2009). Association of mesenteric portovenographic findings with outcome in cats receiving surgical treatment for single congenital portosystemic shunts. *Journal of the American Veterinary Medical Association* 234: 221–228.

Liu, Q., Duan, Z.P., Ha, D.K. et al. (2004). Synbiotic modulation of gut flora: effect on minimal hepatic encephalopathy in patients with cirrhosis. *Hepatology* 39: 1441–1449.

Lockwood, A.H., Finn, R.D., Campbell, J.A., and Richman, T.B. (1980). Factors that affect the uptake of ammonia by the brain: the blood–brain pH gradient. *Brain Research* 181: 259–266.

Lockwood, A.H., McDonald, J.M., Reiman, R.E. et al. (1979). The dynamics of ammonia metabolism in man. Effects of liver disease and hyperammonemia. *Journal of Clinical Investigation* 63: 449–460.

Lowenstein, J.M. (1972). Ammonia production in muscle and other tissues: the purine nucleotide cycle. *Physiological Reviews* 52: 382–414.

Lozeva, V., Tuomisto, L., Sola, D. et al. (2001). Increased density of brain histamine H(1) receptors in rats with portacaval anastomosis and in cirrhotic patients with chronic hepatic encephalopathy. *Hepatology* 33: 1370–1376.

Lozeva, V., Tuomisto, L., Tarhanen, J., and Butterworth, R.F. (2003). Increased concentrations of histamine and its metabolite, tele-methylhistamine and down-regulation of histamine H3 receptor sites in autopsied brain tissue from cirrhotic patients who died in hepatic coma. *Journal of Hepatology* 39: 522–527.

Lux, H.D. and Loracher, C. (1970). Postsynaptic disinhibition by ammonium. *Naturwissenschaften* 57: 456–457.

Maddison, J.E. (1991). Canine congenital portosystemic encephalopathy: a spontaneous animal model of chronic hepatic encephalopathy. In: *Hepatic Encephalopathy and Metabolic Nitrogen Exchange* (ed. F. Bengtsson, B. Jeppsson, T. Almdal and H. Viistrup), 99–104. Boca Raton, FL: CRC Press.

Maddison, J.E. (1992). Hepatic encephalopathy. Current concepts of the pathogenesis. *Journal of Veterinary Internal Medicine* 6: 341–353.

Maddison, J.E., Yau, D., Stewart, P., and Farrell, G.C. (1986). Cerebrospinal fluid gamma-aminobutyric acid levels in dogs with chronic portosystemic encephalopathy. *Clinical Science* 71: 749–753.

Mai, W. (2009). Multiphase time-resolved contrast-enhanced portal MRA in normal dogs. *Veterinary Radiology and Ultrasound* 50: 52–57.

Mai, W. and Weisse, C. (2011). Contrast-enhanced portal magnetic resonance angiography in dogs with suspected congenital portal vascular anomalies. *Veterinary Radiology and Ultrasound* 52: 284–288.

Malaguarnera, M., Gargante, M.P., Malaguarnera, G. et al. (2010). *Bifidobacterium* combined with fructo-oligosaccharide versus lactulose in the treatment of patients with hepatic encephalopathy. *European Journal of Gastroenterology and Hepatology* 22: 199–206.

Malaguarnera, M., Pistone, G., Elvira, R. et al. (2005). Effects of l-carnitine in patients with hepatic encephalopathy. *World Journal of Gastroenterology* 11: 7197–7202.

Malaguarnera, M., Risino, C., Cammalleri, L. et al. (2009). Branched chain amino acids supplemented with l-acetylcarnitine versus BCAA treatment in hepatic coma: a randomized and controlled double blind study. *European Journal of Gastroenterology and Hepatology* 21: 762–770.

Mans, A.M., Biebuyck, J.F., Davis, D.W., and Hawkins, R.A. (1984). Portacaval anastomosis: brain and plasma metabolite abnormalities and the effect of nutritional therapy. *Journal of Neurochemistry* 43: 697–705.

Mans, A.M., Biebuyck, J.F., and Hawkins, R.A. (1983). Ammonia selectively stimulates neutral amino acid transport across blood–brain barrier. *American Journal of Physiology* 245: C74–C77.

Maqsood, S., Saleem, A. et al. (2006). Precipitating factors of hepatic encephalopathy: experience at Pakistan Institute of Medical Sciences Islamabad. *Journal of Ayub Medical College Abbottabad* 18: 58–62.

Marchesini, G., Fabbri, A., Bianchi, G. et al. (1996). Zinc supplementation and amino acid-nitrogen metabolism in patients with advanced cirrhosis. *Hepatology* 23: 1084–1092.

Marchesini, G., Zoli, M., and Forlani, G. (1979). The role of insulin and glucagon in the plasma aminoacid imbalance of chronic hepatic encephalopathy. *Zeitschrift fur Gastroenterologie* 17: 469–476.

Matiasovic, M., Chanoit, G.P.A., Meakin, L.B., and Tivers, M.S. (2020). Outcomes of dogs treated for extrahepatic congenital portosystemic shunts with thin film banding or ameroid ring constrictor. *Veterinary Surgery* 49: 160–171.

Matushek, K.J., Bjorling, D., and Mathews, K. (1990). Generalized motor seizures after portosystemic shunt ligation in dogs: five cases (1981–1988). *Journal of the American Veterinary Medical Association* 196: 2014–2017.

McAlinden, A.B., Buckley, C.T., and Kirby, B.M. (2010). Biomechanical evaluation of different numbers, sizes and placement configurations of ligaclips required to secure cellophane bands. *Veterinary Surgery* 39: 59–64.

Medina, J.H., Peña, C., Levi de Stein, M. et al. (1989). Benzodiazepine-like molecules, as well as other ligands for the brain benzodiazepine receptors, are relatively common constituents of plants. *Biochemical and Biophysical Research Communications* 165: 547–553.

Mehl, M.L., Kyles, A.E., Case, J.B. et al. (2007). Surgical management of left-divisional intrahepatic portosystemic shunts: outcome after partial ligation of, or ameroid ring constrictor placement on, the left hepatic vein in twenty-eight dogs (1995–2005). *Veterinary Surgery* 36: 21–30.

Mehl, M.L., Kyles, A.E., Hardie, E.M. et al. (2005). Evaluation of ameroid ring constrictors for treatment for single extrahepatic portosystemic shunts in dogs: 168 cases (1995–2001). *Journal of the American Veterinary Medical Association* 226: 2020–2030.

Meier, P.J. and Bansky, G. (1990). Current possibilities in the therapy of hepatic encephalopathy. *Schweizerische Medizinische Wochenschrift* 120: 553–556.

Meyer, H.P., Legemate, D.A., van den Brom, W., and Rothuizen, J. (1998). Improvement of chronic hepatic encephalopathy in dogs by the benzodiazepine-receptor partial inverse agonist sarmazenil, but not by the antagonist flumazenil. *Metabolic Brain Disease* 13: 241–251.

Meyer, H.P. and Rothuizen, J. (1992). Management of hepatic encephalopathy (HE) in companion animal medicine. *Tijdschrift voor Diergeneeskunde* 117 (Suppl 1): 14S–15S.

Meyer, H.P., Rothuizen, J., van Sluijs, F.J. et al. (1999). Progressive remission of portosystemic shunting in 23 dogs after partial closure of congenital portosystemic shunts. *Veterinary Record* 144: 333–337.

Michel, K.E. (1995). Nutritional management of liver disease. *Veterinary Clinics of North America Small Animal Practice* 25: 485–501.

Möhler, H., Polc, P., Cumin, R. et al. (1979). Nicotinamide is a brain constituent with benzodiazepine-like actions. *Nature* 278: 563–565.

Monfort, P., Munoz, M.D., ElAyadi, A. et al. (2002). Effects of hyperammonemia and liver failure on glutamatergic neurotransmission. *Metabolic Brain Disease* 17: 237–250.

Monnet, E. and Rosenberg, A. (2005). Effect of protein concentration on rate of closure of ameroid constrictors in vitro. *American Journal of Veterinary Research* 66: 1337–1340.

Morandi, F., Cole, R.C., Tobias, K.M. et al. (2005). Use of $^{99m}TcO_4$-trans-splenic portal scintigraphy for diagnosis of portosystemic shunts in 28 dogs. *Veterinary Radiology and Ultrasound* 46: 153–161.

Morandi, F., Sura, P.A., Sharp, D., and Daniel, G.B. (2010). Characterization of multiple acquired portosystemic shunts using transplenic portal scintigraphy. *Veterinary Radiology and Ultrasound* 51: 466–471.

Morris, J.G. and Rogers, Q.R. (1978). Arginine: an essential amino acid for the cat. *Journal of Nutrition* 108: 1944–1953.

Mullen, K.D. and Howard, R. (2005). Is acarbose an effective drug for treating patients with cirrhosis and hepatic encephalopathy? *Nature Clinical Practice Gastroenterology and Hepatology* 2: 264–265.

Mullins, R.A., Escribano, C.A., Anderson, D.M. et al. (2022). Postattenuation neurologic signs after surgical attenuation of congenital portosystemic shunts in dogs: a review. *Veterinary Surgery* 51: 23–33.

Mullins, R.A., Sanchez, V.C., de Rooster, H. et al. (2019). Effect of prophylactic treatment with levetiracetam on the incidence of postattenuation seizures in dogs undergoing surgical management of single congenital extrahepatic portosystemic shunts. *Veterinary Surgery* 48: 164–172.

Mullins, R.A., Sanchez, V.C., Selmic, L.E. et al. (2020). Prognostic factors for short-term survival of dogs that experience postattenuation seizures after surgical correction of single congenital extrahepatic portosystemic shunts: 93 cases (2005–2018). *Veterinary Surgery* 49: 958–970.

Mumtaz, K., Ahmed, U.S., Abid, S. et al. (2010). Precipitating factors and the outcome of hepatic encephalopathy in liver cirrhosis. *Journal of the College of Physicians and Surgeons Pakistan* 20: 514–518.

Murphy, S.T., Ellison, G.W., Long, M., and Van Gilder, J. (2001). A comparison of the ameroid constrictor versus ligation in the surgical management of single extrahepatic portosystemic shunts. *Journal of the American Animal Hospital Association* 37: 390–396.

Nagasue, N., Kanashima, R., and Inokuchi, K. (1981). Alteration in plasma amino acid concentrations following subtotal hepatectomy in dogs. *Annales Chirurgiae et Gynaecologiae* 70: 50–55.

Neary, J.T., Norenberg, L.O., Gutierrez, M.P., and Norenberg, M.D. (1987). Hyperammonemia causes altered protein phosphorylation in astrocytes. *Brain Research* 437: 161–164.

Nelson, N.C. and Nelson, L.L. (2011). Anatomy of extrahepatic portosystemic shunts in dogs as determined by computed tomography angiography. *Veterinary Radiology and Ultrasound* 52: 498–506.

Niles, J.D., Williams, J.M., and Cripps, P.J. (2001). Hemostatic profiles in 39 dogs with congenital portosystemic shunts. *Veterinary Surgery* 30: 97–104.

Norenberg, M.D., Huo, Z., Neary, J.T., and Roig-Cantesano, A. (1997). The glial glutamate transporter in hyperammonemia and hepatic encephalopathy: relation to energy metabolism and glutamatergic neurotransmission. *Glia* 21: 124–133.

Norenberg, M.D., Jayakumar, A.R., Rama Rao, K.V., and Panickar, K.S. (2007). New concepts in the mechanism of ammonia-induced astrocyte swelling. *Metabolic Brain Disease* 22: 219–234.

O'Connor, J.E. and Costell, M. (1990). New roles of carnitine metabolism in ammonia cytotoxicity. *Advances in Experimental Medicine and Biology* 272: 183–195.

Ono, J., Hutson, D.G., Dombro, R.S. et al. (1978). Tryptophan and hepatic coma. *Gastroenterology* 74: 196–200.

Onstad, G.R. and Zieve, L. (1979). What determines blood ammonia? *Gastroenterology* 77: 803–805.

Otomo, A., Singh, A., Jeong, J. et al. (2020). Long-term clinical outcomes of dogs with single congenital extrahepatic portosystemic shunts attenuated with thin film banding or ameroid ring constrictors. *Veterinary Surgery* 49: 436–444.

Ott, P., Clemmesen, O., and Larsen, F.S. (2005). Cerebral metabolic disturbances in the brain during acute liver failure: from hyperammonemia to energy failure and proteolysis. *Neurochemistry International* 47: 13–18.

Papazoglou, L.G., Monnet, E., and Seim, H.B. III (2002). Survival and prognostic indicators for dogs with intrahepatic portosystemic shunts: 32 cases (1990–2000). *Veterinary Surgery* 31: 561–570.

Pappas, S.C., Ferenci, P., Schafer, D.F., and Jones, E.A. (1984). Visual evoked potentials in a rabbit model of hepatic encephalopathy. II. Comparison of hyperammonemic encephalopathy, postictal coma, and coma induced by synergistic neurotoxins. *Gastroenterology* 86: 546–551.

Park, S.C., Griffith, B.P., Siewers, R.D. et al. (1985). A percutaneously adjustable device for banding of the pulmonary trunk. *International Journal of Cardiology* 9: 477–484.

Parker, J.S., Monnet, E., Powers, B.E., and Twedt, D.C. (2008). Histologic examination of hepatic biopsy samples as a prognostic indicator in dogs undergoing surgical correction of congenital portosystemic shunts: 64 cases (1997–2005). *Journal of the American Veterinary Medical Association* 232: 1511–1514.

Payne, J.T., Martin, R.A., and Constantinescu, G.M. (1990). The anatomy and embryology of portosystemic shunts in dogs and cats. *Seminars in Veterinary Medicine and Surgery (Small Animal)* 5: 76–82.

Payne, J.T., Martin, R.A., Moon, M.L. et al. (1991). Effect of left hepatic vein ligation on hepatic circulation, function, and microanatomy in dogs. *American Journal of Veterinary Research* 52: 774–780.

Peacock, J.T., Fossum, T.W., Bahr, A.M. et al. (2003). Evaluation of gradual occlusion of the caudal vena cava in clinically normal dogs. *American Journal of Veterinary Research* 64: 1347–1353.

Pereg, D., Kotliroff, A., Gadoth, N. et al. (2011). Probiotics for patients with compensated liver cirrhosis: a double-blind placebo-controlled study. *Nutrition* 27: 177–181.

Phear, E.A., Ruebner, B., Sherlock, S., and Summerskill, W.H. (1956). Methionine toxicity in liver disease and its prevention by chlortetracycline. *Clinical Science* 15: 93–117.

Phongsamran, P.V., Kim, J.W., Cupo Abbott, J., and Rosenblatt, A. (2010). Pharmacotherapy for hepatic encephalopathy. *Drugs* 70: 1131–1148.

Pilbeam, C.M., Anderson, R.M., and Bhathal, P.S. (1983a). The brain in experimental portal–systemic encephalopathy. I. Morphological changes in three animal models. *Journal of Pathology* 140: 331–345.

Pilbeam, C.M., Anderson, R.M., and Bhathal, P.S. (1983b). The brain in experimental portal-systemic encephalopathy. II. Water and electrolyte changes. *Journal of Pathology* 140: 347–355.

Plested, M.J., Zwingenberger, A.L., Brockman, D.J. et al. (2020). Canine intrahepatic portosystemic shunt insertion into the systemic circulation is commonly through primary hepatic veins as assessed with CT angiography. *Veterinary Radiology & Ultrasound* 61: 519–530.

Poggi, E., Rubio, D.G., Perez Duarte, F.J. et al. (2022). Laparoscopic portosystemic shunt attenuation in 20 dogs (2018–2021). *Veterinary Surgery* 1: 1–12.

Poo, J.L., Gongora, J., Sanchez-Avila, F. et al. (2006). Efficacy of oral l-ornithine-l-aspartate in cirrhotic patients with hyperammonemic hepatic encephalopathy. Results of a randomized, lactulosec-ontrolled study. *Annals of Hepatology* 5: 281–288.

Proot, S., Biourge, V., Teske, E., and Rothuizen, J. (2009). Soy protein isolate versus meat-based low-protein diet for dogs with congenital portosystemic shunts. *Journal of Veterinary Internal Medicine* 23: 794–800.

Raabe, W. (1981). Ammonia and disinhibition in cat motor cortex by ammonium acetate, monofluoroacetate and insulin-induced hypoglycemia. *Brain Research* 210: 311–322.

Raabe, W. (1987). Synaptic transmission in ammonia intoxication. *Neurochemical Pathology* 6: 145–166.

Raabe, W. and Gumnit, R.J. (1975). Disinhibition in cat motor cortex by ammonia. *Journal of Neurophysiology* 38: 347–355.

Raabe, W. and Lin, S. (1983). Ammonia intoxication and hyperpolarizing postsynaptic inhibition. *Experimental Neurology* 82: 711–715.

Raabe, W. and Onstad, G. (1985). Porta-caval shunting changes neuronal sensitivity to ammonia. *Journal of the Neurological Sciences* 71: 307–314.

Rabinowitz, J.L., Ostermann, L. Jr., Bora, F.W., and Staeffen, J. (1983). Lipid composition and de novo lipid biosynthesis of human palmar fat in Dupuytren's disease. *Lipids* 18: 371–374.

Rabinowitz, J.L., Staeffen, J., Hall, C.L., and Brand, J.G. (1991). A probable defect in the beta-oxidation of lipids in rats fed alcohol for 6 months. *Alcohol* 8: 241–246.

Rama Rao, K.V. and Norenberg, M.D. (2007). Aquaporin-4 in hepatic encephalopathy. *Metabolic Brain Disease* 22: 265–275.

Rama Rao, K.V., Chen, M., Simard, J.M., and Norenberg, M.D. (2003). Increased aquaporin-4 expression in ammonia-treated cultured astrocytes. *Neuroreport* 14: 2379–2382.

Rama Rao, K.V., Reddy, P.V., Hazell, A.S., and Norenberg, M.D. (2007). Manganese induces cell swelling in cultured astrocytes. *Neurotoxicology* 28: 807–812.

Rao, K.V. and Norenberg, M.D. (2001). Cerebral energy metabolism in hepatic encephalopathy and hyperammonemia. *Metabolic Brain Disease* 16: 67–78.

Rao, K.V. and Norenberg, M.D. (2004). Manganese induces the mitochondrial permeability transition in cultured astrocytes. *Journal of Biological Chemistry* 279: 32333–32338.

Rao, K.V., Panickar, K.S., Jayakumar, A.R., and Norenberg, M.D. (2005). Astrocytes protect neurons from ammonia toxicity. *Neurochemical Research* 30: 1311–1318.

Rao, V.L., Audet, R.M., and Butterworth, R.F. (1995). Selective alterations of extracellular brain amino acids in relation to function in experimental portal-systemic encephalopathy: results of an in vivo microdialysis study. *Journal of Neurochemistry* 65: 1221–1228.

Record, C.O., Buxton, B., Chase, R.A. et al. (1976). Plasma and brain amino acids in fulminant hepatic failure and their relationship to hepatic encephalopathy. *European Journal of Clinical Investigation* 6: 387–394.

Rose, C. (2002). Increased extracellular brain glutamate in acute liver failure: decreased uptake or increased release? *Metabolic Brain Disease* 17: 251–261.

Rose, C., Kresse, W., and Kettenmann, H. (2005). Acute insult of ammonia leads to calcium-dependent glutamate release from cultured astrocytes, an effect of pH. *Journal of Biological Chemistry* 280: 20937–20944.

Rossi-Fanelli, F., Freund, H., Krause, R. et al. (1982). Induction of coma in normal dogs by the infusion of aromatic amino acids and its prevention by the addition of branched-chain amino acids. *Gastroenterology* 83: 664–671.

Rothuizen, J., Bunch, B.L., Charles, J.A. et al. (2006). *WSAVA Standards for Clinical and Histological Diagnosis of Canine and Feline Liver Disease*, 41–59. New York: Saunders Elsevier.

Rovira, A., Alonso, J., and Córdoba, J. (2008). MR imaging findings in hepatic encephalopathy. *American Journal of Neuroradiology* 29: 1612–1621.

Rozga, J. (2001). Animal models of liver regeneration. In: *Surgical Research* (ed. W. Souba and D. Wilmore), 703–709. San Diego, CA: Academic Press.

Rozga, J., Jeppsson, B., and Bengmark, S. (1986a). Hepatotrophic effect of portal blood during hepatic arterial recirculation. *European Surgical Research* 18: 302–311.

Rozga, J., Jeppsson, B., and Bengmark, S. (1986b). Portal branch ligation in the rat. Reevaluation of a model. *American Journal of Pathology* 125: 300–308.

Saleem, D.M., Haider, S., Khan, M.M. et al. (2008). Role of tryptophan in the pathogenesis of hepatic encephalopathy. *Journal of the Pakistan Medical Association* 58: 68–70.

Sangameswaran, L., Fales, H.M., Friedrich, P., and De Blas, A.L. (1986). Purification of a benzodiazepine from bovine brain and detection of benzodiazepine-like immunoreactivity in human brain. *Proceedings of the National Academy of Sciences USA* 83: 9236–9240.

Schäfer, K., Ukida, M., Steffen, C. et al. (1985). Effect of ammonia on plasma and cerebrospinal fluid amino acids in dogs with and without portacaval anastomoses. *Research in Experimental Medicine* 185: 35–44.

Schenker, S., McCandless, D.W., Brophy, E., and Lewis, M.S. (1967). Studies on the intracerebral toxicity of ammonia. *Journal of Clinical Investigation* 46: 838–848.

Schermerhorn, T., Center, S.A., Dykes, N.L. et al. (1996). Characterization of hepatoportal microvascular dysplasia in a kindred of cairn terriers. *Journal of Veterinary Internal Medicine* 10: 219–230.

Schliess, F., Görg, B., and Häussinger, D. (2009). RNA oxidation and zinc in hepatic encephalopathy and hyperammonemia. *Metabolic Brain Disease* 24: 119–134.

Schmid, M., Peck-Radosavljevic, M., König, F. et al. (2010). A double-blind, randomized, placebo-controlled trial of intravenous l-ornithine-l-aspartate on postural control in patients with cirrhosis. *Liver International* 30: 574–582.

Schwarz, T., Rossi, F., Wray, J.D. et al. (2009). Computed tomographic and magnetic resonance imaging features of canine segmental caudal vena cava aplasia. *Journal of Small Animal Practice* 50: 341–349.

Seguin, B., Tobias, K.M., Gavin, P.R., and Tucker, R.L. (1999). Use of magnetic resonance angiography for diagnosis of portosystemic shunts in dogs. *Veterinary Radiology and Ultrasound* 40: 251–258.

Sereda, C.W., Adin, C.A., Batich, C.D. et al. (2006). Evaluation of manufacturing variability, diffusion of filling solutions, and long-term maintenance of occlusion in silicone hydraulic occluders. *American Journal of Veterinary Research* 67: 1453–1458.

Sereda, C.W., Adin, C.A., Ginn, P.E., and Farese, J.P. (2005). Evaluation of a percutaneously controlled hydraulic occluder in a rat model of gradual venous occlusion. *Veterinary Surgery* 34: 35–42.

Serrano, G., Charalambous, M., Devriendt, N. et al. (2019). Treatment of congenital extrahepatic portosystemic shunts in dogs: a systematic review and meta-analysis. *Journal of Veterinary Internal Medicine* 33: 1865–1879.

Sharma, P., Sharma, B.C., Puri, V., and Sarin, S.K. (2008). An open-label randomized controlled trial of lactulose and probiotics in the treatment of minimal hepatic encephalopathy. *European Journal of Gastroenterology and Hepatology* 20: 506–511.

Sharma, P., Sharma, B.C., and Sarin, S.K. (2010). Predictors of nonresponse to lactulose in patients with cirrhosis and hepatic encephalopathy. *European Journal of Gastroenterology and Hepatology* 22: 526–531.

Sheth, A.A. and Garcia-Tsao, G. (2008). Probiotics and liver disease. *Journal of Clinical Gastroenterology* 42 (Suppl 2): S80–S84.

Shih, V.E. (1976). Congenital hyperammonemic syndromes. *Clinics in Perinatology* 3: 3–14.

Shores, N.J. and Keeffe, E.B. (2008). Is oral l-acyl-carnitine an effective therapy for hepatic encephalopathy? Review of the literature. *Digestive Diseases and Sciences* 53: 2330–2333.

Siciliano, M., Annicchiarico, B.E., Lucchese, F., and Bombardieri, G. (2006). Effects of a single, short intravenous dose of acetyl-l-carnitine on pattern-reversal visual-evoked potentials in cirrhotic patients with hepatic encephalopathy. *Clinical and Experimental Pharmacology and Physiology* 33: 76–80.

Simert, G., Mobin, A., Rosengren, E., and Vang, J. (1978). Neurotransmittor changes in the rat brain after portacaval anastomosis. *European Surgical Research* 10: 73–85.

Smith, B. and Prockop, D.J. (1962). Central-nervous-system effects of ingestin of l-tryptophan by normal subjects. *New England Journal of Medicine* 267: 1338–1341.

Smith, K.R., Bauer, M., and Monnet, E. (1995). Portosystemic communications: follow-up of 32 cases. *Journal of Small Animal Practice* 36: 435–440.

Soarez, P.C., Oliveira, A.C., Padovan, J. et al. (2009). A critical analysis of studies assessing l-ornithine-l-aspartate (LOLA) in hepatic encephalopathy treatment. *Arquivos de Gastroenterologia* 46: 241–247.

Soeters, P.B. and Fischer, J.E. (1976). Insulin, glucagon, aminoacid imbalance, and hepatic encephalopathy. *Lancet* ii: 880–882.

Sorensen, M. and Keiding, S. (2007). New findings on cerebral ammonia uptake in HE using functional (13)N-ammonia PET. *Metabolic Brain Disease* 22: 277–284.

Specchi, S., Rossi, F., Weisse, C. et al. (2018). Canine and feline abdominal arterioportal communications can be classified based on branching patterns in computed tomographic angiography. *Veterinary Radiology and Ultrasound* 59: 687–696.

Stewart, C.A. and Vella, A. (2005). Acarbose treatment in liver disease: cognitive or glycemic control? *Clinical Gastroenterology and Hepatology* 3: 108–109.

Stewart, P.M., Batshaw, M., Valle, D., and Walser, M. (1981). Effects of arginine-free meals on ureagenesis in cats. *American Journal of Physiology* 241: E310–E315.

Suarez, I., Bodega, G., and Fernández, B. (2002). Glutamine synthetase in brain: effect of ammonia. *Neurochemistry International* 41 (2–3): 123–142.

Sura, P.A., Tobias, K.M., Morandi, F. et al. (2007). Comparison of $^{99m}TcO_4(-)$ trans-splenic portal scintigraphy with per-rectal portal scintigraphy for diagnosis of portosystemic shunts in dogs. *Veterinary Surgery* 36: 654–660.

Swalec, K.M. and Smeak, D.D. (1990). Partial versus complete attenuation of single portosystemic shunts. *Veterinary Surgery* 19: 406–411.

Swart, G.R. and Van den Berg, J.W.O. (1991). Protein turnover in liver disease. In: *Hepatic Encephalopathy and Metabolic Nitrogen Exchange* (ed. F. Bengtsson, B. Jeppsson, T. Almdal and H. Viistrup), 445–455. Boca Raton, FL: CRC Press.

Swennen, K., Courtin, C.M., and Delcour, J.A. (2006). Non-digestible oligosaccharides with prebiotic properties. *Critical Reviews in Food Science and Nutrition* 46: 459–471.

Szatmari, V., van Sluijs, F.J., Rothuizen, J., and Voorhout, G. (2004). Ultrasonographic assessment of hemodynamic changes in the portal vein during surgical attenuation of congenital extrahepatic portosystemic shunts in dogs. *Journal of the American Veterinary Medical Association* 224: 395–402.

Takuma, Y., Nouso, K., Makino, Y. et al. (2010). Clinical trial: oral zinc in hepatic encephalopathy. *Alimentary Pharmacology and Therapeutics* 32: 1080–1090.

Tarter, R.E., Hegedus, A.M., and Van Thiel, D.H. (1984). Neuropsychiatric sequelae of portal–systemic encephalopathy: a review. *International Journal of Neuroscience* 24: 203–216.

Theoret, Y. and Bossu, J.L. (1985). Effects of ammonium salts on synaptic transmission to hippocampal CA1 and CA3 pyramidal cells in vivo. *Neuroscience* 14: 807–821.

Therrien, G., Rose, C., Butterworth, J., and Butterworth, R.F. (1997). Protective effect of l-carnitine in ammonia-precipitated encephalopathy in the portacaval shunted rat. *Hepatology* 25: 551–556.

Thompson, J.S., Schafer, D.F., Haun, J., and Schafer, G.J. (1986). Adequate diet prevents hepatic coma in dogs with Eck fistulas. *Surgery, Gynecology and Obstetrics* 162: 126–130.

Tisdall, P.L., Hunt, G.B., Bellenger, C.R., and Malik, R. (1994). Congenital portosystemic shunts in Maltese and Australian cattle dogs. *Australian Veterinary Journal* 71: 174–178.

Tisdall, P.L., Hunt, G.B., Tsoukalas, G., and Malik, R. (1995). Postprandial serum bile acid concentrations and ammonia tolerance in Maltese dogs with and without hepatic vascular anomalies. *Australian Veterinary Journal* 72: 121–126.

Tisdall, P.L., Hunt, G.B., Youmans, K.R., and Malik, R. (2000). Neurological dysfunction in dogs following attenuation of congenital extrahepatic portosystemic shunts. *Journal of Small Animal Practice* 41: 539–546.

Tivers, M.S., Handel, I., Gow, A.G. et al. (2014). Hyperammoniemia and systemic inflammatory response syndrome predicts presence of hepatic encephalopathy in dogs with congenital portosystemic shunts. *PLOS ONE* 9: e82303.

Tivers, M.S., Handel, I., Gow, A.G. et al. (2015). Attenuation of congenital portosystemic shunt reduces inflammation in dogs. *PLOS ONE* 10: e0117557.

Tobias, K.M., Byarlay, J.M., and Henry, R.W. (2004). A new dissection technique for approach to right-sided intrahepatic portosystemic shunts: anatomic study and use in three dogs. *Veterinary Surgery* 33: 32–39.

Tobias, K.M. and Rawlings, C.A. (1996). Surgical techniques for extravascular occlusion of intrahepatic shunts. *Compendium on Continuing Education for the Practicing Veterinarian* 18: 745–755.

Tobias, K.M. and Rohrbach, B.W. (2003). Association of breed with the diagnosis of congenital portosystemic shunts in dogs: 2,400 cases (1980–2002). *Journal of the American Veterinary Medical Association* 223: 1636–1639.

Tobias, K.S., Barbee, D., and Pluhar, G.E. (1996). Intraoperative use of subtraction angiography and an ultrasonic aspirator to improve identification and isolation of an intrahepatic portosystemic shunt in a dog. *Journal of the American Veterinary Medical Association* 208: 888–890.

Toulza, O., Center, S.A., Brooks, M.B. et al. (2006). Evaluation of plasma protein C activity for detection of hepatobiliary disease and portosystemic shunting in dogs. *Journal of the American Veterinary Medical Association* 229: 1761–1771.

Unseld, E., Krishna, D.R., Fischer, C., and Klotz, U. (1989). Detection of desmethyldiazepam and diazepam in brain of different species and plants. *Biochemical Pharmacology* 38: 2473–2478.

van den Ingh, T.S.G.A.M., Rothuizen, J., and Meyer, H.P. (1995). Portal hypertension associated with primary hypoplasia of the hepatic portal vein in dogs. *Veterinary Record* 137: 424–427.

van Leeuwen, P., van der Bofaard, E., Janssen, E. et al. (1984). Ammonia production and glutamine metabolism in the small and large intestine of the rat and the influence of lactulose and neomycin. In: *Advances in Hepatic Encephalopathy and Urea Cycle Diseases* (ed. G. Kleinberger), 154–162. Basel: Karger.

van Steenbeek, F.G., Leegwater, P.A., van Sluijs, F.J. et al. (2009). Evidence of inheritance of intrahepatic portosystemic shunts in Irish wolfhounds. *Journal of Veterinary Internal Medicine* 23: 950–952.

van Straten, G., Spee, B., Rothuizen, J. et al. (2015). Diagnostic value of the rectal ammonia tolerance test, fasting plasma ammonia and fasting plasma bile acids for canine portosystemic shunting. *Veterinary Journal* 204: 282–286.

Van Vechten, B.J., Komtebedde, J., and Koblok, P.D. (1994). Use of transcolonic portal scintigraphy to monitor blood flow and progressive postoperative attenuation of partially ligated single extrahepatic portosystemic shunts in dogs. *Journal of the American Veterinary Medical Association* 204: 1770–1774.

Vaquero, J., Chung, C., and Blei, A.T. (2003). Brain edema in acute liver failure. A window to the pathogenesis of hepatic encephalopathy. *Annals of Hepatology* 2: 12–22.

Vogt, J.C., Krahwinkel, D.J. Jr., Bright, R.M. et al. (1996). Gradual occlusion of extrahepatic portosystemic shunts in dogs and cats using the ameroid constrictor. *Veterinary Surgery* 25: 495–502.

Walker, C.O. and Schenker, S. (1970). Pathogenesis of hepatic encephalopathy: with special reference to the role of ammonia. *American Journal of Clinical Nutrition* 23: 619–632.

Walker, M.C., Hill, R.C., Guilford, W.G. et al. (2001). Postprandial venous ammonia concentrations in the diagnosis of hepatobiliary disease in dogs. *Journal of Veterinary Internal Medicine* 15: 463–466.

Wallace, M.L., Ellison, G.W., Giglio, R.F. et al. (2016). Assessment of the attenuation of an intra-abdominal vein by use of a silicone-polyacrylic acid gradual venous occlusion device in dogs and cats. *American Journal of Veterinary Research* 77: 653–657.

Wallace, M.L., Ellison, G.W., Giglio, R.F. et al. (2018a). Gradual attenuation of a congenital extrahepatic portosystemic shunt with a self-retaining polyacrylic acid-silicone device in 6 dogs. *Veterinary Surgery* 47: 722–728.

Wallace, M.L., Grimes, J.A., Edwards, L. et al. (2022). Dogs >/= five years of age at the time of congenital extrahepatic portosystemic shunt diagnosis have better long-term outcomes with surgical attenuation than with medical management alone. *Journal of the American Veterinary Medical Association* 260: 758–764.

Wallace, M.L., MacPhail, C.M., and Monnet, E. (2018b). Incidence of postoperative neurologic complications in pugs following portosystemic shunt attenuation surgery. *Journal of the American Animal Hospital Association* 54: 46–49.

Watanabe, A., Takei, N., Higashi, T. et al. (1984). Glutamic acid and glutamine levels in serum and cerebrospinal fluid in hepatic encephalopathy. *Biochemical Medicine* 32: 225–231.

Watson, P.J. and Herrtage, M.E. (1998). Medical management of congenital portosystemic shunts in 27 dogs: retrospective study. *Journal of Small Animal Practice* 39: 62–68.

Weber, F.L. Jr., Minco, D., Fresard, K.M., and Banwell, J.G. (1985). Effects of vegetable diets on nitrogen metabolism in cirrhotic subjects. *Gastroenterology* 89: 538–544.

Weisse, C., Mondschein, J.I., Itkin, M. et al. (2005). Use of a percutaneous atrial septal occluder device for complete acute occlusion of an intrahepatic portosystemic shunt in a dog. *Journal of the American Veterinary Medical Association* 227 (249–252): 236.

Weisse, C., Schwartz, K., Stronger, R. et al. (2002). Transjugular coil embolization of an intrahepatic portosystemic shunt in a cat. *Journal of the American Veterinary Medical Association* 221 (1287–1291): 1266–1267.

Weisse, C., Solomon, J.A., Berent, A. et al. (2006). Percutaneous transvenous coil embolization (PTCE) of canine intrahepatic shunts: experience in 33 dogs. *Journal of Veterinary Internal Medicine* 20: 753.

White, R.N., Burton, C.A., and McEvoy, F.J. (1998). Surgical treatment of intrahepatic portosystemic shunts in 45 dogs. *Veterinary Record* 142: 358–365.

Wildmann, J., Möhler, H., Vetter, W. et al. (1987). Diazepam and N-desmethyldiazepam are found in rat brain and adrenal and may be of plant origin. *Journal of Neural Transmission* 70: 383–398.

Wildmann, J., Niemann, J., and Matthaei, H. (1986). Endogenous benzodiazepine receptor agonist in human and mammalian plasma. *Journal of Neural Transmission* 66: 151–160.

Wiles, C.E. Jr., Schenk, W.G. Jr., and Lindenberg, J. (1952). The experimental production of portal hypertension. *Annals of Surgery* 136: 811–817.

Windsor, R.C. and Olby, N.J. (2007). Congenital portosystemic shunts in five mature dogs with neurological signs. *Journal of the American Animal Hospital Association* 43: 322–331.

Windus-Podehl, G., Lyftogt, C., Zieve, L., and Brunner, G. (1983). Encephalopathic effect of phenol in rats. *Journal of Laboratory and Clinical Medicine* 101: 586–592.

Winkler, J.T., Bohling, M.W., Tillson, D.M. et al. (2003). Portosystemic shunts: diagnosis, prognosis, and treatment of 64 cases (1993–2001). *Journal of the American Animal Hospital Association* 39: 169–185.

Wolpert, E., Phillips, S.F., and Summerskill, W.H. (1971). Transport of urea and ammonia production in the human colon. *Lancet* ii: 1387–1390.

Wolschrijn, C.F., Mahapokai, W., Rothuizen, J. et al. (2000). Gauged attenutation of congenital portosystemic shunts: results in 160 dogs and 15 cats. *Veterinary Quarterly* 22: 94–98.

Worley, D.R. and Holt, D.E. (2008). Clinical outcome of congenital extrahepatic portosystemic shunt attenuation in dogs aged five years and older: 17 cases (1992–2005). *Journal of the American Veterinary Medical Association* 232: 722–727.

Wrigley, R.H., Macy, D.W., and Wykes, P.M. (1983). Ligation of ductus venosus in a dog, using ultrasonographic guidance. *Journal of the American Veterinary Medical Association* 183: 1461–1464.

Wrigley, R.H., Park, R.D., Konde, L.J., and Lebel, J.L. (1987). Subtraction portal venography. *Veterinary Radiology* 28: 208–212.

Youmans, K.R. and Hunt, G.B. (1998). Cellophane banding for the gradual attenuation of single extrahepatic portosystemic shunts in eleven dogs. *Australian Veterinary Journal* 76: 531–537.

Youmans, K.R. and Hunt, G.B. (1999). Experimental evaluation of four methods of progressive venous attenuation in dogs. *Veterinary Surgery* 28: 38–47.

Yurdaydin, C., Karavelioglu, D., Onaran, O. et al. (1998). Opioid receptor ligands in human hepatic encephalopathy. *Journal of Hepatology* 29: 796–801.

Yurdaydin, C., Li, Y., Ha, J.H. et al. (1995). Brain and plasma levels of opioid peptides are altered in rats with thioacetamide-induced fulminant hepatic failure: implications for the treatment of hepatic encephalopathy with opioid antagonists. *Journal of Pharmacology and Experimental Therapeutics* 273: 185–192.

Zauner, A., Bullock, R., Di, X., and Young, H.F. (1995). Brain oxygen, CO_2, pH, and temperature monitoring: evaluation in the feline brain. *Neurosurgery* 37: 1168–1176.

Zieve, F.J., Zieve, L., Doizaki, W.M., and Gilsdorf, R.B. (1974a). Synergism between ammonia and fatty acids in the production of coma: implications for hepatic coma. *Journal of Pharmacology and Experimental Therapeutics* 191: 10–16.

Zieve, L. (1979a). Amino acids in liver failure. *Gastroenterology* 76: 219–221.

Zieve, L. (1979b). Hepatic encephalopathy summary of present knowledge with an elaboration on recent developments. *Progress in Liver Disease* 6: 327–341.

Zieve, L. (1981). The mechanism of hepatic coma. *Hepatology* 1: 360–365.

Zieve, L. (1986). Conditional deficiencies of ornithine or arginine. *Journal of the American College of Nutrition* 5: 167–176.

Zieve, L., Doizaki, W.M., and Zieve, J. (1974b). Synergism between mercaptans and ammonia or fatty acids in the production of coma: a possible role for mercaptans in the pathogenesis of hepatic coma. *Journal of Laboratory and Clinical Medicine* 83: 16–28.

Zieve, L. and Olsen, R.L. (1977). Can hepatic coma be caused by a reduction of brain noradrenaline or dopamine? *Gut* 18: 688–691.

Zwingenberger, A. (2009). CT Diagnosis of portosystemic shunts. *Veterinary Clinics of North America. Small Animal Practice* 39: 783–792.

Zwingenberger, A., McLear, R., and Wiesse, C. (2005a). Diagnosis of arterioportal fistulae in four dogs using computed tomographic angiography. *Veterinary Radiology and Ultrasound* 46: 472–477.

Zwingenberger, A.L., Schwarz, T., and Saunders, H.M. (2005b). Helical computed tomographic angiography of canine portosystemic shunts. *Veterinary Radiology and Ultrasound* 46: 27–32.

Zwingenberger, A.L. and Shofer, F.S. (2007). Dynamic computed tomographic quantitation of hepatic perfusion in dogs with and without portal vascular anomalies. *American Journal of Veterinary Research* 68: 970–974.

Zwingmann, C. and Butterworth, R. (2005). An update on the role of brain glutamine synthesis and its relation to cell-specific energy metabolism in the hyperammonemic brain: further studies using NMR spectroscopy. *Neurochemistry International* 47: 19–30.

14

Liver Lobe Torsion and Abscess

Daniel A. Degner and Jitender Bhandal

Liver Lobe Torsion

Liver lobe torsion is a rare condition, but has been reported in dogs, cats, horses, pigs, rabbits, otters, and humans (Tomlinson & Black 1983; Tate 1993; McConkey *et al.* 1997; Downs *et al.* 1998; Sato & Solano 1998; Sonnenfield *et al.* 2001; Swann & Brown 2001; Martin *et al.* 2003; Schwartz *et al.* 2006; von Pfeil *et al.* 2006; Schenk 2007; Bhandal *et al.* 2008; Lee *et al.* 2009; Massari *et al.* 2012; Sargent *et al.* 2013; Tubby 2013; Nazarali *et al.* 2015; Park *et al.* 2016; Khan *et al.* 2016; Knight & Kovak-McClaran 2020; Cordella & Bertolini 2021; Picavet *et al.* 2021; Tallaj *et al.* 2021). Currently, only 36 dogs and 6 cats are reported with this condition in the veterinary literature. No sex or breed predilection is seen with the condition, although most cases involve medium to large body size and middle-aged to geriatric patients. Torsion of one liver lobe from any division results in strangulation of vessels of the torsed lobe, which may lead to infarction and necrosis. Most often a single lobe is affected; however, simultaneous torsion of two liver lobes has been reported in 16.7% of cases (7 of 42 dogs and cats) or the entire liver is reported in domestic animals and humans (Picavet *et al.* 2021; Cordella & Bertolini 2021; Massari *et al.* 2012; Bhandal *et al.* 2008; Lee *et al.* 2009).

A paucity of feline liver lobe torsion reports has been noted. Two of six were associated with tumors; one cat had undiagnosed multiple liver masses; another cat had a hepatocellular carcinoma (Swann & Brown 2001; Nazarali *et al.* 2015). A case report of a 10-week-old cat with a complete caudate liver lobe torsion has been cited (Tallaj *et al.* 2021). In another case report, a 11-month-old cat

had torsion of the central division of the liver (quadrate and right medial liver lobes) and gallbladder (Picavet *et al.* 2021). A 5-year old British blue shorthair cat was reported to have a torsed papillary process of the caudate lobe (Knight & Kovak-McClaran 2020). A 6-year-old cat had left lateral liver lobe torsion with concurrent moderate pectus excavatum (Haider *et al.* 2015).

Etiology and Pathophysiology

The liver lobes are suspended by their attachments to the diaphragm and body wall by a number of ligaments. The left and right lateral liver lobes are attached to the diaphragm by their triangular ligaments and the left medial, quadrate, and right medial liver lobes are attached to the diaphragm by the coronary ligaments. The caudate process of the caudate lobe is supported by the hepatorenal ligament. Conjoined parenchyma of adjacent liver lobes also stabilizes the liver lobes and makes them more resistant to torsion. Elongation or traumatic rupture of hepatic ligaments may increase the mobility of a liver lobe and predispose it to torsion (Swann & Brown 2001). In addition, if there is a paucity of conjoined liver parenchyma between various liver lobes due to individual variation or anomalies, the stability of the lobe is further compromised. Diaphragmatic herniation may also accompany disruption of hepatic ligaments and displacement of a liver lobe within the chest with resultant torsion. One malamute had a torsion of the caudate process of the caudate lobe associated with rupture of the hepatogastric ligament (McConkey *et al.* 1997). Gastric volvulus was reported to be potentially the causative factor of left lateral liver lobe torsion in a 4-year-old female

Small Animal Soft Tissue Surgery, Second Edition. Edited by Eric Monnet.
© 2023 John Wiley & Sons, Inc. Published 2023 by John Wiley & Sons, Inc.
Companion website: www.wiley.com/go/monnet/small

Irish setter due to stretching of the triangular ligament of the left lateral lobe (Tomlinson & Black 1983).

A hepatocellular carcinoma was reported to be associated with a right medial liver lobe torsion in one cat and multiple undiagnosed tumors in another cat (Swann & Brown 2001; Nazarali *et al.* 2015). A dog was reported to have hemangiosarcoma within a torsed liver lobe (Park *et al.* 2016).

Left lateral liver lobe torsion is reported to be the most common lobe affected in one study, accounting for nearly 50% of all cases (Swann & Brown 2001). This may be due to its large size, pendulous anatomic shape, and lack of conjoined parenchyma to adjacent liver lobes. By combining the results of a series of reports in the literature that noted which liver lobe was torsed (42 cases with a total of 46 known torsed lobes and 2 undocumented locations of torsed lobes), the left lateral, left medial, quadrate, right medial, right lateral, caudate process of the caudate lobe, and papillary process of the caudate lobe accounted for 28%, 20%, 13%, 9%, 2%, 11%, and 17% of all torsed lobes, respectively (Tomlinson & Black 1983; Tate 1993; McConkey *et al.* 1997; Downs *et al.* 1998; Sato & Solano 1998; Sonnenfield *et al.* 2001; Swann & Brown 2001; Martin *et al.* 2003; Schwartz *et al.* 2006; von Pfeil *et al.* 2006; Schenk 2007; Bhandal *et al.* 2008; Lee *et al.* 2009; Massari *et al.* 2012; Sargent *et al.* 2013; Tubby 2013; Nazarali *et al.* 2015; Park *et al.* 2016; Khan *et al.* 2016; Knight & Kovak-McClaran 2020; Cordella & Bertolini 2021; Picavet *et al.* 2021; Tallaj *et al.* 2021).

Liver lobe torsion initially results in obstruction of low-pressure vessels such as the hepatic and portal veins. Because arterial perfusion is initially maintained, the liver lobe becomes engorged with blood, which results in effusion and diapedesis of red blood cells through the thin peritoneal capsule. Stagnation of blood within the venous drainage of the liver lobe results in thrombosis of these vessels. In addition, arterial perfusion is no longer maintained due to increased hydrostatic pressure and arterial thrombosis ensues. Necrosis of the liver lobe and toxemia of the patient occur (Martin *et al.* 2003).

Clinical signs

Nonspecific clinical signs are typical of liver lobe torsion. Presenting clinical signs are either acute or chronic, with a reported duration ranging from 4 hours to 22 days (McConkey *et al.* 1997; Downs *et al.* 1998; Sato & Solano 1998; Sonnenfield *et al.* 2001; Swann & Brown 2001; Martin *et al.* 2003; Schwartz *et al.* 2006; von Pfeil *et al.* 2006; Bhandal *et al.* 2008; Lee *et al.* 2009). Signs observed by the pet owner may include lethargy, anorexia, polyuria/polydipsia, respiratory distress, lateral recumbency, vomiting, diarrhea, acute collapse, and abdominal distension. Physical examination findings may include a combination of fever or hypothermia, dehydration, weak thready pulses, tachycardia, abdominal fluid wave, abdominal mass, and abdominal pain. The electrocardiogram (ECG) may show sinus tachycardia, ventricular tachycardia, or ventricular premature contraction, and hypotension may be noted on measurement of blood pressure.

Diagnostics

Hematologic abnormalities in animals with liver lobe torsion may include mature neutrophilia, leukocytosis, and anemia (McConkey *et al.* 1997; Downs *et al.* 1998; Sato & Solano 1998; Sonnenfield *et al.* 2001; Swann & Brown 2001; Martin *et al.* 2003; Schwartz *et al.* 2006; von Pfeil *et al.* 2006; Bhandal *et al.* 2008; Lee *et al.* 2009). Most patients have elevations of alanine aminotransferase on blood biochemistry. In decreasing frequency, elevated alanine aminotransferase and aspartate aminotransferase, hypoalbuminemia, hyperbilirubinemia, hyponatremia, hypochloridemia, elevated blood urea nitrogen, hypercholesterolemia, and hyperphosphatemia are seen (Schwartz *et al.* 2006). Amylase and lipase may also be elevated. Coagulation profile results are usually within the reference limits. Mild alterations of activated partial thromboplastin time are reported, although no clinical abnormalities in gross coagulation are typically noted during surgery (Schwartz *et al.* 2006).

Thoracic radiography may show microcardia and contracted intrathoracic vasculature due to hypovolemia. Occasionally, the sternal lymph nodes may be enlarged with a chronic liver torsion. The most common finding on abdominal radiograph is a cranial abdominal mass. Other radiographic signs may include loss of abdominal detail due to peritoneal effusion and gas in the stomach and small intestine (Tomlinson & Black 1983; Tate 1993; McConkey *et al.* 1997; Downs *et al.* 1998; Sato & Solano 1998; Sonnenfield *et al.* 2001; Swann & Brown 2001; Martin *et al.* 2003; Schwartz *et al.* 2006; von Pfeil *et al.* 2006; Bhandal *et al.* 2008; Lee *et al.* 2009). A less common finding is gas within the liver, which is due to gas-forming bacteria within the necrotic liver lobe (McConkey *et al.* 1997).

Ultrasound is a sensitive imaging modality used to diagnose liver lobe torsion. The most common ultrasonographic findings include abdominal effusion and hypoechogenicity of the affected liver lobe with decreased blood flow. Thrombosis and distension of the hepatic and portal veins may also be visualized (Figure 14.1). Some torsed liver lobes have a heterogeneous echogenicity (Tate 1993; Sato & Solano 1998; Sonnenfield *et al.* 2001; Swann & Brown 2001; Schwartz *et al.* 2006; von Pfeil *et al.* 2006; Bhandal *et al.* 2008; Lee

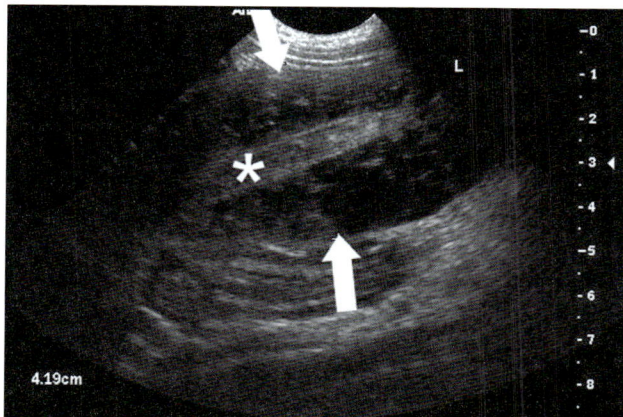

Figure 14.1 Ultrasound image demonstrates a hypoechoic torsed liver lobe (arrows) and a distended thrombosed hepatic vein (asterisk).

et al. 2009). Further evaluation of liver perfusion can be performed using contrast-enhanced ultrasonography and has been described in a rabbit with liver lobe torsion (Stock *et al.* 2020).

Pre- and postcontrast computed tomography (CT) are also useful for diagnosing liver lobe torsion. Precontrast CT images may show deviation or malangulation of the affected liver lobe, or fissures in the liver parenchyma. Postcontrast images typically do not show any contrast enhancement of the torsed liver lobe, indicating thrombosis of the vessels and tissue infarction (Lee *et al.* 2009). Multiplanar CT reconstruction may further assist in localizing the torsed liver lobe (Lee *et al.* 2009). In a recent study five dogs with liver lobe torsion were evaluated with three-phase contrast CT scans and all were definitively diagnosed correctly with this modality. Vascular signs seen with CT scan showed a "whirl sign" and vascular interruption. The "whirl sign" is due to concentric twisting of vessels around the torsed liver lobe pedicle (Cordella & Bertolini 2021).

Treatment and complications

Liver lobe torsion and subsequent hemoabdomen constitute a surgical emergency and should be dealt with immediately, otherwise death can occur due to hypovolemic shock and anemia. The patient should be adequately fluid resuscitated with crystalloids, colloids, or blood products, and hemodynamically stabilized prior to any surgical procedure. During surgery, the torsed liver lobe may have a dark appearance, firm consistency, and evidence of tissue necrosis (Figure 14.2). The extent of the liver torsion varies from 180° to 360°, and the direction of torsion can be in a clockwise or counterclockwise direction. The nontorsed liver lobes should be thoroughly examined for adequate blood supply because

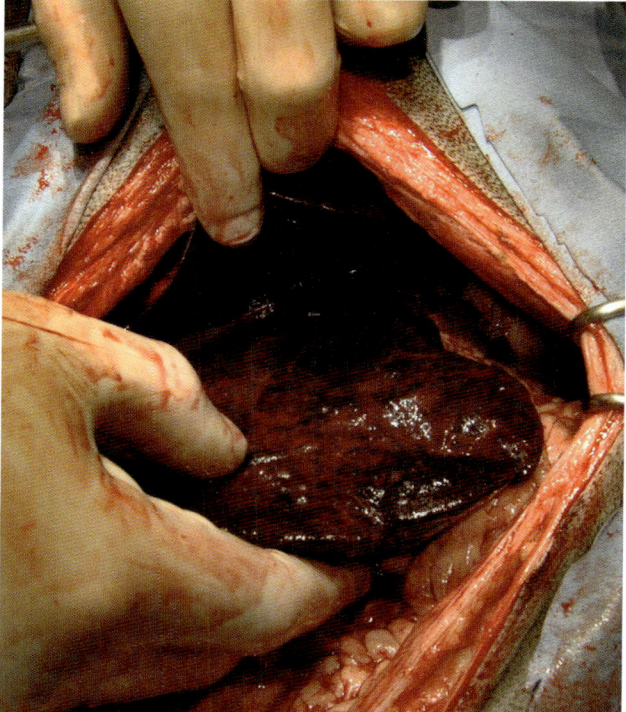

Figure 14.2 Intraoperative view. Note the congested, torsed liver lobe.

of risk of infarction to the adjacent liver lobes. Examination of unaffected liver lobes can be conducted after removal of the affected liver. The torsed liver lobe should not be untwisted before resection to prevent release of bacteria, bacterial toxins, and emboli (thrombi) into the circulation. Removal of the torsed liver lobe can be quickly executed with a V3 thoracoabdominal (TA) 30 or 2.5–3.5 mm endovascular gastrointestinal anastomosis (Endo GIA™, Covidien, Dublin, Ireland) stapler (30–60 mm) or with suture ligation.

Complications following surgery are commonly seen and include anemia, arrhythmia, progressive hypoalbuminemia, vomiting, and aspiration pneumonia. Acute death in the postoperative period may be associated with continued hemorrhage from the stump of the removed liver lobe (slippage of ligature) or secondary to disseminated intravascular coagulation (DIC).

Histologic examination of the torsed or infarcted liver lobe commonly reveals diffuse and marked congestion with prominent dilation of the sinusoids, resulting in compression of the adjacent hepatocellular cords. The hepatocytes may appear diffusely hypereosinophilic and there may be variable degrees of nuclear pyknosis suggestive of coagulation necrosis. A band of neutrophils may border the zone of necrosis. These changes are typical of hepatic infarction. An aerobic and anaerobic culture should be performed, as at least half of these torsed liver lobes have concurrent bacterial infection. The most commonly isolated bacteria include *Staphylococcus intermedius*, *Klebsiella pneumoniae*, *Pasteurella* spp., *Escherichia coli*, *Clostridium* spp., and/or *Bacillus* spp., and Gram-negative nonfermenting rods (Swann & Brown 2001).

Postoperative care

Postoperatively, the patient may develop cardiac arrhythmias and therefore the heart should be monitored with continuous ECG and a plan formulated to treat arrhythmias if needed. Blood pressure should be monitored for a day or two after surgery. Daily bloodwork should be completed including coagulation profile or activated clotting time, platelet count, electrolytes, blood gases, glucose, albumin, urea nitrogen, hematocrit, and total protein. Intravenous fluid therapy is continued until the patient is well enough to eat and drink.

Fresh frozen plasma or colloid should be administered if serum albumin levels are below 2.0 g/dL. Initial empiric intravenous antibiotic administration followed by oral antibiotic administration based on bacterial sensitivity is recommended for at least 7 days after surgery.

Prognosis

Barring no fatal internal hemorrhage, DIC, pneumonia, or other life-threatening complications after surgery, the prognosis for survival is generally very good. Overall, survival of patients with liver lobe torsion that have surgery is 84% (Tate 1993; Sato & Solano 1998; Sonnenfield *et al.* 2001; Swann & Brown 2001; Schwartz *et al.* 2006; von Pfeil *et al.* 2006; Bhandal *et al.* 2008; Lee *et al.* 2009).

Liver abscess

Liver abscesses are uncommon in dogs and cats. In a retrospective study of 1800 cases of canine liver disease, only 0.27% of these had liver abscesses (Center 1990). Concurrent disease is associated with liver abscesses in 50% of patients. This includes diabetes mellitus, chronic recurrent urinary tract infection with concurrent septicemia, pancreatitis, pneumonia, gallbladder rupture, and previous liver biopsy (Lord *et al.* 1982; Grooters *et al.* 1994, 1995; Schwarz *et al.* 1998). Other contributing factors may include neoplasia, long-term phenobarbital or glucocorticoid administration, and hyperadrenocorticism (Farrar *et al.* 1996; Zatelli *et al.* 2005).

Clinical signs

The age of dogs afflicted with liver abscesses typically ranges from 4 to 16 years, with a mean age of 10.6 years; however, puppies have also been reported to develop this condition (Hargis & Thomassen 1980; Schwarz *et al.* 1998). The mean age of cats with liver abscesses is 10.1 years (Zatelli *et al.* 2005). No sex predilection has been substantiated. Clinical signs common to liver abscessation include lethargy, anorexia, vomiting, diarrhea, trembling, abdominal pain, fever, and dehydration. Cats generally have a much lower incidence of fever (23% vs. 86%) and abdominal pain (31% vs. 57%) than dogs (Schwarz *et al.* 1998; Sergeeff *et al.* 2002).

Laboratory

Leukocytosis is found in 75–85% of patients (Farrar *et al.* 1996; Schwarz *et al.* 1998). Neutrophilia with left shift, monocytosis, anemia, and thrombocytopenia are common hematologic abnormalities (Schwarz *et al.* 1998). Elevated serum alkaline phosphatase is uniformly seen in canine patients, and elevated alanine aminotransferase and aspartate aminotransferase levels are common. In cats, alkaline phosphatase is elevated in 18% of cases; however, alanine aminotransferase is elevated in 45% of cases (Sergeeff *et al.* 2002). Hyperbilirubinemia is seen in 36% of affected dogs and is not a negative prognostic indicator as it is in humans (Farrar *et al.* 1996; Schwartz *et al.* 2006). In cats, elevated bilirubin is seen in 27% of cases (Sergeeff *et al.* 2002). Hypoalbuminemia is seen in 64% of dogs and 79% of cats (Farrar *et al.* 1996; Sergeeff *et al.* 2002).

Bacterial infection is present in 69–90% of cats and dogs with liver abscesses (Farrar *et al.* 1996; Schwarz *et al.* 1998; Sergeeff *et al.* 2002). Isolated bacteria include *E. coli*, *Staphylococcus* spp., *Enterococcus* spp., *Micrococcus*, *Proteus mirabilis*, *K. pneumoniae*, *Staphylococcus epidermidis*, *S. intermedius*, *Clostridium* spp., *Lactobacillus*, *Serratia* sp. and *Citrobacter freundi* (Center 1990; Schwarz *et al.* 1998). More than one organism is found in about 55% of cases (Schwarz *et al.* 1998). Because the most common organism isolated is *E. coli*, an ascending biliary infection is suggested (Zatelli *et al.* 2005).

Imaging

In earlier studies, the diagnosis of liver abscessation was based on necropsy findings (Thornburg 1988). Abdominal radiography typically demonstrates nonspecific signs of a problem, including regional hepatomegaly, rounded liver margins, abdominal effusion, and rarely gas shadows within the liver parenchyma (Figure 14.3) (Schwarz *et al.* 1998).

Ultrasound is considered the diagnostic modality of choice, as it is economical, provides a rapid diagnosis, can be used for diagnostic and therapeutic needle aspiration of the abscess, and permits evaluation of regional lymph nodes (Figure 14.4). It is a very good tool for monitoring the lesion following treatment. Multiphase

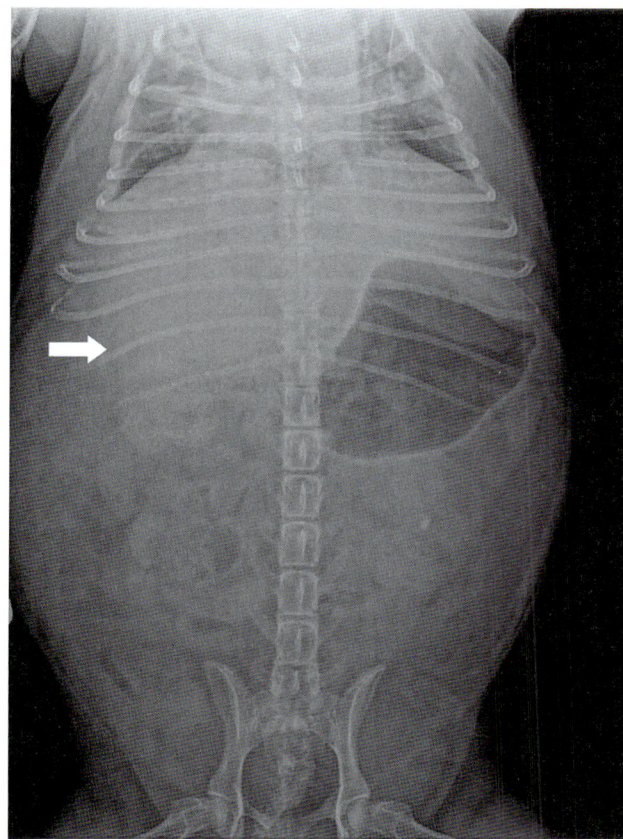

Figure 14.3 Ventrodorsal abdominal radiograph. A mass effect in the right cranial abdomen (arrow) represents a large liver abscess.

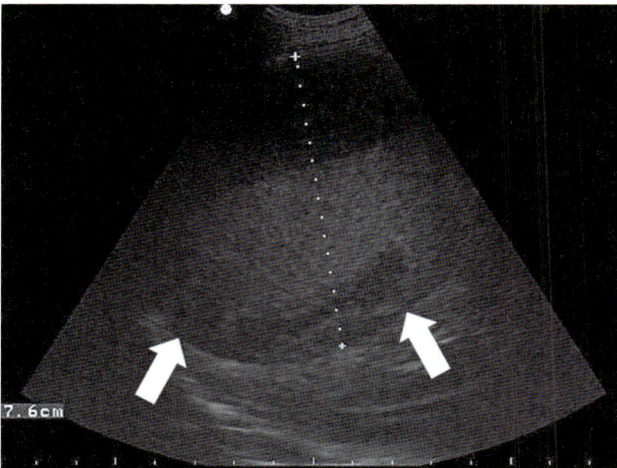

Figure 14.4 Transverse view. The ultrasound image demonstrates hypoechoic material closest to the transducer and hyperechoic sludge in the dependent portion of a liver abscess (arrows).

contrast CT scan has identified a dog with liver lobe torsion and abscessation (Cordella & Bertolini 2021).

In dogs, 77% of all liver abscesses are solitary. Multiple and compartmentalized abscesses are much less common

in dogs (Schwarz *et al.* 1998). In cats, the majority of liver abscesses are either multiple macroscopic or multiple microscopic (Sergeeff *et al.* 2002). The majority of liver abscesses are located in the left lobes in dogs and in the right lobes in cats. The shape, size, and echogenicity of liver abscesses are variable. Some have an echogenic rim representing the wall of the abscess and a central anechoic region. In general, three echo patterns are common to liver abscesses: anechoic, hypoechoic or poorly echogenic, and mixed echogenic lesions. Other ultrasonographic signs may include far enhancement artifact, gas within the abscess, abdominal effusion, and hyperechogenic perihepatic fat (Schwarz *et al.* 1998).

Cytology

Aspiration of a liver lesion and cytology of the exudate are essential for confirming a diagnosis of liver abscess. Cytologically, the cellular population will demonstrate suppurative inflammation with degenerate neutrophils. Phagocytosed bacteria may also be seen within neutrophils.

Treatment

Liver abscesses are drained via an ultrasound-guided percutaneous approach using 14–20-gauge needles. Most dogs only need to have the abscess drained once, but about 25% of cases require repeated treatment (25%) (Schwarz *et al.* 1998).

In humans, ultrasound-guided percutaneous drainage and alcoholization of liver abscesses resulted in reduced hospital stay and satisfactory results (Alberti *et al.* 2002). This technique is also described in feline and canine patients (Zatelli *et al.* 2005). The volume of 95% ethanol injected into the drained abscess is 50% of the aspirated exudate volume. The ethanol is aspirated from the abscess cavity after a period of three minutes. In this series of cases, enrofloxacin was prescribed for one month. Resolution of clinical signs occurs within 2–3 days after treatment. Potential complications of drainage of liver abscesses may include abscess rupture with localized or generalized peritonitis.

Selection of antibiotics for treatment of liver abscesses should be based on culture and sensitivity; however, empirical treatment may include a combination of penicillin, clindamycin, or metronidazole and an aminoglycoside or fluoroquinolone (Farrar *et al.* 1996).

Surgical treatment of liver abscesses is generally via hepatic lobectomy (Figure 14.5), although surgical drainage of the abscess followed by omentalization could also be considered. The former is the best treatment, as some of these patients have a tumor associated with the abscess.

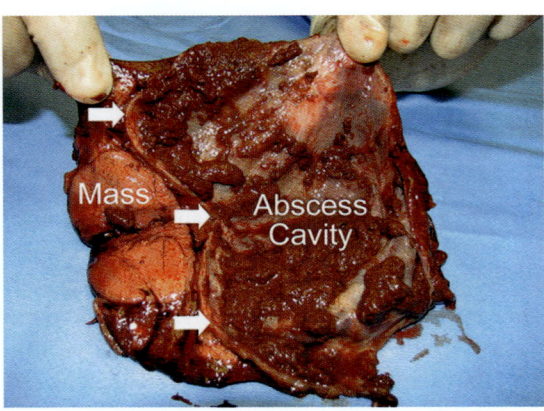

Figure 14.5 Excised liver abscess has been cut in cross-section and exudate has been removed; arrows denote the capsule of the abscess. A liver mass is located adjacent to the abscess cavity.

Prognosis

One study that included patients that had abscesses treated with ultrasound-guided drainage, antibiotic treatment alone, or surgical treatment had a 77% long-term survival rate (Schwarz *et al.* 1998). In contrast, Zatelli *et al.* (2005) reported 100% resolution of abscesses and survival of patients following alcoholization of abscesses, with no complications in a series of five dogs and one cat.

Survival following surgery is reported to be 71% in dogs; however, about 50% of the patients in this study did not have any surgical intervention, as they died on their own or were euthanized (Farrar *et al.* 1996). Cats treated surgically for hepatic abscesses had a 79% mortality rate and this may be due to diffuse involvement of the liver (Sergeeff *et al.* 2002).

References

Alberti, D., Borsellino, A., Locatelli, C. et al. (2002). Percutaneous transhepatic alcoholization: a new therapeutic strategy in children with chronic granulomatous disease and liver abscess. *Pediatric Infectious Disease Journal* 21: 1081–1083.

Bhandal, J., Kuzma, A., and Starrak, G. (2008). Spontaneous left medial liver lobe torsion and left lateral lobe infarction in a Rottweiler. *Canadian Veterinary Journal* 49: 1002–1004.

Center, S.A. (1990). Hepatobiliary infections. In: *Infectious Diseases of the Dog and Cat* (ed. C.E. Green), 146–155. Philadelphia, PA: WB Saunders.

Cordella, A. and Bertolini, G. (2021). Multiphase multidetector-row computed tomographic and ultrasonographic findings in dogs with spontaneous liver lobe torsion. *Research in Veterinary Science* 135: 192–199.

Downs, M.O., Miller, M.A., Cross, A.R. et al. (1998). Liver lobe torsion and liver abscess in a dog. *Journal of the American Veterinary Medical Association* 212: 678–680.

Farrar, E.T., Washabau, R.J., and Saunders, M. (1996). Hepatic abscesses in dogs: 14 cases (1982–1994). *Journal of the American Veterinary Medical Association* 208: 243–247.

Grooters, A.M., Sherding, R.G., Biller, D.S., and Johnson, S.E. (1994). Hepatic abscesses associated with diabetes mellitus in two dogs. *Journal of Veterinary Internal Medicine* 8: 203–206.

Grooters, A.M., Sherding, R.G., and Johnson, S.E. (1995). Hepatic abscesses in dogs. *Compendium of Continuing Education for the Practicing Veterinarian* 6: 833–839.

Haider, G., Dokic, Z., Petritsch, B. et al. (2015). Left lateral liver lobe torsion in a cat with moderate pectus excavatum. *Journal of Feline Medicine and Surgery* 17 (12): 1077–1079. https://doi.org/10.1177/1098612X15573561.

Hargis, A.M. and Thomassen, R.W. (1980). Hepatic abscesses in beagle puppies. *Laboratory Animal Science* 30: 689–693.

Khan, Z., Gates, K., and Simpson, S.A. (2016). Bicavitary effusion secondary to liver lobe torsion in a dog. *Veterinary Medicine (Auckland, N.Z.)* 20 (7): 53–38. https://doi.org/10.2147/VMRR.S83608.

Knight, R. and Kovak-McClaran, J. (2020). Hemoperitoneum secondary to liver lobe torsion in a cat. *Journal of the American Animal Hospital Association* 56 (1): e561–e502. 10.5326/JAAHA-MS-6758.

Lee, K.J., Yamada, K., Hirokawa, H. et al. (2009). Liver lobe torsion in a shih-tzu dog. *Journal of Small Animal Practice* 50: 157.

Lord, P.F., Carb, A., Halliwell, W.H., and Prieter, J. (1982). Emphysematous hepatic abscess associated with trauma, necrotic hyperplasia and adenoma in a dog: a case report. *Veterinary Radiology* 23: 46–49.

Martin, R.A., Lanz, O.I., and Tobias, K.M. (2003). Liver and biliary system. In: *Textbook of Small Animal Surgery*, 3e (ed. D. Slatter), 709. Philadelphia, PA: WB Saunders.

Massari, F., Verganti, S., Secciero, B. et al. (2012). *Australian Veterinary Journal* 90 (1–2): 44–47. https://doi.org/10.1111/j.1751-0813.2011.00869.x.

McConkey, S., Briggs, C., Solano, M.O., and Illanes, O. (1997). Liver torsion and associated bacterial peritonitis in a dog. *Canadian Veterinary Journal* 38: 438–439.

Nazarali, A., Singh, A., Chalmers, H. et al. (2015). Chronic liver lobe torsion in a cat. *Journal of the American Animal Hospital Association* 50 (2): 119–123. https://doi.org/10.5326/JAAHA-MS-5969.

Park, J., Lee, H.B., and Jeong, S.M. (2016). Liver lobe torsion with hemangiosarcoma in a dog. *Journal of Veterinary Clinics* 33 (6): 376–380. https://doi.org/10.17555/jvc.2016.12.33.6.376.

von Pfeil, D.J.F., Jutkowitz, L.A., and Hauptman, J. (2006). Left lateral and left middle liver lobe torsion in a Saint Bernard puppy. *Journal of the American Animal Hospital Association* 42: 381–385.

Picavet, P.P., Vidal, P.A., Bolen, G. et al. (2021). Gallbladder and liver lobe torsion in a young cat presented with hemoabdomen. *Journal of the American Animal Hospital Association* 57 (5): 247–251. 10.5326/JAAHA-MS-7090.

Sargent, J.M., Dennis, S., and Fuentes, V.L. (2013). ECG of the month. Liver lobe torsion. *Journal of the American Veterinary Medical Association* 242 (6): 748–750. 10.2460/javma.242.6.748.

Sato, A.F. and Solano, M. (1998). Radiographic diagnosis: liver lobe entrapment and associated emphysematous hepatitis. *Veterinary Radiology and Ultrasound* 39: 123–124.

Schenk, M.G. (2007). Liver lobe torsion in a dog. *Canadian Veterinary Journal* 48 (4): 423–425.

Schwartz, S.G.H., Mitchell, S.L., Keating, J.H., and Chan, D.L. (2006). Liver lobe torsion in dogs: 13 cases (1995–2004). *Journal of the American Veterinary Medical Association* 228: 242–247.

Schwarz, L.A., Penninck, D.G., and Leveille-Webster, C. (1998). Hepatic abscesses in 13 dogs: a review of ultrasonographic findings, clinical data and therapeutic options. *Veterinary Radiology and Ultrasound* 39: 357–365.

Sergeeff, J.S., Armstrong, J., and Bunch, S.E. (2002). Hepatic abscesses in cats: 14 cases (1985–2002). *Journal of Veterinary Internal Medicine* 18: 295–300.

Sonnenfield, J.M., Armbrust, L.J., Radlinsky, M.A. et al. (2001). Radiographic and ultrasonographic findings of liver lobe torsion in a dog. *Veterinary Radiology and Ultrasound* 42: 344–346.

Stock, E., Vanderperren, K., Moerenans, I. et al. (2020). Use of contrast-enhanced ultrasonography in the diagnosis of a liver lobe torsion in a rabbit (*Oryctolagus cuniculus*). *Veterinary Radiology & Ultrasound* 61 (4): 31–35. 10.1111/vru.12709.

Swann, H.M. and Brown, D.C. (2001). Hepatic lobe torsion in 3 dogs and a cat. *Veterinary Surgery* 30: 482–486.

Tallaj, K.M., Cortes, Y., Kristi, M.G. et al. (2021). Acute liver lobe torsion in a kitten. *Journal of Feline Medicine & Surgery* 7 (1): https://doi.org/10.1177/2055116921990295.

Tate, P. (1993). Hepatic torsion and dislocation with hypotension and colonic obstruction. *American Journal of Surgery* 59: 455–458.

Thornburg, L.P. (1988). A study of canine hepatobiliary diseases. Part 6: Infectious hepatopathies. *Companion Animal Practice* 2: 13–20.

Tomlinson, J. and Black, A. (1983). Liver lobe torsion in a dog. *Journal of the American Veterinary Medical Association* 183: 225–226.

Tubby, K.G. (2013). Concurrent gall bladder, liver lobe torsion, and bile peritonitis in a German shepherd dog 2 months after gastric dilatation/volvulus gastropexy and splenectomy. *Canadian Veterinary Journal* 54 (8): 784–786.

Zatelli, A., Bonfanti, U., Zini, E. et al. (2005). Percutaneous drainage and alcoholization of hepatic abscess in five dogs and a cat. *Journal of the American Animal Hospital Association* 41: 34–38.

15

Liver Tumors and Partial Hepatectomy

Daniel A. Degner and Richard Walshaw

Primary liver tumors constitute 0.6–2.6% of all tumors in dogs (Strombeck 1978; Patnaik *et al.* 1980; Trigo *et al.* 1982; Balkman 2009) and 1.5–2.3% of all tumors in cats (Engle & Brodey 1969; Balkman 2009). They originate from the cells that constitute the liver: hepatocytes, bile duct epithelial cells, neuroendocrine cells, and connective tissue cells. Hepatocytes can transform into hepatocellular carcinomas, adenomas, and hyperplastic nodules. The epithelium that lines bile ducts may become bile duct carcinomas or adenomas. Neuroendocrine cells can transform into carcinoids or carcinomas. Sarcomas develop from connective tissue cells.

Primary liver tumors may also be characterized by their gross morphologic characteristics (Patnaik *et al.* 1981a,b). Massive tumors are large tumors that involve one liver lobe. Of this type, hepatocellular carcinoma is the most common. Nodular tumors are smaller masses that involve multiple lobes. Diffuse tumors such as lymphoma, mastocytosis, and histiocytic sarcoma infiltrate the entire liver (Patnaik *et al.* 1980, 1981a,b; Magne & Withrow 1985; Liptak *et al.* 2004).

Specific tumor types

Hepatocellular tumors

Hepatocellular adenomas are uncommon benign tumors in dogs, but are more common in cats (Trigo *et al.* 1982; Lawrence *et al.* 1994; Balkman 2009). The most common primary liver tumor in dogs is the hepatocellular carcinoma (Figures 15.1–15.3). These are

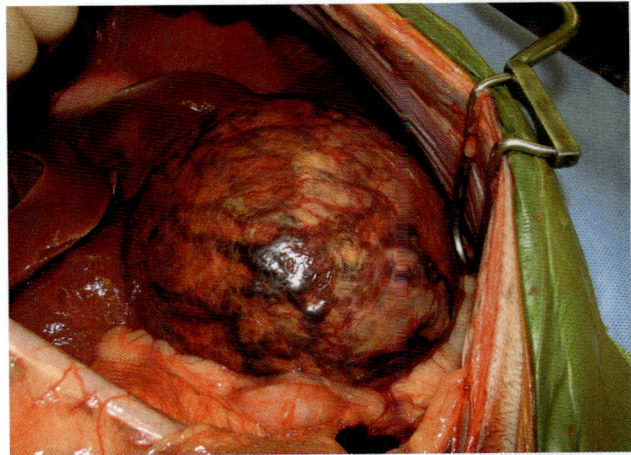

Figure 15.1 Intraoperative view of a large hepatocellular carcinoma of the left lateral lobe. Note the large superficial vessels that can tear easily if the tumor is manipulated.

usually amenable to surgical excision (Patnaik *et al.* 1980, 1981a,b; Magne & Withrow 1985; Kosovsky *et al.* 1989; Liptak *et al.* 2004).

The distribution of hepatocellular carcinoma by location is 68.3% in the left division, 19.5% in the central division, and 12.2% in the right division (Liptak *et al.* 2004). The increased incidence in the left and central lobes is also reported in other studies (Patnaik *et al.* 1980; Kosovsky *et al.* 1989). Histopathology of hepatocellular carcinoma includes well differentiated

Small Animal Soft Tissue Surgery, Second Edition. Edited by Eric Monnet.
© 2023 John Wiley & Sons, Inc. Published 2023 by John Wiley & Sons, Inc.
Companion website: www.wiley.com/go/monnet/small

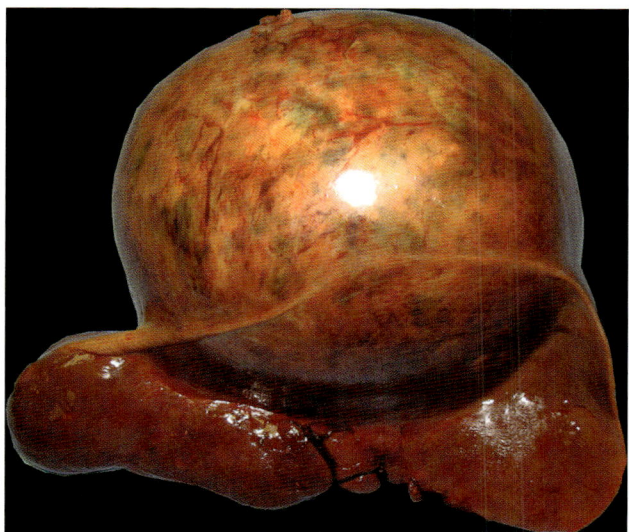

Figure 15.2 Resected hepatocellular carcinoma with a border of normal hepatic parenchyma.

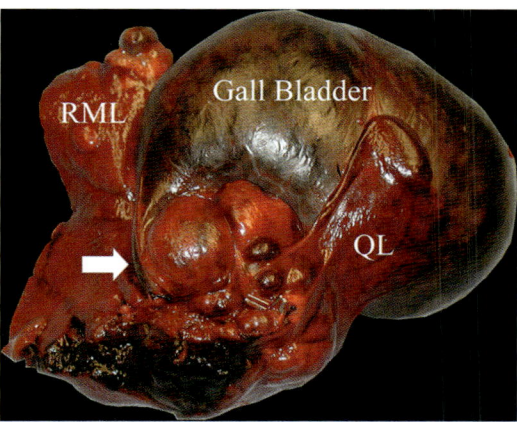

Figure 15.3 Central division hepatocellular carcinoma that is obstructing the cystic duct (arrow) of the gallbladder. QL, quadrate liver lobe; RML, right medial liver lobe.

in 78% of cases, moderately differentiated in 19%, and poorly differentiated in 3% (Liptak *et al.* 2004).

One study reported survival times of more than 300 days, with no disease-related deaths (Kosovsky *et al.* 1989). The median survival time for dogs that had surgery is not reached in another study (>1460 days) (Liptak *et al.* 2004). Dogs in another study also did not reach their median survival time (Kinsley *et al.* 2015). A median survival time of 270 days is seen in dogs that have no surgery (Liptak *et al.* 2004).

Intraoperative mortality rate is 4.8% due to exsanguination. Metastasis was found in 4.8% of patients in one study (Liptak *et al.* 2004). In another study, the metastatic rate was 36.6% (Patnaik *et al.* 1981a,b). Negative prognostic indicators include high levels of

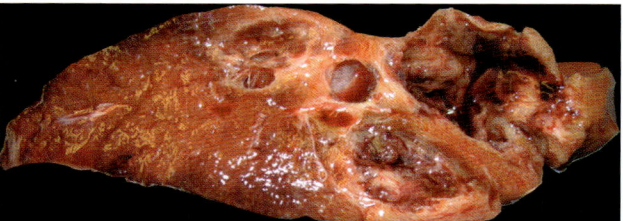

Figure 15.4 Cross-sectional view of a biliary adenocarcinoma in a dog. Note the cystic structures within the liver parenchyma.

alanine aminotransferase (ALT) and aspartate aminotransferase (AST), and right-division tumors (Liptak *et al.* 2004). Tumor size and tumor grade do not affect survival times (Liptak *et al.* 2004).

Biliary tumors

Bile duct tumors are more common in cats and are rarely identified in dogs (Trigo *et al.* 1982; Post & Patnaik 1992; Lawrence *et al.* 1994) (Figure 15.4). In dogs, bile duct adenocarcinomas are more common than adenomas and have a 66–88% incidence of metastasis to local lymph nodes, lungs, abdominal organs, and bones (Patnaik *et al.* 1980; Trigo *et al.* 1982).

Biliary cystadenomas (i.e., biliary adenomas, cholangiocellular adenomas) are the most common liver tumor in cats (Post & Patnaik 1992; Lawrence *et al.* 1994). These tumors are locally invasive, frequently very large at the time of presentation, and commonly recur following resection. The second most common primary liver tumor in cats is bile duct adenocarcinoma, which invariably metastasizes in almost all cases (Post & Patnaik 1992).

Carcinoids (neuroendocrine tumors)

Neuroendocrine tumors in dogs are rare and usually diffuse (Patnaik *et al.* 1981a,b, 2005a,b). This tumor may also affect the gallbladder. Cholecystectomy has been performed in a few cases, but long-term follow-up data are not available (Willard *et al.* 1988; Morrell *et al.* 2002; Lippo *et al.* 2008). In cats, this tumor may affect the liver parenchyma, bile ducts, or gallbladder. Metastasis is common to the lymph nodes, lungs, intestines, and peritoneal cavity (Patnaik *et al.* 2005b).

Sarcomas

In dogs, sarcomas of the liver comprise less than 13% of all primary liver tumors (Patnaik *et al.* 1980; Trigo *et al.* 1982). These tumors include hemangiosarcoma, leiomyosarcoma, fibrosarcoma, osteosarcomas, malignant mesenchymoma, and chondrosarcoma (Patnaik *et al.* 1976; Jeraj *et al.* 1981; McDonald & Helman 1986; Kapatkin *et al.* 1992; Chikata *et al.* 2006). These tumors are most commonly metastatic lesions from a primary tumor elsewhere in the body. In cats, it is uncommon for these tumors to be a primary hepatic tumor.

Clinical signs

Liver tumors are typically seen in geriatric dogs and cats between 9 and 12 years of age (Strombeck 1978; Patnaik *et al.* 1980; Trigo *et al.* 1982; Magne & Withrow 1985; Liptak *et al.* 2004). The median age of dogs affected by carcinoids is 8 years (Patnaik *et al.* 1980, 2005b). There is no specific breed predilection, although the golden retriever, mixed, Australian cattle dog, chow chow, miniature schnauzer, shar-pei, Siberian husky, keeshond, Labrador retriever, Airedale, Alaskan malamute, Australian shepherd, bassett hound, beagle, border collie, bulldog, Chesapeake Bay retriever, English springer spaniel, Hungarian puli, Samoyed, shih tzu, spitz, Jack Russell terrier, and Australian terrier breeds have been reported to develop liver tumors (Schmidt & Langham 1967; Engle & Brodey 1969; Strombeck 1978; Patnaik *et al.* 1980, 1981a,b, 2005a; Trigo *et al.* 1982; Magne & Withrow 1985; Liptak *et al.* 2004).

Clinical signs are reported in 28–71% of all dogs with liver tumors and generally are nonspecific (Kosovsky *et al.* 1989; Liptak *et al.* 2004). Signs include weight loss, inappetence, lethargy, vomiting, polyuria, polydipsia, and seizures (Strombeck 1978; Patnaik *et al.* 1980; Trigo *et al.* 1982; Magne & Withrow 1985; Liptak *et al.* 2004). Only 45% of dogs have a detectable abdominal mass (Liptak *et al.* 2004). Specific signs related to liver disease such as abdominal pain, icterus, and ascites are not typically present unless there is diffuse liver disease (Patnaik *et al.* 1980). Cats with malignant liver tumors commonly have anorexia, vomiting, and lethargy. Cats with benign liver masses are usually not clinically ill (Post & Patnaik 1992; Lawrence *et al.* 1994; Patnaik *et al.* 2005a).

Laboratory findings

Complete blood count abnormalities include anemia in 54%, microcytosis in 31%, leukocytosis in 27%, and thrombocytosis in 46.2% of cases (Liptak *et al.* 2004). In other studies leukocytosis is uncommon (Patnaik *et al.* 1980; Kosovsky *et al.* 1989). Thrombocytosis has been associated with a multitude of malignancies in humans, and has been previously reported in 46.2% of dogs with liver tumors (Liptak *et al.* 2004). Thrombocytosis may be associated with anemia, inflammation, iron deficiency, and cytokine production. In Liptak's study, there was no association found between thrombocytosis, anemia, and inflammation and tumor size (Liptak *et al.* 2004).

The serum concentrations of one or more of total protein, albumin, alkaline phosphatase, and ALT are elevated in all dogs with primary liver tumors. Elevation of AST and ALT may be associated with biologically aggressive liver tumors, but this was not substantiated in Liptak's study. Prothrombin time and activated partial thromboplastin time are abnormal in 21% of cases (Liptak *et al.* 2004).

Imaging modalities

Abdominal radiography and ultrasonography

Because these tumors are typically large, they can usually be visualized on abdominal radiography (Figures 15.5 and 15.6). Abdominal ultrasonography is an ideal diagnostic modality that will allow detection of a liver tumor in most cases (Evans 1987; Liptak *et al.* 2004). This diagnostic modality may help determine if diffuse or nodular tumors or a single massive tumor is present within the liver. Typical ultrasonographic signs of hepatocellular carcinoma include a nonuniform mass that has mixed hyperechoic and hypoechoic properties (Figure 15.7). Ultrasound typically cannot differentiate the degree of invasion of tumor into adjacent liver lobes and major vessels. Contrast ultrasonography has been shown to be beneficial in differentiating malignant metastatic masses from benign tumors in dogs (Kanemoto *et al.* 2009).

Ultrasound-guided fine-needle biopsy is helpful in arriving at a diagnosis in 14–86% of cases. Multiple core biopsies or a surgical wedge biopsy usually provides a definitive diagnosis (Roth 2001; Cole *et al.* 2002; Wang *et al.* 2004). Normal coagulation profile and platelet count are essential if a biopsy is performed (Bigge *et al.* 2001). If a single massive tumor is present, histopathology is usually performed after the tumor has been

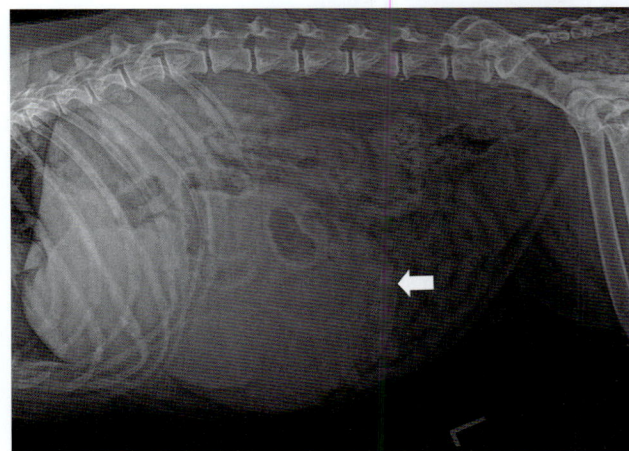

Figure 15.5 Lateral abdominal radiograph reveals a very large central division liver mass (arrow denotes caudal border of tumor).

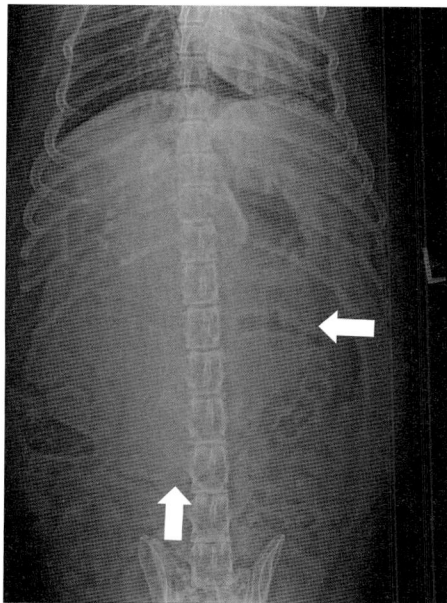

Figure 15.6 Ventrodorsal abdominal radiograph reveals a very large liver mass (arrows denote the caudal and left sides of the tumor).

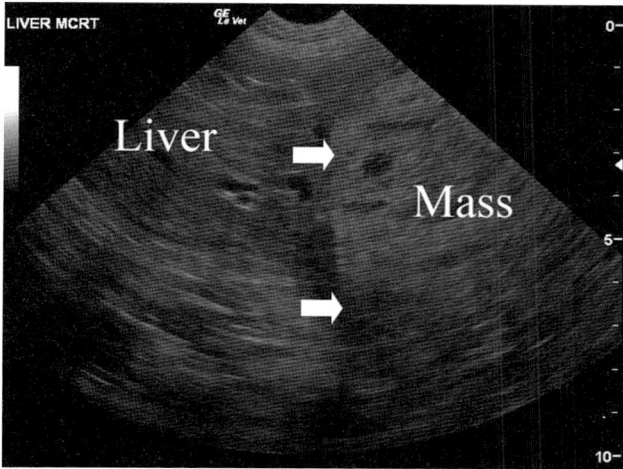

Figure 15.7 Ultrasonographic image of liver tissue with a solitary hepatocellular carcinoma (arrows).

removed, as these most commonly are hepatocellular carcinomas (Liptak *et al.* 2004).

Computed tomography

In humans, computed tomography (CT) is more commonly used and may be beneficial in surgical planning (Coakley & Schwartz 2001; Befeler & Bisceglie 2002; Burti *et al.* 2021). CT scan is becoming more adopted as an important tool to help differentiate hepatocellular carcinoma from nodular hyperplasia and for surgical planning. Contrast ultrasound has not shown a reliable

correlation with malignant versus benign liver masses (Burti *et al.* 2020). Although some large liver tumors may seem ominous and nonresectable on CT scan, in the author's and others' experience these cases frequently are operable (Liptak *et al.* 2004). Three-view chest radiography or chest CT should be used to rule out macroscopic pulmonary metastasis and lymphadenopathy.

Surgical treatment

Surgery is the treatment of choice for the resection of different primary liver tumors. Even large, seemingly inoperable massive liver tumors usually can be successfully removed with meticulous dissection techniques (Liptak *et al.* 2004).

Preoperative considerations

Experimentally, normal dogs can tolerate removal of 70% of the total liver, as the organ is capable of rapid regeneration (Francavilla *et al.* 1978). In clinical patients that undergo liver lobectomy, the remaining liver is frequently not normal and liver enzyme levels commonly do not return to normal. Hypotension is the main concern in the patient undergoing hepatic lobectomy. The primary cause of hypotension in these patients is compression of the vena cava by a large tumor. Once anesthetized, the patient should be placed in lateral recumbency while the abdomen is being clipped to minimize occlusion of the vena cava. Once placed on the operating table in dorsal recumbency, the patient should be tilted to the left if there is a left-sided tumor and to the right if the tumor is primarily on the right side of the liver. Blood products should be available in the event of profound intraoperative hemorrhage. One study including 72 dogs and cats demonstrated the need for transfusion in 17% of dogs and 44% of cats undergoing liver lobectomy (Hanson *et al.* 2017). Patients that have significant clotting abnormalities may require fresh frozen plasma transfusions prior to surgery.

Surgical approach to the liver

A cranial two-thirds, midline celiotomy is adequate for most cases requiring liver lobectomy. Additional exposure to the right division of the liver may be achieved with a right paracostal approach. However, if the right division of the liver is contained within the confines of the ribcage due to breed variation (deep-chested), a paracostal approach will not provide additional visualization of the liver. Rather, a midline celiotomy and partial median sternotomy with partial ventrodorsal splitting of the diaphragm along its midline provide much better exposure of both the right and central divisions of the liver. The incision in the diaphragm shifts the abdominal contents caudally by eliminating negative intrathoracic pressure. Furthermore, the liver can be caudally displaced for better exposure by placing a malleable retractor on the thoracic side of the diaphragm through the incision made in the ventral diaphragm. A left paracostal incision is rarely of benefit for exposing the hilus of the left division of the liver.

Methods of liver lobectomy

A number of techniques have been described to remove liver lobes (Bjorling *et al.* 1985; Martin *et al.* 2003). In the early literature, placement of mattress sutures through a liver lobe or a guillotine ligature at the base of the liver lobe was recommended (Martin *et al.* 2003). This technique should be reserved for left lateral or left medial liver lobectomy in cats and small dogs. It is not used in large dogs, as the ligature may become dislodged in the postoperative period and result in severe or even fatal hemorrhage.

Another technique involves digital fracturing of the liver and ligation of encountered vasculobiliary structures. In humans, a cavitational ultrasonic surgical aspirator has been used to reduce bleeding and help isolate vessels and bile ducts (Nuzzo *et al.* 2001; Takayama *et al.* 2001; Bachellier *et al.* 2007; Gayet *et al.* 2007).

Lewis *et al.* (1990) described the use of a thoracoabdominal stapling device (TA55) in dogs. This device delivers two rows of staggered staples that span a total width of 55 mm. Each staple is 4.0 mm wide and has a leg length of 3.5 mm with a closed height of 1.5 mm (Tobias 2007). Most lobar hepatic arteries are 1.5 mm or less in diameter, and therefore significant arterial hemorrhage is possible using this stapler. This stapler is best used for liver lobes that are pendulous and easily amputated at the hilus. The V3 TA30 stapler is much better suited for achieving good hemostasis of small vessels including hepatic lobar arteries, as these have three staggered rows of staples that are 3.0 mm wide, 2.5 mm open leg length, and 1.0 mm closed staple height (Tobias 2007). The disadvantage of this stapler is that it is only 30 mm wide and has a narrow opening of its anvil, so that thick tissues cannot be inserted into the stapler. A new design of the V3 TA30 (Multifire Premium™ TA, Covidien Autosuture, Norwalk, CT, USA) has been released that can accommodate thicker tissues. The total staple length is 30 mm, which is inadequate for a complete lobectomy in large-breed dogs. Furthermore, TA30 staplers have become less available for purchase.

Endo GIA™ staplers (Covidien, Minneapolis, MN, USA) with a leg length of 2.5 mm are ideal to perform liver lobectomy in medium to large dogs, and those at 2.0 mm are useful in small dogs and cats. The length of the staple line available includes 30 mm, 45 mm, and 60 mm. A significant benefit of the Endo GIA over the V3 TA30 stapler is that it has six rows of staples and cuts between the third and fourth rows of staples. Thus, no back bleeding is present from the stump of the liver lobe. This is more important when the liver lobe cannot be completely stapled with one cartridge, and this is the case when performing a hilar liver lobectomy. Frequently, using our current technique of liver lobectomy, a 30 mm Endo GIA is utilized on inflow vascular structures and conjoining liver parenchyma is divided with a Poole suction tip or a vessel sealing device, followed by utilizing an appropriately sized Endo GIA stapler for the hepatic lobar vein.

We have developed techniques to dissect the liver at the hilus by isolating, ligating, and dividing vasculobiliary structures using a combination of suture ligatures, hemostatic clips, and Endo GIA staples (Covey *et al.* 2009). Based on our clinical use of the hilar liver dissection technique, a more complete lobectomy and less intraoperative bleeding can be achieved (thus blood transfusions are much less commonly needed). The hilar liver lobe resection technique can be utilized in experimental auxiliary liver transplantation (de Jonge *et al.* 2003).

Minimizing intraoperative hemorrhage

When performing resective liver surgery, hemorrhage is a major concern. Large liver tumors are commonly very vascular and tear easily, which can result in profound intraoperative hemorrhage. For this reason, the affected liver lobe should be minimally manipulated during the lobectomy. If possible, the hilus of the lobe of interest should be exposed by retraction of adjacent normal liver lobes. Also if possible, inflow lobar vascular structures should be isolated, ligated, and divided prior to blunt division of conjoined parenchyma between liver lobes. As a final step, the hepatic veins of the liver lobe are ligated and divided. Profound intraoperative hemorrhage is typically due to inadvertent tearing or penetration of large blood vessels during lobectomy. The Pringle technique, which involves occluding the portal vein and hepatic artery with digital pressure or a preplaced Rummel tourniquet, can be used to temporarily reduce blood flow to the liver lobes until the source of bleeding can be arrested.

General anatomy of the liver

The liver consists of six lobes: left lateral, left medial, quadrate, right medial, right lateral, and caudate (Figure 15.8) (Evans 1979). The caudate lobe is subdivided into two processes, but these likely should be considered as separate lobes because each process has a distinctly separate blood supply and biliary duct. The left division, which includes the left lateral and

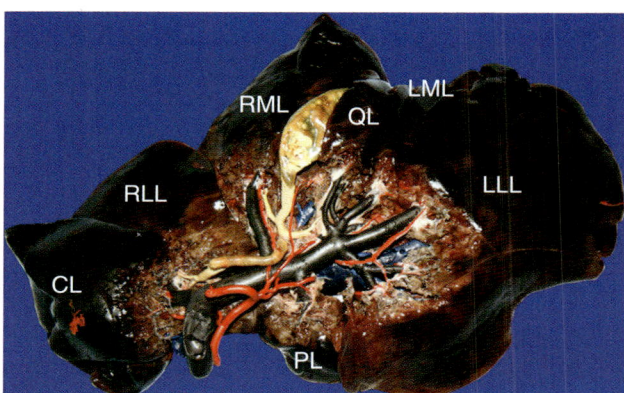

Figure 15.8 Visceral view of the liver. Red vasculature indicates hepatic arteries, purple vasculature portal veins, blue vasculature hepatic veins, and yellow the biliary tree. CL, caudate process of the caudate lobe; LLL, left lateral lobe; LML, left medial lobe; PL, papillary process of the caudate lobe; QL, quadrate lobe; RML, right medial lobe; RLL, right lateral lobe.

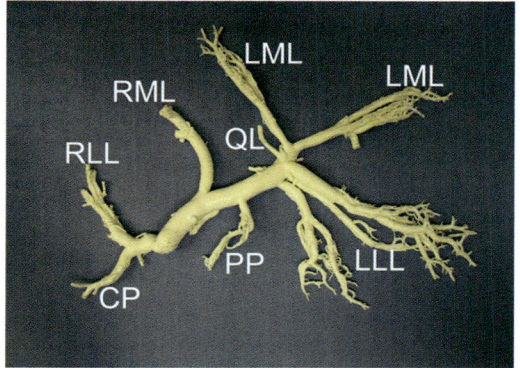

Figure 15.9 Ventral view of a cast of a portal vein in a dog. CP, caudate process of the caudate lobe; LLL, left lateral lobe; LML, left medial lobe; PP, papillary process of the caudate lobe; QL, quadrate lobe; RML, right medial lobe; RLL, right lateral lobe.

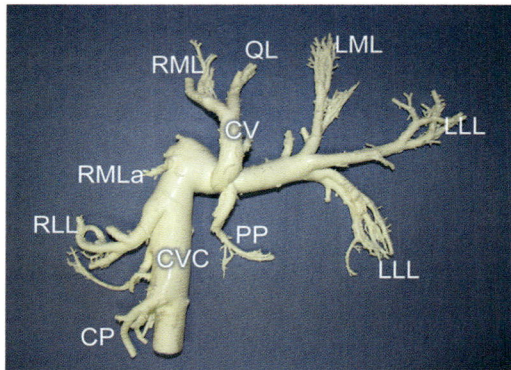

Figure 15.10 Ventral view of a cast of a caudal vena cava and hepatic veins. CP, caudate process of the caudate lobe; LLL, left lateral lobe; LML, left medial lobe; PP, papillary process of the caudate lobe; QL, quadrate lobe; RML, right medial lobe; RMLa, accessory vein to right medial lobe; RLL, right lateral lobe.

left medial lobes, typically constitutes about half the total liver mass. The left lateral liver lobe is usually the largest and covers the left side of the stomach. It has shared parenchyma with the left medial liver lobe at the hilus. The quadrate and right medial liver lobes, constituting the central division, have conjoined hepatic parenchyma with the gallbladder nestled between the two lobes. The quadrate lobe has a conjoined parenchyma with the left medial liver lobe. The right division consists of the right lateral and the caudate lobes, which are attached to the vena cava and have conjoined parenchyma.

The liver lobes are suspended within the abdomen by attachments to the abdominal vena cava, diaphragm, and a series of peritoneal folds called the hepatic ligaments. The cranial aspect of the liver has a peritoneal reflection that forms a crown around the cranial aspect of the left and central division liver lobes, called the coronary ligament. The left lateral lobe has a broad triangular ligament that suspends this lobe to the left aspect of the central diaphragmatic tendon. The left medial liver lobe has a relatively small triangular ligament that attaches the lobe to the diaphragm. The quadrate and right medial liver lobes do not have any triangular ligaments, but are flanked by the coronary ligament. The right lateral liver lobe has a small triangular ligament that is attached to the right side of the diaphragm. The hepatorenal ligament suspends the caudate process of the caudate lobe to the right kidney. The liver has left and right portal veins, which then further branch into lobar portal veins (Figure 15.9). Hepatic veins extend directly off the liver lobes and join the vena cava (Figure 15.10) (Evans 1979).

Left lateral lobectomy

The left lateral biliary duct and left lateral lobar hepatic artery are typically located superficial (ventral and to the left) to the left lateral lobar portal vein and may run in the leading edge of the hepatoduodenal ligament (Figure 15.11). The portal blood supply typically consists of two lobar portal veins that enter the hilus of the lobe. The hepatic veins of the left lateral and left medial liver lobes join together to form the left hepatic vein within the hilar sulcus between these two lobes. Lobar hepatic veins from the left medial and lateral liver lobes join to form the left hepatic vein. The left hepatic vein extends from the left division of the liver and runs in a left-to-right direction along the diaphragm within the parenchyma of the liver. The left hepatic vein is partially visible within the fissure between the left medial and lateral liver lobes.

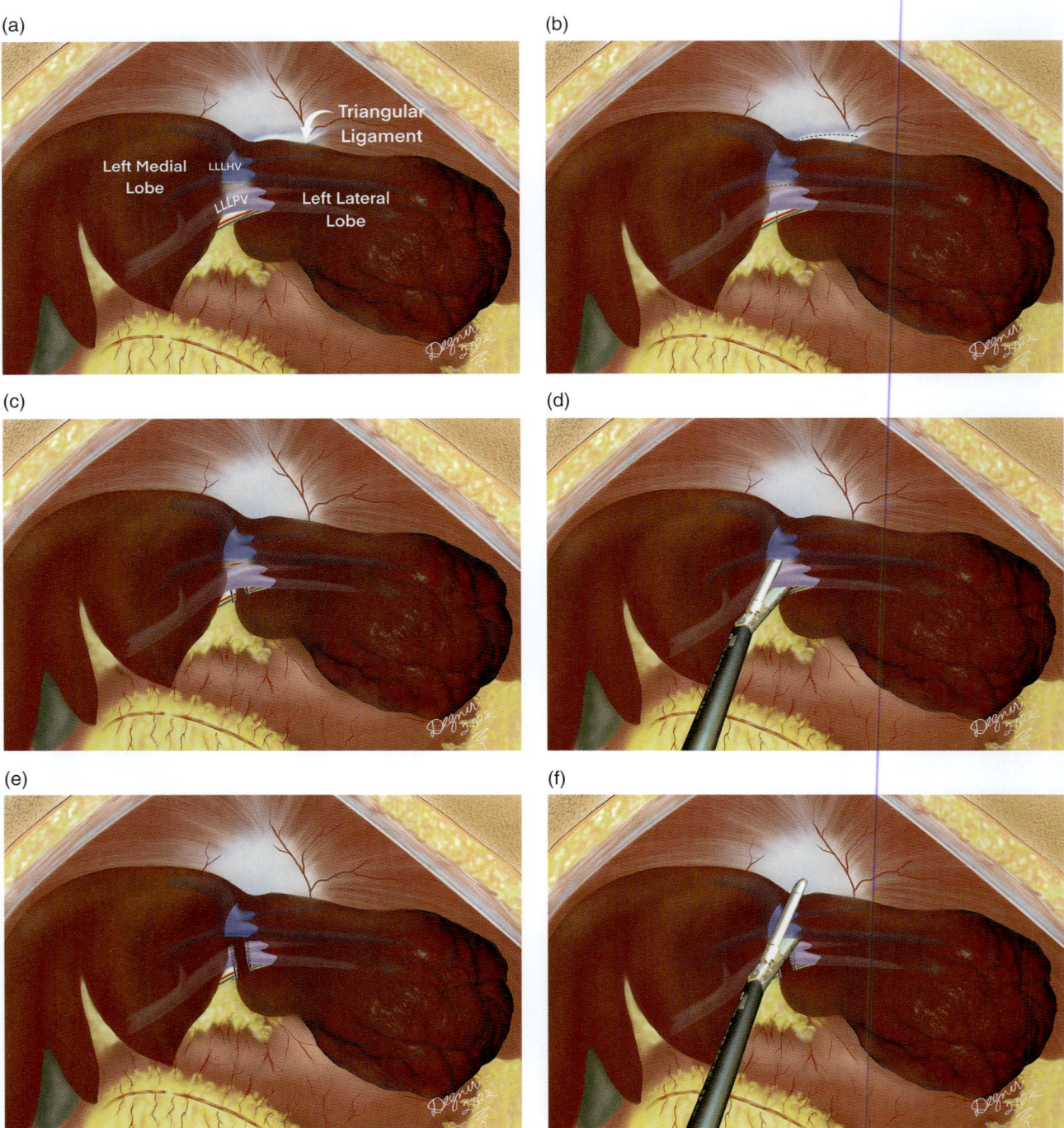

Figure 15.11 (a) Visceral view of liver with left lateral and left medial lobes separated to expose the hilus. (b) Dashed lines denote incisions to divide the triangular ligament, to incise the peritoneum between the left lateral lobar portal vein and the left lateral hepatic vein, and to divide the hepatoduodenal ligament that contains the left lateral lobar hepatic duct and the left lateral lobar hepatic artery. (c) Hemoclips are applied to the hepatic duct and artery and structures divided. An incision is made in the peritoneum in the hilus to allow blunt separation of lobar portal and hepatic veins with forceps. (d) An Endo GIA stapler is used to staple and divide the left lateral lobar portal vein. (e) The left lateral lobar portal vein is stapled and divided. (f) An Endo GIA stapler is used to staple and divide the lobar hepatic vein. (g) All vascular structures and conjoining liver parenchyma at the level of the hilus are divided in preparation for removal of the lobe. (h) The left lateral liver lobe is removed. LLLHV, left lateral lobar hepatic vein; LLLPV, left lateral lobar portal vein.

(g)

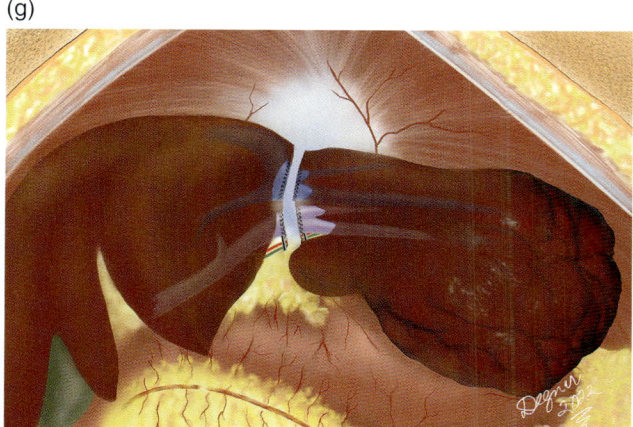

(h)

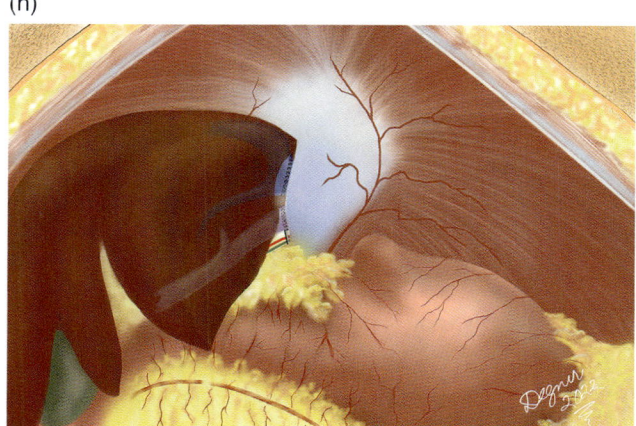

Figure 15.11 (Continued)

The left medial liver lobe is retracted to the right to expose the hilar region of the left lateral liver lobe. The triangular ligament of the left lateral liver lobe is divided. The hepatoduodenal ligament is identified, containing the left lateral lobar artery and left lateral bile duct, extending off the visceral aspect of the hilus of the left lateral lobe. A window is made in this ligament adjacent to the left lateral lobar portal vein at the base of the left lateral liver lobe, and the left lateral lobar hepatic artery and left lateral lobar hepatic biliary duct are isolated, occluded with hemoclips or suture, and divided. In order to allow safe separation of the left lateral portal vein from the left lateral hepatic lobar veins, the peritoneum between these vessels is carefully incised with fine Metzenbaum scissors. A natural cleavage between the left lateral portal and hepatic veins is identified with a blunt instrument such as the inner cannula of a Poole suction tip or Lahey gallbladder forceps. The instrument will easily fall between these vessels with minimal resistance when guided through the correct surgical plane. The surgeon's index finger is placed beneath the hilus (dorsal) to palpate the tip of the blunt instrument as it is passed between the vessels. The lobar portal vein is then stapled and divided with an Endo GIA. The conjoining parenchyma between the left lateral and left medial lobes is divided using a blunt instrument and interlobar vessels are sealed and divided with a vessel sealant device as they are encountered. An Endo GIA stapler is placed across the remaining parenchyma and base of the left lateral hepatic vein from the visceral side (caudal to cranial), staples deployed, and the liver lobe amputated.

In medium-sized to small dogs, the triangular ligament is divided, the parenchyma crushed with Carmalt forceps between the left lateral and left medial liver lobes, and a V3 TA30 stapler or 2.0 mm Endo GIA stapler of appropriate length is used to perform the lobectomy in a single step.

Left medial lobectomy

Generally, one lobar portal vein enters the base of the left medial liver lobe, but two lobar portal veins may supply the lobe (Figure 15.12). Its lobar hepatic artery and bile duct usually run deep to the portal lobar vein. One or two hepatic lobar veins join the lobar veins of the left lateral lobe to form the left hepatic vein. For the most part, these hepatic veins are covered by parenchyma.

The hilus of the left medial liver lobe is exposed by retracting the lobe cranially. The inflow vasculature (lobar portal vein and artery) and lobar hepatic duct are isolated by bluntly creating a tunnel through the parenchyma with a right-angle forceps just deep to these structures, followed by stapling and division of these structures with an Endo GIA stapler. Care must be taken to avoid compromising the left lateral portal vein during the ligation process. Parenchyma conjoining the left medial and quadrate liver lobes is bluntly divided using the inner cannula of a Poole suction tip. Parenchyma conjoining the left medial and left lateral liver lobes is also bluntly divided using the inner cannula of a Poole suction tip. As interlobar vessels between the lobes are encountered, they are ligated or sealed and divided with a vessel sealant device. Division of the parenchyma can also be done solely with a vessel sealant device; however, inadvertent partial division of the left hepatic vein and marked hemorrhage may occur (as experienced by the author). Therefore this method must be used with caution. The left medial lobar hepatic vein(s) is ligated with suture material or stapled with an Endo GIA stapler and the lobe is removed.

Left division resection (left lateral and left medial lobes)

A tumor that encroaches into the hilus between the left lateral and left medial lobes is removed by resecting the entire left division of the liver *en bloc* (Figure 15.13).

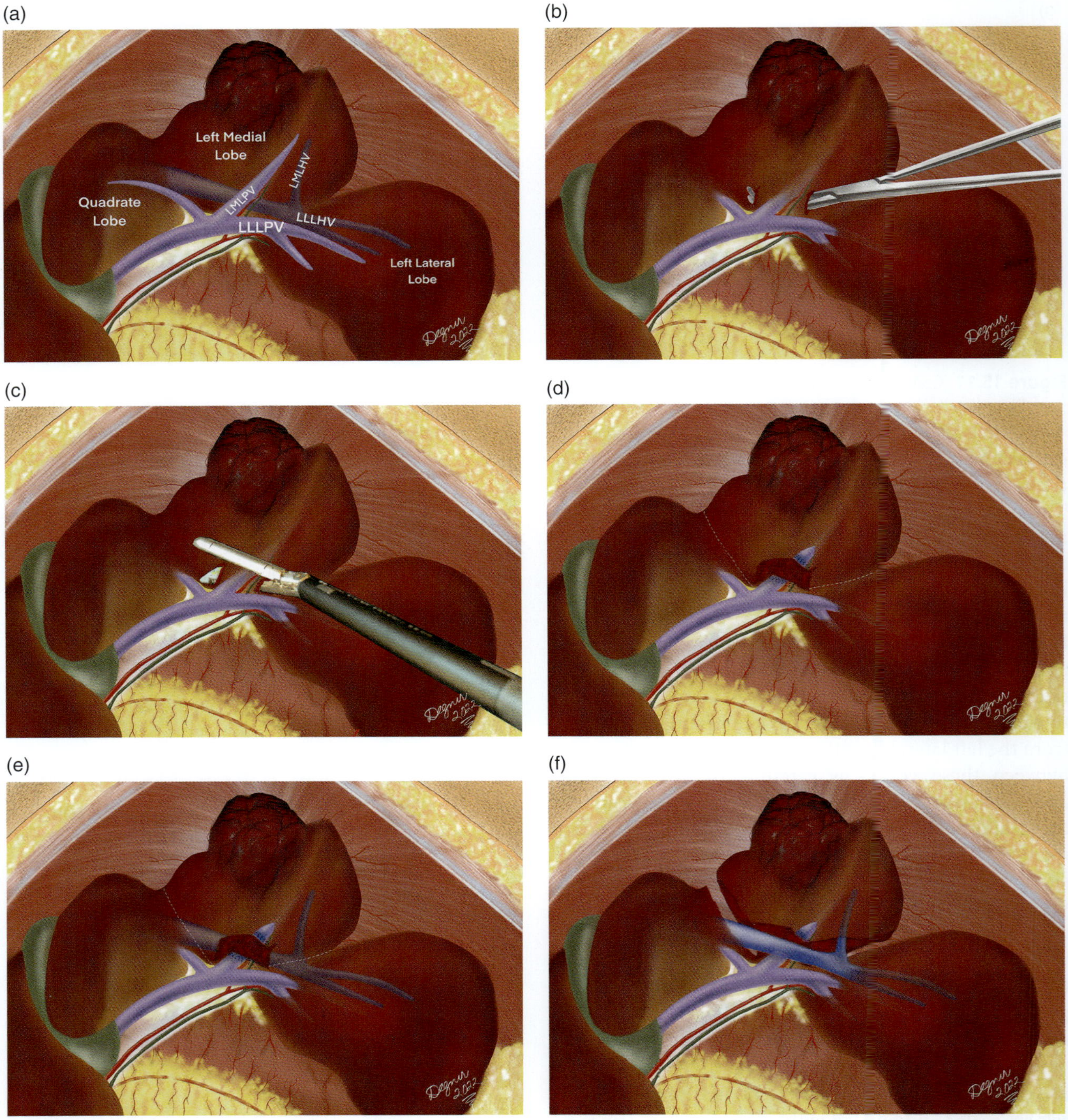

(a)

(b)

(c)

(d)

(e)

(f)

Figure 15.12 (a) Visceral view of liver with left medial liver lobe elevated to expose its hilus. (b) Right-angle forceps are used to bluntly penetrate through the liver parenchyma to create a tunnel for the Endo GIA stapler for occlusion and division of inflow vascular structures and lobar hepatic duct. The path made around these structures should be met with minimal resistance. (c) An Endo GIA stapler is passed around inflow vascular structures and the lobar hepatic duct. (d) The inflow vascular structures and lobar hepatic duct are occluded with staples and divided. (e) Dashed lines in the fissures between the left medial and adjacent lobes are the location for division of the parenchyma. Care is exercised to prevent damage to the left hepatic vein, which lies dorsal and cranially within the base of the left medial lobe. (f) Blunt dissection of parenchyma exposes the left hepatic vein. The left medial lobar hepatic vein is typically located on the left aspect of the left medial liver lobe. (g) The left medial lobar hepatic vein is stapled and divided with an Endo GIA. (h) The left medial lobe is removed from its bed. LLLHV, left lateral lobar hepatic vein; LLLPV, left lateral lobar portal vein; LMLHV, left medial lobar hepatic vein; LMLPV, left medial lobar portal vein.

(g)

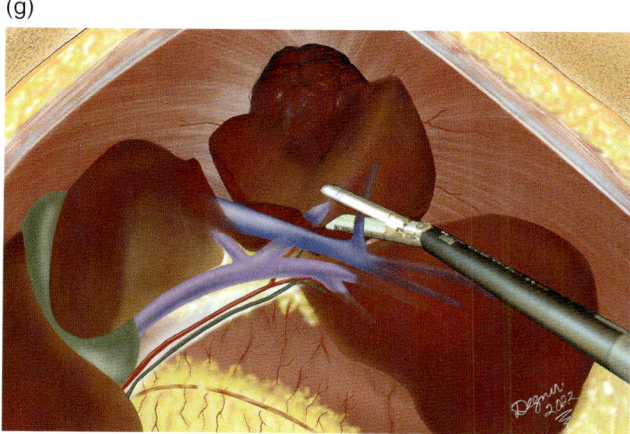

(h)

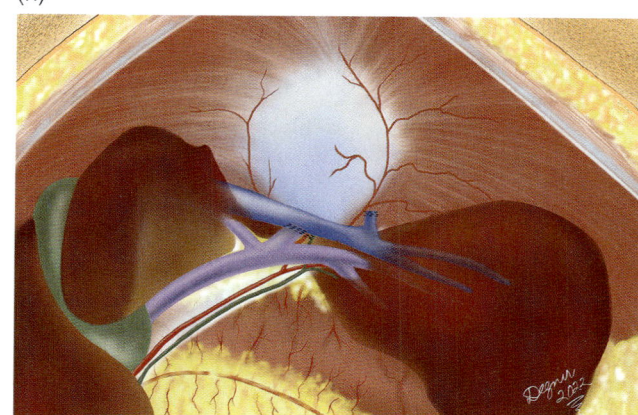

Figure 15.12 (Continued)

A window is made in the hepatoduodenal ligament adjacent to the portal vein that supplies the left liver division (containing the lobar hepatic artery and the lobar biliary duct) and these structures are ligated and divided. Blunt dissection through the parenchyma immediately cranial to the left portal vein between the quadrate and the left medial liver lobes is made with right-angle forceps in a ventral-to-dorsal direction. An Endo GIA stapler is placed through the parenchymal tunnel to encompass the inflow vascular structures, staples deployed, and vessels divided. The conjoined parenchyma between left medial and quadrate lobes is separated using the tip of the inner cannula of a Poole suction instrument. As interlobar vessels are encountered, they are sealed with a vessel sealant device and divided. Once the parenchyma has separated adequately to reach the left hepatic vein, the left triangular ligament adjacent to the left lateral liver lobe is divided and a V3 TA30 stapler or Endo GIA stapler is passed around the remaining tissue and left hepatic vein and the staples are fired into the tissue. The entire left division of the liver is removed.

In small to medium-sized dogs and cats, the left division of the liver can be removed by incising the triangular ligament of the left lateral lobe, crushing the parenchyma between the quadrate and left medial lobes with Carmalt forceps, and deploying an Endo GIA stapler on the vasculobiliary structures. The stapler is placed from caudal to cranial to ensure that all vasculobiliary lobar structures are within the stapler before the staples are deployed. A curved-tip Endo GIA is useful to ensure complete division of all structures.

Central division

The central division of the liver consists of the quadrate and right medial liver lobes (Figure 15.14). The gallbladder is nestled between the visceral surfaces of the central

division lobes. The quadrate liver lobe typically has one main lobar portal vein and cystic duct that enter the lobe to the left of the gallbladder, but may have additional accessory portal vein branches. The quadrate lobar hepatic artery and lobar bile duct consistently enter the base of the lobe, on the right side of the lobar portal vein. The right medial liver lobe has one lobar portal vein located to the right of the gallbladder and the cystic duct. The right medial lobar bile duct and lobar hepatic artery enter the lobe between the lobar portal vein and the neck of the gallbladder. The hepatic veins of the quadrate and the right medial liver lobes are located within the parenchyma immediately deep to the gallbladder fossa. They join together to form the central hepatic vein at the level of the neck of the gallbladder. The central lobar hepatic vein then runs through the parenchyma for 1–3 cm and joins the vena cava at the base of the left hepatic vein. The right medial liver lobe has an accessory hepatic lobar vein that is visible on the right side of its visceral surface. If it is not visible from the visceral surface of the lobe, it can usually be seen on the diaphragmatic surface of the right medial lobe as it joins the vena cava.

Although the quadrate and right medial liver lobes can be resected individually, complete removal of the central division of the liver necessitates removal of both lobes together. The gallbladder can be preserved if the tumor is not associated with this structure; however, in most cases the gallbladder is sacrificed. If the gallbladder is to be preserved, the peritoneum around the gallbladder is incised with a Metzenbaum scissors and small blood vessels are cauterized. Using a Poole suction tip, the gallbladder is bluntly liberated from its bed. To prevent penetration of the central hepatic veins during dissection of the gallbladder, a plane of dissection is maintained outside the liver parenchyma. The biliary lobar duct, lobar portal vein, and lobar hepatic artery of

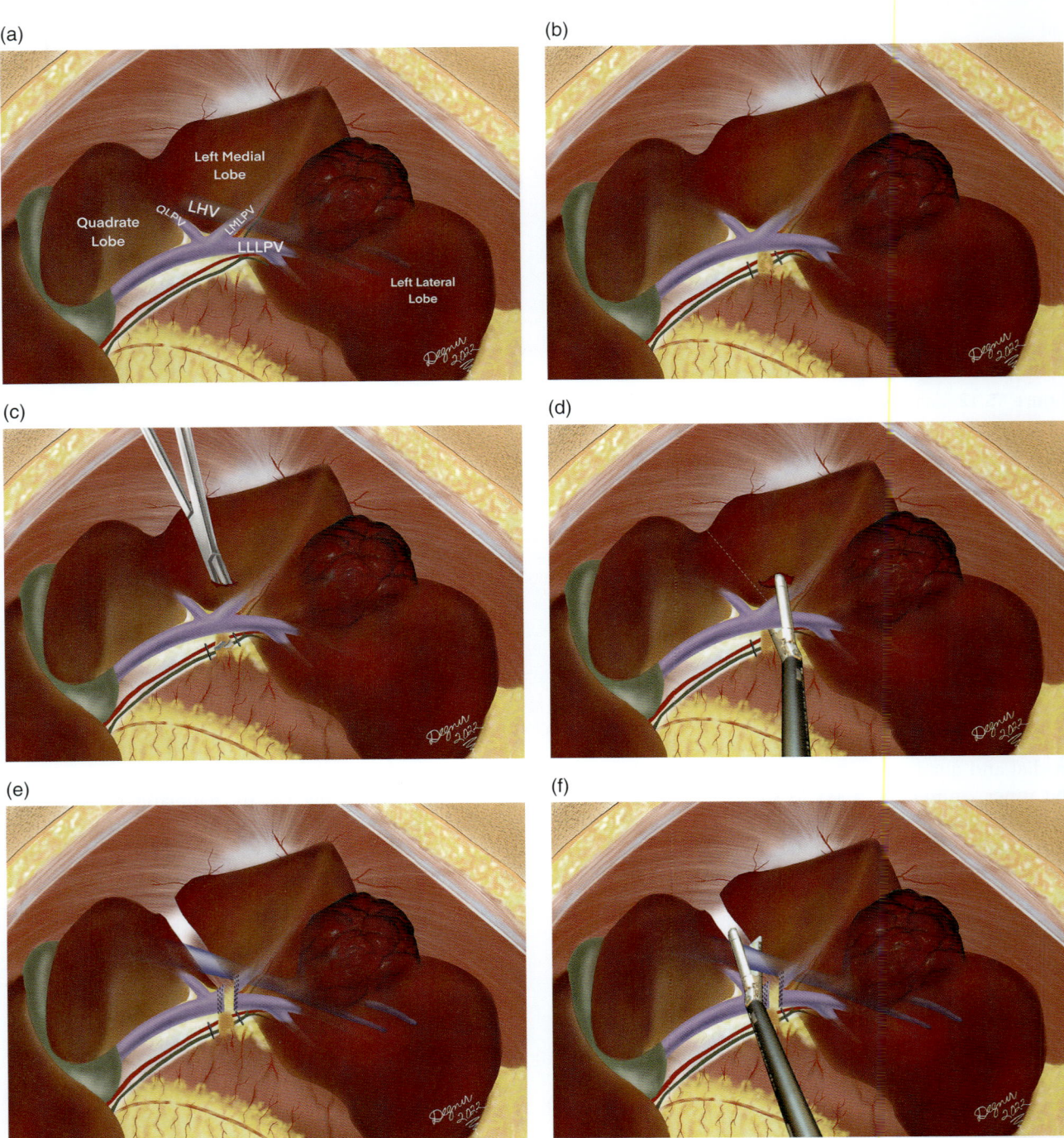

Figure 15.13 (a) Visceral view of the liver. (b) The hepatoduodenal ligament with associated left hepatic duct and left lobar hepatic artery are divided after hemoclips are applied. (c) Right-angle forceps are used to bluntly penetrate through the liver parenchyma, just cranial to the left portal vein and to the left of the quadrate lobar portal vein, to create a path for the Endo GIA stapler for occlusion and division of the left portal vein. The path around the portal vessel structures should be met with minimal resistance. (d) An Endo GIA stapler is placed to encompass the left portal vein. (e) All inflow vascular structures are occluded with staples and divided. The parenchyma between the left medial and quadrate lobes is bluntly divided with a Poole suction tip and interlobar vessels sealed with LigaSure™ (Medtronic, Minneapolis, MN, USA), which then exposes the left hepatic vein. (f) An Endo GIA stapler is placed to encompass the left hepatic vein. (g) The left hepatic vein is occluded with staples and divided. (h) The left division of the liver has been removed. LHV, left hepatic vein; LLLPV, left lateral lobar portal vein; LMLPV, left medial lobar portal vein; QLPV, quadrate lobar portal vein.

(g)

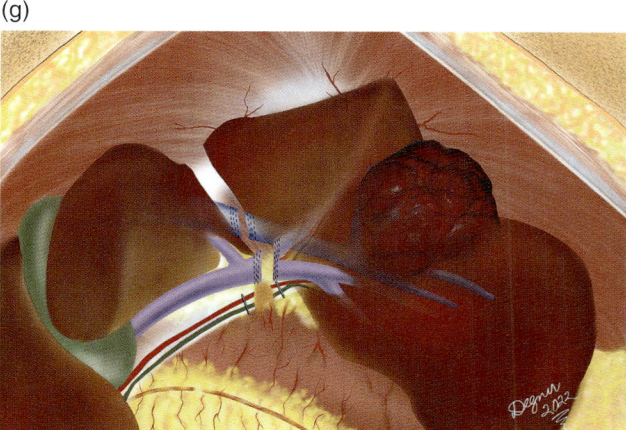

(h)

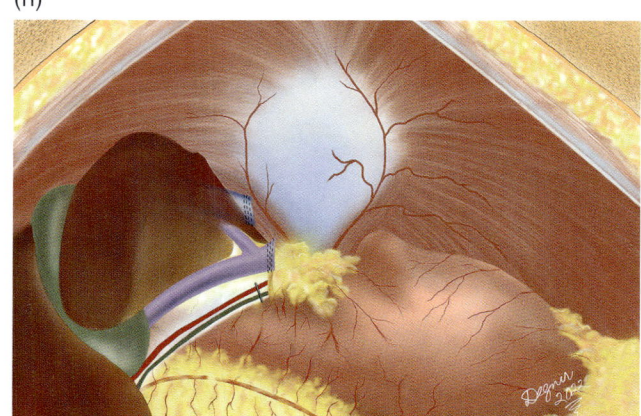

Figure 15.13 (Continued)

the quadrate lobe are identified and a blunt instrument is passed through adjacent liver parenchyma to isolate these structures. Vasculobiliary structures are stapled and divided with an Endo GIA. The process is repeated for the inflow vessels and biliary duct of the right medial liver lobe. The accessory hepatic vein of the right medial liver lobe is identified on the visceral (or diaphragmatic) surface of the lobe, isolated, doubly ligated (or stapled), and divided. The parenchyma between the quadrate and left medial liver lobes is divided with the cannula of a Poole suction tip. The remaining liver parenchyma is separated off the vena cava using a suction cannula. Once the base of the central liver division has been adequately skeletonized, a V3 TA30 or Endo GIA stapler is used to staple the remaining tissue and central hepatic vein. If the gallbladder has been preserved, the fundus of the gallbladder is pexied to the diaphragm using two partial-thickness simple interrupted absorbable sutures. The greater omentum is packed in the space and tacked with a few sutures to reduce the risk of torsion of adjacent liver lobes.

Right lateral and caudate process of the caudate liver lobe

The right division of the liver consists of the right lateral lobe and the caudate process of the caudate liver lobe (Figures 15.15–15.17). The right lateral liver lobe has no conjoined parenchyma with the right medial liver lobe and the caudal vena cava is bare between the two lobes. The right lateral and the caudate process of the caudate lobe have conjoined parenchyma. The caudate and papillary processes of the caudate liver lobe have conjoined parenchyma. The right portal vein supplies blood to these liver lobes. The right portal vein typically divides into two veins: the right lateral lobar portal vein and the caudate lobar portal vein. The lobar hepatic artery is

cranial and deep to the lobar portal vein. The lobar bile duct is typically superficial (ventral) and cranial to the right lateral lobar portal vein. The right lateral lobe commonly has two hepatic veins, one of which is usually more dominant and leaves the cranial part of the lobe to join the vena cava; the smaller vein typically exits the caudal part of the lobe. The caudate process typically has one lobar portal vein, but occasionally will have two. The caudate lobar hepatic artery is located caudal and ventral to its lobar portal vein. The lobar biliary duct of this lobe may run parallel to the lobar hepatic artery or it may run dorsal and cranial to the caudate lobar portal vein. The caudate lobe has one primary hepatic lobar vein and one to two smaller hepatic veins.

Exposure of the right lateral liver lobe is achieved with retraction of the central division of the liver and the descending duodenum to the left. The right triangular ligament is divided to improve the mobility of the lobe. Right-angle forceps are bluntly passed through the parenchyma of the liver just cranial to the right lateral lobar portal vein, and then passed around all inflow vascular structures and bile ducts to exit just caudal to the right lobar portal vein. An Endo GIA is placed through this tunnel, staples deployed, and structures divided. Starting from the cranial aspect of the right lateral liver lobe, the parenchyma is divided off the vena cava. Typically at the cranial extent of the right lateral lobe a hepatic vein is encountered and it is ligated and divided. The dissection is continued caudally until all hepatic venous branches have been isolated, ligated, and divided (using an Endo GIA or ligatures). A similar process is used to remove the caudate process. The hepatorenal ligament is divided and the conjoining parenchyma to the papillary process is bluntly divided. If the entire right division is to be removed *en bloc*, the right portal vein, lobar artery, and biliary duct are ligated and divided and

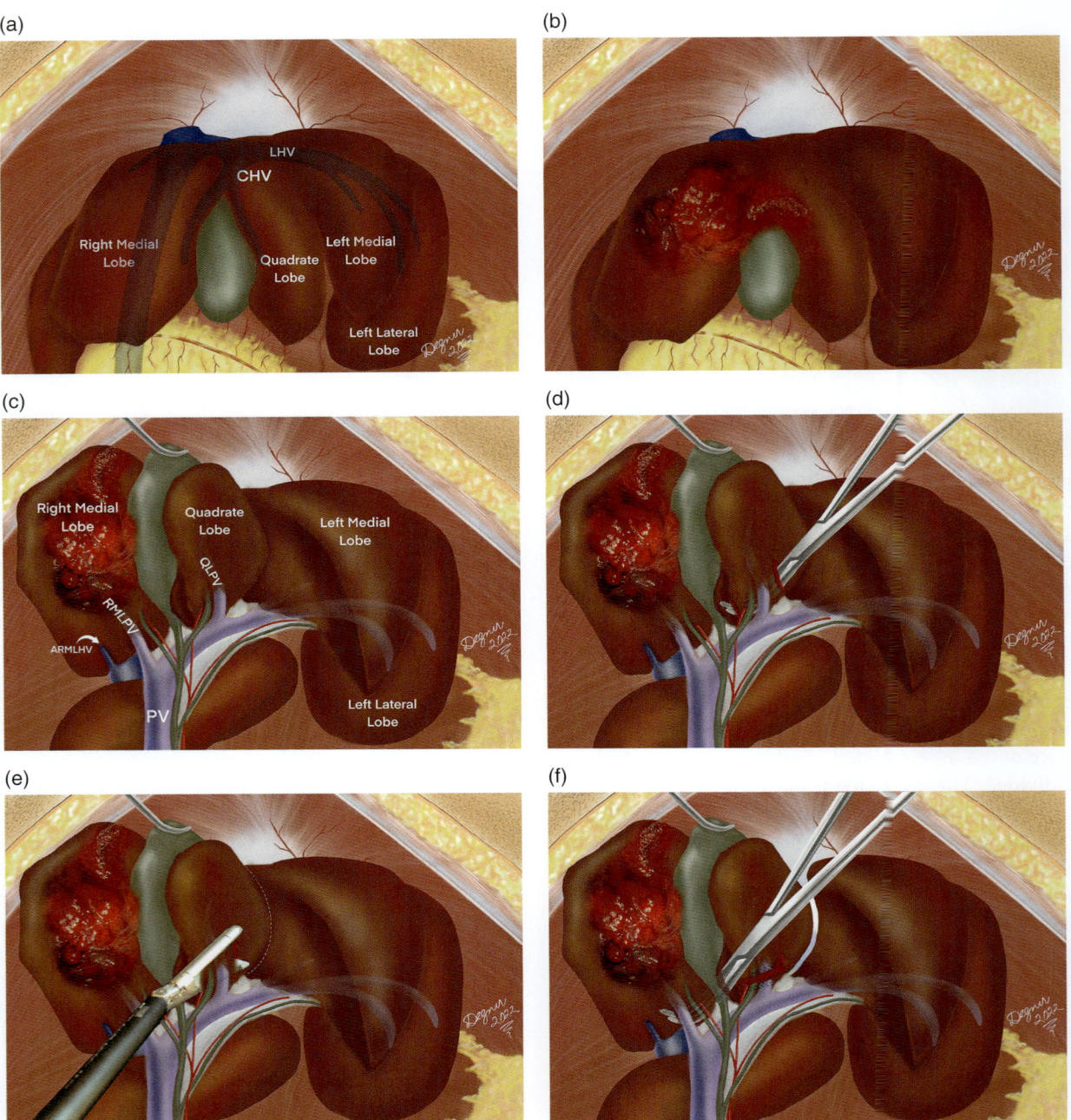

Figure 15.14 (a) Ventral and diaphragmatic surface of the liver. (b) Tumors involving either quadrate or right medial lobe or both are usually more easily and completely removed by removing the entire central division. The illustration depicts a tumor that involves both lobes. (c) In order to expose the visceral surface of the central division of the liver, the gallbladder is grasped with forceps (if it is also removed with the central division) to elevate the central division of the liver. Note: the accessory right medial lobar hepatic vein may be located on either the visceral or diaphragmatic surface of the right medial lobe and less commonly is completely encompassed by parenchyma. (d) Right-angle forceps are used to bluntly penetrate through the liver parenchyma at the hilus of the quadrate lobe, just cranial to the quadrate lobar portal vein, to create a tunnel for an Endo GIA stapler for occlusion and division of the inflow structures and hepatic duct of this lobe. (e) An Endo GIA is passed through the parenchymal tunnel to encompass the inflow vascular structures and lobar hepatic duct of the quadrate lobe. (f) The inflow structures and hepatic duct of the quadrate lobe are stapled and divided. Right-angle forceps are passed through the parenchyma just to the left of the cystic duct of the gallbladder and around the inflow structures and hepatic duct of the right medial liver lobe. (g) An Endo GIA is passed through the parenchymal tunnel to encompass the inflow vascular structures and lobar hepatic duct of the right medial liver lobe. (h) The inflow structures and hepatic duct of the right medial liver lobe are stapled and divided. Right-angle forceps are passed through the parenchyma around the accessory right medial lobar hepatic vein. (i) An Endo GIA is passed through the parenchymal tunnel to encompass the accessory right medial hepatic vein, staples deployed, and vein divided. (j) The parenchyma between the left medial liver lobe and the quadrate lobe is bluntly divided with a Poole suction tip and interlobar vessels are sealed and divided as they are encountered with LigaSure to expose the central hepatic vein. Care is taken to avoid damage to the left hepatic vein. (k) An Endo GIA is placed on the central hepatic vein. (l) The central vein is stapled and divided. (m) As mentioned previously, the accessory hepatic vein may be located on the diaphragmatic surface of the right medial liver lobe. (n) The central division of the liver is removed. ARMLHV, accessory right medial lobar hepatic vein; CHV, central hepatic vein; LHV, left hepatic vein; PV, portal vein; QLPV, quadrate lobar portal vein; RMLPV, right medial lobar portal vein.

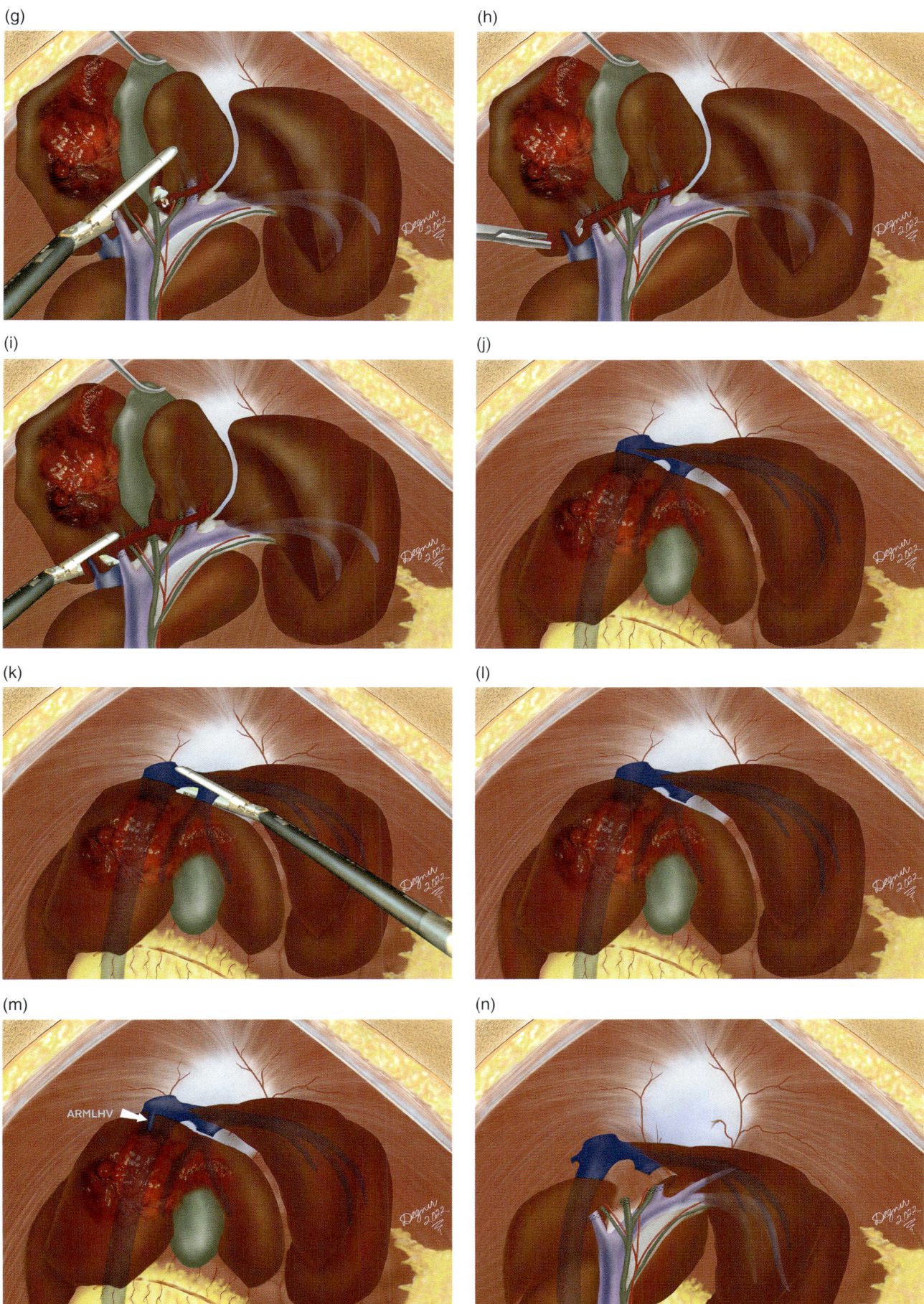

(g)

(h)

(i)

(j)

(k)

(l)

(m)

ARMLHV

(n)

Figure 15.14 (Continued)

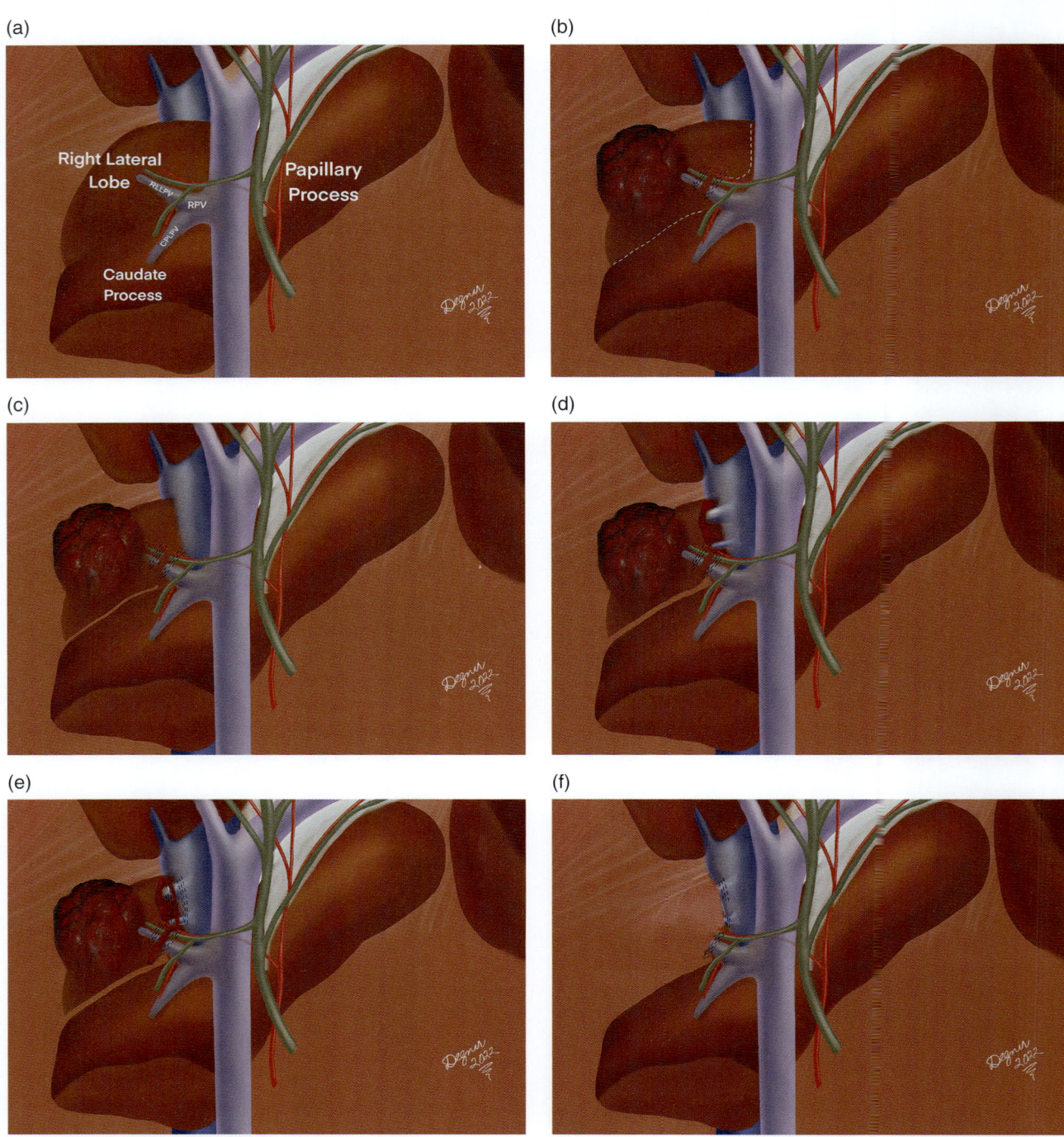

Figure 15.15 (a) Ventral view of the right division of the liver. (b) After bluntly creating a tunnel through the parenchyma around the inflow structures and lobar hepatic duct of the right lateral liver lobe, an Endo GIA stapler is used to occlude and divide these structures. The dotted lines depict the location of blunt dissection of the liver parenchyma. (c) The parenchyma of this lobe is divided from the caudal vena cava and the caudate process. (d) The hepatic veins of the right lateral lobe are exposed with further blunt parenchymal dissection. (e) An Endo GIA is used to staple and divide the hepatic lobar veins of this lobe. (f) The right medial liver lobe is removed. CPLPV, caudate process lobar portal vein; RLLPV, right lateral lobar portal vein; RPV, right portal vein.

(a)

(b)

(c)

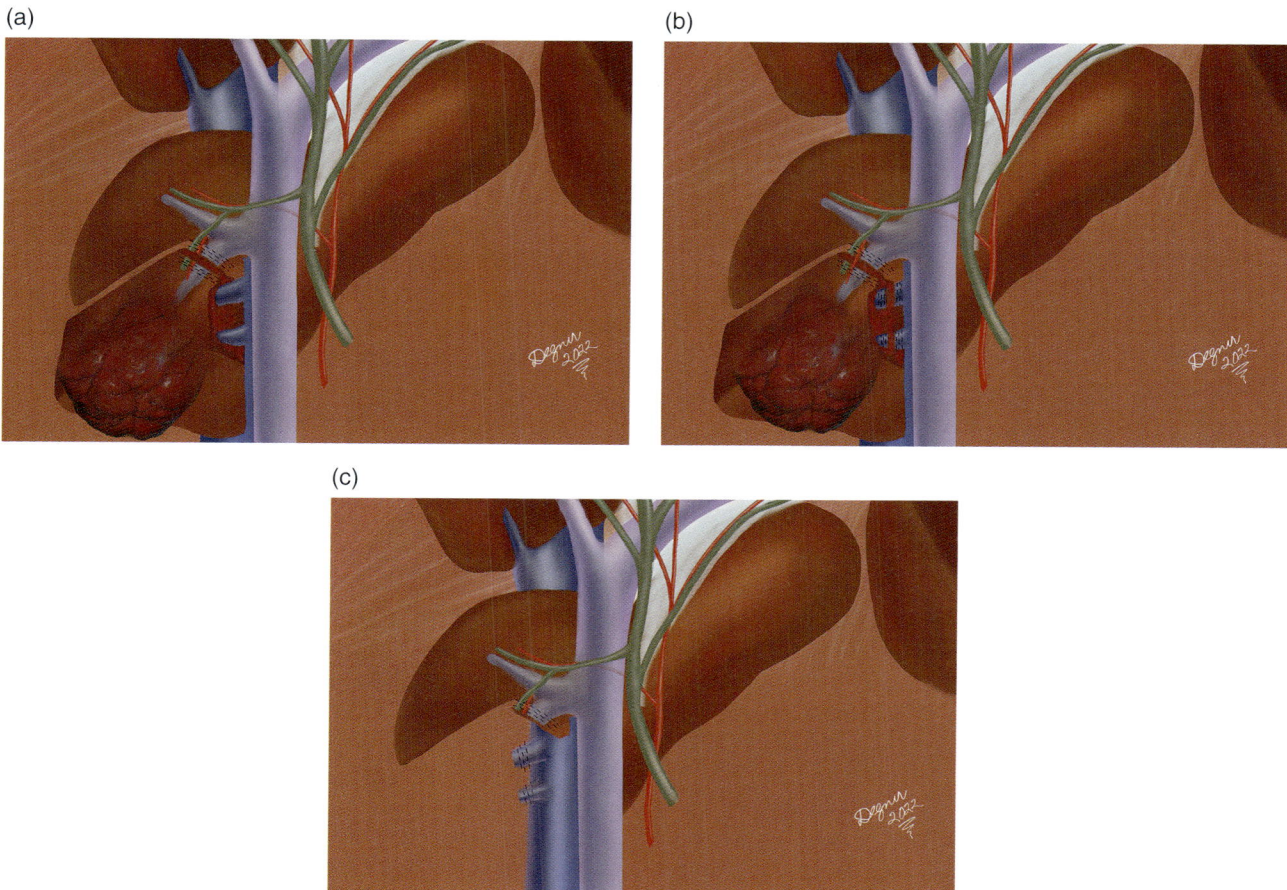

Figure 15.16 (a) After bluntly creating a tunnel through the parenchyma around the inflow structures and lobar hepatic duct of the caudate process of the caudate liver lobe, an Endo GIA stapler is used to staple and divide these structures. The parenchyma between the right lateral liver lobe and caudate process is bluntly separated, sealing and dividing the interlobar vessels with LigaSure as they are encountered. The lobar hepatic veins of this lobe extending off the caudal vena cava are exposed with blunt dissection, as the caudate process is bluntly divided from the accessory process. (b) The hepatic lobar veins of the caudate process are stapled and divided with an Endo GIA. (c) The caudate process is removed.

the parenchymal dissection is performed in a cranial-to-caudal direction, with ligation and division of lobar hepatic veins as they are encountered.

Papillary process of the caudate lobe

The papillary process of the caudate lobe is covered by the lesser omentum and is nestled within the lesser curvature of the stomach (Figure 15.18). Typically this lobe has one lobar portal vein that extends caudally off the left portal vein between the left portal lobar veins of the quadrate and right medial lobes. The lobar hepatic artery is usually superficial to the papillary lobar portal vein, but can also run dorsally. The lobar biliary duct enters the lobe dorsal to the lobar portal vein. The papillary lobar hepatic vein is deep (dorsal) to the papillary lobar portal vein and joins the left hepatic vein at the level of the bifurcation of the central and left hepatic

veins. Less commonly, the papillary hepatic vein may also directly join the vena cava. The papillary process of the caudate lobe and the caudate process of the caudate lobe typically have conjoined parenchyma.

The lesser omentum is opened and the lesser curvature of the stomach is retracted caudally to expose the papillary process of the caudate lobe. Right-angle forceps are passed through liver parenchyma adjacent to the lobar portal vein, lobar artery, and bile duct of the papillary process. These structures are then stapled and divided with an Endo GIA. The hepatic vein, which is cranial and to the left of the lobar portal vein, is isolated with a blunt instrument, stapled, and divided with an Endo GIA. The conjoined parenchyma between the two papillary and caudate processes is divided with a Poole suction tip, as conjoining vessels are sealed and divided using a vessel sealant device.

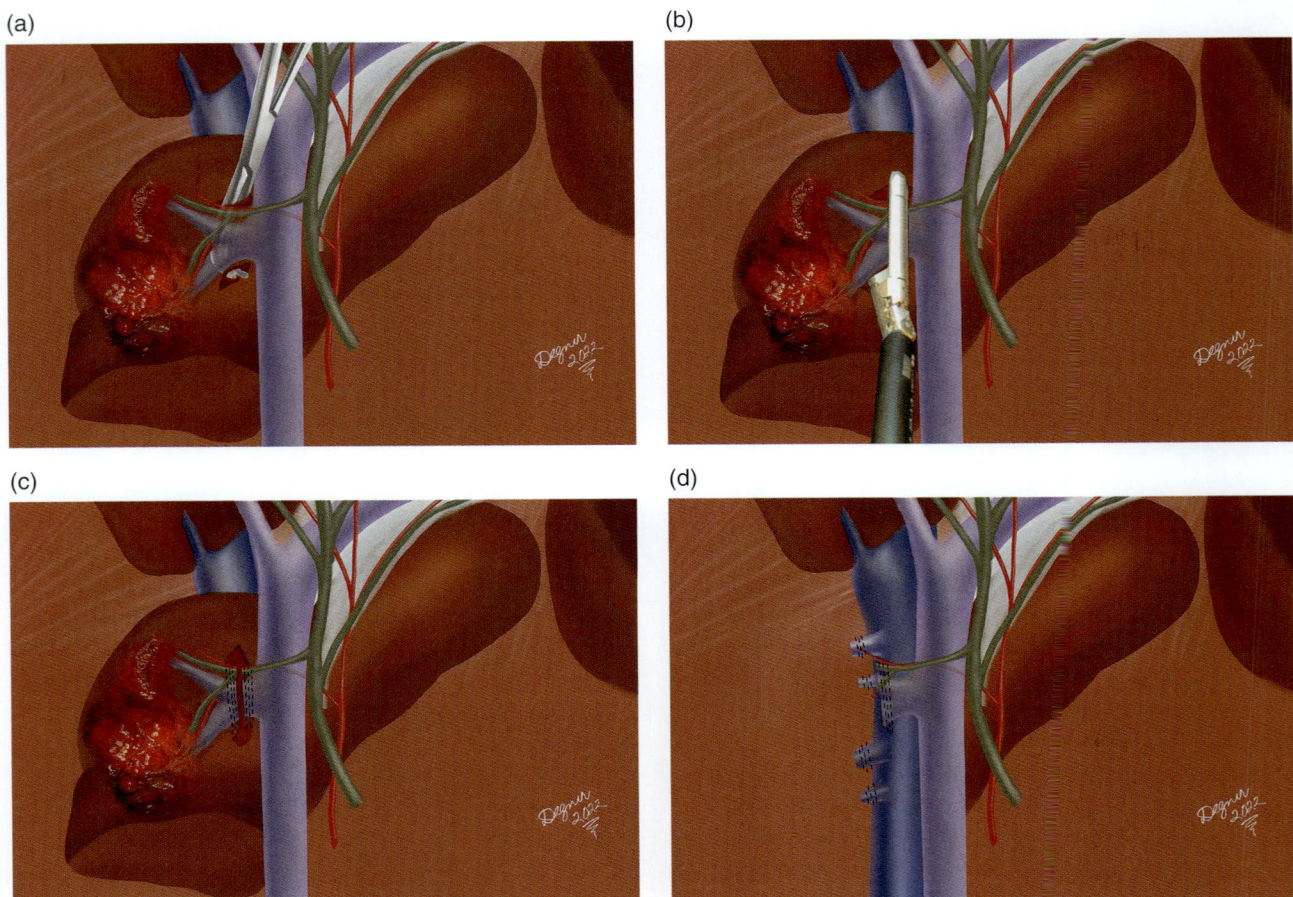

Figure 15.17 (a) Right-angle forceps are bluntly passed through the parenchyma to create a tunnel around the right portal vein, bile ducts, and lobar arteries. (b) An Endo GIA is placed through the parenchymal tunnel to encompass the vascular inflow structures and bile duct of the right division. (c) The inflow vascular structures and hepatic lobar duct of the right division are stapled and divided with an Endo GIA. The dotted line denotes the location of the blunt division of the liver parenchyma to expose the caudal vena cava and hepatic lobar veins. (d) The right division of the liver has been removed following stapling and division of the lobar hepatic veins with an Endo GIA.

Postoperative care

Supportive care is essential following liver lobectomy to ensure a stable cardiovascular status and control of pain. Rectal temperature, pulse, respiration, urinary output, and blood pressure are monitored until the patient is discharged from the hospital. At minimum, the hematocrit and total solids should be measured daily. Ideally, albumin, electrolytes, blood urea nitrogen and glucose, blood gases, and platelet count should also be evaluated daily. Analgesia can be achieved with a number of protocols, which may include a constant-rate intravenous infusion of fentanyl, or administration of morphine or buprenorphine via intramuscular or subcutaneous injection. Intravenous fluid therapy is administered for 1–2 days after surgery. Colloids such as hetastarch or plasma should be administered if serum albumin levels drop below 2.0 g/dL or if needed to treat hypotension.

Cardiovascular support with vasopressor medications is rarely indicated following routine liver lobectomy, but may be needed if blood pressure cannot be maintained with fluid and colloid therapy. In such cases, underlying causes of hypotension such as internal bleeding, systemic inflammatory response syndrome, or cardiac disease (arrhythmias) should be ruled out. Antibiotics should be administered for about 5 days to prevent growth of clostridial bacteria that normally reside in the liver.

Complications

The primary intraoperative complications include acute severe bleeding and hypotension. Bleeding risks may be minimized by understanding the vascular anatomy of the liver prior to attempting this type of surgery, and ensuring that the patient has a normal clotting profile, platelet count, and platelet function. Hypotension during

(a)

(b)

(c)

(d)

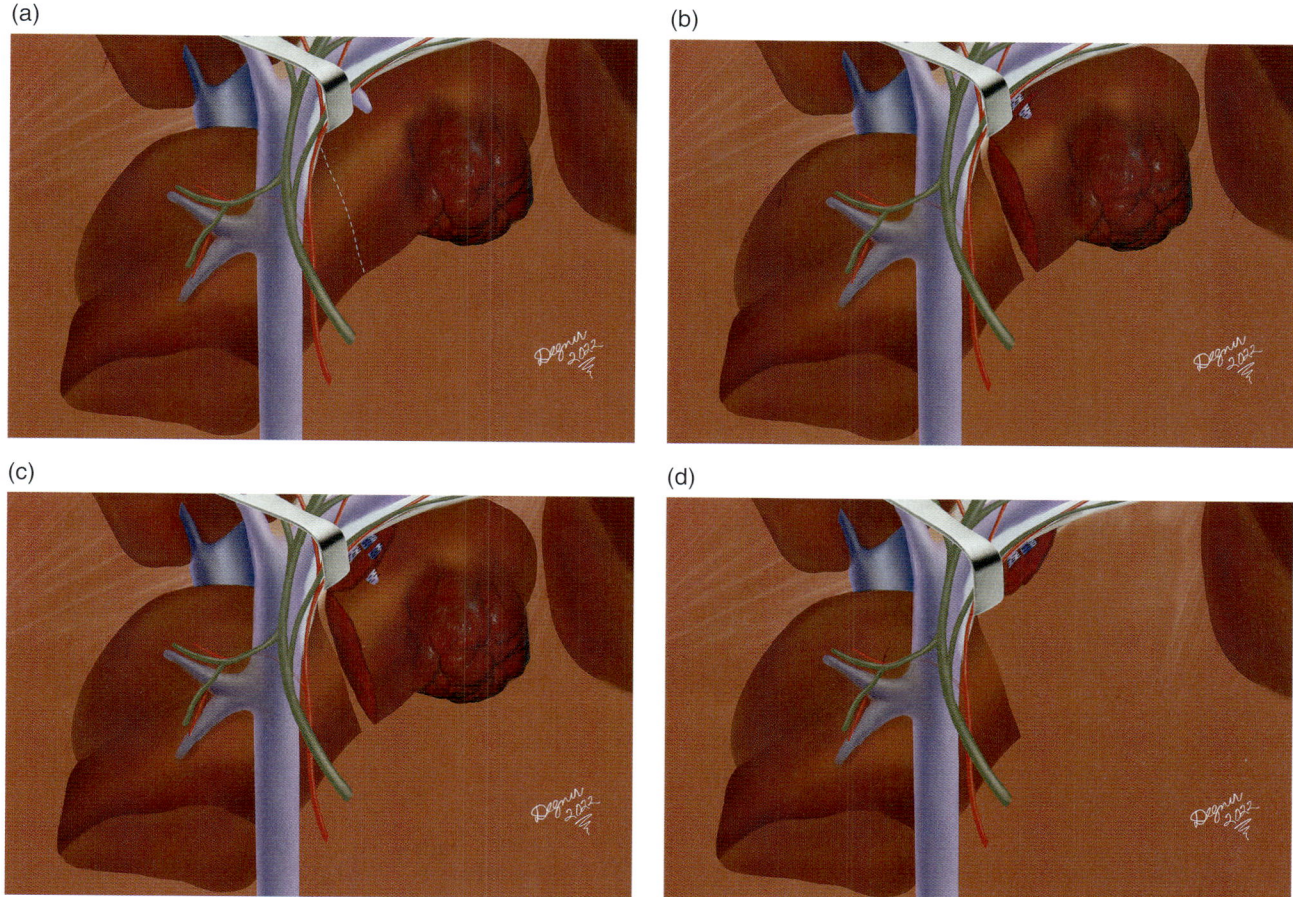

Figure 15.18 (a) The lesser omentum has been removed for illustrative purposes. The portal vein is retracted to the right and cranially. The dotted line demonstrates the line of parenchymal division of the papillary process. (b) The lobar portal vein, lobar hepatic artery, and bile duct of the papillary process are isolated *en bloc* by creating a blunt path of dissection through the surrounding parenchyma. These structures are stapled and divided with an Endo GIA. The parenchyma of the lobe is divided from the caudate process with blunt dissection and smaller vessels sealed and divided as they are encountered. (c) The hepatic lobar vein is exposed with deeper parenchymal dissection. (d) The papillary process is removed after the hepatic lobar vein is stapled and divided with an Endo GIA.

surgery should be managed with fluid support and tilting the patient to reduce compression of the vena cava. Reported intraoperative complications include hemorrhage and compromise of the blood supply of an adjacent liver lobe during lobar resection (left lateral lobe compromised with left medial resection) (Liptak *et al.* 2004). Torsion of an adjacent liver lobe is an infrequent complication after surgery. The greater omentum may be packed between lobes to reduce the risk of this complication. Tumor recurrence is an uncommon complication following hepatocellular carcinoma removal, but may occur with tumors that cannot be resected due to deep invasion of the tumor within the liver. Metastatic disease may also occur with some liver tumors. Therefore, chest radiography and abdominal ultrasound should be performed every 3–4 months.

References

Bachellier, P., Ayav, A., Pai, M. et al. (2007). Laparoscopic liver resection assisted with radiofrequency. *American Journal of Surgery* 193: 427–430.

Balkman, C. (2009). Hepatobiliary tumors in dogs and cats. *Veterinary Clinics of North America: Small Animal Practice* 39: 617–625.

Befeler, A.S. and Bisceglie, A.M. (2002). Hepatocellular carcinoma: diagnosis and treatment. *Gastroenterology* 122: 1609–1619.

Bigge, L.A., Brown, D.J., and Penninck, D.G. (2001). Correlation between coagulation profile findings and bleeding complications after ultrasound-guided biopsies: 434 cases (1993–1996). *Journal of the American Animal Hospital Association* 37: 228–233.

Bjorling, D.E., Prasse, K.W., and Holmes, R.A. (1985). Partial hepatectomy in dogs. *Compendium on Continuing Education for the Practicing Veterinarian* 7: 257–266.

Burti, S., Zotti, A., Contiero, B., and Banzato, T. (2021). Computed tomography features for differentiating malignant and benign focal liver lesions in dogs: a meta-analysis. *Veterinary Journal* 278: 105773.

Burti, S., Zotti, A., Rubini, G. et al. (2020). Contrast-enhanced ultrasound features of malignant focal liver masses in dogs. *Scientific Reports* 10: 6076.

Chikata, S., Nakamura, S., Katayama, R. et al. (2006). Primary chondrosarcoma in the liver of a dog. *Veterinary Pathology* 43: 1033–1036.

Coakley, F.V. and Schwartz, L.H. (2001). Imaging of hepatocellular carcinoma: a practical approach. *Seminars in Oncology* 28: 460–473.

Cole, T.L., Center, S.A., Flood, S.N. et al. (2002). Diagnostic comparison of needle and wedge biopsy specimens of the liver in dogs and cats. *Journal of the American Veterinary Medical Association* 220: 1483–1490.

Covey, J.L., Degner, D.A., Jackson, A.H. et al. (2009). Hilar liver resection in dogs. *Veterinary Surgery* 38: 104–111.

Engle, G.C. and Brodey, R.S. (1969). A retrospective study of 395 feline neoplasms. *Journal of the American Animal Hospital Association* 5: 21–31.

Evans, H.E. (1979). Digestive apparatus and abdomen. In: *Miller's Anatomy of the Dog*, 2e (ed. M.E. Miller, H.E. Evans and G.C. Christensen), 777–778. Philadelphia, PA: WB Saunders.

Evans, S.M. (1987). The radiographic appearance of primary liver neoplasia in dogs. *Veterinary Radiology* 28: 192–196.

Francavilla, A., Porter, K.A., Benichou, J. et al. (1978). Liver regeneration in dogs: morphologic and chemical changes. *Journal of Surgical Research* 25: 409–419.

Gayet, B., Cavaliere, D., Vibert, E. et al. (2007). Totally laparoscopic right hepatectomy. *American Journal of Surgery* 194: 685–689.

Hanson, R.K., Pigott, A.M., and Linklater, A.K.J. (2017). Incidence of blood transfusion requirement and factors associated with transfusion following liver lobectomy in dogs and cats: 72 cases (2007–2015). *Journal of the American Veterinary Medical Association* 251 (8): 929–934.

Jeraj, K., Yano, B., Osborne, C.A. et al. (1981). Primary hepatic osteosarcoma in a dog. *Journal of the American Veterinary Medical Association* 179: 1000–1003.

de Jonge, J., Zondervan, P.E., Kooi, P.P. et al. (2003). Directing portal flow is essential for graft survival in auxiliary partial heterotopic liver transplantation in the dog. *European Surgical Research* 35: 14–21.

Kanemoto, H., Ohno, K., Nakashima, K. et al. (2009). Characterization of canine focal liver lesions with contrast-enhanced ultrasound using a novel contrast agent, sonazoid. *Veterinary Radiology and Ultrasound* 50: 188–194.

Kapatkin, A.S., Mullen, H.S., Matthiesen, D.T., and Patnaik, A.K. (1992). Leiomyosarcoma in dogs: 44 cases (1883–1988). *Journal of the American Veterinary Medical Association* 201: 1077–1079.

Kinsley, J.R., Gilson, S.D., Hauptman, J. et al. (2015). Factors associated with long-term survival in dogs undergoing liver lobectomy as treatment for liver tumors. *Canadian Veterinary Journal* 56: 598–604.

Kosovsky, J.E., Manfra-Marretta, S., Matthiesen, D.T., and Patnik, A.K. (1989). Results of partial hepatectomy in 18 dogs with hepatocellular carcinoma. *Journal of the American Animal Hospital Association* 25: 203–206.

Lawrence, H.J., Erb, H.N., and Harvey, H.J. (1994). Nonlymphomatous hepatobiliary masses in cats: 41 cases (1972 to 1991). *Veterinary Surgery* 23: 365–368.

Lewis, D.D., Bellenger, C.R., Lewis, D.T., and Latter, M.R. (1990). Hepatic lobectomy in the dog: a comparison of stapling and ligation techniques. *Veterinary Surgery* 19: 221–225.

Lippo, N.J., Williams, J.E., Brawer, R.S., and Sobel, K.E. (2008). Acute hemobilia and hemocholecyst in 2 dogs with gall bladder carcinoid. *Journal of Veterinary Internal Medicine* 22: 1249–1252.

Liptak, J.M., Dernell, W.S., Monnet, E. et al. (2004). Massive hepatocellular carcinoma in dogs: 48 cases (1992–2002). *Journal of the American Veterinary Medical Association* 225: 1225–1230.

Magne, M.L. and Withrow, S.J. (1985). Hepatic neoplasia. *Veterinary Clinics of North America: Small Animal Practice* 15: 243–256.

Martin, R.A., Lanz, O.I., and Tobias, K.M. (2003). Liver and biliary system. In: *Textbook of Small Animal Surgery*, 3e (ed. D.H. Slatter), 716–717. Philadelphia, PA: WB Saunders.

McDonald, R.K. and Helman, R.G. (1986). Hepatic mesenchymoma in a dog. *Journal of the American Veterinary Medical Association* 188: 1052–1053.

Morrell, C.N., Volk, M.V., and Mankowski, J.L. (2002). A carcinoid tumor in the gall bladder of a dog. *Veterinary Pathology* 39: 756–758.

Nuzzo, G., Giulante, F., Giovannini, I. et al. (2001). Liver resection with or without pedicle clamping. *American Journal of Surgery* 181: 238–246.

Patnaik, A.K., Hurvitz, A.I., and Lieberman, P.H. (1980). Canine hepatic neoplasms: a clinicopathologic study. *Veterinary Pathology* 17: 553–564.

Patnaik, A.K., Hurvitz, A.I., Lieberman, P.H., and Johnson, G.F. (1981a). Canine hepatocellular carcinoma. *Veterinary Pathology* 18: 427–438.

Patnaik, A.K., Lieberman, P.H., Hurvitz, A.I., and Johnson, G.F. (1981b). Canine hepatic carcinoids. *Veterinary Pathology* 18: 445–453.

Patnaik, A.K., Lieberman, P.H., Erlandson, R.A., and Antonescu, C. (2005a). Hepatobiliary neuroendocrine carcinoma in cats: a clinicopathologic, immunohistochemical, and ultrastructural study of 17 cases. *Veterinary Pathology* 42: 331–338.

Patnaik, A.K., Liu, S., and Johnson, G.F. (1976). Extraskeletal osteosarcoma of the liver in a dog. *Journal of Small Animal Practice* 17: 365–370.

Patnaik, A.K., Newman, S.J., Scase, T. et al. (2005b). Canine hepatic neuroendocrine carcinoma: an immunohistochemical and electron microscopic study. *Veterinary Pathology* 42: 140–146.

Post, G. and Patnaik, A.K. (1992). Nonhemopoietic hepatic neoplasms in cats: 21 cases (1983–1988). *Journal of the American Veterinary Medical Association* 201: 1080–1082.

Roth, L. (2001). Comparison of liver cytology and biopsy diagnoses in dogs and cats: 56 cases. *Veterinary Clinical Pathology* 30: 35–38.

Schmidt, R.E. and Langham, R.F. (1967). A survey of feline neoplasms. *Journal of the American Veterinary Medical Association* 151: 1325–1328.

Strombeck, D.R. (1978). Clinicopathologic features of primary and metastatic neoplastic disease of the liver in dogs. *Journal of the American Veterinary Medical Association* 173: 267–269.

Takayama, T., Makuuchi, M., Kubota, K. et al. (2001). Randomized comparison of ultrasonic vs. clamp transection of the liver. *Archives of Surgery* 136: 922–928.

Tobias, K.M. (2007). Surgical stapling devices in veterinary medicine: a review. *Veterinary Surgery* 36: 341–349.

Trigo, F.J., Thompson, H., Breeze, R.G., and Nash, S. (1982). The pathology of liver tumors in the dog. *Journal of Comparative Pathology* 92: 21–39.

Wang, K.Y., Panciera, D.L., Al-Rukibat, R.K., and Radi, Z.A. (2004). Accuracy of ultrasound-guided fine-needle aspiration of the liver and cytologic findings in dogs and cats: 97 cases (1990–2000). *Journal of the American Veterinary Medical Association* 224: 75–78.

Willard, M.D., Dunstan, R.W., and Faulkner, J. (1988). Neuroendocrine carcinoma of the gall bladder in a dog. *Journal of the American Veterinary Medical Association* 192: 926–928.

16

Gallbladder Mucocele

Steve J. Mehler and Philipp D. Mayhew

Etiology

A biliary mucocele is the distension of a bile-containing structure or cavity by an inappropriate accumulation of mucus (Newell *et al.* 1995; Pike *et al.* 2004a,b; Worley *et al.* 2004; Cornejo & Webster 2005; Aguirre *et al.* 2007; Center 2009). Biliary stasis, decreased gallbladder motility, and altered absorption of water from the gallbladder lumen are predisposing factors to biliary sludge. Biliary sludge may be a precipitating factor for the development of canine biliary mucoceles. Primary extrahepatic biliary tract (EHBT) obstruction does not appear to play a primary role in the formation of gallbladder mucoceles. However, the presence and progression of gelatinous material in the gallbladder may lead to EHBT obstruction. It has been our experience that in the majority of dogs with gallbladder mucoceles, the disease is contained within the gallbladder and cystic duct and does not involve the hepatic ducts or the common bile duct.

Gallbladder mucoceles have recently received much attention in the veterinary literature and have been perceived as a relatively new disease. It is interesting that in a retrospective study evaluating all diseases leading to surgery of the EHBT, no mention of gallbladder mucocele was made (Mehler *et al.* 2004). At the time of its writing, the pathologists at the institution represented in the report were not using the terminology "gallbladder mucocele" to describe the common histologic changes seen in the gallbladder wall. Instead, the histologic abnormalities associated with "gallbladder mucoceles" were being described, but under the morphologic diagnosis of acalculous necrotizing cholecystitis. There are many surgeons, internists, and pathologists who agree that

gallbladder mucoceles are not a new disease or condition, but instead develop along the continuum of progressive cholecystitis, somewhere between acute cholecystitis and chronic necrotizing cholecystitis with rupture. In fact, most histopathologic descriptions of gallbladder mucocele presently focus on the mucosal hyperplasia and less on the description associated with cholecystitis. Histopathology reports detailed the cellular and vascular changes associated with transmural ischemic necrosis and briefly mentioned the cystic mucosal hyperplasia seen in the mucosa of the gallbladder wall.

The underlying lesion has been described as cystic mucosal hyperplasia. Hypersecretion of mucus leads to an accumulation of thick gelatinous bile within the gallbladder. Increased viscosity over a period of weeks or months leads to thick gelatinous material eventually occupying the entire lumen of the gallbladder, and in some cases also being present in the common bile duct and hepatic ducts. This can lead to EHBT obstruction or development of bile peritonitis secondary to gallbladder rupture. The cause of the condition remains largely unknown, but recent evidence has linked gallbladder mucocele to certain intercurrent diseases with a focus on endocrinopathies and other metabolic abnormalities. Particular genetic predispositions may play a role, as Shetland sheepdogs have been shown to be predisposed to gallbladder disease, albeit not specifically gallbladder mucocele formation (Aguirre *et al.* 2007). Several previous studies have commented anecdotally on the relatively high incidence of endocrinopathies that are present in dogs with gallbladder mucocele (Pike *et al.* 2004a; Worley *et al.* 2004; Aguirre *et al.* 2007). In a

Small Animal Soft Tissue Surgery, Second Edition. Edited by Eric Monnet.
© 2023 John Wiley & Sons, Inc. Published 2023 by John Wiley & Sons, Inc.
Companion website: www.wiley.com/go/monnet/small

report evaluating a possible association between gallbladder mucocele and hyperadrenocorticism and hypothyroidism, both conditions were found to have an association with gallbladder mucocele (Mesich *et al.* 2009). Dogs diagnosed with hypothyroidism were three times more likely to have gallbladder mucocele than dogs without hypothyroidism, and the odds of having a mucocele in dogs with hyperadrenocorticism were 29 times greater than for dogs without hyperadrenocorticism. In all, 21% of dogs with gallbladder mucocele had hyperadrenocorticism compared to 2% in the control group. In the case of hypothyroidism, 14% of gallbladder mucocele dogs had the condition compared with 5% in the control group. Certain limitations were present in this study and no causal relationship can be proven from these data (Mesich *et al.* 2009).

Diagnosis

History and physical examination

Patients with gallbladder mucocele can be asymptomatic. However, most patients are presented for vomiting (70%), anorexia (65%), lethargy (65%), and diarrhea (12.5%) (Cornejo & Webster 2005). Shetland sheepdogs may be predisposed to gallbladder mucocele (Aguirre *et al.* 2007). On physical examination, animals exhibit pain on abdominal palpation and are icteric. Rectal temperature is elevated if perforation of the mucocele is present.

Bloodwork

On bloodwork an inflammatory leukogram is present. Alkaline phosphatase is elevated in 81% of cases, followed by elevation of alanine aminotransferase (79%), augmentation of γ-glutamyltransferase (67%), and augmentation of total bilirubin (69%) (Worley *et al.* 2004; Cornejo & Webster 2005; Mayhew *et al.* 2008). Dogs with gallbladder mucocele have decreased levels of serum 25-hydroxyvitamin D; it is unknown whether this a cause or an effect of the disease (Jaffey *et al.* 2020). Coagulation parameters are also abnormal in patients with gallbladder mucoceles, especially elevations in protein C and thromboelastography (TEG) amplitude (Pavlick *et al.* 2021).

Urinalysis

A recent publication identified proteinuria as a common finding associated with gallbladder mucocele. Bloodwork should be concurrently performed to evaluate kidney health (Lindaberry *et al.* 2021).

Ultrasonography

Ultrasonography has been useful in diagnosing gallbladder mucoceles and is 86% sensitive and 100% specific in diagnosing gallbladder rupture associated with mucoceles

(Figure 16.1) (Besso *et al.* 2000). On ultrasound the gallbladder mucocele is heterogeneous, with the center more echodense than the periphery. Very often a stellate pattern is observed in the center of the gallbladder, commonly referred to as a "kiwi fruit" appearance. The presence of false negatives is likely due to some gallbladder ruptures being temporarily sealed with liver or omentum. Also, some patients with chemical or septic peritonitis that are severely dehydrated and cardiovascularly unstable at presentation may have little peritoneal effusion until they are fluid resuscitated. A third reason for this finding may be due to the lack of an actual fluid component within the markedly organized and chronic mucocele. Up to half of patients with gallbladder mucoceles have gallbladder rupture at the time of diagnosis (Besso *et al.* 2000; Pike *et al.* 2004a,b; Worley *et al.* 2004). Most ruptured mucoceles contain semisolidified bile and leak slowly, causing an acute, but local chemical, sterile peritonitis.

Treatment

The treatment of choice for a dog with EHBT obstruction or peritonitis due to a gallbladder mucocele is surgical. If the diagnosis of the mucocele is incidental or the dog does not show obvious clinical signs related to an obstruction of the biliary system, medical treatment might be attempted with ursodeoxycholic acid (15 mg/kg per day orally [p.o.]). Ursodeoxycholic acid is a choleretic that will increase the secretion of bile, although it is contraindicated in EHBT obstruction. The patient should be monitored with bloodwork and ultrasound every six weeks to evaluate the progression of the mucocele. If liver enzymes or bilirubin keep increasing or the ultrasonographic changes are getting worse, it is an indication that medical treatment is failing. There is a report of two cases of gallbladder mucocele regressing on medical treatment (Walter *et al.* 2008).

The surgical treatment of choice for gallbladder mucocele is cholecystectomy (Pike *et al.* 2004a,b; Worley *et al.* 2004). Given that this is a disease of the gallbladder and that many of the gallbladders submitted for histopathology have evidence of necrosis, it is advised not to perform a cholecystotomy or cholecystoenteric anastomosis. Before removing the gallbladder, the surgeon should assess the bile duct to be certain there is no obstruction. An irresolvable obstruction of the common bile duct would preclude a cholecystectomy, and a cholecystoenterostomy may have to be performed in such rare cases. It has been our experience that many dogs with gallbladder mucoceles have gelatinous material within the cystic duct, the hepatic ducts, or the common bile duct. Given that this is a disease of the gallbladder,

(a)   (b)

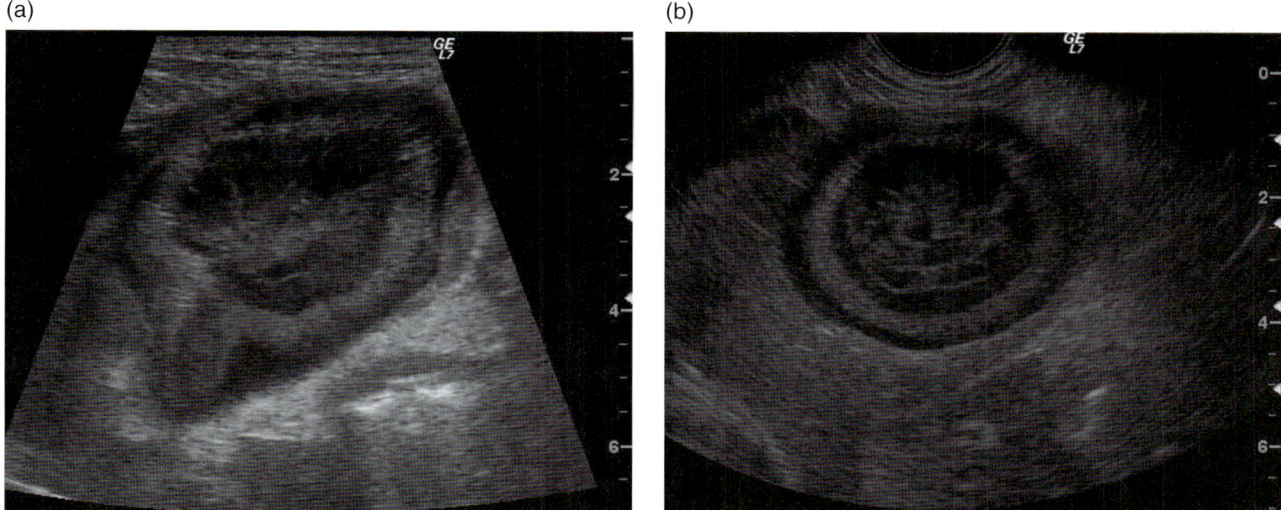

Figure 16.1 Abdominal ultrasound images of a dog with a gallbladder mucocele demonstrating the typical (a) "kiwi fruit" (or "strawberry" in this case) or (b) stellate pattern. Source: Courtesy of Dr. Jennifer Bouma.

many surgeons recommend performing a cholecystectomy and external evaluation of the extrahepatic ducts by direct palpation. In some cases, this technique will fail to identify sludge within the hepatic ducts and/or the common bile duct, and postoperative obstruction of the bile duct is likely to occur (Figure 16.2).

It is our recommendation that in all dogs with long-standing or clinical gallbladder mucoceles, the extrahepatic bile ducts be externally palpated and internally flushed with saline to assure the patency of the system. This can be accomplished by either antegrade or retrograde access and flushing. Retrograde catheterization has been associated with more complications, including postoperative pancreatitis (Putterman *et al.* 2021). Catheterization of the bile duct in either direction is associated with a higher risk for pancreatitis compared to noncatheterized bile duct patients (Piegols *et al.* 2021). An antegrade approach is performed by utilizing a cholecystotomy incision that has been made to evacuate the sludge from the gallbladder. A 5 or 8 Fr catheter is advanced from the cholecystotomy into the cystic duct and the bile duct. The duct is then flushed with sterile saline. Patency is assessed by direct visualization of saline at the major duodenal papilla or by palpating the flow of lavage solution entering the proximal duodenum. A second method of confirming a patent extrahepatic duct system is by retrograde catheterization. The major duodenal papilla is identified by making a duodenotomy over the papilla at the antimesenteric surface of the proximal descending duodenum. Once the papilla is identified, a red rubber catheter is introduced and a gentle flush with sterile saline is performed. Because the EHBT is a closed system, when flushing retrogradely it is

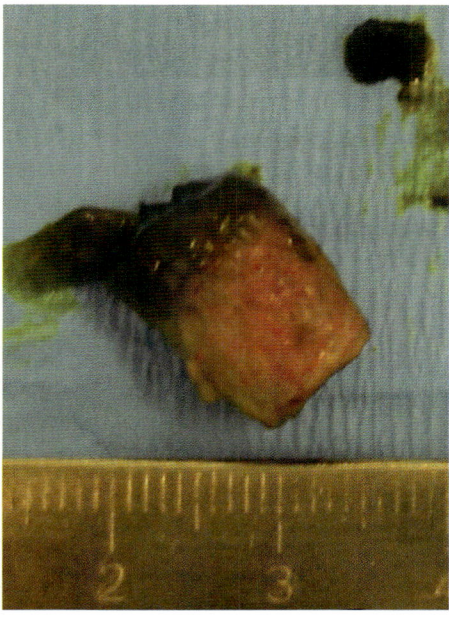

Figure 16.2 A large mucobiliary plug that was removed from the common bile duct of a dog with a gallbladder mucocele. This plug was removed by a choledochotomy incision.

possible to exert enough force that sludge or concretions may enter the hepatic ducts or intrahepatic biliary system. One method to avoid this is to complete the cholecystectomy after making sure that the bile duct is patent and to leave the transected cystic duct open, as described for antegrade flushing (Figure 16.3). Therefore the sludge will come through the open cystic duct instead of being pushed into the hepatic ducts. Some surgeons have also recommended using a red rubber catheter that is half or less the diameter of the major duodenal papilla,

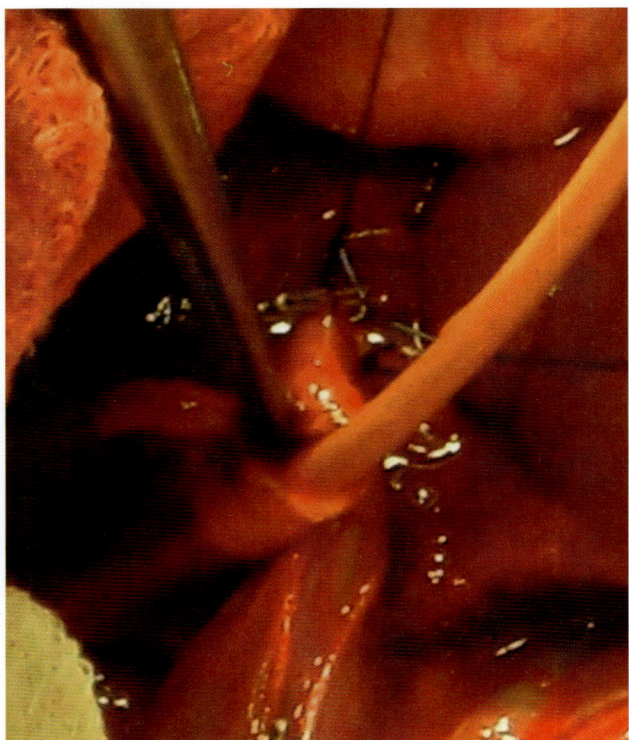

Figure 16.3 An intraoperative image of a dog with a gallbladder mucocele. The gallbladder has been removed from the cystic duct and the cystic artery has been ligated with vascular clips and 4-0 polydioxanone sutures. The cystic duct is catheterized with a 5 Fr red rubber catheter and a gentle antegrade flush is being performed. Saline is observed in the duodenum through the duodenotomy incision.

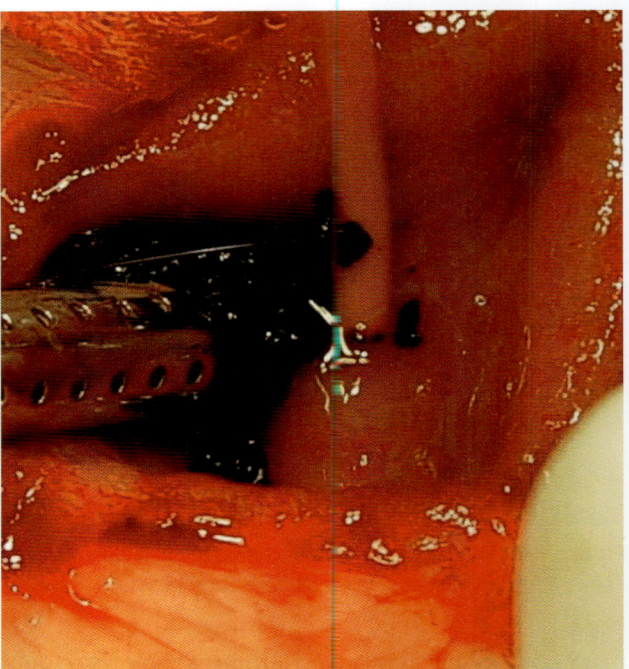

Figure 16.4 An intraoperative image of a dog with a gallbladder mucocele. Flushing of the biliary tract with sterile saline is being performed retrogradely via catheterization of the major duodenal papilla from a duodenotomy incision.

so that retrograde flushing against a closed EHBT will allow excess saline to leak out around the catheter at the papilla. The catheter is inserted retrogradely through the major duodenal papilla to the level of the cystic duct. This is performed with great care, as iatrogenic rupture of the bile duct may occur. With this retrograde technique the seal of the cystic duct can be tested after closure of the cystic duct.

The cystic artery is double ligated. Biliary sludge within the cystic duct is milked into the gallbladder and vascular clips or encircling sutures are used to close off the cystic duct. The cystic duct is then transected between the two sutures or clips. The cystic duct remnant is inspected, and if the duct appears friable a distally placed transfixation suture or an oversew of the duct is required. After completion of ligation of the cystic duct, gentle lavage with a retrograde catheter allows testing of the security of the ligatures on the cystic duct remnant, as well as permitting evacuation of the extrahepatic bile ducts (Figure 16.4).

Dogs with biliary mucoceles that undergo cholecystectomy and survive the immediate perioperative period have an excellent long-term prognosis. Overall mortality rates are reported to be 20–39% for this disease (Pike et al. 2004a,b; Worley et al. 2004; Aguirre et al. 2007); however, early surgical intervention may significantly reduce mortality rate to 2% (Aguirre et al. 2007; Mayhew et al. 2008; Youn et al. 2018). The resected gallbladder is submitted for histopathology and a piece of the mucosa for microbiologic testing. Liver biopsies and cultures should also be obtained and submitted. Bacteria commonly found in a gallbladder mucocele are enteric organisms (*Escherichia coli*, *Enterobacter* spp., *Enterococcus* spp., *Staphylococcus* spp., and *Streptococcus* spp.) (Besso et al. 2000; Pike et al. 2004a,b). Cholecystitis is a common comorbidity associated with gallbladder mucocele (Rogers et al. 2020).

There have been some sporadic case reports regarding the medical dissolution and resolution of gallbladder mucoceles (Walter et al. 2008; Center 2009). We agree that a proactive course should be taken in most patients with gallbladder mucoceles, and that patients with an incidental mucocele or "premucocele" on ultrasound should be considered as candidates for cholecystectomy. A current trend is to wait to perform a cholecystectomy on these patients until they have failed medical management, have become systemically ill, or the gallbladder has ruptured. This "wait and see" philosophy has yielded mortality rates of 20–30% in dogs with gallbladder mucoceles (Pike *et al.* 2004a,b; Worley *et al.* 2004). Many surgeons are now recommending that a cholecystectomy be performed in patients with gallbladder mucoceles at initial presentation or if found as an incidental finding on abdominal ultrasound. Laparoscopic cholecystectomy in the clinically unaffected gallbladder mucocele patient has been found to have an excellent outcome and rapid return to normal function in the small number of cases reported (see Chapter 17 for a description of the technique).

References

Aguirre, A.L., Center, S.A., Randolph, J.F. et al. (2007). Gallbladder disease in Shetland sheepdogs: 38 cases (1995–2005). *Journal of the American Veterinary Medical Association* 231: 79–88.

Besso, J.G., Wrigley, R.H., Gliatto, J.M., and Webster, C.R. (2000). Ultrasonographic appearance and clinical findings in 14 dogs with gallbladder mucocele. *Veterinary Radiology and Ultrasound* 41: 261–271.

Center, S.A. (2009). Diseases of the gallbladder and biliary tree. *Veterinary Clinics of North America Small Animal Practice* 39: 543–598.

Cornejo, L. and Webster, C.R.L. (2005). Canine gallbladder mucoceles. *Compendium on Continuing Education for the Practicing Veterinarian* 27: 912–930.

Jaffey, J.A., Matheson, J., Shumway, K. et al. (2020). Serum 25-hydroxyvitamin D concentrations in dogs with gallbladder mucocele. *PLOS ONE* 15: e0244102.

Lindaberry, C., Vaden, S., Aicher, K.M. et al. (2021). Proteinuria in dogs with gallbladder mucocele formation: a retrospective case control study. *Journal of Veterinary Internal Medicine* 35: 878–886.

Mayhew, P.D., Mehler, S.J., and Radhakrishnan, A. (2008). Laparoscopic cholecystectomy for management of uncomplicated gall bladder mucocele in six dogs. *Veterinary Surgery* 37: 625–630.

Mehler, S.J., Mayhew, P.D., Drobatz, K.J., and Holt, D.E. (2004). Variables associated with outcome in dogs undergoing extrahepatic biliary surgery: 60 cases (1988–2002). *Veterinary Surgery* 33: 644–649.

Mesich, M.L.L., Mayhew, P.D., Paek, M. et al. (2009). Gall bladder mucoceles and their association with endocrinopathies in dogs: a retrospective case–control study. *Journal of Small Animal Practice* 50: 630–635.

Newell, S.M., Selcer, B.A., Mahaffey, M.B. et al. (1995). Gallbladder mucocele causing biliary obstruction in two dogs: ultrasonographic, scintigraphic, and pathological findings. *Journal of the American Animal Hospital Association* 31: 467–472.

Pavlick, M., DeLaforcade, A., Penninck, D.G. et al. (2021). Evaluation of coagulation parameters in dogs with gallbladder mucoceles. *Journal of Veterinary Internal Medicine* 35: 1763–1772.

Piegols, H.J., Hayes, G.M., Lin, S. et al. (2021). Association between biliary tree manipulation and outcome in dogs undergoing cholecystectomy for gallbladder mucocele: a multiinstituional retrospective study. *Veterinary Surgery* 50: 767–774.

Pike, F.S., Berg, J., King, N.W. et al. (2004a). Gallbladder mucocele in dogs: 30 cases (2000–2002). *Journal of the American Veterinary Medical Association* 224: 1615–1622.

Pike, F.S., Berg, J., King, N.W. et al. (2004b). Revision to gallbladder mucocele article. *Journal of the American Veterinary Medical Association* 224: 1916–1917.

Putterman, A.B., Selmic, L.E., Kindra, C. et al. (2021). Influence of normograde versus retrograde catheterization of bile ducts in dogs treated for gallbladder mucocele. *Veterinary Surgery* 50: 784–793.

Rogers, E., Jaffey, J.A., Grahm, A. et al. (2020). Prevalence and impact of cholecystitis on outcome in dogs with gallbladder mucocele. *Journal of Veterinary Internal Medicine* 30: 97–101.

Walter, R., Dunn, M.E., d'Anjou, M.A., and Lécuyer, M. (2008). Nonsurgical resolution of gallbladder mucocele in two dogs. *Journal of the American Veterinary Medical Association* 232: 1688–1693.

Worley, D.R., Hottinger, H.A., and Lawrence, H.J. (2004). Surgical management of gallbladder mucoceles in dogs: 22 cases (1999–2003). *Journal of the American Veterinary Medical Association* 225: 1418–1422.

Youn, G., Waschak, M.J., Kunkel, K.A.R., and Gerard, P.D. (2018). Outcome of elective cholecystectomy for the treatment of gallbladder disease in dogs. *Journal of the American Veterinary Medical Association* 252: 970–975.

17

Extrahepatic Biliary Tract Obstruction

Steve J. Mehler and Philipp D. Mayhew

The earliest known disease of the extrahepatic biliary tract (EHBT) is gallstones, which date back to the twenty-first Egyptian Dynasty (1085–945 BC) and were discovered in the mummy of the Priestess of Amen (Gordon-Taylor 1937). The mummy was destroyed in the bombing of England during World War II, but the description and the radiograph of the ancient specimen survived. Cholelithiasis was also the earliest biliary tract disease described by the Greek physician Alexander Trallianus in the fifth century, and the earliest recorded cholecystectomy performed in a living patient was in 1882 by Carl Langenbuch of Berlin (Shehadi 1979).

Surgical diseases of the EHBT in small animals are not uncommon. As we are evolving into better diagnosticians and clinicians, we as a profession are recognizing the clinical signs of EHBT disease more frequently and earlier. This, accompanied by technological advances in diagnostic modalities (imaging especially), has provided us with a unique opportunity to greatly impact the outcome of our patients with EHBT disease. However, a review of the recent veterinary literature provides a bleak insight into the overall outcome of dogs and cats undergoing surgery for diseases of the EHBT. When study numbers are combined, the overall survival rate for dogs is 63.6% (140 of 220) and for cats is 41% (28 of 68) (Martin *et al.* 1986; Fahie & Martin 1995; Ludwig *et al.* 1997; Mayhew *et al.* 2002, 2006; Bacon & White 2003; Mehler *et al.* 2004; Pike *et al.* 2004a,b; Worley *et al.* 2004; Amsellem *et al.* 2006; Buote *et al.* 2006; Mayhew & Weisse 2008; Morrison *et al.* 2008). These numbers are appalling and should provide a great

impetus for us as scientists to ask why. Many veterinarians read or hear about the common outcome for our patients with biliary diseases (surgical or otherwise) and become reluctant to persuade clients to send them for aggressive diagnostics and surgery. The assumption that surgery of the EHBT alone is the cause of the high mortality rates continues to drive some clinicians to avoid surgical intervention. This thought process may be contributing to a worsening trend in outcome for our patients with EHBT disease. A better understanding of the normal physiology of the EHBT and the pathophysiology of diseases of the EHBT, accompanied by a more aggressive diagnostic and therapeutic approach to patients with EHBT disease, will likely provide an improved outcome for our patients.

A simple example of how a shift in our clinical philosophy regarding EHBT disease may improve a patient's outcome can be borrowed from human medicine. The most common biliary tract surgery performed in humans today is cholecystectomy due to cholelithiasis. Historically, cholelithiasis was treated medically until the patient suffered severe abdominal pain or when obstructive jaundice developed. Morbidity and mortality rates in human EHBT surgery were also around 30% when surgical intervention was viewed as a last resort (Pitt *et al.* 1981; Dixon *et al.* 1983, 1984a,b). The current trend for patients with potentially surgically amenable EHBT disease is to provide interventional, and often definitive, surgical therapy as soon as possible, and preferentially before the patient is ill. The common use of cholecystectomy to treat human patients with

Small Animal Soft Tissue Surgery, Second Edition. Edited by Eric Monnet.
© 2023 John Wiley & Sons, Inc. Published 2023 by John Wiley & Sons, Inc.
Companion website: www.wiley.com/go/monnet/small

nonobstructive cholelithiasis has significantly lowered the morbidity and mortality rates in humans undergoing EHBT surgery (Pitt *et al.* 1999). Although veterinary medicine is lacking scientific evidence of a paradigm shift in how these patients should be dealt with, it is likely that performing definitive surgical procedures early in the course of EHBT disease will provide better short- and long-term outcomes for our patients.

As a profession, we are evolving our abilities to provide therapeutic modalities on a minimally invasive level; unfortunately, sometimes "minimally invasive" is changed to "minimalistic." As already stated, the poor outcome of small animal patients with EHBT disease has led us as clinicians to seek other therapeutic avenues to treat these patients without pursuing surgery. A recent collection of publications involving a small number of cases with EHBT obstruction has provided some alternative techniques to surgery, mostly involving drainage of bile via intermittent or continuous cholecystocentesis until the cause of the obstruction has resolved or until the patient is more stable for surgery (Nakeeb & Pitt 1995; Herman *et al.* 2005; Murphy *et al.* 2007; Mayhew 2009). On a physiologic level this is not a rational course of therapy, as a major component of the patient's systemic alterations is due to the absence of bile within the small intestine.

Human medicine has gone through, and in some cases is still going through, this trend of preoperative biliary drainage and decompression or definitive extracorporeal drainage (Pitt 1986; Nakeeb & Pitt 1995). Most of the human literature agrees that removing bile from the system, preoperative biliary decompression, and attempts at avoiding surgery for these diseases have led to prolonged hospitalization, increased morbidity, and in some instances an increase in mortality (Pitt 1986; Nakeeb & Pitt 1995; Sung *et al.* 1995; Nagino *et al.* 2007; Walter *et al.* 2008). Granted, dogs and cats are not people and veterinary medicine is lacking in clinical evidence that suggests one method over another; however, it would appear that early surgical intervention may provide at least part of the solution to this long-standing problem. A simple veterinary example would be the nonruptured gallbladder mucocele. The current trend is to wait to perform a cholecystectomy on these patients until they have failed medical management, have become systemically ill, or the gallbladder ruptures. This "wait and see" philosophy has yielded mortality rates of 20–30% in dogs with gallbladder mucocele (Pike *et al.* 2004a,b; Worley *et al.* 2004). Many surgeons, intensivists, criticalists, and internists are now recommending that a cholecystectomy be performed in patients with gallbladder mucocele at initial presentation or if found as an incidental finding on abdominal ultrasound.

Others recommend that alterations in diet and medical management of gallbladder mucocele are appropriate, and there is some reported success using this methodology (Walter *et al.* 2008).

The incidence of disorders restricted to the gallbladder and biliary tree is low compared with the many parenchymal hepatic conditions that occur in animals. The diseases of the EHBT are often confused with other intra-abdominal disorders because their course and clinical signs are similar. The diseases that lead to a need for surgery of the EHBT in dogs are primarily acquired conditions and include EHBT obstruction, gallbladder mucocele, traumatic injury, and cholecystitis. The main goal of surgery is to confirm the underlying disease process, establish a patent biliary system, and minimize perioperative complications.

Physiology of the biliary system

Taurocholate and taurocholic acid are the primary salt and acid in canine bile. Bile acids are synthesized from cholesterol, conjugated in the hepatocytes, and secreted continuously into bile canaliculi (Chiang 2013). They are secreted into the duodenum and reabsorbed in the ileum, then carried back to the liver for reexcretion. Up to 90% of the bile in dogs and cats is recirculated bile salts (Chiang 2013). Bilirubin is the major bile pigment and is a product of hemoprotein catabolism (Center 1996, 2009). The average lifespan of the red blood cell is 90–120 days; at the end of their life they rupture and the released hemoglobin is phagocytosed by the reticuloendothelial system (RES) (Guyton & Hale 2006). The hemoglobin is split into globin and heme, the heme being converted into biliverdin. This is rapidly converted to free bilirubin, which is released into the plasma and readily binds with albumin. The albumin-bound bilirubin enters the hepatocyte and most of it is conjugated into bilirubin glucuronide, which is then excreted into the bile canaliculi and eventually into the duodenum (Guyton & Hale 2006). Once in the intestine, bacteria convert about half of the conjugated bilirubin into urobilinogen, of which some is absorbed into the portal blood and reexcreted back into the intestine; however, a small percentage is excreted by the kidneys into the urine. The urobilinogen that remains in the intestine is converted by oxidation into stercobilinogen, which gives feces their color (Guyton & Hale 2006).

Filling of the gallbladder with bile occurs continuously via hepatic secretion and passive gallbladder distension. This is a low-flow, low-pressure system. The sphincter of Oddi is the functional sphincter at the terminal portion of the bile duct (Center 2009). Rhythmic contractions of the sphincter regulate duodenal bile flow as spurts rather than continuous flow and it functions as a one-way valve that can regulate pressure within the biliary tract. It also provides resistance against retrograde passage of duodenal contents or pancreatic secretions into the biliary tree.

Cholecystokinin is a hormone produced and secreted by the duodenal mucosa. It is the principal hormone responsible for the stimulation of gallbladder contraction.

Cholecystectomy, ileal resection, and a rise in cholestyramine increase the release of cholecystokinin. Motilin and the cholinergic pathway also stimulate gallbladder contraction and bile flow (Center 1996).

Unconjugated bile acids are cytotoxic and induce tissue inflammation (Center 1996). They alter the permeability of vascular structures within the peritoneal membranes, resulting in the transudation of fluid and the transmural migration of enteric organisms into the peritoneal cavity. Although virtually all bile acids derived from the biliary tree are conjugated, a bacterial infection or a low pH within the biliary tree will result in bile acid deconjugation (Center 1996).

Bile salts enhance the absorption of the fat-soluble vitamins A, D, E, and K. Decreased production, biliary obstruction, or inactivation of bile salts can contribute to a clinically relevant decrease in vitamin K-dependent coagulation factors (Center 1996). The decreased circulating levels of vitamin K-dependent coagulation factors in affected patients lead to alterations in the intrinsic and extrinsic pathways.

Another clinically important role of bile salts is to function as a natural detergent within the small intestine. Bile salts bind bacteria and endotoxin within the small intestinal lumen, decreasing the amount of free endotoxin in portal and systemic circulation (Evans & Christensen 1979). It is thought that the lack of a detergent within the small intestine of patients with EHBT obstruction is one of the important causes of severe systemic illness. Coagulopathy, thrombopathy, acute tubular degeneration and necrosis, and myocardial depression are some of the documented systemic changes observed in patients with EHBT obstruction. Endotoxemia in obstructive jaundice has been documented in humans and has been experimentally produced in multiple animal models (Pitt *et al.* 1981, 1999; Pain *et al.* 1985, 1987, 1991; Pain & Bailey 1986, 1987, 1988).

Clinical signs of extrahepatic biliary disease

Clinical signs in dogs with surgical diseases of the biliary tree are nonspecific and mimic other abdominal disorders. Signs may wax and wane for several weeks before presentation. In humans, biliary system pain is severe and can be difficult to distinguish from esophageal pain and angina. Such discomfort in animal patients seems to be rare, although occasionally animals with cholelithiasis are examined for episodic abdominal discomfort, vomiting, and diarrhea. Most animals with bile duct obstruction are not likely examined until clinical signs of icterus develop. Clinical icterus becomes evident when serum bilirubin levels are greater than 1.5–2.0 mg/dL (Center 1996; Guyton & Hale 2006). The detection of acholic feces (a lack of stercobilinogen in the intestine) in an icteric animal is consistent with a diagnosis of bile duct obstruction.

Diagnostic evaluation

The primary diagnostic problem in evaluating dogs with icterus is differentiating between an extrahepatic obstructive lesion and a primary hepatic parenchymal disease process. The first requires surgical intervention and the latter is managed medically. One of the difficulties in diagnosing a biliary tract obstruction is that animals may not demonstrate clinical signs or hematologic abnormalities for weeks to months after the obstruction. This has been documented in experimental ligation studies (Washizu *et al.* 1994)

Bloodwork

Bile duct obstruction causes an increase in total serum bilirubin, with more than 50% being direct or conjugated bilirubin along with a corresponding bilirubinuria. Bilirubinuria may be the first sign of bile duct obstruction in dogs and may precede the development of jaundice (Center 2009). Dogs have a low renal threshold for excretion of conjugated bilirubin and, with obstruction of the bile duct, renal excretion of bilirubin becomes important for elimination of the pigment. If the obstruction is complete, urobilinogen will be absent from the urine. Because its detection in urine depends on many variables (exposure to light, drugs, sensitivity of detection methods), the absence of urobilinogen should be interpreted with caution.

Acute experimental biliary obstruction in dogs results in rapid elevation of serum alkaline phosphatase and bilirubin after a latent period of up to six hours (Nyland 1982; Washizu *et al.* 1994). However, the magnitude of some serum liver enzyme elevations has no correlation with the degree of hepatobiliary injury or obstruction. If a dog is septic or if necrotizing cholecystitis is present, a fever and leukocytosis with a left shift are often present. A mild to moderate nonregenerative anemia may also be observed.

Abnormalities in coagulation tests commonly coincide with the absence of, or decrease in the ability for, vitamin K absorption due to decreased amounts of bile salts in the small intestine. Given that factor VII has the shortest half-life of the routinely measured coagulation factors in dogs and cats, it would be expected that pro-thrombin time (PT) would commonly be elevated in patients with EHBT obstruction; however, in many chronic cases of EHBT obstruction partial thromboplas-tin time (PTT) is elevated, and this finding may be asso-ciated with a worse short-term outcome in dogs (Mehler *et al.* 2004). The prolongation in PTT that is frequently seen may be related to the binding of coagulation factors XI and XII by endotoxin (Hunt *et al.* 1982). This should be countered with parenteral supplementation with vita-min K and, if needed, fresh frozen plasma transfusions.

In humans, severe complications from vagal stimula-tion, which have progressed to cardiac arrest, have been described in patients with acute cholecystitis undergo-ing vigorous diagnostic or therapeutic manipulations of the gallbladder. Similar problems have been observed in dogs undergoing simple gallbladder aspiration, palpa-tion, and manipulation (vanSonnenberg *et al.* 1986; Center 1996; Rivers *et al.* 1997).

Imaging modalities
Radiography

Radiography should be undertaken in veterinary patients with clinical signs and laboratory abnormali-ties consistent with biliary disease. In dogs and cats, up to half of choleliths are mineralized and therefore radiopaque (Figure 17.1) (Smith 1998). Gas within the biliary structures is likely to be due to emphysematous cholecystitis, cholangitis, choledochitis, or an abscess, and warrants prompt surgical and antimicrobial therapy.

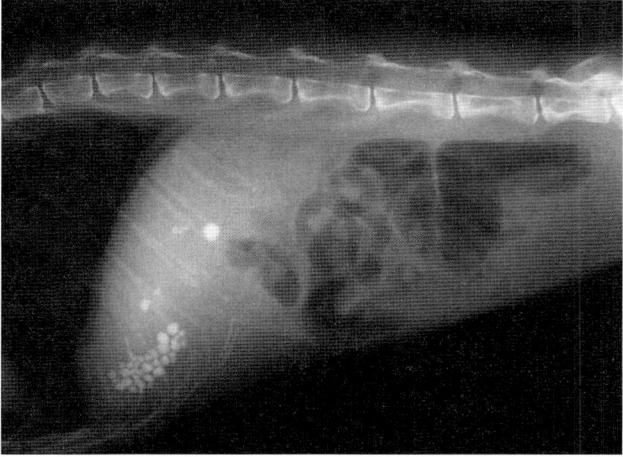

Figure 17.1 Lateral radiograph of a cat with multiple radiopaque stones in the gallbladder and a large stone likely present in the terminal bile duct.

Ultrasound

Ultrasound is a sensitive and specific indicator of the cause of EHBT obstruction (Nyland *et al.* 1989, 1999; Smith 1998). Gallstones are readily identified with abdominal ultrasound. Abdominal ultrasound is cur-rently the most useful and practical technique for dem-onstrating gallbladder and bile duct dilatation associated with obstruction in small animals. Ultrasonographic findings of bile duct distension secondary to obstruction may be identified in up to 100% of cases involving dogs and cats (Figure 17.2) (Washizu *et al.* 1994; Smith 1998; Besso *et al.* 2000). It is important to note that biliary obstruction may be diagnosed before the onset of clini-cal icterus with the use of abdominal ultrasonography, and that minimal intrahepatic duct distension is a subtle abnormality but is identified on ultrasound as early as four hours after experimental biliary occlusion (Zeman *et al.* 1981; Washizu *et al.* 1994; Smith 1998; Besso *et al.* 2000). The absence of gallbladder dilatation does not exclude EHBT obstruction, since the gallbladder may be contracted due to inflammation. The degree of biliary tract dilatation in obstructed dogs is variable. Therefore, duct size would allow only a crude estimation of the duration of obstruction.

Contrast study

Oral, intravenous, and cholangiographic contrast stud-ies can be performed, but are rarely used in veterinary medicine given that safer and less invasive imaging modalities are more sensitive (Smith 1998). If present, high serum bilirubin concentrations, hypoalbuminemia, icterus, hepatocellular disease, pancreatitis, peritonitis, biliary obstruction, cholecystitis, or concurrent sulfona-mide and salicylate administration cause decreased hepatic concentration of the contrast that results in poor opacification of the EHBT. The older techniques of intravenous cholangiocystography and percutaneous transhepatic cholangiocystography are rarely used today, as they are both invasive and have been largely super-seded by ultrasonography for the diagnosis of extrahe-patic bile duct obstruction (Figure 17.3) (Carlisle 1977; Wrigley & Reuter 1982).

Hepatobiliary scintigraphy

Hepatobiliary scintigraphy in animals with hepatic and biliary disease has been investigated and used clinically in patients with EHBT obstruction and may be a valua-ble diagnostic tool for differentiating EHBT obstruction from hepatocellular disease (Boothe *et al.* 1992; Newell *et al.* 1996; Smith 1998; Kerr & Hornof 2005). Various radiopharmaceutical agents have been used for hepato-biliary scintigraphy in both dogs and cats, but most are

(a)   (b)

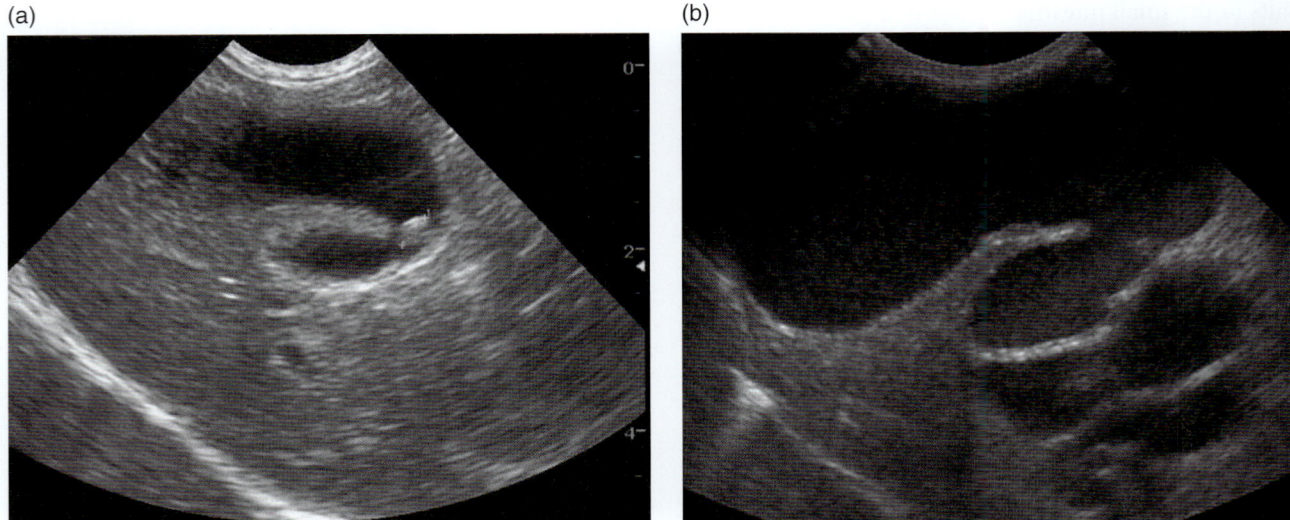

Figure 17.2 (a, b) Focal ultrasound images of the extrahepatic biliary tract. There is a cholelith in the cystic duct with minimal acoustic shadowing and distension of the cystic duct is present.

(a)   (b)

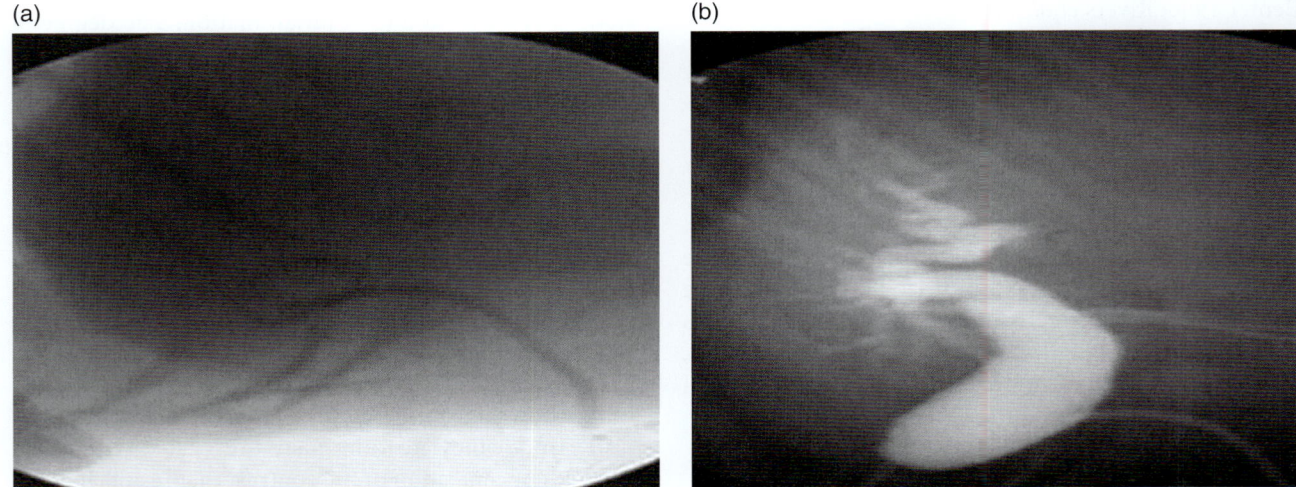

Figure 17.3 (a) A pigtail catheter has been placed percutaneously into the gallbladder using fluoroscopic guidance. A dilute contrast agent has been injected into the cholecystostomy tube to evaluate the patency the extrahepatic biliary tract. (b) A torturous and dilated bile duct is observed in the image with minimal contrast entering the proximal duodenum. Retrograde filling of hepatic ducts and pancreatic ducts is also visualized.

derivatives of technetium-99m iminodiacetic acid (mebrofenin or disofenin) (Boothe *et al.* 1992; Newell *et al.* 1994, 1996; Head & Daniel 2005; Kerr & Hornof 2005). After intravenous injection, excretion of these compounds through the biliary system occurs, followed by their passage into the duodenum through the major duodenal papilla. Most reports have concluded that in dogs and cats if the intestines cannot be visualized within three hours of the injection of the agent, it is generally considered likely that EHBT obstruction is present (Boothe *et al.* 1992; Head & Daniel 2005). The main disadvantages of scintigraphy are that it does not give accurate information as to the exact site or cause of obstruction, the patient must be housed in a radiation-safe area until no longer radioactive (usually within 24 hours), and the test itself takes much longer to perform than most ultrasound examinations of the biliary system.

Microbiology

Partial or complete EHBT obstruction leads to bile stasis and can promote aerobic and anaerobic bacterial growth. Bile is thought to be sterile in normal dogs and cats. In humans, infections of the biliary tree usually begin in the gallbladder and spread into the biliary system, rather than ascending from the gut through the bile ducts into an obstructed biliary system. In dogs with septic bile peritonitis, the most common bacterial isolates have been *Escherichia coli*, followed by *Enterococcus* spp., *Enterobacter* spp., *Klebsiella* spp., *Streptococcus* spp., *Pseudomonas* spp., *Bacteroides* spp., and *Actinobacter* spp. (Ludwig *et al.* 1997; Mehler *et al.* 2004).

Pathology affecting the biliary system

Causes of EHBT obstruction in small animals include cholelithiasis, neoplasia, pancreatitis, inspissated bile, gallbladder mucoceles, parasites, duodenal foreign body, and diaphragmatic hernia (Martin & Page 1951; Razin *et al.* 1965; Schall *et al.* 1973; Barsanti *et al.* 1976; Matthiesen & Lammerding 1984; Martin *et al.* 1986; Matthiesen & Rosin 1986; Cribb *et al.* 1988; Neer & Hedlend 1989; Neer 1992; Fahie & Martin 1995; Center 1996, 2009; Smith 1998; Mayhew *et al.* 2002, 2006; Bacon & White 2003; Mehler *et al.* 2004; Pike *et al.* 2004a,b; Worley *et al.* 2004; Herman *et al.* 2005; Amsellem *et al.* 2006; Buote *et al.* 2006; Mayhew & Weisse 2008; Morrison *et al.* 2008; Papazoglou *et al.* 2008; Baker *et al.* 2009). Animals with obstructive jaundice are often some of the most critically ill patients presented to veterinarians. There are many physiologic explanations for this, but two of the most relevant include the build-up of bilirubin in the blood and the lack of bile salts in the small intestine. The formation of bilirubin is the mechanism by which the body rids itself of old heme from the natural degradation of red blood cells. When bilirubin is not removed from the body, as stercobilino-gen in the feces or urobilinogen in the urine, it will lead to accumulation in the blood and downregulation of the RES (Drivas *et al.* 1976; Pain *et al.* 1991). The latter effect of EHBT obstruction is due to the lack of bile salts in the small intestine, leading to deficiencies in the absorption of fat and fat-soluble vitamins, secondary coagulopathies, and the lack of a detergent effect on bacteria and endotoxin within the lumen of the small intestine. When these two changes occur, bacteria and endotoxin are delivered to the liver unbound and the failing RES is unable to process them accordingly. This leads to severe systemic changes, including acute tubular necrosis, hypotension, coagulopathy, decreased wound healing, gastrointestinal hemorrhage, systemic and portal endotoxemia and bacteremia, continued gastrointestinal bacterial translocation, systemic inflammatory response syndrome, sepsis, disseminated intravascular coagulation (DIC), and myocardial damage (O'Brien & Mitchum 1970; Bayer & Ellis 1976; Drivas *et al.* 1976; Evans & Christensen 1979; Pain *et al.* 1985, 1987;

Jorgensen *et al.* 1987; Radberg *et al.* 1988; Neer & Hedlend 1989; Rege *et al.* 1990; Washizu *et al.* 1994; Rege 1995; Utkan *et al.* 2000; Mehler *et al.* 2004).

The incidence of biliary tract obstruction in the dog is much less than in humans because intraluminal extrahepatic obstruction due to cholelithiasis is rare in dogs. There are a number of other disorders that cause EHBT obstruction in dogs. The most common is mechanical obstruction of the duct due to neoplastic diseases of surrounding tissue or inflammatory/infectious conditions of similar origin.

Pancreatic disease is one of the most common causes of EHBT obstruction in dogs and cats (Fahie & Martin 1995; Mayhew *et al.* 2002, 2006; Bacon & White 2003; Mehler *et al.* 2004; Mayhew & Weisse 2008). Scar tissue formation can occur in or around the bile duct, or the duct can be compressed by fibrotic or inflamed pancreatic tissue, pancreatic cysts, or pancreatic abscesses. In a study evaluating all dogs undergoing surgery of the EHBT, 17 of 60 cases were caused by EHBT obstruction; of these, 5 were due to neoplasia and 12 were secondary to pancreatitis. Half of the pancreatitis patients died intraoperatively or in the immediate postoperative period (Mehler *et al.* 2004).

Intraluminal obstruction is less common, but may be caused by cholelithiasis, choledocholithiasis, or inspissated bile. In the presence of complete bile duct obstruction, bile may become colorless (white bile) due to reduced secretion of bilirubin and increased production of mucin (Center 1996; Jones *et al.* 1997).

Cholelithiasis

Until recently, cholelithiasis has been considered an uncommon disease in dogs and cats. It has been reported that cholelithiasis and choledocholithiasis account for less than 1% of dogs with liver/biliary tract disease. Although most choledocholiths are believed to form in the gallbladder, some may form in the ducts (Figure 17.4). Calcium salts are the major component of pigmented gallstones, and therefore the availability of ionized calcium may be important in the formation of gallstones in dogs and cats (Rege *et al.* 1990; Rege 1995). Cholelithiasis is often an incidental finding on abdominal or thoracic radiography or at necropsy. As a clinical problem, cholelithiasis has a high incidence in the miniature schnauzer and miniature poodle, but up to 75% of the reported cases of cholelithiasis in small animals have been diagnosed at necropsy with no association with clinical signs (Schall *et al.* 1973). The rarity of canine cholelithiasis may be due to decreased concentrations of cholesterol in canine bile compared with human bile.

Gallstones are readily diagnosed using abdominal ultrasonography. There is great variation in the size,

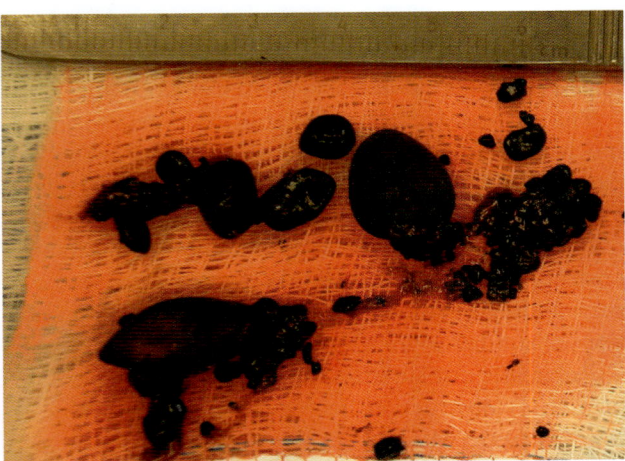

Figure 17.4 Calcium bilirubinate stones removed from the gall-bladder and cystic duct of the cat shown in Figure 17.1.

shape, number, and composition of choleliths. The mechanism of formation is thought to be similar to that of urinary calculi. Solid particles comprising dead cells or inspissated material act as a nidus for crystallization and some constituents of bile are reabsorbed during biliary stasis more easily than others, leaving highly desiccated residues. The cholesterol composition of bile influences risk for bile lithogenicity in mammals. High cholesterol saturation in bile increases risk for cholelithiasis, as seen in humans. Dogs do not have much cholesterol saturation in their bile and therefore do not form cholesterol-based stones. There are some limited reports of cats having cholesterol-based choleliths (Morrison *et al.* 2008). Ursodeoxycholate (ursodiol) is often prescribed for cholelith dissolution in humans because the drug helps prevent cholesterol saturation and build-up in bile. The use of this drug for cholelith dissolution in dogs is inappropriate physiologically and should not be justified as a primary method of stone dissolution. However, its use in cats may be beneficial as some cats produce cholesterol-based stones (O'Brien & Mitchum 1970; Jorgensen *et al.* 1987).

There are many proposed mechanisms and risks for the development of cholelithiasis. Pregnancy in humans has been associated with gallstone formation and this is likely linked to the decrease in the total bile acids pool. A dramatic decrease in the total bile acids pool (35%) has also been linked to pregnancy in the cat, but no increase in cholelith formation has been noted (Radberg *et al.* 1987, 1988). Other induced causes of cholelith formation in humans, dogs, and cats include primary intestinal disease and resection of the ileum and/or colon (Anon. 1969; Mair *et al.* 1974, 1975; Pitt *et al.* 1984; Noshiro *et al.* 1996). Although the prevalence of gallstone formation in cats that have undergone subtotal

colectomy is not known, we have seen cholelith formation in two such patients.

Pancreatitis

We have reported a 50% mortality rate in dogs with pancreatitis that undergo biliary tract surgery, although a mortality rate as high as 100% has been documented in the veterinary literature (Mayhew *et al.* 2002; Mehler *et al.* 2004). Cats with pancreatitis and secondary bile duct obstruction fare similarly (Mayhew *et al.* 2002; Bacon & White 2003; Mayhew & Weisse 2008). The high mortality rate is likely due to the systemic effects of pancreatitis and is not simply because of the local disease process. Other conditions associated with the pancreas that cause EHBT obstruction are pancreatic neoplasia, abscesses, cysts, and granulomas. These causes are less common than obstruction caused by chronic pancreatitis. In a recent publication evaluating dogs with EHBT obstruction secondary to pancreatitis, 76% of dogs survived to discharge and azotemia, elevated body temperature at presentation, and ultrasonographic evidence of gallbladder distention were all associated with a significantly greater risk of death than those patients without azotemia, elevated body temperature, or gallbladder distention (Palermo *et al.* 2020). In another study, 79% of dogs with a bile duct obstruction secondary to pancreatitis survived, and 94% of the surviving patients were treated with medical management alone (Wilkinson *et al.* 2020).

Neoplasia

Primary neoplasms of the gallbladder and bile duct are rare in domestic animals. Bile duct tumors often present with signs of complete EHBT obstruction and are typically nonresectable; however, cholecystoenterostomy may palliate clinical signs for months (Nakeeb *et al.* 2002; Mehler *et al.* 2004).

Mucocele

A biliary mucocele is the distension of a bile-containing structure or cavity by inappropriate accumulation of mucus (Pike *et al.* 2004a,b; Worley *et al.* 2004; Aguirre *et al.* 2007). EHBT obstruction does not appear to play a primary role in the formation of gallbladder mucoceles. However, the presence and progression of gelatinous material in the gallbladder may lead to EHBT obstruction. It has been our experience that in many dogs with gallbladder mucoceles, the disease is not contained within the gallbladder and cystic duct and sludge is found within the hepatic ducts or the bile duct. Overall mortality rates are reported to be 20–39% for this disease (Pike *et al.* 2004a,b; Worley *et al.* 2004; Amsellem *et al.* 2006; Aguirre *et al.* 2007); however, early surgical intervention may significantly reduce mortality rate to 2% (Youn *et al.* 2018) (see Chapter 46 for more information).

Bile peritonitis

Bile peritonitis, or bilious ascites, is the inflammatory response of the peritoneum to the presence of bile. Bile peritonitis is caused by rupture of the extrahepatic bile ducts, the gallbladder, or tears in liver lobes and their intralobar ducts. Rupture may be due to blunt trauma, neoplasia, mucocele formation, necrotizing cholecystitis, obstruction from cholelithiasis, neoplasia, or parasites. The poorly vascularized fundus is the most susceptible area to rupture in the canine gallbladder (Neer & Hedlend 1989; Parchman & Flanders 1990). If the bilirubin concentration of the abdominal effusion is more than twice the serum concentration, it is diagnostic for bile peritonitis. The survival rate for dogs with septic bile peritonitis is 27–45% and for dogs with sterile bile peritonitis is 87–100% (Ludwig *et al.* 1997; Mehler *et al.* 2004). Humans with sterile biliary effusion may have vague symptoms that last for an average of 30 days before surgical treatment, and have a mortality rate of less than 10%; in contrast, humans with septic bile peritonitis have an acute presentation with abdominal pain and shock, and a greater than 20% mortality (Ibragimov *et al.* 1992).

The onset of clinical signs in dogs with a ruptured biliary tract and the degree of peritonitis present are likely dependent on the volume of liquid bile, the concentration of bile salts, and the presence or absence of bacteria. Clinical signs include vomiting, anorexia, diarrhea, weight loss, icterus, abdominal distension, fever, and abdominal pain.

Bile salts are toxic to tissues and cause permeability changes and tissue necrosis, which encourages the growth of bacteria. Sources of bacteria are thought to be endogenous anaerobic bacteria from the liver and intestine as well as hematogenous spread (Martin *et al.* 1986).

Medical management and perioperative therapeutics

There is some evidence to suggest that in patients with EHBT obstruction, therapies aimed at decreasing systemic endotoxin levels should be attempted. Lactulose, enteral bile salts, lidocaine, polymyxin B, and other reported endotoxin scavengers have been shown to help reduce portal and systemic endotoxin levels, but the effect of these medications on morbidity and mortality in human and veterinary patients is controversial (Wardle & Wright 1970; Pain *et al.* 1985; Pain & Bailey 1987).

Surgery related to the biliary system

The diseases that lead to a need for surgery of the extrahepatic biliary system in dogs and cats are primarily acquired conditions and include EHBT obstruction, gallbladder mucoceles, traumatic injury, and cholecystitis. The main goal of surgery is to confirm the underlying disease process, establish a patent biliary system, and minimize perioperative complications. Three traditional surgical approaches to the extrahepatic biliary system have been described. A ventral midline celiotomy is most commonly performed. This approach can be extended through the sternum or paracostally on the right side. A third approach involves a thoracotomy through the right seventh or eighth intercostal space, but we do not recommend this (Matthiesen 1989; Martin *et al.* 2003). A laparoscopic approach to the biliary system has been also described (Mayhew *et al.* 2008).

Surgery of the gallbladder

A cholecystectomy is preferred over a cholecystotomy for stone removal, as this will remove the reservoir for subsequent stone formation (Harkema *et al.* 1982).

Cholecystotomy

Indications include full-thickness biopsy of the gallbladder or mucosal cultures, exploration of the inside of the gallbladder and cystic duct, removal of choleliths and sludge, antegrade flushing and assessment of patency of the extrahepatic biliary ducts, and placement of a cholecystostomy tube (Martin *et al.* 2003). In most circumstances there is no need to dissect the gallbladder from the hepatic fossa when performing a cholecystotomy. If the gallbladder is dissected from the hepatic fossa, great care must be taken not to damage the cystic artery supplying the gallbladder, as the artery branches from the left hepatic artery.

In some deep-chested dogs or in patients with a gallbladder that is hard to exteriorize, moistened laparotomy pads can be placed between the liver and the diaphragm, which will displace the liver and gallbladder caudally in the abdomen. Also the cranial aspect of the ventral midline incision has to be extended to the level of the xiphoid. The gallbladder is isolated from the rest of the abdominal cavity with moistened laparotomy pads. If the gallbladder is left within the hepatic fossa, stay sutures are often not needed. Stay sutures in the gallbladder wall can induce tearing injury.

The contents of the gallbladder can be aspirated with an 18-gauge, or if the bile is thick a 16-gauge, needle before making an incision. An attempt is made to incorporate the needle hole into the incision to minimize the number of holes in the gallbladder. The contents can also be removed with a Poole suction tip after the incision is made.

The gallbladder is stabilized between the thumb and first finger and a no. 11 blade is used to create a stab incision on the ventral surface of the gallbladder, midway between the fundus and the entrance of the cystic duct, or infundibulum, and extending into the infundibulum. The incision is made at this level because the fundus has a limited blood supply compared with the rest of the gallbladder (Church & Matthiesen 1988; Parchman & Flanders 1990; Martin *et al.* 2003). The size of the incision is made only as large as needed. If more exposure is required, the incision is continued ventral toward the fundus.

Closure of the incision is performed with a fine synthetic monofilament suture on a tapered needle in a simple continuous or inverting pattern. Some surgeons prefer a two-layer inverting closure, but this is not necessary or recommended in most cases (Martin *et al.* 2003). Full-thickness bites are recommended to ensure that the submucosa is incorporated in the closure. After a thorough local lavage of the gallbladder incision, the omentum can be placed over the incision.

Cholecystectomy with laparotomy

There are few side effects of cholecystectomy, although episodic abdominal pain and diarrhea associated with fat malabsorption have been described in humans and induced in normal dogs and cats after cholecystectomy (Mahour *et al.* 1968; Friman *et al.* 1990). Cholecystectomy results in loss of the fasting reservoir where bile is concentrated, increasing the volume of bile and significantly reducing the volume of the bile acid pool (Friman *et al.* 1990). A cholecystectomy should not be performed until patency of the EHBT has been assessed and deemed patent. Removal of the gallbladder in a patient with bile duct obstruction is contraindicated and could be a life-threatening surgical error. Indications include any primary disease of the gallbladder (cholecystitis, cholelithiasis, mucocele, neoplasia, infarction) or if severe structural changes have occurred secondary to other diseases or conditions.

Cholelithiasis is mostly a disease of the gallbladder, although primary choledocholithiasis is possible. In most cases, recurrence can be prevented by cholecystectomy. Some surgeons prefer to leave the gallbladder after stone removal so that it may be used for rerouting procedures in the future, if needed (Mahour *et al.* 1968; Center 1996; Martin *et al.* 2003; Walter *et al.* 2008).

Before performing a cholecystectomy, patency of the EHBT must be assured. This is done via a duodenotomy or from a cholecystotomy after removal of the gallbladder contents. Assessing the patency of the biliary tract

after completing the cholecystectomy defeats the purpose, as the lack of a patent system may indicate the need for a cholecystoenterostomy. There are two techniques for initiating a routine cholecystectomy. The first involves dissection of the gallbladder out of the hepatic fossa and the second begins with identification and isolation of the cystic duct and cystic artery (Figure 17.5) (Website Chapter 17: Liver and gall bladder/cholecystectomy). We prefer in most cases to isolate the cystic duct and artery first. This is performed by applying gentle traction to the gallbladder and hepatic fossa in a cranial direction. Mixter or right-angle forceps are used to gently dissect dorsally around the cystic duct and artery. Two encircling or one encircling and one distally placed transfixation sutures are used to securely close the cystic duct and ligate the cystic artery. In most cases, the artery and duct are included in the same ligature. If they can be separated from each other, individual ligation is more secure. A third encircling suture, hemostat, or clip is placed distal to the last suture and the cystic duct is transected immediately proximal to this clip. If the bile duct is very large or friable, it is necessary to oversew the end of the bile duct (Figure 17.5). The end of the cystic duct that is still connected to the gallbladder is used as a handle to apply gentle traction to the gallbladder to facilitate its removal from the hepatic fossa.

Dissection of the hepatic visceral peritoneum from the gallbladder can be initiated with Metzenbaum scissors, electrosurgery, or blunt dissection. The further away the dissection plane is from the liver, the less hemorrhage will occur (Figure 17.5). Once a plane is established, the index finger or tip of a hemostat wrapped in gauze square is used to carefully remove the gallbladder from the hepatic fossa. In chronic cases where the serosa of the gallbladder is adherent to the serosal hepatic surface, electrosurgery or a vessel-sealing device may be used to remove a small rim of liver parenchyma with the gallbladder, to minimize the risk of rupturing the gallbladder wall during cholecystectomy.

Hemorrhage from the hepatic fossa can be controlled with direct pressure applied with a lap sponge or by application of a hemostatic agent (Gelfoam or Surgicel). There is some previously reported risk of abscess formation using hemostatic agents in this area, but we have not observed this clinically (Martin *et al.* 2003).

If a duodenotomy has been used to assess patency of the biliary ducts, a small amount of sterile saline can be flushed gently into the bile duct to assess the security of the ligatures placed on the cystic duct remnant. Aggressive flushing and excessive manipulation of a catheter in this area have led to rupture of the bile ducts and should be avoided.

(a)

(b)

(c)

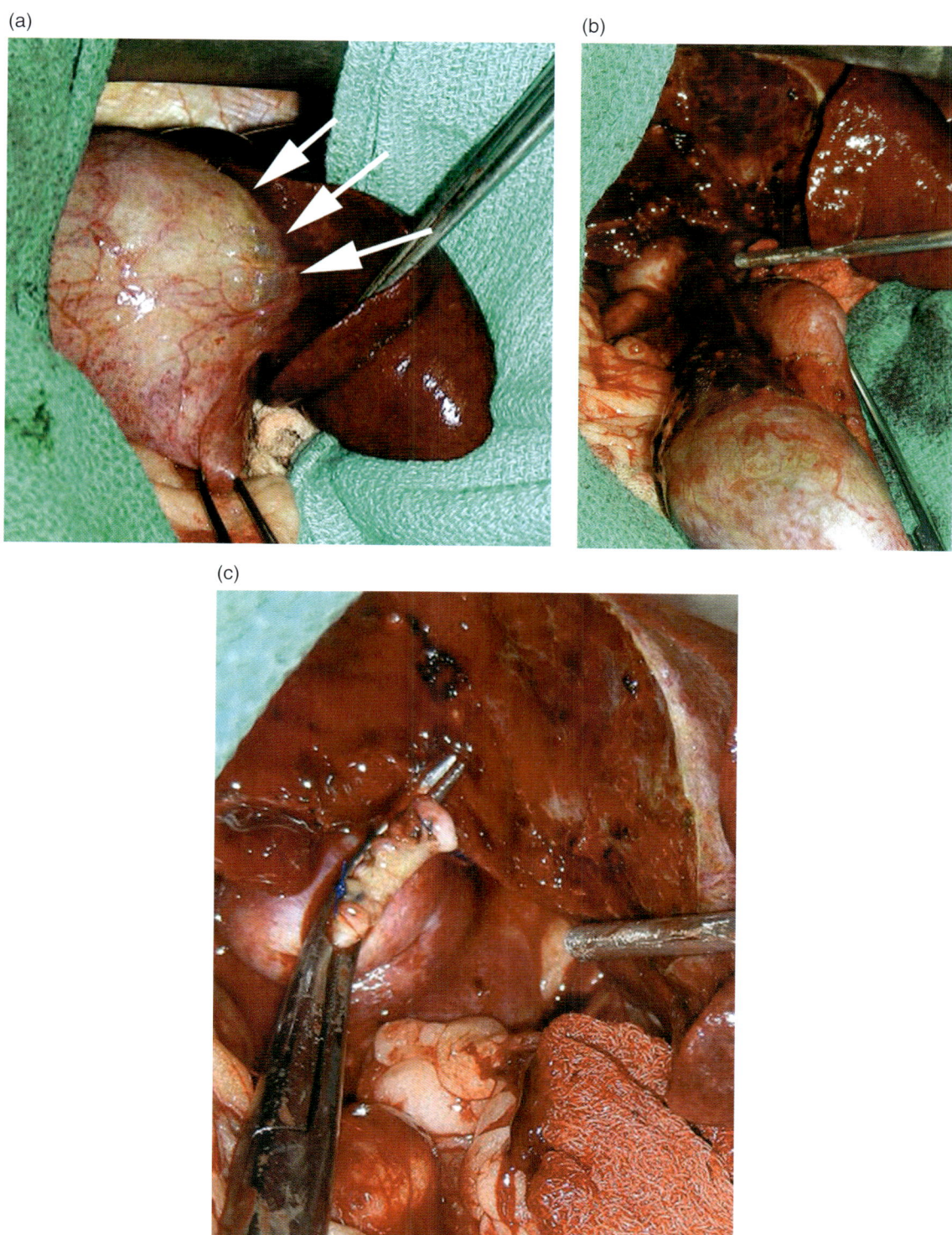

Figure 17.5 (a) A good plane of dissection (arrows) is at the junction between the liver parenchyma and the gallbladder. (b) Mild hemorrhage can occur from the liver parenchyma after completion of the cholecystectomy. (c) The bile duct was very large and friable. A suture was placed to oversew the stump of the bile duct.

Cholecystectomy with laparoscopy

The decision to perform elective cholecystectomy in dogs with gallbladder disease (mucoceles or stones) that is neither ruptured nor obstructed is controversial. This is especially true when patients are not clinical and the condition is found incidentally when an examination is performed for another reason. In humans, laparoscopic cholecystectomy has been performed since the early 1980s and now represents the treatment of choice for gallstone disease and acute cholecystitis. Approximately 75% of all cholecystectomies are performed laparoscopically and almost all elective cholecystectomies are performed this way. This has proven to be a very safe method for cholecystectomy in people and has a very small percentage of conversion to open laparotomy (Lane *et al.* 1967).

In cats and dogs the most common indications for traditional "open" cholecystectomy are necrotizing cholecystitis, gallbladder trauma or neoplasia, symptomatic cholelithiasis, and gallbladder mucocele. Laparoscopic cholecystectomy can only be considered in a subgroup of these cases. An uncomplicated gallbladder mucocele is probably the most suitable indication for laparoscopic cholecystectomy in veterinary patients at this time (Mayhew *et al.* 2008; Scott *et al.* 2016; Simon & Monnet 2020; Kanai *et al.* 2018). Other possible but as yet undescribed indications include symptomatic cholelithiasis without bile duct stones or associated EHBT obstruction and primary gallbladder neoplasia. At present, the following should be considered contraindications to laparoscopic cholecystectomy: uncontrolled coagulopathy, presence of bile peritonitis, EHBT obstruction, small body size (<4 kg), presence of conditions that make a patient poorly tolerant of anesthesia, and pneumoperitoneum (e.g., severe cardiorespiratory diseases and diaphragmatic hernia).

The dog is positioned in dorsal recumbency. A four-ports technique is used, with a subumbilical camera port and three instrument ports: one placed 5–8 cm lateral and 3–5 cm cranial to the umbilicus on the left side and two located 3–5 cm and 5–8 cm lateral to the umbilicus on the right side. A single access port can be used, also with an extra port placed on the right side of the middle (Mayhew *et al.* 2008; Scott *et al.* 2016; Kanai *et al.* 2018, Simon & Monnet 2020). The single access port is placed caudal to the umbilicus (Simon & Monnet 2020). Cranial retraction of the gallbladder is performed with a 5 mm fan retractor placed through the left-sided port to elevate the gallbladder so that the cystic duct is visible. Right-angle dissecting forceps or an articulated forceps are used to dissect around the cystic duct. Two to three extracorporeally tied modified Roeder knots of 0 or 2-0 polydioxanone or nonabsorbable monofilament suture or large hemoclips are placed around the cystic duct (Mayhew *et al.* 2008; Scott *et al.* 2016; Kanai *et al.* 2018; Marvel & Monnet 2014). Sharp sectioning of the cystic duct between sutures/clips is then performed, leaving one to two ligatures/clips in place around the cystic duct. The gallbladder is then dissected out of its fossa with the aid of a vessel-sealing device or electrocautery. Once dissected free, the gallbladder is placed into a specimen retrieval bag passed through the subumbilical port (Figure 17.6) (Website Chapter 17: Liver and gall bladder/laparoscopic

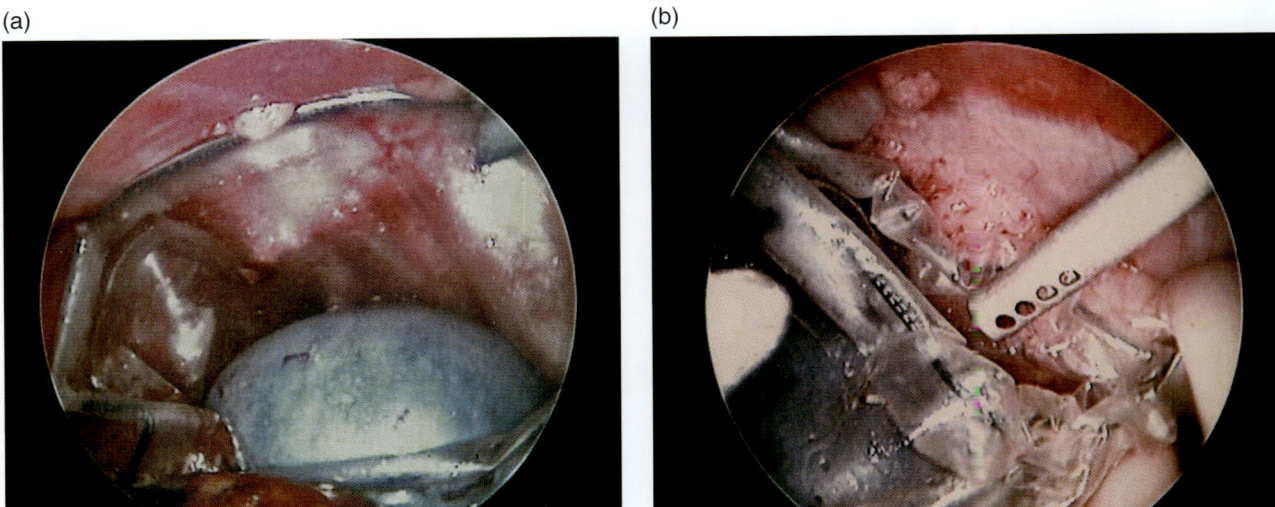

(a) (b)

Figure 17.6 (a) The gallbladder has been removed and placed into a retrieval bag. (b) The contents of the gallbladder are being removed within the retrieval bag using a 5 mm laparoscopic suction device in order to facilitate removal of the gallbladder and retrieval bag through a 10 mm port.

cholecystectomy). The retrieval bag is partially retracted through the camera port and tension is created by lifting the bag upward until a small area of the gallbladder can be directly visualized (while still in the bag) through the small subumbilical port incision. A stab incision is made with the tip of a scalpel blade into the gallbladder to release the bile, allowing it to be suctioned from within the bag using a suction/irrigation device (Figure 17.6). Once bile has been suctioned, the now empty gallbladder can be removed from the abdomen by firm upward traction on the specimen retrieval bag. If a single-port access is used, the gall bladder can be removed from the abdominal cavity without suctioning the bile out of it (Simon & Monnet 2020). Thorough abdominal lavage of the gallbladder fossa is performed followed by aspiration of fluid. The gallbladder should be submitted for histopathologic examination and the gallbladder wall/bile should be submitted for aerobic and anaerobic bacterial culture and sensitivity.

If significant bile leakage, excessive hemorrhage, or anesthetic complications occur, conversion to an open approach should be considered. The conversion rate is between 4% and 30% (Scott *et al.* 2016; Kanai *et al.* 2018; Simon & Monnet 2020). Inadequate ligation of the cystic duct causing bile peritonitis can occur postoperatively, as it can with an "open" cholecystectomy. Postoperative EHBT obstruction can develop as a result of inadequate flushing of residual biliary sludge in the bile duct in dogs with gallbladder mucocele. Avoidance of these latter complications is based on careful case selection and the decision not to perform laparoscopic cholecystectomy in dogs with gallbladder mucocele with preoperative biochemical or imaging evidence of EHBT obstruction.

Perioperative complications

Excessive bleeding can occur following blunt dissection and retraction of the gallbladder from the hepatic fossa, particularly in dogs with bleeding diathesis secondary to vitamin K_1 deficiency, DIC, coagulopathy, or primary hepatic disease. Assessment of coagulation factors and platelet deficiency or dysfunction should be performed preoperatively. In dogs with hemorrhage from the hepatic fossa, hemostatic agents can be placed in the fossa or an omental pedicle can be sutured over the area. In dogs with potential bleeding diathesis, freeing the gallbladder from the fossa can be partially or completely avoided, provided that a duodenal or jejunal loop can be anatomically positioned adjacent to the gallbladder and the biliary–enteric anastomosis successfully performed with minimal tension on the sutures.

Surgery of the biliary ducts

Primary repair of ruptured hepatic ducts, cystic duct, or bile duct can be performed (Martin *et al.* 1986; Church & Matthiesen 1988; Parchman & Flanders 1990; Mayhew *et al.* 2002; Papazoglou *et al.* 2008; Baker *et al.* 2009). There are well-developed intrahepatic and extrahepatic communications between divisions of the liver that allow collateral bile drainage. Given that dogs have between two and six extrahepatic ducts (Evans & Christensen 1979), sacrifice of one or more ducts is acceptable independent of removing the liver lobe being drained by the affected duct. Choledochotomy is commonly performed in humans.

A report of choledochotomy and primary repair of ruptured biliary ducts in dogs and cats described successful outcomes in 10 cases, with only one report of dehiscence and reoperation. A very fine small-diameter suture material is required and microsurgical instruments and techniques are recommended in many cases. A ruptured hepatic duct can be sacrificed, as collateral drainage will develop in the dog. If a large tear or defect exists in the cystic duct, a cholecystectomy can be performed.

Choledochotomy

Incising into the bile duct is indicated for removal of stones, sludge, and masses, for performing a biopsy, or for obtaining access to the EHBT when cannulation of the major duodenal papilla is contraindicated or has failed. Several techniques have been described that create a successful choledochotomy and achieve closure without leakage or stricture (Martin *et al.* 1986; Breznock 1998; Baker *et al.* 2009). The use of red rubber catheters as an internal strut for choledochal repairs has been described in veterinary medicine (Mayhew *et al.* 2006; Mayhew & Weisse 2008; Baker *et al.* 2009).

The bile duct is isolated using the thumb and index finger of the nondominant hand. Using a no. 11 blade, a full-thickness longitudinal incision is made in a dilated portion of the bile duct. The incision is made only as long as needed to accomplish the task. A blunt-ended instrument, an Allis or Babcock tissue forceps, is placed into the incision and gently opened to retract the sides of the incision. We have also used an eyelid retractor to maintain exposure of the bile duct. Closure is performed with a monofilament 4-0 to 6-0 suture in a simple interrupted or continuous pattern. An inverting or two-layer closure is avoided to prevent excessive narrowing of the luminal diameter (Figure 17.7) (Website Chapter 17: Liver and gall bladder/choledochotomy). If the longitudinal incision is relatively short, it can be closed in a transverse direction to limit narrowing of the luminal diameter.

(a)

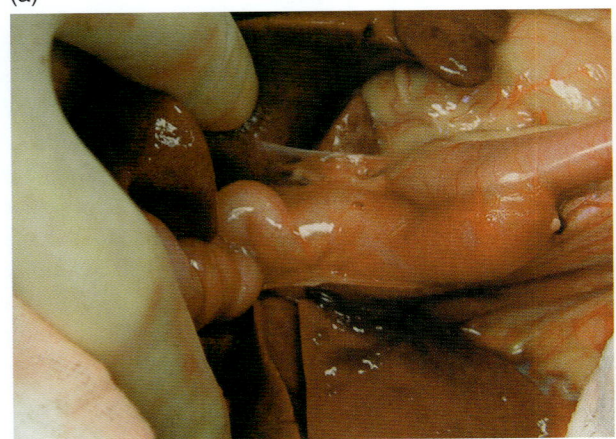

(b)

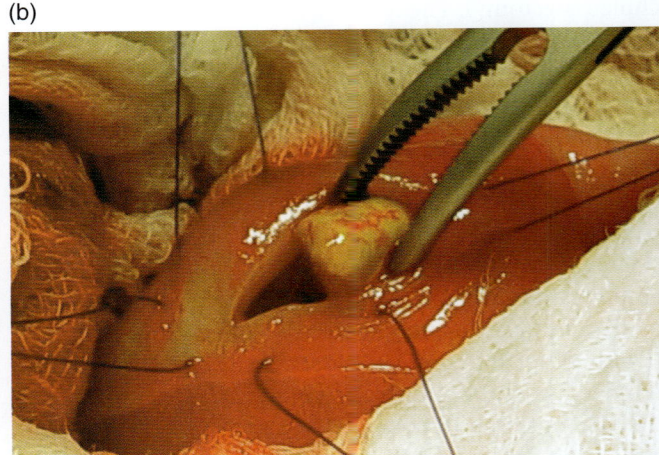

(c)

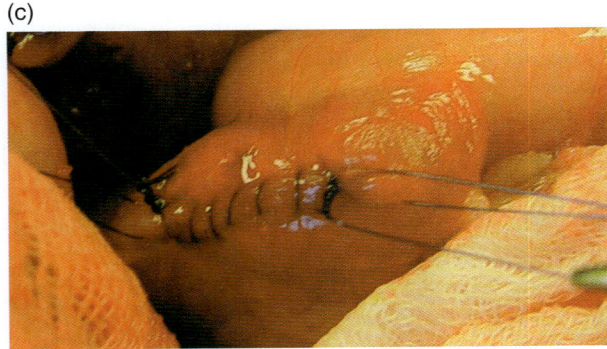

Figure 17.7 (a) Intraoperative view of a cat with distal bile duct obstruction from a large cholelith. The bile duct is larger in diameter than the duodenum. (b) A choledochotomy is being performed and the cholelith is removed. (c) The choledochotomy incision is closed with 5-0 monofilament absorbable suture in a simple continuous pattern.

Omentum is wrapped around the closed incision. A closed-suction drain can be placed as a diagnostic aid to help detect early dehiscence of the choledochotomy. The drain is removed in 3–5 days or when appropriate.

A variety of biomaterials have been investigated with the goal of providing additional biomechanical support and decreasing the risk of biliary leakage following iatrogenic biliary duct injuries or end-to-end bile duct anastomoses (Capper 1957, 1961; Worley *et al.* 2004; Jameel *et al.* 2008).

Choledochoduodenostomy

Choledochoduodenostomy was first described in 1892 and is a commonly performed rerouting procedure in human medicine. Because of the size of the canine bile duct (3 mm) compared with the human bile duct (10 mm), a choledochoenteric anastomosis is technically challenging. A chronically dilated bile duct may facilitate choledochoduodenostomy (Breznock 1998). Choledochoduodenostomy has been reported in the dog as an alternative to cholecystoduodenostomy to reroute the biliary system (Amsellem *et al.* 2006).

This procedure is performed using a routine end-to-side or side-to-side anastomosis (Karaayvaz *et al.* 1998; Wills *et al.* 2002; Zografakis *et al.* 2003; Vazquez 2008). For the end-to-side anastomosis, the bile duct is ligated and transected as close to the duodenum as possible to limit the amount of tension on the anastomosis. A 5-0 stay suture is placed full thickness into the lumen of the free end of the bile duct. A full-thickness, longitudinal, antimesenteric duodenotomy is performed over the major duodenal papilla and extending 3–4 cm aborad. A 0.5 cm stab incision is made immediately adjacent and lateral to the midline of the mesenteric attachment of the duodenum. A mosquito hemostat is placed from the luminal side of the stab incision through to the serosal side of the duodenum. The ends of the stay sutures are grasped and the free end of the bile duct is gently pulled into the lumen of the duodenum (Figure 17.8a). The anastomosis is completed using absorbable monofilament synthetic 5-0 to 8-0 suture in a simple interrupted or simple continuous pattern full thickness through the bile duct and into the mucosa and submucosa of the duodenum (Figure 17.8b). Because the sphincter

(a)

(b)

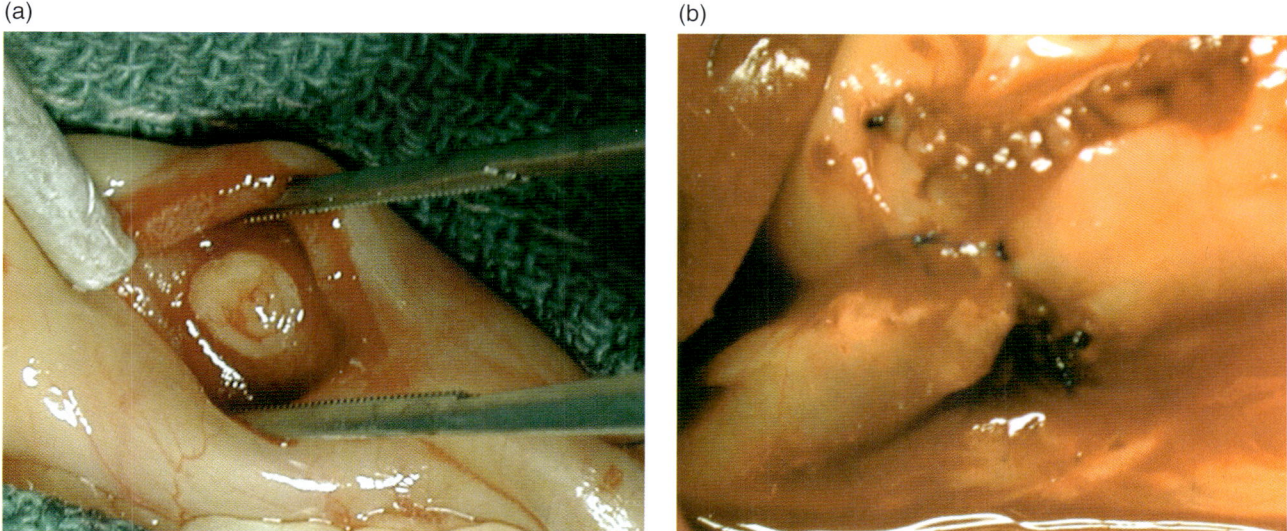

Figure 17.8 (a) The bile duct has been introduced into the duodenum through a small stab incision along the mesenteric border of the duodenum. (b) The choledochoduodenostomy has been completed with full-thickness simple interrupted sutures placed from within the duodenum.

(a)

(b)

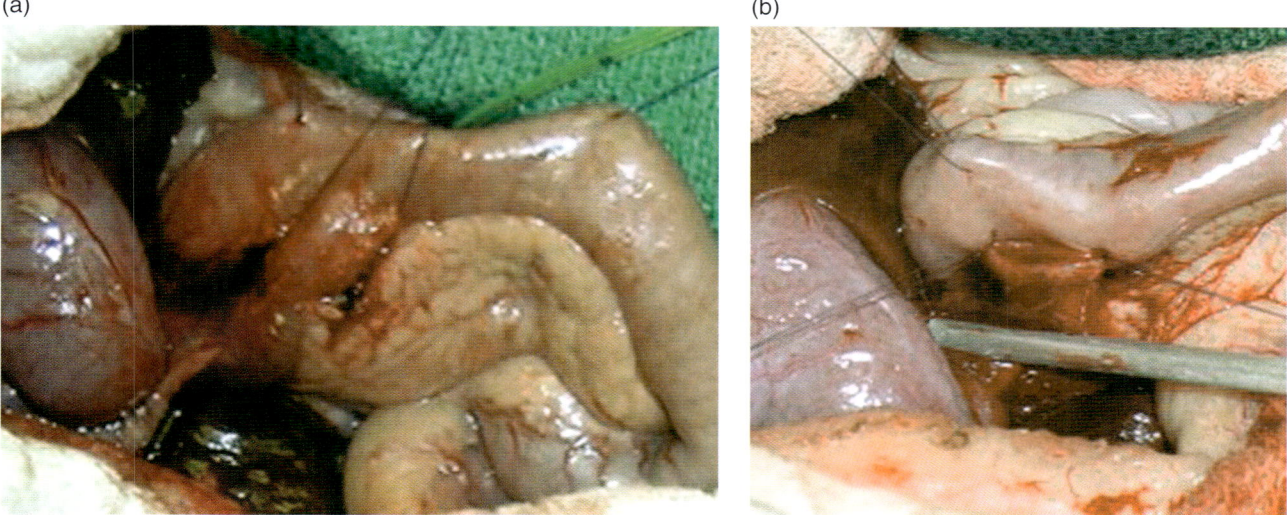

Figure 17.9 (a) A large bile duct that is ligated as close as possible to the duodenum. (b) The end of the bile duct has been spatulated and will be sutured onto the side of the duodenum after creating an incision in the duodenal wall.

mechanism is not included in the anastomosis, enteric reflux into the bile duct is expected.

The side-to-side anastomosis can be performed as a sphincteroplasty technique (described shortly) or as a true side-to-side anastomosis. The bile duct is ligated and transected as close to the duodenum as possible to limit the amount of tension on the anastomosis (Figure 17.9a). A 1.5–2 cm full-thickness incision is made into the antimesenteric surface of the proximal duodenum, or halfway between the mesenteric and antimesenteric border, over the suspected location of the

major duodenal papilla. The free end of the transected bile duct is spatulated on its ventromedial side, beginning from the open end and directed 1.5–2 cm toward the hepatic ducts. Using an absorbable monofilament 5-0 to 8-0 synthetic suture, a simple continuous pattern is used to attach the bile duct to the small intestine. Two separate suture lines are placed and the knots are made on the outside of the lumen. Two stay sutures are placed and will be used to perform the anastomosis (Figure 17.9b). An interrupted suture pattern may also be used to complete the anastomosis. A closed-suction

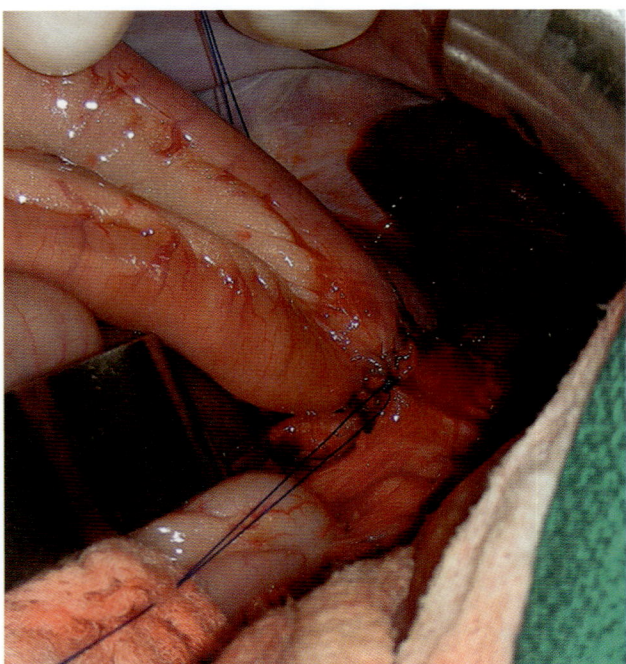

Figure 17.10 Choledochojejunostomy has been performed because excessive tension was present to reimplant the bile duct to the duodenum.

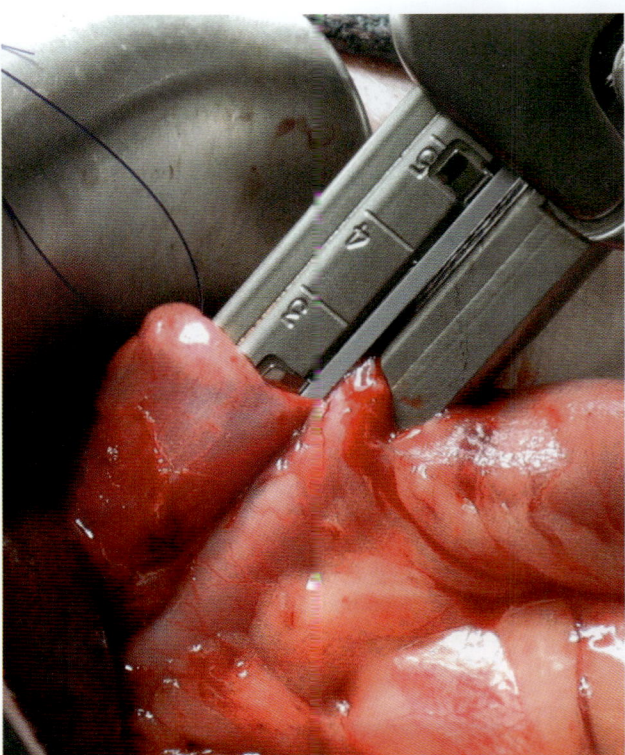

Figure 17.11 Intraoperative view of a large-breed dog undergoing cholecystojejunostomy because of malignant bile duct obstruction. The GIA 55 is being used to create a side-to-side anastomosis.

drain can be placed as a diagnostic aid to help detect early dehiscence of the biliary–enteric anastomosis. The drain is removed in 3–5 days or when appropriate.

If a choledochoduodenostomy cannot be performed because the bile duct is too short and too much tension is present to bring the bile duct to the duodenum, a choledochojejunostomy can be performed instead. A loop of jejunum is brought close to the bile duct and the anastomosis is performed as just described (Figure 17.10).

Stapling equipment can also be used to perform the cholecystoduodenostomy or cholecystojejunostomy. A gastrointestinal stapler is used for the anastomosis (Figure 17.11) and the entry site of the stapler is closed with sutures.

Surgery to palliate acute and chronic biliary outflow acute obstruction: cholecystostomy and choledochal stenting

Biliary decompression by means of a cholecystostomy tube, placed by percutaneous, laparoscopic, or open methods, may be indicated in critically ill patients until they are stable enough for a more complicated procedure. However, preoperative decompression is controversial in humans, and in some studies has led to an increase in morbidity and mortality (Lane *et al.* 1967;

Pitt *et al.* 1981; Pitt 1985, 1986; Lois *et al.* 1987; Nagino *et al.* 2007). Percutaneous and laparoscopic methods for biliary tract drainage have been published for a small number of veterinary patients (Lawrence *et al.* 1992; Herman *et al.* 2005; Murphy *et al.* 2007; Mayhew 2009). Extracorporeal decompression and drainage of bile and its constituents in a patient with EHBT obstruction will facilitate the lowering of systemic bilirubin levels, but will also eliminate the positive effects of bile salts from the body. Without bile salts, fat absorption will continue to fail, as will the absorption of the fat-soluble vitamins. Given the natural detergent and endotoxin-binding properties of bile salts, portal blood flow will continue to carry endotoxin and bacteria to the liver with a compromised RES. It is likely that the lack of bile salts in the small intestine has much to do with the severe and critical systemic illnesses often observed in patients with EHBT obstruction (Pitt 1985, 1986; Pitt *et al.* 1985; Sung *et al.* 1992; Mehler *et al.* 2004; Nagino *et al.* 2007). It is important to remember that treatment of biliary tract sepsis without biliary tract decompression will be ineffective, because no antibiotics will achieve adequate levels in the biliary tree in the presence of EHBT obstruction.

Choledochal stenting

Choledochal stenting is frequently performed in humans to provide a conduit for bile flow into the duodenum across an area of obstruction, or to provide support to maintain an open lumen in the face of ductal stricturing or malignant ingrowth. In dogs and cats, clinical scenarios where temporary reversible EHBT obstruction caused by pancreatitis and/or cholangiohepatitis are more frequently encountered. Candidates for stenting are those with functional EHBT obstruction (demonstrated by laboratory and imaging evidence), but where intraoperatively a stent can be passed across the area of obstruction. Treatment of traumatic bile duct injury with subsequent bile leakage in addition to primary ductal repair can be supported by a choledochal stent, although it remains unclear in small animals whether stents are beneficial or detrimental to healing in these situations. Other indications for choledochal stenting may include palliation of malignancy and temporary drainage of the biliary system prior to definitive surgical repair in severely compromised animals.

Prior to considering choledochal stent placement, the EHBT should be thoroughly evaluated for any evidence of biliary tract perforation, intraluminal or extraluminal masses, or pancreatic abnormalities. An antimesenteric duodenotomy is performed over the anticipated location of the major duodenal papilla. A red rubber catheter of appropriate size (usually 3.5–5 Fr for cats and 8–12 Fr for larger dogs) is used to catheterize the major duodenal papilla to assess patency of the duct. Care should be taken not to enter the pancreatic duct; this can occur especially in cats due to the conjoined nature of the ductal systems in this species. If passage of even a small catheter is impossible, choledochal stenting is not an option in that patient and a technique for biliary rerouting should be considered. The largest stent size that does not completely fill the bile duct lumen should be chosen. If using a red rubber catheter, a section is cut long enough to leave 2–4 cm of stent in the duodenum, with the other end passing into the papilla and crossing the area of constriction within the bile duct. Several more fenestrations can be cut into each end of the stent (Figure 17.12). The duodenal end can be sutured to the duodenal submucosa with one or two 2-0 or 3-0 monofilament absorbable sutures. If available, human polyethylene biliary stents can be used for this purpose, although their use in clinical veterinary patients has not yet been reported. In a report detailing the outcome in 13 dogs where choledochal stenting was employed to treat a variety of causes of EHBT obstruction, no EHBT reobstructions occurred in those that survived the perioperative period (Mayhew *et al.* 2006). However, in a report of seven cats, two reobstructed within one week

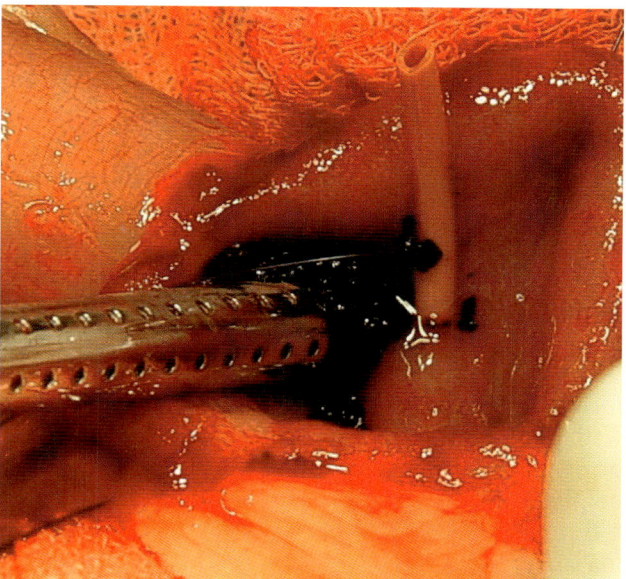

Figure 17.12 Intraoperative view of a dog with extrahepatic bile duct obstruction secondary to pancreatitis. A 5 Fr red rubber catheter has been cut to a shorter length and new fenestrations have been made in the catheter. The stent will be sutured to the mesenteric mucosal surface with 4-0 PDS® (Ethicon, Raritan, NJ, USA) before closing the duodenotomy incision.

of surgery. The small size of the catheter lumen used in cats may predispose to early reobstruction. Care should therefore be taken when using this technique in cats, as morbidity in this species may be higher than in dogs. Spontaneous passage of the stent in the feces was documented in four of five dogs and two of three cats in cases that survived to discharge and where the fate of the stent could be confirmed. In cases where the underlying pathology resolves (especially pancreatitis), stent removal by endoscopy 2–4 months postoperatively is advised due to the possibility for obstruction and ascending cholangiohepatitis. Endoscopic placement of choledochal stents using a side-view endoscope has been evaluated in experimental dogs only, but may hold promise for minimally invasive placement of choledochal stents in the future.

Cholecystostomy tubes

Cholecystostomy tubes provide temporary diversion of bile from the gallbladder to an extracorporeal closed collection system. Similarly to choledochal stenting, if used to treat a temporary and reversible cause of EHBT obstruction, they will not result in any long-term anatomic alteration to the EHBT, unlike biliary rerouting procedures. In some cases judged to be poor candidates for prolonged anesthesia, establishing temporary biliary drainage may be of value. The use of preoperative biliary drainage in high-risk patients prior to definitive surgical intervention is established in humans, but remains controversial. One disadvantage of cholecystostomy tubes is that bile does not drain into the intestines, resulting in a lack of endotoxin-binding capacity, as previously mentioned. If a feeding tube is in place, it may be possible to return the drained bile into the intestine through the tube, as most patients in which cholecystostomy tubes are indicated will be too systemically compromised to accept fluids by mouth.

"Open" cholecystostomy tube placement is performed after thorough evaluation of the gallbladder wall confirms that gallbladder necrosis is not present prior to tube placement. A purse-string suture should be placed in the apex of the gallbladder using 2-0 to 4-0 monofilament absorbable suture material, allowing enough space within it to accommodate either a pigtail or Foley catheter. A small stab incision is made into the gallbladder and the catheter previously passed through the abdominal wall on the right side just caudal to the costal arch is passed through the incision and used to completely drain the gallbladder of bile (Figure 17.13). It is secured to the outside of the body wall with a finger-trap suture using 0 or 2-0 nonabsorbable suture material and attached to a sterile collection system.

Laparoscopic-assisted cholecystostomy tube placement has recently been shown to be technically feasible in dogs. Similar to open cholecystostomy tube placement, the patient is placed in dorsal recumbency. First, a subumbilical port is established for creation of a pneu-

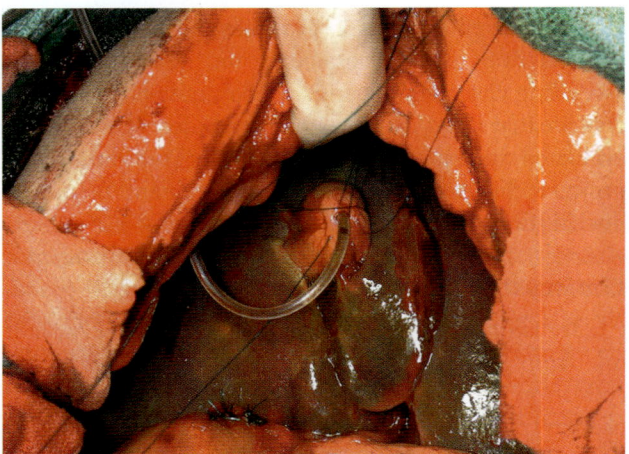

Figure 17.13 A cholecystostomy has been performed with an 8 Fr infant feeding tube. A purse-string suture was placed at the apex of the gallbladder and four pexy sutures are placed between the gallbladder and the abdominal wall.

moperitoneum and exploration of the peritoneal cavity. An instrument port is then placed under direct visualization in the left or right cranial quadrant of the abdomen (the exact location is not critical). Catheter entry in a right paraxiphoid position has been described with a high success rate (Murphy et al. 2007). Entry in a slightly more caudal and right-sided location just caudal to the costal arch has also been described (Murphy et al. 2007). An 8–10 Fr locking loop catheter is normally recommended. A stab incision is made through the skin and using the sharp stylet of the catheter the body wall is penetrated. A blunt probe is placed through the instrument port to manipulate the gallbladder into a position that ensures the catheter enters the apex of the gallbladder. A transhepatic trajectory can also be chosen, although it is uncertain what significance this has. One study found that leak point pressures of nontranshepatically placed cholecystostomy tubes were significantly higher than previously reported intracholic pressures in dogs (Murphy et al. 2007; Mayhew 2009). The importance of transhepatic passage of the tube in humans also appears to be uncertain (Garber et al. 1994). Once the stylet has penetrated the gallbladder and the catheter has been advanced such that all fenestrations reside within the gallbladder lumen, the string to fix the locking loop in place is tightened. The gallbladder is then completely emptied to reduce bile spillage around the catheter site and the gallbladder is gently pulled up against the body wall. At this point it may be helpful to partially or fully evacuate the pneumoperitoneum to minimize tension and ensure the gallbladder can be pulled snugly against the body wall. The catheter is then secured to the outer body wall with a Chinese finger-trap suture using 2-0 nonabsorbable suture material and is attached to a sterile collection system.

The main complications of cholecystostomy tubes are premature obstruction and dislodgment. Obstruction as early as 12 hours postoperatively has been described in a cat (Murphy et al. 2007). Early dislodgment with subsequent intraperitoneal bile leakage has also been reported. Despite some suggestions that 5–10 days is sufficient for catheter tract maturation and leakage prevention, recent evidence suggests that maintenance of the catheters for 3–4 weeks may be more appropriate (Murphy et al. 2007; Mayhew 2009). Follow-up cholangiography in cases of pancreatitis or other potentially reversible conditions are performed every 2–3 days to evaluate biliary tract patency. If patency is reestablished, the cholecystostomy tube can be capped, wrapped, and left in place for approximately one month to prevent leakage. If obstruction remains after 10–14 days, consideration should be given to biliary rerouting for long-term biliary drainage.

Chronic obstruction: biliary–enteric anastamoses (cholecystoenterostomy)

Indications include (i) any underlying disease that has led to permanent complete obstruction of the bile duct, major duodenal papilla, or proximal duodenum such that bile is prevented from exiting the EHBT or (ii) where resection of the proximal duodenum including the bile duct is required. Common causes include cholelithiasis, neoplasia of the bile duct, pancreas, or duodenum, and pancreatitis. The gallbladder must be in good health and the cystic artery must not be damaged during dissection and manipulation of the gallbladder out of the hepatic fossa. If cholecystoenterostomy is being performed because of bile duct rupture or secondary to proximal duodenal resection, it is imperative that the bile duct remnant remaining in the body be ligated securely. If the rerouting procedure is being performed secondary to a blockage of the bile duct and there is little chance of the bile duct rupturing or leaking, ligation of the bile duct is not needed.

The preferred gallbladder rerouting procedure in humans is the cholecystojejunoduodenostomy (jejunal limb interposition or Roux-en-Y procedure), because of the decreased enterobiliary reflux compared with other types of cholecystoenteric anastomosis and the limited derangement in gastrointestinal physiology, but it does require the interposition of a 40 cm segment of jejunum, which might be too long for dogs and cats (Hillis *et al.* 1977; Rokkjaer & Marqversen 1979; Donovan *et al.* 1982; Tatsumi 1984; Gustavsson *et al.* 1988; Lally *et al.* 1989; Martin 1993). It is suspected that dogs and cats will develop clinical short bowel syndrome after utilizing 40–50 cm of jejunum for this procedure, especially in small animals. Since it has been shown in human patients that the interposition of a 40 cm limb of jejunum may lead to stagnant chyme and small intestinal bacterial overgrowth (Ramus *et al.* 1982; Gustavsson *et al.* 1988; Le Blanc-Louvry *et al.* 1999), it might be possible to perform the Roux-en-Y with a shorter segment of jejunum in the smaller animal. Although cholecystoduodenostomy is an acceptable technique, cholecystojejunoduodenostomy with a shorter jejunal limb should be evaluated further in small animal patients.

Clinically useful gallbladder rerouting techniques are limited to cholecystoduodenostomy and cholecystojejunostomy. The mucosal appositional technique of cholecystoduodenostomy is currently the recommended technique for biliary redirection in dogs (Martin *et al.* 2003). The technique involves creating a permanent stoma between the small bowel and the gallbladder. This can be done with hand suturing or with automatic stapling devices (Buote *et al.* 2006; Morrison *et al.* 2008).

The most critical factor in biliary–enteric anastomosis is creating a large enough opening to permit drainage of refluxed intestinal contents from the biliary tract back into the intestine. Numerous surgery texts recommend that the length of the cholecystoenterostomy opening should be 2.5–4 cm to minimize postoperative problems such as cholangitis associated with inadequate draining of refluxed intestinal contents (Blass & Seim 1985; Matthiesen & Rosin 1986; Matthiesen 1989). It is recommended that a large stoma is made, because contraction is expected to be about 50% of the original stoma size. We recommend creating an incision in the gallbladder that extends from the fundus to the beginning of the cystic duct and a corresponding incision in the intestine of equivalent length to minimize the effect of postoperative stoma contraction.

Two main factors must be considered when deciding which part of the small bowel to attach to the gallbladder. It is ideal to be as proximal in the small intestine as possible without creating tension on the biliary–enteric anastomosis. This will allow bile to enter the gastrointestinal tract as close to its normal anatomic location as possible without leading to dehiscence of the anastomosis. Two techniques that assist in decreasing the tension on a proximal anastomosis include release of the duodenocolic ligament and careful dissection of the gallbladder from the hepatic fossa. The surgeon must be careful not to damage, twist, or stretch the cystic artery when removing the gallbladder from the hepatic fossa or when the gallbladder is sutured to the intestine, as dehiscence will occur. In balancing the pros and cons of physiologic location against potential tension and damage of the cystic artery, many surgeons prefer to leave the gallbladder within the hepatic fossa or partially dissect it and perform a cholecystojejunostomy.

The proposed section of bowel that will be used for the anastomosis is brought up to the gallbladder to ensure that there will be minimal tension (Figure 17.14). A full-thickness incision is made in the ventral surface of the gallbladder from the fundus to the beginning of the cystic duct at the infundibulum. A full-thickness longitudinal incision is made on the antimesenteric border of the small intestine the same length as the gallbladder incision. An absorbable synthetic monofilament 3-0 to 5-0 suture is used in a simple continuous pattern to attach the gallbladder to the small intestine. Two separate suture lines are placed and the knots are made on the outside of the lumen. It is important to note that a common spot for leakage is where the knots of both suture lines come together at the oral and aboral ends of the anastomosis. We recommend placing a simple interrupted suture at each end between the knots of the continuous suture lines, as needed. A watertight seal is

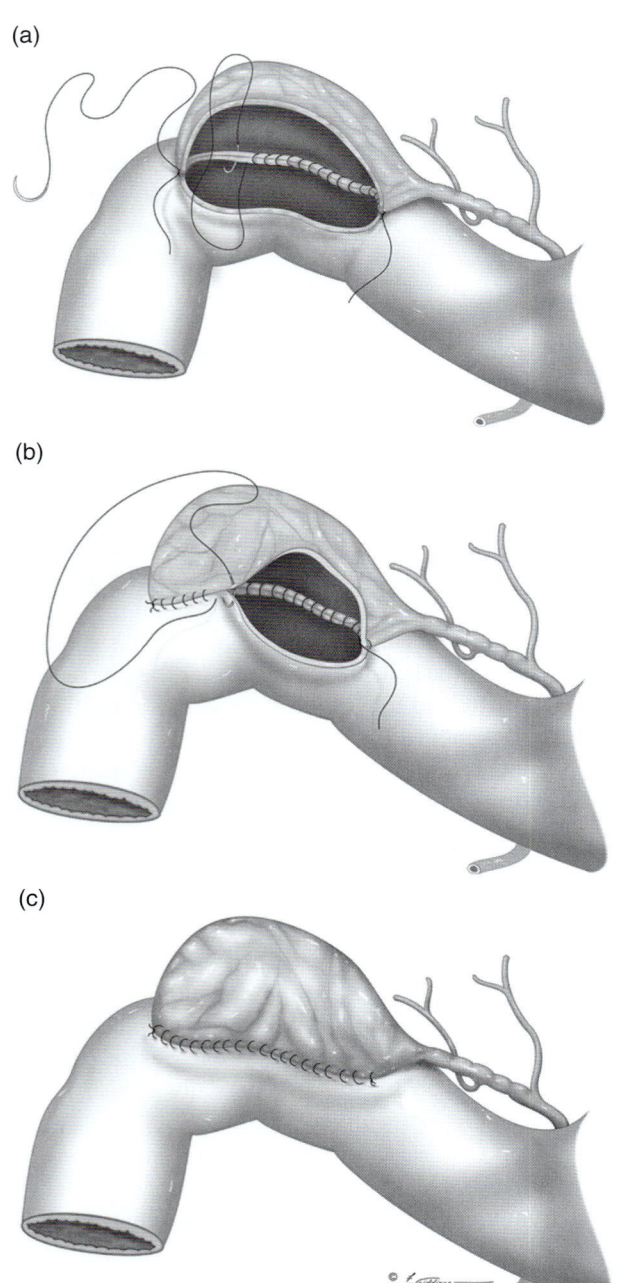

Figure 17.14 Cholecystoenterostomy. (a) A full-thickness incision is made on the antimesenteric border of a loop of intestine. The incision should be at least 2.5 cm long to prevent stenosis and allow adequate drainage from the gallbladder. The gallbladder is also incised along its long axis. A simple continuous apposition pattern with 4-0 monofilament suture is applied to anastomose the gallbladder to the enterostomy site. Two stay sutures are pre-placed to help manipulate the gallbladder during the procedure. The back side of the anastomosis is performed first. (b) Another simple continuous apposition suture is applied on the side of the anastomosis. There is a tendency for leakage to occur at each end of the anastomosis. (c) A one-layer closure is sufficient to achieve a safe cholecystoenterostomy.

difficult to assess, as injected saline will flow into the gallbladder and into the biliary tract. Omentum is brought to and wrapped around the surgical anastomosis following thorough lavage of the area and abdomen. A closed-suction drain can be placed as a diagnostic aid to help detect early dehiscence of the biliary–enteric anastomosis. The drain is removed in 3–5 days or when appropriate.

The use of surgical stapling devices has also been described to accomplish a biliary-enteric anastomosis in dogs and cats (Lehur *et al.* 1986; Morrison *et al.* 2008). The benefits of using a surgical stapling device for this procedure include minimizing the trauma and inflammation caused by multiple manipulations of the bowel and providing a rapid increase in tensile strength compared with sutured anastomoses (Hess *et al.* 1981; Ballantyne *et al.* 1985; Singer *et al.* 2004). The use of stapling equipment also reduces surgical time. Bile-duct anastomoses using titanium staples result in less fibrosis than sutured anastomoses. Titanium staples also promote healing by primary intention and reduce the lag phase of healing (Ballantyne *et al.* 1985). The disadvantages include cost, availability, and the learning curve associated with the correct use of surgical stapling equipment. Endovascular gastrointestinal anastomosis (Endo GIA™, Covidien, Dublin, Ireland) devices are preferred for biliary–enteric anastomosis because of the smaller diameter and shorter tips compared with a linear cutting stapler or GIA, but the GIA has been used successfully in large dogs. Most Endo GIA staplers also have six rows of staggered staples instead of the four rows in most GIA staplers. A stay suture is placed from the fundus of the gallbladder to the location in the small intestine where the biliary–enteric anastomosis will be made. An incision large enough to accommodate the tip of the Endo GIA is made in the fundus of the gallbladder using a no. 11 blade. A similarly sized incision is made in the small intestine and one tip of the Endo GIA is placed into the gallbladder and directed toward the infundibulum, while the other tip is inserted into the incision in the small intestine and directed in an oral direction. Once the stapler has been secured and fired, it is removed to reveal the side-to-side biliary–enteric anastomosis. The remaining hole in the gallbladder and small intestine can be closed with a TA™ (Covidien) stapler or, to minimize the reduction in stoma size, hand suturing with a simple interrupted or continuous pattern is performed.

Cholecystoduodenostomy and cholecystojejunostomy predispose a patient to enterobiliary reflux. Cholecystojejunostomy may decrease the chances of enterobiliary reflux, but increases the risk of peptic ulceration of the duodenum due to the altered physiology of the gastrointestinal tract (Tatsumi 1984; Davies *et al.* 1985; Tsuchiya *et al.* 1986). This is because the bile is a major source of HCO_3^-, which acts to neutralize gastric acid leaving the stomach and entering the duodenum. Other complications of biliary–enteric anastomosis commonly include leakage, dehiscence, stricture, and cholangiohepatitis if the biliary–enteric stoma is too small.

When bile is diverted from the duodenum to the jejunum via a rerouting procedure, fat digestion is decreased, gastric acid secretion is increased, and neutralization of gastric acid in the duodenum is decreased (Shin & Enquist 1970; Tatsumi 1984; Davies *et al.* 1985; Tsuchiya *et al.* 1986). Duodenal ulcers may develop as a sequela and postoperative treatment with a proton pump inhibitor is recommended. Owners should monitor these patients for fever, inappetence, and vomiting, and seek veterinary assistance if cyclic illness is suspected. A complete blood count and serum biochemistry profile (liver enzymes) should be monitored as needed.

Dehiscence of the anastomosis can occur with improper suture placement, ischemic injury to the gallbladder, or excessive tension across the anastomosis site. An early postoperative diagnosis of bile leakage can be difficult due to the insidious onset of clinical signs associated with bile in the abdomen. We routinely place a closed-suction drain intraoperatively close to the cholecystoenteric anastomosis for early detection of dehiscence and leakage of bile.

Pancreatitis can result from excessive intraoperative traction and manipulation of the pancreas, which causes iatrogenic injury to the pancreatic parenchyma, ductal system, or blood supply. The pancreas is also a target organ for ischemic damage resulting from systemic disturbances such as shock and sepsis. Thus, the development of pancreatitis after surgery may be unrelated to manipulation of the pancreas.

Given the potential physiologic consequences of a distal cholecystoduodenostomy or a cholecystojejunostomy in humans and small animals, cholecystojejunoduodenostomy is used in humans and should be evaluated in veterinary surgery.

Prognosis for patients with extrahepatic biliary tract obstruction

Factors affecting prognosis in humans undergoing EHBT surgery include malignancy, age (>60 years), fever, leukocytosis, azotemia, hypoalbuminemia, hyperbilirubinemia, anemia, and increased serum alkaline phosphatase (Dixon *et al.* 1983, 1984a). Humans with obstructive jaundice are at increased risk of acute renal failure that develops as a result of bacterial endotoxemia (Mahour *et al.* 1968; Wardle & Wright 1970; Schall

et al. 1973; Wardle 1982; Pain & Bailey 1986, 1987, 1988; Cahill *et al.* 1987; Pain 1987; Cahill & Pain 1988). The same sequelae are seen in experimental animals with obstructive jaundice (Wardle & Wright 1970; Schall *et al.* 1973; Brady & King 2000). The mortality rate for humans with obstructive jaundice is significantly higher in those with acute renal failure than in those without renal failure (Wilkinson *et al.* 1976; Pain & Bailey 1986). In a rat model, the absence of bile salts in the small intestine enables the absorption of endotoxin (Bayer & Ellis 1976; Cahill *et al.* 1987; Deitch *et al.* 1990). Gut-derived endotoxins are powerful renal vasoconstrictors and cause a decrease in intrarenal blood flow and glomerular filtration rate, and subsequent degeneration of the renal tubular epithelium (Mahour *et al.* 1968; Wardle & Wright 1970; Schall *et al.* 1973; Wardle 1982; Pain & Bailey 1986, 1987, 1988; Cahill *et al.* 1987; Pain 1987).

In dogs and cats, many authors have evaluated the risk factors associated with outcome in patients undergoing surgery of the EHBT (Martin *et al.* 1986; Fahie & Martin 1995; Mayhew *et al.* 2002; Mehler *et al.* 2004; Amsellem *et al.* 2006; Buote *et al.* 2006). Factors besides renal azotemia include the presence of septic bile peritonitis, leukocytosis, prolongation of PTT, hypotension, sepsis, and DIC. Surgical biliary intervention in cats with EHBT obstruction has about a 50% mortality rate overall and almost a 100% mortality when neoplasia is involved (Mayhew *et al.* 2002; Buote *et al.* 2006; Mayhew & Weisse 2008; Morrison *et al.* 2008). Causes of death in these cats included clinical deterioration, enterostomy dehiscence, and cardiopulmonary arrest.

Endotoxin absorption is likely an important factor in the pathophysiology of extrahepatic biliary disease in small animals. Despite advances in preoperative evaluation and postoperative care in human medicine, interventions for relief of obstructive jaundice still carry high morbidity and mortality rates associated with sepsis and renal dysfunction. Endotoxin and bacteria from the gastrointestinal tract gain access to the portal circulation because of a derangement in immunologic, biologic, and anatomic barriers. Elevated systemic bilirubin levels overwhelm and paralyze the RES in the liver and the absence of bile salts in the small intestine deprives the gut of most of its secretory immunoglobulin (Ig)A and the natural detergent properties of bile (Brown & Kloppel 1989; Sung *et al.* 1992; Wells *et al.* 1995). The presence of bile prevents bacterial adherence to intestinal mucosa and binds to endotoxin liberated from Gram-negative bacteria. If any bacteria or endotoxin are able to get into the portal blood, the RES is able to detoxify the blood before it is returned to the systemic circulation. In addition, the lack of bile in the small intestine prevents the absorption of fat-soluble vitamins and therefore the vitamin K-dependent coagulation factors are not adequately activated, leading to disturbances in intrinsic, extrinsic, and common coagulation pathways. With the RES debilitated, a deranged coagulation system, and without bile salts and IgA in the small intestine, it becomes obvious why so many of our patients succumb to their disease. This stresses the need for early stabilization, diagnosis, and surgical intervention to rapidly restore the flow of bile to the small intestine and remove bilirubin from systemic circulation.

References

Aguirre, A.L., Center, S.A., Randolph, J.F. et al. (2007). Gallbladder disease in Shetland sheepdogs: 38 cases (1995–2005). *Journal of the American Veterinary Medical Association* 231: 79–88.

Amsellem, P.M., Seim, H.B., Macphail, C. et al. (2006). Long-term survival and risk factors associated with biliary surgery in dogs: 34 cases (1994–2004). *Journal of the American Veterinary Medical Association* 229: 1451–1457.

Anon. (1969). *Toxocara canis* as a support for cholelithiasis in the dog. *Veterinary Record* 85: 98–99.

Bacon, N.J. and White, R.A. (2003). Extrahepatic biliary tract surgery in the cat: a case series and review. *Journal of Small Animal Practice* 44: 231–235.

Baker, S.G., Mayhew, P.D., and Mehler, S.J. (2009). Choledochotomy and primary repair of extrahepatic biliary duct tears in dogs and cats. *Veterinary Surgery* 38: E25.

Ballantyne, G.H., Burke, J.B., Rogers, G. et al. (1985). Accelerated wound healing with stapled enteric suture lines. An experimental study comparing traditional sewing techniques and a stapling device. *Annals of Surgery* 201: 360–364.

Barsanti, J.A., Higgins, R.J., Spano, J.S., and Jones, B.D. (1976). Adenocarcinoma of the extrahepatic bile duct in a cat. *Journal of Small Animal Practice* 17: 599–605.

Bayer, I. and Ellis, H. (1976). Jaundice and wound healing: an experimental study. *British Journal of Surgery* 63: 392–396.

Besso, J.G., Wrigley, R.H., Gliatto, J.M., and Webster, C.R. (2000). Ultrasonographic appearance and clinical findings in 14 dogs with gallbladder mucocele. *Veterinary Radiology and Ultrasound* 41: 261–271.

Blass, C.E. and Seim, H.B. III (1985). Surgical techniques for the liver and biliary tract. *Veterinary Clinics of North America Small Animal Practice* 15: 257–275.

Boothe, H.W., Boothe, D.M., Komkov, A., and Hightower, D. (1992). Use of hepatobiliary scintigraphy in the diagnosis of extrahepatic biliary obstruction in dogs and cats: 25 cases (1982–1989). *Journal of the American Veterinary Medical Association* 201: 134–141.

Brady, C.A. and King, L.G. (2000). Postoperative management of the emergency surgery small animal patient. *Veterinary Clinics of North America. Small Animal Practice* 30: 681–698.

Breznock, E.M. (1998). Surgical procedures of the hepatobiliary system. In: *Current Techniques in Small Animal Surgery*, 4e (ed. M.J. Bojrab, B. Slocum and G. Ellison), 298–313. Baltimore, MD: Williams & Wilkins.

Brown, W.R. and Kloppel, T.M. (1989). The liver and IgA: immunological, cell biological and clinical implications. *Hepatology* 9: 763–784.

Buote, N.J., Mitchell, S.L., Penninck, D. et al. (2006). Cholecystoenterostomy for treatment of extrahepatic biliary tract obstruction in cats: 22 cases (1994–2003). *Journal of the American Veterinary Medical Association* 228: 1376–1382.

Cahill, C.J. and Pain, J.A. (1988). Obstructive jaundice. Renal failure and other endotoxin-related complications. *Surgery Annual* 20: 17–37.

Cahill, C.J., Pain, J.A., and Bailey, M.E. (1987). Bile salts, endotoxin and renal function in obstructive jaundice. *Surgery Gynecology and Obstetrics* 165: 519–522.

Capper, W.M. (1957). Choledochoduodenostomy. *British Medical Journal* 1: 1417–1418.

Capper, W.M. (1961). External choledochoduodenostomy. An evaluation of 125 cases. *British Journal of Surgery* 49: 292–300.

Carlisle, C.H. (1977). A comparison of techniques for cholecystography in cats. *Journal of the American Veterinary Radiology Society* 18: 173–176.

Center, S.A. (1996). Diseases of the gallbladder and biliary tree. In: *Strombeck's Small Animal Gastroenterology*, 3e (ed. W.G. Guilford, S.A. Center, C.R. Strombeck, et al.), 860–888. Philadelphia, PA: WB Saunders.

Center, S.A. (2009). Diseases of the gallbladder and biliary tree. *Veterinary Clinics of North America Small Animal Practice* 39: 543–598.

Chiang, J.Y. (2013). Bile acid metabolism and signaling. *Comprehensive Physiology* 3: 1191–1212.

Church, E.M. and Matthiesen, D.T. (1988). Surgical treatment of 23 dogs with necrotizing cholecystitis. *Journal of the American Animal Hospital Association* 24: 305–310.

Cribb, A.E., Burgener, D.C., and Reimann, K.A. (1988). Bile duct obstruction secondary to chronic pancreatitis in seven dogs. *Canadian Veterinary Journal* 29: 654–657.

Davies, H.A., Wheeler, M.H., Psaila, J. et al. (1985). Bile exclusion from the duodenum. Its effect on gastric and pancreatic function in the dog. *Digestive Diseases and Sciences* 30: 954–960.

Deitch, E.A., Sittig, K., Li, M. et al. (1990). Obstructive jaundice promotes bacterial translocation from the gut. *American Journal of Surgery* 159: 79–84.

Dixon, J.M., Armstrong, C.P., Duffy, S.W., and Davies, G.C. (1983). Factors affecting morbidity and mortality after surgery for obstructive jaundice: a review of 373 patients. *Gut* 24: 845–852.

Dixon, J.M., Armstrong, C.P., Duffy, S.W. et al. (1984a). Factors affecting mortality and morbidity after surgery for obstructive jaundice. *Gut* 25: 104.

Dixon, J.M., Armstrong, C.P., Duffy, S.W. et al. (1984b). Upper gastrointestinal bleeding. A significant complication after surgery for relief of obstructive jaundice. *Annals of Surgery* 199: 271–275.

Donovan, I.A., Fielding, J.W., Bradby, H. et al. (1982). Bile diversion after total gastrectomy. *British Journal of Surgery* 69: 389–390.

Drivas, G., James, O., and Wardle, N. (1976). Study of reticuloendothelial phagocytic capacity in patients with cholestasis. *British Medical Journal* 1: 1568–1569.

Evans, H.E. and Christensen, G.C. (1979). The digestive apparatus and abdomen. In: *Miller's Anatomy of the Dog*, 2e (ed. M.E. Miller, H.E. Evans and G.C. Christensen), 411–506. Philadelphia, PA: WB Saunders.

Fahie, M.A. and Martin, R.A. (1995). Extrahepatic biliary tract obstruction: a retrospective study of 45 cases (1983–1993). *Journal of the American Animal Hospital Association* 31: 478–482.

Friman, S., Radberg, G., Bosaeus, I., and Svanvik, J. (1990). Hepatobiliary compensation for the loss of gallbladder function after cholecystectomy. An experimental study in the cat. *Scandinavian Journal of Gastroenterology* 25: 307–314.

Garber, S.J., Mathieson, J.R., Cooperberg, P.L., and MacFarlane, J.K. (1994). Percutaneous cholecystostomy: safety of the transperitoneal route. *Journal of Vascular and Interventional Radiology* 5: 295–298.

Gordon-Taylor, G. (1937). On gallstones and their sufferers. *British Journal of Surgery* 25: 241–251.

Gustavsson, S., Ilstrup, D.M., Morrison, P., and Kelly, K.A. (1988). Roux-Y stasis syndrome after gastrectomy. *American Journal of Surgery* 155: 490–494.

Guyton, A.C. and Hale, J.E. (2006). Secretion of bile by the liver, function of the biliary tree. In: *Textbook of Medical Physiology*, 801–804. Philadelphia, PA: Elsevier Saunders.

Harkema, J.R., Mason, M.J., Kusewitt, D.F., and Pickrell, J.A. (1982). Cholecystotomy as treatment for obstructive jaundice in a dog. *Journal of the American Veterinary Medical Association* 181: 815–816.

Head, L.L. and Daniel, G.B. (2005). Correlation between hepatobiliary scintigraphy and surgery or postmortem examination findings in dogs and cats with extrahepatic biliary obstruction, partial obstruction, or patency of the biliary system: 18 cases (1995–2004). *Journal of the American Veterinary Medical Association* 227: 1618–1624.

Herman, B.A., Brawer, R.S., Murtaugh, R.J., and Hackner, S.G. (2005). Therapeutic percutaneous ultrasound-guided cholecystocentesis in three dogs with extrahepatic biliary obstruction and pancreatitis. *Journal of the American Veterinary Medical Association* 227 (1782–1786): 1753.

Hess, J.L., McCurnin, D.M., Riley, M.G., and Koehler, K.J. (1981). Pilot study for comparison of chromic catgut suture and mechanically applied staples in enteroanastomoses. *Journal of the American Animal Hospital Association* 17: 409–414.

Hillis, T.M., Westbrook, K.C., Caldwell, F.T., and Read, R.C. (1977). Surgical injury of the common bile duct. *American Journal of Surgery* 134: 712–716.

Hunt, D.R., Allison, M.E., Prentice, C.R., and Blumgart, L.H. (1982). Endotoxemia, disturbance of coagulation, and obstructive jaundice. *American Journal of Surgery* 144: 325–329.

Ibragimov, E.T., Ordabekov, S.O., and Ongarbaev, S.Z. (1992). Diagnosis and treatment of postoperative bile peritonitis. *Khirurgiia (Moscow)* 1: 86–88.

Jameel, M., Darmas, B., and Baker, A.L. (2008). Trend towards primary closure following laparoscopic exploration of the common bile duct. *Annals of the Royal College of Surgeons of England* 90: 29–35.

Jones, T.C., Hunt, R.D., and King, N.W. (1997). Gallbladder. In: *Veterinary Pathology*, 1103–1105. Baltimore, MD: Williams & Wilkins.

Jorgensen, L.S., Pentlarge, V.W., Flanders, J.A., and Harvey, H.J. (1987). Recurrent cholelithiasis in a cat. *Compendium on Continuing Education for the Practicing Veterinarian* 9: 265–270.

Kanai, H., Hagiwara, K., Nukaya, A. et al. (2018). Short term outcome of laparoscopic cholecystectomy for benign gall bladder diseases in 76 dogs. *Journal of Veterinary Medical Sciences* 80: 1747–1753.

Karaayvaz, M., Uğraş, S., Güler, O. et al. (1998). Use of an autologous vein graft and stent in the repair of common bile defects: an experimental study. *Surgery Today* 28: 830–833.

Kerr, L.Y. and Hornof, W.J. (2005). Quantitative hepatobiliary scintigraphy using ^{99m}Tc-DISIDA in the dog. *Veterinary Radiology and Ultrasound* 27: 173–177.

Lally, K.P., Kanegaye, J., Matsumura, M. et al. (1989). Perioperative factors affecting the outcome following repair of biliary atresia. *Pediatrics* 83: 723–726.

Lane, T.C., Johnson, H.C., and Walker, H.S. Jr. (1967). Extrahepatic biliary decompression in traumatized canine livers. *Surgery* 62: 1039–1043.

Lawrence, D., Bellah, J.R., Meyer, D.J., and Roth, L. (1992). Temporary bile diversion in cats with experimental extrahepatic bile duct obstruction. *Veterinary Surgery* 21: 446–451.

Le Blanc-Louvry, I., Ducrotté, P., Lemeland, J.F. et al. (1999). Motility in the Roux-Y limb after distal gastrectomy: relation to the length of the limb and the afferent duodenojejunal segment. An experimental study. *Neurogastroenterology and Motility* 11: 365–374.

Lehur, P.A., Gaillard, F., and Visset, J. (1986). Value of absorbable stapling in digestive surgery? Experimental study comparing TA metallic stapling, TA absorbable stapling and manual sutures. *Journal de Chirurgie* 123: 563–569.

Lois, J.F., Gomes, A.S., Grace, P.A. et al. (1987). Risks of percutaneous transhepatic drainage in patients with cholangitis. *American Journal of Roentgenology* 148: 367–371.

Ludwig, L.L., McLoughlin, M.A., Graves, T.K., and Crisp, M.S. (1997). Surgical treatment of bile peritonitis in 24 dogs and 2 cats: a retrospective study (1987–1994). *Veterinary Surgery* 26: 90–98.

Mahour, G.H., Wakim, K.G., Soule, E.H., and Ferris, D.O. (1968). Effect of cholecystectomy on the biliary ducts in the dog. *Archives of Surgery* 97: 570–574.

Mair, W.S., Hill, G.L., and Goligher, J.C. (1974). Proceedings: cholelithiasis: a metabolic consequence of ileostomy. *Gut* 15: 830.

Mair, W.S., Hill, G.L., and Goligher, J.C. (1975). Proceedings: cholelithiasis: a metabolic consequence of ileostomy. *British Journal of Surgery* 62: 161–162.

Martin, R.A. (1993). Liver and biliary system. In: *Textbook of Small Animal Surgery* (ed. D.H. Slatter), 645–659. Philadelphia, PA: WB Saunders.

Martin, R.A., Lanz, O.I., and Tobias, K.M. (2003). Liver and biliary system. In: *Textbook of Small Animal Surgery* (ed. D.H. Slatter), 708–726. Philadelphia, PA: Elsevier.

Martin, R.A., MacCoy, D.M., and Harvey, H.J. (1986). Surgical management of extrahepatic biliary tract disease: a report of eleven cases. *Journal of the American Animal Hospital Association* 22: 301–307.

Martin, W.F. and Page, G.D. (1951). Carcinoma of the extrahepatic bile duct: review of recent literature and a case report. *Southern Medical Journal* 44: 109–114.

Marvel, S. and Monnet, E. (2014). Use of a vessel sealant device for cystic duct ligation in the dog. *Veterinary Surgery* 43: 983–987.

Matthiesen, D.T. (1989). Complications associated with surgery of the extrahepatic biliary system. *Problems in Veterinary Medicine* 1: 295–315.

Matthiesen, D.T. and Lammerding, J. (1984). Gallbladder rupture and bile peritonitis secondary to cholelithiasis and cholecystitis in a dog. *Journal of the American Veterinary Medical Association* 184: 1282–1283.

Matthiesen, D.T. and Rosin, E. (1986). Common bile duct obstruction secondary to chronic fibrosing pancreatitis: treatment by use of cholecystoduodenostomy in the dog. *Journal of the American Veterinary Medical Association* 189: 1443–1446.

Mayhew, P.D. (2009). Advanced laparoscopic procedures (hepatobiliary, endocrine) in dogs and cats. *Veterinary Clinics of North America Small Animal Practice* 39: 925–939.

Mayhew, P.D., Holt, D.E., McLear, R.C., and Washabau, R.J. (2002). Pathogenesis and outcome of extrahepatic biliary obstruction in cats. *Journal of Small Animal Practice* 43: 247–253.

Mayhew, P.D., Mehler, S.J., and Radhakrishnan, A. (2008). Laparoscopic cholecystectomy for management of uncomplicated gall bladder mucocele in six dogs. *Veterinary Surgery* 37: 625–630.

Mayhew, P.D., Richardson, R.W., Mehler, S.J. et al. (2006). Choledochal tube stenting for decompression of the extrahepatic portion of the biliary tract in dogs: 13 cases (2002–2005). *Journal of the American Veterinary Medical Association* 228: 1209–1214.

Mayhew, P.D. and Weisse, C.W. (2008). Treatment of pancreatitis-associated extrahepatic biliary tract obstruction by choledochal stenting in seven cats. *Journal of Small Animal Practice* 49: 133–138.

Mehler, S.J., Mayhew, P.D., Drobatz, K.J., and Holt, D.E. (2004). Variables associated with outcome in dogs undergoing extrahepatic biliary surgery: 60 cases (1988–2002). *Veterinary Surgery* 33: 644–649.

Morrison, S., Prostredny, J., and Roa, D. (2008). Retrospective study of 28 cases of cholecystoduodenostomy performed using endoscopic gastrointestinal anastomosis stapling equipment. *Journal of the American Animal Hospital Association* 44: 10–18.

Murphy, S.M., Rodriguez, J.D., and McAnulty, J.F. (2007). Minimally invasive cholecystostomy in the dog: evaluation of placement techniques and use in extrahepatic biliary obstruction. *Veterinary Surgery* 36: 675–683.

Nagino, M., Takada, T., Kawarada, Y. et al. (2007). Methods and timing of biliary drainage for acute cholangitis: Tokyo guidelines. *Journal of Hepato-Biliary-Pancreatic Surgery* 14: 68–77.

Nakeeb, A. and Pitt, H.A. (1995). The role of preoperative biliary decompression in obstructive jaundice. *Hepato-Gastroenterology* 42: 332–337.

Nakeeb, A., Tran, K.Q., Black, M.J. et al. (2002). Improved survival in resected biliary malignancies. *Surgery* 132: 555–563: discussion 563–554.

Neer, T.M. (1992). A review of disorders of the gallbladder and extrahepatic biliary tract in the dog and cat. *Journal of Veterinary Internal Medicine* 6: 186–192.

Neer, T.M. and Hedlend, C.S. (1989). Vitamin K-dependent coagulopathy in a dog with bile and cystic duct obstructions. *Journal of the American Animal Hospital Association* 25: 461–464.

Newell, S.M., Selcer, B.A., Roberts, R.E. et al. (1994). Use of hepatobiliary scintigraphy in clinically normal cats. *American Journal of Veterinary Research* 55: 762–768.

Newell, S.M., Selcer, B.A., Roberts, R.E. et al. (1996). Hepatobiliary scintigraphy in the evaluation of feline liver disease. *Journal of Veterinary Internal Medicine* 10: 308–315.

Noshiro, H., Hotokezaka, M., Higashijima, H. et al. (1996). Gallstone formation and gallbladder bile composition after colectomy in dogs. *Digestive Diseases and Sciences* 41: 2423–2432.

Nyland, T.G. (1982). Sonographic evaluation of experimental bile duct ligation in the dog. *Veterinary Radiology and Ultrasound* 23: 252–260.

Nyland, T.G., Hager, D.A., and Herring, D.S. (1989). Sonography of the liver, gallbladder, and spleen. *Seminars in Veterinary Medicine and Surgery (Small Animal)* 4: 13–31.

Nyland, T.G., Koblik, P.D., and Tellyer, S.E. (1999). Ultrasonographic evaluation of biliary cystadenomas in cats. *Veterinary Radiology and Ultrasound* 40: 300–306.

O'Brien, T.R. and Mitchum, G.D. (1970). Cholelithiasis in a cat. *Journal of the American Veterinary Medical Association* 156: 1015–1017.

Pain, J.A. (1987). Reticulo-endothelial function in obstructive jaundice. *British Journal of Surgery* 74: 1091–1094.

Pain, J.A. and Bailey, M.E. (1986). Experimental and clinical study of lactulose in obstructive jaundice. *British Journal of Surgery* 73: 775–778.

Pain, J.A. and Bailey, M.E. (1987). Measurement of operative plasma endotoxin levels in jaundiced and non-jaundiced patients. *European Surgical Research* 19: 207–216.

Pain, J.A. and Bailey, M.E. (1988). Prevention of endotoxaemia in obstructive jaundice: a comparative study of bile salts. *HPB Surgery* 1: 21–27.

Pain, J.A., Cahill, C.J., and Bailey, M.E. (1985). Perioperative complications in obstructive jaundice: therapeutic considerations. *British Journal of Surgery* 72: 942–945.

Pain, J.A., Cahill, C.J., Gilbert, J.M. et al. (1991). Prevention of postoperative renal dysfunction in patients with obstructive jaundice: a multicentre study of bile salts and lactulose. *British Journal of Surgery* 78: 467–469.

Pain, J.A., Collier, D.S., and Ritson, A. (1987). Reticuloendothelial system phagocytic function in obstructive jaundice and its modification by a muramyl dipeptide analogue. *European Surgical Research* 19: 16–22.

Palermo, S.M., Brown, D.C., Mehler, S.J. et al. (2020). Clinical and prognostic findings in dogs with suspected extrahepatic biliary obstruction and pancreatitis. *Journal of the American Animal Hospital Association* 56: 270–279.

Papazoglou, L.G., Mann, F.A., Wagner-Mann, C., and Song, K.J.E. (2008). Long-term survival of dogs after cholecystoenterostomy: a retrospective study of 15 cases (1981–2005). *Journal of the American Animal Hospital Association* 44: 67–74.

Parchman, M.B. and Flanders, J.A. (1990). Extrahepatic biliary tract rupture: evaluation of the relationship between the site of rupture and the cause of rupture in 15 dogs. *Cornell Veterinarian* 80: 267–272.

Pike, F.S., Berg, J., King, N.W. et al. (2004a). Gallbladder mucocele in dogs: 30 cases (2000–2002). *Journal of the American Veterinary Medical Association* 224: 1615–1622.

Pike, F.S., Berg, J., King, N.W. et al. (2004b). Revision to gallbladder mucocele article. *Journal of the American Veterinary Medical Association* 224: 1916–1917.

Pitt, H.A. (1985). General surgery preoperative biliary tract drainage. *Western Journal of Medicine* 142: 541.

Pitt, H.A. (1986). The use of percutaneous decompression in the jaundiced patient. *Current Surgery* 43: 460–463.

Pitt, H.A., Cameron, J.L., Postier, R.G., and Gadacz, T.R. (1981). Factors affecting mortality in biliary tract surgery. *American Journal of Surgery* 141: 66–72.

Pitt, H.A., Gomes, A.S., Lois, J.F. et al. (1985). Does preoperative percutaneous biliary drainage reduce operative risk or increase hospital cost? *Annals of Surgery* 201: 545–553.

Pitt, H.A., Lewinski, M.A., Muller, E.L. et al. (1984). Ileal resection-induced gallstones: altered bilirubin or cholesterol metabolism? *Surgery* 96: 154–162.

Pitt, H.A., Murray, K.P., Bowman, H.M. et al. (1999). Clinical pathway implementation improves outcomes for complex biliary surgery. *Surgery* 126: 751, discussion 756–758–756.

Radberg, G., Friman, S., Samsioe, G., and Svanvik, J. (1987). Direct measurements of enterohepatic circulation of bile acids in the cat. Influence of contraceptive steroids and oophorectomy. *Scandinavian Journal of Gastroenterology* 22: 827–832.

Radberg, G., Friman, S., Samsioe, G., and Svanvik, J. (1988). Enterohepatic bileacid circulation in the pregnant cat. *Acta Physiologica Scandinavica* 133: 19–24.

Ramus, N.I., Williamson, R.C., and Johnston, D. (1982). The use of jejunal interposition for intractable symptoms complicating peptic ulcer surgery. *British Journal of Surgery* 69: 265–268.

Razin, E., Feldman, M.G., and Dreiling, D.A. (1965). Studies on biliary flow and composition in man and dog. *Journal of the Mount Sinai Hospital, New York* 32: 42–50.

Rege, R.V. (1995). Adverse effects of biliary obstruction: implications for treatment of patients with obstructive jaundice. *American Journal of Roentgenology* 164: 287–293.

Rege, R.V., Dawes, L.G., and Moore, E.W. (1990). Biliary calcium secretion in the dog occurs primarily by passive convection and diffusion and is linked to bile flow. *Journal of Laboratory and Clinical Medicine* 115: 593–602.

Rivers, B.J., Walter, P.A., Johnston, G.R. et al. (1997). Acalculous cholecystitis in four canine cases: ultrasonographic findings and use of ultrasonographic-guided, percutaneous cholecystocentesis in diagnosis. *Journal of the American Animal Hospital Association* 33: 207–214.

Rokkjaer, M. and Marqversen, J. (1979). Intestino-gastric reflux in dogs: spontaneous, after gastrojejunostomy, and after Roux-en-Y gastrojejunostomy with various lengths of the defunctioning loop. *Scandinavian Journal of Gastroenterology* 14: 199–203.

Schall, W.D., Chapman, W.L. Jr., Finco, D.R. et al. (1973). Cholelithiasis in dogs. *Journal of the American Veterinary Medical Association* 163: 469–472.

Scott, J., Singh, A., Mayhew, P.D. et al. (2016). Preoperative complications and outcome of laparoscopic cholecystectomy in 20 dogs. *Veterinary Surgery* 45 (S1): O49–O59.

Shehadi, W.H. (1979). The biliary system through the ages. *International Surgery* 64: 63–78.

Shin, C.S. and Enquist, I.F. (1970). Effect of cholecystojejunostomy, Roux-Y, on intestinal absorption of labelled fat, labelled protein and xylose. *Bulletin de la Société Internationale de Chirurgie* 29: 21–27.

Simon, A. and Monnet, E. (2020). Laparoscopic cholecystectomy with single port access system in 15 dogs. *Veterinary Surgery* 49 (Suppl 1): O156–O162.

Singer, M.A., Cintron, J.R., Benedetti, E. et al. (2004). Hand-sewn versus stapled intestinal anastomoses in a chronically steroid-treated porcine model. *American Surgeon* 70: 151–156. discussion 156.

Smith, S.A. (1998). Diagnostic imaging of biliary obstruction. *Compendium on Continuing Education for the Practicing Veterinarian* 20: 1225–1234.

Sung, J.J., Leung, J.C., Tsui, C.P. et al. (1995). Biliary IgA secretion in obstructive jaundice: the effects of endoscopic drainage. *Gastrointestinal Endoscopy* 42: 439–444.

Sung, J.Y., Leung, J.W., Shaffer, E.A. et al. (1992). Ascending infection of the biliary tract after surgical sphincterotomy and biliary stenting. *Journal of Gastroenterology and Hepatology* 7: 240–245.

Tatsumi, M. (1984). Influences of the biliary reconstructions by Roux-en Y method and jejunal interposition method on the gastric acid secretion in dogs. *Nippon Geka Gakkai Zasshi. Journal of Japan Surgical Society* 85: 705–718.

Tsuchiya, T., Sasaki, I., Imanura, M., and Naito, H. (1986). The influence of biliary diversion on canine gastric acid secretion and gut hormones. *Nippon Geka Gakkai Zasshi. Journal of Japan Surgical Society* 87: 659–670.

Utkan, Z.N., Utkan, T., Sarioglu, Y., and Gönüllü, N.N. (2000). Effects of experimental obstructive jaundice on contractile responses of dog isolated blood vessels: role of endothelium and duration of bile duct ligation. *Clinical and Experimental Pharmacology and Physiology* 27: 339–344.

vanSonnenberg, E., Wittich, G.R., Casola, G. et al. (1986). Diagnostic and therapeutic percutaneous gallbladder procedures. *Radiology* 160: 23–26.

Vazquez, R.M. (2008). Common sense and common bile duct injury: common bile duct injury revisited. *Surgical Endoscopy* 22: 1743–1745.

Walter, R., Dunn, M.E., d'Anjou, M.A., and Lecuyer, M. (2008). Nonsurgical resolution of gallbladder mucocele in two dogs. *Journal of the American Veterinary Medical Association* 232: 1688–1693.

Wardle, E.N. (1982). The importance of anti-lipid A (anti-endotoxin): prevention of "shock lung" and acute renal failure. *World Journal of Surgery* 6: 616–623.

Wardle, E.N. and Wright, N.A. (1970). Endotoxin and acute renal failure associated with obstructive jaundice. *British Medical Journal* 4: 472–474.

Washizu, T., Ishida, T., Washizu, M. et al. (1994). Changes in bile acid composition of serum and gallbladder bile in bile duct ligated dogs. *Journal of Veterinary Medical Science* 56: 299–303.

Wells, C.L., Jechorek, R.P., and Erlandsen, S.L. (1995). Inhibitory effect of bile on bacterial invasion of enterocytes: possible mechanism for increased translocation associated with obstructive jaundice. *Critical Care Medicine* 23: 301–307.

Wilkinson, A.R., DeMonaca, S.M., Panciera, D.L. et al. (2020). Bile duct obstruction associated with pancreatitis in 46 dogs. *Journal of Veterinary Internal Medicine* 34: 1794–1800.

Wilkinson, S.P., Moodie, H., Stamatakis, J.D. et al. (1976). Endotoxaemia and renal failure in cirrhosis and obstructive jaundice. *British Medical Journal* 2: 1415–1418.

Wills, V.L., Gibson, K., Karihaloot, C., and Jorgensen, J.O. (2002). Complications of biliary T-tubes after choledochotomy. *ANZ Journal of Surgery* 72: 177–180.

Worley, D.R., Hottinger, H.A., and Lawrence, H.J. (2004). Surgical management of gallbladder mucoceles in dogs: 22 cases (1999–2003). *Journal of the American Veterinary Medical Association* 225: 1418–1422.

Wrigley, R.H. and Reuter, R.E. (1982). Percutaneous cholecystography in normal dogs. *Veterinary Radiology* 23: 239–242.

Youn, G., Waschak, M.J., Kunkel, K.A.R., and Gerard, P.D. (2018). Outcome of elective cholecystectomy for the treatment of gallbladder disease in dogs. *Journal of the American Veterinary Medical Association* 252: 970–975.

Zeman, R.K., Taylor, K.J., Rosenfield, A.T. et al. (1981). Acute experimental biliary obstruction in the dog: sonographic findings and clinical implications. *American Journal of Roentgenology* 136: 965–967.

Zografakis, J.G., Jones, B.T., Ravichardran, P. et al. (2003). Endoluminal reconstruction of the canine common bile duct. *Current Surgery* 60: 437–441.

18

Other Surgical Diseases of the Gallbladder and Biliary Tract: Cholecystitis, Neoplasia, Infarct, and Trauma

Steve J. Mehler and Philipp D. Mayhew

Trauma

Trauma to the biliary tract is one of the most common causes of sterile bile peritonitis in veterinary patients (Watkins *et al.* 1983; Ludwig *et al.* 1997). The most common traumatic etiology is being hit by a car, but gunshot wounds, bite wounds, and other penetrating abdominal wounds are also potential causes. Blunt trauma causes rupture of the common bile duct more frequently than rupture of the gallbladder. The most common site of common bile duct rupture is just distal to the entrance of the last hepatic duct, but the distal common bile duct, cystic duct (Figure 18.1), and hepatic ducts may also be injured (Martin *et al.* 1986; Parchman & Flanders 1990; Neer 1992; Mehler *et al.* 2004). The proposed mechanism of bile duct rupture from trauma involves rapid gallbladder emptying at the time of impact and a simultaneous shearing force applied to a relatively short duct system. Recognition of biliary tract trauma is frequently delayed, sometimes for weeks, and clinical signs result from the ensuing bile peritonitis. Bile peritonitis is the usual cause of death in cases of traumatic extrahepatic biliary tract (EHBT) rupture; however, reported cases of bile peritonitis secondary to trauma commonly have an excellent outcome (Mehler *et al.* 2004).

Successful repair of ruptured ducts has recently been reported using fine suture and either an interrupted or simple continuous pattern (Baker *et al.* 2009). In some cases it may be necessary to place a choledochal stent as an internal strut to facilitate healing of the bile duct.

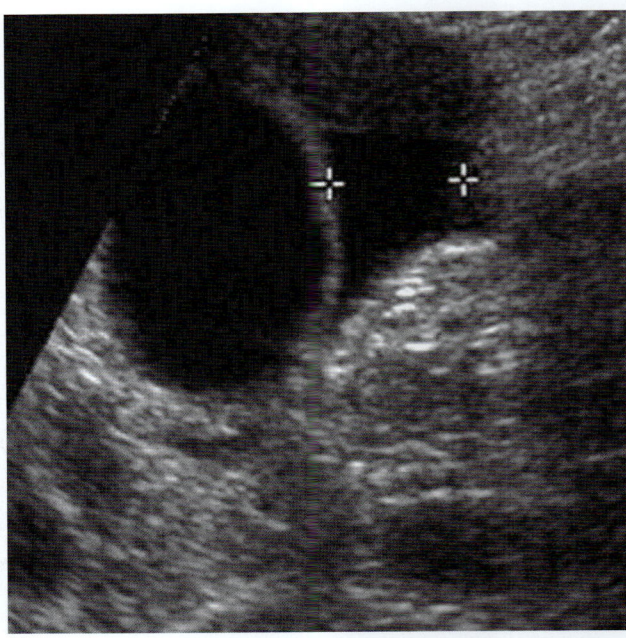

Figure 18.1 An abdominal ultrasound image of a cat that sustained unknown trauma. There is fluid around the outside of the gallbladder within the hepatic fossa. A fluid sample was obtained with ultrasound guidance and was determined to be bile. This cat had a cystic duct rupture at surgery and a cholecystectomy was performed.

Necrotizing cholecystitis and cystic artery infarction

Necrotizing cholecystitis has been reported to be a common cause of gallbladder rupture in dogs. Impaired cystic artery circulation by occlusion, bacterial infection, or cystic duct obstruction from choleliths, neoplasia, or an adjacent inflammatory process may lead to cholecystitis. Necrotizing cholecystitis has been classified in the human and veterinary literature into three categories (Church & Matthiesen 1988). Class I includes patients with necrotizing cholecystitis without gallbladder rupture. Class II includes patients with acute necrotizing cholecystitis with gallbladder perforation and peritonitis. Class III identifies patients with chronic cholecystitis with cholecystic and omental hepatic adhesions with fistulas to other abdominal structures.

Necrotizing cholecystitis leading to gallbladder rupture is very common, manifested in up to 78% of reported cases of bile peritonitis, and is often the reason for presentation (Ludwig *et al.* 1997; Mehler *et al.* 2004; Rogers *et al.* 2020). This disease is associated with a high mortality rate and it is likely that delay in diagnosis and treatment of necrotizing cholecystitis is directly related to poor prognosis. Underlying endocrine dysfunction, especially Cushing disease, may be a contributing factor in the development of necrotizing cholecystitis in dogs. There is some evidence to suggest that gallbladder wall infarction is a cause for necrotizing cholecystitis in dogs. Thrombus formation in the cystic artery, atheromatous vascular changes, and underlying endocrine disease may be involved in the disease process (Holt *et al.* 2004). Cystic artery thrombosis, if diagnosed on histopathology, justifies an aggressive diagnostic approach for causes of a hypercoagulopathic state (Pavlick *et al.* 2021). A presumptive diagnosis of necrotizing cholecystitis, with or without gallbladder rupture, is an indication for emergency surgical intervention and cholecystectomy. Because necrotizing cholecystitis is often associated with gallbladder mucocele, we recommend early intervention and cholecystectomy.

Emphysematous cholecystitis

Emphysematous cholecystitis has been reported infrequently in dogs. This inflammatory condition induces the formation of gas within the wall and/or the lumen of the gallbladder, and is thought to be secondary to a combination of gallbladder wall ischemia and proliferation of gas-forming bacteria such as *Escherichia coli* and *Clostridium perfringens*. Emergency surgical exploration, cholecystectomy, and histopathologic evaluation and culture of the gallbladder wall and liver are indicated.

Neoplasia

Primary neoplasms of the gallbladder and common bile duct are rare in domestic animals, comprising 2% of all canine hepatic tumors (Martin *et al.* 1986; Neer 1992;

Jones *et al.* 1997). It should be remembered that neoplasia affecting surrounding organs, especially the pancreas, can often cause clinical signs attributable to the biliary tract. One study identified that in 20% of animals with EHBT obstruction, the obstruction was due to neoplasia of the pancreas or the bile duct (Patnaik *et al.* 1980). Primary cholangiocellular neoplasia is usually diagnosed in dogs over 9 years old (Balkman 2009).

Most patients demonstrate nonspecific clinical signs such as lethargy, anorexia, weight loss, and vomiting (Patnaik *et al.* 1980; Trigo *et al.* 1982). Physical examination may reveal a palpable abdominal mass, especially with the massive form of cholangiocellular carcinoma. Other signs may be secondary to EHBT obstruction and include icterus and evidence of hemodynamic compromise such as lethargy, anorexia, weak peripheral pulse quality, cold extremities, and collapse.

Plain radiography gives limited information. A cranial abdominal mass effect may be seen in cases with large focal lesions. Abdominal ultrasound is probably the most useful noninvasive modality for imaging of the biliary tract and in most cases the size and location of masses affecting the EHBT will be evident (Lamb 1991; Lamb *et al.* 1995; Gaschen 2009). Computed tomography and magnetic resonance imaging can also be used to characterize lesions of the EHBT.

For specific tissue diagnosis the advantages and disadvantages of fine-needle aspiration, needle core biopsy, laparoscopic exploration and biopsy, or "open" surgical biopsy must be weighed. Percutaneous fine-needle aspiration or needle core biopsy are the least invasive way of procuring a cytologic or histopathologic specimen, respectively. They must be performed under imaging guidance, most commonly using ultrasound. In some cases where masses are small or located deep within the liver, it may be difficult or impossible to obtain diagnostic samples. In these cases more invasive techniques may be required for tissue diagnosis.

Cholangiocellular adenomas are benign tumors of the bile duct epithelium that account for 12% of primary liver tumors in dogs (Trigo *et al.* 1982). Cholangiocellular carcinoma comprised 22% of primary liver tumors in dogs in one study (Patnaik *et al.* 1980). Of these, 4–21% were extrahepatic and 1–4% emanated from the gallbladder, the rest being primarily hepatic in origin (Patnaik *et al.* 1981). Prognosis is considered poor, since at necropsy metastatic disease was present in 88% of cases. Cholangiocellular carcinomas are reported to be of massive type in 46–50%, nodular in 28–54%, and diffuse in 22% of dogs. An association between cholangiocellular carcinoma and Chinese liver fluke infestation exists in humans and this has been described in a canine case (Parkin *et al.* 1993). In cats benign bile duct adenomas, also known as biliary cystadenomas, are approximately twice as common as bile duct carcinomas (Lawrence *et al.* 1994; Adler & Wilson 1995; Nyland *et al.* 1999). The prognosis for benign cystadenoma is very good with surgical excision, and even in incidentally diagnosed cases this may be justified, as precancerous lesions have been observed in these tumors (Adler & Wilson 1995; Trout *et al.* 1995). Prognosis for malignant biliary tumors in cats is poor, with a metastatic rate of 67% in one necropsy study (Patnaik 1992) and 100% perioperative mortality in a study of surgically treated cases (Lawrence *et al.* 1994).

Neuroendocrine carcinomas arise from cells of the neuroendocrine system that are distributed in many different organs (Patnaik *et al.* 1981). They are generally aggressive tumors associated with a very poor prognosis. Most canine cases involving the hepatobiliary system are diffusely spread throughout the liver, although small numbers of cases involving the gallbladder have also been described (Patnaik *et al.* 1981, 2005; Morrell *et al.* 2002; Lippo *et al.* 2008). Metastasis was present in over 90% of dogs in one study (Patnaik *et al.* 1981). In cats a greater proportion of cases are extrahepatic, with most cases arising from the bile ducts, although cases involving the gallbladder have also been described. Tumors are diffuse and metastases are often present in almost all feline cases reported. In cats, longer-term survival has been reported in a small percentage of cases where surgical excision of the extrahepatic form of the disease was possible. Prolonged survival may be seen with cases affecting the gallbladder where only cholecystectomy is performed (Willard *et al.* 1988; Lippo *et al.* 2008).

References

Adler, R. and Wilson, D.W. (1995). Biliary cystadenoma of cats. *Veterinary Pathology* 32: 415–418.

Baker, S.G., Mayhew, P.D., and Mehler, S.J. (2009). Choledochotomy and primary repair of extrahepatic biliary duct tears in dogs and cats. *Veterinary Surgery* 38: E25.

Balkman, C. (2009). Hepatobiliary neoplasia in dogs and cats. *Veterinary Clinics of North America: Small Animal Practice* 39: 617–625.

Church, E.M. and Matthiesen, D.T. (1988). Surgical treatment of 23 dogs with necrotizing cholecystitis. *Journal of the American Animal Hospital Association* 24: 305–310.

Gaschen, L. (2009). Update on hepatobiliary imaging. *Veterinary Clinics of North America: Small Animal Practice* 39: 439–467.

Holt, D.E., Mehler, S.J., Mayhew, P.D., and Hendrick, M.J. (2004). Canine gallbladder infarction: 12 cases (1993–2003). *Veterinary Pathology* 41: 416–418.

Jones, T.C., Hunt, R.D., and King, N.W. (1997). Gallbladder. In: *Veterinary Pathology*, 1103–1105. Baltimore, MD: Williams & Wilkins.

Lamb, C.R. (1991). Ultrasonography of the liver and biliary tract. *Problems in Veterinary Medicine* 3: 555–573.

Lamb, C.R., Simpson, K.W., Boswood, A., and Matthewman, L.A. (1995). Ultrasonography of pancreatic neoplasia in the dog: a retrospective review of 16 cases. *Veterinary Record* 137: 65–68.

Lawrence, H.J., Erb, H.N., and Harvey, H.J. (1994). Nonlymphomatous hepatobiliary masses in cats: 41 cases (1972–1991). *Veterinary Surgery* 23: 365–368.

Lippo, N.J., Williams, J.E., Brawer, R.S., and Sobel, K.E. (2008). Acute hemobilia and hemocholecyst in 2 dogs with gallbladder carcinoid. *Journal of Veterinary Internal Medicine* 22: 1249–1252.

Ludwig, L.L., McLoughlin, M.A., Graves, T.K., and Crisp, M.S. (1997). Surgical treatment of bile peritonitis in 24 dogs and 2 cats: a retrospective study (1987–1994). *Veterinary Surgery* 26: 90–98.

Martin, R.A., MacCoy, D.M., and Harvey, H.J. (1986). Surgical management of extrahepatic biliary tract disease: a report of eleven cases. *Journal of the American Animal Hospital Association* 22: 301–307.

Mehler, S.J., Mayhew, P.D., Drobatz, K.J., and Holt, D.E. (2004). Variables associated with outcome in dogs undergoing extrahepatic biliary surgery: 60 cases (1988–2002). *Veterinary Surgery* 33: 644–649.

Morrell, C.N., Volk, M.V., and Mankowski, J.L. (2002). A carcinoid tumor in the gallbladder of a dog. *Veterinary Pathology* 39: 756–758.

Neer, T.M. (1992). A review of disorders of the gallbladder and extrahepatic biliary tract in the dog and cat. *Journal of Veterinary Internal Medicine* 6: 186–192.

Nyland, T.G., Koblik, P.D., and Tellyer, S.E. (1999). Ultrasonographic evaluation of biliary cystadenomas in cats. *Veterinary Radiology and Ultrasound* 40: 300–306.

Parchman, M.B. and Flanders, J.A. (1990). Extrahepatic biliary tract rupture: evaluation of the relationship between the site of rupture and the cause of rupture in 15 dogs. *Cornell Veterinarian* 80: 267–272.

Parkin, D.M., Ohshima, H., Srivatanakul, P., and Vatanasapt, V. (1993). Cholangiocarcinoma: epidemiology, mechanisms of carcinogenesis and prevention. *Cancer Epidemiology, Biomarkers and Prevention* 2: 537–544.

Patnaik, A.K. (1992). A morphologic and immunocytochemical study of hepatic neoplasms in cats. *Veterinary Pathology* 29: 405–415.

Patnaik, A.K., Hurvitz, A.I., and Lieberman, P.H. (1980). Canine hepatic neoplasms: a clinicopathologic study. *Veterinary Pathology* 17: 553–564.

Patnaik, A.K., Hurvitz, A.I., Lieberman, P.H., and Johnson, G.F. (1981). Canine bile duct carcinoma. *Veterinary Pathology* 18: 439–444.

Patnaik, A.K., Lieberman, P.H., Erlandson, R.A., and Antonescu, C. (2005). Hepatobiliary neuroendocrine carcinoma in cats: a clinicopathologic, immunohistochemical, and ultrastructural study of 17 cases. *Veterinary Pathology* 42: 331–337.

Pavlick, M., DeLaforcade, A., Penninck, D.G. et al. (2021). Evaluation of coagulation parameters in dogs with gallbladder mucoceles. *Journal of Veterinary Internal Medicine* 35: 1763–1772.

Rogers, E., Jaffey, J.A., Grahm, A. et al. (2020). Prevalence and impact of cholecystitis on outcome in dogs with gallbladder mucocele. *Journal of Veterinary Internal Medicine* 30: 97–101.

Trigo, F.J., Thompson, H., Breeze, R.G., and Nash, A.S. (1982). The pathology of liver tumours in the dog. *Journal of Comparative Pathology* 92: 21–39.

Trout, N.J., Berg, R.J., McMillan, M.C. et al. (1995). Surgical treatment of hepatobiliary cystadenomas in cats: five cases (1988–1993). *Journal of the American Veterinary Medical Association* 206: 505–507.

Watkins, P.E., Pearson, H., and Denny, H.R. (1983). Traumatic rupture of the bile duct in the dog. A report of seven cases. *Journal of Small Animal Practice* 24: 731–740.

Willard, M.D., Dunstan, R.W., and Faulkner, J. (1988). Neuroendocrine carcinoma of the gallbladder in a dog. *Journal of the American Veterinary Medical Association* 192: 926–928.

19

Pancreatitis

Panagiotis G. Xenoulis, Jörg M. Steiner, and Eric Monnet

Pancreatitis, an inflammation of the pancreas, is commonly seen in clinical practice and is associated with significant morbidity and mortality in both dogs and cats. In the past, its overall clinical prevalence had been estimated at about 0.8% for dogs and 0.6% for cats, although certain canine and possibly feline breeds might have a higher prevalence of pancreatitis (Steiner & Williams 1999; Steiner 2010). However, with the more widespread use of more sensitive diagnostic tools for pancreatitis, the prevalence of a diagnosis of pancreatitis has been increasing. Histopathologic evidence of pancreatitis is very common, even among clinically healthy animals, and has been reported to be as high as about 90% and 65% for dogs and cats, respectively (Newman et al. 2004; De Cock et al. 2007). It remains to be determined whether any degree of histopathologic pancreatitis is clinically important. The mortality rates for dogs and cats with pancreatitis also vary widely; most animals with mild pancreatitis will recover within a few days and have a very good prognosis, while mortality rates for more severe acute pancreatitis have been reported to be as high as 20–42% in dogs (Cook et al. 1993; Ruaux & Atwell 1998; Thompson et al. 2009; Weatherton & Streeter 2009) and approximately 9% in cats (Klaus et al. 2009). Clinical diagnosis of pancreatitis is often challenging, and many cases remain undiagnosed. Finally, although new directions are being explored, treatment of pancreatitis remains almost exclusively supportive and symptomatic. Surgical intervention for pancreatitis is rarely required and is used most frequently to treat pancreatic complications of pancreatitis (e.g., local fluid collections).

Pathogenesis

The pathogenesis of pancreatitis is very complex and still poorly understood. Most of our understanding regarding the pathogenesis of pancreatitis is based on animal models and some clinical studies in humans. There is mounting evidence that both genetic and environmental factors play a crucial role in the development of pancreatitis (Pandol et al. 2007; Gaisano & Gorelick 2009; Mayerle et al. 2019). Several mutations in genes that are involved in digestive protease/antiprotease homeostasis support the notion that pancreatitis is a disease of autodigestion (Mayerle et al. 2019). Regardless of the actual etiology, there appears to be a relatively uniform pathogenetic mechanism in most cases of acute pancreatitis. Evidence from clinical and experimental studies confirm that the initiating events that lead to pancreatic inflammation take place in the acinar cell. Two well-documented early intracellular events that have been shown to precede the development of acute pancreatitis are retention and premature intracellular activation of zymogens (Pandol et al. 2007; Gaisano & Gorelick 2009; Mayerle et al. 2019). Zymogens are precursors of pancreatic enzymes stored together with actual digestive enzymes in zymogen granules and are normally secreted into the pancreatic duct through the apical membrane of the acinar cell. The factors that lead to retention of these zymogen granules and premature intra-acinar cell activation of the zymogens are not fully elucidated. One of the most popular hypotheses, which has however not been definitively proven, is the colocalization theory (Pandol et al. 2007; Gaisano & Gorelick 2009; Mayerle et al. 2019). Based on this theory,

Small Animal Soft Tissue Surgery, Second Edition. Edited by Eric Monnet.
© 2023 John Wiley & Sons, Inc. Published 2023 by John Wiley & Sons, Inc.
Companion website: www.wiley.com/go/monnet/small

zymogen granules that accumulate in the acinar cell colocalize with lysosomes. In turn, lysosomal enzymes, such as cathepsin B, are believed to activate trypsinogen into trypsin, which subsequently activates other zymogens. Evidence from other studies indicates that the cytosolic free ionized calcium concentration also plays an important role in the intracellular activation of zymogens (Ward *et al.* 1995, 1996; Kruger *et al.* 2000; Mayerle *et al.* 2019). In addition to decreased secretion and intracellular activation of pancreatic enzymes, there is evidence of disruption of the paracellular barrier in the pancreatic duct that allows its contents to leak into the paracellular space, and also redirection of secretion of zymogen granules from the apical pole to the basolateral region of acinar cells and into the interstitial space (Figure 19.1) (Gaisano & Gorelick 2009). However, none of these pathogenetic mechanisms has been conclusively proven.

Once intracellular activation of pancreatic enzymes has taken place, autodigestion of the acinar cell follows and activated enzymes escape initially into the pancreatic tissue (leading to local effects) and subsequently into the peritoneal cavity and systemic circulation, potentially contributing to systemic effects. Local effects vary and can range from mild interstitial edema to severe acinar cell necrosis, hemorrhage, and peripancreatic fat necrosis. The extent and severity of local effects determine to a large degree the systemic response. Acinar cell injury leads to recruitment and activation of a variety of inflammatory cells (mostly neutrophils and macrophages), which release proinflammatory cytokines and other inflammatory mediators, such as interleukin (IL)-1, IL-2, IL-6, IL-18, tumor necrosis factor (TNF)-α, substance P, and platelet activating factor (PAF), which play a crucial role in modulating systemic manifestations (Norman 1998; Pandol *et al.* 2007; Mayerle *et al.* 2019). Such manifestations include cardiovascular shock, disseminated intravascular coagulation (DIC), systemic inflammatory response syndrome (SIRS), and multiple organ failure, and are seen in cases of severe acute pancreatitis (Norman 1998; Pandol *et al.* 2007; Mayerle *et al.* 2019).

Other forms of pancreatitis, such as chronic, autoimmune, and hereditary pancreatitis, seem to have different pathophysiologic bases from that of acute pancreatitis (Gardner & Chari 2008; Whitcomb 2010; Mayerle *et al.* 2019). Chronic pancreatitis occurs frequently in both dogs and cats, but it remains to be determined whether chronic pancreatitis should be considered an extension of acute pancreatitis or a separate disease entity. Both autoimmune and hereditary pancreatitis have been suspected to occur in dogs and autoimmune pancreatitis also in cats, but their clinical impact has not been definitively proven, and therefore discussion of the associated pathophysiologic mechanisms is not part of this chapter.

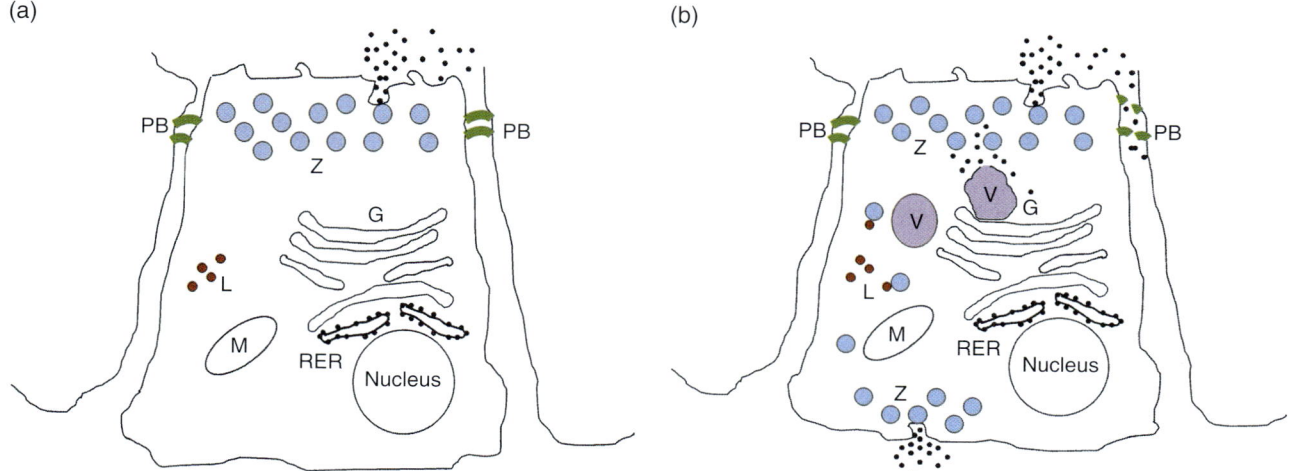

(a)

(b)

Figure 19.1 Proposed pathogenesis of acute pancreatitis. (a) A normal acinar cell. Zymogen granules are found in the apical region of the cell and their contents are excreted exclusively through the apical surface. Lysosomes are stored separately from zymogen granules and the paracellular barriers are intact. (b) An acinar cell during acute pancreatitis. Secretion of the zymogen granules is redirected from the apical pole to the basolateral region of the acinar cell and into the interstitial space. Retention of zymogen granules is followed by colocalization with lysosomes and the formation of large vacuoles. This, in turn, leads to premature intracellular activation of pancreatic zymogens. There is also disruption of the paracellular barrier in the pancreatic duct that allows its contents to leak into the paracellular space. G, Golgi apparatus; L, lysosome; M, mitochondrion; PB, paracellular barrier; RER, rough endoplasmic reticulum; V, vacuole; Z, zymogen granule. Source: From Xenoulis, Panagiotis G. and Steiner, Joerg M. (2013). Necrosis and inflammation: canine. In: *Canine and Feline Gastroenterology* (eds R.J. Washabau and M.J. Day). St. Louis, O: Elsevier, with permission.

Etiology and risk factors

In contrast to humans, in whom an etiology of pancreatitis can be identified in almost 90% of cases, the etiology of pancreatitis in dogs and cats usually remains unknown (idiopathic pancreatitis) (Frossard *et al.* 2008; Xenoulis & Steiner 2008; Steiner 2010). Currently, very few definitive causes of pancreatitis have been described for dogs and even fewer for cats (Xenoulis & Steiner 2008; Steiner 2010). The main causes of human pancreatitis (i.e., biliary obstruction and alcoholism) are of little relevance in small animals (Pandol *et al.* 2007; Frossard *et al.* 2008). Some other well-defined causes of pancreatitis in humans (e.g., hereditary pancreatitis, autoimmune pancreatitis) have currently not been described in dogs and cats.

Recently, two well-described causes of human pancreatitis have been reported as possible causes of pancreatitis in dogs, but not in cats. Two studies have suggested that hypertriglyceridemia, which is a known risk factor for pancreatitis in humans, might also be a risk factor for pancreatitis in miniature schnauzers (Xenoulis *et al.* 2010, 2011). It remains to be determined if such an association is also true for dogs of other breeds. Miniature schnauzers have a high prevalence of idiopathic hypertriglyceridemia, which is often rather severe (Xenoulis *et al.* 2007). As for humans, the severity of hypertriglyceridemia appears to be important. A recent report suggested that miniature schnauzers with serum triglyceride concentrations above 862 mg/dL were at increased risk for pancreatitis (Xenoulis *et al.* 2010). Interestingly, hypertriglyceridemia seems to be present before the development of pancreatitis and persists after resolution of pancreatitis, unless a low-fat diet is being fed (Xenoulis *et al.* 2011). The exact role of hypertriglyceridemia in the development of pancreatitis remains to be determined as, similar to human patients with severe hypertriglyceridemia, not all miniature schnauzers with severe hypertriglyceridemia develop pancreatitis.

In another recent report, a combination of three variants of the serine protease inhibitor Kazal type 1 (SPINK1) gene – also called the pancreatic secretory trypsin inhibitor (PSTI) gene – were identified in miniature schnauzers, and an association of these variants with pancreatitis was identified (Bishop *et al.* 2010). Mutations of the *SPINK1* gene (although different from those found in miniature schnauzers) have also been described and associated with pancreatitis in humans (Whitcomb 2010). However, a more recent study genotyping a larger population of the miniature schnauzer breed than the previous study showed that the *SPINK1* variants are common polymorphisms in the schnauzer lineage and no relationship between these variants and clinically detectable pancreatitis was found (Furrow *et al.* 2012). Thus, the exact role of this gene in the development of pancreatitis remains to be determined. Based on the fact that some breeds have been found to be overrepresented in some reports, genetic causes of pancreatitis are also suspected in other breeds (e.g., Yorkshire terriers) (Hess *et al.* 1998).

Several other pathologic conditions have been identified as potential risk factors for pancreatitis in dogs. Endocrinopathies such as hyperadrenocorticism, hypothyroidism, and diabetes mellitus have all been reported as risk factors for pancreatitis in dogs, although strong evidence is lacking and observations are conflicting (Hess *et al.* 1998).

A history of drug administration in conjunction with compatible clinical findings should raise concern for drug-induced pancreatitis. Medications that have been associated with pancreatitis most commonly in dogs include potassium bromide and/or phenobarbital, L-asparaginase, azathioprine and meglumine antimonate (Aste *et al.* 2005; Steiner *et al.* 2008b; Wright *et al.* 2009).

Diets with a very high fat content may also be a risk factor for pancreatitis in dogs (Lindsay *et al.* 1948; Williams 1996). In a recent retrospective study in dogs, dietary factors (e.g., getting into the trash, consuming table scraps, ingestion of "unusual" food) and surgery at any time prior to the diagnosis of pancreatitis were found to be associated with increased odds for pancreatitis (Lem *et al.* 2008). A relationship between obesity and pancreatitis has been suggested, but has not been definitively demonstrated (Hess *et al.* 1998). Hypotension (e.g., during anesthesia), hypercalcemia, trauma, certain infections (e.g., with certain *Babesia* strains), certain snake envenomations, and pancreatic ductal obstruction are also suspected risk factors for pancreatitis in dogs, but scientific evidence is weak or lacking at this point (Forman *et al.* 2021; Mohr *et al.* 2000; Steiner 2010).

In cats, several studies have shown an association between pancreatitis, inflammatory bowel disease (IBD), and biliary tract disease (e.g., cholangitis) (Weiss *et al.* 1996). Different combinations of these three disorders may occur, and the term triaditis has been used to describe the coexistence of these three disorders in a given patient. In general, 50–67% of cats with pancreatitis have triaditis (Forman *et al.* 2004; Fragkou *et al.* 2016; Twedt *et al.* 2014). Also, 50–80% of cats with cholangitis have pancreatitis with or without IBD (Forman *et al.* 2004; Fragkou *et al.* 2016; Twedt *et al.* 2014). However, it remains unclear which condition occurs first and whether there are any cause-and-effect relationships between these conditions. An association between diabetes mellitus and pancreatitis has also been identified in several studies. The exact nature of this association has not been determined yet, but it is likely that pancreatitis may be predisposing to diabetes mellitus, as the inflammation does not spare the islets of Langerhans. Several viral and parasitic agents have been shown or suspected to occasionally be associated with pancreatitis in cats, but none has been reported as an important or common cause of pancreatitis in this species (Macy 1989; Swift *et al.* 2000; Gerhardt *et al.* 2001; Ferreri *et al.* 2003; Forman *et al.* 2004; Xenoulis *et al.* 2008). Other reported or suspected causes of pancreatitis that are also identified in a small number of cats with pancreatitis include abdominal trauma (e.g., traffic accidents or high-rise syndrome), ischemia (e.g., hypotension), acute hypercalcemia, organophosphate intoxication (e.g., fenthion), pharmacologic substances, tumors of the pancreas, and pancreatic ductal obstruction (Xenoulis & Steiner 2008).

Diagnosis

Signalment

Dogs and cats of any age, breed, or sex can develop pancreatitis. Most animals are middle-aged to old (Anderson & Low 1965; Berman *et al.* 2020; Owens *et al.* 1975; Cook *et al.* 1993; Hess *et al.* 1999; Gerhardt *et al.* 2001). Miniature schnauzers and Yorkshire terriers might be at increased risk for pancreatitis, while the predisposition of other breeds is less clear (Hess *et al.* 1998; Lem *et al.* 2008; Steiner 2010). Domestic shorthair and Siamese breeds have been reported to be at increased risk in some studies, but this has not been confirmed by other studies (Hill & Van Winkle 1993; Gerhardt *et al.* 2001; Ferreri *et al.* 2003). No clear sex predisposition has been identified for either species.

Clinical signs and physical examination findings

It is now recognized that dogs and cats with pancreatitis can present with a wide variety of clinical signs, ranging from asymptomatic to mild partial anorexia with no apparent gastrointestinal signs to cardiovascular shock and DIC. There is no single clinical sign or combination of clinical signs that is pathognomonic for pancreatitis in dogs or cats. In one recent study, clinical signs included lethargy (88%), anorexia (86%), vomiting (83%), and abdominal pain (59%) (Berman *et al.* 2020). Many of the clinical signs reported in dogs with pancreatitis are likely to be the result of systemic complications of pancreatitis or concurrent diseases rather than pancreatitis *per se* (e.g., polyuria and polydipsia are more likely to be the result of concurrent diabetes mellitus than a clinical sign of pancreatic inflammation). Cases with less severe or chronic pancreatitis are believed to

have less profound clinical signs, such as anorexia and/or depression, or they might be subclinical. The most common physical examination findings that have been reported in dogs with severe acute pancreatitis include dehydration (97%), abdominal pain (58%), fever (32%), and icterus (26%) (Hess *et al.* 1998). The combination of vomiting and abdominal pain, though suggestive of pancreatitis, is also seen with other diseases (e.g., gastrointestinal foreign bodies). Other possible findings include shock, hypothermia, cardiac murmur, tachycardia, bleeding diathesis or DIC, ascites, a palpable abdominal mass, and harsh lung sounds (Hess *et al.* 1998). Depending on the severity of pancreatitis, physical examination findings can range from depression and mild dehydration to shock.

The most common clinical signs reported in cats with pancreatitis do not specifically indicate gastrointestinal disease and include complete or partial anorexia (63–97%) and lethargy (28–100%) (Hill & Van Winkle 1993; Gerhardt *et al.* 2001; Saunders *et al.* 2002; Ferreri *et al.* 2003; Forman *et al.* 2004; Klaus *et al.* 2009). Other clinical signs include vomiting (35–76%), weight loss (20–61%), and diarrhea (11–33%) (Hill & Van Winkle 1993; Gerhardt *et al.* 2001; Saunders *et al.* 2002; Ferreri *et al.* 2003; Forman *et al.* 2004; Klaus *et al.* 2009). The combination of vomiting and cranial abdominal pain has not been as commonly reported in cats as it has been in dogs (Hess *et al.* 1998, 1999). Anecdotal evidence suggests that abdominal pain is common in cats with pancreatitis (up to 75% of cases) and is likely being missed during routine physical examination rather than not being present (Zoran 2006). The most common physical examination findings include dehydration (33–96%), pallor (30%), and icterus (16–24%) (Hill & Van Winkle 1993; Gerhardt *et al.* 2001; Saunders *et al.* 2002; Ferreri *et al.* 2003; Forman *et al.* 2004; Klaus *et al.* 2009). Tachypnea and/or dyspnea, hypothermia or fever, tachycardia, signs of abdominal pain, and a palpable abdominal mass may also be noted (Macy 1989; Hill & Van Winkle 1993; Simpson *et al.* 1994; Steiner & Williams 1999; Ferreri *et al.* 2003). Severe systemic complications may occasionally be seen in cats with severe pancreatitis and may include DIC, pulmonary thromboembolism, cardiovascular shock, and multiorgan failure (Williams 1996; Schermerhorn *et al.* 2004; Estrin *et al.* 2006). In two recent studies, 26% of 46 cats diagnosed with DIC and 11.8% of 17 cats with pulmonary thromboembolism had pancreatitis as an underlying condition (Schermerhorn *et al.* 2004; Estrin *et al.* 2006). Finally, other clinical signs may be seen as a consequence of complications of pancreatitis or concurrent disease (e.g., diarrhea and weight loss in cats with concurrent IBD) (Goossens *et al.* 1998).

Clinical pathology

Results of a complete blood count, serum biochemistry profile, and urinalysis are nonspecific and thus of limited usefulness for the diagnosis of pancreatitis in dogs and cats (Akol *et al.* 1993; Hill & Van Winkle 1993; Hess *et al.* 1998; Kimmel *et al.* 2001; Simpson *et al.* 2001; Ferreri *et al.* 2003; Klaus *et al.* 2009; Weatherton & Streeter 2009). However, these tests should always be performed in animals with suspected pancreatitis, because they are useful for the diagnosis or exclusion of other differential diseases, and give important information about the general condition of the animal.

Often, especially in mild cases, the complete blood count, serum biochemistry profile, and urinalysis are normal. At the same time, dogs or cats with pancreatitis, especially when severe, may present with almost any hematologic or biochemical abnormality. Possible hematologic findings in dogs and cats with pancreatitis include anemia or hemoconcentration, leukocytosis or leucopenia, and thrombocytopenia. Evidence of coagulopathy, such as prolonged activated clotting time (ACT), prothrombin time (PT), and partial thromboplastin time (PTT), is seen in some cases, and may or may not be associated with spontaneous clinical bleeding. In other patients there might be evidence suggestive of DIC, such as thrombocytopenia, prolongation of clotting times (i.e., ACT, PT, PTT), and/or an increase in D-dimers. Different combinations of elevated liver enzyme activities (i.e., ALT, AST, ALP) and hyperbilirubinemia are common in both dogs and cats, and might erroneously direct the clinician to suspect primary liver disease. In some cases, these findings might be associated with extrahepatic biliary duct obstruction. Increases in serum creatinine, blood urea nitrogen, and/or symmetric dimethylarginine (SDMA) concentrations are variably present and most often associated with dehydration due to vomiting, diarrhea, and/or decreased water intake (prerenal azotemia). In severe cases, azotemia may indicate secondary kidney injury, which would be supported by a decrease in urine specific gravity in the face of azotemia. Other possible findings include hypoalbuminemia, hypertriglyceridemia, hypercholesterolemia, and hyperglycemia or hypoglycemia. Electrolyte abnormalities are commonly present and variable, with hypokalemia, hypochloremia, and hyponatremia being the most typical. Hypocalcemia is much more commonly seen in cats than in dogs, and has been suggested as a prognostic indicator of severe disease in this species, although it does not seem to accurately predict the outcome in clinical patients (Kimmel *et al.* 2001).

Laboratory tests for pancreatitis

Pancreatic lipase immunoreactivity

Pancreatic lipase is produced exclusively by pancreatic acinar cells. Immunoassays for the specific measurement of pancreatic lipase have been developed and analytically validated for dogs and cats (Steiner *et al.* 2003, 2004). Pancreatic lipase immunoreactivity (PLI) assays are currently considered the most sensitive and specific serum tests for the diagnosis of pancreatitis in dogs and cats. The main advantage of PLI assays over traditional lipase activity assays is based on the fact that, in contrast to the traditional activity assays for lipase that indiscriminately measure the activities of lipases of multiple cellular origins, immunoassays that are used to measure pancreatic lipase concentration in serum (i.e., the PLI assays) quantify exclusively lipase of pancreatic acinar cell origin based on its unique three-dimensional structure (Xenoulis 2015). Therefore, PLI assays have inherent advantages over the traditional serum lipase activity assays that make them more suitable for specific evaluation of the exocrine pancreas in dogs and cats. The originally developed and analytically validated immunoassays for the specific measurement of serum pancreatic lipase in dogs (canine PLI) and cats (feline PLI) (Steiner & Williams 1999; Steiner *et al.* 2003, 2004) have been replaced by more widely available, fully validated immunoassays (Spec cPL® for dogs and Spec fPL® for cats) that demonstrate a similar clinical performance to the original PLI assays and are available through IDEXX Laboratories (Westbrook, ME, USA) and the Gastrointestinal Laboratory at Texas A&M University (Huth *et al.* 2010; Steiner *et al.* 2008a,b). In addition to these validated assays, several other assays measuring PLI in dogs and cats are available, including the Laboklin PLI assay (Batt Laboratories, Coventry, UK), the Abaxis VETSCAN Canine Pancreatic Lipase Rapid Test (Zoetis, Parsipanny, NJ, USA), and the VCheck cPL and fPL assays (Bionote, Big Lake, MN, USA). However, for most of these assays, either analytic validation is not available, or they have failed analytic validation. Therefore, these assays cannot currently be recommended for clinical use.

Both clinical (McCord *et al.* 2012) and histopathologic (Aupperle-Lellbach *et al.* 2020; Steiner *et al.* 2008a,b; Trivedi *et al.* 2011; Watson *et al.* 2010) studies concerning cPLI for canine pancreatitis have been published and all generally agree that serum cPLI is the most sensitive and specific serum marker for pancreatitis in dogs to date. In a large clinical study that included 84 dogs, the sensitivity of cPLI as measured by Spec cPL was reported to range between 72% and 78% (McCord *et al.* 2012). In a recent necropsy study, the sensitivity of the cPLI was reported at 91% for moderate or severe pancreatitis (Aupperle-Lellbach *et al.* 2020). The sensitivity of cPLI is believed to be lower in mild or chronic pancreatitis.

The measurement of serum cPLI concentration is also considered to have the highest specificity for pancreatitis compared to any other serum test currently available, with specificities ranging between 81% and 100% (Aupperle-Lellbach *et al.* 2020; Mansfield & Jones 2000; Mansfield *et al.* 2012; McCord *et al.* 2012; Neilson-Carley *et al.* 2011; Simpson *et al.* 1989; Steiner *et al.* 2010; Strombeck *et al.* 1981; Trivedi *et al.* 2011). In the clinical study already mentioned, the specificity of cPLI was reported to range between 81% and 88% (McCord *et al.* 2012).

A rapid, in-clinic, semi-quantitative, visually read test for the estimation of canine pancreatic lipase in serum is available (Beall *et al.* 2011). One study showed that there is a 90–100% agreement between the SNAP cPL and the reference Spec cPL (Beall *et al.* 2011). Another study reported that SNAP cPL has a sensitivity for pancreatitis between 91% and 94% and a specificity between 71% and 78% (McCord *et al.* 2012). However, the main use of this diagnostic tool is to rule out pancreatitis (i.e., a normal result makes a diagnosis of pancreatitis very unlikely) and thus the sensitivity of the SNAP cPL is more important than its specificity.

Multiple studies in cats with both experimental and spontaneous pancreatitis have reported that serum fPLI concentration is the most sensitive and specific serum marker for feline pancreatitis currently available (Allen *et al.* 2006; Forman *et al.* 2004, 2009; Gerhardt *et al.* 2001; Lee *et al.* 2020; Parent *et al.* 1995; Schnauss *et al.* 2019; Swift *et al.* 2000; Torner *et al.* 2020; Zavros *et al.* 2008). In a recent retrospective study of 274 cats, Spec fPL was reported to have a sensitivity of about 76% in cats with definite or probable pancreatitis (Lee *et al.* 2020). In another clinical study in abstract form that included 182 cats, the sensitivity of serum Spec fPL concentration was reported at 79% (Forman *et al.* 2009). Similar to its sensitivity, the specificity of serum fPLI concentration for feline pancreatitis is very high, with reported values ranging between 67% and 100% (Forman *et al.* 2004, 2009; Lee *et al.* 2020). In a recent clinical study that included 274 cats, Spec fPL had a specificity of about 90% (Lee *et al.* 2020). In another clinical study in abstract form that included 182 cats, the specificity of fPLI was 82% (Forman *et al.* 2009). In a recent study, azotemia as a result of experimentally induced chronic renal failure did not have any clinically significant effect on serum fPLI concentrations (Xenoulis *et al.* 2021).

A rapid, in-clinic, semi-quantitative test for the estimation of feline pancreatic lipase in serum is available (Xenoulis 2015). In a recent clinical study, the agreement between SNAP fPL and Spec fPL was reported to be 97.5% for negative results and 90% for positive results, suggesting that overall there is a high agreement between these two methods (Schnauss *et al.* 2019). In that study, it was concluded that the SNAP fPL was a valuable tool to exclude or include pancreatitis as a differential diagnosis in an emergency setting (Schnauss *et al.* 2019).

Serum amylase and lipase activities

Serum amylase and lipase activities have long been considered markers for pancreatitis in dogs, but several studies have shown that they are not good markers for spontaneous canine pancreatitis due to their low sensitivity and specificity (Strombeck *et al.* 1981; Jacobs *et al.* 1985). Many tissues other than the exocrine pancreas synthesize amylases and lipases (Simpson *et al.* 1991). Traditional catalytic assays are not able to differentiate amylases and lipases according to their tissue of origin. In one study, about 50% of dogs with increased activity of either serum amylase or lipase had no histopathologic evidence of pancreatitis (Strombeck *et al.* 1981). This means that a large proportion of dogs that have diseases other than pancreatitis (e.g., certain renal, hepatic, intestinal, and neoplastic diseases) have increased serum lipase and/or amylase activities (Strombeck *et al.* 1981). Even significant increases in amylase and lipase activities can result from nonpancreatic disorders, and should always be followed by the use of more specific and sensitive tests (Strombeck *et al.* 1981; Polzin *et al.* 1983; Williams 1996; Mansfield & Jones 2000). In addition, the sensitivity of serum amylase and lipase activities for spontaneous canine pancreatitis varies, but is generally low (14–73% for lipase and 18–69% for amylase) (Hess *et al.* 1998; Steiner *et al.* 2001, 2008b). Therefore, pancreatitis cannot be diagnosed or ruled out based on serum amylase and/or lipase activities alone (Strombeck *et al.* 1981; Hess *et al.* 1998).

Although well-designed clinical studies are lacking, both serum lipase and amylase activities do not appear to be of any clinical value for the diagnosis of spontaneous feline pancreatitis (Hill & Van Winkle 1993; Simpson *et al.* 1994; Parent *et al.* 1995). Therefore, these two tests are not recommended for the diagnosis of pancreatitis in cats (Hill & Van Winkle 1993; Simpson *et al.* 1994).

More recently developed colorimetric lipase activity assays, such as those based on DGGR as a substrate, have been reported to show better performance than traditional catalytic assays. Supposedly, this substrate is more specific for pancreatic lipase than traditional catalytic assays, but such increased analytic specificity was not found in humans (Beisson *et al.* 2000). Some studies have compared DGGR-based assays with PLI assays and have suggested similar performance between the two (Kook *et al.* 2014; Oppliger *et al.* 2013, 2014, 2016). A study in 142 dogs found high agreement between a specific DGGR-based lipase assay and the Spec cPL assay, with the best agreement (κ = 0.80) for a cutoff of this DGGR-based lipase activity assay of >216 U/L (Kook *et al.* 2014). In cats, when specific cutoffs are used there was good agreement between one of these assays and the Spec fPL assay (Oppliger *et al.* 2013). Specifically, in this study of 250 cats, the best agreement (κ = 0.755) was found for a cutoff of DGGR lipase of >34 U/L. However, it should be noted that an agreement of 0.755 is not very high for two assays that supposedly measure the same analyte. Also, there are various DGGR-based assays for the measurement of serum lipase activity and they differ dramatically due to changes in added compounds (e.g., colipase, bile acids) and assay conditions (e.g., pH). Moreover, the analyzer used can have an impact on test results. Regardless, none of the currently available DGGR-based assays has been shown to be consistently any more specific for the measurement of pancreatic lipase than more traditional serum lipase activity assays. For example, a recent experimental study in both dogs and cats showed that DGGR is hydrolyzed not only by pancreatic lipase, but also by lipoprotein lipase, hepatic lipase, or both (Lim *et al.* 2020). These extrapancreatic lipases may contribute to a lack of analytic specificity of this assay (Lim *et al.* 2020). In the same study, no significant effect was shown for serum cPLI or fPLI concentrations (Lim *et al.* 2020). Further, it should be noted that different studies have reported vastly different results. For example, one study reported a specificity of a DGGR lipase assay of 53% when a cutoff value at the upper limit of the reference interval was used (Graca *et al.* 2005). A cutoff value that is lower than this would be expected to show a lower specificity, but another study reported a specificity of 100% at a cutoff value of approximately one-third of the upper limit of the reference interval (Hope *et al.* 2021). Thus, the results of these studies cannot be reconciled and further studies are needed before DGGR lipase assays can be recommended for the routine diagnosis of pancreatitis in either dogs or cats.

Serum trypsin-like immunoreactivity

Assays for serum trypsin-like immunoreactivity (TLI) are species-specific immunoassays that measure trypsinogen and trypsin in serum. The sensitivity of serum cTLI concentration for the diagnosis of canine spontaneous pancreatitis is low (36–47%), probably due to its short half-life (Mansfield & Jones 2000; Steiner *et al.* 2001, 2008a). Although there was strong evidence that trypsinogen is exclusively of pancreatic origin

(Simpson *et al.* 1991), it is believed that there might be some extrapancreatic expression under certain conditions and that TLI is cleared by glomerular filtration in dogs, thus increased serum cTLI concentrations have been seen in dogs with renal failure and also in those with chronic enteropathies, limiting its usefulness for the diagnosis of pancreatitis (Simpson *et al.* 1989; Mansfield & Jones 2000).

Feline TLI (fTLI) has been evaluated for the diagnosis of spontaneous pancreatitis in cats and several cutoff values have been suggested (Swift *et al.* 2000; Gerhardt *et al.* 2001; Allen *et al.* 2006). When cutoff values allowing adequate specificity of the assay are used (e.g., 100 μg/L), the sensitivity of fTLI for the diagnosis of pancreatitis in cats is generally low (28–33%), with the highest reported sensitivity for this cutoff value being 64% (Swift *et al.* 2000; Gerhardt *et al.* 2001; Allen *et al.* 2006). In addition, the specificity of fTLI has been questioned, because high serum fTLI concentrations have been reported in cats with no demonstrable pancreatic disease that had other gastrointestinal disorders (e.g., IBD or gastrointestinal lymphoma) or azotemia (Swift *et al.* 2000; Simpson *et al.* 2001; Allen *et al.* 2006).

In summary, cTLI and fTLI are currently considered to be of limited usefulness for diagnosing pancreatitis in dogs and cats.

Diagnostic imaging
Abdominal radiography

Conclusive diagnosis or exclusion of pancreatitis is not possible based on abdominal radiography alone (Akol *et al.* 1993; Hill & Van Winkle 1993; Williams 1996; Hess *et al.* 1998; Gerhardt *et al.* 2001; Ferreri *et al.* 2003). In the majority of dogs and cats with pancreatitis, abdominal radiography is normal or only shows nonspecific findings. Despite this, radiography remains a logical initial approach for patients suspected of having pancreatitis, because it is useful for the diagnosis and/or exclusion of other differential diagnoses. However, if such a differential diagnosis is not reached, radiography should always be followed by use of more sensitive and specific diagnostic tests for the definitive diagnosis or exclusion of pancreatitis.

Possible radiographic findings in dogs and cats with pancreatitis include an increased soft tissue opacity and decreased serosal detail in the cranial right abdomen, displacement of the stomach and/or duodenum from their normal positions, dilation of bowel loops adjacent to the pancreas, abdominal effusion, and the presence of a cranial abdominal mass (Hill & Van Winkle 1993; Hess *et al.* 1998; Gerhardt *et al.* 2001; Saunders *et al.* 2002; Ferreri *et al.* 2003).

Abdominal ultrasound

Abdominal ultrasound is considered the imaging method of choice for the diagnosis of pancreatitis in both dogs and cats. Both the quality of ultrasound machines and expertise have greatly advanced over the last two decades and ultrasonography is now routinely used for the investigation of dogs and cats suspected of having pancreatitis. However, abdominal ultrasonography is highly dependent on the skill and experience of the ultrasonographer and the equipment available. An older study reported a sensitivity of 68% for detecting fatal acute pancreatitis in dogs (Hess *et al.* 1998). In a recent study that included both healthy dogs and dogs with clinical pancreatitis, it was shown that the sensitivity and specificity of ultrasound for pancreatitis depend on the definition of ultrasonographic evidence of pancreatitis (Cridge *et al.* 2020). If only one criterion was applied (e.g., pancreatic enlargement or changes in peripancreatic echogenicity), the sensitivity was 89% but the specificity was only 43%. In contrast, if stringent criteria were applied (i.e., pancreatic enlargement, hypoechoic areas within the pancreas due to pancreatic necrosis, increased echogenicity of the surrounding mesentery due to peripancreatic fat necrosis), the sensitivity decreased to 43% and the specificity increased to 92% (Cridge *et al.* 2020). Therefore, when stringent criteria are applied to ensure high specificity, the sensitivity of ultrasound for pancreatitis can be low and pancreatitis cannot be excluded based on a normal ultrasound examination. The reported sensitivity of abdominal ultrasonography for the diagnosis of feline pancreatitis is generally low (11–35%), with only one study reporting a sensitivity of 67% (Swift *et al.* 2000; Saunders *et al.* 2002; Ferreri *et al.* 2003; Forman *et al.* 2004). However, it needs to be noted that the studies mentioned are a decade old or even older. Other more recent studies have evaluated the agreement between serum fPLI concentration and ultrasonography. The results of these studies often show conflicting results. In one study, the sensitivity and specificity of pancreatic ultrasonography in cats with increased serum fPLI and clinical signs indicative of pancreatitis were 84% and 75%, respectively (Williams *et al.* 2013).

It should also be noted that there may be a delay in the appearance of imaging findings in comparison to the actual disease process, which may require repeat ultrasonography 24–48 hours after initial presentation (Puccini *et al.* 2020). In one study of 38 dogs suspected of having acute pancreatitis in which abdominal ultrasound was performed at presentation and again 40–52 hours later, 12 dogs (32%) had no ultrasonographic changes at either examination, 14 dogs (37%) showed changes only at the second ultrasonographic examination, and only 12 dogs (32%) showed changes at both ultrasonographic exams (Puccini *et al.* 2020). Finally, there is currently no convincing evidence that repeated ultrasonography is useful for disease monitoring and response to treatment. It should be noted that ultrasonographic changes in dogs and cats with chronic pancreatitis are far less obvious than in those with acute disease.

The most important ultrasonographic findings suggestive of pancreatitis in dogs include hypoechoic areas within the pancreas, increased echogenicity of the surrounding mesentery (because of necrosis of the peripancreatic fat), and enlargement and/or irregularity of the pancreas (Figure 19.2) (Cridge *et al.* 2020; Xenoulis 2015).

It is important to note that a normal pancreas on ultrasound examination does not rule out pancreatitis in either dogs or cats (Hess *et al.* 1998; Swift *et al.* 2000; Saunders *et al.* 2002; Ferreri *et al.* 2003; Forman *et al.* 2004).

Abdominal ultrasonography is also very useful for the diagnosis of complications of pancreatitis, such as pancreatic and peripancreatic fluid accumulations (Figure 19.3) or biliary obstruction (Hecht & Henry 2007). In addition, ultrasound-guided fine-needle aspiration (FNA) is a useful tool for the management of noninfectious fluid accumulations of the pancreas (e.g., pancreatic pseudocyst) and for obtaining pancreatic specimens for cytology (Lamb 1999).

Pathology

Certain gross pancreatic lesions identified during surgery, laparoscopy, or necropsy are highly suggestive of pancreatitis and are preferred sites for the collection of a

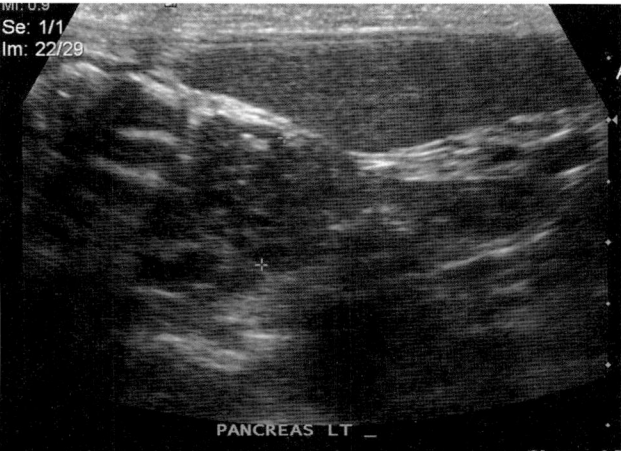

Figure 19.2 Ultrasonographic appearance of the pancreas in a cat with pancreatitis. The pancreas is enlarged and appears heterogeneous, with hypoechoic areas and hyperechoic surrounding fat. These findings are highly suggestive of pancreatitis. Source: Courtesy of Dr. Benjamin Young, Texas A&M University.

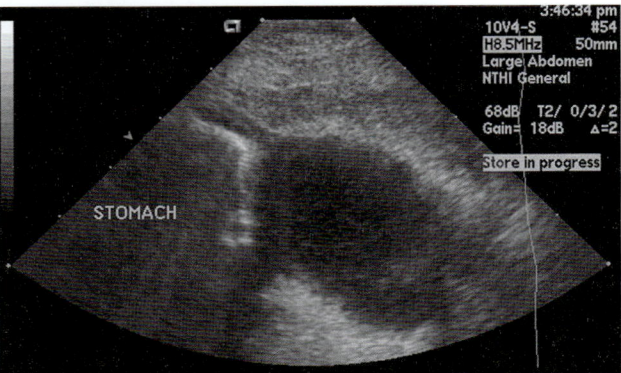

Figure 19.3 Ultrasonographic appearance of the pancreas of a dog with a pancreatic abscess. This lesion appears as a large hypoechoic area within the pancreas surrounded by a hyperechoic area. Source: Courtesy of Dr. Benjamin Young, Texas A&M University.

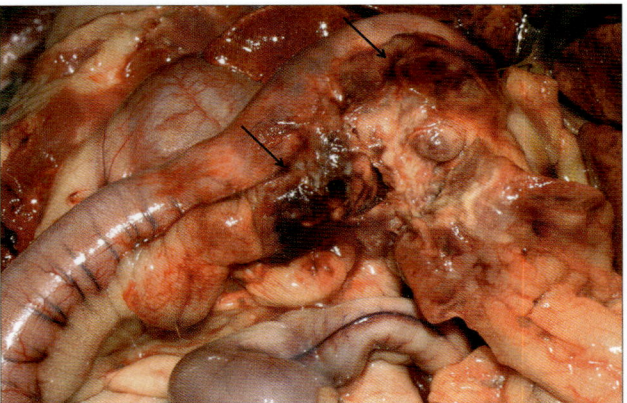

Figure 19.4 Gross appearance of the pancreas in a dog with acute pancreatitis. The pancreas appears severely edematous, hemorrhagic, and necrotic (arrows). Such appearance is highly suggestive of acute pancreatitis with pancreatic necrosis. Source: Courtesy of Dr. Dharani Ajithdoss, Texas A&M University.

tissue specimen (Hill & Van Winkle 1993; Saunders *et al.* 2002; Steiner *et al.* 2008a). Gross pancreatic lesions suggestive of pancreatitis may include peripancreatic fat necrosis, pancreatic hemorrhage or congestion, and a dull granular capsular surface (Figure 19.4) (Hill & Van Winkle 1993; Saunders *et al.* 2002; Steiner *et al.* 2008a). However, gross pathologic lesions may not always be apparent in dogs and cats with pancreatitis, and in some cases they might be difficult to differentiate from nodular hyperplasia or neoplasia (Hill & Van Winkle 1993; Saunders *et al.* 2002; Newman *et al.* 2004).

Histopathologic examination of pancreatic tissue is considered the gold standard for a definitive diagnosis of pancreatitis in both dogs and cats. Histopathology is also the only way to definitively differentiate acute from chronic pancreatitis. Although not clearly defined in veterinary species, the presence of permanent histopathologic changes (such as fibrosis and acinar atrophy) is considered suggestive of chronic pancreatitis (Williams 1996; Newman *et al.* 2004). Acute pancreatitis is characterized by the absence of such permanent histopathologic changes (Acute Pancreatitis Classification Working Group 2008). The predominant inflammatory cellular infiltrate (neutrophils or lymphocytes) is often used to describe pancreatitis as suppurative or lymphocytic, respectively, and a significant degree of necrosis is usually used to characterize the pancreatitis as necrotizing (Hill & Van Winkle 1993; Ferreri *et al.* 2003).

Several limitations are associated with pancreatic histopathology as a definitive diagnostic tool for pancreatitis. First, determining the clinical significance of histopathologic findings may be challenging. For example, in a recent study, histopathologic lesions of pancreatitis were identified in 67% of all cats examined, including 45% of healthy cats (De Cock *et al.* 2007). At the same time, exclusion of pancreatitis based on histopathology is difficult because inflammatory lesions of the pancreas are often highly localized and can easily be missed (Hill & Van Winkle 1993; Saunders *et al.* 2002; Newman *et al.* 2004; De Cock *et al.* 2007). Therefore, multiple sections of the pancreas must be evaluated in order to increase the likelihood of finding microscopic lesions, although this is not always feasible in clinical practice (Newman *et al.* 2004; De Cock *et al.* 2007). Finally, although pancreatic biopsy *per se* is considered to be safe, it requires invasive procedures that are expensive and potentially detrimental in patients that are hemodynamically unstable (Webb & Trott 2008).

Because concurrent inflammation of the intestines and/or liver appears to be a common problem in cats and in some dogs, intestinal and hepatic biopsies should be collected in patients (especially cats) suspected of having pancreatitis that are undergoing exploratory laparotomy or laparoscopy. Likewise, cats with IBD and/or cholangitis that undergo laparotomy or laparoscopy should also have their pancreas evaluated.

Cytology

FNA of the pancreas and cytologic examination of the aspirated material is a minimally invasive technique that can be used for the diagnosis and differentiation of pancreatitis and other exocrine pancreatic diseases in dogs and cats. It should be performed either under ultrasonographic guidance (in which case specimen collection is quite demanding) or during laparotomy (Bjorneby & Kari 2002).

In the only available study in dogs, ultrasound-guided pancreatic aspiration was described retrospectively in 92 dogs and was found to be safe and the aspirated material was reported to be diagnostic in 74% of the samples obtained (Cordner *et al.* 2015). In the same study, there was 91% agreement with histopathology in the small number of dogs for which histopathology was also available (Cordner *et al.* 2015). In another study in which ultrasound-guided pancreatic aspiration was performed in 73 cats, the procedure was found to be safe and the aspirated material was diagnostic in 67% of the samples obtained (Crain *et al.* 2015). In the same study, there was 86% agreement with histopathology in the small number of cats for which histopathology was also available (Crain *et al.* 2015).

Pancreatic acinar cells constitute the majority of cells found in FNA smears from a normal pancreas (Bjorneby & Kari 2002). In patients with acute pancreatitis, the cytologic picture is mainly characterized by hypercellularity and the presence of intact and degenerated neutrophils and degenerated pancreatic acinar cells. It should be noted that, as for histopathology, highly localized lesions might be missed. Therefore, negative results are not sufficient to rule out pancreatitis. FNA cytology might also be useful in differentiating other conditions of the pancreas (e.g., neoplasia) from pancreatitis.

Treatment

Treatment of the cause

The etiology of pancreatitis remains unknown in the majority of cases in both dogs and cats, and therefore treatment of pancreatitis remains almost exclusively supportive and symptomatic. It is expected that better characterization of this disease in the future will allow the development of new and specific treatments for different forms of pancreatitis that are currently being classified as idiopathic pancreatitis. Until then, the presence of possible risk factors should be investigated in all animals with pancreatitis. If any of these factors are present, they should be removed or treated. Dogs should be investigated for the presence of factors such as hypertriglyceridemia. Dogs and cats should be investigated for hypercalcemia, concurrent endocrine diseases, obesity, certain toxicities (e.g., zinc), evidence of certain infectious diseases (e.g., babesiosis, feline infectious peritonitis, toxoplasmosis), and inflammatory diseases of the intestine and the hepatobiliary system. Important information from the medical history of the animal includes drugs administered (especially potassium bromide, phenobarbital, and azathioprine), diet offered (especially high-fat diets), and recent surgery or trauma. Concurrent diseases that may have an etiologic association with pancreatitis, such as IBD and inflammatory hepatobiliary disease, should also be investigated.

Fluid therapy

Early and adequate fluid administration is the cornerstone of management of acute pancreatitis and aggressive fluid therapy has been shown to improve outcome in humans with severe acute pancreatitis (Lee & Papachristou 2019). Dogs with severe pancreatitis are often presented with variable degrees of dehydration, hypovolemia, or both, due to ongoing anorexia, vomiting, diarrhea, and/or third-space losses. However, close monitoring is required in order not to overhydrate the animal, as, at least in humans, overly aggressive fluid therapy may be associated with an increased risk of acute kidney injury and/or acute respiratory distress syndrome (Gad & Simons-Linares 2020). Tissue hypoperfusion and especially diminished pancreatic microcirculation are believed to contribute to the development of major local and systemic complications (Talukdar & Vege 2009). Studies in experimental acute pancreatitis in dogs suggest that hypertonic saline–dextran solutions may be more efficacious than crystalloid solutions in restoring tissue perfusion (Horton *et al.* 1989). However, studies in dogs and cats with spontaneous pancreatitis are lacking and current recommendations in humans favor crystalloid use in most cases (Talukdar & Vege 2009). Thus, replacement isotonic solutions (e.g., lactated Ringer, 0.9% NaCl) given intravenously are the treatment of choice for dehydrated animals with pancreatitis. Mild dehydration (<5%) can be treated by subcutaneous fluid administration, but severe dehydration must be corrected by intravenous fluid administration. Administration of colloid fluids (e.g., hetastarch) might be indicated in cases of severe hypoalbuminemia or hypotension.

Electrolyte and acid–base therapy

Electrolyte abnormalities are common in animals with acute pancreatitis. Various combinations and degrees of hypokalemia, hyponatremia, and hypochloremia can be present as a result of diarrhea, vomiting, fluid therapy, and/or anorexia (Schaer 1979; Hill & Van Winkle 1993; Simpson *et al.* 1994; Hess *et al.* 1998). Hyperkalemia, hypernatremia, and hypocalcemia or hypercalcemia have also been reported, but much less frequently (Schaer 1979; Hill & Van Winkle 1993; Hess *et al.* 1998; Kimmel *et al.* 2001). Unfortunately, electrolyte abnormalities in dogs and cats with pancreatitis cannot be accurately predicted and serum potassium, sodium, chloride, and ionized calcium concentrations should always be measured and corrected in these animals. Hypokalemia is often present as a result of potassium loss due to a combination of diarrhea, vomiting, fluid therapy, and anorexia. Therefore, serum potassium should be monitored throughout hospitalization, and potassium must be added to the intravenous fluids where necessary. Hypocalcemia can also be seen in patients with pancreatitis (more commonly in cats than in dogs), but clinical signs attributable to hypocalcemia are rarely noted (Hess *et al.* 1998; Kimmel *et al.* 2001). The value of supplementing calcium has not been evaluated in either dogs or cats. In cats, low serum ionized calcium concentration (<1.0 mmol/L) has been associated with a worse prognosis and calcium supplementation might be beneficial in these cases (Kimmel *et al.* 2001). Hypocalcemia can be treated with 10% calcium gluconate at a dose of 5–10 mg/kg per hour of elemental calcium given in the crystalloid infusion.

Acid–base disturbances are also common in small animal patients with pancreatitis and could occur as a result of vomiting, diarrhea, and/or hypoperfusion. Unfortunately, the nature of acid–base disorders in patients with pancreatitis cannot be accurately predicted and blood gas analysis is recommended in those with severe disease.

Nutrition

It is now recognized that both parenteral and enteral routes of alimentation are superior to providing no supplementary nutrition, and thus providing early and adequate nutritional support has become a priority in the treatment of human patients with acute pancreatitis (Petrov *et al.* 2008a). In addition, several studies in humans have shown that enteral nutrition is superior in many ways compared with parenteral nutrition, and enteral nutrition is now the preferred method of alimentation for patients with acute pancreatitis (Petrov *et al.* 2008a,b). Jejunal feeding is considered by many to be the method of choice, but studies in humans have shown that nasojejunal feeding offers no advantages compared with nasogastric feeding (Eatock *et al.* 2005; Petrov *et al.* 2008a).

In a pilot study, early enteral nutrition in five dogs with naturally occurring severe acute pancreatitis delivered proximal to the pylorus was well tolerated and resulted in fewer complications than parenteral nutrition (Mansfield *et al.* 2011). In another study of 34 dogs with pancreatitis, feeding within 48 hours of hospitalization had a positive impact on return to voluntary intake and reduced the incidence of gastrointestinal signs (Harris *et al.* 2017).

Unfortunately, there are currently no clinical trials evaluating different nutritional approaches in cats with pancreatitis and therefore evidence-based recommendations for cats cannot be made. However, given the evidence available from studies in humans, dogs, and experimental animals, it appears safe to assume that cats

with pancreatitis likely also benefit from early enteral nutrition. This is particularly important because cats have considerably higher dietary protein requirements than dogs or humans, and therefore are more prone to protein malnutrition during anorexia or prolonged fasting. In addition, because the vast majority of cats with acute pancreatitis are presented with a history of anorexia of several days' duration, additional food restriction could induce or worsen hepatic lipidosis. In the only study evaluating the use of feeding tubes in cats with pancreatitis, nasogastric tube feeding was tolerated well with no worsening of clinical signs (Klaus *et al.* 2009).

In general, cats with pancreatitis that do not vomit should be fed orally. In cats that do not vomit but are anorectic, some form of feeding tube should be used (see later). Appetite stimulants might be used in anorectic cats, but might not lead to adequate caloric intake, especially in severe cases. In cases of severe vomiting there is a risk of aspiration pneumonia and oral intake of food or feeding tube placement should probably be delayed until vomiting is controlled with antiemetics. This period should be as short as possible and thus antiemetic treatment should be aggressive. After vomiting has been controlled, small amounts of water or food can be introduced and if vomiting does not recur a feeding tube can be placed if needed.

It is important to note that there is no evidence to support the use of postpyloric feeding in either humans or animals with acute pancreatitis (Eatock *et al.* 2000, 2005; Kumar *et al.* 2006) and therefore achieving postpyloric feeding should not be an absolute goal in dogs and cats with acute pancreatitis. Nasogastric or nasoesophageal tubes are easily placed and do not require general anesthesia. Thus, they can be used for short-term nutritional support in severely ill patients in which general anesthesia is contraindicated. They have been reported to be well tolerated and associated with only a few clinically significant complications (Klaus *et al.* 2009). The main disadvantage of these tubes is their small diameter, which results in frequent obstructions. Placement of esophagostomy tubes requires only a short general anesthesia and represents an excellent option for both dogs and cats with pancreatitis. Complications are uncommon and usually mild, provided that tube placement is confirmed both visually and radiographically or endoscopically prior to anesthetic recovery. In a recent study, complications were reported in 35% of 248 cats and included stoma site infection (12%), removal of the tube (17%), and tube blockage (3%) (Klaus *et al.* 2009). Gastrostomy tube placement requires a longer anesthesia and endoscopy (or potentially surgery), and might be associated with more complications. Therefore, less invasive methods are preferred by the author and gastrostomy tubes are typically reserved for animals that undergo surgery or endoscopy for other reasons (e.g., exploratory laparotomy, biopsies, biliary tract obstruction). However, because of the larger-diameter tube, they can be used for longer periods of time when necessary. Finally, jejunostomy tubes offer the theoretical advantage that they are placed distal to the site of pancreatic stimulation and might also be better tolerated in animals with intractable vomiting. As with gastrostomy tubes, placement of a jejunostomy tube typically requires laparotomy and therefore these tubes are typically reserved for animals that might require laparotomy for other reasons.

With regard to the appropriate diet that should be used in dogs and cats with pancreatitis, evidence-based information is lacking. Hyperlipidemia, high-fat diets, obesity, and dietary indiscretion are considered risk factors for pancreatitis in dogs, and life-long fat restriction is usually recommended in dogs with pancreatitis. A relationship between pancreatitis and hyperlipidemia or obesity has not been reported in cats. Cats have higher protein requirements and appear to digest and use high levels of dietary fat better than dogs. In a retrospective study of 55 cats with acute pancreatitis, a liquid high-lipid diet (45% of caloric density as lipids) fed through a nasogastric tube was well tolerated (Klaus *et al.* 2009). Having said this, anecdotally, there is a group of cats that will develop pancreatitis a few weeks after having been switched to a high-fat diet and improve with switching to a diet with a lower fat content. Therefore, it would appear prudent to avoid diets that are particularly high in fat, but more studies on the subject are needed and are ongoing to more clearly delineate the impact of dietary fat in cats with acute or chronic pancreatitis.

If vomiting cannot be controlled, administration of parenteral nutrition has been frequently reported in dogs and cats, but in our practice has only been infrequently used in clinical patients, mainly because of data from human studies (see earlier), the unproven efficacy in animals with pancreatitis, and the potential for serious complications (Lippert *et al.* 1993; Freeman *et al.* 1995; Chan *et al.* 2002; Pyle *et al.* 2004).

Plasma and blood transfusion

The use of fresh frozen plasma (10–15 mg/kg once daily) is recommended by some authors in dogs with severe pancreatitis because it contains useful components, such as protease inhibitors (e.g., α_1-proteinase inhibitor, α_2-macroglobulin), albumin, and both coagulation and antithrombotic factors (Williams 1996; Logan *et al.* 2001). Protease inhibitors were once believed to protect from the development or worsening of pancreatitis, and depletion of protease inhibitors has been

reported in dogs with both experimental and spontaneous pancreatitis (Murtaugh & Jacobs 1985; Williams 1996; Ruaux & Atwell 1999). However, in one study α_2-macroglobulin concentrations did not correlate with severity of pancreatitis in dogs (Ruaux & Atwell 1999). Studies in humans have shown no benefit of plasma administration in the clinical outcome of patients with acute pancreatitis, despite the increase in plasma concentrations of protease inhibitors (Leese *et al.* 1991). Therefore fresh frozen plasma is generally not recommended for the treatment of humans with pancreatitis. In addition, in a recent retrospective study, dogs with pancreatitis that received fresh frozen plasma had a worse outcome than dogs that did not receive fresh frozen plasma (Weatherton & Streeter 2009). In this study there was no significant difference in the severity of pancreatitis before treatment, although treatments were not controlled in the two groups and group allocation was not randomized (Weatherton & Streeter 2009). Thus, the actual value of plasma administration remains controversial in dogs with pancreatitis and has never been studied in cats.

Analgesic therapy

Pain is believed to accompany virtually all cases of pancreatitis in dogs and cats, even when pain is not clinically detected. Pain induces several physiologic changes, including decreased appetite, decreased gastrointestinal tone, decreased regional blood flow to several abdominal organs (including the pancreas), tachycardia, and production of a catabolic state (Asfar *et al.* 2006; Muir 2009). Therefore, analgesic therapy is extremely important in animals with pancreatitis and should be used in all patients with this condition.

Pain in dogs and cats with pancreatitis can range from mild to excruciating. Opioid administration (e.g., buprenorphine, fentanyl, hydromorphone, morphine) is often necessary in the management of pain in acute pancreatitis, and the intravenous route is usually preferred because it provides fast relief. Multimodal pain management might be indicated in some cases with severe pain, because it seems to be more effective and associated with fewer side effects due to lower doses of each of the drugs being administered. Lidocaine and ketamine are commonly used together with opioids.

Antiemetic therapy

Maropitant (1 mg/kg every [q]24 h orally [p.o.] or subcutaneously [s.c.]), a neurokinin-1 receptor antagonist, is a very potent and safe antiemetic that is often used as a first-line antiemetic in dogs with pancreatitis. There is also evidence that maropitant has analgesic properties, making this drug very attractive for use in pancreatitis patients. Furthermore, recent evidence in experimental models of pancreatitis has suggested that maropitant may also have anti-inflammatory properties. Other good antiemetic choices include 5-HT3 antagonists, such as ondansetron (0.1–0.2 mg/kg slow intravenously [i.v.], q6–12 h). Dopaminergic antagonists (e.g., metoclopramide, 0.2–0.5 mg/kg i.v., intramuscularly [i.m.], s.c., or p.o. q6–8 h) are considered less effective in treating nausea and vomiting, but might be useful in enhancing upper gastrointestinal motility, although constant-rate infusion of metoclopramide (1–2 mg/kg/day i.v.) may be more effective than intermittent dosing. In cases of intractable vomiting, combinations of different antiemetics can be used.

Appetite stimulants

Dogs and cats with acute pancreatitis often have a reduced appetite. Many of these animals have nausea, leading to anorexia. Thus, treatment with an antiemetic may have a positive impact on appetite, but many patients remain hyporexic. These patients may benefit from an appetite stimulant. In hospitalized patients capromorelin is likely the most effective treatment option for dogs (3 mg/kg p.o. q24 h) and cats (1–3 mg/kg p.o. q24 h). Mirtazapine (1.88 mg/cat p.o. every other day or 7.5 mg transdermally applied aurally) is a good option for cats and may also be used in dogs (1.1–1.3 mg/kg p.o. q24 h in dogs; not to exceed 30 mg/dog/day). Mirtazapine might also have antiemetic properties.

Antibiotics

The goal of antibiotic prophylaxis in human patients with necrotizing pancreatitis is to prevent bacterial translocation from the intestine, prevent or decrease pancreatic colonization, and reduce mortality (Hart et al. 2008; Jafri et al. 2009). However, meta-analyses in humans have often have shown conflicting results, with most studies demonstrating no benefit of routine use of antibiotics (Pandol et al. 2007; Hart et al. 2008; Jafri et al. 2009; Talukdar & Vege 2009). This is likely due to the fact that infectious complications of severe acute pancreatitis in humans usually occur rather late in the course of the disease, often after the patient has spent many weeks in intensive care. Thus, based on this recognized timeline and the fact that multicenter, double-blind, placebo-controlled, and meta-analysis studies have failed to show a clear advantage of prophylactic antibiotic use in humans with severe necrotizing pancreatitis, recent practice guidelines published by the American Gastroenterological Association do not provide any recommendations for prophylactic antibiotic (American Gastroenterological Association Institute on "Management of Acute Pancreatitis" Clinical Practice and Economics

Committee 2007; Forsmark & Baillie 2007). However, antibiotics should be used on demand, based on evidence of infection (American Gastroenterological Association Institute on "Management of Acute Pancreatitis" Clinical Practice and Economics Committee 2007; Forsmark & Baillie 2007; Pandol et al. 2007; Talukdar & Vege 2009).

Studies on prophylactic antibiotic use in dogs and cats with spontaneous pancreatitis of any severity are lacking. However, use of antibiotics is recommended in cases where infectious complications have been identified (e.g., infected pancreatic abscess, sepsis, aspiration pneumonia) or are strongly suspected (e.g., toxic neutrophils, severe neutropenia, persistent fever). Animals with severe pancreatitis should be closely monitored for infectious complications. Antibiotic selection should be based on culture and sensitivity, but cefotaxime ciprofloxacin, metronidazole, clindamycin, and chloramphenicol have all been shown to achieve therapeutic levels in the pancreas in experimental pancreatitis (Trudel et al. 1994; Greene 2006).

Glucocorticoids

Glucocorticoids were once believed to cause pancreatitis in both humans and dogs. However, the scientific basis for this hypothesis is weak and in humans glucocorticoids are no longer considered as a risk factor for pancreatitis (Frick et al. 1993). A recent, uncontrolled study in 45 client-owned dogs suggested that 1 mg/kg prednisolone (s.c. q24 h), given from diagnosis to discharge, decreased hospitalization time, time to decrease of serum C-reactive protein (CRP) concentration, and one-month survival (Okanishi et al. 2019). However, further studies are needed before routine use of corticosteroids in dogs with severe acute pancreatitis can be recommended.

Surgery for pancreatitis

Surgery is not indicated for acute pancreatitis unless a complete biliary obstruction needs to be corrected or a feeding tube needs to be placed. Most of the procedures can be performed via laparoscopy. Peritoneal lavage can also be performed at the end of the procedure, but the clinical benefit of this procedure has not been established.

Temporary bile diversion

Extrahepatic biliary duct obstruction (EHBO) (Mayhew et al. 2002, 2006; Mayhew & Weisse 2008) has been reported as a result of pancreatitis in both dogs and cats. It usually results from compression of the bile duct by the inflamed pancreas and can lead to severe icterus and distension of the biliary system. If obstruction occurs, the biliary system might need to be decompressed. Surgical treatment of EHBO is described in detail in Chapter 17. The gallbladder can be drained intermittently using needle aspiration under ultrasound guidance (Herman et al. 2005). This technique has been described in three clinical dogs without inducing bile peritonitis. Although needle aspiration is less invasive than other methods of decompression, it does not provide continuous drainage. The effect of repeated cholecystostocentesis is unknown. However, it should be noted that most patients with pancreatitis and EHBO do not have a complete obstruction and thus intermittent decompression may be sufficient.

Continuous decompression of the biliary system can be accomplished with a catheter placed retrogradely from the duodenum into the common bile duct or through the apex of the gallbladder. If a catheter is placed retrogradely through the duodenal papilla, a 5 Fr infant feeding tube is used. The tube is first placed similarly to a jejunostomy feeding tube, but in the distal duodenum and then advanced into the common bile duct. This technique requires a duodenotomy in order to guide the feeding tube through the duodenal papilla and into the common bile duct, which increases the risk of contamination of the peritoneal cavity.

A cholecystostomy tube can be placed during laparotomy, laparoscopy, or by ultrasound guidance. With these techniques the biliary system is decompressed without increasing the risk of infection. The catheter can also be used to perform a cholangiogram. The apex of the gallbladder can be pexied to the abdomen wall during laparotomy if the gallbladder is severely distended, and a 5 Fr infant feeding tube can be advanced percutaneously into the apex of the gallbladder.

Percutaneous placement of a cholecystostomy tube is possible under ultrasound guidance or laparoscopy. Placement of the tube with laparoscopic guidance appears superior to placement with ultrasound in cadavers (Murphy et al. 2007).

Feeding tube placement

Jejunostomy feeding tubes can be placed during a laparotomy or laparoscopy in dogs or cats that have refractory vomiting, but as already noted the notion that a jejunostomy tube is preferable over a more proximally placed tube has not been substantiated. If other procedures are not required, a laparoscopic approach is desirable for the recovery of the patient (Rawlings et al. 2002).

Peritoneal lavage

The peritoneal exudate that develops during severe pancreatitis contains several harmful substances such as trypsin and inflammatory cytokines (Platell et al. 2001; Dong et al. 2010). Peritoneal lavage was once hypothesized to be beneficial to patients with severe acute pancreatitis by reducing intraperitoneal concentrations of these factors (Dong et al. 2010). Although initial studies were encouraging, recent well-designed and meta-analysis studies have shown that the use of peritoneal lavage is not associated with any significant improvement in mortality, morbidity, or hospital stay in humans with severe acute pancreatitis (Platell et al. 2001; Dong et al. 2010). Therefore, peritoneal lavage is generally not recommended in human patients with pancreatitis (Platell et al. 2001; Dong et al. 2010).

The usefulness of peritoneal lavage has been evaluated in a single study of experimental canine pancreatitis (Bassi et al. 1989). No data are available for its benefit in dogs and cats with spontaneous disease and it is currently not recommended.

Pancreatic and peripancreatic fluid collections

In humans, pancreatic and peripancreatic fluid collections are classified either as collections composed of fluid alone or collections that contain a necrotic material (Banks et al. 2013). Although in humans the classification and terminology of these collections have been standardized, in dogs and cats this is not the case, and this leads to confusion. In this chapter we use the terminology adapted from humans, but also correlate that with the older terminology used in the veterinary literature.

Walled-off necrosis (previously termed pancreatic abscess)

Walled-off necrosis consists of necrotic tissue that has been encapsulated within an enhancing wall of reactive tissue (Banks et al. 2013). Usually this is the result of necrotizing pancreatitis and occurs weeks after the onset of pancreatitis. Most cases of a pancreatic abscess described in the veterinary literature should probably be considered to represent a walled-off necrosis. A pancreatic abscess (Salisbury et al. 1988; Edwards et al. 1990; Simpson et al. 1994; Stimson et al. 1998; Coleman & Robson 2005; Johnson & Mann 2006; Anderson et al. 2008) is the most commonly reported pancreatic complication of pancreatitis in dogs, with a reported prevalence of 1.4–6.5%, but should generally be considered to be rare. It has only been reported in one cat (Nemoto et al. 2017). In people a walled-off necrosis can be sterile or infected, but in dogs only very few cases reported with an abscess had evidence of an infection (Salisbury et al. 1988; Stimson et al. 1998).

Clinical signs and diagnosis

Clinical signs of a walled-off necrosis (pancreatic abscesses) are nonspecific and generally do not differ from those of pancreatitis, although they may persist despite treatment of pancreatitis. Common clinicopathological findings are neutrophilia with a left shift, elevation of serum lipase activity or PLI concentration, elevations of hepatic enzyme activities, and hyperbilirubinemia. A mass in the cranial abdomen may be identified upon abdominal palpation in a small number of cases. Indirect visualization of the abscess is usually achieved ultrasonographically (a hypoechoic structure that can be of variable size) or, less commonly, radiographically. The diagnosis is usually based on cytologic and bacteriologic analysis of material obtained through an ultrasound-guided FNA (which is usually the initial approach) or surgery. The cytologic picture is usually highly cellular and characterized by degenerate neutrophils. This picture may be difficult to distinguish from acute pancreatitis and histopathology may be required for a definitive diagnosis. Bacteria may or may not be present. Walled-off necrosis is usually sterile, but on rare occasions it might be infected in both humans and dogs. In dogs only 0–22% of the reported cases yield bacterial growth, although many of these dogs had received antibiotics prior to admission. In one cat *Staphylococcus aureus* was isolated from a pancreatic abscess (Nemoto et al. 2017).

Management

In humans intervention is required when the walled-off necrosis is infected, but in cases of sterile walled-off necrosis the need for intervention is less clear and when undertaken is usually done by a minimally invasive procedure. The goals of surgical treatment are to débride the abscess, collect samples for culture, and provide drainage of the abscess and the peritoneal cavity if peritonitis is present (Salisbury et al. 1988; Edwards et al. 1990; Stimson et al. 1998; Thompson et al. 2009). Partial pancreatectomy of the left limb of the pancreas can be performed in order to remove a pancreatic abscess. A splenectomy may be required at the same time if the splenic artery cannot be preserved (Salisbury et al. 1988). Partial gastrectomy may also be required if the pancreatic abscess is adherent to the greater curvature of the stomach (Figure 19.5). Partial pancreatectomy is performed with gentle dissection across the pancreatic parenchyma and ligation of the pancreatic duct. Absorbable suture is usually used to ligate the pancreatic duct, but staples can also be used. If the pancreatic abscess is localized in the right limb or the body of the pancreas, the partial pancreatectomy might be more

complicated because of the close relationship between the pancreas, the pancreaticoduodenal artery, the duodenum, and the bile duct. A resection of the duodenum might be required (Figure 19.6). Drainage of an unresectable abscess has been established in the stomach or the duodenum (Bellenger e al. 1989). A cholecystojejunostomy or a choledochoduodenostomy might be required to maintain the normal flow of bile (see Chapter 17). If the pancreatic abscess cannot be débrided completely, the omentum can be used to provide further drainage of the pancreatic abscess.

Closed-suction drains can be placed at the end of the surgery if the amount of contamination of the peritoneal cavity is not too severe. An open abdomen has been used to provide adequate drainage of the abdominal cavity, especially if the abscess has ruptured at the time of surgery (see Chapter 20) (Salisbury et al. 1988; Edwards et al. 1990; Stimson et al. 1998; Thompson et al. 2009).

Antibiotics should be used in cases of infected abscesses, but their use in patients with a sterile abscess is questionable.

Prognosis

Reported mortality rates in dogs with a pancreatic abscess range from 50% to 36%, making the presence of a pancreatic abscess a poor prognostic indicator. Also, the dogs that survived to discharge had a mean hospitalization time of 12.4 days, highlighting the importance of preparing the owner for a guarded prognosis and a prolonged recovery period (Anderson et al. 2008).

Pancreatic pseudocyst

A pancreatic pseudocyst (Wolfsheimer et al. 1991; Hines et al. 1996; Smith & Biller 1998; VanEnkevort et al. 1999; Jerram et al. 2004; Coleman & Robson 2005) is defined as a collection of sterile fluid containing mainly pancreatic juice and no solid material that is enclosed by a wall of fibrous or granulation tissue. Pancreatic pseudocysts have been reported in dogs and a small number of cats as a complication of pancreatitis (both acute and chronic), but they appear to be rather uncommon. Their exact pathogenesis is unknown.

Clinical signs and diagnosis

Clinical signs reported usually include different combinations of vomiting, anorexia, depression, and abdominal pain, although it might be difficult to determine if they are due to the pancreatitis or the pseudocyst *per se*. Occasionally, pancreatic pseudocysts may cause extrahepatic biliary tract obstruction. Detection of a pseudocyst is usually achieved during abdominal ultrasonography or

(a)

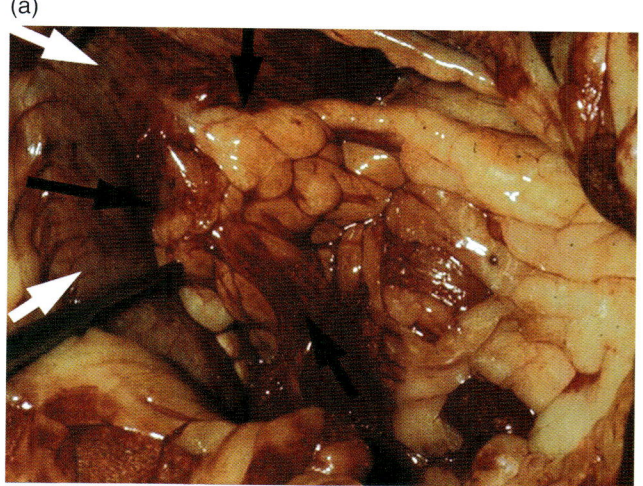

(b)

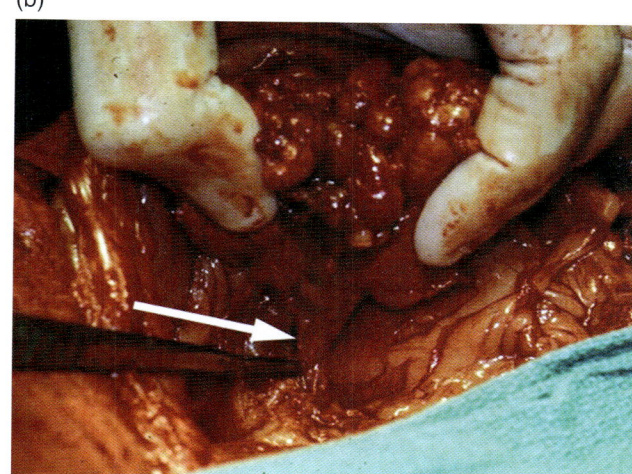

(c)

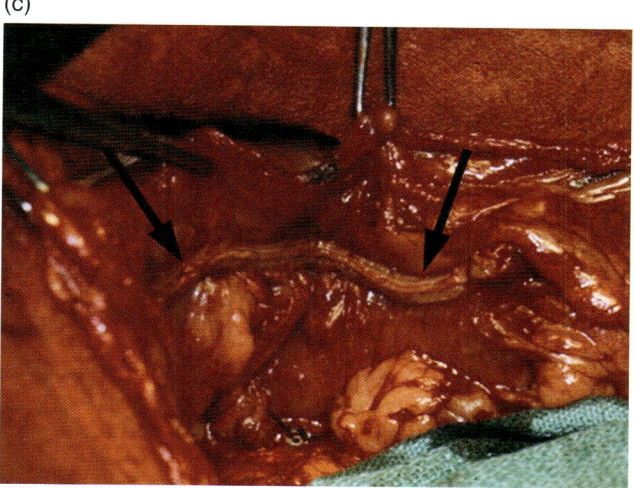

Figure 19.5 (a) A pancreatic walled-off necrosis (abscess; black arrows) is in the left limb of the pancreas and is well adhered to the wall of the stomach (white arrows). (b) The splenic artery (white arrow) is incorporated in the walled-off necrosis. A splenectomy is required. (c) A gastrectomy (black arrow) along the greater curvature has been performed with the splenectomy in order to excise the walled-off necrosis.

with abdominal computed tomography, where a cystic structure in close proximity to the pancreas can be identified. In most cases described so far, the cystic structure was associated with the left lobe of the pancreas. The diagnosis can be made via cytologic examination of fluid from the lesion collected through an ultrasound-guided FNA or surgery. In contrast to walled-off necrosis, cytologic examination of fluid from a pseudocyst is characterized by low cellularity. High amylase and lipase activities and PLI concentrations in the cyst fluid are also suggestive of a pseudocyst. Definitive diagnosis may require histopathology in some cases. The clinical signs may resolve with medical management for pancreatitis despite persistence of the pseudocyst. In some cases, small pseudocysts may spontaneously resolve.

Management

Ultrasound-guided FNA of the cystic fluid may be used for management of small pseudocysts. Repeated ultrasound-guided aspiration may be required in some cases (Smith & Biller 1998). In other cases, however, clinical signs may persist or worsen despite treatment and enlargement of the pseudocyst occurring over time. In these cases surgical intervention is usually recommended, although surgical techniques are poorly described in veterinary medicine. Internal drainage seems to be the treatment of choice in humans.

The surgical treatment of a pseudocyst is similar to that of a walled-off necrosis. The goals are to resect the cyst, collect tissue for histopathologic analysis and culture, and provide drainage if needed. The omentum has been used successfully in one case report to drain a pseudocyst (Jerram *et al.* 2004). Drainage of the cyst can be achieved into the duodenum or the stomach if the capsule is thick to prevent leakage (Bellenger *et al.* 1989).

Acute peripancreatic fluid collection

This kind of fluid collection usually develops during the early stages of edematous pancreatitis and does not

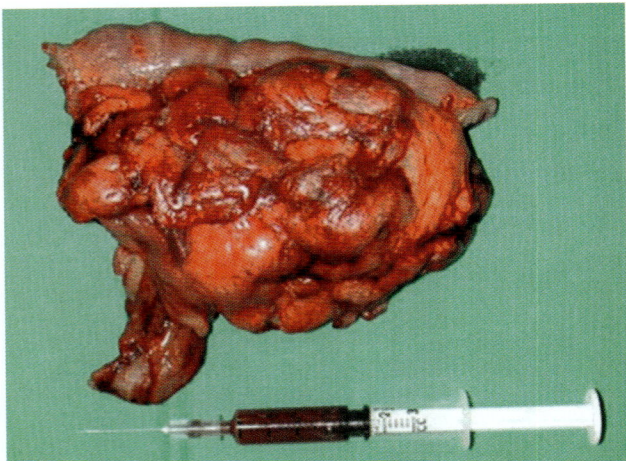

Figure 19.6 Walled-off necrosis in the right limb of the pancreas. A resection anastomosis of the distal part of the duodenum was required. The bile duct was preserved.

contain any solid components or a solid wall structure (Banks *et al.* 2013). Most of these acute peripancreatic fluid collections have been reported to be sterile in humans and are likely also sterile in dogs and cats. Ultrasonographically, these fluid collections appear as homogenously hypoechogenic structures without a clear wall. Most of these acute peripancreatic fluid collections will resolve spontaneously and do not require any intervention.

Acute necrotic fluid collection

An acute necrotic fluid collection arises during acute necrotizing pancreatitis when necrotic debris undergoes liquefaction and can be located entirely within the pancreatic parenchyma or in the immediate peripancreatic space (Banks *et al.* 2013). Most acute necrotic fluid collections are sterile, but they can also be infected. Ultrasonographically, these fluid collections appear as hypoechoic structures of mixed echogenicity without a solid wall. Sterile acute fluid collections have not been described as such in dogs or cats, but in humans are usually considered a part of pancreatic necrosis in patients with severe pancreatitis. Acute necrotic fluid collections do not require surgical intervention unless they are infected, in which case the patient should be treated systemically with antimicrobials based on sensitivity testing, when available. Surgical débridement has not been extensively studied in small animals, but in one report all five dogs that underwent débridement and drainage for an acute necrotic fluid collection died or were euthanized during the postoperative period (Edwards *et al.* 1990).

References

Acute Pancreatitis Classification Working Group (2008). Revision of the Atlanta classification of acute pancreatitis. www.pancreasclub.com/wp-content/uploads/2017/10/AtlantaClassification.pdf (accessed September 21, 2022).

Akol, K.G., Washabau, R.J., Saunders, H.M., and Hendrick, M.J. (1993). Acute pancreatitis in cats with hepatic lipidosis. *Journal of Veterinary Internal Medicine* 7: 205–209.

Allen, H.S., Steiner, J., Broussard, J. et al. (2006). Serum and urine concentrations of trypsinogen-activation peptide as markers for acute pancreatitis in cats. *Canadian Journal of Veterinary Research* 70: 313–316.

American Gastroenterological Association (AGA) Institute on "Management of Acute Pancreatits" Clinical Practice and Economics Committee (2007). AGA institute medical position statement on acute pancreatitis. *Gastroenterology* 132: 2019–2021.

Anderson, N.V. and Low, D.G. (1965). Diseases of the canine pancreas: a comparative summary of 103 cases. *Animal Hospital* 1: 189–194.

Anderson, J.R., Cornell, K.K., Parnell, N.K., and Salisbury, S.K. (2008). Pancreatic abscess in 36 dogs: a retrospective analysis of prognostic indicators. *Journal of the American Animal Hospital Association* 44: 171–179.

Asfar, P., Hauser, B., Radermacher, P., and Matejovic, M. (2006). Catecholamines and vasopressin during critical illness. *Critical Care Clinics* 22: 131–149.

Aste, G., Di Tommaso, M., Steiner, J.M. et al. (2005). Pancreatitis associated with *N*-methyl-glucamine therapy in a dog with leishmaniasis. *Veterinary Research Communications* 29 (Suppl 2): 269–272.

Aupperle-Lellbach, H., Torner, K., Staudacher, M. et al. (2020). Histopathological findings and canine pancreatic lipase immunoreactivity in normal dogs and dogs with inflammatory and neoplastic diseases of the pancreas. *Journal of Veterinary Internal Medicine* 34: 1127–1134.

Banks, P.A., Bollen, T.L., Dervenis, C. et al. (2013). Classification of acute pancreatitis – 2012: revision of the Atlanta classification and definitions by international consensus. *Gut* 62: 102–111.

Bassi, C., Briani, G., Vesentini, S. et al. (1989). Continuous peritoneal dialysis in acute experimental pancreatitis in dogs. Effect of aprotinin in the dialysate medium. *International Journal of Pancreatology* 5: 69–75.

Beall, M.J., Cahill, R., Pigeon, K. et al. (2011). Performance validation and method comparison of an in-clinic enzyme-linked immunosorbent assay for the detection of canine pancreatic lipase. *Journal of Veterinary Diagnostic Investigation* 23: 115–119.

Beisson, F., Tiss, A., Riviere, C., and Verger, R. (2000). Methods for lipase detection and assay: a critical review. *European Journal of Lipid Science and Technology* 102: 133–153.

Bellenger, C.R., Ilkiw, J.E., and Malik, R. (1989). Cystogastrostomy in the treatment of pancreatic abscess in two dogs. *Veterinary Record* 125: 181–184.

Berman, C.F., Lobetti, R.G., and Lindquist, E. (2020). Comparison of clinical findings in 293 dogs with suspect acute pancreatitis: different clinical presentation with left lobe, right lobe or diffuse involvement of the pancreas. *Journal of the South African Veterinary Association* 91: e1–e10.

Bishop, M.A., Xenoulis, P.G., Levinski, M.D. et al. (2010). Identification of variants of the SPINK1 gene and their association with pancreatitis in Miniature Schnauzers. *American Journal of Veterinary Research* 71: 527–533.

Bjorneby, J.M. and Kari, S. (2002). Cytology of the pancreas. *Veterinary Clinics of North America: Small Animal Practice* 32: 1293–1312.

Chan, D.L., Freeman, L.M., Labato, M.A., and Rush, J.E. (2002). Retrospective evaluation of partial parenteral nutrition in dogs and cats. *Journal of Veterinary Internal Medicine* 16: 440–445.

Coleman, M. and Robson, M. (2005). Pancreatic masses following pancreatitis: pancreatic pseudocysts, necrosis, and abscesses. *Compendium on Continuing Education for the Practicing Veterinarian* 27: 147–154.

Cook, A.K., Breitschwerdt, E.B., Levine, J.F. et al. (1993). Risk factors associated with acute pancreatitis in dogs: 101 cases (1985–1990). *Journal of the American Veterinary Medical Association* 203: 673–679.

Cordner, A.P., Sharkey, L.C., Armstrong, P.J., and McAteer, K.D. (2015). Cytologic findings and diagnostic yield in 92 dogs undergoing fine-needle aspiration of the pancreas. *Journal of Veterinary Diagnostic Investigation* 27: 236–240.

Crain, S.K., Sharkey, L.C., Cordner, A.P. et al. (2015). Safety of ultrasound-guided fine-needle aspiration of the feline pancreas: a case–control study. *Journal of Feline Medicine and Surgery* 17: 858–863.

Cridge, H., Sullivant, A.M., Wills, R.W., and Lee, A.M. (2020). Association between abdominal ultrasound findings, the specific canine pancreatic lipase assay, clinical severity indices, and clinical diagnosis in dogs with pancreatitis. *Journal of Veterinary Internal Medicine* 34: 636–643.

De Cock, H.E., Forman, M.A., Farver, T.B., and Marks, S.L. (2007). Prevalence and histopathologic characteristics of pancreatitis in cats. *Veterinary Pathology* 44: 39–49.

Dong, Z., Petrov, M.S., Xu, J. et al. (2010). Peritoneal lavage for severe acute pancreatitis: a systematic review of randomized trials. *World Journal of Surgery* 34: 2103–2108.

Eatock, F.C., Brombacher, G.D., Steven, A. et al. (2000). Nasogastric feeding in severe acute pancreatitis may be practical and safe. *International Journal of Pancreatology* 28: 23–29.

Eatock, F.C., Chong, P., Menezes, N. et al. (2005). A randomized study of early nasogastric versus nasojejunal feeding in severe acute pancreatitis. *American Journal of Gastroenterology* 100: 432–439.

Edwards, D.F., Bauer, M.S., Walker, M.A. et al. (1990). Pancreatic masses in seven dogs following acute pancreatitis. *Journal of the American Animal Hospital Association* 26: 189–198.

Estrin, M.A., Wehausen, C.E., Jessen, C.R., and Lee, J.A. (2006). Disseminated intravascular coagulation in cats. *Journal of Veterinary Internal Medicine* 20: 1334–1339.

Ferreri, J.A., Hardam, E., Kimmel, S.E. et al. (2003). Clinical differentiation of acute necrotizing from chronic nonsuppurative pancreatitis in cats: 63 cases (1996–2001). *Journal of the American Veterinary Medical Association* 223: 469–474.

Forman, M.A., Marks, S.L., De Cock, H.E. et al. (2004). Evaluation of serum feline pancreatic lipase immunoreactivity and helical computed tomography versus conventional testing for the diagnosis of feline pancreatitis. *Journal of Veterinary Internal Medicine* 18: 807–815.

Forman, M.A., Shiroma, J., Armstrong, P.J. et al. (2009). Evaluation of feline pancreas-specific lipase (Spec fPLTM) for the diagnosis of feline pancreatitis [Abstract]. *Journal of Veterinary Internal Medicine* 23: 733–734.

Forman, M.A., Steiner, J.M., Armstrong, P.J. et al. (2021). ACVIM consensus statement on pancreatitis in cats. *Journal of Veterinary Internal Medicine* 35: 703–723.

Forsmark, C.E. and Baillie, J. (2007). AGA institute technical review on acute pancreatitis. *Gastroenterology* 132: 2022–2044.

Fragkou, F.C., Adama-Moraitou, K.K., Poutahidis, T. et al. (2016). Prevalence and clinicopathological features of triaditis in a pro-spective case series of symptomatic and asymptomatic cats. *Journal of Veterinary Internal Medicine* 30: 1031–1045.

Freeman, L.M., Labato, M.A., Rush, J.E., and Murtaugh, R.J. (1995). Nutritional support in pancreatitis: a retrospective study. *Journal of Veterinary Emergency and Critical Care* 5: 32–40.

Frick, T.W., Speiser, D.E., Bimmler, D., and Largiadèr, F. (1993). Drug-induced acute pancreatitis: further criticism. *Digestive Diseases* 11: 113–132.

Frossard, J.L., Steer, M.L., and Pastor, C.M. (2008). Acute pancreatitis. *Lancet* 371: 143–152.

Furrow, E., Armstrong, P.J., and Patterson, E.E. (2012). High prevalence of the c.74A>C SPINK1 variant in miniature and standard Schnauzers. *Journal of Veterinary Internal Medicine* 26: 1295–1299.

Gad, M.M. and Simons-Linares, C.R. (2020). Is aggressive intravenous fluid resuscitation beneficial in acute pancreatitis? A meta-analysis of randomized control trials and cohort studies. *World Journal of Gastroenterology* 26: 1098–1106.

Gaisano, H.Y. and Gorelick, F.S. (2009). New insights into the mechanisms of pancreatitis. *Gastroenterology* 136: 2040–2044.

Gardner, T.B. and Chari, S.T. (2008). Autoimmune pancreatitis. *Gastroenterology Clinics of North America* 37: 439–460.

Gerhardt, A., Steiner, J.M., Williams, D.A. et al. (2001). Comparison of the sensitivity of different diagnostic tests for pancreatitis in cats. *Journal of Veterinary Internal Medicine* 15: 329–333.

Goossens, M.M., Nelson, R.W., Feldman, E.C., and Griffey, S.M. (1998). Response to insulin treatment and survival in 104 cats with diabetes mellitus (1985–1995). *Journal of Veterinary Internal Medicine* 12: 1–6.

Graca, R., Messick, J., McCullough, S. et al. (2005). Validation and diagnostic efficacy of a lipase assay using the substrate 1,2-o-dilauryl-rac-glycero glutaric acid-(6′ methyl resorufin)-ester for the diagnosis of acute pancreatitis in dogs. *Veterinary Clinical Pathology* 34: 39–43.

Greene, C.E. (2006). Gastrointestinal and intraabdominal infections. In: *Infectious Diseases of the Dog and Cat*, 3e (ed. C.E. Greene), 883–912. St Louis, MO: Saunders Elsevier.

Harris, J.P., Parnell, N.K., Griffith, E.H., and Saker, K.E. (2017). Retrospective evaluation of the impact of early enteral nutrition on clinical outcomes in dogs with pancreatitis: 34 cases (2010–2013). *Journal of Veterinary Emergency and Critical Care* 27: 425–433.

Hart, P.A., Bechtold, M.L., Marshall, J.B. et al. (2008). Prophylactic antibiotics in necrotizing pancreatitis: a meta-analysis. *Southern Medical Journal* 101: 1126–1131.

Hecht, S. and Henry, G. (2007). Sonographic evaluation of the normal and abnormal pancreas. *Clinical Techniques in Small Animal Practice* 22: 115–121.

Herman, B.A., Brawer, R.S., Murtaugh, R.J., and Hackner, S.G. (2005). Therapeutic percutaneous ultrasound-guided cholecystocentesis in three dogs with extrahepatic biliary obstruction and pancreatitis. *Journal of the American Veterinary Medical Association* 227: 1782–1786.

Hess, R.S., Saunders, H.M., Van Winkle, T.J. et al. (1998). Clinical, clinicopathologic, radiographic, and ultrasonographic abnormalities in dogs with fatal acute pancreatitis: 70 cases (1986–1995). *Journal of the American Veterinary Medical Association* 213: 665–670.

Hess, R.S., Kass, P.H., Shofer, F.S. et al. (1999). Evaluation of risk factors for fatal acute pancreatitis in dogs. *Journal of the American Veterinary Medical Association* 214: 46–51.

Hill, R.C. and Van Winkle, T.J. (1993). Acute necrotizing pancreatitis and acute suppurative pancreatitis in the cat. A retrospective study of 40 cases (1976–1989). *Journal of Veterinary Internal Medicine* 7: 25–33.

Hines, B.L., Salisbury, S.K., Jakovljevic, S., and DeNicola, D.B. (1996). Pancreatic pseudocyst associated with chronic active necrotizing pancreatitis in a cat. *Journal of the American Animal Hospital Association* 32: 147–152.

Hope, A., Bailen, E.L., Shiel, R.E., and Mooney, C.T. (2021). Retrospective study evaluation of DGGR lipase for diagnosis, agreement with pancreatic lipase and prognosis in dogs with suspected acute pancreatitis. *Journal of Small Animal Practice* 62: 1092–1100.

Horton, J.W., Dunn, C.W., Burnweit, C.A., and Walker, P.B. (1989). Hypertonic saline-dextran resuscitation of acute canine bile-induced pancreatitis. *American Journal of Surgery* 158: 48–56.

Huth, S.P., Relford, R., Steiner, J.M. et al. (2010). Analytical validation of an ELISA for the measurement of canine pancreas-specific lipase. *Veterinary Clinical Pathology* 39: 346–353.

Jacobs, R.M., Murtaugh, R.J., and DeHoff, W.D. (1985). Review of the clinicopathological findings of acute pancreatitis in the dog: use of an experimental model. *Journal of the American Animal Hospital Association* 21: 795–800.

Jafri, N.S., Mahid, S.S., Idstein, S.R. et al. (2009). Antibiotic prophylaxis is not protective in severe acute pancreatitis: a systematic review and meta-analysis. *American Journal of Surgery* 197: 806–813.

Jerram, R.M., Warman, C.G., Davies, E.S. et al. (2004). Successful treatment of a pancreatic pseudocyst by omentalisation in a dog. *New Zealand Veterinary Journal* 52: 197–201.

Johnson, M.D. and Mann, F.A. (2006). Treatment for pancreatic abscesses via omentalization with abdominal closure versus open peritoneal drainage in dogs: 15 cases (1994–2004). *Journal of the American Veterinary Medical Association* 228: 397–402.

Kimmel, S.E., Washabau, R.J., and Drobatz, K.J. (2001). Incidence and prognostic value of low plasma ionized calcium concentration in cats with acute pancreatitis: 46 cases (1996–1998). *Journal of the American Veterinary Medical Association* 219: 1105–1109.

Klaus, J.A., Rudloff, E., and Kirby, R. (2009). Nasogastric tube feeding in cats with suspected acute pancreatitis: 55 cases (2001–2006). *Journal of Veterinary Emergency and Critical Care* 19: 337–346.

Kook, P.H., Kohler, N., Hartnack, S. et al. (2014). Agreement of serum Spec cPL with the 1,2-o-dilauryl-rac-glycero glutaric acid-(6'-methylresorufin) ester (DGGR) lipase assay and with pancreatic ultrasonography in dogs with suspected pancreatitis. *Journal of Veterinary Internal Medicine* 28: 863–870.

Kruger, B., Albrecht, E., and Lerch, M.M. (2000). The role of intracellular calcium signaling in premature protease activation and the onset of pancreatitis. *American Journal of Pathology* 157: 43–50.

Kumar, A., Singh, N., Prakash, S. et al. (2006). Early enteral nutrition in severe acute pancreatitis: a prospective randomized controlled trial comparing nasojejunal and nasogastric routes. *Journal of Clinical Gastroenterology* 40: 431–434.

Lamb, C.R. (1999). Recent developments in diagnostic imaging of the gastrointestinal tract of the dog and cat. *Veterinary Clinics of North America: Small Animal Practice* 29: 307–342.

Lee, P.J. and Papachristou, G.I. (2019). New insights into acute pancreatitis. *Nature Reviews Gastroenterology & Hepatology* 16: 479–496.

Lee, C., Kathrani, A., and Maddison, J. (2020). Retrospective study of the diagnostic utility of Spec fPL in the assessment of 274 sick cats. *Journal of Veterinary Internal Medicine* 34: 1406–1412.

Leese, T., Holliday, M., Watkins, M. et al. (1991). A multicentre controlled clinical trial of high-volume fresh frozen plasma therapy in prognostically severe acute pancreatitis. *Annals of the Royal College of Surgeons of England* 73: 207–214.

Lem, K.Y., Fosgate, G.T., Norby, B., and Steiner, J.M. (2008). Associations between dietary factors and pancreatitis in dogs. *Journal of the American Veterinary Medical Association* 233: 1425–1431.

Lim, S.Y., Xenoulis, P.G., Stavroulaki, E.M. et al. (2020). The 1,2-o-dilauryl-rac-glycero-3-glutaric acid-(6'-methylresorufin) ester (DGGR) lipase assay in cats and dogs is not specific for pancreatic lipase. *Veterinary Clinical Pathology* 49: 607–613.

Lindsay, S., Entenmann, C., and Chaikoff, I.L. (1948). Pancreatitis accompanying hepatic disease in dogs fed a high fat, low protein diet. *Archives of Pathology* 45: 635–638.

Lippert, A.C., Fulton, R.B., and Parr, A.M. (1993). A retrospective study of the use of total parenteral nutrition in dogs and cats. *Journal of Veterinary Internal Medicine* 7: 52–64.

Logan, J.C., Callan, M.B., Drew, K. et al. (2001). Clinical indications for use of fresh frozen plasma in dogs: 74 dogs (October through December 1999). *Journal of the American Veterinary Medical Association* 218: 1449–1455.

Macy, D.W. (1989). Feline pancreatitis. In: *Current Veterinary Therapy X: Small Animal Practice* (ed. R.W. Kirk and J.D. Bonagure), 893–896. Philadelphia, PA: WB Saunders.

Mansfield, C.S. and Jones, B.R. (2000). Plasma and urinary trypsinogen activation peptide in healthy dogs, dogs with pancreatitis and dogs with other systemic diseases. *Australian Veterinary Journal* 78: 416–422.

Mansfield, C.S., James, F.E., Steiner, J.M. et al. (2011). A pilot study to assess tolerability of early enteral nutrition via esophagostomy tube feeding in dogs with severe acute pancreatitis. *Journal of Veterinary Internal Medicine* 25: 419–425.

Mansfield, C.S., Anderson, G.A., and O'Hara, A.J. (2012). Association between canine pancreatic-specific lipase and histologic exocrine pancreatic inflammation in dogs: assessing specificity. *Journal of Veterinary Diagnostic Investigation* 24: 312–318.

Mayerle, J., Sendler, M., Hegyi, E. et al. (2019). Genetics, cell biology, and pathophysiology of pancreatitis. *Gastroenterology* 156: 1951–1968.

Mayhew, P.D. and Weisse, C.W. (2008). Treatment of pancreatitis-associated extrahepatic biliary tract obstruction by choledochal stenting in seven cats. *Journal of Small Animal Practice* 49: 133–138.

Mayhew, P.D., Holt, D.E., McLear, R.C., and Washabau, R.J. (2002). Pathogenesis and outcome of extrahepatic biliary obstruction in cats. *Journal of Small Animal Practice* 43: 247–253.

Mayhew, P.D., Richardson, R.W., Mehler, S.J. et al. (2006). Choledochal tube stenting for decompression of the extrahepatic portion of the biliary tract in dogs: 13 cases (2002–2005). *Journal of the American Veterinary Medical Association* 228: 1209–1214.

McCord, K., Morley, P.S., Armstrong, J. et al. (2012). A multi-institutional study evaluating the diagnostic utility of the spec cPL and SNAP(R) cPL in clinical acute pancreatitis in 84 dogs. *Journal of Veterinary Internal Medicine* 26: 888–896.

Mohr, A.J., Lobetti, R.G., and Van der Lugt, J.J. (2000). Acute pancreatitis: a newly recognised potential complication of canine babesiosis. *Journal of the South African Veterinary Association* 71: 232–239.

Muir, W.W. (2009). Pain and stress. In: *Handbook of Veterinary Pain Management*, 2e (ed. J.S. Gaynor and W.W. Muir), 42–59. St Louis, MO: Mosby Elsevier.

Murphy, S.M., Rodriguez, J.D., and McAnulty, J.F. (2007). Minimally invasive cholecystostomy in the dog: evaluation of placement techniques and use in extrahepatic biliary obstruction. *Veterinary Surgery* 36: 675–683.

Murtaugh, R.J. and Jacobs, R.M. (1985). Serum antiprotease concentrations in dogs with spontaneous and experimentally induced acute pancreatitis. *American Journal of Veterinary Research* 46: 80–83.

Neilson-Carley, S.C., Robertson, J.E., Newman, S.J. et al. (2011). Specificity of a canine pancreas-specific lipase assay for diagnosing pancreatitis in dogs without clinical or histologic evidence of the disease. *American Journal of Veterinary Research* 72: 302–307.

Nemoto, Y., Haraguchi, T., Shimokawa Miyama, T. et al. (2017). Pancreatic abscess in a cat due to *Staphylococcus aureus* infection. *Journal of Veterinary Medical Science* 79: 1146–1150.

Newman, S., Steiner, J., Woosley, K. et al. (2004). Localization of pancreatic inflammation and necrosis in dogs. *Journal of Veterinary Internal Medicine* 18: 488–493.

Norman, J. (1998). The role of cytokines in the pathogenesis of acute pancreatitis. *American Journal of Surgery* 175: 76–83.

Okanishi, H., Nagata, T., Nakane, S., and Watari, T. (2019). Comparison of initial treatment with and without corticosteroids for suspected acute pancreatitis in dogs. *Journal of Small Animal Practice* 60: 298–304.

Oppliger, S., Hartnack, S., Riond, B. et al. (2013). Agreement of the serum Spec fPL and 1,2-o-dilauryl-rac-glycero-3-glutaric acid-(6′-methylresorufin) ester lipase assay for the determination of serum lipase in cats with suspicion of pancreatitis. *Journal of Veterinary Internal Medicine* 27: 1077–1082.

Oppliger, S., Hartnack, S., Reusch, C.E., and Kook, P.H. (2014). Agreement of serum feline pancreas-specific lipase and colorimetric lipase assays with pancreatic ultrasonographic findings in cats with suspicion of pancreatitis: 161 cases (2008–2012). *Journal of the American Veterinary Medical Association* 244: 1060–1065.

Oppliger, S., Hilbe, M., Hartnack, S. et al. (2016). Comparison of serum Spec fPL and 1,2-o-dilauryl-rac-glycero-3-glutaric acid-(6′-methylresorufin) ester assay in 60 cats using standardized assessment of pancreatic histology. *Journal of Veterinary Internal Medicine* 30: 764–770.

Owens, J.M., Drazner, F.H., and Gilbertson, S.R. (1975). Pancreatic disease in the cat. *Journal of the American Animal Hospital Association* 11: 83–89.

Pandol, S.J., Saluja, A.K., Imrie, C.W., and Banks, P.A. (2007). Acute pancreatitis: bench to the bedside. *Gastroenterology* 132: 1127–1151.

Parent, C., Washabau, R.J., Williams, D.A. et al. (1995). Serum trypsin-like immunoreactivity, amylase and lipase in the diagnosis of feline acute pancreatitis [Abstract]. *Journal of Veterinary Internal Medicine* 9: 194.

Petrov, M.S., Pylypchuk, R.D., and Emelyanov, N.V. (2008a). Systematic review: nutritional support in acute pancreatitis. *Alimentary Pharmacology and Therapeutics* 28: 704–712.

Petrov, M.S., van Santvoort, H.C., Besselink, M.G. et al. (2008b). Enteral nutrition and the risk of mortality and infectious complications in patients with severe acute pancreatitis: a meta-analysis of randomized trials. *Archives of Surgery* 143: 1111–1117.

Platell, C., Cooper, D., and Hall, J.C. (2001). A meta-analysis of peritoneal lavage for acute pancreatitis. *Journal of Gastroenterology and Hepatology* 16: 689–693.

Polzin, D.J., Osborne, C.A., Stevens, J.B., and Hayden, D.W. (1983). Serum amylase and lipase activities in dogs with chronic primary renal failure. *American Journal of Veterinary Research* 44: 404–410.

Puccini Leoni, F., Pelligra, T., Citi, S. et al. (2020). Ultrasonographic monitoring in 38 dogs with clinically suspected acute pancreatitis. *Veterinary Science* 7: 180.

Pyle, S.C., Marks, S.L., and Kass, P.H. (2004). Evaluation of complications and prognostic factors associated with administration of total parenteral nutrition in cats: 75 cases (1994–2001). *Journal of the American Veterinary Medical Association* 225: 242–250.

Rawlings, C.A., Howerth, E.W., Bement, S., and Canalis, C. (2002). Laparoscopic-assisted enterostomy tube placement and full-thickness biopsy of the jejunum with serosal patching in dogs. *American Journal of Veterinary Research* 63: 1313–1319.

Ruaux, C.G. and Atwell, R.B. (1998). A severity score for spontaneous canine acute pancreatitis. *Australian Veterinary Journal* 76: 804–808.

Ruaux, C.G. and Atwell, R.B. (1999). Levels of total α-macroglobulin and trypsin-like immunoreactivity are poor indicators of clinical severity in spontaneous canine acute pancreatitis. *Research in Veterinary Science* 67: 83–87.

Salisbury, S.K., Lantz, G.C., Nelson, R.W., and Kazacos, E.A. (1988). Pancreatic abscess in dogs: six cases (1978–1986). *Journal of the American Veterinary Medical Association* 193: 1104–1108.

Saunders, H.M., Van Winkle, T.J., Drobatz, K. et al. (2002). Ultrasonographic findings in cats with clinical, gross pathologic, and histologic evidence of acute pancreatic necrosis: 20 cases (1994–2001). *Journal of the American Veterinary Medical Association* 221: 1724–1730.

Schaer, M. (1979). A clinicopathologic survey of acute pancreatitis in 30 dogs and 5 cats. *Journal of the American Animal Hospital Association* 15: 681–687.

Schermerhorn, T., Pembleton-Corbett, J.R., and Kornreich, B. (2004). Pulmonary thromboembolism in cats. *Journal of Veterinary Internal Medicine* 18: 533–535.

Schnauss, F., Hanisch, F., and Burgener, I.A. (2019). Diagnosis of feline pancreatitis with SNAP fPL and Spec fPL. *Journal of Feline Medicine and Surgery* 21: 700–707.

Simpson, K.W., Batt, R.M., McLean, L., and Morton, D.B. (1989). Circulating concentrations of trypsin-like immunoreactivity and activities of lipase and amylase after pancreatic duct ligation in dogs. *American Journal of Veterinary Research* 50: 629–632.

Simpson, K.W., Simpson, J.W., Lake, S. et al. (1991). Effect of pancreatectomy on plasma activities of amylase, isoamylase, lipase and trypsin-like immunoreactivity in dogs. *Research in Veterinary Science* 51: 78–82.

Simpson, K.W., Shiroma, J.T., Biller, D.S. et al. (1994). Ante mortem diagnosis of pancreatitis in four cats. *Journal of Small Animal Practice* 35: 93–99.

Simpson, K.W., Fyfe, J., Cornetta, A. et al. (2001). Subnormal concentrations of serum cobalamin (vitamin B12) in cats with gastrointestinal disease. *Journal of Veterinary Internal Medicine* 15: 26–32.

Smith, S.A. and Biller, D.S. (1998). Resolution of a pancreatic pseudocyst in a dog following percutaneous ultrasonographic-guided drainage. *Journal of the American Animal Hospital Association* 34: 515–522.

Steiner, J.M. (2010). Canine pancreatic disease. In: *Textbook of Veterinary Internal Medicine*, 7e (ed. S.J. Ettinger and E.C. Feldman), 1965–1704. St Louis, MO: Saunders Elsevier.

Steiner, J.M. and Williams, D.A. (1999). Feline exocrine pancreatic disorders. *Veterinary Clinics of North America: Small Animal Practice* 29: 551–575.

Steiner, J.M., Broussard, J., Mansfield, C.S. et al. (2001). Serum canine pancreatic lipase immunoreactivity (cPLI) concentrations in dogs with spontaneous pancreatitis [Abstract]. *Journal of Veterinary Internal Medicine* 15: 274.

Steiner, J.M., Teague, S.R., and Williams, D.A. (2003). Development and analytic validation of an enzyme-linked immunosorbent assay for the measurement of canine pancreatic lipase immunoreactivity in serum. *Canadian Journal of Veterinary Research* 67: 175–182.

Steiner, J.M., Wilson, B.G., and Williams, D.A. (2004). Development and analytical validation of a radioimmunoassay for the measurement of feline pancreatic lipase immunoreactivity in serum. *Canadian Journal of Veterinary Research* 68: 309–314.

Steiner, J.M., Newman, S., Xenoulis, P. et al. (2008a). Sensitivity of serum markers for pancreatitis in dogs with macroscopic evidence of pancreatitis. *Veterinary Therapeutics* 9: 263–273.

Steiner, J.M., Xenoulis, P.G., Anderson, J.A. et al. (2008b). Serum pancreatic lipase immunoreactivity concentrations in dogs treated with potassium bromide and/or phenobarbital. *Veterinary Therapeutics* 9: 37–44.

Steiner, J.M., Finco, D.R., and Williams, D.A. (2010). Serum lipase activity and canine pancreatic lipase immunoreactivity (cPLI) concentration in dogs with experimentally induced chronic renal failure. *Veterinary Research* 3: 58–63.

Stimson, E.L., Espada, Y., Moon, M., and Troy, C. (1998). Pancreatic abscess in nine dogs [Abstract]. *Journal of Veterinary Internal Medicine* 9: 202.

Strombeck, D.R., Farver, T., and Kaneko, J.J. (1981). Serum amylase and lipase activities in the diagnosis of pancreatitis in dogs. *American Journal of Veterinary Research* 42: 1966–1970.

Swift, N.C., Marks, S.L., MacLachlan, N.J., and Norris, C.R. (2000). Evaluation of serum feline trypsin-like immunoreactivity for the diagnosis of pancreatitis in cats. *Journal of the American Veterinary Medical Association* 217: 37–42.

Talukdar, R. and Vege, S.S. (2009). Recent developments in acute pancreatitis. *Clinical Gastroenterology and Hepatology* 7: S3–S9.

Thompson, L.J., Seshadri, R., and Raffe, M.R. (2009). Characteristics and outcomes in surgical management of severe acute pancreatitis: 37 dogs (2001–2007). *Journal of Veterinary Emergency and Critical Care* 19: 165–173.

Torner, K., Staudacher, M., Tress, U. et al. (2020). Histopathology and feline pancreatic lipase immunoreactivity in inflammatory, hyperplastic and neoplastic pancreatic diseases in cats. *Journal of Comparative Pathology* 174: 63–72.

Trivedi, S., Marks, S.L., Kass, P.H. et al. (2011). Sensitivity and specificity of canine pancreas-specific lipase (cPL) and other markers for pancreatitis in 70 dogs with and without histopathologic evidence of pancreatitis. *Journal of Veterinary Internal Medicine* 25: 1241–1247.

Trudel, J.L., Wittnich, C., and Brown, R.A. (1994). Antibiotics bioavailability in acute experimental pancreatitis. *Journal of the American College of Surgeons* 178: 475–479.

Twedt, D.C., Cullen, J., McCord, K. et al. (2014). Evaluation of fluorescence in situ hybridization for the detection of bacteria in feline inflammatory liver disease. *Journal of Feline Medicine and Surgery* 16: 109–117.

VanEnkevort, B.A., O'Brien, R.T., and Young, K.M. (1999). Pancreatic pseudocysts in 4 dogs and 2 cats: ultrasonographic and clinicopathologic findings. *Journal of Veterinary Internal Medicine* 13: 309–313.

Ward, J.B., Petersen, O.H., Jenkins, S.A., and Sutton, R. (1995). Is an elevated concentration of acinar cytosolic-free ionized calcium the trigger for acute-pancreatitis? *Lancet* 346: 1016–1019.

Ward, J.B., Sutton, R., Jenkins, S.A., and Petersen, O.H. (1996). Progressive disruption of acinar cell calcium signaling is an early feature of cerulein-induced pancreatitis in mice. *Gastroenterology* 111: 481–491.

Watson, P.J., Archer, J., Roulois, A.J. et al. (2010). Observational study of 14 cases of chronic pancreatitis in dogs. *Veterinary Record* 167: 968–976.

Weatherton, L.K. and Streeter, E.M. (2009). Evaluation of fresh frozen plasma administration in dogs with pancreatitis: 77 cases (1995–2005). *Journal of Veterinary Emergency and Critical Care* 19: 617–622.

Webb, C.B. and Trott, C. (2008). Laparoscopic diagnosis of pancreatic disease in dogs and cats. *Journal of Veterinary Internal Medicine* 22: 1263–1266.

Weiss, D.J., Gagne, J.M., and Armstrong, P.J. (1996). Relationship between inflammatory hepatic disease and inflammatory bowel disease, pancreatitis, and nephritis in cats. *Journal of the American Veterinary Medical Association* 209: 1114–1116.

Whitcomb, D.C. (2010). Genetic aspects of pancreatitis. *Annual Review of Medicine* 61: 413–424.

Williams, D.A. (1996). The pancreas. In: *Strombeck's Small Animal Gastroenterology*, 3e (ed. W.G. Guilford, S.A. Center, D.R. Strombeck, et al.), 381–410. Philadelphia, PA: WB Saunders.

Williams, J.M., Panciera, D.L., Larson, M.M., and Were, S.R. (2013). Ultrasonographic findings of the pancreas in cats with elevated serum pancreatic lipase immunoreactivity. *Journal of Veterinary Internal Medicine* 7: 913–918.

Wolfsheimer, K.J., Hedlund, C.S., and Pechman, R.D. (1991). Pancreatic pseudocyst in a dog with chronic pancreatitis. *Canine Practice* 16: 6–9.

Wright, Z., Steiner, J., Suchodolski, J. et al. (2009). A pilot study evaluating changes in pancreatic lipase immunoreactivity concentrations in canines treated with l-asparaginase (ASNase), vincristine, or both for lymphoma. *Canadian Journal of Veterinary Research* 73: 103–110.

Xenoulis, P.G. (2015). Diagnosis of pancreatitis in dogs and cats. *Journal of Small Animal Practice* 56: 13–26.

Xenoulis, P.G. and Steiner, J.M. (2008). Current concepts in feline pancreatitis. *Topics in Companion Animal Medicine* 23: 185–192.

Xenoulis, P.G., Suchodolski, J.S., Levinski, M.D., and Steiner, J.M. (2007). Investigation of hypertriglyceridemia in healthy miniature schnauzers. *Journal of Veterinary Internal Medicine* 21: 1224–1230.

Xenoulis, P.G., Suchodolski, J.S., and Steiner, J.M. (2008). Chronic pancreatitis in dogs and cats. *Compendium on Continuing Education for the Practicing Veterinarian* 30: 166–180.

Xenoulis, P.G., Suchodolski, J.S., Ruaux, C.G., and Steiner, J.M. (2010). Association between serum triglyceride and canine pancreatic lipase immunoreactivity concentrations in Miniature Schnauzers. *Journal of the American Animal Hospital Association* 46: 229–234.

Xenoulis, P.G., Levinski, M.D., Suchodolski, J.S., and Steiner, J.M. (2011). Serum triglyceride concentrations in Miniature Schnauzers with and without a history of probable pancreatitis. *Journal of Veterinary Internal Medicine* 25: 20–25.

Xenoulis, P.G., Moraiti, K.T., Finco, D.R. et al. (2021). Serum feline pancreatic lipase immunoreactivity and trypsin-like immunoreactivity concentrations in cats with experimentally induced chronic kidney disease. *Journal of Veterinary Internal Medicine* 35: 2821–2827.

Zavros, N.S., Rallis, T.S., Koutinas, A.F., and Vlemmas, I. (2008). Clinical and laboratory investigation of experimental acute pancreatitis in the cat. *European Journal of Inflammation* 6: 105–114.

Zoran, D.L. (2006). Pancreatitis in cats: diagnosis and management of a challenging disease. *Journal of the American Animal Hospital Association* 42: 1–9.

Section 3

Peritoneal Cavity

20

Peritonitis

Lori Ludwig

Etiology

Peritonitis is inflammation of the peritoneum and can result from a variety of causes, which may be classified as septic or aseptic. Aseptic peritonitis can be caused by endogenous chemical contamination of the peritoneum with sterile bile, urine, lymph, or pancreatic enzymes. Exogenous chemical contamination with talc or irritating lavage solutions and mechanical irritation from manipulation of organs during surgery or trauma can also result in aseptic peritonitis (Kirby 2003). More commonly peritonitis is associated with infection and is classified as primary, secondary, or tertiary septic peritonitis.

Primary peritonitis

Primary peritonitis, also commonly referred to as spontaneous bacterial peritonitis, is infection of the peritoneal cavity that is not related to an identifiable intraperitoneal source of contamination or history of penetrating trauma. The route of infection is believed to be hematogenous or via bacterial translocation (Culp et al. 2009). Feline infectious peritonitis (FIP), associated with coronavirus infection, is the most common form of primary peritonitis identified in small animals (Kirby 2003). A few case reports have identified other organisms such as Clostridium, Chlamydia, Salmonella, and Neospora (Holmberg et al. 2006; Culp et al. 2009). In a retrospective study on primary peritonitis not associated with FIP, infection was most commonly caused by a single organism and, overall, Gram-positive organisms predominated (Culp et al. 2009). This is in contrast to patients with secondary peritonitis, where Gram-negative

bacteria predominate and polymicrobial infection is frequently found (Mueller et al. 2001; Bonczynski et al. 2003). The most common organisms identified in cats with primary peritonitis were Escherichia coli, Streptococcus, and Clostridium, while Enterococcus, Clostridium, and E. coli were found more frequently in dogs. Patients with primary peritonitis are often taken to surgery because they present with abnormalities on history and physical examination similar to those with secondary peritonitis. Unfortunately, this has resulted in a worse prognosis in dogs (Culp et al. 2009). The recommended treatment for any species with primary peritonitis is supportive care and antimicrobials.

Secondary peritonitis

Secondary peritonitis is associated with intra-abdominal leakage of bacteria into the peritoneum or disruption of the body wall, resulting in the introduction of external bacteria. Rupture, perforation, or leakage of bacteria from the gastrointestinal tract is the most common cause of secondary peritonitis in dogs and cats (King 1994; Mueller et al. 2001; Bentley et al. 2007). Intra-abdominal infection can also occur from leakage of bacteria from an infection or abscess of the liver, gallbladder, pancreas, spleen, lymph node, or genitourinary tract. Rarely, secondary peritonitis results from infection with fungal organisms (Gilroy et al. 2020).

Tertiary peritonitis

Tertiary peritonitis has been reported in humans and is defined as severe persistent or recurrent infection after adequate source control of secondary peritonitis (Laroche & Harding 1998).

Sclerosing encapsulating peritonitis

Sclerosing encapsulating peritonitis (SEP) is a rarely reported condition in which the abdominal organs are encased in a thick fibrous membrane resembling a cocoon (Figure 20.1) (Hardie *et al.* 1994; Adamama-Moraitou *et al.* 2004; Yang *et al.* 2009). The etiology is unknown, but in humans it has been associated with congenital abnormalities, long-term propranolol usage, peritoneal dialysis, previous abdominal surgery, neoplasia, and intra-abdominal infection (Eltoum *et al.* 2006; Yang *et al.* 2009). In dogs and cats, steatitis, fiberglass ingestion, bacterial peritonitis, and leishmaniasis have been associated with SEP (Hardie *et al.* 1994; Adamama-Moraitou *et al.* 2004). Veterinary patients with SEP most often present with anorexia, vomiting, diarrhea, and ascites. SEP has also been recently reported to cause pyloric outflow obstruction (Carroll *et al.* 2020). Diagnosis can be challenging and patients may be explored based on the presence of gathered intestinal loops found with radiography or ultrasonography and the presence of a septic abdominal effusion or a copious sterile effusion that has an unexplained cause. Computed tomography (CT) has been used to aid diagnosis in human patients, but it is not often definitive and patients are usually explored based on the lack of response to conservative treatment (Yang *et al.* 2009).

Recommended treatment in humans with SEP is surgical débridement of the fibrocollagenous membrane and intestinal adhesions and resection of necrotic small bowel (Xu *et al.* 2007; Yang *et al.* 2009). In addition, corticosteroids and tamoxifen have been commonly recommended (Jagirdar *et al.* 2019). The mechanism of action of tamoxifen is believed to be related to its antifibrotic action through an effect on transforming growth factor (TGF)-β. Successful treatment of SEP in veterinary patients has been rarely reported. Surgery may involve transection of adhesions and small intestinal resection and anastomosis, but hemorrhage and severe intestinal perforation have been reported with these techniques (Hardie *et al.* 1994; Adamama-Moraitou *et al.* 2004). Additional treatment with corticosteroids may reduce inflammation and slow effusion. Successful treatment of a German shepherd dog with SEP has been reported with a combination of enterolysis, open abdominal lavage, and tamoxifen after failure of treatment with surgery and methylprednisolone alone (Etchepareborde *et al.* 2010).

Pathophysiology

The peritoneum is a serous membrane consisting of flattened mesothelial cells and loose connective tissue with vascular and lymphatic capillaries, nerves, lymphocytes, and macrophages. The peritoneal lining covers the abdominal wall and diaphragm (parietal layer) and the abdominal organs (visceral layer). A small amount of fluid (<1 mL/kg) is normally present in the peritoneal cavity (Swann & Hughes 2000).

Peritoneal injury results in vasodilation, increased vascular permeability, and formation of a protein-rich exudate. Lymphatics of the parietal peritoneum, diaphragm, and omentum work to clear the noxious stimulus and associated peritoneal fluid. Fibrin formation acts to wall off infectious substances, but can result in inhibition of lymphatic drainage.

Hypovolemia results from massive fluid loss into the peritoneal cavity and may be exacerbated by vomiting, diarrhea, and anorexia. The result of hypovolemia is decreased cardiac output and poor tissue perfusion, which can compromise the intestinal mucosa and result in bacterial translocation.

Mesothelial cells secrete proinflammatory and other mediators as a defense response (Broche & Tellado 2001). White blood cells migrate from the peritoneal capillaries to the mesothelial surface in order to opsonize or lyse bacteria that contaminate the peritoneal cavity. Lysis of

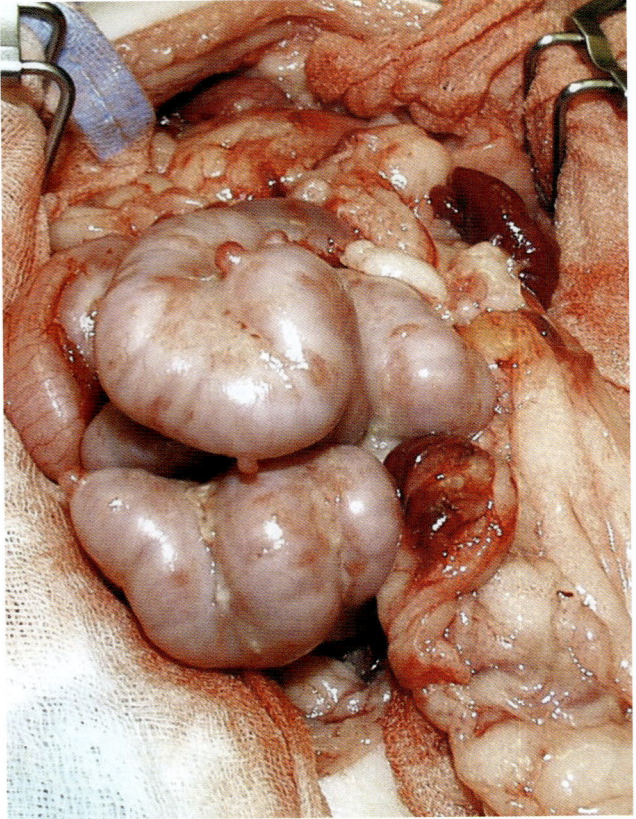

Figure 20.1 Intraoperative photograph of a dog with sclerosing peritonitis. Notice the white fibrous coating on several intestinal loops that are adhered to each other.

bacteria results in the release of cellular proteases and endotoxins, and in activation of the arachidonic acid pathway, complement system, and coagulation cascade (Dulisch 1993).

The amount of bacterial contamination, the virulence of the organism, the presence of adjuvants, and the adequacy of local and systemic host defenses determine the response of the body to infection. An adjuvant such as bile, blood, or foreign material will result in destruction of mesothelial cells and impair local host defenses. The response of the body to the resulting cascade of inflammatory mediators is called the systemic inflammatory response syndrome (SIRS), and when infection is involved it is defined as sepsis. Ultimately, circulatory collapse, hypoxemia, and inflammation lead to tissue ischemia, reduced mitochondrial and cell function, and multiple organ dysfunction.

Diagnosis

History, clinical signs, and physical examination

The clinical signs in patients with peritonitis are often nonspecific and range from mild signs of lethargy and anorexia to signs consistent with septic shock. The clinician should question the owner about potential risk factors, including a recent history of trauma or surgery, access to foreign bodies, previous medical conditions, and whether or not the patient is intact. Information should be obtained on the administration and dosing of medications, especially the use of nonsteroidal and steroidal anti-inflammatory medications, which may result in gastroduodenal perforation. Unfortunately, the presence of mild chronic signs does not exclude the possibility of peritonitis. Patients with gastroduodenal perforation rarely present with signs of shock and acute collapse, and according to one retrospective study the diagnosis of this condition may take days to weeks from the onset of clinical signs (Hinton *et al.* 2002). This is also true for patients with bile peritonitis, especially if the biliary effusion is sterile (Ludwig *et al.* 1997). Blunt abdominal trauma may result in bile peritonitis, septic peritonitis, and uroabdomen. It can take up to 5–7 days to detect septic peritonitis in patients with mesenteric avulsion resulting from blunt abdominal trauma (Rollings *et al.* 2001). Patients with uroabdomen may not show evidence of severe illness for 2–3 days after the traumatic incident and are not always anuric (Aumann *et al.* 1998). Urine is not an aggressive chemical and should be sterile, so the peritonitis that is triggered is very mild during the first 2–3 days.

Physical examination may reveal a normal body temperature, fever, or hypothermia. Signs of shock in these patients may include tachycardia, tachypnea, and pale or injected mucous membranes, with a rapid or prolonged capillary refill time and weak or bounding pulses. Unlike dogs, cats with septic shock may be bradycardic (Costello *et al.* 2004; Parsons *et al.* 2009). The abdomen may be distended and should be palpated to assess for pain, masses, a fluid wave, and tympany from a gas-filled gastrointestinal tract or severe pneumoperitoneum. Cats with septic peritonitis are less likely than dogs to show signs of abdominal pain during palpation (Costello *et al.* 2004). An oral examination may reveal pale, injected, or icteric mucous membranes. The mucous membranes should also be evaluated for petechiae and the base of the tongue should be examined for the presence of a string foreign body. Rectal palpation may reveal ingested foreign material, melena, hematochezia, prostatomegaly, and masses or uroliths in the pelvic urethra. Intact females may have a vaginal discharge.

Abdominocentesis

Cytologic and biochemical evaluation of a peritoneal effusion can provide a definitive diagnosis of peritonitis. In patients with a large effusion, the fluid can be retrieved by aseptically introducing a single needle blindly into the abdomen near the umbilicus. The likelihood of retrieving fluid may be increased by using multiple needles, which can be placed using a four-quadrant approach or under ultrasound guidance. It has been reported that at least 5 mL/kg of abdominal fluid must be present to obtain a fluid sample with abdominocentesis (Swann & Hughes 2000). Therefore, fluid may not be retrieved if abdominocentesis is performed soon after the onset of peritonitis, in a dehydrated patient, or in a patient with localized peritonitis. Abdominocentesis can be repeated after the patient is rehydrated or diagnostic peritoneal lavage can be performed if the clinical suspicion of peritonitis is high and no fluid is retrieved. Radiography and abdominal ultrasonography should be performed to document the presence of abdominal fluid prior to diagnostic peritoneal lavage. Because the abdominal fluid retrieved with diagnostic peritoneal lavage has been diluted, chemical analysis of the fluid is not accurate.

Cytology should be performed immediately on any fluid retrieved. The presence of intracellular bacteria and degenerate neutrophils is an indication for emergency surgical exploration (Figure 20.2a). The presence of extracellular bacteria without white blood cells is more likely a result of penetration of the gastrointestinal tract with the needle rather than gastrointestinal tract rupture (Figure 20.2b). In this instance, abdominocentesis should be carefully repeated or performed under ultrasound guidance. If intracellular bacteria are not seen, fluid can be submitted in an ethylenediaminetetraacetic acid (EDTA; purple top) tube for analysis and

(a)　(b)

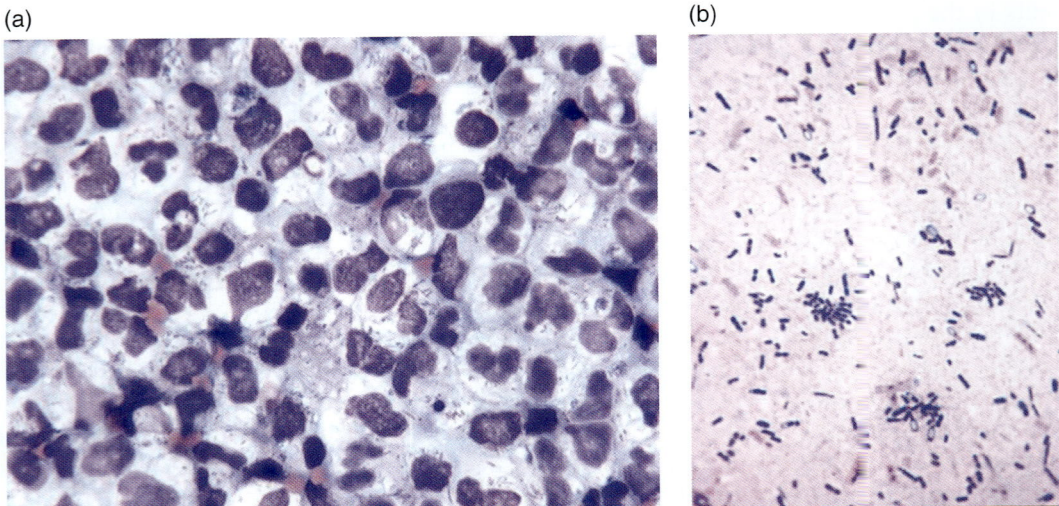

Figure 20.2 (a) Cytology of an abdominal effusion from a dog with septic peritonitis. Intracellula bacteria can be seen in several neutrophils. (b) Cytology demonstrating a large number of bacteria without white blood cells. This slide demonstrates inadvertent penetration of a distended bowel loop during abdominocentesis.

cell counts. Patients with fewer than 13 000 white blood cells in their effusion are more likely to have a nonseptic peritonitis (Bonczynski *et al.* 2003). However, if the total white blood cell count of the effusion is less than 13 000 but the majority of neutrophils in the effusion are degenerate, septic peritonitis is likely present (Botte & Rosin 1983). Cytology may also reveal the presence of bilirubin crystals (yellow or green pigment) that are free floating and within macrophages, indicating bile peritonitis.

Chemical evaluation of the fluid compared with similar tests on the blood is useful for the diagnosis of peritonitis. In patients with suspected septic effusions, the fluid should be collected by abdominocentesis. Unfortunately, fluid collected from closed-suction abdominal drains may not be accurate for the diagnosis of septic peritonitis following intestinal surgery (Guieu *et al.* 2016). In patients with septic effusions, the glucose concentration in the blood should be higher than that in the fluid due to utilization of glucose by bacteria and phagocytic cells in the effusion. In one study, patients with nonseptic effusions had a blood glucose concentration that was similar to or lower than the fluid glucose concentration, whereas in dogs with septic peritonitis, the blood glucose concentration was always at least 20 mg/dL greater than the fluid glucose concentration (Bonczynski *et al.* 2003). The test was slightly less accurate in cats. The presence of a large amount of blood in the effusion or recent intravenous glucose administration will make this test inaccurate. A false-negative result may also be found when performing this test in patients if the onset of bacterial

contamination of the peritoneum is acute, or if the infection is localized. Patients with acute gastric perforation may have a false-negative result because of the low number of bacteria present in what is often a large volume of effusion. This test has also been shown to be insensitive when whole blood glucose concentration is compared to peritoneal fluid glucose concentration using a veterinary point-of-care glucometer instead of a blood chemistry analyzer (Koenig & Verlander 2015). In that study, comparing plasma glucose concentration to peritoneal fluid or peritoneal fluid supernatant glucose concentration and using a higher cutoff value (≥38 mg/dL) provided an accurate diagnosis.

An additional test that has been reported to aid in the diagnosis of septic peritonitis is comparison of the lactate concentrations in the blood and fluid; however, in one study this test was not as accurate as comparing the fluid to blood glucose concentrations (Levin *et al.* 2004). The lactate concentration of a septic abdominal effusion may be increased because of the anaerobic microenvironment in the abdomen, the presence of bacterial metabolites, and the production of lactate by neutrophils. In one study, all dogs with septic peritonitis had a fluid lactate concentration greater than 2.5 mmol/L and the lactate concentration was higher in the effusion than in the blood (Levin *et al.* 2004). However, dogs with nonseptic effusions also frequently had increased fluid lactate concentrations compared with blood lactate concentrations. When the blood lactate concentration was subtracted from the fluid lactate concentration, a difference of less than −1.5 mmol/L was 90% accurate for diagnosing a septic effusion in dogs (88% sensitivity and 91%

specificity). This test was only 78% accurate for detecting septic peritonitis in cats. A lactate difference of less than −0.5 mmol/L had 78% sensitivity and 78% specificity. Recently, a study evaluated the ability of several biomarkers (glucose, lactate, cytokines, procalcitonin, etc.) to discriminate septic peritonitis from nonseptic ascites (Martiny & Goggs 2019). Effusion lactate concentration was the marker that best differentiated between the two conditions, but no single biomarker provided 100% sensitivity and specificity. For this reason, a combination of the historical evidence, the clinical findings, the cytologic evaluation, and the biochemical evaluation of the blood and effusion should be used together to make a diagnosis of a septic effusion.

Additional biochemical testing should be performed if bile peritonitis or uroabdomen is suspected. A diagnosis of bile peritonitis can be made if the bilirubin concentration in the effusion is greater than the bilirubin concentration in the serum (Ludwig *et al.* 1997). The abdominal effusion in patients with a ruptured gallbladder mucocele may not have a bilirubin concentration that is greater than that in the serum because the inspissated bile stays localized. In addition, some dogs with gallbladder rupture will not be icteric (Guess *et al.* 2015). In these patients, the presence of a gallbladder mucocele and an abdominal effusion on ultrasonography may aid in the diagnosis of gallbladder rupture. A comparison of serum to peritoneal fluid bile acid concentrations may provide additional support for the diagnosis of gallbladder rupture in anicteric patients. A diagnosis of uroabdomen can be made when the potassium concentration of the abdominal effusion is greater than the concentration in the blood (>1.4:1 in dogs or >1.9:1 in cats). A creatinine concentration of the effusion that is higher than in the blood (>2:1) is also diagnostic of uroabdomen (Stafford & Bartges 2013).

Diagnostic imaging

Abdominal radiography most commonly reveals decreased abdominal detail indicating the presence of an abdominal effusion (Figure 20.3). In patients with pancreatitis, this decreased detail may be seen as a ground-glass appearance localized to the right cranial abdomen. Widening of the angle between the pyloric antrum and duodenum may also be seen with pancreatitis.

Pneumoperitoneum may be present as a result of penetrating trauma or rupture of an abdominal viscus and can often be visualized caudal to the diaphragm outlining the crura (Figure 20.4). Presence of free air in the abdomen without penetrating trauma usually results from the rupture of the stomach, duodenum, or colon. Free air in the abdomen may also be seen normally for weeks after abdominal surgery, complicating the

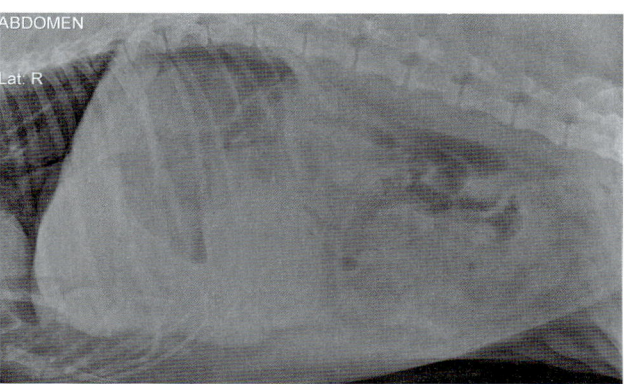

Figure 20.3 Lateral abdominal radiograph of a dog with a ruptured gastroduodenal ulcer. Notice the poor abdominal detail and ground-glass appearance.

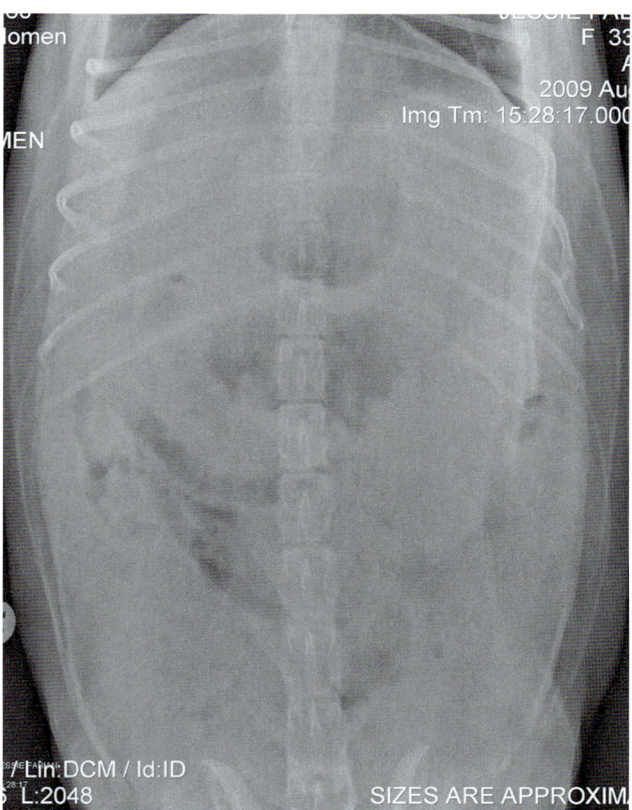

Figure 20.4 Ventrodorsal radiograph of a dog with septic peritonitis and pneumoperitoneum. Free air can be seen along the caudal surface of the diaphragm.

diagnosis of a leaking intestinal anastomosis. Air seen within the parenchyma of an organ is an indication of necrosis or infection with gas-producing bacteria.

Organomegaly may indicate the presence of an abdominal mass or abscess and an extremely dilated bowel may be seen with an obstructing foreign body or

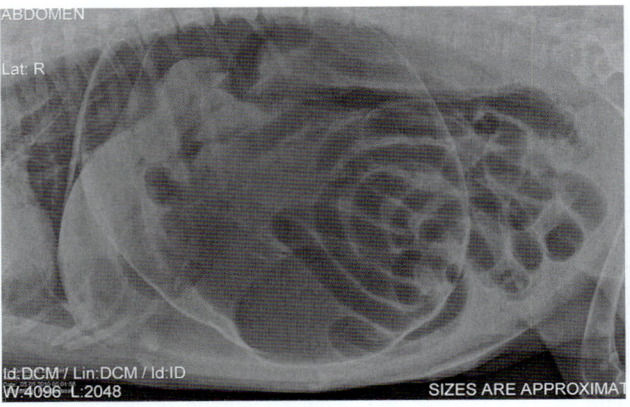

Figure 20.5 Lateral abdominal radiograph of a dog with gastric dilatation volvulus and gastric necrosis. Pneumoperitoneum indicates gastric rupture.

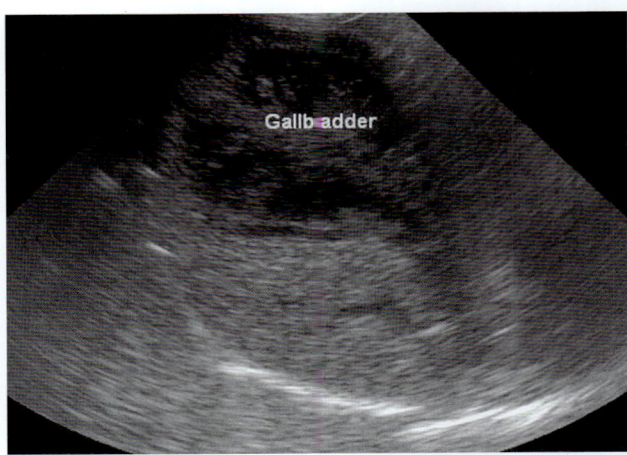

Figure 20.6 Abdominal ultrasound image of a ruptured gallbladder mucocele. There is loss of gallbladder wall continuity and a small amount of free fluid outside the gallbladder wall.

volvulus (Figure 20.5). Organ malpositioning can also be seen with volvulus, torsion, or neoplasia of abdominal organs.

Thoracic radiography should be performed in patients with a history of trauma or if neoplasia is suspected. Positive contrast radiography is most helpful in determining the site of leakage with rupture of the urinary tract. Cystography and retrograde urethrography are used to evaluate the integrity of the bladder and urethra. False-negative results may be obtained if an inadequate amount of contrast agent is administered. Excretory urography is useful for demonstrating rupture of the kidney or ureter. Gastrointestinal evaluation can be performed with a water-soluble contrast agent if intestinal perforation is suspected. Barium should be avoided in these patients because it acts as an adjuvant for peritonitis and increases the risk of mortality (Kirby 2003). This test may not be accurate for the diagnosis of peritonitis if the perforation has been walled off by the omentum.

Abdominal ultrasonography is valuable for detecting an abdominal effusion. The FAST (focused assessment with sonography for trauma) technique involves obtaining specific views that aid in rapid detection of abdominal fluid (Boysen et al. 2004). Transverse and longitudinal images of the subxiphoid region, the midline position over the bladder, and the right and left flank are obtained and guided fluid aspiration can be achieved with this technique (see Chapter 33). Abdominal ultrasound is also useful for the diagnosis of intra-abdominal pathology such as organ abscessation or neoplasia. Decreased pancreatic echogenicity with hyperechogenicity in the peripancreatic region is indicative of pancreatitis (Steiner 2010). Gallbladder rupture can be reliably identified with ultrasound when there is loss of gallbladder wall continuity, free fluid around the gallbladder,

hyperechoic fat attached or adjacent to the gallbladder wall, or, if striated, echogenic material is found outside the gallbladder lumen indicating a ruptured gallbladder mucocele (Figure 20.6) (Aguirre 2010).

CT has been found to be more sensitive and specific than ultrasonography in evaluating the entire abdomen in humans with peritonitis, and it has been demonstrated recently to be useful for the diagnosis of gastrointestinal ulceration with perforation in dogs (Evans et al. 2001; Fitzgerald et al. 2017). Unfortunately, the need for general anesthesia and cost have prohibited the use of this imaging modality in most veterinary patients. As in human patients, the future of the diagnosis and treatment of peritonitis may also include laparoscopy. Laparoscopy has been found to be more accurate than diagnostic peritoneal lavage in humans for the diagnosis of intra-abdominal infection and has also been used for the diagnosis and treatment of gastric perforation (Evans et al. 2001).

Laboratory testing

Results of laboratory testing on blood obtained from patients with peritonitis may aid in diagnosis, guide treatment, and provide information about prognosis. Neutrophilia with a left shift is seen frequently in patients with peritonitis, but neutropenia can also be found. The white blood cell count and band neutrophil count may increase normally in dogs after intestinal surgery; however, an increasing band neutrophil count 4–6 days after surgery may be predictive of small intestinal dehiscence (Allen et al. 1992). An increased hematocrit may be seen in patients with peritonitis at initial presentation due to dehydration or splenic contraction. Anemia is frequently found and may be related to blood loss, hemolysis, the inhibition of erythroid precursor cells by inflammatory mediators, and decreased red blood cell lifespan with inflammation and oxidative damage (Costello *et al.* 2004). Thrombocytopenia and evidence of coagulopathy including increased prothrombin time, partial thromboplastin time, fibrin degradation product, and D-dimer concentrations with decreased protein C and antithrombin concentrations have also been reported in dogs and cats with peritonitis and sepsis (DeLaforcade *et al.* 2003; Klainbart *et al.* 2017).

Serum chemical analysis is often indicative of the source of peritonitis. Increased liver enzyme and total bilirubin concentrations are usually seen in patients with bile peritonitis. In addition, patients with a gallbladder mucocele should be suspected of having gallbladder rupture if there is a marked increase in total bilirubin, alanine aminotransferase, and alkaline phosphatase concentrations and a leukocytosis is found (Pike *et al.* 2004). As a result of decreased hepatosplanchnic perfusion, patients with septic peritonitis may also have increased liver enzyme concentrations. Increased creatinine, blood urea nitrogen, and potassium concentrations are usually seen in patients with uroabdomen, but can also be seen in patients with urinary obstruction and acute renal failure. Although an increase in serum amylase and lipase activities has been used to aid in the diagnosis of pancreatitis in dogs, this test has low sensitivity and specificity in this species and has no clinical usefulness in cats (Steiner 2010). Canine pancreatic lipase immunoreactivity concentration (cPLI) and feline pancreatic lipase immunoreactivity (fPLI) are the most sensitive and specific laboratory tests for diagnosing pancreatitis (see Chapter 19) (Schnaub *et al.* 2019). Serum glucose concentrations vary from hyperglycemic to hypoglycemic in dogs and cats with peritonitis, but the presence of hypoglycemia should make the clinician suspicious of a septic process. Most animals with peritonitis will be hypoalbuminemic due to loss of albumin into the effusion, poor nutritional status, and the underlying disease process.

Treatment

The treatment of choice for secondary peritonitis is surgery. The goals of surgery are to find and correct the source of contamination, remove as much necrotic or infected material as possible, prevent recurrent infection, and provide a means for postoperative nutrition if it is believed that the patient will not eat or will continue to vomit after surgery. However, before surgery is started preoperative stabilization has to be performed as soon as possible.

Preoperative management

Most patients with peritonitis will be hypovolemic on presentation and this should be corrected prior to surgery. Sepsis and septic shock, which are often seen in patients with peritonitis, have recently been redefined by the human sepsis-3 guidelines (Singer *et al.* 2016). Sepsis is defined as life-threatening organ dysfunction caused by a dysregulated host response to infection. Patients are considered to have septic shock when vasopressors are needed to maintain a mean arterial pressure of ≥65 mmHg and when they have a serum lactate level >2 mmol/L in the absence of hypovolemia. A diagnosis of SIRS is based on the presence of at least two of four criteria: hyperthermia or hypothermia, tachycardia or bradycardia (cats), tachypnea, and leukocytosis or leukopenia (Hauptman *et al.* 1997). Guidelines have been proposed in humans for the management of sepsis and septic shock, and these recommendations include goal-directed resuscitation that occurs as soon as possible after presentation (Rivers *et al.* 2001). These goals can also be applied to the treatment of veterinary patients (Table 20.1).

Rapid volume resuscitation with isotonic crystalloids should be given as an intravenous bolus in increments of 10–20 mL/kg over 10–15 minutes (up to 90 mL/kg/h in dogs and 40–60 mL/kg/h in cats) until perfusion parameters have normalized. Balanced crystalloids should be chosen over 0.9% saline to avoid hyperchloremia and the risk of worsening kidney function (Londono 2019). In addition, fluid overload should be avoided, as it has been associated with an increased mortality rate in

Table 20.1 Physical examination and laboratory parameters to be used as goals of resuscitation.

Parameter	Target value
Mucous membrane	Color pink
Capillary refill time	1–2 s
Heart rate	Dog: 80–120 bpm
	Cat: 160–200 bpm
Blood pressure	Mean: >65 mmHg
	Systolic: ≥90 mmHg
Central venous pressure	5–8 cmH$_2$O
Urinary output	>1–2 mL/kg/h
Colloid osmotic pressure	15–20 mmHg
Oxygen saturation	>95%
Packed cell volume	>25%
Albumin	>2.0 g/dL
Lactate	<2 mmol/L
Body temperature	37.8–39.2 °C (100–102.5 °F)

humans and dogs (Caavanagh *et al.* 2016). If the patient is hypoproteinemic and/or has low colloid osmotic pressure, a synthetic colloid, such as hydroxyethyl starch, can be considered. The use of synthetic colloids in people with sepsis has been associated with higher mortality rates, acute kidney injury, and coagulopathies, and is no longer recommended. The use of colloids in veterinary patients with critical illness has become controversial. If a synthetic colloid is used, it can be given in boluses of 5 mL/kg, up to a maximum of 20 mL/kg in the dog and 15 mL/kg in the cat. Colloid boluses can be given rapidly to dogs, but should be given over 15–20 minutes in cats because of the potential for hypotension to worsen in some cats with rapid infusion (Devey 2010). Hypertonic saline (7.5% sodium chloride) is another fluid alternative that leads to rapid volume expansion at doses of 4 mL/kg and has been shown experimentally to decrease mortality and improve healing of colonic anastomoses in rats with peritonitis (Shih *et al.* 2008). The effects of hypertonic saline are short-lived but may be prolonged by concurrent colloid administration.

If volume resuscitation does not normalize perfusion parameters, vasopressor therapy is instituted. Norepinephrine (0.05–2 µg/kg/min) is an α-adrenoceptor agonist that can be used to improve blood pressure through vasoconstriction. Vasopressin can be used with norepinephrine to lower the dose of norepinephrine required. Vasopressin stimulates vasoconstriction through V_1 receptors in vascular smooth muscle and can be given at a dose of 0.5–5 mU/kg/min administered as a constant-rate infusion (Scroggin & Quandt 2009). The positive inotrope dobutamine increases cardiac output and myocardial contractility through β_1-adrenoceptors and can be given at doses ranging from 2.5 to 10 µg/kg/min. Dopamine use has fallen out of favor in humans with septic shock, but is still often used in small animal patients (Silverstein & Santoro Beer 2015). A dose of 5–20 µg/kg/min will increase blood pressure through effects on β_1-adrenoceptors (improved myocardial contractility) and α_1-adrenoceptors (vasoconstriction). The lowest effective dose should be used, because the vasopressor effect predominates at higher doses and can result in vasoconstriction of splanchnic blood vessels.

Blood transfusions should be given to maintain a packed cell volume above 25% and plasma should be given to patients with a coagulopathy or pancreatitis. Plasma may be beneficial to patients with pancreatitis because it provides a source of α-macroglobulin, which binds activated proteases. Serum glucose and electrolyte concentrations should be monitored and deficits corrected during fluid replacement.

Broad-spectrum antibiotic therapy should be instituted in any patient suspected of having septic peritonitis. The choice of antibiotic should be based on the suspected cause of peritonitis and the most likely types of organisms involved. Abdominal fluid obtained from abdominocentesis can be submitted for culture prior to administering antibiotics, but the use of antibiotics should not be delayed until cultures are taken at surgery. In human patients with peritonitis, the most profound decrease in mortality is associated with immediate and adequate antibiotic treatment (Boermeester 2007). Each hour delay in treating human patients with septic shock with effective antibiotics is associated with an increase in mortality (Dellinger *et al.* 2008). A meta-analysis in humans with secondary peritonitis found no conclusive evidence to suggest that one antibiotic regimen is preferable to another (Wong *et al.* 2005). However, the combination of fluoroquinolones/anti-anaerobes and cephalosporins/β-lactamase inhibitors appeared to be more effective clinically than other regimens. In veterinary patients, combination therapy that provides both aerobic and anaerobic coverage should be considered. Ampicillin, ampicillin/sulbactam, or metronidazole will provide anaerobic coverage and can be used in combination with a fluoroquinolone or aminoglycoside. Patients receiving an aminoglycoside should be monitored for nephrotoxicity. Alternatively, a third-generation cephalosporin such as cefotaxime or ceftazidime or a carbapenem, such as meropenem, may be effective alone. Treatment may be modified once culture and sensitivity results are available.

In patients with uroabdomen, hyperkalemia and acidosis should be corrected prior to anesthesia to limit the risk of fatal arrhythmias. If serum potassium levels are <7.5 mEq/L, urinary diversion and fluid therapy alone may correct hyperkalemia. A urethral catheter is adequate for diversion in some patients with urethral or bladder rupture. If a urethral catheter cannot be passed, the abdomen can be drained temporarily with a peritoneal dialysis catheter or other multifenestrated catheter placed percutaneously into the abdomen and attached to a fluid collection system. When potassium levels exceed 7.5 mEq/L, additional treatments should be instituted (Stafford & Bartges 2013). Intravenous administration of regular insulin (0.1–0.25 units/kg i.v.) with a dextrose bolus (1–2 g/unit of insulin i.v.) followed by a continuous-rate infusion of dextrose will decrease serum potassium concentration. Following insulin administration, blood glucose should be monitored for 24 hours. After injection of insulin, potassium is exchanged with protons, resulting in acidosis. Administration of sodium bicarbonate (1–2 mEq/kg i.v. over 15 min) may be considered if severe acidosis is present. To counteract the effects of potassium on the heart, 10% calcium gluconate

(0.5–1.5 mL/kg i.v. over 5–10 min) can be administered. An electrocardiogram should be monitored during the administration of calcium gluconate and if a prolonged PR interval, widened QRS complex, shortened QT interval, shortened or absent ST segment, and/or widened T wave are noted, the rate of infusion should be slowed.

Anesthesia

Anesthetic time should be kept to a minimum in critical patients with peritonitis. Multiple peripheral intravenous catheters or a central multilumen catheter should be placed and emergency drug dosages calculated prior to induction of anesthesia. Opioids and benzodiazepines are used for premedication because they have minimal cardiorespiratory effects and can be reversed if needed. Propofol is less than ideal for induction of anesthesia due to its vasodilatory effects, but it is often used. Alfalaxone, a neurosteroid induction agent, may have fewer cardiovascular depressant effects (Bazzle & Brainard 2019). Fentanyl can also be considered for induction. Isoflurane and sevoflurane are good choices for maintenance anesthesia, but cause dose-dependent hypotension. A balanced anesthetic protocol to reduce minimum alveolar concentration (MAC) by the use of lidocaine, ketamine, and/or narcotic constant-rate infusions (CRI) may be desirable to address inhalation agent–induced hypotension. A lidocaine CRI may also be beneficial due to its analgesic and inflammatory modulator properties in septic patients. A recent study in dogs showed a significant increase in short-term survival when patients with septic peritonitis were administered a 2 mg/kg intravenous bolus of lidocaine followed by a CRI of 50 μg/kg/min during surgery (Bellini & Seymour 2016).

Surgery

After a midline approach to the abdominal cavity, a complete abdominal exploration is required to evaluate every organ. If the infection is localized, the surgeon should make every effort to keep the infection from spreading throughout the abdomen by packing the area with sterile laparotomy sponges and limiting lavage to the affected site. Abscessed organs are removed if possible or débrided, lavaged, and omentalized in cases of pancreatic and prostatic abscesses. Omentalization of pancreatic abscesses with abdominal closure has been associated with improved survival compared with pancreatic abscesses treated by open abdominal drainage (Johnson & Mann 2006). Compromised bowel is repaired or removed and anastomotic sites may be additionally treated with a serosal patch or wrapped in omentum. Recent reports have found that a stapled anastomosis may be preferred to a hand-sewn anastomosis if there is preoperative septic peritonitis (Davis et al. 2018; DePompeo et al. 2018). If a functional end-to-end stapled anastomosis is performed, the transverse staple line should be oversewn to reduce the chances of postoperative dehiscence (Sumner et al. 2019). Cholecystectomy, ligation of a torn hepatic duct, repair of a common bile duct rupture, or biliary diversion are all procedures that may be required in patients with bile peritonitis. A ruptured kidney should be removed, while a ruptured ureter can be removed, primarily repaired, or transposed. Primary repair of bladder or urethral ruptures can be supported with urine diversion through a tube cystostomy or urethral catheter.

Lavage

Lavage of the abdomen with sterile saline has been recommended for removal of bacteria and material such as blood that may promote bacterial proliferation. Much debate still exists about the effectiveness of lavage and the ideal lavage solution. Bacteria adhere to mesothelial cells in the peritoneal cavity and are resistant to removal by lavage (Platell et al. 2000). In addition, if lavage fluid is not cleared from the abdomen, the ability of the peritoneal defense mechanisms to localize infection and absorb bacteria is impaired. Potentially beneficial inflammatory mediators such as opsonic proteins, complement, proteases, and immunoglobulins may also be removed with the lavage fluid. A meta-analysis of the effect of lavage on survival in experimental peritonitis in animals concluded that lavage was beneficial in decreasing mortality (Qadan et al. 2010). In this study, animals that had lavage performed with antiseptics such as povidone iodine and chlorhexidine added to the fluid had the highest mortality rates. In contrast, improved survival was seen when antibiotics were added to the lavage solution compared with saline lavage alone. Other studies have shown no advantage to adding antibiotics to the lavage solution if systemic antibiotics are used (Platell et al. 2000). Clinical veterinary studies have reported a difference in pre- and post-lavage culture results for patients having surgery for septic peritonitis, but this did not appear to affect survival (Swayne et al. 2012; Kalafut et al. 2018). Another study showed that the same organism was isolated in pre- and post-lavage cultures in some dogs and a new bacterial isolate detected in others, with an overall decrease in the total number of bacterial isolates in post-lavage cultures (Marshall et al. 2019). This study also showed a significant decrease in the likelihood of isolating a multidrug-resistant organism following peritoneal lavage. Until further clinical research provides more information, it is generally recommended that the surgeon lavages the abdomen with large volumes of warm sterile saline as needed to remove gross contamination followed by complete removal of all lavage fluid.

Drainage

Abdominal drainage has been recommended for clearing established intra-abdominal infection in patients with severe generalized peritonitis, facilitating reexploration of the abdomen in patients with questionable control of the source of contamination, aiding in the treatment of anaerobic infection, and decreasing intra-abdominal pressure (IAP) to counteract the effects of abdominal compartment syndrome. Patients with peritonitis can be expected to have postoperative abdominal fluid accumulation and this fluid may allow proliferation of bacteria and limit the ability of the peritoneal defense mechanisms to fight infection. As the volume of fluid increases, abdominal pressure can increase, leading to abdominal compartment syndrome. Abdominal compartment syndrome is impaired organ function resulting from increased IAP, which is assessed by measuring urinary bladder pressure. Abdominal compartment syndrome has been documented in humans with peritonitis, and the life-threatening systemic effects of abdominal compartment syndrome have been demonstrated experimentally in dogs (Drellich 2000). The negative effects of increased IAP include impaired pulmonary and cardiovascular function, increased intracranial pressure, and decreased blood flow to abdominal organs, resulting in oliguria, renal failure, splanchnic ischemia, and facilitation of bacterial translocation (De Backer 1999). There is limited clinical information on the measurement of IAP in veterinary patients, but an IAP of $30\,cmH_2O$ or more has been reported to be associated with anuria in two dogs with abdominal pathology. The anuria in these patients resolved after surgical decompression and the authors recommended surgical decompression when IAP approaches $30\,cmH_2O$ (Conzemius et al. 1995). Abdominal drainage provides a means for decompression of the abdomen in patients with peritonitis.

In order to provide abdominal drainage, the normal subatmospheric pressure of the peritoneal cavity must be overcome by allowing air to enter the peritoneal cavity or by the use of a vacuum system (Hosgood et al. 1989). Open abdominal drainage involves closing the linea alba with nonabsorbable suture in a simple continuous pattern, allowing a gap of 2–6 cm (depending on patient size) in the body wall. An alternative technique involves placing loops of suture on either side of the abdominal incision in the external rectus sheath and using umbilical tape placed through these loops in a crisscross fashion (Staatz et al. 2002). In males, the parapreputial incision can be closed routinely and a urinary catheter can be placed to divert urine away from the incision. A sterile bandage consisting of laparotomy sponges and surgical towels is placed over the open incision and covered with a water-impermeable drape. The bandage is changed at least once daily with the patient sedated or anesthetized. During the bandage change, fluid is collected for cytologic evaluation and the abdomen can be explored or lavaged as needed. The abdomen is usually closed within 2–3 days and the decision to close the incision is based on gross and cytologic improvement of the abdominal effusion.

Although open abdominal drainage has been regarded as an effective means of drainage, mortality rates as high as 48% have been reported in dogs with peritonitis treated by this technique (Woolfson & Dulisch 1986). One study comparing open abdominal drainage to primary closure of the incision found no significant difference in survival between the two groups; however, animals with open abdominal drainage spent more time in the critical care unit and a higher number were treated with blood products and jejunostomy tubes (Staatz et al. 2002). The potential disadvantages of open abdominal drainage include hypoproteinemia and nosocomial infection, but the clinical significance of these complications is unknown. Patients with peritonitis are often hypoproteinemic and in one study the severity of hypoproteinemia was not different between animals treated with open abdominal drainage 48 hours after surgery and those treated with primary closure (Staatz et al. 2002). In addition, growth of a different type of bacteria on cultures obtained from abdominal fluid at the time of closure has not been associated with increased mortality (Woolfson & Dulisch 1986; Greenfield & Walshaw 1987). The use of open abdominal drainage in humans has been discouraged (Boermeester 2007; Robledo et al. 2007). A randomized clinical trial comparing open versus closed management of the abdomen for the treatment of severe secondary peritonitis was terminated at the first interim analysis because of the increased risk of death in patients treated with open abdominal drainage (Robledo et al. 2007). Current recommendations in humans are that the use of open abdominal drainage should be reserved for patients who are expected to need more than one laparotomy because of the inability to provide adequate source control at the first surgery, for those with hemodynamic instability during surgery, or for those where the abdominal wall cannot be closed without risking intra-abdominal hypertension (Peralta et al. 2010).

Active drainage of the abdomen is used frequently in patients with peritonitis and involves applying an external vacuum to an abdominal drain to create negative pressure. The most commonly used type of

(a)

(b)

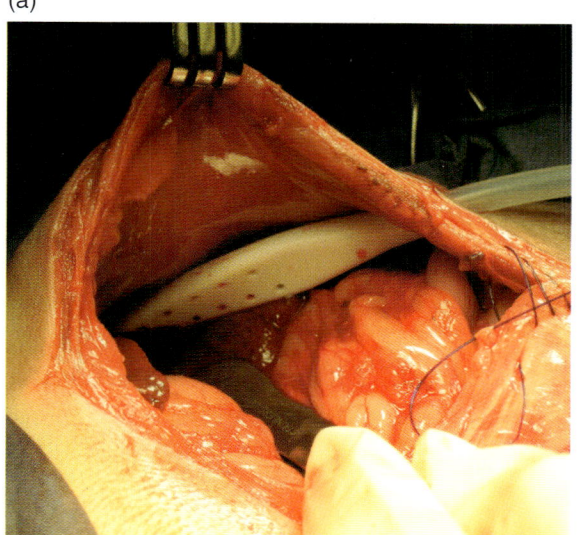

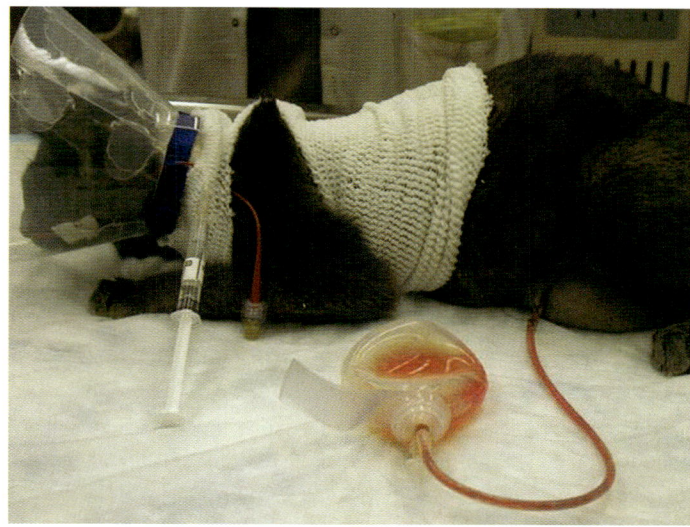

Figure 20.7 (a) Intraoperative photograph of placement of a Jackson–Pratt drain in a dog with peritonitis. The drain is less likely to be occluded by omentum if it is placed between the liver and diaphragm. If a second drain is used it should be placed in the caudal abdomen. (b) Postoperative photograph of a cat treated for septic peritonitis by closed-suction drain placement.

closed-suction drain is the Jackson–Pratt drain (Cardinal Health, Dublin, OH, USA) (Figure 20.7). The fenestrated portion of the drain is placed in a dependent position in the abdomen between the liver and the diaphragm. An additional drain can be placed in the caudal abdomen. The drain is connected to a bulb reservoir that creates negative pressure when it is compressed. The exit site of the drain is covered by a bandage and kept as clean as possible to prevent ascending infection. The bulb reservoir is emptied at least every 6 hours and the fluid volume recorded. The decision to remove the drain is based on criteria similar to those used with open abdominal drainage. Advantages of this technique over open abdominal drainage include less intensive postoperative care, elimination of the need for a second surgical procedure to close the abdomen, the ability to quantify the volume of effusion, and the ease of access for fluid samples for cytologic and biochemical analysis. Hypoproteinemia, nosocomial infection, and occlusion of the drain with omentum, fibrin, and clots are potential complications. In addition, these drains may not provide drainage of the entire peritoneal cavity if they become encased in omentum and visceral adhesions, as has been demonstrated experimentally in normal dogs with sump Penrose drains (Hosgood *et al.* 1991). One clinical study of patients with peritonitis treated with closed-suction drains reported that the abdominal drains remained patent until removal and that no deleterious effects were seen when fluid cultures obtained from the drain at the time of removal grew bacteria different from those cultured at the initial surgery (Mueller

et al. 2001). The survival rate (70%) in this study was similar to that reported with other techniques. Another study evaluating the use of closed-suction drains for the treatment of septic peritonitis of gastrointestinal origin had an even higher survival rate (85%) and all drains remained patent until removal (Adams *et al.* 2014)

The use of a vacuum-assisted closure device has been reported to provide controlled drainage of the abdomen while increasing local blood flow and accelerating granulation tissue formation (Perez *et al.* 2007; Buote *et al.* 2009; Peralta *et al.* 2010). With this technique, the abdominal incision is left open and a permeable layer is placed over the incision and covered with a polyurethane sponge. This permeable layer can be mesh that is sutured to the abdominal incision or a perforated plastic barrier that is placed over the abdomen and extends laterally under the abdominal wall. An aspiration system connected to a low-level suction device and drainage canister is placed between the sponge and an adherent airtight plastic sheet. In dogs, a modification of this technique involves inserting a sterile red rubber catheter into a piece of polyethylene foam that is placed over the open abdominal incision (Figure 20.8). The open abdomen and foam are covered with a sterile sealant drape and soft padded bandage after the red rubber catheter is attached to a sterile suction unit. Intermittent suction is applied to the wound to allow drainage of abdominal fluid. The advantages of the vacuum-assisted closure device over closed-suction drainage are that the pressure applied to the drainage tubing can be controlled and the abdominal incision is left open, potentially resulting in

(a)

(b)

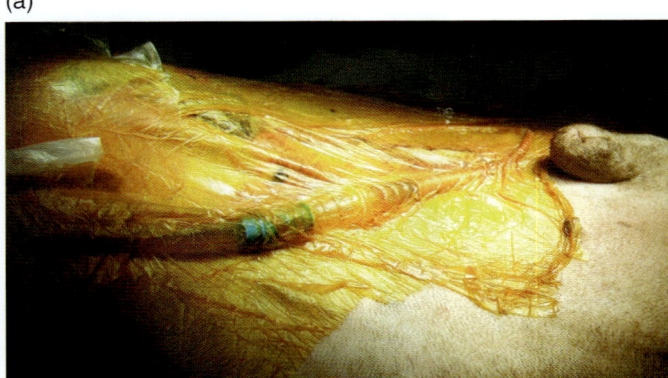

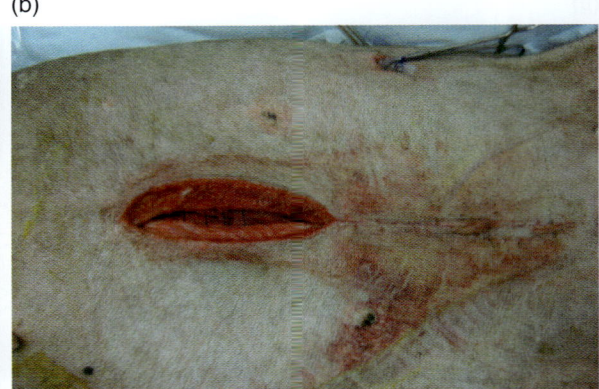

Figure 20.8 (a) Immediate postoperative photograph after placing a vacuum-assisted closure (VAC) device. The abdominal incision has been left open and has been covered by a piece of polyethylene foam. A red rubber catheter is inserted into the foam and attached to a sterile suction unit after the abdomen is covered with a sealant drape. (b) Appearance of the abdomen two days after treatment for septic peritonitis with a VAC device. The VAC has been removed and the abdomen is prepared for closure. Source: Courtesy of Dr. Nicole Buote.

more effective drainage of the entire peritoneal cavity. The advantages over open abdominal drainage include the ability to quantify the amount of drainage and a decreased number of bandage changes. The disadvantage of this technique is that a second surgery is required to close the abdomen. A preliminary study of vacuum-assisted closure in dogs with septic peritonitis demonstrated that it is well tolerated and provides effective abdominal drainage, but had no survival advantage (Buote *et al.* 2009). Another study comparing passive open abdominal drainage to negative-pressure abdominal drainage (NPAD) showed no difference in survival or postoperative complications, but NPAD eliminated the need for frequent bandage changes and showed improved local healing response on biopsy of abdominal tissue (Spillebeen *et al.* 2017).

There is still no definitive evidence in human or veterinary medicine that mortality rate is decreased by providing postoperative abdominal drainage in patients with peritonitis. Death in patients with septic peritonitis most often occurs less than 24 hours from surgery (Mueller *et al.* 2001). Mortality in these patients most likely results from the effects of sepsis, refractory hypotension, and multiple organ dysfunction syndrome (MODS) rather than ineffective drainage. The peritoneal cavity is capable of absorbing fluid through stomata in the mesothelial cells of the visceral and parietal peritoneum and through the omentum, which may make postoperative drainage unnecessary once the source of contamination has been corrected. Reports of patients with bile peritonitis, uroperitoneum, and septic peritonitis have documented survival without postoperative drainage (Ludwig *et al.* 1997; Aumann *et al.* 1998; Lanz *et al.* 2001). A mortality rate of 46% was reported in one study of septic peritonitis treated without postoperative

drainage, even though most of the cases were caused by gastrointestinal leakage (Lanz *et al.* 2001). Another study comparing open abdominal drainage to primary closure found no significant difference in survival (Staatz *et al.* 2002). Currently, surgeons must use their assessment of the ability to provide source control, the severity of peritonitis, and the possibility of the development of intra-abdominal hypertension to decide if postoperative drainage is needed.

Postoperative treatment

Patients with peritonitis lose large amounts of fluid, electrolytes, and proteins into the abdominal cavity. Fluid replacement requirements should take this into account and the amount of fluid collected from abdominal drains or lost into abdominal bandages must be replaced. Urine output should be measured every few hours and insensible losses (10–20 mL/kg daily) must also be considered when calculating fluid requirements. Measurement of blood pressure, urine specific gravity, and body weight can be used to determine fluid therapy needs. A loss of 1 kg of body weight is equivalent to a loss of 1 L of water. Usually, patients with peritonitis will initially need a fluid rate that is at least twice normal maintenance requirements.

Patients may become hypokalemic and hypoglycemic from decreased intake of nutrients and increased losses from vomiting or sepsis. Potassium and glucose should be monitored daily in critically ill animals and supplementation provided as needed. Excessive glucose administration should be avoided because hyperglycemia disrupts immune function, promotes inflammation, and has been associated with a worse prognosis in humans with sepsis (Dellinger *et al.* 2008). Hypocalcemia has been correlated with an increased mortality rate in humans and dogs with sepsis, but not in cats with septic peritonitis (Kellett-Gregory et al. 2010). It has been recommended that ionized calcium concentrations should be evaluated in all critically ill animals, because normalization of ionized calcium may improve survival (Holowaychuk & Martin 2007). Patients with refractory hypocalcemia or hypokalemia may also have hypomagnesemia. Ionized magnesium levels should be measured in these patients and magnesium supplementation provided as needed.

Vasopressors may continue to be needed after surgery and should be provided as indicated in preoperative treatment. Hypotension that is refractory to fluid resuscitation and vasopressor therapy may be related to a relative adrenal insufficiency and this has been documented in humans and dogs with sepsis (Ashton & Simmons 2008; Dellinger et al. 2008). This syndrome is characterized by normal basal serum cortisol concentrations but inadequate response to adrenocorticotropic hormone (ACTH) administration. In humans, low-dose hydrocortisone therapy is recommended for adult patients with septic shock if their blood pressure is poorly responsive to fluid resuscitation and vasopressor therapy (Dellinger et al. 2008). Critical illness-related corticosteroid insufficiency (CIRCI) has been reported in a cat suffering from trauma, prepubic tendon rupture, and possible sepsis, a cat with septic peritonitis due to a ruptured pyometra, and a dog with septic shock due to aspiration pneumonia (Durkan et al. 2007; Pisano et al. 2017; Peyton & Burkitt 2009). In these patients, hypotension that was refractory to fluids and vasopressors responded to low doses of dexamethasone (0.08 mg/kg) or hydrocortisone (1–2 mg/kg/day). High-dose glucocorticoid therapy has not been shown to be successful for the treatment of human patients with septic shock and because of immune suppression and the risk of gastrointestinal complications it should be avoided in veterinary patients.

Hypoalbuminemia and decreased colloid osmotic pressure (COP) are common in patients with peritonitis and can lead to delayed wound healing, tissue edema, hypoperfusion, and organ failure. Synthetic colloids are commonly used to help maintain intravascular fluid volume in these patients, but their use is controversial. The use of plasma to replace serum albumin is impractical because of the cost and the large doses required: a plasma dose of 20 mL/kg is required to increase serum albumin by 0.5 g/dL (Devey 2010). The use of 25% human serum albumin (HSA) has been shown to increase albumin, total protein, and COP in hypoalbuminemic dogs with septic peritonitis (Horowitz et al. 2015). However, its administration has been associated with potentially life-threatening complications such as fluid overload and

immediate or delayed type III hypersensitivity reactions (Trow et al. 2008; Mazzaferro et al. 2020). Also, dogs will develop anti-has antibodies, so repeated infusion is not recommended. Alternatively, canine-specific albumin (administered as a 5% solution at a dose of 800 mg/kg over 6 h) has been reported to increase albumin, COP, and blood pressure in dogs with septic peritonitis, with only minimal adverse events (Craft & Powell 2012).

Nutritional support is critical for wound healing and immune function. Enteral nutrition (EN) is preferred to parenteral nutrition (PN) to decrease bacterial translocation. One study showed that dogs with septic peritonitis that received PN were less likely to survive and those that survived were hospitalized longer than those receiving EN (Smith et al. 2019). An esophagostomy, gastrostomy, jejunostomy, or gastrojejunostomy tube should be placed at the time of surgery to support critically ill patients (Cavanaugh et al. 2008; Mazzaferro 2010). Tube feeding should be instituted as soon as possible after surgery. Animals that are not vomiting should be encouraged to eat and administration of an appetite stimulant may be considered. If the animal is not eating on its own but is not vomiting, then an esophagostomy or gastrostomy tube can be used. If a feeding tube was not placed at the time of surgery, a nasogastric tube can be placed without the need for general anesthesia. The daily resting energy requirement (RER) in kcal/day is estimated in dogs and cats weighing between 2 and 45 kg by multiplying the body weight in kilograms by 30 and adding 70 to the total. It is no longer recommended to multiply the RER by an "illness factor" of 1.1–2 because of the risks of overfeeding and the refeeding syndrome (Marks 2010). Tube feeding is initiated at one-fourth the RER divided over 4–6 feedings per day, and is increased by 25% each day until the RER is reached. When feeding through a jejunostomy tube, continuous feeding is preferable to avoid cramping associated with bolus feeding. Feeding with a jejunostomy tube can be initiated in patients that are vomiting or in those under heavy sedation. If a feeding tube was not placed in these patients at surgery, transpyloric tube insertion can be facilitated with fluoroscopy or endoscopy. Alternatively, PN can be used. Gastrointestinal protectants, antacids, and antiemetics are helpful to treat ileus, control vomiting, protect against ulcers, and prevent bacterial translocation.

Analgesia is essential after surgery and can be provided through the use of opiates or a combined infusion of lidocaine, ketamine, and morphine in dogs. Nonsteroidal anti-inflammatory agents should be avoided because of the potential for gastrointestinal ulceration. Patients should be kept clean and dry and should be protected from decubital ulcers with frequent turning and adequate bedding. A urinary catheter should be placed in most patients to monitor urine output and prevent discomfort associated with urine retention and soiling.

Empiric antibiotic therapy is continued until the results of cultures are known. The type of antibiotic will be modified based on culture results as they become available. The antibiotic therapy will be continued for at least 2–4 weeks after surgery. Critically ill patients are at risk of aspiration pneumonia. Lung auscultation, pulse oximetry, and/or arterial blood gas analysis should be monitored in patients suspected of having respiratory compromise and oxygen supplementation provided as needed. Cardiac arrhythmias may develop as a result of excessive sympathetic stimulation, hypovolemia, and hypoxia. Electrocardiography is indicated if an abnormal heart rhythm is auscultated or asynchronous pulses are noted. Initial treatment should involve controlling the source of the arrhythmia (pain, hypovolemia, hypoxia, or electrolyte abnormalities). Antiarrhythmic therapy is only instituted if the arrhythmia is affecting perfusion and after extracardiac causes of the arrhythmia have been eliminated. Red blood cell count and coagulation parameters should be monitored in anemic patients or in those suspected of having a coagulopathy. White blood cell counts can be monitored to determine the effectiveness of treatment and to indicate the possible presence of SIRS or intestinal dehiscence (Allen et al. 1992; Hauptman et al. 1997). Chemistry panels should be monitored to evaluate for organ dysfunction. Lactate measurements will provide information about response to fluid therapy and tissue perfusion and will decrease over time in patients being treated successfully (Karagiannis et al. 2006).

Prognosis

Prognosis for veterinary patients with peritonitis depends on the source of peritoneal inflammation and the presence or absence of infection. The survival rate for dogs and cats with primary peritonitis not associated with FIP was 40–44% (Culp et al. 2009). In this study, dogs with primary peritonitis that were taken to surgery were more likely to die than those that were not taken to surgery. This finding was not true for cats.

The prognosis for patients with uroperitoneum depends on the severity and presence of concomitant injuries, the ability to correct electrolyte abnormalities and restore renal perfusion, and healing of the urinary tract without leakage or stricture formation (Stafford & Bartges 2013). Outcomes in dogs with uroperitoneum are good, with a reported 79% survival rate and no identified preoperative risk factors in one study (Grimes et al. 2018). Uroperitoneum has been reported to be

associated with a 61.5–74% survival rate in cats, with death attributed to concurrent injuries and acute kidney injury (Aumann et al. 1998; Hornsey et al. 2020).

The prognosis for patients with bile peritonitis depends on the presence of infection, with survival rates of 27–45% for patients with septic biliary effusions compared with 87–100% for those with a sterile effusion (Ludwig et al. 1997; Mehler et al. 2004). A prolonged duration of biliary effusion has been reported prior to treatment and may not be associated with a poor prognosis if the effusion is sterile (Ludwig et al. 1997).

Survival rates reported for dogs and cats with septic peritonitis from any cause are variable and range from 14% to 80% (Hinton et al. 2002; Staatz et al. 2002; Bentley et al. 2007; Kenney et al. 2010). The lowest survival rates have been associated with gastroduodenal perforation (31–63% in dogs, 14% in cats) and intestinal dehiscence in dogs (15–26%) (Allen et al. 1992; Hinton et al. 2002; Ralphs et al. 2003; Lascelles et al. 2005). The risk of dehiscence and death in dogs having gastric or intestinal surgery has been reported to increase with an American Society of Anesthesiology (ASA) status ≥ 3 (Gill et al. 2019). In addition, the risk of death increased with higher preoperative plasma lactate concentrations (4.6 ± 3.7 mmol/L for nonsurvivors and 2.4 ± 1.7 mmol/L for survivors). The postoperative dehiscence (10%) and mortality rate (17%) for full-thickness large intestinal incisions in dogs are similar to those for small intestinal surgery (Latimer et al. 2019).

In two retrospective studies, cats with septic peritonitis had a lower survival rate (14–40%) than dogs with septic peritonitis (63–80%) (Mueller et al. 2001; Hinton et al. 2002). Other retrospective studies of cats with septic peritonitis report survival rates of 46–70% (Costello et al. 2004; Parsons et al. 2009; Scotti et al. 2019). A recent study of cats with septic peritonitis found that those that received appropriate empirical antimicrobial therapy and had a lower blood glucose concentration on presentation were more likely to survive (Scotti et al. 2019).

Several biomarkers have been associated with survival in patients with septic peritonitis. A lower preoperative and postoperative serum albumin concentration, serum lactate >4 mmol/L at admission, persistent postoperative hyperlactatemia, and lactate clearance <42% at 12 hours have been reported to be poor prognostic indicators for dogs with peritonitis (King 1994; Bentley et al. 2007; Declue 2010; Cortellini et al. 2015; Bush et al. 2016). Preoperative protein C and antithrombin deficiencies and mean platelet volume above the reference interval have also been associated with increased mortality in dogs with septic peritonitis (Bentley et al. 2013; Llewellyn et al. 2017).

A retrospective study that compared the treatment and outcome of dogs with septic peritonitis from two time periods failed to find an improvement in survival despite the addition of new antibiotics, colloids, and better pain management (Bentley *et al.* 2007). In this study, the survival rate for dogs treated between 1988 and 1993 was 64% compared with 57% for those treated between 1999 and 2003. Poor prognostic indicators for dogs and cats with septic peritonitis include the development of respiratory disease or disseminated intravascular coagulation and refractory hypotension (King 1994; Bentley *et al.* 2007). For septic dogs, the development of MODS, defined as dysfunction of at least two organ systems, is associated with a significant decrease in survival. Only 30% of dogs with MODS survived compared with 70% in those without MODS (Kenney *et al.* 2010). In this study, age, cause of gastrointestinal tract perforation, and presence of hepatic dysfunction were not associated with outcome, while dysfunction of the respiratory, cardiovascular, renal, or coagulation systems significantly increased the risk of death. Overall, animals with septic peritonitis that do not survive usually die or are euthanized within the first 48 hours of surgery (Mueller *et al.* 2001; Bentley *et al.* 2007).

References

Adamama-Moraitou, K.K., Prassinos, N.N., Patsikas, M.N. et al. (2004). Sclerosing encapsulating peritonitis in a dog with leishmaniasis. *Journal of Small Animal Practice* 45: 117–121.

Adams, R.J., Doyle, R.S., Bray, J.P., and Burton, C.A. (2014). Closed suction drainage for treatment of septic peritonitis of confirmed gastrointestinal origin in 20 dogs. *Veterinary Surgery* 43: 843–851.

Aguirre, A. (2010). Diseases of the gallbladder and extrahepatic biliary system. In: *Textbook of Veterinary Internal Medicine*, 7e, vol. 2 (ed. S.J. Ettinger and E.C. Feldman), 1689–1695. St Louis, MO: WB Saunders.

Allen, D.A., Smeak, D.D., and Schertel, E.R. (1992). Prevalence of small intestinal dehiscence and associated clinical factors: a retrospective study of 121 dogs. *Journal of the American Animal Hospital Association* 28: 70–76.

Ashton, J.A. and Simmons, J.P. (2008). Relative adrenal insufficiency in critically ill patients. *Standards of Care: Emergency and Critical Care Medicine* 10: 7–11.

Aumann, M., Worth, L.T., and Drobatz, K.J. (1998). Uroperitoneum in cats: 26 cases (1986–1995). *Journal of the American Animal Hospital Association* 34: 315–324.

Bazzle, L.J. and Brainard, B.M. (2019). Anesthesia and analgesia in the emergency room: an overview. In: *Textbook of Small Animal Emergency Medicine*, vol. 2 (ed. K.J. Drobatz, K. Hopper, E. Rozanski and D.C. Silverstein), 1225–1229. Hoboken, NJ: Wiley.

Bellini, L. and Seymour, C.J. (2016). Effect of intraoperative constant rate infusion of lidocaine on short-term survival of dogs with septic peritonitis: 75 cases (2007–2011). *Journal of the American Veterinary Medical Association* 248: 422–429.

Bentley, A.M., Otto, C.M., and Shofer, F.S. (2007). Comparison of dogs with septic peritonitis: 1988–1993 versus 1999–2003. *Journal of Veterinary Emergency and Critical Care* 17: 391–398.

Bentley, A.M., Mayhew, P.D., Culp, W.T., and Otto, C.M. (2013). Alterations in the hemostatic profiles of dogs with naturally occurring septic peritonitis. *Journal of Veterinary Emergency and Critical Care* 23: 14–22.

Boermeester, M.A. (2007). Surgical approaches to peritonitis. *British Journal of Surgery* 94: 1317–1318.

Bonczynski, J.J., Ludwig, L.L., Barton, L.J. et al. (2003). Comparison of peritoneal fluid and peripheral blood pH, bicarbonate, glucose and lactate concentration as a diagnostic tool for septic peritonitis in dogs and cats. *Veterinary Surgery* 32: 161–166.

Botte, R.J. and Rosin, E. (1983). Cytology of peritoneal effusion following intestinal anastomosis and experimental peritonitis. *Veterinary Surgery* 12: 20–23.

Boysen, S.R., Rozanski, E.A., Tidwell, A.S. et al. (2004). Evaluation of a focused assessment with sonography for trauma protocol to detect free abdominal fluid in dogs involved in motor vehicle accidents. *Journal of the American Veterinary Medical Association* 225: 1198–1204.

Broche, F. and Tellado, J.M. (2001). Defense mechanisms of the peritoneal cavity. *Current Opinion in Critical Care* 7: 105–116.

Buote, N., Havig, M., and Hackner, S. (2009). Vacuum-assisted laparostomy in septic peritonitis. Symposium of the American College of Veterinary Surgeons (October 8, 2009). Washington, DC.

Bush, M., Carno, M.A., Germaine, L.S., and Hoffmann, D.E. (2016). The effect of time until surgical intervention on survival in dogs with secondary septic peritonitis. *Canadian Veterinary Journal* 57: 1267–1273.

Caavanagh, A.A., Sullivan, L.A., and Hansen, B.D. (2016). Retrospective evaluation of fluid overload and relationship outcome in critically ill dogs. *Journal of Veterinary Emergency and Critical Care* 26: 578–586.

Carroll, K.A., Wallace, M.L., Hill, T.L. et al. (2020). Pyloric outflow obstruction secondary to sclerosing encapsulating peritonitis in a dog. *Australian Veterinary Journal* 98: 11–16.

Cavanaugh, R.P., Kovak, J.R., Fischetti, A.J. et al. (2008). Evaluation of surgically placed gastrojejunostomy feeding tubes in critically ill dogs. *Journal of the American Veterinary Medical Association* 232: 380–388.

Conzemius, M.G., Sammarco, J.L., Holt, D.E., and Smith, D.K. (1995). Clinical determination of preoperative and postoperative intraabdominal pressures in dogs. *Veterinary Surgery* 24: 195–201.

Cortellini, S., Seth, M., and Kellett-Gregory, L.M. (2015). Plasma lactate concentrations in septic peritonitis: a retrospective study of 83 dogs (2007–2012). *Journal of Veterinary Emergency and Critical Care* 25: 388–395.

Costello, M.F., Drobatz, K.J., Aronson, L.R., and King, L.G. (2004). Underlying cause, pathophysiologic abnormalities, and response to treatment in cats with septic peritonitis: 51 cases (1990–2001). *Journal of the American Veterinary Medical Association* 225: 897–902.

Craft, E.M. and Powell, L.L. (2012). The use of canine-specific albumin in dogs with septic peritonitis. *Journal of Veterinary Emergency and Critical Care* 22: 631–639.

Culp, W.T.N., Zeldis, T.E., Reese, M.S., and Drobatz, K.J. (2009). Primary bacterial peritonitis in dogs and cats: 24 cases (1990–2006). *Journal of the American Veterinary Medical Association* 234: 906–913.

Davis, D.J., Demianiuk, R.M., Musser, J. et al. (2018). Influence of peroperative septic peritonitis and anastomotic technique on the dehiscence of enterectomy sites in dogs: a retrospective review of 210 anastomoses. *Veterinary Surgery* 47: 125–129.

De Backer, D. (1999). Abdominal compartment syndrome. *Critical Care* 3: R103–R104.

Declue, A. (2010). Sepsis and the systemic inflammatory response syndrome. In: *Textbook of Veterinary Internal Medicine*, 7e, vol. 1 (ed. S.J. Ettinger and E.C. Feldman), 523–527. St Louis, MO: WB Saunders.

DeLaforcade, A.M., Freeman, L.M., Shaw, S.P. et al. (2003). Hemostatic changes in dogs with naturally occurring sepsis. *Journal of Veterinary Internal Medicine* 17: 674–679.

Dellinger, R.P., Levy, M.M., Carlet, J.M. et al. (2008). Surviving sepsis campaign: international guidelines for management of severe sepsis and septic shock: 2008. *Critical Care Medicine* 36: 296–327.

DePompeo, C.M., Bond, L., George, Y.E. et al. (2018). Intra-abdominal complications following intestinal anastomoses by suture and staple techniques in dogs. *Journal of the American Veterinary Medical Association* 253: 437–443.

Devey, J.J. (2010). Crystalloid and colloid fluid therapy. In: *Textbook of Veterinary Internal Medicine*, 7e, vol. 1 (ed. S.J. Ettinger and E.C. Feldman), 487–496. St Louis, MO: WB Saunders.

Drellich, S. (2000). Intraabdominal pressure and abdominal compartment syndrome. *Compendium on Continuing Education for the Practicing Veterinarian* 22: 764–769.

Dulisch, M.L. (1993). Peritonitis. In: *Disease Mechanisms in Small Animal Surgery*, 2e (ed. M.J. Bojrab), 109–112. Philadelphia, PA: Lea & Febiger.

Durkan, S., DeLaforcade, A., Rozanski, E., and Rush, J.E. (2007). Suspected relative adrenal insufficiency in a critically ill cat. *Journal of Veterinary Emergency and Critical Care* 17: 197–201.

Eltoum, M.A., Wright, S., Atchley, J., and Mason, J.C. (2006). Four consecutive cases of peritoneal dialysis-related encapsulating peritoneal sclerosis treated successfully with tamoxifen. *Peritoneal Dialysis International* 26: 203–206.

Etchepareborde, S., Heimann, M., Cohen-Solal, A., and Hamaide, A. (2010). Use of tamoxifen in a German Shepherd dog with sclerosing encapsulating peritonitis. *Journal of Small Animal Practice* 51: 649–653.

Evans, H.L., Raymond, D.P., Pelletier, S.J. et al. (2001). Diagnosis of intra-abdominal infection in the critically ill patient. *Current Opinion in Critical Care* 7: 117–121.

Fitzgerald, E., Barfield, D., Lee, K.C.L., and Lamb, C.R. (2017). Clinical findings and results of diagnostic imaging in 82 dogs with gastrointestinal ulceration. *Journal of Small Animal Practice* 58: 211–218.

Gill, S.S., Buote, N.J., Peterson, N.W., and Bergman, P.J. (2019). Factors associated with dehiscence and mortality rates following gastrointestinal surgery in dogs. *Journal of the American Veterinary Medical Association* 255: 569–573.

Gilroy, C., Raab, O., and Hanna, P. (2020). Pathology in practice. *Journal of the American Veterinary Medical Association* 257: 161–164.

Greenfield, C.L. and Walshaw, R. (1987). Open peritoneal drainage for treatment of contaminated peritoneal cavity and septic peritonitis in dogs and cats: 24 cases (1980–1986). *Journal of the American Veterinary Medical Association* 191: 100–105.

Grimes, J.A., Fletcher, J.M., and Schmiedt, C.W. (2018). Outcomes in dogs with uroabdomen: 43 cases (2006–2015). *Journal of the American Veterinary Medical Association* 252: 92–97.

Guess, S.C., Harkin, K.R., and Biller, D.S. (2015). Anicteric gallbladder rupture in dogs: 5 cases (2007–2013). *Journal of the American Veterinary Medical Association* 247: 1412–1414.

Guieu, L.V., Bersenas, A.M., Brisson, B.A. et al. (2016). Evaluation of peripheral blood and abdominal fluid variables as predictors of intestinal surgical site failure in dogs with septic peritonitis following celiotomy and the placement of closed-suction abdominal drains. *Journal of the American Veterinary Medical Association* 249: 515–525.

Hardie, E.M., Rottman, J.B., and Levy, J.K. (1994). Sclerosing encapsulating peritonitis in four dogs and a cat. *Veterinary Surgery* 23: 107–114.

Hauptman, J.G., Walshaw, R., and Olivier, N.B. (1997). Evaluation of the sensitivity and specificity of diagnostic criteria for sepsis in dogs. *Veterinary Surgery* 26: 393–397.

Hinton, L.E., McLoughlin, M.A., Johnson, S.E., and Weisbrode, S.E. (2002). Spontaneous gastroduodenal perforation in 16 dogs and seven cats (1982–1999). *Journal of the American Animal Hospital Association* 38: 176–187.

Holmberg, T.A., Vernau, W., Melli, A.C., and Conrad, P.A. (2006). *Neospora caninum* associated with septic peritonitis in an adult dog. *Veterinary Clinical Pathology* 35: 235–238.

Holowaychuk, M.K. and Martin, L.G. (2007). Review of hypocalcemia in septic patients. *Journal of Veterinary Emergency and Critical Care* 17: 348–358.

Hornsey, S.J., Halfacree, Z., Kulendra, E. et al. (2020). Factors affecting survival to discharge in 53 cats diagnosed with uroabdomen: a single-centre retrospective analysis. *Journal of Feline Medicine and Surgery* 23: 115–120.

Horowitz, F.B., Read, R.L., and Powell, L.L. (2015). A retrospective analysis of 25% human serum albumin supplementation in hypoalbuminemic dogs with septic peritonitis. *Canadian Veterinary Journal* 56: 591–597.

Hosgood, G., Salisbury, S.K., Cantwell, H.D., and DeNicola, D.B. (1989). Intraperitoneal circulation and drainage in the dog. *Veterinary Surgery* 18: 261–268.

Hosgood, G., Salisbury, S.K., and DeNicola, D.B. (1991). Open peritoneal drainage versus sump-Penrose drainage: clinicopathological effects in normal dogs. *Journal of the American Animal Hospital Association* 27: 115–121.

Jagirdar, R.M., Bozikas, A., Zarogiannis, S.C. et al. (2019). Encapsulating peritoneal sclerosis: pathophysiology and current treatment options. *International Journal of Molecular Sciences* 20: 1–21.

Johnson, M.D. and Mann, F.A. (2006). Treatment for pancreatic abscesses via omentalization with abdominal closure versus open peritoneal drainage in dogs: 15 cases (1994–2004). *Journal of the American Veterinary Medical Association* 228: 397–402.

Kalafut, S.R., Schwartz, P., Currao, R.L. et al. (2018). Comparison of initial and postlavage bacterial culture results of septic peritonitis in dogs and cats. *Journal of the American Animal Hospital Association* 54: 257–266.

Karagiannis, M.H., Reniker, A.N., Kerl, M.E., and Mann, F.A. (2006). Lactate measurement as an indicator of perfusion. *Compendium on Continuing Education for the Practicing Veterinarian* 28: 287–298.

Kellett-Gregory, L.M., Mittleman Boller, E., Brown, D.C., and Silverstein, D.C. (2010). Ionized calcium concentrations in cats with septic peritonitis: 55 cases (1990–2008). *Journal of Veterinary Emergency and Critical Care* 20: 398–405.

Kenney, E.M., Rozanski, E.A., Rush, J.F. et al. (2010). Association between outcome and organ system dysfunction in dogs with sepsis: 114 cases (2003–2007). *Journal of the American Veterinary Medical Association* 236: 83–87.

King, L.G. (1994). Postoperative complications and prognostic indicators in dogs and cats with septic peritonitis: 23 cases (1989–1992). *Journal of the American Veterinary Medical Association* 204: 407–414.

Kirby, B.M. (2003). Peritoneum and peritoneal cavity. In: *Textbook of Small Animal Surgery*, vol. 1 (ed. D. Slatter), 414–445. Philadelphia, PA: WB Saunders.

Klainbart, S., Agi, L., Bdolah-Abram, T. et al. (2017). Clinical, laboratory, and hemostatic findings in cats with naturally occurring sepsis. *Journal of the American Veterinary Medical Association* 251: 1025–1034.

Koenig, A. and Verlander, L.L. (2015). Usefulness of whole blood, plasma, peritoneal fluid, and peritoneal fluid supernatant glucose concentrations obtained by a veterinary point of care glucometer to identify septic peritonitis in dogs with peritoneal effusion. *Journal of the American Veterinary Medical Association* 247: 1027–1032.

Lanz, O.I., Ellison, G.W., Bellah, J.R. et al. (2001). Surgical treatment of septic peritonitis without abdominal drainage in 28 dogs. *Journal of the American Animal Hospital Association* 37: 87–92.

Laroche, M. and Harding, G. (1998). Primary and secondary peritonitis: an update. *European Journal of Clinical Microbiology and Infectious Diseases* 17: 542–550.

Lascelles, B.D., Blikslager, A.T., Fox, S.M., and Reece, D. (2005). Gastrointestinal tract perforation in dogs treated with a selective cyclooxygenase-2 inhibitor: 29 cases (2002–2003). *Journal of the American Veterinary Medical Association* 227: 1112–1117.

Latimer, C.R., Lux, C.N., Grimes, J.A. et al. (2019). Evaluation of short-term outcomes and potential risk factors for death and intestinal dehiscence following full-thickness large intestinal incisions in dogs. *Journal of the American Veterinary Medical Association* 255: 915–925.

Levin, G.M., Bonczynski, J.J., Ludwig, L.L. et al. (2004). Lactate as a diagnostic test for septic peritoneal effusions in dogs and cats. *Journal of the American Animal Hospital Association* 40: 364–371.

Llewellyn, E.A., Todd, J.M., Sharkey, L.C., and Rendahl, A. (2017). A pilot study evaluating the prognostic utility of platelet indices in dogs with septic peritonitis. *Journal of Veterinary Emergency and Critical Care* 27: 569–578.

Londono, L. (2019). Fluid therapy in critical care. *Today's Veterinary Practice* 9: 43–50.

Ludwig, L.L., McLoughlin, M.A., Graves, T.K., and Crisp, M.S. (1997). Surgical treatment of bile peritonitis in 24 dogs and 2 cats: a retrospective study (1987–1994). *Veterinary Surgery* 26: 90–98.

Marks, S.L. (2010). The principles and implementation of enteral nutrition. In: *Textbook of Veterinary Internal Medicine*, 7e, vol. 1 (ed. S.J. Ettinger and E.C. Feldman), 715–717. St Louis, MO: WB Saunders.

Marshall, H., Sinnott-Stutzman, V., Ewing, P. et al. (2019). Effect of peritoneal lavage on bacterial isolates in 40 dogs with confirmed septic peritonitis. *Journal of Veterinary Emergency and Critical Care* 29: 635–642.

Martiny, P. and Goggs, R. (2019). Biomarker guided diagnosis of septic peritonitis in dogs. *Frontiers in Veterinary Science* 6: 1–13.

Mazzaferro, E.M. (2010). Enteral nutrition. In: *Mechanisms of Disease in Small Animal Surgery*, 3e (ed. M.J. Bojrab and E. Monnet), 24–31. Jackson, WY: Teton New Media.

Mazzaferro, E.M., Balekrishnan, A., Hackner, S.G. et al. (2020). Delayed type 111 hypersensitivity reaction with acute kidney injury in two dogs following administration of concentrated human albumin during treatment for hypoalbuminemia secondary to septic peritonitis. *Journal of Veterinary Emergency and Critical Care* 30: 574–580.

Mehler, S.J., Mayhew, P.D., Drobatz, K.J., and Holt, D.E. (2004). Variables associated with outcome in dogs undergoing extrahepatic biliary surgery: 60 cases (1988–2002). *Veterinary Surgery* 33: 644–649.

Mueller, M.G., Ludwig, L.L., and Barton, L.J. (2001). Use of closed suction drains to treat generalized peritonitis in dogs and cats: 40

cases (1997–1999). *Journal of the American Veterinary Medical Association* 219: 789–794.

Parsons, K.J., Owen, L.J., Lee, K. et al. (2009). A retrospective study of surgically treated cases of septic peritonitis in the cat (2000–2007). *Journal of Small Animal Practice* 50: 518–524.

Peralta R, Genuit T, Napolitano LM (2010) Peritonitis and abdominal sepsis: treatment. WebMD, 1–9.

Perez, D., Wildi, S., Demartines, N. et al. (2007). Prospective evaluation of vacuum-assisted closure in abdominal compartment syndrome and severe abdominal sepsis. *Journal of the American College of Surgeons* 205: 586–592.

Peyton, J.L. and Burkitt, J.M. (2009). Critical illness-related corticosteroid insufficiency in a dog with septic shock. *Journal of Veterinary Emergency and Critical Care* 3: 262–268.

Pike, F.S., Berg, J., King, N.W. et al. (2004). Gallbladder mucocele in dogs: 30 cases (2000–2002). *Journal of the American Veterinary Medical Association* 224: 1615–1622.

Pisano, S.R.R., Howard, J., Posthaus, H. et al. (2017). Hydrocortisone therapy in a cat with vasopressor-refractory septic shock and suspected critical illness-related corticosteroid insufficiency. *Clinical Case Reports* 7: 1123–1129.

Platell, C., Papadimitriou, J.M., and Hall, J.C. (2000). The influence of lavage on peritonitis. *Journal of the American College of Surgeons* 191: 672–679.

Qadan, M., Dajani, D., Dickinson, A., and Polk, H.C. Jr. (2010). Meta-analysis of the effect of peritoneal lavage on survival in experimental peritonitis. *British Journal of Surgery* 97: 151–159.

Ralphs, S.C., Jessen, C.R., and Lipowitz, A.J. (2003). Risk factors for leakage following intestinal anastomosis in dogs and cats: 115 cases (1991–2000). *Journal of the American Veterinary Medical Association* 223: 73–77.

Rivers, E.R., Nguyen, B., Havstad, S. et al. (2001). Early goal-directed therapy in the treatment of severe sepsis and septic shock. *New England Journal of Medicine* 345: 1368–1377.

Robledo, F.A., Luque-de-León, E., Suárez, R. et al. (2007). Open versus closed management of the abdomen in the surgical treatment of severe secondary peritonitis: a randomized clinical trial. *Surgical Infections* 8: 63–71.

Rollings, C., Rozanski, E.A., DeLaforcade, A. et al. (2001). Traumatic mesenteric avulsion and subsequent septic peritonitis in a dog. *Journal of Veterinary Emergency and Critical Care* 11: 211–215.

Schnaub, F., Hanisch, F., and Burgener, A. (2019). Diagnosis of feline pancreatitis with SNAP FPL and Spec fPL. *Journal of Feline Medicine and Surgery* 21: 700–707.

Scotti, K.M., Koenigshof, A., Sri-Jayantha, L.S.H. et al. (2019). Prognostic indicators in cats with septic peritonitis (2002–2015): 83 cases. *Journal of Veterinary Emergency and Critical Care* 29: 647–652.

Scroggin, R.D. and Quandt, J. (2009). The use of vasopressin for treating vasodilatory shock and cardiopulmonary arrest. *Journal of Veterinary Emergency and Critical Care* 19: 145–157.

Shih, C.C., Chen, S.J., Chen, A. et al. (2008). Therapeutic effects of hypertonic saline on peritonitis induced septic shock with multiple organ dysfunction syndrome in rats. *Critical Care Medicine* 36: 1864–1872.

Silverstein, D.C. and Santoro Beer, K.A. (2015). Controversies regarding choice of vasopressor therapy for management of septic shock in animals. *Journal of Veterinary Emergency and Critical Care* 25: 48–54.

Singer, M., Deutchman, C.S., and Seymour, C.W. (2016). The third international consensus definitions for sepsis and septic shock (sepsis-3). *Journal of the American Medical Association* 315: 801–810.

Smith, K.M., Rendahl, A., Sun, Y., and Todd, J.M. (2019). Retrospective evaluation of the route and timing of nutrition in dogs with septic peritonitis: 68 cases (2007–2016). *Journal of Veterinary Emergency and Critical Care* 29: 288–295.

Spillebeen, A.L., Robben, J.H., Thomas, R. et al. (2017). Negative pressure therapy versus passive open abdominal drainage for the treatment of septic peritonitis in dogs: a randomized, prospective study. *Veterinary Surgery* 46: 1086–1097.

Staatz, A.J., Monnet, E., and Seim, H.B. (2002). Open peritoneal drainage versus primary closure for the treatment of septic peritonitis in dogs and cats: 42 cases (1993–1999). *Veterinary Surgery* 31: 174–180.

Stafford, J.R. and Bartges, J.W. (2013). A clinical review of pathophysiology, diagnosis, and treatment of uroabdomen in the dog and cat. *Journal of Veterinary Emergency and Critical Care* 23: 216–229.

Steiner, J.M. (2010). Canine pancreatic disease. In: *Textbook of Veterinary Internal Medicine*, 7e, vol. 2 (ed. S.J. Ettinger and E.C. Feldman), 1695–1704. St Louis, MO: WB Saunders.

Sumner, S.M., Regier, P.J., Case, J.B., and Ellison, G.W. (2019). Evaluation of suture reinforcement for stapled intestinal anastomoses: 77 dogs (2008–2018). *Veterinary Surgery* 48: 1188–1193.

Swann, H. and Hughes, D. (2000). Diagnosis and management of peritonitis. *Veterinary Clinics of North America: Small Animal Practice* 30: 603–615.

Swayne, S.L., Brisson, B., Scott Weese, J., and Sears, W. (2012). Evaluating the effect of intraoperative peritoneal lavage on bacterial culture in dogs with suspected septic peritonitis. *Canadian Veterinary Journal* 53: 971–977.

Trow, A.V., Rozanski, E.A., DeLaforcade, A.M., and Chan, D.L. (2008). Evaluation of use of human albumin in critically ill dogs: 73 cases (2003–2006). *Journal of the American Veterinary Medical Association* 233: 607–612.

Wong, P.F., Gilliam, A.D., Kumar, S. et al. (2005). Antibiotic regimens for secondary peritonitis of gastrointestinal origin in adults. *Cochrane Database of Systematic Reviews* 2005, 2: CD004539. https://doi.org/10.1002/14651858.CD004539.pub2.

Woolfson, J.M. and Dulisch, M.L. (1986). Open abdominal drainage in the treatment of generalized peritonitis in 25 dogs and cats. *Veterinary Surgery* 15: 27–32.

Xu, P., Chen, L.H., and Li, Y.M. (2007). Idiopathic sclerosing encapsulating peritonitis (or abdominal cocoon): a report of 5 cases. *World Journal of Gastroenterology* 13: 3649–3651.

Yang, W., Ding, J., Jin, X. et al. (2009). The plication and splinting procedure for idiopathic sclerosing encapsulating peritonitis. *Journal of Investigative Surgery* 22: 286–291.

21

Hemoperitoneum

Jennifer Prittie and Lori Ludwig

Hemoperitoneum, defined as free blood within the peritoneal cavity, is a common clinical presentation in dogs (rare in cats) with potentially devastating consequences. Intra-abdominal hemorrhage results in hypovolemic shock and anemia, contributing to tissue hypoperfusion, organ dysfunction, and possibly death. Rapid diagnosis, restoration of effective circulating fluid volume (ECFV), and cessation of bleeding are paramount for a successful outcome.

Etiology

Hemoperitoneum is broadly categorized as naturally occurring (spontaneous) or traumatic. Most commonly in small animals, spontaneous hemoperitoneum is associated with rupture of intra-abdominal neoplasia (i.e., spleen, liver, or adrenal gland) (Whittemore *et al.* 2001; Aronsohn *et al.* 2009).

In one study, 75% of dogs with hemangiosarcoma presented with concurrent hemoperitoneum, and the presence of free abdominal blood was strongly associated with malignant cancer (Hammond & Pesillo-Crosby 2008). About 30% of these dogs had hemoperitoneum associated with benign disease (Hammond & Pesillo-Crosby 2008). Other reported etiologies of naturally occurring disease in dogs include anticoagulant rodenticide, organ malposition (i.e., liver lobe torsion, splenic torsion, mesenteric volvulus, or gastric dilatation/volvulus), gastrointestinal perforation, massive hepatic necrosis, and exercise-induced iliopsoas trauma in racing greyhounds (Brockman *et al.* 1995; Hardie *et al.* 1995; Neath *et al.* 1997; Sheafor & Couto 1999; Swann &

Cimino Brown 2001; Pintar *et al.* 2003; Beal *et al.* 2008; Hammond & Pesillo-Crosby 2008; Aronsohn *et al.* 2009; Morey-Matamalas *et al.* 2020; Kook *et al.* 2019). Recently, spontaneous hemoperitoneum was reported in a dog with severe anaphylaxis (Caldwell *et al.* 2018). The mechanisms are not completely elucidated, but believed to be multifactorial, secondary to coagulopathy, hyperfibrinolysis, and vasculitis.

Both blunt and penetrating abdominal trauma can result in hemoperitoneum. In dogs, motor vehicle accidents are the primary cause, with hemoperitoneum reported in 5–40% of cases (Mongil *et al.* 1995; Boysen *et al.* 2004; Simpson *et al.* 2009). Other less commonly reported etiologies in dogs include being hit by a train, being in a dog fight, and falling down stairs (Mongil *et al.* 1995). The spleen is the primary source of injury (58%), with damage to the liver (50%), kidneys (23%), or external iliac artery (8%) contributing to blood loss less frequently (Mongil *et al.* 1995). Iatrogenic intra-abdominal hemorrhage has also been reported in dogs and cats following renal and hepatic ultrasound-guided biopsy, especially in coagulopathic animals, and as a complication of surgery (Bigge *et al.* 2001).

Hemoperitoneum is rarely reported in cats, with an incidence of 0.3% (Mapstone *et al.* 2003; Culp *et al.* 2010). One study documented that the most common cause of naturally occurring hemoperitoneum in this species was rupture of hepatocellular neoplasia (carcinoma or mast cell tumor). However, a more recent investigation found that while 30 of 65 cats had neoplasia (in the spleen, most commonly), 35 cats had hemoperitoneum from nonneoplastic causes, including

Small Animal Soft Tissue Surgery, Second Edition. Edited by Eric Monnet.
© 2023 John Wiley & Sons, Inc. Published 2023 by John Wiley & Sons, Inc.
Companion website: www.wiley.com/go/monnet/small

coagulopathy (23%) and hepatic necrosis (23%) (Culp *et al.* 2010). Other documented etiologies include liver lobe torsion, hepatic amyloidosis, rupture of intestinal mast cell tumor, gastric or duodenal ulcer, splenic or urinary bladder lymphosarcoma, feline infectious peritonitis-induced liver rupture or nephritis, perinephric pseudocyst, and necrotic hemorrhagic cystitis (Knight & Kovak McClaran 2020; Mapstone *et al.* 2003; Culp *et al.* 2010).

Diagnosis

Clinical presentation

Historical findings are vague and nonspecific, and include anorexia, lethargy, weight loss, vomiting, abdominal discomfort, vocalizing, or collapse. Owners may report exercise intolerance, progressive abdominal distension, previous collapse episodes, recent trauma or surgery, or exposure to rodenticides. Breed predispositions for bleeding abdominal masses (golden retriever, Labrador) or splenic torsion (German shepherd) may aid in achieving a diagnosis (Aronsohn *et al.* 2009; Herold *et al.* 2008).

Triage physical examination may reveal signs of hypovolemic shock (i.e., dull mentation, prolonged capillary refill time, tachycardia or bradycardia, poor pulses, and hypothermia), recumbency, and abdominal distension or discomfort. Weakness, pallor, tachypnea, tachycardia, and hyperdynamic pulse quality characterize clinical anemia. Low systolic blood pressure (SBP) accompanies hypovolemic (and possibly hemorrhagic) shock. Recently, the shock index (SI) (heart rate/SBP) was demonstrated to be higher in dogs with hemorrhagic shock than in healthy dogs (Peterson *et al.* 2013). In this study, 20 of 38 dogs had shock secondary to a bleeding abdominal mass. An SI of >0.9 assisted in identifying bleeding patients.

Concurrent injuries occur in more than 80% of dogs with traumatic hemoperitoneum (Mongil *et al.* 1995; Boysen *et al.* 2004). Pulmonary contusions and pneumothorax are the most common associated injuries. Rib, long bone, and pelvic fractures, traumatic brain or spinal injury, proptosis, epistaxis, and skin lacerations are also reported (Mongil *et al.* 1995).

Physical examination is insensitive for diagnosis of abdominal injury, with false-positive and false-negative results reported in 6% and 59% of small animal patients, respectively (Crowe & Dewey 1994). In one review of feline hemoperitoneum, only 1 of 16 cats was suspected to have abdominal effusion on physical examination (Mapstone *et al.* 2003). In another, 28% of cats had abdominal distention and 8% had a palpable abdominal mass (Culp *et al.* 2010).

Definitive diagnosis requires retrieval and analysis of fluid from the abdominal cavity. Approximately 40 mL/kg of free intra-abdominal fluid is necessary for a palpable fluid wave (Crowe & Crane 1976). Ancillary diagnostic tests are therefore typically indicated.

Imaging

Various imaging modalities with increased sensitivity over physical examination, namely abdominal radiography, abdominal ultrasonography, and computed tomography (CT), can aid in fluid detection. Abdominal fluid is then retrieved for analysis via needle or catheter centesis or diagnostic peritoneal lavage (DPL).

Abdominal radiography

Abdominal radiography is a relatively insensitive test for the presence of abdominal effusion. Approximately 9 mL/kg of fluid must be present for detection, an amount that may take several hours to evolve (Henley *et al.* 1989). Poor serosal detail is reported in most cats with hemoperitoneum that undergo this test (Mapstone *et al.* 2003; Culp *et al.* 2010). In selected cases, abdominal radiography is also indicated to evaluate for an underlying cause, such as gastric dilatation volvulus or abdominal/retroperitoneal soft tissue mass effect.

Thoracic radiography is indicated in patients with trauma to evaluate for concurrent injuries and in patients with neoplasia to evaluate for metastasis.

Abdominal ultrasonography

Abdominal ultrasonography can confirm the presence of fluid in the abdominal cavity and aid in sample retrieval. Ultrasound can also be utilized to identify abnormalities of the abdominal viscera. Abdominal assessment with sonography for trauma (AFAST) has become standard of care in human emergency rooms (ERs), and is performed within minutes of triage to identify or exclude free intra-abdominal fluid. The advantages of AFAST include noninvasiveness, use of portable equipment, and rapidity/repeatability. Additionally, when performed by human emergency doctors with limited ultrasound experience, AFAST has sensitivities and specificities above 80% for detection of free fluid (Shackford *et al.* 1999; Boysen *et al.* 2004).

While a full abdominal ultrasound is likely indicated in all veterinary hemoperitoneum cases, AFAST is routinely incorporated into the initial evaluation of bleeding patients in the ER. For AFAST exam, patients are placed in lateral recumbency and transverse and longitudinal ultrasonographic views are obtained at four sites (caudal to the xiphoid process, at midline over the urinary bladder, and in the left and right flank regions)

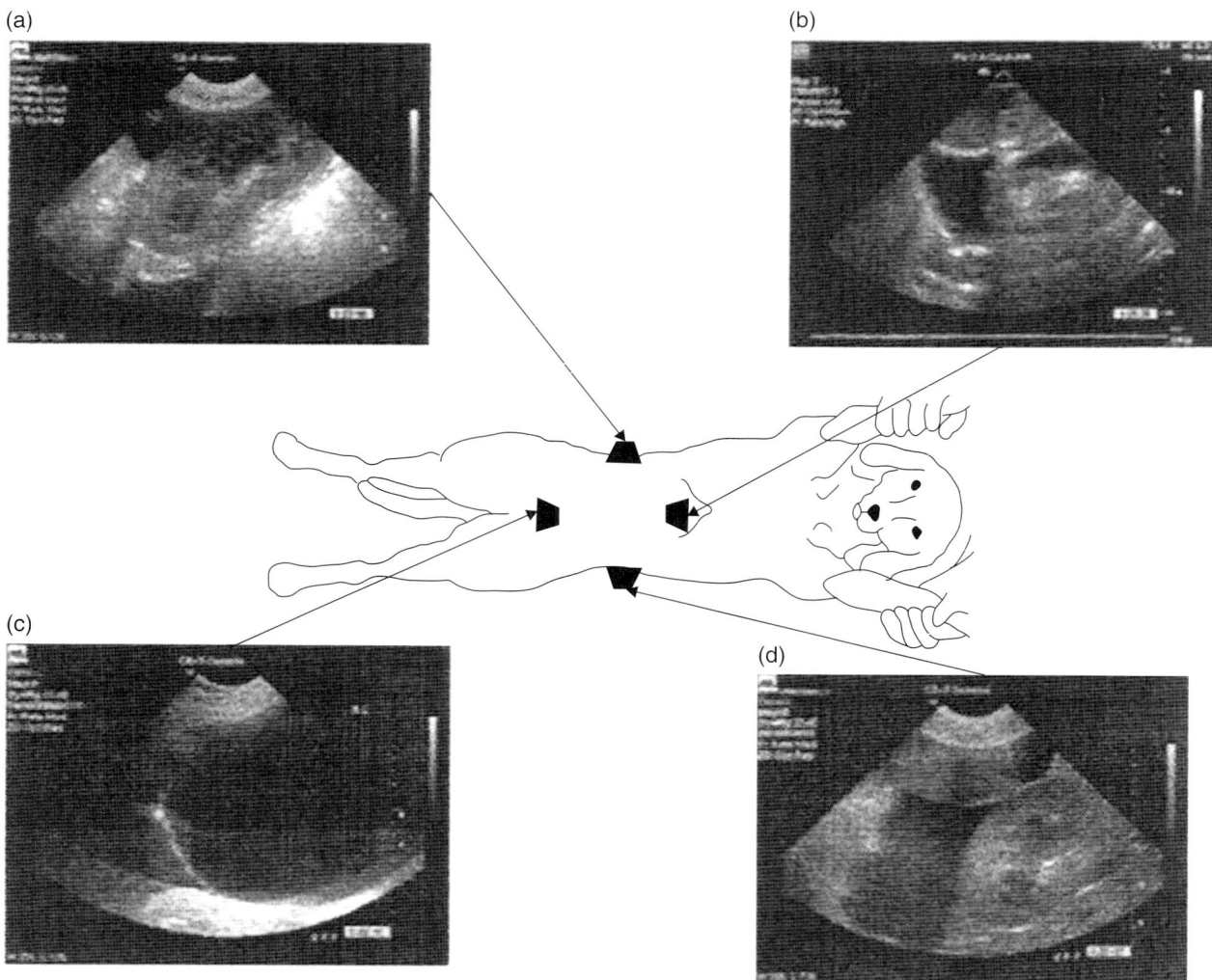

Figure 21.1 (a–d) Views obtained during FAST (focused assessment with sonography for trauma): right flank longitudinal, subxiphoid transverse, longitudinal midline over bladder, and left flank longitudinal. Source: From *Journal of Veterinary Emergency and Critical Care* (2008) 18:47.

(Figure 21.1). In dogs following motor vehicle trauma, AFAST was a simple, rapid, and efficacious means of diagnosing abdominal effusion. Median duration of AFAST exam was 6 minutes, and the most successful view for detection of free abdominal fluid was the gravity-dependent flank view (Boysen *et al.* 2004).

There are several limitations to AFAST, including lack of ultrasound equipment/expertise, cost, requirement for centesis to confirm abdominal fluid type, and limited ability of this modality to detect intestinal injury. False-negative results are predicted in human patients with concurrent pelvic or spinal injuries, subcutaneous emphysema, and obesity (Gaarder *et al.* 2009). Hemodynamic instability also reduces test sensitivity (Gaarder *et al.* 2009). In patients with hypotension, an initial negative FAST (focused assessment with sonography for trauma) exam cannot exclude intra-abdominal bleeding, and serial examinations are recommended.

Degree (and progression) of hemorrhage can be assessed by inclusion of an abdominal fluid score (AFS) into the AFAST examination. This has also been reported in dogs following motor vehicle trauma, utilizing a four-point system (AFS 1–4) to document fluid in one, two, three, or four quadrants, respectively (Lisciandro *et al.* 2009). In this population 27% of dogs were AFS positive; 6/27 (22%) were positive only on serial evaluation. A higher AFS predicted a greater packed cell volume (PCV) drop and need for blood transfusion.

Contrast enhanced ultrasonography (CEUS) has been described for use in humans and dogs for the detection of active abdominal hemorrhage. With this technique, ultrasonography is performed after injection of an advanced sonographic contrast agent. An experimental study using CEUS revealed active bleeding in traumatic splenic lesions, either as contrast medium extravasation or pooling in the spleen and outside the capsule (Lin *et al.* 2013). CEUS has also been used in a clinical case to diagnose active renal hemorrhage in a dog with kidney rupture (Gerboni *et al.* 2015).

Computed tomography and magnetic resonance imaging

In humans with suspected intra-abdominal hemorrhage, CT has been utilized to quantitate blood loss, grade severity of solid-organ injury, and assess patients as candidates for nonoperative management. Advantages of CT include ability to delineate retroperitoneal injuries and specificity for organ injury type and grade. Disadvantages include lack of availability of necessary equipment or personnel, expense, need for patient transport and general anesthesia, and risk associated with administration of ionic contrast agent (Block 1999). In human patients with hemoperitoneum, magnetic resonance imaging (MRI) offers no advantage over CT (Block 1999).

Recently, whole body CT utilization in dog and cat blunt polytrauma patients was investigated. This imaging modality was deemed safe and useful. One of 16 patients had abdominal fluid detected on CT that was not seen on AFAST (Dozeman *et al.* 2020). With CT angiography, extravasation of contrast medium is an indication of active hemorrhage and the "sentinel clot sign" (highest-attenuation hematoma adjacent to the bleeding organ) can be used to identify the organ that is bleeding (Specchi *et al.* 2017; Brooks *et al.* 2019)

Clinical pathology

Blood loss causes anemia and hypoproteinemia (or decreased total solids), and may result in a high anion gap metabolic acidosis and hyperlactatemia consistent with tissue hypoperfusion. Serial evaluation of patient hematocrit is warranted, as hemoconcentration from intravascular dehydration and splenic contraction initially increases measured hematocrit. A normal hematocrit with a concurrent decrease in total solids in a patient with compatible clinical signs is consistent with acute blood loss.

Assessment of patient coagulation status via coagulogram and/or viscoelastic testing (thromboelastography) is indicated if anticoagulant rodenticide toxicity or disseminated intravascular coagulation is suspected, in the face of ongoing bleeding, and when invasive procedures are planned. Hemoperitoneum is frequently accompanied by a hypocoagulable state and possibly hyperfibrinolysis.

Fluid retrieval and analysis

Two- or four-quadrant needle centesis (with 20- or 22-gauge needles) can be performed utilizing an open technique (no syringe) or a closed technique (attachment of a 1 or 3 mL syringe and application of mild negative pressure). An isolated report documented improved sensitivity utilizing the open compared with the closed technique (Crowe 1984). A "blind" tap is performed 2–3 cm to the right and caudal to the umbilicus with the patient in lateral recumbency.

A minimum of 5–6 mL/kg of free fluid must be present in the abdomen to obtain a sample using needle centesis, and the overall sensitivity of this test approximates 50% (Crowe 1984). False-positive results are associated with solid-organ or vessel penetration. Exacerbation of bleeding in coagulopathic patients, vessel laceration, introduction or spreading of infection (ruptured hollow viscus or penetration of intra-abdominal abscess or pyometra), and iatrogenic pneumoperitoneum are potential complications.

Methods of improving diagnostic yield include ultrasound-guided needle centesis, an over-the-needle catheter technique (utilizing a 16–20 gauge, 1.5–3 cm long catheter), and DPL. The over-the-needle technique has a sensitivity of 83%, and requires a minimum of 1–4.4 mL/kg of free fluid for diagnostic yield (Kolata 1976; Crowe 1984; Walters 2003). DPL has a reported 95% sensitivity, and can detect as little as 0.8 mL/kg of free fluid (Kolata 1976; Crowe 1984; Walters 2003). Larger catheter diameter and numerous side holes that increase surface area for contact with abdominal fluid account for the improved sensitivity of these latter two techniques. Additionally, lavage allows collection of a fluid sample that is more representative of all areas within the peritoneal cavity. Prior to the advent of AFAST, DPL was the gold-standard diagnostic modality in human trauma patients with hemodynamic instability or suspected hollow viscus perforation (Block 1999). Disadvantages of DPL include the need for sedation and/or local anesthesia, the possibility of overlooking retroperitoneal injuries, and complications like urinary bladder or intestinal perforation, laceration of solid organs or vessels, introduction of air or infection, subcutaneous leakage of lavage fluid, and hematoma formation. The techniques outlined are well described elsewhere (Kolata 1976; Crowe 1984; Walters 2003).

Cytology and fluid analysis, measurement of PCV, total protein, and biochemical tests are performed following fluid retrieval. A diagnosis of hemoperitoneum is made if the hemorrhagic fluid does not clot and has a PCV at least 25% that of peripheral blood. An exception to this rule is fluid obtained via DPL, for which a PCV above 2–5% signifies significant hemorrhage (Connally 2003). Clotting of blood in the fluid sample suggests inadvertent aspiration of the spleen, other abdominal organ, or blood vessel.

Cytologically, hemoperitoneum is typically classified as a modified transudate or exudate. The presence of erythrophagocytosis is suggestive of chronicity. Ancillary biochemical tests, including creatinine, potassium, and bilirubin, may be indicated in cases of traumatic hemoperitoneum to evaluate for concurrent injury to the urinary and biliary tracts. Comparison of abdominal fluid values with those of peripheral blood may provide definitive diagnoses in such cases (Connally 2003).

Emergency treatment

Choice of fluid to restore effective circulating fluid volume

The two primary initial goals of resuscitation in the bleeding patient are to restore ECFV and stop hemorrhage. Intravenous fluid administration is essential in this effort. However, ideal resuscitation fluid and appropriate resuscitation endpoints remain controversial.

Historically, large-volume resuscitation with isotonic crystalloids was the hallmark of human trauma care (Alam & Rhee 2007). In the last 50 years, many deleterious effects associated with this intervention have been elucidated, such as exacerbation of tissue edema (lung, gastrointestinal tract, and heart) and resultant organ hypoxia and dysfunction, and development of intra-abdominal hypertension. Additionally, aggressive fluid administration may disrupt blood clots, reduce blood viscosity, and dilute clotting factors, thereby exacerbating bleeding (Santry & Alam 2010).

Administration of synthetic colloids as an alternative or adjunct to isotonic crystalloids has several *theoretical* advantages, including the ability to maintain plasma oncotic pressure (thereby minimizing interstitial fluid extravasation), and the requirement of less volume and time to restore ECFV. In one veterinary study, incorporation of hydroxyethyl starch (HES) (with hypertonic saline [HTS]) to resuscitate clinical canine spontaneous hemoperitoneum patients resulted in faster stabilization of hemodynamic parameters than did resuscitation with large-volume isotonic crystalloid resuscitation (Hammond *et al.* 2014). Limited fluid volume resuscitation (LFVR) to normal endpoints may avoid the deleterious effects of fluid overload.

Synthetic colloids have historically been utilized for treatment of hypovolemic shock. However, superior efficacy (to isotonic crystalloids) is not evident, and use of these fluids in critically ill human patients has recently been scrutinized. Several human studies have discounted the previously touted volume-sparing effect afforded by synthetic colloids (Brunkhorst *et al.* 2008; Wiedermann & Joannidis 2014). Further, reported adverse effects are common, including anaphylactoid reactions, pruritus, and coagulation disorders (i.e., decreased platelet function and fibrin polymerization) (Cazzolli & Prittie 2015; Innerhofer *et al.* 2002). More recently, acute kidney injury in human patients with sepsis or septic shock has been described (Schortgen *et al.* 2001; Zarychanski *et al.* 2013). HES solutions are currently banned in the European market, and their use in septic patients is recommended against in the current Surviving Sepsis Campaign Guidelines (Cazzolli & Prittie 2015; Dellinger *et al.* 2013).

A single retrospective veterinary study demonstrated an increased risk of both kidney injury and death in dogs admitted to the intensive care unit (ICU) that received HES (Hayes *et al.* 2016). The clinical significance of these findings remains to be elucidated in larger prospective studies. Despite the recent data warning against the prolonged use of synthetic colloids (at higher doses), judicious and thoughtful administration of these fluids to veterinary shock patients (with possible avoidance in select populations such as those with sepsis or underlying kidney disease) remains standard of care in many practices. Balanced isotonic crystalloids and synthetic colloids are bolused in increments of 15–20 mL/kg and 5 mL/kg, respectively, to achieve and maintain desired resuscitation endpoints.

Both isotonic crystalloid and synthetic colloid solutions can potentiate hemorrhage-induced inflammation and immune modulation via increased expression of neutrophil adhesion molecules, facilitation of the neutrophil oxidative burst, and induction of apoptosis (Alam & Rhee 2007; Santry & Alam 2010). This "resuscitation injury," in addition to the adverse consequences of fluid overload, has sparked an interest in hypertonic fluid alternatives. Unlike other fluids, HTS results in downregulation of neutrophil function and inflammatory cytokine release, and attenuation of cellular injury (Alam & Rhee 2007; Santry & Alam 2010). Furthermore, the ability of HTS to rapidly increase ECFV after a small-volume infusion makes it an attractive fluid for incorporation into LFVR strategies.

A meta-analysis evaluating HTS as an initial treatment for people with hypovolemic shock demonstrated improved survival compared with conventional resuscitation, particularly in patients with more severe hypotension or traumatic brain injury (Wade *et al.* 1997). Other investigators have shown either no benefit or harm associated with its administration (Rotondo *et al.* 1993; Bulger *et al.* 2008). Complications from HTS include hypernatremia, hypokalemia, hyperchloremic metabolic acidosis, bleeding exacerbation, and cellular dehydration. When added to a LFVR protocol, a bolus of 2–4 mL/kg HTS (7.5% solution) can be administered concurrently with synthetic colloid or isotonic crystalloid fluids.

Methodology for emergency treatment

Cessation of ongoing bleeding remains central to successful resuscitation. Reestablishment of normotension before achieving hemorrhage control negatively impacts outcome in experimental animal studies (Kowalenko *et al.* 1992; Stern *et al.* 1993; Santry & Alam 2010). This is attributed to clot disruption and bleeding exacerbation from increased hydrostatic pressure. Withholding intravenous fluids until hemorrhage control is achieved reduces blood loss and improves outcome in experimental animal models and in specific human trauma populations (penetrating torso trauma) (Bickell *et al.* 1994; Holmes *et al.* 2002; Santry & Alam 2010). However, this approach is not universally accepted and is not currently a recommended standard of care for veterinary patients (Mandell & Drobatz 1993; Santry & Alam 2010).

Hypotensive resuscitation reduces acidemia, hemodilution, coagulopathy, apoptosis, and bleeding in experimental animals subjected to hemorrhage (Mandell & Drobatz 1993; Santry & Alam 2010). In a swine model, rebleeding following fluid resuscitation occurred at an average mean arterial pressure (MAP) of 64 mmHg and SBP of 94 mmHg (Sondeen *et al.* 2003). Human and animal studies have demonstrated that targeting MAPs between 40 and 60 mmHg or SBPs between 80 and 90 mmHg improves outcome compared with large-volume or delayed resuscitation (Sondeen *et al.* 2003; Lu *et al.* 2007; Santry & Alam 2010). An alternative approach in hemorrhagic shock is maintenance of a fixed predetermined fluid rate unlikely to achieve normotension (i.e., 60–80 mL/kg per hour) (Santry & Alam 2010). Either of these strategies is reasonable in the veterinary patient with hemoperitoneum. However, prolonged hypotension (>8 hours) will compromise vital organ perfusion and increase mortality and is inadvisable (Skarda *et al.* 2008; Santry & Alam 2010).

Endpoints of emergency treatment

Traditional endpoints of resuscitation for patients in hypovolemic shock include restoration of normal clinical perfusion parameters (i.e., mentation, capillary refill time, heart rate, pulse quality, and rectal temperature), blood pressure, and urine output. Additionally, normalization of blood lactate, base deficit, and central venous oxygen saturation are indicators of repaid oxygen debt.

In animals presenting with hemorrhagic shock from hemoperitoneum, vital organ perfusion must be restored while minimizing risk of further bleeding. Full shock reversal may be harmful in these patients. Hemorrhage triggers a series of compensatory mechanisms designed to reestablish normal tissue perfusion. Various hormone systems are activated that help to preserve blood flow via increased heart rate and contractility, peripheral vasoconstriction, water and sodium retention, and fluid shifts from the interstitium to the vasculature. In the absence of traumatic brain injury, goal-directed resuscitation (hypotensive and possibly limited volume) is currently recommended in human patients with hemorrhagic shock to augment these physiologic responses, targeting systolic and MAPs of 80–90 and 40–60 mmHg, respectively (Alam & Rhee 2007).

Asanguinous fluid alternatives

Emergency treatment of the bleeding patient may also include blood product administration, external counterpressure, and pharmacologic therapy. Blood components constitute an important therapy for hemoperitoneum patients. Fresh whole blood is the most effective fluid for hemorrhagic shock resuscitation, but is not readily available (Alam & Rhee 2007). Allogeneic red blood cell (RBC) transfusion augments oxygen-carrying capacity, and is indicated in hemoperitoneum patients with clinical signs referable to anemia. Bleeding animals with PCV below 25–30% are candidates for transfusion. Packed RBCs are warmed to room temperature, diluted with saline, and administered through an inline filter over a period of 4–6 hours with careful monitoring. Transfusion rate can be increased in patients with active life-threatening hemorrhage. An initial dose of 10 mL/kg is expected to increase patient PCV by 10% in the absence of ongoing blood loss. History of previous transfusion and confirmation of donor–recipient compatibility are necessary prior to transfusion. If transfusion is performed without donor–recipient compatibility testing, transfusion of blood from a dog erythrocyte antigen 1.1 negative donor is recommended (Herold *et al.* 2008). Adverse transfusion-related events include acute lung injury, immunosuppression, hypothermia, infectious disease transmission, allergy, and hemolysis.

Autotransfusion provides RBCs and replenishes intravascular volume in the bleeding patient, and may be considered during life-threatening hemorrhage when RBC products are not available. Blood is collected from the peritoneal cavity aseptically into sterile syringes via centesis or suctioned into sterile containers (intraoperatively) and reinfused into the patient via an inline filter. Anticoagulation is unnecessary, as blood is defibrinated when contact is made with the peritoneal surface. Techniques in canine and feline patients with hemoperitoneum have been described (Higgs *et al.* 2015; Robinson *et al.* 2016; Cole & Humm 2019). Advantages include lack of disease transmission or incompatibility, immediate availability, and decreased cost. Possible associated complications include hypocalcemia, hemolysis, and prolonged clotting times (Higgs *et al.* 2015). The concurrent presence of septic peritonitis is a contraindication.

Coagulopathy is a common complication of both naturally occurring and traumatic hemoperitoneum, and its etiology is multifactorial. Hypothermia results in altered platelet function and slowed kinetics of clotting factor enzymatic activity. Bleeding results in clotting factor consumption and thrombocytopenia, and aggressive fluid resuscitation and/or massive transfusion with RBC products dilute remaining factors and platelets. Animals with hemoperitoneum from trauma may additionally experience acute traumatic coagulopathy (ATC), postulated causes of which include initiation of the tissue factor pathway of coagulation from tissue damage and systemic inflammation, and hyperfibrinolysis resulting from endothelial injury (Hess *et al.* 2008; Palmer & Martin 2013). ATC is reported in 25% of human patients with active abdominal hemorrhage. These patients have coagulopathy at the time of presentation to the ER. This syndrome is rarely reported in veterinary patients (Brohi *et al.* 2003; Abelson *et al.* 2013; Gottlieb *et al.* 2017). One veterinary study failed to demonstrate hypocoagulability in 30 severely traumatized dogs, while another reported ATC in 1/18 dogs and 1/19 cats, respectively (Abelson *et al.* 2013; Gottlieb *et al.* 2017).

Coagulopathic human trauma patients transfused with fresh frozen plasma (FFP)/pRBC ratios of 1:1 or 1:2 demonstrate a survival advantage compared with patients receiving these products in a 1:4 ratio, and these higher ratios are now recommended (Duchesue *et al.* 2008; Santry & Alam 2010). Similar data are not available for veterinary patients. However, FFP transfusion (10–20 mL/kg) is indicated in the coagulopathic small animal patient with active abdominal bleeding and/or prior to invasive surgery. An experimental animal study demonstrated that administration of FFP not only early during blood volume restoration but also for an additional hour during continued hemorrhage without shock prevents reduction of clotting factors and may be beneficial in cessation of bleeding in the veterinary patient with hemoperitoneum (Ledgerwood & Lucas 2003).

Circumferential external counterpressure may be used in patients with hemoperitoneum to help achieve hemostasis. Pressure applied to the ventral abdomen from xiphoid to pubis utilizing layers of cotton roll and Elastikon® (Johnson & Johnson, New Brunswick, NJ, USA) may slow hemorrhage and increase blood pressure through several mechanisms: reduction of bleeding vessel radius and subsequent flow, production of a tamponade effect on bleeding abdominal organs, decreased size of the peritoneal space and hemorrhage volume, augmentation of venous return via fluid shifts, and increased cardiac afterload (McAnulty & Smith 1986). An experimental dog model of intra-abdominal hemorrhage evaluating abdominal wraps demonstrated that dogs with compressive bandaging had less of a decline in MAP and increased survival compared with unwrapped controls (McAnulty & Smith 1986). A similar survival advantage has not been demonstrated in human or veterinary patients. The use of counterpressure devices may result in increased intrathoracic, central venous, and intracranial pressures. Therefore, compressive bandaging may not be appropriate for animals with concurrent injuries including traumatic brain injury or respiratory distress from pulmonary contusions or pleural space disease. An additional consequence of external counterpressure is development of intra-abdominal hypertension and abdominal compartment syndrome, which may result in organ ischemia and dysfunction. Staged removal of the compressive wrap is advisable to avoid bleeding exacerbation and resultant hypotension. The wrap is loosened in a cranial to caudal direction at 15–30-minute intervals while carefully monitoring perfusion parameters. Shock recurrence requires reintroduction of resuscitative efforts and consideration of emergency surgery.

A number of pharmacologic agents have been evaluated as adjuncts to fluid resuscitation in patients with hemorrhagic shock. Drugs that impact coagulation include the anti-fibrinolytic agents tranexamic acid (TXA) and aminocaproic acid, and recombinant factor VIIa (Levi *et al.* 2005). The latter agent functions locally at the site of tissue injury or vascular wall disruption to activate the tissue factor pathway of coagulation and platelets. In humans, this drug has documented efficacy in control of life-threatening bleeding associated with hemophilia, thrombocytopathia, and severe trauma (Levi *et al.* 2005). The most serious potential adverse effect, aggravated systemic microvascular thrombosis, is reported infrequently (Levi *et al.* 2005). Lack of availability, potential antigenicity, and cost have precluded evaluation of recombinant factor VIIa in bleeding veterinary patients.

TXA and epsilon-aminocaproic acid (EACA) are antifibrinolytic agents. These drugs are lysine analogs, blocking lysine binding sites on plasminogen, thereby preventing its activation. This antiplasmin action results in reduced fibrinolysis and increased clot strength. A large, randomized controlled trial evaluating the use of TXA in human victims of trauma reported a reduction in death due to bleeding if the drug was administered within three hours of presentation (Roberts *et al.* 2013). There are a few veterinary studies evaluating TXA and EACA, with conflicting results. In an *in vitro* hyperfibrinolysis model using viscoelastic testing, TXA at varying dosages and routes improved clot strength and reduced fibrinolysis in healthy dog blood (Osekavage *et al.* 2018). Another investigation concluded that while administration of TXA to healthy dogs was safe, the drug's antifibrinolytic effects were unpredictable (Kelmer *et al.* 2015). The most common complication was vomiting, especially with higher doses. A retrospective review concluded that administration of EACA to dogs with hemoperitoneum did not reduce the need for packed RBC transfusion (Davis & Bracker 2016). Concurrent administration of Yunnan Baiyao and EACA to dogs bleeding from right atrial masses did not delay recurrence of clinical signs or extend survival (Murphy *et al.* 2017). However, aminocaproic acid administration to greyhounds undergoing gonadectomy did reduce prevalence of postoperative bleeding via improved clot strength (as measured via thromboelastography) (Marin *et al.* 2012). TXA or EACA can be considered in hemoperitoneum cases. Recommended dosages in dogs are 10–20 mg/kg and 15–40 mg/kg, respectively, intravenously three times a day (Kelmer *et al.* 2015; Marin *et al.* 2012). Data regarding use of antifibrinolytics in cats are lacking.

Sex steroids (estrogen), phosphodiesterase inhibitors (pentoxifylline), and opiate antagonists (naloxone) have been shown in experimental animal hemorrhagic shock models to reduce neutrophil activation, augment reticuloendothelial function, and limit oxidative tissue injury and apoptotic cell death (Santry & Alam 2010). The role of the histone deacetylase inhibitor valproic acid in hemorrhagic shock treatment has also been investigated (Li *et al.* 2008). Histone deacetylase inhibitors modulate histone proteins at the level of chromatin, altering gene transcription to create a "prosurvival" phenotype (Alam & Rhee 2007; Li *et al.* 2008; Santry & Alam 2010). In experimental animal shock models, valproic acid has been shown to protect neurons from hypoxia-induced apoptosis and improve survival, not from improved resuscitation but rather from better tolerance of shock by cells (Li *et al.* 2008).

Additional therapies

Concurrent life-threatening injuries following blunt trauma include airway obstruction, pleural space disease (pneumothorax, hemothorax, or diaphragmatic hernia), pulmonary or myocardial contusions, flail chest, and traumatic brain injury. Early recognition and prompt treatment of these comorbidities are essential. Provision of oxygen is recommended for all bleeding patients regardless of respiratory status to maximize oxygen-carrying capacity. Pain stimulates the sympathetic nervous system and magnifies the stress response; titration of reversible μ-agonist opioids can provide analgesia in painful animals. Ventricular arrhythmias may accompany hemoperitoneum from organic splenic disease, adrenal mass, gastric dilatation/volvulus, or trauma (among other causes). Continuous electrocardiogram monitoring in these patients is indicated for the first 24–48 hours. Hypothermia impairs vasoreactivity and blood clotting and rapid passive external rewarming targeting a temperature of 37.2 °C (99 °F) is recommended to prevent these complications. Fluid therapy following initial resuscitative efforts is individualized to replenish the interstitial fluid compartment, maintain normal plasma oncotic pressure and intravascular hydration, and provide oxygen-carrying capacity when indicated. Combinations of isotonic crystalloids, colloids, and blood products will meet those needs.

Shock and emergency treatment sequelae

Both the accumulation of a large volume of blood within the peritoneal cavity and high-volume fluid resuscitation place hemoperitoneum patients at risk for development of abdominal compartment syndrome. Attempts at external counterpressure exacerbate this risk. Compartment syndrome occurs when the pressure within a closed anatomic space increases to a point where vascular inflow is compromised, threatening the viability of tissues within that compartment (Cheatham 1999; Cheatham *et al.* 2007). Abdominal compartment syndrome is associated with increased intracranial pressure, acute kidney injury, impaired portal blood flow and splanchnic ischemia, hypoxemia, and decreased cardiac output (Cheatham 1999; Cheatham *et al.* 2007).

Massive transfusion – delivery of a blood transfusion volume that exceeds the patient's blood volume within 24 hours or half the patient's blood volume within 3 hours – is sometimes indicated in animals with hemoperitoneum. This intervention may lead to delayed wound healing, acute lung injury, and infectious disease transmission. People and dogs receiving massive transfusions have developed hypocalcemia from citrate chelation of calcium, which may cause tetany. Additionally, administration of blood products devoid of clotting factors and platelets can contribute to the development of a hypocoagulable state in these patients (Corazza & Hranchook 2000; Jutkowitz *et al.* 2002).

Both shock from hemorrhage and resuscitation efforts may lead to a potentially lethal triad of acidosis, hypothermia, and coagulopathy (the "triad of death"). Lactic acidosis and acidemia are well-recognized consequences of hemorrhagic shock, arising from persistent tissue hypoperfusion and a shift to anaerobic metabolism. Severe acidemia (arterial pH <7.2) results in cardiac arrhythmias, impaired inotropy and reduced cardiac output, and decreased systemic vascular resistance (Mitchell *et al.* 1972). Hypothermia may result from impaired thermoregulation and administration of unwarmed fluids or blood products and is an independent risk factor for death in human trauma patients (Ku *et al.* 1999). Hypothermia is exacerbated in surgical patients from anesthesia and opening of the peritoneal cavity. Adverse effects include cardiac arrhythmias, reduced cardiac output, impaired oxygen extraction from a left-shifted oxyhemoglobin saturation curve, and coagulopathy (Ku *et al.* 1999). In human patients, the triangle of death results in shock progression, cardiovascular collapse, and increased risk of death (Ku *et al.* 1999). Early recognition and treatment of this syndrome are paramount for a successful outcome. Reversal of cellular anaerobic metabolism via LFVR and administration of blood products, avoidance of hypothermia, and replenishment of clotting factors through plasma transfusion can all assist in this effort.

Surgical intervention

Nonoperative management of trauma-induced hemoperitoneum in human patients is usually possible (e.g., in more than 95% of pediatric cases), and is associated with decreased blood transfusion requirements, complication rate, and length of hospital stay, and improved outcome (Ozturk *et al.* 2004). Similarly, the majority of small animal patients suffering from traumatic hemoperitoneum can be successfully managed medically (Mongil *et al.* 1995). Progressive hemodynamic instability during emergency treatment or the need to transfuse more than half the patient's blood volume in the first 24 hours typically mandates laparotomy.

Indications for surgical management in patients with hemoperitoneum include progressive abdominal effusion with serial FAST examinations or a decreasing peripheral PCV concurrent with an increasing abdominal fluid PCV, pneumoperitoneum, septic or bile peritonitis, penetrating abdominal trauma, diaphragmatic or abdominal wall hernia, organ ischemia, and hemorrhage from an abdominal mass.

The goals of surgery are to arrest hemorrhage, remove ischemic or neoplastic tissue, and obtain a diagnosis. The patient and operating room should be prepared for surgery as much as possible before induction of anesthesia. Additional intravenous catheters may be placed in anticipation of transfusions or constant-rate infusions of vasopressors or anesthetic agents during surgery. Blood products, crystalloids, colloids, and emergency drugs should be readily available and dosages calculated so that institution of treatment can be provided rapidly if needed during surgery. The abdomen is clipped cranially to allow for the possibility of extension of the incision by caudal sternotomy, caudally to the pubis, and laterally to allow the creation of a paracostal incision. In patients with catastrophic hemorrhage, the surgeon should be gowned and gloved in the operating room preparing the instrument table while the patient is being induced and sterilely prepared for surgery.

The abdomen is entered quickly and blood can be immediately collected for autotransfusion if necessary. If the source of bleeding is known before surgery or is quickly identified on entering the abdomen, the surgeon's attention is immediately focused on that area. If bleeding is known to be associated with a previous surgery, all previously ligated vessels and pedicles are examined and additional ligatures applied. For patients with a bleeding splenic mass, the spleen can be exteriorized and removed rapidly by using multiple hemostats to double clamp the short gastric vessels, splenic artery and vein, and omental attachments. The spleen is removed by transecting the vessels between the clamps. Ligatures are applied to the vessels occluded by hemostats remaining in the abdomen after the spleen has been removed. Alternatively, stapling equipment (LDS stapler, US Surgical Corporation, Norwalk, CT, USA) or vessel sealant devices (LigaSure™, Covidian/Medtronic, Mansfield, MA, USA) can be used (Sirochman *et al.* 2020). Care should be taken to avoid the left limb of the pancreas when performing rapid ligation of the splenic vessels (Figure 21.2) (for a more detailed description of splenectomy, see Chapter 88). Evaluation for abdominal metastasis can be performed more safely after the hemorrhaging spleen has been removed.

If the source of hemorrhage is not known before surgery, the liver, spleen, kidneys, and adrenal glands are examined first, because these organs are the most common source of hemorrhage (Martin 1993; Herold *et al.* 2008). After initial examination of these organs, a thorough and systematic abdominal exploratory is performed. Laceration of organs may be controlled by application of hemostatic agents or omentum and digital pressure. If this is unsuccessful or for deeper lacerations, the bleeding area can be sutured with 3-0 to 5-0 monofilament absorbable suture material placed in a cruciate, mattress, or simple continuous pattern. For severely traumatized organs or neoplasia, partial or complete organ removal will be required.

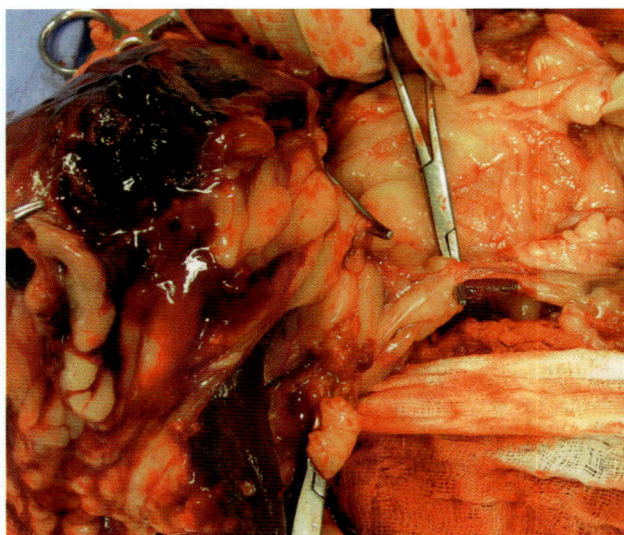

Figure 21.2 Intraoperative photograph of method for rapid splenectomy. Multiple hemostats have been used to double clamp the short gastric vessels and omental attachments. The spleen and associated mass are to the left of a hemostat that is placed between the splenic artery and vein. The proximity of the left limb of the pancreas is noted to the right of the hemostat.

If hemorrhage is ongoing, laparotomy sponges can be used to pack the abdomen in areas that are not being directly examined for hemorrhage. Temporary occlusion of major blood vessels may be helpful in identifying the source of bleeding and in slowing or arresting hemorrhage until definitive control is achieved. Atraumatic temporary occlusion can be accomplished with digital pressure, Satinsky tangential vascular clamps, Debakey bulldog clamps, or a Rumel tourniquet (Figure 21.3). The aorta can be occluded at the level of the celiac artery just cranial and medial to the left adrenal gland to control hemorrhage from the celiac artery caudally. The Pringle maneuver (occlusion of the hepatic artery, portal vein, and common bile duct as they course through the hepatoduodenal ligament in the epiploic foramen) may aid in slowing hemorrhage from the liver, but will not control hemorrhage from the hepatic veins or vena cava. The Pringle maneuver should not be performed for more than 10–20 minutes because of the risk of hepatic ischemia–reperfusion injury, portal hypertension, and bacterial translocation (Martin 1993). The hepatic artery, renal artery and vein, caudal vena cava (caudal to the liver), and abdominal aorta can be occluded for up to 30 minutes while preserving organ function (Herold et al. 2008).

In a minority (10%) of human trauma patients requiring surgical intervention, damage control surgery is recommended (Brasel & Weigelt 2000; Riddez et al. 2002). Patients with arterial pH below 7.2, body temperature under 35 °C, prothrombin or partial thromboplastin times more than twice normal, and those requiring massive transfusion in the ER are potential candidates. The most common indication for damage control surgery is the development of a coagulopathy that is resistant to blood component therapy (Brasel et al. 1999). Shock and hypothermia must be aggressively treated in these patients to correct coagulopathy. Other indications for damage control surgery include inaccessible major venous injury, anticipated need for a lengthy procedure, inability to approximate the abdominal wall fascia, and desire to serially evaluate abdominal contents (Brasel et al. 1999). Damage control involves a two-stage approach to the treatment of severe trauma. Stage 1 is an abbreviated surgical exploration with the goals of arresting hemorrhage and controlling contamination. This is followed by temporary abdominal closure and continued resuscitative efforts in the ICU. Definitive surgery and closure (stage 2) are delayed 24–72 hours and proceed with improved patient condition. Complications of damage control surgery include missed injuries and ongoing bleeding, abdominal compartment syndrome, and sepsis (Brasel et al. 1999). Additionally, damage control surgery is a risk factor for increased transfusion requirements, multiple organ failure, and death (Nicholas et al. 2003). Temporary abdominal packing has been described for the management of three dogs with persistent hemorrhage after liver lobectomy (Evans et al. 2019). For this technique, a sterile polyethylene sheet was placed over the bleeding sites and three 4×8 gauze sponges and five laparotomy sponges were placed over the sheet and conformed to the bleeding liver lobes. The abdomen was closed and a second laparotomy was planned within 24–72 hours. The technique was successful for controlling bleeding in all three patients, but only one dog survived to discharge. This technique should only be considered when surgical hemostasis cannot be achieved in unstable patients not able to tolerate prolonged anesthesia.

Prognosis

The short-term prognosis for small animal patients with hemoperitoneum depends on rapid diagnosis, support of ECFV and vital organ perfusion with limited-volume fluid resuscitation and blood product administration, control of bleeding, and surgical readiness when indicated. Long-term prognosis is dependent on underlying etiology. Dogs with traumatic hemoperitoneum have reported overall mortality rates of 6–27% (Mongil et al. 1995; Boysen et al. 2004). Outcome for small animals with naturally occurring disease is variable, but one study showed that surgical treatment of hemoperitoneum,

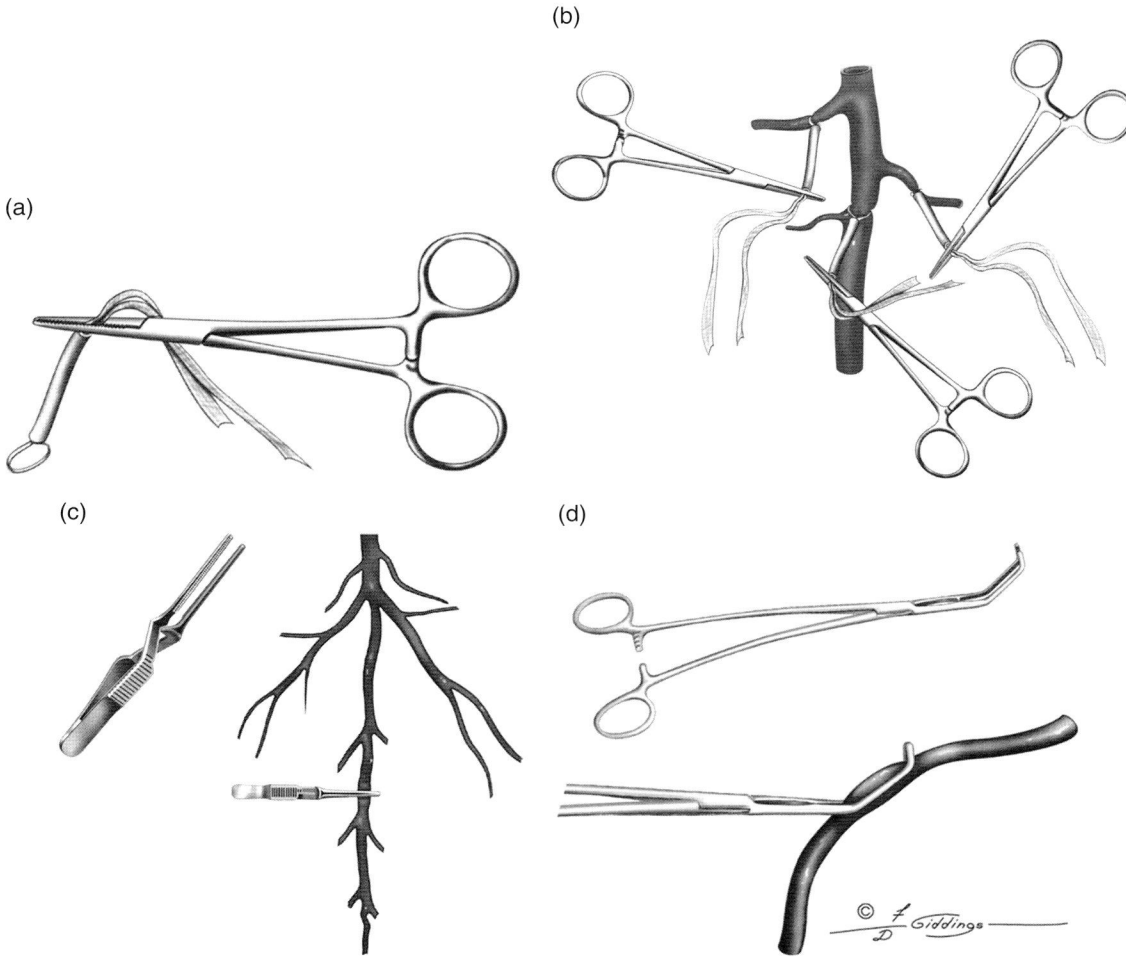

(b)

(a)

(c)

(d)

© D. Giddings

Figure 21.3 (a) Rumel tourniquet. Cotton umbilical tape is placed around the vessel to be occluded and the free ends of the tape are drawn through a short piece of rubber tubing. (b) The vessel is occluded by sliding the rubber tubing down the umbilical tape and applying a hemostat to the ends of the tape. (c) Debakey bulldog clamp. (d) Satinsky vascular clamp. © D. Giddings.

regardless of etiology, resulted in 84% of dogs being discharged from the hospital (Lux *et al.* 2013). Factors associated with death included tachycardia, a massive transfusion with blood products, bicavitary effusion, and severe respiratory disease believed to be related to pulmonary thromboembolism or acute respiratory distress syndrome.

References

Abelson, A.L., O'Toole, T.E., Johnston, A. et al. (2013). Hypoperfusion and acute traumatic coagulopathy in severely traumatized canine patients. *Journal of Veterinary Emergency and Critical Care* 23: 395–401.

Alam, H.B. and Rhee, P. (2007). New developments in fluid resuscitation. *Surgical Clinics of North America* 78: 55–72.

Aronsohn, M.G., Dubiel, B., Roberts, B., and Powers, B.E. (2009). Prognosis for acute nontraumatic hemoperitoneum in the dog: a retrospective analysis of 60 cases (2003–2006). *Journal of the American Animal Hospital Association* 45: 72–77.

Beal, M.W., Doherty, A.M., and Curcio, K. (2008). Peliosis hepatis and hemoperitoneum in a dog with diphacinone intoxication. *Journal of Veterinary Emergency and Critical Care* 18: 388–392.

Bickell, W.H., Wall, M.J. Jr., Pepe, P.E. et al. (1994). Immediate versus delayed resuscitation for hypotensive patients with penetrating torso injuries. *New England Journal of Medicine* 331: 1105–1109.

Bigge, L.A., Brown, D.J., and Penninck, D.G. (2001). Correlation between coagulation profile findings and bleeding complications after ultrasound-guided biopsies: 434 cases (1993–1996). *Journal of the American Animal Hospital Association* 37: 228–233.

Block, E.F.J. (1999). Diagnostic modalities in acute trauma. *New Horizons: The Science and Practice of Acute Medicine* 7: 10–25.

Boysen, S.R., Rozanski, E.A., Tidwell, A.S. et al. (2004). Evaluation of a focussed assessment with sonography for trauma protocol to detect free abdominal fluid in dogs involved in motor vehicle accidents. *Journal of the American Veterinary Medical Association* 225: 1198–1204.

Brasel, K.J. and Weigelt, J.A. (2000). Damage control in trauma surgery. *Current Opinion in Critical Care* 6: 276–280.

Brasel, K.J., Ku, J., Baker, C.C. et al. (1999). Damage control in the critically ill and injured patient. *New Horizons: The Science and Practice of Acute Medicine* 7: 73–86.

Brockman, D.J., Washabau, R.J., and Drobatz, K.J. (1995). Canine gastric dilatation/volvulus syndrome in a veterinary critical care unit: 295 cases (1986–1992). *Journal of the American Veterinary Medical Association* 207: 460–464.

Brohi, S., Singh, J., Heron, M., and Coats, T. (2003). Acute traumatic coagulopathy. *Journal of Trauma* 54: 1127–1130.

Brooks, J.J., Oliveira, C.R., McHenry, K.M. et al. (2019). What is your diagnosis. *Journal of the American Veterinary Medical Association* 254: 203–205.

Brunkhorst, F.M., Engel, C., Bloos, F. et al. (2008). Intensive insulin therapy and pentastarch resuscitation in severe sepsis. *New England Journal of Medicine* 358: 125–139.

Bulger, E.M., Jurkovich, G.J., Nathens, A.B. et al. (2008). Hypertonic resuscitation of hypovolemic shock after blunt trauma: a randomized controlled trial. *Archives of Surgery* 143: 139–148.

Caldwell, D.J., Petras, K.E., Mattison, B.L. et al. (2018). Spontaneous hemoperitoneum and anaphylactic shock associated with hymenoptera envenomation in a dog. *Journal of Veterinary Emergency and Critical Care* 19: 476–482.

Cazzolli, D. and Prittie, J. (2015). The crystalloid-colloid debate: consequences of resuscitation fluid selection in veterinary critical care. *Journal of Veterinary Emergency and Critical Care* 25: 6–19.

Cheatham, M.L. (1999). Intra-abdominal hypertension and abdominal compartment syndrome. *New Horizons: The Science and Practice of Acute Medicine* 7: 96–115.

Cheatham, M.L., Malbrain, M.L.N.G., Kirkpatrick, A. et al. (2007). Results from the international conference of experts on intra-abdominal hypertension and abdominal compartment syndrome. II recommendations. *Intensive Care Medicine* 33: 951–962.

Cole, L.P. and Humm, K. (2019). Twelve autologous blood transfusions in eight cats with haemoperitoneum. *Journal of Feline Medicine and Surgery* 21: 481–487.

Connally, H.E. (2003). Cytology and fluid analysis of the acute abdomen. *Clinical Techniques in Small Animal Practice* 18: 39–44.

Corazza, M.L. and Hranchook, A.M. (2000). Massive blood transfusion therapy. *AANA Journal* 68: 311–314.

Crowe, D.T. (1984). Diagnostic abdominal paracentesis techniques: clinical evaluation in 129 dogs and cats. *Journal of the American Animal Hospital Association* 20: 223–230.

Crowe, D.T. and Crane, S.W. (1976). Diagnostic abdominal paracentesis and lavage in the evaluation of abdominal injuries in dogs and cats: clinical and experimental investigations. *Journal of the American Veterinary Medical Association* 168: 700–705.

Crowe, D.T. and Dewey, J.J. (1994). Assessment and management of the hemorrhaging patient. *Veterinary Clinics of North America: Small Animal Practice* 24: 434–461.

Culp, W.T.N., Weisse, C., Kellogg, M.E. et al. (2010). Spontaneous hemoperitoneum in cats: 65 cases (1994–2006). *Journal of the American Veterinary Medical Association* 236: 978–982.

Davis, M. and Bracker, K. (2016). Retrospective study of 122 dogs that were treated with the antifibrinolytic drug aminocaproic acid: 2010–2012. *Journal of the American Animal Hospital Association* 52: 144–148.

Dellinger, R.P., Levy, M.M., Rhodes, A. et al. (2013). Surviving sepsis campaign: international guidelines for management of severe sepsis and septic shock: 2012. *Critical Care Medicine* 41: 580–637.

Dozeman, E.T., Prittie, J.P., and Fischetti, A.J. (2020). Utilization of whole body computed tomography in polytrauma patients. *Journal of Veterinary Emergency and Critical Care* 30: 28–33.

Duchesue, J.C., Hunt, J.P., Wahl, G. et al. (2008). Review of current blood transfusion strategies in a mature level 1 trauma center: were we wrong for the last 60 years? *Journal of Trauma* 65: 272–276.

Evans, N.A., Hardie, R.J., Walker, J. et al. (2019). Temporary abdominal packing for management of persistent hemorrhage after liver lobectomy in three dogs with hepatic neoplasia. *Journal of Veterinary Emergency and Critical Care* 29: 535–541.

Gaarder, C., Kroepelien, C.F., Loekke, R. et al. (2009). Ultrasound performed by radiologists: confirming the truth about FAST in trauma. *Journal of Trauma* 67: 323–329.

Gerboni, G.M., Capra, G., Ferro, S. et al. (2015). The use of contrast-enhanced ultrasonography for the detection of active renal hemorrhage in a dog with spontaneous kidney rupture resulting in hemoperitoneum. *Journal of Veterinary Emergency and Critical Care* 25: 751–758.

Gottlieb, D.L., Prittie, J., Buriko, Y. et al. (2017). Evaluation of acute traumatic coagulopathy in dogs and cats following blunt force trauma. *Journal of Veterinary Emergency and Critical Care* 27: 35–43.

Hammond, T.N. and Pesillo-Crosby, S.A. (2008). Prevalence of hemangiosarcoma in anemic dogs with a splenic mass and hemoperitoneum requiring a transfusion: 71 cases (2003–2005). *Journal of the American Veterinary Medical Association* 232: 553–558.

Hammond, T.N., Holm, J.L., and Sharp, C.R. (2014). A pilot study of limited versus large fluid volume resuscitation in canine spontaneous hemoperitoneum. *Journal of the American Animal Hospital Association* 50: 159–166.

Hardie, E.M., Vaden, S.L., Spaulding, K., and Malarkey, D.E. (1995). Splenic infarction in 16 dogs: a retrospective study. *Journal of Veterinary Internal Medicine* 9: 141–148.

Hayes, G., Benedicenti, L., and Mathews, K. (2016). Retrospective cohort study on the incidence of acute kidney injury and death following hydroxyethyl starch (HES 10% 250/0.5/5:1) administration in dogs (2007–2010). *Journal of Veterinary Emergency and Critical Care* 26: 35–40.

Henley, R.K., Hager, D.A., and Ackerman, N.A. (1989). A comparison of two-dimensional ultrasonography and radiography for the detection of small amounts of free peritoneal fluid in the dog. *Veterinary Radiology* 30: 121–124.

Herold, L.V., Devey, J.J., Kirby, R., and Rudloff, E. (2008). Clinical evaluation and management of hemoperitoneum in dogs. *Journal of Veterinary Emergency and Critical Care* 18: 40–53.

Hess, J.R., Brohi, K., and Dutton, R.P. (2008). The coagulopathy of trauma: a review of mechanisms. *Journal of Trauma* 65: 748–754.

Higgs, V.A., Rudloff, E., Kirby, R. et al. (2015). Autologous blood transfusion in dogs with thoracic or abdominal hemorrhage: 25 cases (2007–2012). *Journal of Veterinary Emergency and Critical Care* 25: 731–738.

Holmes, J.F., Sakles, J.C., Lewis, G., and Wisner, D.H. (2002). Effects of delaying fluid resuscitation on an injury to the systemic arterial vasculature. *Academic Emergency Medicine* 9: 267–274.

Innerhofer, P., Fries, D., Margreiter, J. et al. (2002). The effects of perioperatively administered colloids and crystalloids on primary platelet-mediated hemostasis and clot formation. *Anesthesia and Analgesia* 95: 858–865.

Jutkowitz, L.A., Rozanski, E.A., Moreau, J.A., and Rush, J.E. (2002). Massive transfusion in dogs: 15 cases (1997–2001). *Journal of the American Veterinary Medical Association* 220: 1664–1669.

Kelmer, E., Segev, G., Papashvilli, V. et al. (2015). Effects of intravenous administration of tranexamic acid on hematological, hemostatic, and thromboelastographic analytes in healthy adult dogs. *Journal of Veterinary Emergency and Critical Care* 25: 495–501.

Knight, R. and Kovak McClaran, J. (2020). Hemoperitoneum secondary to liver lobe torsion in a cat. *Journal of the American Animal Hospital Association* 56: e56102.

Kolata, R.J. (1976). Diagnostic abdominal paracentesis and lavage: experimental and clinical evaluations in the dog. *Journal of the American Veterinary Medical Association* 168: 697–699.

Kook, P.H., Baumstark, M., and Ruetten, M. (2019). Clinical and histologic outcome in a dog surviving massive hepatic necrosis. *Journal of Veterinary Internal Medicine* 33: 879–884.

Kowalenko, T., Stern, S., Dronen, S., and Wang, X. (1992). Improved outcome with hypotensive resuscitation of uncontrolled hemorrhagic shock in a swine model. *Journal of Trauma* 33: 349–353.

Ku, J., Brasel, K.J., Baker, C.C. et al. (1999). Triangle of death: hypothermia, acidosis, and coagulopathy. *New Horizons: The Science and Practice of Acute Medicine* 7: 61–72.

Ledgerwood, A.M. and Lucas, C.E. (2003). A review of studies on the effects of hemorrhagic shock and resuscitation on the coagulation profile. *Journal of Trauma* 54: S68–S74.

Levi, M., Peters, M., and Buller, H.R. (2005). Efficacy and safety of recombinant factor VIIa for treatment of severe bleeding: a systematic review. *Critical Care Medicine* 33: 883–890.

Li, Y., Liu, B., Sailhamer, E.A. et al. (2008). Cell protective mechanism of valproic acid in lethal hemorrhagic shock. *Surgery* 144: 217–224.

Lin, Q., Luo, Y., Song, Q. et al. (2013). Contrast-enhanced ultrasound for detection of traumatic splenic bleeding in a canine model during hemorrhagic shock and resuscitation. *Journal of Medical Ultrasound* 21: 207–212.

Lisciandro, G.R., Lagutchik, M.S., Mann, K.A. et al. (2009). Evaluation of an abdominal fluid scoring system determined using abdominal focused assessment with sonography for trauma in 101 dogs with motor vehicle trauma. *Journal of Veterinary Emergency and Critical Care* 19: 426–437.

Lu, Y.Q., Cai, X.J., Gu, L.H. et al. (2007). Experimental study of controlled fluid resuscitation in the treatment of severe and uncontrolled hemorrhagic shock. *Journal of Trauma* 63: 798–804.

Lux, C.N., Culp, W.T.N., Mayhew, P.D. et al. (2013). Perioperative outcome in dogs with hemoperitoneum: 83 cases (2005–2010). *Journal of the American Veterinary Medical Association* 242: 1385–1391.

Mandell, D.C. and Drobatz, K.J. (1993). Feline hemoperitoneum: 16 cases (1986–1993). *Journal of Veterinary Emergency and Critical Care* 5: 93–97.

Mapstone, J., Roberts, I., and Evans, P. (2003). Fluid resuscitation strategies: a systematic review of animal trials. *Journal of Trauma* 55: 571–589.

Marin, L., Iazbik, M., Zaldivar-Lopez, S. et al. (2012). Epsilon aminocaproic acid for the prevention of delayed postoperative bleeding in retired racing greyhounds undergoing gonadectomy. *Veterinary Surgery* 41: 594–603.

Martin, R.A. (1993). Liver and biliary system. In: *Textbook of Small Animal Surgery* (ed. D.H. Slatter), 708–709. Philadelphia, PA: WB Saunders.

McAnulty, J.F. and Smith, G.K. (1986). Circumferential external counterpressure by abdominal wrapping and its effect on simulated intraabdominal hemorrhage. *Veterinary Surgery* 15: 270–274.

Mitchell, J.H., Wildenthal, K., and Johnson, R.L. Jr. (1972). The effects of acid–base disturbances on cardiovascular and pulmonary function. *Kidney International* 1: 375–389.

Mongil, C.M., Drobatz, K.J., and Hendricks, J.C. (1995). Traumatic hemoperitoneum in 28 cases: a retrospective review. *Journal of the American Animal Hospital Association* 31: 217–222.

Morey-Matamalas, A., Corbetta, D., Waine, K. et al. (2020). Exercise-induced acute abdominal haemorrhage due to iliopsoas trauma in racing greyhounds. *Journal of Comparative Pathology* 177: 42–46.

Murphy, L.A., Panek, C.M., Bianco, D. et al. (2017). Use of Yunnan Baiyo and epsilon aminocaproic acid in dogs with right atrial masses and pericardial effusion. *Journal of Veterinary Emergency and Critical Care* 27: 121–126.

Neath, P.J., Brockman, D.J., and Saunders, H.M. (1997). Retrospective analysis of 19 cases of isolated torsion of the splenic pedicle in dogs. *Journal of Small Animal Practice* 38: 387–392.

Nicholas, J.M., Rix, E.P., Easley, K.A. et al. (2003). Changing patterns in the management of penetrating abdominal trauma: the more things change, the more they stay the same. *Journal of Trauma* 55: 1095–1110.

Osekavage, K., Brainard, B., Lane, S. et al. (2018). Pharmacokinetics of tranexamic acid in healthy dogs and assessment of its antifibrinolytic properties in canine blood. *American Journal of Veterinary Research* 79: 1057–1063.

Ozturk, H., Dokucu, A.I., Onen, A. et al. (2004). Nonoperative management of isolated solid organ injuries due to blunt trauma in children: a fifteen-year experience. *European Journal of Pediatric Surgery* 14: 29–34.

Palmer, L. and Martin, L. (2013). Traumatic coagulopathy—part 1: pathophysiology and diagnosis. *Journal of Emergency and Critical Care* 24: 63–74.

Peterson, K.L., Hardy, B.T., and Hall, K. (2013). Assessment of shock index in healthy dogs and dogs with hemorrhagic shock. *Journal of Veterinary Emergency and Critical Care* 23: 545–550.

Pintar, J., Breitschwerdt, E.B., Hardie, E.M., and Spaulding, K.A. (2003). Acute nontraumatic hemoabdomen in the dog: a retrospective analysis of 39 cases (1987–2001). *Journal of the American Animal Hospital Association* 39: 518–522.

Riddez, L., Drobin, D., Sjöstrand, F. et al. (2002). Lower dose of HTS dextran reduces the risk of lethal rebleeding in uncontrolled hemorrhage. *Shock* 17: 377–382.

Roberts, I., Shakur, H., Coats, T. et al. (2013). The CRASH-2 trial: a randomized controlled trial and economic evaluation of the effects of tranexamic acid on death, vascular occlusive events and transfusion requirement in bleeding trauma patients. *Health Technology Assessment* 17: 1–79.

Robinson, D.A., Kiefer, K., Bassett, R. et al. (2016). Autotransfusion in dogs using a 2-syringe technique. *Journal of Veterinary Emergency and Critical Care* 26: 766–774.

Rotondo, M.F., Schwab, C.W., McGonigal, M.D. et al. (1993). "Damage control": an approach for improved survival in exsanguinating penetrating abdominal injury. *Journal of Trauma* 35: 375–382.

Santry, H.P. and Alam, H.B. (2010). Fluid resuscitation: past, present, and the future. *Shock* 33: 229–241.

Schortgen, R., Lacherade, J.C., Bruneel, F. et al. (2001). Effects of hydroxyethyl starch and gelatin on renal function in severe sepsis: a multicenter randomized study. *Lancet* 357: 911–916.

Shackford, S.R., Rogers, F.B., Osler, T.M. et al. (1999). Focussed abdominal sonogram for trauma: the learning curve of nonradiologist clinicians in detecting hemoperitoneum. *Journal of Trauma* 46: 553–564.

Sheafor, S.E. and Couto, C.G. (1999). Anticoagulant rodenticide toxicity in 21 dogs. *Journal of the American Animal Hospital Association* 35: 38–46.

Simpson, S.A., Syring, R., and Otto, C.M. (2009). Severe blunt trauma in dogs: 235 cases (1997–2003). *Journal of Veterinary Emergency and Critical Care* 19: 588–602.

Sirochman, A.L., Milovancev, M., Townsend, K. et al. (2020). Influence of use of a bipolar vessel sealing device on short-term postoperative mortality after splenectomy: 203 dogs (2005–2018). *Veterinary Surgery* 49: 291–303.

Skarda, D.E., Mulier, K.E., George, M.E., and Bellman, G.J. (2008). Eight hours of hypotensive versus normotensive resuscitation in a porcine model of uncontrolled hemorrhagic shock. *Academic Emergency Medicine* 15: 845–852.

Sondeen, J.L., Coppes, V.G., and Holcomb, J.B. (2003). Blood pressure at which rebleeding occurs after resuscitation in swine with aortic injury. *Journal of Trauma* 54: S110–S117.

Specchi, S., Auriemma, E., Morabito, S. et al. (2017). Evaluation of the computed tomographic "sentinel clot sign" to identify bleeding abdominal organs in dogs with hemoabdomen. *Veterinary Radiology and Ultrasound* 58: 18–22.

Stern, S.A., Dronen, S.C., Birrer, P., and Wang, X. (1993). Effect of blood pressure on hemorrhage volume and survival in a near-fatal hemorrhage model incorporating a vascular injury. *Annals of Emergency Medicine* 22: 155–163.

Swann, H.M. and Cimino Brown, D. (2001). Hepatic lobe torsion in 3 dogs and a cat. *Veterinary Surgery* 30: 482–486.

Wade, C.E., Kramer, G.C., Grady, J.J. et al. (1997). Efficacy of hypertonic 7.5% saline and 6% dextran-70 in treating trauma: a meta-analysis of controlled clinical studies. *Surgery* 122: 609–616.

Walters, J.M. (2003). Abdominal paracentesis and diagnostic peritoneal lavage. *Clinical Techniques in Small Animal Practice* 18: 32–38.

Whittemore, J.C., Preston, C.A., Kyles, A.E. et al. (2001). Nontraumatic rupture of an adrenal gland tumor causing intra-abdominal or retroperitoneal hemorrhage in four dogs. *Journal of the American Veterinary Medical Association* 219: 329–333.

Wiedermann, C.J. and Joannidis, M. (2014). Accumulation of hydroxyethyl starch in human and animal tissues: a systematic review. *Intensive Care Medicine* 40: 160–170.

Zarychanski, R., Abou-Setta, A.M., Turgeon, A.F. et al. (2013). Association of hydroxyethyl starch administration with mortality and acute kidney injury in critically ill patients requiring volume resuscitation: a systematic review and meta-analysis. *Journal of the American Medical Association* 309: 678–688.

22

Pneumoperitoneum

Jennifer Prittie and Lori Ludwig

Pneumoperitoneum refers to the presence of free air within the peritoneal cavity. This syndrome may be spontaneous or traumatic in origin, is typically readily diagnosed via survey radiography, and, in most situations, necessitates immediate abdominal exploration. Prognosis is variable and dependent on underlying etiology, comorbidities, and treatment.

Etiology

In both human and veterinary patients, recent abdominal surgery is a common reason for detection of free air within the peritoneal cavity (Mezghebe *et al.* 1994; Lykken *et al.* 2003). The severity of air accumulation is dependent on the total volume present at the time of surgical closure. The reported durations of postoperative pneumoperitoneum in humans and dogs are 28 and 34 days, respectively (Samuel *et al.* 1963; Probst *et al.* 1986). This condition is typically benign and self-limiting, and warrants no intervention.

In human patients, underlying causes of pathologic pneumoperitoneum are spontaneous (associated with severe disease of the gastrointestinal, respiratory, or urogenital tracts) or traumatic (penetrating gunshot or knife wounds, traumatic pneumothorax with diaphragmatic herniation, positive-pressure ventilation, or peritoneal dialysis) (Hillman 1982). Perforation of a hollow viscus (most often the gastrointestinal tract) accounts for over 90% of pneumoperitoneum cases in human patients (Hillman 1982; Mezghebe *et al.* 1994).

Both spontaneous (64%) and traumatic (36%) pneumoperitoneum cases have been reported in dogs and cats (Saunders & Tobias 2003). As with humans, perforation of the gastrointestinal tract accounts for the majority (74–77%) of pneumoperitoneum cases in small animal patients, and approximately 30% of spontaneous gastrointestinal perforations are associated with gastrointestinal neoplasia (Saunders & Tobias 2003; Smelstoys *et al.* 2004; Mellanby *et al.* 2002). Spontaneous rupture of the gastrointestinal tract and associated free abdominal air has also been reported in association with gastric dilatation and volvulus (i.e., splenic necrosis and infection with a gas-producing organism, gastric necrosis, and leakage of gas through an intact distended stomach wall) and gastrointestinal ulceration (Wong 1981; Probst *et al.* 1984; Hinton *et al.* 2002; Saunders & Tobias 2003; Smelstoys *et al.* 2004; Mellanby *et al.* 2002; Simpson 2010). Diseases associated with gastrointestinal ulceration in small animals include:

- Gastrointestinal neoplasia, i.e., mast cell tumor or gastrinoma (dog)
- Inflammatory bowel disease
- Intestinal parasitism
- Intestinal foreign body
- Severe hepatic disease
- Uremia
- Polytrauma
- Shock
- Toxicity (i.e., cholecalciferol)
- Endocrinopathy (i.e., hypoadrenocorticism)
- Concurrent use of glucocorticoids and nonsteroidal anti-inflammatory drugs (NSAIDs).

Additional risk factors for NSAID-associated gastrointestinal ulceration are increasing age, dose and duration of administration, neurologic disease, and shock

Small Animal Soft Tissue Surgery, Second Edition. Edited by Eric Monnet.
© 2023 John Wiley & Sons, Inc. Published 2023 by John Wiley & Sons, Inc.
Companion website: www.wiley.com/go/monnet/small

(Godshalk *et al.* 1992; Jones *et al.* 1992; Schenck *et al.* 2006; Simpson 2010).

Idiopathic gastrointestinal perforation is an additional cause of spontaneous pneumoperitoneum in small animals, with a reported incidence of 4–32% (Saunders & Tobias 2003; Smelstoys *et al.* 2004; Itoh *et al.* 2005). Perforations have been observed in the stomach, duodenum, and ileum of affected small animal patients, with no evidence of histopathologic *in situ* disease. Disruption of the urinary conduit, a ruptured splenic abscess, and leakage of air into the peritoneal cavity from abdominal drain sites are also reported causes of spontaneous pneumoperitoneum in small animals (Saunders & Tobias 2003; Smelstoys *et al.* 2004; Rubanick *et al.* 2020; Heslin & Malt 1964). Reasons for urinary bladder rupture in the two reported cases were entrapment of the urinary bladder within a perineal hernia and urethral obstruction (Saunders & Tobias 2003).

Traumatic rupture of the gastrointestinal tract in small animals has been most frequently reported in association with motor vehicle accidents, gunshot wounds, and abdominal bite wounds (Saunders & Tobias 2003). A single case report in a dog with blunt force trauma to the chest described subsequent development of nonsurgical pneumoperitoneum (Simmonds *et al.* 2011). Successful nonsurgical management of traumatic pneumoperitoneum has also recently been reported in a cat (Philip & Hammond 2018). Patients with blunt trauma that causes pneumothorax and/or pneumomediastinum can develop pneumoperitoneum due to air leakage into the abdomen. Postulated mechanisms of air transfer from the thorax to the abdomen include direct passage through diaphragmatic and pleural defects and indirect movement via the mediastinum (along portals such as the esophageal hiatus), first to the retroperitoneum and ultimately to the abdomen (Simmonds *et al.* 2011). Another proposed mechanism of air leakage in patients with blunt trauma is through intestinal microperforations that subsequently seal (Philip & Hammond 2018). Less frequently in veterinary (and human) patients, pneumoperitoneum, subcutaneous emphysema, and/or pneumoretroperitoneum can be a complication of endoscopic gastrointestinal biopsy, placement of a gastrostomy tube, or the use of high positive-pressure and/or end-expiratory pressure ventilation (Altman & Johnson 1979; Gottfried *et al.* 1986; Mason & Michel 2000; Woolhead *et al.* 2020).

Idiopathic pneumoperitoneum is diagnosed following exclusion of a perforated gastrointestinal tract, penetrating abdominal wounds, peritonitis, or other known causes of free intra-abdominal air. Idiopathic disease is nonsurgical and is reported infrequently in human patients. Other nonsurgical causes of pneumoperitoneum in human patients (5–15%) are grouped into the following categories: postoperative; thoracic (i.e., positive-pressure ventilation or pulmonary tuberculosis); abdominal (i.e., pneumocystoides intestinalis); and gynecologic. Idiopathic pneumoperitoneum has been reported rarely in veterinary patients (Rowe *et al.* 1998; Mularski *et al.* 2000; Mehl *et al.* 2001).

Presentation

Compatible historical and clinical signs in dogs and cats with pneumoperitoneum depend on the underlying cause and include lethargy, inappetence, weight loss, vomiting/diarrhea, abdominal pain and/or distension, hematemesis, melena, and evidence of dehydration and/or hypoperfusion. Patients with traumatic pneumoperitoneum may exhibit other signs referable to trauma (i.e., epistaxis, subcutaneous emphysema, and/or evisceration). Other injuries reported in trauma patients with pneumoperitoneum include degloving injuries, tracheal trauma, pneumothorax, and pelvic or rib fractures (Saunders & Tobias 2003; Smelstoys *et al.* 2004).

Laboratory abnormalities are nonspecific, and include most frequently hypoalbuminemia (69%), hyperbilirubinemia (64%), elevated transaminases (55%), leukocytosis (52%), and elevated blood urea nitrogen (49%). Alterations in hepatic enzymes and bilirubin concentrations are more frequently reported in small animals with trauma-associated pneumoperitoneum, and may be reflective of either concurrent hepatic injury or shock (Saunders & Tobias 2003; Smelstoys *et al.* 2004).

Diagnosis

In small animal patients, survey abdominal radiography has high sensitivity (100% in one retrospective study) in securing a diagnosis of pneumoperitoneum (Figure 22.1) (Saunders & Tobias 2003). However, when only a small amount of free air is present in the abdomen, the smaller gas bubbles formed are oftentimes superimposed over the gastrointestinal tract. This complicates the clinician's ability to differentiate between intraluminal and extraluminal locations of air. Small-volume pneumoperitoneum may necessitate postural radiography (i.e., horizontal beam). Such techniques promote identification of the fluid–gas interface and may aid in confirmatory diagnoses in less straightforward cases. For horizontal beam projections, the patient is placed in left lateral recumbency with the x-ray tube head and detector positioned horizontally to obtain a ventrodorsal view. Performing horizontal beam radiography with the patient in right lateral recumbency should be avoided, as the gas in the fundus can be misinterpreted as pneumoperitoneum (Ferrel & Graham 2002). Although horizontal

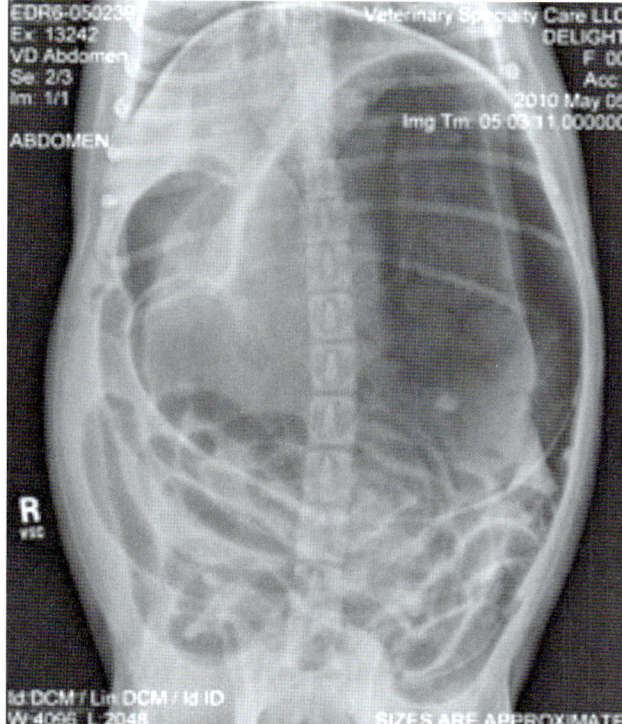

Figure 22.1 Ventrodorsal radiograph of a dog with gastric dilatation volvulus and pneumoperitoneum resulting from gastric necrosis. Free air can be seen between the stomach and diaphragm.

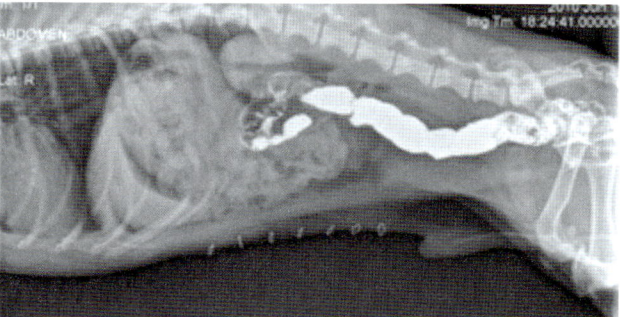

Figure 22.2 Lateral radiograph of a dog taken four days after surgery to remove an intestinal foreign body. A large amount of air is seen surrounding the liver and bowel loops and can be normal after surgery. Barium is noted in the colon from a radiographic study performed before surgery. Poor abdominal detail indicates an effusion, which in this patient resulted from dehiscence of the previous enterotomy site. The diagnosis of dehiscence was made by examination of fluid collected by abdominocentesis.

beam radiography has been recommended for patients with small-volume pneumoperitoneum, a recent experimental study found that the left lateral projection was comparable to horizontal beam radiography for detecting pneumoperitoneum in dogs with ≤10 mL of air in the abdomen (Ng *et al.* 2020). Additional radiographic findings consistent with disease processes that result in free intra-abdominal air include loss of serosal detail associated with concurrent abdominal effusion (most common), diffuse intestinal distension, abdominal soft tissue mass effect or foreign body, subcutaneous emphysema, or concurrent pneumothorax, pneumomediastinum, or pneumoretroperitoneum (Figure 22.2). Short-term outcomes in small animal patients are not influenced by radiographic severity of pneumoperitoneum or by the detection of concurrent radiographic abnormalities in affected patients (Edwards *et al.* 1994; Saunders & Tobias 2003; Smelstoys *et al.* 2004).

In human patients, upright and horizontal beam radiographs are limited to a diagnostic sensitivity of 50–75% (Rob *et al.* 1983; Chen *et al.* 2002). Ultrasound has demonstrated superior sensitivity (86–92%) in detection of free peritoneal gas in humans (Chen *et al.* 2002). On ultrasonography, free air in the peritoneal cavity produces an attenuation artifact known as acoustic shadowing, and

this modality may aid in the diagnosis of pneumoperitoneum when radiography is inconclusive (Ferrel & Graham 2002). This has not consistently been found in small animals and in a recent study of dogs and cats with ileocecocolic perforations associated with endoscopy, radiography was more diagnostic than ultrasonography in detecting free air (Woolhead *et al.* 2020).

Computed tomography (CT) is reported to be a sensitive modality for the diagnosis of pneumoperitoneum in people and it has recently been shown to be useful to diagnose both nonperforating and perforating gastrointestinal ulcers with pneumoperitoneum in dogs (Fitzgeral *et al.* 2017). In this study, CT had 93% sensitivity in detecting the ulcer and signs of perforation, such as gas bubbles within the intestinal wall, free air in the abdomen, and peritoneal fluid.

Abdominocentesis is an important ancillary test when gastrointestinal leakage and peritonitis are suspected concurrent with pneumoperitoneum. In retrospective veterinary studies, abdominocentesis has been positive in the majority of cases in which it was undertaken, and has yielded a variety of fluid types, including septic and nonseptic exudates, pure transudates with spermatozoa, and normal fluid. Culture of peritoneal fluid is advisable (positive in 75% of cases in one report), as cytologic examination may not reflect underlying disease. The most common organisms reported to be cultured from the abdominal fluid in patients with concurrent pneumoperitoneum are *Escherichia coli*, *Enterococcus* spp., and *Clostridium perfringens*, and the presence of polymicrobial infections is common (Saunders & Tobias 2003; Smelstoys *et al.* 2004). Relative contraindications to abdominocentesis include coagulopathy, diaphragmatic hernia, organomegaly, and extreme

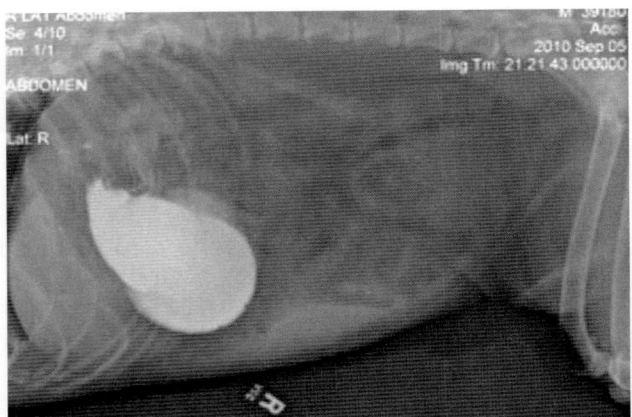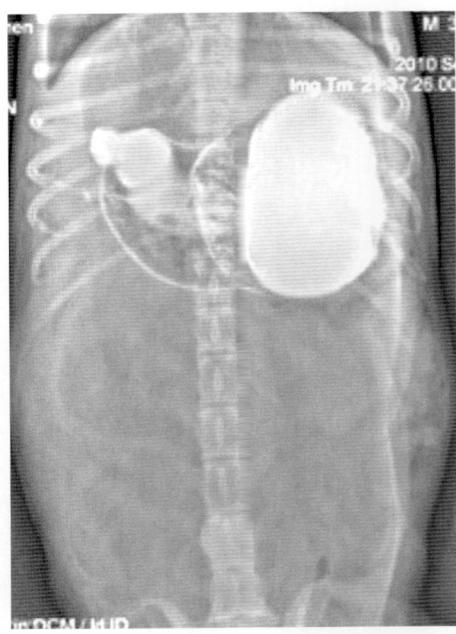

Figure 22.3 Barium series of a dog with a history of abdominal pain and chronic administration of a nonsteroidal anti-inflammatory medication. These radiographs were taken one hour after barium administration. Poor abdominal detail is the result of a duodenal perforation and peritonitis. Free air can be seen along the diaphragm and ventral to the liver on the lateral view and between the diaphragm and stomach on the ventrodorsal view. The site of perforation was sealed by omentum and the pancreas, preventing barium leakage.

distension of a hollow viscus. Negative abdominocentesis does not exclude a ruptured hollow viscus. Gastrointestinal ulcers may seal after air leak due to patching via the omentum or pancreas (Figure 22.3).

Sequelae

Tension pneumoperitoneum is the presence of massive free intra-abdominal air compromising cardiorespiratory function. Forceful ventilation and/or continued aerophagia contribute to the progression of peritoneal gas accumulation. Tympanic abdominal distension and evidence of respiratory distress and/or cardiovascular collapse are typically evident on physical examination, and are due to an increase in intra-abdominal pressure (Malbrain *et al.* 2006). Severe intra-abdominal hypertension results in abdominal compartment syndrome, threatening the viability of tissues within the peritoneal cavity (see Chapters 25 and 26). Tension pneumoperitoneum is well documented in human patients and requires immediate needle decompression to restore hemodynamic stability and abdominal perfusion pressure (Lal *et al.* 1995; Devine & McCarter 2001). Tension pneumoperitoneum has also been reported in a cat. This patient presented with signs referable to hypovolemic shock and respiratory distress, which improved immediately following abdominocentesis for air removal. Subsequent surgical exploration revealed gastric perforation and

mild generalized peritonitis, and the cat made a full recovery (Teruo *et al.* 2005).

Definitive treatment

Standard of care for the majority of cases of pneumoperitoneum in both humans and animals remains prompt surgical exploration. In one veterinary study evaluating dogs and cats with pneumoperitoneum (spontaneous or traumatic), 59% of patients were managed surgically, and 65% of these patients lived. Conversely, only 1 of 16 animals managed medically survived to hospital discharge. In a second veterinary study of small animals with pneumoperitoneum and no history of penetrating trauma, 1 of 14 animals that did not undergo surgery survived hospitalization, whereas 40 of 5? surgical patients survived (Saunders & Tobias 2003; Smelstoys *et al.* 2004).

For a small percentage of humans with free intra-abdominal air not referable to gastrointestinal tract perforation (5–15%), surgical intervention is not necessary for a successful outcome. Examples of pneumoperitoneum in humans not treated surgically include complications associated with bronchoscopy, gastroscopy, or percutaneous endoscopic gastrostomy (PEG) tube placement and idiopathic pneumoperitoneum (Mularski *et al.* 2000). Pneumoretroperitoneum and/or pneumoperitoneum following PEG tube placement in humans are treated with broad-spectrum antibiotics, and free intra-abdominal air typically resolves within one week (Gottfried *et al.* 1986). In contrast, surgery was recommended in a cat with subcutaneous emphysema, pneumoperitoneum, and pneumoretroperitoneum after PEG tube placement. Abdominal exploration in this cat revealed a perforated gastric fundus, and peritoneal fluid obtained during surgery cultured *Pasteurella multocida* and *Enterobacter* spp., suggestive of leakage of gastric contents from the perforation (Mehl *et al.* 2001). It is unknown whether cases of small animal pneumoperitoneum not associated with penetrating trauma, severe clinical signs, peritonitis, or progressive abdominal distension would be amenable to medical management. However, the available veterinary studies suggest that medical management of pneumoperitoneum is not successful in disease reversal and patient survival, and that surgery is advised in all dogs and cats with pneumoperitoneum that is not associated with blunt trauma, postoperative, or subsequent to abdominal procedures such as abdominocentesis.

Prognosis

In one veterinary study, animals that survived pneumoperitoneum had significantly higher albumin concentrations than animals that died or were euthanized (Saunders & Tobias 2003). Although a number of other variables have been evaluated, including sex, age, breed, medical history, duration of illness, clinical signs, radiographic findings, results of peritoneal fluid analysis, time from presentation until surgery, and location of gastrointestinal compromise, no additional prognostic factors have been identified (Smelstoys *et al.* 2004).

In small animal patients, reported survival following surgical treatment of pneumoperitoneum with no history of trauma is 58%. Survival rate for pneumoperitoneum of all causes has been reported to be 65% and survival rates in these patients were no different in animals with traumatic versus spontaneous disease. A recent report showed a good outcome (93% survival to discharge) in patients treated surgically for ileocecocolic perforations associated with endoscopy (Woolhead *et al.* 2020). Prognosis associated with medical management appears to be poor unless it is associated with blunt trauma, and this therapeutic modality must be used cautiously in a select subset of veterinary patients (Saunders & Tobias 2003; Smelstoys *et al.* 2004; Philip & Hammond 2018).

References

Altman, A.R. and Johnson, T.H. (1979). Pneumoperitoneum and pneumoretroperitoneum. Consequences of positive end-expiratory pressure therapy. *Archives of Surgery* 114: 208–211.

Chen, S.C., Yen, Z.S., Wang, H.P. et al. (2002). Ultrasonagraphy is superior to plain radiography in the diagnosis of pneumoperitoneum. *British Journal of Surgery* 89: 351–354.

Devine, J.F. and McCarter, T.G. (2001). Images in clinical medicine. Tension pneumoperitoneum. *New England Journal of Medicine* 344: 1985.

Edwards, N.J., Mead, W.W., and Haviland, D.G. (1994). Radiographic diagnosis: spontaneous pneumoperitoneum in a cat. *Veterinary Radiology and Ultrasound* 35: 428–429.

Ferrel, E.A. and Graham, J.P. (2002). Ultrasound corner diagnosis of pneumoperitoneum. *Veterinary Radiology and Ultrasound* 44: 307–308.

Fitzgeral, E., Barfield, K.C., Lee, C.L., and Lamb, C.R. (2017). Clinical findings and results of diagnostic imaging in 82 dogs with gastrointestinal ulceration. *Journal of Small Animal Practice* 58: 211–218.

Godshalk, C.P., Roush, J.K., Fingland, R.B. et al. (1992). Gastric perforation associated with administration of ibuprofen in a dog. *Journal of the American Veterinary Medical Association* 201: 1734–1736.

Gottfried, E.B., Plumser, A.B., and Clair, M.R. (1986). Pneumoperitoneum following percutaneous gastrostomy. A prospective study. *Gastrointestinal Endoscopy* 32: 397–399.

Heslin, J.D. and Malt, R.A. (1964). Progressive postoperative pneumoperitoneum: air entering through drain sites. *American Journal of Roentgenology* 92: 1166–1168.

Hillman, K.M. (1982). Pneumoperitoneum: a review. *Critical Care Medicine* 10: 476–481.

Hinton, H.E., McLoughlin, M.A., Johnson, S.E., and Weisbrode, S.E. (2002). Spontaneous gastroduodenal perforation in 16 dogs and seven cats (1982–1999). *Journal of the American Animal Hospital Association* 38: 176–187.

Itoh, T., Nibe, K., and Naganobu, K. (2005). Tension pneumoperitoneum due to gastric perforation in a cat. *Journal of Veterinary Medicine Science* 67: 617–619.

Jones, R.D., Baynes, R.E., and Nimitz, C.T. (1992). Nonsteroidal antiinflammatory drug toxicosis in dogs and cats: 240 cases (1989–1990). *Journal of the American Veterinary Medical Association* 201: 475–477.

Lal, A.B., Kumar, N., and Sami, K.A. (1995). Tension pneumoperitoneum from tracheal tear during pharyngolaryngoesophagectomy. *Anesthesia and Analgesia* 80: 408–409.

Lykken, J.D., Brisson, B.A., and Etue, S.M. (2003). Pneumoperitoneum secondary to a perforated gastric ulcer in a cat. *Journal of the American Veterinary Medical Association* 222: 1713–1716.

Malbrain, M.L.N.G., Cheatham, M.L., Kirkpatrick, A. et al. (2006). Results from the international conference of experts on intra-abdominal hypertension and abdominal compartment syndrome. I. Definitions. *Intensive Care Medicine* 32: 1722–1732.

Mason, N.J. and Michel, K.E. (2000). Subcutaneous emphysema, pneumoperitoneum, and pneumoretroperitoneum after gastrostomy tube placement in a cat. *Journal of the American Veterinary Medical Association* 216: 1096–1099.

Mehl, M.L., Seguin, B., Norrdin, R.W. et al. (2001). Idiopathic pneumoperitoneum in a dog. *Journal of the American Animal Hospital Association* 37: 549–551.

Mellanby, R.J., Baines, E.A., and Herrtage, M.E. (2002). Spontaneous pneumoperitoneum in two cats. *Journal of Small Animal Practice* 43: 543–546.

Mezghebe, H.M., Leffall, L.D., Siram, S.M., and Syphax, B. (1994). Asymptomatic pneumoperitoneum: diagnostic and therapeutic dilemma. *American Surgeon* 60: 691–694.

Mularski, R.A., Sippel, H.M., and Osborne, M.L. (2000). Pneumoperitoneum: a review of nonsurgical causes. *Critical Care Medicine* 28: 2638–2644.

Ng, J., Linn, K.A., Shmon, C.L. et al. (2020). The left lateral projection is comparable to horizontal beam radiography for identifying experimental small volume pneumoperitoneum in the canine abdomen. *Veterinary Radiology and Ultrasound* 61: 130–136.

Philip, H.S. and Hammond, G.J.C. (2018). Nonsurgical management of traumatic pneumoperitoneum in a cat. *Journal of Veterinary Emergency and Critical Care* 28: 591–595.

Probst, C.W., Bright, R.M., Ackerman, N. et al. (1984). Spontaneous pneumoperitoneum subsequent to volvulus in two dogs. *Veterinary Radiology and Ultrasound* 25: 37–42.

Probst, C.W., Stickle, R.L., and Barlett, P.C. (1986). Duration of pneumoperitoneum in the dog. *American Journal of Veterinary Research* 47: 176–178.

Rob, J.J., Thompson, J.S., Harned, R.K., and Hodgson, P.E. (1983). Value of pneumoperitoneum in the diagnosis of visceral perforation. *American Journal of Surgery* 146: 830–883.

Rowe, N.M., Kahn, F.B., Acinapura, A.J., and Cunningham, J.N. Jr. (1998). Nonsurgical retroperitoneum: a case report and review. *American Surgeon* 64: 313–322.

Rubanick, J.V., Breiteneicher, A.H., and Thieman-Mankin, K. (2020). Large-volume pneumoperitoneum and septic peritonitis secondary to splenic abscess rupture in a dog. *Canadian Veterinary Journal* 61: 138–141.

Samuel, E., Duncan, J.G., Philip, T., and Sumerling, M.D. (1963). Radiology of the postoperative abdomen. *Clinical Radiology* 14: 133–148.

Saunders, W.B. and Tobias, K.M. (2003). Pneumoperitoneum in dogs and cats: 39 cases (1983–2002). *Journal of the American Veterinary Medical Association* 223: 462–468.

Schenck, P.A., Chew, D.J., Nagode, L.A. et al. (2006). Disorders of calcium: hypercalcemia and hypocalcemia. In: *Fluid, Electrolyte and Acid–Base Disorders in Small Animal Practice*, 3e (ed. S.P. DiBartola), 122–194. St Louis, MO: Elsevier.

Simmonds, S.L., Whelan, M.F., and Basseches, J. (2011). Nonsurgical pneumoperitoneum in a dog secondary to blunt force trauma to the chest. *Journal of Veterinary Emergency and Critical Care* 21: 552–557.

Simpson, K.W. (2010). Diseases of the stomach. In: *Textbook of Veterinary Internal Medicine* 7e, vol. 2 (ed. S.J. Ettinger and E.C. Feldman), 1504–1526. St Louis, MO: WB Saunders.

Smelstoys, J.A., Davis, G.J., Learn, A.E. et al. (2004). Outcome of and prognostic indicators for dogs and cats with pneumoperitoneum and no history of penetrating trauma: 54 cases (1988–2002). *Journal of the American Veterinary Medical Association* 225: 251–255.

Teruo, I., Kazumi, N., and Kiyokaza, N. (2005). Tension pneumoperitoneum due to gastric perforation in a cat. *Journal of Veterinary Medical Science* 67: 617–619.

Wong, P.L. (1981). Pneumoperitoneum associated with splenic necrosis and clostridial peritonitis in a dog. *Journal of the American Animal Hospital Association* 17: 466–467.

Woolhead, V.L., Whittemore, J.C., and Stewart, S.A. (2020). Multicenter retrospective evaluation of ileocecal perforations associated with diagnostic lower gastrointestinal endoscopy in dogs and cats. *Journal of Veterinary Internal Medicine* 34: 684–690.

23

Retroperitoneal Diseases

Amelia M. Simpson

Diseases of the retroperitoneal space include retroperitonitis, hemoretroperitoneum, uroretroperitoneum, pneumoretroperitoneum, and primary or metastatic retroperitoneal neoplasia. The retroperitoneal space is defined as a potential space within the abdominal cavity. Included in this space are fat, loose connective tissue, nerves, blood vessels (aorta and caudal vena cava), iliac and sublumbar lymph nodes, and organs (kidneys, ureters, and adrenal glands) (Johnston & Christie 1990). The borders of the retroperitoneum include the diaphragm cranially, anus caudally, peritoneum ventrally, epaxial muscles and vertebral bodies dorsally, and quadratus lumborum muscles laterally. The retroperitoneal space is also continuous with the retropleural space and the mediastinum in the dog (Johnston & Christie 1990).

Pathogenesis

Hemorrhage and urine leakage are the most common causes of fluid accumulation in the retroperitoneal space (Smallwood & Spaulding 2000).

Hemoretroperitoneum

Retroperitoneal hemorrhage often results from blunt abdominal or pelvic trauma, but can also occur with retroperitoneal tumor rupture (Whittemore *et al.* 2001). Coagulopathy should be considered in cases of spontaneous hemorrhage with no history of trauma.

Uroretroperitoneum

Urine leakage can occur from proximal ureteral rupture, kidney rupture, or ureteral avulsion from the kidney.

Perirenal effusion has also been reported in dogs and cats with acute renal failure (Holloway & O'Brien 2007).

Retroperitonitis

Inflammation and abscessation of the retroperitoneal space may be caused by migrating grass awns, penetrating wounds, foreign bodies, inflammatory reaction to ovariohysterectomy ligatures, and perforation of the urethra during catheterization (Smallwood & Spaulding 2000).

Pneumoretroperitoneum

Pneumoretroperitoneum can occur secondary to extension of free air from a pneumomediastinum. It can also be caused by gas-producing bacteria in the retroperitoneal space, penetrating wounds to the retroperitoneum, or perforation of the genitourinary tract during catheterization (Kirby 2003).

Retroperitoneal tumors

Primary retroperitoneal tumors are tumors that are located in the retroperitoneal space but that do not arise from the kidneys, adrenal glands, ureters, or lymph nodes. Lipomas are the most common retroperitoneal tumor in small animals (Kirby 2003) (Figure 23.1). Many primary retroperitoneal sarcomas have been described, including hemangiosarcoma, osteosarcoma, chondrosarcoma, leiomyosarcoma, myxoid-type peripheral nerve sheath tumor, hemangiopericytoma, and fibrosarcoma (Kirby 2003; Liptak *et al.* 2004). Hemangiosarcoma is the most commonly diagnosed primary retroperitoneal sarcoma (Liptak *et al.* 2004). A primary retroperitoneal

(a)

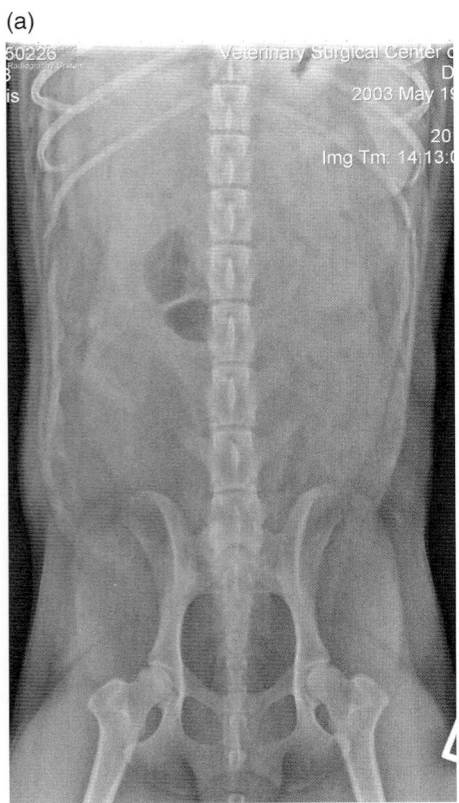

(b)

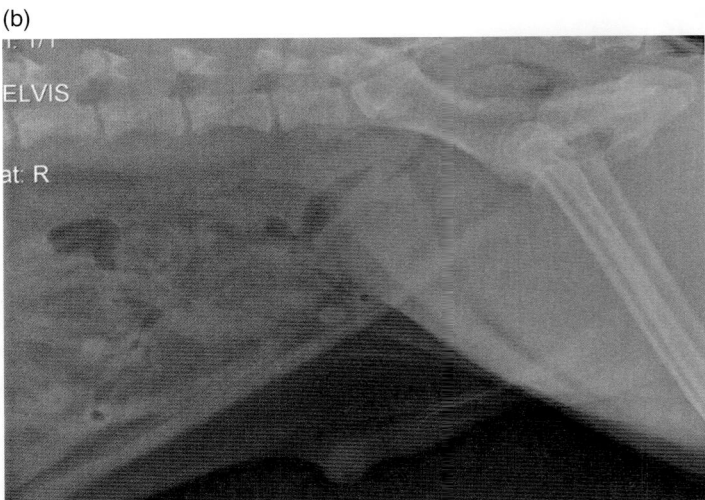

Figure 23.1 (a) Ventrodorsal and (b) lateral radiographs of a dog with a retroperitoneal lipoma. This dog was presented for evaluation of right hindlimb lameness, but was also noted to have a soft tissue swelling in the dorsolateral aspect of the right flank that was uncomfortable on palpation. Radiographs and surgery were suggestive of a lipoma and histopathologic evaluation confirmed the diagnosis.

teratoma and seminoma have also been reported (Nagashima *et al.* 2000; Wang *et al.* 2001). Metastatic tumors that may involve structures within the retroperitoneal space include lymphoma, anal sac adenocarcinoma, mammary and prostatic neoplasia, perianal adenocarcinoma, and mast cell tumors.

History and clinical signs

Dogs and cats with retroperitoneal disease may be presented with a history of recent trauma. Clinical signs can range from asymptomatic to severe illness or shock. Retroperitoneal infections or uroretroperitoneum can cause dogs and cats to be febrile and show signs of pain. Dogs with retroperitoneal tumors can have nonspecific signs of illness including weight loss, lethargy, and inappetence, or hindleg lameness with or without associated neurologic abnormalities (Liptak *et al.* 2004). Periumbilical discoloration (Cullen sign) has been reported with retroperitoneal hemorrhage (Kirby 2003).

Diagnostics

Survey radiography is an excellent modality for evaluating the retroperitoneal space for evidence of disease. Loss of contrast and detail in the retroperitoneal space is an indication of fluid accumulation and less commonly

inflammation. Fluid accumulation within this space gives the appearance of "streaking" as the fluid dissects between the fascial planes of the fat and soft tissues (Figure 23.2). Visualization of the left kidney may be obscured on a lateral projection and there may be an appearance of retroperitoneal displacement ventrally into the abdominal space (Smallwood & Spaulding 2000). An excretory urogram can be performed to diagnose urine leakage from traumatic rupture of the kidney or ureter (Weisse *et al.* 2002).

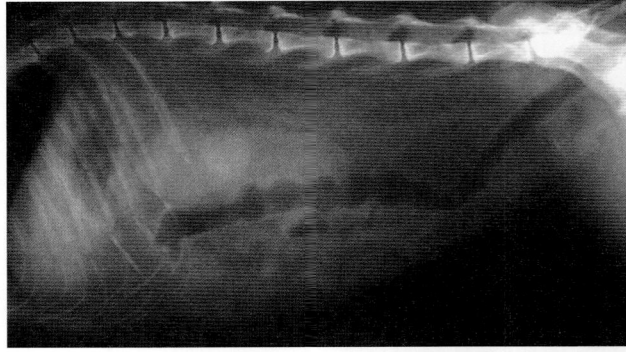

Figure 23.2 Lateral radiograph of a cat with uroretroperitoneum as a result of a ureteral tear. Note the classic "streaking" appearance of the tissues in the retroperitoneal space.

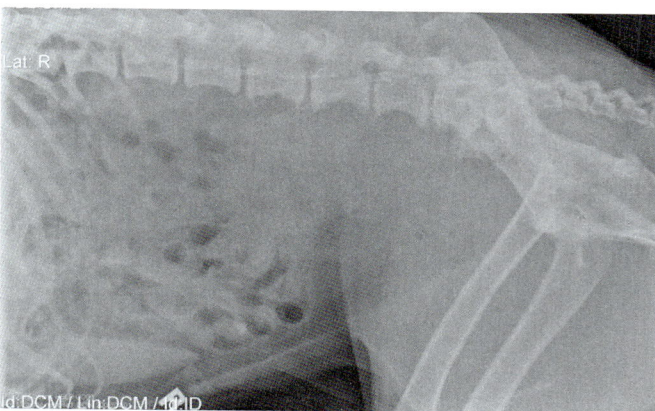
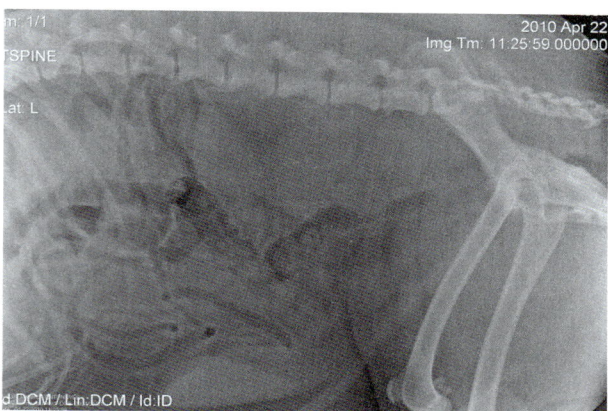

Figure 23.3 Lateral radiograph of two dogs with anal sac adenocarcinoma metastasis to the sublumbar and iliac lymph nodes. Note the ventral deviation of the colon in both cases.

A retroperitoneal mass may be seen on a lateral radiograph as a soft tissue opacity located below the lumbar vertebral bodies. Often these masses can be large enough to cause ventral deviation of the colon or rectum (Figure 23.3). Ultrasonography and computed tomography of the abdomen can help to differentiate between renal and other retroperitoneal masses.

Because of the communication of the mediastinum with the neck and retroperitoneal space, pneumomediastinum can develop into subcutaneous emphysema or pneumoretroperitoneum (Smallwood & Spaulding 2000). On survey radiographs, retroperitoneal gas enhances detail in the dorsal abdomen, with the aorta and right kidney becoming clearly visible (Graham *et al.* 2000).

Treatment

Although treatment for retroperitoneal diseases varies with the primary cause, surgical exploration via ventral abdominal midline incision is often indicated (Figure 23.4). The surgeon may be required to perform an adrenalectomy, ureteronephrectomy, or lymphadenectomy for retroperitoneal neoplasia.

Uroretroperitoneum caused by trauma to the kidney or ureter may be managed by ureteronephrectomy, primary repair, or ureteral reimplantation. Traumatic urethral rupture that results in retroperitoneal urine or air leakage may be managed conservatively with urine diversion through a urethral catheter or tube cystostomy, primary repair, or urethrostomy.

Pneumoretroperitoneum resulting from pneumomediastinum will usually resolve once the source of air leakage into the mediastinum resolves or is corrected. Duration of a pneumoretroperitoneum has not been evaluated in small animals, but resolution of experimentally induced pneumoperitoneum in dogs took 15–34 days (Kirby 2003).

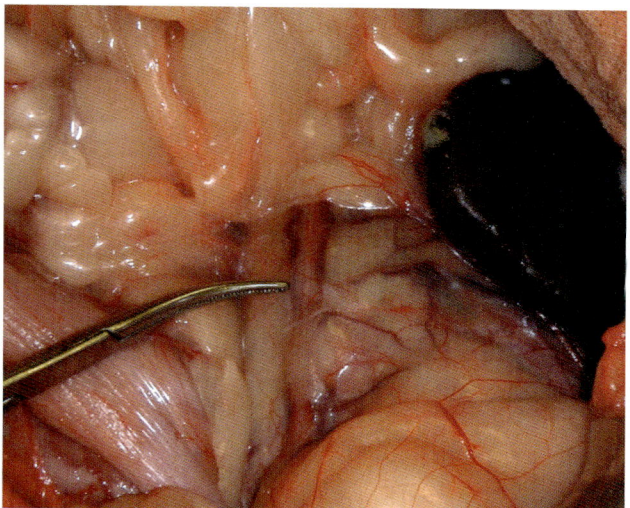

Figure 23.4 Intraoperative picture of left medial iliac lymphadenectomy for treatment of metastatic anal sac adenocarcinoma. Note the ventral displacement of the left ureter as it courses around the enlarged lymph node.

Conservative management is recommended for patients with coagulopathy-related retroperitoneal hemorrhage. Retroperitoneal hemorrhage caused by trauma can also often be managed conservatively, although patients should be monitored closely and given supportive care, to include blood transfusions if necessary. Retroperitoneal hemorrhage resulting from neoplasia warrants organ removal and biopsy.

Prognosis

Prognosis for dogs and cats with primary or metastatic retroperitoneal tumors depends on the tumor type and staging. A recent study of dogs with retroperitoneal sarcomas found a median survival time of 37.5 days (range 2–498 days) (Liptak *et al.* 2004). The clinical impression is that dogs and cats with early and accurate diagnosis of retroperitoneal diseases such as retroperitonitis, retroperitoneal hemorrhage or urine leakage, and pneumoretroperitoneum can be managed successfully with appropriate surgery or conservative treatment.

References

Graham, J.P., Berry, C.R., and Thrall, D.E. (2000). Technical issues and interpretation principles relating to the canine and feline abdomen. In: *Textbook of Veterinary Diagnostic Radiology*, 2e (ed. D.E. Thrall), 626–644. St Louis, MO: Saunders Elsevier.

Holloway, A. and O'Brien, R. (2007). Perirenal effusion in dogs and cats with acute renal failure. *Veterinary Radiology and Ultrasound* 48: 574–579.

Johnston, D.E. and Christie, B.A. (1990). The retroperitoneum in dogs: anatomy and clinical significance. *Compendium on Continuing Education for the Practicing Veterinarian* 12: 1027–1033.

Kirby, B.M. (2003). Peritoneum and peritoneal cavity. In: *Textbook of Small Animal Surgery*, 3e (ed. D. Slatter), 414–445. Philadelphia, PA: WB Saunders.

Liptak, J.M., Dernell, W.S., Earhart, E.J. et al. (2004). Retroperitoneal sarcomas in dogs: 14 cases (1992–2002). *Journal of the American Veterinary Medical Association* 224: 1471–1477.

Nagashima, Y., Hoshi, K., Tanaka, R. et al. (2000). Ovarian and retroperitoneal teratomas in a dog. *Journal of Veterinary Medical Science* 62: 793–795.

Smallwood, J.E. and Spaulding, K.A. (2000). Radiographic anatomy of the abdomen. In: *Textbook of Veterinary Diagnostic Radiology*, 2e (ed. D.E. Thrall), 647–666. St Louis, MO: Saunders Elsevier.

Wang, F.I., Liang, S.L., and Chin, S.C. (2001). A primary retroperitoneal seminoma invading the kidneys of a cryptorchid dog. *Experimental Animals* 50: 341–344.

Weisse, C., Aronson, L.R., and Drobatz, K. (2002). Traumatic rupture of the ureter: 10 cases. *Journal of the American Animal Hospital Association* 38: 188–192.

Whittemore, J.C., Preston, C.A., Kyles, A.E. et al. (2001). Nontraumatic rupture of an adrenal gland tumor causing intra-abdominal or retroperitoneal hemorrhage in four dogs. *Journal of the American Veterinary Medical Association* 219: 329–333.

24

Congenital Abdominal Wall Hernia

Amelia M. Simpson

Abdominal wall hernias are abnormal openings in the muscle wall of the abdominal cavity that allow the protrusion or projection of intra-abdominal fat or organs into the subcutaneous or intramuscular space. In general, there are three parts to a hernia: the ring, the sac, and the contents. In abdominal wall hernias the ring is the actual defect in the abdominal wall, the hernia contents are the organs and structures that are permitted to pass through the ring into the abnormal location, and the sac surrounds the hernia contents. True abdominal hernias, most often congenital, have a peritoneal sac surrounding the hernia contents. False hernias do not have a peritoneal sac. In traumatic or acquired abdominal wall hernias, the contents usually do not have a peritoneal sac initially, although peritonealization may occur later if the hernia is left untreated (Read & Bellenger 2003; Shaw *et al.* 2003).

Abdominal wall hernias can be reducible or irreducible/incarcerated. In general, reducible abdominal wall hernias appear as small, soft, nonpainful swellings with hernia contents that can be gently manipulated back into the abdominal cavity. If the hernia is firm and the tissues within it are not freely movable, the hernia is classified as incarcerated or irreducible.

Congenital abdominal wall hernias include umbilical and ventral midline hernias as well as inguinal, femoral, and scrotal hernias (Figure 24.1). Inguinal hernias, femoral hernias, and rarely umbilical hernias can be either congenital or trauma-induced defects.

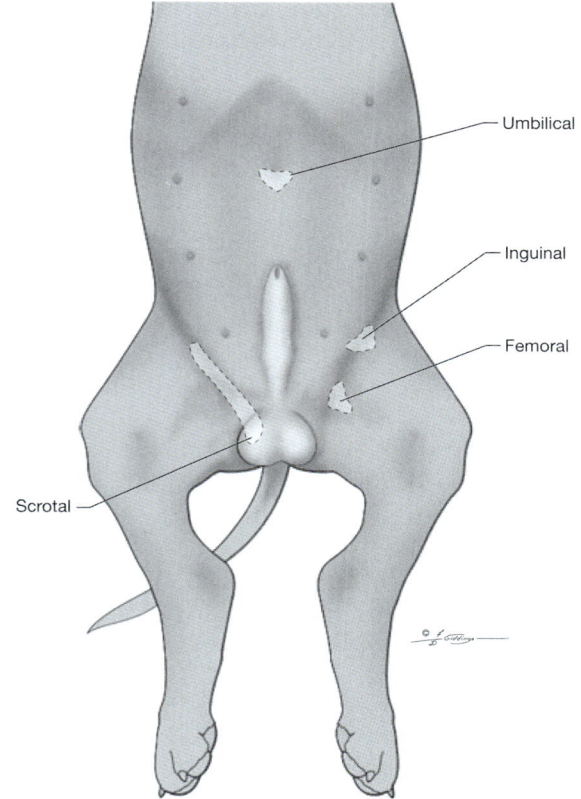

Figure 24.1 Ventral abdominal wall hernias: umbilical, inguinal, scrotal, femoral. © D. Giddings.

Umbilical and ventral midline hernias

Anatomy and etiology

Umbilical hernias are the most common hernia in small animals. They occur on the ventral abdominal midline through the umbilical ring. The abdominal wall is formed in the embryo by the migration and eventual fusion of the cephalic, caudal, and lateral folds. Normally the umbilical aperture remains open in the embryo, serving as a passageway for the umbilical cord and closing down shortly after birth, leaving an umbilical scar. Most umbilical hernias result from failure of fusion of the lateral folds at the umbilicus and as such are considered to be congenital anomalies (Smeak 2003). The result is an abnormal opening in the abdominal wall through which fat, omentum, and other abdominal organs may herniate (Figure 24.2).

It is widely accepted that umbilical hernias are hereditary, although the exact mechanism has yet to be elucidated. Cryptorchidism is often seen in male dogs with umbilical hernias and some breeds seem predisposed: Airedales, basenjis, Pekingese, pointers, and Weimaraners (Smeak 2003). Early neutering is recommended for affected cats and dogs for these reasons.

Traumatic umbilical hernias are uncommon. They can be caused during the birthing process if there is excessive traction on the umbilical cord at parturition or iatrogenically with ligation of the umbilical cord too close to the abdominal wall (Smeak 2003).

Omphalocele and gastroschisis are two rare types of congenital abdominal wall defect. An omphalocele is a large midline umbilical and skin defect caused by an error in the embryonic development of the intestinal tract. Failure of the midgut to reenter the abdomen inhibits the proper migration and fusion of the abdominal wall folds. The result is a large hernia of abdominal contents that is covered by two thin transparent membranes: the amniotic tissue and the peritoneum. Gastroschisis occurs when abdominal organs herniate through the base of the umbilical cord and into the amniotic fluid. A gastroschisis looks similar to an omphalocele, but it is always paramedian in location and not covered by the peritoneum. Children with these congenital abdominal wall malformations have a high mortality rate, with only 60% alive at the end of the first year (Chircor et al. 2009). The mortality rate in dogs and cats with these malformations is not known, but it is suspected to be very high.

Clinical signs

The most common clinical sign of an umbilical hernia is a soft swelling/mass effect at the umbilical scar. Generally seen in young animals, these hernias are often nonpainful and easily reducible. Patients with umbilical hernias should be thoroughly evaluated for other congenital abnormalities.

Diagnostics

Although an umbilical hernia is the most likely diagnosis for a soft swelling at the umbilical scar, other differentials include neoplasia, hematomas, seromas, and abscesses. Radiographs may help if gas trapped in obstructed intestines is seen outside the body wall. In general, aspiration is not recommended, since cytology rarely changes the decision to go to surgery in these cases. However, I have seen a mast cell tumor mimic an umbilical hernia, so fine-needle aspiration may be prudent in middle-aged to older dogs with a history of recent mass development.

Treatment

Soft nonpainful umbilical hernias with a very large or very small hernia ring are generally left untreated, as spontaneous closure may occur as late as 6 months of age (Fossum 2007). If closure does not occur spontaneously, repair is recommended during ovariohysterectomy or neutering procedures.

Intestinal strangulation or obstruction should be considered in patients with warm, painful umbilical hernias that cannot be reduced. Emergency surgery is warranted in these cases and should be performed as soon as the patient is stabilized. In efforts to avoid potential

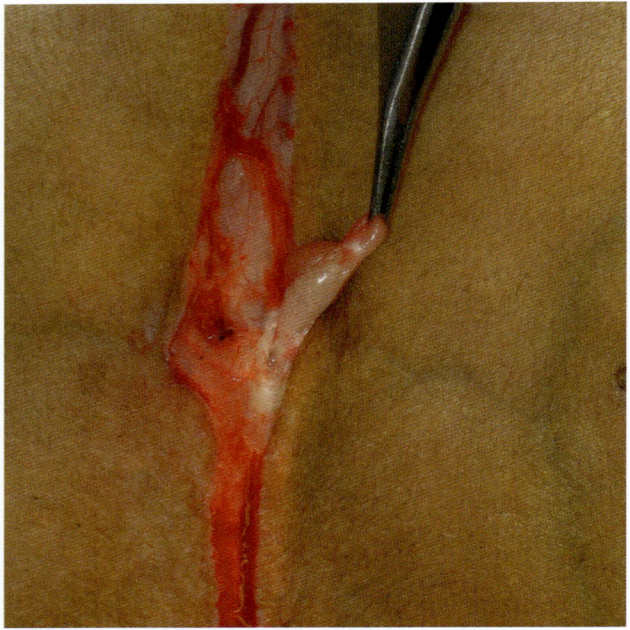

Figure 24.2 Umbilical hernia with abdominal fat in the hernia.

herniation, prompt treatment is also recommended in patients with umbilical hernias that have a hernia ring about the size of a finger (10–12 mm). An opening this size may be just large enough for a loop of intestine to slip through and become incarcerated.

For small umbilical hernias, an incision is made in the skin on the ventral midline over the hernia after it has been reduced. The hernia sac is inverted and the hernia ring is closed without débriding the edges of the ring. A simple interrupted suture pattern is recommended using synthetic monofilament absorbable or nonabsorbable suture. The use of a synthetic mesh graft in umbilical hernia repair is rarely indicated.

If the hernia contents cannot be reduced, then extreme care is taken not to incise the contents as the skin incision is made. Alternatively, the incision can be made around the hernia contents. If the hernia contains incarcerated fat and/or omentum, these are ligated at the base of the hernia and removed, and the hernia ring is closed routinely. If the herniated contents contain intestines or other abdominal organs, the hernia ring should be enlarged cranially and caudally along the linea alba for a routine abdominal exploratory. Intestines and other organs should be examined for viability, and resection and anastomosis or organ removal should be performed as indicated, followed by routine abdominal wall closure and herniorrhaphy as previously stated.

Aftercare and prognosis

Patients should be kept quiet at home for two weeks following surgical repair of an umbilical hernia. They should be confined to a crate or small area in the house and walks should be limited to short leash walks only. Elizabethan collars should be worn as necessary to prevent patients from licking or otherwise bothering their incisions. Incisions should be evaluated daily by owners. Swelling, redness, and serosanguinous discharge around the incision may indicate infection, or may be early signs of impending dehiscence. Patients who develop postoperative fever, inappetence, lethargy, or vomiting should be evaluated for possible peritonitis or incisional abscess.

In young patients with reducible hernias and a routine repair, the prognosis is generally excellent. In complicated cases, the prognosis is usually dictated by the concurrent disease or injury.

Inguinal, scrotal, and femoral hernias

Anatomy and etiology

Inguinal hernias occur when abdominal contents slip through a defect in the inguinal ring (Figure 24.3). The cause is not well understood. Congenital inguinal hernias do occur, although they are most commonly associated with trauma or thought to be a result of weakening of normal tissues. Pregnancy, obesity, and other causes of increased abdominal pressure can predispose animals to inguinal hernia formation. The basenji, Pekingese, poodle, basset hound, Cairn terrier, Cavalier King Charles spaniel, cocker spaniel, dachshund, Pomeranian, Maltese, and West Highland white terrier breeds are predisposed to the formation of congenital inguinal hernias (Smeak 2003). Such hernias can form in male or female dogs and can occur as direct or indirect hernias. In a direct inguinal hernia, abdominal fat and organs pass through the inguinal ring adjacent to the vaginal process. An indirect hernia exists if the abdominal organs enter the cavity of the vaginal process and protrude through the inguinal ring (Figures 24.4 and 24.5). An indirect inguinal hernia is referred to as a scrotal hernia in male dogs.

Femoral hernias, rare in the dog and cat, occur when fat or abdominal contents protrude through the femoral canal. Differentiating a femoral hernia from an inguinal hernia can be challenging due to the close proximity of the two structures (Figure 24.6). The inguinal ring is located medially and cranially to the pelvic brim, whereas the femoral canal is located caudal to the inguinal ligament and ventrolateral to the pelvic brim. Although femoral hernias can be congenital in origin, they are usually caused by blunt trauma in which both the prepubic tendon (also known as the cranial pubic tendon) and inguinal ligaments are avulsed. These hernias can also occur iatrogenically by transection of the origin of the pectineus muscle directly off the pubis.

Clinical signs

Physical examination on presentation can vary widely. Animals with direct inguinal hernias usually present with a soft, painless, unilateral, or bilateral swelling in the inguinal area. These swellings can be relatively small with abdominal fat protrusion or very large, as in the case of a female with a gravid uterus or pyometra in the hernia sac. Unilateral inguinal hernias occur more commonly on the left side in dogs (Smeak 2003).

Generally, a healthy young pet with a soft nonpainful inguinal swelling is likely only to have abdominal fat or omentum in the hernia sac. An animal should be suspected of having incarcerated, strangulated, and possibly necrotic intestines in the hernia if they are presented with a firm, painful, inguinal swelling and history of vomiting, inappetence, and lethargy. In a study of 35 dogs with inguinal hernias, vomiting for 2–6 days predicted strangulated small intestines. In this study, all the dogs with nonviable intestines vomited, whereas none of the dogs with healthy intestines vomited (Waters *et al.* 1993).

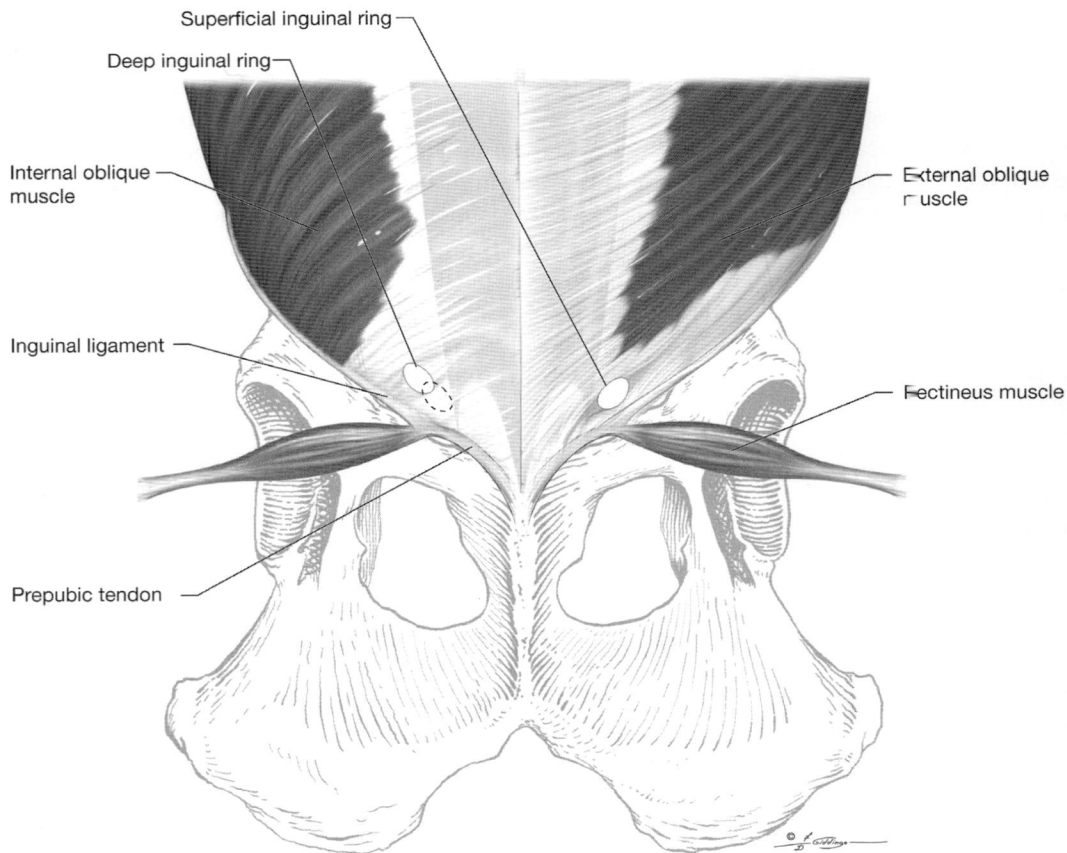

Figure 24.3 Inguinal ring anatomy. The external abdominal oblique muscle has been removed on the left side of the figure to reveal the internal abdominal oblique muscle. © D. Giddings.

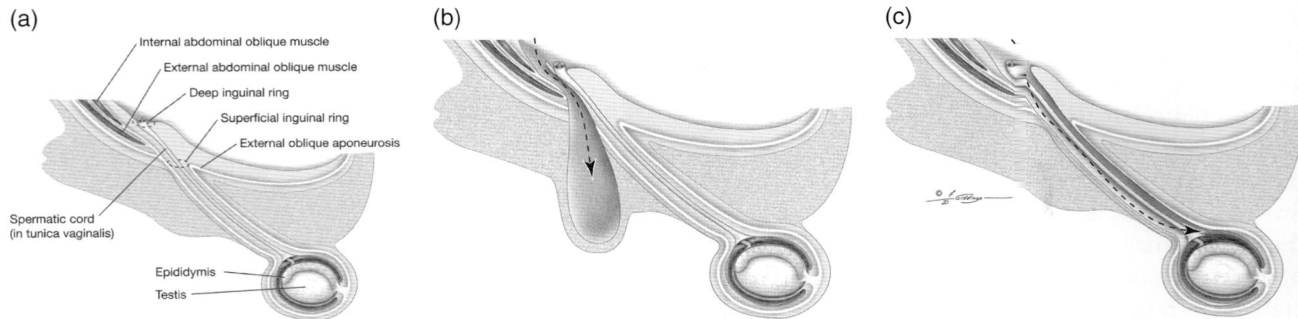

Figure 24.4 (a) Inguinal canal anatomy. (b) Direct inguinal hernia. (c) Indirect inguinal hernia or scrotal hernia. © D. Giddings.

Diagnostics

Differential diagnoses for patients with a swelling in the inguinal area include abscesses, enlarged lymph nodes, and neoplastic masses such as mammary masses, lymphoma, mast cell tumors, or sarcomas. Radiographs may provide a diagnostic aid if gas-filled intestinal loops are seen outside the body wall or if fetal skeletons are seen, as in the case of a herniated gravid uterus. A contrast cystourethrogram may confirm urinary bladder herniation. In general, palpation of the inguinal ring after reduction of the hernia confirms the diagnosis. It is difficult to distinguish an inguinal hernia from a scrotal or femoral hernia by palpation alone if the contents of the hernia are incarcerated.

Treatment

Surgery is recommended soon after the diagnosis of an inguinal, scrotal, or femoral hernia. For patients who are subclinical at the time of presentation, immediate repair will mitigate the possibility of life-threatening herniation.

(a)

(b)

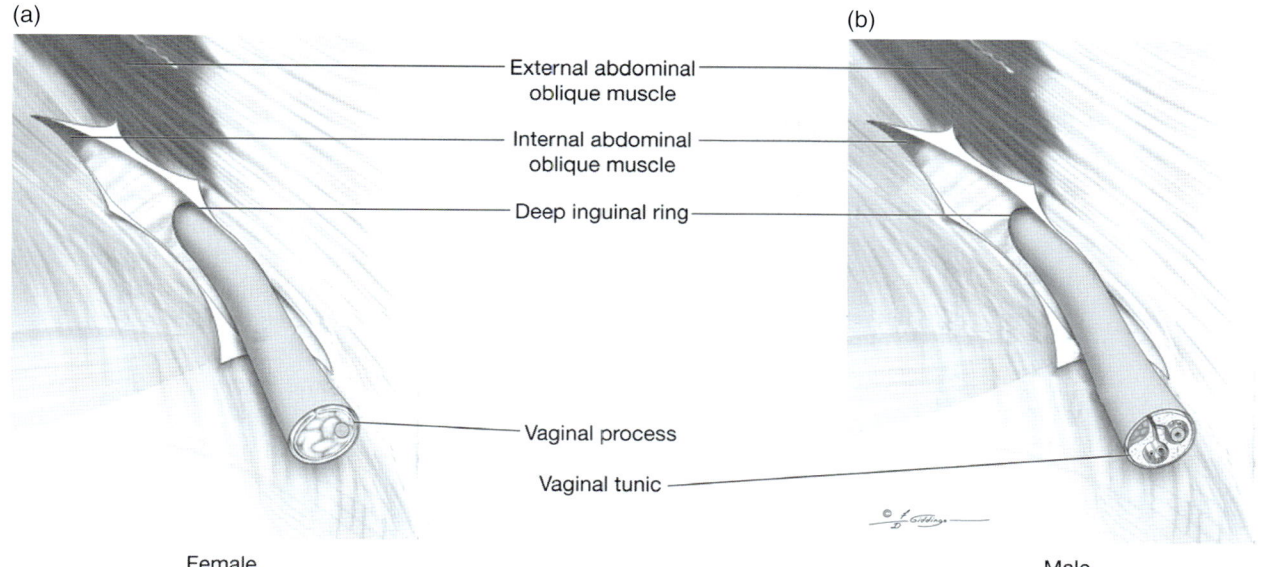

External abdominal oblique muscle

Internal abdominal oblique muscle

Deep inguinal ring

Vaginal process

Vaginal tunic

Female

Male

Figure 24.5 (a, b) Vaginal process anatomy. © D. Giddings.

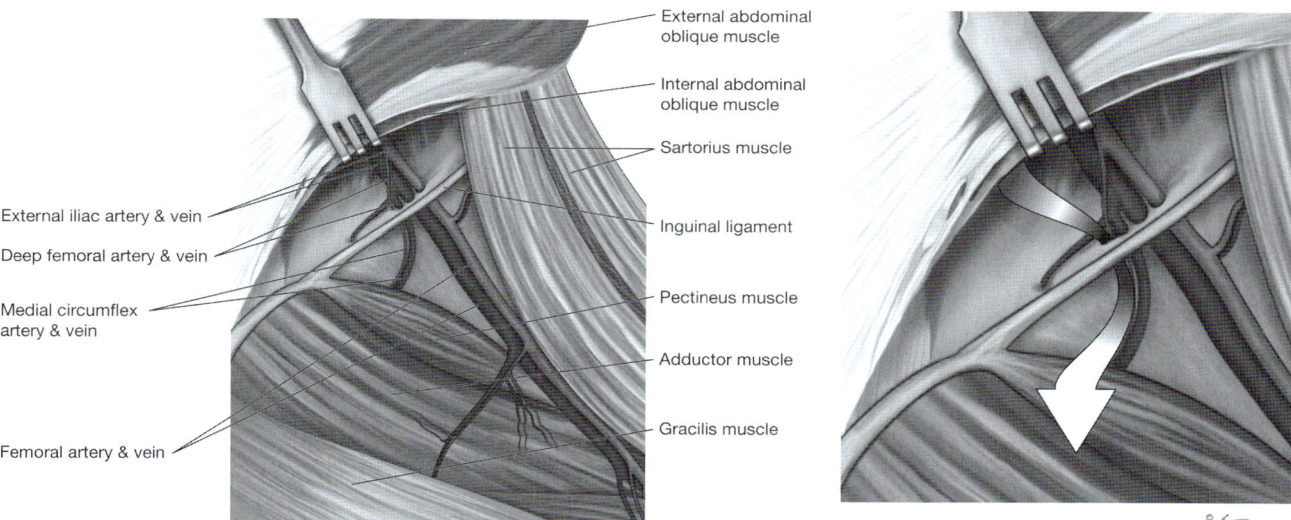

External abdominal oblique muscle

Internal abdominal oblique muscle

Sartorius muscle

Inguinal ligament

External iliac artery & vein

Deep femoral artery & vein

Pectineus muscle

Medial circumflex artery & vein

Adductor muscle

Gracilis muscle

Femoral artery & vein

Figure 24.6 Vital structures of the femoral canal. The arrow shows the pathway for a femoral hernia. © D. Giddings.

Patients with complicated hernias should be taken to emergency surgery after stabilization.

Inguinal hernia repair

There are several repair options for inguinal hernias. In general, uncomplicated inguinal hernias are approached over the inguinal rings or through a ventral midline incision, while complicated hernias are approached through a ventral midline incision and celiotomy. For the direct approach to an inguinal hernia, an incision is made parallel to the flank fold over the lateral aspect of the hernia. The hernia sac is dissected from the surrounding mammary and subcutaneous tissues and the hernia contents are gently pushed back through the canal into the abdomen. If the hernia cannot be reduced, then the hernia sac is opened and the inguinal ring is enlarged in the craniomedial direction to facilitate reduction. Alternatively, a hernia sac containing abdominal fat can be ligated and transected at the base to facilitate inguinal ring closure. Some surgeons prefer to amputate the hernia sac at the base, while others prefer to reduce the sac along with the hernia contents. If the hernia sac is amputated, the base is closed with an inverting suture pattern such as a Cushing or Connell, or with a horizontal mattress in a simple continuous pattern. The inguinal ring is then closed using a synthetic absorbable or nonabsorbable monofilament suture in a simple interrupted suture pattern. During inguinal ring closure, care is taken to protect the vital structures that exit at the caudomedial aspect of the inguinal ring (Figure 24.7). These include the external pudendal vessels, genitofemoral nerve, and spermatic cord in the male dog.

For the abdominal midline approach, a caudoventral abdominal midline incision is made that extends from the umbilicus to the brim of the pubis. The mammary and subcutaneous tissues are elevated from the body wall to expose the inguinal rings. Both inguinal rings are evaluated, since these hernias can occur bilaterally and small hernias may be difficult to palpate on physical examination. The hernia is reduced as stated earlier or, if a celiotomy is indicated, reduction is achieved by gentle traction on the herniated tissues from inside the abdomen. The inguinal ring is closed routinely.

Inguinal hernia repair from inside the abdominal cavity has been described. Sutures are placed through the parietal peritoneum, the aponeurosis of the transversalis muscle, and the rectus abdominis and internal abdominal oblique muscles (Smeak 2003). Bilateral inguinal herniorrhaphy via natural orifice transluminal endoscopic surgery (NOTES) has also recently been investigated in dogs (Sherwinter & Eckstein 2009).

Ovariohysterectomy followed by inguinal hernia repair is the recommended treatment for a herniated pyometra. Several options exist for animals with a herniated gravid uterus. In cats and dogs, ovariohysterectomy can be performed followed by herniorrhaphy. In dogs, up to the seventh week of gestation, it is possible to replace the uterus into the abdomen and then perform herniorrhaphy; after the seventh week, cesarean section can be performed followed by ovariohys-

terectomy or replacement of the uterus into the abdomen (Smeak 2003).

Scrotal hernia repair

Surgical correction of a scrotal hernia is performed as soon as possible after diagnosis, since the risk of intestinal and organ strangulation is high (Smeak 2003). Extra-abdominal repair is considered for reducible scrotal hernias, whereas intra-abdominal repair is indicated with incarcerated or complicated scrotal hernias.

For reducible scrotal hernias, an incision is made lateral to the inguinal swelling and parallel to the flank fold (Figure 24.8). Minimal dissection of the sac or inguinal rings is performed to preserve the integrity of surrounding structures. Castration is recommended during herniorrhaphy (Figure 24.9). Hernia contents are reduced, the hernia sac (parietal vaginal tunic) is incised, the spermatic cord is ligated, and the testicle is removed. The hernia sac is ligated at the internal inguinal ring and the external inguinal ring is closed as for an inguinal hernia repair. If the patient is not to be neutered, the hernia sac is incised, the hernia contents are reduced and a transfixation ligature is placed to close down the enlarged vaginal orifice. This is followed by routine herniorrhaphy.

Femoral hernia repair

The uncomplicated femoral hernia is approached externally, with an incision made parallel to the inguinal ligament to expose the hernia sac. The contents are reduced or the sac is ligated as high as possible in the femoral canal. Herniorrhaphy is achieved by placing sutures between

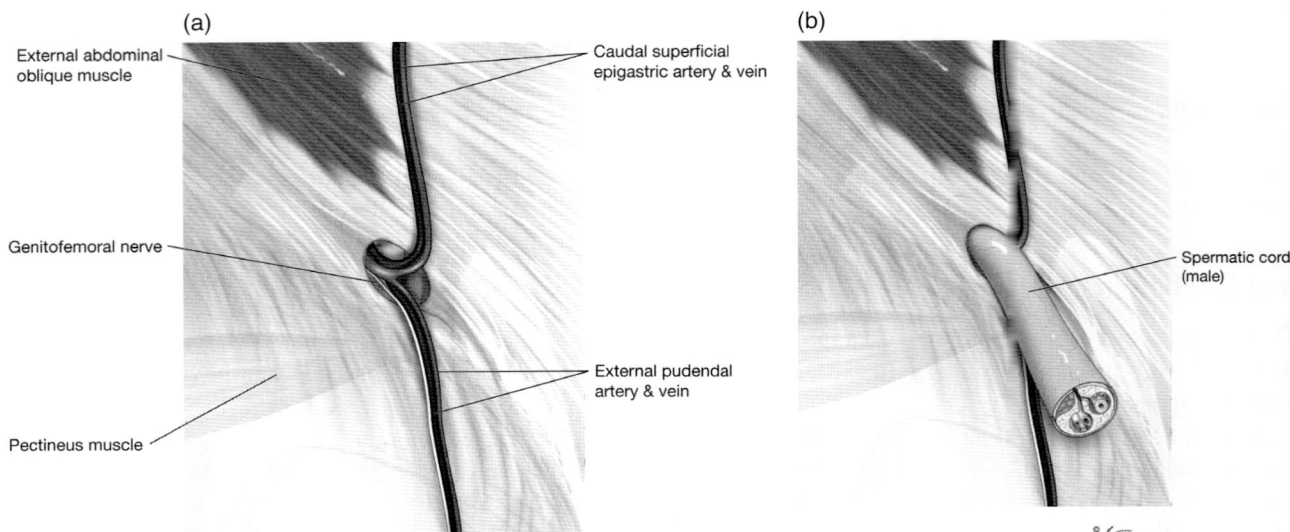

Figure 24.7 (a) Vital structures near the inguinal ring. (b) The arrow indicates the path of femoral herniation. The inguinal canal is cranial and medial to the inguinal ligament. © D. Giddings.

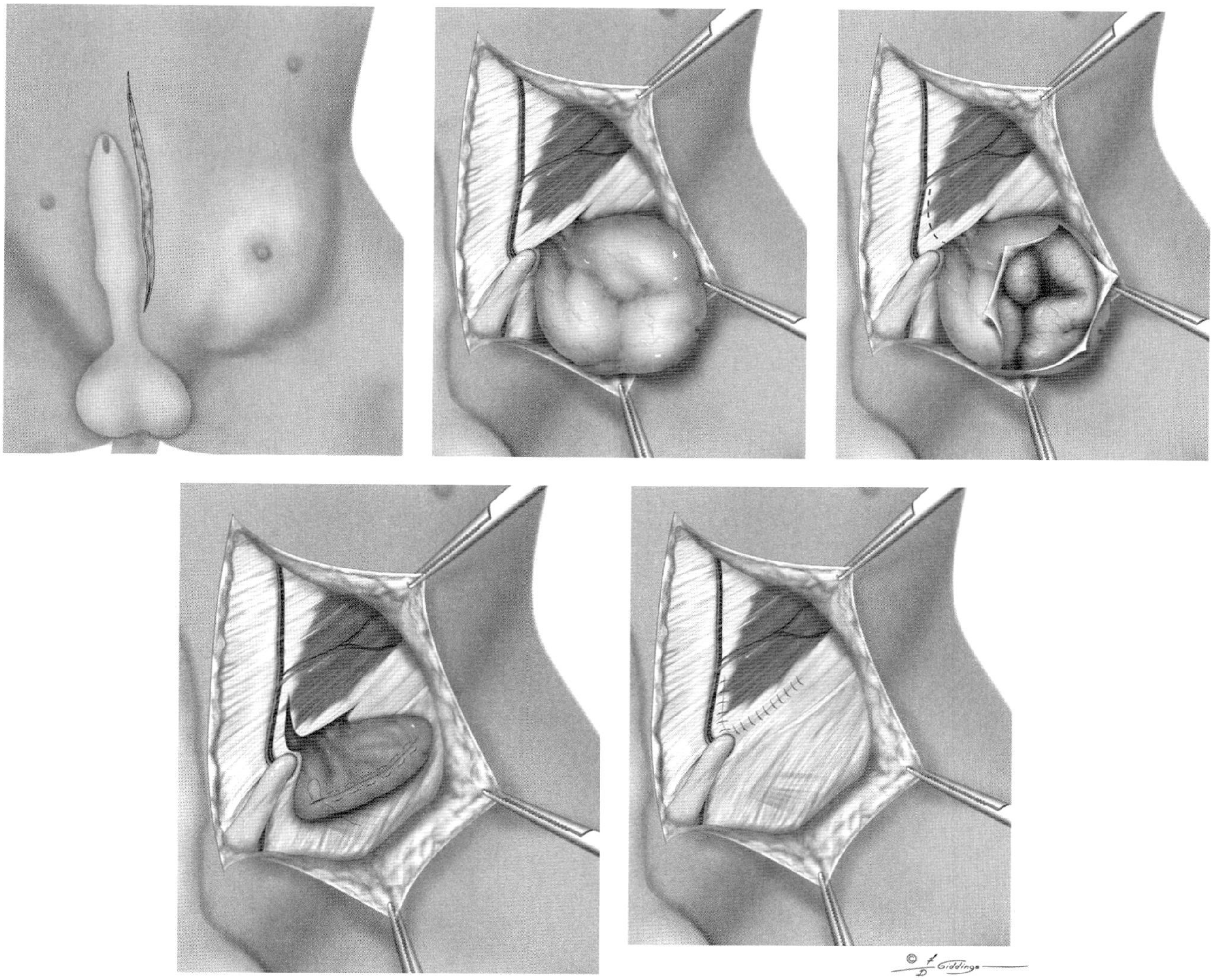

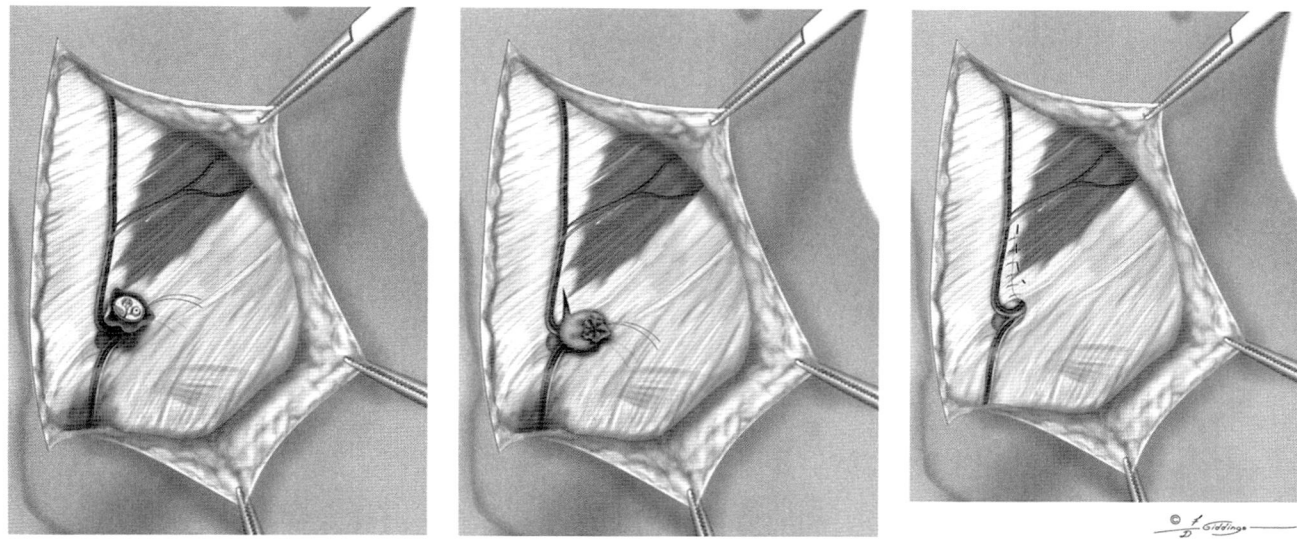

Figure 24.8 Repair of a scrotal hernia without castration. © D. Giddings.

Figure 24.9 Repair of a scrotal hernia with castration. © D. Giddings.

the inguinal ligament and pectineal fascia. Special care is taken to avoid damaging the neurovascular structures in the femoral canal.

Aftercare and prognosis

Patients should be kept inside with limited activity for 2–3 weeks following surgery. Incisions should be evaluated daily by owners. As mentioned previously, swelling, redness, and serosanguinous discharge around the incision may indicate infection or be early signs of impending dehiscence. Peritonitis or incisional abscess should be suspected in patients who develop postoperative fever, inappetence, lethargy, or vomiting.

In young patients with reducible hernias and a routine repair, the prognosis is generally excellent. In a study of 35 dogs with inguinal hernias, the overall complication rate was 17% and the mortality rate was 3% (Waters *et al.* 1993). In complicated cases, the prognosis is usually dictated by the extent of concurrent disease.

References

Chircor, L., Mehedinţi, R., and Hîncu, M. (2009). Risk factors related to omphalocele and gastroschisis. *Romanian Journal of Morphology and Embryology* 50: 645–649.

Fossum, T.W. (2007). Surgery of the abdominal cavity. In: *Small Animal Surgery*, 3e (ed. T.W. Fossum), 317–338. St Louis, MO: Mosby.

Read, R.A. and Bellenger, C.R. (2003) Hernias. In: *Textbook of Small Animal Surgery*, 3e (ed. D. Slatter), 446–448. Philadelphia, PA: WB Saunders.

Shaw, S.P., Rozanski, E.A., and Rush, J.E. (2003). Traumatic body wall herniation in 36 dogs and cats. *Journal of the American Animal Hospital Association* 39: 35–46.

Sherwinter, D.A. and Eckstein, J.G. (2009). Feasibility study of natural orifice transluminal endoscopic surgery inguinal hernia repair. *Gastrointestinal Endoscopy* 70: 126–130.

Smeak, D. (2003). Abdominal hernias. In: *Textbook of Small Animal Surgery*, 3e (ed. D. Slatter), 449–470. Philadelphia, PA: WB Saunders.

Waters, D.J., Roy, R.G., and Stone, E.A. (1993). A retrospective study of inguinal hernia in 35 dogs. *Veterinary Surgery* 22: 44.

25

Acquired Abdominal Wall Hernia

Amelia M. Simpson

Acquired abdominal wall hernias occur when abdominal contents protrude through a trauma-induced defect in the abdominal wall. Overall incidence in small animals is low (Shaw *et al.* 2003).

Traumatic hernias

Anatomy and etiology

Traumatic abdominal wall hernias have traditionally been defined by their location, with common sites including the paracostal, lateral, inguinal, femoral, prepubic, and ventral areas. The inguinal and prepubic areas along with the paracostal regions are the most common areas of herniation due to blunt trauma (Smeak 2003).

In the dog, the prepubic tendon is composed of fibers from the rectus abdominis muscle, pectineus muscle, and external abdominal oblique muscles. It is firmly attached to the brim of the pubis (Constantinescu *et al.* 2007). Cats do not have a prepubic tendon, but it is suspected that in this species the strong attachments of the crura of the superficial inguinal ring and aponeurosis of the external abdominal oblique muscle serve a similar function to the prepubic tendon in the dog (Beittenmiller *et al.* 2009).

Traumatic body wall hernias occur from bite wounds, postsurgical dehiscence, or severe blunt trauma, as seen when small animals are hit by a car or kicked. Shearing forces that are distributed across the bony prominences of the pubis result in the shearing or tearing of muscles or tendons that attach in this area (Shaw *et al.* 2003).

According to recent literature, 44–75% of animals with an abdominal wall hernia are diagnosed with concurrent injuries (Smeak 2003; Beittenmiller *et al.* 2009). Orthopedic injuries are common, but soft tissue injuries such as intestinal perforation, mesenteric avulsion, or compromise of the genitourinary system are also seen (Beittenmiller *et al.* 2009).

History and clinical signs

Most patients with traumatic abdominal wall hernias present with a history of recent trauma. Occasionally the hernia is not recognized initially as the patient is stabilized and life-threatening issues are treated. Abdominal wall hernias usually result in asymmetry of the body wall (Figure 25.1). As the intestines and abdominal organs move into the subcutaneous space, they can create a mass effect.

Diagnostics

Traumatic body wall hernias are usually diagnosed on physical examination as a soft swelling under the skin through which intestines or other organs can be palpated. Radiographs of the abdomen and thorax are recommended and can be helpful in identifying abdominal wall hernias, showing gas-filled intestines within the subcutaneous or intramuscular space, displacement of abdominal organs, or partial or complete loss of the abdominal wall outline (Figures 25.2 and 25.3). Thoracic radiography can be useful for identifying the presence of pulmonary contusions, pleural effusion, rib or spinal fractures, diaphragmatic hernias, and pneumothorax.

Small Animal Soft Tissue Surgery, Second Edition. Edited by Eric Monnet.
© 2023 John Wiley & Sons, Inc. Published 2023 by John Wiley & Sons, Inc.
Companion website: www.wiley.com/go/monnet/small

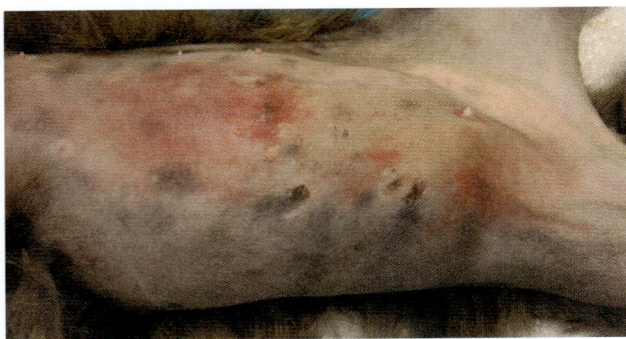

Figure 25.1 Traumatic abdominal wall hernias causing loss of abdominal wall symmetry. Cranial is to the left.

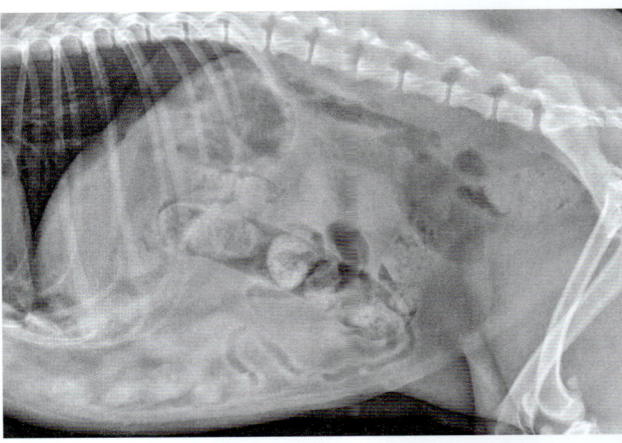

Figure 25.3 Lateral radiograph of a dog with a paracostal abdominal wall hernia.

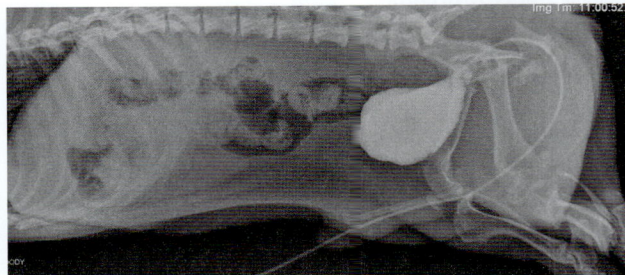

Figure 25.4 Radiographs of a dog with a prepubic tendon hernia. This dog was hit by a car and suffered a pelvic fracture. A cystogram was performed to evaluate the integrity of the lower urinary tract.

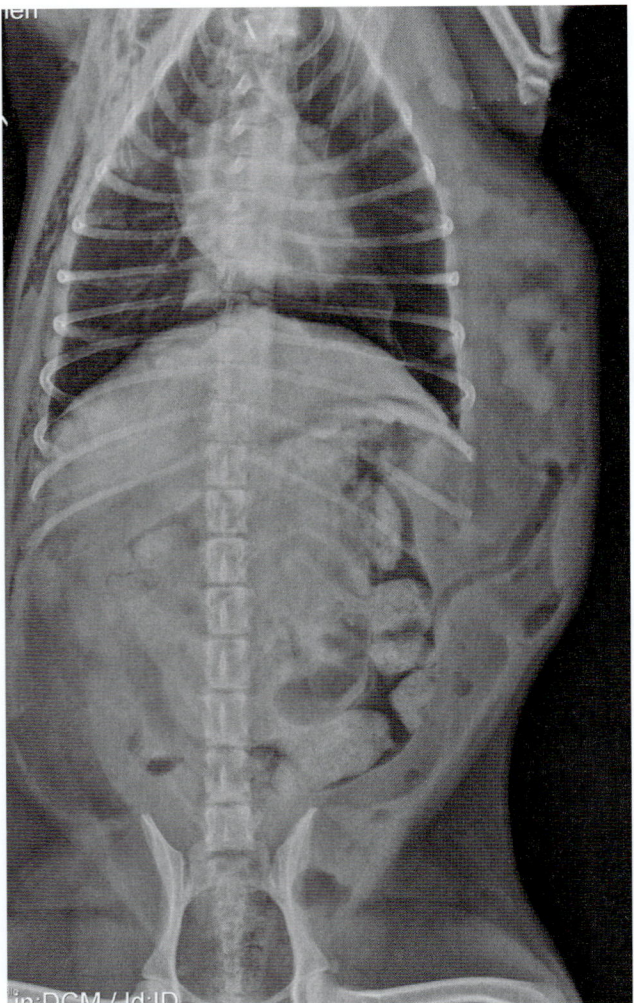

Figure 25.2 Ventro-dorsal radiography of a dog with a paracostal hernia.

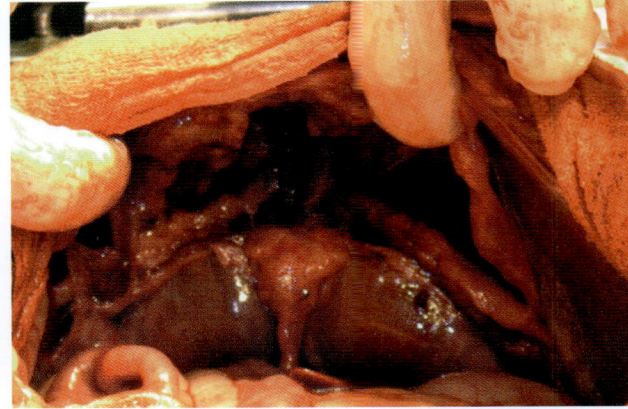

Figure 25.5 Intraoperative view of a large paracostal abdominal wall hernia.

It is important to evaluate the entire radiograph, since many animals with traumatic abdominal wall hernias may have serious concurrent injuries (Figure 25.4) (Beittenmiller *et al.* 2009).

Treatment

Surgery is aimed at reconstruction of the abdominal wall (Figure 25.5). Most often abdominal hernias can be repaired by suturing torn muscle or reattaching the torn portion of the abdominal wall to the pubis or ribs. A ventral abdominal midline incision is preferred to allow thorough evaluation of the abdominal contents. Alternatively, for large defects in the lateral abdominal wall, an incision can be made directly over the herniated contents and an abdominal exploratory performed through the hernia. The hernia is reduced by placing gentle traction on the intestines or herniated organs. If necessary the hernia can be enlarged to facilitate reduction.

Abdominal exploratory surgery is performed and damaged organs and intestines are treated accordingly. The muscle layers are then apposed and sutured with an interrupted or continuous suture pattern using a synthetic nonabsorbable monofilament suture. The use of nylon and polypropylene is recommended because they provide long-lasting support to the tissues. For paracostal hernia repair, a rib is incorporated into the suture line when the abdominal wall has been avulsed from the costal arch. Prepubic tendon ruptures are repaired by suturing the avulsed portion of the tendon to the pubis through predrilled holes in the cranial brim if there is not enough tissue caudally for primary repair (Figure 25.6). Occasionally the tissue is devitalized or the damage so severe that reconstruction is impossible without a mesh graft to close the defect. In this case synthetic Prolene® (Ethicon, Raritan, NJ, USA) or Marlex mesh (CR Bard, Murray Hill, NJ, USA) is used. The edges are folded over and the mesh is sutured to viable tissues using a simple interrupted or horizontal mattress pattern. Alternatively, a biosynthetic mesh such as porcine small intestinal submucosa can be used (Clarke *et al.* 1996).

In patients with traumatic femoral hernias, often the prepubic tendon is torn, the inguinal ligament is not intact, and/or the pectineal muscle attachments are compromised. In these patients primary reconstruction of the tissues is attempted (Figures 25.7 and 25.8). If the damage is too severe, a cranial sartorious muscle flap can be used to close the defect or a mesh graft may be used (Smeak 2003).

Aftercare and prognosis

Strict rest and decreased activity are absolutely necessary for 2–4 weeks after surgery. This will minimize stress on the repair, decrease seroma formation, and allow rapid healing of the tissues. A patient with a femoral hernia repair may benefit from having hobbles placed on the back legs to prevent tearing of the repair if the patient should slip early in the recovery. If necessary a light wrap can be placed over the affected area for a couple of weeks to minimize dead space in the subcutaneous layer. Elizabethan collars are recommended until suture removal to prevent licking or bothering of the incision.

Complications are generally dependent on the amount and type of tissue trauma. Postoperative seromas and

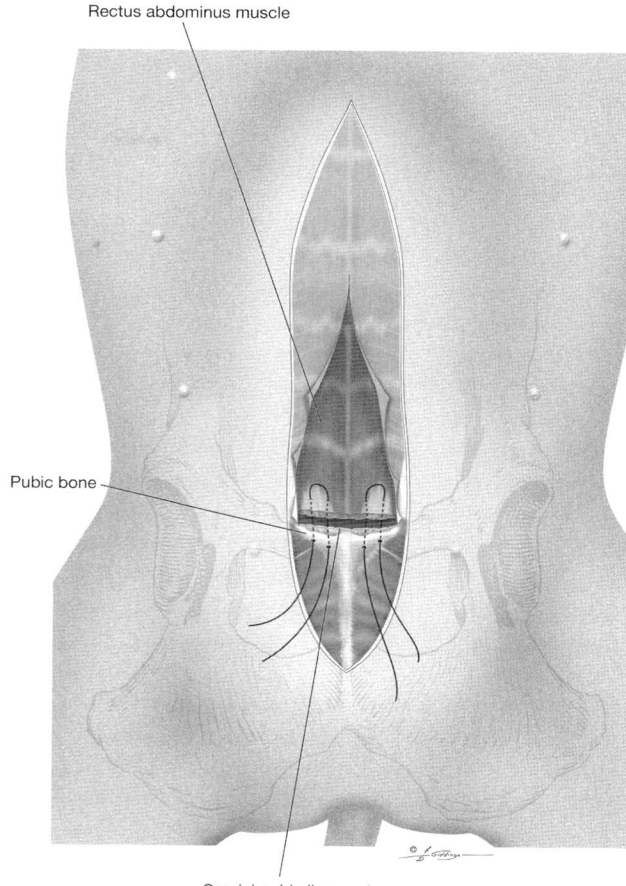

Rectus abdominus muscle

Pubic bone

Cranial pubic ligament

Figure 25.6 Diagram of a prepubic tendon repair. © D. Giddings.

hematomas are not uncommon. The use of closed suction drains is recommended when large subcutaneous defects exist after closure of the abdominal wall. Drains, if placed, are removed in 3–5 days. Incisional and body wall infections can occur with any repair, but are more common when the hernia is caused by bite wounds. Breakdown of the herniorrhaphy is uncommon with a tension-free closure and strict adherence to surgical principles.

Studies show an overall mortality rate of 9–25% in dogs and cats with traumatic body wall hernia (Shaw *et al.* 2003). Prognosis depends on the extent of the injuries, and death is usually attributed to coexisting injuries and not the herniorrhaphy itself (Smeak 2003; Beittenmiller *et al.* 2009).

Incisional hernias in abdominal wall closures

Abdominal incisional hernias occur when the suture line of an abdominal incision breaks down. Incisional hernias in people are a frequent complication of abdominal wall closure, with a reported incidence of 5–15% following vertical midline incisions at one-year follow-up

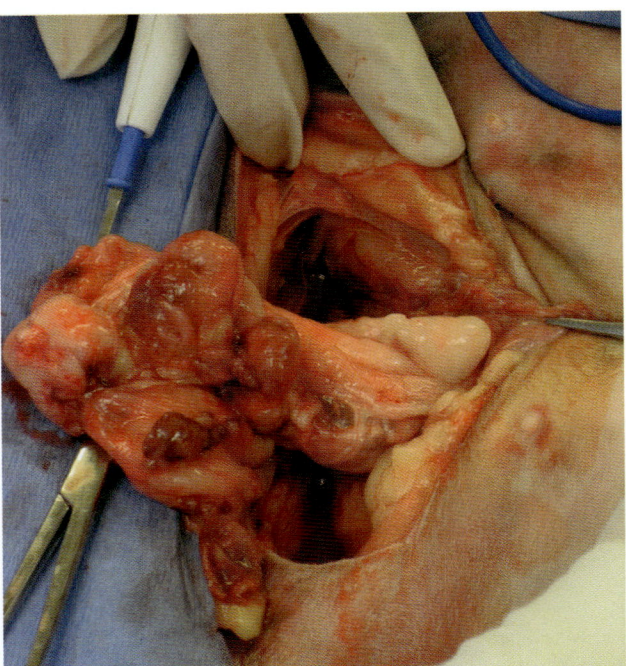

Figure 25.7 Intraoperative views of a femoral hernia associated with a prepubic tendon rupture.

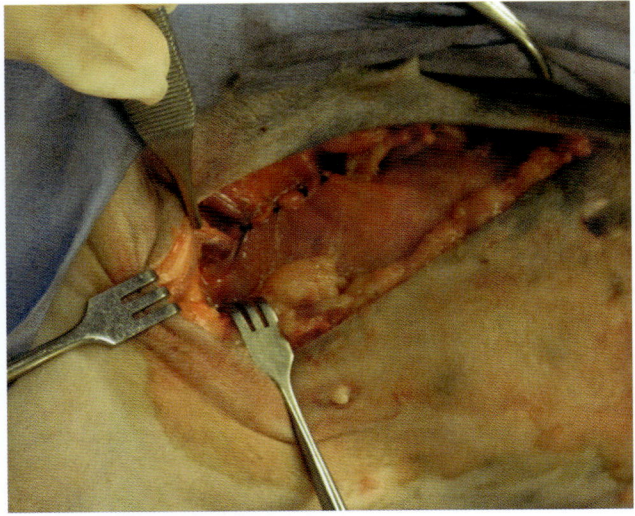

Figure 25.8 The hernia in Figure 25.7 has been reduced and the pectineal muscle reattached.

(O'Dwyer & Courtney 2003). Although incisional dehiscence is less common in small animals, it is nonetheless associated with increased morbidity and mortality in the patient and increased cost for the owners. Abdominal evisceration occurs if there is herniation through both the body wall and skin. In one study, this occurred most commonly after ovariohysterectomy (Gower et al. 2009).

Poor surgical technique is the most common cause of acute incisional dehiscence (Smeak 2003). Other factors that contribute to dehiscence of an abdominal wall incision include infection, increased tension on the incision as a result of increased intra-abdominal pressure due to pain, fat entrapped between incision edges, chronic steroid use, metabolic derangement (e.g., diabetes mellitus or hyperadrenocorticism), and poor patient care during the convalescent period with self-inflicted trauma (Gower et al. 2009).

Anatomy and etiology

In general, abdominal wall incisional hernias occur because of excessive tension placed on the incision or because of poor holding strength of the wound. A hernia is considered acute if it occurs within 7 days of surgery, whereas chronic hernias can occur weeks to years later.

Clinical signs and diagnostics

Acute abdominal wall incisional hernias usually occur 3–5 days after surgery when the holding strength of the tissues is at its weakest. In cases where the suture breaks or knots fail, the hernia can occur soon after the patient recovers from the procedure. Serosanguinous drainage from the incision is often an indicator of impending acute abdominal wound dehiscence.

Patients with abdominal wall incisional hernias commonly have a soft swelling at the site of the incision. In the case of a large reducible hernia, there is usually minimal associated pain or discomfort noted in the patient. If the hernia sac is not reducible and intestines or organs are strangulated or incarcerated, the swelling is typically firm, warm, and painful on palpation.

When the surgery is recent, the hernia is large, and abdominal contents can be palpated under the skin, additional diagnostics are usually not required to confirm incisional dehiscence. Radiographs can be taken to confirm the presence of the abdominal wall hernia.

Smaller hernias, or hernias in which just omentum or falciform fat is herniated, may provide a diagnostic challenge, as it can be difficult to distinguish these hernias from postoperative inflammation and/or edema, a suture reaction, seroma, or incisional abscess. Palpation of the abdominal wall suture line may reveal a defect. Abdominal ultrasound may be useful in these cases as well. Aspiration of the swelling may reveal seroma fluid or purulent material, thereby diagnosing seroma or abscess. Consideration for surgical exploration should be made in cases with a persistent swelling along the incision.

In patients with incisional hernias, the skin layer will often remain intact; however, if the skin layer dehisces as well, evisceration will occur with abdominal contents protruding through the skin incision. These patients require immediate supportive care and emergency surgery following stabilization.

Treatment

Acute incisional hernias are usually repaired without delay. In cases where the dehisced incision is not a ventral midline celiotomy, an approach is carefully made over the original incision. If strangulation or incarceration of the abdominal organs is suspected, then a routine abdominal midline incision is made for abdominal exploratory surgery and damaged intestines or organs are repaired as necessary before herniorrhaphy.

The original incision is evaluated and the cause for dehiscence is determined. If a suture has broken or a knot failed, then the entire incision is resutured using an appropriate-gauge suture with strict adherence to surgical principles for abdominal wall closure. The strength-holding tissue layer is the external rectus fascia, so it is of paramount importance to incorporate this layer in the closure. A simple continuous suture pattern is acceptable, but more throws on the knot are required at the ends to secure this type of closure than are required with individual knots in a simple interrupted suture pattern. In general, five throws are recommended for the initial knot and six or seven for the final knot. Sutures should be placed approximately 5 mm from the skin edge.

If excessive tension is the suspected cause for the original dehiscence, then placement of a prosthetic or biosynthetic mesh graft is indicated. In humans there are many problems associated with the use of prosthetic mesh grafts (Cavallaro *et al.* 2010). Complications include infection, fistula formation, and skin erosion, which lead to a high rate of removal. Prosthetic mesh grafts are removed in the majority of cases when applied in a contaminated surgical field. Bovine pericardium grafts, porcine dermal collagen, and porcine submucosa grafts have been used in humans in the reconstruction of abdominal wall defects (Armellino *et al.* 2006; Franklin *et al.* 2008; Cavallaro *et al.* 2010). These biosynthetic mesh grafts provide a collagen and extracellular matrix scaffold that allows host fibroblasts to create angiogenesis and deposit new collagen, thereby incorporating the graft as healing takes place. It is thought that they are more resistant to infections since they are not synthetic (Cavallaro *et al.* 2010).

Treatment for patients with eviscerated intestines and abdominal organs is initiated immediately. In these patients, a moistened sterile dressing should be placed over the exposed organs while the patient is treated for shock and prepared for surgery. Extension of the abdominal rent may be necessary to prevent vascular compromise to herniated organs. The intestines and eviscerated organs should be copiously lavaged with saline to eliminate gross contamination. Samples should be obtained for aerobic and anaerobic culture and sensitivity, and broad-spectrum antibiotic treatment instituted. The abdomen should be closed with an abdominal drain in place, or the abdomen can be maintained open with closure scheduled in the near future.

Aftercare and prognosis

Routine postoperative care is recommended for these patients, with special emphasis on activity restrictions during the convalescent period. There is a good prognosis for animals with an incisional dehiscence due to suture failure in which the skin layer remains intact. Animals with evisceration have previously been considered to have a guarded prognosis as postoperative infection rates are high in these cases. However, a recent retrospective study found that all animals survived to discharge from the hospital (Gower *et al.* 2009). As with the other complicated abdominal wall hernias, prognosis usually depends on the extent of the injuries.

References

Armellino, M.F., De Stefano, G., Scardi, F. et al. (2006). Use of Permacol in complicated incisional hernia. *Chirurgia Italiana* 58: 627–630.

Beittenmiller, M.R., Mann, F.A., Constantinescu, G.M., and Luther, J.K. (2009). Clinical anatomy and surgical repair of prepubic hernia in dogs and cats. *Journal of the American Animal Hospital Association* 45: 284–290.

Cavallaro, A., Lo Menzo, E., Di Vita, M. et al. (2010). Use of biological meshes for abdominal wall reconstruction in highly contaminated fields. *World Journal of Gastroenterology* 16: 1928–1933.

Clarke, K.M., Lantz, G.C., Salisbury, S.K. et al. (1996). Intestine submucosa and polypropylene mesh for abdominal wall repair in dogs. *Journal of Surgical Research* 60: 107–114.

Constantinescu, G.M., Beittenmiller, M.R., Mann, F.A. et al. (2007). Clinical anatomy of the prepubic tendon in the dog and a comparison with the cat. *Cercetări Experimentale Medico-Chirurgicale* XIV: 81–85.

Franklin, M.E. Jr., Treviño, J.M., Portillo, G. et al. (2008). The use of porcine small intestinal submucosa as a prosthetic material for laparoscopic hernia repair in infected and potentially contaminated fields: long-term follow-up. *Surgical Endoscopy* 22: 1941–1946.

Gower, S.B., Weisse, C.W., and Brown, D.C. (2009). Major abdominal evisceration injuries in dogs and cats: 12 cases (1998–2008). *Journal of the American Veterinary Medical Association* 234: 1566–1571.

O'Dwyer, P.J. and Courtney, C.A. (2003). Factors involved in abdominal wall closure and subsequent incisional hernia. *The Surgeon* 1: 17–22.

Shaw, S.P., Rozanski, E.A., and Rush, J.E. (2003). Traumatic body wall herniation in 36 dogs and cats. *Journal of the American Animal Hospital Association* 39: 35–46.

Smeak, D. (2003). Abdominal hernias. In: *Textbook of Small Animal Surgery*, 3e (ed. D. Slatter), 449–470. Philadelphia, PA: WB Saunders.

26

Diaphragmatic and Peritoneopericardial Diaphragmatic Hernias

Janet Kovak McClaran

The diaphragm serves as a physical barrier between the pleural and peritoneal cavities. It is a tendino-muscular septum that functions in assisting ventilation and movement of lymphatic fluid. Innervation of the diaphragm is via the phrenic nerve, which arises from the fifth to seventh cervical nerves. The diaphragm is divided into a weaker left crus and stronger right crus at the level of the aortic hiatus. There is a central tendinous portion and a peripheral muscular portion of the diaphragm. The muscular portion consists of sternal, costal, and lumbar regions. The right phrenic nerve and the caudal vena cava reach the diaphragm in the plica of the vena cava. The caudal vena cava passes through the caval foramen. The dorsally located aortic hiatus allows passage of the aorta, thoracic duct, and right azygous vein. The slit-like esophageal hiatus lies in the muscular portion of the diaphragm and allows transit for the esophagus, as well as the accompanying dorsal and ventral vagal trunks (Budras & Fricke 1994).

Diaphragmatic hernia

Herniation of abdominal contents through the diaphragm may be a result of either a congenital or a traumatic event. True congenital or pleuroperitoneal hernias are rare in dogs and cats and involve the dorsolateral diaphragm (Voges et al. 1995; Hunt & Johnson 2003). They are thought to be a result of failure of fusion of the pleuroperitoneal membrane, with an autosomal recessive mode of inheritance for the defect (Noden & De Lahunta 1985; Valentine et al. 1988).

Trauma is the most common cause for diaphragmatic hernias and is usually the result of a motor vehicle accident (Spackman et al. 1984; Gibson et al. 2005; Worth & Machon 2005). Trauma has been reported as the cause of diaphragmatic hernia in 77–85% of the cases reported (Wilson & Hayes 1986; Boudrieau & Muir 1987; Worth & Machon 2005). Orthopedic injury has been reported in up to 33% of dogs and 14% of cats with diaphragmatic hernia (Gibson et al. 2005). In cases of traumatic diaphragmatic injury, 41% of cats and 27% of dogs sustained other soft tissue injury (Gibson et al. 2005).

Hernias occur following the creation of a large pleuroperitoneal pressure gradient, with trauma to the abdominal wall increasing abdominal pressure and rapid deflation of the lungs lowering pleural pressure (Boudrieau & Muir 1987; Worth & Machon 2005).

Rents in the diaphragm tend to occur in the weaker, muscular portions. While distribution of tears in diaphragmatic hernias is uniform left to right, 15% may be bilateral or multiple (Hunt & Johnson 2003; Schmiedt et al. 2003; Minihan et al. 2004; Gibson et al. 2005; Worth & Machon 2005). In one study, dogs were noted to tear costal muscles circumferentially (40%), radially (40%), or a combination of both (20%). Cats more commonly had circumferential tears (59%) rather than radial tears (18%) (Figures 26.1 and 26.2) (Garson et al. 1980; Schmiedt et al. 2003; Minihan et al. 2004; Gibson et al. 2005; Worth & Machon 2005). The liver is the most frequently herniated organ (64–82%), followed by the intestines or stomach (47–56%), spleen (32–44%), omentum (26–44%), and pancreas (4–8%) (Schmiedt

Small Animal Soft Tissue Surgery, Second Edition. Edited by Eric Monnet.
© 2023 John Wiley & Sons, Inc. Published 2023 by John Wiley & Sons, Inc.
Companion website: www.wiley.com/go/monnet/small

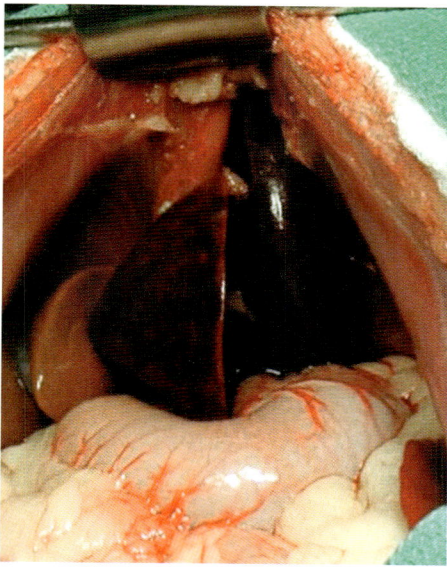

Figure 26.1 Feline diaphragmatic hernia: circumferential tear with one liver lobe and the spleen herniated in the pleural space. Source: Courtesy of Dr. Chick Weisse.

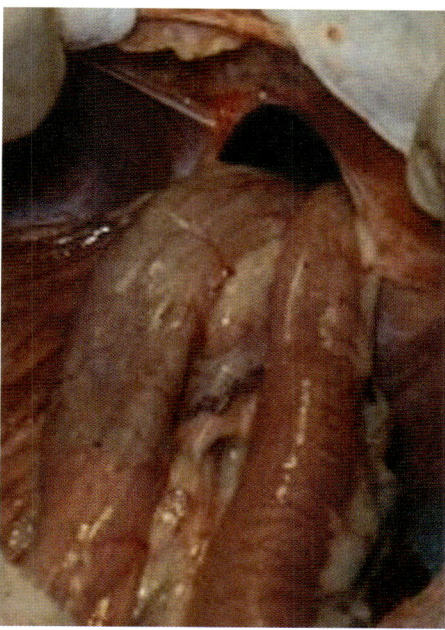

Figure 26.2 Canine diaphragmatic hernia: radial tear with loops of jejunum herniated.

et al. 2003; Minihan *et al.* 2004; Gibson *et al.* 2005; Worth & Machon 2005). The side of the tear influences which abdominal viscera are likely to herniate. With right-sided tears, the liver, small intestine, and pancreas are most likely to herniate, while left-sided hernias more commonly contain stomach, spleen, and small intestine (Garson *et al.* 1980).

Pathophysiology

Respiratory and cardiac functions are altered after a traumatic diaphragmatic hernia, resulting in reduction of oxygen delivery. Hypoxemia results from hypoventilation because of the lack of a functional diaphragm, accumulation of air and fluid in the pleural space, atelectasis, and pulmonary contusion. Atelectasis results from the presence of herniated organs in the pleural space. It results in a low ventilation–perfusion mismatch that does not respond well to oxygenation. If a pneumothorax or hemothorax is present with a diaphragmatic hernia, it should be treated aggressively to allow reexpansion of the lungs (Worth & Machon 2005). Rib fractures and pain also compromise thoracic expansion and ventilation, and therefore analgesia is important for the emergency treatment of those cases (Boudrieau & Muir 1987). Herniated organs interfere with venous return, which will induce a reduction in cardiac output. Cardiac dysrhythmias may occur due to the effects of hypovolemia and traumatic myocarditis. Hypoxemia and reduction of cardiac output result in severe reduction of oxygen delivery.

Incarceration of herniated abdominal viscera may occur, which can lead to gastrointestinal obstruction or necrosis of the affected organ and further exacerbate systemic signs of illness. Gastric dilatation and volvulus with associated diaphragmatic hernia have been reported in three cats (Formaggini *et al.* 2008).

Other organs and tissues can be injured during formation of a traumatic hernia, including kidney damage, rupture of ureters, laceration of the spleen, fracture of extremities, and pelvic fractures (Gibson *et al.* 2005). Liver herniation can occur with a hernia on the left or the right side. Liver herniation can result in hepatic vein obstruction, hepatic necrosis, and biliary tract obstruction (Figure 26.3). Following herniation, hepatic venous

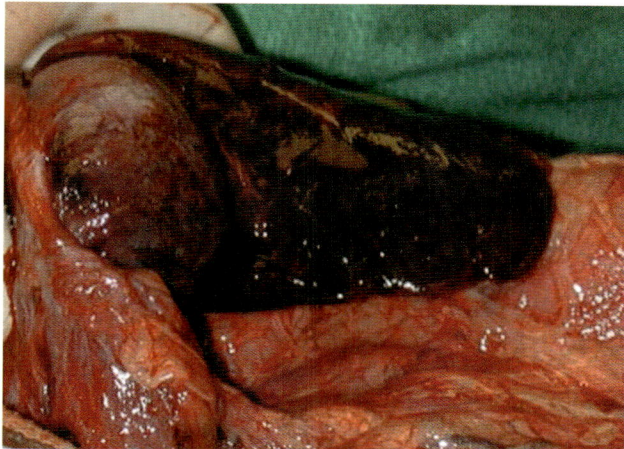

Figure 26.3 Necrosis of the left medial liver lobe in a dog with a diaphragmatic hernia.

outflow is easily compromised. A slight increase in the pressure in the hepatic vein can induce severe liver congestion (Laine *et al.* 1979; Johnson 1987). The lymphatic vessels increase in diameter and a large quantity of hepatic lymph can accumulate in the pleural space, the pericardium (if the pericardium is incomplete), and the abdominal cavity. Usually pleural effusion will develop when the diaphragm is healing around a herniated liver lobe.

Clinical presentation

Diaphragmatic hernia should always be suspected for a dog or cat following trauma. Even if there are no pathognomonic signs of diaphragmatic hernia, most animals present with acute signs and symptoms associated with respiratory distress. Animals with more chronic symptoms have also been reported (Stokhof 1986; Schmiedt *et al.* 2003; Minihan *et al.* 2004; Gibson *et al.* 2005; Worth & Machon 2005). Additionally, gastrointestinal signs such as vomiting may be observed as abdominal contents within the thoracic cavity may be compromised.

Physical examination can be normal in some patients. However, auscultation most commonly reveals abnormally located and/or muffled heart sounds. Tachycardia with weak femoral pulses can be documented in animals presenting in shock following acute trauma (Minihan *et al.* 2004; Gibson *et al.* 2005). On palpation, the abdomen may feel empty because most of the abdominal organs are herniated.

Diagnostic imaging

Thoracic and abdominal radiography is recommended for confirming the diagnosis of a diaphragmatic hernia. Abdominal radiographs may display an absence or cranial displacement of normal viscera. Thoracic radiographs may show the following: loss of the diaphragmatic line in the ventral portion (mostly due to the presence of pleural effusion), loss of the cardiac silhouette, cranial and dorsal displacement of lung fields and heart, and pleural effusion. Additionally, gas (related to the gastrointestinal tract) may be present in the thoracic cavity (Figure 26.4) (Williams *et al.* 1998; Park 2002; Milson 2007).

Pleural effusion is usually present with a chronic diaphragmatic hernia that involves entrapment of a liver lobe. As many patients may have suffered from past vehicular trauma, additional findings such as rib fractures or lung contusions may be present radiographically. Abdominal radiographs may show the absence of certain organs from the abdominal cavity and/or a forward shift of the gastric axis. Additional imaging, such as administration of barium sulfate per os, positional radiographic views, or peritoneography (Figure 26.5),

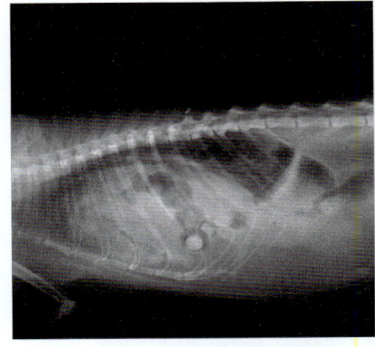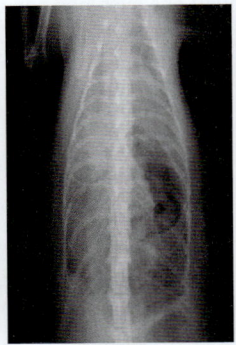

Figure 26.4 Lateral and ventrodorsal thoracic radiograph of a diaphragmatic hernia in a cat. The ventral border of the diaphragm is not visible. A loop of intestine is visible in the thoracic cavity. Source: Courtesy of Dr. Chick Weisse.

(a)

(b)

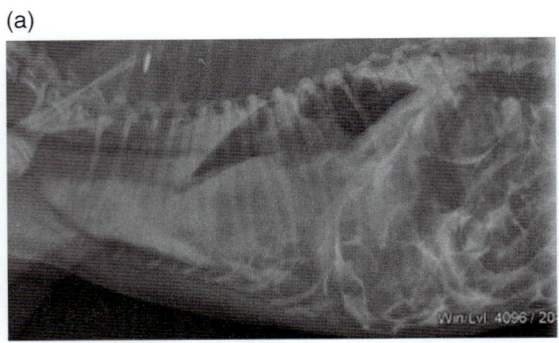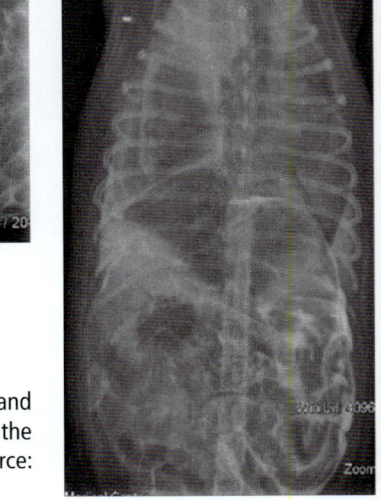

Figure 26.5 Peritoneography: (a) lateral radiograph and (b) ventrodorsal radiograph with contrast material in the cranial thorax confirming a diaphragmatic hernia. Source: Courtesy of Dr. Chick Weisse.

(a)

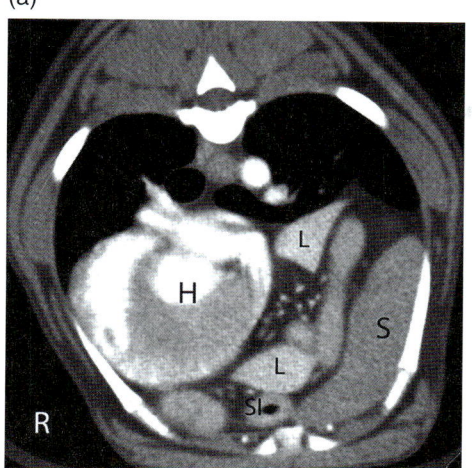

(b)

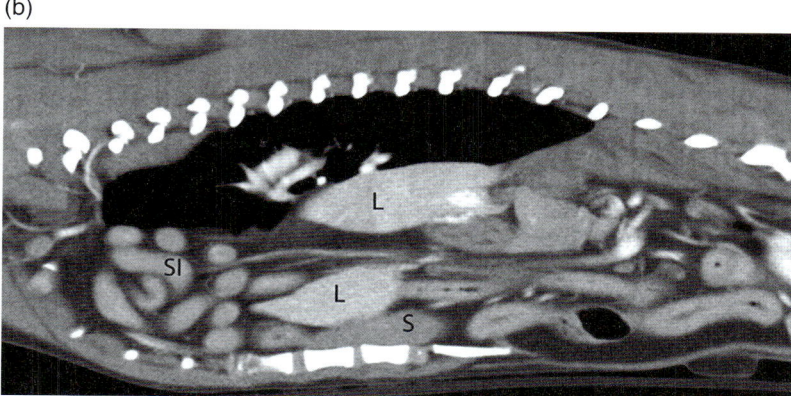

Figure 26.6 (a) Transverse and (b) sagittal computed tomography images after intravenous contrast administration, in a dog with a chronic traumatic diaphragmatic hernia noted several years after a known trauma (motor vehicle accident). Herniation of abdominal contents spans a large area of the left thorax and includes multiple liver lobes (L), spleen (S), small intestine (SI), mesenteric fat, and associated blood vessels. Source: Courtesy of Dr. Anthony J. Fischetti.

may confirm the diagnosis (Rendano 1979; Park 2002). An erect ventrodorsal radiograph is usually helpful to show the migration of different abdominal organs into the abdominal cavity (Williams *et al.* 1998).

Imaging techniques such as ultrasonography, angiography, portography, positive contrast pleurography, and cholecystography have also been reported to aid in the diagnosis (Williams *et al.* 1998; Park 2002). Additionally, computed tomography (CT) can be a useful modality to add in diagnosis. Sagittal and transverse CT images are included of a dog with a traumatic diaphragmatic hernia (Figure 26.6a,b).

Treatment

Preoperative management and timing of surgery

A patient with an acute traumatic diaphragmatic hernia presents a high anesthetic risk and often needs to be treated for hypovolemic shock, cardiac arrhythmias, and hypoxemia. Patients with a chronic diaphragmatic hernia are usually more stable. However, chronic diaphragmatic hernias can cause acute decompensation when several abdominal organs herniate into the thoracic cavity, inducing severe atelectasis. Hypovolemic shock should be treated with adequate amounts of fluid. Atelectasis, lung contusions, and the presence of pleural fluid may increase the risk of reexpansion pulmonary edema (Schertel *et al.* 1996; Worth & Machon 2005). Therefore, a combination of colloids and crystalloid therapy for low-volume resuscitation should be the goal (Schertel *et al.* 1996). Dyspnea, cyanosis, tachypnea, and

tachycardia are signs of hypoxia and should be treated aggressively with oxygen by a mask, intranasal cannula, or oxygen cage. Endotracheal intubation may be required for cases with severe pulmonary contusions. Ventilation with positive end-expiratory pressure and 100% oxygen may be required to expand alveoli and help control the contusions (Van Pelt *et al.* 1993a,b). If pleural effusion or a pneumothorax is present, either should be evacuated by thoracocentesis or placement of a chest tube. This will facilitate ventilation and correction of atelectasis. If a gas- or fluid-filled stomach is within the thoracic cavity, a nasogastric tube may be placed to provide decompression.

There is some controversy over the timing of surgical intervention with these patients. An early study reported a significantly higher mortality in patients that had surgery performed within 24 hours or more than 1 year from the time of the initial traumatic event when compared with dogs undergoing surgery at any other time (Boudrieau & Muir 1987). A more recent study, however, suggests that early surgical intervention for acute diaphragmatic hernia in dogs and cats is possible (Gibson *et al.* 2005). In this study, a 93.7% survival rate was found in patients with acute diaphragmatic hernia that received surgical intervention within 24 hours of admission to the hospital, with an overall survival rate of 89.7% for the entire population. The odds ratio (OR) for perioperative survival was no different between cases admitted earlier than 24 hours and cases admitted later than 24 hours after trauma (OR 0.51, 95% confidence interval [CI] 0.06–2.92; $P = 0.67$), or between cases receiving surgical correction of acute diaphragmatic hernia earlier than 24 hours and those receiving surgical correction later than 24 hours after trauma (OR 0.83, 95% CI 0.14–4.90; $P = 1.00$) (Gibson *et al.* 2005). The higher survival rate may be due to advancements in anesthetic protocols and intensive care practices. It is important to recognize that injuries to other organs and tissues might be more life-threatening than the diaphragmatic hernia and may need to be treated before surgical correction of the diaphragmatic hernia itself (Schmiedt *et al.* 2003). Specific indications for more rapid surgical intervention include gastric herniation with gastric tympany that cannot be relieved with a stomach tube (Figure 26.7), a large volume of herniated abdominal organs that are prohibiting lung expansion, and the presence of compromised bowel within the hernia. In addition, patients not responding to aggressive medical treatment should be taken to surgery, realizing that they are at higher risk for complications.

Schmiedt *et al.* (2003) reported a 17% mortality rate in a study on 34 cats with traumatic diaphragmatic hernia. Postoperative complications developed in 50% of the cats. The mortality rate was not associated with duration of the herniation, but was associated with concurrent injuries (rib fractures and abdominal herniation). Younger cats had a better outcome than older cats. The organs that were herniated had no effect on survival. Reexpansion pulmonary edema developed in one cat.

Surgical technique

Surgical repair is most often through a midline celiotomy, although a median sternotomy may be included for an irreducible hernia if needed (Hunt & Johnson 2003). Positioning of the patient in slight reverse Trendelenburg orientation may facilitate organ reduction, as well as alleviate compression of pulmonary parenchyma. More recently, a single paracostal approach has been reported for repair when a midline celiotomy was unsuccessful

(O'Byrne *et al.* 2021). Assisted positive-pressure ventilation is important in these patients during the surgical procedure; however, the anesthetist should not attempt to overinflate the lungs and should maintain an airway pressure below 20 cmH$_2$O to prevent the development of reexpansion pulmonary edema in cats. Full abdominal exploration is recommended to evaluate all viscera. Inspection of the entire diaphragm should be performed to assess for multiple tears or rents. With traumatic hernias, reduction can generally be achieved through gentle traction of herniated organs caudally (Figure 26.8). Enlargement of the hernia ring may be performed to remove incarcerated viscera. If enlargement is performed, it should be directed ventrally with caution to avoid trauma to the herniated organs, lungs, vena cava, phrenic nerve, and esophagus. Evaluation of the pulmonary parenchyma should be performed before closure of the diaphragm. Lavage of the thoracic cavity to check for air leakage should be performed if compromised pulmonary parenchyma is suspected. A thoracostomy tube is placed before closure of the diaphragm. With chronic injury, adhesions may be present between herniated organs and the lungs or the pericardium. In a study evaluating 50 cases of diaphragmatic hernia, 28% of the cases required a caudal median sternotomy to break down adhesions (Minihan *et al.* 2004).

It has been recommended that the edges of the diaphragm are débrided before repair. This will increase the size of the defect, although the diaphragm is very compliant and it will not compromise closure of the hernia. Repair with either nonabsorbable suture or 3-0 to 0 polydioxanone or polyglactin 910 is recommended

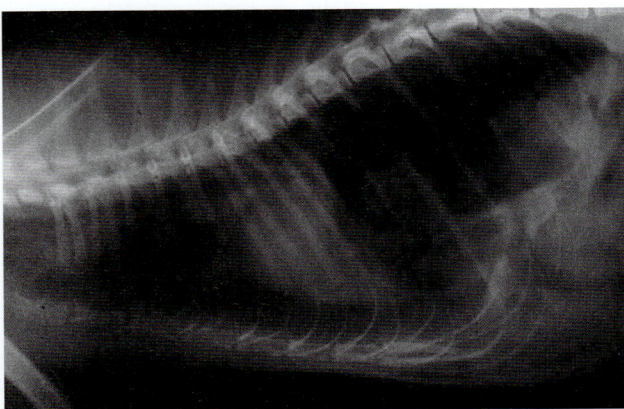

Figure 26.7 Lateral radiograph of a cat with a diaphragmatic hernia. The stomach is dilated inside the thoracic cavity.

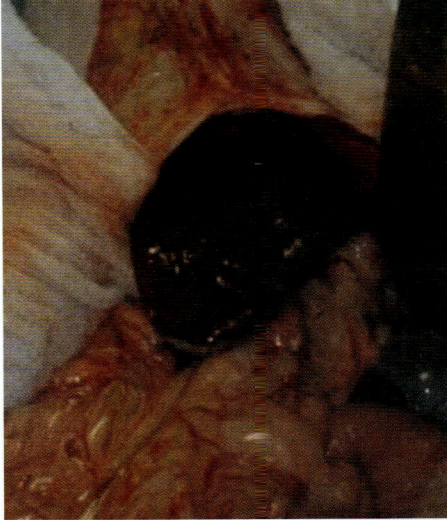

Figure 26.8 A spleen that was herniated in the thoracic cavity is being reduced after incising the diaphragm in a ventral direction from the hernia.

(Figure 26.9) (Hunt & Johnson 2003). A continuous suture pattern is preferred to an interrupted pattern because it is rapid (Figure 26.10). Care is taken to avoid damage to, or constriction of, structures such as the esophagus, vena cava, and aorta that travel through the normal diaphragmatic hiatus. It might be indicated to preplace simple interrupted sutures to close the defect near those structures to prevent stenosis of the hiatus or foramen. In patients with circumferential tears, there may not be enough tissue to allow for direct apposition of the torn edges of the diaphragm. In these patients, sutures may be placed through the body wall or around the ribs/sternum. For defects that cannot be completely closed, patching has been reported using omentum, muscle, liver, polypropylene mesh, and silicon rubber sheeting (Hunt & Johnson 2003) (Figure 26.11).

All repositioned abdominal organs are assessed for viability prior to closure and resected as needed. Minihan *et al.* (2004) performed 14 resections of different organs during reduction of diaphragmatic hernia in 50 cases. Partial or complete liver lobectomy has been performed for severe hemorrhage from the liver lobes after breakdown of adhesions, or for liver lobe necrosis (Minihan *et al.* 2004).

Minimally invasive methods, including thoracoscopic or laparoscopic repair of hernias, have been reported in human medicine. Thoracoscopic congenital hernia repair was associated with a lower morbidity and quicker recovery than traditional open repair in a study of 33 newborn patients (Gourlay *et al.* 2009). There are few reports of minimally invasive repair of hernias in veterinary medicine, but include a report of laparoscopic herniorrhaphy, with documented reoccurrence in a cat with peritoneopericardial diaphragmatic hernia (PPDH) (Fransson 2021), and successful short-term outcome in two dogs (Sharf *et al.* 2021).

Complications and prognosis

The most frequent reported complications following surgical repair of diaphragmatic hernias are pneumothorax, hypothermia, vomiting, and hypoxemia. Reexpansion pulmonary edema is a rare complication that is more common in cats than in dogs. Reexpansion pulmonary edema results from mechanical disruption

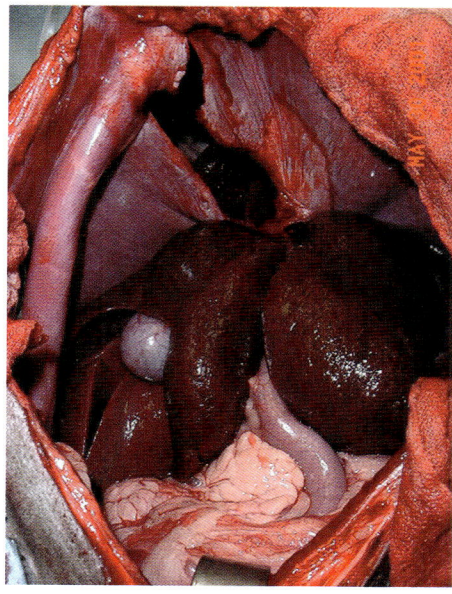

Figure 26.9 Diaphragmatic hernia after débridement of the edges ready for closure. Source: Courtesy of Dr. Chick Weisse.

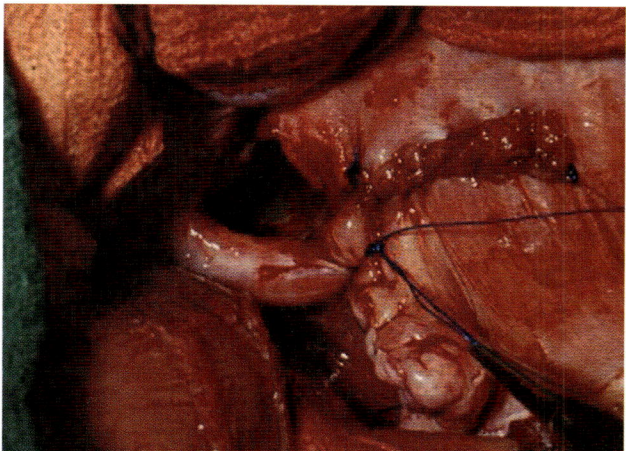

Figure 26.10 Diaphragmatic hernia being closed with three different simple continuous suture lines. A third simple continuous suture line will be required.

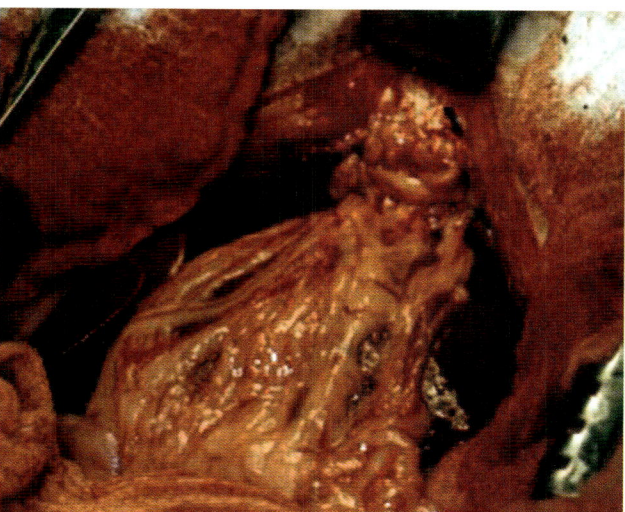

Figure 26.11 Omentum has been used to patch a defect left in the diaphragm. The closure could not be completed primarily without having too much tension on the edges of the diaphragm.

of vessels during reexpansion, surfactant abnormalities, change in pulmonary artery pressure, and the direct effect of hypoxemia on blood vessels. Atelectasis of a lung lobe is associated with a 72% reduction in blood flow because of hypoxemic pulmonary vasoconstriction (Glasser *et al.* 1983). It is recommended that attempts are not made to reinflate completely chronically collapsed lungs during surgery (Worth & Machon 2006). It has been suggested that air should not be completely evacuated from the thorax after surgery to avoid this complication (Worth & Machon 2006).

A recent case report documented acquired portosystemic shunts in a dog that had repair of a traumatic diaphragmatic four months following initial injury (Hoe & Sakals 2020).

An overall good prognosis for survival has been reported in 89.7% of patients that received surgical intervention within 24 hours of admission in a study of 92 dogs and cats with both acute and chronic traumatic diaphragmatic hernias (Gibson *et al.* 2005). In a study of animals with chronic hernias (>2 weeks duration), 86% of patients survived surgery and 79% were discharged with complete resolution of clinical signs. Postoperative complications included pneumothorax (10%), hypothermia (8%), vomiting (6%), anemia (6%), fever (4%), shock (2%), cardiac arrhythmia (2%), and respiratory arrest (2%) (Minihan *et al.* 2004). Cats have a reported survival rate following surgery of 82.4%, with a higher mortality rate in older cats with higher respiratory rates and the presence of concurrent injuries at admission (Schmiedt *et al.* 2003).

Peritoneopericardial diaphragmatic hernia

A PPDH is a congenital communication between the abdomen and the pericardial sac. Pathogenesis is attributed to a failure of normal development of the septum transversum, the embryologic structure that forms the ventral portion of the diaphragm. This may be due to failure of closure of the septum transversum itself or due to failure of fusion of the septum transversum and the pleuroperitoneal folds (the embryologic structures that form the dorsolateral portion of the diaphragm) (Reimer *et al.* 2004). Other cardiac or sternal deformities may occur concomitantly with PPDH, including ventricular septal defects, sternal defects, umbilical hernia, as well as polycystic kidneys in cats (Evans & Biery 1980; Hunt & Johnson 2003).

Clinical presentation

Organs herniated into the pericardial sac may include the liver, gallbladder, falciform ligament, omentum, spleen, stomach, small intestine, and colon (Hunt &

Johnson 2003; Reimer *et al.* 2004). Domestic longhair and Himalayan cats were overrepresented in a feline study (Reimer *et al.* 2004). Additionally, Weimaraners represented 30.8% of the affected dogs in one study (Evans & Biery 1980). Animals may present asymptomatically, with PPDH diagnosed as an incidental finding on imaging. Alternatively, respiratory, gastrointestinal, or nonspecific signs such as anorexia, lethargy, or exercise intolerance may be seen (Reimer *et al.* 2004). Physical examination findings may be normal or may reveal muffled heart sounds or signs attributable to cardiac tamponade (Hunt & Johnson 2003).

Although herniated viscera do not enter the pleural cavity, they may still cause signs of respiratory insufficiency due to indirect compression. Similar to traumatic diaphragmatic hernia, there may be strangulation or entrapment of herniated viscera. Signs of cardiac tamponade and right-sided heart failure may occur due to diminished venous return. Reported associated disease processes attributed to congenital PPDH include chylothorax in one dog (Schmiedt *et al.* 2009), pericardial pseudocysts (Cabon *et al.* 2017; Hennink *et al.* 2021) in two dogs and intrapericardial cyst formation in dogs and one cat (Hunt & Johnson 2003).

Diagnostic imaging

Radiographic findings associated with PPDH include cardiomegaly, convex projection of the caudal cardiac silhouette, abdominal organs identified within the pericardial sac, and a confluent silhouette between the diaphragm and the heart (Figures 26.12 and 26.13). Diagnosis may be difficult with herniation of solid organs such as the liver or spleen, as they will lack radiographic contrast (Park 2002; Chalkley *et al.* 2006). Additional radiographic studies include barium administration per os or nonselective angiography. Peritoneography may be used, but is often less diagnostic since contrast material may not flow through a small or obstructed defect (Park 2002).

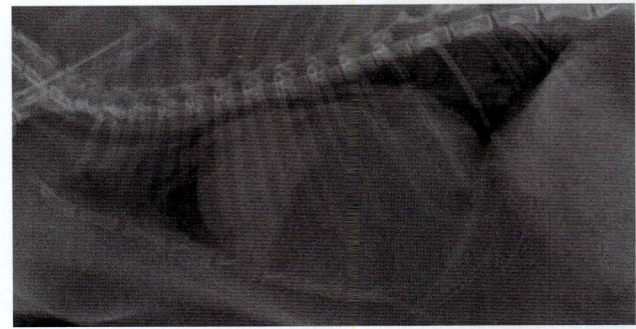

Figure 26.12 Lateral radiograph of a peritoneopericardial hernia.

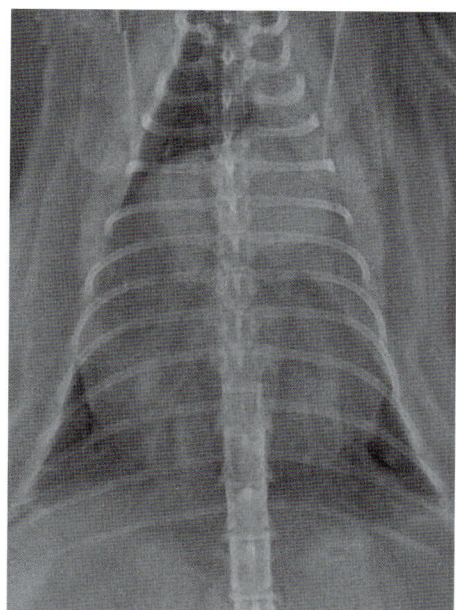

Figure 26.13 Ventrodorsal radiograph of a peritoneopericardial hernia.

Ultrasonography, echocardiography, and CT may aid in diagnosis and help to rule out any other congenital defects (Evans & Biery 1980; Williams *et al.* 1998). CT images of a cat with a clinically incidental PPDH are included (Figure 26.14).

Treatment

The principles of medical stabilization and surgical treatment are similar to those for traumatic diaphragmatic hernias. Median celiotomy generally provides adequate exposure of these midline defects. If needed, the diaphragm is incised to reduce herniated organs. Because the pericardial sac is joined with the diaphragmatic defect, suturing the pericardial sac from dorsal to ventral results in closure of the hernia. Débridement of the edges of the hernia is indicated and will result in opening of the pleural space. For larger defects under significant tension, the pericardium may be incised cranially and used to close the diaphragm as a flap or free graft. A thoracostomy tube is placed since the pleural space has been entered (Hunt & Johnson 2003).

Complications and prognosis

A recent retrospective multi-institutional report evaluated the outcomes of both surgical and conservative treatment of PPDH in 128 dogs. Overall, surgically treated dogs had a good survival rate, with 97% of dogs discharged from the hospital, and no recurrences reported. Postoperative complications were reported in 42 of 88 (47.7%) dogs that survived surgery. The most common postoperative complications were pneumothorax (8) and pneumopericardium (2), although only two cases required therapeutic thoracocentesis and/or pericardiocentesis. Major complications included a case of hepatic failure secondary to obstructive portal hypertension attributed to surgery. Deaths could be attributed to PPDH in five dogs treated surgically and four dogs treated conservatively (Morgan *et al.* 2020).

In a study of cats, intraoperative complications developed in 38% of cases and included hypotension, respiratory

(a)

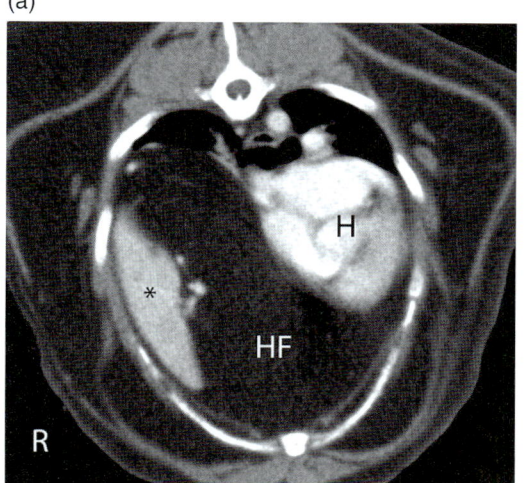

(b)

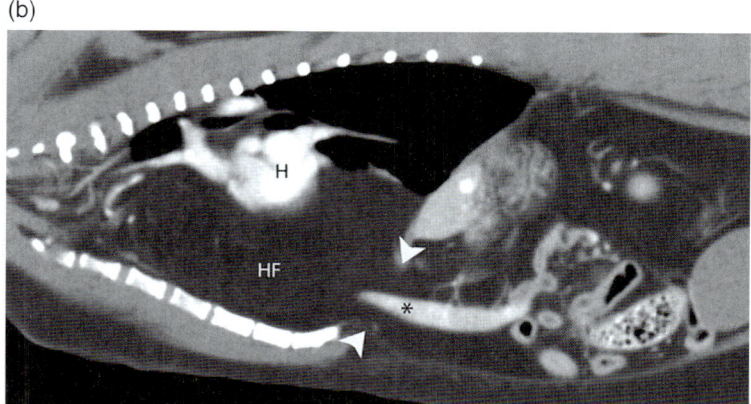

Figure 26.14 (a) Transverse and (b) sagittal computed tomography images after intravenous contrast administration in a cat with a clinically incidental peritoneopericardial diaphragmatic hernia (PPDH). PPDH tends to arise from a defect in the ventral diaphragm, close to the midline at the level of the xiphoid process. The defect is denoted by the white arrowheads. A large amount of falciform and mesenteric fat herniated (HF) into the ventral thorax, displacing the heart (H) dorsally. In this image the spleen (*) is also herniated cranial to the limits of the diaphragm. Source: Courtesy of Dr. Anthony J. Fischetti.

acidosis, hypoventilation, hypoxia, loss of palpable pulses, and ventricular premature contractions (Reimer *et al.* 2004). Postoperative complications developed in 78% of cats and included hyperthermia, tachypnea, dyspnea, hypoventilation, persistent acidemia, partial blindness, hypoxia, and refractory pneumothorax. Overall, the prognosis for surgical correction is good, with 9 of 11 (81%) dogs surviving in one study (Evans & Biery 1980) and 86% of cats surviving in another (Reimer *et al.* 2004).

Deciding between surgical and conservative treatment in patients with PPDH can be challenging. It has been reported that cats with historical problems attributed to PPDH had episodes of recurrent clinical signs with conservative treatment. Owner satisfaction with treatment choice and outcome was rated as very satisfied in 88% of those with cats that underwent surgical treatment and in 68% of those with conservatively treated cats (Reimer *et al.* 2004). In the recent retrospective study of 128 dogs, as anticipated, dogs receiving surgical treatment were younger and more likely to have clinical signs associated with herniation. The cases that did not have surgery were either asymptomatic or had severe concurrent diseases that precluded surgical intervention. Both conservative and surgically treated cases had good long-term survival times of 5 years and 8.2 years, respectively (Morgan *et al.* 2020). Future prospective studies will aid in decision making about the correction of incidentally discovered PPDH.

References

Boudrieau, R.J. and Muir, W.W. (1987). Pathophysiology of traumatic diaphragmatic hernia in dogs. *Compendium on Continuing Education for the Practicing Veterinarian* 9: 379–385.

Budras, K.-D. and Fricke, W. (1994). *Anatomy of the Dog: An Illustrated Text*, 3e. London: Mosby-Wolfe.

Cabon, Q., Carmel, E.N., and Cabassu, J. (2017). Cholecystopexy and pericardial pseudocyst removal in a dog with a congenital peritoneopericardial diaphragmatic hernia. *Journal of the American Animal Hospital Association* 53 (5): 270–276.

Chalkley, J., Salinardi, B.J., and Bulmer, B.J. (2006). What is your diagnosis? Peritoneopericardial diaphragmatic hernia (PPDH). *Journal of the American Veterinary Medical Association* 228: 695–696.

Evans, S.M. and Biery, D.N. (1980). Congenital peritoneopericardial diaphragmatic hernia in the dog and cat: a literature review and 17 additional case histories. *Veterinary Radiology* 21: 108–116.

Formaggini, L., Schmidt, K., and De Lorenzi, D. (2008). Gastric dilatation–volvulus associated with diaphragmatic hernia in three cats: clinical presentation, surgical treatment and presumptive aetiology. *Journal of Feline Medicine and Surgery* 10: 198–201.

Fransson, B (2021) Peritoneal pericardial diaphragmatic hernia repair in a cat. Scientific Presentation Abstracts Veterinary Endoscopy Society 17th Annual Society Meeting. *Veterinary Surgery* 50: O138–O160.

Garson, H.L., Dodman, N.H., and Baker, G.J. (1980). Diaphragmatic hernia: analysis of fifty-six cases in dogs and cats. *Journal of Small Animal Practice* 21: 469–481.

Gibson, T.W., Brisson, B.A., and Sears, W. (2005). Perioperative survival rates after surgery for diaphragmatic hernia in dogs and cats: 92 cases (1990–2002). *Journal of the American Veterinary Medical Association* 227: 105–109.

Glasser, S.A., Domino, K.B., Lindgren, L. et al. (1983). Pulmonary blood flow during atelectasia in the dog. *Anesthesiology* 58: 225–231.

Gourlay, D.M., Cassidy, L.D., Sato, T.T. et al. (2009). Beyond feasibility: a comparison of newborns undergoing thoracoscopic and open repair of congenital diaphragmatic hernias. *Journal of Pediatric Surgery* 44: 1702–1707.

Hennink, I., Düver, P., Rytz, U. et al. (2021). Case report: unusual peritoneopericardial diaphragmatic hernia in an 8-month-old German Shepherd dog, associated with a pericardial pseudocyst and coexisting severe pericardial effusion resulting in right-sided heart failure. *Frontiers in Veterinary Science* 8: 673543.

Hoe, S. and Sakals, S. (2020). Multiple acquired portosystemic shunts subsequent to traumatic diaphragmatic hernia in a dog. *Canadian Veterinary Journal* 61 (2): 153–156.

Hunt, G.B. and Johnson, K.A. (2003). Diaphragmatic, pericardial and hiatal hernia. In: *Textbook of Small Animal Surgery*, 3e (ed. D.H. Slatter), 471–487. Philadelphia, PA: WB Saunders.

Johnson, S.E. (1987). Portal hypertension. Part 1. Pathophysiology and clinical consequences. *Compendium on Continuing Education for the Practicing Veterinarian* 9: 741–748.

Laine, G.A., Hall, J.T., Laine, S.H., and Granger, J. (1979). Transsinusoidal fluid dynamics in canine liver during venous hypertension. *Circulation Research* 45: 317–323.

Milson, M.B. (2007). Diaphragmatic hernia. In: *Clinical Veterinary Advisor*, 293–294. St Louis, MO: Mosby Elsevier.

Minihan, A.C., Berg, J., and Evans, R.L. (2004). Chronic diaphragmatic hernia in 34 dogs and 16 cats. *Journal of the American Animal Hospital Association* 40: 51–63.

Morgan, K.R.S., Singh, A., Giuffrida, M.A. et al. (2020). Outcome after surgical and conservative treatments of canine peritoneopericardial diaphragmatic hernia: a multi-institutional study of 128 dogs. *Veterinary Surgery* 49 (1): 138–145.

Noden, D.M. and De Lahunta, A.D. (1985). *The Embryology of Domestic Animals. Developmental Mechanisms and Malformations*. Baltimore, MD: Williams & Wilkins.

O'Byrne, K.L., Smalle, T., and Ryan, S.D. (2021). Repair of a delayed, traumatic dorsal diaphragmatic hernia using a single paracostal approach in a dog. *New Zealand Veterinary Journal* 70: 55–62.

Park, R.D. (2002). The diaphragm. In: *Textbook of Veterinary Diagnostic Radiology*, 4e (ed. D.E. Thrall), 359–375. Philadelphia, PA: WB Saunders.

Reimer, S.B., Kyles, A.E., Filipowicz, D.E., and Gregory, C.R. (2004). Long-term outcome of cats treated conservatively or surgically for peritoneopericardial diaphragmatic hernia: 66 cases (1987–2002). *Journal of the American Veterinary Medical Association* 224: 728–732.

Rendano, V.T. Jr. (1979). Positive contrast peritoneography: an aid in the radiographic diagnosis of diaphragmatic hernia. *Veterinary Radiology* 20: 67–73.

Schertel, E.R., Allen, D.A., Muir, W.W., and Hansen, B.D. (1996). Evaluation of a hypertonic sodium chloride/dextran solution for treatment of traumatic shock in dogs. *Journal of the American Veterinary Medical Association* 208: 366–370.

Schmiedt, C.W., Tobias, K.M., and Stevenson, M.A. (2003). Traumatic diaphragmatic hernia in cats: 34 cases (1991–2001). *Journal of the American Veterinary Medical Association* 222: 1237–1240.

Schmiedt, C.W., Washabaugh, K.F., Rao, D.B., and Stepien, R.L. (2009). Chylothorax associated with a congenital peritoneopericardial diaphragmatic hernia in a dog. *Journal of the American Animal Hospital Association* 45: 134–137.

Sharf, V., Anciano, C., Iannettoni, M. (2021). Laparoscopic peritoneopericardial herniorrhaphy in two dogs. Scientific Presentation Abstracts Veterinary Endoscopy Society 17th Annual Society Meeting. *Veterinary Surgery* 50: O138–O160.

Spackman, C.J., Caywood, D.D., Feeney, D.A., and Johnston, G.R. (1984). Thoracic wall and pulmonary trauma in dogs sustaining fractures as a result of motor vehicle accidents. *Journal of the American Veterinary Medical Association* 185: 975–977.

Stokhof, A.A. (1986). Diagnosis and treatment of acquired diaphragmatic hernia by thoracotomy in 49 dogs and 72 cats. *Veterinary Quarterly* 8: 177–183.

Valentine, B.A., Cooper, B.J., Dietze, A.E., and Noden, D.M. (1988). Canine congenital diaphragmatic hernia. *Journal of Veterinary Internal Medicine* 2: 109–112.

Van Pelt, D.R., Wingfield, W.E., Hackett, T.B., and Martin, L.G. (1993a). Application of airway pressure therapy in veterinary critical care. Part 1: Respiratory mechanics and hypoxemia. *Journal of Veterinary Emergency and Critical Care* 3: 63–70.

Van Pelt, D.R., Wingfield, W.E., Hackett, T.B., and Martin, L.G. (1993b). Application of airway pressure therapy in veterinary critical care. Part 2: Airway pressure therapy. *Journal of Veterinary Emergency and Critical Care* 3: 71–81.

Voges, A.K., Bertrand, S., Hill, R.C. et al. (1995). True diaphragmatic hernia in a cat. *Veterinary Radiology and Ultrasound* 38: 116–119.

Williams, J., Leveille, R., and Myer, C.W. (1998). Imaging modalities used to confirm diaphragmatic hernia in small animals. *Compendium on Continuing Education for the Practicing Veterinarian* 20: 1199–1209.

Wilson, G.P. and Hayes, H.M.J. (1986). Diaphragmatic hernia in the dog and cat: a 25-year overview. *Seminars in Veterinary Medicine and Surgery (Small Animal)* 1: 318–326.

Worth, A.J. and Machon, R.G. (2005). Traumatic diaphragmatic herniation: pathophysiology and management. *Compendium on Continuing Education for the Practicing Veterinarian* 27: 178–191.

Worth, A.J. and Machon, R.G. (2006). Prevention of reexpansion pulmonary edema and ischemia–reperfusion injury in the management of diaphragmatic herniation. *Compendium on Continuing Education for the Practicing Veterinarian* 28: 531–539.

27

Perineal Hernia

F.A. (Tony) Mann and Carlos Henrique de Mello Souza

Perineal hernia develops when pelvic or abdominal contents protrude (herniate) through the muscles that form the pelvic diaphragm, after weakening or atrophy of these muscles has occurred. Four anatomic locations of perineal herniation were described by Dorn *et al.* (1982): (i) sciatic (between the sacrotuberous ligament and coccygeus muscle); (ii) dorsal (between the coccygeus and levator ani muscles); (iii) caudal (between the levator ani muscle and external anal sphincter); and (iv) ventral (ventral to the ischiourethralis muscle). The latter was noted in only one female dog. Subsequently, two cases of sciatic hernia were reported (Rochat & Mann 1998). Most canine perineal hernias are caudal hernias, although differentiating between dorsal and caudal hernias is difficult when the levator ani muscle is unidentifiable, as is common. Unilateral or bilateral subcutaneous bulging occurs lateral or ventrolateral to the anus. The clinical signs vary depending on the size of the hernia and the organs involved. The rectum commonly herniates in one of three forms: deviation (flexure); dilatation (sacculation); or diverticulum, the latter being the least common (Krahwinkel 1983; Mann & Boothe 1985). Other commonly herniated structures include retroperitoneal fat, prostate, and urinary bladder. Rarely, the small intestine becomes part of the contents of the hernia.

Etiology

Perineal hernia has been reported in humans as well as dogs, cats, and other domestic species, but is most common in dogs (Dorn *et al.* 1982; Welches *et al.* 1992; Skipworth *et al.* 2007; Augustin *et al.* 2009; El-Gazzaz *et al.* 2009). In people, where the condition is rare, predisposing factors include female sex, pregnancy, and previous perineal or rectal surgery for treatment of neoplasia (Skipworth *et al.* 2007; Augustin *et al.* 2009; El-Gazzaz *et al.* 2009). A few case reports and one retrospective study describing 40 cases of feline perineal hernia have been published (Ashton 1976; Johnson & Gourley 1980; Welches *et al.* 1992; Risselada *et al.* 2003; Benitah *et al.* 2004; Pratschke & Martin 2014; Vnuk *et al.* 2005; Moreira *et al.* 2020; Swieton *et al.* 2020). Perineal hernia seems to be more common in queens than in bitches. In the retrospective study already mentioned, the largest reported to date, 25% of the affected cats were females. Predisposing conditions such as previous perineal urethrostomy, megacolon, and perineal masses were reported in 50% of the affected cats. The condition is bilateral in the majority of feline cases (Welches *et al.* 1992). The remaining discussion of perineal hernia in this chapter will refer to the condition in dogs, unless otherwise noted.

Factors that have been associated with the development of perineal hernia in dogs include the male anatomy, breed, tail-docking surgery, hormonal imbalances, prostatic disease, and persistent straining due to constipation, diarrhea, or lower urinary disease. The majority of dogs with perineal hernia are males between 7 and 9 years of age. Dogs younger than 5 years of age are rarely affected (Dorn *et al.* 1982). A single report of perineal hernia has been described in a 4-month-old puppy (Vyacheslav & Ranen 2009). Perineal hernia is rare in female dogs. In a large retrospective study of 771 dogs, only 7% of affected animals were females (Hayes 1978).

Small Animal Soft Tissue Surgery, Second Edition. Edited by Eric Monnet.
© 2023 John Wiley & Sons, Inc. Published 2023 by John Wiley & Sons, Inc.
Companion website: www.wiley.com/go/monnet/small

A later study reported that 4% of the dogs with perineal hernia were female (Hayashi *et al.* 2016). That study investigated comorbidities and found that aged female dogs with chronic cough or previous pelvic trauma were potentially at risk for development of perineal hernia (Hayashi *et al.* 2016). A single case of perineal hernia in a pregnant bitch has been reported (Sontas *et al.* 2008).

The cause for the much greater frequency in male dogs is not completely understood. Differences in the weight of the levator ani and coccygeus muscles between males and females were found in some studies, but this difference does not seem to be consistent among the breeds studied (Moltzen-Nielsen 1953; Desai 1982). An anatomic study of the pelvic diaphragm of male and female dogs concluded that the levator ani was significantly longer, larger, and heavier in the female. The authors correlated these differences with the extra load that must be accommodated by the muscles of the pelvic diaphragm during parturition (Desai 1982). Dog breeds found to be overrepresented in two or more studies include the Boston terrier, boxer, corgi, collie, kelpie, dachshunds, Old English sheepdog, and Pekingese (Burrows & Harvey 1973; Hayes 1978; Bellenger 1980; Weaver & Omamegbe 1981; Sjollema *et al.* 1993; Hosgood *et al.* 1995; Ragni & Moore 2011). The right side is thought by some to be more commonly affected than the left, but the clinical significance of right-side preponderance is unknown, and not all studies support a side predilection for the occurrence of perineal hernia in dogs (Mann *et al.* 2014).

Pathogenesis

Perineal herniation is thought to occur after deterioration of the muscles forming the pelvic diaphragm. The muscle most severely affected is the levator ani muscle, which can be completely absent or atrophied to such a degree that only its cranial remnants are found during surgery. Various degrees of atrophy may also be found in the coccygeus and internal obturator muscles. Electromyography of the levator ani and coccygeus muscles performed in 40 dogs revealed four types of spontaneous potentials in 35 of those dogs: fibrillation potentials, positive sharp waves, complex repetitive discharges, and fasciculations. The authors concluded that atrophy of the muscles of the pelvic diaphragm is likely to be of neurogenic origin. Nerve damage was localized to the sacral plexus proximal to the muscular branches of the pudendal nerve or in the muscular branches separately (Sjollema *et al.* 1993).

Chronic straining to urinate or defecate due to prostatic disease has been suggested as a cause of perineal hernia. This link seems to exist in cats, but in dogs the same is not as evident (Welches *et al.* 1992). In dogs, rectal dilatation or deviation may be the initial event followed by constipation and tenesmus, or a consequence of prostatomegaly, chronic straining, and weakening of the pelvic diaphragm. In a group of 30 dogs evaluated with abdominal radiographs for rectal dilation/deviation after oral barium, 18 dogs had rectal deviation and an additional 12 had a combination of deviation and dilation (Hosgood *et al.* 1995). The levator ani and coccygeus muscles participate in tail movement in such a way that constant tail movement exercise can lead to strong pelvic diaphragm muscles. Deficient tail muscle strength due to lack of exercise could be part of the reason why so many short-tailed dog breeds such as Boston terrier, Old English sheepdog, boxer, and corgi are overrepresented in perineal hernia studies. However, no study to date has shown statistically significant differences between the pelvic diaphragm muscles of short- and long-tailed dogs of the same breed. A study comparing the weight of muscles of the pelvic diaphragm in long- and short-tailed corgis in relation to thigh circumference revealed a trend for greater muscle weight in long-tailed corgis (Head & Francis 2002).

Hormonal imbalances have been associated with perineal hernia development. In addition, prostatomegaly and prostatic disease, which may or may not be a consequence of these imbalances, may also play a role in perineal hernia development. One large study revealed that the recurrence rate after perineal hernia repair without orchiectomy was 2.7 times greater than if orchiectomy was performed (Hayes 1978). Furthermore, prostatomegaly can lead to tenesmus, which, theoretically, can cause excessive tension and progressive weakening of the pelvic diaphragm. In cases of benign prostatic hyperplasia, orchiectomy leads to decrease in size of the prostate; thus, both prostatomegaly and hormonal imbalances could play roles in the development of perineal hernia in dogs. The presence of prostatomegaly and prostatic disease was evaluated by radiographs for enlargement using the ratio of prostatic diameter to pubis–promontory distance in 43 dogs. Only three dogs were considered to have significant prostatomegaly. In addition, of the dogs undergoing prostatic biopsy, only 50% showed histologic abnormalities (Hosgood *et al.* 1995).

The greater incidence of perineal hernia in sexually intact versus castrated male dogs suggests that anatomic differences or hormonal influences may play a role in the pathogenesis. Perineal hernia has been described concurrently with testicular tumors. The combination was found to be more frequent with seminomas and interstitial cell tumors (19% and 15% of cases, respectively) than with sertoliomas (2% of cases), and suggested that increased concentrations of systemic estrogens likely do not play a role in the herniation process (Lipowitz *et al.* 1973).

The serum concentrations of testosterone and estradiol-17β and the serum testosterone-to-estradiol ratio were analyzed in mature dogs with perineal hernia and mature normal dogs without perineal hernia and significant differences were not detected (Mann *et al.* 1989). Subsequently, androgen and estrogen receptor analyses in the levator ani and coccygeus muscles of mature dogs with perineal hernia were compared with those from mature healthy control beagles. These receptors were again measured in the contralateral levator ani and coccygeus muscles two months after orchiectomy in control dogs. The results showed that androgen receptors increased two months after orchiectomy compared with prior to castration. More importantly, the concentrations of androgen receptors were significantly lower in dogs with perineal hernia (intact and castrated) compared with controls at both times. Estrogen receptors were not detected (Mann *et al.* 1995).

Another hormone that has been implicated in the development of perineal hernia in dogs is relaxin (Ragni & Moore 2011). Some of the effects of relaxin were first discovered after observing relaxation of interpubic ligament in nonpregnant guinea pigs by injection of serum from pregnant ones. Years later the hormone was positively identified and named relaxin (Merchav *et al.* 2005). The highest production of relaxin takes place in reproductive organs during pregnancy. In males, the prostate is the primary site for relaxin production (Merchav *et al.* 2005). Relaxin is thought to alter connective tissue components by its effects on collagen metabolism and, in addition, has various effects on cardiovascular and renal tissues (Teichman *et al.* 2010). When immunohistochemistry for relaxin was performed on the prostate of dogs with perineal hernia and compared with that in age-matched intact and neutered dogs, there was greater staining intensity in dogs with perineal hernia, suggesting that weakening of the pelvic diaphragm caused by relaxin could predispose dogs to perineal hernia (Niebauer *et al.* 2005). In another study the expression of relaxin receptor, relaxin, and relaxin-like factor were detected by real-time polymerase chain reaction in dogs with perineal hernia and compared with control dogs. The expression of relaxin receptor was found to be significantly higher in dogs with perineal hernia than in control dogs, but unfortunately the controls were not age matched (Merchav *et al.* 2005). A more recent study failed to detect differences in the expression of relaxin in testicular samples of dogs with and without perineal hernia (Pirker *et al.* 2009). If the prostate is the crucial site for relaxin production, it is possible that castration leads to prostatic atrophy and consequent decrease in relaxin. While not all studies support a protective effect of castration, the results of the two largest studies published to date strongly suggest that castration will decrease the chances of perineal hernia recurrence in dogs (Hayes 1978; Weaver & Omamegbe 1981).

Historical findings and clinical signs

Perineal swelling in an otherwise clinically normal dog is a common reason for presentation. The swelling is usually lateral and both sides of the perineum can be affected (Figure 27.1). Perineal hernia may also occur with ventral herniation and bladder retroflexion (Niles & Williams 1999; Sontas *et al.* 2008). Cats have a high incidence (95%) of bilateral perineal herniation (Welches *et al.* 1992). In contrast to dogs, the largest case series of perineal hernia in cats showed that previous surgery or perineal disease is common. In the 40 cats presented, 50% had a predisposing condition, such as previous perineal urethrostomy surgery in 10 cats, megacolon in 5 cats, perineal mass in 4 cats, and fibrosing colitis in 1 cat (Welches *et al.* 1992). Pelvic trauma has also been implicated as a possible predisposing factor in cats (Risselada *et al.* 2003).

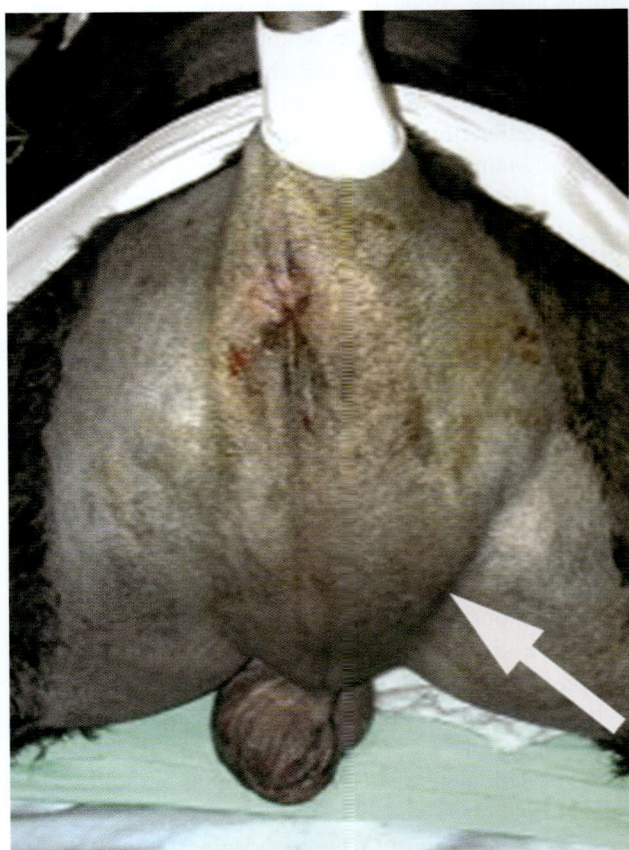

Figure 27.1 A male dog with right perineal hernia. Notice the marked ventrolateral bulging of the perineal area (arrow).

Constipation, obstipation, tenesmus, dyschezia (painful defecation), and fecal incontinence can also be present. These signs are probably secondary to a combination of rectal dilation or flexure and prostatomegaly (Burrows & Harvey 1973; Bellenger 1980; Hosgood et al. 1995). Tenesmus and constipation are the most common clinical signs in cats, and perineal hernia should be part of the differential diagnosis when these clinical signs are present (Welches et al. 1992). In the previously mentioned study, queens were more frequently affected (25%) than has been reported in bitches (7%) (Hayes 1978; Welches et al. 1992). Bladder retroflexion has also been reported in a queen postpartum. In that case, a previous acetabular fracture that led to pelvic narrowing was a likely aggravating condition (Risselada et al. 2003).

Diagnosis

Physical examination

A complete physical examination should be performed in all patients and must include careful rectal examination. The initial rectal examination will help define the presence of unilateral versus bilateral disease, the condition of the pelvic diaphragm, and the presence of rectal dilatation and/or flexure; determine which structures are herniated; and detect the presence of prostatomegaly or perineal masses. Urethral catheterization may be necessary in cases of bladder retroflexion and urinary obstruction. The bladder will be repositioned more easily if small. Occasionally, retrograde urinary catheterization may not be possible and cystocentesis should be performed. If deemed necessary, ultrasonography will also facilitate catheterization of the urinary bladder and fine-needle aspiration of the prostate if indicated. Bladder retroflexion occurs in 14–25% of dogs with perineal hernia and may result in clinical signs secondary to partial or complete urinary obstruction, such as oliguria or anuria, stranguria, anorexia, vomiting, collapse, and urinary incontinence. Dogs with bladder retroflexion are significantly more likely to have elevations in serum urea nitrogen, creatinine, potassium, and phosphate (Bellenger 1980; White & Herrtage 1986; Dupre et al. 1993; Hosgood et al. 1995). In both dogs and cats, complete urinary obstruction associated with bladder retroflexion should be treated as an emergency.

Radiographic and ultrasound examination

Radiographs and/or ultrasound of the caudal abdomen can also be performed to detect caudal displacement of the bladder, rectal dilatation and/or flexure, prostatomegaly, and paraprostatic cysts.

Treatment

Medical treatment

Medical treatment of perineal hernia includes high-fiber diet or fiber supplement (bulk-forming laxatives), docusates, periodic enemas or manual rectal evacuation, and bladder catheterization. Concurrent conditions such as benign prostatic hyperplasia and prostatitis, urinary tract obstruction/infection, and megacolon must also be addressed. Medical treatment should be used to palliate the clinical signs until surgery is performed. Clients who refuse surgical treatment for perineal hernia should be advised of the risk of visceral entrapment even when animals are initially presented without clinical signs (Burrows & Harvey 1973).

In patients presented with severe constipation/obstipation, digital rectal evacuation or a water enema may be performed until surgery can be scheduled. If a water enema is employed, it should be performed no later than 12 hours before the herniorrhaphy to decrease the possibility of rectal leakage during surgery (Bellenger 1980; Hosgood et al. 1995; Head & Francis 2002). If possible, enemas should be avoided altogether. Instead, it is recommended to perform digital rectal evacuation with the animal under general anesthesia immediately before the herniorrhaphy procedure (Mann et al. 2014).

Surgical treatment

Surgical treatment is indicated for most cases, and multiple techniques have been described (Gill & Barstad 2018). Prophylactic antibiotics (cefazolin 22 mg/kg or cefoxitin 20–30 mg/kg) are administered after induction of anesthesia. The surgical area is clipped from the entire perineal area, the base of the tail, and the proximal caudolateral thigh bilaterally. The rectum is manually evacuated as needed, a gauze tampon is inserted, and a purse-string suture placed around the anus to minimize contamination of the surgical field. The dog is positioned in sternal recumbence with the pelvic limbs hanging over the edge of the surgical table. The edge of the table should be cushioned by a thick towel or foam to prevent damage to the femoral nerve. The tail is pulled cranially and secured to the table with adhesive tape.

After antiseptic preparation, the surgical site is isolated with quarter drapes followed by a fenestrated drape. An additional adhesive drape such as Ioban® (3M, St. Paul, MN, USA) is used by some surgeons in an attempt to prevent fecal contamination of the incision site. Another method used to decrease fecal contamination is to suture towels to the incision edges. Draping is done in such a way that the anus is covered and the surgical site includes the lateral aspect of the base of the tail and the ischial table. The standard technique for surgical correction of perineal hernia relies on apposition of the pelvic diaphragm muscles. Due to atrophy of these muscles, simple apposition of the coccygeus, levator ani, and external anal sphincter muscles may predispose to recurrence (Hosgood *et al.* 1995). Transposition of the internal obturator muscle is regarded by many veterinary surgeons as the preferred method for surgical repair of perineal hernia (Hardie *et al.* 1983; Orsher 1986; Van Sluijs & Sjollema 1989; Sjollema & Van Sluijs 1989; Brissot *et al.* 2004; Szabo *et al.* 2007; Vnuk *et al.* 2008; Mann *et al.* 2014; Wolberg 2014). Techniques using polypropylene mesh, fascia lata, swine intestinal submucosa, and semitendinosus and gluteal muscle flaps have been reported in combination with internal obturator muscle transposition or alone with varied results, although mostly good (Weaver & Omamegbe 1981; Chambers & Rawlings 1991; Stoll *et al.* 2002; Bongartz *et al.* 2005; Vnuk *et al.* 2006; Szabo *et al.* 2007; Theil *et al.* 2010; Gill & Barstad 2018; Swieton *et al.* 2020). Use of swine intestinal submucosa has yielded promising results in clinically normal research dogs (Stoll *et al.* 2002) and in dogs with perineal hernia (Theil *et al.* 2010; Swieton *et al.* 2020).

Surgical anatomy

The perineum covers the caudal aspect of the pelvic outlet, bordered dorsally by the first coccygeal vertebra, laterally by the sacrotuberous ligament (not present in cats), and ventrally by the internal obturator muscle and ischium. The pelvic diaphragm, which provides support to the caudal rectum, is formed by the paired levator ani and coccygeus muscles, lateral to the anus (Figure 27.2). The levator ani muscle lies medial to the coccygeus muscle and originates on the medial edge of the shaft of the ilium and the dorsal surface of the pubis and pelvic symphysis. The levator ani, divided into iliocaudalis and pubocaudalis portions, inserts on caudal vertebrae 3–7. The coccygeus muscle arises from the ischiatic spine and inserts on the transverse processes of caudal vertebrae 1–4 (Constantinescu 2018). The ischiorectal fossa is the deep wedge-shaped depression located lateral to the terminal portions of the digestive and urogenital tracts. The boundaries of the ischiorectal fossa are formed by the levator ani and coccygeus muscles medially, the superficial gluteal muscle dorsolaterally, and the internal obturator muscle ventrally. Variable amounts of fat are present in the fossa.

Additional structures that are important to the understanding of perineal hernia anatomy include the pudendal nerve and internal pudendal artery and vein and the sciatic nerve. The pudendal nerve and the internal pudendal artery and vein lie lateral to the coccygeus muscle and cross its dorsolateral aspect into the ischiorectal fossa in a ventral and medial direction. The pudendal nerve branches into the caudal rectal nerve, which innervates the external anal sphincter and dorsal nerve of the penis or clitoris. The internal pudendal artery and vein originate from the corresponding internal iliac vessels and branch into three vessels each: the caudal rectal artery and vein, the ventral perineal artery and vein, and the artery and vein of the penis or clitoris. The sciatic nerve is located dorsolateral to the sacrotuberous ligament exiting the pelvis toward the thigh (Dorn *et al.* 1982).

Transposition of internal obturator

The repair of perineal hernia in the dog by transposition of the internal obturator muscle is described here based on the initial report by Van Sluijs and Sjollema (1989) (Figures 27.2–27.5). A vertical curvilinear incision is made starting just distal and lateral to the base of the tail and ending 2–3 cm distal to the ischial table. The hernia sac will then become evident filling the ischiorectal fossa. The sac is usually filled with fluid and multiple approximately 1 cm fatty nodules, which are sometimes necrotic. Once the hernia sac is open and fluid has been removed, the herniated contents can be inspected for abnormalities, pushed cranially, and packed with gauze or a laparotomy sponge. The gauze packing is helpful in keeping the herniated contents reduced while inspecting the anatomy and preplacing the repair sutures; however, care must be taken to ensure that the packing is removed before tying the preplaced sutures to avoid complications of a retained sponge (Forster *et al.* 2011). The following anatomic structures must be identified before beginning the hernia repair: the external anal sphincter, levator ani, coccygeus, and internal obturator muscle; the pudendal artery, vein, and nerve; and the caudal rectal nerve. Often, only remnants of the levator ani muscle can be identified or this muscle may be altogether absent. As such, the levator ani muscle rarely contributes to the repair.

The periosteum is incised caudal to the internal obturator muscle but cranial to the ischiourethralis muscle, and subperiosteal elevation of the internal obturator muscle is performed. Subperiosteal elevation decreases the chance of iatrogenic damage to the pudendal nerves. The internal obturator is elevated medially, cranially, and laterally until its tendon can be seen coursing ventral to the sacrotuberous ligament. The tendon of the internal obturator is severed to relieve tension and provide optimal transposition as the internal obturator is

(a)

Pudendal
nerve & artery

Perineal
nerve & artery

Coccygeus
muscle

Sacrotuberous
ligament

External
anal spnincter

Obturator
internus

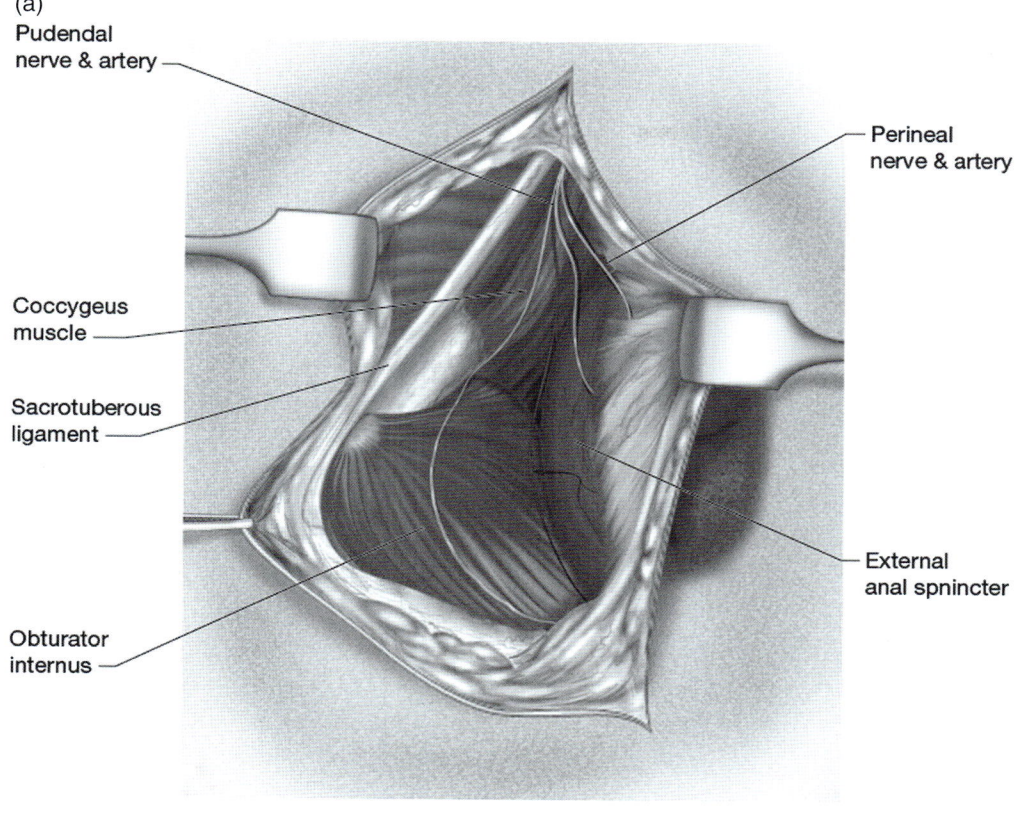

(b)

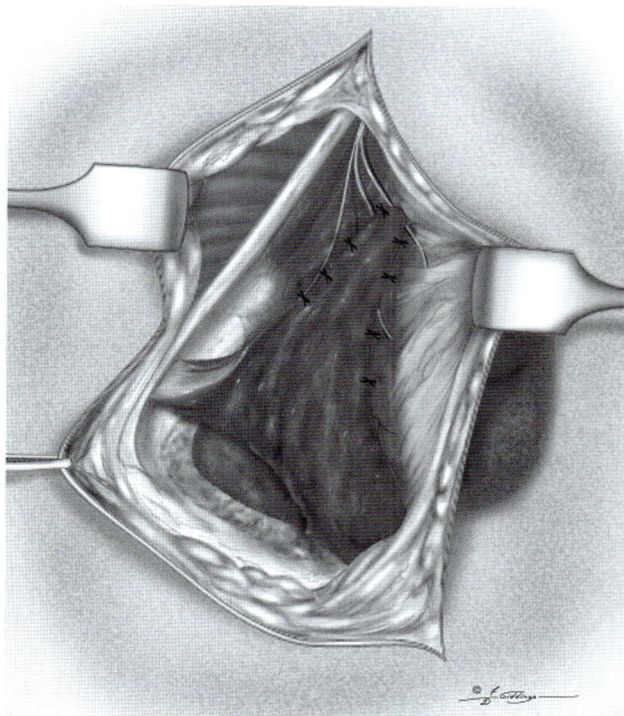

Figure 27.2 (a) Surgical anatomy of the left pelvic diaphragm. (b) The left internal obturator muscle has been transposed to repair the hernia. © D. Giddings.

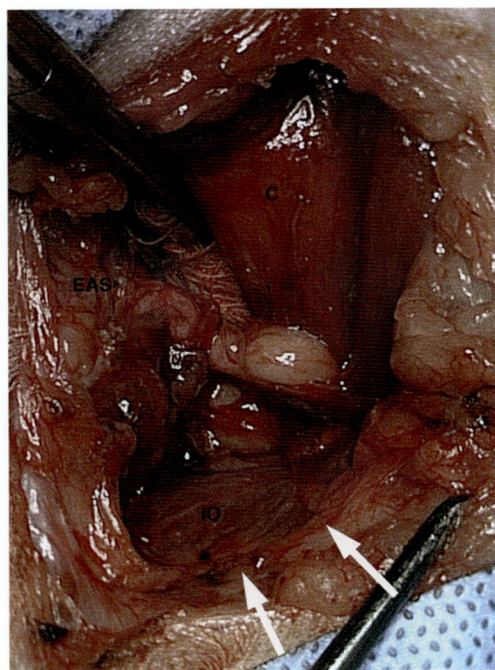

Figure 27.3 Surgery for transposition of the right internal obturator muscle. The pudendal artery and nerves are outlined by the white arrows. C, coccygeus muscle; EAS, external anal sphincter; IO, internal obturator muscle.

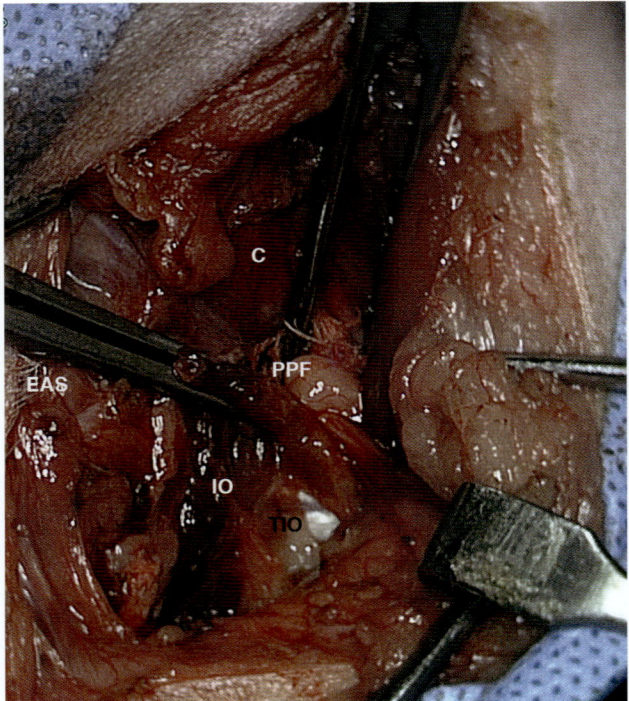

Figure 27.4 Elevation of the right internal obturator muscle. It is recommended that a periosteal elevator is used. C, coccygeus muscle; EAS, external anal sphincter; IO, internal obturator muscle; PPF, periprostatic fat; TIO, tendon of the internal obturator muscle.

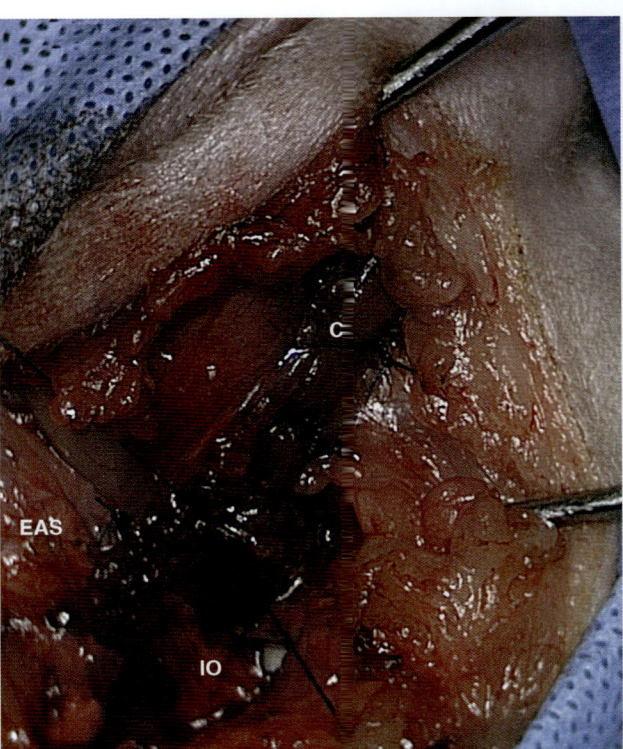

Figure 27.5 Suture of the hernia defect (right perineum) has been completed with sutures between the coccygeal muscle (C), internal obturator muscle flap (IO), and external anal sphincter (EAS).

apposed to the sacrotuberous ligament, coccygeus (and levator ani, if present), and external anal sphincter. Care must be taken to avoid trauma to the pudendal nerve on the dorsal surface of the internal obturator muscle during internal obturator tenotomy. In a ventral to dorsal order, preplace sutures from the internal obturator muscle to the sacrotuberous ligament and coccygeus and levator ani muscles laterally, and to the external anal sphincter medially. Avoid damage to the nearby sciatic nerve by passing the needle through the sacrotuberous ligament rather than around the ligament. It is safer to transfix the sacrotuberous ligament than to place the suture around the ligament. The most dorsal suture is placed through the apex of the internal obturator muscle and the coccygeus muscle and the external anal sphincter. Care is taken to avoid rectal penetration when engaging the external anal sphincter. Depending on the size of the animal and the preference of the surgeon, 2-0 or 3-0 polypropylene, polydioxanone, or polyglyconate sutures are used. As described earlier, all of these sutures are preplaced. The gauze or laparotomy sponge is then removed, the wound is thoroughly lavaged with warm saline, and the sutures are tied. The subcutaneous tissues are closed in a routine manner. Intradermal sutures without skin sutures may be used to prevent postoperative contamination of the incision due to fecal accumulation on the suture tags. The purse-string suture is removed and rectal palpation is performed to ensure that reconstruction of the muscular support has been achieved and that sutures were not placed through the rectal wall.

Castration can be performed immediately before (preferred) or after the herniorrhaphy. Caudal castration with the dog in the same ventrally recumbent position used for perineal herniorrhaphy allows castration and hernia repair to proceed without changing the animal's position between the two procedures (Knecht 1976; Mann *et al.* 2014).

Various studies have reported the results following transposition of the internal obturator muscle in dogs. Three studies reported recurrence rates of 5% (Sjollema & Van Sluijs 1989), 3% (Wolberg 2014), and 2% (Hardie *et al.* 1983). In a fourth study, which evaluated 31 dogs for 11 months or longer, 67% of the operated pelvic diaphragms were considered intact, whereas only 6 (12.5%) had perineal swelling (Orsher 1986). Failure of the ventral pelvic diaphragm was present in approximately 19% and failure of both dorsal and ventral pelvic diaphragm was present in approximately 15% of the cases. The outcome of surgery was affected by the severity of preoperative clinical signs or if the hernia was bilateral (Orsher 1986). The experience of the surgeon was significantly associated with better success rates in two studies (Burrows & Harvey 1973; Orsher 1986). In the study by Hardie *et al.* (1983), a difference related to experience was not observed.

Overall, the authors of these and other studies report that advantages of internal obturator muscle transposition include decreased tension on the anal sphincter compared with primary suture of the pelvic diaphragm, decrease in wound dehiscence compared with superficial gluteal muscle flap, and decrease in recurrence compared with both primary suturing and superficial gluteal muscle technique. Because of variations in technique, the criteria for evaluation of success rate, method and time of follow-up evaluation, in addition to the retrospective nature of almost all studies, direct comparison of results from these studies is very difficult (Knecht 1976; Hayes 1978; Bellenger 1980; Weaver & Omamegbe 1981; Hardie *et al.* 1983; Orsher 1986; White & Herrtage 1986; Sjollema & Van Sluijs 1989; Dupre *et al.* 1993; Hosgood *et al.* 1995; Brissot *et al.* 2004; Szabo *et al.* 2007; Wolberg 2014). In a long-term study, a recurrence rate of 27.4% has been reported after internal obturator transposition (Shaughnessy & Monnet 2015). In that study dogs were followed up for four years and showed recurrence as long as one year after surgery. Postoperative tenesmus was identified as a risk factor for recurrence, with a hazard ratio of 2.29 (Shaughnessy & Monnet 2015). Table 27.1 summarizes important information provided by some of the largest studies. In a retrospective study from Weaver and Omamegbe (1981), apposition of the pelvic diaphragm muscles (standard technique) was compared with the superficial gluteal flap. Success rate criteria (i.e., remission of clinical signs) was higher with the conventional technique (81%) than with the gluteal flap (64%). In addition, recurrence rate was higher with the superficial gluteal flap technique (14.3%) compared with the standard technique (8.7%).

Colopexy, cystopexy, and vasopexy

Colopexy, and cystopexy or vasopexy (fixation of deferens to the abdominal wall), can be performed when there is a need to delay primary repair or in other circumstances where primary repair is not feasible (D'Asis *et al.* 2010; Mann *et al.* 2014). These procedures prevent herniation of a commonly herniated organ (i.e., the rectum) and an organ (i.e., the urinary bladder) that could become acutely obstructed if herniated (Bilbrey *et al.* 1990; Mann *et al.* 2014). Vasopexy, like cystopexy, prevents herniation of both the prostate and urinary bladder (Figure 27.6).

Some authors have advocated these procedures for the treatment of bilateral perineal hernia (Orsher 1986; Bilbrey *et al.* 1990; Popovitch *et al.* 1994; Gilley *et al.* 2003; Brissot *et al.* 2004). The intention is to create adhesions of these organs to the abdominal wall to impair caudal organ displacement, improving clinical results. However, results of a study by White and Herrtage (1986) suggest that effective surgical repair of the hernia will preclude movement of the bladder. In this study, cystopexy was performed in only 1 of 12 dogs with bladder retroflexion and recurrence was not detected. Cystopexy was successfully performed with a laparoscopic-assisted technique in three dogs with retroflexion of the bladder (Rawlings *et al.* 2002). In another study (Bilbrey *et al.* 1990), vasopexy was performed in nine dogs with bladder retroflexion in addition to herniorrhaphy. In two dogs, vasopexy was the only procedure performed and recurrence of clinical signs was not observed during a follow-up period of 5 and 29 months (Bilbrey et al. 1990). In another study (Maute *et al.* 2001), the authors performed colopexy, vasopexy or cystopexy, and castration in 32 dogs with perineal hernia. Herniorrhaphy was not performed. The perineal hernia recurrence rate was 22%, which is higher than most reports (see Table 27.1); however, the authors questioned the absolute need for herniorrhaphy (Maute *et al.* 2001). With this recurrence risk in mind, some dog owners may elect against herniorrhaphy after

Table 27.1 Presence of bladder retroflexion, surgical procedures performed, hernia recurrence rate, and follow-up time in different studies of canine perineal hernia.

Reference	Number of dogs	Bladder retroflexion	Surgical procedures	Hernia recurrence rate	Follow-up
Burrows & Harvey (1973)	72	18%	Conven	46%	>1 year
Bellenger (1980)	35	14%	Conven	15.4%	>6 months
Weaver & Omamegbe (1981)	101	NA	Conven, SGF		>12 months
Hardie et al. (1983)	42	NA	IOMT	2.4%	>1 year
Orsher (1986)	31	NA	IOMT	33%	>11 months
White & Herrtage (1986)	61	20%	Conven		NA
Sjollema & van Sluijs (1989)	100	13%	IOMT	5.0%	16 months (mean)
Hosgood et al. (1995)	100	20%	Conven, IOMT	8.0%	8 months (mean)
Brissot et al. (2004)	41	25%	Conven, various[a]	10%	>6 months
Szabo et al. (2007)	59	NA	IOMT with polypro mesh	14%	29 months (mean)
Maute et al. (2001)	32	28%	Colo, cysto, vaso, and castration	22%	>1 month
Bongartz et al. (2005)	12	17%	AFLG	0%	>1 month
Vnuk et al. (2008)	40	7.5	Conven (n = 22), IOMT (n = 18)	27% (Conven), 11% (IOMT)	>6 months
Pekcan et al. (2010)	41	NA	IOMT	7.3%	>4 months
Theil et al. (2010)	15	27%	SIS	9.5%	>6 months
Grand et al. (2013)	41	24%	IOMT (n = 41), including colo or cysto before IOMT (n = 21)	9.7%	>6 months
Wolberg (2014)	60	1.7%	Modified IOMT	3.0%	>6 months
Morello et al. (2015)	14	NA	SSMT (n = 14), including IOMT with SSMT (n = 11)	1.4%	>19 months
Shaughnessy & Monnet (2015)	34	NA	IOMT	27.4%	4 years
Agrawal et al. (2020)	12	NA	PgPp mesh (n = 6), diaph scaff (n = 6)	0%	3 months
Guerios et al. (2020)	7	NA	Tunica vaginalis graft	0%	>9 months
Swieton et al. (2020)	11	9.0%	SIS (n = 11), including SIS with IOMT (n = 8)	18.2%	>4 months

AFLG, autogenous fascia lata graft; colo, colopexy; conven, conventional pelvic diaphragm muscle apposition; cysto, cystopexy; diaph scaff, decellularized bubaline diaphragmatic scaffold; IOMT, internal obturator muscle transposition; NA: not assessed; PgPp, polyglactin/polypropylene composite; polypro, polypropylene; SGF, superficial gluteal flap; SIS, swine intestinal submucosa; SSMT, split semitendinosus muscle transposition; vaso, vasopexy.

[a] Includes one or more of cystopexy, vasopexy, colopexy, and prostatic omentalization or cyst resection.

cystopexy and vasopexy or cystopexy to avoid additional surgery. Brissot et al. (2004) described 41 patients with complicated perineal hernia treated by staged celiotomy and herniorrhaphy. The criteria used by the authors to define complicated perineal hernia were bilateral disease, unilateral disease with major rectal dilation, perineal hernia with concurrent surgical prostatic disease, and perineal hernia with bladder retroflexion. Procedures performed during celiotomy included colopexy (41 dogs), vasopexy (32 dogs), cystopexy (6 dogs), and prostatic surgery (omentalization or cyst resection, 9 dogs). Herniorrhaphy was performed 2–15 days after celiotomy. Recurrence was detected in 10% of patients and all recurred within six months after surgery (Brissot et al. 2004). Minimally invasive techniques for cystopexy have been described

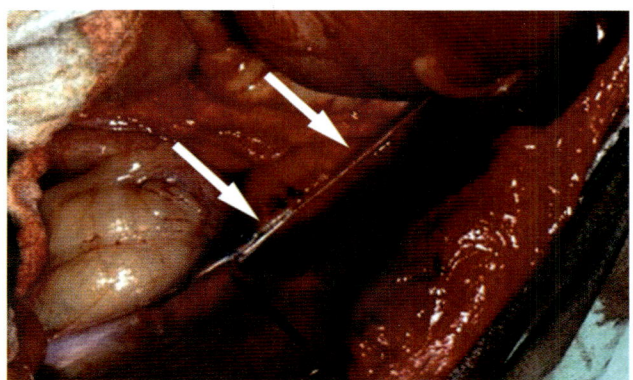

Figure 27.6 Vasopexy performed in a dog with a recurrent perineal hernia. The right vas deferens (white arrow) has been looped around a flap in the transverse abdominalis muscle (black arrow) under slight tension. The procedure is performed bilaterally.

and may be helpful in decreasing surgical time and morbidity when single-stage surgery is to be performed (Rawlings *et al.* 2002; Bray *et al.* 2009; Zhang *et al.* 2010).

Postoperative management

Antibiotics can be continued for the first 24 hours after surgery, but are routinely discontinued as soon as surgery is finished, unless treating an infection. There is no evidence to support continuing antibiotic therapy beyond 24 hours. If gross fecal contamination of the

wound is detected during surgery, copious lavage of the wound is usually sufficient to prevent a wound infection. Culture and susceptibility are reserved for when signs of infection ensue. Analgesic opioids and nonsteroidal anti-inflammatory drugs are recommended for the first 24–48 hours after surgery. Oral analgesic medications are administered thereafter. Urination and defecation must be monitored during the convalescence period. Stool softeners, such as lactulose, may be used in selected cases to achieve soft but formed stools and facilitate defecation, but watery fecal material must be avoided since it will predispose to wound contamination. A prudent approach is to wait for the first episode or two of defecation to see if stool softeners are warranted. The perineum can be cleaned daily with soft wipes to avoid accumulation of fecal material on the surgical site. Clients should be instructed that the animal must wear an Elizabethan collar at all times when unsupervised to avoid licking and chewing of the area.

Complications after perineal herniorrhaphy range from the expected and manageable postoperative pain to the rare and severe sciatic nerve entrapment. Possible complications include perineal swelling, partial or complete wound dehiscence, infection, tenesmus, urinary incontinence, fecal incontinence, rectal prolapse, and sciatic neuropraxia or paralysis (Table 27.2). Hemorrhage and urethral damage have been rarely reported. Bladder necrosis has been rarely reported to occur in severe cases

Table 27.2 Complications after surgical treatment of perineal hernia in dogs.

Reference	Overall complication rate	Wound dehiscence	Wound infection	Sciatic injury	Tenesmus	Rectal prolapse	Urinary incontinence	Fecal incontinence
Burrows & Harvey (1973)	NR	26%[a]	10%	5.5%	21%	2%	20%[b]	22%
Bellenger (1980)	57%	8.5%	20%	0%	8.5%	8.5%	9%	6%
Weaver & Omamegbe (1981)	NR	29%	NR	3%	NR	14%	NR	0%
Hardie *et al.* (1983)	19%	4.7%	12%	NR	NR	2.3%	NR	NR
White & Herrtage (1986)	5%	NR	NR	NR	NR	NR		5%
Orsher (1986)	68%	0%	6.5%	NR	NR	6.5%	NR	6.5%
Sjollema & van Sluijs (1989)	53%	NR	43%	NR	3%	NR	5%	15%
Hosgood *et al.* (1995)	20%	3%	11%	NR	8%	9%	4%	3%
Maute *et al.* (2001)	16%	NR	NR	NR	9%	NR	NR	3%
Brissot *et al.* (2004)	NR	NR	17%	NR	43%	NR	NR	37%
Bongartz *et al.* (2005)	30%	NR	NR	NR	NR	17%	NR	NR
Vnuk *et al.* (2006)	25%	NR	12.5% (noted as "suture sinus")	NR	6% (noted as "obstipation")	NR	NR	NR

(*Continued*)

Table 27.2 (Continued)

Reference	Overall complication rate	Wound dehiscence	Wound infection	Sciatic injury	Tenesmus	Rectal prolapse	Urinary incontinence	Fecal incontinence
Szabo et al. (2007)	39%	NR	6%	NR	NR	NR	NR	NR
Vnuk et al. (2008)	75%	3.3%	NR	NR	20%	3.3%	3.3%	3.3%
Pekcan et al. (2010)	14%	NR	NR	NR	7%	NR	NR	7%
Grand et al. (2013)	22%	NR	NR	NR	7%	NR	NR	7%
Morello et al. (2015)	42%	21%	NR	NR	14%	7%	NR	NR
Shaughnessy & Monnet (2015)	30%	NR	NR	NR	26%	NR	NR	NR
Wolberg (2014)	20%	2%	NR	NR	4%	2%	NR	NR
Swieton et al. (2020)	81%	NR	NR	NR	63%	9%	1%	2%

NR, not reported.

Percentages are approximate. Surgical method employed, complications and their rates, and follow-up methods are reported differently among references. Some authors report transient and permanent complications, whereas others do not. Due to differences in the way the results are reported, a direct comparison of different studies cannot be made.

[a] Included wound dehiscence, leakage, and infection.

[b] Reported as "urinary problems," not specifically urinary incontinence.

of bladder retroflexion. In many studies the distinction between postoperative complications and lack of resolution of preoperative clinical signs is not made. Some of the clinical signs, such as tenesmus and urinary and fecal incontinence, may persist, especially in the most severe cases (Burrows & Harvey 1973; Hayes 1978; Bellenger 1980; Weaver & Omamegbe 1981; Orsher 1986; White & Herrtage 1986; Dupre et al. 1993; Hosgood et al. 1995; Brissot et al. 2004; Szabo et al. 2007; Shaughnessy & Monnet 2015).

References

Agrawal, S., Shahi, A., Singh, R. et al. (2020). Comparison of decellularized bubaline diaphragmatic scaffold with synthetic polyglactin and polypropylene composite mesh for perineal hernioplasty in dogs. *Journal of Animal Research* 10: 205–213.

Ashton, D.G. (1976). Perineal in the cat – a description of two cases. *Journal of Small Animal Practice* 17: 473–477.

Augustin, G., Matosevic, P., Kekez, T. et al. (2009). Abdominal hernias in pregnancy. *Journal of Obstetrics and Gynaecology Research* 35: 203–211.

Bellenger, C.R. (1980). Perineal hernia in dogs. *Australian Veterinary Journal* 56: 434–438.

Benitah, N., Matousek, J.L., Barnes, R.F. et al. (2004). Diaphragmatic and perineal hernias associated with cutaneous asthenia in a cat. *Journal of the American Veterinary Medical Association* 224: 706–709.

Bilbrey, S.A., Smeak, D.D., and DeHoff, W. (1990). Fixation of the deferent ducts for retrodisplacement of the urinary bladder and prostate in canine perineal hernia. *Veterinary Surgery* 19: 24–27.

Bongartz, A., Carofiglio, F., and Balligand, M. (2005). Use of autogenous fascia lata graft for perineal herniorrhaphy in dogs. *Veterinary Surgery* 34: 405–413.

Bray, J.P., Doyle, R.S., and Burton, C.A. (2009). Minimally invasive inguinal approach for tube cystostomy. *Veterinary Surgery* 38: 411–416.

Brissot, H.N., Dupre, G.P., and Bouvy, B.M. (2004). Use of laparotomy in a staged approach for resolution of bilateral or complicated perineal hernia in 41 dogs. *Veterinary Surgery* 33: 412–421.

Burrows, C.F. and Harvey, C.E. (1973). Perineal hernia in the dog. *Journal of Small Animal Practice* 14: 315–332.

Chambers, J.N. and Rawlings, C.A. (1991). Application of a semitendinosus muscle flap in two dogs. *Journal of the American Veterinary Medical Association* 199: 84–86.

Constantinescu, G.M. (2018). *Illustrated Veterinary Anatomical Nomenclature*, 4e. Stuttgart: Georg Thieme.

D'Asis, M.J.M.H., da Costa Neto, J.M., da Sliva, E.-L.A. et al. (2010). Colopexy and deferentopexy associated with omentopexy in the treatment of perineal hernia in dogs: study of thirty cases. *Ciência Rural* 40: 371–377.

Desai, R. (1982). An anatomical study of the canine male and female pelvic diaphragm and the effect of testosterone on the status of the levator ani of male dogs. *Journal of the American Animal Hospital Association* 18: 195–202.

Dorn, A.S., Cartee, R.E., and Richardson, D.C. (1982). A preliminary comparison of perineal hernias in the dog and man. *Journal of the American Animal Hospital Association* 18: 624–632.

Dupre, G.P., Prat, N., and Bouvy, B. (1993). Perineal hernia in the dog: evaluation of associated lesions and results in 60 dogs [Abstract]. *Veterinary Surgery* 22: 250.

El-Gazzaz, G., Kiran, R.P., and Lavery, I. (2009). Wound complications in rectal cancer patients undergoing primary closure of the perineal wound after abdominoperineal resection. *Diseases of the Colon and Rectum* 52: 1962–1966.

Forster, K., Anderson, D., Yool, D.A. et al. (2011). Retained surgical swabs in 13 dogs. *Veterinary Record Case Reports* 1 (1): ed4396.

Gill, S.S. and Barstad, R.D. (2018). A review of the surgical management of perineal hernias in dogs. *Journal of the American Animal Hospital Association* 54: 179–187.

Gilley, R.S., Caywood, D.D., Lulich, J.P., and Bowersox, T.S. (2003). Treatment with a combined cystopexy–colopexy for dysuria and rectal prolapse after bilateral perineal herniorrhaphy in a dog. *Journal of the American Veterinary Medical Association* 222: 1717–1721.

Grand, J.G., Bureau, S., and Monnet, E. (2013). Effects of urinary bladder retroflexion and surgical technique on postoperative complication rates and long-term outcome in dogs with perineal hernia: 41 cases (2002–2009). *Journal of the American Veterinary Medical Association* 243: 1442–1447.

Guerios, S., Orms, K., and Serrano, M.A. (2020). Autologous tunica vaginalis graft to repair perineal hernia in shelter dogs. *Veterinary and Animal Science* 9: 100122.

Hardie, E.M., Kolata, R.J., Earley, T.D. et al. (1983). Evaluation of internal obturator muscle transposition in treatment of perineal hernia in dogs. *Veterinary Surgery* 12: 69–72.

Hayashi, A.M., Rosner, S.A., de Assumpção, T.C.A. et al. (2016). Retrospective study (2009–2014): perineal hernias and related comorbidities in bitches. *Topics in Companion Animal Medicine* 31: 130–133.

Hayes, H.M. Jr. (1978). The epidemiologic features of perineal hernia in 771 dogs. *Journal of the American Animal Hospital Association* 14: 703–707.

Head, L.L. and Francis, D.A. (2002). Mineralized paraprostatic cyst as a potential contributing factor in the development of perineal hernias in a dog. *Journal of the American Veterinary Medical Association* 221: 533–535.

Hosgood, G., Hedlund, C.S., and Dean, P.W. (1995). Perineal herniorrhaphy: perioperative data from 100 dogs. *Journal of the American Animal Hospital Association* 31: 331–342.

Johnson, M.S. and Gourley, I.M. (1980). Perineal hernia in a cat: a possible complication of perineal urethrostomy. *Veterinary Medicine, Small Animal Clinician* 75: 241–243.

Knecht, C.D. (1976). An alternative approach for castration of the dog. *Veterinary Medicine, Small Animal Clinician* 71: 469–472.

Krahwinkel, D.J. (1983). Rectal diseases and their role in perineal hernia. *Veterinary Surgery* 12: 160–165.

Lipowitz, A.J., Schwartz, A., Wilson, G.P., and Ebert, J.W. (1973). Testicular neoplasms and concomitant clinical changes in the dog. *Journal of the American Veterinary Medical Association* 163: 1364–1368.

Mann, F.A. and Boothe, H.W. (1985). Rectal diverticulum in a dog with perineal hernia. *California Veterinary* 39: 8–10.

Mann, F.A., Boothe, H.W., Amoss, M.S. et al. (1989). Serum testosterone and estradiol 17–beta concentrations in 15 dogs with perineal hernia. *Journal of the American Veterinary Medical Association* 194: 1578–1580.

Mann, F.A., Constantinescu, G.M., and Anderson, M.A. (2014). Surgical techniques for treatment of perineal hernia. In: *Current Techniques in Small Animal Surgery*, 5e (ed. M.J. Bojrab, D. Waldron and J.P. Toombs), 569–584. Jackson, WY: Teton NewMedia.

Mann, F.A., Nonneman, D.J., Pope, E.R. et al. (1995). Androgen receptors in the pelvic diaphragm muscles of dogs with and without perineal hernia. *American Journal of Veterinary Research* 56: 134–139.

Maute, A.M., Koch, D.A., and Montavon, P.M. (2001). Perineale hernie beim hund: colopexie, vasopexie, cystopexie, und kastration als therapy der wahl bei 32 hunden. *Schweizer Archiv für Tierheilkunde* 143: 360–367.

Merchav, R., Feuermann, Y., Shamay, A. et al. (2005). Expression of relaxin receptor LRG7, canine relaxin, and relaxin-like factor in the pelvic diaphragm musculature of dogs with and without perineal hernia. *Veterinary Surgery* 34: 476–481.

Moltzen-Nielsen, H. (1953). Perineal hernia. In: *Proceedings of the 15th International Veterinary Congress*, vol. 1, 971. Stockholm: World Veterinary Congress.

Moreira, S., Silva, F.L., da Silva, C.R.A. et al. (2020). Hérnia perineal bilateral em uma gata: relato de caso. *PUBVET* 14: 128–131.

Morello, E., Martano, M., Zabarino, S. et al. (2015). Modified semitendinosus muscle transposition to repair ventral perineal hernia in 14 dogs. *Journal of Small Animal Practice* 56: 370–376.

Niebauer, G.W., Shibli, S., Seltenhammer, M. et al. (2005). Relaxin of prostatic origin may be linked to perineal hernia formation in dogs. *Annals of the New York Academy of Sciences* 1041: 415–422.

Niles, J.D. and Williams, J.M. (1999). Perineal hernia with bladder retroflexion in a female cocker spaniel. *Journal of Small Animal Practice* 40: 92–94.

Orsher, R.J. (1986). Clinical and surgical parameters in dogs with perineal hernia. Analysis of results of internal obturator transposition. *Veterinary Surgery* 15: 253–258.

Pekcan, Z., Besalti, O., Sirin, Y.S., and Caliskan, M. (2010). Clinical and surgical evaluation of perineal hernia in dogs: 41 cases. *Kafkas Üniversitesi Veteriner Fakültesi Dergisi* 16: 573–578.

Pirker, A., Brandt, S., Seltenhammer, M. et al. (2009). Relaxin expression in the testes of dogs with and without perineal hernia. *Wiener Tierärztliche Monatsschrift* 96: 34–38.

Popovitch, C.A., Holt, D., and Bright, R. (1994). Colopexy as a treatment for rectal prolapse in dogs and cats: a retrospective study of 14 cases. *Veterinary Surgery* 23: 115–118.

Pratschke, K. and Martin, L. (2014). Bilateral perineal hernia in three cats: case studies. *Veterinary Times* 18: 10–13.

Ragni, R.A. and Moore, A.H. (2011). Perineal hernia. *Companion Animal* 16: 21–29.

Rawlings, C.A., Howerth, E.W., Mahaffey, M.B. et al. (2002). Laparoscopic-assisted cystopexy in dogs. *American Journal of Veterinary Research* 63: 1226–1231.

Risselada, M., Kramer, M., Van de Velde, B. et al. (2003). Retroflexion of the urinary bladder associated with a perineal hernia in a female cat. *Journal of Small Animal Practice* 44: 508–510.

Rochat, M.C. and Mann, F.A. (1998). Sciatic perineal hernia in two dogs. *Journal of Small Animal Practice* 39: 240–243.

Shaughnessy, M. and Monnet, E. (2015). Internal obturator muscle transposition for treatment of perineal hernia in dogs: 34 cases (1998–2012). *Journal of the American Veterinary Medical Association* 246: 321–326.

Sjollema, B.E. and van Sluijs, F.J. (1989). Perineal hernia repair in the dog by transposition of the internal obturator muscle. II Complications and results in 100 patients. *Veterinary Quarterly* 11: 18–23.

Sjollema, B.E., Venker-van Haagen, A.J., van Sluijs, F. et al. (1993). Electromyography of the pelvic diaphragm and anal sphincter in dogs with perineal hernia. *American Journal of Veterinary Research* 54: 185–190.

Skipworth, R.J.E., Smith, G.H.M., and Anderson, D.N. (2007). Secondary perineal hernia following open abdominoperineal excision of the rectum: report of a case and review of the literature. *Hernia* 11: 541–545.

Sontas, B.H., Apaydin, S.O., Toydemir, T.S. et al. (2008). Perineal hernia because of retroflexion of the urinary bladder in a Rottweiler bitch during pregnancy. *Journal of Small Animal Practice* 49: 421–425.

Stoll, M.R., Cook, J.L., Pope, E.R. et al. (2002). The use of porcine small intestinal submucosa as a biomaterial for perineal herniorrhaphy in the dog. *Veterinary Surgery* 31: 379–390.

Swieton, N., Singh, A., Lopez, D. et al. (2020). Retrospective evaluation on the outcome of perineal herniorrhaphy augmented with porcine small intestinal submucosa in dogs and cats. *Canadian Veterinary Journal* 61: 629–637.

Szabo, S., Wilkens, B., and Radasch, R.M. (2007). Use of polypropylene mesh in addition to internal obturator transposition: a review of 59 cases. *Journal of the American Animal Hospital Association* 43: 136–142.

Teichman, S.L., Unemori, E., Teerlink, J.R. et al. (2010). Relaxin: review of biology and potential role in treating heart failure. *Current Heart Failure Reports* 7: 75–82.

Theil, C., Fischer, A., Kramer, M., and Lautersack, O. (2010). Surgical therapy of perineal hernia in dogs by the use of small intestinal submucosa (SIS™). *Tierärztliche Praxis* 38: 71–78.

Van Sluijs, F.J. and Sjollema, B.E. (1989). Perineal hernia repair in the dog by transposition of the internal obturator muscle. I. Surgical technique. *Veterinary Quarterly* 11: 12–17.

Vnuk, D., Babić, T., Stejskal, M. et al. (2005). Application of a semitendinosus muscle flap in the treatment of perineal hernia in a cat. *Veterinary Record* 156: 182–183.

Vnuk, D., Lipar, M., Matičić, D. et al. (2008). Comparison of standard perineal herniorrhaphy and transposition of the internal obturator muscle for perineal hernia repair in the dog. *Veterinarski Arhiv* 78: 197–207.

Vnuk, D., Maticic, D., Kreszinger, M. et al. (2006). A modified salvage technique in surgical repair of perineal hernia in dogs using polypropylene mesh. *Veterinární Medicína* 51: 111–117.

Vyacheslav, H. and Ranen, E. (2009). Perineal hernia with retroflexion of the urinary bladder in a 4 month old puppy. *Journal of Small Animal Practice* 50: 625.

Weaver, A.D. and Omamegbe, J.O. (1981). Surgical treatment of perineal hernia in the dog. *Journal of Small Animal Practice* 22: 749–758.

Welches, C.D., Scavelli, T.D., Aronsohn, M.G. et al. (1992). Perineal hernia in the cat: a retrospective study of 40 cases. *Journal of the American Animal Hospital Association* 28: 431–438.

White, R.A.S. and Herrtage, M.E. (1986). Bladder retroflexion in the dog. *Journal of Small Animal Practice* 27: 735–746.

Wolberg, I.W.K. (2014). Perineal hernia repair in the dog by a modified technique of transposition of the internal obturator muscle. Long term results in 60 patients. Doctoral thesis, Faculty of Veterinary Medicine, Utrecht University.

Zhang, J.T., Wang, H.B., Shi, J. et al. (2010). Laparoscopy for percutaneous tube cystostomy in dogs. *Journal of the American Veterinary Medical Association* 236: 975–977.

Section 4

Chest Wall

28

Pectus Excavatum

Raymond K. Kudej

Pectus excavatum (PE) is an uncommon skeletal deformity resulting from a dorsal intrusion of the sternum and costal cartilages into the thoracic cavity. The cause of PE is unknown. Most of the reported cases are congenital and involve the caudal aspect of the sternum and xiphoid process; however, atypical cases involving the cranial portion of the sternum have been described (Ellison & Halling 2004; Hassan *et al.* 2018; Bedu *et al.* 2012). The severity of the deformity is variable (Figure 28.1), as is the presence of clinical signs. Many animals are asymptomatic.

Pectus carinatum (keeled breast) is the opposite of PE and involves a ventral protrusion of the sternum out from the thoracic cavity. Synonyms include pectus gallinatum (hen breast), chicken breast, and pigeon breast. Pectus carinatum is less common than PE in humans and animals, and has been described infrequently in the veterinary literature (Souza *et al.* 2009).

Incidence

PE has been described in humans, dogs, cats, sheep, cows, and nondomestic animals (sea otter, ruffed lemur, and nonhuman primate) (Ellison & Halling 2004). In the veterinary literature, there are only 31 well-documented cases of PE in dogs, with 2 others mentioned (total 33 dogs), and 37 well-documented cases in cats, with 5 others mentioned (total 42 cats). The incidence of PE in animals is unknown, although it is considered to be uncommon. In humans, PE is the most common chest wall deformity and has an incidence of approximately 1 in 400 births, occurring four times more frequently in

boys than in girls (Cartoski *et al.* 2006). However, in the veterinary literature there is no sex predilection in dogs or in cats. In humans, PE is commonly associated with connective tissue disorders such as Marfan and Ehlers–Danlos syndromes (Creswick *et al.* 2006). In dogs, cranial PE was acquired in 23 of 44 retrievers with muscular dystrophy and was likely secondary to muscle contracture (Bedu *et al.* 2012).

Etiology

The cause of PE is unknown. Proposed etiologies include mechanical forces, upper airway obstruction, and genetic predisposition. Any of these potential causes on their own, or in combination, may result in the development of PE. However, affected animals should be spayed or neutered due to a strong genetic component apparent in the literature.

Mechanical forces have been implicated in many hypotheses. Thickened substernal ligaments, shortening of the central tendon of the diaphragm, and a deficiency in the muscular development of the ventral portion of the diaphragm have each been proposed to cause an inward pull on the xiphoid during development resulting in PE. These theories are supported somewhat by a 30% occurrence of acquired PE following neonatal congenital diaphragmatic hernia repair in humans (Peetsold *et al.* 2009). However, an abnormal substernal ligament has not been noted in any veterinary report, was specifically not found in one study (Smallwood & Beaver 1977), and is refuted as a cause of PE in the human literature (Kelly 2008). Abnormal intrauterine pressures have been

Small Animal Soft Tissue Surgery, Second Edition. Edited by Eric Monnet.
© 2023 John Wiley & Sons, Inc. Published 2023 by John Wiley & Sons, Inc.
Companion website: www.wiley.com/go/monnet/small

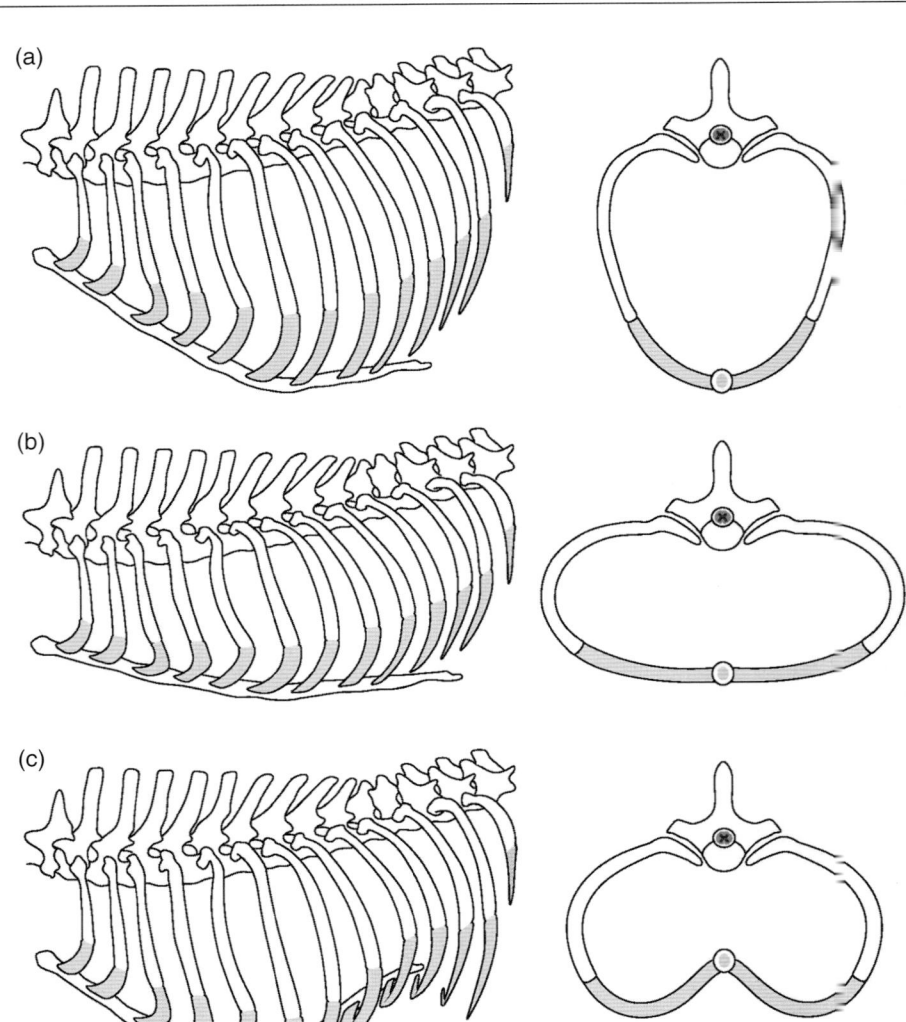

Figure 28.1 Variable severity of pectus excavatum (PE) deformity. (a) Normal thorax. (b) Mild PE deformity or flat chest. (c) More severe PE with dorsal intrusion of caudal sternum and xiphoid into the thorax. © D. Giddings.

theorized to cause PE (Boudrieau *et al.* 1990). A history of dystocia was associated with PE in a recent case report (Fournier 2008); however, the abnormality had resolved in this dog without treatment by 2 months of age. In a large population of Burmese cats with increased incidence of flat chest and PE, the defects were usually not present at birth (Sturgess *et al.* 1997). Prolonged external pressure on the chest has also been documented as a cause of PE in humans (Kloetzel *et al.* 1973). Prolonged external pressure may play a role in the development of PE in dogs with swimmer's syndrome (Fossum *et al.* 1989a), where an animal is unable to adduct the forelimbs (Fournier 2008; Gifford & Flanders 2010).

A mechanical etiology is also suggested in children with upper airway obstruction, where abnormally large negative intrathoracic pressures and a compliant chest resulted in PE (Olsen *et al.* 1980; Fan & Murphy 1981). Similarly, a case of acquired PE in a dog secondary to laryngeal paralysis has been described (Kurosawa *et al.* 2012). Although upper airway obstruction is not relevant to the vast majority of human cases, it may be a more prominent contributing factor for PE in animals, because brachycephalic breeds account for 58% (19 of 33) of the documented cases in dogs.

In a recent multicenter study on the surgical management of a series of 327 humans with PE, 43% of the patients had a familial history of PE (Kelly *et al.* 2007). In humans, the mode of inheritance has been shown to be autosomal dominant, autosomal recessive, X-linked, and multifactorial in different families (Creswick *et al.* 2006). In the veterinary literature, 11 of 33 dogs (33%) and 4 of 42 cats (10%) with PE had an affected littermate. Oriental breeds account for 50% (21/42) of feline cases of PE in the literature. Burmese and Bengal kittens in the UK have been reported to have an increased incidence of thoracic wall deformities and PE occurring within these groups, although bias in these populations is possible (Sturgess *et al.* 1997; Charlesworth & Sturgess 2012; Charlesworth *et al.* 2016).

Pathophysiology

Narrowing of the distance between the caudal sternum and thoracic vertebrae can cause cardiac compression, resulting in decreased stroke volume and cardiac output (Beiser *et al.* 1972). Common electrocardiographic abnormalities noted in humans are right-axis deviation and depressed ST segments, each related to rotation of the heart within the thorax. Cardiac displacement in both dogs and cats is most frequently to the left side of the thoracic cavity. Compression of the right ventricular outflow tract causing a systolic murmur occurs in approximately 18% of human patients (Fonkalsrud *et al.* 2002). Cardiac murmurs associated with right ventricular outflow tract stenosis have been documented in the veterinary literature (Fournier 2008; Gifford & Flanders 2010); however, murmurs associated with intrinsic cardiac abnormalities can also occur in animals with PE and must be ruled out (Fossum *et al.* 1989a).

Although thoracic volume is decreased, many recent studies of pulmonary function in human PE patients demonstrate lung volumes within the normal range (Koumbourlis & Stolar 2004; Kelly *et al.* 2007). However, symptomatic patients frequently have extensive phrenic excursions that cause them to use more energy and experience early exercise fatigue. Under exercise conditions, surgical repair of PE has been shown to significantly improve maximum voluntary ventilation, maximum oxygen utilization, total lung capacity, and total exercise time (Cahill *et al.* 1984).

Despite the lack of extensive cardiopulmonary function data in veterinary patients, PE is believed to have a similar effect on cardiac and pulmonary function to that in humans (Boudrieau *et al.* 1990). This belief is supported by the demonstration of improvement of clinical signs and cardiac abnormalities following surgical repair of PE in animals (Shires *et al.* 1988; Fossum *et al.* 1989b; McAnulty & Harvey 1989; Gifford & Flanders 2010).

Clinical signs

Many affected animals are asymptomatic and there has been no demonstration that clinical signs are related to the severity of the anatomic abnormality. Most of the symptomatic animals are presented prior to 3 months of age. Clinical signs include dyspnea, exercise intolerance, lack of weight gain, hyperpnea, cyanosis, inappetence, inability to walk or thoracic limb splaying, recurrent pulmonary infections, mild upper respiratory disease, mild inspiratory stridor, vomiting, and persistent productive cough. The disease process may be progressive, as some cases have documented a worsening of clinical signs following the initial presentation.

Diagnosis

Even asymptomatic patients have typically a visible or palpable caudal sternal defect (Figure 28.2). Increased inspiratory effort is evident in symptomatic patients. Thoracic auscultation commonly denotes inspiratory stridor, moist rales if infection is present, and a cardiac murmur.

Heart sounds are frequently muffled unilaterally due to cardiac displacement, which is more frequently to the left in dogs and almost always to the left in cats. Echocardiography must be used to rule out intrinsic cardiac abnormalities when murmurs, cardiomegaly, or any cardiac abnormalities are noted. Baseline laboratory data (complete blood count, serum biochemistries, urinalysis) are typically unremarkable in uncomplicated cases.

Thoracic radiography will show decreased thoracic volume, especially on lateral projections, due to dorsal displacement of the caudal sternum (Figure 28.3). Objective assessment of the degree of the deformity has been made by determining the frontosagittal or vertebral indexes (Figure 28.3) (Fossum *et al.* 1989a). However, the severity of the clinical signs has not been shown to be associated with the degree of deformity.

The frontosagittal index is calculated by dividing the width of the chest at the tenth thoracic vertebra (measured on a dorsoventral radiograph; Figure 28.3a, length *a*) by the distance between the sternum and the center of the ventral surface of the vertebral body nearest the deformity

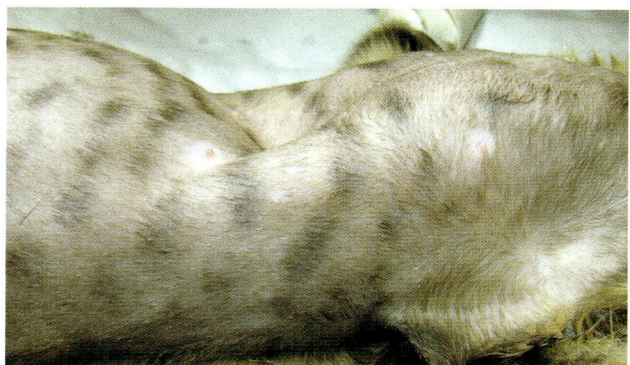

Figure 28.2 Caudal sternal pectus excavatum deformity in a cat (thorax and head are to the right).

(a)

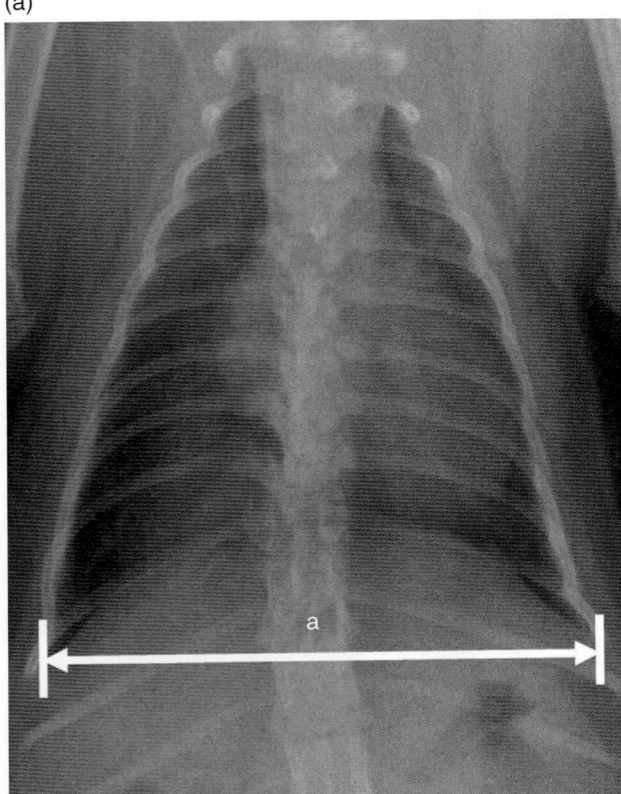

(b)

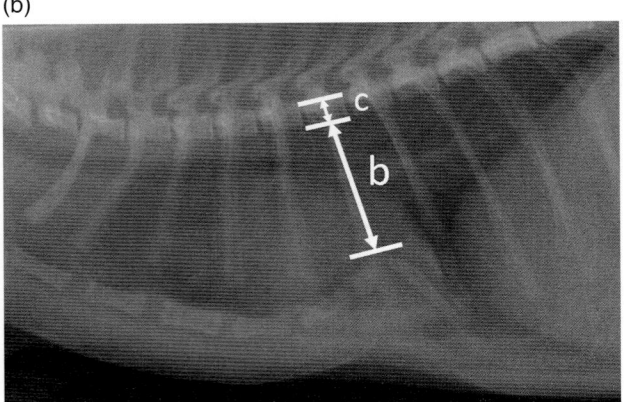

Figure 28.3 (a) Dorsoventral and (b) lateral thoracic radiographs used to calculate the degree of pectus excavatum deformity. The frontosagittal index is calculated by dividing the width of the chest at the tenth thoracic vertebra [measured on a dorsoventral radiograph; (a) length a] by the distance between the sternum and the center of the ventral surface of the vertebral body nearest the deformity [measured on a lateral radiograph; (b) length b]. The vertebral index is calculated by dividing the distance between the sternum and the center of the dorsal surface of the vertebral body nearest the deformity [measured on a lateral radiograph; (b) length $b+c$] by the dorsoventral diameter of the center of the same vertebral body [(b) length c].

(measured on a lateral radiograph; Figure 28.3b, length b). Normal values for dogs and cats range between 0.7 and 1.5. Suggested values for determining the severity of PE are mild, <2; moderate, 2–3; and severe, >3 (Boudrieau et al. 1990). Similar to the frontosagittal index, the Haller index is used in humans and is calculated from computed tomography (Haller et al. 1987).

The vertebral index is calculated by dividing the distance between the sternum and the center of the dorsal surface of the vertebral body nearest the deformity (measured on a lateral radiograph; Figure 28.3b, length $b+c$) by the dorsoventral diameter of the center of the same vertebral body (Figure 28.3b, length c). Normal values for dogs and cats range between 11.8 and 19.6. Suggested values for determining the severity of PE are mild, >9; moderate, 6–9; and severe, <6 (Boudrieau et al. 1990).

Cardiac displacement will likely be present. Cardiac displacement may result in apparent cardiomegaly, which has resolved following surgical correction of the chest wall (Fossum et al. 1989). Additionally, the lung fields should be assessed for the presence of pneumonia or other abnormalities.

Treatment

The variable expression of PE (i.e., degree of pathologic involvement) results in a variety of treatment options. The technique selected may be dictated by the presence of clinical signs, severity of the defect, age of the animal, rigidity of the costal arches, and ability to retract the sternal defect.

Conservative management

Young animals with mild PE or a flat chest may develop a normal or near-normal chest wall without surgical intervention. However, lateral-to-medial compression of the chest should not be used with more severe cases of PE, because this may exacerbate dorsal intrusion of the sternum into the thoracic cavity. It remains undetermined whether an asymptomatic animal with moderate or severe PE should undergo a corrective surgical procedure; however, the owners should be advised that the disease process may be progressive.

Surgery

In the majority of cases, an external splinting technique can be used to correct the sternal defect and alleviate the clinical signs. The efficacy of external splinting is dependent on the pliability of the costal cartilage and sternum in young animals (usually <4 months of age). Because of this flexibility, percutaneous circumsternal sutures can be used to place traction on the sternum and secure it in a more normal position with the aid of an external splint. Any soft tissues that may have been contributing to the defect should be ruptured by the repositioning of the sternum. Subsequent mineralization of the costal cartilages then provides adequate stiffness for the sternum to maintain the more normal position after splint removal. However, a standard external splinting technique cannot be used in older animals because the sternum is noncompliant. Corrective surgery in symptomatic animals over 5 months of age has been described (Bennett 1973; Shires *et al.* 1988; Crigel & Moissonnier 2005; Risselada *et al.* 2006). Older animals probably require a sternal wedge ostectomy, multiple chondrectomies, and some form of internal and/or external fixation; however, a partial sternectomy has been described (Bennett 1973).

External splinting technique

Prior to surgery, a moldable splinting material is used to create a U-shaped splint fashioned to fit the normal contour of the ventral thorax (Figure 28.4). The cranial aspect of the splint should be shaped or cut to accommodate movement of the thoracic limbs. A small Steinmann pin is used to make two rows of holes in the splint, parallel to the ventral midline with the midline in between them. The rows should be slightly farther apart than the width of the sternum. The inner surface and edges of the splint should be lightly padded to minimize skin trauma.

After anesthetic induction, the animal is placed in dorsal recumbency and the ventral thorax is clipped and prepared for aseptic surgery. Large (2) monofilament nonabsorbable (polypropylene or nylon) suture material with a swaged-on half-circle taper-point needle is used for the circumsternal sutures. It is important that the sutures be placed in the area with the greatest concavity. The needle is blindly and carefully passed through the skin and around the sternum. The needle point should be walked off the lateral aspect of the sternum and advanced as close as possible to the dorsal sternum (to avoid trauma to the heart or lungs) prior to exiting the skin on the opposite side. A towel clamp can be used to place ventral traction on the xiphoid process to help protect internal structures while passing the needle around the sternum (Figure 28.5). Advancement of the needle during expiration may help prevent lung laceration. It has also been recommended that sutures be passed at a 45° angle to include costocartilage and prevent the possibility of sutures pulling through fragile sternal cartilage (Figure 28.6) (Boudrieau *et al.* 1990). After each of the sutures has been preplaced, the suture ends are advanced through corresponding holes in the splint (Figure 28.7). The sutures are then tied together with tension sufficient to oppose and fix the caudal sternum into a normal position adjacent to the splint (Figure 28.8). The suture ends can be left long, tied into a bow, and

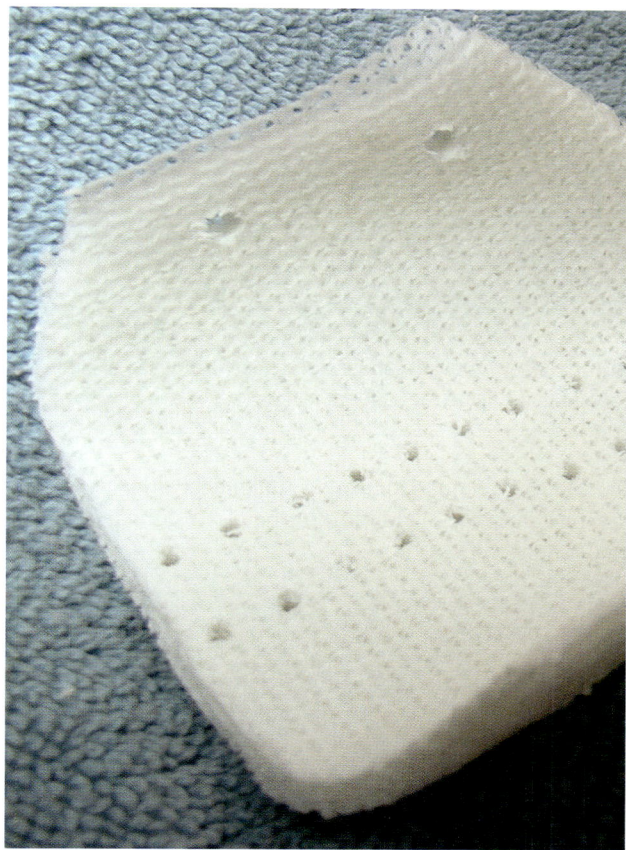

Figure 28.4 A U-shaped splint fashioned to fit the normal contour of the ventral thorax.

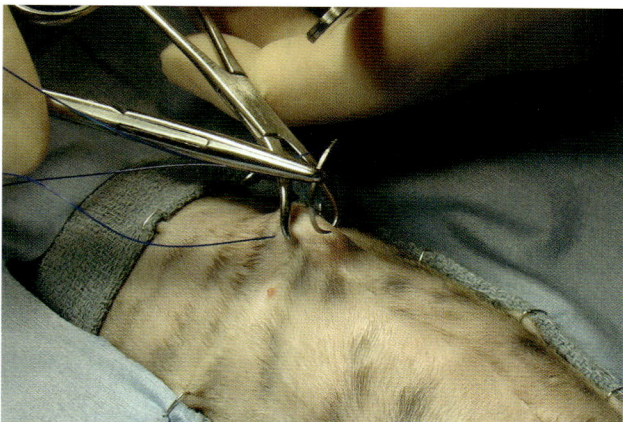

Figure 28.5 A towel clamp can be used to place ventral traction on the xiphoid process to help protect internal structures while passing the needle around the sternum.

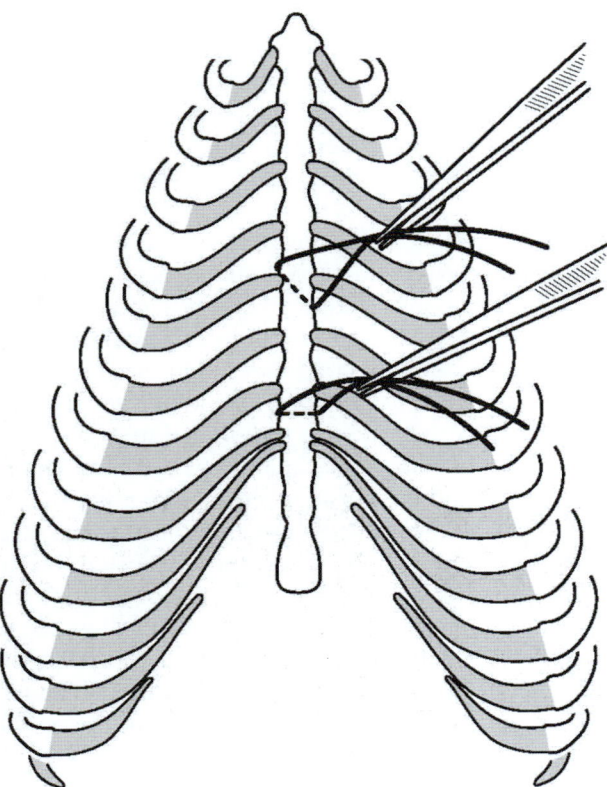

Figure 28.6 Sutures can be passed perpendicular to the sternum, or at a 45° angle to include costocartilage and prevent the possibility of the sutures pulling through fragile sternal cartilage. © D. Giddings.

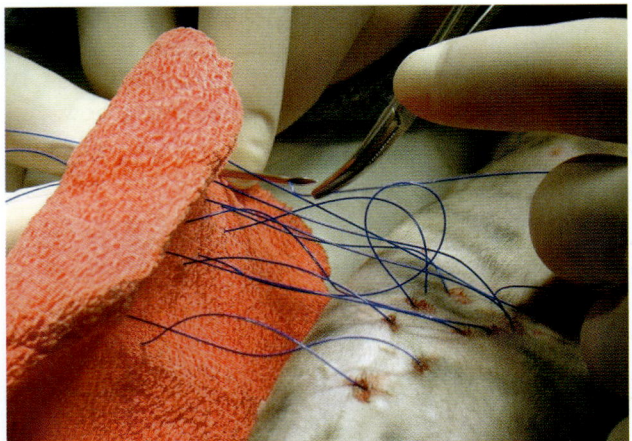

Figure 28.7 After each of the sutures has been preplaced, the suture ends are advanced through corresponding holes in the splint. It is important that the sutures be placed in the area with the greatest concavity.

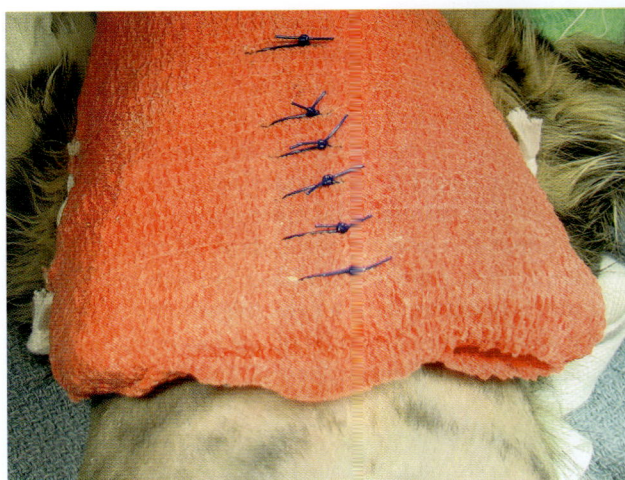

Figure 28.8 The sutures are tied with tension sufficient to oppose and fix the caudal sternum into a normal position adjacent to the splint.

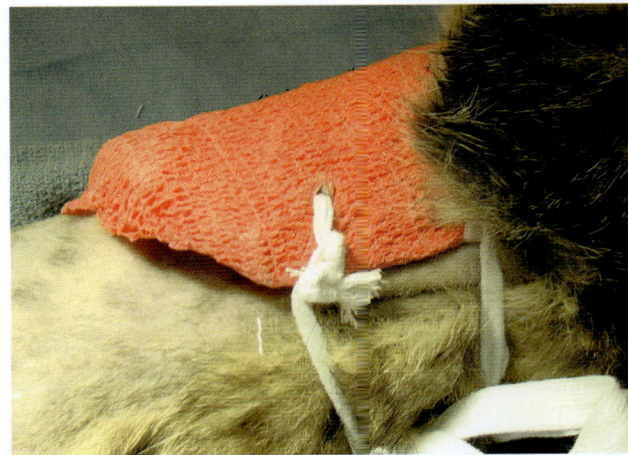

Figure 28.9 Tie-overs can be fashioned with gauze or umbilical tape to help secure the splint dorsally.

adhered ventrally to accommodate splint removal, adjustment, and reapplication. Tie-overs can be fashioned with gauze or umbilical tape to help secure the splint dorsally (Figure 28.9). Postoperative radiographs should be taken to document normal positioning of the sternum and for evaluation of the heart, lungs, and thorax (Figure 28.10).

Complications

Potential major complications associated with suture placement include laceration of the heart, lung, or internal vessels. Reexpansion pulmonary edema following PE surgery in a kitten has been described (Soderstrom *et al.* 1995). Minor expected complications include suture abscesses, mild skin abrasions, and superficial dermatitis (Figure 28.11), which heal rapidly following splint removal.

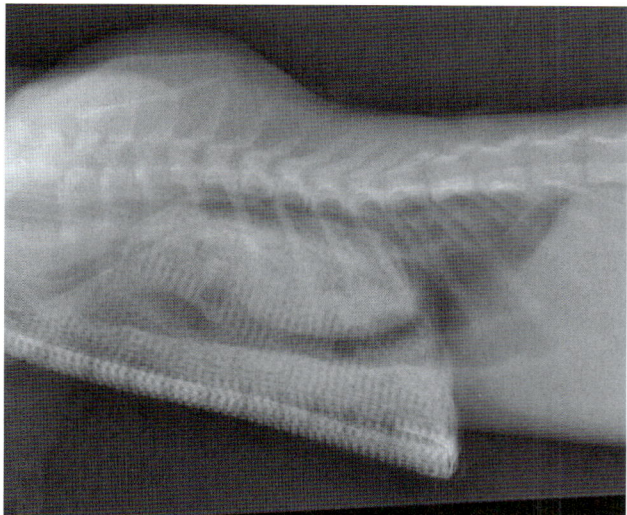

Figure 28.10 Postoperative radiographs should be taken to document normal positioning of the sternum and for evaluation of the heart, lungs, and thorax.

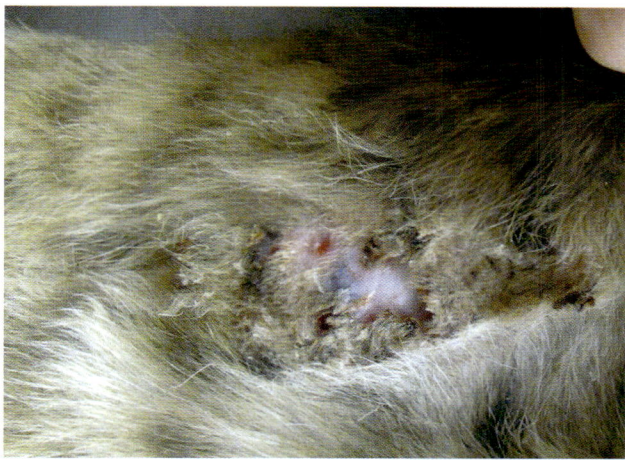

Figure 28.11 Mild skin abrasions and superficial dermatitis secondary to splint application. These lesions heal rapidly following splint removal.

Postoperative management

The animal should be monitored closely for evidence of hemothorax or pneumothorax. Body temperature and blood glucose should also be monitored and supported, if necessary, until full recovery. The length of time the splint is left in place should be between two and three weeks. However, successful outcomes have been described in a dog (Fossum *et al.* 1989a) and cat (Johnston *et al.* 1993) following one-week splint applications.

References

Bedu, A.-S., Labruyere, J.J., Thibaud, J.L. et al. (2012). Age-related thoracic radiographic changes in golden and labrador retriever muscular dystrophy. *Veterinary Radiology & Ultrasound* 53: 492–500.

Beiser, G.D., Epstein, S.E., Stampfer, M. et al. (1972). Impairment of cardiac function in patients with pectus excavatum, with improvement after operative correction. *New England Journal of Medicine* 287: 267–272.

Bennett, D. (1973). Successful surgical correction of pectus excavatum in a cat. *Veterinary Medicine, Small Animal Clinician* 68: 936.

Boudrieau, R.J., Fossum, T.W., Hartsfield, S.M. et al. (1990). Pectus excavatum in dogs and cats. *Compendium on Continuing Education for the Practicing Veterinarian* 12: 341–355.

Cahill, J.L., Lees, G.M., and Robertson, H.T. (1984). A summary of preoperative and postoperative cardiorespiratory performance in patients undergoing pectus excavatum and carinatum repair. *Journal of Pediatric Surgery* 19: 430–433.

Cartoski, M.J., Nuss, D., Goretsky, M.J. et al. (2006). Classification of the dysmorphology of pectus excavatum. *Journal of Pediatric Surgery* 41: 1573–1581.

Charlesworth, T.M. and Sturgess, C.P. (2012). Increased incidence of thoracic wall deformities in related Bengal kittens. *Journal of Feline Medicine and Surgery* 14: 365–368.

Charlesworth, T.M., Schwarz, T., and Sturgess, C.P. (2016). Pectus excavatum: computed tomography and medium-term surgical outcome in a prospective cohort of 10 kittens. *Journal of Feline Medicine and Surgery* 18: 613–619.

Creswick, H.A., Stacey, M.W., Kelly, R.E. Jr. et al. (2006). Family study of the inheritance of pectus excavatum. *Journal of Pediatric Surgery* 41: 1699–1703.

Crigel, M.H. and Moissonnier, P. (2005). Pectus excavatum surgically repaired using sternum realignment and splint techniques in a young cat. *Journal of Small Animal Practice* 46: 352–356.

Ellison, G. and Halling, K.B. (2004). Atypical pectus excavatum in two Welsh terrier littermates. *Journal of Small Animal Practice* 45: 311–314.

Fan, L. and Murphy, S. (1981). Pectus excavatum from chronic upper airway obstruction. *American Journal of Diseases of Children* 135: 550–552.

Fonkalsrud, E.W., DeUgarte, D., and Choi, E. (2002). Repair of pectus excavatum and carinatum deformities in 116 adults. *Annals of Surgery* 236: 304–312.

Fossum, T.W., Boudrieau, R.J., and Hobson, H.P. (1989a). Pectus excavatum in eight dogs and six cats. *Journal of the American Animal Hospital Association* 25: 595–605.

Fossum, T.W., Boudrieau, R.J., Hobson, H.P., and Rudy, R.L. (1989b). Surgical correction of pectus excavatum, using external splintage in two dogs and a cat. *Journal of the American Veterinary Medical Association* 195: 91–97.

Fournier, T.E. (2008). Dynamic right ventricular outflow tract (infundibular) stenosis and pectus excavatum in a dog. *Canadian Veterinary Journal* 49: 485–487.

Gifford, A.T. and Flanders, J.A. (2010). External splinting for treatment of pectus excavatum in a dog with right ventricular outflow obstruction. *Journal of Veterinary Cardiology* 12: 53–57.

Haller, J.A. Jr., Kramer, S.S., and Lietman, S.A. (1987). Use of CT scans in selection of patients for pectus excavatum surgery: a preliminary report. *Journal of Pediatric Surgery* 22: 904–906.

Hassan, E.A., Hassan, M.H., and Torad, F.A. (2018). Correlation between clinical severity and type and degree of pectus excavatum in twelve brachycephalic dogs. *Journal of Veterinary Medical Science* 80: 766–771.

Johnston, S.A., Moon, M.L., Atkinson, R.N., and Eyster, G.E. (1993). Pectus excavatum and left to right intracardiac shunt in a kitten. *Journal of Small Animal Practice* 34: 577–581.

Kelly, R.E. Jr. (2008). Pectus excavatum: historical background, clinical picture, preoperative evaluation and criteria for operation. *Seminars in Pediatric Surgery* 17: 181–193.

Kelly, R.E. Jr., Shamberger, R.C., Mellins, R.B. et al. (2007). Prospective multicenter study of surgical correction of pectus excavatum: design, perioperative complications, pain, and baseline pulmonary function facilitated by internet-based data collection. *Journal of the American College of Surgeons* 205: 205–216.

Kloetzel, K., Cassetari, L., and Lopes, J.A. (1973). Pectus excavatum (funnel chest) as an occupational disease. *Journal of Occupational Medicine* 15: 118–119.

Koumbourlis, A.C. and Stolar, C.J. (2004). Lung growth and function in children and adolescents with idiopathic pectus excavatum. *Pediatric Pulmonology* 38: 339–343.

Kurosawa, T.A., Ruth, J.D., Steurer, J. et al. (2012). Imaging diagnosis-acquired pectus excavatum secondary to laryngeal paralysis in a dog. *Veterinary Radiology & Ultrasound* 53: 329–332.

McAnulty, J.F. and Harvey, C.E. (1989). Repair of pectus excavatum by percutaneous suturing and temporary external coaptation in a kitten. *Journal of the American Veterinary Medical Association* 194: 1065–1067.

Olsen, K.D., Kern, E.B., and O'Connell, E.J. (1980). Pectus excavatum: resolution after surgical removal of upper airway obstruction. *Laryngoscope* 90: 832–837.

Peetsold, M.G., Heij, H.A., Kneepkens, C.M. et al. (2009). The long-term follow-up of patients with a congenital diaphragmatic hernia: a broad spectrum of morbidity. *Pediatric Surgery International* 25: 1–17.

Risselada, M., de Rooster, H., Liuti, T. et al. (2006). Use of internal splinting to realign a noncompliant sternum in a cat with pectus excavatum. *Journal of the American Veterinary Medical Association* 228: 1047–1052.

Shires, P.K., Waldron, D.R., and Payne, J. (1988). Pectus excavatum in three kittens. *Journal of the American Animal Hospital Association* 24: 203–208.

Smallwood, J.E. and Beaver, B.V. (1977). Congenital chondrosternal depression (pectus excavatum) in the cat. *Veterinary Radiology* 18: 141–146.

Soderstrom, M.J., Gilson, S.D., and Gulbas, N. (1995). Fatal reexpansion pulmonary edema in a kitten following surgical correction of pectus excavatum. *Journal of the American Animal Hospital Association* 31: 133–136.

Souza, D.B., Andrade Junior, P.S.C., Mariano, C.M.A. et al. (2009). Pectus carinatum in a dog. *Arquivo Brasileiro de Medicina Veterinária e Zootecnia* 61: 276–279.

Sturgess, C.P., Waters, L., Gruffyd-Jones, T.J. et al. (1997). Investigation of the association between whole blood and tissue taurine levels and the development of thoracic deformities in neonatal Burmese kittens. *Veterinary Record* 141: 566–570.

29

Surgery of the Thoracic Wall

Julius M. Liptak, Eric Monnet, and Kristin Zersen

Thoracic surgery requires a good understanding of pulmonary and cardiac physiology. Perioperative management of cases is very important for a successful outcome. In addition, management of postoperative pain is an important component of the procedure.

Perioperative monitoring and management

All animals undergoing thoracic surgery should be monitored closely in the perioperative period. This should include respiratory monitoring and cardiovascular monitoring. At a minimum, respiratory monitoring should include monitoring of ventilation and oxygenation. Cardiovascular monitoring should include monitoring of blood pressure, electrocardiography (ECG), and lactate.

Respiratory monitoring

Respiratory monitoring is required in the perioperative thoracic surgery patient. While blood gas analysis is invaluable, the importance of a physical examination and thoracic auscultation should not be discounted. Frequent thoracic auscultation will help identify patients who have developed respiratory complications such as pleural space disease and pulmonary disease. Pleural space disease, like pleural effusion or pneumothorax, may be suspected in patients with decreased lung sounds and short, shallow breathing patterns. Pulmonary disease, such as aspiration pneumonia, may be suspected in patients with crackles on auscultation. Frequent reassessment of the postoperative patient by physical exam and thoracic auscultation cannot be replaced by other diagnostic modalities.

Ventilation

Monitoring for hypoventilation in the perioperative period is extremely important. In order to understand the causes and pathophysiology of hypoventilation, a foundational knowledge of the definitions of minute ventilation (MV), tidal volume (TV), and alveolar ventilation (VA) is required.

- Minute ventilation (MV): total volume of gas exhaled per minute; equal to the respiratory rate times the tidal volume ($MV = RR \times TV$).
- Tidal volume (TV): volume of air that enters the lung with each normal inspiration; includes dead space volume and alveolar volume.
- Alveolar ventilation (VA): volume of inspired air available for gas exchange; this does not include the volume of air in dead space.
- Dead space ventilation: portion of air that does not participate in gas exchange; may include anatomic, alveolar, physiologic, and apparatus dead space.

Hypoventilation is due to inadequate alveolar ventilation given the amount of CO_2 produced via aerobic metabolism (Luks & West 2016). The alveolar ventilation equation explains the relationship between the alveolar partial pressure of CO_2 (P_ACO_2) and alveolar ventilation. The alveolar ventilation equation is:

$$P_ACO_2 = \frac{V_{CO2} \times K}{V_A}$$

where $V_{CO2} = CO_2$ production, VA = alveolar ventilation, and K = constant.

This equation shows that the $PACO_2$ is inversely proportional to alveolar ventilation. If alveolar ventilation is halved, the $PACO_2$ doubles. CO_2 diffuses 20 times more quickly than oxygen (Luks & West 2016), which is important because this means the $PACO_2$ will roughly equal the arterial partial pressure of CO_2 ($PaCO_2$). Therefore, hypoventilation always causes a rise in the $PaCO_2$.

Diagnosing hypoventilation

Hypoventilation can be diagnosed by assessing the $PaCO_2$, venous partial pressure of CO_2 ($PvCO_2$), or end-tidal CO_2 ($ETCO_2$). The gold standard for diagnosing hypoventilation is through the measurement of $PaCO_2$, and hypoventilation is defined as a $PaCO_2$ greater than 40–45 mmHg. More specifically, it has been defined as a $PaCO_2$ greater than 36 mmHg in the cat and a $PaCO_2$ greater than 42 mmHg in the dog (Hopper & Haskins 2008). $PvCO_2$ can also be used to diagnose hypoventilation. The $PvCO_2$ is roughly 3–5 mmHg higher than the $PaCO_2$, but this can vary significantly in patients with altered tissue perfusion (Hopper & Haskins 2008). Hypoventilation can also be diagnosed using capnography to assess the $ETCO_2$. $ETCO_2$ is measured using a mainstream or side-stream $ETCO_2$ monitor that displays a capnograph and $ETCO_2$ value. $ETCO_2$ monitoring is most commonly used in intubated patients, and the $ETCO_2$ has been shown to be strongly correlated to the $PaCO_2$ in healthy, anesthetized dogs (Hightower *et al.* 1980). The $ETCO_2$ is approximately 2–6 mmHg lower than the $PaCO_2$ in normal dogs (Hightower *et al.* 1980).

Clinical signs and complications of hypoventilation

There is no specific breathing pattern associated with hypoventilation. The patient may have a rapid, shallow breathing pattern, they may be taking slow, deep breaths, or they may appear dyspneic. Hypoventilation causes a respiratory acidosis, so other clinical signs and complications may be due to the altered acid–base status. A respiratory acidosis can affect cardiovascular, neurologic, and metabolic functions (Johnson 2012). Hypoventilation stimulates sympathetic tone, so tachycardia, tachyarrhythmias, and hypertension may also be seen (Johnson 2012). In experimental models, respiratory acidosis increases heart rate and cardiac output (CO) but decreases myocardial contractility and systemic vascular resistance (SVR) (Johnson 2012). Hypoventilation will cause cerebral vasodilation and subsequently an increase in cerebral blood flow, which may result in elevated intracranial pressure. Neurologic signs including anxiety, disorientation, obtundation, or coma may be

seen when the $PaCO_2$ acutely rises to greater than 70–100 mmHg (Johnson 2012). Metabolic effects of hypoventilation may include acute kidney injury due to afferent renal artery vasoconstriction. Hypoventilation may also cause sodium and water retention and hyperkalemia (Johnson 2012).

Causes of hypoventilation

There are many potential causes of hypoventilation that can be broadly described as hypoventilation due to (i) decreased minute ventilation; (ii) increased dead space ventilation; (iii) increased carbon dioxide production with fixed tidal volume (uncommon); or (iv) increased inspired carbon dioxide due to expired CO_2 adsorbent in the anesthesia circuit (uncommon) (Daly 2015). The most common causes of hypoventilation in patients who have thoracic surgery include:

- Decreased minute ventilation due to:
  - Central respiratory depression: due to administration of general anesthetics, opioids.
  - Abnormal respiratory mechanics: due to respiratory fatigue from prolonged increased work of breathing, pleural space disease, loss of chest wall or lung elasticity, loss of structural integrity of the chest wall, decreased functional residual capacity, increased airway resistance.
- Increased dead space ventilation due to:
  - High V/Q mismatch: due to poor cardiac output, shock, pulmonary emboli, pulmonary bulla.
  - Increased anatomic dead space: due to excessive dead space in the anesthetic circuit or endotracheal tube.

Hypoventilation due to central respiratory depression is most likely to affect the patient under general anesthesia during surgery, but this may persist due to high-dose opioid administration postoperatively. Prolonged work of breathing associated with pulmonary or pleural space disease may result in respiratory fatigue and hypoventilation. Loss of the structural integrity of the chest wall and the pain associated with thoracic surgery may result in the patient taking very short, shallow breaths in order to minimize pain associated with expanding the chest wall. If a patient is in shock or has poor cardiac output, this may result in increased dead space ventilation and subsequent hypoventilation (Daly 2015).

Treatment of hypoventilation

Hypoventilation is treated by addressing the underlying cause. After thoracic surgery, many patients will hypoventilate because of the pain associated with expanding the chest wall. Ensuring adequate pain control is imperative so the patient can generate adequate tidal volumes.

Consider limiting opioids in patients that are hypoventilating. Placement of a thoracostomy tube intraoperatively will ensure that the patient does not have a pneumothorax or pleural effusion postoperatively. This will enable the patient to expand their lungs and generate adequate tidal volumes. The thoracostomy tube should be aspirated regularly to check that pleural space disease has not developed. Mechanical ventilation may be indicated in cases of severe hypoventilation ($PaCO_2 > 60$ mmHg) that does not respond to treatment. Shock should be treated immediately in all cases. Intravenous fluids can be used for hypovolemic patients, and vasopressors can be used for hypotensive patients that are euvolemic. Ensure that the anesthetic circuit and endotracheal tube are appropriate for the patient to prevent dead space ventilation.

The administration of sodium bicarbonate is contraindicated in the treatment of respiratory acidosis or hypoventilation. Bicarbonate is converted to CO_2 and will worsen hypercarbia (Johnson 2012).

Oxygenation

Hypoxemia may be a perioperative complication of thoracic surgery and is defined as a PaO_2 of less than 80 mmHg or a hemoglobin saturation (SpO_2 or SaO_2) of less than 95% (Haskins 2015). Severe hypoxemia is defined as a PaO_2 of less than 60 mmHg or a hemoglobin saturation (SpO_2 or SaO_2) of less than 90% (Haskins 2015).

Diagnosing hypoxemia

The gold standard for assessing oxygenation and diagnosing hypoxemia is through measuring PaO_2, which requires an arterial blood sample. Although a venous sample can be used to assess ventilation, it cannot be used to assess oxygenation because venous blood is more representative of tissue function as opposed to pulmonary function (Haskins 2015). It is also important to note that the PaO_2 represents the dissolved oxygen in blood, not the oxygen bound to hemoglobin.

Hemoglobin saturation may also be used to assess oxygenation and to diagnose hypoxemia through measurement of SaO_2, or more commonly SpO_2, using pulse oximetry. The SpO_2 is directly associated with the PaO_2 and this relationship is described via the oxyhemoglobin dissociation curve. Through this curve, we know that an SpO_2 of 95% equates to a PaO_2 of 80 mmHg, and an SpO_2 of 90% equates to a PaO_2 of 60 mmHg. Although there can be difficulties in obtaining an SpO_2 with a pulse oximeter, it is generally considered easier than collecting an arterial blood sample.

Causes of hypoxemia

There are five general causes of hypoxemia: (i) decreased partial pressure of inspired oxygen (PiO_2); (ii) hypoventilation; (iii) ventilation–perfusion mismatch (V/Q mismatch); (iv) diffusion impairment; and (v) shunts. When considering the five causes of hypoxemia, it is important to note whether the cause of hypoxemia is oxygen responsive and whether or not it results in an increased alveolar–arterial gradient (A–a gradient) (West 2012).

Oxygen responsiveness can be determined by assessing the PaO_2/FiO_2 ratio, also called the P/F ratio or oxygen index. The PaO_2 should be approximately four to five times the FiO_2 at sea level. For example, a patient breathing room air (FiO_2 21%) should have a PaO_2 of approximately 84–105 mmHg, whereas a patient breathing 100% oxygen (FiO_2 100%) should have a PaO_2 of 400–500 mmHg. The normal P/F ratio is 400–500 mmHg. A P/F ratio less than 200 mmHg may indicate acute respiratory distress syndrome (ARDS) (Haskins 2015).

By assessing the patient's P/F ratio on room air, then again with oxygen supplementation, you can determine if the patient is responding to oxygen. If a patient is oxygen responsive, their P/F ratio should increase with oxygen supplementation. If they are not oxygen responsive, the P/F ratio will not increase. Assessing for clinical improvement in your patient is also important.

Measuring the A–a gradient can also help narrow down the list of differentials for hypoxemia. It should only be calculated on patients breathing room air. The first step to calculating the A–a gradient is to calculate the PAO_2 using the alveolar gas equation:

$$P_AO_2 = \left[FiO_2 \left(PB - P_{H2O} \right) \right] - \left[PaCO_2 / 0.8 \right]$$

where P_B = barometric pressure, P_{H2O} = water vapor pressure (= 47 mmHg), and 0.8 = respiratory exchange ratio constant.

You then subtract the PaO_2 from the PAO_2 to determine the A–a gradient. A normal A–a gradient is less than 10 mmHg; an A–a gradient greater than 20 mmHg suggests venous admixture.

Decreased PiO$_2$

Decreased PiO_2 is an uncommon cause of hypoxemia and is due to either a decreased fraction of inspired oxygen (FiO_2) or a decrease in barometric pressure. A decrease in FiO_2 is most commonly due to human error, when someone forgets to turn on the oxygen source for a patient attached to an anesthetic circuit or in an enclosed oxygen cage. At altitude, the barometric pressure decreases and this results in a decreased PiO_2. Subsequently, people and animals living at altitude have a lower PaO_2, which they compensate for by hyperventilating (Haskins 2015). Hypoxemia due to a decreased PiO_2 is oxygen responsive and has a normal A–a gradient.

Hypoventilation

Hypoxemia due to hypoventilation is common in postoperative thoracic surgery patients. The definition and causes of hypoventilation were discussed previously in this chapter. For every 1 mmHg increase in $PaCO_2$, there is an approximately 1 mmHg decrease in PaO_2 (West 2012). Therefore, hypoventilation generally results in mild hypoxemia. For instance, if a patient's $PaCO_2$ increases to 80 mmHg, this will result in a PaO_2 of approximately 60 mmHg. This patient is more likely to suffer complications of hypoventilation before they suffer significant complications of hypoxemia. Hypoxemia due to hypoventilation is oxygen responsive, but oxygen supplementation will not correct the underlying hypoventilation and the A–a gradient is normal.

Ventilation–perfusion (V/Q) mismatch

V/Q mismatch occurs when ventilation and blood flow are not appropriately matched to maximize oxygenation of blood. V/Q mismatch is the most common cause of hypoxemia and it is most commonly described as either high V/Q mismatch or low V/Q mismatch.

High V/Q mismatch is associated with adequate ventilation but compromised perfusion. A pulmonary thromboembolism (PTE) is a classic example of high V/Q mismatch. In cases of PTE, the alveoli are being appropriately ventilated, but there is no blood flow to those alveoli.

Low V/Q mismatch is associated with normal perfusion but compromised ventilation, so in these cases blood is flowing through regions of lung that are poorly oxygenated. Low V/Q mismatch is most commonly associated with fluid (blood, transudate, exudate) filling the alveoli and impairing gas exchange. It may also be due to small airway narrowing or bronchospasm. Hypoxemia due to low V/Q mismatch may be seen in postoperative thoracotomy patients that develop aspiration pneumonia.

Depending on the cause, V/Q mismatch may or may not be oxygen responsive. The A–a gradient is elevated.

Diffusion impairment

Diffusion impairment occurs when equilibrium is not reached between the PaO_2 and the PAO_2 (West 2012). This is most commonly due to thickening of the blood–gas barrier. In dogs and cats, this is an uncommon cause of hypoxemia, but may be due to diseases affecting the

Table 29.1 Causes of hypoxemia.

Cause of hypoxemia	Oxygen responsive?	A–a gradient
Decreased PiO_2	Yes	Normal
Hypoventilation	Yes	Normal
V/Q mismatch	Variable	Elevated
Diffusion impairment	Partially	Elevated
Shunt	No	Elevated

pulmonary interstitial space, including interstitial pneumonia and pulmonary fibrosis. In humans, emphysema is one of the more common causes of diffusion impairment. Hypoxemia due to diffusion impairment is partially oxygen responsive and results in an elevated A–a gradient.

Shunts

Hypoxemia due to shunts is usually due to congenital right-to-left cardiac shunts (i.e., reverse patent ductus arteriosus), but can also include right-to-left pulmonary shunts (see Table 29.1). In cases of right-to-left cardiac or pulmonary shunts, blood enters the arterial system without being oxygenated because all alveoli are bypassed. Hypoxemia due to shunts are not oxygen responsive and have an elevated A–a gradient.

The most common causes of hypoxemia in patients who have thoracic surgery include:

- Low V/Q mismatch due to:
  - Fluid accumulation in the alveoli: due to pneumonia (exudate), hemorrhage, transudate.
  - Atelectasis.
  - Small airway narrowing or bronchoconstriction.
- High V/Q mismatch due to PTE.
- Hypoventilation due to:
  - Decreased minute ventilation: due to central respiratory depression, respiratory fatigue, pleural space disease, pain.
  - Increased dead space ventilation: due to high V/Q mismatch or increased anatomic dead space.

Treatment of hypoxemia

Hypoxemia is treated by addressing the underlying cause and providing oxygen supplementation. There are many techniques for supplementing oxygen, including flow-by oxygen, use of a face mask, use of an oxygen hood, placement in an oxygen cage, use of nasal or nasopharyngeal catheters, or high-flow nasal oxygen.

Flow-by oxygen is convenient during examination of the patient, but is a temporary modality and only provides approximately 30% FiO_2 when the oxygen source is held within 2 cm of the patient's nose (Mazzaferro 2015). A tight-fitting face mask may also be used temporarily, but oftentimes patients are not amenable to their use. An oxygen hood can be created by placing an Elizabethan collar on the patient, covering approximately three-quarters of the front opening of the Elizabethan collar with saran wrap, then feeding an oxygen line through the back of the Elizabethan collar and taping it in place inside of the collar. Approximately one-quarter of the front opening of the Elizabethan collar should be left open to allow for carbon dioxide removal. This provides approximately 30–40% FiO_2 (Mazzaferro 2015). An oxygen cage is the most commonly used modality for providing up to 60% FiO_2 for patients. Benefits of an oxygen cage include the ability to control the FiO_2, humidification, and temperature. Unfortunately, oxygen cages are expensive and they do limit the ability to handle the patient.

Oxygen may also be provided via nasal or nasopharyngeal catheters. Human nasal prongs can be used in dogs and are generally well tolerated, but there can be some difficulty keeping them in place. A red rubber catheter can be placed in the nasal cavity to the level of the lateral canthus of the eye. The nasal passage should be anesthetized (commonly with proparacaine), then the catheter should be lubricated and inserted into the ventral nasal meatus, directing the catheter ventral and medially. The catheter can be secured with suture or staples. Placement of a nasopharyngeal catheter is similar, but the catheter is advanced to the ramus of the mandible. These techniques can provide an FiO_2 of 30–70%, depending on flow rate (Mazzaferro 2015).

High-flow nasal oxygen is a newer modality of oxygen support in veterinary medicine. It is a noninvasive ventilation system that delivers a medical air and oxygen mixture through a humidifier and circuit to the patient via nasal prongs (Jagodich *et al.* 2019). One can deliver up to 60 L/min of the air–oxygen mixture and up to 100% FiO_2 using these systems (Jagodich *et al.* 2019). High-flow nasal oxygen has been shown to be well tolerated in veterinary patients and may be especially useful in hypoxemic patients where mechanical ventilation is not an option.

Cardiovascular monitoring

Cardiovascular monitoring of the perioperative thoracic surgery patient is also required. Ultimately, the cardiovascular assessment of the patient should be based on many factors, including physical examination, blood pressure, and lactate measurement. Other techniques may include measurement of central venous pressure, central or mixed venous oxygen saturation, and cardiac

output. ECG should also be monitored in the perioperative period. Again, the importance of physical examination for monitoring the cardiovascular status of a patient should not be discounted. Shock can be identified in a patient by assessing the six perfusion parameters: mentation, heart rate, pulse quality, mucous membrane color, capillary refill time, and core to toe web temperature gradient.

Blood pressure monitoring

Blood pressure monitoring for perioperative thoracic surgery patients is essential because blood pressure ultimately drives blood flow (Cooper 2015). It is important to note that although blood pressure contributes to tissue perfusion, it is not a direct assessment of perfusion. Arterial blood pressure is a function of cardiac output (CO) and SVR, such that BP = CO × SVR (Cooper 2015). A patient can have a normal blood pressure, but have poor perfusion. An example of this would be a patient who is hemorrhaging. That patient will increase SVR by vasoconstriction, and this vasoconstriction may decrease perfusion although it maintains a normal blood pressure.

Techniques for monitoring blood pressure include direct and indirect measurements. Direct blood pressure monitoring is the gold standard technique and requires placement of an arterial catheter. Indirect techniques, including Doppler and oscillometry techniques, are technically easier to perform but have limitations to their use and they are not as accurate as direct measurement, especially in patients with high or low blood pressure. While direct measurement of blood pressure is preferred in the perioperative monitoring of thoracic surgery patients, indirect measurements are considered an acceptable alternative as long as the limitations of their use are understood.

Lactate

Blood lactate measurement is a useful marker of decreased oxygen delivery. Lactate is produced via anaerobic metabolism and hyperlactatemia most commonly represents a relative or absolute decrease in oxygen delivery, called type A hyperlactatemia (Rosenstein 2018). Less commonly, hyperlactatemia can be due to other underlying diseases, drugs, toxins, or metabolic defects (Rosenstein *et al.* 2018). Hyperlactatemia due to causes other than decreased oxygen delivery is called type B hyperlactatemia.

Regular monitoring of lactate should be used to help guide fluid resuscitation, and normalization of lactate should be considered an endpoint of resuscitation. In addition, lactate values can be used to separate patients into higher and lower risk categories (Rosenstein et al. 2018). However, human and veterinary literature has demonstrated that in most cases, consecutive lactate measurements are more beneficial than single measurements and lactate clearance is more important than initial values (Rosenstein et al. 2018).

Electrocardiography

ECG should be used to monitor heart rate and rhythm in the perioperative period. Monitoring heart rate is important, as tachycardia may be an indication of shock, acid–base abnormalities, electrolyte abnormalities, anemia, hypoxemia, or pain (Wright 2015). All of these potential causes of tachycardia should be addressed immediately. Uncommonly, increased vagal tone due to respiratory disease may lead to bradycardia in a perioperative thoracic surgery patient (Pariaut & Reynolds 2015). Bradycardia due to increased vagal tone does not need to be treated unless the patient is suffering from hypotension or cardiovascular compromise.

Although patients under general anesthesia can suffer from a number of cardiac arrhythmias, ventricular arrhythmias are most common. It is important to note that not all patients with ventricular arrhythmias require treatment. The following are indications for treating ventricular arrhythmias: sustained ventricular tachycardia (heart rate greater than 160–180 bpm); hemodynamic compromise; polymorphic ventricular arrhythmias; R-on-T phenomenon; and ventricular fibrillation (Pariaut & Reynolds 2015).

There are many potential causes of ventricular premature contractions (VPCs) and ventricular tachycardia in the perioperative thoracic surgery patient. Noncardiac causes may include hypoxemia, acid–base disturbances, electrolyte abnormalities, and sympathetic stimulation (Pariaut & Reynolds 2015). Cardiac causes may include heart failure, cardiac tumors, myocarditis, and ischemia (Pariaut & Reynolds 2015).

The first step in treating VPCs or ventricular tachycardia is to identify and treat the underlying cause, if possible. If determined that the patient requires further treatment, lidocaine is the first-line antiarrhythmic of choice for treating VPCs or ventricular tachycardia. In dogs, the recommended dose is 2 mg/kg intravenously (i.v.) to effect, up to a total of 8 mg/kg (Pariaut & Reynolds 2015). Doses higher than 8 mg/kg may result in significant side effects. If the arrhythmia is responsive to lidocaine, a continuous rate infusion of 25–80 μg/kg/h can also be used in dogs (Pariaut & Reynolds 2015). Cats are much more sensitive to lidocaine, so it should be used with caution. Other options for treatment include procainamide, mexiletine, β-blockers, sotalol, amiodarone, and magnesium sulfate (Pariaut & Reynolds 2015).

Thoracoscopy

Thoracoscopy is a minimally invasive operative procedure for the examination of the pleural cavity and its organs (Hsin & Yim 2010). With the development of high-resolution microcameras, video optics, and fiberoptic light delivery systems, clear magnified images of the surgical field can be transferred to a video screen. The ability to perform diagnostic and advanced therapeutic procedures is possible with minimally invasive video-assisted endoscopy in combination with minimally invasive surgical instruments.

Thoracoscopy is indicated for thoracic exploration, evaluation of pleural effusion of unknown origin, prevention of cardiac tamponade due to pericardial effusion with the creation of a pericardial window, lung lobectomy, correction of persistent right aortic arch, ligation of thoracic duct, and ligation of patent ductus arteriosus (Jackson et al. 1999; MacPhail et al. 2001; Kovak et al. 2002; Borenstein et al. 200–; Lansdowne et al. 2005; Allman et al. 2010). Biopsy of the pleural surface, lymph nodes, pericardium, and lungs can be performed during exploration of the thoracic cavity (Website Chapter 29: Thoracic wall/thoracoscopy: exploration and biopsy).

Thoracoscopy is a safe and effective method for evaluating pathology without the expense and morbidity of open thoracotomy (Mehta et al. 2010; Nagasawa & Johnson 2010; Yamamoto et al. 2010). The view obtained via thoracoscopy is often superior to that obtained via open thoracotomy because the thoracoscope can be placed directly on the lesion(s) under investigation. The thoracoscope also provides excellent lighting and magnification, both of which help visualize different lesions or structures.

Anesthetic considerations

Thoracoscopy can be performed with or without mechanical ventilation. Utilization of closed cannulas with controlled pneumothorax is required for cases in which thoracoscopic surgery is performed without mechanical ventilation. It is very important to monitor ventilation with a capnograph and oxygen saturation measurements. The benefit of this approach is that a mechanical ventilator is not required and a thoracic drain may not be needed, since the pneumothorax is limited during the procedure. In the vast majority of cases, open cannulas are used to gain access to the thoracic cavity. With this technique, a pneumothorax invariably results and mechanical ventilation is therefore required. The creation of a pneumothorax induces partial collapse of the lungs, creating sufficient space to explore the thoracic cavity and perform biopsies of the pleura, lymph nodes, or lung.

One-lung ventilation, with selective intubation of either the left or the right lung, will allow better exposure of specific areas of the thoracic cavity (Fischer & Cohen 2010; Nakanishi *et al.* 2010). Selective intubation is used commonly in humans to achieve one-lung ventilation and its utilization has been reported in dogs (Mayhew & Friedberg 2008; Fischer & Cohen 2010). A bronchial blocker (Arnsdt endobronchial blocker, Cook, Bloomington, IN, USA) can be used instead of selective intubation to achieve one-lung ventilation (Website Chapter 29: Thoracic wall/Thoracic surgery: approaches Figure W29.1) (Lansdowne *et al.* 2005). Another type of blocker has been used to induce one-lung ventilation in dogs (EZ blocker, Teleflex, Morrisville, NC, USA) (Mayhew *et al.* 2020). It is our experience that an endobronchial blocker is more appropriate for dogs than selective intubation as a result of their anatomy. The placement of the endobronchial blocker requires bronchoscopy to visualize the position of the blocker while being manually placed in the lung lobe that needs to stay deflated. When one-lung ventilation is used, the non-ventilated lung will collapse.

Arterial blood gases need to be performed to monitor the oxygenation of the patient. Positive end-expiratory pressure (PEEP) can be used to maintain expanded alveoli and prevent atelectasia of the dependent lung (Kudnig *et al.* 2004, 2006; Riquelme *et al.* 2005a,b). The application of $5\,cmH_2O$ PEEP in one-lung ventilation during thoracoscopy in normal dogs does not affect cardiac output (Kudnig *et al.* 2006). Therefore, any gain in oxygen saturation observed with the application of PEEP will translate into an augmentation in oxygen delivery.

Insufflation of the pleural space with carbon dioxide has been used to collapse the lung and increase the working space (Kaneko *et al.* 2010). If this technique is used, the pressure of insufflation should not be above 3–5 mmHg. Higher pressure will increase the risk of severe atelectasia of the lungs and reduce ventilation.

Surgical technique

Thoracoscopy can be performed using either a transdiaphragmatic or an intercostal approach. The transdiaphragmatic approach provides a long-axis view of the thorax and allows visualization of both hemithoraces. This is the approach of choice for exploration of the thoracic cavity and biopsy (Kovak *et al.* 2002). The intercostal approach allows visualization of only a specific area of the thoracic cavity and is most commonly used for surgical procedures (MacPhail *et al.* 2001; Borenstein *et al.* 2004; Lansdowne *et al.* 2005).

Transdiaphragmatic subxiphoid approach

The patient is positioned in a dorsal recumbency. A small skin incision is created caudal to the xiphoid. A screw-in cannula is inserted from a subxiphoid position, oriented in a cranial direction. The cannula is screwed into the thoracic cavity under thoracoscopic visualization. After penetration of the thoracic cavity by the cannula, the thoracoscope is advanced in the thoracic cavity. After an initial exploration of the thoracic cavity, two other cannulas are placed under thoracoscopic visualization to allow the use of instruments. These cannulas are placed through intercostal spaces according to the location of the lesion(s) that require exploration or treatment. Cannulas need to be placed as ventral as possible to allow maximum mobility of the instruments. A vessel-sealant device is used in to dissect the mediastinum from the sternum. It is important to visualize the internal thoracic artery during the dissection. This will allow exploration of both hemithoraces. A 0° telescope is used at the beginning of the exploration.

Intercostal approach

The patient is placed in either right or left lateral or sternal recumbency. Sternal recumbency is used for exposure of the dorsal part of the pleural space to visualize the thoracic duct (Radlinsky *et al.* 2002; Allman *et al.* 2010).

Cannulas can be placed from the third to the ninth or tenth intercostal space. Cranial to the third intercostal space the scapula is covering the thoracic wall and caudal to the ninth or tenth intercostal space the diaphragm would interfere with visualization. Cannulas should preferably be placed in the ventral two-thirds of the intercostal space because the ribs are too stiff dorsally, making manipulation of the instruments very difficult.

The intercostal space used to introduce the cannula is selected according to the location of the pathology. It is important to place the cannulas as far as possible from the lesion. This allows easier manipulation of the instruments. For example, if a cranial lung is removed, cannulas are better placed in the eighth or ninth intercostal space. After a skin incision, the subcutaneous tissue, the muscle of the thoracic wall, and the intercostal musculature are bluntly dissected to facilitate placement of the blunt cannulas.

After completion of the procedure, a thoracostomy tube is placed under thoracoscopic guidance. The drain should not be placed through a cannula hole because of the difficulty in establishing and maintaining a seal around the tube. The cannulas are removed one by one and the portal sites should be inspected for bleeding. It is possible to damage an intercostal artery during placement of the cannulas. While the cannulas are in place the intercostal artery is compressed and no bleeding is visible. If the intercostal artery bleeds after removal of the cannula, either electrocoagulation or a suture ligature can be used to control hemorrhage. The cannula used for the thoracoscope is removed last. Negative pressure is established after removal of the cannulas and closure of the portals. The thoracostomy tube is maintained for 12–24 hours.

Thoracotomy

Lateral or intercostal thoracotomy

A lateral or intercostal thoracotomy is the standard approach for many intrathoracic diseases and provides good exposure for a specifically defined region. For instance, a left fourth or fifth intercostal thoracotomy is recommended for surgical treatment of cardiovascular conditions such as patent ductus arteriosus, vascular anomalies like a persistent right aortic arch, and pulmonic stenosis. The cranial lung lobes are exposed through a left or right fourth to fifth intercostal thoracotomy, the right middle lung lobe through a right fifth intercostal thoracotomy, and the caudal lung lobes through a left or right fifth intercostal thoracotomy. The cranial esophagus is exposed through a right third or fourth intercostal thoracotomy and the caudal esophagus through either a left or right seventh to ninth intercostal thoracotomy. The thoracic duct is ligated through a right eighth to tenth intercostal thoracotomy in dogs and a left eighth to tenth intercostal thoracotomy in cats. However, access to structures not in the immediate area of the thoracotomy is limited and, as a general rule, an intercostal thoracotomy allows access to approximately one-third of the ipsilateral thoracic cavity (Orton 1995, 2003; Moores *et al.* 2007).

Surgical technique

The animal is positioned in lateral recumbency. An incision is made through the skin, subcutaneous tissue, and cutaneous trunci muscle parallel to the long axis of the ribs over the desired intercostal space, extending from the costovertebral junction dorsally to the sternum ventrally (Website Chapter 29: Thoracic wall/Thoracic surgery: approaches Figure W29.2). The latissimus dorsi and pectoral muscles are incised parallel to the skin incision across their muscle fibers (Website Chapter 29: Thoracic wall/Thoracic surgery: approaches Figure W29.3). The desired intercostal space for the thoracotomy is identified by counting ribs and intercostal spaces, usually from the first rib caudally, and/or identifying the fifth rib. The external abdominal oblique muscle originates from the fifth rib and the scalenus muscle inserts

on the fifth rib. One of these muscles is incised depending on whether the intercostal thoracotomy is cranial (scalenus muscle) or caudal (external abdominal oblique muscle) to the fifth rib. The serratus ventralis muscle is separated between its muscle bellies or incised parallel to its fibers to expose the intercostal space (Website Chapter 29: Thoracic wall/Thoracic surgery: approaches Figure W29.4). The external and internal intercostal muscles are then incised in the middle of the intercostal space to avoid iatrogenic trauma to the intercostal vessels coursing over the caudal aspect of the ribs (Website Chapter 29: Thoracic wall/Thoracic surgery: approaches Figure W29.5). The pleura is a distinct structure and is penetrated by blunt puncture and then opened to the extent of the thoracotomy using scissors (Website Chapter 29: Thoracic wall/Thoracic surgery: approaches Figures W29.6 and W29.7). The edges of the intercostal thoracotomy incision should be protected with moistened laparotomy sponges and Finochietto rib retractors are recommended to maintain retraction of the ribs and maximize exposure of the thoracic cavity (Website Chapter 29: Thoracic wall/Thoracic surgery: approaches Figure W29.8). Although rarely required, exposure can be increased by approximately 33% with dorsal and ventral osteotomies of the rib either cranial or caudal to the intercostal incision (Orton 1995, 2003).

Following completion of the surgical procedure, a thoracostomy tube is inserted to evacuate intrathoracic fluid or air accumulation in the postoperative period (Website Chapter 29: Thoracic wall/Thoracic surgery: approaches Figure W29.9). For diseases in which this is unlikely, a temporary thoracostomy tube, such as an 8 FG urinary catheter, can be placed through the intercostal thoracotomy incision. The thoracostomy tube should be kept open to the atmosphere during closure of the thoracotomy to prevent tension pneumothorax. Once an airtight closure is achieved, air and fluid are evacuated from the pleural space, negative intrathoracic pressure is reestablished, and the thoracostomy tube is then capped (Orton 1995, 2003).

The intercostal thoracotomy incision is closed with either circumcostal or transcostal sutures. The traditional circumcostal suture technique involves preplacing large-gauge (2-0 to 2 depending on the size of the animal) absorbable or nonabsorbable suture material around the cranial and caudal ribs in either a simple interrupted or cruciate suture pattern (Website Chapter 29: Thoracic wall/Thoracic surgery: approaches Figure W29.10). The needle should be passed as close as possible to the ribs to avoid entrapping soft tissues between the suture material and the ribs. In one study, the intercostal nerve was entrapped by circumcostal sutures in 70% and 100% of cases when the blunt and sharp end of the needle was passed around the caudal rib, respectively (Rooney *et al.* 2004). In this same study, it was shown that dogs in which intercostal thoracotomies were closed with circumcostal sutures experienced significantly more pain and had significantly greater requirements for fentanyl in the first 24 hours postoperatively than dogs in which the ribs were closed using a transcostal technique (Rooney *et al.* 2004). For the transcostal technique, holes are drilled in the mid-body of the caudal rib (Website Chapter 29: Thoracic wall/ Thoracic surgery: approaches Figure W29.11) so that the suture material is passed through the rib rather than around the rib, thus avoiding entrapment of the intercostal nerve (Website Chapter 29: Thoracic wall/ Thoracic surgery: approaches Figure W29.12) (Rooney *et al.* 2004). Regardless of whether a circumcostal or transcostal technique is used, the preplaced sutures are used by an assistant to approximate the ribs while the surgeon ties the sutures (Orton 1995, 2003). The serratus ventralis, scalenus, external abdominal oblique, latissimus dorsi, and cutaneous trunci muscles are closed individually with either interrupted or continuous suture patterns to prevent air leakage postoperatively (Orton 1995, 2003). Following routine closure of the subcutaneous layer and skin, the thoracostomy tube is secured with a finger-trap suture pattern.

Complications

Short-term complications are reported in up to 47% of cats and dogs following lateral intercostal thoracotomy (Moores *et al.* 2007). Hemorrhage, pain, air leakage, seroma, infection, wound dehiscence, and ipsilateral thoracic limb lameness are all rare but potential complications following intercostal thoracotomy (Orton 1995, 2003; Bonath 1996; Tattersall & Welsh 2006; Moores *et al.* 2007). Hemorrhage is most often caused by inadvertent trauma to the internal thoracic artery during the approach for an intercostal thoracotomy (Bonath 1996). Postoperative air leakage, which can manifest as pneumothorax, pneumomediastinum, or subcutaneous emphysema, is caused by problems with either the thoracotomy closure (e.g., insufficient apposition resulting in failure to achieve an airtight closure, incisional dehiscence, infection, or self-mutilation) or the thoracostomy tube (e.g., leakage from the stoma, leakage from the seals between the thoracostomy tube and three-way stopcock) (Bonath 1996). Intercostal thoracotomy is a painful procedure. An effective multimodality analgesia is required to ameliorate the negative effects of pain on recovery.

Modified rib pivot lateral thoracotomy

The modified rib pivot lateral thoracotomy (Appelgrein & Hosgood 2018) is a modification of the standard lateral thoracotomy technique.

Surgical technique

The animal is positioned in lateral recumbency. An incision is made through the skin, subcutaneous tissue, and cutaneous trunci muscle from the costovertebral junction dorsally to the sternum ventrally and running parallel to the ribs over the desired intercostal space. The ventral aspect of the latissimus dorsi muscle is identified, freed with an incision extending cranially and caudally, and elevated dorsally. The muscle bellies of the serratus ventralis muscle are separated over the designated rib. If the designated rib is the fifth rib, then the insertion of the scalenus muscle on this rib is also incised. The lateral periosteum is incised and circumferentially reflected off the rib using a periosteal elevator from the costovertebral articulation to the costochondral junction (Appelgrein & Hosgood 2018). Once the rib is isolated, two holes are drilled with a Kirschner wire, one 1.0 cm dorsal to the costochondral junction and the second 1.5 cm dorsal to the first hole. The rib is transected between these two holes with either a bone cutter or oscillating saw. The rib is pivoted cranially, hinged on the costovertebral articulation (Appelgrein & Hosgood 2018). The pleura is then incised to expose the hemithorax and area of interest.

Following completion of the surgical procedure, 2-0 to 0 absorbable suture material is preplaced through the previously drilled holes in the transected rib. The external fascia of the intercostal muscles, periosteum, and parietal pleura is closed with appropriately sized suture material in a simple continuous pattern, taking care to avoid including the neurovascular structures along the caudal aspect of the periosteal sleeve in this closure (Appelgrein & Hosgood 2018). The rib is then pivoted back into its normal position and the suture material through the two holes is tightened to appose the osteotomized ends of the rib. The remainder of the closure is the same as described for a standard intercostal thoracotomy.

Median sternotomy

A median sternotomy is the only approach that provides exposure to the entire thoracic cavity and is recommended for diseases involving both hemithoraces (e.g., cranial mediastinal tumors, pyothorax, and penetrating thoracic injuries) and for exploratory thoracotomies (e.g., spontaneous pneumothorax) (Orton 1995, 2003; Tattersall & Welsh 2006). Access to structures in the dorsal thoracic cavity, such as the great vessels and bronchial hilus, can be difficult, particularly in deep-chested dogs (Orton 1995, 2003). If required, a median sternotomy can be combined with either a ventral midline cervical incision or celiotomy.

Surgical technique

Animals are positioned in dorsal recumbency. The skin and subcutaneous tissues are incised along the ventral midline over the sternum (Website Chapter 29: Thoracic wall/Thoracic surgery: approaches Figure W29.13). The

pectoral muscles are sharply incised along the sternal midline (Website Chapter 29: Thoracic wall/Thoracic surgery: approaches Figure W29.14). A sternotomy is

then performed along the midline with an oscillating saw (Website Chapter 29: Thoracic wall/Thoracic surgery: approaches Figure W29.15). Care should be taken to avoid iatrogenic damage to the lungs and heart during the sternal osteotomy by limiting penetration of the saw blade (Orton 1995, 2003). Once a segment of the sternotomy has been completed, a malleable retractor can be inserted into the thorax to protect the intrathoracic structures during completion of the remainder of the median sternotomy. The manubrium and/or xiphoid should be preserved if possible (Orton 1995, 2003; Burton & White 1996), but occasionally a complete median sternotomy is required (e.g., when excising large cranial mediastinal masses). Some surgeons have expressed concerns that complete median sternotomy will result in sternal instability and an increased risk of postoperative complications (Orton 1995, 2003), but these are not supported by the findings of other investigators provided that the median sternotomy is closed appropriately (Burton & White 1996). The edges of the sternotomy incision should be protected with moistened laparotomy sponges, and Finochietto rib retractors are recommended to maintain retraction of the sternum and maximize exposure of the thoracic cavity (Website

Chapter 29: Thoracic wall/Thoracic surgery: approaches Figure W29.16).

Following completion of the surgical procedure, a thoracostomy tube should be inserted into one or both hemithoraces. The thoracostomy tube should be kept open to the atmosphere during closure of the thoracotomy to prevent tension pneumothorax. Once an airtight closure is achieved, air and fluid are evacuated from the pleural space, negative intrathoracic pressure is reestablished, and the thoracostomy tube is then capped.

Stable closure of the median sternotomy is imperative to avoid postoperative pain, pneumothorax, and sternal nonunion. A figure-of-eight technique over the sternal synchondrosis is preferred, with either heavy-gauge suture material (Website Chapter 29: Thoracic wall/Thoracic surgery: approaches Figure W29.17) or orthopedic wire (Website Chapter 29: Thoracic wall/Thoracic surgery: approaches Figures W29.18 and W29.19) being passed around each sternebra so that each costosternal junction is incorporated in the closure (Pelsue *et al.* 2002;

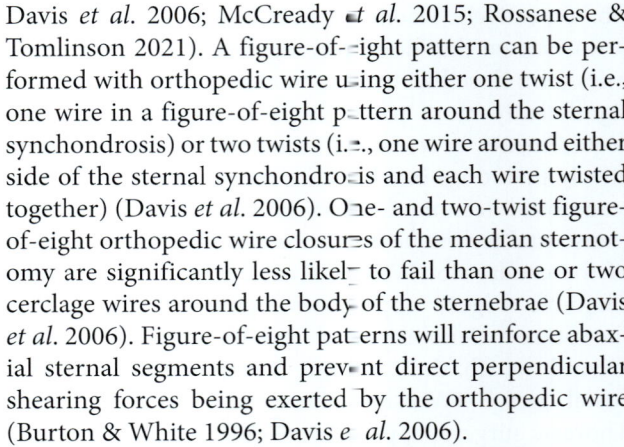

Davis *et al.* 2006; McCready et al. 2015; Rossanese & Tomlinson 2021). A figure-of-eight pattern can be performed with orthopedic wire using either one twist (i.e., one wire in a figure-of-eight pattern around the sternal synchondrosis) or two twists (i.e., one wire around either side of the sternal synchondrosis and each wire twisted together) (Davis *et al.* 2006). One- and two-twist figure-of-eight orthopedic wire closures of the median sternotomy are significantly less likely to fail than one or two cerclage wires around the body of the sternebrae (Davis *et al.* 2006). Figure-of-eight patterns will reinforce abaxial sternal segments and prevent direct perpendicular shearing forces being exerted by the orthopedic wire (Burton & White 1996; Davis e al. 2006).

There are no significant differences in either postoperative pain or wound complication rates between suture and wire closure of sternotomies (Pelsue *et al.* 2002). Closure with suture material is significantly faster than orthopedic wire closure, but orthopedic wire closure is recommended for large-breed dogs because sternal stability and osseous healing are superior compared with suture material closure (Pelsue *et al.* 2002). Closure with orthopedic wire results in less radiographic evidence of displacement of sternebrae at 28 days after sternotomy compared with suture closure. Furthermore, closure with orthopedic wire results in better long-term sternal stability because of chondral or osteochondral union between the osteotomized sternebrae, whereas suture closure only results in fibrous union (Pelsue *et al.* 2002). In an *in vitro* study comparing sutures and wires for the closure of a sternotomy, the utilization of suture could not be recommended because the loading for failure was superior with wires (Gines *et al.* 2011).

Following closure of the sternotomy, the pectoral muscles, subcutaneous tissue, and skin are closed routinely in separate layers (Website Chapter 29: Thoracic wall/Thoracic surgery: approaches Figure W29.20). The thoracostomy tube is secured with a finger-trap suture pattern (Website Chapter 29: Thoracic wall/Thoracic surgery: approaches Figure W29.21) and the thoracic cavity is evacuated until negative intrathoracic pressure has been reestablished.

Complications

Complications are reported in 0–78% of cats and dogs following median sternotomy. Median sternotomy is a painful procedure. Effective multimodality analgesia is required to ameliorate the negative effects of pain on recovery. Complications are rare in cats surviving more than 14 days after surgery (Burton & White 1996), and are more common in cats and dogs with pyothorax (Tattersall & Welsh 2006). Short-term complications are reported in 19–40% of dogs surviving longer than 14 days, including hemorrhage, incisional seroma, wound infection, thoracic limb neurologic deficits, and excessive postoperative pain (Burton & White 1996; Pelsue et al. 2002; Tattersall & Welsh 2006). Heavier dogs are predisposed to short-term complications, but not long-term complications (Burton & White 1996). Wound complications are significantly more likely in dogs treated with median sternotomy compared with lateral intercostal thoracotomy (Tattersall & Welsh 2006). Long-term complications occur in 22% of dogs and include hemorrhage, sternal fracture, sternal osteomyelitis, and delayed wound healing (Burton & White 1996). Sternal osteomyelitis is the most common long-term complication and causes sternal discomfort, bilateral thoracic limb lameness, recurrent ventral thoracic edema, pyrexia, inappetence, and depression. Other reported complications include unstable sternebrae repair, transient iatrogenic chylothorax, incisional edema, and incisional dehiscence (Burton & White 1996).

Postoperative management

Postoperative management is dependent on the surgical procedure and the underlying pathology. Intercostal thoracotomy or median sternotomy leads to postoperative pain because of rib separation during the procedure and stretching of the intercostal muscles or splitting of the sternum. Thoracoscopy is significantly less painful than open thoracotomy procedures (Walsh et al. 1999). Pain after thoracic surgery will contribute to hypoventilation, atelectasia, and hypoxemia, because the patient cannot take deep breaths to reexpand the lungs. Therefore, ensuring the animal has adequate pain control, but is not oversedated to the point of causing hypoventilation, is important. A multimodal approach to pain management, as well as addition of sedation protocols, may be necessary in some of these patients. Adequate pain control after thoracic surgery should be provided with a combination of techniques to minimize the negative effect of each technique. Epidural analgesia, intrapleural administration of bupivacaine and lidocaine, and systemic administration of opioid analgesics have been recommended in the postoperative period (Berg & Orton 1986; Popilskis et al. 1991; Thompson & Johnson 1991; Conzemius et al. 1994; Stobie et al. 1995). In a study of 134 dogs that were treated for lung lobectomy, 41 dogs (31%) underwent median sternotomy and 93 dogs (69%) underwent intercostal thoracotomy. Fluid production from the chest tube ($P = 0.0061$), alveolar arterial pressure gradient ($P = 0.0001$), and complications requiring

intervention ($P = 0.0245$) were more common in the median sternotomy group than the intercostal thoracotomy group. Pain management and all other short-term outcome factors did not differ between procedures (Bleakley et al. 2018).

Oxygen saturation should be closely monitored in animals recovering from any type of thoracic surgery. If hypoxemia is present with an A–a gradient above 20 mmHg, supplemental oxygen should be administered to the patient. It is important to keep FiO_2 below 60% during this time to prevent oxygen toxicity (Tobin 2006). Ventilation should be taken into consideration and $PaCO_2$ should ideally be below 45 mmHg, although most animals do not need to be mechanically ventilated unless $PaCO_2$ is above 55–60 mmHg or there is severe respiratory acidosis. Partial reversal of pure opioids with low-dose butorphanol or low-dose naloxone can help with opioid-induced hypoventilation while maintaining analgesia. Arterial blood gases should be measured every 2–6 hours initially until the animal is oxygenating and ventilating adequately. Monitoring blood gases every 6–12 hours thereafter is usually adequate. Pulse oximetry may be useful for monitoring oxygenation, but can be difficult to accurately measure in the awake patient.

Thoracic auscultation needs to be performed immediately postoperatively and repeated every 1–2 hours initially. If a sudden change in respiratory rate or pattern occurs, respiratory auscultation should be the first diagnostic test performed. A restrictive breathing pattern (quick, shallow breathing) is indicative of pleural space disease (i.e., pleural effusion or pneumothorax). Aspirating the thoracostomy tube should be performed every 2–4 hours initially. Aspiration of the pleural space frequently after surgery will allow better ventilation, reexpansion of the lung, and correction of hypoxemia. If a patient is hypoxemic, it is important first to aspirate the thoracostomy tube and then rotate the animal. Turning the patient every 4–6 hours after surgery will help reduce atelectasia and reestablish a better V/Q ratio.

Heart rate, ECG, temperature, and blood pressure should be monitored in the immediate postoperative period and are frequently continued on a regular basis for 24–48 hours. Animals seem to recovery quickly once the thoracostomy tube is removed, the time of which is usually determined by the degree of fluid or air production. If the thoracostomy tube is negative for air over a 6–8-hour period and is producing minimal fluid, then the thoracostomy tube is frequently removed. Most animals are eating and on oral analgesics within 48–72 hours following open thoracic surgery.

References

Allman, D.A., Radlinsky, M.G., Ralph, A.G., and Rawlings, C.A. (2010). Thoracoscopic thoracic duct ligation and thoracoscopic pericardectomy for treatment of chylothorax in dogs. *Veterinary Surgery* 39: 21–27.

Appelgrein, C. and Hosgood, G. (2018). Modified rib pivot lateral thoracotomy: a case series. *Australian Veterinary Journal* 96: 28–32.

Berg, R.J. and Orton, E.C. (1986). Pulmonary function in dogs after intercostal thoracotomy: comparison of morphine, oxymorphone, and selective intercostal nerve block. *American Journal of Veterinary Research* 47: 471–474.

Bleakley, S., Phipps, K., Petrovsky, B., and Monnet, E. (2018). Median sternotomy versus intercostal thoracotomy for lung lobectomy: a comparison of short-term outcome in 134 dogs. *Veterinary Surgery* 47: 104–113.

Bonath, K.H. (1996). Thoracic wall closure. In: *Complications in Small Animal Surgery* (ed. A.J. Lipowitz, D.D. Caywood, C. Newton, et al.), 229–239. Baltimore, MD: Williams & Wilkins.

Borenstein, N., Behr, L., Chetboul, V. et al. (2004). Minimally invasive patent ductus arteriosus occlusion in 5 dogs. *Veterinary Surgery* 33: 309–313.

Burton, C.A. and White, R.N. (1996). Review of the technique and complications of median sternotomy in the dog and cat. *Journal of Small Animal Practice* 37: 516–522.

Conzemius, M.G., Brockman, D.J., King, L.G., and Perkowski, S.Z. (1994). Analgesia in dogs after intercostal thoracotomy: a clinical trial comparing intravenous buprenorphine and interpleural bupivacaine. *Veterinary Surgery* 23: 291–298.

Cooper, E. (2015). Hypotension. In: *Small Animal Critical Care Medicine*, 2e (ed. D.C. Silverstein and K. Hopper), 46–50. St. Louis: Elsevier Saunders.

Daly, M.L. (2015). Hypoventilation. In: *Small Animal Critical Care Medicine*, 2e (ed. D.C. Silverstein and K. Hopper), 86–92. St. Louis: Elsevier Saunders.

Davis, K.M., Roe, S.C., Mathews, K.G., and Mente, P.L. (2006). Median sternotomy closure in dogs: a mechanical comparison of technique stability. *Veterinary Surgery* 35: 271–277.

Fischer, G.W. and Cohen, E. (2010). An update on anesthesia for thoracoscopic surgery. *Current Opinion in Anaesthesiology* 23: 7–11.

Gines, J.A., Friend, E.J., Vives, M.A. et al. (2011). Mechanical comparison of median sternotomy closure in dogs using polydioxanone and wire sutures. *Journal of Small Animal Practice* 52: 582–586.

Haskins, S.C. (2015). Hypoxemia. In: *Small Animal Critical Care Medicine*, 2e (ed. D.C. Silverstein and K. Hopper), 81–86. St. Louis, MO: Elsevier Saunders.

Hightower, C.E., Kiorpes, A.L., Butler, H.C., and Fedde, M.R. (1980). End-tidal partial pressure of CO_2 as an estimate of arterial partial pressure of CO_2 during various ventilator regimens in halothane-anesthetized dogs. *American Journal of Veterinary Research* 41: 610–612.

Hopper, K. and Haskins, S.C. (2008). A case-based review of a simplified quantitative approach to acid-base analysis. *Journal of Veterinary Emergency and Critical Care* 18 (5): 467–476.

Hsin, M.K. and Yim, A.P. (2010). Management of complications of minimally invasive thoracic surgery. *Respirology* 15: 6–18.

Jackson, J., Richter, K.P., and Launer, D.P. (1999). Thoracoscopic partial pericardiectomy in 13 dogs. *Journal of Veterinary Internal Medicine* 13: 529–533.

Jagodich, T.A., Bersenas, A.M.E., Bateman, S.W., and Kerr, C.L. (2019). Comparison of high flow nasal cannula oxygen administration to traditional nasal cannula oxygen therapy in healthy dogs. *Journal of Veterinary Emergency and Critical Care* 29 (3): 246–255.

Johnson, R.A. (2017). A quick reference on respiratory acidosis. *Veterinary Clinics of North America. Small Animal Practice* 47: 185–189.

Kaneko, K., Ono, Y., Tainaka, T. et al. (2010). Thoracoscopic lobectomy for congenital cystic lung diseases in neonates and small infants. *Pediatric Surgery International* 26: 361–365.

Kovak, J.R., Ludwig, L.L., Bergman, P. et al. (2002). Use of thoracoscopy to determine the etiology of pleural effusion in dogs and cats: 18 cases (1998–2001). *Journal of the American Veterinary Medical Association* 221: 990–994

Kudnig, S.T., Monnet, E., Riquelme, M. et al. (2004). Cardiopulmonary effect of thoracoscopy in anesthetized normal dogs. *Veterinary Anaesthesia and Analgesia* 31: 121–128.

Kudnig, S.T., Monnet, E., Riquelme, M. et al. (2006). Effect of positive end-expiratory pressure on oxygen delivery during one-lung ventilation for thoracoscopy in normal dogs. *Veterinary Surgery* 35: 534–542.

Lansdowne, J.L., Monnet, E., Twedt, D.C., and Dernell, W.S. (2005). Thoracoscopic lung lobectomy for treatment of lung tumors in dogs. *Veterinary Surgery* 34: 530–535.

Luks, A. and West, J.B. (2016). *West's Respiratory Physiology: The Essentials*. Amsterdam: Wolters Kluwer.

MacPhail, C.M., Monnet, E., and Twedt, D.C. (2001). Thoracoscopic correction of persistent right aortic arch in a dog. *Journal of the American Animal Hospital Association* 37: 577–581.

Mayhew, P.D. and Friedberg, J.S. (2008). Video-assisted thoracoscopic resection of noninvasive thymoma using one-lung ventilation in two dogs. *Veterinary Surgery* 37: 756–762.

Mayhew, P.D., Chohan, A., Hardy, B.T et al. (2020). Cadaveric evaluation of fluoroscopy-assisted placement of one-lung ventilation devices for video-assisted thoracoscopic surgery in dogs. *Veterinary Surgery* 49 (Suppl 1): O93–O101.

Mazzaferro, E.M. (2015). Oxygen therapy. In: *Small Animal Critical Care Medicine*, 2e (ed. D.C. Silverstein and K. Hopper), 77–80. St. Louis, MO: Elsevier Saunders.

McCready, D.J., Bell, J.C., Ness, M.G., and Tarlton, J.F. (2015). Mechanical comparison of monofilament nylon leader and orthopaedic wire for median sternotomy closure. *Journal of Small Animal Practice* 56: 510–515.

Mehta, K.D., Gundappa, R., Contractor, R. et al. (2010). Comparative evaluation of thoracoscopy versus thoracotomy in the management of lung hydatid disease. *World Journal of Surgery* 34: 1828–1831.

Moores, A.L., Halfacree, Z.J., Baines, S.J., and Lipscomb, V.J. (2007). Indications, outcomes and complications following lateral thoracotomy in dogs and cats. *Journal of Small Animal Practice* 48: 695–698.

Nagasawa, K.K. and Johnson, S.M. (2010). Thoracoscopic treatment of pediatric lung abscesses. *Journal of Pediatric Surgery* 45: 574–578.

Nakanishi, R., Fujino, Y., Oka, S., and Odate, S. (2010). Video-assisted thoracic surgery involving major pulmonary resection for central tumors. *Surgical Endoscopy* 24: 16 –169.

Orton, C.E. (1995). Disorders of the thoracic wall. In: *Small Animal Thoracic Surgery* (ed. C.E. Orton, T.O. McCracken and C.C. Cann), 75. Malvern, PA: Williams & Wilkins.

Orton, C.E. (2003). Thoracic wall. In: *Textbook of Small Animal Surgery*, 3e (ed. D.H. Slatter), 373–387. Philadelphia, PA: WB Saunders.

Pariaut, R. and Reynolds, C. (2015). Bradyarrhythmias and conduction disturbances. In: *Small Animal Critical Care Medicine*,

2e (ed. D.C. Silverstein and K. Hopper), 246–249. St. Louis, MO: Elsevier Saunders.

Pelsue, D.H., Monnet, E., Gaynor, J.S. et al. (2002). Closure of median sternotomy in dogs: suture versus wire. *Journal of the American Animal Hospital Association* 38: 569–576.

Popilskis, S., Kohn, D., Sanchez, J.A., and Gorman, P. (1991). Epidural vs. intramuscular oxymorphone analgesia after thoracotomy in dogs. *Veterinary Surgery* 20: 462–467.

Radlinsky, M.G., Mason, D.E., Biller, D.S., and Olsen, D. (2002). Thoracoscopic visualization and ligation of the thoracic duct in dogs. *Veterinary Surgery* 31: 138–146.

Riquelme, M., Monnet, E., Kudnig, S.T. et al. (2005a). Cardiopulmonary changes induced during one-lung ventilation in anesthetized dogs with a closed thoracic cavity. *American Journal of Veterinary Research* 66: 973–977.

Riquelme, M., Monnet, E., Kudnig, S.T. et al. (2005b). Cardiopulmonary effects of positive end-expiratory pressure during one-lung ventilation in anesthetized dogs with a closed thoracic cavity. *American Journal of Veterinary Research* 66: 978–983.

Rooney, M.B., Mehl, M., and Monnet, E. (2004). Intercostal thoracotomy closure: transcostal sutures as a less painful alternative to circumcostal suture placement. *Veterinary Surgery* 33: 209–213.

Rosenstein, P.G., Tennent-Brown, B.S., and Hughes, D. (2018). Clinical use of plasma lactate concentration. Part 1: Physiology, pathophysiology, and measurement. *Journal of Veterinary Emergency and Critical Care* 28 (2): 85–105.

Rossanese, M. and Tomlinson, A. (2021). Crimped monofilament nylon leader for median sternotomy closure in 10 dogs. *Veterinary Surgery* 50: 402–409.

Stobie, D., Caywood, D.D., Rozanski, E.A. et al. (1995). Evaluation of pulmonary function and analgesia in dogs after intercostal thoracotomy and use of morphine administered intramuscularly or intrapleurally and bupivacaine administered intrapleurally. *American Journal of Veterinary Research* 56: 1098–1109.

Tattersall, J.A. and Welsh, E. (2006). Factors influencing the short-term outcome following thoracic surgery in 98 dogs. *Journal of Small Animal Practice* 47: 715–720.

Thompson, S.E. and Johnson, J.M. (1991). Analgesia in dogs after intercostal thoracotomy. A comparison of morphine, selective intercostals nerve block, and interpleural regional analgesia with bupivacaine. *Veterinary Surgery* 20: 73–77.

Tobin, M.J. (2006). *Principles and Practices of Mechanical Ventilation*, 2e. New York: McGraw-Hill.

Walsh, P.J., Remedios, A.M., Ferguson, J.F. et al. (1999). Thoracoscopic versus open partial pericardectomy in dogs: comparison of postoperative pain and morbidity. *Veterinary Surgery* 28: 472–479.

Wright, K.N. (2015). Supraventricular tachyarrhythmias. In: *Small Animal Critical Care Medicine, 2e* (ed. D.C. Silverstein and K. Hopper), 250–255. St. Louis, MO: Elsevier Saunders.

Yamamoto, K., Ohsumi, A., Kojima, F. et al. (2010). Long-term survival after video-assisted thoracic surgery lobectomy for primary lung cancer. *Annals of Thoracic Surgery* 89: 353–359.

30

Tumors of the Thoracic Wall

Julius M. Liptak

Chest wall tumors include primary tumors of the ribs and sternum, invasion of adjacent tumors into the chest wall, and metastasis from distant tumors. Primary rib tumors are the most common tumors of the chest wall and are frequently malignant sarcomas (Ling *et al.* 1974; Feeney *et al.* 1982; Matthiesen *et al.* 1992; Montgomery *et al.* 1993; Pirkey-Ehrhart *et al.* 1995; Baines *et al.* 2002; Liptak *et al.* 2008a,b). Osteosarcoma (OSA) is the most common primary rib tumor, accounting for 28–63% of cases. Chondrosarcoma (CSA) is the second most common primary rib tumor and accounts for 28–35% of cases. Other primary bone tumors, such as fibrosarcoma and hemangiosarcoma, are uncommon (Matthiesen *et al.* 1992; Montgomery *et al.* 1993; Pirkey-Ehrhart *et al.* 1995; Baines *et al.* 2002; Liptak *et al.* 2008a,b).

Diagnosis

Signalment

The signalment is typically older large-breed dogs, with no breed or sex predilection. Age is an inconsistent finding in dogs with rib tumors, with dogs reported to be either young (median 2.0–4.5 years) or old (median 7.0–9.0 years) at presentation (Matthiesen *et al.* 1992; Montgomery *et al.* 1993; Pirkey-Ehrhart *et al.* 1995; Baines *et al.* 2002; Liptak *et al.* 2008a,b).

Presenting signs

Common presenting signs include a visible or palpable chest wall mass, thoracic limb lameness, and dyspnea. Thoracic limb lameness can be caused by mechanical interference or muscular or brachial plexus invasion

from primary rib tumors arising from the first to fourth ribs (Baines *et al.* 2002).

Causes for dyspnea include decreased lung volume and expansion because of the intrapleural extent of the chest wall tumor, or pleural effusion. Rib tumors are usually evenly distributed from ribs 2 to 8 and either the left or right chest wall can be affected. The majority of rib tumors arise from or near to the costochondral junction (Brodey *et al.* 1959; Feeney *et al.* 1982; Matthiesen *et al.* 1992; Montgomery *et al.* 1993; Pirkey-Ehrhart *et al.* 1995; Baines *et al.* 2002; Liptak *et al.* 2008a,b).

Imaging

Radiography can confirm the presence of a mass arising from the ribs (Figures 30.1 and 30.2). However, radiographic changes cannot be used to determine tumor type because there are no significant differences in the distribution of lytic, productive, and mixed patterns between OSA, CSA, and other rib tumors (Feeney *et al.* 1982; Liptak *et al.* 2008a).

Computed tomography (CT) is recommended for both local and distant staging of chest wall tumors (Incarbone & Pastorino 2001). Local staging assists in surgical planning by determining tumor size and location, the extent of rib involvement (both the number of ribs and the dorsal and ventral extent of the tumor), and whether there is adhesion or invasion into adjacent structures such as the lungs, pericardium, sternum, and vertebra (Figures 30.3–30.5) (Incarbone & Pastorino 2001; Liptak *et al.* 2008a,b). The detection of metastatic pulmonary lesions is also significantly more sensitive using

---

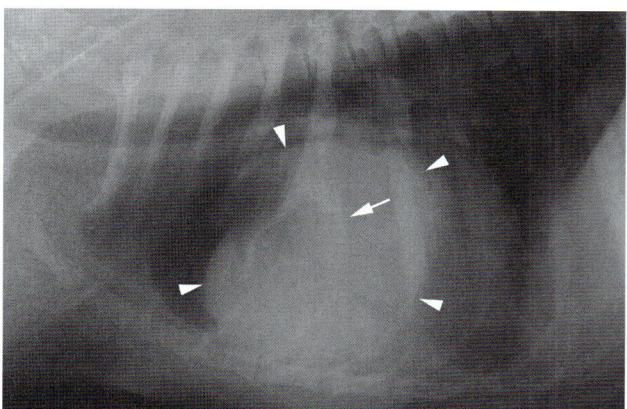

Figure 30.1 Lateral thoracic radiograph showing a large soft tissue mass (arrowheads) arising from the mid aspect of the fifth rib with bone lysis (arrow) and obscuring the cardiac silhouette. The radiographic pattern of rib tumors (lytic, blastic, or mixed) does not assist in differentiating tumor types.

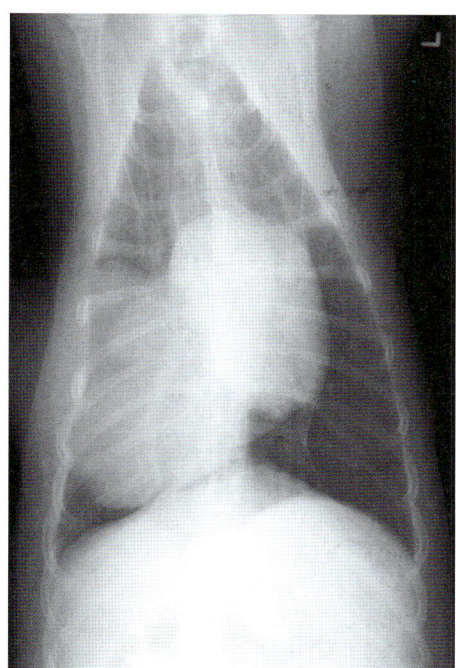

Figure 30.2 A ventrodorsal thoracic radiograph showing a large, primarily intrathoracic mass arising from the right fifth rib, resulting in separation of the adjacent fourth and sixth ribs, and displacing the cardiac silhouette to the left side.

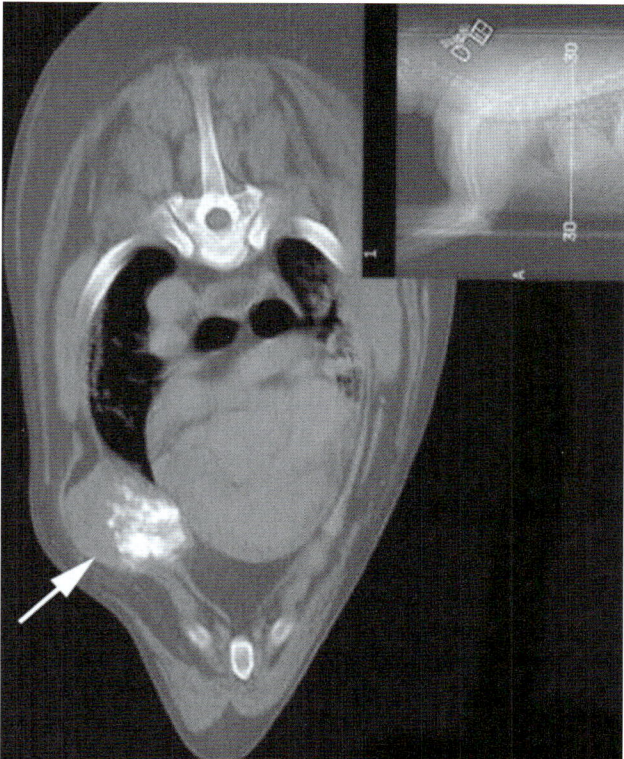

Figure 30.3 Computed tomography scan of the thorax of a dog with a mineralized mass arising from the costochondral junction of the fifth rib (arrow). The mass is causing mild displacement of the heart.

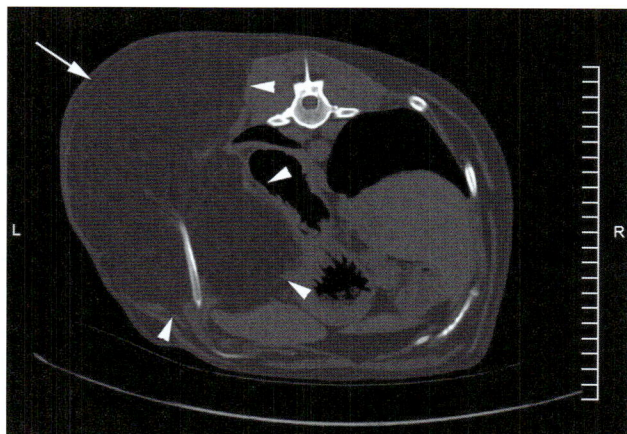

Figure 30.4 Computed tomography scans are very useful for determining the extent of disease and then planning the surgical approach and resection. In this case, an infiltrative lipoma (arrow) extends from the epaxial musculature dorsally to the pectoral muscles ventrally and through the intercostal spaces into the thoracic and abdominal cavities (arrowheads). Although this is benign, wide surgical resection with a minimum of 3 cm margins is required to minimize the risk of local recurrence of infiltrative lipomas.

helical CT compared with survey radiography. This may be more pertinent in dogs with rib tumors, because of superimposition of the lungs by the chest wall mass and because pleural effusion may make detection of metastatic lesions more difficult (Figure 30.5) (Incarbone & Pastorino 2001; Nemanic *et al.* 2006; Liptak *et al.* 2008a,b).

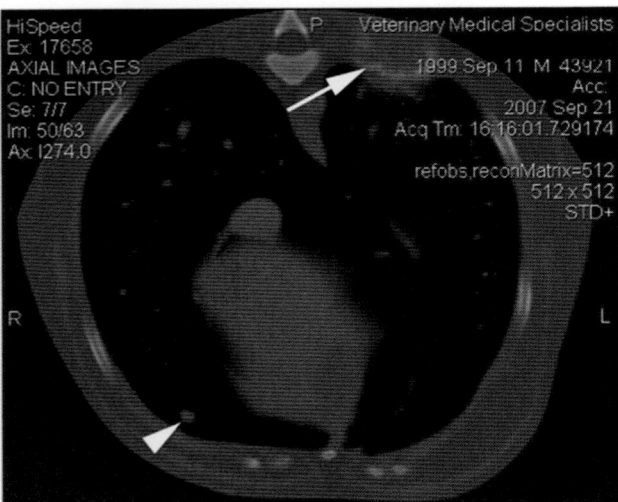

Figure 30.5 Computed tomography scans are significantly more sensitive for the diagnosis of pulmonary metastasis than three-view thoracic radiographs. Computed tomography is more important for the assessment of pulmonary metastasis in dogs with rib tumors because the rib mass can obscure visualization and assessment of the lungs. In this case, a dog with a lytic dorsal rib osteosarcoma (arrow) also has evidence of suspected pulmonary metastasis (arrowhead). Source: Courtesy of Dr. Nick Brebner.

Magnetic resonance imaging (MRI) provides excellent soft tissue detail, as well as an accurate method of determining intramedullary extension of bone tumors, but the quality of images is adversely affected by respiratory movements and hence CT is preferred for advanced imaging of the thoracic cavity.

There is a relatively high incidence of bone metastasis in dogs with primary rib OSA (16%) and, similar to appendicular OSA in dogs, whole-body bone scans are recommended for the detection of occult synchronous or metastatic disease, and possibly for determination of dorsal and ventral surgical margins for rib resection.

Biopsy

A preoperative biopsy is recommended to determine tumor type, whether adjuvant chemotherapy is required, and prognosis. The biopsy results will not change the need for chest wall resection and reconstruction for treatment of the local tumor, or the extent of this surgery, but it may change the willingness of the owner to pursue definitive treatment. Dogs with rib OSA have a worse prognosis than dogs with rib CSA, and adjuvant chemotherapy is recommended for dogs with rib OSA but not rib CSA (Pirkey-Ehrhart *et al.* 1995; Liptak *et al.* 2008a). If the owner decides to pursue definitive treatment regardless of tumor type and prognosis, then a preoperative biopsy is not required.

Treatment: chest wall resection and reconstruction

Chest wall resection is most commonly performed in dogs for the management of rib tumors and in cats for the management of injection-site sarcomas.

Chest wall resection

Surgical technique

Surgical excision of rib tumors should include one rib cranial and caudal to the tumor, 3 cm of grossly normal bone dorsal and ventral to the tumor in the affected rib(s), and 3 cm lateral margins around all contiguous soft tissues, including biopsy tracts, pleura, muscle, and fascia (Website Chapter 30: Thoracic wall/thoracic wall reconstruction: tumor: Figures W30.1 and W30.2) (Matthiesen *et al.* 1992; Montgomery *et al.* 1993; Pirkey-Ehrhart *et al.* 1995; Baines *et al.* 2002; Liptak *et al.* 2008a,b). Noninvolved muscle should be preserved for autogenous reconstruction (Website Chapter 30: Thoracic wall/thoracic wall reconstruction: tumor: Figure W30.2) (Incarbone & Pastorino 2001). The caudal intercostal thoracotomy incision should be performed first, one rib caudal to the tumor based on preoperative imaging, to assist in determining ventral and dorsal margins (Website Chapter 30: Thoracic wall/thoracic wall reconstruction: tumor: Figures W30.3 and W30.4). The intercostal vessels are ligated dorsally, either individually or with a heavy-gauge circumcostal ligature (Website Chapter 30: Thoracic wall/thoracic wall reconstruction: tumor: Figure W30.5). The internal thoracic artery should be identified and ligated. The ribs are ostectomized dorsally and ventrally with bone cutters (Website Chapter 30: Thoracic wall/thoracic wall reconstruction: tumor: Figures W30.6 and W30.7), a sagittal saw, or an oscillating saw. An oscillating saw is preferred if a partial sternectomy is required to achieve adequate ventral margins (Website Chapter 30: Thoracic wall/thoracic wall reconstruction: tumor: Figure W30.8).

In some human and veterinary reports, excision of the entire affected rib has been recommended for treatment of primary malignant sarcomas because of intramedullary spread of the tumor beyond the grossly palpable extent of the tumor (Incarbone & Pastorino 2001; Halfacree *et al.* 2007). Intramedullary extension is common in dogs with appendicular OSA. Advanced imaging modalities such as CT, magnetic resonance imaging (MRI), and whole-body bone scans are recommended prior to limb-sparing surgery to determine surgical margins because of the increased accuracy of these modalities compared with radiography (Leibman *et al.* 2001; Davis *et al.* 2002; Wallack *et al.* 2002). Intramedullary extension of a rib tumor resulting in incomplete excision has been reported in one dog (Halfacree *et al.* 2007), so excision of the entire affected rib(s) may be a more prudent approach rather than 3 cm margins based on the palpable tumor (Website Chapter 30: Thoracic wall/thoracic wall reconstruction: tumor: Figure W30.9), especially when the completeness of excision of the tumor has such an important impact on postoperative survival. If there is evidence of either adhesion or invasion of the rib tumor into adjacent structures, such as the lungs, pericardium, diaphragm, or vertebrae (Matthiesen *et al.* 1992), then these should be resected *en bloc* with the rib tumor (Website Chapter 30: Thoracic wall/thoracic wall reconstruction: tumor: Figures W30.10 and W30.11). Adhesions should be excised *en bloc* rather than broken down, because 57% of tumor-associated adhesions in people have histologic evidence of invasion (Nogueras & Jagelman 1993). In one series of chest wall resection for rib tumors in dogs, *en bloc* partial lung lobectomy was reported in 25.6% of dogs and partial pericardiectomy in 7.7% of dogs (Liptak *et al.* 2008b). Concurrent resection of any volume of lung with the rib tumor is associated with a significantly higher risk of respiratory complications and perioperative mortality in people (Weyant *et al.* 2006). However, respiratory complications are rare in dogs following chest wall resection (Mathes 1995; Novoa *et al.* 2005; Halfacree *et al.* 2007) and *en bloc* partial lung lobectomy is not associated with an increased risk of postoperative complications in dogs (Pirkey-Ehrhart *et al.* 1995; Liptak *et al.* 2008b).

Number of ribs resected

The maximum number of ribs that can be safely resected in cats and dogs is unknown. Six ribs can be safely resected in dogs without the need for rigid reconstruction of the thoracic wall. Furthermore, the number of ribs resected does not significantly increase the risk of postoperative complications (Matthiesen *et al.* 1992; Pirkey-Ehrhart *et al.* 1995; Liptak *et al.* 2008b). Eight ribs have been resected in one dog, but this dog died because of ventilatory failure (Dr. Kudnig, personal communication). However, this dog also had pulmonary metastasis and this may have contributed its postoperative complications and death. To the best of the author's knowledge, seven ribs have not been resected in dogs and hence it is unknown whether seven ribs can be resected and safely reconstructed with standard autogenous or prosthetic techniques. Furthermore, it is unknown whether chest wall reconstruction with more rigid techniques, such as spinal plates or rib grafts (Nogueras & Jagelman 1993; Pirkey-Ehrhart *et al.* 1995), may prevent ventilatory complications if seven or more ribs are resected in dogs.

Location of rib tumor

Rib tumors can occur in any rib. It has previously been reported that chest wall resection should not be attempted in dogs with tumors arising from the first rib because of the risk of postoperative complications (Baines *et al.* 2002). However, in one retrospective series of 42 dogs, the first rib was safely resected in 5 dogs and only 1 of these had complications (Liptak *et al.* 2008b). Excision of rib tumors with complete histologic margins is the most important risk factor for local tumor recurrence and survival in both dogs and people (Pirkey-Ehrhart *et al.* 1995), and hence chest wall resection should not be compromised by either the location of the affected rib(s) or the number of ribs that require resection.

Sternal tumors and resections

Sternal resection and reconstruction present a greater challenge compared with rib resection and reconstruction because of the role of the sternum in chest wall stability and the increased risk of complications following sternal reconstruction with standard autogenous and prosthetic techniques in dogs (Liptak *et al.* 2008b). Reconstruction of partial and total sternectomy defects is also associated with a higher rate of complications compared with rib defects in people (Galli *et al.* 1995; Chapelier *et al.* 2004; Weyant *et al.* 2006; Liptak *et al.* 2008b). Autogenous muscle flaps alone may be sufficient for reconstruction of sternal defects (Galli *et al.* 1995; Mathes 1995; Incarbone & Pastorino 2001; Chapelier *et al.* 2004). However, mesh–methylmethacrylate sandwiches are preferred by most surgeons for sternal reconstruction in people, particularly following total sternectomy, because this provides additional rigidity to the chest wall and protection of intrathoracic structures, and more closely mimics the anatomy and function of the normal sternum (Sabanathan *et al.* 1997; Incarbone & Pastorino 2001; Mansour *et al.* 2002; Losken *et al.* 2004; Haraguchi *et al.* 2006; Skoracki & Chang 2006). Composite reconstructions, using mesh sandwiches containing either methylmethacrylate or corticocancellous bone, have been successfully used to reconstruct clinical and experimental sternal defects in a cat and a series of dogs (Johnson & Goldsmid 1993; Di Meo *et al.* 1996). Sternal defects should be reconstructed with autogenous muscle flaps, composite techniques such as prosthetic mesh with either autogenous muscle flaps or omental pedicle flaps, or more rigid prosthetic techniques such as mesh– methylmethacrylate sandwiches (Johnson & Goldsmid 1993; Di Meo *et al.* 1996; Liptak *et al.* 2008a,b).

Chest wall reconstruction

Surgical technique

Primary repair of chest wall defects is rarely possible because of the large size of the resultant defect (Website Chapter 30: Thoracic wall/thoracic wall reconstruction: tumor: Figures W30.12–W30.14). As a result, a number of autogenous and prosthetic techniques have been reported for reconstructing chest wall defects. The aim of chest wall reconstruction is to fill the defect and reduce dead space, establish an airtight seal of the pleural cavity, and provide sufficient rigidity to prevent respiratory compromise and protect intrathoracic structures (Sabanathan et al. 1997; Incarbone & Pastorino 2001; Mansour et al. 2002; Losken et al. 2004; Skoracki & Chang 2006; Halfacree et al. 2007).

In people, the reconstruction technique is primarily determined by the location and size of the chest wall defect. Autogenous techniques alone are sufficient for anterolateral chest wall defects less than 5 cm diameter or fewer than three resected ribs, and for posterior chest wall defects less than 10 cm diameter (Mathes 1995; Sabanathan et al. 1997; Incarbone & Pastorino 2001; Mansour et al. 2002; Losken et al. 2004; Novoa et al. 2005; Weyant et al. 2006). However, greater rigidity is recommended for reconstruction of sternal and larger chest wall defects (Sabanathan et al. 1997; Incarbone & Pastorino 2001; Mansour et al. 2002; Losken et al. 2004; Novoa et al. 2005; Weyant et al. 2006). Meshes and mesh–methylmethacrylate sandwiches are preferred for these reconstructions as the additional rigidity reduces paradoxical chest wall motion and resultant ventilatory compromise, and provides superior protection of intrathoracic organs and vessels (Sabanathan et al. 1997; Incarbone & Pastorino 2001; Mansour et al. 2002; Losken et al. 2004; Novoa et al. 2005). However, the necessity for rigid chest wall reconstruction in dogs is questionable, as paradoxical chest wall motion does not affect ventilatory function in experimental models of traumatic flail chest and in clinical reports of chest wall reconstruction in dogs (Craven et al. 1979; Cappello et al. 1995; Gyhra et al. 1996; Halfacree et al. 2007).

In dogs, the selection of chest wall reconstructive technique depends on the size and location of the defect. Surgical techniques to reconstruct chest wall defects in dogs include autogenous latissimus dorsi muscle and myocutaneous flaps, deep pectoral muscle flaps, external abdominal oblique muscle flaps, omental pedicle flaps, diaphragmatic advancement, prosthetic mesh, mesh–methylmethacrylate sandwich, and rib replacement with rib grafts or spinal plates (Brasmer 1971; Bright 1981; Bright et al. 1982; Aronsohn 1984; Runnels & Trampel 1986; Matthiesen et al. 1992; Johnson &

Goldsmid 1993; Kroll et al. 1993; Pirkey-Ehrhart et al. 1995; Di Meo et al. 1996; Bowman et al. 1998; Baines et al. 2002; Gradner et al. 2008; Liptak et al. 2008b). The latissimus dorsi muscle or myocutaneous flap is the most commonly utilized autogenous technique for reconstruction of chest wall defects (Matthiesen et al. 1992; Pirkey-Ehrhart et al. 1995; Baines et al. 2002; Liptak et al. 2008b). However, this may not be a viable option for some defects because the pedicled flap may be too small to completely fill large chest wall defects; the arc of rotation of the latissimus dorsi muscle flap may not reach ventral and caudal chest wall defects; and either the dominant vascular pedicle, the thoracodorsal artery and vein, or the muscle itself may be involved in the neoplastic process or wide excision of the rib tumor (Bowman et al. 1998). In such cases, prosthetic mesh is commonly employed to reconstruct chest wall defects (Pirkey-Ehrhart et al. 1995; Bowman et al. 1998; Baines et al. 2002; Liptak et al. 2008b).

Primary rib suturing

Suturing of the ribs without supplemental reconstruction is only possible following resection of a small number of ribs (Montgomery et al. 1993; Pirkey-Ehrhart et al. 1995). Primary suturing is acceptable if wide excision of the tumor is possible with minimal rib resection, but wide excision of the tumor should not be compromised because of concerns regarding closure of the defect, especially with the numerous options available for reconstruction of large chest wall defects. This is highlighted by an early report of chest wall resection for treatment of primary rib sarcomas in dogs, in which the survival rate was decreased when chest wall defects were closed with primary rib suture (0% 44-week survival rate) compared with reconstructive techniques (40% 44-week survival rate) (Montgomery et al. 1993).

Diaphragmatic advancement

Chest wall defects involving the ninth to thirteenth ribs do not necessarily require reconstruction, as normal thoracic physiology and function can be restored by advancement of the diaphragm cranially (Aronsohn 1984; Matthiesen et al. 1992; Pirkey-Ehrhart et al. 1995; Baines et al. 2002; Liptak et al. 2008b). Following resection of the caudal chest wall tumor, the free edge of the diaphragm is sutured to the ribs and chest wall defect with absorbable suture material in either a continuous or interrupted suture pattern (Website Chapter 30: Thoracic wall/thoracic wall reconstruction: tumor: Figures W30.15–W30.17). Rarely, caudal lung lobectomy may be required to allow sufficient intrathoracic volume for lung expansion following advancement of the diaphragm (Website Chapter 30: Thoracic wall/thoracic

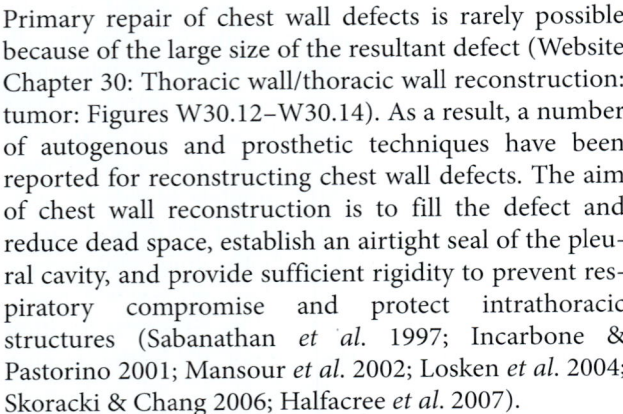

wall reconstruction: tumor: Figures W30.18–W30.21). The resultant abdominal wall defect can be repaired primarily, or reconstructed with autogenous muscle flaps (e.g., latissimus dorsi and/or external abdominal oblique muscle flaps) or prosthetic mesh (Website Chapter 30: Thoracic wall/thoracic wall reconstruction: tumor: Figures W30.22 and W30.23).

Muscle flaps

Pedicled muscle flaps are ideal for reconstruction of chest wall defects because of their large size and good survival rates.

Latissimus dorsi muscle flap and myocutaneous flap

The latissimus dorsi muscle is the most common autogenous flap used for reconstruction of chest wall defects in both dogs and people (Matthiesen *et al.* 1992; Pirkey-Ehrhart *et al.* 1995; Sabanathan *et al.* 1997; Baines *et al.* 2002; Skoracki & Chang 2006; Liptak *et al.* 2008b). The latissimus dorsi flap can be harvested either as a muscle alone or as a myocutaneous flap (Halfacree *et al.* 2007). The latissimus dorsi is a flat triangular muscle covering the dorsal half of the lateral chest wall. This muscle flap is commonly used for reconstruction of chest wall defects because of its location relative to the chest wall, large size, good arc of rotation to permit coverage of the majority of chest wall defects, and excellent flap survival based on the thoracodorsal artery and extensive anastomoses between its intercostal and thoracodorsal pedicles (Purinton *et al.* 1992). The latissimus dorsi muscle flap is a type V muscle flap based on the thoracodorsal artery arising at the level of the caudal depression of the shoulder (Gregory *et al.* 1988; Purinton *et al.* 1992). The thoracodorsal artery is the dominant pedicle of the latissimus dorsi muscle, but the lateral thoracic, intercostal, and subscapular arteries also provide minor contributions to the vascular supply of the latissimus dorsi muscle (Purinton *et al.* 1992). Furthermore, perfusion of the middle segment of the latissimus dorsi muscle is significantly better when the perforating artery from the fifth intercostal space and thoracodorsal artery were preserved compared with the thoracodorsal artery alone (Monnet *et al.* 2003). The muscle covers the dorsal half of the lateral thoracic wall, originates from the aponeurosis of the triceps muscle, and inserts on the tendinous superficial leaf of the lumbodorsal fascia associated with spinous processes of thoracic and lumbar vertebrae. The dorsal border of the flap extends from ventral to the acromion and caudal border of the triceps muscle to the head of the thirteenth rib (Gregory *et al.* 1988; Purinton *et al.* 1992). The ventral border is either the ventral border of the muscle, if intact, or the

incised edge if part of the latissimus dorsi is excised *en bloc* with the rib tumor (Website Chapter 30: Thoracic wall/thoracic wall reconstruction: tumor: Figure W30.24). Perforating intercostal vessels are ligated and divided, allowing elevation of the flap and rotation into the chest wall defect (Website Chapter 30: Thoracic wall/thoracic wall reconstruction: tumor: Figure W30.25). The muscle flap is sutured to the cranial and caudal ribs of the chest wall defect and the ventral pectoral musculature with an interrupted or continuous suture pattern using monofilament absorbable suture material (Website Chapter 30: Thoracic wall/thoracic wall reconstruction: tumor: Figure W30.26). Chest wall defects of up to six ribs have been reconstructed with latissimus dorsi muscle flaps in dogs. For larger defects, the latissimus dorsi muscle flap can be used to reconstruct part of the defect and a prosthetic mesh for the remainder of the defect (Website Chapter 30: Thoracic wall/thoracic wall reconstruction: tumor: Figures W30.27 and W30.28).

Deep pectoral muscle flap

The deep pectoral muscle is a suitable muscle flap for reconstruction of ventral chest wall and sternal defects in dogs because of its accessibility and favorable vascular pattern (Purinton *et al.* 1992; Liptak *et al.* 2008b). The deep pectoral muscle is a type V muscle flap that can be rotated cranially and dorsally based on its lateral thoracic pedicle, or ventrally across the midline based on segmental branches of the internal thoracic artery (Purinton *et al.* 1992). The latter is more commonly used for reconstruction of chest wall defects. In such cases, the deep pectoral muscle flap is elevated by incising its sternal attachment, undermining the muscle belly while preserving the cranial portion of the sternal attachment and as many branches of the internal thoracic artery as possible, and rotating the muscle flap across the ventral midline into the contralateral chest wall or sternal defect (Purinton *et al.* 1992; Liptak *et al.* 2008b).

External abdominal oblique muscle flap

The external abdominal oblique muscle has been suggested as an autogenous muscle flap for the reconstruction of caudal thoracic wall defects. The external abdominal oblique muscle has costal and lumbar components. The costal part originates segmentally from the fourth or fifth ribs to the thirteenth rib, and the lumbar part originates from lumbosacral fascia along the iliocostalis muscle. The aponeurosis of the external abdominal oblique muscle contributes to the external rectus sheath, external inguinal ring, and prepubic tendon. The external abdominal oblique muscle is supplied by the cranial branch of the cranial abdominal artery and the deep branch of the deep circumflex artery. The cranial branch of the cranial abdominal artery supplies the middle zone of the lateral wall. The deep branch of the deep circumflex artery anastomoses with the cranial and caudal abdominal arteries and supplies the caudodorsal quarter of the abdominal wall. The fascial edges of the lumbar portion of the external abdominal oblique muscle are divided ventrally and caudally, leaving a 0.5 cm margin of fascia along the muscular edge. The lumbar portion of the external abdominal oblique muscle is then undermined and the neurovascular pedicle (cranial abdominal artery, cranial hypogastric nerve, and satellite vein) is identified craniodorsal to the thirteenth rib and preserved. The dorsal fascial attachment is divided and the lumbar part of the external abdominal oblique muscle is severed at level of the thirteenth rib. The lumbar external abdominal oblique musculofascial island flap, tethered by its neurovascular pedicle, can be rotated into caudal thoracic wall defects.

Prosthetic mesh

Prosthetic meshes are commonly used to reconstruct chest wall defects, either alone or in combination with muscle flaps and/or omental pedicle flaps (Pirkey-Ehrhart *et al.* 1995; Bowman *et al.* 1998; Baines *et al.* 2002; Liptak *et al.* 2008b). Composite autogenous–prosthetic reconstruction techniques are used if the chest wall defect is too large to be reconstructed with an autogenous muscle flap alone (Website Chapter 30: Thoracic wall/thoracic wall reconstruction: tumor: Figures W30.27 and W30.28). Prosthetic meshes are used for reconstruction of larger chest wall defects in humans because they provide additional rigidity when sutured under tension, and as a result are associated with a significantly decreased rate of respiratory complications and shorter hospital stays when compared with autogenous muscle flap reconstructions (Kroll *et al.* 1993; Sabanathan *et al.* 1997; Losken *et al.* 2004; Novoa *et al.* 2005).

Nonabsorbable polypropylene mesh (Marlex®, Chevron Phillips Chemical, The Woodlands, TX, USA) is the most commonly used prosthetic mesh for reconstruction of chest wall defects in dogs (Bright 1981; Bright *et al.* 1982; Matthiesen *et al.* 1992; Pirkey-Ehrhart *et al.* 1995; Baines *et al.* 2002; Liptak *et al.* 2008b), but prolene, polytetrafluoroethylene (PTFE), and vicryl mesh are also used to reconstruct chest wall defects in people (Sabanathan *et al.* 1997; Incarbone & Pastorino 2001; Skoracki & Chang 2006). The ideal characteristics of prosthetic material for chest wall reconstruction include rigidity, malleability, inertness, radiolucency, and resistance to infection (Trostle & Rosin 1994; Mansour *et al.* 2002; Losken *et al.* 2004).

Marlex mesh is constructed of knitted nonabsorbable monofilament polypropylene (Trostle & Rosin 1994). It has a high tensile strength and low permeability to liquids and gases (Trostle & Rosin 1994; Bowman *et al.* 1998). By six months, Marlex mesh is incorporated with no loss of tensile strength or fragmentation of mesh material (Usher & Gannon 1959; Watkins & Gerard 1960; Parrish *et al.* 1978).

Prolene mesh is often preferred to Marlex mesh in humans, despite both being constructed from polypropylene, because prolene mesh is constructed from double-knitted polypropylene and thus resists stretching in all directions, rather than in a single direction such as with Marlex mesh (Sabanathan *et al.* 1997; Incarbone & Pastorino 2001). Vicryl is an absorbable mesh and is indicated for reconstruction of contaminated wounds (Skoracki & Chang 2006).

PTFE is strong, resistant to infection, and impervious to air and fluids, and hence has ideal characteristics for chest wall reconstruction; however, it is very expensive (Trostle & Rosin 1994; Sabanathan *et al.* 1997). Marlex and prolene meshes, while not impervious to air and fluids, are just as effective as PTFE for chest wall reconstruction (Sabanathan *et al.* 1997; Incarbone & Pastorino 2001).

When being used for chest wall reconstruction, the size of the prosthetic mesh is tailored to the size of the chest wall defect so that the edges are doubled over to provide a double layer of thickness for suturing to adjacent host tissue (Bright 1981). The mesh is sutured under mild tension to either the pleural or lateral surface of the defect using either absorbable or nonabsorbable monofilament suture material (Figure 30.6) (Bright 1981). If possible, the mesh should be sutured to the ribs. Although it is rarely required, prosthetic mesh can be supported with autogenous split rib grafts, allogeneic free rib grafts, or plastic spinal plates between the ends of the resected ribs following extensive resections. If a composite reconstruction is planned, then omental pedicle grafts should cover the pleural surface of the mesh and autogenous muscle flaps should be sutured over the lateral surface of the mesh (Website Chapter 30: Thoracic wall/thoracic wall reconstruction: tumor: Figures W30.22 and W30.23).

Omental pedicle flap

The omental pedicle flap is a supplementary technique to other autogenous or prosthetic reconstructions of the thoracic wall (Website Chapter 30: Thoracic wall/thoracic wall reconstruction: tumor: Figures W30.22 and W30.23). It should not be used for primary reconstruction of chest wall defects. In people, omental pedicle

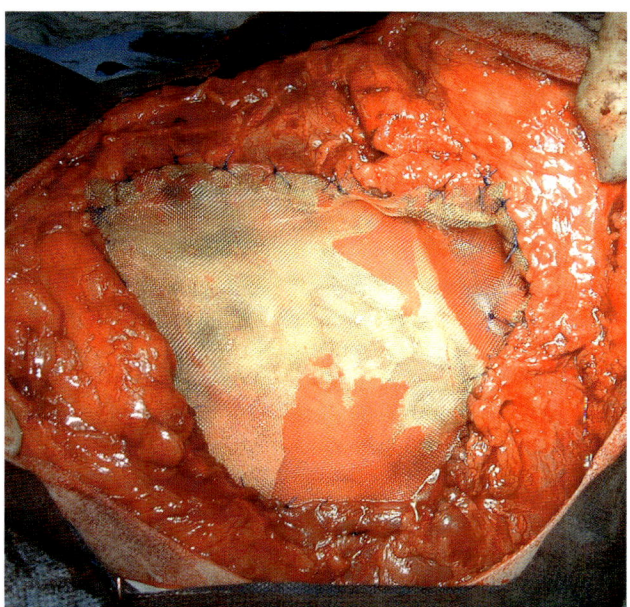

Figure 30.6 Prosthetic polypropylene (Marlex) mesh has been used to reconstruct a chest wall defect following resection of a primary rib osteosarcoma. The edges of the mesh are doubled over and sutured to the chest wall defect using either an interrupted (depicted) or continuous suture pattern under mild tension.

flaps are used to cover the pleural surface of the mesh to minimize mesh-induced pleuritis, promote local healing and enhance neovascularity, and provide an airtight seal (Sabanathan *et al.* 1997). The omental pedicle graft involves lengthening the bursal portion of the greater omentum based on either the left or right gastroepiploic arteries (Ross & Pardo 1993).

Complications

Complications following chest wall resection and reconstruction are reported in up to 50% of dogs; however, the majority of these complications are minor and require no to minimal intervention for effective management. Respiratory complications are common in people and include prolonged mechanical ventilation, pneumonia, acute respiratory distress syndrome, and pulmonary hypofunction (Kroll *et al.* 1993; Mansour *et al.* 2002; Losken *et al.* 2004; Weyant *et al.* 2006). In contrast, respiratory complications are very rare in dogs (Bright *et al.* 1982; Halfacree *et al.* 2007; Liptak *et al.* 2008b). Paradoxical motion of the reconstructed chest wall is common for 3–7 days after surgery, but paradoxical motion in the absence of underlying pulmonary trauma does not result in pulmonary hypofunction in dogs in both experimental and clinical studies (Craven *et al.* 1979; Cappello *et al.* 1995; Gyhra *et al.* 1996; Halfacree *et al.* 2007; Liptak *et al.* 2008b).

Wound problems are the most common complications following chest wall resection in dogs (Brasmer 1971; Bright 1981; Bowman *et al.* 1998; Baines *et al.* 2002; Halfacree *et al.* 2007; Liptak *et al.* 2008b). Incisional seromas are reported in up to 40% of dogs following chest wall reconstruction. Seromas are common because of the aggressive resection and degree of dead space following reconstruction. Seroma formation may also indicate partial failure of the latissimus dorsi muscle flap, and therefore distal flap necrosis should be investigated if the seroma does not resolve spontaneously within two weeks (Liptak *et al.* 2008b). The incidence of incisional seromas may be decreased with the use of either active or passive drains and bandaging the chest postoperatively (Bright 1981; Bright *et al.* 1982; Bowman *et al.* 1998). Early wound infection, incisional wound dehiscence, and muscle flap necrosis and failure are rare (Figure 30.7).

Infection rates of 0% and 2.3% have been reported in two retrospective studies with long-term follow-up of chest wall reconstruction with prosthetic mesh (Bowman *et al.* 1998; Liptak *et al.* 2008b). The majority of these

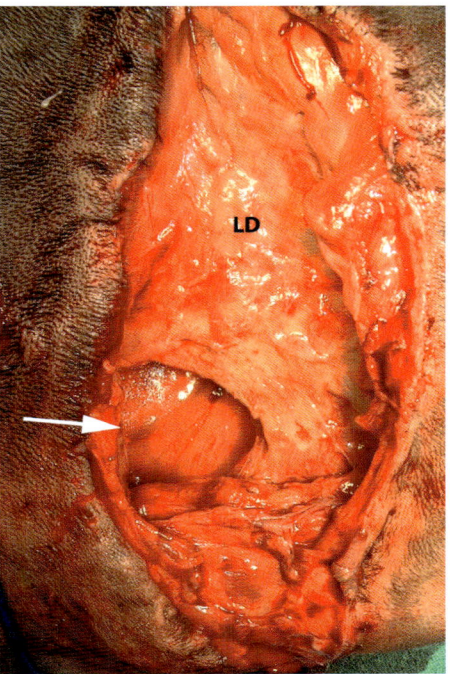

Figure 30.7 Distal necrosis of a latissimus dorsi (LD) muscle flap resulting in a chest wall defect (arrow). This complication has also been noted following use of the latissimus dorsi muscle flap for treatment of dogs with dilated cardiomyopathy, and for this reason some surgeons prefer a latissimus dorsi myocutaneous flap, because preservation of the choke anastomoses between the overlying skin and latissimus dorsi muscle may maximize blood supply to the distal aspect of the flap.

infections are deep-seated and usually occur late in the postoperative period, with infection reported in one dog 767 days postoperatively (Liptak *et al.* 2008b). In people, infected meshes are managed with surgical removal and culture-directed antimicrobial therapy (Skoracki & Chang 2006). Fibrous ingrowth into Marlex mesh results in a stable fibrous wall within six weeks (Usher & Gannon 1959) and removal of the mesh does not compromise the integrity or strength of the reconstructed chest wall (Skoracki & Chang 2006).

Postoperative pleural effusion and peripheral edema are uncommon complications. These complications were reported in 5 of 54 dogs in one retrospective series (9.3%), but resolved without specific treatment in all 5 dogs (Pirkey-Ehrhart *et al.* 1995). In contrast, 3 of 42 dogs (7.1%) developed pleural effusion in another study and these did not resolve spontaneously (Liptak *et al.* 2008b). One dog died due to hemothorax secondary to disruption of the internal thoracic artery, and two dogs developed a serosanguineous pleural effusion secondary to pleuritis because of a large surface area of contact between the lungs and Marlex mesh following large sternal reconstructions (Website Chapter 30: Thoracic wall/thoracic wall reconstruction: tumor: Figures W30.29–W30.32) (Liptak *et al.* 2008b).

Prognosis

Primary rib osteosarcoma

Primary rib OSA is the most common rib tumor in dogs. The median survival time (MST) for dogs with primary rib OSA treated with chest wall resection alone is 35–120 days, with six-month survival rates of 25% or less and 240–290 days when treated with surgery and adjuvant chemotherapy (Feeney *et al.* 1982; Matthiesen *et al.* 1992; Montgomery *et al.* 1993; Pirkey-Ehrhart *et al.* 1995; Baines *et al.* 2002; Liptak *et al.* 2008a). Postoperative chemotherapy significantly improves the median disease-free interval and MST for dogs with primary rib OSA from 60 to 225 days and from 90 to 240 days, respectively (Pirkey-Ehrhart *et al.* 1995). Histologic subtype and histologic grade do not appear to be prognostic for dogs with primary rib OSA (Liptak *et al.* 2008a); however, similar to dogs with appendicular OSA (Ehrhart *et al.* 1998; Garzotto *et al.* 2000), total serum alkaline phosphatase (ALP) is a prognostic factor in dogs with primary rib OSA (Liptak *et al.* 2008a). The MST for dogs with total ALP within and greater than the reference range is 675 and 210 days, respectively, with tumor-related deaths 7.9 times more likely in dogs with increased total ALP (Liptak *et al.* 2008a). Metastasis is reported in 75% of dogs with rib OSA and 17% of dogs with CSA (Liptak *et al.* 2008a).

Primary rib chondrosarcoma

The MSTs reported for dogs with primary rib CSA range from 1080 to 1750 days. In two studies the MST was not reached (>3820 days, with mean survival times of 1301 and 3097 days) because less than 50% of dogs died from their tumor (Pirkey-Ehrhart *et al.* 1995; Baines *et al.* 2002; Waltman *et al.* 2007; Liptak *et al.* 2008a). The prognosis for dogs with primary rib CSA is significantly better than for other primary rib tumors (Pirkey-Ehrhart *et al.* 1995; Liptak *et al.* 2008a). Histologic grade has prognostic importance in dogs and people with appendicular CSA, but histologic grade does not appear to be prognostic for primary rib CSA in either dogs or people (Waltman *et al.* 2007; Liptak *et al.* 2008a). Chemotherapy is unlikely to provide a survival benefit in dogs with rib CSA because the metastatic rate is low to moderate (8–50%), and when metastasis does occur it usually does so late in the course of disease (Matthiesen *et al.* 1992; Pirkey-Ehrhart *et al.* 1995; Waltman *et al.* 2007; Liptak *et al.* 2008a). Chemotherapy has no benefit in preventing metastasis or prolonging survival in people with CSA (Malawer *et al.* 2005).

Prognostic factors

Prognostic factors in dogs with primary rib tumors include tumor type, completeness of excision, local tumor recurrence, and metastasis. Dogs with primary rib CSA have a significantly better MST than dogs with rib OSA or other types of rib tumors (Figure 30.8) (Pirkey-Ehrhart *et al.* 1995; Liptak *et al.* 2008a). Local tumor recurrence is up to 6.7 times more likely when there is histologic evidence of tumor cells at the surgical margins (Pirkey-Ehrhart *et al.* 1995; Liptak *et al.* 2008a). Decreased body weight significantly increases the risk of local tumor recurrence, most likely because it is more difficult to achieve appropriate surgical margins in smaller dogs (Liptak *et al.* 2008a). Local tumor recurrence is reported in 10–25% of dogs with primary rib tumors treated with chest wall resection (Montgomery *et al.* 1993; Pirkey-Ehrhart *et al.* 1995; Bowman *et al.* 1998; Baines *et al.* 2002; Liptak *et al.* 2008a). In one study, local tumor recurrence was reported in 25% of dogs with incompletely excised tumors (but this may be underrepresentative because 50% of dogs with incompletely excised tumors lived less than 120 days and hence may not have had time to develop local tumor recurrence) and 13.3% of dogs with completely excised tumors (Liptak *et al.* 2008a).

Complete surgical margins is the most important prognostic factor for determining local tumor recurrence and overall survival following chest wall resection of rib tumors in both dogs and humans (Figure 30.9)

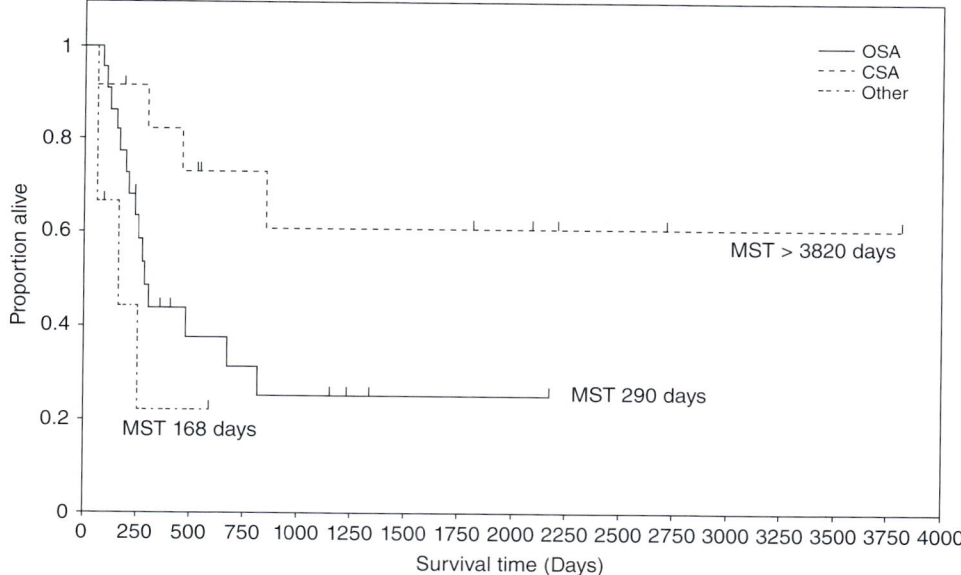

Figure 30.8 Kaplan–Meier survival curve for dogs with rib tumors. Dogs with chondrosarcomas (CSA) had a significantly better estimated median survival time (MST; >3820 days) than dogs with either osteosarcoma (OSA, 290 days) or other tumor types (256 days for hemangiosarcoma and 168 days overall). Source: Reproduced with permission from Liptak *et al.* (2008a).

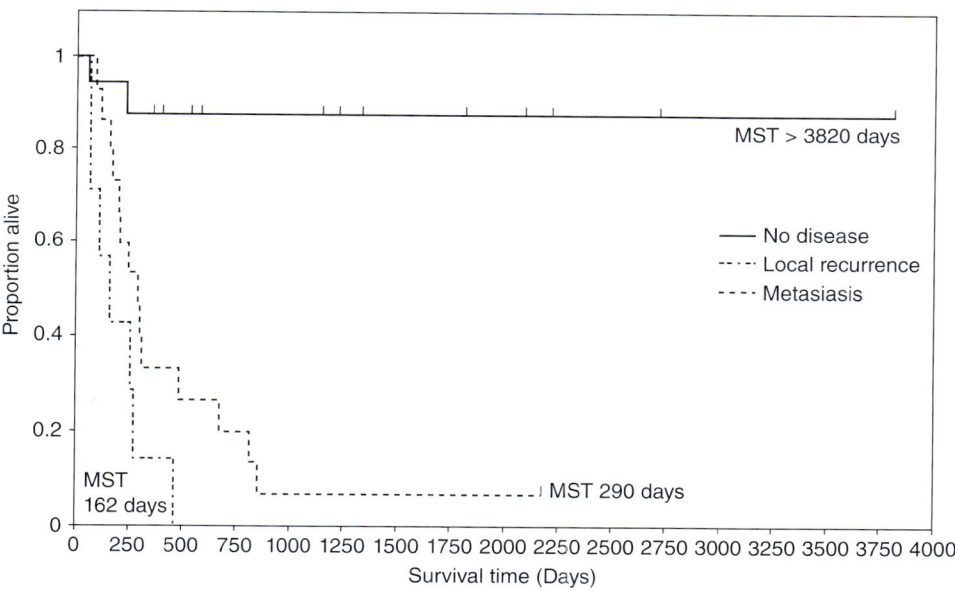

Figure 30.9 Kaplan–Meier survival curve for dogs with local tumor recurrence, distant metastasis, and no local tumor recurrence or distant metastasis. The estimated median survival times (MST) are significantly worse for dogs with local tumor recurrence (162 days) and metastasis (290 days) than for dogs with no disease-related events (>3820 days). Tumor-related deaths were 28.0 and 55.6 times greater in dogs with local tumor recurrence and metastasis, respectively. Source: Reproduced with permission from Liptak *et al.* (2008a).

(Pirkey-Ehrhart *et al.* 1995; Incarbone & Pastorino 2001; Baines *et al.* 2002; Liptak *et al.* 2008a). As a result, aggressive chest wall resection is essential in achieving the optimum postoperative survival for dogs with rib tumors. Furthermore, intraoperative and postoperative morbidity associated with chest wall resection and reconstruction is relatively low (Matthiesen *et al.* 1992; Pirkey-Ehrhart *et al.* 1995; Liptak *et al.* 2008b). The estimated overall MST for dogs with no evidence of disease, local tumor recurrence, and distant metastasis is over 3820, 162, and 290 days, respectively (Figure 30.9) (Liptak *et al.* 2008a). Furthermore, tumor-related deaths are 28.0 times more likely with local tumor recurrence and 55.6 times more likely with metastasis (Pirkey-Ehrhart *et al.* 1995; Liptak *et al.* 2008a). This highlights the necessity of appropriate preoperative staging and aggressive surgical resection to excise rib tumors with complete histologic margins, and the use of postoperative chemotherapy for rib tumors that are associated with a high risk of metastasis, such as OSA.

References

Aronsohn, M. (1984). Diaphragmatic advancement for defects of the caudal thoracic wall in the dog. *Veterinary Surgery* 13: 26–28.

Baines, S.J., Lewis, S., and White, R.A. (2002). Primary thoracic wall tumours of mesenchymal origin in dogs: a retrospective study of 46 cases. *Veterinary Record* 150: 335–339.

Bowman, K.L., Birchard, S.J., and Bright, R.M. (1998). Complications associated with the implantation of polypropylene mesh in dogs and cats: a retrospective study of 21 cases (1984–1996). *Journal of the American Animal Hospital Association* 34: 225–233.

Brasmer, T.H. (1971). Thoracic wall reconstruction in dogs. *Journal of the American Veterinary Medical Association* 159: 1758–1762.

Bright, R.M. (1981). Reconstruction of thoracic wall defects using Marlex mesh. *Journal of the American Animal Hospital Association* 17: 415–420.

Bright, R.M., Birchard, S.J., and Long, G.G. (1982). Repair of thoracic wall defects in the dog with an omental pedicle flap. *Journal of the American Animal Hospital Association* 18: 277–282.

Brodey, R.S., McGrath, J.T., and Reynolds, H. (1959). A clinical and radiological study of canine bone neoplasms. *Journal of the American Veterinary Medical Association* 134: 53–71.

Cappello, M., Yuehua, C., and De Troyer, A. (1995). Rib cage distortion in a canine model of flail chest. *American Journal of Respiratory and Critical Care Medicine* 151: 1481–1485.

Chapelier, A.R., Missana, M.C., Couturaud, B. et al. (2004). Sternal resection and reconstruction for primary malignant tumors. *Annals of Thoracic Surgery* 77: 1001–1007.

Craven, K.D., Oppenheimer, L., and Wood, L.D. (1979). Effects of contusion and flail chest on pulmonary perfusion and oxygen exchange. *Journal of Applied Physiology* 47: 729–737.

Davis, G.J., Kapatkin, A.S., Craig, L.E. et al. (2002). Comparison of radiography, computed tomography, and magnetic resonance imaging for evaluation of appendicular osteosarcoma in dogs. *Journal of the American Veterinary Medical Association* 220: 1171–1176.

Di Meo, A., Pepe, M., Bellezza, E. et al. (1996). Experimental use of Kiel bone after subtotal sternectomy in the dog. *Veterinary and Comparative Orthopaedics and Traumatology* 9: 172–176.

Ehrhart, N., Dernell, W.S., Hoffmann, W.E. et al. (1998). Prognostic importance of alkaline phosphatase activity in serum from dogs with appendicular osteosarcoma: 75 cases (1990–1996). *Journal of the American Veterinary Medical Association* 213: 1002–1006.

Feeney, D.A., Johnston, G.R., Grindem, C.B. et al. (1982). Malignant neoplasia of canine ribs: clinical, radiographic, and pathologic findings. *Journal of the American Veterinary Medical Association* 180: 927–933.

Galli, A., Raposio, E., and Santi, P. (1995). Reconstruction of full-thickness defects of the thoracic wall by myocutaneous flap transfer: latissimus dorsi compared with transverse rectus abdominis. *Scandinavian Journal of Plastic and Reconstructive Surgery and Hand Surgery* 29: 39–43.

Garzotto, C.K., Berg, J., Hoffmann, W.E., and Rand, W.M. (2000). Prognostic significance of serum alkaline phosphatase activity in canine appendicular osteosarcoma. *Journal of Veterinary Internal Medicine* 14: 587–592.

Gradner, G., Weissenböck, H., Kneissl, S. et al. (2008). Use of latissimus dorsi and abdominal external oblique muscle for reconstruction of a thoracic wall defect in a cat with feline osteochondromatosis. *Journal of Feline Medicine and Surgery* 10: 88–94.

Gregory, C.R., Gourley, I.M., Koblik, P.D., and Patz, J.D. (1988). Experimental definition of latissimus dorsi, gracilis, and rectus abdominus musculocutaneous flaps in the dog. *American Journal of Veterinary Research* 49: 878–884.

Gyhra, A., Torres, P., Pino, J. et al. (1996). Experimental flail chest: ventilatory function with fixation of flail segment in internal and external position. *Journal of Trauma* 40: 977–979.

Halfacree, Z.J., Baines, S.J., Lipscomb, V.J. et al. (2007). Use of a latissimus dorsi myocutaneous flap for one-stage reconstruction of the thoracic wall after en bloc resection of primary rib chondrosarcoma in five dogs. *Veterinary Surgery* 36: 587–592.

Haraguchi, S., Hioki, M., Hisayoshi, T. et al. (2006). Resection of sternal tumors and reconstruction of the thorax: a review of 15 patients. *Surgery Today* 36: 225–229.

Incarbone, M. and Pastorino, U. (2001). Surgical treatment of chest wall tumors. *World Journal of Surgery* 25: 218–230.

Johnson, K.A. and Goldsmid, S.E. (1993). Methyl methacrylate and polypropylene mesh reconstruction of ventral thoracic wall deficit following sternal liposarcoma resection. *Veterinary and Comparative Orthopaedics and Traumatology* 6: 62–65.

Kroll, S.S., Walsh, G., Ryan, B., and King, R.C. (1993). Risks and benefits of using Marlex mesh in chest wall reconstruction. *Annals of Plastic Surgery* 31: 303–306.

Leibman, N.F., Kuntz, C.A., Steyn, P.F. et al. (2001). Accuracy of radiography, nuclear scintigraphy, and histopathology for determining the proximal extent of distal radial osteosarcoma in dogs. *Veterinary Surgery* 30: 240–245.

Ling, G.V., Morgan, J.P., and Pool, R.R. (1974). Primary bone tumors in the dog: a combined clinical, radiographic, and histologic approach to early diagnosis. *Journal of the American Veterinary Medical Association* 165: 55–67.

Liptak, J.M., Kamstock, D.A., Dernell, W.S. et al. (2008a). Oncologic outcome after curative-intent treatment in 39 dogs with primary chest wall tumors (1992–2005). *Veterinary Surgery* 37: 488–496.

Liptak, J.M., Dernell, W.S., Rizzo, S.A. et al. (2008b). Reconstruction of chest wall defects following rib tumor resection: a comparison of autogenous, prosthetic, and composite techniques in 44 dogs. *Veterinary Surgery* 37: 479–487.

Losken, A., Thourani, V.H., Carlson, G.W. et al. (2004). A reconstructive algorithm for plastic surgery following extensive chest wall resection. *British Journal of Plastic Surgery* 57: 295–302.

Malawer, M.M., Helman, L.J., and O'Sullivan, B. (2005). Sarcomas of bone. In: *Cancer: Principles and Practice of Oncology*, 7e (ed. V.T. DeVita, S. Hellman and S.A. Rosenberg), 1638–1686. Philadelphia, PA: Lippincott Williams & Wilkins.

Mansour, K.A., Thourani, V.H., Losken, A. et al. (2002). Chest wall resections and reconstruction: a 25-year experience. *Annals of Thoracic Surgery* 73: 1720–1726.

Mathes, S.J. (1995). Chest wall reconstruction. *Clinics in Plastic Surgery* 22: 187–198.

Matthiesen, D.T., Clark, G.N., Orsher, R.J. et al. (1992). En bloc resection of primary rib tumors in 40 dogs. *Veterinary Surgery* 21: 201–204.

Monnet, E., Rooney, M.B., and Chachques, J.C. (2003). in vitro evaluation of the distribution of blood flow within a canine bipedicled latissimus dorsi muscle flap. *American Journal of Veterinary Research* 64: 1255–1259.

Montgomery, R.D., Henderson, R.A., Powers, R.D. et al. (1993). Retrospective study of 26 primary tumors of the osseous thoracic wall in dogs. *Journal of the American Animal Hospital Association* 29: 68–72.

Nemanic, S., London, C.A., and Wisner, E.R. (2006). Comparison of thoracic radiographs and single breath-hold helical CT for detection of pulmonary nodules in dogs with metastatic neoplasia. *Journal of Veterinary Internal Medicine* 20: 508–515.

Nogueras, J.J. and Jagelman, D.G. (1993). Principles of surgical resection. Influence of surgical technique on treatment outcome. *Surgical Clinics of North America* 73: 103–116.

Novoa, N., Benito, P., Jiménez, M.F. et al. (2005). Reconstruction of chest wall defects after resection of large neoplasms: ten-year experience. *Interactive Cardiovascular and Thoracic Surgery* 4: 250–255.

Parrish, F.F., Murray, J.A., and Urquhart, B.A. (1978). The use of polyethylene mesh (Marlex) as an adjunct in reconstructive surgery of the extremities. *Clinical Orthopaedics and Related Research* 137: 276–286.

Pirkey-Ehrhart, N., Withrow, S.J., Straw, R.C. et al. (1995). Primary rib tumors in 54 dogs. *Journal of the American Animal Hospital Association* 31: 65–69.

Purinton, P.T., Chambers, J.N., and Moore, J.L. (1992). Identification and categorization of the vascular patterns to muscles of the thoracic limb, thorax, and neck of dogs. *American Journal of Veterinary Research* 53: 1435–1445.

Ross, W.E. and Pardo, A.D. (1993). Evaluation of an omental pedicle extension technique in the dog. *Veterinary Surgery* 22: 37–43.

Runnels, C.M. and Trampel, D.W. (1986). Full-thickness thoracic and abdominal wall reconstruction in dogs using carbon/polycaprolactone composite. *Veterinary Surgery* 15: 363–368.

Sabanathan, S., Shah, R., Mearns, A.J., and Richardson, J. (1997). Chest wall resection and reconstruction. *British Journal of Hospital Medicine* 57: 255–259.

Skoracki, R.J. and Chang, D.W. (2006). Reconstruction of the chest wall and thorax. *Journal of Surgical Oncology* 94: 455–465.

Trostle, S.S. and Rosin, E. (1994). Selection of prosthetic mesh implants. *Compendium on Continuing Education for the Practicing Veterinarian* 16: 1147–1154.

Usher, F.C. and Gannon, J.P. (1959). Marlex mesh, a new plastic mesh for replacing tissue defects. I. Experimental studies. *A.M.A. Archives of Surgery* 78: 131–137.

Wallack, S.T., Wisner, E.R., Werner, J.A. et al. (2002). Accuracy of magnetic resonance imaging for estimating intramedullary osteosarcoma extent in preoperative planning of canine limb-salvage procedures. *Veterinary Radiology & Ultrasound* 43: 432–441.

Waltman, S.S., Seguin, B., Cooper, B.J., and Kent, M. (2007). Clinical outcome of nonnasal chondrosarcoma in dogs: thirty-one cases (1986–2003). *Veterinary Surgery* 36: 266–271.

Watkins, N.S. Jr. and Gerard, F.P. (1960). Malignant tumors involving chest wall. *Journal of Thoracic and Cardiovascular Surgery* 39: 117–129.

Weyant, M.J., Bains, M.S., Venkatraman, E. et al. (2006). Results of chest wall resection and reconstruction with and without rigid prosthesis. *Annals of Thoracic Surgery* 81: 279–285.

31

Flail Chest

Dennis Olsen and Ronald S. Olsen

Flail chest at one time was considered uncommon in veterinary medicine and therefore much of the previous literature extrapolated data from the human field for pathophysiology and treatment recommendations (Bjorling *et al.* 1982; Dixon 1982; Anderson *et al.* 1993; Olsen *et al.* 2002; Slensky 2009). Increased understanding of the pathophysiology of flail chest and apparent improvements in diagnosis in veterinary patients have decreased the need to rely solely on extrapolated data from the human field. However, there is still considerable valuable information that can be obtained from studies in that field.

When the integrity of the thoracic wall has been compromised such that an isolated section moves in a paradoxic fashion during respiration, a flail chest condition exists. Two situations in veterinary medicine have been reported to result in a flail chest. The first is when multiple adjacent ribs are fractured in two locations, dorsally and ventrally. The other is with dorsal fractures of multiple adjacent ribs and pliable costal cartilages, such as those in young animals, that cannot resist the interpleural pressure changes that occur during respiration (Kolata 1981; Bjorling 1998). The paradoxic motion that characterizes flail chest is inward displacement of the section at inhalation and outward displacement upon exhalation. The erratic thoracic wall motion was, for many years, thought to be the primary cause of severe respiratory distress that accompanied this condition (Trinkle *et al.* 1975; Shackford *et al.* 1976; Kagen 1980; Bjorling *et al.* 1982; Dixon 1982; Anderson *et al.* 1993; Bjorling 1998; Pettiford *et al.* 2007). Therapy was therefore directed primarily to rapid stabilization of the flail segment, despite other potentially life-threatening injuries and conditions overshadowed by the dramatic appearance of the unstable chest wall (Kagen 1980; Dixon 1982; Orton 1993; McAnulty 1995). Consequently, there are many published reports of internal and external fixation methods used for rib stabilization (Kagen 1980; Bjorling *et al.* 1982; Anderson *et al.* 1993; Orton 1993; McAnulty 1995; Bjorling 1998).

Despite the historical recommendations for immediate fixation of the flailing section of the thoracic wall, studies and clinical experience in the veterinary and human field have shown that successful treatment can be achieved with no surgical stabilization. One retrospective study could find no statistically significant differences in outcomes between stabilized and nonstabilized cases (Olsen *et al.* 2002). This study, which evaluated clinical treatment methods, corroborates the changes made in treatment recommendations secondary to increased understanding of the pathophysiology of flail chest. It is now known that the paradoxic motion alone seems to have minimal effect on adequate ventilation (Trinkle *et al.* 1975; Shackford *et al.* 1976; Craven *et al.* 1979; Cappello *et al.* 1995; Bjorling 1998; Smith 2004; Slensky 2009). The main factors contributing to respiratory distress seen with flail chest are the accompanying pulmonary damage, pain, and inflammatory mediators (Trinkle *et al.* 1975; Shackford *et al.* 1976; Parham *et al.* 1978; Craven *et al.* 1979; Bjorling *et al.* 1982; Dixon 1982; Cappello *et al.* 1995; Hackner 1995; Bjorling 1998; Melton *et al.* 1999; Pettiford *et al.* 2007; Bastos *et al.* 2008; Olsen 2010; Donahue & Silverstein 2014).

Pathophysiology

Trauma sufficient to create a flail chest causes tissue damage by transference of the kinetic energy of the inducing object to the chest wall. The more kinetic energy transmitted, the greater potential for damage to the thorax. Blunt trauma produces crush and shear injury to the soft tissues and skeletal structures, depending on the speed of the trauma. Low-speed trauma produces a localized crushing injury to the tissues, whereas high-speed trauma adds shearing injury (Olsen 2010). Penetrating trauma to the thoracic wall can also be seen in flail chest for various reasons. One cause is when bite wounds initiate the trauma, and another is when a fractured rib perforates through soft tissues of the wall. Differences in tissue resilience and tissue specific gravities dictate the degree of trauma incurred by the various tissues of the thorax. Common injuries leading to flail chest are bite wounds, vehicular impact, and other types of blunt trauma (Bjorling *et al.* 1982; Anderson *et al.* 1993; Olsen *et al.* 2002).

Fractures of the thoracic cage most commonly occur from a direct force applied to the lateral body wall. Local bending and shear are the primary loading modes resulting in fracture (Spackman & Caywood 1987; Shen *et al.* 2005). The rate at which a force is applied to the cortical bone of the ribs affects the material characteristics of the bone, a property known as viscoelasticity (Palmer & James 2010; Moreno *et al.* 2017). The ultimate strength of the bone is less when a load is applied slowly than when it is applied quickly. This property affects the amount of kinetic energy absorbed by the bone when the force is applied. The slower the load is applied, the less kinetic energy is absorbed, and when fracture occurs it is likely a simple fracture with minimal associated soft tissue disruption. The faster the load is applied, the more kinetic energy is absorbed, the more complex the fracture will be, and the greater will be the soft tissue injury (Palmer & James 2010; Moreno *et al.* 2017). Fractured ribs and the accompanying soft tissue injury reduce the compliance of the thoracic wall and the work of respiration is increased (McAnulty 1995; Olsen 2010; Tzelepis & McCool 2016).

The most common pulmonary lesion following traumatic incidents that lead to flail chest is contusion (Bjorling *et al.* 1982; Crowe 1983; Spackman *et al.* 1984; Sweet & Waters 1991; Hackner 1995; Ludwig 2000; Smith 2004; Rozanski 2017). Contusions result from parenchymal disruption and rupture of alveoli and vasculature, with subsequent hemorrhage and leakage of plasma components into tissues and airways (Oppenheimer *et al.* 1979; Hackner 1995; Jackson & Drobatz 2004; Olsen 2014; Rozanski 2017). Shortly after injury, interstitial edema increases and there is an accumulation of inflammatory cells that continues over the next 24–48 hours, resulting in near complete loss of pulmonary architecture (Jackson & Drobatz 2004). In addition to the physical damage and cellular infiltrate, there is a release of inflammatory mediators that contribute to localized tissue damage through the effects of oxygen radicals (Hackner 1995; Melton *et al.* 1999). The result of the collective damage leads to progression of gas diffusion compromise and decreased pulmonary compliance, which contribute to hypoventilation and hypoxemia with the ensuing clinical signs (Tamas *et al.* 1985; Jackson & Drobatz 2004; Serrano & Boag 2014).

The pulmonary parenchyma can be directly damaged by the ends of fractured ribs (Cockshutt 1995; Bjorling 1998; Olsen 2010; Donahue & Silverstein 2014; Serrano & Boag 2014). This is self-limiting as long as there is not continued pulmonary damage from fracture segments and a fibrin seal forms over the traumatized parenchyma. An additional result of pulmonary parenchymal damage is pneumothorax. Pneumothorax can result from rupture of alveoli due to increased pressure from thoracic compression while the glottis is closed, as well as tearing of pulmonary structures secondary to tensile and shearing forces created from rapid acceleration and deceleration that occur with sudden impact (Brockman & Puerto 2004). As air escapes into the pleural space, the loss of negative pressure results in varying degrees of pulmonary atelectasis, a further decrease in compliance, and increased work of respiration. Respiratory compromise caused by contusions is exacerbated when pneumothorax exists due to the inability of the lungs to expand.

Pain is recognized as one of the main components in the pathophysiology of respiratory distress that accompanies flail chest (Shackford *et al.* 1976; Anderson *et al.* 1993; Cappello *et al.* 1995; McAnulty 1995; Bjorling 1998; Smith 2004; Pettiford *et al.* 2007; Bastos *et al.* 2008; Slensky 2009; Donahue & Silverstein 2014; Tzelepis & McCool 2016). Pain contributes to hypoventilation due to splinting of the thoracic wall, which results in a lower tidal volume and vital capacity. Pain-induced splinting also inhibits coughing, which leads to the accumulation of pulmonary secretions and in turn increases the potential for pneumonia (Cullen *et al.* 1975; Shackford *et al.* 1976; MacKersie *et al.* 1987; Anderson *et al.* 1993). It has also been shown that there is decreased tone and contractility of the diaphragm due to sensory intercostal nerve reflexes initiated in response to painful stimuli (Vana *et al.* 2014). The decrease in effective ventilatory effort due to pain compounds pulmonary atelectasis, hypoxemia, and hypercapnia (Anderson *et al.* 1993; Smith 2004; Jackson & Drobatz 2004; Vana *et al.* 2014).

Diagnosis

During physical exam, patients with thoracic trauma will often display tachypnea and dyspnea. If noted, it is important that patient stabilization is achieved prior to diagnostic procedures that may compound these findings. The paradoxic motion of the flail segment, classically described with flail chest, may not be apparent on initial evaluation due to splinting by the intercostal muscles that can decrease that motion (Vana *et al.* 2014). However, visualization of the flail segment will become more obvious as intercostal muscles fatigue, with administration of local anesthetics, analgesic therapy, or patient sedation. Lung sounds may be absent on auscultation if there is a pneumothorax or hemothorax. Crackles, if auscultated, may indicate the presence of pulmonary infiltrate secondary to contusion. Thoracic radiographs can be helpful in confirming a diagnosis of flail chest and evaluating the extent of the thoracic wall injury, as well as in evaluating the pleural space and pulmonary parenchyma. However, it should be remembered that pulmonary contusions may not become radiographically evident until 24–48 hours after the injury. Therefore, it is important that the presence of these additional, complicating injuries be presumed in all cases where trauma sufficient to cause rib fractures has occurred, despite initial radiographic appearance. It has been shown that computed tomography with three-dimensional reconstruction of the images has increased sensitivity for identification of a flail segment and comorbidities (Vana *et al.* 2014). However, it comes at the cost of necessitating general anesthesia or at least heavy sedation, which may depress respiratory function (Smith 2004).

Treatment

Medical therapy

Trauma sufficient to cause flail chest has likely produced multisystemic problems, some of which may require more immediate therapy. Triage is essential in order to identify critical abnormalities so that primary therapy will focus on stabilization of the traumatized patient (Jackson & Drobatz 2004; Serrano & Boag 2014). Life-threatening injuries are addressed as soon as they are recognized and the familiar "A, B, C" acronym provides a time-proven guide for evaluation and treatment priority. Following stabilization of conditions that are an immediate threat to life, specific therapy directed at the pathologic consequences of flail chest can be initiated. Severely affected animals may show hemoptysis or an accumulation of a foamy blood-tinged fluid in the airways, which can lead to airway obstruction.

If obstruction is present or imminent, these cases will benefit from immediate endotracheal intubation and ventilator support. Airway suction with a catheter placed through the tube into the mainstem bronchi and intermittent aspiration can remove secretions.

Pneumothorax should be suspected in cases of flail chest regardless of the etiology. Therapy should be initiated immediately if the thoracic wall is open to the environment. A sterile occlusive bandage should be placed over the penetration site to convert the open pneumothorax to closed. Securing the dressing on only three of four sides will allow air to escape and prevent development of a tension pneumothorax. When the patient is stable, surgical closure of the opening can be performed in conjunction with thoracostomy tube placement and rib stabilization. Generally, closed pneumothorax of traumatic origin can be treated conservatively as long as patient ventilatory and respiratory parameters are only minimally affected (Brockman & Puerto 2004). However, the cumulative effects of associated pathologies in flail chest cases mean that even a small amount of pneumothorax may contribute to respiratory compromise and alleviation should be considered (Donahue & Silverstein 2014).

Placing the patient in lateral recumbency with the affected side down will minimize the paradoxic motion of the flail section, which will in turn decrease pain and potential further injury to the lung lobes (Donahue & Silverstein 2014; Reinaro 2017; Monnet 2018). It may also be effective at stopping the progression of ipsilateral pneumothorax, but may not be effective at improving ventilation (Zidulka *et al.* 1982; Brockman & Puerto 2004; Smith 2004).

It is a safe assumption that animals with flail chest have pulmonary contusions (Ludwig 2000; Rozanski 2017). Therapy for pulmonary contusion is considered supportive and the degree of therapy depends on the severity of the lesion (Hackner 1995; Serrano & Boag 2014; Cohn 2017; Rozanski 2017). Basic support starts with maintaining and/or improving blood oxygenation. Oxygen supplementation methods include flow-by, nasal cannulation, oxygen cage, or hoods, and these can be used to maintain arterial oxygen saturation (SpO_2) above 92% and partial pressure of arterial oxygen (PaO_2) above 60 mmHg (Hackner 1995; Rozanski 2017). Continued leaking of plasma components, increasing edema, and inflammatory mediators can contribute to deterioration of blood oxygenation and this must be closely monitored (Hackner 1995; Melton *et al.* 1999; Serrano & Boag 2014). If SpO_2 continues to fall or PaO_2 does not respond to O_2 supplementation, mechanical ventilation may be necessary. Positive-pressure ventilation (PPV) provides oxygen and is effective in treating hypoxemia caused by atelectasis, pain, and blood or tissue fluids within the airways and alveoli. Improving pulmonary function is evidenced by a progressive decrease in peak inspiratory pressure required to maintain adequate oxygenation (Campbell & King 2000). There are other advantages of PPV for the flail chest patient. It stops paradoxic motion of the flail section, which allows better apposition of the fractured ribs and in turn decreases pain. Unfortunately, long-term maintenance of a veterinary patient on mechanical ventilation is difficult and not without complications (Hackner 1995; Bateman 2001). Survival of patients requiring mechanical ventilation has been shown to be only about 30% (Powell *et al.* 1999; Campbell & King 2000). Minimizing pulmonary atelectasis is an important component of maintaining oxygenation. Frequent positional changes can help prevent hypostatic congestion and if the patient's condition permits, then intermittent standing episodes or short walks can improve thoracic expansion (Hackner 1995; Bateman 2001; Rozanski 2017).

Pain management is a very important aspect of medical therapy for flail chest and may contribute to return of normal respiratory mechanics (Pettiford *et al.* 2007; Vana *et al.* 2014). Pain from thoracic wall motion and the inciting trauma leads to reduced ventilatory efforts, which in turn contribute to hypoxia and atelectasis. Pain and the accompanying thoracic splinting tend to decrease the cough response, which leads to accumulation of pulmonary secretions, contributing to airway obstruction and potentially to bacterial infection. Aggressive pain management is one of the major components of medical management and has been shown to improve effective ventilation, decrease atelectasis, improve blood oxygen content, and enhance the ability to cough (Hunt 2017; Pettiford *et al.* 2007; Bastos *et al.* 2008; Slensky 2009; Donahue & Silverstein 2014). The method of pain control selected is important, as some methods can adversely affect ventilation in the compromised patient. Some opioid analgesics are known to significantly depress respiration and are potent antitussives. Caution is therefore advised in their use in flail chest.

Achieving balance between the adverse effects of the drug and effective pain control may be difficult, so alternative methods of pain control are available (Hackner 1995; Slensky 2009; Serrano & Boag 2014; Quandt & Lee 2014). Constant-rate infusions of combinations of drugs such as fentanyl/lidocaine or morphine/lidocaine/ketamine titrated to effect can be useful (Plunkett 2013; Guillaumin & Adin 2015). Intercostal nerve blocks using agents such as bupivacaine hydrochloride have been shown to be effective in controlling pain and improving ventilation (Anderson *et al.* 1993;

Hackner 1995; Tzelepis & McCool 2016; Rozanski 2017). Nerve blocks should be performed for all fractured ribs as well as one rib cranial and caudal to the flail section. Some authors advocate blocking the nerves dorsal to the fractures, while others suggest both dorsal and ventral to the fractures (Figure 31.1) (Spackman & Caywood 1987; Slensky 2009; Guillaumin & Adin 2015; Quandt & Lee 2014). A small-gauge needle (25–27 g) is carefully "walked" off the caudal margin of the rib without entering the pleural space (Figure 31.2). Gentle aspiration of the syringe prior to injection ensures that the drug will not be infused into an intercostal vessel. Approximately 0.25–0.5 cc of the anesthetic is injected at each site. When bupivacaine hydrochloride is used in the canine, the total dose should not exceed 1.5 mg/kg (Rozanski 2017; Monnet 2018). Ventilatory capability may be compromised if excess intercostal nerves are blocked due to local anesthetic agent effect on motor nerves as well as sensory nerves (Rozanski 2017).

Interpleural instillation of local anesthetic agent has also been shown to be an effective method of pain control. Interpleural bupivacaine has been used effectively in cases of human chest trauma as well as post thoracotomy in veterinary patients (Knottenbelt *et al.* 1991; Thompson & Johnson 1991; Conzemius *et al.* 1994). When a chest tube has been placed the drug can be instilled through the chest tube while the patient is in lateral recumbency with the flail side down. This allows the traumatized parietal pleural surface to be bathed with the local anesthetic. Local anesthetics cause short-term pain on injection due to the acidic nature; the addition of sodium bicarbonate to the drug increases the pH and will decrease the pain. It is also theorized that more of the anesthetic agent molecules are converted to

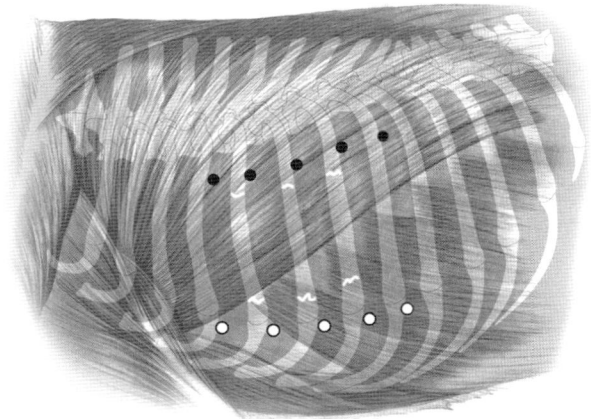

Figure 31.1 Schematic representation of the locations for placement of intercostal nerve blocks for a three-rib flail section. Red dots indicate dorsal location while blue dots indicate the optional ventral location.

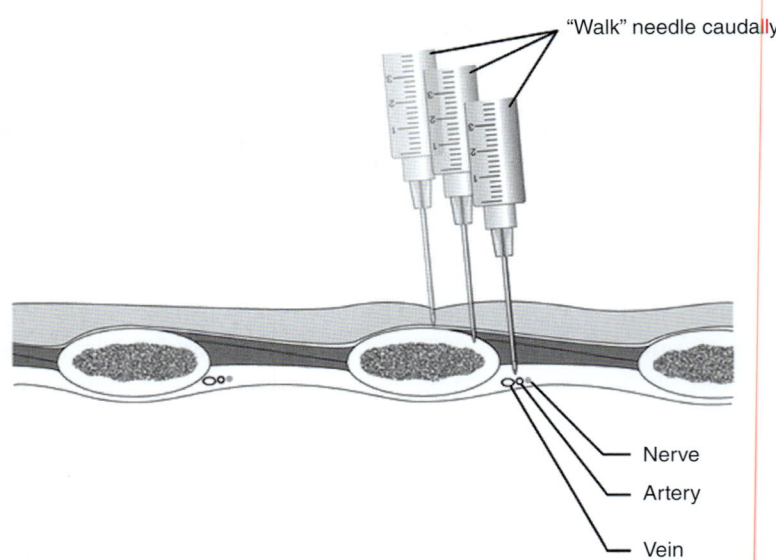

"Walk" needle caudally

Nerve

Artery

Vein

Figure 31.2 Schematic drawing of the technique for instillation of local anesthetic for intercostal nerve block. The rib is located with the hypodermic needle, and the needle is "walked" off the rib in a caudal direction prior to instillation of the anesthetic.

the nonionic form, which increases the rate of penetration and shortens the onset of anesthesia. Unfortunately, a slight increase in the pH of bupivacaine can lead to precipitation and inactivation (Grabinsky 2005). One method to minimize the discomfort of interpleural local anesthesia is to administer a preliminary dose of alkalinized lidocaine (1 cc 8.4% sodium bicarbonate in 10 cc 1% lidocaine) at 1.5 mg/kg, followed by the bupivacaine also at 1.5 mg/kg.

Epidural analgesia can also be an effective pain control method for thoracic trauma (Hackner 1995; Wetmore & Glowaski 2000; Hunt 2017; Rozanski 2017). As previously mentioned, certain opioids given systemically can lead to significant respiratory depression and minimize the protective cough reflex. However, when opioids are administered epidurally, these detrimental side effects are diminished and if they are seen the opioid can be easily reversed (Hackner 1995). Epidural analgesics are administered in the lumbosacral space. Proper epidural technique and appropriate drugs and dosages can be obtained through an appropriate anesthesia or pain management text.

Management of flail chest cases includes fluid therapy due to the potential for significant cardiovascular compromise. However, the presence of the pulmonary contusions that invariably accompany flail chest can complicate fluid therapy. It is important to maintain adequate tissue perfusion and hydration without contributing to fluid overload and pulmonary edema that could occur with the high fluid rates required in cases of shock (Cockshutt 1995; Hackner 1995; Bateman 2001; Mazzaferro 2001; Rozanski 2017). The type of fluid,

crystalloid (isotonic or hypertonic) or colloid, that should be used is a point of debate and controversy (Hackner 1995; Bateman 2001; Serrano & Boag 2014; Rozanski 2017). However, there is agreement that regardless of the fluid type, the therapy should maintain cardiac performance and tissue perfusion. This requires that therapy be titrated to proper effect instead of administering preset amounts at specific rates. Careful monitoring of physiologic parameters such as indicators of perfusion, arterial blood pressure, central venous pressure, urine output, and respiratory function is required. Therefore, whether delivering isotonic crystalloids, hypertonic saline followed by isotonic crystalloids, or hypertonic saline and colloid combinations, the primary aim is to maintain tissue perfusion (Cohn 2017; Rozanski 2017). There is evidence that early treatment with hypertonic saline may prevent neutrophil activation and this may decrease neutrophil-induced injury to the lungs (Bastos et al. 2008). Caution should be exercised with colloid administration, including hemoglobin-based oxygen carriers. These products may be detrimental in therapy of contusions (Cohn et al. 1997).

Antibiotics should be used when cases of flail chest have been caused by penetrating injury such as bite wounds. However, antibiotics are not indicated when pulmonary contusions are the primary concern, because of the low incidence of bacterial pneumonia (Hackner 1995; Beal 2005; Cohn 2017; Rozanski 2017).

Inflammatory mediators elicited in trauma cases are known to exacerbate clinical signs seen with flail chest and another alternative in minimizing pulmonary injury may be to control the inflammatory cascade.

Unfortunately, a generally accepted method to control the cascade is not available. The use of corticosteroids is controversial. Some studies have shown some benefit, while others suggest just the opposite. Because of the overall lack of evidence for improved outcome and the potential for deleterious effects, some authors conclude there are no indications for corticosteroids (Serrano & Boag 2014). Nonsteroidal anti-inflammatory drugs (NSAIDs) may be considered. However, patients should be eating, and renal function should be closely monitored. Severe musculoskeletal trauma may result in myoglobinemia and lead to acute kidney injury at any time within a week of the injury, and NSAID use may exacerbate this damage. There are other approaches to mitigate the effects of inflammatory mediators and many have shown promise in laboratory models and initial clinical trials, but there are many that do not (Hackner 1995; Bateman 2001; Dahlem *et al.* 2004; Kelly *et al.* 2003). Further research is needed before general recommendations regarding anti-inflammatory therapy can be made.

Despite the success of medical therapy for flail chest, there are indications for surgical intervention as soon as the patient is stable. Indications for early surgical intervention include the following scenarios: a thoracotomy or celiotomy is required due to concomitant injury; imminent risk of further trauma to thoracic organs; persistent or increasing loss of pulmonary function that may lead to ventilator support; and unrelenting pain that cannot be controlled.

Surgical therapy

Surgical stabilization of the flail segment has been a key component of the therapeutic recommendations in veterinary medicine for many years because of concerns relative to chest wall instability. Consequently, there are many methods described for stabilization (Kagen 1980; Bjorling *et al.* 1982; Dixon 1982; Anderson *et al.* 1993; Orton 1993; McAnulty 1995; Bjorling 1998). However, it must be emphasized that surgery should only be performed following patient stabilization when one of the previously mentioned indications exists.

When trauma leading to flail chest has also resulted in the need for surgical intervention, open reduction of the fractured ribs and restoration of thoracic wall continuity is indicated. Rib fractures can be repaired with appropriately sized orthopedic pins and wire or plates and screws. It is equally important to reestablish soft tissue integrity such that negative pleural space pressure can be restored. Restoration of soft tissue continuity when one intercostal space has been disrupted can be accomplished in a manner similar to closure of an intercostal thoracotomy following adequate débridement (Orton 1993). If soft tissues of multiple intercostal spaces have been disrupted, it may be necessary to place a series of staggered circumcostal sutures incorporating all adjacent ribs in the affected area and then one rib cranial and caudal to the affected section. This creates a "basket-weave" pattern that becomes a support for soft tissues mobilized to cover the defect. The latissimus dorsi muscle, external abdominal oblique muscles, a flap created from the greater omentum, or a combination of any or all of these can be used over the stabilized segment (Orton 1993). A thoracostomy tube will facilitate reestablishment of negative interpleural pressure and aid in postoperative management.

When surgical stabilization of costal fractures or wound closure is not required, the flail segment should still be stabilized. Common methods for stabilization of a flail section involve percutaneous placement of sutures that encircle ribs within the section, applying traction to the unstable section with those sutures, and attaching the sutures to some form of external brace that uses the adjacent intact thoracic wall to provide counter-traction. Previous intercostal nerve blocks will facilitate placement of the external brace. One method utilizes heat-sensitive plastic or fiberglass casting material that has been molded to fit the thoracic wall over the area of the flail section. It is important that the prosthetic material extend beyond the borders of the flail section so that it rests across nonfractured ribs. Once the material is molded and set, two holes are placed through it in locations that will correspond to the central area of each fractured rib in the flail section. While some researchers describe one set of holes centrally placed, others advocate using two sutures, dorsal and ventral, per rib segment (Spackman & Caywood 1987; Anderson *et al.* 1993). The area for suture placement should be prepared aseptically and monofilament nonabsorbable sutures should be passed around each rib so that the suture ends can be passed through the holes placed through the bracing material. It is important to preplace all of the sutures prior to securing them to the brace in order to avoid interference of the brace with proper suture placement. When passing the suture circumcostally, it is essential that as the needle passes around the rib it remains immediately adjacent to the bone, especially along the caudal and medial borders. This will minimize the potential of encircling the neurovascular bundle caudally and lacerating pulmonary parenchyma (Figure 31.3). Additionally, the authors recommend passing the needle from the caudal aspect of the rib to the cranial, as this will ensure the greatest needle control near the neurovascular bundle.

Intercostal nerve impingement may become a source of chronic pain (Vana et al. 2014). Placement of circumcostal sutures reportedly does not usually damage the underlying lung when pneumothorax exists because of the resulting gap between the visceral and parietal pleura (Bjorling 1998). However, caution should nonetheless be exercised during placement. Light padding can be interposed between the thoracic wall and the bracing material after suture placement. The suture ends are passed medial to lateral through the holes in the brace and secured (Figure 31.4). A loose thoracic bandage (i.e., stockinette) can then be placed to help secure and protect the brace. The bandage should not impede thoracic motion. The bandage should be checked on a periodic basis to ensure proper position and evaluate the skin under the edges of the brace. If cutaneous lesions become evident, the padding may need to be increased around the edges of the brace. The brace should be left in place for 3–4 weeks to allow for soft tissue healing and callus formation around the fractured ribs.

An alternative method of stabilization utilizes one suture passed around the midpoint of each rib in the flail section as previously described. The sutures are then tied around splinting material such as tongue depressors so that the long axis of the splints lies vertically over each rib in the flail section (costal splints). At this point, rigid counterbraces, such as additional tongue depressors, are placed at the dorsal and ventral extents of the costal splints. The counterbraces must rest across stable thoracic wall and are placed beneath and perpendicular (horizontally oriented) to the costal splints so that the flail section cannot be drawn inward. Cotton padding is placed between the costal splint ends and the dorsal and ventral counterbraces to increase traction on the flail section for added stability. This simplified method of stabilization requires materials that are readily available and the placement of only one circumcostal suture (Figure 31.5) (McAnulty 1995; Bjorling 1998). The bracing should be protected from becoming entangled in bedding or being dislodged by covering it with a lightly padded bandage or stockinette. The brace is left in place for 3–4 weeks to allow osseous callus formation and soft tissue healing.

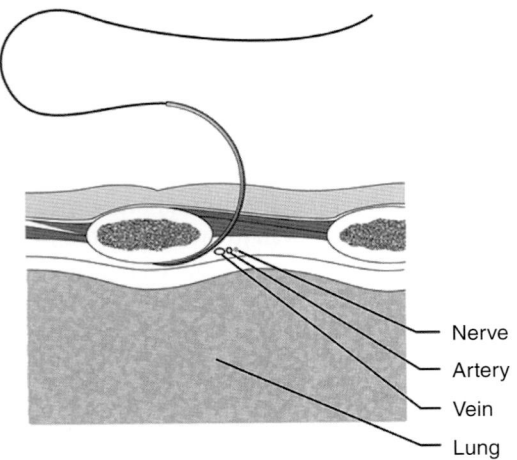

Figure 31.3 Schematic drawing of the technique for passing suture around the rib. The needle should stay adjacent to the bone to avoid the neurovascular bundle and underlying lung.

Nerve

Artery

Vein

Lung

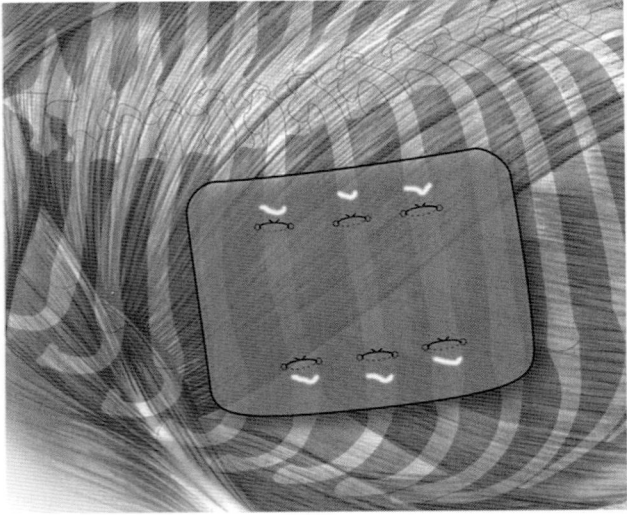

Figure 31.4 Schematic drawing of an external moldable splint for stabilization of a flail section. Two circumcostal sutures are preplaced at the dorsal and ventral extents of each rib of the flail section and then secured to the moldable splint through appropriately placed perforations. The splint extends beyond the flail section to rest on stable thoracic wall.

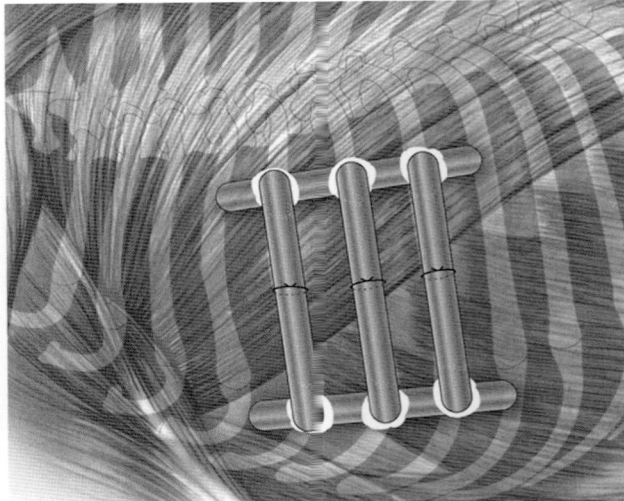

Figure 31.5 Schematic drawing of a simplified bracing of a flail section. One circumcostal suture is placed around the mid-portion of each rib in the flail section and then tied around a tongue depressor. Horizontal counterbraces are placed beneath the dorsal and ventral extents of the tongue depressors and cotton padding is placed between each depressor and counterbrace contact point. Padding is sufficient to result in lateral traction on the flail section to create stability.

References

Anderson, M., Payne, J.T., Mann, F.A., and Constantinescu, G.M. (1993). Flail chest: pathophysiology, treatment, and prognosis. *Compendium on Continuing Education for the Practicing Veterinarian* 15: 65–74.

Bastos, R., Calhoon, J.H., and Baisden, C.E. (2008). Flail chest and pulmonary contusion. *Seminars in Thoracic and Cardiovascular Surgery* 20: 39–45.

Bateman, S.W. (2001). Managing the acutely lung injured patient. In: *Proceedings of the 11th Annual ACVS Symposium*, 559. Chicago, IL: American College of Veterinary Surgeons.

Beal, M.W. (2005). Thoracic trauma. In: *Textbook of Veterinary Internal Medicine*, 6e (ed. S.J. Ettinger and E.C. Feldman), 461–463. St. Louis, MO: Elsevier.

Bjorling, D.E. (1998). Surgical management of flail chest. In: *Current Techniques in Small Animal Surgery*, 4e (ed. M.J. Bojrab, G.W. Ellison and B. Slocum), 421–425. Baltimore, MD: Williams & Wilkins.

Bjorling, D.E., Kolata, R.J., and DeNovo, R.C. (1982). Flail chest: review, clinical experience and new method of stabilization. *Journal of the American Animal Hospital Association* 18: 269–272.

Brockman, D.J. and Puerto, D.A. (2004). Pneumomediastinum and pneumothorax. In: *Textbook of Respiratory Diseases in Dogs and Cats* (ed. L.G. King), 616–621. St. Louis, MO: Elsevier.

Campbell, V.L. and King, L.G. (2000). Pulmonary function, ventilator management, and outcome of dogs with thoracic trauma and pulmonary contusions: 10 cases (1994-1998). *Journal of the American Veterinary Medical Association* 217: 1505–1509.

Cappello, M., Yuehua, C., and DeTroyer, A. (1995). Rib cage distortion in a canine model of flail chest. *American Journal of Respiratory and Critical Care Medicine* 151: 1481–1485.

Cockshutt, J.R. (1995). Management of fracture-associated thoracic trauma. *Small Animal Practice* 25: 1031–1046.

Cohn, L.A. (2017). Diseases of the pulmonary parenchyma. In: *Textbook of Veterinary Internal Medicine: Diseases of the Dog and Cat*, 8e (ed. S.J. Ettinger), 1108–1131. St. Louis, MO: Elsevier.

Cohn, S., Zieg, P., Rosenfield, A., and Fisher, B.T. (1997). Resuscitation of pulmonary contusion: effects of a red cell substitute. *Critical Care Medicine* 25: 484–491.

Conzemius, M.G., Brockman, D.J., King, L.G., and Perkowski, S.Z. (1994). Analgesia in dogs after intercostal thoracotomy: a clinical trial comparing intravenous buprenorphine and interpleural bupivacaine. *Veterinary Surgery* 23: 291–298.

Craven, K.D., Oppenheimer, L., and Wood, L.D. (1979). Effects of contusion and flail chest on pulmonary perfusion and oxygen exchange. *Journal of Applied Physiology* 47: 729–737.

Crowe, D.T. (1983). Traumatic pulmonary contusions, hematomas, pseudocysts, and acute respiratory distress syndrome: an update. Part I. *Compendium on Continuing Education for the Practicing Veterinarian* 5: 396–400.

Cullen, P., Modell, J.H., Kirby, R.R. et al. (1975). Treatment of flail chest. Use of intermittent mandatory ventilation and positive end-expiratory pressure. *Archives of Surgery* 110: 1099–1103.

Dahlem, P., van Aalderen, W.M., de Neef, M. et al. (2004). Randomized controlled trial of aerosolized prostacyclin therapy in children with acute lung injury. *Critical Care Medicine* 32: 1055–1060.

Dixon, J.S. (1982). Use of a slab traction splint to stabilize canine flail chest. *Veterinary Medicine, Small Animal Clinician* 77: 601–605.

Donahue, S. and Silverstein, D.C. (2014). Chest wall disease. In: *Small Animal Critical Care Medicine*, 2e (ed. D.C. Silverstein and K. Hopper), 148–150. St. Louis, MO: Elsevier.

Grabinsky, A. (2005). Mechanisms of neural blockade. *Pain Physician* 8: 411–416.

Guillaumin, J. and Adin, C.A. (2015). Postthoracotomy management. In: *Small Animal Critical Care Medicine*, 2e (ed. D.C. Silverstein and K. Hopper), 703–707. St. Louis, MO: Elsevier.

Hackner, S.G. (1995). Emergency management of traumatic pulmonary contusions. *Compendium on Continuing Education for the Practicing Veterinarian* 17: 677–686.

Hunt, G.B. (2017). Thoracic wall. In: *Veterinary Surgery: Small Animal*, 2e (ed. S.A. Johnston and K.M. Tobias), 2001–2019. St. Louis, MO: Elsevier.

Jackson, C.B. and Drobatz, K.J. (2004). Pulmonary contusion. In: *Textbook of Respiratory Disease in Dogs and Cats* (ed. L.G. King), 472–480. St Louis, MO: Elsevier.

Kagen, K.G. (1980). Thoracic trauma. *Veterinary Clinics of North America. Small Animal Practice* 10: 641–650.

Kelly, M.E., Miller, P.R., Greenhaw, J.J. et al. (2003). Novel resuscitation strategy for pulmonary contusion after severe chest trauma. *Journal of Trauma* 55: 94–105.

Knottenbelt, J.D., James, M.F., and Bloomfield, M. (1991). Intrapleural bupivacaine analgesia in chest trauma: a randomized double-blind controlled trial. *Injury* 22: 114–116.

Kolata, R.J. (1981). Management of thoracic trauma. *Veterinary Clinics of North America. Small Animal Practice* 11: 103–120.

Ludwig, L.L. (2000). Surgical emergencies of the respiratory system. *Veterinary Clinics of North America. Small Animal Practice* 30: 531–553. vi.

MacKersie, R.C., Shackford, S.R., Hoyt, D.B., and Karagianes, T.G. (1987). Continuous epidural fentanyl analgesia: ventilatory function improvement with routine use in treatment of blunt chest injury. *Journal of Trauma* 27: 1207–1212.

Mazzaferro, E.M. (2001). Respiratory emergencies. In: *Veterinary Emergency Medicine Secrets*, 2e (ed. W.E. Wingfield), 60–65. Philadelphia, PA: Hanley & Belfus.

McAnulty, J.F. (1995). A simplified method for stabilization of flail chest injuries in small animals. *Journal of the American Animal Hospital Association* 31: 137–141.

Melton, S.M., Davis, K.A., Moomey, C.B. et al. (1999). Mediator-dependent secondary injury after unilateral blunt thoracic trauma. *Shock* 11: 396–402.

Monnet, E.C. (2018). Thoracic wall. In: *Small Animal Thoracic Surgery* (ed. C.E. Orton and E. Monnet), 65–76. Hoboken, NJ: Wiley Blackwell.

Moreno, M.R., Zambrano, S., Déjardin, L.M., and Saunders, W.B. (2017). Bone biomechanics and fracture biology. In: *Veterinary Surgery: Small Animal*, 2e (ed. S.A. Johnston and K.M. Tobias), 613–649. St. Louis, MO: Elsevier.

Olsen, D.E. (2010). Thoracic wall and sternum. In: *Mechanisms of Disease in Small Animal Surgery*, 3e (ed. M.J. Bojrab and E. Monnet), 325–332. Jackson, WY: Teton NewMedia.

Olsen, D. (2014). Management of flail chest. In: *Current Techniques in Small Animal Surgery*, 5e (ed. M.J. Bojrab, D.R. Waldron and J.P. Toombs), 437–442. Jackson, WY: Teton NewMedia.

Olsen, D., Renberg, W., Perrett, J. et al. (2002). Clinical management of flail chest in dogs and cats: a retrospective study of 24 cases (1989–1999). *Journal of the American Animal Hospital Association* 38: 315–320.

Oppenheimer, L., Craven, K.D., Forkert, L., and Wood, L.D. (1979). Pathophysiology of pulmonary contusion in dogs. *Journal of Applied Physiology* 47: 718–728.

Orton, C.E. (1993). Thoracic wall. In: *Textbook of Small Animal Surgery* (ed. D.H. Slatter), 370–381. Philadelphia, PA: WB Saunders.

Palmer, R.H. and James, S.P. (2010). Fracture biomechanics of the appendicular skeleton. In: *Mechanisms of Disease in Small Animal Surgery*, 3e (ed. M.J. Bojrab and E. Monnet), 669–685. Jackson, WY: Teton NewMedia.

Parham, A.M., Yarbrough, D.R., and Redding, J.S. (1978). Flail chest syndrome and pulmonary contusion. *Archives of Surgery* 113: 900–903.

Pettiford, B.L., Luketich, J.D., and Landreneau, R.J. (2007). The management of flail chest. *Thoracic Surgery Clinics* 17: 25–33.

Plunkett, S.J. (2013). Traumatic emergencies. In: *Emergency Procedures for the Small Animal Veterinarian*, 3e (ed. S.J. Plunkett), 145–159. Edinburgh: Elsevier.

Powell, L.L., Rozanski, E.A., Tidwell, A.S., and Rush, J.E. (1999). A retrospective analysis of pulmonary contusion secondary to motor vehicle accidents in 143 dogs. *Journal of Veterinary Emergency and Critical Care* 9: 127–135.

Quandt, J. and Lee, J.A. (2014). Analgesia and constant rate infusions. In: *Small Animal Critical Care Medicine*, 2e (ed. D.C. Silverstein and K. Hopper), 766–773. St. Louis, MO: Elsevier.

Reinaro, C.R. (2017). Initial evaluation of respiratory emergencies. In: *Textbook of Veterinary Internal Medicine: Diseases of the Dog and Cat*, 8e (ed. S.J. Ettinger), 578–580. St. Louis, MO.

Rozanski, E. (2017). Thoracic trauma. In: *Textbook of Veterinary Internal Medicine: Diseases of the Dog and Cat*, 8e (ed. S.J. Ettinger), 621–627. St. Louis, MO: Elsevier.

Serrano, S. and Boag, A.K. (2014). Pulmonary contusions and hemorrhage. In: *Small Animal Critical Care Medicine*, 2e (ed. D.C. Silverstein and K. Hopper), 138–143. St. Louis, MO: Elsevier.

Shackford, S.R., Smith, D.E., Zarins, C.K. et al. (1976). The management of flail chest. A comparison of ventilatory and nonventilatory treatment. *American Journal of Surgery* 132: 759–762.

Shen, W., Niu, Y., and Stuhmiller, J.H. (2005). Biomechanically based criteria for rib fractures induced by high-speed impact. *Journal of Trauma* 58: 538–545.

Slensky, K. (2009). Thoracic trauma. In: *Small Animal Critical Care Medicine* (ed. D. Silverstein and K. Hopper), 662–666. St Louis, MO: Elsevier.

Smith, M.M. (2004). Flail chest. In: *Textbook of Respiratory Disease in Dogs and Cats* (ed. L.G. King), 647–660. St. Louis, MO: Elsevier.

Spackman, C.J. and Caywood, D.D. (1987). Management of thoracic trauma and chest wall reconstruction. *Veterinary Clinics of North America. Small Animal Practice* 17: 431–447.

Spackman, C.J.A., Caywood, D.D., Feeney, D.A., and Johnston, G.R. (1984). Thoracic wall and pulmonary trauma in dogs sustaining fractures as a result of motor vehicle accidents. *Journal of the American Veterinary Medical Association* 185: 975–977.

Sweet, D.C. and Waters, D.J. (1991). Role of surgery in the management of dogs with pathologic conditions of the thorax. Part II. *Compendium on Continuing Education for the Practicing Veterinarian* 13: 1671–1676.

Tamas, P.M., Paddleford, R.R., and Krahwinkel, D.J. (1985). Thoracic trauma in dogs and cats presented for limb fractures. *Journal of the American Animal Hospital Association* 21: 161–165.

Thompson, S.E. and Johnson, J.M. (1991). Analgesia in dogs after intercostal thoracotomy. A comparison of morphine, selective intercostal nerve block, and interpleural regional analgesia with bupivacaine. *Veterinary Surgery* 20: 73–77.

Trinkle, J.K., Richardson, J.D., Franz, J.L. et al. (1975). Management of flail chest without mechanical ventilation. *Annals of Thoracic Surgery* 19: 355–363.

Tzelepis, G.E. and McCool, F.D. (2016). The respiratory system and chest wall diseases. In: *Murray & Nadel's Textbook of Respiratory Medicine*, 6e (ed. V.C. Broaddus), 1707–1723. Philadelphia, PA: Elsevier.

Vana, P.G., Neubauer, D.C., and Luchette, F.A. (2014). Contemporary management of flail chest. *American Surgeon* 80 (6): 527–535.

Wetmore, L.A. and Glowaski, M.M. (2000). Epidural analgesia in veterinary critical care. *Clinical Techniques in Small Animal Practice* 15: 177–188.

Zidulka, A., Brady, T.F., Rizzi, M.C., and Shiner, R.J. (1982). Position may stop pneumothorax progression in dogs. *American Journal of Respiratory Disease* 126: 51–53.

Section 5

Pleural Space

32

Chylothorax

Jonathan F. McAnulty

Chylothorax is a relatively uncommon, yet devastating condition that is characterized by the accumulation of free chyle within the thoracic cavity. If unable to be resolved, chylothorax can often result in death due to secondary sequelae such as fibrous encapsulation of the lungs, especially in cats, and cachexia from chronic removal of nutrient-rich fluids during long-term management by fluid aspiration. A wide variety of medical and surgical treatments, many of which have not had good success in the long term, have been utilized to treat chylothorax. This chapter will focus on those procedures currently in use and of contemporary interest, as well as areas for future development, and not attempt to provide a comprehensive historical review of treatments for this disease.

Chylothorax can be seen in any breed of dog or cat, but does have some predilection for presentation in Afghan hounds and Shetland sheep dog breeds (Birchard *et al.* 1988, 1998). The Shiba Inu has also been shown to be overrepresented in case series of chylothorax and tends to develop the condition at a younger age compared to most other breeds. Potential etiologies of chylothorax include traumatic or iatrogenic rupture of the thoracic duct, mediastinal neoplasia, cardiac disease (cardiomyopathy, hyperthyroidism, pericardial effusion or restriction, congenital cardiac anomalies, heartworm infection), embolization, occult infections, and lung lobe torsion (Fossum *et al.* 1986; Hodges *et al.* 1993; Fossum 1993; Geizer *et al.* 1997). It is important to recognize that chylothorax in animals is most frequently a chronic disease, unlike the presentation in humans where acute trauma is a significant cause, and thus seldom resolves on its own. Frequently, an inciting cause is not found or able to be

mechanistically linked to the condition and the chylothorax is considered to be idiopathic.

Idiopathic chylothorax is poorly understood and has long carried a guarded prognosis in dogs and cats, although more recent developments in treatment have improved the outlook somewhat. In cases where contrast lymphangiography is performed, it is routinely shown to occur in concert with cranial mediastinal lymphangiectasis, suggesting a chronic lymphatic obstructive pathophysiology (Birchard *et al.* 1982). However, the source of the obstruction is seldom able to be ascertained. Idiopathic chylothorax may be due to a variety of undetected underlying conditions, or it is feasible that more than one condition combines in some cases to result in chylothorax. This variability in the inciting causes of chylothorax may be a central reason why any single therapy has not met with consistently high success in resolving chylothorax. Currently, idiopathic chylothorax is mostly treated in ways that address the common clinical signs of the underlying diseases (pleural accumulation of chylous effusion) and not by directly addressing the causes. In the future, better diagnostic technologies and increased knowledge of the disease in specific subsets of this patient population, such as breed-specific predilections, may expand the options for therapies or promote selective breeding practices to reduce the incidence of the condition in purebred genetic lines.

Diagnosis

The diagnosis of chylothorax is usually fairly straightforward. Affected animals present with a pleural effusion of varying severity. Sequelae secondary to the pleural

Small Animal Soft Tissue Surgery, Second Edition. Edited by Eric Monnet.
© 2023 John Wiley & Sons, Inc. Published 2023 by John Wiley & Sons, Inc.
Companion website: www.wiley.com/go/monnet/small

effusion, such as elevated respiration rate, dyspnea, cyanosis, or muffled heart and lung sounds, are frequently noted upon presentation and physical examination. In some instances, animals may be in severe distress and require emergency thoracocentesis and supportive therapy such as supplemental oxygen and sedation.

The presence of the pleural effusion may be most easily detected and/or confirmed by thoracic radiography or ultrasonography. The specific diagnosis of chylothorax is made by obtaining a sample of pleural fluid and performing biochemical analysis for triglyceride content, which will be elevated relative to the triglyceride content of the serum. The pleural fluid will generally be milky-white in appearance, but may also have a sanguineous or suppurative component, giving it a pink, strawberry milkshake appearance or a yellowish-white color. It has also been suggested that a triglyceride to cholesterol ratio in the pleural fluid sample >1.0 is indicative of a chylous effusion (Birchard et al. 1988). Cytologic evaluation of chylous effusions will reveal a cellular composition primarily composed of lymphocytes, with occasional neutrophils and some red blood cells.

It should be noted that chylous effusions may not always be purely chylous but can be mixed in character. Other pathologies in the thorax may result in some dilutional effect on the chyle so, depending on the severity of these conditions and the diet of the patient, absolute triglyceride values may vary significantly, although they will still exceed that seen in serum. The cytologic character of the effusion may also reflect an underlying pathophysiology, the chronicity of the condition, or effects of previous interventions such as multiple thoracocenteses. In such cases, increases in the relative proportion of neutrophils or macrophages to lymphocyte numbers will be seen. High neutrophil counts in the fluid may support further investigation into possible inflammatory or infectious conditions that warrant treatment if identified.

Further diagnostic testing is targeted at finding any potential causes for the chylothorax. This is supported by numerous case reports where treatment of a specific thoracic pathology, even in the absence of a compelling mechanistic connection to production of chyle in the chest, can result in resolution of the condition. Thus, blood testing for heartworm infestation and similar, and radiographic or ultrasound examination searching for lung pathologies, thoracic masses or other thoracic pathology, should be undertaken. Computed tomographic scans are a better imaging modality than plain radiographs, since the images are less confounded by residual pleural fluid. Echocardiography may also provide key information regarding heart function and evidence on whether there is a restrictive pericardium impairing diastolic filling of the ventricles.

As already noted, infectious agents may play a role in chylothorax. In these cases, the chylous fluid may have a more purulent character or be reflective of a pyogranulomatous process. Bacterial and fungal culture should be considered in cases where a chylous pleural fluid has characteristics suggestive of an infectious process. Atypical mycobacterial organisms have also been seen as a cause of chylothorax and may in some cases be detected only upon polymerase chain reaction amplification. Some clinicians have proposed empirical adjunctive therapy with agents such as azithromycin in such cases, although data on the efficacy of such an approach are currently nonexistent.

Pathophysiology

Chylothorax has been documented in concert with a variety of detectable pathologies of the chest and when these pathologies, such as thoracic masses, heartworm disease, lung lobe torsion, and so on are treated, the chylothorax may resolve and provide a presumptive cause-and-effect connection between the disease and chylous pleural effusion. Thus, diagnostic testing to reveal a feasible causative condition for the chylothorax is always recommended. An interesting example of this approach is described in report of a dog where removal of a rib chondroma resulted in resolution of chylothorax (Watine et al. 2003). However, idiopathic chylothorax remains a conundrum with respect to its pathophysiology. In the majority of cases, idiopathic chylothorax differs markedly from the condition in humans, which is usually acute and secondary to external or surgical trauma. Idiopathic chylothorax in animals seldom seems to involve acute rupture of the chylous lymphatic system or any point source leakage of chyle from this vessel bed. Thus, performing contrast studies to identify the "location of the leak" is nearly uniformly futile. Instead, as inferred from consistent detection of lymphangiectasis in the cranial mediastinum by lymphangiography (Birchard et al. 1982), chylothorax appears most likely to be related to an obstructive condition of these lymphatics, and the chylous effusion occurs due to diffuse leakage of chyle across the wall of the affected lymphatics. Thus, in nearly all instances, idiopathic chylothorax must be viewed as a chronic acquired disease that is unlikely to resolve on its own, in contrast to the acute condition in humans where healing of a lymphatic rupture may occur. It should be noted that there are occasional anecdotal reports of medically managed chylothorax where over time the effusion resolves. In the author's experience, these results are rare, and pose the risk of severe secondary sequelae such as restrictive pleuritis due to long-term irritation of the pleural surfaces by chyle.

Restrictive pericardial disease can play a role in the development of chylothorax. However, the frequency with which restrictive pericardial disease is a primary cause of chylothorax remains unclear. Conclusive evidence supporting a role for restrictive pericardial disease is currently found in one case reported in the veterinary literature (Campbell *et al.* 1995). In that instance, physical signs and cardiac chamber pressure measurements, particularly those from the right ventricle, were indicative of a restrictive pericardial disease. The relationship of this condition and the chylothorax was confirmed by resolution of the cardiac pressure abnormalities along with the pleural effusion after subtotal pericardiectomy (PC). The remaining evidence for restrictive pericardial disease as a cause of chylothorax is indirect and is based upon results obtained after performing PC, which was usually combined with other procedures such as thoracic duct ligation (TDL) (Fossum *et al.* 2004; Carobbi *et al.* 2008; Allman *et al.* 2010; Bussadori *et al.* 2011; McAnulty 2011). High reported success rates in small clinical case series (Fossum *et al.* 2004) have made this an attractive hypothesis that is currently receiving attention in the field. The first manuscript to promote PC as a routine treatment of chylothorax hypothesized that a restrictive pericardial condition occurs secondary to a thickened pericardium that "would increase systemic venous pressures and that abnormal venous pressures would act to impede the drainage of chyle via lymphaticovenous communications into the venous system while increasing lymphatic flow through the thoracic duct" (Fossum *et al.* 2004). However, no data have been published to support this hypothesis. In a recent prospective study, central venous pressure measurements obtained in eight dogs with chylothorax before and after PC showed no change in venous pressures in these dogs (McAnulty 2011). That study also failed to replicate the high success rate of other institutions with this approach, and thus either these findings may be interpreted as not supporting a hypothesis of venous hypertension as a common cause of chylothorax, or the limited patient cohort examined did not include animals with restrictive pericardial disease as a primary factor in the chylothorax. Regardless, these observations indicate that the role of restrictive pericardial disease in preventing resolution of chylothorax may be more complex than previously proposed or apply to a limited patient subcohort with this disease, and not be universally applicable across the chylothorax patient population. More sophisticated data collection, perhaps similar to that of Campbell *et al.* (1995), with respect to cardiac function and chamber pressures in a larger number of animals with spontaneous chylothorax may provide greater clarity with respect to the role of restrictive pericardial disease in the

pathophysiology of chylothorax. In the meantime, clinicians have been forced to rely on mostly weak scientific evidence and anecdotal reports to guide their treatment decisions (Reeves *et al.* 2020).

Lung lobe torsion with chylothorax also presents the clinician with some difficulties in establishing cause and effect. Lung lobe torsion can be an inciting cause of chylothorax and when treated by surgery the chylothorax may resolve. However, it is also feasible that a lung lobe torsion may occur secondarily in animals with a pleural effusion, and thus removal of the affected lung lobe will not affect the cause of the chylothorax. In the absence of data to establish the chronological order of occurrence of these conditions, it may be difficult to predict how effective lung lobe removal will be in any individual patient in terms of resolving a chylothorax condition. A treatment decision in these cases may be based on practical considerations rather than driven by scientific rigor. For example, resection of a torsed lung lobe might be combined with a PC to avoid having to reopen the chest at a later time if the chylothorax were not to resolve with lobectomy alone. This approach emphasizes minimizing overall surgical trauma while its impact on success remains unknown.

Treatment

Secondary chylothorax (nonidiopathic)

Treatment of chylothorax with detectable causative diseases (infectious agents, thoracic masses, heartworm disease, etc.) should be focused on resolving the putative disease process. In many cases, resolution of the inciting cause can result in resolution of the chylothorax. Resolution of the causative disease may require some time, such as for resolution of a chronic infectious/inflammatory process, and thus may need to be combined with symptomatic treatment of the pleural effusion to prevent a potentially fatal respiratory compromise. Periodic thoracocentesis and placement of a subcutaneous port attached to a pleural drainage catheter, as described by Cahalane *et al.* (2007) are both effective means of managing the pleural effusion while waiting for a response to treatment. Long-term drainage is more easily managed by placement of a pleural port drainage system than by thoracocentesis. Placement of a subcutaneous port is a routine part of treatment with this author. It allows for easy and relatively nonstressful pleural drainage over long time periods as the effect of surgery is assessed. Due to detachment of the port tube and the Jackson–Pratt drainage tube during removal in a prior case, this author has modified the Cahalane method by using a short piece of the port drain tubing as a size adaptor on the outlet of the port, and then placing the

Jackson–Pratt tubing over that and securing it to the port outlet with circumferential sutures. In this iteration, the Jackson–Pratt tubing is able to be accessed immediately when the port is exposed for removal and there is no chance of detachment as the tube is extracted.

Idiopathic chylothorax

Conservative medical management

A number of medical therapies to manage chylothorax have been proposed and used in the past. Dietary modification to reduce the amount of fat absorbed in the intestine, and hence the volume of chyle, has been used with varied effects. Low-fat high-fiber diets are one approach that may be utilized (Birchard *et al.* 1998). At one time, the addition of medium-chain triglyceride (MCT) oils to the diet was recommended to attempt to reduce the volume of chyle. MCT oils are seldom used today due to the relatively minimal impact this treatment had on the overall volume of chyle production and detection of MCT in the chyle, suggesting that the hypothesized effects of MCT oils may have been overestimated.

Neutraceuticals have been used with some frequency to attempt to reduce the accumulation of chyle in the thorax. Rutin, one such compound, has been one of the most common medical therapies for chylothorax in the past several decades. Rutin is a bioflavonoid compound with antioxidant properties and effects on macrophage activity. Rutin is recommended at a dose of 50–100 mg/kg three times a day and has been purported to be successful in 25% of animals if used for two months or longer (Thompson *et al.* 1999). However, in many animals the volume of chyle produced may make a two-month period of trial of conservative treatment unfeasible. It has also been suggested that the efficacy of rutin may be increased with concomitant use of hesperidin, a flavanone glycoside, which is purported to be a "sister herb" to rutin. There is currently no objective evidence available that combinations of these herb therapies are effective in animals with chylothorax.

Pycnogenol has also been suggested as a therapeutic agent for chylothorax. The basis for pycnogenol (as well as rutin) is in its use for lymphedema in humans (Cesarone *et al.* 2006). Pycnogenol is an extract of the maritime pine tree and is a natural antioxidant with anti-inflammatory effects that is purported to help boost the immune system and strengthen blood vessel walls and capillaries. It has not been used extensively for treatment of chylothorax in animals and there are no published reports on its efficacy. Dosing in animals is not well described, but has been suggested at 2.5 mg/kg twice a day. Side effects may include gastrointestinal upset and interaction with anticoagulant drugs.

Somatostatin has been shown to be effective in reducing the amount of chyle in humans and in experimental studies in dogs will reduce the flow of thoracic duct lymph (Nakabayashi *et al.* 1981). However, somatostatin has a very short half-life and significant side effects. Octreotide, an analogue of somatostatin, is more potent and has a longer half-life than the parent compound. Octreotide has been shown to reduce chyle output in humans and preliminary data in cats suggest a similar effect (Markham *et al.* 2000). Octreotide is an injectable compound given at 10 µg/kg subcutaneously three times a day. Due to its parenteral route of administration, octreotide is not likely to be useful for long-term therapy for chylothorax, but may be advantageous after surgery to reduce chyle flow while healing and rerouting of chyle drainage are occurring.

Conservative medical therapy is attractive due to its simplicity and relatively low cost for most of the commonly used products. In particular, in those patients where financial or other considerations preclude surgery, medical therapy may be worthwhile to attempt. However, the presence of chyle and repeated thoracocenteses will result in significant pleural fibrosis over time. Thus, prolonged unsuccessful medical therapy may reduce the potential for recovery after surgery due to lung entrapment and collapse within these fibrous layers. This is particularly true for cats, which appear to develop pleural fibrosis more rapidly and more aggressively than do dogs. For these reasons and the lack of efficacy of these therapies in our previous experience, we do not recommend medical therapy as a primary treatment for chylothorax in most animals, unless there are overriding client concerns or limiting patient comorbidities.

Surgical treatment

The current recommended treatment of idiopathic chylothorax is surgical intervention. Surgery is mostly targeted at rerouting of chyle into the venous circulation outside of the thoracic duct system and, as such, is targeted at resolution of the clinical signs rather than the inciting mechanisms of chylothorax. Up until recently, TDL has been the gold standard for treatment of chylothorax since its introduction in 1982 (Birchard *et al.* 1982). In the subsequent period after 1997, new surgical treatment approaches have been introduced that have appeared to increase the success obtainable with TDL. These procedures, cisterna chyli ablation (CCA) (Sicard *et al.* 2005; Hayashi *et al.* 2005; McAnulty 2011), and PC currently enjoy widespread application either alone or in combination with TDL, with published reports regarding their efficacy increasing in number.

Thoracic duct ligation

TDL as a sole treatment of idiopathic chylothorax varies in its success between 50% and 60% in dogs and approximately 25% in cats (Birchard *et al.* 1988, 1998). TDL is performed through a right caudal thoracotomy (ninth or tenth intercostal space) in the dog and a left caudal thoracotomy in the cat. The thoracic duct is found by surgical exploration of the tissues dorsal to the caudal thoracic aorta. This area is accessed by incision of the pleural membrane, which is usually thickened due to the effects of exposure to chyle, and reflection of this membrane to expose the dorsal aorta and fatty tissue between the aorta and azygous vein. The main thoracic duct typically will lie on the dorsal surface of the aorta, but may have multiple channels that may course within the epiaortic fat or lie toward either the left or right lateral surfaces of the aorta. The variability in the anatomy of the thoracic duct and the cisterna chyli has been the focus of numerous studies (Enwiller *et al.* 2003; Naganobu *et al.* 2006; Korpes *et al.* 2021; Chiang *et al.* 2022; Kanai *et al.* 2021, and others). TDL has also been performed successfully using a minimally invasive thoracoscopic approach (Allman *et al.* 2010; Mayhew *et al.* 2012) or by *en bloc* ligation of all of the tissues/fat dorsal to the aorta (MacDonald *et al.* 2008; Kanai *et al.* 2020).

Identification of the thoracic duct is greatly aided by administration of a contrast agent, since the chyle within the duct is frequently insufficiently colored to allow easy identification of the duct or its smaller collateral vessels. In the past, administration of multiple per os dosings of a fatty substrate such as corn oil or heavy cream prior to surgery was used to increase the fat content of the chyle and its contrast from surrounding structures (Birchard *et al.* 1982). This method was incompletely effective and has been replaced by direct injection of methylene blue dye into the lymphatic system (Enwiller *et al.* 2003) by directly injecting into a lacteal, a mesenteric lymph node, or other draining lymph nodes such as the popliteal. More recently, methylene blue has become difficult to obtain or inordinately expensive. Other dyes including indocyanine green or trypan blue have also been used (Coratti *et al.* 2021) in place of methylene blue. Anecdotal reports of clinicians inadvertently using new methylene blue instead of methylene blue with no ill effects have also surfaced, but must be viewed with caution since there are no Material Safety Data Sheet (MSDS) reports on toxicity available for systemic injection of new methylene blue at this time.

Methylene blue dye and other dyes are highly effective in providing visual contrast of the lymphatics from surrounding structures and easing identification of lymphatic vessels. For identification of the thoracic duct, methylene blue is most easily injected into a mesenteric lymph node, typically the ileocecocolic node, via laparotomy or laparoscopy, after which it will flow into the cisterna chyli and thoracic duct within seconds to minutes and persist for variable periods of time, up to an hour or more. Methylene blue can be toxic and is administered at 0.5 mg/kg or less per injection. Dosing of methylene blue at 5 mg/kg has been shown to result in toxicity, which is reflected in reduced packed cell volumes, presumably due to hemolysis (Fingeroth *et al.* 1988). Methylene blue may also induce methemoglobinemia, although this has not been reported as a clinical problem in animals with chylothorax where it has been utilized. Methylene blue can be diluted twofold to fivefold with saline, which allows for larger volumes of injectates and repeated injections without approaching a toxic threshold. An amount of 1–3 mL of diluted methylene blue injected into the mesenteric lymph node is more than sufficient to outline the thoracic duct system to aid in its isolation and ligation. Methylene blue has also been shown to be effective for outlining the thoracic duct when injecting 0.5 mg/kg into a popliteal lymph node using undiluted 1% dye solution (Enwiller *et al.* 2003). However, the popliteal lymph node injection method was not as consistently effective as the use of a mesenteric lymph node, with only 60% of dogs developing adequate coloration of the thoracic duct within 10 minutes of injection. It should also be noted that methylene blue will stain the endothelium of the lymphatics a light blue color that is persistent, and thus is advantageous when dissecting and removing the cisterna chyli.

Indocyanine green comes in powder that is reconstituted with sterile water to a concentration of 2.5 mg/mL. Usually 0.5 mL injected in a mesenteric lymph node is enough to highlight the thoracic duct within 5 minutes. A second injection of another 0.5 mL is always possible. It will diffuse into the lymphatic system and highlight the cisterna chyli and the thoracic duct. When near infrared light is used the indocyanine green becomes fluorescent. The fluorescence can be seen through 5 mm of tissue covering the thoracic duct. It has been most commonly used with thoracoscopy to improve visualization of the thoracic duct and laparoscopy to visualize the cisterna chyli (Steffey & Mayhew, 2018; Dip *et al.* 2015) (Figures 32.1–32.3).

Lymphangiography

The addition of lymphangiography to determine the relevant anatomy of the thoracic duct prior to ligation and to confirm occlusion of the thoracic duct afterward was instrumental in improving outcomes with TDL.

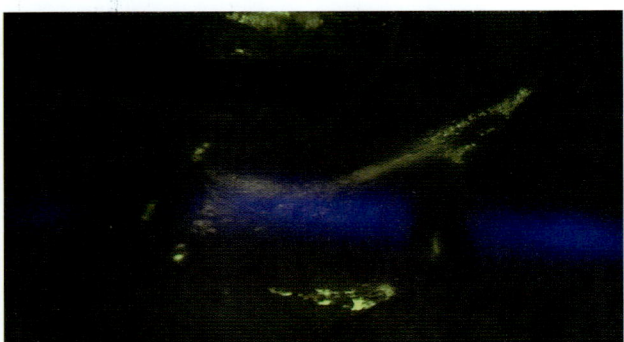

Figure 32.1 Fluorescence of indocyanine green (ICG) in the thoracic duct before dissection of the mediastinum covering the thoracic duct. Near infrared light was used to induce fluorescence.

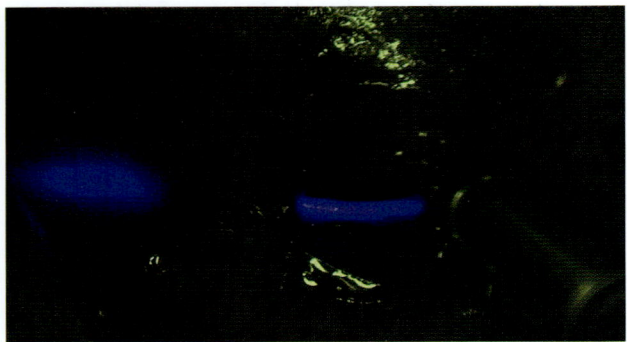

Figure 32.2 Same as Figure 32.1 but after dissection of the mediastinum.

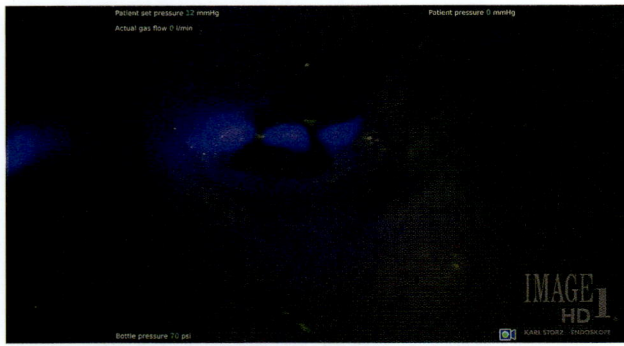

Figure 32.3 Two endoclips have been placed on the thoracic duct after dissection.

Lymphangiography was introduced for use in chylothorax by Birchard *et al.* in 1982. Lymphangiography provided a key quality control step in determining how many channels of the thoracic duct were present in the location of ligation and whether all channels had been identified and obstructed after ligation.

Lymphangiography is currently performed by cannulation of a mesenteric lymphatic and injection of aqueous contrast media directly into the lymphatic system. This is accomplished by injection of a small volume of methylene blue dye into the ileocecocolic lymph node and selection of a relatively straight lymphatic, usually at the base of the duodenum, for cannulation. Once a catheter is placed in a lymphatic (such as with a 1 in. 22-gauge intravenous catheter), the catheter is secured to the mesentery with suture to prevent dislodgment and attached to tubing and stopcocks to facilitate radiographic contrast dye injection. After cannulation, aqueous radiographic contrast, material diluted twofold to reduce its viscosity, is injected and imaged, ideally using digital subtraction radiographic techniques that enhance the contrast detail in the resulting images (Figure 32.4). After the first lymphangiographic study and assessment of the pertinent anatomy, the catheter is reinfused with methylene blue to assist in isolation of the thoracic duct. After isolation of the thoracic duct and collateral channels, thoracic duct ligatures are preplaced and the tubing and cisterna chyli flushed with aqueous radiographic contrast material, to which sufficient methylene blue may be added to allow visual assessment of the location of the contrast in the tubing. Preflushing of the tubing and cisterna chyli with contrast prior to completion of ligation ameliorates the need for larger flush volumes to perform the postligation lymphangiogram, which, in what should now be a closed system, can overpressurize the lymphatics upon injection and cause cisternal or caudal thoracic duct rupture (unpublished observations).

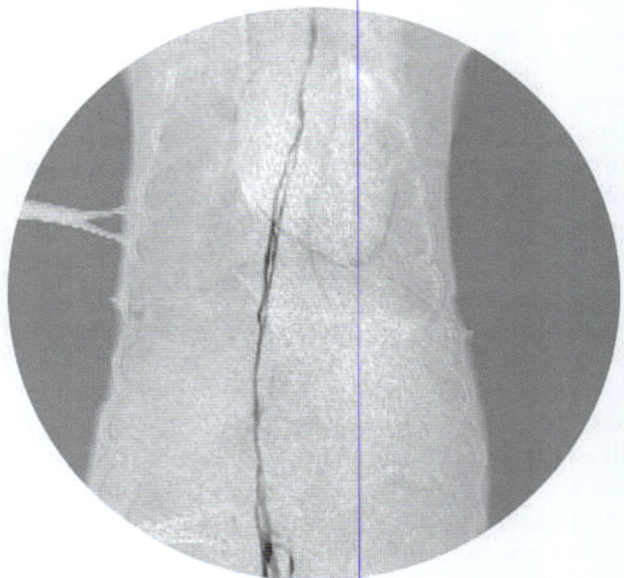

Figure 32.4 Lymphangiogram using aqueous contrast injection of a mesenteric lymphatic and digital subtraction radiography. Note the multiple channels of the thoracic duct as it courses through the thorax.

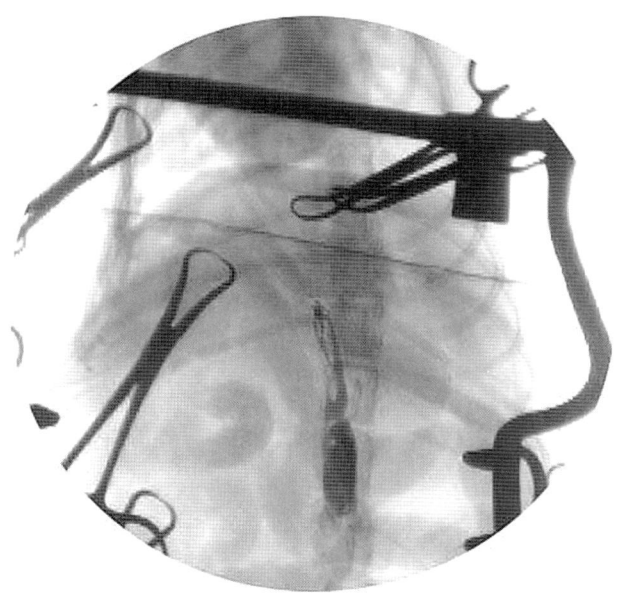

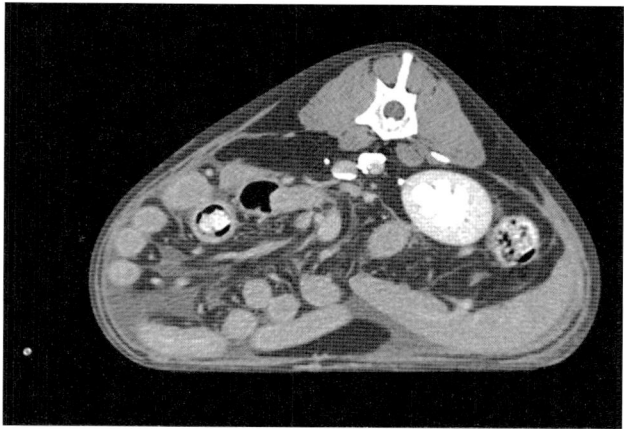

Figure 32.6 Computer tomographic imaging after injection of aqueous contrast material into a popliteal lymph node. The cisterna chyli, filled with contrast material, can be seen clearly covering the dorsal surface of the aorta at this location in the abdomen.

Figure 32.5 Postligation lymphangiogram showing abrupt ending of contrast stream at the site of the thoracic duct ligation. Contrast is also seen pooling within the cisterna chyli in the abdomen.

After completion of the TDL in this scenario, a postligation lymphangiogram can be performed using 3 mL or less of injected contrast material (Figure 32.5). If additional undetected channels of the thoracic duct are present, this process can be repeated until all channels are identified and occluded.

More recently, thoracic duct and cisterna chyli lymphangiography has been described using computed tomography (Figure 32.6). Computed tomography provides much greater detail than digital subtraction radiography (Esterline *et al.* 2005). Contrast may be injected into a mesenteric lymph node, lacteal, or an external site such as the popliteal lymph node, metatarsal pad, or caudal subcutaneous tissue to obtain useful imaging studies (Naganobu *et al.* 2006; Iwanaga *et al.* 2016; Chiang *et al.* 2022). This technique may be easier than by cannulation of a mesenteric lymphatic and does not require a laparotomy incision, but may not provide as detailed a contrast image as can be obtained from direct injection of mesenteric lymphatics. It is also not clear how effective this approach may be in performing postligation lymphangiograms, where lymphatic flow is likely to be considerably slowed.

Lymphangiography can be challenging and may not always be able to be performed successfully (Fossum *et al.* 2004). Further, the best studies may be most easily achieved using digital subtraction radiography in the operating room, a procedure that requires specialized and expensive equipment not available at all surgical

practices. In the current era of high costs and the trend for multiple procedures to be performed at one time for treatment of chylothorax, it is warranted to reevaluate whether all dogs need lymphangiography at first treatment. Going forward, determination of best practices with respect to the relevant available evidence and benefits achievable with lymphangiography should be pursued.

Lymphangiography can provide an important check on the thoroughness of the thoracic duct occlusion by ligation. This was particularly true at the time when methods to outline the duct (feeding of fatty substrates) were not very effective and channels were frequently missed (Birchard *et al.* 1982). In the current era with the use of methylene blue, identification of the thoracic duct is greatly simplified, with a reduced probability of missing additional channels. This is supported by our current clinical experience where over the last 13 years, we have had only one dog out of 46 where lymphangiography affected our treatment by detecting an unligated thoracic duct channel. Further, our observation is that in all dogs where complete occlusion of the thoracic duct is achieved, visual cues to support the conclusion that no significant alternative channels remain unoccluded, such as distension and pressurization of the caudal thoracic duct and cisterna chyli and blockage of transport of methylene blue dye beyond the ligation site upon reinjection, are present and easily observable at the time of surgery. Omission of lymphangiography upon initial treatment of chylothorax where methylene blue is used to identify the lymphatics may allow considerable simplification of the necessary procedures and reduce the cost of treatment. This is an area where further evidence gathering and debate within the field are needed to arrive at a best practices consensus. Regardless, lymphangiography is likely to continue to play an important role when a second surgery is needed after failure of the first treatment to ascertain the conformation of lymphatics, single vessels, or multiple varicosities, bypassing the thoracic duct ligatures. In reoperating on an animal with a previous TDL, it may be difficult to cannulate an abdominal lymphatic vessel to perform the study due to the increased lymph vessel tortuosity and wall thinning that can occur (Sicard et al. 2005). In that situation, a good-quality lymphangiographic study can be obtained by direct injection of the ileocecocolic lymph node with aqueous contrast media. In summary, the role for lymphangiography in chylothorax may be evolving as other methodologies have been introduced. Its use will ultimately depend upon the experience and judgment of the attending surgeon.

Subtotal pericardiectomy

PC has been reported to be successful in resolving chylothorax when used alone or if combined with TDL (Fossum et al. 2004). Initial reported long-term success rates with PC in small case series of spontaneously occurring chylothorax in the dog were 100% (Fossum et al. 2004). However, subsequent reported success rates have varied between 57% and 100% (Carobbi et al. 2008; Allman et al. 2010; Bussadori et al. 2011; McAnulty 2011), with a study in our center achieving 60% success. The proposed rationale for PC is to remove a restrictive pericardium that affects right heart filling and elevates

venous pressures, which subsequently affect the flow of chyle from the thoracic duct to the venous circulation (Fossum et al. 2004). This rationale may also relate to theories related to experiments where partial cranial vena cava ligation produced chylothorax in 70% of normal dogs (Fossum & Birchard 1986). This restrictive pericardium may also be due to epipericardial fibrosis induced by the chylothorax, hence preventing a response to TDL (Figure 32.7), or due to a primary pericardial condition. Documented evidence of a restrictive pericardial disease with effects on right heart pressure dynamics as a cause of chylothorax in animals has been rare, with only a single case reported in the veterinary literature (Campbell et al. 1995). Thus, it remains unclear if the hypothesis regarding the mechanism of benefit of PC for chylothorax is correct for the broader population of patients presented with idiopathic chylothorax. Regardless of the mechanism of effect, current literature suggests there may be a beneficial effect of PC for the treatment of chylothorax in some dogs and cats.

It is unclear why results with PC appear to be highly variable between groups (Fossum et al. 2004; Carobbi et al. 2008; Allman et al. 2010; Bussadori et al. 2011; McAnulty 2011). The reasons for this variance may lie in possible differences in the technical performance of the procedure, differences in the underlying disease in the reported patient cohorts, or natural variances in response to treatment that appear magnified when studies with small patient numbers are reported. With respect to differences in the pericardial excision, the first report on the application of PC with TDL for idiopathic chylothorax

(a)

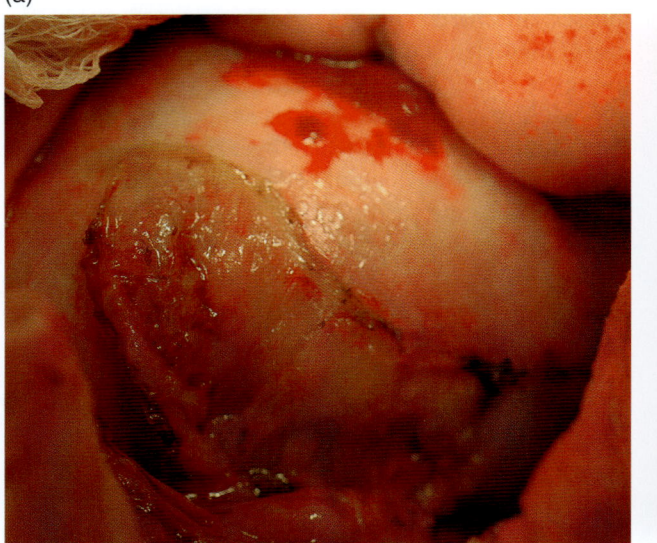

(b)

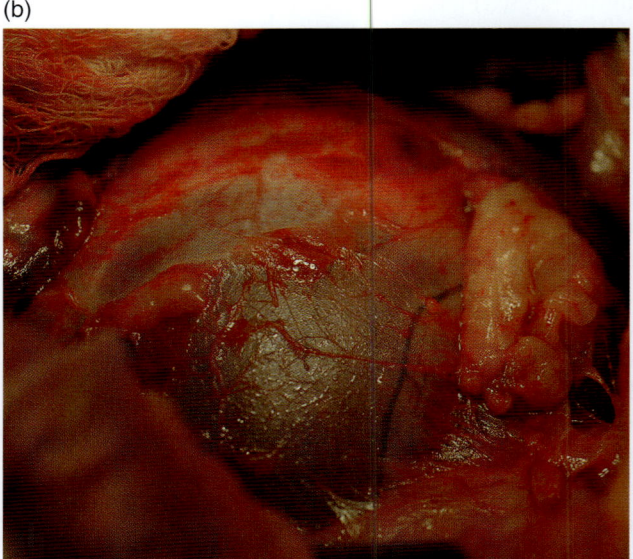

Figure 32.7 (a) Surface of pericardium showing severe fibrous epipericardial reaction due to the chylous effusion. (b) Surface of pericardium after stripping of epipericardial fibrous tissue. The pericardium in these animals is frequently normal in appearance and exhibits only mild inflammatory reaction on histopathology.

did not describe the extent of the PC (Fossum *et al.* 2004). Subsequent reports have been more specific, with either a subphrenic PC (Carobbi *et al.* 2008; Bussadori *et al.* 2011; Mayhew *et al.* 2012, 2019) or creation of a 4 cm pericardial window with "2–3 vertical fenestrations made in the pericardium starting at the phrenic nerve and extending to the apex of the heart" (Allman *et al.* 2010). In our recent study, removal of the pericardium was more extensive, with a subphrenic margin on the contralateral side and removal of the pericardium to the base of the pulmonary arteries, after elevation of the phrenic nerve, on the ipsilateral surface. In addition, this was described to include incising the pericardium to create a "butterfly" opening of the residual pericardium that may have been somewhat analogous to the maneuvers described by Allman *et al.* (2010), where 86% (6 of 7 dogs) achieved resolution of chylothorax. Regardless, the fact that in studies with more rather than less pericardial tissue excision there was variable efficacy likely obviates any argument that a more extensive pericardial resection would potentially resolve the differences in reported outcomes.

It is feasible that differences in response to PC in these case series may lie in differences in the inciting pathology of the chylothorax between the study patient cohorts. Idiopathic chylothorax is a broad-based diagnosis and feasibly includes a range of inciting pathologies. One such difference may be in the incidence of restrictive pericardial disease; a hypothesis that presumes that restrictive pericardial disease plays a significant role in idiopathic chylothorax. However, this potential difference between studies remains speculative due to the difficulty in diagnosing pericardial restriction, lack of such data in past reports, and the lack of knowledge regarding the relative degree of pericardial restriction needed to induce chylothorax.

Diagnosis of pericardial restriction, specifically with reference to chylothorax, may be difficult to achieve with any degree of precision. In the past, pericardial restriction was best ascertained by measurement of right ventricular pressures and recognition of a "square root sign" in the ventricular pressure trace (Campbell *et al.* 1995). This pressure trace is due to early rapid diastolic filling, causing a rapid increase in ventricular pressure, followed by an early diastole termination of flow, resulting in a major increase of diastolic pressures in all four cardiac chambers, with a dip and plateau pattern seen on pressure traces. Doppler ultrasound has subsequently been used to detect a restriction to filling pattern on the Doppler flow velocity curves (Nishimura 2001), but these changes may be subtle and the severity of change needed for pericardial restriction to play a role in idiopathic chylothorax remains unknown.

The supporting hypothesis for the role of PC in the treatment of chylothorax is that a restrictive pericardial condition occurs secondary to a thickened pericardium that "would increase systemic venous pressures" (Fossum *et al.* 2004), although there were no data available to support this hypothesis. In a recent study on PC in idiopathic chylothorax, CVP was measured before and after PC as a simple method to begin to garner data that might provide support for the hypothesized role of increased venous pressures in chylothorax, and to obtain objective data regarding the impact of PC on lowering central venous pressure in dogs with chylothorax (McAnulty 2011). In that study, the average CVP measured under anesthesia in the dogs was 6.9 ± 0.7 mmHg, which is within the range described as normal for both awake and anesthetized dogs (0–8.8 mmHg) (Guyton & Greganti 1956; Oakley *et al.* 1997; Chow *et al.* 2006; Nelson *et al.* 2010). Individually, 12 dogs had averaged CVP values in a normal range, but 2 dogs had averaged CVP measurements that would typically be considered somewhat elevated at 10 and 12.3 mmHg. However, it should be noted that absolute CVP values are a poor measure of right-sided vascular conditions due to the measure's susceptibility to change through factors such as anesthesia, positive-pressure ventilation, and hydration status, as well as disease conditions and measurement variables. CVP is best used as a relative indicator of change after an intervention such as fluid therapy or, in this case, after PC. Eight dogs treated by PC in this study had CVP measurements both before and after PC, but only one showed any change in CVP after PC with a 1.9 mmHg reduction, although both the pre- and post-PC CVP values would be considered to be within a normal range in that dog.

A lack of effect of PC on CVP would argue strongly against a hypothesis of impacts on elevated venous pressures as a mechanism where PC plays a role in resolving chylothorax. However, it is also feasible that other factors, such as chronic myocardial hypoxia, might create an environment where a rapid change in venous pressure after PC might be unlikely to be due to reduced cardiac contractility that may take some time to recover. Further, it is also possible that the cohort of patients in this study were not affected by venous hypertension and that this may also explain the reduced efficacy of PC in this case series (60% success) relative to previous reports in the literature. In the future, better data will be needed to assess the validity of a venous hypertension hypothesis and may include right ventricular pressure measurements or careful comparisons of inflow velocities and other echocardiographic findings. In this study, we attempted in several animals to obtain right ventricular pressure recordings, but found that significant arrhythmias were commonly induced, likely due to an irritable hypoxic myocardium.

In summary, PC does appear to provide benefits in resolving chylothorax in some patients, although the strength of the available evidence is low (Reeves *et al.* 2020). The mechanism behind this effect and the overall efficacy of PC remain unknown. Considering that PC is not a risk-free procedure, future efforts targeted at diagnostic testing to ascertain which patients might best benefit from this procedure, as well as studies examining the relevant mechanisms, would be fruitful in advancing the understanding and treatment of chylothorax.

Cisterna chyli ablation

CCA was first performed on a clinical case in 1997 by McAnulty and subsequently has been studied in a laboratory study, a clinical case series, and a prospective comparative randomized trial (Sicard *et al.* 2005; Hayashi *et al.* 2005; McAnulty 2011). CCA is targeted at alleviating the common primary life-threatening clinical sign of diseases that cause chylothorax (i.e., accumulation of chyle in the pleural space) and does not address potential underlying disease mechanisms. CCA has been applied in combination with TDL in the studies to date and has not been examined as a standalone procedure. The therapeutic goals of CCA are to (i) detach the lymphatic drainage pathways of the abdominal viscera from the thoracic duct as much as possible; (ii) temporarily alleviate lymphatic hypertension induced by TDL and thereby reduce the impetus for development of collateral lymphatics around the TDL suture sites while new lymphaticovenous drainage pathways are forming; and (iii) promote new lymphatic drainage pathways into the venous circulation outside of the thoracic cavity.

The cisterna chyli is a saccular structure that lies dorsal to the abdominal aorta, but may also have portions that are ventral to the aorta, as well as having plexiform distributions in its caudal location (Rengert *et al.* 2021; Chiang *et al.* 2022). CCA was originally performed via a midline laparotomy as the procedure was being developed, but more recent contributions have shown that a right flank approach in the dog can be more efficiently used for both CCA and TDL via a transdiaphragmatic approach using a single abdominal wall incision (Staiger *et al.* 2011). This is currently the more preferred approach. More recently there are also reports where the cisterna chyli may be effectively ablated using a minimally invasive laparoscopic approach (Morris *et al.* 2019). From a midline abdominal incision, the cisterna chyli is best approached by incision of the peritoneum lateral to the left kidney and medial retraction of the kidney to expose the tissues dorsal to the aorta (Figure 32.8). Although the cisterna chyli is positioned slightly more toward the right side, it is obscured by the

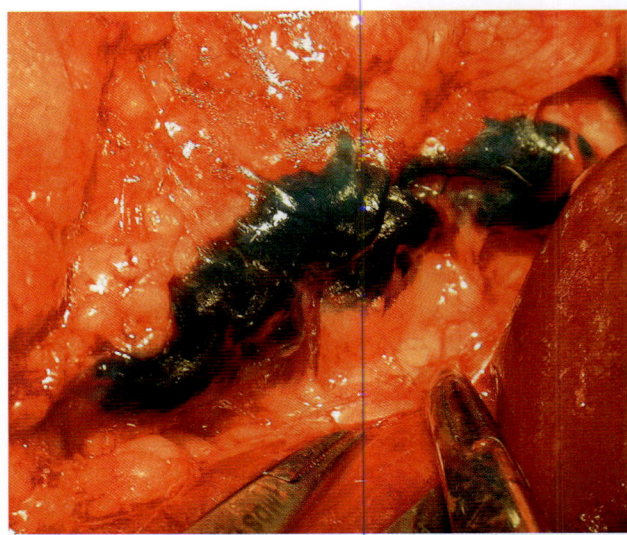

Figure 32.8 Cisterna chyli dorsal and lateral to the aorta, as seen from a midline laparotomy incision on the left side after injection of methylene blue into a mesenteric lymphatic. The cisterna chyli is distended due to prior ligation of the thoracic duct.

vena cava on the right, and thus with a midline abdominal approach it is more advantageous to address from the left side. The vena cava does not present an obstruction from either a flank or laparoscopic approach, and these are more amenable to a right-sided surgery in the dog (Figure 32.9).

The cisterna chyli is easily observed after injection of a mesenteric lymph node with methylene blue. Further, methylene blue will lightly dye the lining membrane of the cisterna chyli and aid in its complete extirpation after it is ruptured. The goal of CCA is to remove all visible cisternal membranes and connections to the thoracic duct to force the lymphatics to develop new lymphaticovenous connections rather than reroute through the thoracic duct. To date, CCA has been done in concert with TDL (which is done first to aid in thoracic duct identification). This necessitates a bicavitary approach to access both structures. A right flank abdominal incision combined with a transdiaphragmatic approach to the thoracic duct achieves these aims.

Clinical results with CCA to date have shown a resolution rate for chylothorax in between 83% and 86% of dogs (Hayashi *et al.* 2005; McAnulty 2011). The proposed hypothetical benefit of CCA, rerouting of chyle into the venous circulation outside of the thorax, is supported by a laboratory study in normal dogs, where 5 of 6 dogs had shunting of chyle into the abdominal venous circulation (Sicard *et al.* 2005) (Figure 32.10). It is not known whether combining CCA with PC in select patients will increase the success rate seen with either procedure. However, in a prospective trial of CCA and

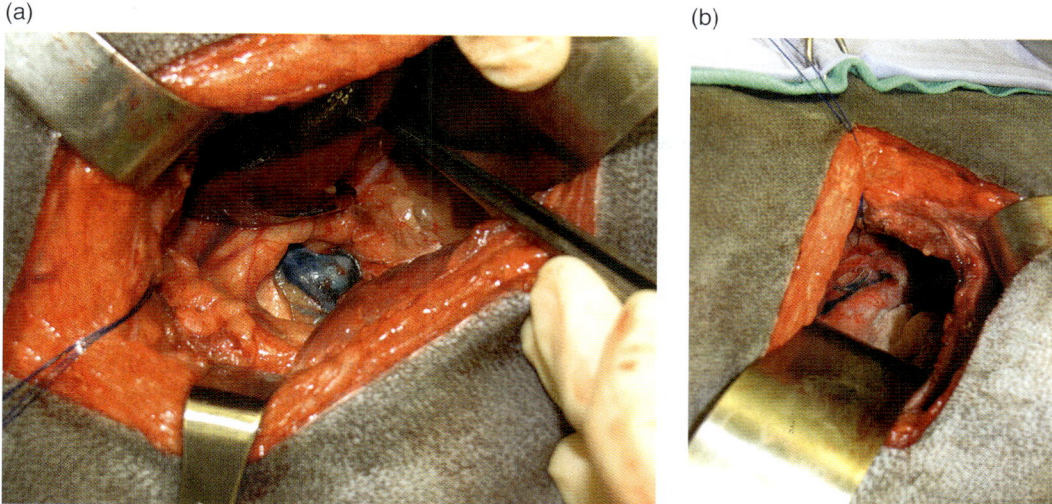

(a)   (b)

Figure 32.9 View of cisterna chyli and thoracic duct via a right flank approach and injection of methylene blue in a mesenteric lymph node. (a) The cisterna chyli is seen dorsal and lateral to the surface of the aorta from the right flank approach. (b) The thoracic duct (with branching) is seen dorsal to the thoracic aorta after a transdiaphragmatic approach. This surgical strategy allows access to both the cisterna chyli and thoracic duct through a single body wall incision.

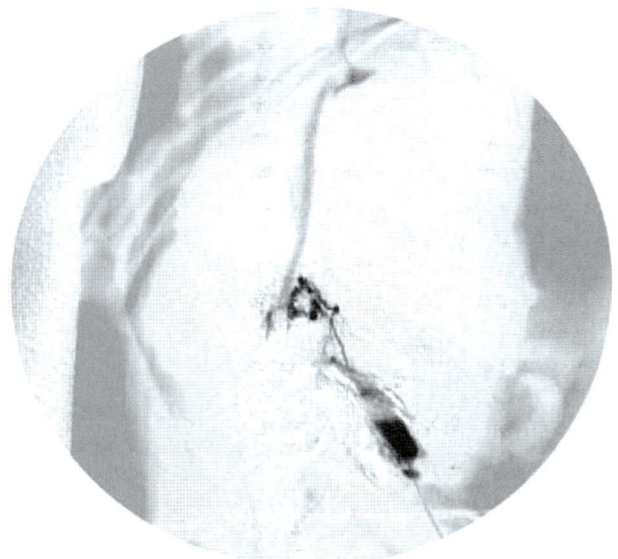

Figure 32.10 Lymphangiographic study using radiographic digital subtraction technique with contrast injection into a mesenteric lymph node one month after cisterna chyli ablation (CCA). Contrast can be seen entering a plexus of lymphatics at the site of the CCA and draining directly into the abdominal vena cava.

PC (McAnulty 2011), there was a limited number of CCA cases that were finally able to resolve the chylothorax after a follow-up PC procedure. This may provide some support for clinicians that perform the "trifecta" of procedures: CCA, TDL, and PC at one time, particularly with clients with limited resources for whom a follow-up

surgery would not be feasible. Future studies in this area may be best focused on the development of less invasive surgical approaches that are able to simplify the overall procedure of TDL–CCA and PC without reducing the rate of success in resolving chylothorax. It should be noted that PC, particularly in a situation with chronic myocardial hypoxia, carries some finite degree of risk for inducing arrhythmias that may potentially be fatal, and thus should be considered carefully within a treatment regimen.

Other procedures

There are several other procedures currently gaining attention for the treatment of chylothorax. Adhesive embolization using cyanoacrylic adhesive (Pardo *et al.* 1989), with the addition of embolizing the cisterna chyli in addition to the thoracic duct, has more recently been reexamined (Clendaniel *et al.* 2014), although outcomes in a large series of cases remain unknown. Omentalization of the thorax by omental draping through a diaphragmatic incision has previously been proposed as a treatment for chylothorax and is sporadically done at various centers (Williams & Niles 1999; Lafond *et al.* 2002; Stewart & Padgett 2010; Bussadori *et al.* 2011; Da Silva & Monnet 2011). However, there is currently no evidence in the published literature that clearly supports a positive effect of omentalization for chylothorax. In all published reports where omentalization was performed, either TDL or surgery in the area of the thoracic duct was also performed. Thus, separation of the effects of the separate procedures is not possible.

Evidence to support a role for omentalization would require a prospective trial where omentalization when combined with TDL was shown to improve on results of TDL alone, or evidence that thoracic omentalization alone results in resolution of chylothorax.

The rationale behind thoracic omentalization for chylothorax is difficult to discern. The omental lymphatics feed back to the cisterna chyli and thoracic duct and thus are not a likely route for lymphatic absorption to the venous circulation. Other mechanisms, such as provision of "healing factors" or direct venous absorption, do not seem plausible. Until such time as objective evidence of efficacy for transdiaphragmatic omental draping can be presented, this treatment cannot be considered a viable therapeutic option for chylothorax. However, it does seem feasible that transdiaphragmatic omental draping may have a role for the treatment of nonchylous effusions where the thoracic duct drainage is not impaired or has been rerouted by a previous treatment.

Outcomes

Treatment of chylothorax can provide life-long resolution of chylothorax. However, in some case series, recurrence of chylothorax has been noted up to 1–2 years after treatment (Bussadori *et al.* 2011). Resolution of restrictive pleural fibrosis has not been documented in detail, but if animals survive initial treatment, pleural fibrosis may resolve to some degree, or at least be tolerated over long time periods.

In some animals, chylothorax may resolve but a significant nonchylous effusion may persist (Smeak *et al.* 1987; Birchard *et al.* 1988; Fossum *et al.* 2004; McAnulty 2011). Nonchylous effusions may be tolerated for very long periods, as they do not appear to induce pleural fibrosis like a chylous effusion and may be managed by intermittent aspiration. Management of chronic effusions may also be eased by placement of a pleural port drain system rather than periodic needle thoracocentesis. The cause of a nonchylous effusion is not known, but may feasibly either represent lymphatic drainage from the head and cranial thorax entering the area of lymphangiectasis in the cranial mediastinum, be secondary to chronic pleural inflammation, or be due to a previously undiscovered pathology such as mesothelioma (Allman *et al.* 2010). The role of inflammation in production of a nonchylous effusion is supported by both cytologic analysis of the effusion and resolution of the effusion in 60% of a limited number of dogs with such an effusion in a recent study after an anti-inflammatory course of steroids (McAnulty 2011). In dogs where a course of steroids is not effective in resolving the effusion, an underlying pathology should be more vigorously pursued via echocardiography, biopsies, or PC if it has not previously been done.

In spite of recent improvements in outcomes, chylothorax remains a difficult clinical problem. The procedures described here appear to improve on historical success rates with TDL alone, but continue to fail to control the chylous effusion in 15–20% of dogs. However, a key observation is our recent case series is that a second "salvage" surgery may frequently be successful and should be recommended. Two dogs in this series that had follow-up second surgeries survived a sufficient time to evaluate outcomes, and both had resolution of the chylothorax. In both dogs, the thoracic duct had reestablished a substantial collateral vessel or vessels that bypassed the original ligature sites. These dogs were treated with a repeat TDL and an additional procedure such as CCA or PC. Due to the fact that each of these dogs had two procedures performed as part of the salvage effort, it cannot be determined whether simply readdressing the thoracic duct would have been sufficient for success, or whether the added procedure of CCA or PC was either necessary or increased the probability of a good outcome in these individuals. Previous cases reported in the literature where success was obtained after failure of an initial surgery also support a recommendation for reoperation, which should at least include thoracic duct reexploration and religation if feasible, to achieve resolution of chylothorax (Fossum *et al.* 2004; Carobbi *et al.* 2008; Bussadori *et al.* 2011; Allman *et al.* 2010). Reoperation of a previously failed surgical treatment for chylothorax would be considered a strong indication for the performance of lymphangiography so that a determination of the location and number of recurrent collateral lymphatics can be made.

Future directions

The study of chylothorax remains a field that is wide open for new investigation. Areas that are in development or in need of study include new methods for resolution of the chylous effusion, studies that better characterize why certain breeds of dog are prone to this condition, and exploration of new approaches to the treatment and development of effective means for medical management.

One such effort is targeted at direct anastomosis of the thoracic duct to the venous circulation. This has been a recent focus within both the human and veterinary medical arenas. Anastomosis has been performed in humans using microvascular suturing techniques (Othman *et al.* 2021; Lindenblatt *et al.* 2020) and successfully in a veterinary experimental study using microvascular anastomotic clips (Shriwise *et al* 2021). Further development on anastomotic techniques using synthetic conduits or vascular grafts warrant study, as well as evaluation of the method in patients with naturally occurring disease. It remains to be determined how effective such measures will be in ameliorating the accumulation of chyle in the pleural space and how durable this solution is over time.

Other avenues for study include why specific breeds, such as Afghan hounds, are prone to chylothorax, or what role impingements on the cranial end of the thoracic duct may play in this disease. One hypothesis may be that these dogs such as Afghan hounds are prone to thoracic duct compression or occlusion due to the extreme conformation of their thorax that creates a very narrow thoracic inlet. The cranial termination of the thoracic duct is variable. It is described as terminating as a single vessel in 50% of dogs, ending at the junction of the left external jugular vein and left subclavian vein, and usually has an ampulla-like dilatation prior to its termination (Hermanson *et al.* 2020). In this conformation, the thoracic duct traverses the thoracic inlet before emptying into the venous circulation, and may be prone to compression in dogs with these extreme thoracic conformations. Possible support for this putative mechanism may be a case report of a single dog with a chondroma lesion of the left first rib (Watine *et al.* 2003) that had resolution of its chylothorax after removal of the rib and expansile lesion. Another case, reported by Suter and Greene (1971), describes chylothorax related to an abnormal termination of the thoracic duct, supporting a role for a terminal obstruction of the thoracic duct as one cause of chylothorax. First rib resection or lateralization may be one avenue to pursue for study in dog breeds with narrow deep chest conformations. It may also be of value to focus study in clinical cases on the ampulla of the thoracic duct where it empties into the jugular vein. Abnormalities in that location may create some degree of obstruction and might be addressed through placement of vascular stents or other maneuvers.

Lastly, the role of medical management remains an area ripe for study. Controlled and blinded studies are needed to determine the efficacy of medical regimens. Further, exploration of new drugs may also be fruitful. However, specific candidate drugs for study are not currently known.

In summary, chylothorax remains a challenging condition and performing high-value studies is difficult at a single institution due to the relatively low number of cases that may be presented. Future studies should focus on multi-institutional efforts to overcome this barrier to progress.

References

Alander, J.T., Villet, O.M., Patilla, T. et al. (2015). Review of indocyanine green for imaging in surgery. In: *Fluorescence Imaging for Surgeons* (ed. F.D. Dip, T. Ishizawa, N. Kokudo, et al.), 35–53. New York: Springer.

Allman, D.A., Radlinsky, M.G., Ralph, A.G., and Rawlings, C.A. (2010). Thoracoscopic thoracic duct ligation and thoracoscopic pericardectomy for treatment of chylothorax in dogs. *Veterinary Surgery* 39: 21–27.

Birchard, S.J., Cantwell, H.D., and Bright, R.M. (1982). Lymphangiography and ligation of the canine thoracic duct: a study in normal dogs and three dogs with chylothorax. *Journal of the American Animal Hospital Association* 18: 769–777.

Birchard, S.J., Smeak, D.D., and Fossum, T.W. (1988). Results of thoracic duct ligation in dogs with chylothorax. *Journal of the American Veterinary Medical Association* 193: 68–71.

Birchard, S.J., Smeak, D.D., and McLoughlin, M.A. (1995). Chylothorax in the dog and cat: a review. *Lymphology* 28: 64–72.

Birchard, S.J., Smeak, D.D., and McLoughlin, M.A. (1998). Treatment of idiopathic chylothorax in dogs and cats. *Journal of the American Veterinary Medical Association* 212: 652–657.

Bussadori, R., Provera, A., Martano, M. et al. (2011). Pleural omentalisation with en bloc ligation of the thoracic duct and pericardiectomy for idiopathic chylothorax in nine dogs and four cats. *Veterinary Journal* 188: 234–236.

Cahalane, A.K., Flanders, J.A., Steffey, M.A., and Rassnick, K.M. (2007). Use of vascular access ports with intrathoracic drains for treatment of pleural effusion in three dogs. *Journal of the American Veterinary Medical Association* 230: 527–531.

Campbell, S.L., Forrester, S.D., Johnston, S.A. et al. (1995). Chylothorax associated with constrictive pericarditis in a dog. *Journal of the American Veterinary Medical Association* 206: 1561–1564.

Carobbi, B., White, R.A.S., and Romanelli, G. (2008). Treatment of idiopathic chylothorax in 14 dogs by ligation of the thoracic duct and partial pericardiectomy. *Veterinary Record* 163: 743–745.

Cesarone, M.R., Belcaro, G., Rohdewald, P. et al. (2006). Rapid relief of signs/symptoms in chronic venous microangiopathy with pycnogenol: a prospective, controlled study. *Angiology* 57: 569–576.

Chiang, C., Chen, K.S., Chiu, H.C. et al. (2022). Computed tomography lymphangiography via intrametatarsal pad injection is feasible in cats with chylothorax. *American Journal of Veterinary Research* 83 (2): 133–139.

Chow, R.S., Kass, P.H., and Haskins, S.C. (2006). Evaluation of peripheral and central venous pressure in awake dogs and cats. *American Journal of Veterinary Research* 67: 1987–1991.

Clendaniel, D.C., Weisse, C., Culp, W.T. et al. (2014). Salvage cisterna chyli and thoracic duct glue embolization in 2 dogs with recurrent idiopathic chylothorax. *Journal of Veterinary Internal Medicine* 28: 672–677.

Coratti, F., Barbato, G., and Cianchi, F. (2021). Thoracic duct identification with indocyanine green fluorescence: a simplified method. *Diseases of the Esophagus* 34 (3): doaa130.

Dip, F.D., Ishizawa, T., Kokudo, N. et al. (ed.) (2015). *Fluorescence Imaging for Surgeons*. New York: Springer.

Enwiller, T.M., Radlinsky, M.G., Mason, D.E., and Roush, J.K. (2003). Popliteal and mesenteric lymph node injection with methylene blue for coloration of the thoracic duct in dogs. *Veterinary Surgery* 32: 359–364.

Esterline, M.L., Radlinsky, M.G., Biller, D.S. et al. (2005). Comparison of radiographic and computed tomography lymphangiography for identification of the canine thoracic duct. *Veterinary Radiology & Ultrasound* 46: 391–395.

Fingeroth, J.M., Smeak, D.D., and Jacobs, R.M. (1988). Intravenous methylene blue infusion for intraoperative indentification of parathyroid gland and pancreatic islet-cell tumors in dogs. Part 1: experimental determination of dose-related staining efficacy and toxicity. *Journal of the American Animal Hospital Association* 24: 165–173.

Fossum, T.W. (1993). Feline chylothorax. *Compendium of Continuing Education* 15: 549–563.

Fossum, T.W. and Birchard, S.J. (1986). Lymphangiographic evaluation of experimentally induced chylothorax after ligation of the cranial vena cava in dogs. *American Journal of Veterinary Research* 47: 967–971.

Fossum, T.W., Birchard, S.J., and Jacobs, R.M. (1986). Chylothorax in 34 dogs. *Journal of the American Veterinary Medical Association* 188: 1315–1317.

Fossum, T.W., Miller, M.W., Rogers, K.S. et al. (1994). Chylothorax associated with right-sided heart failure in five cats. *Journal of the American Veterinary Medical Association* 204: 84–89.

Fossum, T.W., Mertens, M.M., Miller, M.W. et al. (2004). Thoracic duct ligation and pericardectomy for treatment of idiopathic chylothorax. *Journal of Veterinary Internal Medicine* 18: 307–310.

Geizer, A.R.M., Downs, M.O., Newell, S.M. et al. (1997). Accessory lung lobe torsion and chylothorax in an afghan hound. *Journal of the American Animal Hospital Association* 33: 171–176.

Guyton, A.C. and Greganti, F.P. (1956). A physiologic reference point for measuring circulatory pressures in the dog; particularly venous pressure. *American Journal of Physiology* 185: 137–141.

Hayashi, K., Sicard, G., Gellasch, K. et al. (2005). Cisterna chyli ablation with thoracic duct ligation for chylothorax: results in eight dogs. *Veterinary Surgery* 34: 519–523.

Hermanson, J.W., de Lahunta, A., and Evans, H.E. (2020). The lymphatic system. In: *Miller and Evans' Anatomy of the Dog*, 5e, 616–649. Philadelphia, PA: Elsevier.

Hodges, C.C., Fossum, T.W., and Evering, W. (1993). Evaluation of thoracic duct healing after experimental laceration and transection. *Veterinary Surgery* 22: 431–435.

Iwanaga, T., Tokunaga, S., and Momoi, Y. (2016). Thoracic duct lymphography by subcutaneous contrast agent injection in a dog with chylothorax. *Open Veterinary Journal* 6: 238–241.

Kanai, H., Furuya, M., Hagiwara, K. et al. (2020). Efficacy of en bloc thoracic duct ligation in combination with pericardiectomy by video-assisted thoracoscopic surgery for canine idiopathic chylothorax. *Veterinary Surgery* 49 (Suppl 1): O102–O111.

Kanai, H., Furuya, M., Yoneji, K. et al. (2021). Canine idiopathic chylothorax: anatomic characterization of the pre- and postoperative thoracic duct using computed tomography lymphography. *Veterinary Radiology & Ultrasound* 62: 429–436.

Korpes, K., Kolenc, M., Trbojević Vukičević, T., and Đuras, M. (2021). Anatomical variations of the thoracic duct in the dog. *Anatomia, Histologia, Embryologia* 50: 1015–1025.

Lafond, E., Weirich, W.E., and Salisbury, S.K. (2002). Omentalization of the thorax for treatment of idiopathic chylothorax with constrictive pleuritis in a cat. *Journal of the American Animal Hospital Association* 38: 74–78.

Lindenblatt, N., Puippe, G., Broglie, M.A. et al. (2020). Lymphovenous anastomosis for the treatment of thoracic duct lesion: a case report and systematic review of literature. *Annals of Plastic Surgery* 84: 402–408.

MacDonald, N.J., Noble, P.J., and Burrow, R.D. (2008). Efficacy of en bloc ligation of the thoracic duct: descriptive study in 14 dogs. *Veterinary Surgery* 37: 696–701.

Markham, K.M., Glover, J.L., Welsh, R.J. et al. (2000). Octreotide in the treatment of thoracic duct injuries. *American Surgeon* 66: 1165–1167.

Mayhew, P.D., Culp, W.T., Mayhew, K.N., and Morgan, O.D. (2012). Minimally invasive treatment of idiopathic chylothorax in dogs by thoracoscopic thoracic duct ligation and subphrenic pericardiectomy: 6 cases (2007-2010). *Journal of the American Veterinary Medical Association* 241: 904–909.

Mayhew, P.D., Steffey, M.A., Fransson, B.A. et al. (2019). Long-term outcome of video-assisted thoracoscopic thoracic duct ligation and pericardectomy in dogs with chylothorax: a multi-institutional study of 39 cases. *Veterinary Surgery* 48 (S1): O112–O120.

McAnulty, J.F. (2011). Prospective comparison of cisterna chyli ablation to pericardectomy for treatment of spontaneously occurring idiopathic chylothorax in the dog. *Veterinary Surgery* 40: 926–934.

Morris, K.P., Singh, A., Holt, D.E. et al. (2019). Hybrid single-port laparoscopic cisterna chyli ablation for the adjunct treatment of chylothorax disease in dogs. *Veterinary Surgery* 48 (S1): O121–O129.

Naganobu, K., Ohigashi, Y., Akiyoshi, T. et al. (2006). Lymphography of the thoracic duct by percutaneous injection of iohexol into the popliteal lymh node of dogs: experimental study and clinical application. *Veterinary Surgery* 35: 377–381.

Nakabayashi, H., Sagara, H., Usukura, N. et al. (1981). Effect of somatostatin on the flow rate and triglyceride levels of thoracic duct lymp in normal and vagotomized dogs. *Diabetes* 30: 440–445.

Nelson, N.C., Drost, W.T., Lerche, P., and Bonagura, J.D. (2010). Noninvasive estimation of central venous pressure in anesthetized dogs by measurement of hepatic venous blood flow velocity and abdominal venous diameter. *Veterinary Radiology & Ultrasound* 51: 313–323.

Nishimura, R.A. (2001). Constrictive pericarditis in the modern era: a diagnostic dilemma. *Heart* 86: 619–623.

Oakley, R.E., Olivier, B., Eyster, G., and Hauptman, J.G. (1997). Experimental evaluation of central venous pressure monitoring in the dog. *Journal of the American Animal Hospital Association* 33: 77–82.

Othman, S., Azoury, S.C., Klifto, K. et al. (2021). Microsurgical thoracic duct lymphovenous bypass in the adult population. *Plastic and Reconstructive Surgery* 9: e3875.

Pardo, A.D., Bright, R.M., Walker, M.A., and Patton, C.S. (1989). Transcatheter thoracic duct embolization in the dog: an experimental study. *Veterinary Surgery* 18: 279–285.

Reeves, L.A., Anderson, K.M., Luther, J.K., and Torres, B.T. (2020). Treatment of idiopathic chylothorax in dogs and cats: a systematic review. *Veterinary Surgery* 49: 70–79.

Rengert, R., Wilkinson, T., Singh, A. et al. (2021). Morphology of the cisterna chyli in nine dogs with idiopathic chylothorax and in six healthy dogs assessed by computed tomographic lymphangiography. *Veterinary Surgery* 50: 223–229.

Shriwise, G.B., Loeber, S.J., and Hardie, R.J. (2021). Lymphaticovenous anastomosis of the caudal thoracic duct to an intercostal vein: a canine cadaver study. *Veterinary Surgery* 50: 207–212.

Sicard, G.K., Waller, K.R., and McAnulty, J.F. (2005). The effect of cisterna chyli ablation combined with thoracic duct ligation on abdominal lymphatic drainage. *Veterinary Surgery* 34: 64–70.

da Silva, C.A. and Monnet, E. (2011). Long-term outcome of dogs treated surgically for idiopathic chylothorax: 11 cases (1995-2009). *Journal of the American Veterinary Medical Association* 239: 107–113.

Smeak, D.D., Gallagher, L., Birchard, S.J., and Fossum, T.W. (1987). Management of intractable pleural effusion in a dog with a pleuroperitoneal shunt. *Veterinary Surgery* 16: 212–216.

Staiger, B.A., Stanley, B.J., and McAnulty, J.F. (2011). Single paracostal approach to thoracic duct and cisterna chyli: experimental study and case series. *Veterinary Surgery* 40: 786–794.

Steffey, M.A. and Mayhew, P.D. (2018). Use of direct near-infrared fluorescent lymphography for thoracoscopic thoracic duct identification in 15 dogs with chylothorax. *Veterinary Surgery* 47: 267–276.

Stewart, K. and Padgett, S. (2010). Chylothorax treated via thoracic duct ligation and omentalization. *Journal of the American Animal Hospital Association* 46: 312–317.

Suter, P.F. and Greene, R.W. (1971). Chylothorax in a dog with abnormal termination of the thoracic duct. *Journal of the American Veterinary Medical Association* 159: 302–309.

Thompson, M.S., Cohn, L.A., and Jordan, R.C. (1999). Use of rutin for medical management of idiopathic chylothorax in four cats. *Journal of the American Veterinary Medical Association* 215: 345–348.

Watine, S., Hamaide, A., Peeters, D. et al. (2003). Resolution of chylothorax after resection of rib chondroma in a dog. *Journal of Small Animal Practice* 44: 546–549.

Williams, J.M. and Niles, J.D. (1999). Use of omentum as a physiologic drain for treatment of chylothorax in a dog. *Veterinary Surgery* 28: 61–65.

33

Pyothorax in Dogs and Cats

Chad Schmiedt

Pyothorax is an infection of the pleural space. Pyothorax occurs in dogs and cats and is characterized by a septic, suppurative pleural effusion. Pyothorax is reported in about 14–16% of cats and dogs with pleural effusion (Davies & Forrester 1996; Mellanby *et al.* 2002). Animals with pyothorax can have severe systemic signs, and despite a variety of potential causes the principles of therapy are relatively similar between species and etiologies.

Etiology

Pyothorax is most often associated with a bacterial infection. In one study of dogs and cats presenting with suppurative pleural effusion, bacteria were cultured from 47 of 51 dogs (92%) and 45 of 47 cats (96%) (Walker *et al.* 2000). Common causative bacteria are listed in Table 33.1. Obligate anaerobic bacteria are commonly associated with pyothorax, and in one study they were found in 28 of 47 dogs (60%) and 40 of 45 cats (89%) with positive cultures (Walker *et al.* 2000). Facultative anaerobic bacteria are also encountered. Polymicrobial infections occur frequently and have been reported in 58% of patients with pyothorax (Boothe *et al.* 2010). *Candida albicans*, *Spirocerca lupi*, and *Crytococcus gatti* have also been reported as causes of pyothorax in dogs or cats (McCaw *et al.* 1984; Barrs *et al.* 2005; Klainbart *et al.* 2007).

Gram-positive, aerobic, filamentous, branching organisms known as actinomycetes are often implicated as etiologies of pyothorax. These organisms include mycobacteria, corynebacteria, and *Nocardia*. *Actinomyces* spp. and *Filifactor villosus* are also members of the actinobacteria class of bacteria, have a similar morphology and Gram-stain characteristics, but are obligate or facultative anaerobes (Love *et al.* 1982; Walker *et al.* 2000; Malik *et al.* 2006). Bacterial macrocolonies characteristic of actinomycetes may be identified grossly as sulfur-like granules within pleural effusion (Malik *et al.* 2006). *Nocardia* is a ubiquitous environmental saprophyte and may be more common in dogs with pyothorax (Malik *et al.* 2006). While both *Actinomyces* and *Filifactor* are common oropharyngeal bacteria, *Actinomyces*, unlike *Filifactor*, is associated with grass awn foreign bodies in animals with pyothorax (Walker *et al.* 2000).

Most often, the route of infection of the pleural space is not identified. Potential mechanisms of infection include direct inoculation from penetrating thoracic wounds, thoracic surgery, thoracostomy tubes, or thoracocentesis; extension of infection from adjacent structures such as the mediastinum, esophagus, trachea, bronchi, or lung; or hematogenous or lymphatic spread from a distant infected focus (Barrs & Beatty 2009). Animals with pyothorax should be completely evaluated to identify puncture wounds, independent sites of infection, and abnormal structures adjacent to the pleural space that may have resulted in local or distant spread of infection.

In cats, actinomycetes and other obligate or facultative anaerobic bacteria are routinely isolated from pyothorax effusions and are similar to commensal oral flora (Love *et al.* 1990). Most recently, of 55 cats treated for pyothorax, 11 cats cultured positive for *Pasteurella* sp., 6 cats for *Bacteroides* sp., and 3 cats for *Actinomyces* sp. (Krämer *et al.* 2021). This parallel has historically

Table 33.1 Common aerobic and anaerobic bacteria associated with pyothorax in dogs and cats.

Aerobic
  Enteric
    Escherichia coli
    Enterobacter spp.
    Klebsiella pneumoniae
  Nonenteric
    Pasteurella spp.
    Acinetobacter spp.
    Capnocytophaga spp.
    Pseudomonas spp.
  Actinomyces spp.
  Streptococcus spp.
  Enterococcus spp.
  Mycoplasma spp.
  Nocardia spp.
Anaerobic
  Peptostreptococcus anaerobius
  Bacteroides spp.
  Fusobacterium spp.
  Porphyromonas spp.
  Prevotella spp.
  Filifactor villosus
  Clostridium spp.
  Eubacterium spp.
  Propionibacterium spp.
  Fibrobacter succinogenes

Source: Adapted from Walker et al. (2000) and Love et a . (1982).

supported the theory that pleural inoculation was frequently from the oropharynx from bite wounds, foreign bodies migrating from the oropharynx, or esophageal tears (Love *et al*. 1982, 1990; Barrs & Beatty 2009). Circumstantially, this is also supported by suggestions that outdoor intact male cats are at higher risk of pyothorax (Jonas 1983). Additionally, one study found cats with pyothorax to be younger than control animals and 3.8 times more likely to come from multicat households; these findings may also support bite wounds as a common etiology, as territorial defense might cause more inter-cat aggression (Waddell *et al*. 2002). Although bite wounds may be a cause of pyothorax in cats, a history of a bite wound or physical evidence of a bite wound is uncommonly encountered (Waddell *et al*. 2002).

Other authors offer evidence suggesting that parapneumonic spread following oropharyngeal aspiration is more common (Barrs *et al*. 2005; Barrs & Beatty 2009; Krämer *et al*. 2021). In one study of 27 cats with pyothorax, a suspected etiology was documented in 18 patients (Barrs *et al*. 2005). Of these 18 cats, aspiration of oropharyngeal flora was identified as the most likely source in 15 (78%) (Barrs *et al*. 2005). Of these 15 cats, 11 had pneumonia diagnosed radiographically, surgically, or by necropsy examination (Barrs *et al*. 2005). Further, 7 had an upper respiratory tract infection, and 3 of these also had pneumonia (Barrs *et al*. 2005). Broncholithiasis, lower airway inflammation, and pulmonary abscessation were present in one cat diagnosed with pyothorax (Sanchez *et al*. 2018). Potential differences in etiology may be a result of increased neutering of male cats, different husbandry techniques, or may represent geographic differences, as these two studies were of cats from North America and Australia (Waddell *et al*. 2002; Barrs & Beatty 2009). Regardless, in the individual patient, either etiology is a reasonable means of pleural inoculation and each should be investigated as a possibility.

Animals with a recent history of a thoracotomy are also at risk for developing pyothorax. Postoperative pyothorax has also been reported in 6.5% or 15 of 232 dogs that underwent intrathoracic surgery (Meakin *et al*. 2013). Identified risk factors for postoperative pyothorax included a diagnosis of idiopathic chylothorax, preoperative intrathoracic biopsy, and postoperative thoracocentesis (Meakin *et al*. 2013).

Diagnosis

There is no breed predilection for pyothorax in dogs or cats, but younger animals seem to be at higher risk (Waddell *et al*. 2002). Clinical history and physical examination abnormalities in animals with pyothorax relate to respiratory and systemic illness. Clinical signs can be present in animals for weeks to months prior to presentation. One study reported a median clinical sign duration of four weeks prior to presentation (Johnson & Martin 2007). Anorexia, dyspnea, lethargy, and weight loss are commonly identified by owners (Demetriou *et al*. 2002; Waddell *et al*. 2002; Barrs *et al*. 2005; Johnson & Martin 2007; Boothe *et al*. 2010). A history of hypersalivation was reported more frequently in nonsurviving cats in one study (Waddell *et al*. 2002).

Clinically, dogs and cats can be dyspneic, tachypneic, or have increased respiratory effort. Heart and lung sounds may be muffled or otherwise abnormal. Pulse quality may be weak. Animals may be cyanotic or have other abnormal mucous membrane color (Waddell *et al*. 2002). Evidence of a thoracic penetrating injury, an upper respiratory tract infection, pneumonia, or a distant site of infection may be apparent. Clinical signs of systemic illness such as lethargy, malaise, dehydration, hyperthermia, tachycardia, reduced appetite, or poor body condition can also be observed. Patients should be evaluated for signs of sepsis or systemic inflammatory response syndrome. Cats surviving pyothorax have been documented to have lower respiratory rates and higher heart rates compared with cats that did not survive (Waddell *et al.* 2002). Although uncommonly related, cats with pyothorax should be evaluated for feline immunodeficiency virus and feline leukemia virus.

A complete blood count, serum biochemical profile, and urinalysis should be undertaken as part of the minimum database in these patients. Elevated total leukocyte and neutrophil counts may be used to support the initial diagnosis of an infectious or inflammatory process and serially monitored to assess response to therapy. Anemia of inflammatory disease was described in six cats with pyothorax as mild to moderate, frequently nonregenerative, normocytic, and normochromic (Ottenjann *et al.* 2006). Animals with systemic illness may have deviations in electrolytes, which should be corrected. Additionally, biochemical evidence of organ dysfunction may be apparent in severely affected animals.

Because of respiratory historical complaints or clinical signs, chest radiography is indicated in these patients (Figure 33.1). Most animals will have bilateral effusion; unilateral effusion is present in a minority (Demetriou *et al.* 2002; Waddell *et al.* 2002; Barrs *et al.* 2005).

Radiographs should be evaluated for bronchopulmonary disease, including atelectatic lung lobes, bronchoalveolograms, pulmonary or mediastinal masses, tracheal elevation, widened mediastinum, thickening of the pleura, or lymph node enlargement. Restrictive pleuritis is characterized by rounding of the lung margins, especially evident on the caudal margin of the caudal lung lobes. Restrictive pleuritis results from fibrin on pleural surface and may suggest chronicity or increased severity of inflammation. Free air, in the absence of recent surgery or thoracocentesis, may suggest esophageal rupture or leakage from lung or bronchi. Effusion may hinder complete radiographic evaluation of the thorax, so radiography should be repeated following aspiration of pleural effusion.

Thoracic ultrasound examination can confirm pleural effusion, localize abscessed areas, and diagnose thickened pleura. Mediastinal masses or enlarged lymph nodes may also be diagnosed with thoracic ultrasound evaluation. In an emergency setting with severely dyspneic animals, ultrasound may rapidly confirm pleural effusion and guide thoracocentesis without the need to stress the animal during positioning for radiography. A thoracic focused assessment with sonogram for trauma (TFAST) is commonly used to evaluate for pleural effusion through bilateral pericardial sites (PCS) and the diaphragmatic-hepatic (DH) site (Lisciandro 2011).

(a)

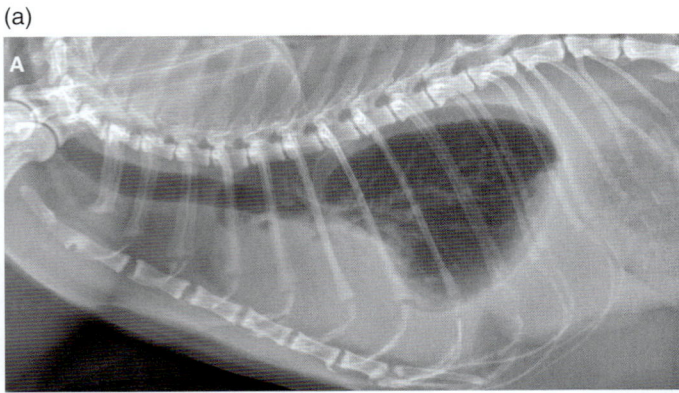

(b)

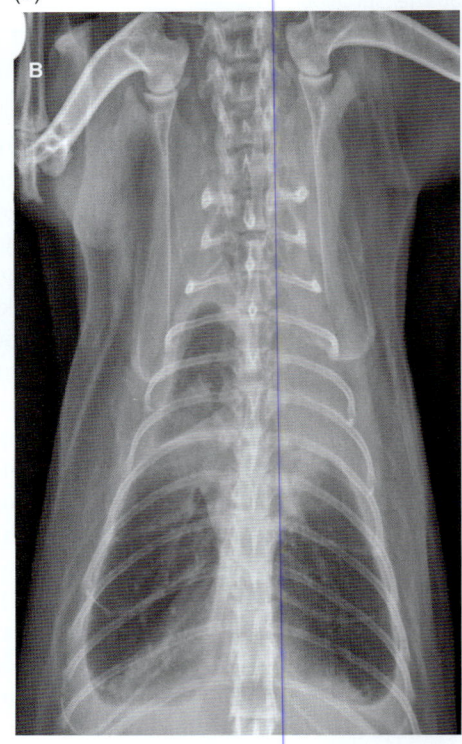

Figure 33.1 (a) Lateral and (b) dorsoventral radiographs of a cat diagnosed with pyothorax. There is a moderate amount of bilateral pleural effusion. There is retraction and rounding of the lung margins, especially the caudal margins of the caudal lung lobes, characteristic of restrictive pleuritis. The left cranial lung lobe is consolidated and an air bronchogram can be observed. It is possible that disease in the left cranial lung (neoplasia, foreign body, pneumonia, or abscess) resulted in pyothorax, or the lung collapsed as a result of the pleural disease. Source: Courtesy of Anthony J. Fischetti DVM, MS, DACVR.

Effusions occurring as a result of pyothorax may be loc-ulated secondary to fibrous tissue and are less echoic, or complex echoic, compared with a transudate (Barrs & Beatty 2009). Echogenic swirling is present secondary to suspended echogenic debris.

A thoracic computed tomography (CT) scan is useful to further define radiographic lesions, identify and direct planning of surgically treatable lesions or foreign material, and establish a definitive radiographic diagno-sis. One study compared lesions identified on CT with those identified during exploratory thoracotomy, and commonly found agreement between the two modalities (Swinbourne *et al.* 2011). However, another study evalu-ating migrating plant awns found that CT was unreliable for identification of the foreign material and did not regularly agree with bronchoscopic findings (Gibson *et al.* 2018).

Other studies compared animals with malignant effusion to those with pleuritic effusion resulting from chylothorax or pyothorax. They concluded that dogs and cats with malignant effusion were older, had more evidence of pleural thickening, particularly of the parietal pleura, and more commonly had nodular dia-phragmatic pleural thickening, costal pleural masses, pulmonary masses, and invasion of the thoracic wall (Reetz *et al.* 2018; Watton *et al.* 2017). Although most cases had some type of imaging abnormality, there was significant overlap in CT-identified lesions between ani-mals with malignant and inflammatory pleural disease.

Aspiration of the suppurative effusion is indicated in patients with pyothorax. Location of thoracic aspiration should be based on thoracic imaging and serves both diagnostic and therapeutic roles. Aspiration should be done in a gravity-dependent position typically between the seventh and ninth ribs, unless otherwise directed by imaging studies. Diagnostically, samples should be col-lected for aerobic and anaerobic culture with antibiotic sensitivity, Gram stain, fluid evaluation, and cytology. Prior to aspiration, clinicians should contact the micro-biology laboratory to optimize handling and transport of specimens for anaerobic culture, as false negatives are common with incorrectly handled anaerobic specimens. Gram stain and cytology will assist in confirming and characterizing the diagnosis, as well as guiding antibiotic therapy prior to receiving final culture and sensitivity results.

Fluid aspirated from the thoracic cavity of animals with pyothorax is an exudate. The color can be pink, yel-low, or white with a turbid appearance. Protein concen-trations are elevated (>3 g/dL) and cell counts are above 15×10^8/L. Cytologically, the hallmarks of diagnosis of pyothorax aspirates are degenerate and nondegenerate neutrophils with intracellular and extracellular bacteria (Figure 33.2). Bacteria may or may not be apparent on cytologic examination; nonetheless, microbial culture is indicated in patients with suppurative exudates. If *Actinomyces* spp., *Nocardia* spp., or *Mycoplasma* spp. are suspected, communication with the microbiology labo-ratory prior to submission is critical to allow appropriate adjustments to culture techniques (Lappin *et al.* 2017). Other cells may be present, including macrophages, eosinophils, lymphocytes, reactive mesothelial cells, and

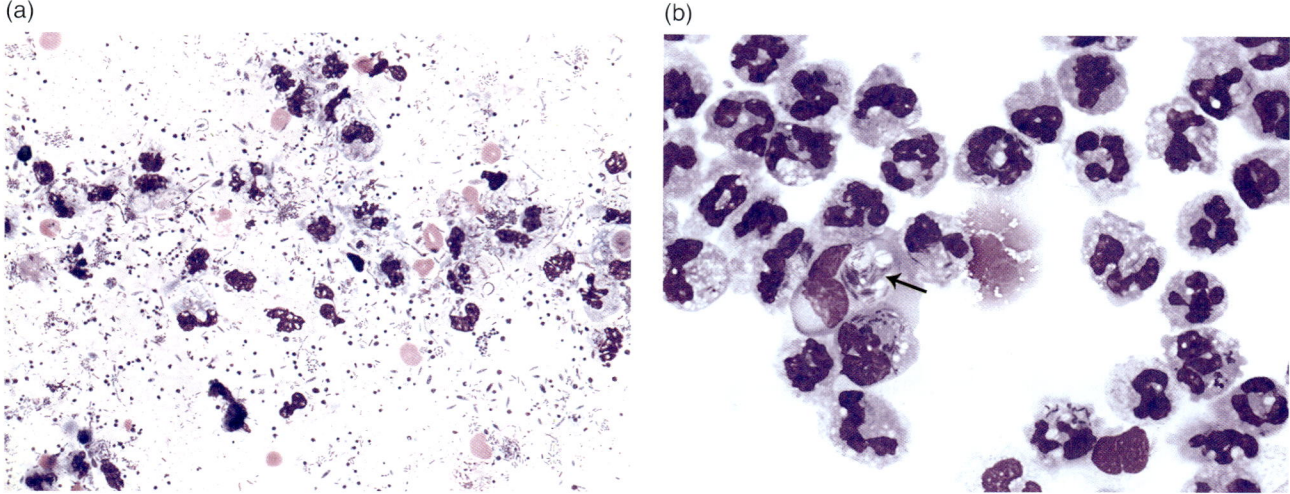

(a) (b)

Figure 33.2 Pleural fluid from (a) a dog and (b) a cat with pyothorax. There are many neutrophils, including degenerate forms. Mixed bacteria are found free (a) and within neutrophils (a, b) and include thin filamentous forms (arrow), likely anaerobic bacteria. Wright's stain. (a) 600×; (b) 1000×. Source: Courtesy of Karen M. Young, University of Wisconsin-Madison.

erythrocytes (Duncan *et al.* 1994). In cases where bacterial macrocolonies or sulfur granules are present, pleomorphic branching filamentous rods surrounded by degenerate neutrophils can be observed (Duncan *et al.* 1994). Observation of this bacterial morphology suggests an infection by an actinomycete organism described earlier. Neutrophils tend to be more degenerate near the colony and less degenerate away from the colony (Duncan *et al.* 1994).

Therapy

The principles of treatment of animals with pyothorax include removal of the septic effusion and long-term treatment with appropriate antibiotics. Removal of necrotic or foreign material is also indicated in some patients. Both medical and surgical strategies are employed to accomplish these goals.

Initial stabilization and medical treatment

Initial stabilization of the patient should include correction of dehydration and electrolyte imbalances, as well as removal of as much thoracic effusion as possible. The quantity of pleural effusion may increase following rehydration in severely debilitated animals. In 15 dogs treated with a single unilateral thoracic aspiration under sedation or general anesthesia, followed by long-term (>6 weeks) antibiotic administration, all dogs recovered and no relapses were documented over a 27-month mean follow-up (Johnson & Martin 2007). Dogs in this study were initially hospitalized as needed for systemic stabilization, and one dog was not included because a pulmonary abscess was diagnosed on thoracic radiographic examination; this dog was treated surgically (Johnson & Martin 2007). These results contrast with another study where a similar treatment regimen resulted in a 29% short- and long-term survival rate, significantly worse than dogs treated with thoracic lavage and/or surgery (Boothe *et al.* 2010). A combination of crystalloids and colloids is required to maintain adequate hydration of the patient without decreasing the oncotic pressure. It is important to replace the fluid loss from the thoracostomy tube. Since the fluids drained with the thoracostomy tube have a high protein content, it is important to monitor the oncotic pressure of the patient and provide appropriate fluid support, plasma, or whole blood, depending on the need for coagulation factors or red blood cells. Monitoring of coagulation times, antithrombin III levels, and platelet count is appropriate, because patients with a pyothorax are at risk for developing disseminated intravascular coagulation.

Antibiotic therapy

Long-term antibiotic therapy is indicated in patients with pyothorax. Initial antibiotic therapy may be guided by the cytology and Gram stain results. Given the frequency with which facultative and obligate anaerobic bacteria are isolated from cats and dogs with pyothorax, initial antibiotic therapy should target these organisms (Walker *et al.* 2000). In a study evaluating the susceptibility of obligate anaerobic bacteria to various antibiotics, bacteria had 100% susceptibility to amoxicillin–clavulanic acid and chloramphenicol, and most bacteria were susceptible to metronidazole (Jang *et al.* 1997). Ampicillin and clindamycin are also efficacious against the majority of these bacteria. The antimicrobial guidelines from the Working Group of the International Society of Infectious Diseases recommend the combination of parenteral enrofloxacin or marbofloxacin with a penicillin or clindamycin (Lappin *et al.* 2017). Until final microbial culture results are available, antibiotic coverage should include Gram-positive and Gram-negative bacteria, as well as aerobic and anaerobic organisms. It is also recommended that treatment against anaerobic bacteria continue regardless of the culture results, because of the potential for fastidious anaerobic bacteria (Lappin *et al.* 2017). Antibiotic treatment should continue for at least 3 weeks and ideally for 4–6 weeks (Lappin *et al.* 2017). Radiographs should be used to monitor response to therapy and guide continuance of therapy.

Thoracostomy tube

While there is some success with the single aspiration strategy described earlier, the standard of care for dogs and cats with pyothorax involves hospitalization and placement of unilateral or bilateral thoracostomy tubes for thoracic drainage and repeated pleural lavage. Dogs with pyothorax that received pleural lavage had higher survival percentages compared with those that did not (Boothe *et al.* 2010). In another study of cats with pyothorax, placement of thoracostomy tubes was more common in cats that survived than in cats that died (Waddell *et al.* 2002). Bilateral thoracostomy tubes allow both hemithoraces to be flushed and maximize the opportunity for removal of bacteria, as well as inflammatory and necrotic debris, although the superior efficacy of bilateral thoracostomy tubes compared with unilateral tubes has not been proven (Boothe *et al.* 2010).

Small-diameter wire-guided thoracostomy tubes have been described as an alternative to larger-bore standard thoracostomy tubes in dogs and cats with pyothorax (Valtolina & Adamantos 2009; Del Magno *et al.* 2020). Patients with viscous pleural exudates may require large-bore tubes. However, in cats with pyothorax, small-bore chest tube occlusion was reported in only 3 of 10 cats, 2 of which were able to be resolved with lavage (Del Magno *et al.* 2020).

The pleural space is lavaged 2–3 times daily with warm, sterile, isotonic fluids. Prior to instillation of lavage fluid, the thoracostomy tubes should be aspirated to remove any residual fluid. Isotonic lavage (20 mL/kg) should be instilled over 5–10 minutes and the respiratory rate should be monitored during the procedure. Instillation should be halted and fluid removed if the animal becomes dyspneic. Heparin (10–15 units/mL) may be added to the flush solution, and has been shown to be associated with better survival in dogs with pyothorax (Boothe *et al.* 2010). Lavage fluid may be left in the thoracic cavity for brief periods of time (<1 h) and removed. The entirety of the instilled lavage may not be removed, but as much as possible should be. Thoracic lavage is continued based on the clinical signs of the patient and changes in gross and cytologic characteristics of the aspirated fluid.

Monitoring of medical treatment

Daily cytologic evaluation of the fluid is a convenient and sensitive way to monitor a patient's response to therapy. The fluid should become clearer and populated with fewer, more healthy-appearing leukocytes and no bacteria. Lavage is generally continued for 3–7 days. However, in healthy dogs with a thoracostomy tube in place, evidence of a pyothorax (septic, suppurative inflammation, and positive microbial cultures) developed in most dogs between days 4 and 6, suggesting that thoracostomy tube removal should be performed as soon as indicated and that ongoing or new cytologic evidence of pyothorax may be related to infection from the thoracostomy tube tract rather than the primary pathology (Hung *et al.* 2016).

Bronchoscopy

Use of bronchoscopy to identify migrating plant awns causing intrathoracic disease has been described in a case series of 37 dogs (Gibson *et al.* 2018). Bronchoscopic abnormalities were commonly observed in all dogs during examination. In this series, bronchoscopic removal of the migrating plant awn was possible in 37% (10 of 27) of dogs. The authors postulate that bronchoscopy may have saved some dogs from lung lobectomy.

Surgical treatment

Deciding whether to treat animals surgically for pyothorax can be difficult. Indications for surgical treatment of pyothorax include evidence of a surgically resectable lesion thought to be responsible for the pyothorax, such

as an abscess, mass, or foreign body, or inadequate response to medical management. Patients who "fail" medical management are usually those that do not have significant resolution of clinical signs or fluid cytology after 3–5 days of appropriate medical therapy. Prior to surgery, patients should be treated medically for several days, or until they are metabolically stabilized and good anesthetic candidates. Patients managed medically have the lowest hospitalization costs, while patients managed medically for a period of time, then taken to surgery, tend to have higher hospitalization costs (Bach & Balakrishnan 2015). If budget is a concern, early surgical intervention may reduce overall costs compared to later intervention (Bach & Balakrishnan 2015).

Thoracoscopic evaluation

Thoracoscopic exploration and débridement of the pleural space are becoming more common in veterinary surgery and offer a minimally invasive means of diagnosing an etiology of pyothorax as well as performing focused débridement and lavage. Thoracoscopic treatment of pyothorax has been reported in a small number of dogs using multiple ports or a single-incision subxiphoid approach (Jiménez Peláez & Jolliffe 2012; Scott *et al.* 2017; Gordo *et al.* 2020). Patients are positioned in dorsal recumbency and a paraxiphoid camera position used initially for exploration. Additional intercostal camera or instrument ports are placed as needed for diagnosis, débridement, and lavage. Adhesions or large amounts of fibrin may impair creation of an adequate optical and working space and necessitate a thoracotomy. In human pediatrics, early thoracoscopic treatment for children with pyothorax from parapneumonic spread resulted in reduced hospital stay and overall costs (Gates *et al.* 2004; Aziz *et al.* 2008). Early thoracoscopic treatment may be a viable treatment strategy for veterinary patients with pyothorax.

Median sternotomy

When open surgery is required in patients with bilateral pleural effusion, a median sternotomy is performed, whereas an intercostal thoracotomy might be appropriate for patients with unilateral disease. Thoracic exploration is performed in an organized and systematic manner. Infected or necrotic material is débrided. Abnormal tissue should be removed and submitted for microbial culture and pathologic analysis. Lung lobectomy or pneumonectomy may be required for consolidated or abscessed lung lobes (Crawford *et al.* 2011; Gibson *et al.* 2018).

The amount of débridement performed likely varies with each patient. Mediastinectomy after median sternotomy has been described in 12 dogs with chronic pyogranulomatous plural disease (Trinterud *et al.* 2014). Six of those dogs had pyothorax, others pleural foreign material, chronic thoracic draining tracks, or imaging findings consistent with chronic granulomatous pleural disease (Trinterud *et al.* 2014). One dog died postoperatively; the remaining 11 dogs had complete resolution of clinical signs.

Copious lavage of the pleural space with warm isotonic fluid is required prior to closure.

Outcomes

In one study of dogs with pyothorax, treatment with medical therapy alone was associated with a 5.4 times increased likelihood of failure (Rooney & Monnet 2002). In that study, the calculated proportions of dogs free from disease at one year after treatment was 25% for medically treated dogs and 78% for surgically treated dogs (Rooney & Monnet 2002). Another study reports an overall survival rate of 74%, with a significant difference in short- and long-term survival in patients treated with single pleural drainage (at discharge, 29% survival; at 12 months, 29% survival), thoracostomy tube placement and pleural lavage (at discharge, 77% survival; at 12 months, 71% survival), and surgical débridement (at discharge, 92% survival; at 12 months, 70% survival) (Boothe *et al.* 2010). Other studies in dogs report an approximately 54–100% survival with medical or surgical treatment (Demetriou *et al.* 2002; Mellanby *et al.* 2002; Rooney & Monnet 2002; Johnson & Martin 2007). Recurrence is reported in 0–20% of dogs, and may be substantially delayed (Demetriou *et al.* 2002; Rooney & Monnet 2002; Johnson & Martin 2007; Boothe *et al.* 2010). Medical treatment with isolation of *Actinomyces* spp. and medical treatment with radiographic detection of mediastinal or pulmonary lesions have been shown to be significantly associated with reductions in disease-free interval in dogs with pyothorax (Rooney & Monnet 2002).

Dogs with postoperative pyothorax have a significantly worse prognosis with a 67% mortality rate (Meakin *et al.* 2013).

In cats which received treatment, survival following diagnosis of pyothorax is reported to be 66–93% (Demetriou *et al.* 2002; Waddell *et al.* 2002; Barrs *et al.* 2005; Ottenjann *et al.* 2008; Krämer *et al.* 2021). One study reported successful medical management (thoracostomy tubes, pleural lavage, antibiotics therapy) in 85% (47/55) of cats with pyothorax (Krämer *et al.* 2021). Recurrence is uncommon and is reported in 0–7% of cats (Demetriou *et al.* 2002; Waddell *et al.* 2002; Barrs *et al.* 2005; Krämer *et al.* 2021).

References

Aziz, A., Healey, J.M., Qureshi, F. et al. (2008). Comparative analysis of chest tube thoracostomy and video-assisted thoracoscopic surgery in empyema and parapneumonic effusion associated with pneumonia in children. *Surgical Infections* 9: 317–323.

Bach, J.F. and Balakrishnan, A. (2015). Retrospective comparison of costs between medical and surgical treatment of canine pyothorax. *Canadian Veterinary Journal* 56: 1140–1143.

Barrs, V.R. and Beatty, J.A. (2009). Feline pyothorax: new insights into an old problem. Part 1. Aetiopathogenesis and diagnostic investigation. *Veterinary Journal* 179: 163–170.

Barrs, V.R., Allan, G.S., Martin, P. et al. (2005). Feline pyothorax: a retrospective study of 27 cases in Australia. *Journal of Feline Medicine and Surgery* 7: 211–222.

Boothe, H.W., Howe, L.M., Boothe, D.M. et al. (2010). Evaluation of outcomes in dogs treated for pyothorax: 46 cases (1983–2001). *Journal of the American Veterinary Medical Association* 236: 657–663.

Crawford, A.H., Halfacree, Z.J., Lee, K.C.L., and Brockman, D.J. (2011). Clinical outcome following pneumonectomy for management of chronic pyothorax in four cats. *Journal of Feline Medicine and Surgery* 13: 762–767.

Davies, C. and Forrester, S.D. (1996). Pleural effusion in cats: 82 cases (1987 to 1995). *Journal of Small Animal Practice* 37: 217–224.

Del Magno, S., Foglia, A., Folinelli, L. et al. (2020). The use of small-bore wire-guided chest drains for the management of feline pyothorax: a retrospective case series. *Open Veterinary Journal* 10: 443–451.

Demetriou, J.L., Foale, R.D., Ladlow, J. et al. (2002). Canine and feline pyothorax: a retrospective study of 50 cases in the UK and Ireland. *Journal of Small Animal Practice* 43: 388–394.

Duncan, J.R., Prasse, K.W., and Mahaffey, E.A. (1994). Cytology. In: *Veterinary Laboratory Medicine*, ch. 12, 3e (ed. J.R. Duncan, K.W. Prasse and E.A. Mahaffey). Ames, IA: Iowa State University Press.

Gates, R.L., Caniano, D.A., Hayes, J.R., and Arca, M.J. (2004). Does VATS provide optimal treatment of empyema in children? A systematic review. *Journal of Pediatric Surgery* 39: 381–386.

Gibson, E.A., Balsa, I.M., Mayhew, P.D. et al. (2018). Utility of bronchoscopy combined with surgery in the treatment and outcomes of dogs with intrathoracic disease secondary to plant awn migration. *Veterinary Surgery* 48: 1309–1317.

Gordo, I., Hubers, M., Bird, F.G. et al. (2020). Feasibility of the single-incision subxiphoid approach for video-assisted thoracoscopic surgery in dogs. *Journal of Small Animal Practice* 61: 480–486.

Hung, G.C., Gaunt, M.C., Rubin, J.E. et al. (2016). Quantification and characterization of pleural fluid in healthy dogs with thoracostomy tubes. *American Journal of Veterinary Research* 77: 1387–1391.

Jang, S.S., Breher, J.E., Dabaco, L.A., and Hirsh, D.C. (1997). Organisms isolated from dogs and cats with anaerobic infections and susceptibility to selected antimicrobial agents. *Journal of the American Veterinary Medical Association* 210: 1610–1614.

Jiménez Peláez, M. and Jolliffe, C. (2012). Thoracoscopic foreign body removal and right middle lung lobectomy to treat pyothorax in a dog. *Journal of Small Animal Practice* 53: 240–244.

Johnson, M.S. and Martin, M.W. (2007). Successful medical treatment of 15 dogs with pyothorax. *Journal of Small Animal Practice* 48: 12–16.

Jonas, L.D. (1983). Feline pyothorax: a retrospective study of twenty cases. *Journal of the American Animal Hospital Association* 19: 865–871.

Klainbart, S., Mazaki-Tovi, M., Auerbach, N. et al. (2007). Spirocercosis-associated pyothorax in dogs. *Veterinary Journal* 173: 209–214.

Krämer, F., Rainer, J., and Bali, M.S. (2021). Short- and long-term outcome in cats diagnosed with pyothorax: 47 cases (2009 – 2018). *Journal of Small Animal Practice* 62 (8): 669–676.

Lappin, M.R., Blondeau, J., Boothe, D. et al. (2017). Antimicrobial use guidelines for treatment of respiratory tract disease in dogs and cats: Antimicrobial Guideline Working Group of the International Society for companion animal infectious diseases. *Journal of Veterinary Internal Medicine* 279–294.

Lisciandro, G.R. (2011). Abdominal and thoracic focused assessment with sonography for trauma, triage, and monitoring in small animals. *Journal of Veterinary Emergency and Critical Care* 21: 104–122.

Love, D.N., Jones, R.F., Bailey, M. et al. (1982). Isolation and characterisation of bacteria from pyothorax (empyaemia) in cats. *Veterinary Microbiology* 7: 455–461.

Love, D.N., Vekselstein, R., and Collings, S. (1990). The obligate and facultatively anaerobic bacterial flora of the normal feline gingival margin. *Veterinary Microbiology* 22: 267–275.

Malik, R., Krockenberger, M.B., O'Brien, C.R. et al. (2006). *Nocardia* infections in cats: a retrospective multi-institutional study of 17 cases. *Australian Veterinary Journal* 84: 235–245.

McCaw, D., Franklin, R., Fales, W. et al. (1984). Pyothorax caused by *Candida albicans* in a cat. *Journal of the American Veterinary Medical Association* 185: 311–312.

Meakin, L.B., Salonene, L.K., Baines, S.J. et al. (2013). Prevalence, outcome, and risk factors for postoperative pyothorax in 232 dogs undergoing thoracic surgery. *Journal of Small Animal Practice* 54: 313–317.

Mellanby, R.J., Villiers, E., and Herrtage, M.E. (2002). Canine pleural and mediastinal effusions: a retrospective study of 81 cases. *Journal of Small Animal Practice* 43: 447–451. *Journal of Veterinary Internal Medicine* 20: 1143–1150.

Ottenjann, M., Weingart, C., Arndt, G., and Kohn, B. (2006). Characterization of the anemia of inflammatory disease in cats with abscesses, pyothorax, or fat necrosis. *Journal of Veterinary Internal Medicine* 20 (5): 1143–1150.

Ottenjann, M., Lubke-Becker, A., Linzmann, H. et al. (2008). Pyothorax in 26 cats: clinical signs, laboratory results and therapy (2000–2007) [German]. *Berliner und Münchener Tierarztliche Wochenschrift* 121: 365–373.

Reetz, J.A., Suran, J.N., and Zwingenberger, A.L. (2018). Nodules and masses are associated with malignant pleural effusion in dogs and cats but many other intrathoracic CT features are poor predictors of effusion type. *Veterinary Radiology and Ultrasound* 60: 289–299.

Rooney, M.B. and Monnet, E. (2002). Medical and surgical treatment of pyothorax in dogs: 26 cases (1991–2001). *Journal of the American Veterinary Medical Association* 221: 86–92.

Sanchez, F.V., Stewart, J., Bovens, C., and Puig, J. (2018). Broncholithiasis associated with lower airway inflammation and subsequent pyothorax in a cat. *Journal of Feline Medicine and Surgery Open Reports* 4: 2055116917746798.

Scott, J., Singh, A., Monnet, E. et al. (2017). Video-assisted thoracic surgery for the management of pyothorax in dogs: 14 cases. *Veterinary Surgery* 46: 722–730.

Swinbourne, F., Baines, E.A., Baines, S.J., and Halfacree, Z.J. (2011). Computed tomographic findings in canine pyothorax and correlation with findings at exploratory thoracotomy. *Journal of Small Animal Practice* 52: 203–208.

Trinterud, T., Nelissen, P., Caine, A.R., and White, R.A.S. (2014). Mediastinectomy for management of chronic pyogranulomatous plural disease in dogs. *Veterinary Record* 174: 607–612.

Valtolina, C. and Adamantos, S. (2009). Evaluation of small-bore wireguided chest drains for management of pleural space disease. *Journal of Small Animal Practice* 50: 290–297.

Waddell, L.S., Brady, C.A., and Drobatz, K.J. (2002). Risk factors, prognostic indicators, and outcome of pyothorax in cats: 80 cases (1986–1999). *Journal of the American Veterinary Medical Association* 221: 819–824.

Walker, A.L., Jang, S.S., and Hirsh, D.C. (2000). Bacteria associated with pyothorax of dogs and cats: 98 cases (1989–1998). *Journal of the American Veterinary Medical Association* 216: 359–363.

Watton, T.C., Lara-Garcia, A., and Lamb, C.R. (2017). Can malignant and inflammatory pleural effusions in dogs be distinguished using computed tomography? *Veterinary Radiology and Ultrasound* 58: 535–541.

34

Pneumothorax

Robert J. Hardie

Definition and classification

Pneumothorax is defined as the presence of air or gas in the pleural space (Noppen & De Keukeleire 2008). Air or gas may enter the pleural space via direct communication with the environment through a defect in the thoracic wall; through defects in the lungs, bronchi, trachea, or esophagus; or from a gas-forming organism present within the pleural space.

Classifications of pneumothorax include traumatic, iatrogenic, and spontaneous. Understanding the general classifications of pneumothorax is important for determining the most accurate diagnostic imaging technique(s) for the suspected cause, the most appropriate methods for treatment, and the overall prognosis.

Traumatic pneumothorax is generally due to some type of blunt or penetrating force to the thorax that results in injury to the lung parenchyma, or less commonly the bronchi, trachea, or esophagus, leading to leakage of air into the pleural space (Figure 34.1). Traumatic pneumothorax can also be classified as either open or closed, depending upon whether a direct communication between the environment and the pleural space was created during the injury.

Iatrogenic pneumothorax is generally the result of a diagnostic or therapeutic procedure such as thoracocentesis, lung biopsy, esophagoscopy, or partial or complete lung lobectomy that results in leakage of air into the pleural space from the site of the procedure. Barotrauma and tracheal lacerations occurring during endotracheal intubation and ventilation during general anesthesia are also causes of iatrogenic pneumothorax (Mitchell et al. 2000; Alderson et al. 2006; Bhandal & Kuzma 2008).

Spontaneous pneumothorax is a form of pneumothorax that occurs in the absence of trauma or direct injury to the lungs. Spontaneous pneumothorax has been further classified into either primary or secondary based on the type or source of the underlying lung pathology (Noppen & De Keukeleire 2008; Tschopp et al. 2006). Traditionally, primary spontaneous pneumothorax has been used to describe pneumothorax arising from pulmonary blebs, bullae, or emphysematous lesions (generally of unknown etiology) (Lipscomb et al. 2003), and secondary spontaneous pneumothorax has been used to describe pneumothorax arising from many different underlying causes, such as migrating or inhaled foreign bodies, neoplasia, parasites, abscesses, lobar emphysema, pulmonary thromboembolism, lower airway inflammation, and asthma (Busch & Noxon 1992; Forrester et al. 1992; Cooper et al. 2003; White et al. 2003; Hopper et al. 2004; Gopalakrishnan & Stevenson 2007; Sobel & Williams 2009). However, as diagnostic imaging and tissue analysis techniques continue to advance, the distinction as to what constitutes a primary versus secondary cause (i.e., inherited α-1 antitrypsin deficiency or low-grade lower airway inflammation due to environmental factors) has become less obvious and the classification system is likely to evolve in the future (Gilday et al. 2021).

The term "tension" pneumothorax refers to the condition where a defect in the parietal or visceral pleural creates a one-way valve that allows air to enter the pleural space on inspiration, but does not allow air to escape on expiration (Barton 1999). This results in progressive accumulation of air within the pleural space that eventually leads to compression of intrathoracic structures (i.e., lungs, heart, vena cava) and subsequent cardiovascular

Small Animal Soft Tissue Surgery, Second Edition. Edited by Eric Monnet.
© 2023 John Wiley & Sons, Inc. Published 2023 by John Wiley & Sons, Inc.
Companion website: www.wiley.com/go/monnet/small

(a)

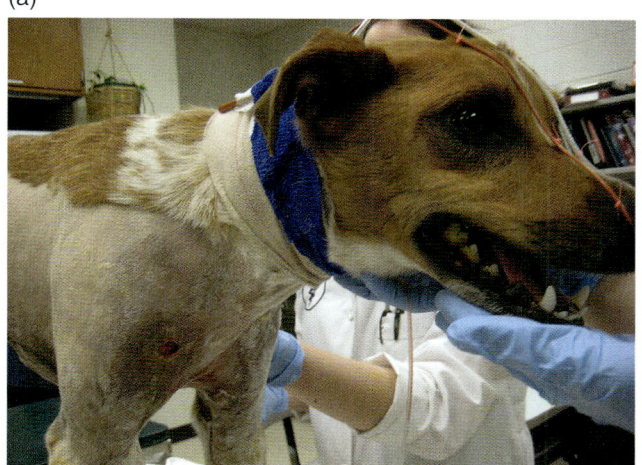

(b)

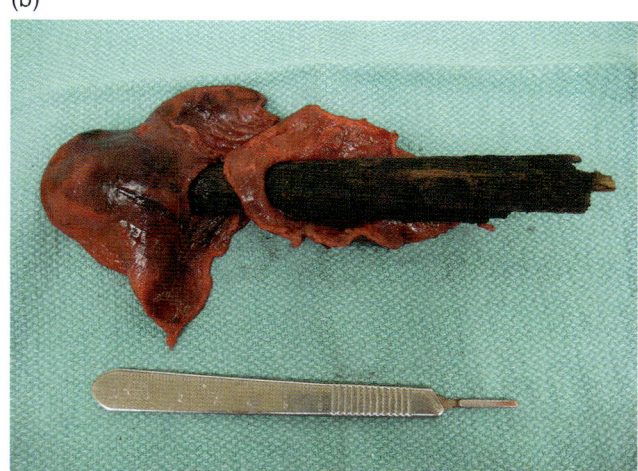

Figure 34.1 (a) Penetrating "stick injury" wound on the right caudal cervical area resulting in direct lung trauma and pneumothorax. (b) The resected right cranial lung lobe with the penetrating stick in place.

collapse if not treated effectively. The severity of tension pneumothorax depends greatly on the rate of air accumulation, the integrity of the mediastinum, and whether pneumothorax is unilateral or bilateral, as well as the degree of trauma or underlying condition of the lungs.

Clinical signs and physical examination findings

Clinical signs from pneumothorax can vary dramatically depending upon the rate and severity of air accumulation and presence of any concurrent injuries or underlying lung disease. Common clinical signs of pneumothorax include tachypnea, increased respiratory effort, dyspnea, anxiousness, flaring of the nostrils, extension of the head and neck, expansion of the chest ("barrel-chested" appearance), increased abdominal effort, paradoxical thoracic and abdominal movement, pale mucous membranes, cyanosis, and collapse. In addition, more nonspecific findings that have been reported with pneumothorax include anorexia, lethargy, vomiting, gagging, and polydipsia and polyuria (Puerto *et al.* 2002; Lipscomb *et al.* 2003; Howes *et al.* 2020; Gilday *et al.* 2021; Dickson *et al.* 2021). On thoracic auscultation, lung and heart sounds are decreased or muffled due to the presence of the air interface within the thorax. Similarly, on percussion of the thoracic wall, auscultated sounds are tympanic or have increased resonance due to the presence of the air within the thorax. Peripheral pulses may be decreased, and capillary refill times increased, if cardiac output becomes affected by the progressive accumulation of air in the thorax. Animals with lesions of the trachea, bronchi, or esophagus may also develop subcutaneous emphysema due to

air leaking through the mediastinum and into the subcutaneous tissue (Bhandal & Kuzma 2008).

Pathophysiology

Pneumothorax causes an increase in intrapleural pressure that disrupts the normal pressure gradients within the thorax, responsible for moving air through the lungs and into the alveoli. It also increases capillary resistance and thus disrupts the pulmonary circulation with each respiratory cycle. The physiologic consequences of increased intrapleural pressure vary depending upon the severity, but generally result in pulmonary collapse, decreased tidal volume, ventilation/perfusion mismatch, compensatory pulmonary vasoconstriction, and intrapulmonary shunting of blood away from poorly ventilated portions of the lungs, and compensatory increase in respiration rate and depth to maintain ventilation and minute volume. If pneumothorax progresses to such a degree that it overcomes normal compensatory responses, additional physiologic changes ensue, including hypoxemia, acidosis, increased pulmonary vascular resistance, increased pulmonary arterial pressure, increased afterload to the right side of the heart, increased central venous pressure, decreased cardiac preload, and ultimately decreased cardiac output and cardiovascular collapse (Bennett *et al.* 1989; Barton 1999; Gilday *et al.* 2021).

The physiologic effects of pneumothorax are relatively well characterized in experimental studies involving various animal species; however, the degree to which the changes described occur varies dramatically depending upon the specific species being studied (i.e., the anatomy of the mediastinum); whether animals were conscious, sedated, or anesthetized; and whether animals were breathing spontaneously or mechanically ventilated during investigation. In addition, due to the inevitable differences in experimental design and research objectives, caution should be exercised when attempting to directly extrapolate results to the clinical situation. For example, in an experimental study involving conscious spontaneously breathing dogs, bilateral pneumothorax created with a volume of air corresponding to 150% of lung volume (V_L) [V_L (L) = 0.032 × body weight (kg)$^{1.05}$] was well tolerated, with minimal changes in cardiovascular parameters (Bennett *et al.* 1989). In contrast, another study involving anesthetized dogs ventilated with either positive-pressure ventilation or high-frequency jet ventilation, bilateral pneumothorax created with 45 mL/kg of nitrogen resulted in significantly decreased cardiac index, which was further exacerbated by the addition of positive end-expiratory pressure (Bjorling & Whitfield 1986). Similarly, in an experimental study involving mechanically ventilated, anesthetized bloodhound dogs with progressively increased pneumothorax ranging from 30 to 60 mL/kg of air (1–2 × functional residual capacity [FRC]), PaO$_2$ consistently decreased and PaCO$_2$ consistently increased with the increased volume of pneumothorax. However, mean arterial pressure and heart rate varied among the dogs despite the increasing pneumothorax, and were considered poor indicators of the severity of pneumothorax in anesthetized dogs (Walker *et al.* 1993).

In the clinical setting, the physiologic effects of pneumothorax are almost certainly exacerbated by the individual circumstances of the animal, including the specific source of the pneumothorax, the degree of direct lung involvement, the presence of concurrent lung pathology such as contusions, pneumonia, fibrosis, emphysema, metastasis, or pleural effusion, and ultimately the overall condition of the animal. Consequently, the decision to treat pneumothorax should be based not only on the immediate clinical status of the patient, but also on the understanding that once compensatory mechanisms are overcome, cardiovascular decompensation can occur rapidly. Unfortunately, the clinical dilemma still lies with the difficulty in accurately and consistently assessing the lungs for underlying pathology with the currently available diagnostic techniques.

Diagnostic imaging

Radiography

Thoracic radiography is currently the most practical technique for diagnosing pneumothorax in small animals. The hallmark signs of pneumothorax include the presence of air density within the thorax and separation of the lungs from the thoracic wall. Depending upon the volume of air and whether pneumothorax is bilateral or unilateral, other radiographic signs include elevation of the heart from the sternum on lateral recumbent views, increased opacity of the lungs due to progressive collapse, shifting of the mediastinum away from the side with the greatest volume, flattening of one or both domes of the diaphragm, and the appearance of an expanded or "barrel-chested" thorax on ventrodorsal or dorsoventral views. Radiographic positions for examining the thorax include left and right lateral, ventrodorsal, and dorsoventral views using standard vertical beam projection, and standing or lateral recumbent views using horizontal beam projection. Radiography is generally very accurate for detecting pneumothorax in small animals, although there is some debate regarding the most accurate views for detecting pneumothorax. In one report, the dorsoventral view is recommended over the ventrodorsal view for detecting small-volume pneumothorax, because of the improved ability to see the margins of the lungs and relative increased density of the lung parenchyma (Aronson & Reed 1995). In another experimental study involving three groups of 24 dogs that were injected with 5, 15, or 45 mL/kg of air into one hemithorax, pneumothorax was readily detected in all dogs (Kern *et al.* 1994). The mean body weight for the dogs (n = 7) in the 5 mL/kg group was 19.5 kg, which corresponded to approximately 100 mL of air injected in each dog in that group. Specific parameters that were evaluated in this study included the degree of separation (distance in mm) of the heart from the sternum on lateral recumbent views using vertical beam projection, and the degree of pleural separation on the lateral recumbent ventrodorsal view using the horizontal beam projection. The most effective views for detecting pneumothorax were the left lateral recumbent view using a vertical beam projection, and the expiratory, right lateral recumbent ventrodorsal view using horizontal beam projection. Additionally, separation of the pleural surfaces on the ventrodorsal view using horizontal beam projection was a better indicator for small amounts of pneumothorax than elevation of the heart from the sternum on the lateral view using vertical beam projection. In this same study, 22 of 24 dogs developed bilateral pneumothorax after injection of only one hemithorax, indicating that the mediastinum is incomplete or permeable in most dogs. Also, the mean time to resolution of pneumothorax (absorption of air) corresponded to the volume of air injected and was 4.9, 6.6, and 12.5 days for each group, respectively.

In general, standard survey radiography is an accurate method for detecting pneumothorax in small animals, even when the volumes of air within the thorax are

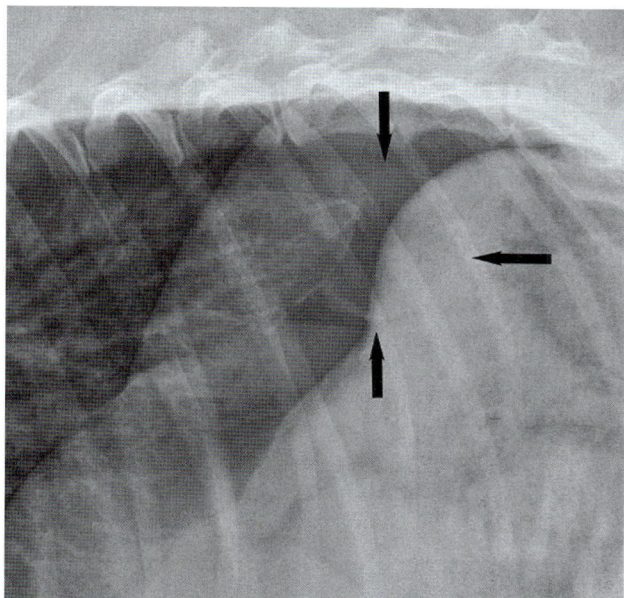

Figure 34.2 Lateral thoracic radiograph of a dog with pneumothorax and a pulmonary bulla lesion on the caudal margin of the lung (black arrows).

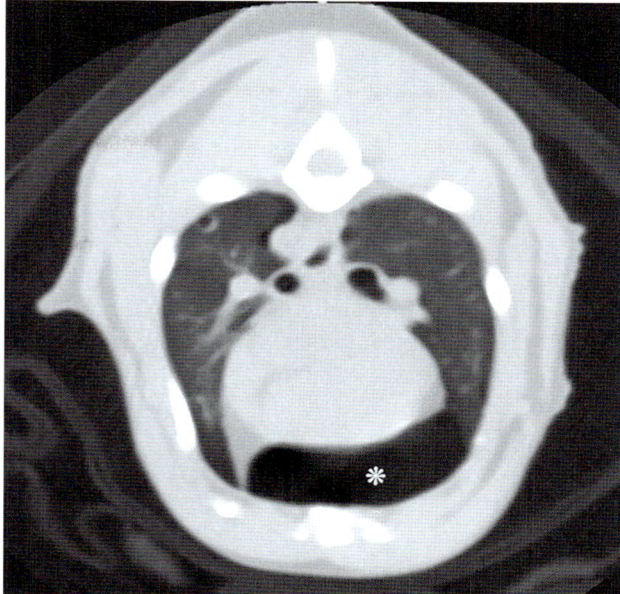

Figure 34.3 Thoracic computed tomographic image (dorsal recumbency) of a cat with a moderate degree of pneumothorax. Note the air present in the ventral aspect of the thorax (asterisk) and the dorsal displacement of the lungs.

relatively small. The value of radiography for diagnosing underlying causes of pneumothorax depends upon the size, location, and type of lesion (Figure 34.2). Obvious limitations of standard radiography include the superimposition of the tissues, the relative inability to resolve different tissue densities, and the inability to detect lesions less than approximately 1 cm in diameter.

Computed tomography

Computed tomography (CT) is currently considered the "gold standard" for diagnosing and evaluating pneumothorax in humans. The advantages of CT over thoracic radiographs for the diagnosis of pneumothorax include the ability to minimize soft tissue superimposition with cross-sectional imaging, to more accurately differentiate different tissue densities, to scan very thin slices at high resolutions, and to view structures in multiple planes or as three-dimensional images allowing for more accurate evaluation (Figure 34.3). The relative disadvantage of CT is the need for general anesthesia to position most animals during scanning.

There are multiple studies in the veterinary literature describing the use of CT for the diagnosis and evaluation of pneumothorax in small animals (Schwarz & Tidwell 1999; Au *et al.* 2006; Johnson & Wisner 2007; Reetz *et al.* 2013; Trempala & Herold 2013; Boudreau *et al.* 2013; Dickson *et al.* 2020; Trehiou *et al.* 2020; Seriot *et al.* 2021). In an experimental study, CT was used to evaluate the relationship between increasing levels of pneumothorax and changes in cross-sectional area of the caudal thorax and lungs in anesthetized, mechanically ventilated bloodhound dogs. It was determined that a 33%, 40%, and 50% reduction in lung area corresponded to approximately 30, 45, and 60 mL of air (pneumothorax) per kg of body weight, or described another way, 30–60 mL of air per kg body weight resulted in pneumothorax that was considered to be of "moderate severity" based on CT examination (Walker *et al.* 1993).

In a clinical study, CT was used for evaluation of 12 dogs with spontaneous pneumothorax due to pulmonary blebs and bulla. In this report, CT was superior to radiography in identifying the affected lung lobe(s) and the correlation of CT and radiography with the surgical findings was (k = 0.735) and (k = 0.306), respectively. In the 10 dogs with lesions confirmed at surgery, CT correctly identified lesions in 9 dogs compared to only 2 with radiography. When looking specifically at the lung lobes involved, CT correctly identified 13 of 17 affected lobes, versus only 4 of 17 for radiography. A potential explanation as to why lesions were missed with CT in some of the dogs was the presence of pneumothorax at the time of the scan, which resulted in displacement and collapse of the lungs that may have interfered with detection of the lesions. Based on this concern, it was recommended that the thorax be completely evacuated or maintained on continuous suction at the time of scanning to minimize artifact caused by persistent pneumothorax (Au *et al.* 2006).

Ultrasonography

The use of ultrasound for the diagnosis of pneumothorax is well established in humans with steadily improving clinical accuracy. Thoracic ultrasound is primarily used in the emergency setting for rapid diagnosis of pneumothorax in trauma patients, or as a bedside technique for serial assessment of patients that have undergone thoracic aspiration or biopsy procedures or are being mechanically ventilated. The advantages of thoracic ultrasound include the ability to rapidly and repeatedly evaluate the pleural space in real time, avoiding the stress and delay encountered with radiography or CT scan; the ability to examine patients while recumbent or in various positions, avoiding the need to sit upright or stand for optimal thoracic radiographs; and the lack of exposure to ionizing radiation compared to radiography or CT scan.

The use of ultrasound for diagnostic evaluation of pneumothorax was first reported in the veterinary literature in 1986 (Rantanen 1986). In that report, the technique for scanning the thorax and the sonographic characteristics of pneumothorax were described, establishing the foundation for the use of ultrasound for the diagnosis and assessment of pneumothorax. Since then, multiple experimental and clinical studies have described the use of ultrasound for diagnosing pneumothorax in small animals and its evolving practicality and accuracy compared to other diagnostic techniques (Tidwell 1998; Boy & Sweeney 2000; Jung & Bostedt 2004; Ramirez et al. 2004; Lisciandro et al. 2008; Moon 2009; Hwang et al. 2018; Boysen 2021; Cole et al. 2021).

Thoracic ultrasound is generally performed with a portable ultrasound machine using a 2–12 MHz convex or linear probe. The technique described in dogs involves examination of the dorsolateral aspect of intercostal spaces 7–9 and the ventrolateral aspect of intercostal spaces 5–6. Dogs are positioned in lateral recumbency for examination of the ipsilateral (nondependent) hemithorax, and then rotated into sternal recumbency for examination of the contralateral hemithorax. Dogs experiencing respiratory distress can also be placed in sternal recumbency, allowing for examination of both hemithoraces (Lisciandro et al. 2008).

The ability of ultrasound to detect pneumothorax is based on the principle that in the normal thorax, the lungs (visceral pleura) are in contact with the chest wall (parietal pleura) and move against each other during expansion and contraction of the chest. The movement of the two pleural surfaces against each other can be readily detected with ultrasound and has been characterized as the "sliding sign" or the "glide sign" (Figure 34.4).

(a)

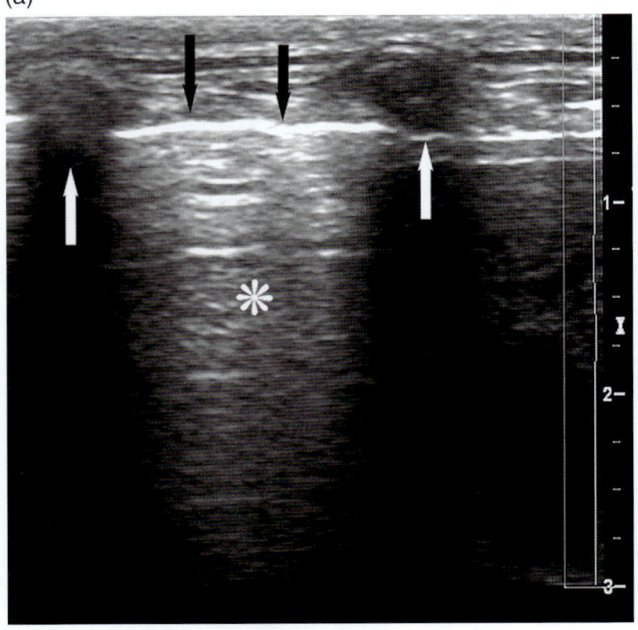

(b)

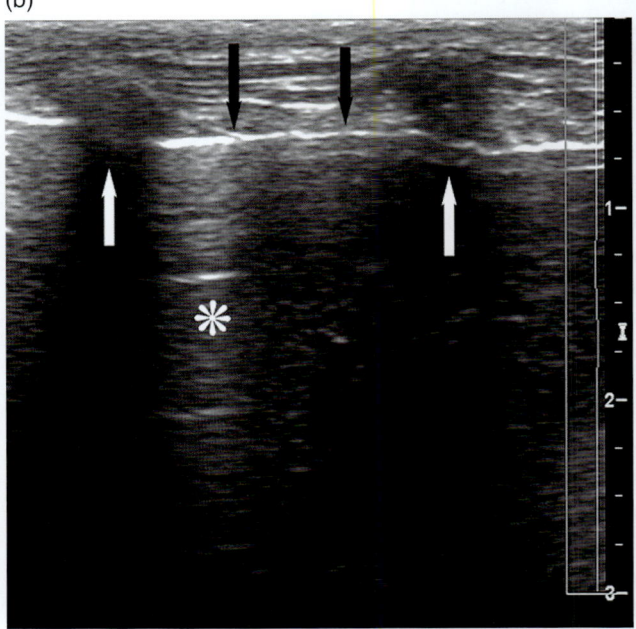

Figure 34.4 (a, b) Ultrasound images of the thoracic cavity in a normal dog. The hyperechoic "pleural line" (black arrows) is created by the visceral pleural of the lung contacting the parietal pleura of the chest wall. Reverberation of the ultrasound signal from the air-filled deeper lung parenchyma is indicated by the asterisk. Imaging of the lung during respiration reveals the pleural line moving back and forth past the ribs (white arrows), creating a "sliding" or "gliding" sign. Note the position and relationship of the pleural line and deeper lung tissue relative to the ribs (a, b). In the presence of pneumothorax, the pleural line is still present; however, the "gliding sign" is eliminated due to the air separating the visceral and parietal pleural surfaces from each other.

In cases of pneumothorax, air in the pleural space creates a hyperechoic interface between the two pleural surfaces, disrupting or eliminating the gliding sign and thereby leading to a positive diagnosis. "B lines" or "comet tail" artifacts are another ultrasound finding that have been used in the diagnosis of pneumothorax. B lines are hyperechoic reverberations that arise from the pleura and extend into the deeper portions of the image. B lines are generally associated with some degree of lung pathology, including pulmonary edema, foreign bodies, calcification, and discrete or focal collections of air on the pleural surface. Similar to the "glide sign," the detection of B lines requires that both pleural surfaces be in close contact with each other for proper transmission of the ultrasound signal. In cases of pneumothorax, the air interface between the pleural surfaces disrupts the transmission of the ultrasound signal and thus eliminates the B lines, leading to a positive diagnosis (Lisciandro et al. 2008; Boysen 2021).

The accuracy of ultrasound for the diagnosis of pneumothorax in humans has improved steadily over time and it has proven to be more accurate than conventional portable radiographs (supine recumbency taken with vertical beam) for detecting small volumes of pneumothorax (Chan et al. 2020). Numerous studies comparing the efficacy of thoracic ultrasound to radiographs and CT for detecting pneumothorax have been performed in humans, and several recent studies revealed sensitivities of 75–99% and specificities of 40–100% when evaluating specific sonographic characteristics (Alrajab et al. 2013; Staub et al. 2018; Dahmarde et al. 2019; Chan et al. 2020; Fei et al. 2021).

Although thoracic ultrasound is highly operator dependent, it appears that when used by various clinical specialists (i.e., radiologists, emergency and critical care clinicians, surgeons) trained in its use, the clinical accuracy is generally high, making it a valuable diagnostic tool for detecting pneumothorax (Abassi et al. 2013; Alrajab et al. 2013; Shumbusho et al. 2020; Chan et al. 2020). There are, however, several factors that can affect the accuracy of ultrasound, resulting in a false-negative or false-positive diagnosis. A false-positive diagnosis of pneumothorax may result from conditions that affect the normal sliding of the pleural surfaces, such as pleural adhesions or pulmonary atelectasis due to inadequate ventilation. Also, B lines are generally associated with some degree of underlying lung pathology and in cases where the lungs are normal or free of direct trauma, the sign may not be readily evident, leading to false-positive diagnosis. False-negative diagnoses may occur when the volume of air in the thorax is very small or located in pockets, such that it is missed on routine examination of the thorax. Another potential cause

for a false-negative diagnosis occurs when contraction and relaxation of the intercostal muscles mimic the appearance of "lung sliding" and interfere with the detection of underlying pneumothorax. In addition, more overt forms of thoracic trauma such as rib fractures, intercostal muscle tears, subcutaneous emphysema, hemothorax, and diaphragmatic hernia can affect the detection of pleural air, resulting in either a false-negative or false-positive diagnosis (Walters et al. 2018; Santorelli et al. 2021).

Treatment

The decision to treat pneumothorax will depend greatly on the cause, extent, and rate of air leakage. Knowing the cause or source of pneumothorax helps in predicting whether a leak is likely to seal spontaneously, and thus what types of treatment(s) may be necessary and most effective. Various treatment options are discussed here and generally range from the least to most invasive.

Conservative management

For animals with mild or moderate pneumothorax that does not appear to be progressing rapidly, conservative management including cage confinement, careful monitoring of vital parameters, oxygen supplementation via cage, nasal or flow-by routes, and intravenous fluid support may be all that is necessary for stabilization. If the site of leakage is known, such as in cases of iatrogenic pneumothorax due to thoracocentesis or lung biopsy, it may be beneficial to place the animal in lateral recumbency with the site of leakage down (dependent position) to potentially reduce leakage and assist in affecting a seal. In an experimental study performed on six dogs with experimentally created pneumothorax using a 20-gauge needle to puncture the lung, the rate of leakage decreased significantly when dogs were placed with the puncture site down compared to up (Zidulka et al. 1982; Zidulka 1987). The proposed benefits of placing the leak in the dependent position include the reduced difference in alveolar and pleural pressures (i.e., equilibration), the reduced alveolar size, and decreased ventilation of the dependent lung compared to the nondependent lung. Also, any hemorrhage or clots arising from the lung may be more effective in sealing the site due to the surface tension on the lung, as well as being less likely to be dislodged while in the dependent position.

Thoracocentesis

Needle thoracocentesis is generally successful for most simple pneumothorax. Basic requirements include an 18–22-gauge needle or intravenous catheter, extension set, syringe, and three-way stopcock. Alternatively, a butterfly needle can be used instead of a standard needle and extension set. The gauge of the needle should be appropriate for the size of the animal and the length of the needle should be adequate to completely penetrate the thoracic wall to avoid false-negative aspiration. In situations where the animal is stable, survey thoracic radiographs should be obtained prior to thoracocentesis to better assess the degree of pneumothorax and any potential underlying cause or concurrent lung or thoracic pathology that may help determine the most appropriate intercostal space to place the needle. If the animal is not stable, and pneumothorax is suspected based on the history and physical examination findings, thoracocentesis should be performed as part of emergency stabilization prior to any further stress being placed on the animal. In preparation for placing the needle, the caudodorsal aspect of the thorax should be adequately clipped and prepped. The site of needle placement is generally between the seventh and ninth intercostal spaces toward the dorsal third of the thorax if the animal is in sternal recumbency, or the uppermost (nondependent) aspect of the thorax if the animal is in lateral recumbency. Placement of the needle should be done carefully to avoid accidental injury to the underlying lungs when penetrating the pleura. The presence of pneumothorax typically displaces the lungs away from the thoracic wall, creating a potential space for the needle to enter safely. However, as the air is removed and the lungs expand, the risk for iatrogenic injury increases and care must be taken to redirect the needle away from the lungs when continuing to aspirate. Depending upon the nature and source of the pneumothorax, aspirating one hemithorax is usually sufficient to alleviate clinical signs; however, if the animal fails to improve or significant air remains, the opposite hemithorax should be aspirated.

Thoracostomy tube drainage

Animals with severe or persistent pneumothorax beyond that which can be adequately managed with repeated thoracocentesis require thoracostomy tube drainage. Thoracostomy tubes allow for more effective intermittent or continuous pleural drainage, while avoiding the risks of repeated needle thoracocentesis. Placement of a thoracostomy tube typically requires heavy sedation or general anesthesia, but can be done using sedation and local analgesia in emergency situations. Preparation and location of tube placement are similar to thoracocentesis. Selecting the appropriate-sized tube should be based on the size of the animal and width of the intercostal space, as well as whether any blood or other fluid is likely to be removed in addition to air.

Small-bore or "mini" thoracostomy tubes have been described for the successful management of

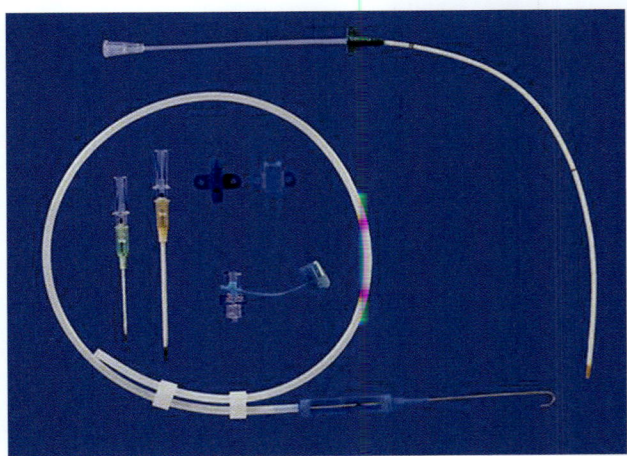

Figure 34.5 Small-bore thoracostomy tube set-up, including an over-the-needle catheter, flexible guidewire, fenestrated thoracostomy tube, and stopcock.

pneumothorax in dogs and cats and have essentially replaced the use of large-bore tubes (Valtolina & Adamantos 2009) (Figure 34.5). Small-bore tubes can be placed using a modified Seldinger technique with minimal disruption to the intercostal muscles and ribs. Potential advantages of smaller-bore tubes include ease of placement, less tissue dissection, and less pain after placement compared to larger-bore tubes. In a canine cadaver study, the efficacy of small-bore thoracostomy tubes (12 Ga) was similar to that of large-bore tubes (16–20 Fr) for removing air and fluid (Fetzer et al. 2017). Similarly, a meta-analysis of catheter type (small bore versus large bore) for management of spontaneous pneumothorax in humans determined that complications were lower, drainage duration was shorter, and hospitalization time was shorter when small-bore catheters were used for management of primary or secondary pneumothorax (Chang et al. 2018).

Large-bore thoracostomy tubes can be placed using either a sharp trocar or with the aid of a mosquito or Kelly hemostat to grip the tube and penetrate the intercostal musculature. To place the tube, a skin incision is made 5–7 cm caudal to the desired intercostal space and the tube tunneled cranially under the latissimus dorsi muscle to provide a seal around the tube and minimize the risk of air leaking into the thorax (Yoon et al. 2009). Alternatively, an assistant can stretch the thoracic skin cranially while the tube is inserted directly over the desired intercostal space. Once the tube is in place, the skin is released, creating a subcutaneous tunnel around the tube as the skin returns to its normal position. The latter technique has the advantage of allowing more complete dissection of the intercostal musculature prior to tube placement. This reduces the force necessary to insert the tube and therefore minimizes the risk of injuring underlying structures in animals with compliant thoracic walls such as cats or small dogs. Once the tube is in place, it is secured with a finger-trap suture anchored firmly to the underlying musculature, combined with either a purse-string suture placed around the skin incision or an encircling suture placed around the tunneled portion of the tube to reinforce the seal and minimize the risk of air leaking around the tube. Aspirating the tube can be done either intermittently or continuously, depending upon the rate of air leakage. Intermittent aspiration of thoracostomy tubes allows for more accurate measurement of the volume of air removed and assessment of the rate of leakage; however, it requires more frequent manipulation of the tube and increases the potential for accidental dislodgment or mishandling of the stopcock mechanism.

Alternatively, a Heimlich valve can be used to provide "continuous" drainage of air provided that the risks and benefits of using a Heimlich valve system are well understood. The use of Heimlich valves for thoracic drainage has been described in a series of 34 dogs (Salci *et al.* 2009). The majority of dogs in this study had undergone a thoracotomy for lung lobectomy or pneumonectomy. Heimlich valves were used successfully for 1–5 days for continuous postoperative drainage of residual air. Complications with the valve system were described in two dogs and included obstruction of the flapper valve mechanism with pleural fluid in one dog, and accidental pneumothorax that developed when one dog accidentally broke and dislodged the valve from the thoracostomy tube. Advantages of Heimlich valves include the relatively simple design and the ability to continually drain pleural air, alleviating the need for intermittent or continuous suction. Disadvantages of Heimlich valves include the ease with which the flapper valve mechanism can become obstructed with blood or other fluid, as already described, and the inability of animals with small tidal volumes (cats and small dogs) or weakened respiratory effort to overcome inherent resistance within the valve mechanism and effectively evacuate the pleural space. A modification to the traditional Heimlich valve system (Pneumostat™, Atrium Medical, Hudson, NH, USA) has been described in retrospective study in 98 humans with overall good outcome and few complications (Ramzisham *et al.* 2009) (Figure 34.6). The device includes a similar one-way valve, with the addition of a collection reservoir (30 mL) that can be emptied periodically, as necessary.

For animals with rapidly accumulating pneumothorax that cannot be practically managed with intermittent drainage, use of continuous suction is necessary. Continuous suction requires the use of house or portable

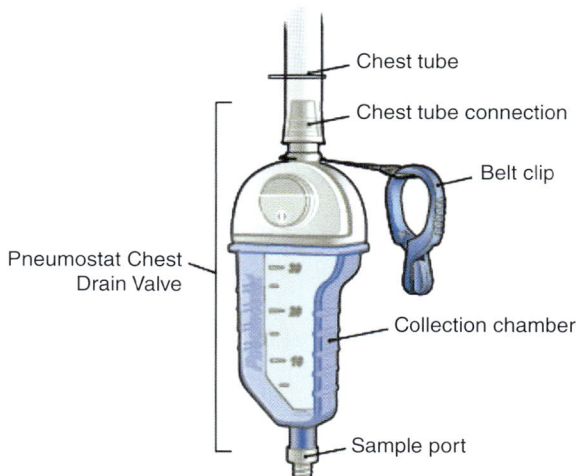

Figure 34.6 Pneumostat thoracic drainage device with a one-way valve and 30 mL fluid reservoir.

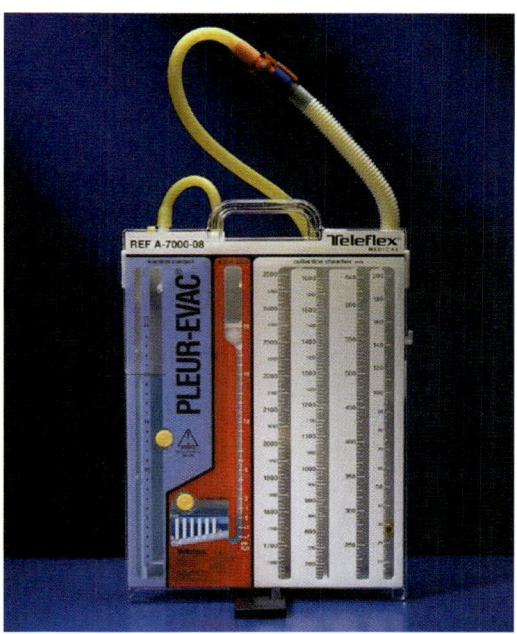

Figure 34.7 Pleur-evac® device for three-chamber continuous thoracic suction. Source: Teleflex Incorporated.

suction, as well as a three-chamber thoracic suction unit (Pleur-evac®, Teleflex Medical, Morrisville, NC, USA) to maintain an "underwater" seal and allow for regulating the degree of negative pressure applied to the tube (maximum 20 cm/H_2O) (Figure 34.7). Advantages of continuous suction include the potential for more rapid sealing of pulmonary leaks due to the increased contact between the visceral and parietal pleural surfaces, facilitating sealing of the parenchyma via adhesion and/or epithelialization. The volume of air removed during continuous suction can be crudely quantified by monitoring the collection chamber for bubbles arising from the tube. When it appears that the degree of air leakage is decreasing, the animal can be switched to intermittent suction to assess the degree of pneumothorax more accurately and determine when tube removal is appropriate based on individual circumstances.

Surgical management of pneumothorax

For animals with severe or persistent pneumothorax that does not resolve with continuous suction, surgical management may be necessary to resect or seal the source of leakage. Choosing the appropriate surgical approach requires knowing the precise source and anatomic location of the leak(s) (i.e., lungs, bronchi, trachea, esophagus). For cases where the source of the leakage is definitively known and confined to one hemithorax (i.e., focal pulmonary abscess), a lateral thoracotomy approach would be appropriate, and generally provides the best access to the lungs and other structures on that side. For cases where the source of leakage is not known or involves both lungs (i.e., multiple pulmonary bullae), a median sternotomy approach would be appropriate to allow access to both lungs.

The most difficult part of the surgical procedure is identifying the source of leakage, because it is not always obvious on initial inspection. Each lung should be carefully examined and palpated to identify any lesion that might be the source of leakage. If a lesion is not readily identified, the pleural space can be filled with sterile saline and each lung submerged, while actively ventilating the patient to help identify the source leakage. However, identifying the precise site of leakage while the lungs are inflated and filling the thoracic cavity can be very difficult, especially if the lesion is on the dorsal medial aspect of the caudal or accessory lung lobes.

Alternatively, thoracoscopy can be used as a less invasive means of examining the thorax and determining the source of leakage (Schmiedt 2009; Singh *et al.* 2019; Gordo *et al.* 2020). Thoracoscopic approaches are performed with the animal in either lateral or dorsal recumbency, depending upon whether one or both sides of the thorax are being examined. Advantages of thoracoscopy include improved lighting and magnification during examination of the thorax. Disadvantages include incomplete visualization of all of the surfaces of all of the lungs, due to the limited maneuverability of the scope and instruments and the constant motion of the lungs. To overcome the interference from the lungs, selective ventilation of one lung can be performed to improve visualization in the hemithorax of the nonventilated lung. Selective ventilation can be accomplished by either blocking the mainstem bronchus of one lung using a bronchial blocker or by selectively intubating one of the mainstem bronchi using a specialized endotracheal tube, thus resulting in the same effect. Placement of these specialized endotracheal tubes generally requires the use of flexible endoscopy to ensure accurate placement. Alternatively, bronchial intubation can be done "blindly," and the positioning of the endobronchial tube assessed at the time of thoracoscopy by evaluating the degree of inflation of the nonintubated lung lobes. Additionally, the use of fluoroscopy has been described for assessment of proper positioning of endobronchial tubes (Mayhew *et al.* 2012a). Use of selective ventilation can result in significant cardiovascular changes that require careful monitoring during anesthesia (Cantwell *et al.* 2000; Kudnig *et al.* 2003).

Other techniques that may be useful for reducing or eliminating pulmonary leaks alone or in combination with surgical resection are described next.

Tissue-sealing devices

The use of bipolar vessel-sealing devices (BVSDs) for the purpose of sealing pulmonary tissue has been reported in humans, as well as in a limited number of clinical, *in vivo*, and *ex vivo* experimental studies in various animal species including pigs, horses, rabbits, and dogs (Sakuragi *et al.* 2008; Relave *et al.* 2010; Mayhew *et al.* 2012b; Marvel & Monnet 2013; Kirschbaum *et al.* 2015; Brückner *et al.* 2019; Oberhaus & McFadden 2020). The experimental studies in animals involved resecting peripheral portions of lung tissue with a BVSD and then leak testing the site by inflating the remaining lung to physiologic, or greater, pressures. Additionally, in some studies, the tissue seal and the extent of thermal injury from the BVSD were examined histologically. The results of these studies demonstrated the BVSD to be generally successful at sealing lung tissue, with histologic evidence of a zone of fused tissue that was within the jaws of the device (seal) and a transition zone of thermal injury (0.9–6.75 mm) adjacent to the seal. However, leakage at the BVSD resection site has been identified in several studies, raising some concern about the use of this technology for partial lung lobectomy in dogs and horses (Relave *et al.* 2010; Marvel & Monnet 2013; Kirschbaum *et al.* 2015). More specifically, guidelines regarding the thickness of the lung tissue that can be safely sealed with bipolar vessel-sealing technology has not been well defined, and to date there have been no reports of a series of clinical case in small animals.

In contrast, there are multiple reports in humans describing the clinical use of BVSD for resection of pulmonary bulla and other lesions in the lungs (Shigemura *et al.* 2004; Santini *et al.* 2006; Sakuragi *et al.* 2008; Linchevskyy *et al.* 2010; Kovacs *et al.* 2009; Li *et al.* 2014).

The BVSD has been used alone or in combination with traditional stapling devices for partial lung lobectomy. In addition, some studies utilized pleural abrasion pleurodesis or tissue sealants (polyglycolic acid [PGA] sheet and fibrin glue) over the resection site to further augment the seal (Sakuragi *et al.* 2008; Linchevskyy *et al.* 2010). The clinical outcomes in humans have been favorable, with few reported complications other than isolated cases of persistent air leakage requiring extended thoracostomy tube drainage. A systematic review of the use of bipolar tissue-sealing technology for sealing tissues in the thoracic and abdominal cavities suggested that its use for pulmonary tissue is feasible, safe, and comparable to established technologies for partial lobectomy (Arya *et al.* 2015).

Tissue sealants

There are a number of topical products that have been developed for use as tissue sealants or patches to reduce leakage from lung tissue after surgical biopsy or resection. Some of the components of different sealants include gelatin, cellulose, alginate, fibrinogen, thrombin, albumin, hydrogel, polyethylene glycol, glutaraldehyde, cyanoacrylate, and, most recently, plant-based pectin (Zhong *et al.* 2021). Assessing the evidence for clinical effectiveness of individual products is challenging, due to the fact that very few studies are randomized or controlled, and most meta-analyses combine various products together, despite the potential for a product to have unique properties that might be more efficacious compared to others. A detailed review of all of the available sealants is beyond the scope of this chapter, but knowledge of the various types of sealants and their functionality is useful when faced with managing intraoperative air leaks so as to potentially minimize postoperative complications.

Currently, the only US Food and Drug Association (FDA)-approved (2012) product for pulmonary application is Progel™ (BD, Franklin Lakes, NJ, USA), which contains human serum albumin and polyethylene glycol, and is applied as a gel using a mixing syringe. The product has been evaluated in multiple studies with overall positive outcomes, demonstrating the ability to seal intraoperative leaks, as well as reduce postoperative leakage, the duration of chest tube use, and hospitalization time (Klijian 2012; Fuller 2013; Ibrahim *et al.* 2016; Park *et al.* 2016; Mortman *et al.* 2018). However, as with many studies, patient variables, the lack of operative standardization, and the lack of control groups make interpretation of these data challenging (Belda-Sanchís *et al.* 2010). Additionally, a more recent study evaluating the prophylactic use of Progel on surgical sites with no active intraoperative leakage showed no difference in

the rate of postoperative air leakage when compared to a control group (Gologorsky *et al.* 2019).

Fibrin sealants are made up of primarily thrombin and fibrinogen (and in some cases other co-factors such as calcium, aprotinin, factor XIII, and fibronectin) incorporated into a scaffold material (Zhong *et al.* 2021). Fibrin sealants were initially approved for use as hemostatic agents, but over time the indications have evolved to include their use as sealants in pulmonary surgery. Two established fibrin sealants that are manufactured in sheet form for direct application over a leaking site include TachoSil® (Baxter, Deerfield, IL, USA) and EVARREST® (Ethicon, Somerville, NJ, USA). Multiple experimental and clinical reports have proven fibrin to be effective at sealing various types of pulmonary leaks (Kawamura *et al.* 2005). However, an evidence-based analysis of various studies concluded that the routine use of fibrin sealants in pulmonary surgery was not indicated, based on the overall incidence of recurrent postoperative pneumothorax, duration of chest tube drainage, duration of hospitalization, and cost with use of fibrin sealants, compared to not using them (Rice & Blackstone 2010).

Combining fibrin with various synthetic agents such as glutaraldehyde-albumin, polyethylene glycol, cyanoacrylate, and collagen fleece has also been described for use in pulmonary surgery, with advantages including improved tissue adherence and greater bursting pressure. However, reports of their use are less extensive and similar concerns have been raised with overall efficacy, as well as the degree of tissue reaction and biocompatibility (Araki *et al.* 2007; Spotnitz & Burks 2008; Petter-Puchner *et al.* 2010).

A novel type of tissue sealant that is recently under investigation is a plant-based pectin polymer (Servais *et al.* 2018; Kuckelman *et al.* 2020; Zheng *et al.* 2021). Pectin is a heteropolysaccharide that has substantial binding affinity to the glycocalyx of the visceral pleura. The polymer is a combination of high methoxyl pectin and carboxymethylcellulose that is formulated into a sheet (100 μm) that is applied directly to the lung. The unique property of the polymer is its ability to adhere to the mesothelial surface of the lung via interlinking of the glycocalyx of the pleura with the polysaccharide of the pectin. The mechanical bond is both strong and flexible, making it an appealing material for a pulmonary sealant. Several experimental studies using mouse and pig lung injury models have investigated the adhesive and sealing properties, as well as the short-term (seven-day) biocompatibility. In an *ex vivo* study in pigs, the pectin polymer was compared to other fibrin sealants and conventional stapling techniques for sealing a standardized lung injury, and it proved superior for immediate seal, return to normal tidal volume, and lack of air leakage after closure of the chest (Kuckelman *et al.* 2020). In an *in vivo* study in mice, the adhesive strength of the pectin polymer was compared to other sealants (cellulose patch, fibrin patch, gelatin sponge, Prolene® mesh [Ethicon], and cyanoacrylate) and was statistically stronger in a load displacement measurement (Servais *et al.* 2018). Although not currently available for clinical use, this class of sealant appears to have promise based on the unique mechanism of adhesion and performance in early studies.

Pleurodesis

Pleurodesis is the creation of adhesions between the visceral and parietal surfaces of the thoracic cavity. The rationale for pleurodesis in the treatment of persistent or recurrent pneumothorax is to create an inflammatory reaction over the pleural surfaces that leads to permanent adhesion of the lung to the thoracic wall, or at least fibrosis and thickening of the visceral pleura that prevent or reduce leakage from the affected portion of the lung. Techniques for pleurodesis include mechanical abrasion or disruption of the pleural surfaces, or instillation of irritating or caustic substances directly into the thorax. In humans, pleurodesis is a well-established treatment, used either alone or in combination with other surgical techniques, for persistent or recurrent pneumothorax caused by pulmonary blebs, bullae, or emphysematous lesions. The most common techniques for pleurodesis in humans include the instillation of talc slurry or tetracycline derivatives via thoracostomy tube, thoracoscopic talc poudrage, or mechanical abrasion of the pleura using dry gauze or pleural abrader, performed via thoracoscopic or conventional surgical approach (Gossot *et al.* 2004; Ramos-Izquierdo *et al.* 2010; Chen *et al.* 2014). There are very few tightly controlled, randomized studies comparing pleurodesis techniques in humans and a consensus as to the most effective treatment has yet to be determined.

A confounding problem with investigating techniques and agents for pleurodesis is that efficacy varies considerably between species, so extrapolation of results from different experimental studies using animal models should be done with caution. There are only few studies that examine the effectiveness of pleurodesis techniques specifically in dogs, and based on these studies, mechanical abrasion, talc slurry, and talc poudrage produced inconsistent or limited adhesions in normal dogs (Bresticker *et al.* 1993; Colt *et al.* 1997; Jerram *et al.* 1999). However, there are no reports describing the use of these techniques specifically for the clinical management of pneumothorax in dogs, and thus it remains unknown whether the degree of fibrosis or thickening of the visceral pleura induced by these techniques would be sufficient to seal leaks from pulmonary blebs, bullae, or other lesions associated with spontaneous pneumothorax.

Blood patch pleurodesis

Blood pleurodesis was first described in humans in 1987 for treatment of persistent spontaneous pneumothorax. Since that time, blood pleurodesis has gradually gained acceptance due to its relative simplicity, general lack of complications, and overall success rate (Lang-Lazdunski & Coonar 2004; Athanassiadi *et al.* 2009; Oliveira *et al.* 2010). The technique involves direct injection of venous peripheral blood (45–250 mL) into the chest via a thoracostomy tube and then rotating body position periodically to distribute the blood throughout the thorax. After injection, thoracic suction is temporarily halted or modified to prevent premature removal of the blood. The proposed mechanism of action includes the direct sealing of pleural leaks via adhesion of clotted blood to the affected pleural surface, and possibly the generalized inflammation of the pleural surfaces leading to pleurodesis. Relative contraindications to blood pleurodesis include active pleural infections or known bacterial contamination of the thoracostomy tube. Potential complications include fever or signs of systemic inflammation, obstruction of the thoracostomy tube with clotted blood, or pyothorax due to growth of bacteria within the injected blood. Although most reports in humans are uncontrolled and lack randomization or comparison with other techniques, blood pleurodesis appears to be very effective at resolving persistent pneumothorax of various underlying causes, with success rates ranging from 70% to 100% (Cao *et al.* 2012; Manley *et al.* 2012; Evman *et al.* 2016; Campisi *et al.* 2022; Karampinis *et al.* 2021).

The use of blood patch pleurodesis for the clinical management of pneumothorax in a dog was first described by Merbl *et al.* in 2010 and since that time an additional 24 cases (21 dogs and 3 cats) have been reported (Oppenheimer *et al.* 2014; Bersenas & Hoddinott 2020; Dickson *et al.* 2021; Théron *et al.* 2021). The causes for pneumothorax in the 21 dogs included pulmonary blebs and bullae (n = 8), trauma (n = 3), bullous emphysema (n = 2), congenital bullae (n = 2), pneumonia (n = 1), lungworm infection (n = 1), bite injury (n = 1), migrating grass awn (n = 1), and unknown (n = 2). Similar to humans, the technique for blood pleurodesis described in dogs involves injecting 5–10 mL/kg of venous blood into the chest via a thoracostomy tube or butterfly catheter. For dogs with bilateral pneumothorax, half of the blood volume was injected into each hemithorax with a 30-minute interval between sides, or alternatively dogs were rotated onto the opposite recumbency to promote distribution of the blood within the thorax. When injecting blood via a thoracostomy tube, 10–20 mL of saline was injected after the blood to flush the tube and minimize the risk of clots obstructing the tube. Additionally, tubes were not evacuated for at least four hours after injection to maintain the volume of blood in the chest for as long as possible. The success rate for the 13 dogs from the two studies by Theron and Oppenheimer, with specific details regarding treatment and follow-up, was 85% (11 of 13). Eight dogs responded to one treatment, two dogs responded to two treatments, one dog responded to three treatments, and two dogs failed to respond after two treatments, resulting in one death and one euthanasia (Oppenheimer *et al.* 2014; Théron *et al.* 2021). An additional eight dogs have been mentioned in a report as having failed blood pleurodesis for treatment of spontaneous pneumothorax due to pulmonary blebs or bulla, although no specific details of the treatment were included. The eight dogs had undergone 1–3 pleurodesis treatments and were part of a retrospective study on surgical treatment of 110 dogs with primary spontaneous pneumothorax (Dickson *et al.* 2021). Complications related to the blood pleurodesis include two cases of positive bacterial cultures (one from a pleural effusion sample and one from a bronchoalveolar lavage sample).

Blood pleurodesis has also been described in three cats for management of postoperative pneumothorax following diaphragmatic herniorrhaphy (Bersenas & Hoddinott 2020). The specific cause for the pneumothorax was not known, but likely due to some type of direct injury to the lungs, barotrauma, or reexpansion injury. The unique difference in these cats compared to dogs was the use of allogenic blood from donor cats (blood type matched), due to concerns for exacerbating cardiovascular instability with autologous blood pleurodesis. In this study 18–24 mL of blood (6.9–7.3 mL/kg) was injected via a thoracostomy tube and thoracic drainage was withheld for at least one hour after injection. Pneumothorax resolved in all three cats within 4–24 hours and no complications were reported. Based on the data from clinical and experimental studies in humans and animals, blood pleurodesis would appear to be a reasonable option for the treatment of pneumothorax in dogs and cats; however, the small number of cases and the variety of underlying causes for pneumothorax preclude any realistic assessment of the efficacy at this time, and further investigation into case selection, volume of blood, timing of administration, and complications is obviously warranted.

Types of pneumothorax

Traumatic pneumothorax

Traumatic pneumothorax is the most common form of pneumothorax in small animals and has been reported to occur in 30–47% of animals that have sustained blunt-force trauma to the body and 69% of dogs with thoracic bite wounds (Powell *et al.* 1999; Sigrist *et al.* 2004; Scheepens *et al.* 2006; Simpson *et al.* 2009). Traumatic pneumothorax can be classified as either open or closed, depending upon whether the thorax has been penetrated and a direct communication exists between the pleural space and the atmosphere. Open pneumothorax may be further characterized as transient or continuous, depending upon whether the communication with the atmosphere seals spontaneously via the surrounding soft tissues, as may occur with some stab or penetrating wounds, or remains open, as with large lacerations or significant tissue loss (Figure 34.8). Initial management of open pneumothorax requires sealing the penetration site with a sterile occlusive dressing and evacuating the residual air from within the thorax to reestablish negative pressure. Definitive treatment depends on the type of injury, but generally requires some degree of lavage and débridement of the puncture site, followed by closure or reconstruction of the thoracic wall. If the

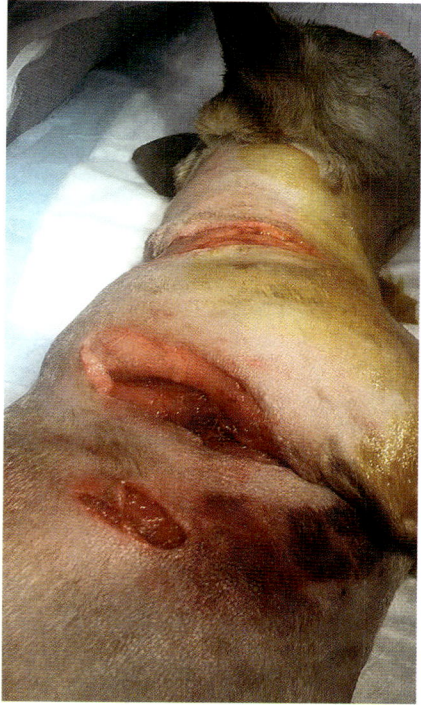

Figure 34.8 Dog-bite injury to the right lateral thorax and cervical area, resulting in "open pneumothorax" partially sealed by the overlying soft tissues.

penetrating injury has led to significant contamination of the thorax or damage to other thoracic structures, additional thoracic lavage and exploration of the thorax may be indicated (Scheepens *et al.* 2006; Risselada *et al.* 2008).

Closed pneumothorax is generally the result of some type of blunt force causing barotrauma or avulsion injury to the pulmonary structures. The source of air is typically the lung parenchyma, but the bronchi and trachea are also potential sites of leakage. If the trachea or bronchi are involved, pneumomediastinum is likely to be present. Traumatic pneumothorax is often accompanied by concurrent thoracic injuries such as pulmonary contusions, diaphragmatic hernia, rib fractures, or hemothorax, which may also impact the extent of respiratory compromise and likewise affect the course of treatment (Powell *et al.* 1999; Sigrist *et al.* 2004; Simpson *et al.* 2009). Treatment for traumatic pneumothorax will vary depending upon the nature of the injury and the rate of air leakage; however, simple needle thoracocentesis or thoracostomy tube drainage is usually sufficient for stabilizing most dogs and cats. Unfortunately, there are no extensive retrospective studies or case series describing the outcome specifically for dogs or cats with traumatic, closed pneumothorax; however, clinical experience and anecdotal evidence indicate that most pulmonary leaks resolve spontaneously over a period of 72 hours and thus rarely require surgical intervention.

Other traumatic injuries such as tracheal or bronchial avulsions or lacerations may result in substantial pneumothorax and mediastinal or subcutaneous emphysema, and potentially require more immediate and aggressive diagnostic and surgical intervention to locate and seal the source of leakage (Lawrence *et al.* 1999; White & Burton 2000; White & Oakley 2001).

Spontaneous pneumothorax

Spontaneous pneumothorax can be further classified as either primary or secondary based on the underlying cause or condition of the lung and whether a lesion is "clinically apparent" or not (Noppen & De Keukeleire 2008). Various causes of spontaneous pneumothorax include migrating or inhaled foreign bodies, parasites, abscesses, lobar emphysema, pulmonary thromboembolism, lower airway inflammation, pulmonary neoplasia, asthma, and pulmonary blebs and bullae (Busch & Noxon 1992; Forrester *et al.* 1992; Lipscomb *et al.* 2003; Cooper *et al.* 2003; White *et al.* 2003; Hopper *et al.* 2004; Gopalakrishnan & Stevenson 2007; Sobel & Williams 2009; Mooney *et al.* 2012; Trempala & Herold 2013; Boudreau *et al.* 2013; Trehiou *et al.* 2020; Seriot *et al.* 2021). Knowledge of the many and various causes of spontaneous pneumothorax aids in the clinical management of affected animals; however, determining the underlying cause is highly dependent on the type and accuracy of the particular diagnostic tests (i.e., survey radiography, CT, thoracoscopy, lung biopsy, bronchial lavage) used to assess the lungs. In addition, classification of the underlying cause as either primary or secondary can be somewhat controversial or a matter of semantics, even with definitive histopathologic information (Cheng *et al.* 2009; Louw *et al.* 2020).

Pulmonary blebs and bullae

Pulmonary blebs and bullae are the most common cause of spontaneous pneumothorax in dogs. Pulmonary blebs are accumulations of air within the layers of the visceral pleura and are most commonly located at the lung apices (Murphy & Fishman 1988). They form when air escapes from within the lung parenchyma, travels to the surface of the lung, and becomes trapped between the layers of the visceral pleura. Grossly, blebs appear as "bubbles" or "blister-like" lesions on the surface of the lung that range in size up to several centimeters in diameter (Figure 34.9a).

Pulmonary bullae are air-filled spaces within the lung parenchyma that result from the destruction, dilatation, and confluence of adjacent alveoli (Murphy & Fishman 1988). Bullae can vary in size, with some being small, involving only a few alveoli, and others being very large, involving the majority of the lung. Bullae are confined by the connective tissue septa within the lung and the internal layer of the visceral pleura. Bullae have been classified into three types based on the size and connection with surrounding lung tissue (Murphy & Fishman 1988; Lipscomb *et al.* 2003) (Figure 34.9b,c).

Pulmonary blebs or bullae have been reported most commonly in healthy, middle-aged, large-breed or deep-chested dogs, with the Siberian husky being highly represented in several studies (Howes *et al.* 2020; Dickson *et al.* 2020, 2021). Clinical signs typically include anorexia, lethargy, coughing, tachypnea, exercise intolerance, increased respiratory effort, and various degrees of respiratory distress or dyspnea. For some dogs, respiratory signs may develop rapidly and be very obvious, whereas for others, initial clinical signs may be very nonspecific (i.e., anorexia, depression) and it is not until the pneumothorax progresses that respiratory signs develop (Holtsinger *et al.* 1993; Puerto *et al.* 2002; Howes *et al.* 2020; Dickson *et al.* 2021). In a recent study, the median duration of clinical signs prior to presentation was 4 days, ranging from 0 to 32 days, highlighting the variability of progression and effect of pneumothorax in dogs (Dickson *et al.* 2021).

The pathogenesis of pulmonary bleb and bulla lesions in both dogs and humans has yet to be completely understood; however, the histopathologic similarities

(a)

(b)

(c)

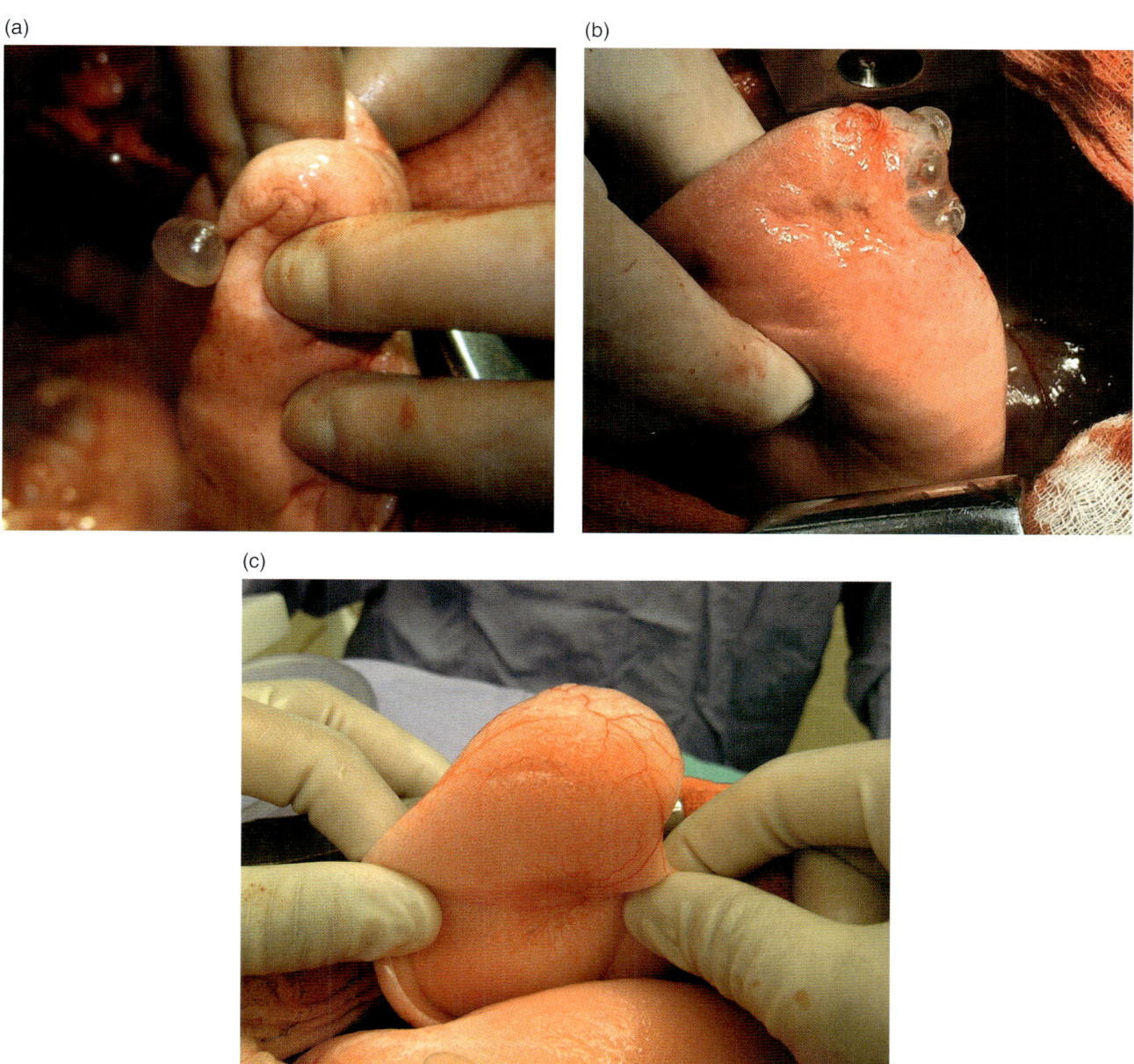

Figure 34.9 (a–c) Intraoperative images of three different dogs with primary spontaneous pneumothorax. (a) Pulmonary bleb; (b) type 1 pulmonary bulla; and (c) type 3 pulmonary bulla.

between species may suggest a similar pathogenesis. A study by Wilke and Robinson revealed decreased levels of α-1 antitrypsin in lung samples from dogs with spontaneous pneumothorax compared to normal dogs (Wilke & Robinson 2010). Using immunohistochemical staining techniques, a significantly decreased level of α-1 antitrypsin was detected in the subpleural cells of surgically resected bullous lesions from dogs with spontaneous pneumothorax compared to lung samples from normal dogs.

In humans, primary spontaneous pneumothorax occurs most commonly in young, tall males with a low body mass index. The hypothesis for pneumothorax in individuals with this body conformation is that there are increased distensive forces at the apices of the lungs, resulting in the formation of blebs and bullae that eventually leak, causing pneumothorax (Vawter *et al.* 1975). Additionally, cigarette smoking has been determined to be a significant risk factor for developing pulmonary bleb and bulla lesions in humans, due to its effect on degradative enzymes in the alveoli and increased inflammation in the lower airways. One study revealed a 22-fold increase in relative risk for developing pneumothorax in male smokers and a 9-fold increase in relative risk in female smokers (Bense *et al.* 1987). Smoking may inactivate α-1 antitrypsin, creating a focal imbalance between elastase and α-1 antitrypsin. This results in increased elastase-induced degradation of elastic fibers and progressive destruction of pulmonary parenchyma (Fukuda *et al.* 1994). Smoking also increases the number of macrophages and neutrophils in the distal airways. This influx of inflammatory cells may create a partial obstruction that acts as a "check valve" leading to increased pressures in the distal air spaces, hyperinflation of alveoli, and eventual bullae formation. Influx of inflammatory cells has also been associated with bronchiolitis, bronchiolar wall fibrosis, and destruction of pulmonary parenchyma, leading to the formation of emphysematous-like changes (Adenisa *et al.* 1991). Bronchoalveolar lavage in humans with primary spontaneous pneumothorax has shown a close relationship between the total cell count, especially macrophages, and the extent of emphysematous-like changes seen on CT (Schramel *et al.* 1995). Another theory suggests that there may be anatomic differences in the lower airways that predispose humans who have never smoked to spontaneous pneumothorax. A significant number of airway anomalies, including abnormal airway branching, smaller-diameter airways, and accessory airways have been identified with bronchoscopy in humans with primary spontaneous pneumothorax (Bense *et al.* 1992). More recently, various connective tissue disorders and genetic syndromes affecting the structural integrity of the lungs have been associated with primary spontaneous pneumothorax (Louw *et al.* 2020). Increases in transpulmonary pressure resulting from changes in atmospheric (weather) conditions have also been implicated as a potential cause for the formation and rupture of pulmonary bleb and bulla lesions. However, this has not been consistently validated and substantial institutional and regional biases exist in most of the studies examining atmospheric conditions, and thus the relationship to spontaneous pneumothorax remains undetermined (Scott *et al.* 1989; Celik *et al.* 2009; Mendogni *et al.* 2020).

Definitive diagnosis of pulmonary blebs and bullae with survey radiography can be difficult, since the lesions are not usually apparent due to their relatively small size and location on the margins of the lungs. However, serial thoracic radiographs should be taken to help rule out other potential causes of pneumothorax, such as pulmonary neoplasia or abscesses. As previously mentioned, CT is currently the most accurate imaging modality for detecting pulmonary blebs and bulla lesions; however, the rate of false positives and false negatives is still relatively high and thus CT cannot be relied upon to definitively identify the number or location of lesions (Figure 34.10).

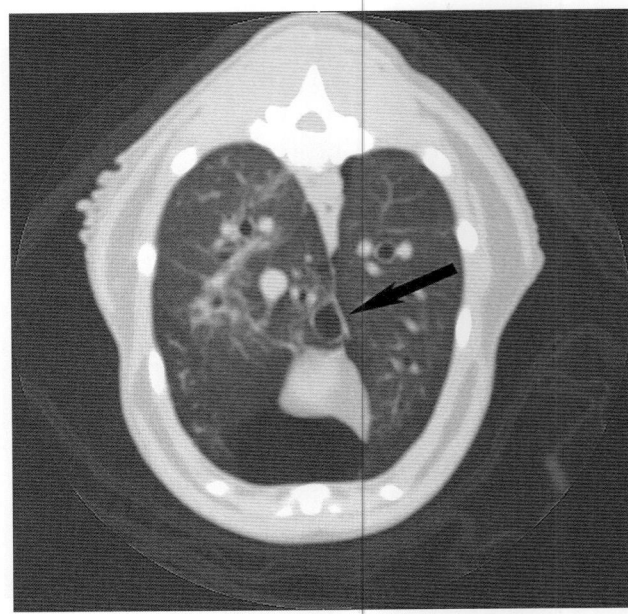

Figure 34.10 Thoracic computed tomographic image of a pulmonary bulla lesion on the accessory lung lobe (black arrow).

In two studies evaluating the ability of CT to accurately detect bullous lesions in dogs with spontaneous pneumothorax, the sensitivity ranged from 42% to 69% (Reetz *et al.* 2013; Dickson *et al.* 2020). Variables such as the degree of pneumothorax, degree of atelectasis, and the size of the lesions were evaluated as potential factors contributing to the accuracy of detecting lesions. The findings varied between studies, but the degree of atelectasis (decreased) and the size of the lesions (increased) were associated with improved accuracy, reinforcing the importance of minimizing the degree of atelectasis induced by anesthesia during CT. Additionally, the accuracy of identifying lesions was improved when CT was performed in both dorsal and sternal recumbency (Dickson *et al.* 2020). The positioning protocol allowed for better assessment of the ventral and dorsal margins of the lungs when in the opposite recumbency, due to the separation of the lung margins from the thoracic wall. In addition, the repositioning protocol allowed for displacement of air trapped between the lungs that may potentially mimic the appearance of bullous lesions, and thus improved the overall accuracy of the scan.

Thoracoscopy may also be used for evaluating suspicious lesions detected on CT to help determine the most appropriate approach to treatment; however, thoroughly evaluating all of the surfaces of the lungs thoracoscopically is challenging, and thus concern for missing lesions should be factored into the decision making. Other diagnostic tests, such as a complete blood count, serum biochemical profile, and urine analysis, are typically not helpful for determining the cause of pneumothorax, although rarely may help identify other concurrent problems or systemic conditions (i.e., peripheral eosinophilia) associated with the primary problem affecting the lungs (i.e., dirofilaria immitis).

Initial treatment of pneumothorax should focus on stabilization with strict rest, oxygen supplementation, and thoracic drainage. Thoracocentesis should be performed as often as necessary to maintain adequate ventilation. For dogs with more rapid accumulation of air, a thoracostomy tube should be placed to allow for more efficient drainage, and if necessary the use of continuous thoracic suction. Unfortunately, thoracic drainage alone is not a reliable means of definitively treating pneumothorax caused by pulmonary blebs and bullae in dogs, due to the persistent and recurrent nature of the leakage (recurrence rate ranging from 25% to 50%) and surgical treatment should be considered once other obvious nonsurgical causes of pneumothorax have been ruled out (Puerto *et al.* 2002; Lipscomb *et al.* 2003). For dogs in which surgical treatment is not an option or when a less invasive treatment is initially prioritized, treatment with blood patch pleurodesis as described earlier may be considered recognizing the current lack of evidence for specific treatment of pulmonary blebs and bullae in dogs.

Definitive treatment for dogs involves resecting the pulmonary blebs and bullae with a partial or complete lung lobectomy. Due to the likelihood of multiple (21–42%) and bilateral (16–58%) lesions, a median sternotomy approach is recommended so that the entire thorax can be explored (Lipscomb *et al.* 2003; Reetz *et al.* 2013; Dickson *et al.* 2020, 2021; Howes *et al.* 2020). Use of a lateral thoracotomy approach is not recommended unless it can be definitively determined that lesions are confined to one hemithorax.

Overall, the results for surgical treatment of pulmonary blebs and bullae are generally very good. Recurrence (or persistence) of pneumothorax is the most common complication, with rates ranging from 0% to 14%, typically occurring within 30 days of surgery (Lipscomb *et al.* 2003; Au *et al.* 2006; Howes *et al.* 2020; Dickson *et al.* 2021). For most cases, it is unknown whether recurrent pneumothorax was due to leakage from a newly developed lesion or from a lesion that was missed at the time of surgery. The early timeframe for recurrence for most dogs suggests that it is more likely to be the result of a missed rather than a new lesion; however, in some of the dogs that have undergone a second surgery, lesions have been found on the cranial lung lobes that are generally very easy to evaluate, and thus it is surprising that lesions in that location would have been missed during the first procedure. In contrast, lesions have also been identified in the accessory lung lobe, which is typically challenging to examine, and thus missing a lesion in that lobe would not be completely unexpected. Additionally, although it has not been specifically described in any of the recent retrospective studies, pneumothorax in the immediate postoperative period could also be due to leakage from a lobectomy site(s), which adds to the challenge of determining the true cause of recurrence and complicates the decision making, regarding additional surgical intervention. There are only a small number of dogs (n = 10) reported to have undergone a second surgical procedure for recurrent pneumothorax due to the fact that many dogs are euthanized without further treatment (Howes *et al.* 2020; Dickson *et al.* 2021). For dogs undergoing a second surgery, the outcomes were generally good if newly identified lesions are successfully removed. However, second episodes of recurrent pneumothorax have been described in two dogs, emphasizing the challenging and dynamic nature of this disease process.

Various risk factors for the recurrence of pneumothorax have been investigated, including age, breed, sex, body weight, surgical approach, number and location of lesions, and lobectomy technique. Thus far, no clear risk factors have been identified, with the possible exception of "giant-breed" dogs having a potentially higher risk for recurrence. However, without a more definitive way of confirming the status of lungs at the time of initial surgical examination, the clinical value of determining risk factors for recurrent pneumothorax remains questionable.

Thoracoscopy has been described in several reports as a minimally invasive approach for treating pulmonary blebs and bullae. In a report by Brissot *et al.* (2003), three dogs with pulmonary bullae were treated with partial lung lobectomy using an endoscopic linear stapling device, without complications or recurrence for 18–29 months after surgery. More recently, the use of video-assisted thoracoscopic surgery (VATS) was described in 12 dogs with pulmonary bullae. Conversion to median sternotomy was performed in 6 dogs and 6 dogs were treated entirely with VATS. The success rate for the dogs treated with VATS was 50% (3/6) and the success rate for dogs treated via median sternotomy was 83% (5/6). Conclusions from the study were that positively identifying and resecting lesions via a thoracoscopic approach is very challenging, and the risk for missing lesions and the need to convert to an open procedure should be considered when determining the surgical approach (Case *et al.* 2015).

Histopathologic examination of bleb and bullae lesions from dogs has revealed a consistent pattern of focal abnormalities, including subpleural emphysema, atelectasis, muscular hypertrophy of the respiratory ducts, increased foreign particulate matter, and varying degrees of inflammation (Lipscomb *et al.* 2003; Howes *et al.* 2020). It is not clear whether the muscular hypertrophy found surrounding the respiratory ducts is the cause or result of bleb and bulla formation; however, it does suggest a chronic change and indicates that the lesions may exist for some time before clinical signs develop. The consistent histologic changes support the idea that focal blebs and bullae represent a distinct or "primary" form of disease in dogs, but with an underlying cause that has yet to be definitively determined. In humans, bleb and bulla lesions exhibit similar focal changes, including emphysema, atelectasis, chronic inflammation, fibrosis, increased particulate foreign material, bronchial lesions, and vascular changes, with the remainder of the lungs appearing macroscopically normal (Lichter & Gwynne 1971; Ohata & Suzuki 1980).

References

Abassi, S., Farsi, D., Hafezimoghadam, P. et al. (2013). Accuracy of emergency physician-performed ultrasound in detecting traumatic pneumothorax after a 2-h training course. *European Journal of Emergency Medicine* 20: 173–177.

Adenisa, A.M., Vallyathan, V., McQuillen, E.N. et al. (1991). Bronchiolar inflammation and fibrosis associated with smoking: a morphologic cross-sectional population analysis. *American Review of Respiratory Disease* 143: 144–149.

Alderson, B., Senior, J.M., and Dugdale, A.H.A. (2006). Tracheal necrosis following tracheal intubation in a dog. *Journal of Small Animal Practice* 47: 754–756.

Alrajab, S., Youssef, A.M., Akkus, N.I. et al. (2013). Pleural ultrasonography versus chest radiography for the diagnosis of pneumothorax: review of the literature and meta-analysis. *Critical Care* 17: R208.

Araki, M., Tao, H., Nakajima, N. et al. (2007). Development of new biodegradable hydrogel glue for preventing alveolar air leakage. *Journal of Thoracic and Cardiovascular Surgery* 134: 1241–1248.

Aronson, E. and Reed, A.L. (1995). Pneumothorax: ventrodorsal or dorsoventral view – does it make a difference? *Veterinary Radiology & Ultrasound* 36: 109–110.

Arya, S., Mackenzie, H., and Hanna, G.B. (2015). Non-vascular experimental and clinical applications of advanced bipolar radiofrequency thermofusion technology in the thorax and abdomen: a systematic review. *Surgical Endoscopy* 29: 1659–1678.

Athanassiadi, K., Bagaev, E., and Haverich, A. (2009). Autologous blood pleurodesis for persistent air leak. *Thoracic and Cardiovascular Surgeon* 57: 476–479.

Au, J.J., Weisman, D.L., Stefanacci, J.D. et al. (2006). Use of computed tomography for evaluation of lung lesions associated with spontaneous pneumothorax in dogs: 12 cases (1999-2002). *Journal of the American Veterinary Medical Association* 228: 733–737.

Barton, E.D. (1999). Tension pneumothorax. *Current Opinion in Pulmonary Medicine* 5: 269–284.

Belda-Sanchís, J., Serra-Mitjans, M., Iglesias Sentis, M. et al. (2010). Surgical sealant for preventing air leaks after pulmonary resections in patients with lung cancer. *Cochrane Database of Systematic Reviews* (1): CD003051. https://doi.org/10.1002/14651858.CD003051.pub3.

Bennett, R.A., Orton, E.C., Tucker, A. et al. (1989). Cardiopulmonary changes in conscious dogs with induced progressive pneumothorax. *American Journal of Veterinary Research* 50: 280–284.

Bense, L., Eklund, G., Odont, D. et al. (1987). Smoking and the increased risk of contracting spontaneous pneumothorax. *Chest* 92: 1009–1012.

Bense, L., Eklund, G., and Winan, L.G. (1992). Bilateral bronchial anomaly. A pathogenic factor in spontaneous pneumothorax. *American Review of Respiratory Disease* 146: 513–516.

Bersenas, A.M. and Hoddinott, K.L. (2020). Allogenic blood patch pleurodesis for continuous pneumothorax in three cats. *Journal of Feline Medicine and Surgery Open Reports* 6: 2055116920945595.

Bhandal, J. and Kuzma, A. (2008). Tracheal rupture in a cat: diagnosis by computed tomography. *The Canadian Veterinary Journal* 49: 595–597.

Bjorling, D.E. and Whitfield, J.B. (1986). High-frequency jet ventilation during pneumothorax in dogs. *American Journal of Veterinary Research* 47: 1984–1987.

Boudreau, B., Nelson, L.L., Carey, S.A. et al. (2013). Spontaneous pneumothorax secondary to reactive bronchopneumopathy in a dog. *Journal of the American Veterinary Medical Association* 242: 658–662.

Boy, M.G. and Sweeney, C.R. (2000). Pneumothorax in horses: 40 cases (1980-1997). *Journal of the American Veterinary Medical Association* 216: 1955–1959.

Boysen, S.R. (2021). Lung ultrasonography for pneumothorax in dogs and cats. *Veterinary Clinics of North America. Small Animal Practice* 51: 1153–1167.

Bresticker, M.A., Oba, J., LoCicero, J. et al. (1993). Optimal pleurodesis: a comparison study. *Annals of Thoracic Surgery* 55: 364–366.

Brissot, H.N., Dupre, G.P., Bouvy, B.M. et al. (2003). Thoracoscopic treatment of bullous emphysema in 3 dogs. *Veterinary Surgery* 32: 524–529.

Brückner, M., Heblinski, N., and Henrich, M. (2019). Use of a novel vessel-sealing device for peripheral lung biopsy and lung lobectomy in a cadaveric model. *Journal of Small Animal Practice* 60: 411–416.

Busch, D.S. and Noxon, J.O. (1992). Pneumothorax in a dog infected with *Dirofilaria immitis*. *Journal of the American Veterinary Medical Association* 201: 1893.

Campisi, A., Dell'Amore, A., Gabryel, P. et al. (2022). Autologous blood patch pleurodesis: a large retrospective multicenter cohort study. *Annals of Thoracic Surgery* 114: 273–279.

Cantwell, S.L., Duke, T., Walsh, P.J. et al. (2000). One-lung versus two-lung ventilation in the closed-chest anesthetized dog: a comparison of cardiopulmonary parameters. *Veterinary Surgery* 29: 365–373.

Cao, G., Kang, J., Wang, F. et al. (2012). Intrapleural instillation of autologous blood for persistent air leak in spontaneous pneumothorax in patients with advanced chronic obstructive pulmonary disease. *Annals of Thoracic Surgery* 93: 1652–1657.

Case, J.B., Mayhew, P.D., and Singh, A. (2015). Evaluation of video-assisted thoracic surgery for treatment of spontaneous pneumothorax and pulmonary bullae in dogs. *Veterinary Surgery* 44: 31–38.

Celik, B., Kefeli, H., Hamzacebi, H. et al. (2009). The role of meteorological conditions on the development of spontaneous pneumothorax. *Thoracic and Cardiovascular Surgeon* 57: 409–412.

Chan, K.K., Joo, D.A., McRae, A.D. et al. (2020). Chest ultrasonography versus supine chest radiography for diagnosis of pneumothorax in trauma patients in the emergency department. *Cochrane Database of Systematic Reviews* 7: CD013031. https://doi.org/10.1002/14651858.cd013031.pub2.

Chang, S.H., Kang, Y.N., Chiu, H.Y. et al. (2018). A systematic review and meta-analysis comparing pigtail catheter and chest tube as the initial treatment for pneumothorax. *Chest* 153: 1201–1212.

Chen, J.S., Chan, W.K., Yang, P.C. et al. (2014). Intrapleural minocycline pleurodesis for the treatment of primary spontaneous pneumothorax. *Current Opinion in Pulmonary Medicine* 20: 371–376.

Cheng, Y.L., Huang, T.W., Lin, C.K. et al. (2009). The impact of smoking in primary spontaneous pneumothorax. *Journal of Thoracic and Cardiovascular Surgery* 138: 192–195.

Cole, L., Pivetta, M., and Humm, K. (2021). Diagnostic accuracy of a lung ultrasound protocol (Vet BLUE) for detection of pleural fluid, pneumothorax and lung pathology in dogs and cats. *Journal of Small Animal Practice* 62: 178–186.

Colt, H.G., Russack, V., Chiu, Y. et al. (1997). A comparison of thoracoscopic talc insufflation, slurry, and mechanical abrasion pleurodesis. *Chest* 111: 442–448.

Cooper, E.S., Syring, R.S., and King, L.G. (2003). Pneumothorax in cats with a clinical diagnosis of feline asthma: 5 cases (1990-2000). *Journal of Veterinary Emergency and Critical Care* 13: 95–101.

Dahmarde, H., Parooie, F., and Salarzaei, M. (2019). Accuracy of ultrasound in diagnosis of pneumothorax: a comparison between neonates and adults - a systematic review and meta-analysis. *Canadian Respiratory Journal* 2019: 5271982.

Dickson, R., Scharf, V.F., Michael, A.E. et al. (2021). Surgical management and outcome of dogs with primary spontaneous pneumothorax: 110 cases (2009–2019). *Journal of the American Veterinary Medical Association* 258: 1229–1235.

Dickson, R., Scharf, V.F., Nelson, N.C. et al. (2020). Computed tomography in two recumbencies aides in the identification of pulmonary bullae in dogs with spontaneous pneumothorax. *Veterinary Radiology & Ultrasound* 61: 641–648.

Evman, S., Alpay, L., Metin, S. et al. (2016). The efficacy and economical benefits of blood patch pleurodesis in secondary spontaneous pneumothorax patients. *Kardiochirurgia i Torakochirurgia Polska* 13: 21–25.

Fei, Q., Lin, Y., and Yuan, T.M. (2021). Lung ultrasound, a better choice for neonatal pneumo-thorax: a systematic review and meta-analysis. *Ultrasound in Medicine & Biology* 47: 359–369.

Fetzer, T.J., Walker, J.M., and Bach, J.F. (2017). Comparison of the efficacy of small and large-bore thoracostomy tubes for pleural space evacuation in canine cadavers. *Journal of Veterinary Emergency and Critical Care* 27: 301–306.

Forrester, S.D., Fossum, T.W., and Miller, M.W. (1992). Pneumothorax in a dog with a pulmonary abscess and suspected infective endocarditis. *Journal of the American Veterinary Medical Association* 200: 351–354.

Fukuda, Y., Haraguchi, S., Tanaka, S. et al. (1994). Pathogenesis of blebs and bullae of patients with spontaneous pneumothorax: an ultrastructural and immunohistochemical study. *American Journal of Respiratory and Critical Care Medicine* 149: A1022.

Fuller, C. (2013). Reduction of intraoperative air leaks with Progel in pulmonary resection: a comprehensive review. *Journal of Cardiothoracic Surgery* 8: 90–97.

Gilday, C., Odunayo, A., and Hespel, A.M. (2021). Spontaneous pneumothorax: pathophysiology, clinical presentation and diagnosis. *Topics in Companion Animal Medicine* 45: 1–8.

Gologorsky, R.C., Alabaster, A.L., Ashiku, S.K. et al. (2019). Progel use is not associated with decreased incidence of postoperative air leak after nonanatomic lung surgery. *Permanente Journal* 23: 18–59.

Gopalakrishnan, G. and Stevenson, G.W. (2007). Congenital lobar emphysema and tension pneumothorax in a dog. *Journal of Veterinary Diagnostic Investigation* 19: 322–325.

Gordo, I., Hubers, M., Bird, F.G. et al. (2020). Feasibility of the single-incision subxiphoid approach for video-assisted thoracoscopic surgery in dogs. *Journal of Small Animal Practice* 61: 480–486.

Gossot, D., Daletta, D., Stern, J.B. et al. (2004). Results of thoracoscopic pleural abrasion for primary spontaneous pneumothorax. *Surgical Endoscopy* 18: 466–471.

Holtsinger, R.H., Beale, B.S., Bellah, J.R. et al. (1993). Spontaneous pneumothorax in the dog: a retrospective analysis of 21 cases. *Journal of the American Animal Hospital Association* 29: 195–210.

Hopper, B.J., Lester, N.V., Irwin, P.J. et al. (2004). Imaging diagnosis: pneumothorax and focal peritonitis in a dog due to migration of an inhaled grass awn. *Veterinary Radiology & Ultrasound* 45: 136–138.

Howes, C.L., Sumner, J.P., Ahlstrand, K. et al. (2020). Long-term clinical outcomes following surgery for spontaneous pneumothorax caused by pulmonary blebs and bullae in dogs – a multicenter (AVSTS Research Cooperative) retrospective study. *Journal of Small Animal Practice* 61: 436–441.

Hwang, T.S., Yoon, Y.M., Jung, D.I. et al. (2018). Usefulness of transthoracic lung ultrasound for the diagnosis of mild pneumothorax. *Journal of Veterinary Science* 19: 660–666.

Ibrahim, M., Pindozzi, F., Menna, C. et al. (2016). Intraoperative bronchial stump air leak control by Progel® application after pulmonary lobectomy. *Interactive Cardiovascular and Thoracic Surgery* 22: 222–224.

Jerram, R.M., Fossum, T.W., Berridge, B.R. et al. (1999). The efficacy of mechanical abrasion and talc slurry as methods of pleurodesis in normal dogs. *Veterinary Surgery* 28: 322–332.

Johnson, E.G. and Wisner, E.R. (2007). Advances in respiratory imaging. *Veterinary Clinics of North America. Small Animal Practice* 37: 879–900.

Jung, C. and Bostedt, H. (2004). Thoracic ultrasonography technique in newborn calves and description of normal and pathological findings. *Veterinary Radiology & Ultrasound* 45: 331–335.

Karampinis, I., Galata, C., and Arani, A. (2021). Autologous blood pleurodesis for the treatment of postoperative air leaks. A systematic review and meta-analysis. *Thoracic Cancer* 12, 2648–2654.

Kawamura, M., Gika, M., Izumi, Y. et al. (2005). The sealing effect of fibrin glue against alveolar air leakage evaluated up to 48 h; comparison between different methods of application. *European Journal of Cardio-Thoracic Surgery* 28: 39–42.

Kern, D.A., Carrig, C.B., and Martin, R.A. (1994). Radiographic evaluation of induced pneumothorax in the dog. *Veterinary Radiology & Ultrasound* 35: 411–417.

Kirschbaum, A., Clemens, A., Steinfeldt, T. et al. (2015). Bipolar sealing of lung parenchyma: tests in an ex vivo model. *Surgical Endoscopy* 29: 127–132.

Klijian, A. (2012). A novel approach to control air leaks in complex lung surgery: a retrospective review. *Journal of Cardiothoracic Surgery* 7: 49–55.

Kovacs, O., Szanto, Z., Krasznai, G. et al. (2009). Comparing bipolar electrothermal device and endostapler in endoscopic lung wedge resection. *Interactive Cardiovascular and Thoracic Surgery* 9: 11–14.

Kuckelman, J., Conner, J., Zheng, Y. et al. (2020). Improved outcomes utilizing a novel pectin-based pleural sealant following acute lung injury. *Journal of Trauma and Acute Care Surgery* 89: 915–919.

Kudnig, S.T., Monnet, E., Riquelme, M. et al. (2003). Effect of one-lung ventilation on oxygen delivery in anesthetized dogs with an open thoracic cavity. *American Journal of Veterinary Research* 64: 443–448.

Lang-Lazdunski, L. and Coonar, A.S. (2004). A prospective study of autologous "blood patch" pleurodesis for persistent air leak after pulmonary resection. *European Journal of Cardio-Thoracic Surgery* 26: 897–900.

Lawrence, D.L., Lang, J., Culvenor, J. et al. (1999). Intrathoracic tracheal rupture. *Journal of Feline Medicine and Surgery* 1: 43–51.

Li, Z., Chen, L., Wang, J. et al. (2014). A single institution experience using the LigaSure vessel sealing system in video-assisted thoracoscopic surgery for primary spontaneous pneumothorax. *Journal of Biomedical Research* 28: 494–497.

Lichter, I. and Gwynne, J.F. (1971). Spontaneous pneumothorax in young subjects, a clinical and pathological study. *Thorax* 26: 409–417.

Linchevskyy, O., Makarov, A., and Getman, V. (2010). Lung sealing using the tissue-welding technology in spontaneous pneumothorax. *European Journal of Cardio-Thoracic Surgery* 37: 1126–1128.

Lipscomb, V.J., Hardie, R.J., and Dubielzig, R.R. (2003). Spontaneous pneumothorax caused by pulmonary blebs and bullae in 12 dogs. *Journal of the American Animal Hospital Association* 39: 435–445.

Lisciandro, G.R., Lagutchik, M.S., Mann, K.A. et al. (2008). Evaluation of a thoracic focused assessment with sonography for trauma (TFAST) protocol to detect pneumothorax and concurrent thoracic injury in 145 traumatized dogs. *Journal of Veterinary Emergency and Critical Care* 18: 258–269.

Louw, E.H., Shaw, J.A., and Koegelenberg, C.F.N. (2020). New insights into spontaneous pneumothorax: a review. *African Journal of Thoracic and Critical Care Medicine* 26: 18–22.

Manley, K., Coonar, A., Wells, F. et al. (2012). Blood patch for persistent air leak: a review of the current literature. *Current Opinion in Pulmonary Medicine* 18: 333–338.

Marvel, S. and Monnet, E. (2013). ex vivo evaluation of canine lung biopsy techniques. *Veterinary Surgery* 42: 473–477.

Mayhew, P.D., Culp, W.T.N., Pascoe, P.J. et al. (2012a). Evaluation of blind thoracoscopic-assisted placement of three double-lumen endobronchial tube designs for one-lung ventilation in dogs. *Veterinary Surgery* 41: 664–670.

Mayhew, P.D., Culp, W.T.N., Pascoe, P.J. et al. (2012b). Use of the ligasure vessel-sealing device for thoracoscopic peripheral lung biopsy in healthy dogs. *Veterinary Surgery* 41: 523–528.

Mendogni, P., Vannucci, J., Ghisalberti, M. et al. (2020). Epidemiology and management of primary spontaneous pneumothorax: a systematic review. *Interactive Cardiovascular and Thoracic Surgery* 30: 337–345.

Merbl, Y., Kelmer, E., Shipov, A. et al. (2010). Resolution of persistent pneumothorax by use of blood pleurodesis in a dog after surgical correction of a diaphragmatic hernia. *Journal of the American Veterinary Medical Association* 237: 299–303.

Mitchell, S.L., McCarthy, R., Rudolff, E. et al. (2000). Tracheal rupture associated with intubation in cats: 20 cases (1996–1998). *Journal of the American Veterinary Medical Association* 216: 1592–1595.

Moon, L.M. (2009). Ultrasound of the thorax (non-cardiac). *Veterinary Clinics of North America. Small Animal Practice* 39: 733–745.

Mooney, E.T., Rozanski, E.A., Ryan, G.P. et al. (2012). Spontaneous pneumothorax in 35 cats (2001–2010). *Journal of Feline Medicine and Surgery* 14: 384–391.

Mortman, K.D., Corral, M., Zhang, X. et al. (2018). Length of stay and hospitalization costs for patients undergoing lung surgery with Progel pleural air leak sealant. *Journal of Medical Economics* 21: 1016–1022.

Murphy, D.M. and Fishman, A.P. (1988). Bullous disease of the lung. In: *Pulmonary Diseases and Disorders*, 2e, 1219–2793. New York: McGraw-Hill.

Noppen, M. and De Keukeleire, T. (2008). Pneumothorax. *Respiration* 76: 121–127.

Oberhaus, A. and Mcfadden, M. (2020). Use of vessel sealing system for multiple partial lung lobectomies for spontaneous pneumothorax. *Canadian Veterinary Journal* 61: 875–879.

Ohata, M. and Suzuki, H. (1980). Pathogenesis of spontaneous pneumothorax with special reference to the ultrastructure of emphysematous bullae. *Chest* 77: 771–777.

Oliveira, F.H.S., Cataneo, D.C., Ruiz, R.L. et al. (2010). Persistent pleuropulmonary air leak treated with autologous blood: results from a university hospital and review of literature. *Respiration* 79: 302–306.

Oppenheimer, N., Klainbart, S., Merbl, Y. et al. (2014). Retrospective evaluation of the use of autologous blood-patch treatment for persistent pneumothorax in 8 dogs (2009–2012). *Journal of Veterinary Emergency and Critical Care* 24: 215–220.

Park, B.J., Snider, J.M., Bates, N.R. et al. (2016). Prospective evaluation of biodegradable polymeric sealant for intraoperative air leaks. *Journal of Cardiothoracic Surgery* 11: 168–176.

Petter-Puchner, A.H., Simunek, M., Redl, H. et al. (2010). A comparison of a cyanoacrylate glue (Glubran) vs. fibrin sealant (Tisseel) in experimental models of partial pulmonary resection and lung incision in rabbits. *Journal of Investigative Surgery* 23: 40–47.

Powell, L.L., Rozanski, E.A., Tidwell, A.S. et al. (1999). A retrospective analysis of pulmonary contusion secondary to motor vehicle accidents in 143 dogs: 1994-1997. *Journal of Veterinary Emergency and Critical Care* 9: 127–136.

Puerto, D.A., Brockman, D.J., Lindquist, C. et al. (2002). Surgical and nonsurgical management of and selected risk factors for spontaneous pneumothorax in dogs: 64 cases (1986-1999). *Journal of the American Veterinary Medical Association* 220: 1670–1674.

Ramirez, S., Lester, G.D., and Roberts, G.R. (2004). Diagnostic contribution of thoracic ultrasonography in 17 foals with rhodococcus equi pneumonia. *Veterinary Radiology & Ultrasound* 45: 172–176.

Ramos-Izquierdo, R., Moya, J., Macia, I. et al. (2010). Treatment of primary spontaneous pneumothorax by videothoracoscopic talc pleurodesis under local anesthesia: a review of 133 procedures. *Surgical Endoscopy* 24: 984–987.

Ramzisham, A.R., Ooi Su, M.J., Fikri, A.M. et al. (2009). Pocket-sized Heimlich valve (Pneumostat) after bullae resection: a 5-year review. *Annals of Thoracic Surgery* 88: 979–981.

Rantanen, N.W. (1986). Diagnostic ultrasound: diseases of the thorax. *Veterinary Clinics of North America. Equine Practice* 2: 49–66.

Reetz, J.A., Caceres, A.V., Suran, J.N. et al. (2013). Sensitivity, positive predictive value, and interobserver variability of computed tomography in the diagnosis of bullae associated with spontaneous pneumothorax in dogs: 19 cases (2003–2012). *Journal of the American Veterinary Medical Association* 243: 244–251.

Relave, F., David, F., Leclere, M. et al. (2010). Thoracoscopic lung biopsies in heaves-affected horses using a bipolar tissue sealing system. *Veterinary Surgery* 39: 839–846.

Rice, T.W. and Blackstone, E.H. (2010). Use of sealants and buttressing material in pulmonary surgery: an evidence-based approach. *Thoracic Surgery Clinics* 20: 377–389.

Risselada, M., de Rooster, H., Taeymans, O. et al. (2008). Penetrating injuries in dogs and cats: a study of 16 cases. *Veterinary and Comparative Orthopaedics and Traumatology* 21: 434–439.

Sakuragi, T., Okazaki, Y., Mitsuoka, M. et al. (2008). The utility of a reusable bipolar sealing instrument, BiClamp® for pulmonary resection. *European Journal of Cardio-Thoracic Surgery* 34: 505–509.

Salci, H., Bayram, A.S., and Gorgul, O.S. (2009). Outcomes of Heimlich valve drainage in dogs. *Australian Veterinary Journal* 87: 148–151.

Santini, M., Vicidomini, G., Baldi, A. et al. (2006). Use of an electro-thermal bipolar tissue sealing system in lung surgery. *European Journal of Cardio-Thoracic Surgery* 29: 226–230.

Santorelli, J.E., Chau, H., Godat, L. et al. (2021). Not so FAST—chest ultrasound underdiagnoses traumatic pneumothorax. *Journal of Trauma and Acute Care Surgery* 92: 44–48.

Scheepens, E.T.F., Peeters, M.E., L'Eplattenier, H.F.L. et al. (2006). Thoracic bite trauma in dogs: a comparison of clinical and radiological parameters with surgical results. *Journal of Small Animal Practice* 47: 721–726.

Schmiedt, C. (2009). Small animal exploratory thoracoscopy. *Veterinary Clinics of North America. Small Animal Practice* 39: 953–964.

Schramel, F.M.N.H., Meyer, C.J.L.M., and Postmus, P.E. (1995). Inflammation as a cause of spontaneous pneumothorax and emphysematous-like changes: results of bronchoalveolar lavage. *European Respiratory Journal* 8: 397–402.

Schwarz, L.A. and Tidwell, A.S. (1999). Alternative imaging of the lung. *Clinical Techniques in Small Animal Practice* 14: 187–206.

Scott, G.C., Berger, R., and McKean, H.E. (1989). The role of atmospheric pressure variation in the development of spontaneous pneumothoraces. *American Review of Respiratory Disease* 139: 659–662.

Seriot, P., Dunie-Merigot, A., Trehiou, C.B. et al. (2021). Treatment and outcome of spontaneous pneumothorax secondary to suspected migrating vegetal foreign body in 37 dogs. *Veterinary Record* 189, e22.

Servais, A.B., Valenzuela, C.D., Kienzle, A. et al. (2018). Functional mechanics of a pectin-based pleural sealant after lung injury. *Tissue Engineering Parts A* 24: 695–702.

Shigemura, N., Akashi, A., Nakagiri, T. et al. (2004). A new tissue-sealing technique using the LigaSure system for nonanatomical pulmonary resection: preliminary results of sutureless and stapleless thoracoscopic surgery. *Annals of Thoracic Surgery* 77: 1415–1419.

Shumbusho, J.P., Duanmu, Y., Kim, S.H. et al. (2020). Accuracy of resident performed point-of-care lung ultrasound versus chest radiography in pneumothorax follow-up after tube thoracostomy in Rwanda. *Journal of Ultrasound in Medicine* 39: 499–506.

Sigrist, N.E., Doherr, M.G., and Spreng, D.E. (2004). Clinical findings and diagnostic value of post-traumatic thoracic radiographs in dogs and cats with blunt trauma. *Journal of Veterinary Emergency and Critical Care* 14: 259–268.

Simpson, S.A., Syring, R., and Otto, C.M. (2009). Severe blunt trauma in dogs: 235 cases (1997–2003). *Journal of Veterinary Emergency and Critical Care* 19: 588–560.

Singh, A., Scott, J., Case, J.B. et al. (2019). Optimization of surgical approach for thoracoscopic-assisted pulmonary surgery in dogs. *Veterinary Surgery* 48: 99–104.

Sobel, K.E. and Williams, J.E. (2009). Pneumothorax secondary to pulmonary thromboembolism in a dog. *Journal of Veterinary Emergency and Critical Care* 19: 120–126.

Spotnitz, W.D. and Burks, S. (2008). Hemostats, sealants, and adhesives: components of the surgical toolbox. *Transfusion* 48: 1502–1516.

Staub, L.J., Biscaro, R.R.M., Kaszubowski, E. et al. (2018). Chest ultrasonography for the emergency diagnosis of traumatic pneumothorax and haemothorax: a systematic review and meta-analysis. *Injury* 49: 457–466.

Théron, M.L., Lahuerta-Smith, T., Sarrau, S. et al. (2021). Autologous blood patch pleurodesis treatment for persistent pneumothorax: a case series of five dogs (2016–2020). *Open Veterinary Journal* 11: 289–294.

Tidwell, A.S. (1998). Ultrasonography of the thorax (excluding the heart). *Veterinary Clinics of North America. Small Animal Practice* 28: 993–1015.

Trehiou, C.B., Gibert, S., Seriot, P. et al. (2020). CT is helpful for the detection and presurgical planning of lung perforation in dogs with spontaneous pneumothorax induced by grass awn migration: 22 cases. *Veterinary Radiology & Ultrasound* 61: 157–166.

Trempala, C.L. and Herold, L.V. (2013). Spontaneous pneumothorax associated with Aspergillus bronchopneumonia in a dog. *Journal of Veterinary Emergency and Critical Care* 23: 624–630.

Tschopp, J.M., Rami-Porta, R., Noppen, M. et al. (2006). Management of spontaneous pneumothorax: state of the art. *European Respiratory Journal* 28: 637–650.

Valtolina, C. and Adamantos, S. (2009). Evaluation of small-bore wire-guided chest drains for management of pleural space disease. *Journal of Small Animal Practice* 50: 290–297.

Vawter, D., Matthews, F.L., and West, J.B. (1975). Effect of shape and size of lung and chest wall on stresses in the lung. *Journal of Applied Physics* 39: 9–17.

Walker, M., Hartsfield, S., Matthews, N. et al. (1993). Computed tomography and blood gas analysis of anesthetized bloodhounds with induced pneumothorax. *Veterinary Radiology & Ultrasound* 34: 93–98.

Walters, A.M., O'Brien, M.A., Selmic, L.E. et al. (2018). Evaluation of the agreement between focused assessment with sonography for trauma (AFAST/TFAST) and computed tomography in dogs and cats with recent trauma. *Journal of Veterinary Emergency and Critical Care* 28: 429–435.

White, H.L., Rozanski, E.A., Tidwell, A.S. et al. (2003). Spontaneous pneumothorax in two cats with small airway disease. *Journal of the American Veterinary Medical Association* 222: 1573–1575.

White, R.N. and Burton, C.A. (2000). Surgical management of intrathoracic tracheal avulsion in cats: long-term results in 9 consecutive cases. *Veterinary Surgery* 29: 430–435.

White, R.N. and Oakley, M.R. (2001). Left principal bronchus rupture in a cat. *Journal of Small Animal Practice* 42: 495–498.

Wilke, V.L. and Robinson, N.A. (2010). Histological characteristics of spontaneous pneumothorax in the dog. *Veterinary Surgery* 39: E60.

Yoon, H.Y., Mann, F.A., Lee, S. et al. (2009). Comparison of the amounts of air leakage into the thoracic cavity associated with four thoracostomy tube placement techniques in canine cadavers. *American Journal of Veterinary Research* 70: 1161–1167.

Zheng, Y., Pierce, A.F., Wagner, W.L. et al. (2021). Functional adhesion of pectin biopolymers to the lung visceral pleura. *Polymers* 13: 2976.

Zhong, Y., Hu, H., Min, N. et al. (2021). Application and outlook of topical hemostatic materials: a narrative review. *Annals of Translational Medicine* 9: 577.

Zidulka, A. (1987). Position may reduce or stop pneumothorax formation in dogs receiving mechanical ventilation. *Clinical and Investigative Medicine* 10: 290–294.

Zidulka, A., Braidy, T.F., Rizzi, M.C. et al. (1982). Position may stop pneumothorax progression in dogs. *American Review of Respiratory Disease* 126: 51–53.

Section 6

Respiratory Surgery

Section 6

Respiratory

35

Oronasal and Oroantral Fistula

Naomi Hoyer

An oronasal fistula (ONF) is a communication between the oral and nasal cavities that is lined by epithelium. An oroantral fistula (OAF) is an epithelium-lined communication between the oral cavity and the maxillary recess. In dogs, the maxillary recess can be found palatal to the maxillary dentition in the caudal portion of the oral cavity. Oronasal communications can be caused by a number of different factors, including congenital maxillofacial clefts, trauma, iatrogenic injury during extraction, oncological surgery, surgical dehiscence, and advanced periodontal disease (Lommer 2020; Peralta & Marretta 2020; Sauve et al. 2019). The chronicity of a lesion allows the epithelium to form, transforming a communication to a fistula. There are a number of repair techniques that can be utilized to repair ONF/OAF defects. The most common is the single-layer mucoperiosteal flap.

Anatomy

ONF are pathologic, epithelium-lined communications between the oral and nasal cavities. OAF are pathologic, epithelium-lined communication between the oral cavity and the maxillary recess. This chapter will focus on acquired ONF that affect the area of the dental arcade at the site of attached gingiva and buccal mucosa. Congenital lesions will not be addressed.

The anatomy of the periodontal structures associated with these structures is critical for understanding and planning repairs of ONFs (Figure 35.1). The attached gingiva, which is immediately adjacent to the teeth, meets the buccal mucosa at the mucogingival junction (MGJ), which is a distinct anatomic structure in both the dog and the cat. The recognition of the MGJ is critical for the creation of the mucoperiosteal flaps associated with repair techniques. The attached gingiva meets the tooth at the sulcus, which is a 1–3 mm deep groove that extends circumferentially around each tooth. Within the dental arcade, the nasal cavity and the oral cavity are separate by very thin alveolar bone (Figure 35.2).

ONF may be associated with clinical signs consistent with rhinitis, such as sneezing, reverse sneezing, nasal discharge, and epistaxis. Patients who present with those clinical signs should be evaluated for disease of the dentition. Additional symptoms may include pawing at the face or oral cavity.

Etiology

The most common cause of ONF/OAF in dogs is periodontal disease. Periodontitis, which involves the presence of inflammatory mediators within the periodontium, results in alveolar bone loss, which can cause a communication. These communications may be masked if the associated tooth is still present in its alveolus. Bone loss due to periodontitis, especially on the palatal aspect of maxillary canine teeth, is a common contributor to OAF/ONF formation. One common feature of ONF associated with maxillary canine teeth is heavy calculus accumulation on the palatal aspect of the maxillary canine teeth (Figure 35.3). Periodontal disease and tooth resorption are often contributing factors in cats as well (Figure 35.4). Dachshunds develop ONF associated with their maxillary canine teeth (Figure 35.5) more frequently than other small breeds of dog because of the anatomic relationship between their maxillary canine tooth roots and the long, narrow configuration of their maxillae.

Small Animal Soft Tissue Surgery, Second Edition. Edited by Eric Monnet.
© 2023 John Wiley & Sons, Inc. Published 2023 by John Wiley & Sons, Inc.
Companion website: www.wiley.com/go/monnet/small

(a)

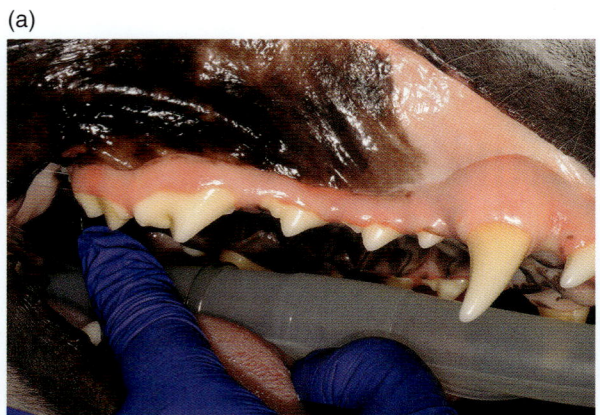

(b)

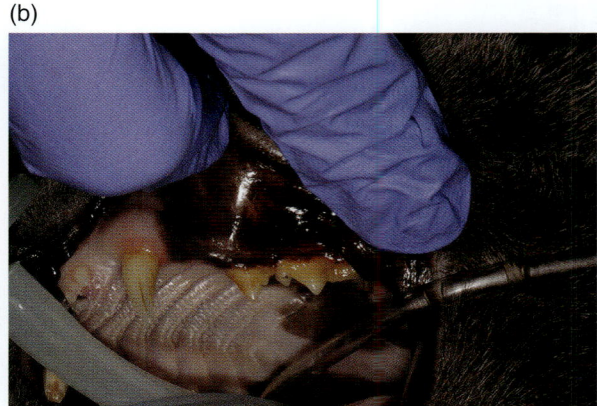

Figure 35.1 Normal periodontal anatomy in (a) the dog and (b) the cat.

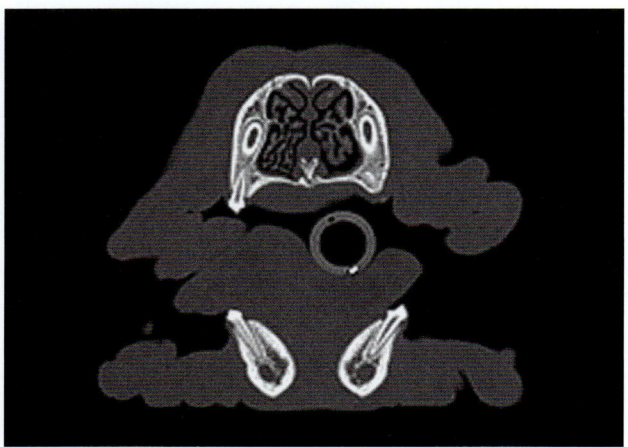

Figure 35.2 Computed tomography cross-section of a dog maxilla showing the thin wall of alveolar bone that exists between the apex of the maxillary canine and the adjacent nasal cavity.

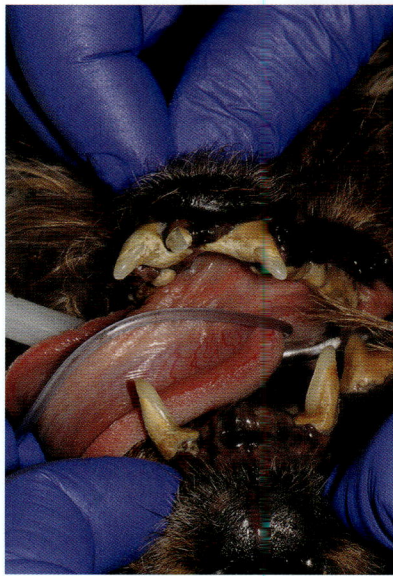

Figure 35.3 Maxillary canine teeth with heavy calculus accumulation on the palatal aspect of the maxillary canine teeth.

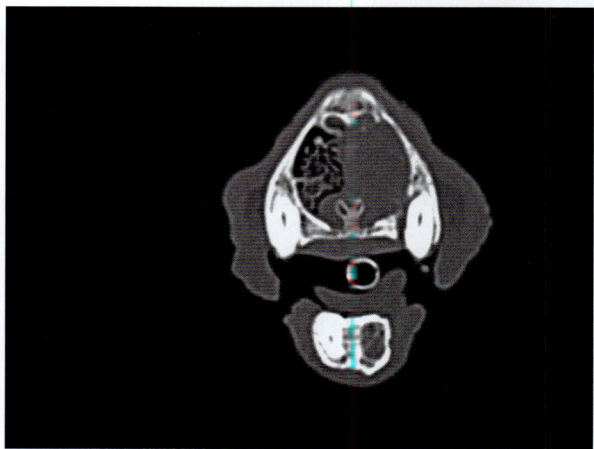

Figure 35.4 Stage 4 periodontal disease and tooth resorption associated with a maxillary canine tooth that led to an oronasal fistula in a cat.

Endodontic disease, which is infection of the pulp, can also cause loss of the nasoalveolar bone integrity, and can contribute to significant clinical signs of rhinitis. Because an ONF/OAF has an epithelial lining, a fistula is not present unless there is also a periodontal pocket that communicates with the periapical lesion.

Another common cause of ONF/OAF formation is inappropriate extraction technique of maxillary teeth. Dental elevators or luxators may be inadvertently inserted into the nasal and maxillary cavity if excessive force is used. If these extraction sites are not closed without a tension-free mucogingival flap, epithelialization of the communication will occur, resulting in a fistula.

Other causes of ONF/OAF include trauma, tumors, and surgical dehiscence from oral surgery (Figures 35.6 and 35.7). Acute traumatic causes of communication can often be repaired without development of an ONF/OAF. If a traumatic lesion causes a defect that can be

(a)

(b)

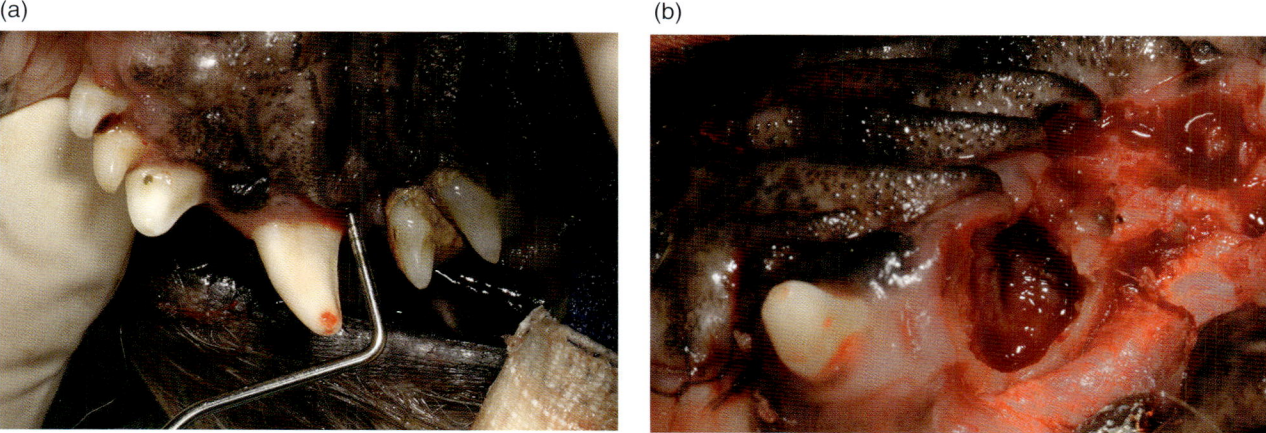

Figure 35.5 (a) A periodontal probe in an oronasal fistula (ONF) on the palatal aspect of a maxillary canine tooth. (b) The same ONF during the surgical repair, showing the defect in the alveolar bone that was identified after extraction of the maxillary canine tooth.

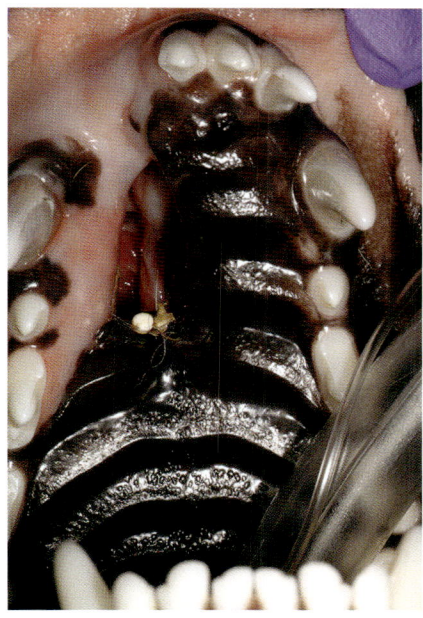

Figure 35.6 A dog who was discovered to have suffered from a gunshot wound as a puppy with a chronic oronasal fistula as a result of the tissue destruction.

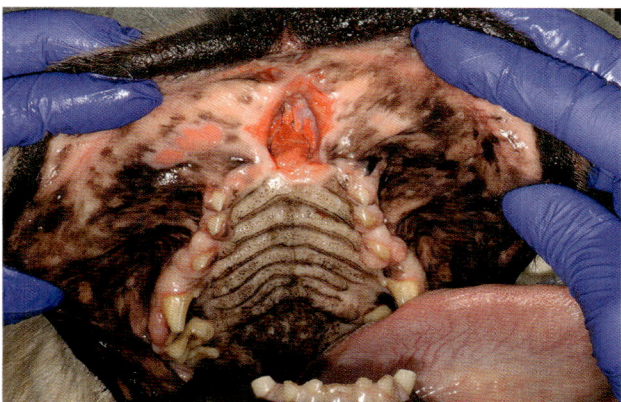

Figure 35.7 A dog with a large oronasal fistula secondary to a rostral maxillectomy.

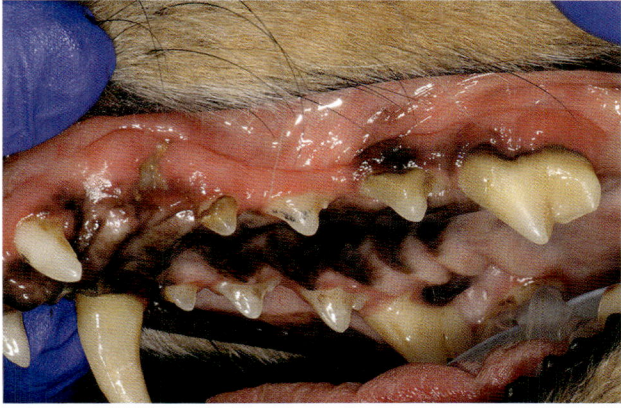

Figure 35.8 Lesions secondary to periodontal disease in a dog.

repaired without a flap, then the repair should be undertaken as soon as the patient is stable after trauma so that the gingival tissues do not recede. If the trauma has caused a large defect or was a high-velocity injury, for example a ballistic injury, then repair may need to be delayed due to the degree of the soft tissue injury.

Diagnosis

Diagnosis of an ONF/OAF is made with a careful, anesthetized oral examination and appropriate imaging techniques. Lesions secondary to periodontal disease may be disguised by the presence of the teeth. Larger more,

obvious lesions will be evident during a visual examination of oral tissues (Figure 35.8).

If the ONF secondary to periodontal disease is discovered during an anesthetized oral examination,

(a)

(b)

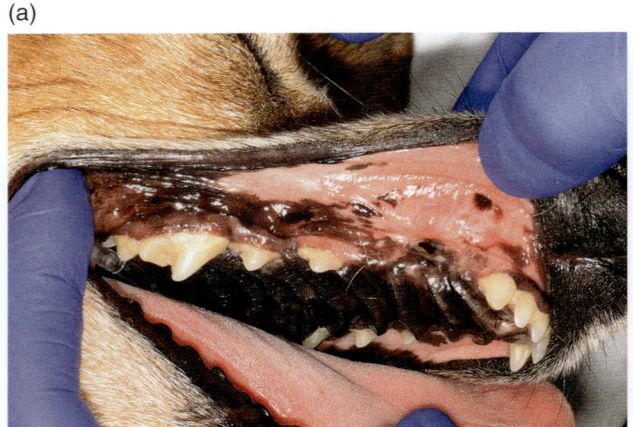
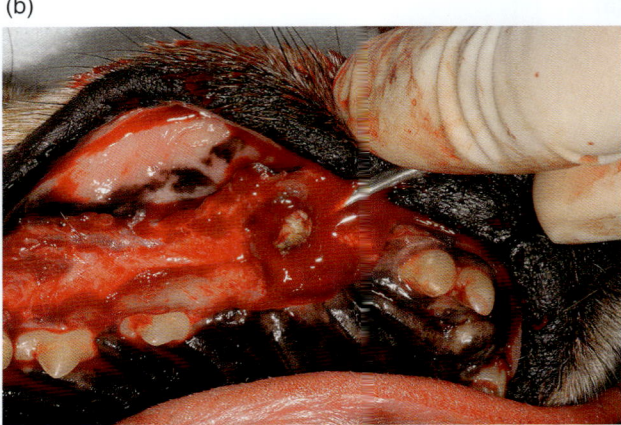

Figure 35.9 (a) A lesion in the oral cavity, (b) after elevation of the flap and visualization of the granulation tissue.

imaging with intraoral radiographs is recommended (Mulherin *et al.* 2018). Extraction of the associated tooth, with development of an appropriate mucoperiosteal or mucogingival flap that can be extended to cover the defect and closed with any tension on the suture line, is the best approach for these fistulae. Collection of a biopsy of the associated bone and soft tissue at the time of repair is also prudent to rule out underlying neoplastic or other causes for the communication. The epithelium lining the defect must be debrided thoroughly in order to minimize chances of dehiscence. This will result in a much larger lesion than was present initially (Figure 35.9).

If the tooth is already missing, then imaging should include computed tomography in order to evaluate the extent of the osseous lesion. If multiple repairs have already been attempted, surgical planning and staged extractions may be necessary in order to obtain adequate tissue.

Repair techniques

While there are several different repair techniques that have met with treatment success, it cannot be stressed enough how important the lack of tension and the apposition of the mucosal edges are for a successful repair (Smith 2000). Another important factor when making treatment decisions about ONF/OAF repair is allowing adequate time between repair techniques. If an initial repair fails, at least 4 weeks should be planned before a second repair is attempted. In addition, using a less invasive repair technique initially should be considered in order to preserve as much tissue as possible.

Single-layer vestibular or mucoperiosteal flaps are the most frequent repair technique used to repair fistulas associated with periodontal lesions (Marretta & Smith 2005). These flaps can be created at the time of extraction, or they can be created after abnormal epithelium is removed from the ONF/OAF site if the tooth is already missing. If there is not adequate tissue for closure, staged extractions of teeth near the defect may be performed in order provide more tissue to use for closure.

In addition to the single layer of closer, there are several other techniques described, depending on the location of the fistula and the extent of the lesion. These include double-flap techniques, rotating and island flap techniques, auricular cartilage grafts, and use of palatal obturators for lesions that are not amenable to surgical repair (Cox 2007; De Souza *et al.* 2005; Lorrain & Legendre 2012; Peralta *et al.* 2015).

References

Cox, H. (2007). Repair of oronasal fistulae using auricular cartilage grafts in five cats. *Veterinary Surgery* 36 (2): 164–169.

De Souza, H.J.M., Amorim, F.V., Corgozinho, K.B., and Tavares, R.R. (2005). Management of the traumatic oronasal fistula in the cat with a conical silastic prosthetic device. *Journal of Feline Medicine and Surgery* 7 (2): 129–133.

Lommer, M.J. (2020). Complications of extractions. In: *Oral and Maxillofacial Surgery in Dogs and Cats*, 2e (ed. F.J.M. Verstraete, M.J. Lommer and B. Arzi), 173–179. St Louis, MO: Elsevier.

Lorrain, R.P. and Legendre, L.F.J. (2012). Oronasal fistula repair using auricular cartilage. *Journal of Veterinary Dentistry* 29 (3): 172–175.

Marretta, S.M. and Smith, M.M. (2005). Single mucoperiosteal flap for oronasal fistula repair. *Journal of Veterinary Dentistry* 22 (3): 200–205.

Mulherin, B.L., Ewing, J.R., and Miles, K. 2018). Diagnostic imaging of oronasal fistulas in a dachshund *Journal of Small Animal Practice* 59 (6): 373–377.

Peralta, S. and Marretta, S.M. (2020). Acquired palatal defects. In: *Oral and Maxillofacial Surgery in Dogs and Cats*, 2e (ed. F.J.M. Verstraete, M.J. Lommer and B. Arzi), 404–414. St Louis, MO: Elsevier.

Peralta, S., Nemec, A., Fiani, N., and Verstraete, F.J.M. (2015). Staged double-layer closure of palatal defects in 6 dogs. *Veterinary Surgery* 44 (4): 423–431.

Sauve, C.P., MacGee, S.E., Crowder, S.E., and Schultz, L. (2019). Oronasal and oroantral fistulas secondary to periodontal disease: a retrospective study comparing the prevalence within dachshunds and a control group. *Journal of Veterinary Dentistry* 36 (4): 236–244.

Smith, M.M. (2000). Oronasal fistula repair. *Clinical Techniques in Small Animal Practice* 15 (4): 243–250.

36

Cleft Lip and Palate

Yoav Bar-Am

Cleft of the lip and palate are congenital deformities of the face reported in dogs and cats. In humans it is the most common facial deformity, with an incidence of 1/1000–2000 live births, and it can be manifested as a sole condition or as a part of a syndrome (Kemp *et al.* 2009a; Arosarena 2007). In dogs and cats, an accurate epidemiologic study of this condition is very difficult due to deaths of affected animals being unreported by their owners; however, one study reports the incidence as 0.5/1000 in dogs and 0.2/1000 in cats (Mulvihill *et al.* 1980). Another more recent study in purebred dogs suggests that the overall incidence of orofacial clefts varies significantly across breeds, ranging from none to a few cases per 1000 live births in some, to several dozen cases per 1000 live births in others (Roman *et al.* 2019). This study also indicates that breed, genetic cluster, and skull type are of importance in the development of orofacial clefts in dogs. Breeds in the mastiff/terrier genetic cluster and brachycephalic breeds are predisposed to orofacial clefts (Roman *et al.* 2019). This is in accordance with the suggestion that the risk for cleft palate increases the more the breed tends toward brachycephaly (Fox 1963). Furthermore, this assumption may be encouraged by the over 40-year notion of the great risk of bulldogs for cleft palate defects and by the low risk of dolichocephalic dogs such as German shepherds and collies. Other reported breeds affected by cleft palate include the American Staffordshire terrier, beagle, Bernese mountain dog, Boston terrier, boxer, English bulldog, French bulldog, bullmastiff, bull terrier, chihuahua, cocker spaniel, Cavalier King Charles spaniel, dachshund, Labrador retriever, Norwegian elkhound, Pekingese, poodle (toy), papillon, and shih-tzu (Padgett *et al.* 1986; Roman *et al.* 2019).

In dogs the cleft is not considered syndromic, although associated congenital defects such as cryptorchidism, hydrocephalus, epidermoid cyst, septal defect, microphthalmia, entropion, malformed bulla tympanica, bifid nose and/or tongue, and polydactyly have been reported (Mulvihill *et al.* 1980; Nemec *et al.* 2015; Arzi & Verstraete 2011).

In cats it seems that the Abyssinian breed is at the highest risk. Other reported breeds include Siamese, Persian, and domestic shorthair (Mulvihill *et al.* 1980).

Classification

Palatal defects are classified primarily as congenital or acquired.

Congenital clefts may occur in the primary palate, secondary palate, or both. The primary palate involves the structures situated rostral to the palatine fissure, while the secondary palate consists of those structures caudal to the palatine fissure (Coleman & Sykes 2001; Harvey & Emily 1993).

Cleft of the primary palate may affect the soft tissue only (cheiloschisis, aka harelip) or involve the alveolar ridge and incisive bone as well. It is most commonly manifested unilaterally with prevalence to the left side; it rarely occurs bilaterally and extremely rare is the medial cleft lip. Cleft of the primary palate may be associated with cleft of the secondary palate (Ellis 2008; Harvey & Emily 1993; Hale 2005; Peralta *et al.* 2017).

Cleft of the secondary palate may involve the hard palate, the soft palate, or both. It usually affects the midline, although left or right cleft of the soft palate has been reported.

Embryology

Facial development that includes the orbital, nasal, and oral regions begins when neural crest cells migrate and combine with the mesoderm to form five facial primordia, which include the single fronto-nasal prominence and the paired maxillary and mandibular prominence. The philtrum, primary palate, and lateral and medial nasal prominences are first to start forming by proliferation and differentiation of the fronto-nasal prominence (Figure 36.1). During the late embryonic phase the maxillary prominences proliferate and increase in size ventro-medially. When the tongue moves ventrally, it clears the way for the maxillary prominences to assume a horizontal position and fuse at the midline, forming the secondary palate (days 30–33 of gestation in dogs and cats) (Figure 36.1). The maxillary prominences fuse rostrally with the medial nasal prominences to form the incisive bones and the upper lip (Arosarena 2007; Johnston & Bronsky 1991; McGeady et al. 2006; Coleman & Sykes 2001; Ellis 2008).

Cleft lip will result from the failure of fusion between the maxillary prominences and the medial nasal prominences (Figure 36.1).

Primary cleft palate is the result of failure or incomplete fusion of the maxillary prominences with the fronto-nasal prominence.

Secondary cleft palate will result from incomplete or failure of the lateral palatine processes (maxillary prominences) to fuse.

Causative factors

Because of the importance of facial clefting in human medicine, the causes of this deformity have been extensively investigated, including in animal models. Although the exact cause of clefting is unknown, it is widely agreed to be multifactorial with a hereditary component (Arosarena 2007). Studies in humans have been able to implicate genetics in only 20–30% of patients with nonsyndromic cleft (Ellis 2008). Most genetic studies of cleft lip and palate in dogs suggest that these defects are inherited as an autosomal recessive trait (Kemp et al. 2009b; Cooper & Mattern 1971; Richtsmeier et al. 1994), while one study has shown this to be an X-linked gene or a sexually influenced autosomal-dominant gene (Sponenberg & Bowling 1985).

Other factors that have been implicated as possible etiologic contributors for the development of facial clefting include mechanical (intrauterine trauma), nutritional (hypervitaminosis A, folic acid deficiency), drugs (corticosteroids), toxins, and viral (Ellis 2008; Arosarena 2007; Warzee et al. 2001).

Problems associated with facial clefting

Feeding

Nursing is the major problem of neonates with facial clefting. A cleft lip deformity does not allow the formation of a tight seal around the mother's nipple, and the communication with the nasal cavity in the cleft of the primary and/or secondary palate does not allow for enough negative pressure to form for effective suckling. Inadequate ability or inability to nurse means a deficit in caloric intake, which leads to a deficit in weight gain. In

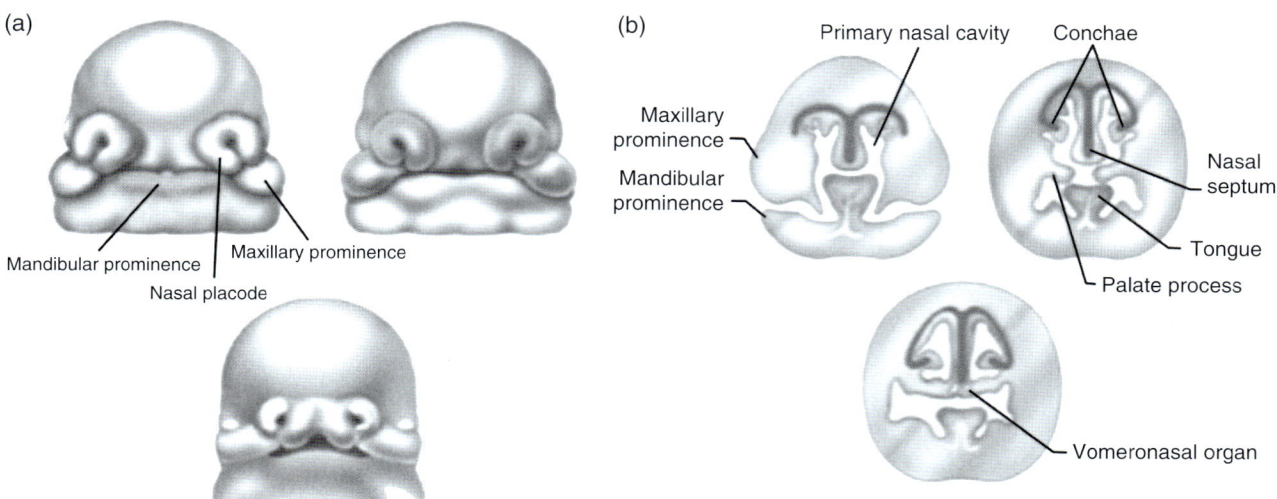

Figure 36.1 (a) Development of the oral and nasal structures. (b) Separation of the oral and nasal cavities by fusion of the palatal processes. © D. Giddings.

fact affected pups are considerably less developed than their normal littermates. The presence of the cleft causes milk to pass into the nasal cavity where it can cause rhinitis, or can be aspirated causing bronchopneumonia and aspiration pneumonia. In these cases the prognosis is poor and the neonate may rapidly succumb to malnutrition and/or respiratory infection.

Dental problems

Hypodontia and malocclusion of the maxillary incisors are common in animals suffering from cleft of the primary palate. In the majority of cases the clefting occurs at the maxillo-incisive suture, situated interproximally at the maxillary third incisor and canine tooth, and extends from the alveolar margin to the palatine fissure. Teeth may be missing, deformed, or displaced. Supernumerary and/or persistent deciduous incisor teeth may be present at the area of the defect and the whole incisive bone is shifted mesially and rostrally due to fusion failure at the embryonic stage (Fiani *et al.* 2016).

Nasal deformity

Deformity of the normal nasal architecture is characteristic of an animal suffering from cleft of the primary palate with or without cleft lip. The bony defect at the floor of the nose allows for the ipsilateral alar cartilage to flare and the philtrum of the nose is pulled toward the noncleft side due to the lack of bony support.

Ear problems

Animals with cleft of the soft palate may develop otitis media. The tensor and levator veli palatini muscles normally insert at the midline into the same muscle of the other side and, with deglutition, allow the opening of the ostium of the eustachian tubes. In animals with cleft palate, opening of the tubes does not occur due to dysfunction of these muscles leaving the middle ear without a draining outlet that may lead to serous or suppurative otitis media (Gregory 2000).

Diagnosis

Diagnosis of cleft palate is straightforward and can be confirmed by history and physical examination findings. Affected animals demonstrate poor growth due to difficulty nursing. Milk discharge from the nostrils, coughing, sneezing, and gagging are often observed during or after nursing. On oral examination cleft lip can be immediately observed. Cleft of the primary palate, secondary palate, involvement of the soft palate, and assessing the extent of the defect require opening the animal's mouth and examination of the oral cavity. Thoracic auscultation is indicated to detect abnormal

breathing sounds that may suggest respiratory tract infection due to aspiration. Thoracic radiographs are necessary for the diagnosis of aspiration pneumonia. Thorough physical examination is important to detect congenital malformations associated with cleft lip and palate defects (Sherwood *et al.* 1971).

Management of cleft lip and palate

The objectives of cleft lip and palate management are:

- To provide adequate caloric intake.
- To ensure safe delivery of nutritional support.
- To prevent/treat respiratory tract infections.
- To perform surgical repair of the defects at the optimal timing.
- To reduce the occurrence of the defect (spay/neuter).

Presurgical management

Cleft lip

Neonates presenting only cleft lip are easier to manage. The defect may result in being strictly esthetic or may cause ineffective suckling. These animals may be bottle fed, with a nipple long enough to be able to create negative pressure between the tongue and the hard palate. The nipple should have a big enough hole to deliver milk under relatively low negative pressure. After weaning these animals usually have no difficulties prehending, chewing, and swallowing food.

Cleft palate

Management of neonates with cleft of the primary and/or secondary palate is challenging. Clients should be well informed and aware of the treatment plan, risks, and complications. Clients should also be aware that the management and treatment of the condition may be protracted over months and that their compliance and dedication are imperative to its success.

Upon presentation, most affected animals suffer from caloric intake deficit, and may present signs of respiratory tract infection or aspiration pneumonia. Bypassing the oral cavity is necessary in these cases to ensure adequate and safe caloric intake and prevent food contamination and infections due to aspiration. Oro-esophageal or naso-esophageal feeding are usually well tolerated and may be implemented until weaning. As the animal grows, and requires larger amounts of food, an esophagostomy feeding tube can be placed and kept until surgical healing is confirmed (this could take several months).

Palatal obturators can be custom made, either by a dental laboratory or in clinics from acrylic, composite materials or silicon. Their purpose is to provide a temporary separation between the oral and nasal cavity until corrective surgery is performed (Hale *et al.* 1997; Lee *et al.* 2006). Their major disadvantage is the accumulation of debris along the edges of the obturator causing a foul smell and inflammation of the tissues in contact, which require frequent removal and cleaning.

Broad-spectrum antibiotic therapy with an anaerobic component is indicated in cases with signs of respiratory tract infection, especially in those with aspiration pneumonia.

Surgical management

Timing of surgery

In humans, for the last three decades, the timing of surgery for the repair of cleft of the primary and secondary palate has been a source of serious debate between those who favor late intervention with better surgical results, fewer complications, and fewer facial deformities, and those favoring early surgical correction to minimize the social, emotional, and psychological problems associated with these defects (Ellis 2008; Liao & Mars 2006; Tollefson *et al.* 2008).

In veterinary medicine there are no guidelines on the optimal timing for performing such surgeries. The suggested time of surgical interventions varies between 6 and 12 weeks of age (Waldron & Martin 1991). This is based on the size of the animal to allow access to the palate and on the notion that anesthesia risks are greater at an earlier age.

Factors that may influence timing of palatal surgery include the following:

- Younger animals are more prone to drug overdose, hyperthermia, and hypoglycemia, so they have increased odds of anesthetic-related death (Brodbelt *et al.* 2008).
- The palatal mucosa is much thinner and the periosteum much thicker the younger the animal is (Wijdeveld *et al.* 1991), thus the younger the animal the less keratinized epithelium there is to support the sutures, which increases the chance of dehiscence.
- The palatal defect gets proportionally larger as the animal grows.
- Surgical correction of palatal defects in growing animals using mucoperiosteal flaps and/or denudation of bone causes palatal growth and occlusion deformations. It was therefore suggested that performing the surgical correction after eruption of the permanent dentition would prevent such deformations (Wijdeveld *et al.* 1989, 1991; Leenstra *et al.* 1995).
- Owners' commitment and dedication. The more dedicated and committed the owner is, the later the surgery can be delayed.

In the author's opinion and experience, delaying the performance of cleft palate repair, preferably after the eruption of the permanent dentition (between 7 and 8 months of age) carries a better prognosis. At that age the maxilla has exerted most of its growing potential and the permanent maxillary premolar and molar teeth are in place, so disruption of the periosteum during corrective surgery will not alter maxillary growth nor cause tipping of the teeth. In addition, the size of the animal at this age allows a good approach to the palate and poses considerably less anesthetic risk than at an earlier age.

General considerations

Patients should be screened for other congenital abnormalities.

Surgery should be performed only on animals free from lower respiratory tract infections and thoracic radiographs are indicated to rule out aspiration pneumonia.

Patients with cleft palate should be spayed/neutered.

Surgical considerations

Surgical technique should be determined after careful evaluation of advanced imaging of the affected area. Computed tomography, multiplanar views, and tridimensional reconstruction images are recommended. It has been shown that orofacial clefts are quite complex and variable and that the extent of the bony defect is often larger than the mucosal defect (Nemec *et al.* 2015; Peralta *et al.* 2017; Peralta *et al.* 2018).

The employment of proper surgical technique and gentle tissue handling is extremely important for the success of the procedure. Use stay sutures or skin hooks, and avoid tissue crushing and overstretching. Avoid the use of electrocautery.

Preserve the blood supply by creating muco-periosteal flaps.

Plan and create flaps that are larger than the defects. This will result in a relaxed flap with no tension at the suture line (flaps sutured under tension are more likely to dehisce).

Cleft lip

Surgical anatomy

The lip consists of the skin, muco-cutaneous junction, orbicularis oris muscle, and oral mucosa.

Objectives

The objective of the surgical correction of cleft lip (cheilorrhaphy) is mainly cosmetic, and defect closure and reconstruction of the upper lip margin continuity are the ultimate goals.

Surgical technique

The animal is positioned in sternal recumbency with the neck and chin supported.

A regional nerve block is performed at the infraorbital foramen of the affected side.

Both the affected and normal sides are clipped and aseptically prepped.

The incisions are carefully designed, keeping in mind the following principles: every defect is different; no one pattern fits all. The unaffected side serves as a reference for symmetry and lip length. Z-plasty techniques using a no. 11 scalpel blade should be employed in order to free enough tissues for defect closure and lip reconstruction. These techniques serve also to break up lines so that with scar formation, fibrosis, and contracture, minimal deformation will occur (Figure 36.2).

Closure is done in 2–3 layers of simple interrupted sutures: absorbable synthetic monofilament for oral mucosa and subcutaneous; nylon 4-0 for skin.

Postoperative management and complications

An Elizabethan collar should be placed to prevent the animal from rubbing the sutures.

A soft food diet should be fed for 14 days and chewing, carrying, or playing hard objects should be prevented. Suture removal is done 10–14 days postoperatively.

Complications may consist of surgical infection and suture dehiscence.

Cleft of the primary palate

Surgical anatomy

Tissues used for a rostral palatorrhaphy are the nasal mucosa and the palatal mucosa.

Objectives

The objective of the palatorrhaphy is to create a separation between the oral and nasal cavity, preferably by reconstruction of the floor of the nasal cavity and the roof of the oral cavity.

Surgical technique

Supernumerary, maloccluding, or incisor teeth that may interfere with the surgery are extracted several weeks prior to the corrective surgery.

The animal may be positioned in dorsal or sternal recumbency. A mouth gag is used to keep the mouth wide open.

A maxillary nerve block of the affected side should be performed.

The rostral maxilla and nose are rinsed with 0.12% chlorhexidine gluconate.

Pedicle mucosal flaps are created using no. 11 or 15 scalpel blades, first in the nasal mucosa to form the nasal floor, and then repeated in the oral mucosa to form the roof of the mouth. If there is not enough tissue to create separate nasal floor and oral roof then the nasal mucosal flap can be sutured to the oral mucosal flap, forming a one-layer separation.

Monofilament absorbable 4-0 or 5-0 suture on a reverse cutting needle in a simple interrupted fashion is recommended.

(a)

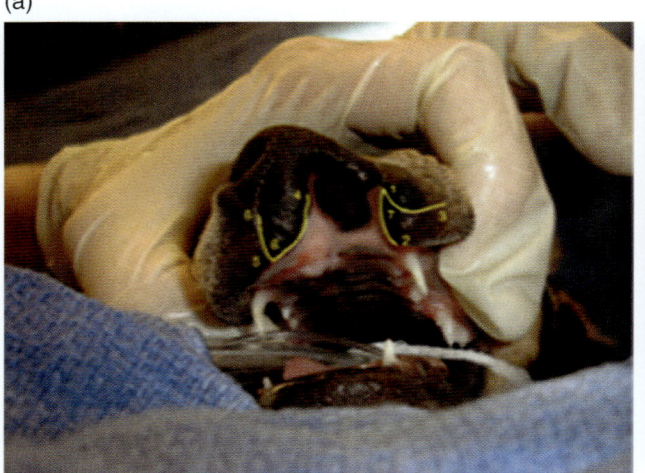

(b)

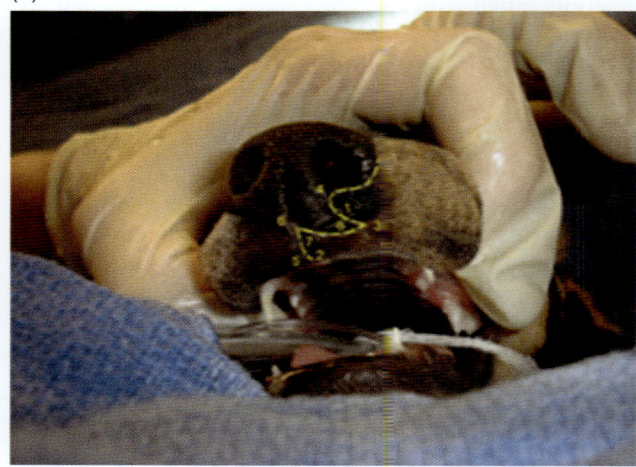

Figure 36.2 Modified Z-plasty technique for repair of cleft lip.

If the primary cleft is associated with cleft lip, the defect in the primary palate is fixed first and then the defect in the lip.

Postoperative management and complications

The animal should be fed a soft food diet for 14 days. If the animal already has a feeding tube, feeding through the tube is recommended for 2 weeks postoperatively. Disinfection of the surgical site should be performed twice daily with 0.12% chlorhexidine gluconate oral rinse or gel.

Chewing, carrying, or playing with hard objects should be prevented.

Complications may consist of surgical infection and suture dehiscence.

Cleft of the secondary palate

Surgical anatomy

The bony part of the secondary palate consists of the horizontal laminae of the maxillary and palatine bones. The mucosa of the hard palate is a masticatory mucosa that consists of keratinized stratified squamous epithelium in which the lamina propria is firmly and directly attached to the periosteum. The major palatine artery is the main blood vessel of the hard palate. It originates from the major palatine foramen situated approximately halfway between the maxillary fourth premolar and the midline on both sides, and runs rostrally parallel to the dental arch in the palatine groove.

The oral aspect of the soft palate consists of non-keratinized squamous epithelium and is considered lining mucosa, which is much more elastic and loose than masticatory mucosa. Dorsally situated are the paired palatine muscles and the levator and tensor veli palatini muscles. On the naso-pharyngeal aspect, nasal mucosa lines the soft palate musculature. The minor palatine artery is the main blood vessel of the soft palate. Originating from the minor palatine foramen situated caudally to the major palatine foramen halfway between the maxillary first molar and the midline on both sides, it runs caudally to supply the soft palate.

Objectives

For the hard palate the objective of the surgical correction is to close the communication between the oral and nasal cavities.

Reconstruction is the surgical objective for the soft palate

Surgical technique

The animal is positioned in dorsal recumbency. To maximize visibility and accessibility the mouth is kept fully opened, the tongue is secured to the mandible with tape, and pharyngotomy or transmylohyoid (Soukup & Snyder 2015) intubation is recommended.

Bilateral maxillary nerve block should be performed.

The hard and soft palate are rinsed with 0.12% chlorhexidine gluconate.

Hard palate repair

There are two principal techniques used for the correction of cleft of the hard palate: (i) the Von Langenbeck technique; and (ii) the overlapping (or inversion flap) technique (Howard *et al.* 1974; Sinibaldi 1979; Waldron & Martin 1991).

The Von Langenbeck technique consists of the formation of bipedicle mucoperiosteal flaps by performing a longitudinal full-thickness incision in the hard palate mucosa parallel to the maxillary teeth on both sides. The elevation and releasing of the mucoperiosteal flaps are done with a periosteal elevator. Care should be taken to preserve the palatine artery. The medial borders of each flap are incised to create a fresh wound, then apposed and sutured in a simple interrupted fashion, using 4-0 or 5-0 absorbable synthetic monofilament suture on a reverse cutting needle (Figure 36.3).

Notes:

- The length of the incision should not be less than the defect length.
- The incision should be placed in the hard palate mucosa between the teeth and the major palatine artery.
- The mucoperiosteal flaps should include the major palatine artery.
- The apposition and suture of the flaps should be done without any tension.
- This technique is suitable for relatively narrow defects.
- One report describes that about 58% of dogs with cleft palate treated with this technique required second and some even third surgical attempts before clinical cure was achieved (Howard *et al.* 1974).

The overlapping (or inversion flap) technique consists of a rectangular pedicle flap that is pivoted 180° on its attached medial border and its free border inserted between the hard palate mucosa and bone of the opposite side. A full-thickness incision extending the full length of the defect is made in the hard palate mucosa on one side, parallel to the defect and close to the maxillary teeth, without involving the palatal aspect of the gingiva. Two full-thickness perpendicular incisions to the first one are then made from the rostral and caudal ends of the longitudinal incision to the defect. A fine periosteal elevator is used to elevate the mucoperiosteum in a latero-medial direction, leaving only the medial border

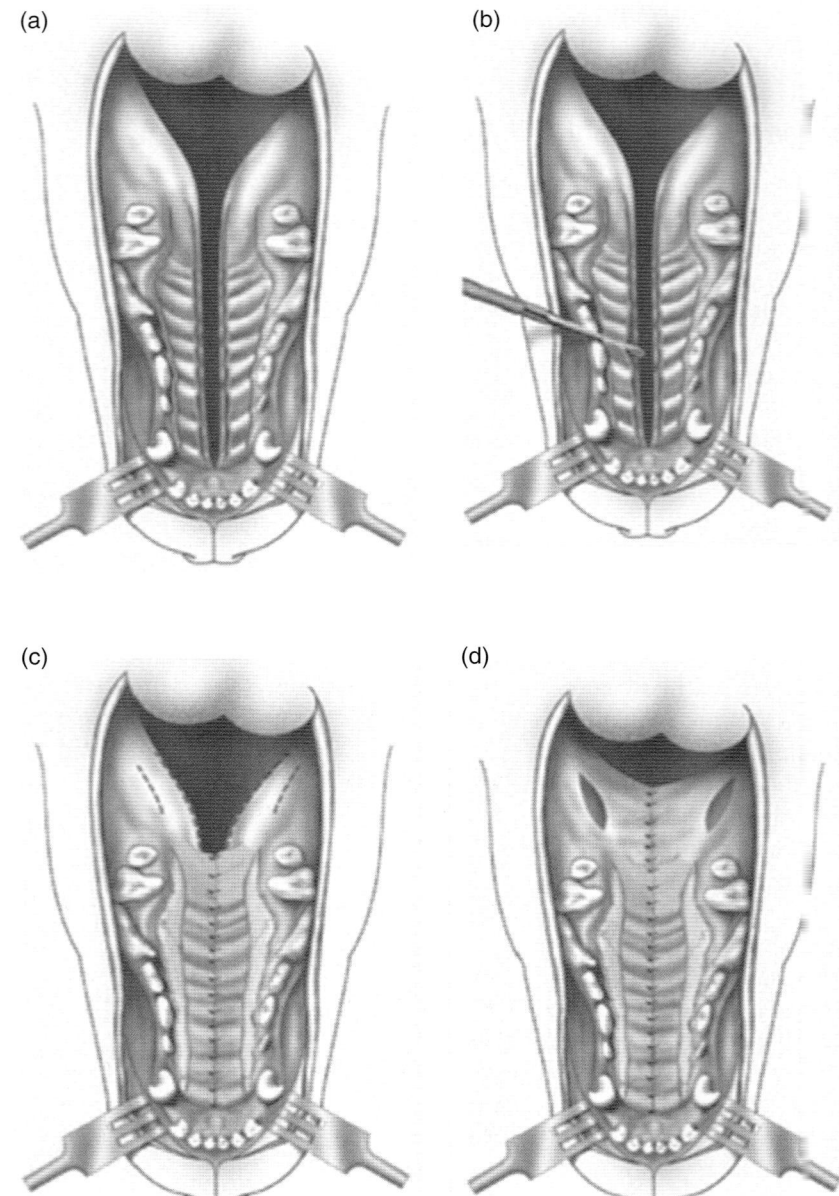

(a)   (b)

(c)   (d)

Figure 36.3 Repair of cleft of the hard palate. (a) Full-thickness releasing incisions in the hard palate mucosa. (b) Release of the flap with periosteal elevator (preserve palatine artery). (c) Suture of bipedicle flap. (c, d) Repair of cleft of soft palate: partial-thickness releasing incisions and mucosal incision of medial margins of soft palate (c, dotted lines). Suture in two or three layers. © D. Giddings.

of the defect still attached. With a fine periosteal elevator the mucoperiosteum is separated from the bone on the other side of the defect. The rectangle pedicle flap is then pivoted 180° on its attached medial border and its free border is laid flat on the other side of the defect, sandwiched between the bone and the mucoperiosteum, with the palatal rugae now facing the nasal cavity. Vertical mattress sutures are preplaced in a caudo-rostral direction using 4-0 or 5-0 absorbable synthetic monofilament suture on a reverse cutting needle (Figure 36.4).

Notes:

- The major palatine artery should be preserved and incorporated in the pedicle flap. If the caudal vertical incision is made rostral to the maxillary fourth premolar, care should be taken not to damage the palatine artery.
- In large defects, in order to ensure adequate flap coverage, extraction of the maxillary premolar and molar teeth can be performed on the side designated for flap

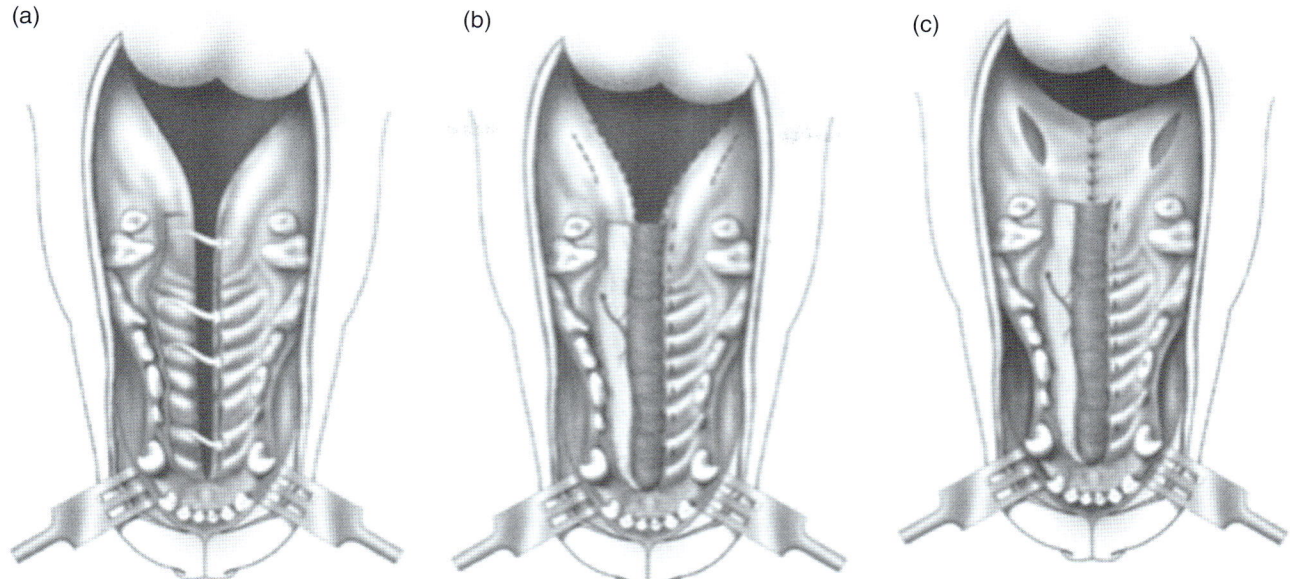

Figure 36.4 (a) Hard palate mucoperiosteal flap is created on one side by full-thickness rostral, buccal, and distal incisions (palatal aspect stays intact). On the other side, hard palate mucosa is separated from underlying bone with a periosteal elevator. (b) The flap is flipped 180°, its edges tucked between palatal mucosa and bone of the other side, and sutured with preplaced mattress sutures. Note that the palatine arteries should be preserved on both sides. (c) Complete repair of cleft of the secondary palate. © D. Giddings.

formation 4–6 weeks prior to the corrective surgery. This will provide several additional millimeters to the flap width by incorporating the palatal gingiva and gingival margin.

- The apposition and suture of the flap should be done without any tension.
- This technique is suitable for relatively wide defects.
- The exposed bone and mucosa will form granulation tissue and will epithelialize.
- In cases of cleft of the caudal part of the hard palate, advancement of the pedicle flap technique was described. Care should be taken not to cause shortening of the soft palate while advancing the flap rostrally to cover the defect.

Soft palate repair

Placing stay sutures in the caudo-medial point of each side of the defect allows for good manipulation without damaging the tissues. Partial-thickness releasing incisions are performed on the lateral aspect of the soft palate on each side of the defect. A horizontal incision is made in the mucosa over the medial border of each side of the defect to separate the nasal from the oral mucosa and expose the palatal musculature. Sutures for apposition should be placed in three layers, preferably in a simple interrupted pattern using 4-0 or 5-0 absorbable synthetic monofilament suture material on a reverse cutting needle. First the nasal mucosa is sutured together, then the muscles, and last the oral mucosa. The sutures

should be placed in a caudo-rostral direction for each layer. In cases in which three layers cannot be distinguished, two layers, one comprising the muscles and one the oral mucosa, should be performed.

In cases of unilateral palate defect, a pedicle flap can be created as a shelf from the mucosa of the pharyngeal wall on the defect side and sutured to the incised medial edge of the soft palate (Hammer & Sacks 1971; Griffiths & Sullivan 2001). One should recognize that this technique only provides physical separation between the oral and nasal pharynx. The lack of palatine musculature (especially the levator veli palatini) in the flap will pull on deglutition and the reconstructed soft palate in the direction of the existing soft palate without occluding the naso-pharynx on the repaired side, thus although cosmetically repaired, the symptoms may persist.

Postoperative management and complications

The animal should be fed a soft food diet for 14 days. If it already has a feeding tube, feeding through the tube is recommended for 2 weeks postoperatively. Disinfection of the surgical site should be performed twice daily with 0.12% chlorhexidine gluconate oral rinse or gel.

Chewing hard objects should be prevented.

Complications may consist of surgical infection and suture dehiscence. Dehiscence of the most rostral point of the flap just caudal to the incisive papilla is very common, but is rarely symptomatic. The general approach to palatal dehiscence is not to intervene if there are no associated symptoms such as active infection of the area, purulent discharge, coughing/sneezing/gagging, or food entrapment. In any case, the decision to surgically correct a dehiscence should be postponed until the wound healing process is complete.

Prognosis

The first surgical attempt is the one with the highest chances of succeeding. Therefore, careful planning and meticulous execution of the surgery are paramount. Every additional intervention to correct a palatal defect has a decreased prognosis due to increased scar tissue and decreased blood supply and healthy tissue.

The reported success rate of congenital hard and soft palate repair in dogs is approximately 85%, but revision surgery to address oro-nasal fistulas is often necessary (up to 50% of cases) to achieve a successful functional outcome (Peralta et al. 2018). This study also concludes that dogs older than 8 months at the time of surgical repair may be at increased risk for oro-nasal fistula formation in the hard palate or at the junction between the hard and soft palate. Also dogs weighing less than 1 kg at the time of surgery have a poorer prognosis than heavier dogs (Peralta et al. 2018).

The success rate of cleft lip and cleft of the primary palate in dogs as well as the success rate of cleft of the secondary palate in cats are unknown. However, as long as adequate technique is used and surgical principles are followed, a high success rate should be expected.

References

Arosarena, O.A. (2007). Cleft lip and palate. *Otolaryngologic Clinics of North America* 40: 27–60, vi.

Arzi, B. and Verstraete, F.J.M. (2011). Repair of a bifid nose combined with cleft of the primary palate in a one year old dog. *Veterinary Surgery* 40: 865–869.

Brodbelt, D.C., Pfeiffer, D.U., Young, L.E., and Wood, J.L. (2008). Results of the confidential enquiry into perioperative small animal fatalities regarding risk factors for anesthetic-related death in dogs. *Journal of the American Veterinary Medical Association* 233: 1096–1104.

Coleman, J.R. and Sykes, J.M. (2001). The embryology, classification, epidemiology, and genetics of facial clefting. *Facial Plastic Surgery Clinics of North America* 9: 1–13.

Cooper, H.K. Jr. and Mattern, G.W. (1971). Genetic studies of cleft lip and palate in dogs. *Birth Defects Original Article Series* 7: 98–100.

Ellis, E. (2008). Management of patients with orofacial clefts. In: *Contemporary Oral and Maxillofacial Surgery* (ed. J.R. Hupp, E. Ellis and M.Y. Tucker), 583–603. St. Louis, MO: Mosby.

Fiani, N., Verstraete, F.J.M., and Arzi, B. (2016). Reconstruction of congenital nose, cleft primary palate, and lip disorders. *Veterinary Clinics of North America: Small Animal Practice* 46: 663–675.

Fox, M.W. (1963). Developmental abnormalities of the canine skull. *Canadian Journal of Comparative Medicine and Veterinary Science* 27: 219–222.

Gregory, S.P. (2000). Middle ear disease associated with congenital palatine defects in seven dogs and one cat. *Journal of Small Animal Practice* 41: 398–401.

Griffiths, L.G. and Sullivan, M. (2001). Bilateral overlapping mucosal single-pedicle flaps for correction of soft palate defects. *Journal of the American Animal Hospital Association* 37: 183–186.

Hale, F.A. (2005). Juvenile veterinary dentistry. *Veterinary Clinics of North America: Small Animal Practice* 35: 789–817. v–vi.

Hale, F.A., Sylvestre, A.M., and Miller, C. (1997). The use of a prosthetic appliance to manage a large palatal defect in a dog. *Journal of Veterinary Dentistry* 14: 61–64.

Hammer, D.L. and Sacks, M. (1971). Surgical closure of cleft soft palate in a dog. *Journal of the American Veterinary Medical Association* 158: 342–345.

Harvey, C.E. and Emily, P.P. (1993). Oral Surgery. *Small Animal Dentistry*, 340–345. St. Louis, MO: Mosby-Year Book.

Howard, D.R., Davis, D.G., Merkley, D.F. et al. (1974). Mucoperiosteal flap technique for cleft palate repair in dogs. *Journal of the American Veterinary Medical Association* 165: 352–354.

Johnston, M.C. and Bronsky, P.T. (1991). Animal models for human craniofacial malformations. *Journal of Craniofacial Genetics and Developmental Biology* 11: 277–291.

Kemp, C., Thiele, H., Dankof, A. et al. (2009a). Cleft lip and/or palate with monogenic autosomal recessive transmission in Pyrenees shepherd dogs. *Cleft Palate-Craniofacial Journal* 46: 81–88.

Lee, J.I., Kim, Y.S., Kim, M.J. et al. (2006). Application of a temporary palatal prosthesis in a puppy suffering from cleft palate. *Journal of Veterinary Science* 7: 93–95.

Leenstra, T.S., Kuijpers-Jagtman, A.M., Maltha, J.C., and Freihofer, H.P. (1995). Palatal surgery without denudation of bone favours dentoalveolar development in dogs. *International Journal of Oral and Maxillofacial Surgery* 24: 440–444.

Liao, Y.F. and Mars, M. (2006). Hard palate repair timing and facial growth in cleft lip and palate: a systematic review. *Cleft Palate-Craniofacial Journal* 43: 563–570

McGeady, T.A., Quinn, P.J., Fitzpatrick, E.S., and Ryan, M.T. (2006). Structures in the head and neck. In: *Veterinary Embryology* (ed. T.A. McGeady), 268–283. Ames, IA: Blackwell.

Mulvihill, J.J., Mulvihill, C.G., and Priester, W.A. (1980). Cleft palate in domestic animals: epidemiologic features. *Teratology* 21: 109–112.

Nemec, A., Daniaux, L., Johnson, E. et al. (2015). Cranio-maxillofacial abnormalities in dogs with congenital palatal defects: computed tomographic findings. *Veterinary Surgery* 44: 417–422.

Padgett, G.A., Bell, T.G., and Patterson, W.R. (1986). Genetic disorders affecting reproduction and periparturient care. *Veterinary Clinics of North America: Small Animal Practice* 16: 577–586.

Peralta, S., Fiani, N., Kahn-Rohrer, K.H., and Verstraete, F.J.M. (2017). Morphological evaluation of clefts of the lip, palate, or both in dogs. *American Journal of Veterinary Research* 78: 926–933.

Peralta, S., Campbell, R.D., Fiani, N. et al. (2018). Outcomes of surgical repair of congenital palatal defects in dogs. *Journal of the American Veterinary Medical Association* 253 (11): 1445–1551.

Richtsmeier, J.T., Sack, G.H. Jr., Grausz, H.M., and Cork, L.C. (1994). Cleft palate with autosomal recessive transmission in Brittany spaniels. *Cleft Palate-Craniofacial Journal* 31: 364–371.

Roman, N., Carney, P.C., Fiani, N., and Peralta, S. (2019). Incidence patterns of orofacial clefts in purebred dogs. *PLOS ONE* 14 (11).

Sherwood, B.F., Vakilzadeh, J., and Lemay, J.C. (1971). Observations on the pathology in a colony of cleft palate and cleft lip dogs. *Cleft Palate Journal* 8: 56–60.

Sinibaldi, K.R. (1979). Cleft palate. *Veterinary Clinics of North America: Small Animal Practice* 9: 245–257.

Soukup, J.W. and Snyder, C.J. (2015). Transmylohyoid orotracheal intubation in surgical management of canine maxillofacial fractures: an alternative to pharyngotomy endotracheal intubation. *Veterinary Surgery* 44: 432–436.

Sponenberg, D.P. and Bowling, A.T. (1985). Heritable syndrome of skeletal defects in a family of Australian shepherd dogs. *Journal of Heredity* 76: 393–394.

Tollefson, T.T., Senders, C.W., and Sykes, J.M. (2008). Changing perspectives in cleft lip and palate: from acrylic to allele. *Archives of Facial Plastic Surgery* 10: 395–400.

Waldron, D.R. and Martin, R.A. (1991). Cleft palate repair. *Problems in Veterinary Medicine* 3: 142–152.

Warzee, C.C., Bellah, J.R., and Richards, D. (2001). Congenital unilateral cleft of the soft palate in six dogs. *Journal of Small Animal Practice* 42: 338–340.

Wijdeveld, M.G., Grupping, E.M., Kuijpers-Jagtman, A.M., and Maltha, J.C. (1989). Maxillary arch dimensions after palatal surgery at different ages on beagle dogs. *Journal of Dental Research* 68: 1105–1109.

Wijdeveld, M.G., Maltha, J.C., Grupping, E.M. et al. (1991). A histological study of tissue response to simulated cleft palate surgery at different ages in beagle dogs. *Archives of Oral Biology* 36: 837–843.

37

Brachycephalic Airway Syndrome

Dorothee Krainer and Gilles Dupré

Brachycephalic airway syndrome (BAS) is an established cause of respiratory distress in brachycephalic breeds (Hendricks 1992). Their shortened skull is accompanied by shortening and compression of nasal and nasopharyngeal passages, which leads to increased inspiratory resistance (Leonard 1957; Cook 1964; Aron & Crowe 1985; Hobson 1995; Koch *et al.* 2003). Additional mucosal hyperplasia and collapse of the upper airway secondary to the increased respiratory effort contribute to a multilevel obstruction with a gradual worsening of clinical signs. Breeds most affected are English and French bulldogs, pugs, and Boston terriers; however, Pekingese, shih tzu, Lhasa apsos, Cavalier King Charles spaniels, boxers, dogue de Bordeaux, Brussels griffon, and bullmastiffs are also categorized as brachycephalic dogs (Meola 2013). Clinical signs include snoring, inspiratory dyspnea, exercise intolerance, stridor, sleep disturbances, cyanosis, and even syncopal episodes in more severe cases. Labored breathing is accompanied by overdilatation of the chest, since a higher intrathoracic negative pressure tends to suck the abdomen into the thoracic cavity. These problems are usually aggravated by stress, exercise, or heat. Affected animals suffer from lifelong respiratory distress, particularly in elevated ambient temperatures. Gastrointestinal signs such as vomiting, regurgitation, and dysphagia are particularly common in French bulldogs, and many owners describe these gastrointestinal signs occurring when their brachycephalic dog becomes excited or is in respiratory distress (Poncet *et al.* 2005, 2006; Lecoindre & Richard 2004; Kaye *et al.* 2018; Eivers *et al.* 2019).

Anatomy and pathophysiology

Airway obstruction in brachycephalic dogs is described to occur at multiple levels, but stenotic nares and a hyperplastic soft palate are described as the major contributors to the upper airway obstruction (Harvey 1982b,c; Ohnishi & Ogura 1969; Negus *et al.* 1970). Primary static anomalies such as skull conformation, aberrant conchae, stenotic nares, hyperplastic soft palate, macroglossia, glottis narrowing, and tracheal hypoplasia lead to decreased airway dimensions and subsequent increased respiratory effort in order to obtain sufficient oxygen. The consequence of this increased negative pressure during the breathing cycle is that the soft tissues are drawn into the lumen and subsequent collapse of the upper airway (Thews 1983). These dynamic changes affect the airway at multiple levels and lead to secondary manifestations of brachycephalic syndrome, such as everted laryngeal saccules, partial collapse of the dorsonasal pharynx, laryngeal collapse, and even collapse of other parts of the cartilaginous respiratory tract. All these properties contribute to the clinical signs and lead to further deterioration, which may ultimately cause syncopal episodes and death from suffocation (Cook 1964; Aron & Crowe 1985).

Primary static anomalies of the airway

Stenotic nares

The openings of the nostrils (nares) are bounded medially by the nasal septum and laterally by the most mobile portion of the nose, the wing of the nostril (ala nasi), which contains most of the dorsolateral and accessory

---

Small Animal Soft Tissue Surgery, Second Edition. Edited by Eric Monnet.
© 2023 John Wiley & Sons, Inc. Published 2023 by John Wiley & Sons, Inc.
Companion website: www.wiley.com/go/monnet/small

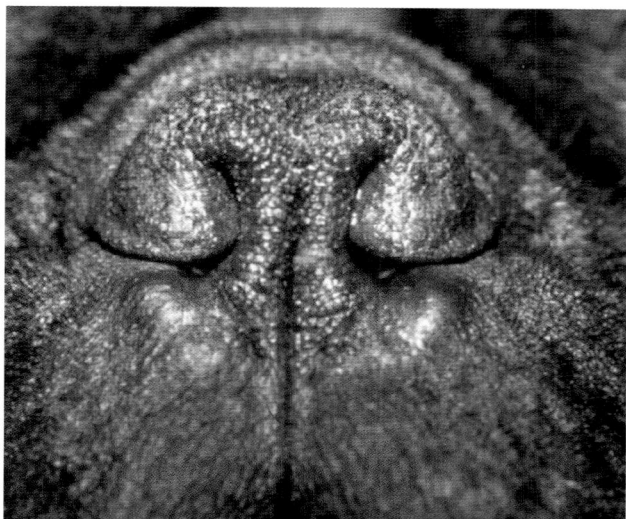

Figure 37.1 Stenotic nares in a 1-year-old French bulldog. Note the almost complete closure of the nasal opening.

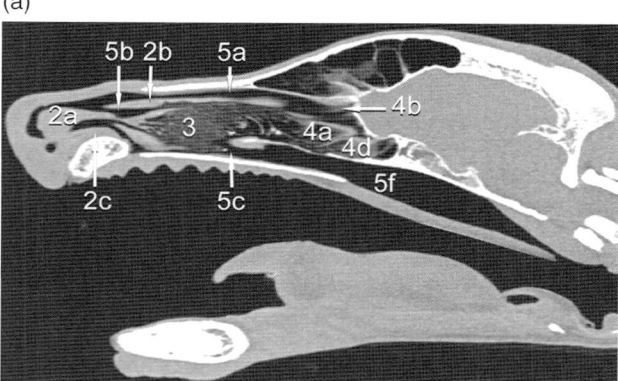

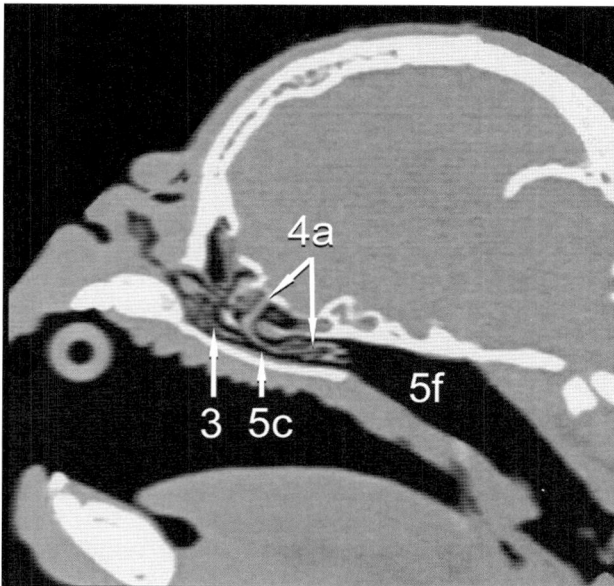

Figure 37.2 Comparison of sagittal computed tomographic images of the head of (a) a German shepherd dog and (b) a pug. In the pug, caudal aberrant turbinates originating from the middle nasal concha (4a) extend caudally and obstruct the air passage (5c) as well as the nasopharyngeal meatus (5f).

nasal cartilages. Dogs affected with BAS have stenotic nares, which reduce each nostril, often to a vertical slit (Figure 37.1). This typical and easily recognized primary anatomic component of the BAS is widely accepted as a major cause of upper airway obstruction in these breeds (Harvey 1982b). The nares are filled to a large extent by the ala nasi, which then merges into the plica alaris. In brachycephalic animals, in relation to the nose, the ala is too large and presses against the septum from the lateral aspect, leading to obstruction of the nasal vestibule. In dogs without brachycephalia, the nasal wing or ala nasi is very mobile; during inspiration it can be abducted to facilitate airflow into the nose. In brachycephalic animals, its size appears to greatly restrict this mobility by impeding abduction.

Stenotic nares can be described with the following grading system (Liu *et al.* 2017a):

- 0 = open = wide open
- 1 = mild = slightly narrowed, lateral nostril wall not in contact with septum
- 2 = moderate = lateral nostril wall in contact with septum dorsally but nostrils open ventrally
- 3 = severe = nostrils almost closed

Aberrant conchae, and nasopharyngeal turbinates

Abnormal conchal growth obstructing the intranasal airways and the nasopharyngeal meatus (Figure 37.2) are common findings (43%) in extreme brachycephalic breeds such as pugs, French bulldogs, and English bulldogs (Billen *et al.* 2006; Oechtering *et al.* 2007; Ginn *et al.* 2008). However, their impact on airway obstruction

is difficult to assess and remains unclear. Vilaplana *et al.* (2015) reported aberrant caudal turbinates in 100% of English bulldogs with no or mild clinical signs of BAS. Other studies evaluating the intranasal airway obstruction with computed tomography (CT) and rhinoscopy state that the presence of aberrant conchae contribute to the heat and exercise intolerance of brachycephalic breeds (Schuenemann & Oechtering 2014a). Pugs seem to be most affected by rostral aberrant turbinates (90.9%) and nasal septum deviation compared to French bulldogs (56.4%) and English bulldogs (36.4%), which might be due to the dorsorotation of their skull (Billen *et al.* 2006; Oechtering *et al.* 2007; Ginn *et al.* 2008). These abnormal turbinates are thought to be more present in these breeds, as their growth fails to stop. Interconchal and intrachonal contact points were found in 91.7% of brachycephalic and 24% of normocephalic dogs. Regrowth of aberrant turbinates is reported as a common complication after laser-assisted turbinectomy (LATE) and revision surgery was required in 20% of French bulldogs and pugs (Schuenemann & Oechtering 2014b).

Soft palate hyperplasia

Although the literature originally described an elongated soft palate (Torrez & Hunt 2006; Riecks *et al.* 2007; Ginn *et al.* 2008), fluttering, and obstructing the rima glottidis (Figure 37.3) as a primary component of BAS, it is now commonly agreed that an additional pathologic thickening of the soft palate plays a major role in the nasopharyngeal obstruction (Findji & Dupré 2009; Grand & Bureau 2011; Pichetto *et al.* 2011; Heidenreich *et al.* 2016). Radiographic, CT, fluoroscopic, and histologic examinations demonstrated hypertrophy of the soft palate (Figure 37.4) (Grand & Bureau 2011; Pichetto *et al.* 2011; Heidenreich *et al.* 2016; Crosse *et al.* 2015). Grand and Bureau (2011) found a positive correlation between the thickness of the soft palate and the severity of the clinical signs. A CT study evaluating the upper airway dimension in pugs and French bulldogs showed that French bulldogs have a significantly thicker soft palate compared with pugs. Pugs, however, have a smaller nasopharyngeal airway space, with a complete airway obstruction dorsal to the soft palate in 81% (Heidenreich *et al.* 2016).

Further primary anomalies of the airway

In addition to soft palate hyperplasia, nasopharyngeal mucosa hyperplasia (Poncet *et al.* 2006), hypertrophy and eversion of the tonsils (Fasanella *et al.* 2010), and an

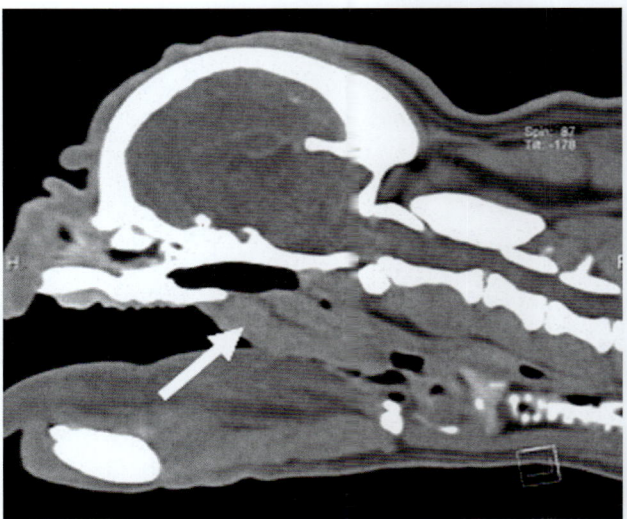

Figure 37.4 Soft palate thickening and nasopharyngeal obstruction. Midsagittal computed tomographic image of a 2-year-old French bulldog with thickening of the soft palate.

overlong and thickened tongue (macroglossia) (Fox 1963) further contribute to the nasopharyngeal obstruction (Figure 37.5). The oversized tongue displaces the soft palate dorsally (Herdt 1997). Recent anatomic CT-aided measurements of the tongue size and its extent within the oro- and nasopharynx describe a relative macroglossia and an associated reduction of upper airway space in extreme brachycephalic breeds (Jones *et al.* 2020). Pugs were found to have smaller tongues compared to French and English bulldogs (Siedenburg & Dupré 2021). However, the effect of tongue size on the air volume in the upper airway is difficult to assess, as its position and the dynamic changes of the oropharynx space during a breathing circle can vary significantly. French bulldogs were reported to have abnormally shaped basishyoid bones, with a more acute curvature and greater ventrodorsal thickness compared to mesaticephalic dogs. This hyoid malformation can complicate the BAS treatment as reported in a French bulldog (De Bruyn & Hosgood 2022).

Pugs were found to have a more oval-shaped and narrower glottis than English and French bulldogs (Caccamo *et al.* 2014), and the cricoid cartilage was also found to be more oval-shaped in pugs and French bulldogs compared to mesaticephalic dogs (Rutherford *et al.* 2017). A recent report of a Pekinese and a French bulldog with BAS describes difficulties during tracheal intubation due to narrowing of the cricoid cartilage and a thickened mucous membrane (Tamura *et al.* 2021). The English bulldog has the highest incidence of tracheal hypoplasia among brachycephalic breeds and tracheal hypoplasia in this breed has been defined as a ratio of the tracheal

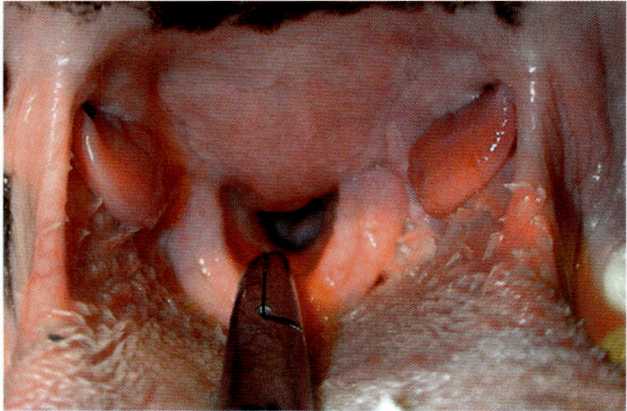

Figure 37.3 Macroscopic view of the pharyngolaryngeal region of a 2-year-old English bulldog. The tonsils are everted and the soft palate flutters in the rima glottidis well beyond the tip of the epiglottic cartilage.

(a)

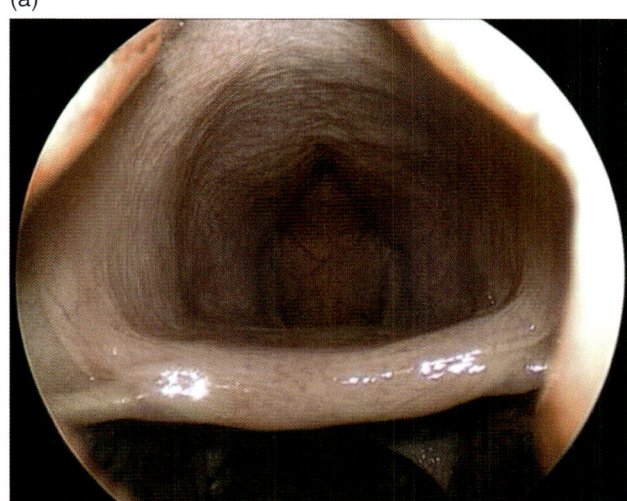

(b)

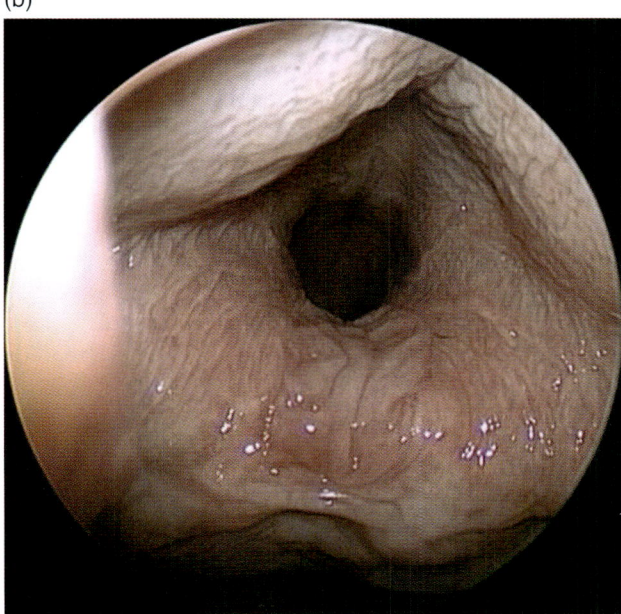

Figure 37.5 Retrograde endoscopic view of the nasopharynx of (a) a poodle and (b) a French bulldog. Note the differences in soft palate thickness and the effect on the diameter of the nasopharynx.

diameter to the thoracic inlet of less than 0.12. Tracheal hypoplasia was found to occur more often in screw-tailed brachycephalic dogs compared to non-screw-tailed brachycephalics (Komsta *et al.* 2019). A comparison of tracheal dimensions assessed with radiography, CT, and thoracoscopy showed that the latter was the most reliable technique to identify tracheal hypoplasia and did not correlate with the two other imaging techniques. CT measurements were 19% greater than those assessed with radiographs (Kaye *et al.* 2015).

Although tracheal hypoplasia increases airway resistance, its contribution to the syndrome is likely minimal and tracheal hypoplasia was found not to improve after surgical correction for BAS (Regier *et al.* 2020).

Incidental middle ear effusion is common in brachycephalic dogs (Milne *et al.* 2020), and French bulldogs and Cavalier King Charles spaniels appear to be most affected (Hayes *et al.* 2010; Krainer & Dupré 2021). The middle ears of brachycephalic dogs have a smaller luminal size (Salguero *et al.* 2016; Foster *et al.* 2015; Mielke *et al.* 2017), an abnormal shape and rostral position of the tympanic bulla (Mielke *et al.* 2017), and an increased thickness of the ventral tympanic wall (Salgüero *et al.* 2016; Krainer & Dupré 2021). A decreased pharyngeal aperture was found to be related to middle ear effusion in Cavalier King Charles spaniels (Hayes *et al.* 2010) but not in French bulldogs or pugs (Krainer & Dupré 2021). However, a correlation of soft palate hyperplasia and middle ear effusion was found in bulldogs, French bulldogs, and pugs (Salgüero *et al.* 2016). French bulldogs were reported to be more commonly affected with middle ear effusion and inflammation (41.6%) compared to pugs 5.0%. These dogs also showed an increased incidence of regurgitation, which might contribute to middle ear effusion and inflammation (Krainer & Dupré 2021).

Secondary dynamic changes of the airway

Nasopharyngeal obstruction and collapse

Static CT measurements of the nasopharynx showed that its smallest airway space is located dorsal to the caudal end of the soft palate and was smaller in pugs compared to French bulldogs, who have a significant thicker soft palate (Heidenreich *et al.* 2016). The increased thickness of the soft palate was also identified as the most relevant pharyngeal CT parameter in dogs severely affected by BAS (Grand & Bureau 2011). The maximal nasopharyngeal occlusion was found to be located about 1 cm caudal to the hamuli pterygoidei, which is a useful landmark during soft palate resection (Sarran *et al.* 2018).

Dynamic nasopharyngeal collapse is common in brachycephalic dogs and most likely secondary to long-term negative pressure of the upper airway (Pollard *et al.* 2018). It is most accompanied by bronchial or tracheal collapse, but also seen in dogs with brachycephalic syndrome (Rubin *et al.* 2015). Recent dynamic CT studies identified the order of the pharyngeal motion during inspiration as pharyngeal collapse followed by pharyngeal contraction and laryngospasm (Hara *et al.* 2020). Factors that might influence nasopharyngeal collapsibility are thickening of the soft palate, weight gain, or epiglottis location (Noh *et al.* 2021).

Tonsillar eversion and hypertrophy

Palatine tonsillar enlargement and eversion have been reported in up to 56% of BAS-affected dogs and is thought to occur secondary to an increased negative pressure during inspiration (Fasanella *et al.* 2010). Histopathology of these excised tonsils showed mild to marked inflammation and edema (Belch *et al.* 2017) and inflammation of the tonsils was also thought to be secondary to gastroesophageal reflux (Poncet *et al.* 2005). Enlarged tonsils can contribute to the upper airway obstruction and tonsillectomy is performed routinely as part of a multilevel surgical approach by some surgeons (Belch *et al.* 2017; Liu *et al.* 2017b). Other surgeons prefer not to remove the tonsils, as they expect the tonsillar inflammation to resolve after treating the primary anomalies of these dogs.

Laryngeal collapse

Laryngeal diseases associated with BAS include mucosal edema, everted laryngeal saccules, and laryngeal collapse. They are thought to be secondary to the turbulent airflow and chronic high negative pressures in the pharynx (Figure 37.6) (Koch *et al.* 2003; Monnet 2003; Pink *et al.* 2006; Torrez & Hunt 2006; Riecks *et al.* 2007).

In one early classification, everted laryngeal saccules were considered the first degree of laryngeal collapse (Leonard 1960). In this classification, stage 2 was characterized by medial displacement of the cuneiform processes of the arytenoid cartilages, and stage 3 by collapse of the corniculate processes of the arytenoid cartilages, with loss of the dorsal arch of the rima glottidis. However, laryngeal collapse can be more accurately

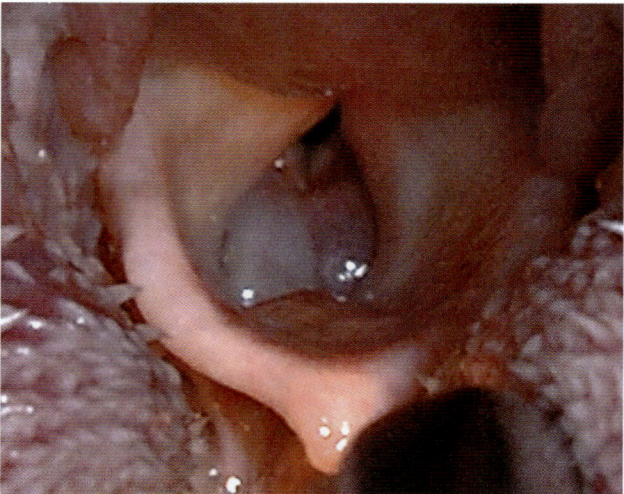

Figure 37.6 Macroscopic view of laryngeal saccule eversion in a 1-year-old French bulldog. The everted laryngeal saccules completely obstruct the ventral part of the rima glottidis and hide the ventral folds.

defined as loss of mechanical rigidity of the laryngeal cartilages (chondromalacia), making it incapable of withstanding high pharyngeal negative pressures without collapsing. Chondromalacia seems to be a particular problem in pugs. A recent histologic and mechanical examination of the larynx identified a cartilage degeneration and mechanical weakness in brachycephalic dogs compared to nonbrachycephalic dogs (Tokunaga *et al.* 2020). Everted saccules, or laryngoceles, are formed by eversion of the mucosa of the laryngeal ventricles. The everted saccules are swollen from inflammation and edema, which obstructs the ventral half of the rima glottidis.

Laryngeal collapse was initially reported to affect mainly middle-aged to older dogs, although younger dogs were found to be affected (Harvey 1982a). More recently, laryngeal collapse has been described in very young, immature dogs (Pink *et al.* 2006). Altogether, the incidence of laryngeal collapse in brachycephalic dogs varies considerably depending on the type of examination, the type of grading, and the examiner's expertise. It might be found in from 50% (Wilson *et al.* 1960; Wegner 1987) to as many as 95% of patients (De Lorenzi *et al.* 2009). Pugs seem to be overrepresented.

Endoscopically, the larynx of different brachycephalic dogs can differ from each other. For instance, in pugs, the predominant picture is one of laryngeal collapse, due to lack of rigidity of the cartilage. On endoscopic examination of the laryngeal inlet, sections of the arytenoids (cuneiform and corniculate processes) appear to enter the lumen. In these cases, manipulation can demonstrate severe flaccidity of the epiglottis and of the arytenoid cartilage. The abnormally enlarged cuneiform processes may overlap, additionally hindering the incoming air. The redundant, frequently edematous, excess mucous membrane in the region of the corniculate process may be sucked into the narrow rima glottidis on inspiration. Other breeds, like French bulldogs, seem to have more rigid laryngeal cartilage and less redundant mucosal membrane at the laryngeal inlet (Oechtering 2010). It can therefore be postulated that in some breeds such as pugs, laryngeal collapse is a primary condition (i.e., congenital malacia of the laryngeal cartilages) that may worsen due to the high negative pressures in the pharynx, whereas in some other breeds it would be a secondary condition. Unfortunately, endoscopic examination under anesthesia may not reflect the actual situation of the laryngeal cartilages during inspiration under an increased negative pressure situation such as exercise, heat, or excitement. Ultrasonography has been evaluated as an alternative way to objectivate laryngeal collapse (Rudorf *et al.* 2001). Whereas some authors describe laryngeal collapse as a negative prognostic indicator for the surgical outcome (Liu *et al.* 2017b), other authors found no correlation between the severity of laryngeal collapse and overall respiratory signs or prognosis (Haimel & Dupré 2015).

Other reported abnormalities of the larynx associated with BAS are epiglottic cysts and laryngeal granulomas (Bernaerts *et al.* 2010).

Tracheal and bronchial collapse

Tracheal and bronchial collapse was found to be significantly correlated with the severity of the laryngeal collapse, and pugs were found to be most severely affected. With tracheal and bronchial collapse, a degeneration of the cartilage (chondromalacia) leads to flattening of the cartilage rings and to marked broadening of the paries membranaceus. Left-side bronchi were generally more affected by bronchial collapse (52.1%) than the right, with the cranial left bronchus most commonly collapsed (De Lorenzi *et al.* 2009). Whether the etiology is loss of rigidity, increased negative pressure, or compression within the chest remains to be investigated. Rubin *et al.* (2015) found an association of bronchial and tracheal collapse with dynamic pharyngeal collapse, which is likely secondary to increased negative gradients during inspiration.

Gastroesophageal disease associated with brachycephalic airway syndrome

Dysphagia, vomiting, and regurgitation are common clinical signs in brachycephalic breeds (Koch *et al.* 2003). The prevalence of gastrointestinal disease in BAS-affected dogs has been reported to be as high as 97% (Poncet *et al.* 2005; Fasanella *et al.* 2010; Meola 2013) and investigations of these dogs showed concurrent esophageal, gastric, or duodenal anomalies (Poncet *et al.* 2005). The correlation between respiratory and digestive disorders suggests an influence of upper respiratory tract diseases on gastroesophageal diseases, and vice versa. Gastroesophageal disorders (ptyalism, regurgitation, vomiting, and reflux) can aggravate the respiratory signs by encumbering the pharyngeal region and stimulating persistent inflammation. Conversely, chronic respiratory depression promotes gastroesophageal reflux. Brachycephaly was found to be significantly associated with esophageal dysmotility, prolonged esophageal transit time, and gastroesophageal reflux (Eivers *et al.* 2019). The negative intrathoracic pressures generated by increased inspiratory effort is believed to be a major cause of gastroesophageal reflux (Hardie *et al.* 1998; Boesch *et al.* 2005). The associated regurgitation and vomiting can contribute to upper esophageal, pharyngeal, laryngeal, and middle ear inflammation (White *et al.* 2002). French bulldogs exhibit significantly more frequent and more severe digestive signs than pugs

(Poncet *et al.* 2005; Roedler *et al.* 2013; Haimel & Dupré 2015; Kaye *et al.* 2018). A recent comparison of three brachycephalic dog breeds showed an overall prevalence of gastrointestinal signs in 56%, with 93% of French bulldogs, 58% of English bulldogs, and 16% of pugs affected (Kaye *et al.* 2018). Gastrointestinal signs, gastritis, and regurgitation significantly improved following surgical treatment of stenotic nares and soft palate hyperplasia (Poncet *et al.* 2006; Haimel & Dupré 2015; Kaye *et al.* 2018), especially in French bulldogs, whereas pugs and English bulldogs showed little alleviation – most likely due to the small number of pugs affected with gastrointestinal disease (Kaye *et al.* 2018).

Gastroesophageal reflux and hiatal hernia

Brachycephalic dogs are predisposed to hiatal hernia and accompanied gastroesophageal reflux (Freiche & Poncet 2007), which is thought to be secondary to increased negative intrathoracic pressure and increased inspiratory effort (Lorinson *et al.* 1997; Hardie *et al.* 1998; Boesch *et al.* 2005). The increased inspiratory effort leads to a reduction of intraesophageal and intrapleural pressures, with subsequent axial displacement of the distal esophagus and stomach into the thoracic cavity during inspiration (Hardie *et al.* 1998). In a recent esophageal imaging study, 8 of 8 dogs diagnosed with hiatal hernia were brachycephalic (Eivers *et al.* 2019) and the prevalence of sliding hiatal hernia in French bulldogs with BAS was found to be 44% (Reeve *et al.* 2017). Transient manual obstruction of the endotracheal tube to increase the trans-diaphragmatic pressure gradient was found helpful to identify gastroesophageal junction abnormalities in BAS-affected dogs (Broux *et al.* 2018; Reeve *et al.* 2017; Vangrinsven *et al.* 2021).

Aspiration pneumonia is a common complication of reflux and regurgitation, which should be investigated before anesthesia (see perioperative treatment).

Diagnosis

Diagnosis of upper airway compromise is usually based on owners' reports, clinical examination, and diagnostic imaging. Conformational risk factors for BAS are stenotic nostrils, high body condition score, thick neck girth, and a relative short muzzle length (Packer *et al.* 2015; Liu *et al.* 2017a).

Additional respiratory function testing and scoring to document the severity of BAS can be performed.

Clinical signs

Owners usually report heat, stress, and exercise intolerance. Clinical signs include snoring, inspiratory dyspnea, exercise intolerance, sleep disturbances, cyanosis, and, in the most severe cases, syncopal episodes. On inspection, stenotic nares and inspiratory efforts with even abdominal breathing can be observed. A particular attention shall be paid to respiratory sounds. These can be more apparent during exercise tests. Whereas snoring is most likely caused by air turbulences in the oropharyngeal region, the high-pitched sound associated with extreme inspiratory effort is related to more severe airway compromise when turbulent air is passing through the collapsed larynx or nasopharynx.

In addition, many owners describe signs of regurgitation, vomiting, and dysphagia when their brachycephalic dog becomes excited or is in respiratory distress.

Grading systems, clinical scores, and respiratory function testing

To classify the severity of BAS, several grading systems and forms of function testing have been introduced, including exercise tolerance tests and whole-body barometric plethysmography (WBBP).

The Poncet-Dupré score is a grading system based on the frequency of respiratory and digestive clinical signs (Poncet et al. 2005). Bernaerts et al. (2010) also introduced a respiratory scoring system, which is a combination of a symptom score (noisy breathing and exercise intolerance) and lesion score based on anatomic abnormalities of the nose, soft palate, ventricle, larynx, trachea, and lower airways. Similar grading systems assess the upper airway dimensions and obstruction at the different anatomic levels. These include evaluation of nares, nasopharyngeal turbinate protrusion, soft palate elongation, narrowed pharyngeal dimensions (dorsoventral flattening, thickness of base of tongue, tonsillar protrusion, diffuse pharyngeal oedema), and narrowed laryngeal dimensions (laryngeal hypoplasia, laryngeal collapse) (Vilaplana et al. 2015; Liu et al. 2016; Seneviratne et al. 2020; Erjavec et al. 2021). Most of these systems describe the severity as mild, moderate, or severe.

A functional grading system based on respiratory signs (respiratory noise, inspiratory effort, dyspnea/cyanosis/syncope) combined with an exercise tolerance test was established by Liu et al. (2015). A three-minute slow trot test should be included in the clinical examination to identify dogs that display respiratory noise only when stressed or exercised (Riggs et al. 2019). Other suggested exercise tests assess how far dogs can walk and if they can walk 1000 m in 6 minutes (Villedieu et al. 2019) or the time taken to walk 1000 m (Lilja-Maula et al. 2017).

WBBP can be used for respiratory function testing. A dog is placed in a sealed chamber with biased air flow moving across it. Changes in the air pressure within the chamber that result from the humidification and expansion of air on breathing are detected by a pressure transducer.

These WBBP flow traces are 93% specific and 90% sensitive to identify respiratory obstruction and has been validated to discriminate BAS-affected versus nonaffected brachycephalic dogs. With WBBP a BAS index can be calculated, which allows an objective evaluation of BAS severity, risk for BAS, and effectiveness of surgical treatment (Liu et al. 2015, 2016).

Diagnostic imaging

Radiographic, fluoroscopic, CT, and endoscopic studies all contribute to the evaluation of the static and dynamic obstruction of the respiratory tract. In a clinical practice setting, a proper evaluation of BAS patients should include at least neck and thoracic radiographs, and endoscopic examination of the upper airways.

Radiologic examination

Thoracic radiography is performed to document secondary heart or lung diseases and to rule out aspiration pneumonia. On occasion a sliding hiatal hernia can also be found on a lateral radiograph. When CT scan is not available, lateral radiography of the neck can help to assess the soft palate thickness (Hendricks 1992).

Computed tomography

CT examination should include the entire respiratory tract. It allows a detailed assessment of the nostrils, vestibule, nasal cavity, naso- and oropharynx, and cricoid and tracheal size. Additionally a hiatal hernia might be identified. CT enables estimation of the level of obstruction and a detailed assessment of the nostrils, vestibule, nasal cavity, and nasopharynx and oropharynx (Oechtering et al. 2007; Grand & Bureau 2011; Heidenreich et al. 2016; Rutherford et al. 2017).

Endoscopic examination

Endoscopic examination provides more information on the dynamic changes within the upper airways. With the dog intubated, retrograde rhinoscopy can be performed with a 120° rigid scope or flexible endoscope to assess the nasopharynx for tissue hyperplasia, collapse, or nasopharyngeal turbinates (Figure 37.5). Rhinoscopy is a complementary method to assess cranial aberrant turbinates in the nasal cavity (Schuenemann & Oechtering 2014a) (Figure 37.7). With the dog extubated, a laryngoscopic examination is performed to assess the laryngeal saccules and laryngeal dynamics (Figure 37.6). In the case of laryngeal collapse, lack of abduction during inspiration or even paradoxical movements of the arytenoid cartilages can occur. In pugs and other dogs affected by laryngeal chondromalacia, the dorsal border of the cuneiform process of the arytenoid cartilages can even invert into the laryngeal lumen.

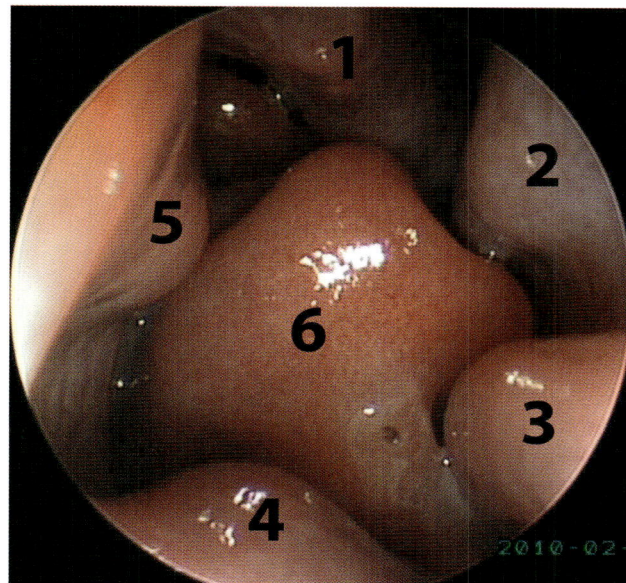

Figure 37.7 Endoscopic view of nasal cavity of an English bulldog. (1) Plica recta; (2) plica alaris; (3) plica basalis; (4) ventral septal swell body; (5) dorsal septal swell body; (6) rostral aberrant turbinate obstructing the main nasal meatus.

Tracheoscopy was reported to be more accurate for diagnosing tracheal hypoplasia compared to radiography and CT (Kaye *et al.* 2015).

Treatment

Medical therapy

Patients presented with acute signs of respiratory distress should be treated accordingly, with cooling, tranquilizers, oxygen therapy, and anti-inflammatory drugs. However, relief of upper airway obstruction is the mainstay of treatment. Whenever digestive signs are observed in dogs with BAS, medical treatment including inhibition of hydrogen ion secretion and gastric prokinetic drugs is recommended before and immediately after surgery.

Surgical therapy

According to the pathophysiology of the syndrome, early relief of the proximally located obstruction should be attempted, because it is postulated that early correction could prevent or even reverse more deeply located tissue collapse (Harvey 1982b). However, the optimal time to correct upper airway obstruction has not yet been determined and was recommended to be performed after the age of 6 months. Recent studies suggest that improvement in clinical signs is still obtained when surgery is performed on mature and middle-aged dogs (Haimel & Dupré 2015).

Pre- and perioperative treatment

To reduce the risk of perioperative aspiration pneumonia and reflux esophagitis, medical treatment to reduce the incidence of gastroesophageal reflux should be administered. Especially younger dogs and those with a history of regurgitation seem to be predisposed to postoperative regurgitation and should receive preventive treatment (Fenner *et al.* 2020). At least dogs with gastrointestinal signs should receive omeprazole (1 mg/kg twice daily orally [p.o.]) and metoclopramide (0.2–0.5 mg/kg three times daily p.o.) for 1–2 weeks prior to surgery. Pre- and postoperative antacid treatment was found to positively influence the digestive clinical signs and was recommended to be administered to all dogs scheduled for BAS surgery, even those without digestive clinical signs (Vangrinsven *et al.* 2021). Other combinations of perioperative prokinetics (metoclopramide, cisapride), gastroprotectants (famotidine, omeprazole, sucralfate), and antiemetics (metoclopramide, ondansetron) can also be given to reduce postoperative regurgitation (Poncet *et al.* 2006; Mercurio 2011; Costa *et al.* 2020). However, adverse reactions after administration of histamine-2 blockers (famotidine) to French and English bulldogs have been reported anecdotally.

General considerations of anesthesia

Brachycephalic dogs have a 1.57 times higher risk for complications during anesthesia and need to be monitored closely during the recovery phase to address any potential postanesthetic complications such as acute airway blockage, regurgitation, vomiting, aspiration pneumonia, prolonged recovery, and stertorous breathing. Brachycephalic dogs are also 4.33 times more likely to have postanesthetic complications, with aspiration pneumonia being the most common complication (Gruenheid *et al.* 2018). To minimize the critical recovery phase, the airway assessment and corrective surgery should be performed under the same anesthetic. In-depth descriptions of anesthesia in brachycephalic dogs can be found elsewhere, but important aspects to consider are the following.

A light meal of wet food 3–4 hours before anesthesia was found to decrease the incidence of gastroesophageal reflux in dogs (Savvas *et al.* 2016). Intravenous lidocaine (2 mg/kg i.v. 2%) was found to reduce coughing during endotracheal intubation compared to locally applied lidocaine. This might also aid in reducing the risk of regurgitation during induction and intubation (Thompson & Rioja 2016). The patient should be preoxygenated for 3 minutes (McNally *et al.* 2009), and induction and intubation should be rapid and smooth (Koch *et al.* 2003). Anticholinergic drugs need to be available to combat bradycardic effects of vagal stimulation secondary to glottic handling (Aron & Crowe 1985). Extubation should be delayed until the endotracheal tube is not tolerated any more (Hobson 1995). While dogs used to be monitored for at least 12–24 hours after BAS surgery in an intensive care unit, a newer, less stressful practice is to have the dogs recover with the owner present and to discharge them the same day. The complication rate of a subsequent anesthetic after corrective BAS surgery was found to be reduced by 79% (Doyle *et al.* 2020).

Controversy of which surgical techniques to apply

Surgical treatment options to address upper airway obstruction are manifold, and there is a discrepancy over whether to perform multilevel surgery or to focus on the two most relevant primary obstructions – the nares and the elongated, hypertrophic soft palate. Traditionally, BAS surgery consisted of alarplasty, staphylectomy, and sacculectomy if the laryngeal saccules were everted. Nowadays there is an ongoing debate regarding the additional improvement in airflow achieved by sacculectomy, particularly when balanced against concerns regarding increased risk of complications such as laryngeal webbing or regrowth (Matushek & Bjorling 1988; Mehl *et al.* 2008). A higher complication rate was found in patients undergoing additional sacculectomy compared with patients undergoing nares resection and staphylectomy alone (Hughes *et al.* 2018). However, the theory that the saccules return to their original position once the negative inspiratory pressure has resolved was also found to be unrealistic (Cantatore *et al.* 2012). A recent study evaluating the short-term outcome of two-level BAS surgery found that 70.7% of dogs improved after alarplasty and staphylectomy. This improvement was associated with the severity of inspiratory effort, but not with any other clinical sign or anatomic abnormality. This study also found an association between snoring and pharyngeal dimensions, but not with soft palate length (Seneviratne *et al.* 2020). This strengthens the argument that the thickness of the soft palate needs to be corrected, either by a palatoplasty reducing its thickness or by a rostrally extending staphylectomy.

Comparison of two types of multilevel surgery – a traditional one consisting of vertical wedge resection alaplasty, staphylectomy, sacculectomy, and partial tonsillectomy; and a modified one that included a modified rhinoplasty technique combining a Trader's alaplasty and nasal vestibuloplasty, folded flap palatoplasty, bilateral sacculectomy, partial cuneiformectomy, and partial tonsillectomy – was in favor of the modified version. Treated dogs showed improvement of their BAS index by 10%, but were not clinically normal (Liu *et al.* 2017b). Laser-assisted turbinectomy (LATE) was added to the treatment for severely affected dogs and those that did not improve enough after the multilevel surgery (Liu *et al.* 2019).

Stenotic nares

Stenotic nares are considered to be primary anatomic components of brachycephalic syndrome, and their early correction has been advocated to minimize exacerbation of obstructive disease at other sites such as the soft palate and larynx (Aron & Crowe 1985; Wykes 1991; Harvey 1985). Surgical treatment include amputation of the ala nasi, various alaplasty techniques (wedge and punch resections), alapexy, and vestibuloplasty.

Amputation of the ala nasi

The first surgical treatment for stenotic nares consisted of the simple amputation of the ala nasi and was reported by Trader in 1949. It has since been largely abandoned, but it may be easier than alaplasty techniques in very small or immature animals (Tobias 2010b).

Alaplasty

Alaplasty is the most used procedure and consists of the excision of a wedge of the ala nasi with primary closure of the defect. This wedge can be vertical, horizontal, or lateral. Incisions are made with a no. 11 or 15 scalpel blade or alternatively with a punch (Trostel & Frankel 2010). Hemorrhage is usually brisk on incision and may impair visibility of the surgical field to some extent, but it resolves quickly when the wound is sutured. Two to four sutures are placed in a simple interrupted pattern, using absorbable monofilament material.

Vertical wedge technique

In the vertical wedge technique, incisions are started at the apex of the wedge, which is positioned slightly dorsolaterally to the dorsal limit of the slit-like opening of the stenotic naris (Figure 37.5) (Website Chapter 37: Respiratory tract/BAS/stenotic nares). The medial border of the wedge is parallel to the medial wall of the ala nasi. The lateral border of the wedge is made at an angle (40–70°) from the medial border. The degree of postoperative opening of the naris will be grossly proportional to the angle chosen. It is important that incisions be deep enough and include a portion of the alar fold to fully relieve the obstruction and not limit the opening to the rostral part of the nostril. Care must be taken to obtain a symmetric opening on both sides.

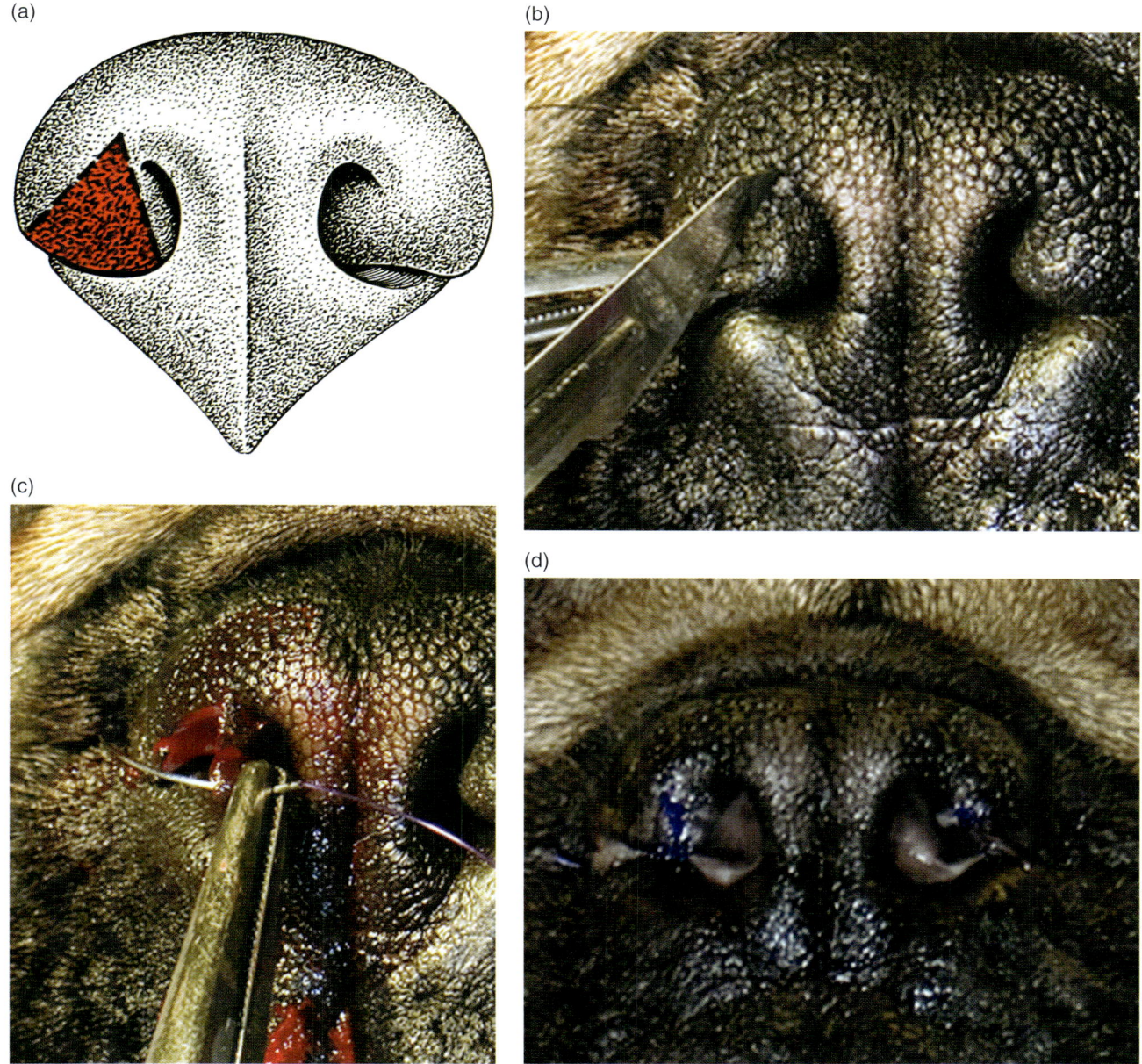

Figure 37.8 (a) Schematic view of a vertical wedge alaplasty. (b) The scalpel blade is held first vertically and then at a 60° angle in order to remove a pyramidal piece of tissue. The cut should be as deep as possible. (c) The two edges are brought together and sutured with absorbable monofilament suture material. (d) Vertical wedge alaplasty technique three weeks after surgery. An important opening of the nasal cavity should be observed.

Horizontal wedge technique

The horizontal wedge technique has been described with various approaches. Hobson (1995) describes a right-angled wedge technique with the tip of the wedge positioned laterally. Harvey (1982b) describes a wide wedge with a medial tip, which is similar to a wide vertical wedge.

Lateral wedge technique

The lateral wedge resection technique consists of the excision of a vertical wedge of tissue from the caudolateral aspect of the external nose, at the junction between the nose and the skin. The wedge can include a portion of skin (Nelson 1993; Monnet 2003) or not (Aron & Crowe 1985). The wedge is made deep enough to include a portion of the alar fold (Wykes 1991). When the wound edges are sutured together, the ala nasi is displaced caudolaterally and fixed in an abducted position, thereby opening the nostril.

Punch resection alaplasty

A technique of punch resection alaplasty has been reported (Trostel & Frankel 2010), in which a dermatologic punch biopsy is used to incise the portion of the ala nasi to be resected, down to the level of the alar fold. The diameter of the punch biopsy instrument used varies from 2 mm for puppies and cats to 3–6 mm for dogs. The size of the punch is chosen so that 2–3 mm of ala nasi tissue remains medially and laterally to the resected portion.

Alapexy

Alapexy is an alternative technique that could be considered when excessive flaccidity of the nasal cartilages has led, or is anticipated to lead, to recurrence of stenosis after conventional wedge alapasty (Ellison 2004). In this technique the ala nasi is fixed abducted by creation of a permanent adhesion between the ventral edge of the lateral aspect of the ala nasi and the skin lateral to it. The ventral edge of the lateral aspect of the ala nasi is amputated, leading to an elliptical wound along the alar groove. A matching elliptical incision is made in the skin, 3–5 mm laterally to the alar wound. The two wounds are sutured together in two layers (medial and lateral). As the ala nasi is held abducted by the created adhesion to the skin, the opening of the naris is not dependent on the rigidity of the nasal cartilages and long-term failure is believed to be less likely (Ellison 2004).

Vestibuloplasty

Vestibuloplasty has been advocated instead of alaplasty to further improve airflow (Oechtering & Schuenemann 2010). It involves the dorsomedial and caudal portion of the ala and its transition into the bulbous connection to the alar fold, and results in a wide and open vestibule.

Turbinectomy

Turbinectomy (Tobias 2010a,b) and its laser-assisted variation (LATE) (Oechtering *et al.* 2016) are applied to remove malformed obstructive parts of the ventral and medial nasal turbinates. The LATE, combined with vestibuloplasty and staphylectomy, resulted in a decrease of 55% of intranasal resistance 3–6 months after surgery compared with preoperative values (Hueber *et al.* 2007). When LATE was performed 2–6 months after modified multilevel surgery, an addi-

tional improvement of the BAS index by 25% (Liu *et al.* 2019) was observed. Complications were reverse sneezing, nasal noise, and hemorrhage. Partial regrowth of the removed turbinates but with less mucosal contact points is also being reported (Schuenemann & Oechtering 2014b). The long-term positive effects of turbinectomy on intranasal resistance and adverse effects on thermoregulation require further investigation.

Elongated hyperplastic soft palate

Common surgical techniques for correction of elongated soft palate are aimed at shortening the soft palate by simple resection of its caudal portion (staphylectomy), to prevent it from obstructing the rima glottidis on inspiration. Different landmarks have been recommended, varying from the tip of the epiglottis to the middle to caudal aspect of the palatine tonsils. A more recent trend is to extend the staphylectomy rostrally to the level of the rostral end of the tonsils (Brdecka *et al.* 2008; Dunie-Merigot *et al.* 2010; Seneviratne *et al.* 2020). The hamuli pterygoidei was found useful as a landmark to identify the maximal nasopharyngeal occlusion intraoperatively (Sarran *et al.* 2018). Staphylectomies are performed through an oral approach (Website Chapter 37: Respiratory tract/BAS/ soft palate resection). The caudal border of the soft palate is grasped and held with Allis forceps (Bright & Wheaton 1983; Brdecka *et al.* 2007, 2008). Alternatively, stay sutures are used to retract the soft palate. Resection of excessive length of soft palate can be performed with a scalpel blade, scissors, monopolar electrocoagulation, carbon dioxide laser, diode laser, or bipolar sealing device (LigaSure®, Valleylab, Covidien, Boulder, CO, USA).

As these palate-trimming techniques may not address the soft palate hyperplasia, other techniques designed to more extensively shorten and thin the soft palate have been described (Brdecka *et al.* 2008; Findji & Dupré 2008, 2009; Dunié-Merigot *et al.* 2010). The folded flap palatoplasty has been developed to correct both the excessive length and excessive thickness of the soft palate (Findji & Dupré 2008, 2009). In this technique, the soft palate is made thinner by excision of a portion of its oropharyngeal mucosa and soft tissues and made shorter by being folded on itself (Figures 37.9– 37.14). These techniques leave only a few centimeters of soft palate by using the cranial commissure of the tonsillar crypt as a landmark for simple palatal resection (Brdecka *et al.* 2008; Dunié-Mérigot *et al.* 2010), or by folding the soft palate on itself enough for the caudal opening of the nasopharynx to be directly visible transorally (Findji & Dupré 2008). Postoperative adverse

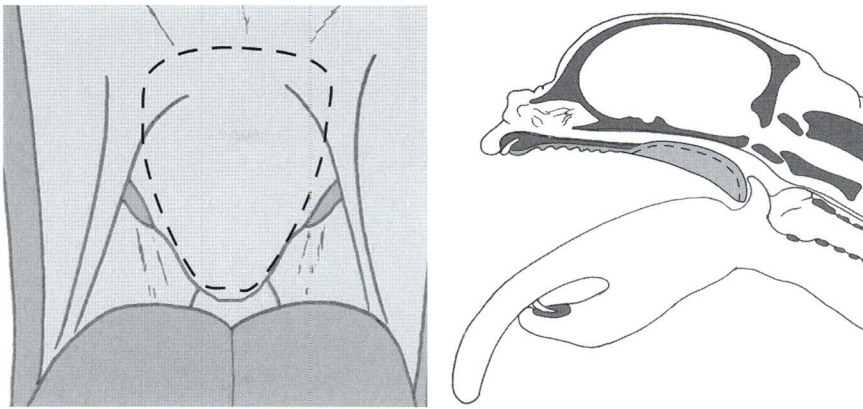

Figure 37.9 Folded flap palatoplasty: incision lines for the thinning process of soft palate hyperplasia.

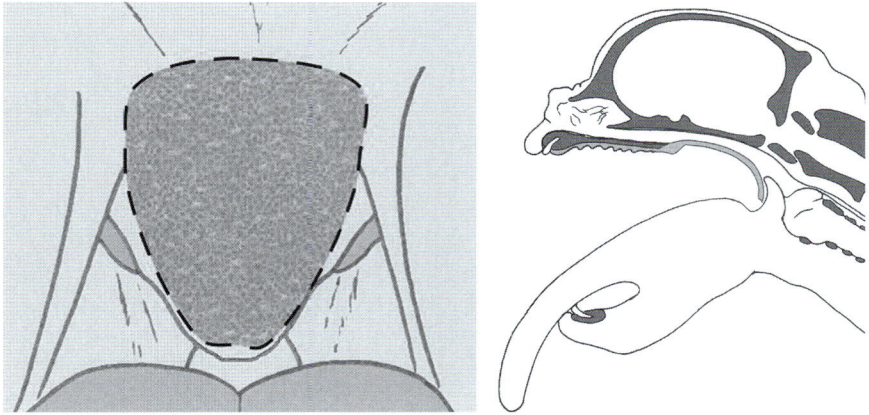

Figure 37.10 Folded flap palatoplasty: end of dissection of the soft palate.

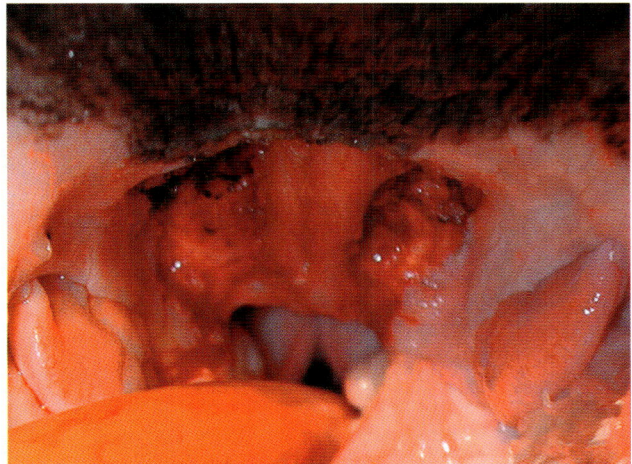

Figure 37.11 Folded flap palatoplasty: intraoperative views after excavation of the oral mucosa and of the hyperplastic tissues.

effects or pharyngonasal regurgitation have not been observed with this technique (Brdecka *et al.* 2008; Findji & Dupré 2008, 2009; Dunié-Mérigot *et al.* 2010),

apart from one dog reported with soft palate necrosis and two dogs with dehiscence (Findji & Dupré 2008; Haimel & Dupré 2015; Stordalen *et al.* 2020). Whatever technique is chosen, a telescope and high-definition camera system for magnification and illumination of the surgical field (VITOM™, Karl Storz Endoscopy, Tuttlingen, Germany) are helpful.

Laryngeal diseases

Everted laryngeal ventricles (often named saccules, or laryngoceles) are formed by eversion of the mucosa of the laryngeal ventricles. The everted saccules may obstruct the ventral half of the rima glottidis. In the past, their excision has been recommended as a routine procedure when they are found (Harvey 1982a,d; Aron & Crowe 1985; Hendricks 1992; Torrez & Hunt 2006). It is performed via an oral approach using electrocautery, scissors, tonsil snares, or laryngeal biopsy cup forceps (Wykes 1991; Hedlund 1998). To perform a complete and safe resection of everted lateral ventricles, magnification and endoscopic assistance are recommended. Diode

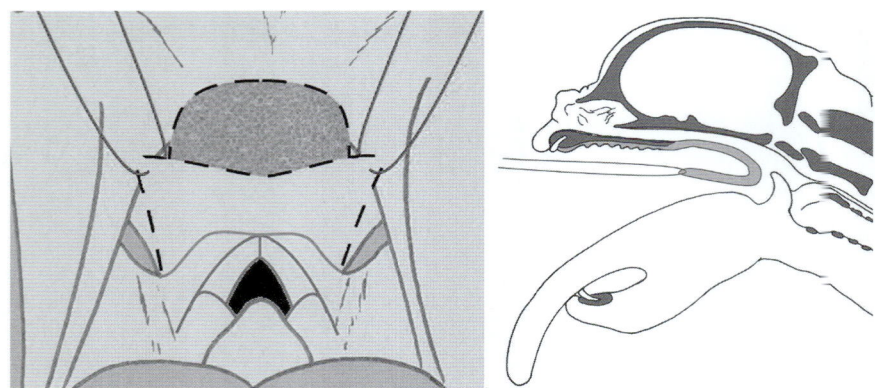

Figure 37.12 Folded flap palatoplasty: schematic view once the thinned soft palate is folded upon itself.

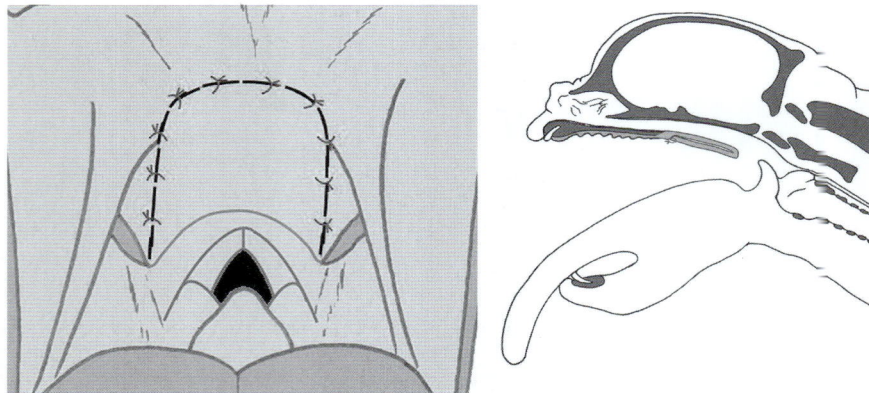

Figure 37.13 Folded flap palatoplasty: after the flap has been sutured.

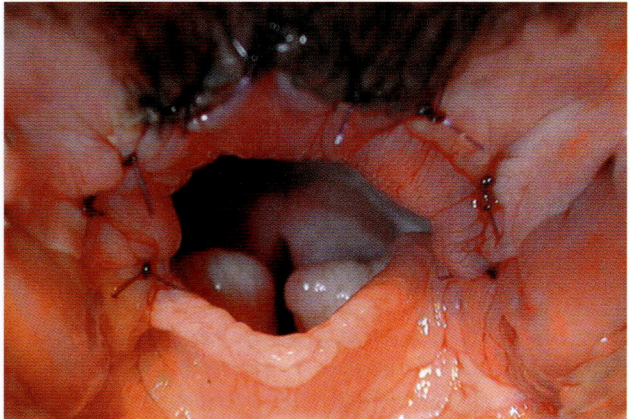

Figure 37.14 Folded flap palatoplasty: intraoperative view after the flap has been sutured.

laser-assisted ventriculectomy seems to carry a lesser risk of laryngeal webbing.

Overall, the problem of laryngeal collapse deserves specific attention. Laryngeal mucosal edema, everted saccules, and laryngeal collapse are thought to develop secondary to airway obstructions (stenotic nares, aberrant conchae, elongated soft palate). Therefore, addressing these primary conditions may improve laryngeal diseases and obviate the need to surgically address them (Pink *et al.* 2006; Torrez & Hunt 2006; Riecks *et al.* 2007; Seim 2010). Indeed, in several recent studies, everted laryngeal saccules were not, or were rarely, addressed, with similar positive outcomes compared with studies where everted laryngeal saccules were excised (Poncet *et al.* 2006; Findji & Dupré 2008; Dunié-Mérigot *et al.* 2010; Seneviratne *et al.* 2020). In one study, everted laryngeal saccule excision was even associated with a poorer outcome (Ducarouge 2002). However, reevaluation of everted laryngeal ventricles after single-side resection revealed no regression of the nonremoved site was found, despite treatment of nares and soft palate. Histopathology of the removed saccules identified edema and inflammation (Cantatore *et al.* 2012). In most cases, the relief in airway obstruction will be sufficient for laryngeal diseases to stabilize and not require later surgical treatment. If such treatment is required, despite appropriate surgical correction of primary obstructive conditions, then surgical treatment should be considered.

Early reports describe treatment of laryngeal collapse by partial laryngectomy (Harvey & Venker-von Haagan 1975). This was later found to be associated with unacceptable (50%) mortality rates, and is no longer recommended (Harvey 1983). Arytenoid lateralization can be performed (Ducarouge 2002; Pink *et al.* 2006; White 2012), but its efficacy is questionable when laryngeal cartilages are extremely flaccid (Poncet *et al.* 2006). In these cases, laser-assisted partial arytenoidectomy has been recommended, and might offer a safer and more efficient approach. Laser-assisted partial arytenoidectomy as recommended for treatment of laryngeal paralysis might provide some relief, but needs to be further investigated (Olivieri *et al.* 2009). In one study, dogs with advanced laryngeal collapse treated with partial cuneiformectomy did not show greater improvement compared to those that did not receive partial cuneiformectomy (Liu *et al.* 2017b). Further, handling of the larynx can lead to severe bradycardia secondary to vagal stimulation, which should be balanced against the benefits of partial laryngeal resection. Alternatively, a permanent tracheostomy (Harvey 1982a,e; Aron & Crowe 1985; Wykes 1991; Hendricks 1992; Hedlund 1998; Koch *et al.* 2003; Monnet 2003) has been advocated as a palliative possibility.

Excision of the edematous mucosa of the aryepiglottic folds has been advocated in the past (Hedlund 1998). Although it seems rarely to be indicated, it can be useful in some breeds, where the laryngeal mucosa is very hyperplastic and is sucked into the rima glottidis during inspiration.

Tonsillectomy and removal of other hyperplastic tissues

In brachycephalic dogs, the chronically increased negative pressures, turbulent airflow in the pharynx, and regurgitation frequently cause the palatine tonsils to be inflamed and enlarged, and to protrude from their crypts. Their excision has been recommended when they seem to contribute to the pharyngeal obstruction (Singleton 1962; Harvey & Venker-von Haagan 1975; Aron & Crowe 1985). Other surgeons remove them when everted as part of a multilevel surgery strategy (Liu *et al.* 2017b). The improvement after tonsillectomy is thought to result from direct removal of the obstructive tissue, but also from the lateral tension exerted on the soft palate after suture of the tonsillar crypts (Singleton 1962). Tonsillectomy does carry the risk of postoperative hemorrhage and thorough hemostasis is mandatory. As other authors consider it unnecessary, the advantages of tonsillectomy warrant further investigation (Hobson 1995; Koch *et al.* 2003; Fasanella *et al.* 2010).

Similarly, excision of redundant soft tissues located in the pharynx, especially in its dorsal aspect, has been suggested (Hobson 1995), but more data are needed to evaluate which of the pharyngeal tissues are involved in the obstruction process and the optimal surgical method to remove the hyperplastic tissue.

Tracheostomy

Although it has been advocated in the past (Hendricks 1992; Orsher 1993), a preoperative temporary tracheostomy is not necessary. Postoperative temporary tracheostomy has been reported in the past in 5–28% of cases (Harvey 1982a,e; Harvey & O'Brien 1982; Poncet *et al.* 2006; Torrez & Hunt 2006; Findji & Dupré 2008, 2009). As the complication rate of temporary tracheostomy in brachycephalic dogs is very high (86–95.2%) (Nicholson & Baines 2012; Stordalen *et al.* 2020), it should be reserved for cases not responding to routine postoperative care. The small tracheal diameter and abundant mucus production can cause the tracheostomy tube to become easily obstructed and require continuous monitoring. The narrow diameter of the trachea of English bulldogs, as well as the flaccidity of the trachea of pugs, may make them more prone to secondary stenosis. The most commonly reported complications are tracheostomy tube obstruction or dislodgment, and coughing (Stordalen *et al.* 2020). Risk factors for temporary tracheostomy tube placement following BAS surgery were higher age, corticosteroid use, and pneumonia (Worth *et al.* 2018). A modified temporary tracheostomy that included a Penrose drain sling dorsal to the trachea was reported to simplify tracheostomy care, improve tracheostomy outcome, and reduce tube-associated mortality compared with the standard procedure (Bird *et al.* 2018). Ideally, postoperative tracheostomy should be avoided and used only in severe cases. To palliate the effects of local swelling after surgery, it seems beneficial to rouse the patient with the upper jaw hung. This enables temporary breathing through the mouth. Placement of a nasotracheal tube immediately after surgery, allowing flow of oxygen beyond the rima glottidis, is also helpful (Senn *et al.* 2011).

Permanent tracheostomy is also associated with a high rate (50–80%) of major complications (aspiration pneumonia, stoma stenosis, and skinfold occlusion); however, long-term survival with a good quality of life is possible. Reported median survival times were 328 (Occhipinti & Hauptman 2014) and 1825 days (Grimes *et al.* 2019), respectively. Acute death at home most likely secondary to tube obstruction was reported in 26% of patients (Occhipinti & Hauptman 2014). Older dogs with preoperative administration of corticosteroids or tracheal collapse had a shorter survival time (Grimes *et al.* 2019). Dorsal skin resection to prevent skinfold occlusion and intermittent placement of plastic tubes into redilatated stomas were found to be useful long-term treatments of these complications (Bernardé *et al.* 2021). Overall, permanent tracheostomy seems to be a valuable salvage procedure for those dogs with severe laryngeal collapse not responsive to more conservative surgeries (Occhipinti & Hauptman 2014; Grimes *et al.* 2019; Gobbetti *et al.* 2018; Bernardé *et al.* 2021).

Surgical management of hiatal hernia

Gastrointestinal clinical signs are reported to dramatically improve after corrective BAS surgery (Poncet *et al.* 2006; Haimel & Dupré 2015; Kaye *et al.* 2018). Brachycephalic dogs with persistent regurgitation despite correction of the upper airway obstruction or gastroesophageal reflux secondary to hiatal hernia are potentially surgical candidates for hernia repair. Circumferential esophageal hiatal rim reconstruction and esophagopexy were reported to substantially reduce the regurgitation frequency and allow discontinuation of medical treatment (Hosgood *et al.* 2021). Mayhew *et al.* (2017) reported surgical treatment of sliding hiatal hernia in nine brachycephalic dogs after applying hiatal plication, esophagopexy, and left-sided incisional gastropexy through a celiotomy. The clinical signs of sliding hiatal hernia improved in most dogs after surgery, but did not consistently resolve. A laparoscopic technique for treatment of sliding hiatal hernia in 18 brachycephalic dogs was recently described. Hiatal plication and esophagopexy were performed with intracorporeal suturing, combined with a left-sided laparoscopic or laparoscopic-assisted gastropexy. Regurgitation improved significantly after surgery, but did not resolve the clinical signs completely (Mayhew *et al.* 2021).

Postoperative care

The challenge during the postoperative period is to enable adequate airflow in a not yet fully awake patient with potentially swollen airway mucosa. It is critical that BAS-affected dogs are monitored constantly after extubation to determine if ventilation is inadequate. Several methods can be combined or used independently to help relieve upper airway obstruction or improve ventilation after surgical repair.

Firstly, the dog can be recovered with the upper jaw hung up, which allows the lower jaw to drop, opening the airway further. Placement of a small nasotracheal tube immediately after surgery but before the dog is awake is a very simple technique of insufflating oxygen, allowing oxygen delivery beyond the rima glottis (Senn *et al.* 2011).

Stress, panting, and barking should be avoided, as they can lead to life-threatening pharyngeal edema and/or regurgitation. Some authors encourage owners to be present during the recovery phase after the dog has been extubated to minimize stress. This technique seems to reduce the need for hospitalization after recovery and is currently being used by several surgeons. Life-threatening pharyngeal edema can be treated with nebulized or sprayed adrenalin to avoid tracheostomy (Ellis & Leece 2017; Debuigne & Chesnel 2021). Nebulized epinephrine also decreases respiratory clinical signs and might be useful to treat acute respiratory distress (Franklin *et al.* 2021).

Complications

The overall major complication rate after BAS surgery was reported to be 7% and pneumonia was associated with the development of major postoperative complications (Ree *et al.* 2016). The most important complications after BAS surgery are airway swelling, regurgitation, and aspiration pneumonia.

Dyspnea secondary to pharyngeal swelling is reported to occur in 1.6–23.4% of dogs (Haimel & Dupré 2015; Hughes *et al.* 2018; Tarricone *et al.* 2019; Fenner *et al.* 2020; Lindsay *et al.* 2020) and treatment options are supplemental oxygen, corticosteroid administration, and nebulization with adrenalin or epinephrine. Reintubation and temporary tracheostomy are further treatment options if the swelling does not resolve. Age, corticosteroid use, and pneumonia were identified as risk factors for temporary tracheostomy (Worth *et al.* 2018). Postoperative regurgitation is reported to occur in 4.7–14.5% of brachycephalic dogs (Poncet *et al.* 2006; Haimel & Dupré 2015; Ree *et al.* 2016; Fenner *et al.* 2020; Lindsay *et al.* 2020) and younger dogs and those with a history of regurgitation are reported to be at increased risk (Fenner *et al.* 2020). Perioperative administration of metoclopramide and famotidine was found to reduce the risk of post-operative regurgitation from 35% to 9% (Costa *et al.* 2020).

Darcy *et al.* (2018) reported that English and French bulldogs are at high risk for aspiration pneumonia. Preoperative aspiration pneumonia has been identified in 1.6–8.3% of dogs (Ree *et al.* 2016; Kirsch *et al.* 2019; Lindsay *et al.* 2020) and in 0.8–5.5% following surgery (Haimel & Dupré 2015; Ree *et al.* 2016; Kirsch *et al.* 2019; Fenner *et al.* 2020; Lindsay *et al.* 2020). Brachycephalic dogs have a 3.77 times higher risk for aspiration pneumonia compared to other dogs and gastrointestinal clinical signs are risk factors to develop aspiration pneumonia (Darcy *et al.* 2018). Postoperative aspiration pneumonia was found to be associated with temporary tracheostomy and death (Ree *et al.* 2016; Worth *et al.* 2018; Kirsch *et al.* 2019).

A brachycephalic risk (BRisk) score for predicting complications following BAS surgery has been recently introduced (Tarricone *et al.* 2019).

Prognosis

The objective determination of the prognosis associated with brachycephalic syndrome from the data in the veterinary literature is hindered by several difficulties. Most studies are retrospective and involve different populations of dogs in terms of breed and conformation, and these populations underwent several concurrent treatments in various combinations, performed at variable ages, using variable techniques and instruments. Furthermore, many studies only rate the outcome in terms of improvement compared with the preoperative condition, but this preoperative condition is either ungraded, graded according to scales that are not consistent between preoperative and postoperative assessments, or described at the population level, which poorly reflects the severity of affected individuals (Harvey 1982e; Clark & Sinibaldi 1994; Lorinson *et al.* 1997; Davidson *et al.* 2001; Pink *et al.* 2006; Torrez & Hunt 2006; Riecks *et al.* 2007; Trostel & Frankel 2010). Other studies use grading systems in an effort to objectively compare preoperative and postoperative clinical signs, but these scales are not consistent between studies (Brdecka *et al.* 2008; Findji & Dupré 2008; Huck *et al.* 2008; Dunié-Mérigot *et al.* 2010; Seneviratne *et al.* 2020). Lastly, follow-up times are also quite variable and in most cases long-term follow-up is obtained by way of a questionnaire.

Keeping in mind these methodologic limitations, it is clear that most dogs suffering from brachycephalic syndrome benefit from surgery. In one study, younger age has been significantly associated with a poor treatment outcome (Liu *et al.* 2017b) and with an increased risk of postoperative regurgitation (Fenner *et al.* 2020). Another study comparing pre- and postoperative treatments in different breeds that underwent the same diagnostic work-up, treatment, and evaluation methods found no correlations between the severity of laryngeal collapse and overall respiratory signs or prognosis (Haimel & Dupré 2015). Yet others identified laryngeal collapse as a negative prognostic indicator for a good outcome post surgery (Liu *et al.* 2017b). Despite inherent study limitations, late studies report that around 70–90% of BAS dogs are significantly improved with surgery (Poncet *et al.* 2006; Riecks *et al.* 2007; Findji & Dupré 2008; Dunié-Mérigot *et al.* 2010; Haimel & Dupré 2015; Seneviratne *et al.* 2020), which is better than earlier reports (Harvey 1982e; Lorinson *et al.* 1997). Similarly, perioperative mortality rates have improved from around 15% in earlier reports (Harvey 1982e; Lorinson *et al.* 1997) to less than 4% in more recent studies (Poncet *et al.* 2006; Torrez & Hunt 2006; Riecks *et al.* 2007; Brdecka *et al.* 2008; Findji & Dupré 2008; Dunié-Mérigot *et al.* 2010). Postoperative improvement is most often observed immediately after surgery (Poncet *et al.* 2006; Findji & Dupré 2008). Concurrent laryngeal collapse is a major determinant of long-term prognosis. As described, it is thought to be mainly a secondary disease (although in the pug, congenital chondromalacia can be suspected) and palliation is provided by surgical relief of other components of airway obstruction. In one study, dogs with mild to severe laryngeal collapse undergoing surgical correction of stenotic nares, elongated soft palate, and everted laryngeal saccules had good long-term outcomes without additional surgery (Torrez & Hunt 2006). However, laryngeal collapse resulting in signs of airway obstruction, despite surgical relief of other sites of obstruction, carries a more guarded prognosis. Conversely, in some other studies, concurrent tracheal hypoplasia did not influence clinical outcome after surgical treatment (Pink *et al.* 2006; Riecks *et al.* 2007).

In some studies, long-term recurrence of clinical signs has been described as occurring in up to 100% of cases, although 89% of dogs remained improved, compared with their preoperative status (Torrez & Hunt 2006). Such recurrence may require additional surgery, possibly using alternative corrective techniques (Ellison 2004). Although these numbers seem high, long-term evaluation using appropriate grading systems is warranted to appreciate the late treatment improvements.

Although a better understanding of the current anatomic and functional changes associated with brachycephalic syndrome has led to improvement in surgical techniques and results, a radical rethinking regarding brachycephalic breeding is warranted.

References

Aron, D.N. and Crowe, D.T. (1985). Upper airway obstruction. General principles and selected conditions in the dog and cat. *Veterinary Clinics of North America. Small Animal Practice* 15: 891–917.

Belch, A., Matiasovic, M., Rasotto, R. et al. (2017). Comparison of the use of LigaSure versus a standard technique for tonsillectomy in dogs. *Veterinary Record* 180 (8): 196.

Bernaerts, F., Talavera, J., Leemans, J. et al. (2010). Description of original endoscopic findings and respiratory functional assessment using barometric whole-body plethysmography in dogs suffering from brachy-cephalic airway obstruction syndrome. *Veterinary Journal* 183: 95–102.

Bernardé, A., Matres-Lorenzo, L., and Carcia-Rodriguez, M. (2021). Long-term management of stenosis after tube-less permanent tracheostomy in brachycephalic dogs: 19 cases. Unpublished data.

Billen, F., Day, M.J., and Clercx, C. (2006). Diagnosis of pharyngeal disorders in dogs: a retrospective study of 67 cases. *Journal of Small Animal Practice* 47: 122–129.

Bird, F.G., Vallefuoco, R., Dupré, G. et al. (2018). A modified temporary tracheostomy in dogs: outcome and complications in 21 dogs (2012 to 2017). *Journal of Small Animal Practice* 59 (12): 769–776.

Boesch, R.P., Shah, P., Vaynblat, M. et al. (2005). Relationship between upper airway obstruction and gastroesophageal reflux in a dog model. *Journal of Investigative Surgery* 18: 241–245.

Brdecka, D., Rawlings, C., Howerth, E. et al. (2007). A histopathological comparison of two techniques for soft palate resection in normal dogs. *Journal of the American Animal Hospital Association* 43: 39–44.

Brdecka, D.J., Rawlings, C.A., Perry, A.C., and Anderson, J.R. (2008). Use of an electrothermal, feedback-controlled, bipolar sealing device for resection of the elongated portion of the soft palate in dogs with obstructive upper airway disease. *Journal of the American Veterinary Medical Association* 233: 1265–1269.

Bright, R.M. and Wheaton, L.G. (1983). A modified surgical technique for elongated soft palate in dogs. *Journal of the American Animal Hospital Association* 19: 288–292.

Broux, O., Clercx, C., Etienne, A.L. et al. (2018). Effects of manipulations to detect sliding hiatal hernia in dogs with brachycephalic airway obstructive syndrome. *Veterinary Surgery* 47 (2): 243–251.

Caccamo, R., Buracco, P., La Rosa, G. et al. (2014). Glottic and skull indices in canine brachycephalic airway obstructive syndrome. *BMC Veterinary Research* 10: 12.

Cantatore, M., Gobbetti, M., Romussi, S. et al. (2012). Medium term endoscopic assessment of the surgical outcome following laryngeal saccule resection in brachycephalic dogs. *Veterinary Record* 170: 518.

Clark, G.N. and Sinibaldi, K.R. (1994). Use of a carbon dioxide laser for treatment of elongated soft palate in dogs. *Journal of the American Veterinary Medical Association* 204: 1779–1781.

Cook, W.R. (1964). Observations on the upper respiratory tract of the dog and cat. *Journal of Small Animal Practice* 5: 309–329.

Costa, R.S., Abelson, A.L., Lindsey, J.C. et al. (2020). Postoperative regurgitation and respiratory complications in brachycephalic dogs undergoing airway surgery before and after implementation of a standardized perianesthetic protocol. *Journal of the American Veterinary Medical Association* 256 (8): 899–905.

Crosse, K.R., Bray, J.P., Orbell, G. et al. (2015). Histological evaluation of the soft palate in dogs affected by brachycephalic obstructive airway syndrome. *New Zealand Veterinary Journal* 63 (6): 319–325.

Darcy, H.P., Humm, K., and Ter Haar, G. (2018). Retrospective analysis of incidence, clinical features, potential risk factors, and prognostic indicators for aspiration pneumonia in three brachycephalic dog breeds. *Journal of the American Veterinary Medical Association* 253 (7): 869–876.

Davidson, E.B., Davis, M.S., Campbell, G.A. et al. (2001). Evaluation of carbon dioxide laser and conventional incisional techniques for resection of soft palates in brachycephalic dogs. *Journal of the American Veterinary Medical Association* 219: 776–781.

De Bruyn, B.W. and Hosgood, G. (2022). Abnormal hyoid conformation in French bulldogs: case report and computed tomographic anatomical comparison. *Australian Veterinary Journal* 100: 63–66.

De Lorenzi, D., Bertoncello, D., and Drigo, M. (2009). Bronchial abnormalities found in a consecutive series of 40 brachycephalic dogs. *Journal of the American Veterinary Medical Association* 235: 835–840.

Debuigne, M. and Chesnel, M. (2021). Life-threatening pharyngeal oedema secondary to severe per-anaesthetic regurgitation in a French bulldog: management with topical adrenaline and nasotracheal tube. *Veterinary Record Case Reports* 9: e2179.

Doyle, C.R., Aarnes, T.K., Ballash, G.A. et al. (2020). Anesthetic risk during subsequent anesthetic event in brachycephalic dogs that have undergone corrective airway surgery: 45 cases (2007–2019). *Journal of the American Veterinary Medical Association* 257 (7): 744–749.

Ducarouge, B. (2002). Le syndrome obstructif des voies respiratoires supèrieures chez les chiens brachycéphales. Etude clinique à propos de 27 cas. Doctoral thesis, University of Lyon.

Dunié-Mérigot, A., Bouvy, B., and Poncet, C. (2010). Comparative use of CO_2 laser, diode laser and monopolar electrocautery for resection of the soft palate in dogs with brachycephalic airway obstruction syndrome. *Veterinary Record* 167: 700–704.

Eivers, C., Chicon Rueda, R., Liuti, T. et al. (2019). Retrospective analysis of esophageal imaging features in brachycephalic versus non-brachycephalic dogs based on videofluoroscopic swallowing studies. *Journal of Veterinary Internal Medicine* 33 (4): 1740–1746.

Ellis, J. and Leece, E.A. (2017). Nebulized adrenaline in the postoperative management of brachycephalic obstructive airway syndrome in a pug. *Journal of the American Animal Hospital Association* 53 (2): 107–110.

Ellison, G.W. (2004). Alapexy: an alternative technique for repair of stenotic nares in dogs. *Journal of the American Animal Hospital Association* 40: 484–489.

Erjavec, V., Vovk, T., and Svete, A.N. (2021). Evaluation of oxidative stress parameters in dogs with brachycephalic obstructive airway syndrome before and after surgery. *Journal of Veterinary Research* 65 (2): 201–208.

Fasanella, F.J., Shivley, J.M., Wardlaw, J.L., and Givaruangsawat, S. (2010). Brachycephalic airway obstructive syndrome in dogs: 90 cases (1991–2008). *Journal of the American Veterinary Medical Association* 237: 1048–1051.

Fenner, J.V.H., Quinn, R.J., and Demetriou, J.L. (2020). Postoperative regurgitation in dogs after upper airway surgery to treat brachycephalic obstructive airway syndrome: 258 cases (2013–2017). *Veterinary Surgery* 49 (1): 53–60.

Findji, L. and Dupré, G. (2008). Folded flap palatoplasty for treatment of elongated soft palates in 55 dogs. *Wiener Tierärztliche Monatsschrift* 95: 56–63.

Findji, L. and Dupré, G. (2009). Folded flap palatoplasty for treatment of elongated soft palates in 55 dogs. *European Journal of Companion Animal Practice* 19: 125–132.

Foster, A., Morandi, F., and May, E. (2015). Prevalence of ear disease in dogs undergoing multidetector thin-slice computed tomography of the head. *Veterinary Radiology & Ultrasound* 56: 18–24.

Fox, M.W. (1963). Developmental abnormalities of the canine skull. *Canadian Journal of Comparative Medicine and Veterinary Science* 27 (9): 219–222.

Franklin, P.H., Liu, N.C., and Ladlow, J.F. (2021). Nebulization of epinephrine to reduce the severity of brachycephalic obstructive airway syndrome in dogs. *Veterinary Surgery* 50 (1): 62–70.

Freiche, V. and Poncet, C. (2007). Upper airway and gastrointestinal syndrome in brachycephalic dogs. *Veterinary Focus* 17 (2): 4–10.

Ginn, J.A., Kumar, M.S.A., McKiernan, B.C., and Powers, B.E. (2008). Nasopharyngeal turbinates in brachycephalic dogs and cats. *Journal of the American Animal Hospital Association* 44: 243–249.

Gobbetti, M., Romussi, S., Buracco, P. et al. (2018). Long-term outcome of permanent tracheostomy in 5 dogs with severe laryngeal collapse secondary to brachycephalic airway obstructive syndrome. *Veterinary Surgery* 47 (5): 648–653.

Grand, J.G. and Bureau, S. (2011). Structural characteristics of the soft palate and meatus nasopharyngeus in brachycephalic and non-brachycephalic dogs analysed by CT. *Journal of Small Animal Practice* 52: 232–239.

Grimes, J.A., Davis, A.M., Wallace, M.L. et al. (2019). Long-term outcome and risk factors associated with death or the need for revision surgery in dogs with permanent tracheostomies. *Journal of the American Veterinary Medical Association* 254 (9): 1086–1093.

Gruenheid, M., Aarnes, T.K., McLoughlin, M.A. et al. (2018). Risk of anesthesia-related complications in brachycephalic dogs. *Journal of the American Veterinary Medical Association* 253 (3): 301–306.

Haimel, G. and Dupré, G. (2015). Brachycephalic airway syndrome: a comparative study between pugs and French bulldogs. *Journal of Small Animal Practice* 56 (12): 714–719.

Hara, Y., Teshima, K., Seki, M. et al. (2020). Pharyngeal contraction secondary to its collapse in dogs with brachycephalic airway syndrome. *Journal of Veterinary Medical Science* 82 (1): 64–67.

Hardie, E.M., Ramirez, O. III, Clary, E.M. et al. (1998). Abnormalities of the thoracic bellows: stress fractures of the ribs and hiatal hernia. *Journal of Veterinary Internal Medicine* 12: 279–287.

Harvey, C.E. (1982a). Upper airway obstruction surgery. 4: partial laryngectomy in brachycephalic dogs. *Journal of the American Animal Hospital Association* 18: 548–550.

Harvey, C.E. (1982b). Upper airway obstruction surgery. 1: stenotic nares surgery in brachycephalic dogs. *Journal of the American Animal Hospital Association* 18: 535–537.

Harvey, C.E. (1982c). Upper airway obstruction surgery. 2: soft palate resection in brachycephalic dogs. *Journal of the American Animal Hospital Association* 18: 538–544.

Harvey, C.E. (1982d). Upper airway obstruction surgery. 3: everted laryngeal saccule surgery in brachycephalic dogs. *Journal of the American Animal Hospital Association* 18: 545–547.

Harvey, C.E. (1982e). Upper airway obstruction surgery. 8: overview of results. *Journal of the American Animal Hospital Association* 18: 567–569.

Harvey, C.E. (1983). Review of results of airway obstruction surgery in the dog. *Journal of Small Animal Practice* 24: 555–559.

Harvey, C.E. (1985). Surgical correction of stenotic nares in a cat. *Journal of the American Animal Hospital Association* 22: 31–32.

Harvey, C.E. and O'Brien, J.A. (1982). Upper airway obstruction surgery. 7: tracheotomy in the dog and cat: analysis of 89 episodes in 79 animals. *Journal of the American Animal Hospital Association* 18: 563–566.

Harvey, C.E. and Venker-von Haagan, A. (1975). Surgical management of pharyngeal and laryngeal airway obstruction in the dog. *Veterinary Clinics of North America: Small Animal Practice* 5: 515–535.

Hayes, G.M., Friend, E.J., and Jeffery, N.D. (2010). Relationship between pharyngeal conformation and otitis media with effusion in Cavalier King Charles spaniels. *Veterinary Record* 167: 55–58.

Hedlund, C.S. (1998). Brachycephalic syndrome. In: *Current Techniques in Small Animal Surgery*, 4e (ed. M.J. Bojrab, G.W. Ellison and B. Slocum), 357–362. Baltimore: Williams & Wilkins.

Heidenreich, D., Gradner, G., Kneissl, S. et al. (2016). Nasopharyngeal dimensions from computed tomography of pugs and French bulldogs with brachycephalic airway syndrome. *Veterinary Surgery* 45 (1): 83–90.

Hendricks, J.C. (1992). Brachycephalic airway syndrome. *Veterinary Clinics of North America. Small Animal Practice* 22: 1145–1153.

Herdt, T. (1997). Movements of the gastrointestinal tract. In: *Textbook of Veterinary Physiology*, 2e (ed. J.G. Cunningham), 272–289. Philadelphia, PA: WB Saunders.

Hobson, H.P. (1995). Brachycephalic syndrome. *Seminars in Veterinary Medicine and Surgery (Small Animal)* 10: 109–114.

Hosgood, G.L., Appelgrein, C., and Gelmi, C. (2021). Circumferential esophageal hiatal rim reconstruction for treatment of persistent regurgitation in brachycephalic dogs: 29 cases (2016–2019). *Journal of the American Veterinary Medical Association* 258 (10): 1091–1097.

Huck, J.L., Stanley, B.J., and Hauptman, J.G. (2008). Technique and outcome of nares amputation (trader's technique) in immature shih tzus. *Journal of the American Animal Hospital Association* 44: 82–85.

Hueber, J.P., Smith, H.J., Reinhold, P. et al. (2007). Brachycephalic airway syndrome: effects of partial turbinectomy on intranasal airway resistance. *Paper presented at 25th Symposium of the Veterinary Comparative Respiratory Society*, Lafayette, IN, USA.

Hughes, J.R., Kaye, B.M., Beswick, A.R. et al. (2018). Complications following laryngeal sacculectomy in brachycephalic dogs. *Journal of Small Animal Practice* 59 (1): 16–21.

Jones, B.A., Stanley, B.J., and Nelson, N.C. (2020). The impact of tongue dimension on air volume in brachycephalic dogs. *Veterinary Surgery* 49 (3): 512–520.

Kaye, B.M., Boroffka, S.A., Haagsman, A.N. et al. (2015). Computed tomographic, radiographic, and endoscopic tracheal dimensions in English bulldogs with grade 1 clinical signs of brachycephalic airway syndrome. *Veterinary Radiology & Ultrasound* 56 (6): 609–616.

Kaye, B.M., Rutherford, L., Perridge, D.J. et al. (2018). Relationship between brachycephalic airway syndrome and gastrointestinal signs in three breeds of dog. *Journal of Small Animal Practice* 59 (11): 670–673.

Kirsch, M.S., Spector, D., Kalafut, S.R. et al. (2019). Comparison of carbon dioxide laser versus bipolar vessel device for staphylectomy for the treatment of brachycephalic obstructive airway syndrome. *Canadian Veterinary Journal* 60 (2): 160–166.

Koch, D.A., Arnold, S., Hubler, M., and Montavon, P.M. (2003). Brachycephalic syndrome in dogs. *Compendium on Continuing Education for the Practicing Veterinarian* 25: 48–55.

Komsta, R., Osinski, Z., Debiak, P. et al. (2019). Prevalence of pectus excavatum (PE), pectus carinatum (PC), tracheal hypoplasia, thoracic spine deformities and lateral heart displacement in thoracic radiographs of screw-tailed brachycephalic dogs. *PLoS One* 14 (10): e0223642.

Krainer, D. and Dupré, G. (2021). Influence of computed tomographic dimensions of the nasopharynx on middle ear effusion and inflammation in pugs and French bulldogs with brachycephalic airway syndrome. *Veterinary Surgery* 50 (3): 517–526.

Lecoindre, P. and Richard, S. (2004). Digestive disorders associated with the chronic obstructive syndrome of brachycephalic dogs: 30 cases. *Revue de medécine vétérinaire* 155: 141–146.

Leonard, H.C. (1957). Eversion of the lateral ventricles of the larynx in dogs: five cases. *Journal of the American Veterinary Medical Association* 131: 83–84.

Leonard, H.C. (1960). Collapse of the larynx and adjacent structures in the dog. *Journal of the American Veterinary Medical Association* 137: 360–363.

Lilja-Maula, L., Lappalainen, A.K., Hyytiainen, H.K. et al. (2017). Comparison of submaximal exercise test results and severity of brachycephalic obstructive airway syndrome in English bulldogs. *Veterinary Journal* 219: 22–26.

Lindsay, B., Cook, D., Wetzel, J.M. et al. (2020). Brachycephalic airway syndrome: management of post-operative respiratory complications in 248 dogs. *Australian Veterinary Journal* 98 (5): 173–180.

Liu, N.C., Sargan, D.R., Adams, V.J. et al. (2015). Characterisation of brachycephalic obstructive airway syndrome in French bulldogs using whole- body barometric plethysmography. *PLoS One* 10: e0130741.

Liu, N.C., Adams, V.J., Kalmar, L. et al. (2016). Whole-body barometric plethysmography characterizes upper airway obstruction in 3 brachycephalic breeds of dogs. *Journal of Veterinary Internal Medicine* 30 (3): 853–865.

Liu, N.C., Troconis, E.L., Kalmar, L. et al. (2017a). Conformational risk factors of brachycephalic obstructive airway syndrome (BOAS) in pugs, French bulldogs, and bulldogs. *PLoS One* 12 (8): e0181928.

Liu, N.C., Oechtering, G.U., Adams, V.J. et al. (2017b). Outcomes and prognostic factors of surgical treatments for brachycephalic obstructive airway syndrome in 3 breeds. *Veterinary Surgery* 46 (2): 271–280.

Liu, N.C., Genain, M.A., Kalmar, L. et al. (2019). Objective effectiveness of and indications for laser-assisted turbinectomy in brachycephalic obstructive airway syndrome. *Veterinary Surgery* 48 (1): 79–87.

Lorinson, D., Bright, R.M., and White, R.A.S. (1997). Brachycephalic airway obstruction syndrome: a review of 118 cases. *Canine Practice* 22: 18–21.

Matushek, K.J. and Bjorling, D.E. (1988). A mucosal flap technique for correction of laryngeal webbing results in four dogs. *Veterinary Surgery* 17: 318–320.

Mayhew, P.D., Marks, S.L., Pollard, R. et al. (2017). Prospective evaluation of surgical management of sliding hiatal hernia and gastroesophageal reflux in dogs. *Veterinary Surgery* 46 (8): 1098–1109.

Mayhew, P.D., Balsa, I.M., Marks, S.L. et al. (2021). Clinical and videofluoroscopic outcomes of laparoscopic treatment for sliding hiatal hernia and associated gastroesophageal reflux in brachycephalic dogs. *Veterinary Surgery* 50 (Suppl 1): O67–O77.

McNally, E.M., Robertson, S.A., and Pablo, L.S. (2009). Comparison of time to desaturation between preoxygenated and nonpreoxygenated dogs following sedation with acepromazine maleate and morphine and induction of anesthesia with propofol. *American Journal of Veterinary Research* 70 (11): 1333–1338.

Mehl, M.L., Kyles, A.E., Pypendop, B.H. et al. (2008). Outcome of laryngeal web resection with mucosal apposition for treatment of airway obstruction in dogs: 15 cases (1992–2006). *Journal of the American Veterinary Medical Association* 233: 738–742.

Meola, S.D. (2013). Brachycephalic airway syndrome. *Topics in Companion Animal Medicine* 28: 91–96.

Mercurio, A. (2011). Complications of upper airway surgery in companion animals. Review. *Veterinary Clinics of North America. Small Animal Practice* 41 (5): 969–980.

Mielke, B., Lam, R., and Ter Haar, G. (2017). Computed tomographic morphometry of tympanic bulla shape and position in brachycephalic and mesaticephalic dog breeds. *Veterinary Radiology & Ultrasound* 58 (5): 552–558.

Milne, E., Nuttall, T., Marioni-Henry, K. et al. (2020). Cytological and microbiological characteristics of middle ear effusions in brachycephalic dogs. *Journal of Veterinary Internal Medicine* 34 (4): 1454–1463.

Monnet, E. (2003). Brachycephalic airway syndrome. In: *Textbook of Small Animal Surgery*, 3e (ed. D.H. Slatter), 808–813. Philadelphia, PA: WB Saunders.

Negus, V.E., Oram, S., and Banks, D.C. (1970). Effect of respiratory obstruction on the arterial and venous circulation in animals and man. *Thorax* 25: 1–10.

Nelson, A. (1993). Upper respiratory system. In: *Textbook of Small Animal Surgery*, 2e (ed. D.H. Slatter), 733–776. Philadelphia, PA: WB Saunders.

Nicholson, I. and Baines, S. (2012). Complications associated with temporary tracheostomy tubes in 42 dogs (1998 to 2007). *Journal of Small Animal Practice* 53: 108–114.

Noh, D., Choi, S., Choi, H. et al. (2021). Dynamic computed tomography evaluation of the nasopharynx in normal Beagle dogs. *Journal of Veterinary Medical Science* 83 (9): 1356–1362.

Occhipinti, L.L. and Hauptman, J.G. (2014). Long-term outcome of permanent tracheostomies in dogs: 21 cases (2000–2012). *Canadian Veterinary Journal* 55 (4): 357–360.

Oechtering, G.U. (2010). Brachycephalic syndrome: new information on an old congenital disease. *Veterinary Focus* 20: 2–9.

Oechtering, G.U. and Schuenemann, R. (2010). Brachycephalics: trapped in a man made misery? *Paper presented at the Association of Veterinary Soft Tissue Surgeons, Autumn Scientific Meeting: Congenital and Hereditary Diseases of Dogs and Cats*, Cambridge, UK.

Oechtering, T.H., Oechtering, G.U., and Nöller, C. (2007). Structural characteristics of the nose in brachycephalic dog breeds analysed by computed tomography. *Tierärtliche Praxis. Ausgabe K, Kleintiere/Heimtiere* 35: 177–187.

Oechtering, G.U., Pohl, S., Schlueter, C. et al. (2016). A novel approach to brachycephalic syndrome. 2. Laser-assisted turbinectomy (LATE). *Veterinary Surgery* 45 (2): 173–181.

Ohnishi, T. and Ogura, J.H. (1969). Partitioning of pulmonary resistance in the dog. *Laryngoscope* 79: 1847–1878.

Olivieri, M., Voghera, S., and Fossum, T. (2009). Video-assisted left partial arytenoidectomy by diode laser photoablation for treatment of canine laryngeal paralysis. *Veterinary Surgery* 38: 439–444.

Orsher, R. (1993). Brachycephalic airway disease. In: *Disease Mechanisms in Small Animal Surgery* (ed. M. Bojrab), 369–370. Philadelphia, PA: Lea & Febiger.

Packer, R.M.A., Hendricks, A., Tivers, M.S. et al. (2015). Impact of facial conformation on canine health—brachycephalic obstructive airway syndrome. *PLOS ONE* 10: e0137496.

Pichetto, M., Arrighi, S., Roccabianca, P. et al. (2011). The anatomy of the dog soft palate. II. Histological evaluation of the caudal soft palate in brachycephalic breeds with grade I brachycephalic airway obstructive syndrome. *Anatomical Record (Hoboken)* 294: 1267–1272.

Pink, J.J., Doyle, R.S., Hughes, J.M.L. et al. (2006). Laryngeal collapse in seven brachycephalic puppies. *Journal of Small Animal Practice* 47: 131–135.

Pollard, R.E., Johnson, L.R., and Marks, S.L. (2018). The prevalence of dynamic pharyngeal collapse is high in brachycephalic dogs undergoing videofluoroscopy. *Veterinary Radiology & Ultrasound* 59 (5): 529–534.

Poncet, C.M., Dupré, G.P., Freiche, V.G. et al. (2005). Prevalence of gastrointestinal tract lesions in 73 brachycephalic dogs with upper respiratory syndrome. *Journal of Small Animal Practice* 46: 273–279.

Poncet, C.M., Dupré, G.P., Freiche, V.G. and Bouvy, B.M. (2006). Long-term results of upper respiratory syndrome surgery and gastrointestinal tract medical treatment in 51 brachycephalic dogs. *Journal of Small Animal Practice* 47: 137–142.

Ree, J.J., Milovancev, M., MacIntyre, L.A. et al. (2016). Factors associated with major complications in the short-term postoperative period in dogs undergoing surgery for brachycephalic airway syndrome. *Canadian Veterinary Journal* 57 (9): 976–980.

Reeve, E.J., Sutton, D., Friend, E.J. et al. (2017). Documenting the prevalence of hiatal hernia and oesophageal abnormalities in brachycephalic dogs using fluoroscopy. *Journal of Small Animal Practice* 58 (12): 703–708.

Regier, P.J., Grosso, F.V., Stone, H.K. et al. (2020). Radiographic tracheal dimensions in brachycephalic breeds before and after surgical treatment for brachycephalic airway syndrome. *Canadian Veterinary Journal* 61 (9): 971–976.

Riecks, T.W., Birchard, S.J., and Stephens, J.A. (2007). Surgical correction of brachycephalic syndrome in dogs: 62 cases (1991–2004). *Journal of the American Veterinary Medical Association* 230: 1324–1328.

Riggs, J., Liu, N.C., Sutton, D.R. et al. (2019). Validation of exercise testing and laryngeal auscultation for grading brachycephalic obstructive airway syndrome in pugs, French bulldogs, and English bulldogs by using whole-body barometric plethysmography. *Veterinary Surgery* 48 (4): 488–496.

Roedler, F.S., Pohl, S., and Oechtering, G.U. (2013). How does severe brachycephaly affect dog's lives? Results of a structured preoperative owner questionnaire. *Veterinary Journal* 198: 606–610.

Rubin, J.A., Holt, D.E., Reetz, J.A. et al. (2015). Signalment, clinical presentation, concurrent diseases, and diagnostic findings in 28 dogs with dynamic pharyngeal collapse (2008–2013). *Journal of Veterinary Internal Medicine* 29: 815–821.

Rudorf, H., Barr, F.J., and Lane, J.G. (2001). The role of ultrasound in the assessment of laryngeal paralysis in the dog. *Veterinary Radiology & Ultrasound* 42 (4): 338–343.

Rutherford, L., Beever, L., Bruce, M. et al. (2017). Assessment of computed tomography derived cricoid cartilage and tracheal dimensions to evaluate degree of cricoid narrowing in brachycephalic dogs. *Veterinary Radiology & Ultrasound* 58 (6): 634–646.

Salguero, R., Herrtage, M., Holmes, M. et al. (2016). Comparison between computed tomographic characteristics of the middle ear in non-brachycephalic and brachycephalic dogs with obstructive airway syndrome. *Veterinary Radiology & Ultrasound* 57 (2): 137–143.

Sarran, D., Caron, A., Testault, I. et al. (2018). Position of maximal nasopharyngeal maximal occlusion in relation to hamuli pterygoidei: use of hamuli pterygoidei as landmarks for palatoplasty in brachycephalic airway obstruction syndrome surgical treatment. *Journal of Small Animal Practice* 59 (10): 625–633.

Savvas, I., Raptopoulos, D., and Rallis, T. (2016). A "light meal" three hours preoperatively decreases the incidence of gastro-esophageal reflux in dogs. *Journal of the American Animal Hospital Association* 52 (6): 357–363.

Schuenemann, R. and Oechtering, G.U. (2014a). Inside the brachycephalic nose: intranasal mucosal contact points. *Journal of the American Animal Hospital Association* 50: 149–158.

Schuenemann, R. and Oechtering, G. (2014b). Inside the brachycephalic nose: conchal regrowth and mucosal contact points after laser-assisted turbinectomy. *Journal of the American Animal Hospital Association* 50 (4): 237–246.

Seim, H.B. (2010). Surgical management of brachycephalic syndrome. *Paper presented at the North American Veterinary Conference*, Orlando, FL, USA.

Seneviratne, M., Kaye, B.M., and Ter Haar, G. (2020). Prognostic indicators of short-term outcome in dogs undergoing surgery for brachycephalic obstructive airway syndrome. *Veterinary Record* 187 (10): 403.

Senn, D., Sigrist, N., Forterre, F. et al. (2011). Retrospective evaluation of postoperative nasotracheal tubes for oxygen supplementation in dogs following surgery for brachycephalic syndrome: 36 cases (2003–2007). *Journal of Veterinary Emergency and Critical Care* 21: 261–267.

Siedenburg, J.S. and Dupré, G. (2021). Tongue and upper airway dimensions: a comparative study between three popular brachycephalic breeds. *Animals (Basel)* 11: 662.

Singleton, W.B. (1962). Partial velum palatiectomy for relief of dyspnea in brachycephalic breeds. *Journal of Small Animal Practice* 3: 215–216.

Stordalen, M.B., Silveira, F., Fenner, J.V.H. et al. (2020). Outcome of temporary tracheostomy tube-placement following surgery for brachycephalic obstructive airway syndrome in 42 dogs. *Journal of Small Animal Practice* 61 (5): 292–299.

Tamura, J., Oyama, N., Matsumoto, S. et al. (2021). Unrecognized difficult airway management during anesthesia in two brachycephalic dogs with narrow cricoid cartilage. *Journal of Veterinary Medical Science* 83 (2): 234–240.

Tarricone, J., Hayes, G.M., Singh, A. et al. (2019). Development and validation of a brachycephalic risk (BRisk) score to predict the risk of complications in dogs presenting for surgical treatment of brachycephalic obstructive airway syndrome. *Veterinary Surgery* 48 (7): 1253–1261.

Thews, G. (1983). Lungenatmung. In: *Physiologie des Menschen* (ed. F. Schmidt and G. Thews), 500–536. Berlin: Springer.

Thompson, K.R. and Rioja, E. (2016). Effects of intravenous and topical laryngeal lidocaine on heart rate, mean arterial pressure and cough response to endotracheal intubation in dogs. *Veterinary Anaesthesia and Analgesia* 43 (4): 371–378.

Tobias, K.M. (2010a). Elongated soft palate. In: *Manual of Small Animal Soft Tissue Surgery* (ed. K.M. Tobias), 407–415. Oxford: Wiley Blackwell.

Tobias, K.M. (2010b). Stenotic nares. In: *Manual of Small Animal Soft Tissue Surgery* (ed. K.M. Tobias), 401–406. Oxford: Wiley Blackwell.

Tokunaga, S., Ehrhart, E.J., and Monnet, E. (2020). Histological and mechanical comparisons of arytenoid cartilage between 4 brachycephalic and 8 non-brachycephalic dogs: a pilot study. *PLOS ONE* 15 (9): e0239223.

Torrez, C.V. and Hunt, G.B. (2006). Results of surgical correction of abnormalities associated with brachycephalic airway obstruction syndrome in dogs in Australia. *Journal of Small Animal Practice* 47: 150–154.

Trader, R.L. (1949). Nose operation. *Journal of the American Veterinary Medical Association* 114: 210–211.

Trostel, C.T. and Frankel, D.J. (2010). Punch resection alaplasty technique in dogs and cats with stenotic nares: 14 cases. *Journal of the American Animal Hospital Association* 46: 5–11.

Vangrinsven, E., Broux, O., Massart, L. et al. (2021). Diagnosis and treatment of gastro-oesophageal junction abnormalities in dogs with brachycephalic syndrome. *Journal of Small Animal Practice* 62 (3): 200–208.

Vilaplana Grosso, F., Haar, G.T., and Boroffka, S.A. (2015). Gender, weight, and age effects on prevalence of caudal aberrant nasal turbinates in clinically healthy English bulldogs: a computed tomographic study and classification. *Veterinary Radiology & Ultrasound* 56 (5): 486–493.

Villedieu, E., Rutherford, L., and Ter Haar, G. (2019). Brachycephalic obstructive airway surgery outcome assessment using the 6-minute walk test: a pilot study. *Journal of Small Animal Practice* 60 (2): 132–135.

Wegner, W. (1987). Genetisch bedingte zahnanomalien. *Der Praktische Tierarzt* 68: 19–22.

White, R.N. (2012). Surgical management of laryngeal collapse associated with brachycephalic airway obstruction syndrome in dogs. *Journal of Small Animal Practice* 53: 44–50.

White, D.R., Heavner, S.B., Hardy, S.M. et al. (2002). Gastroesophageal reflux and eustachian tube dysfunction in an animal model. *Laryngoscope* 112: 955–961.

Wilson, F.D., Rajendran, E.I., and David, G. (1960). Staphylotomy in a dachshund. *Indian Veterinary Journal* 37: 639–642.

Worth, D.B., Grimes, J.A., Jimenez, D.A. et al. (2018). Risk factors for temporary tracheostomy tube placement following surgery to alleviate signs of brachycephalic obstructive airway syndrome in dogs. *Journal of the American Veterinary Medical Association* 253 (9): 1158–1163.

Wykes, P.M. (1991). Brachycephalic airway obstructive syndrome. *Problems in Veterinary Medicine* 3: 88–197.

38

Laryngeal Paralysis

Eric Monnet

Laryngeal paralysis is characterized by the lack of abduction of the arytenoid cartilages during inspiration. During expiration the arytenoid cartilages are passive, so the expiration phase is not affected by laryngeal paralysis. The functions of the larynx are to regulate airflow, produce the voice, and prevent inhalation of food. If the intrinsic muscles and/or the nerve supply of the larynx are not normal, laryngeal function is abnormal. The cricoarytenoideus dorsalis muscle abducts the arytenoid cartilages at each inspiration. The recurrent laryngeal nerve innervates this muscle. Lesions to the recurrent laryngeal nerve or to the cricoarytenoideus dorsalis muscle result in laryngeal paralysis in dogs and cats. Laryngeal paralysis is a clinical sign of an underlying disease or syndrome.

Etiology

Congenital and acquired forms of laryngeal paralysis have been recognized in dogs and cats.

Congenital laryngeal paralysis

Congenital laryngeal paralysis has been reported in bouvier des Flandres, bull terrier, Dalmatian, Rottweiler, and huskies (O'Brien & Hendriks 1986; Braund et al. 1989, 1994; Bennett & Clarke 1997; Eger et al. 1998; Mahony et al. 1998). The bouvier des Flandres and bull terrier have mostly been reported in Europe, while the Dalmatian and husky are commonly reported in the USA. In the bouvier des Flandres, laryngeal paralysis is transmitted as an autosomal dominant trait (Venker-van Haagen 1982; Greenfield 1987; Braund et al. 1989;

Ubbink et al. 1992). Wallerian degeneration of the recurrent laryngeal nerves and abnormalities of the nucleus ambiguus are both present (Braund et al. 1994; Bennett & Clarke 1997). Dogs with congenital laryngeal paralysis present clinically at an earlier age (before 1 year old) than dogs with acquired laryngeal paralysis. Most of the time dogs with congenital laryngeal paralysis have other central neurologic abnormalities.

Acquired laryngeal paralysis

Acquired laryngeal paralysis is most commonly reported in the Labrador retriever, golden retriever, Saint Bernard, and Irish setter at an age of 9 years (Wykes 1983a; Gaber et al. 1985; White et al. 1986; Greenfield 1987; Burbidge 1995; LaHue 1995; MacPhail & Monnet 2001). It has also been reported in cats (Hardie et al. 1981; Campbell & Holmberg 1984; White et al. 1986; Busch et al. 1992; Venker-van Haagen 1992; Schachter & Norris 2000).

Since the recurrent laryngeal nerve is the motor nerve of the larynx and is responsible for the abduction of the arytenoid cartilages during inspiration, any lesions of this nerve will induce laryngeal paralysis. In order to be symptomatic the majority of dogs need to have bilateral paralysis, except if they are performing heavy exercise (Burbidge 1995).

Trauma to the recurrent laryngeal nerve during dogfights or during surgery in the neck is a cause of laryngeal paralysis. Laryngeal paralysis in the cat has been diagnosed after bilateral thyroidectomy (Mallery et al. 2003). A cranial mediastinal or neck mass

Small Animal Soft Tissue Surgery, Second Edition. Edited by Eric Monnet.
© 2023 John Wiley & Sons, Inc. Published 2023 by John Wiley & Sons, Inc.
Companion website: www.wiley.com/go/monnet/small

stretching or compressing the recurrent laryngeal nerve can induce laryngeal paralysis (Salisbury *et al.* 1990; Klein *et al.* 1995).

Any form of polyneuropathy can induce laryngeal paralysis (Burbidge 1995). Endocrine, infectious, or immune-mediated polyneuropathy can be the cause of laryngeal paralysis (Jaggy & Oliver 1994; Jaggy *et al.* 1994; Gaynor *et al.* 1997). Most commonly the polyneuropathy is idiopathic, because a cause cannot be identified. More likely dogs with acquired laryngeal paralysis are suffering from a generalized progressive idiopathic polyneuropathy (Shelton 2010; Stanley *et al.* 2010). Stanley *et al.* (2010) reported severe progressive esophageal dysfunction in dogs with laryngeal paralysis. None of the dogs had evidence of megaesophagus when entered in the study, but 25% of the dogs had neurologic signs at the time of enrollment. At six months and one year after enrollment, 58% and 100%, respectively, had neurologic signs (ataxia, decreased proprioception, weakness, muscle atrophy). Esophageal dysfunction evaluated by esophagram was related to polyneuropathy and the severity of esophageal dysfunction seemed to correlate with the development of aspiration pneumonia. The cervical and cranial thoracic esophagus seemed more affected than the distal part of the esophagus. It is interesting to note in this study that two dogs in the control group had an elevated score for their esophagrams and subsequently developed laryngeal paralysis five and six months later (Stanley *et al.* 2010).

A myopathy involving the intrinsic muscle of the larynx is another cause of laryngeal paralysis in the adult dog.

Clinical findings

History

Dogs presented for laryngeal paralysis manifest either a chronic or an acute-on-chronic presentation. Dogs presented as an emergency only exhibit an exacerbation of their chronic laryngeal paralysis. Most of the time it is associated with an increase in ambient temperature and heat stroke. The clinical signs of these dogs will be different from those dogs presented for chronic laryngeal paralysis.

Progression of signs is often slow; months to years may pass before an animal develops severe respiratory distress (Greenfield 1987). Early signs include change in voice, followed by gagging and coughing, especially during eating or drinking. Endurance decreases and exercise intolerance develops. Often owners think the reduction in exercise is age related or due to worsening of degenerative joint disease. Laryngeal stridor during inspiration increases as the airway occlusion worsens.

Moderate airway obstruction is exacerbated by laryngeal edema and inflammation secondary to turbulent airflow in the larynx. Episodes of severe difficulty breathing, cyanosis, or syncope occur in severely affected patients (Greenfield 1987; Burbidge 1995). Male dogs are approximately two to three times more affected than female dogs (Gaber *et al.* 1985; Burbidge 1995; MacPhail & Monnet 2001). Laryngeal paralysis can be accompanied by various degrees of dysphagia and megaesophagus, which significantly enhance the probability of aspiration after surgical correction of the laryngeal paralysis.

Physical examination

The presenting signs are similar for the congenital and acquired forms. Dogs with congenital laryngeal paralysis usually have other neurologic signs in addition to laryngeal paralysis. The physical examination of dogs with laryngeal paralysis is fairly unremarkable. Dogs have an inspiratory dyspnea that is not alleviated with open-mouth breathing. Mild lateral compression of the larynx significantly increases inspiratory dyspnea. Mild exercise can exacerbate the clinical signs if they are not very obvious at the time of presentation.

Since dogs regulate their temperature by panting, some patients can be hyperthermic if the difficulty in breathing is severe. Dogs can present with heat stroke, especially in the spring or early summer when the ambient temperature is rising.

Referred upper airway sounds are present during auscultation of the thoracic cavity. Auscultation of the thoracic cavity and lung fields may reveal the presence of a pneumonia in the cranial lung lobes due to aspiration.

Palpation of the muscle mass may reveal skeletal muscle atrophy in cases of polyneuropathy. A complete neurologic examination is required to evaluate the animal for a polyneuropathy.

Laboratory findings

Complete blood count and chemistry profile are usually within normal limits. An elevation of the white blood cell count might be an indicator of aspiration pneumonia. Hypercholesterolemia, hyperlipidemia, and augmentation of liver enzyme activity are present on the chemistry profile of dogs with hypothyroidism. A thyroid profile with endogenous thyroid-stimulating hormone and free T_4 is then required to further define the diagnosis. Laryngeal paralysis has an inconsistent correlation with hypothyroidism.

Radiographic examination and ultrasonography

It is necessary to perform a radiographic examination of the thoracic cavity for the evaluation of the lung parenchyma and the esophagus. Aspiration pneumonia is a common finding preoperatively in dogs with laryngeal paralysis. If aspiration pneumonia is present, surgical intervention should be delayed until the aspiration pneumonia has resolved. Presence of aspiration pneumonia prior to surgery increases the risk of postoperative complications by 2.75 times for dogs treated with unilateral lateralization (MacPhail & Monnet 2001). Acute pulmonary edema can also be present, especially in patients with an acute-on-chronic presentation. If pulmonary edema is present, surgery should not be delayed. Megaesophagus may be present in dogs with laryngeal paralysis, especially if the paralysis is due to polyneuropathy or polymyopathy (Stanley *et al.* 2010). Megaesophagus places the animal at greater risk for aspiration pneumonia after surgery. MacPhail and Monnet (2001) showed that the development of megaesophagus in the postoperative period increased the risk of postoperative complications by 5.5 times after arytenoid lateralization. Radiographic examination of the larynx is unremarkable. Ultrasonography has been used to evaluate the larynx and laryngeal function (Rudorf *et al.* 2001).

Laryngeal examination

Laryngeal examination is required for the diagnosis of laryngeal paralysis. It can be performed with a routine laryngoscope, transnasal laryngoscopy, or ultrasound (Rudorf *et al.* 2001; Radlinsky *et al.* 2004, 2009). A light plane of anesthesia is required to be able to evaluate laryngeal function during each inspiration with laryngoscopy (Wykes 1983b; Gaber *et al.* 1985; Greenfield 1987; Kuehn 1995; LaHue 1995; Miller *et al.* 2002; Jackson *et al.* 2004). If the plane of anesthesia is too deep, then every dog will appear to have laryngeal paralysis. Therefore the patient has to be sufficiently lightly anesthetized to be able to open its mouth and for the larynx to be visualized. Ultrasound does not require sedation, so there is no risk of inducing a false laryngeal paralysis. The dog is placed in ventral recumbency for the laryngeal examination. A laryngoscope or a video-endoscope can be used to visualize the motion of the arytenoid cartilages during inspiration (Radlinsky *et al.* 2004, 2009; Tobias *et al.* 2004).

In the normal dog, the arytenoid cartilages should abduct at each inspiration and the vocal cords should remain under slight tension during inspiration and expiration. In dogs with laryngeal paralysis, the edges of the arytenoid cartilages are swollen and edematous with areas of ulceration (Figure 38.1) (Gaber *et al.* 1985; Greenfield 1987; Kuehn 1995; Miller *et al.* 2002; Jackson *et al.* 2004). Also, the vocal cords are distended and vibrating during expiration and inspiration (Website

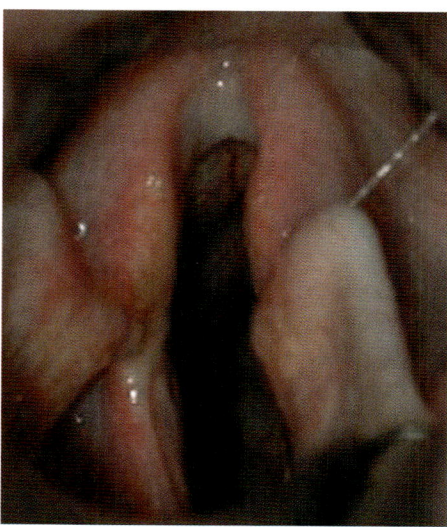

Figure 38.1 Laryngeal examination in a dog with laryngeal paralysis. The corniculate process of both arytenoids are edematous and ulcerated. The arytenoid cartilages are in a neutral position.

Chapter 38: Respiratory tract/laryngeal paralysis, laryngeal examination). Paradoxic motion of the arytenoid cartilages can be noticed and may confuse the diagnosis. During paradoxic motion the arytenoid cartilages are pulled into the rima glottidis at inspiration and return to normal position during expiration. The paradoxic motion is due to the Venturi effect: when air travels through a narrow tube its velocity increases, inducing a decrease in pressure that can pull the two arytenoid cartilages together. Therefore, it is important to time the motion of the arytenoid cartilages with inspiration and expiration. It is imperative that this is measured accurately, otherwise the motion of the arytenoid cartilages will appear adequate when actually the reverse is the case.

Jackson *et al.* (2004) evaluated different anesthetic protocols for use during the diagnosis of laryngeal paralysis. They measured the motion of the arytenoid cartilages during the recovery phase of anesthesia when the patient was not in apnea. Arytenoid motion was significantly greater when thiopental was used as an anesthetic than when propofol, ketamine with diazepam, acepromazine with thiopental, or acepromazine with propofol were used. Since the addition of acepromazine may abolish arytenoid motion even in normal dogs, its utilization during laryngeal examination is not recommended (Jackson *et al.* 2004). Therefore, thiopental and propofol are both used for laryngeal examination because both provide adequate evaluation, but the motion of the arytenoid cartilages seems weaker with propofol (Jackson *et al.* 2004).

Use of doxapram at a dose of 1 mg/kg intravenously during a laryngeal examination has been shown to improve motion of the arytenoids and aid in the diagnosis of laryngeal paralysis. Doxapram stimulates the respiratory center of the medulla, increasing respiratory rate and the amplitude of each inspiration, thereby increasing tidal volume (Miller *et al.* 2002; Yost 2006). The surface area of the rima glottidis increased by 57% during inspiration after injection of doxapram in normal dogs (Miller *et al.* 2002). However, doxapram may induce or exacerbate paradoxic motion of the arytenoid cartilages in dogs with laryngeal paralysis (Tobias *et al.* 2004). The paradoxic motion may be so severe that it completely occludes the rima glottidis and necessitates tracheal intubation (Tobias *et al.* 2004).

Ultrasound evaluation can be used to evaluate laryngeal function and diagnose laryngeal paralysis (Rudorf *et al.* 2001). The advantage of this technique is that the motion of the arytenoid cartilages can be performed in an awake animal. In a study on 30 dogs with laryngeal paralysis diagnosed by laryngeal examination, the ultrasonographer was able to diagnose asymmetry or absence of motion of the cuneiform processes in 100% of cases (Rudorf *et al.* 2001). However, in another study by Radlinsky *et al.* (2009) ultrasound was not found to be as accurate as oral laryngoscopy. Three dogs with bilateral laryngeal paralysis on oral laryngoscopy were diagnosed with unilateral paralysis by ultrasound. Three dogs with paradoxic motion of the arytenoid cartilages during oral or transnasal laryngoscopy were diagnosed as normal with ultrasound.

Electromyography

Electromyography of the intrinsic laryngeal muscle has been used to demonstrate denervation potentials in suspected cases of laryngeal paralysis (Venker-van Haagen 1992). The abductor muscles of the larynx should be evaluated. In an experimental study, denervation potentials were recorded five days after trauma to the recurrent laryngeal nerves (Peterson *et al.* 1999).

Treatment

Medical (emergency) treatment

Animals are usually presented with acute cyanosis or collapse as a result of upper airway obstruction. Most animals in a cyanotic crisis precipitated by upper airway obstruction recover initially with medical therapy. Excitement or increase in ambient temperature can trigger an acute onset of inspiratory dyspnea. Excitement or increase in ambient temperature increases the respiratory rate, which results in trauma to the mucosa of the arytenoid cartilages. Inflammation and acute swelling of

the mucosa of the arytenoid cartilages can exacerbate the chronic airway obstruction and induce an acute onset of inspiratory dyspnea. A vicious circle is then initiated.

First the animals should be placed in a cool environment with supplemental oxygen. Oxygen can be administered by mask or with an oxygen cage and will help correct hypoxemia. If the patient is still hyperthermic (>40.6 °C, 105 °F), an iced-water bath can be used. Sedation with acepromazine intravenously is indicated (0.1 mg/kg, maximum dose 3 mg) if the animal is still stressed. Corticosteroids are given intravenously (dexamethasone 0.2–1.0 mg/kg once) to reduce laryngeal inflammation and edema. Fluid therapy is administered with caution, because some animals with severe upper respiratory tract obstruction develop pulmonary edema; diuretics are indicated in these patients. If the patient's condition is deteriorating, an emergency tracheostomy is recommended to bypass the upper airway. In a study by MacPhail and Monnet (2001) on 140 dogs presented for the treatment of laryngeal paralysis, it has been shown that a temporary tracheostomy was a negative prognostic indicator for surgical complications (hazard ratio [HR] 10.4) and for long-term survival (HR 9.17). It is likely that dogs that required a temporary tracheostomy were more compromised in their pulmonary function prior to presentation than dogs that did not require a temporary tracheostomy. Temporary tracheostomies interfere with mucociliary clearance and resolution of pneumonia.

Surgical treatment

Laryngeal surgery is directed at removing or repositioning laryngeal cartilages that obstruct the rima glottidis in order to decrease airway resistance. The surgical procedures described to correct laryngeal paralysis are (i) unilateral or bilateral arytenoid cartilage lateralization; (ii) ventricular cordectomy and partial arytenoidectomy via the oral or ventral laryngotomy approach; (iii) modified castellated laryngofissure; and (iv) permanent tracheostomy (Rosin & Greenwood 1982; Gourley *et al.* 1983; Harvey 1983b; Smith *et al.* 1986; LaHue 1989; Lozier & Pope 1992; Lussier *et al.* 1996; Greenberg *et al.* 2007; Schofield *et al.* 2007). Lozier and Pope (1992) evaluated the effect of the different techniques on the rima glottidis in cadavers. They showed that bilateral lateralization increased the surface area of the rima glottidis the most, followed by castellated laryngofissure and unilateral lateralization. Castellated laryngofissure is rarely performed, while unilateral lateralization is recognized as the gold standard technique because of its very consistent outcome. Since it is not necessary to overabduct the arytenoid cartilage to reduce airway resistance, it seems that unilateral lateralization should be sufficient to palliate the clinical signs (Bureau & Monnet 2002; Greenberg *et al.* 2007). Reinnervation of the laryngeal muscles has been described for the treatment of recurrent laryngeal nerve injury (Sato & Ogura 1978; Greenfield *et al.* 1988). Reinnervation is not used currently in small animal surgery because it does not provide immediate relief of the upper airway obstruction.

Arytenoid cartilage lateralization

This procedure has been used successfully to treat laryngeal paralysis in cats and dogs (Rosin & Greenwood 1982; White *et al.* 1986; LaHue 1989; White 1989a,b; Griffiths *et al.* 2001; Schofield *et al.* 2007). Arytenoid lateralization has been performed bilaterally or unilaterally. The procedure was originally described as bilateral (Rosin & Greenwood 1982). However, since bilateral lateralization seems to be associated with more complications, unilateral lateralization is most commonly performed. In a study of 140 dogs treated for laryngeal paralysis, MacPhail and Monnet (2001) showed that dogs treated with bilateral lateralization had a 55.12 times greater chance of complications than dogs treated with unilateral lateralization ($P < 0.001$) (Figure 38.2). In this study, dogs treated with bilateral lateralization had a 46.69 times greater chance of dying than dogs treated with unilateral lateralization ($P < 0.001$). Unilateral arytenoid lateralization is sufficient to reduce clinical signs of laryngeal paralysis (White 1989a,b; MacPhail & Monnet 2001).

Bilateral arytenoid lateralization is performed through a ventral midline incision, while unilateral lateralization can be performed through a ventral or a lateral incision. It is the author's preference to perform lateralization through a lateral incision. The animal is positioned in lateral recumbency for a unilateral lateralization, and a skin incision is made over the larynx just ventral to the jugular groove and caudal to the vertical ramus of the mandible (Figure 38.3a–c) (Website Chapter 38: Respiratory tract/laryngeal paralysis, arytenoid lateralization). A small incision (2–3 cm) is usually sufficient to approach the larynx. If needed, the incision can be extended to be better centered over the larynx. After dissection through the subcutaneous tissue and the platysma muscle, the dissection is continued ventral to the jugular vein. After dissection into adipose tissue, the dorsal edge of the thyroid cartilage can be palpated. The larynx is rotated to expose the thyropharyngeal muscle, which is transected at the dorsocaudal edge of the thyroid cartilage. The wing of the thyroid cartilage is retracted laterally with a stay suture (Figure 38.3a–c). It is not necessary to separate the cricothyroid junction. Separation of the cricothyroid junction might destabilize the larynx and decrease the diameter of the rima glottidis, which typically occurs when the surgery is bilateral (Lozier & Pope 1992; Bureau & Monnet 2002). Incision of the cricothyroid joint may give better exposure, but it is rarely needed. The muscular process of the arytenoid cartilage is then palpated. The cricoarytenoideus dorsalis muscle or the fibrous tissue left is dissected and transected at its insertion on the muscular process of the arytenoid cartilage (Figure 38.4).

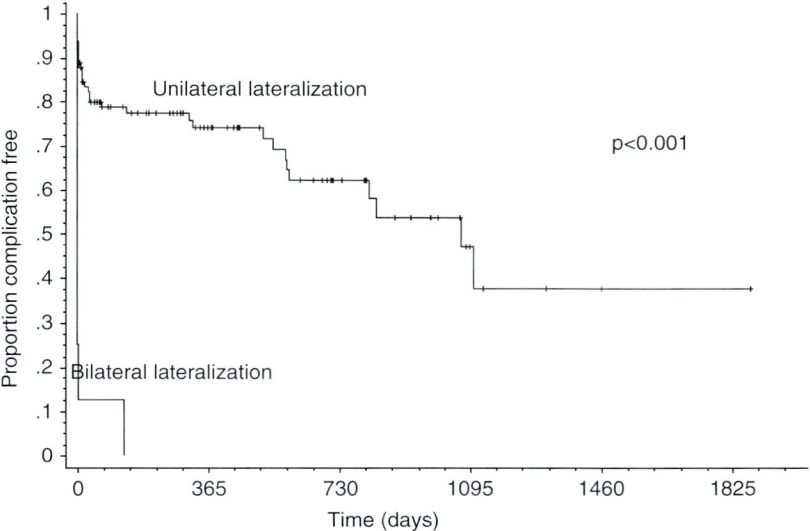

Figure 38.2 Actuarial Kaplan–Meier curve showing the proportion of dogs free of complications after unilateral and bilateral lateralization.

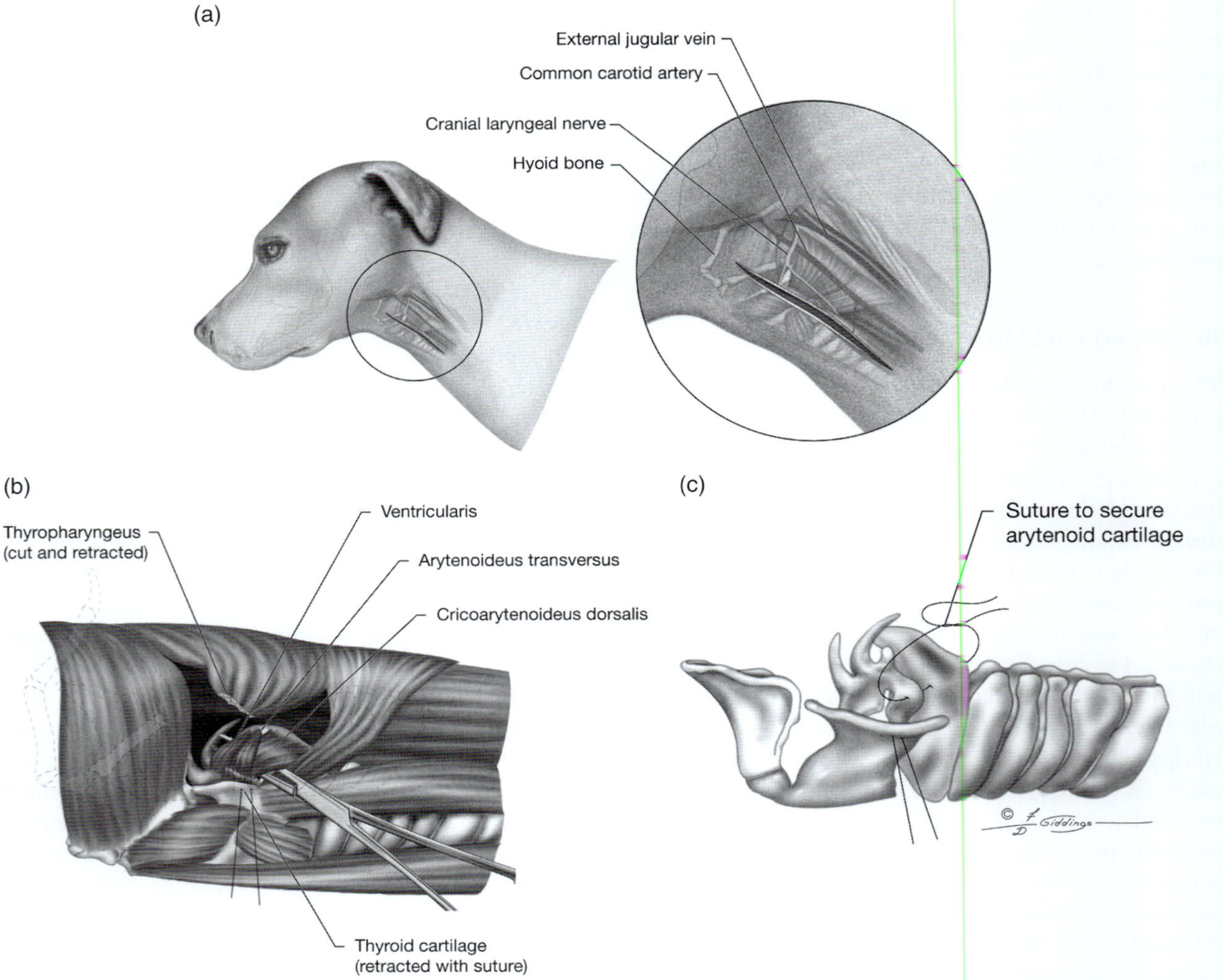

(a)

External jugular vein

Common carotid artery

Cranial laryngeal nerve

Hyoid bone

(b)

Thyropharyngeus
(cut and retracted)

Ventricularis

Arytenoideus transversus

Cricoarytenoideus dorsalis

Thyroid cartilage
(retracted with suture)

(c)

Suture to secure
arytenoid cartilage

© D. Giddings

Figure 38.3 Unilateral lateralization. (a) The dog is placed in lateral recumbency and an incision is made ventral to the jugular vein. (b) After dissection through the subcutaneous tissue, the thyropharyngeal muscle is incised along the dorsal edge of the wing of the thyroid cartilage. The thyropharyngeal muscle has been incised. (c) A stay suture is placed in the wing of the thyroid cartilage for retraction. © D. Giddings.

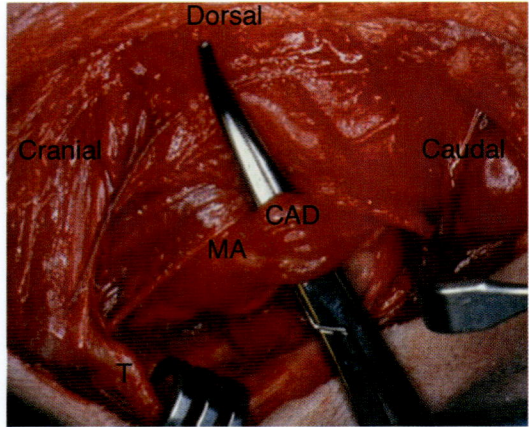

Figure 38.4 The cricoarytenoideus dorsalis muscle (CAD) has been dissected. T, thyroid cartilage; MA, muscular process of the arytenoid cartilage.

The cricoarytenoid articulation is opened caudally with Metzenbaum scissors. The opening should be large enough to just see the joint cartilage to confirm the location and to place a needle. The limited opening of the joint capsule should prevent abduction of the arytenoid cartilage. The sesamoid band connecting the arytenoid cartilages dorsally is left intact. Transection of the band can distort the rima glottidis (Lussier *et al*. 1996). A nonabsorbable 2-0 suture is placed between the caudodorsal border of the cricoid cartilage and the muscular process of the arytenoid cartilage (Figure 38.3c). The suture is first passed around the caudal border of the cricoid cartilage (Figure 38.5a) and then through the muscular process of the arytenoid cartilage from the cricoarytenoid joint surface (Figure 38.5b). The placement of two simple interrupted sutures instead of one

(a)   (b)

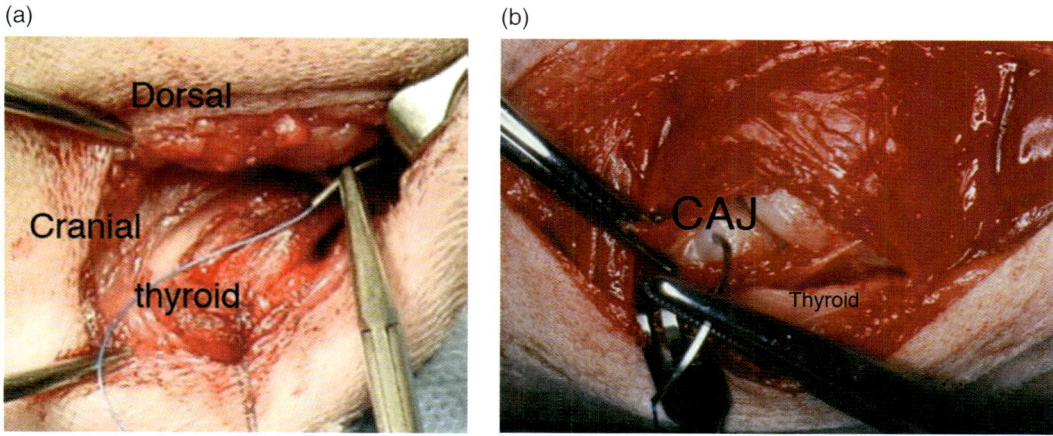

Figure 38.5 (a) A suture is placed around the caudodorsal border of the cricoid cartilage and (b) through the muscular process of the arytenoid cartilage in a medio-lateral direction. CAJ, cricoarytenoid joint.

has also been described (LaHue 1989). Griffiths *et al.* (2001) described placement of the suture around the caudal border of the thyroid cartilage instead of around the cricoid cartilage. Demetriou and Kirby (2003) reported placing a cricoarytenoid and a thyroarytenoid suture to maximize the opening of the rima glottidis. The reason for using a thyroarytenoid suture was to achieve lateral displacement of the arytenoid and not just caudal displacement with the cricoarytenoid suture. Schofield *et al.* (2007) described the placement of a mattress suture through the muscular process and the cuneiform process of the arytenoid cartilage. The suture was placed in the thyroid cartilage. A mineralized aryt- enoid cartilage may crumble if a suture needle is forced through it; therefore, holes can be predrilled in the carti- lage with a sharp 18-gauge hypodermic needle before the suture is passed. Even with predrilling, the cartilage may break during the operation or later. An assistant can observe through the mouth the size of the laryngeal opening achieved to ensure that adequate abduction of the laryngeal cartilages has been obtained.

By pulling the arytenoid cartilage, the surface area of the rima glottidis is increased (Lozier & Pope 1992; Lussier *et al.* 1996; Griffiths *et al.* 2001; Greenberg *et al.* 2007). The degree of clinical improvement has not been related to augmentation of the surface area of the rima glottidis. In one study on clinical cases, the surface area of the rima glottidis was significantly greater after cricoarytenoid lateralization (207%) than following thy- roarytenoid lateralization (140%); however, there was no difference clinically between dogs treated with either technique (Griffiths *et al.* 2001). No correlation seems to exist between the increase in surface area of the rima glottidis and the clinical signs. According to Poiseuille's law, airway resistance is proportional to the fourth power of the radius of the airway, and thus a small increase in

the radius or surface area significantly reduces the clini- cal signs. It has been shown that if the surface area of the rima glottidis is increased beyond the edges of the epi- glottis, then a segment of the rima glottidis is not cov- ered by the epiglottis, which may increase the risk of aspiration (Figure 38.6) (Bureau & Monnet 2002). Therefore, it would seem logical to limit the amount of abduction of the arytenoid cartilage. Greenberg *et al.* (2007) showed in a cadaver study that limited displace- ment of the arytenoid cartilages can significantly reduce laryngeal resistance with the epiglottis open (Figure 38.7). With limited displacement of the arytenoid cartilage, the epiglottis can still almost completely cover the rima glot- tidis, which should limit the risk of aspiration pneumo- nia (Figure 38.6) (Greenberg *et al.* 2007). To limit the caudal displacement of the arytenoid cartilage and avoid exposure of the rima glottidis with a closed epiglottis, the suture for the lateralization after being placed cau- dally and dorsally around the cricoid cartilage should exit the cricoid cartilage just caudal to the cricoaryte- noid joint (Gauthier & Monnet 2014). The surgery site is closed by suturing the thyropharyngeal muscle and rou- tinely closing the subcutaneous tissue and skin.

Complication rates after unilateral lateralization have been reported to range from 10% to 58% (Gaber *et al.* 1985; MacPhail & Monnet 2001; Hammel *et al.* 2006; Wilson & Monnet 2016). Complications associated with laryngeal lateralization include intramu- ral hematoma, aspiration pneumonia, persistent cough exacerbated after drinking, seroma, breaking of the suture, and fragmentation of the arytenoid cartilage. Factors significantly associated with development of aspiration pneumonia after unilateral lateralization include preoperative pneumonia (HR 2.75), postopera- tive megaesophagus (HR 5.55), and temporary tracheos- tomy (HR 3.41) (MacPhail & Monnet 2001). Presence of

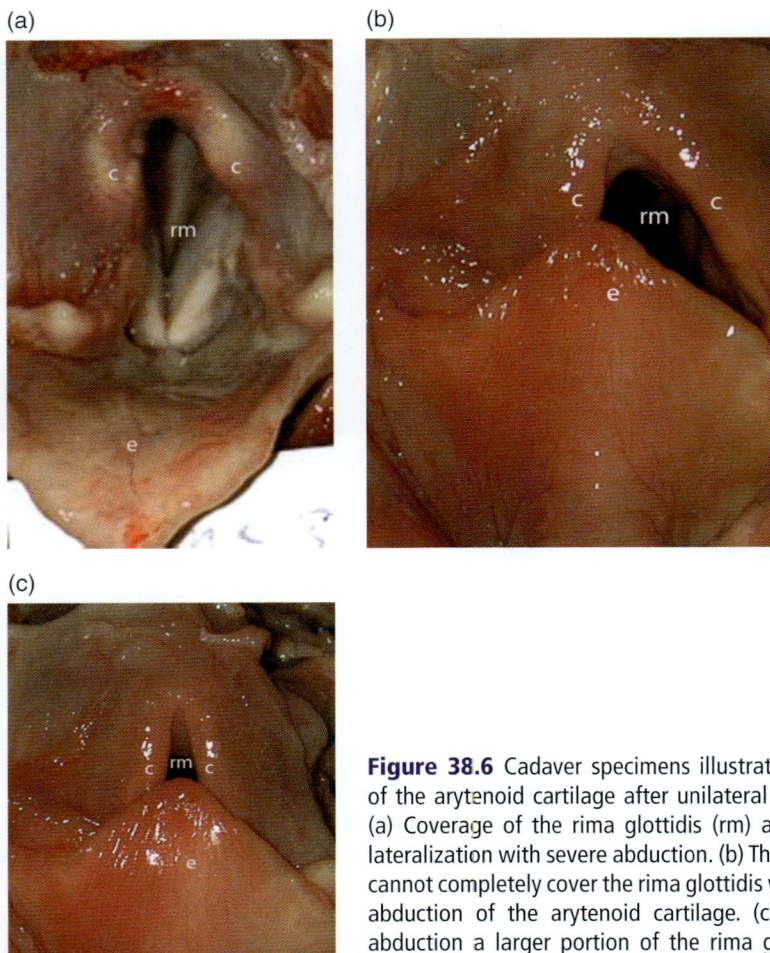

(a)

(b)

(c)

Figure 38.6 Cadaver specimens illustrating abduction of the arytenoid cartilage after unilateral lateralization. (a) Coverage of the rima glottidis (rm) after unilateral lateralization with severe abduction. (b) The epiglottis (e) cannot completely cover the rima glottidis with moderate abduction of the arytenoid cartilage. (c) With severe abduction a larger portion of the rima glottidis is left uncovered by the epiglottis, exposing more of the airway for potential aspiration pneumonia. c, corniculate process of the arytenoid cartilage.

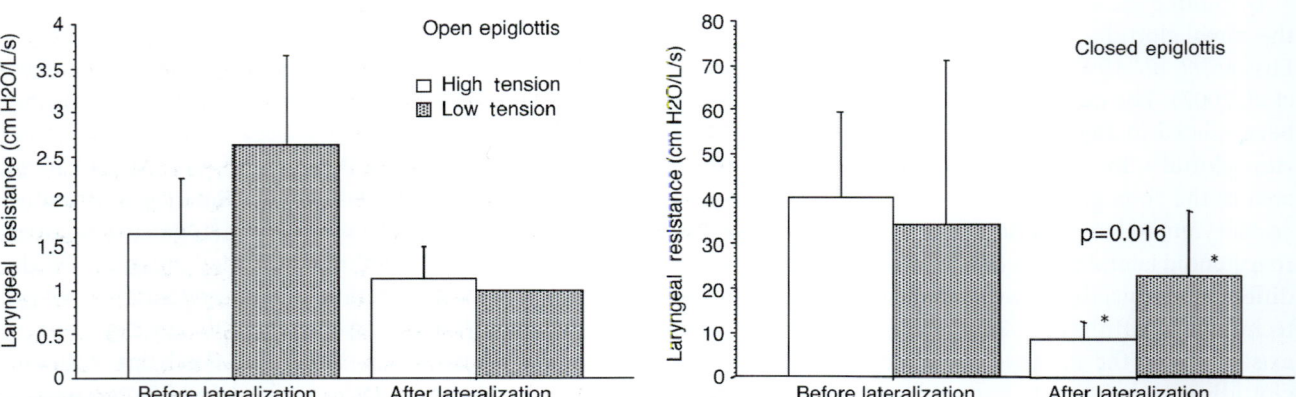

Figure 38.7 Laryngeal resistance with open and closed glottis after unilateral lateralization. The lateralization was performed with more or less displacement of the arytenoid cartilage.

a megaesophagus after unilateral lateralization was associated with a significant risk of death after surgery (HR 13.88) (MacPhail & Monnet 2001). In a more recent study, Wilson *et al.* (Wilson & Monnet 2016) reported that 30% of the dogs will develop aspiration pneumonia within four years after surgery. Breaking of the suture or fragmentation of the cartilage induced recurrence of the clinical signs of laryngeal paralysis. MacPhail and Monnet (2001) reported a 4% incidence rate for suture failure. Laryngeal lateralization should then be performed on the other side. Seroma formation is very common and is self-limiting. The incidence of aspiration pneumonia is more common in dogs with bilateral laryngeal lateralization. MacPhail and Monnet (2001) showed that dogs treated with bilateral lateralization had more complications and were less likely to survive than dogs treated with unilateral lateralization. Aspiration pneumonia after unilateral lateralization has been reported in 10–21% of cases (MacPhail & Monnet 2001; Demetriou & Kirby 2003; Hammel *et al.* 2006).

Schofield *et al.* (2007) showed a good outcome with bilateral lateralization when combined with vocal cord resection. The authors hypothesized that the low incidence of complications (15%), with only three dogs (7.5%) with aspiration pneumonia, was the result of reduced abduction of the arytenoid cartilages. The vocal cord resection also helped to reduce airway resistance.

Water and food should be completely withdrawn after surgery until the patient is fully awake. Two or three meatballs should be delivered 24 hours after surgery under constant direct supervision. However, it has never been shown that the type of food has any effect on the rate of aspiration pneumonia after surgery. If the animal can handle meatballs without aspirating, water can be delivered. After surgery, the risk of aspiration is lifelong.

Partial laryngectomy per os

Partial laryngectomy for the treatment of laryngeal paralysis involves removal of one or both vocal folds and unilateral or bilateral resection of the corniculate and vocal processes of the arytenoid cartilage (Figure 38.8) (Petersen *et al.* 1991; Holt & Harvey 1994a; Trout *et al.* 1994; Olivieri *et al.* 2009). The procedure is relatively simple to perform and is effective in medium to large dogs if laryngeal collapse is not present (Harvey & O'Brien 1982; Petersen *et al.* 1991; Holt & Harvey 1994a; Trout *et al.* 1994; Olivieri *et al.* 2009). However, the outcome is not very consistent (Ross *et al.* 1991; Holt & Harvey 1994a; Trout *et al.* 1994; Olivieri *et al.* 2009).

A temporary tracheostomy may be required during the procedure or the postoperative period. Ross *et al.*

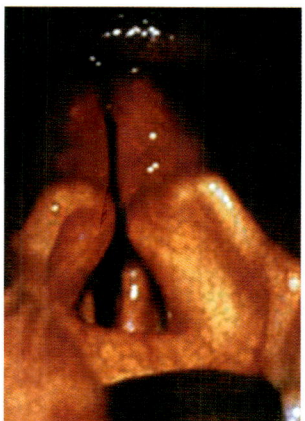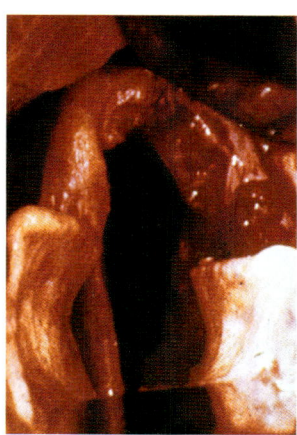

Figure 38.8 Vocal cordectomy per os and partial arytenoidectomy.

(1991) performed a temporary tracheostomy in 14 of 45 cases prior to surgery. It was required as an emergency treatment to palliate an acute upper airway obstruction.

With the animal in sternal recumbency, the head is suspended by the maxilla, the mandible is held open with a mouth gag or with tape to the table, and the tongue is held extended. The rima glottidis is observed while the soft palate is elevated and the base of the tongue is depressed with malleable retractors. The surgical procedure for laryngeal paralysis is initially limited to one side of the larynx. Unilateral resection of the vocal fold and the corniculate processes of the arytenoid cartilage usually provides an adequate airway opening. Harvey (1983b) showed that the surface area of the rima glottidis increased by 70–80% after bilateral vocal fold resection and unilateral partial arytenoidectomy. Unilateral resection minimizes scar tissue webbing across the glottis, and reduces aspiration. The cuneiform process of the arytenoid and the aryepiglottic folds are preserved. The opposite side can be resected after healing is complete and there is evidence of an inadequate airway.

Long thumb forceps (20–25 cm), Metzenbaum scissors, a long scalpel handle, and 30–35 cm long cup biopsy forceps are useful surgical instruments (Petersen *et al.* 1991; Ross *et al.* 1991; Holt & Harvey 1994a). The corniculate process is grasped and retracted medially with the biopsy forceps, and the long-handled scalpel is used to excise the corniculate process in a smooth arc. The aryepiglottic fold and the cuneiform process are left intact. The vocal process is removed with the biopsy forceps. The entire vocal fold and vocal muscle are removed as close as possible to the cricoid cartilage with the Metzenbaum scissors and biopsy forceps. Remnants of soft tissue and cartilage are removed to provide a smooth surface. If both vocal cords are removed, the ventral and dorsal commissures of the glottis, where the vocal folds meet ventrally and the arytenoid cartilages join dorsally, are preserved to minimize scar tissue webbing across the rima glottidis. However, bilateral resection is not recommended (Ross *et al.* 1991).

The objective is to resect sufficient tissue to provide a functional airway without significantly affecting laryngeal function (Harvey 1983a). Resection of excessive tissue results in a laryngeal closure defect and aspiration. Vocal fold resection alone produces satisfactory results in 83% of cases, with fewer complications than when partial arytenoidectomy is performed (Holt & Harvey 1994a). Several surgeries may be required before there is significant reduction in laryngeal resistance and the palliation of clinical signs (Ross *et al.* 1991).

The use of electrocautery for resection of laryngeal structures should be avoided in order to reduce postoperative swelling and granulation tissue formation (Petersen *et al.* 1991). Bleeding can be controlled by direct pressure with gauze sponges in conjunction with topical 1 in 10 000 epinephrine (Petersen *et al.* 1991). Mucosal suturing is not feasible with an oral approach. Diode laser has been successfully used to perform partial arytenoidectomy in dogs (Olivieri *et al.* 2009).

Harvey and O'Brien (1982) reported a 49% complication rate, with a 36% incidence of death due to airway disease. Petersen *et al.* (1991) reported a 58% complication rate after bilateral vocal fold resection in dogs with laryngeal paralysis. Complications reported after partial laryngectomy per os include aspiration pneumonia, persistent cough, increased respiratory stridor, exercise intolerance, and difficulty cooling off after exercise (Ross *et al.* 1991). This technique is associated with a 30% chance of aspiration pneumonia in the short term and a 16% chance in the long term (Ross *et al.* 1991). Trout *et al.* (1994) reported a 2% rate of aspiration pneumonia on postoperative radiographs. Narrowing of the rima glottidis because of scar tissue formation has been reported in 66% of cases 4.2 weeks after surgery (Trout *et al.* 1994). Narrowing of the rima glottidis and development of scar tissue were not present one and six months after surgery when a diode laser was used for the resection (Olivieri *et al.* 2009). Laryngeal webbing is the most common complication with the per os approach, especially if bilateral vocal fold resection has been performed (Holt & Harvey 1994a,b; Mehl *et al.* 2008). If special attention is taken to preserve the dorsal and ventral commissures, the incidence of webbing may be reduced to 14% (Holt & Harvey 1994b). Prednisolone may be given perioperatively to reduce scar tissue formation. Prednisolone has been given at a dose of 0.25–1 mg/kg in the first three days and tapered down over two weeks to prevent scar tissue (Holt & Harvey 1994b). Mitomycin C has shown promise in

reducing scarring and stenosis in the larynx in humans (Greenfield *et al.* 1988). Cicatrix formation across the larynx can be life-threatening in extreme cases. Laryngeal webbing requires a second surgery in most cases to open the airway. A ventral laryngotomy is then required to expose the scar tissue and surgically resect it (Mehl *et al.* 2008). The mucosa is closed over to prevent scar tissue formation.

Ventral laryngotomy approach

A ventral approach to the larynx can be used to perform bilateral vocal fold resection (Schofield *et al.* 2007; Mehl *et al.* 2008). It can be combined with bilateral lateralization (Schofield *et al.* 2007). This approach provides better exposure for the procedure and allows primary closure of the mucosa to prevent scar tissue formation. The animal is positioned in dorsal recumbency, and the head is extended and secured to the operating table. A ventral midline skin incision is made over the larynx. The underlying sternohyoid muscles are separated and retracted laterally with Gelpi retractors. The cricothyroid membrane and thyroid cartilage are incised on the midline, and the edges are retracted with small Gelpi retractors to expose the arytenoid cartilages and vocal folds. The mucosa is incised over the corniculate, cuneiform, and vocal processes of one arytenoid cartilage to facilitate their removal as well as removal of the entire vocal fold. Any redundant mucosa is excised, and the mucosal defect sutured to reduce granulation tissue formation and increase the size of the healed airway. The opposite vocal cord and process can be removed and the mucosal defect sutured. Mucosal closures are made with 5-0 or 6-0 absorbable suture in a continuous pattern. The thyroid cartilage incision is sutured with interrupted nonabsorbable sutures that do not penetrate the laryngeal lumen to prevent overriding of the cartilage edges. The subcutaneous tissue and skin are routinely closed.

When combined with arytenoid lateralization, a mattress suture is placed through the mid-body of the thyroid cartilage and the cuneiform process of the arytenoid cartilage before closure of the thyroid cartilage. The knot is placed on the lateral side of the thyroid cartilage (Schofield *et al.* 2007).

Schofield *et al.* (2007) performed a ventral approach for bilateral vocal fold resection and bilateral lateralization in 65 dogs. Quality of life of the dogs was significantly improved and three dogs developed aspiration pneumonia within a year. Since a ventriculocordectomy was performed the lateralization was limited, so limiting the risk for aspiration. However, 13 dogs had recurrence of their clinical signs within a year of surgery. On laryngeal examination the rima glottidis of these dogs seemed narrow. Bilateral partial arytenoidectomy (four dogs), permanent tracheostomy (four dogs), unilateral partial arytenoidectomy (four dogs), and soft palate resection (one dog) were performed to palliate the clinical signs in a second procedure.

Castellated laryngofissure

Castellated laryngofissure entails a stepped, or castellated, incision through the thyroid cartilage. A tracheostomy tube needs to be placed before surgery. The patient is placed in dorsal recumbency and a ventral approach to the larynx is performed. The thyroid cartilage is measured and divided in three segments. The middle segment is the base for the square central flap. Cautery can be used to mark the castellated line on the ventral part of the thyroid cartilage. The thyroid is incised along the line with a no. 11 blade. Castellated laryngofissure is associated with severe postoperative laryngeal bleeding and edema that requires a temporary tracheostomy for 2–3 days. It opens the rima glottidis as much as bilateral arytenoid lateralization. Castellated laryngofissure does not seem to be very efficient at reducing airway resistance (Burbidge *et al.* 1991).

Permanent tracheostomy

Permanent tracheostomy is a surgical option for the treatment of dogs with laryngeal paralysis. The permanent tracheostomy bypasses the upper airway obstruction without inducing any modification in the size of the rima glottidis. This surgical technique is therefore more valuable for dogs at high risk of aspiration pneumonia (myopathy, megaesophagus, hiatal hernia, gastrointestinal disorder). Animals are responding well to the treatment. Permanent tracheostomy requires attention and maintenance from the owners.

Prognosis

The long-term outcome for dogs surgically treated for laryngeal paralysis is good with a survival rate of 75% at five years after surgery (Figure 38.9) (Wilson & Monnet 2016). After unilateral lateralization, the risk of aspiration pneumonia is 31% four years after surgery. After partial laryngectomy, 59% of dogs are alive five years after surgery (MacPhail & Monnet 2001; Wilson & Monnet 2016). The development of aspiration pneumonia increases the mortality rate. The four-year survival rate has been reported at 25.8% for dogs that developed aspiration pneumonia after surgery (Figure 38.10) (Wilson & Monnet 2016). Prognostic indicators of long-term survival that have been identified include the presence of pneumonia before surgery, the development of megaesophagus after surgery, and the need for a temporary tracheostomy (MacPhail & Monnet 2001; Wilson & Monnet 2016). Dogs treated for laryngeal paralysis are at lifelong risk of aspiration pneumonia (Figure 38.11) (Wilson & Monnet 2016). The development of a generalized polyneuropathy and esophageal dysfunction may influence the long-term prognosis (Stanley *et al.* 2010).

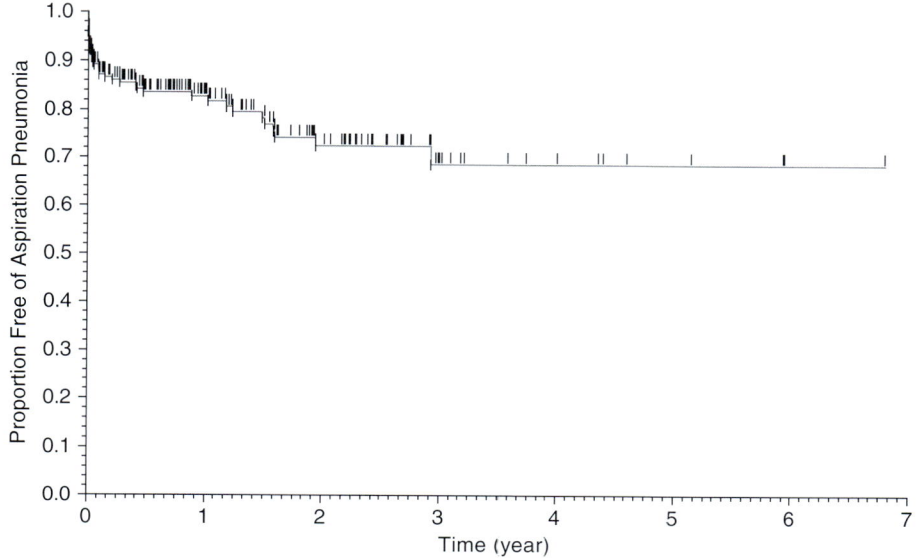

Figure 38.9 Distribution of survival for dogs with laryngeal paralysis treated with unilateral lateralization. Dotted lines represent the 95% confidence interval.

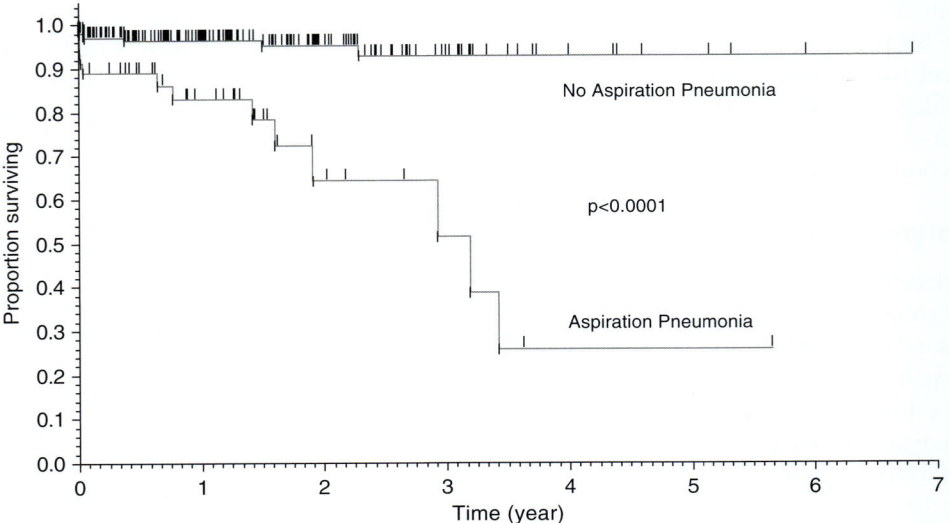

Figure 38.10 Effect of the diagnosis of aspiration pneumonia on distribution of survival for dogs with laryngeal paralysis treated with unilateral lateralization ($P < 0.0001$).

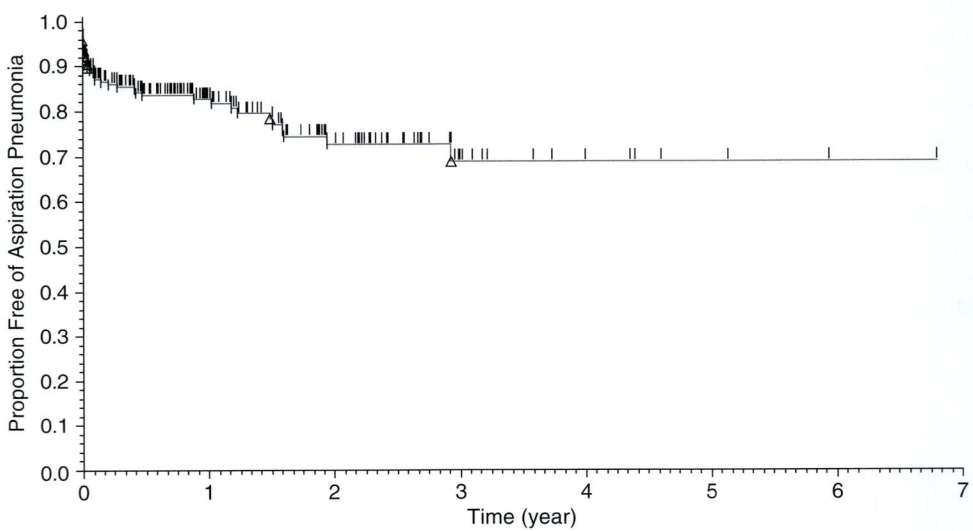

Figure 38.11 Distribution of the diagnosis of aspiration pneumonia over time for dogs with laryngeal paralysis treated with unilateral lateralization.

References

Bennett, P.F. and Clarke, R.E. (1997). Laryngeal paralysis in a Rottweiler with neuroaxonal dystrophy. *Australian Veterinary Journal* 75: 784–786.

Braund, K.G., Shores, A., Cochrane, S. et al. (1994). Laryngeal paralysis/polyneuropathy complex in young Dalmatians. *American Journal of Veterinary Research* 55: 534–541.

Braund, K.G., Steinberg, H.S., Shores, A. et al. (1989). Laryngeal paralysis in immature and mature dogs as one sign of a more diffuse polyneuropathy. *Journal of the American Veterinary Medical Association* 194: 1735–1740.

Burbidge, H.M. (1995). A review of laryngeal paralysis in dogs. *British Veterinary Journal* 151: 71–82.

Burbidge, H.M., Goulden, B.E., and Jones, B.R. (1991). An experimental evaluation of castellated laryngofissure and bilateral arytenoid lateralisation for the relief of laryngeal paralysis in dogs. *Australian Veterinary Journal* 68: 268–272.

Bureau, S. and Monnet, E. (2002). Effects of suture tension and surgical approach during unilateral arytenoid lateralization on the rima glottidis in the canine larynx. *Veterinary Surgery* 31: 589–595.

Busch, D.S., Noxon, J.O., and Miller, L.D. (1992). Laryngeal paralysis and peripheral vestibular disease in a cat. *Journal of the American Animal Hospital Association* 28: 82–86.

Campbell, D. and Holmberg, D.L. (1984). Surgical treatment of laryngeal paralysis in a cat. *Canadian Veterinary Journal* 25: 414–416.

Demetriou, J.L. and Kirby, B.M. (2003). The effect of two modifications of unilateral arytenoid lateralization on rima glottidis area in dogs. *Veterinary Surgery* 32: 62–68.

Eger, C.E., Huxtable, C.R., Chester, Z.C., and Summers, B.A. (1998). Progressive tetraparesis and laryngeal paralysis in a young Rottweiler with neuronal vacuolation and axonal degeneration: an Australian case. *Australian Veterinary Journal* 76: 733–737.

Gaber, C.E., Amis, T.C., and LeCouteur, R.A. (1985). Laryngeal paralysis in dogs: a review of 23 cases. *Journal of the American Veterinary Medical Association* 186: 377–380.

Gauthier, C.M. and Monnet, E. (2014). in vitro evaluation of anatomic landmarks for the placement of suture to achieve effective arytenoid cartilage abduction by means of unilateral cricoarytenoid lateralization in dogs. *American Journal of Veterinary Research* 75: 602–606.

Gaynor, A.R., Shofer, F.S., and Washabau, R.J. (1997). Risk factors for acquired megaesophagus in dogs. *Journal of the American Veterinary Medical Association* 211: 1406–1412.

Gourley, I.M., Paul, H., and Gregory, C. (1983). Castellated laryngofissure and vocal fold resection for the treatment of laryngeal paralysis in the dog. *Journal of the American Veterinary Medical Association* 182: 1084–1086.

Greenberg, N.J., Bureau, S., and Monnet, E. (2007). Effects of suture tension during unilateral cricoarytenoid lateralization on canine laryngeal resistance in vitro. *Veterinary Surgery* 36: 526–532.

Greenfield, C.L. (1987). Canine laryngeal paralysis. *Compendium on Continuing Education for the Practicing Veterinarian* 9: 1011–1017.

Greenfield, C.L., Walshaw, R., Kumar, K. et al. (1988). Neuromuscular pedicle graft for restoration of arytenoid abductor function in dogs with experimentally induced laryngeal hemiplegia. *American Journal of Veterinary Research* 49: 1360–1366.

Griffiths, L.G., Sullivan, M., and Reid, S.W. (2001). A comparison of the effects of unilateral thyroarytenoid lateralization versus cricoarytenoid laryngoplasty on the area of the rima glottidis and clinical outcome in dogs with laryngeal paralysis. *Veterinary Surgery* 30: 359–365.

Hammel, S.P., Hottinger, H.A., and Novo, R.E. (2006). Postoperative results of unilateral arytenoid lateralization for treatment of idiopathic laryngeal paralysis in dogs: 39 cases (1996–2002). *Journal of the American Veterinary Medical Association* 228: 1215–1220.

Hardie, E.M., Kolata, R.J., Stone, E.A., and Steiss, J.E. (1981). Laryngeal paralysis in three cats. *Journal of the American Veterinary Medical Association* 179: 879–882.

Harvey, C.E. (1983a). Partial laryngectomy in the dog. I: Healing and swallowing function in normal dogs. *Veterinary Surgery* 12: 192–197.

Harvey, C.E. (1983b). Partial laryngectomy in the dog. II: Immediate increase in glottic area obtained and compared with other laryngeal surgical procedures. *Veterinary Surgery* 12: 197–201.

Harvey, C.E. and O'Brien, J.A. (1982). Treatment of laryngeal paralysis in dogs by partial laryngectomy. *Journal of the American Animal Hospital Association* 18: 551–556.

Holt, D. and Harvey, C.E. (1994a). Idiopathic laryngeal paralysis: results of treatment by bilateral vocal fold resection in 40 dogs. *Journal of the American Animal Hospital Association* 30: 389–395.

Holt, D. and Harvey, C.E. (1994b). Glottic stenosis secondary to vocal fold resection: results of scar removal and corticosteroid treatment in nine dogs. *Journal of the American Animal Hospital Association* 30: 396–400.

Jackson, A.M., Tobias, K., Long, C. et al. (2004). Effects of various anesthetic agents on laryngeal motion during laryngoscopy in normal dogs. *Veterinary Surgery* 33: 102–106.

Jaggy, A. and Oliver, J.E. (1994). Neurologic manifestations of thyroid disease. *Veterinary Clinics of North America* 24: 487–494.

Jaggy, A., Oliver, J.E., Ferguson, D.C. et al. (1994). Neurological manifestations of hypothyroidism: a retrospective study of 29 dogs. *Journal of Veterinary Internal Medicine* 8: 328–336.

Klein, M.K., Powers, B.E., Withrow, S.J. et al. (1995). Treatment of thyroid carcinoma in dogs by surgical resection alone: 20 cases (1981–1989). *Journal of the American Veterinary Medical Association* 206: 1007–1009.

Kuehn, N.F. (1995). Diagnostic methods for upper airway disease. *Seminars in Veterinary Medicine and Surgery (Small Animals)* 10: 70–76.

LaHue, T.R. (1989). Treatment of laryngeal paralysis in dogs by unilateral cricoarytenoid laryngoplasty. *Journal of the American Animal Hospital Association* 25: 317–324.

LaHue, T.R. (1995). Laryngeal paralysis. *Seminars in Veterinary Medicine and Surgery (Small Animals)* 10: 94–100.

Lozier, S. and Pope, E. (1992). Effects of arytenoid abduction and modified castellated laryngofissure on the rima glottidis in canine cadavers. *Veterinary Surgery* 21: 195–200.

Lussier, B., Flanders, J.A., and Erb, H.N. (1996). The effect of unilateral arytenoid lateralization on rima glottidis area in canine cadaver larynges. *Veterinary Surgery* 25: 121–126.

MacPhail, C.M. and Monnet, E. (2001). Outcome of and postoperative complications in dogs undergoing surgical treatment of laryngeal paralysis: 140 cases (1985–1998). *Journal of the American Veterinary Medical Association* 218: 1949–1956.

Mahony, O.M., Knowles, K.E., Braund, K.G. et al. (1998). Laryngeal paralysis/polyneuropathy complex in young Rottweilers. *Journal of Veterinary Internal Medicine* 12: 330–337.

Mallery, K.F., Pollard, R.E., Nelson, R.W. et al. (2003). Percutaneous ultrasound-guided radiofrequency heat ablation for treatment of hyperthyroidism in cats. *Journal of the American Veterinary Medical Association* 223: 1602–1607.

Mehl, M.L., Kyles, A.E., Pypendop, B.H. et al. (2008). Outcome of laryngeal web resection with mucosal apposition for treatment of airway obstruction in dogs: 15 cases (1992–2006). *Journal of the American Veterinary Medical Association* 233: 738–742.

Miller, C.J., McKiernan, B.C., Pace, J., and Fettman, M.J. (2002). The effects of doxapram hydrochloride (dopram-V) on laryngeal function in healthy dogs. *Journal of Veterinary Internal Medicine* 16: 524–528.

O'Brien, J.A. and Hendriks, J. (1986). Inherited laryngeal paralysis. Analysis in the husky cross. *Veterinary Quarterly* 8: 301–302.

Olivieri, M., Voghera, S.G., and Fossum, T.W. (2009). Video-assisted left partial arytenoidectomy by diode laser photoablation for treatment of canine laryngeal paralysis. *Veterinary Surgery* 38: 439–444.

Petersen, S.W., Rosin, E., and Bjorling, D.E. (1991). Surgical options for laryngeal paralysis in dogs: a consideration of partial laryngectomy. *Compendium on Continuing Education for the Practicing Veterinarian* 13: 1531–1540.

Peterson, K.L., Graves, M., Berke, G.S. et al. (1999). Role of motor unit number estimate electromyography in experimental canine laryngeal reinnervation. *Otolaryngology Head and Neck Surgery* 121: 180–184.

Radlinsky, M.G., Mason, D.E., and Hodgson, D. (2004). Transnasal laryngoscopy for the diagnosis of laryngeal paralysis in dogs. *Journal of the American Animal Hospital Association* 40: 211–215.

Radlinsky, M.G., Williams, J., Frank, P.M., and Cooper, T.C. (2009). Comparison of three clinical techniques for the diagnosis of laryngeal paralysis in dogs. *Veterinary Surgery* 38: 434–438.

Rosin, E. and Greenwood, K. (1982). Bilateral arytenoid cartilage lateralization for laryngeal paralysis in the dog. *Journal of the American Veterinary Medical Association* 180: 515–518.

Ross, J.T., Matthiesen, D.T., Noone, K.E., and Scavelli, T.A. (1991). Complications and long term results after partial laryngectomy for the treatment of idiopathic laryngeal paralysis in 45 dogs. *Veterinary Surgery* 20: 169–173.

Rudorf, H., Barr, F.J., and Lane, J.G. (2001). The role of ultrasound in the assessment of laryngeal paralysis in the dog. *Veterinary Radiology and Ultrasound* 42: 338–343.

Salisbury, S.K., Forbes, S., and Blevins, W.E. (1990). Peritracheal abscess associated with tracheal collapse and bilateral laryngeal paralysis in a dog. *Journal of the American Veterinary Medical Association* 196: 1273–1275.

Sato, F. and Ogura, J.H. (1978). Functional restoration for recurrent laryngeal paralysis: an experimental study. *Laryngoscope* 88: 855–871.

Schachter, S. and Norris, C.R. (2000). Laryngeal paralysis in cats: 16 cases (1990–1999). *Journal of the American Veterinary Medical Association* 216: 1100–1103.

Schofield, D.M., Norris, J., and Sadanaga, K.K. (2007). Bilateral thyro-arytenoid cartilage lateralization and vocal fold excision with mucosoplasty for treatment of idiopathic laryngeal paralysis: 67 dogs (1998–2005). *Veterinary Surgery* 36: 519–525.

Shelton, G.D. (2010). Acquired laryngeal paralysis in dogs: evidence accumulating for a generalized neuromuscular disease. *Veterinary Surgery* 39: 137–138.

Smith, M.M., Gourley, I.M., Kurpershoek, C.J., and Amis, T.C. (1986). Evaluation of a modified castellated laryngofissure for alleviation of upper airway obstruction in dogs with laryngeal paralysis. *Journal of the American Veterinary Medical Association* 188: 1279–1283. [Published erratum appears in *Journal of the American Veterinary Medical Association* (1986) 189: 304].

Stanley, B.J., Hauptman, J.G., Fritz, M.C. et al. (2010). Esophageal dysfunction in dogs with idiopathic laryngeal paralysis: a controlled cohort study. *Veterinary Surgery* 39: 139–149.

Tobias, K.M., Jackson, A.M., and Harvey, R.C. (2004). Effects of doxapram HCl on laryngeal function of normal dogs and dogs with naturally occurring laryngeal paralysis. *Veterinary Anaesthesia and Analgesia* 31: 258–263.

Trout, N.J., Harpster, N.K., Berg, J., and Carpenter, J. (1994). Long term results of unilateral ventriculocordectomy and partial arytenoidectomy for the treatment of laryngeal paralysis in 60 dogs. *Journal of the American Animal Hospital Association* 30: 401–407.

Ubbink, G.J., Knol, B.W., and Bouw, J. (1992). The relationship between homozygosity and the occurrence of specific diseases in Bouvier Belge des Flandres dogs in The Netherlands. *Veterinary Quarterly* 14: 137–140.

Venker-van Haagen, A.J. (1982). Laryngeal paralysis in Bouviers Belge des Flandres and breeding advice to prevent this condition. *Tijdschrift Voor Diergeneeskunde* 107: 21–22.

Venker-van Haagen, A.J. (1992). Diseases of the larynx. *Veterinary Clinics of North America* 22: 1155–1172.

White, R.A.S. (1989a). Arytenoid lateralization: an assessment of technique, complications and long-term results in 62 dogs with laryngeal paralysis [Abstract]. *Veterinary Surgery* 18: 72.

White, R.A.S. (1989b). Unilateral arytenoid lateralisation: an assessment of technique and long term results in 62 dogs with laryngeal paralysis. *Journal of Small Animal Practice* 30: 543–549.

White, R.A.S., Littlewood, J.D., Herrtage, M.E., and Clarke, D.D. (1986). Outcome of surgery for laryngeal paralysis in four cats. *Veterinary Record* 118: 103–104.

Wilson, D. and Monnet, E. (2016). Risk factors for the development of aspiration pneumonia after unilateral arytenoid lateralization in dogs with laryngeal paralysis: 232 cases (1987–2012). *Journal of the Veterinary Medical Association* 248: 188–194.

Wykes, P.M. (1983a). Canine laryngeal diseases. Part I. Anatomy and disease syndromes. *Compendium on Continuing Education for the Practicing Veterinarian* 5: 8–13.

Wykes, P.M. (1983b). Canine laryngeal diseases. Part II. Diagnosis and treatment. *Compendium on Continuing Education for the Practicing Veterinarian* 5: 105–110.

Yost, C. (2006). A new look at the respiratory stimulant doxapram. *CNS Drug Reviews* 12: 236–249.

39

Laryngeal Neoplasia

Eric Monnet

Laryngeal neoplasia is rare in dogs and cats, with most information coming from case reports. Tumor types reported include rhabdomyoma (oncocytoma), osteosarcoma, chondrosarcoma, melanoma, undifferentiated carcinoma, fibrosarcoma, mast cell, adenocarcinoma, and squamous cell carcinoma (McConnell et al. 1971; Beaumont et al. 1979; Pass et al. 1980; Wheeldon et al. 1982; Stann & Bauer 1985; Neer & Zeman 1987; Venker-van Haagen 1992; Clercx et al. 1998; O'Hara et al. 2001; Slensky et al. 2003; Hayes et al. 2007; Rossi et al. 2007). No breed or sex predilection has been documented in small animals. Dogs from 2 to 12 years of age have been presented with laryngeal tumors. Oncocytoma can appear in younger mature animals (Pass et al. 1980; Saik et al. 1986). Most laryngeal tumors are locally invasive with a potential to metastasize. Oncocytoma is locally very aggressive and does not readily metastasize (Pass et al. 1980). Lymphoma and squamous cell carcinoma have been reported in cats (Saik et al. 1986; Withrow 2001). Benign polyps or inflammatory polyps have also been diagnosed in brachycephalic breeds.

Clinical signs

Animals with laryngeal tumors are presented with dyspnea that does not improve with open-mouth breathing, respiratory stridor, exercise intolerance, dysphagia, and progressive voice change (Saik et al. 1986; Withrow 2001). Acute upper airway obstruction can occur with inflammation, edema, and accumulation of airway secretions in the trachea. A temporary tracheostomy might be required to bypass the upper airway and stabilize the patient while further diagnosis is conducted.

Diagnosis

Diagnosis is confirmed with a laryngeal examination and a biopsy of the mass. Radiographic evaluation of the neck may show a mass in the upper airway. Thoracic radiography is recommended for the evaluation of metastasis and aspiration pneumonia.

Surgical treatment

Local resection

Small benign masses can be resected by mucosal resection via an oral approach or a ventral laryngotomy (Withrow 2001). As the tumor becomes larger or more aggressive, partial or complete laryngectomy can be performed (Harvey & Venker-von Haagan 1975; Henderson et al. 1991; Block et al. 1995).

Partial laryngectomy

Partial or segmental laryngectomy is performed for a tumor invading one side of the larynx and one vocal cord. A ventral midline incision is performed to expose the larynx. The thyroid cartilage is incised on the midline to gain access to the lumen of the larynx. After establishing the limit of the tumor, a segmental resection is performed with removal of the vocal cord and a segment of the thyroid cartilage. Small defects can be primarily closed by sliding the cranial part of the thyroid cartilage caudally. If the defect is too large for primary closure, a local muscle flap can be used to patch the defect. A "rotary door" procedure has been used to bring vascularized epidermis into the laryngeal defect with the support of a myocutaneous flap (Mathias 1975; Eliachar et al. 1986, 1987).

Small Animal Soft Tissue Surgery, Second Edition. Edited by Eric Monnet.
© 2023 John Wiley & Sons, Inc. Published 2023 by John Wiley & Sons, Inc.
Companion website: www.wiley.com/go/monnet/small

Complete laryngectomy

When the tumor is large and involves both sides of the larynx, a complete laryngectomy combined with a permanent tracheostomy is required to palliate the clinical signs (Crowe *et al.* 1986; Henderson *et al.* 1991; Block *et al.* 1995). Complete laryngectomy has limited utilization in veterinary surgery and the success rate of this surgery is not known in dogs. After a midline incision, the thyropharyngeal, cricopharyngeal, and sternohyoid muscles are detached from the larynx. The sternohyoid muscle is left intact. Four stay sutures are placed in the fourth tracheal ring. The trachea is detached from the cricoid cartilage and a sterile endotracheal tube is inserted in the distal trachea. The larynx is then dissected from the surrounding tissue without damaging the wall of the esophagus and its innervation. The dissection is carried out from caudal to cranial. The larynx is detached from the hyoid apparatus and the oral mucosa is incised around the rima glottidis. The oral mucosa is closed with an inverting suture pattern with 3-0 monofilament absorbable suture. The paired thyropharyngeal and cricopharyngeal muscles are sutured ventral to the esophagus without compressing the esophagus. The trachea is trimmed and brought to the skin. A simple continuous suture pattern is used to perform the permanent tracheostomy. The subcutaneous tissue and skin are closed routinely.

References

Beaumont, P.R., O'Brien, J.B., Allen, H.L., and Tucker, J.A. (1979). Mast cell sarcoma of the larynx in a dog: a case report. *Journal of Small Animal Practice* 20: 19–25.

Block, G., Clarke, K., Salisbury, S.K., and DeNicola, D.B. (1995). Total laryngectomy and permanent tracheostomy for treatment of laryngeal rhabdomyosarcoma in a dog. *Journal of the American Animal Hospital Association* 31: 510–513.

Clercx, C., Desmecht, D., Michiels, L. et al. (1998). Laryngeal rhabdomyoma in a golden retriever. *Veterinary Record* 143: 196–198.

Crowe, D.T.J., Goodwin, M.A., and Greene, C.E. (1986). Total laryngectomy for laryngeal mast cell tumor in a dog. *Journal of the American Animal Hospital Association* 22: 809–816.

Eliachar, I., Levine, S., Broniatowski, M. et al. (1986). Combined rotary door flap and epiglottic laryngoplasty for reconstruction of large laryngotracheal defects in dogs. *Laryngoscope* 96: 1154–1158.

Eliachar, I., Roberts, J.K., Hayes, J.D. et al. (1987). Laryngotracheal reconstruction: sternohyoid myo utaneous rotary door flap. *Archives of Otolaryngology Head and Neck Surgery* 113: 1094–1097.

Harvey, C.E. and Venker-von Haagen, A. (1975). Surgical management of pharyngeal and laryngeal airway obstruction in the dog. *Veterinary Clinics of North America* 5: 515–535.

Hayes, A.M., Gregory, S.P., Murphy, S. et al. (2007). Solitary extramedullary plasmacytoma of the canine larynx. *Journal of Small Animal Practice* 48: 288–291.

Henderson, R.A., Powers, R.D., and Perry, L. (1991). Development of hypoparathyroidism after excision of laryngeal rhabdomyosarcoma in a dog. *Journal of the American Veterinary Medical Association* 198: 639–643.

Mathias, D. (1975). Skin and homograft cartilage reconstruction. *Archives of Otolaryngology* 101: 301–304.

McConnell, E.E., Smit, J.D., and Venter H.J. (1971). Melanoma in the larynx of a dog. *Journal of the South African Veterinary Medical Association* 42: 189–191.

Neer, T.M. and Zeman, D. (1987). Tracheal adenocarcinoma in a cat and review of the literature. *Journal of the American Animal Hospital Association* 23: 377–380.

O'Hara, A.J., McConnell, M., Wyatt, K., and Huxtable, C. (2001). Laryngeal rhabdomyoma in a dog. *Australian Veterinary Journal* 79: 817–821.

Pass, D.A., Huxtable, C.R., Cooper, B.J. et al. (1980). Canine laryngeal oncocytomas. *Veterinary Pathology* 17: 672–677.

Rossi, G., Tarantino, C., Taccini, E. et al. (2007). Granular cell tumour affecting the left vocal cord in a dog. *Journal of Comparative Pathology* 136: 74–78.

Saik, J.E., Toll, S.L., Diters, R.W., and Goldschmidt, M.H. (1986). Canine and feline laryngeal neoplasia. *Journal of the American Animal Hospital Association* 22: 359–365.

Slensky, K.A., Volk, S.W., Schwarz, T. et al. (2003). Acute severe hemorrhage secondary to arterial invasion in a dog with thyroid carcinoma. *Journal of the American Veterinary Medical Association* 223 (649–653): 636.

Stann, S.E. and Bauer, T.G. (1985). Respiratory tract tumors. *Veterinary Clinics of North America: Small Animal Practice* 15: 535–556.

Venker-van Haagen, A. (1992). Diseases of the larynx. *Veterinary Clinics of North America: Small Animal Practice* 22: 1155–1172.

Wheeldon, E.B., Suter, P.F., and Jenkins, T. (1982). Neoplasia of the larynx in the dog. *Journal of the American Veterinary Medical Association* 180: 642–647.

Withrow, S.J. (2001). Tumors of the respiratory system. In: *Small Animal Clinical Oncology*, 3e (ed. S.J. Withrow and E.G. MacEwen), 354–377. Philadelphia PA: WB Saunders.

40

Tracheal Surgery

Catriona M. MacPhail

The primary function of the trachea is to serve as a conduit for air into and away from the bronchial tree. Disease mechanisms potentially amenable to surgical intervention include collapse, tears, and obstruction. Tracheal obstruction can occur from foreign body inhalation or by occlusion from inflammatory or neoplastic masses. In addition, the trachea can be accessed to alleviate life-threatening upper airway obstruction through temporary tracheotomy. Permanent tracheostomy may provide palliative relief for upper airway obstruction that may not otherwise be amenable to treatment.

Tracheal collapse

Canine tracheal collapse syndrome is a challenging condition to diagnose and treat. Diagnosis is complicated by concurrent illnesses that exacerbate clinical signs, while treatment standards of care have not been established. Appropriate medical management may alleviate clinical signs in a large percentage of affected dogs, although those refractory to pharmacologic intervention may benefit from extraluminal or endoluminal support.

Pathophysiology

Tracheal collapse results from structural abnormalities of the cartilage rings and secondary changes in the dorsal tracheal membrane. Histopathologic and ultrastructural analysis of tracheal cartilage in dogs with tracheal collapse has found hypocellularity leading to decreased chondroitin sulfate and glycosaminoglycans and transformation of normal hyaline cartilage to fibrous cartilage. This chondromalacia makes the trachea less rigid and less able to withstand external pressures, resulting in dorsoventral flattening. In the normal dog, the peritracheal nerve plexus may be more complex than in other small animals, potentially playing an important role in airway regulation and in the pathogenesis of tracheal collapse. The specific etiology of tracheal collapse is unknown, but is thought to be multifactorial with a congenital or inheritable component.

Tracheal collapse may be confined to an isolated segment or may involve the entire trachea and bronchial tree. The thoracic inlet is the most commonly involved area (Figure 40.1). Collapse typically occurs in a dorsoventral direction, as the cartilages weaken and the dorsal tracheal membrane thins and lengthens (traditional type); however, static and rigid W-shaped collapse (malformation type) and rigid lateral collapse have also been described.

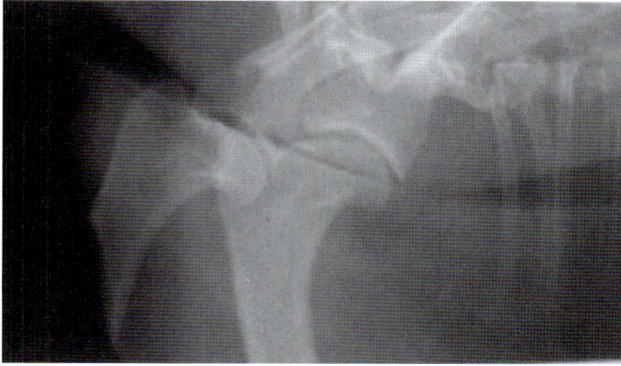

Figure 40.1 Lateral radiograph of the thoracic inlet in a 2-year-old Yorkshire terrier showing significant tracheal collapse.

Small Animal Soft Tissue Surgery, Second Edition. Edited by Eric Monnet.
© 2023 John Wiley & Sons, Inc. Published 2023 by John Wiley & Sons, Inc.
Companion website: www.wiley.com/go/monnet/small

Traditional-type tracheal collapse is graded by its appearance on fluoroscopy or bronchoscopy. This grading scheme allows determination of the severity of the collapse, establishes a baseline from which to assess disease progression, and identifies or eliminates the potential for surgical intervention. Grades range from I to IV, mild to severe, reflective of 25% interval losses of luminal diameter:

- Grade 1: relatively normal tracheal cartilage anatomy; redundant dorsal tracheal membrane decreases luminal diameter up to 25%.
- Grade 2: mild to moderate flattening of tracheal cartilages; 50% loss of luminal diameter.
- Grade 3: severe flattening of tracheal cartilages; 75% loss of luminal diameter.
- Grade 4: complete tracheal collapse; lumen is obliterated; W-shaped malformation (Maggiore 2020).
- Grade 5: this grade was used to classify lateral collapse in one study (Buback et al. 1996).

Collapse in the cervical and thoracic inlet trachea classically occurs on inspiration, as pressure within the lumen drops and the walls are susceptible to atmospheric pressure; intrathoracic tracheal collapse occurs on expiration. Although pressure within the trachea decreases on inspiration, luminal pressure still exceeds intrapleural pressure, keeping airways open. On expiration, intrapleural pressure becomes less negative and exceeds intraluminal pressure. Dogs with weakened cartilages lack sufficient strength to withstand the increased intrapleural pressure. The thoracic inlet is most susceptible to tracheal collapse, as this is the site of the equal-pressure point where intrapleural pressure equals intraluminal airway pressure and where the transition from intrapleural to atmospheric pressure occurs.

Signalment and presentation

Tracheal collapse is typically associated with middle-aged toy and miniature-breed dogs. Classic breeds include Yorkshire terriers, toy poodles, miniature poodles, Pomeranians, chihuahuas, and pugs. This condition has also been occasionally described in young large-breed dogs. In cats, tracheal collapse has been associated with intraluminal, extraluminal, or nasal masses.

Most dogs are diagnosed around 6–7 years of age, although dogs presenting with rigid tracheal malformation tend to be younger. Affected dogs have an easily solicited cough that most often described as a "goose-honk," while severely affected dogs may have exercise intolerance, respiratory distress, and syncope. Clinical signs are exacerbated by heat, stress, or excitement.

Dogs with tracheal collapse may suffer from a variety of concurrent problems. Almost 50% of dogs suffer from a degree of obesity that will worsen clinical signs (Johnson 2000). Laryngeal paresis or paralysis has been reported in 20–30% of dogs, while around 33% of dogs have concurrent systolic heart murmurs consistent with mitral valve insufficiency. Upper respiratory signs may be aggravated by an enlarged left atrium putting pressure on the carina and mainstem bronchi.

At least 40% of dogs are thought to have a degree of dental or periodontal disease (Johnson 2000; Pardali et al. 2010). Aspiration of oral bacteria into diseased airways is hypothesized to contribute to exacerbation of clinical signs due to increased airway inflammation or increased coughing. In a study of 37 dogs with tracheal collapse, 83% had a positive large airway culture, with 59% growing more than one species of bacteria (Johnson & Fales 2001). This is of interest, as oropharyngeal flora have been found in the trachea of normal dogs, but only 17% had multiple mixed colonization. Concurrent cytologic inflammation, however, was not consistently found in a population of dogs with tracheal collapse. Therefore, an association between bacterial colonization of large airways and clinical signs has not yet been proven.

Concurrent hepatomegaly and hepatopathy are also common in dogs with tracheal collapse. In a study of 26 dogs, 46% had increased serum activity of two or more liver enzymes, with 92% having elevated serum basal bile acid concentrations (Bauer et al. 2006). The reason for this association is still unclear, although speculative hypotheses include passive hepatic congestion or centrilobular liver cell necrosis secondary to chronic hypoxia.

Diagnosis

The diagnosis of tracheal collapse is often suspected based on signalment, history, and physical examination findings. Physical examination findings include tracheal stridor, marked difficulty in breathing, spontaneous paroxysmal coughing, cyanosis, and exercise intolerance. Lateral survey radiographs of the neck and thorax may confirm this diagnosis. Views should be taken of the cervical and thoracic trachea on both inspiration and expiration. The cervical trachea narrows during inspiration due to negative pressure within the trachea, while the intrathoracic trachea collapses during expiration due to increased intrapleural pressure. Static radiographs may only detect collapse in 59–92% of cases (Tangner & Hobson 1982; White & Williams 1994; Macready et al. 2007; Johnson & Pollard 2010), but radiographs should be closely evaluated for signs of concurrent airway pathology or cardiac disease. In a study of 60 dogs with tracheal collapse, a 30% incidence of bronchiectasia associated with the tracheal collapse was reported (Marolf et al. 2007). Dynamic evaluation of the trachea can be performed using fluoroscopy and is particularly helpful for identification of intrathoracic collapse. When comparing fluoroscopy and standard radiographic evaluation, radiography has been found to underestimate the frequency and degree of tracheal collapse (Macready *et al.* 2007). Detection of tracheal collapse using ultrasonography has also been described (Rudorf *et al.* 1997).

Bronchoscopy allows direct visualization and evaluation of the entire tracheobronchial tree. In particular, it allows evaluation of the mainstem bronchi. Airway samples for cytology and bacterial culture can be obtained by tracheal brushing or bronchoalveolar lavage, as tracheobronchitis or bronchopneumonia may play a role in the severity of clinical signs. Normal bronchoalveolar lavage in a dog is composed of 70–80% macrophages, 6% lymphocytes, and 6% neutrophils (Johnson 2000). If degenerative neutrophils are present with intracellular bacteria, then infection is likely present. It is not unusual to have bronchopneumonia associated with tracheal collapse, as septic inflammation has been reported in 23% of cases (Buback *et al.* 1996). The disadvantage of bronchoscopy is that general anesthesia is required. However, it provides an opportunity to assess laryngeal anatomy and function. Bronchoscopy also allows evaluation of the bronchi for signs of bronchomalacia, as this condition has been diagnosed in 50% of dogs with lower airway disease (Johnson & Pollard 2010). Bronchial collapse without tracheal collapse was diagnosed in 59% of the patients evaluated. For dogs with tracheal collapse, lobar bronchial collapse was present in 83% of cases, while sublobar collapse was present in 38%. Bronchial collapse involved both the left and right principal bronchi, as well as being present in the right middle lung lobe (59%) and the left cranial lung lobe (52%). The diagnosis of bronchomalacia was performed more readily with bronchoscopy than with radiography and inflammation did not appear to be a risk factor for its development.

Treatment

Conservative treatment

Medical management of tracheal collapse results in improvement of clinical signs in most dogs. Weight loss is critical to the success of other medical therapies. Environmental modifications, such as the use of a harness instead of a collar and creation of a nonsmoking atmosphere, may help some dogs, as will management of concurrent underlying conditions. It has also been advocated to perform dental prophylaxis in affected dogs to decrease the bacterial load that can be aspirated into the trachea (Johnson 2000). Frequently used medications include antitussives, bronchodilators, anti-inflammatories, and antibiotics. Butorphanol or dihydrocodeinone (hydrocodone) is recommended as an oral antitussive medication.

Butorphanol injectable can also be used in an emergency. If the patient is cyanotic, oxygen supplementation is required with or without humidification. Steroids might be indicated in cases with extreme inflammation of the upper airway and the trachea. Bronchodilators (e.g., aminophylline) are indicated to improve mucociliary clearance and reduce ventilatory work of the diaphragm. When theophylline was used as a first-line treatment in a cohort of dogs, clinical improvements were seen in 98% of dogs with tracheal collapse (Jeung *et al.* 2019). Use of antibiotics is controversial because the role of infection in tracheal collapse is not known. A transtracheal wash or bronchoalveolar lavage can be performed to obtain samples for culture and sensitivity, and antibiotherapy can be instituted based on the results. The utilization of doxycycline (3–5 mg/kg orally [p.o.] twice daily), clindamycin (5–11 mg/kg p.o. twice daily), or enrofloxacin (2.5–11 mg/kg p.o. twice daily) has been recommended in the initial phase of medical treatment (Johnson 2000).

Surgical/interventional treatment

Intervention is suggested in patients with moderate to severe tracheal collapse that are refractory to medical management. It is not recommended in patients with underlying laryngeal disease or concurrent cardiopulmonary disease; studies conflict on whether mainstem bronchi collapse influences outcome. Treatment of tracheal collapse is currently achieved by either surgical placement of extraluminal ring prostheses or fluoroscopic placement of endoluminal stents. Results reported in the literature regarding treatment of clinical cases are summarized in Table 40.1.

Extraluminal stents

Extraluminal tracheal ring or spiral prostheses can be implanted in dogs with cervical tracheal collapse or proximal intrathoracic tracheal collapse. The technique requires careful dissection of the trachea while preserving the segmental blood supply and both recurrent laryngeal nerves. Good to excellent outcomes have been reported in 75–96% of patients; however, this technique is limited by candidate selection and surgical complications. Following surgery, laryngeal paralysis, laryngeal necrosis, and postoperative distress requiring permanent tracheostomy have been reported. In a study of 25 dogs treated for tracheal collapse with prosthetic ring placement, White and Williams (1994) performed a unilateral lateralization in each case as a preventive measure. The success rate of the procedure was 75%. Dogs older than 6 years appear to have worse outcomes compared with younger dogs, regardless of the degree of collapse (Buback *et al.* 1996). Becker *et al.* (2012) placed

Table 40.1 Results reported in the literature regarding surgical or interventional treatment of clinical cases.

Reference	No. of cases	Complications	Outcome
Extraluminal prostheses			
Suematsu *et al.* (2019)	54	Laryngeal paralysis in one dog; no tracheal necrosis	12-, 24-, and 36-month survival = 96%, 86%, 86%
Tinga *et al.* (2015)	73	Major complications 42%; laryngeal paralysis 15%	MST = 1460 days
Chisnell & Pardo (2015)	23	Laryngeal paralysis 17%	96% survived to discharge
Becker *et al.* (2012)	33	Laryngeal paralysis 21%; no tracheal necrosis	91% survived to discharge; 88% survived >6 months; MST = 1680 days
Ayres & Holmberg (1999)	4	Coughing 50%	4 months to 11 years
Buback *et al.* (1996)	90	Laryngeal paralysis; dyspnea requiring permanent tracheostomy	85% clinical success; 5% mortality
Spodnick & Nwadike (1997)	2	Not reported	Not reported
White (1995)	25	Perioperative complications 4%	75% very satisfactory six months to three years
Endoluminal stents			
Congiusta *et al.* (2021)	75	Not reported	MST = 1913 days
Violette *et al.* (2019)	52	Major complications 56%	11% mortality within 60 days
Weisse *et al.* (2019)	75	Major complications 47%	MST = 1005 days
Raske *et al.* (2018)	50	No significant stent migration	Not reported
Rosenheck *et al.* (2017)	29	Major complications 37%	MST = 502 days
Tinga *et al.* (2015)	30	Major complications 43%	MST = 365 days
Beranek *et al.* (2014)	26	Fracture 26.7%; granuloma 11.5%; stent shortening 11.5%	MST = 20 months
Durant *et al.* (2012)	18	Fracture 22.2%; postoperative aspiration pneumonia 16.7%	11.1% mortality within 60 days
Sura & Krahwinkel (2008)	12	Fracture 41.7%	83% clinical success >1 year
Kim *et al.* (2008)	4	None reported	100% technical success
Moritz *et al.* (2004)	24	Stent shortening; granuloma formation	91.3% clinical success; 8.3% mortality
Woo *et al.* (2007)	1	Fracture	4-week survival
Ouellet *et al.* (2006)	1	Fracture	8-month survival
Mittleman *et al.* (2004)	1	Fracture	>1 year survival
Gellasch *et al.* (2002)	1	None reported	>10-month survival

MST, median survival time.

cervical extraluminal prosthetic rings in dogs with or without intrathoracic or mainstem bronchi collapse and found no significant difference in median survival time. This is in contrast to Tinga *et al.* (2015), who found that dogs with mainstem bronchi collapse had shorter survival times following extraluminal ring placement.

Endoluminal stents

Endoluminal stents are placed under general anesthesia using fluoroscopy and are used for rapid relief of clinical signs in dogs with moderate to severe intrathoracic tracheal collapse or diffuse tracheal collapse. Good immediate-, short-, and long-term outcomes have been reported. Complications include stent fracture, stent migration, aspiration pneumonia, and tissue ingrowth. Endoluminal stenting has been reported in a variety of settings using a large array of materials. In a study by Radlinsky *et al.* (1997), 19 Palmaz stents were first placed in 10 normal dogs. These stents require balloon insufflation for deployment. Stents were placed in the thoracic trachea, the cervical trachea, and/or one mainstem bronchi. Of the 19 stents, 10 migrated, 7 collapsed, and pulmonary edema developed in 2 dogs.

Self-expanding stainless steel biliary stents (Wallstent™, Boston Scientific, Marlborough, MA, USA) were implanted in 24 clinical dogs (median age 12 years) to support the cervical and thoracic trachea (Moritz et al. 2004); 54% of the cases had grade 4 collapse, while 33.3% were grade 3. In 79% of the cases the entire trachea was collapsed, and bronchial collapse was present in 45% of the cases. The median survival time was 681 days; death was unrelated to the respiratory system in 75% of the cases.

Sura and Krahwinkel (2008) reported the implantation of 17 single-stranded self-expanding nitinol stents in 12 cases. Of these, 9 cases had collapse of the cervical and thoracic trachea, and 1 case had only cervical collapse. The diameter of the stent was determined on lateral radiographs under anesthesia. The diameter of the trachea at the level of the collapse was measured with a positive pressure of 20 cmH$_2$O, and the diameter of the stent implanted was 10–20% larger than the maximal tracheal diameter. The length of the stent was based on the length of the collapse plus 1–2 cm; therefore, the entire trachea was not stented. Median survival time after stent placement was 19 months. Stent fracture at the level of the thoracic inlet was recorded in 41% of the cases; stent migration occurred in one dog. Granuloma formation partially occluding the airway was present in two dogs and was successfully treated with steroids.

Kim et al. (2008) reported 100% success between four and seven months after surgery on four dogs treated for cervical and thoracic tracheal collapse. They used self-expandable nitinol stents 10–15% larger than the diameter of the trachea, measured caudal to the larynx on lateral radiographs in awake animals. The length of the stent was from mid-cervical to mid-thoracic trachea.

Durant et al. (2012) described endoluminal stent placement using bronchoscopy with fair to good outcomes despite significant stent foreshortening. Stenting the entire length of the trachea regardless of degree of tracheal collapse has been described to possibly decrease the risk of caudal stent fracture (Figure 40.2), although a

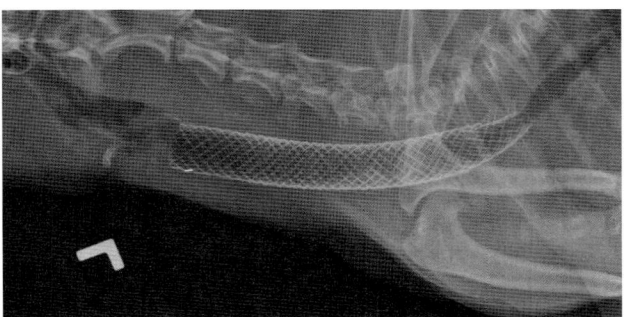

Figure 40.2 Lateral cervical radiograph of a 9-year-old Yorkshire terrier with an endoluminal tracheal stent and stent fracture at the caudal extent.

fracture still occurred in over 25% of dogs in that study (Beranek et al. 2014). More recent studies have considered that dogs with the malformation type of collapse and/or large variation in the diameter of the trachea along its length may have a higher risk of fracture (Violette et al. 2019).

Tracheal obstruction

Tracheal tumors

Intratracheal obstruction, although uncommon, is most often the result of neoplastic masses. Tumor types reported include adenocarcinoma, adenoma, carcinoma, lymphoma, fibrosarcoma, squamous cell carcinoma, mast cell tumor, leiomyoma, chondroma, osteosarcoma, extramedullary plasmacytoma, rhabdomyosarcoma, chondrosarcoma, and fibrosarcoma. In addition, several cases of osteochondroma and osteochondromal dysplasia have been reported in young dogs.

Surgical excision is considered the treatment of choice for solitary nonlymphomatous tumors without evidence of metastatic disease. Excision typically involves tracheal resection and anastomosis, although debulking the mass by tracheoscopy may provide palliative relief for slow-growing tumors.

Inflammatory tracheal masses

Non-neoplastic differentials for intraluminal obstruction include a variety of inflammatory nodules, including lymphoplasmacytic inflammation, lymphoid hyperplasia, granulomatous tracheitis, and tissue reaction to *Oslerus osleri*. Aside from nematode infection or reaction to intraluminal stents, the underlying etiology of inflammatory lesions in the upper airway is unknown, although other infectious agents or trauma are suspected. Regardless, the prognosis is guarded, but successful outcomes have been described with a combination of medical treatment and surgical debulking (Jakubiak et al. 2005).

Tracheal foreign body

Inhalation of foreign bodies into the respiratory tree is an uncommon clinical scenario. However, tracheal foreign bodies appear to be more common in cats, while bronchial foreign bodies are more common in dogs. This difference is likely due to the small diameter of the feline trachea that entraps foreign material before it reaches the bronchial tree. Animals present with respiratory distress of varying severity and duration. Plain radiography is often sufficient for diagnosis (Figure 40.3), although advanced imaging could also be considered. Removal can be performed by a variety of methods. Most often tracheoscopy is utilized, and the foreign

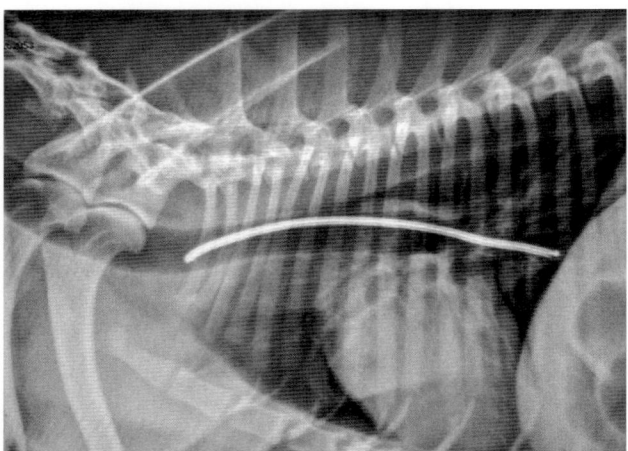

Figure 40.3 Lateral thoracic radiograph of a 3-year-old beagle with a tracheal foreign body: esophageal thermometer bitten off and aspirated during anesthetic recovery.

body is grasped with forceps or retrieval basket. This method has been shown to be successful in 79% of cases (Tenwolde *et al.* 2010).

Use of a Foley catheter has also been described: the balloon is inflated caudal to the obstruction and the foreign body is recovered as the catheter is gently pulled out (Pratschke *et al.* 1999). Fluoroscopic-guided retrieval may be of particular benefit in small dogs or cats, as it minimizes further obstruction of the airway with equipment. This technique has been successfully reported in 12 cats (Tivers & Moore 2006). With failure of these methods, thoracotomy can be performed to facilitate tracheotomy or tracheal resection with reconstruction to achieve foreign body retrieval.

Tracheal trauma

External injury

The cervical and thoracic trachea is relatively well protected from blunt trauma. However, tracheal separation may occur in the thoracic trachea due to violent stretching or hyperextension. Otherwise, injury to the trachea most often occurs in the cervical region due to bite wounds or other penetrating injury (e.g., gunshot wounds). Animals present with obvious skin trauma in the neck area, with varying degrees of subcutaneous emphysema that is identified visually or by feeling crackling of the tissues during gentle palpation. These animals may present with respiratory distress due to pneumomediastinum or if there are large tracheal defects or tracheal avulsion. Unstable animals may require rapid establishment of a patent airway. A small-diameter endotracheal tube can be inserted through large tracheal tears to ensure patency of the distal trachea. The location

of the tear is typically found at wound exploration, as there is likely to be extensive tissue damage due to the nature of the injury. Small tears may be self-limiting. Larger tears may be primarily sutured with small monofilament nonabsorbable suture or a tracheal resection and anastomosis may be performed.

Internal injury

Overinflation of endotracheal tube cuffs can result in tracheal tears or tracheal rupture, and this most often occurs in cats (Mitchell *et al.* 2000). Iatrogenic tracheal tears are also commonly associated with general anesthesia for dental procedures, presumably due to overinflation of the cuff to prevent aspiration of fluid or debris (Hardie *et al.* 1999). Often these cats can be managed with conservative treatment, with resolution of subcutaneous emphysema about two weeks on average. Surgery may be indicated in cases with progressive respiratory distress or subcutaneous emphysema, or in chronic cases that develop severe circumferential luminal stenosis at the proximal and distal ends of the tracheal avulsion (White & Burton 2000) (Figure 40.4).

(a)

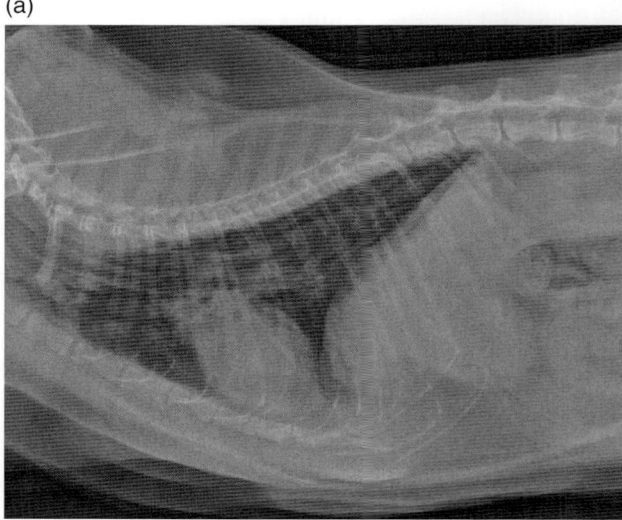

(b)

Figure 40.4 (a) Lateral thoracic radiograph of a 3-year-old cat with a cervical tracheal tear demonstrating severe pneumomediastinum and subcutaneous emphysema. (b) 3D computed tomography reconstruction of the same cat's trachea showing marked disruption of the dorsal tracheal membrane.

Tracheal resection and anastomosis

Tracheal resection and anastomosis may be indicated in cases of tracheal trauma, tracheal avulsion, or for removal of tracheal masses. Tracheal segment removal can be challenging due to concerns about dehiscence and stenosis. The goal of this procedure is to achieve precise anatomic apposition while preserving blood supply and avoiding excessive tension. The amount of trachea that can be resected is dependent on the age of the animal as well as the affected location. Historical experimental studies found that resection of 20–25% of the trachea in a puppy and 25–50% of the trachea in an adult dog can be tolerated (Hsieh *et al.* 1988). This translates to approximately 8–10 rings that can be safely removed. A more recent *ex vivo* study compared the influence of age on tracheal anastomoses to withstand distraction; tracheal anastomoses failed at lower forces but sustained more elongation in immature dogs than adult dogs (Brisimi *et al.* 2022). A degree of luminal stenosis is expected following anastomosis, although clinical signs of respiratory obstruction are not expected until there is at least 50% attenuation of the cross-sectional area. Imprecise anastomosis and tension across the suture site are considerable risk factors in the development of stenosis. Therefore, accurate and meticulous surgical technique is paramount for tracheal reconstruction. Additional procedures may be used to prevent anastomotic stenosis, including tracheal mobilization, tension-relieving sutures, and head–neck immobilization.

For the anastomotic technique, sutures are placed either through or around the tracheal rings, but the latter is most commonly performed. Both simple continuous and simple interrupted patterns have been described. Although a simple continuous pattern is associated with less but clinically insignificant apposition, it is more rapidly performed and is associated with pullout strength similar to that seen with a simple interrupted pattern reinforced with horizontal mattress sutures (Fingland *et al.* 1995; Demetriou *et al.* 2006). A variety of suture materials can be utilized for suturing the trachea, but multifilament nonabsorbable suture material is associated with an unacceptably high incidence of granuloma formation, submucosal inflammation, and fibrosis (Lau *et al.* 1980; Dallman & Bojrab 1982).

Replacement of large segment defects with prosthetic materials has only been evaluated experimentally in dogs (Zang *et al.* 2010; Ueda *et al.* 2021). It is associated with a higher complication rate and prosthetic failure, such that further investigation is required prior to clinical application.

Palliative tracheal surgery

Upper airway obstruction is a life-threatening condition that may require aggressive intervention. In emergency situations, temporary redirection of airflow through the cervical trachea allows the veterinarian to gain control of the airway status of the patient. Permanent bypass of the larynx and proximal trachea may provide palliative relief from upper airway obstruction that cannot be otherwise treated.

Temporary tracheostomy

The use of a temporary tracheostomy tube is far more common than creation of a permanent stoma. Temporary tracheostomies can be used on a planned or an emergency basis. The most common indication for emergency tracheostomy is upper airway obstruction. Risk factors for need of temporary tracheostomy tube placement in dogs with brachycephalic obstructive airway syndrome were increasing age, the need to administer corticosteroids, and the presence of pneumonia (Worth *et al.* 2018). Most emergency situations can be handled by anesthetizing the animal and passing an endotracheal tube orally to allow placement of a tracheostomy tube in a controlled and calm manner. However, situations can occur that require immediate tracheotomy or tracheostomy to save the life of the animal. Such circumstances would include laryngeal or tracheal foreign bodies, advanced neoplasia, or severe swelling.

Temporary tracheostomies may also be preplaced for certain surgeries if postoperative oropharyngeal or laryngeal swelling is anticipated. Advanced reconstructive procedures in the oral cavity, such as cleft palate correction, may also be facilitated by placing the endotracheal tube through a temporary tracheostomy rather than standard oral intubation. Temporary tracheostomies may also be used in animals requiring long-term positive-pressure ventilation. By using a tracheostomy tube, the animal can be free from the heavy sedation or anesthesia that would otherwise be necessary to maintain an oral endotracheal tube.

The incision in the trachea to facilitate tube placement can be performed transversely (horizontally) or longitudinally (vertically). Instead of a simple incision, the surgeon may also choose to create a transverse or longitudinal flap. A transverse incision is most commonly utilized, as it is simple to perform and allows easy removal and replacement of tracheostomy tubes. A small midline incision is made through skin and subcutaneous tissue along the ventral neck. The paired sternohyoideus muscles lie directly over the ventral aspect of the trachea, and they are divided using blunt dissection. A horizontal tracheotomy is performed between the third and fourth or fourth and fifth rings, with no more than half of the circumference of the trachea incised. A monofilament nonabsorbable suture is placed around the ring distal to the tracheostomy site. This suture is used to open the tracheal incision to facilitate tube placement, particularly if the tube has been removed accidentally.

A variety of tubes are available for use in tracheostomies: single or double lumen, cuffed or noncuffed. In an emergency, a standard endotracheal tube can be used, but care must be taken to ensure that the tube is not inserted too far into the respiratory tree, and that the cuff is not inflated. Single-lumen tracheostomy tubes are easier to place, particularly in smaller animals; however, the entire tube must be removed when cleaning is required, and this may cause distress to the animal. Double-lumen tubes have an inner cannula that is amenable to easier cleaning and maintenance, as the outer cannula stays in place, providing an airway for the animal. Cuffed tubes should only be utilized in animals requiring mechanical ventilation, and proper cuff inflation is important to avoid damage to the tracheal mucosa from pressure necrosis. The size of tracheostomy tube placed is based on the luminal diameter of the trachea at that level, and is typically only 50% of the tracheal lumen diameter. The tube extends into the trachea approximately 6–7 tracheal rings. Once placed, the tube is secured to the patient by tying umbilical tape or rolled gauze to the tube and around the animal's neck. Once a tracheostomy tube is deemed no longer necessary, the tube is removed, and the surgical site is left to heal by second intention.

Temporary tracheostomies are not without potentially significant complications. The presence of a tube within the tracheal lumen causes epithelial erosion, submucosal inflammation, and inhibition of the mucociliary apparatus from the level of the tracheostomy to the bifurcation. Mucus production dramatically increases, and the tube must be suctioned or cleaned at very frequent intervals to prevent tube obstruction. In dogs, one study found 16 types of complications occurring in 86% of cases (Nicholson & Baines 2012). Major complications (occlusion, dislodgment, pneumonia) were found in 25%, but successfully managed tracheostomy tubes occurred in 81%. English bulldogs were shown to be more at risk for tube dislodgment as well as unsuccessful tube outcome. In a study specifically looking at outcome following temporary tracheostomy placement in brachycephalic dogs, 83% of dogs had major complications (Stordalen et al. 2020).

Major complications have been reported in 44% of cats with temporary tracheostomies, with an overall complication rate of 87% (Guenther-Yenke & Rozanski 2007). Therefore, intensive monitoring of a patient with a temporary tracheostomy tube is required to avoid life-threatening complications, particularly in smaller animals. A small degree of luminal stenosis does occur following tracheostomy, but it is typically clinically insignificant if the procedure has been performed properly.

Permanent tracheostomy

Permanent tracheostomy is most often performed for dogs with laryngeal paralysis, brachycephalic dogs with severe laryngeal collapse, or dogs and cats with laryngeal neoplasia or inflammatory disease. Before creating a permanent stoma in the trachea, owners should be counseled regarding the care and attention their animal will require, although a study regarding owner perception of outcome in dogs following permanent tracheostomy found satisfaction to be high in approximately 90% of owners despite the high level of intensive care required (Davis et al. 2018). The stoma must be kept clean and clipped free of hair at frequent intervals. Dogs are also no longer allowed to swim.

The most common method of performing permanent tracheostomy is to create a window in the ventral trachea encompassing 3–5 tracheal rings longitudinally and one-third of the circumference transversely. Tracheal collapse can occur if the created stoma is too large. Ideally, only the tracheal rings are removed, leaving the mucosa intact (Figure 40.5). An I-shaped incision is then made in the mucosa and the edges are sutured directly to the skin using 4-0 to 5-0 monofilament nonabsorbable suture in a simple interrupted or simple continuous pattern. To minimize tension on the newly created stoma, some surgeons prefer to bring the trachea to a more superficial location by suturing the paired sternohyoideus muscles together dorsally to the trachea for the length of the proposed stoma.

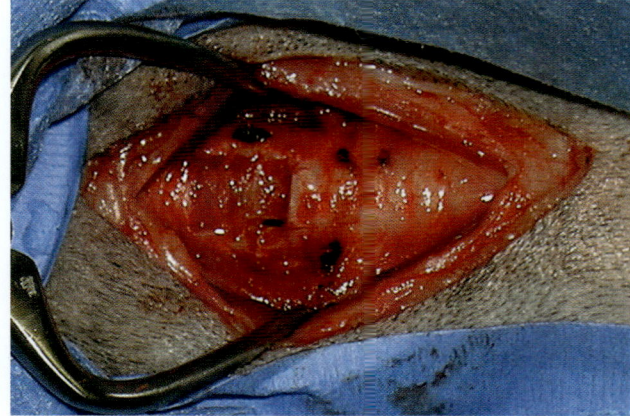

Figure 40.5 Intraoperative photograph of a permanent tracheostomy: the ventral third of three tracheal rings have been removed, leaving the tracheal mucosa intact.

An alternative method for performing a permanent tracheostomy is to make a full-thickness H-shaped incision in the ventral trachea, which then creates two tracheal flaps that are reflected cranially and caudally and sutured directly to the skin.

The most significant complication associated with permanent tracheostomy comes from accumulation of mucus and secretions that may obstruct the trachea or stoma. Animals must be observed extremely closely in the first few days following surgery. They are also at increased risk for drowning, aspiration pneumonia, and hyperthermia. Other complications include stoma stricture or occlusion of the stoma by excessive skin folds.

Reported outcomes following permanent tracheostomy are associated with high complication and mortality rates, primarily due to aspiration pneumonia or the occlusion of the stoma from skinfolds, mucus, blood, or stricture. In one study median survival in dogs undergoing permanent tracheostomies was 328 days, with 50% having major complications and 20% requiring revision surgery (Occhipinti & Hauptman 2014). A separate study found a median survival time in dogs with permanent tracheostomies to be 1825 days, with 61% having major complications and 35% requiring revision surgery (Grimes et al. 2019). Worse survival was associated with increasing age, need for corticosteroids, or concurrent tracheal collapse. Revision surgery most often occurred in brachycephalic breeds. In a study evaluating permanent tracheostomy in dogs with severe laryngeal collapse due to brachycephalic obstructive airway syndrome, median survival time was 100 days, with 80% of dogs having major complications (Gobbetti et al. 2018).

Median survival in cats undergoing permanent tracheostomy for upper airway obstruction was reported to be 20.5 days in one study (Stepnik et al. 2009). In that same study it was found that cats with inflammatory laryngeal disease were 6.61 times as likely to die as cats that underwent permanent tracheostomy for any other reason. A separate study of seven cats with permanent tracheostomy reports one cat with granulomatous laryngitis alive at over 1600 days (Guenther-Yenke & Rozanski 2007). However, the remaining six cats died or were euthanized 2–281 days postoperatively due to stoma occlusion or disease progression.

References

Ayres, S.A. and Holmberg, D.L. (1999). Surgical treatment of tracheal collapse using pliable total ring prostheses: results in one experimental and 4 clinical cases. *Canadian Veterinary Journal* 40: 787–791.

Bauer, N.B., Schneider, M.A., Neiger, R., and Moritz, A. (2006). Liver disease in dogs with tracheal collapse. *Journal of Veterinary Internal Medicine* 20: 845–849.

Becker, W.M., Beal, M., Stanley, B.J., and Hauptman, J.G. (2012). Survival after surgery for tracheal collapse and the effect of intrathoracic collapse on survival. *Veterinary Surgery* 41: 501–506.

Beranek, J., Jaresova, H., and Rytz, U. (2014). Use of nitinol self-expandable stents in 26 dogs with tracheal collapse. *Schweizer Archiv für Tierheilkunde* 156: 91–98.

Brisimi, N.G., Papazoglou, L.G., Terzopoulou, A.K. et al. (2022). Influence of age on resistance to distraction after tracheal anastomoses in dogs: an ex vivo study. *Veterinary Surgery* 51 (5): 827–832.

Buback, J.L., Boothe, H.W., and Hobson, H.P. (1996). Surgical treatment of tracheal collapse in dogs: 90 cases. *Journal of the American Veterinary Medical Association* 208: 380–384.

Chisnell, H.K. and Pardo, A.D. (2015). Long-term outcome, complications and disease progression in 23 dogs after placement of tracheal ring prostheses for treatment of extrathoracic tracheal collapse. *Veterinary Surgery* 44: 103–113.

Congiusta, M., Weisse, C., Berent, A.C., and Tozier, E. (2021). Comparison of short-, intermediate-, and long-term results between dogs with tracheal collapse that underwent multimodal medical management alone and those that underwent tracheal endoluminal stent placement. *Journal of the American Veterinary Medical Association* 258: 279–289.

Dallman, M.J. and Bojrab, M.J. (1982). Large-segment tracheal resection and interannular anastomosis with a tension relieving technique in the dog. *American Journal of Veterinary Research* 43: 217–223.

Davis, A.M., Grimes, J.A., Wallace, M.L. et al. (2018). Owner perception of outcome following permanent tracheostomy in dog. *Journal of the American Animal Hospital Association* 54: 285–290.

Demetriou, J.L., Hughes, R., and Sissener, T.R. (2006). Pullout strength for three suture patterns used for canine tracheal anastomosis. *Veterinary Surgery* 35: 278–283.

Durant, A.M., Suraa, P., Rohrback, B., and Bohling, M.W. (2012). Use of nitinol stents for end-stage tracheal collapse in dogs. *Veterinary Surgery* 41: 807–817.

Fingland, R.B., Layton, C.I., Kennedy, G.A., and Galland, J.C. (1995). A comparison of simple continuous versus simple interrupted suture patterns for tracheal anastomosis after large-segment tracheal resection in dogs. *Veterinary Surgery* 24: 320–330.

Gellasch, K.L., Dá Costa Gómez, T., McAnulty, J.F., and Bjorling, D.E. (2002). Use of intraluminal nitinol stents in the treatment of tracheal collapse in a dog. *Journal of the American Veterinary Medical Association* 221: 1719–1723.

Gobbetti, M., Romussi, S., Buracco, P. et al. (2018). Long-term outcome of permanent tracheostomy in 15 dogs with severe laryngeal collapse secondary to brachycephalic airway obstructive syndrome. *Veterinary Surgery* 47: 648–653.

Grimes, J.A., Davis, A.M., Wallace, M.L. et al. (2019). Long-term outcome and risk factors associated with death or the need for revision surgery in dogs with permanent tracheostomies. *Journal of the American Veterinary Medical Association* 254: 1086–1093.

Guenther-Yenke, C.L. and Rozanski, E.A. (2007). Tracheostomy in cats: 23 cases (1998–2006). *Journal of Feline Medicine and Surgery* 9: 451–457.

Hardie, E.M., Spodnick, G.J., Gilson, S.D. et al. (1999). Tracheal rupture in cats: 16 cases (1983–1998). *Journal of the American Veterinary Medical Association* 214: 508–512.

Hsieh, C.M., Tomita, M., Ayabe, H. et al. (1988). Influence of suture on bronchial anastomosis in growing puppies. *Journal of Thoracic and Cardiovascular Surgery* 95: 998–1002.

Jakubiak, M.J., Siedlecki, C.T., Zenger, E. et al. (2005). Laryngeal, laryngotracheal, and tracheal masses in cats: 27 cases (1998–2003). *Journal of the American Animal Hospital Association* 41: 310–316.

Jeung, S.Y., Sohn, S.J., An, J.H. et al. (2019). A retrospective study of theophylline-based therapy with tracheal collapse in small-breed dogs: 47 cases (2013–2017). *Journal of Veterinary Science* 20: e57.

Johnson, L.R. (2000). Tracheal collapse. Diagnosis and medical and surgical treatment. *Veterinary Clinics of North America. Small Animal Practice* 30: 1253–1266.

Johnson, L.R. and Fales, W.H. (2001). Clinical and microbiologic findings in dogs with bronchoscopically diagnosed tracheal collapse: 37 cases (1990–1995). *Journal of the American Veterinary Medical Association* 219: 1247–1250.

Johnson, L.R. and Pollard, R.E. (2010). Tracheal collapse and bronchomalacia in dogs: 58 cases (7/2001–1/2008). *Journal of Veterinary Internal Medicine* 24: 298–305.

Kim, J.Y., Han, H.J., Yun, H.Y. et al. (2008). The safety and efficacy of a new self-expandable intratracheal nitinol stent for the tracheal collapse in dogs. *Journal of Veterinary Science* 9: 91–93.

Lau, R.E., Schwartz, A., and Buergelt, C.D. (1980). Tracheal resection and anastomosis in dogs. *Journal of the American Veterinary Medical Association* 176: 134–138.

Macready, D.M., Johnson, L.R., and Pollard, R.E. (2007). Fluoroscopic and radiographic evaluation of tracheal collapse in dogs: 62 cases (2001–2006). *Journal of the American Veterinary Medical Association* 230: 1870–1876.

Maggiore, A.D. (2020). An update on tracheal and airway collapse in dogs. *Veterinary Clinics of North America: Small Animal Practice* 50: 419–430.

Marolf, A., Blaik, M., and Specht, A. (2007). A retrospective study of the relationship between tracheal collapse and bronchiectasis in dogs. *Veterinary Radiology & Ultrasound* 8: 199–203.

Mitchell, S.L., McCarthy, R., Rudloff, E., and Pernell, R.T. (2000). Tracheal rupture associated with intubation in cats: 20 cases (1996–1998). *Journal of the American Veterinary Medical Association* 216: 1592–1595.

Mittleman, E., Weisse, C., Mehler, S.J., and Lee, J.A. (2004). Fracture of an endoluminal nitinol stent used in the treatment of tracheal collapse in a dog. *Journal of the American Veterinary Medical Association* 225: 1217–1221.

Moritz, A., Schneider, M., and Bauer, N. (2004). Management of advanced tracheal collapse in dogs using intraluminal self-expanding biliary wallstents. *Journal of Veterinary Internal Medicine* 18: 31–42.

Nicholson, I. and Baines, S. (2012). Complications associated with temporary tracheostomy tubes in 42 dogs (1998 to 2007). *Journal of Small Animal Practice* 53: 108–114.

Occhipinti, L.L. and Hauptman, J.G. (2014). Long-term outcome of permanent tracheostomies in dogs: 21 cases (2000–2012). *Canadian Veterinary Journal* 55: 357–360.

Ouellet, M., Dunn, M.E., Lussier, B. et al. (2006). Noninvasive correction of a fractured endoluminal nitinol tracheal stent in a dog. *Journal of the American Animal Hospital Association* 42: 467–471.

Pardali, D., Adamama-Moraitou, K.K., Rallis, T.S. et al. (2010). Tidal breathing flow–volume loop analysis for the diagnosis and staging of tracheal collapse in dogs. *Journal of Veterinary Internal Medicine* 24: 832–842.

Pratschke, K.M., Hughes, J.M., Guerin, S.R., and Bellenger, C.R. (1999). Foley catheter technique for removal of a tracheal foreign body in a cat. *Veterinary Record* 144: 181–182.

Radlinsky, M.G., Fossum, T.W., Walker, M.A. et al. (1997). Evaluation of the Palmaz stent in the trachea and mainstem bronchi or normal dogs. *Veterinary Surgery* 26: 99–107.

Raske, M., Weisse, C., Berent, A.C. et al. (2018). Immediate, short-, and long-term changes in tracheal stent diameter, length, and positioning after placement in dogs with tracheal collapse syndrome. *Journal of Veterinary Internal Medicine* 32: 782–791.

Rosenheck, S., Davis, G., Sammarco, C.D., and Bastian, R. (2017). Effect of variations in stent placement on outcome of endoluminal stenting for canine tracheal collapse. *Journal of the American Animal Hospital Association* 53: 150–158.

Rudorf, H., Herrtage, M.E., and White, R.A. (1997). Use of ultrasonography in the diagnosis of tracheal collapse. *Journal of Small Animal Practice* 38: 513–518.

Spodnick, G.J. and Nwadike, B.S. (1997). Surgical management of extrathoracic tracheal collapse in two large-breed dogs. *Journal of the American Veterinary Medical Association* 211: 1545–1548.

Stepnik, M.W., Mehl, M.L., Hardie, E.M. et al. (2009). Outcome of permanent tracheostomy for treatment of upper airway obstruction in cats: 21 cases (1990–2007). *Journal of the American Veterinary Medical Association* 234: 638–643.

Stordalen, M.B., Silveira, F., Fenner, J.V.H., and Demetriou, J.L. (2020). Outcome of temporary tracheostomy tube-placement following surgery for brachycephalic obstructive airway syndrome in 42 dogs. *Journal of Small Animal Practice* 61: 292–299.

Suematsu, M., Suematsu, H., Minamoto, T. et al. (2019). Long-term outcomes of 54 dogs with tracheal collapse treated with a continuous extraluminal tracheal prosthesis. *Veterinary Surgery* 48: 825–834.

Sura, P.A. and Krahwinkel, D.J. (2008). Self-expanding nitinol stents for the treatment of tracheal collapse in dogs: 12 cases (2001–2004). *Journal of the American Veterinary Medical Association* 232: 228–236.

Tangner, C.H. and Hobson, H.P. (1982). A retrospective study of 20 surgically managed cases of collapsed trachea. *Veterinary Surgery* 11: 146–149.

Tenwolde, A.C., Johnson, L.R., Hunt, G.B. et al. (2010). The role of bronchoscopy in foreign body removal in dogs and cats: 37 cases (2000–2008). *Journal of Veterinary Internal Medicine* 24: 1063–1068.

Tinga, S., Thieman Mankin, K.M., Peycke, L.E., and Cohen, N.D. (2015). Comparison of outcome after use of extra-luminal rings and intra-luminal stents for treatment of tracheal collapse in dogs. *Veterinary Surgery* 44: 858–865.

Tivers, M.S. and Moore, A.H. (2006). Tracheal foreign bodies in the cat and the use of fluoroscopy for removal: 12 cases. *Journal of Small Animal Practice* 47: 155–159.

Ueda, Y., Sato, T., Yutaka, Y. et al. (2021). Replacement of a 5-cm intra-thoracic trachea with a tissue-engineered prosthesis in a canine model. *Annals of Thoracic Surgery* 113 (6): 1891–1900.

Violette, N.P., Weisse, C., Berent, A.C., and Lamb, K.E. (2019). Correlations among tracheal dimensions, tracheal stent dimensions, and major complications after endoluminal stenting of tracheal collapse syndrome in dogs. *Journal of Veterinary Internal Medicine* 33: 2209–2216.

Weisse, C., Berent, A., Violette, N. et al. (2019). Short-, intermediate-, and long-term results for endoluminal stent placement in dogs with tracheal collapse. *Journal of the American Veterinary Medical Association* 254: 380–392.

White, R.N. (1995). Unilateral arytenoid lateralisation and extraluminal polypropylene ring prostheses for correction of tracheal collapse in the dog. *Journal of Small Animal Practice* 36: 151–158.

White, R.N. and Burton, C.A. (2000). Surgical management of intra-thoracic tracheal avulsion in cats: long-term results in 9 consecutive cases. *Veterinary Surgery* 29: 430–435.

White, R.A.S. and Williams, J.M. (1994). Tracheal collapse in the dogs: is there really a role for surgery? A survey of 100 cases. *Journal of Small Animal Practice* 35: 191–196.

Woo, H.-M., Kim, M.-J. et al. (2007). Intraluminal tracheal stent fracture in a Yorkshire terrier. *Canadian Veterinary Journal* 48: 1063–1066.

Worth, D.B., Grimes, J.A., Jiménez, D.A. et al. (2018). Risk factors for temporary tracheostomy tube placement following surgery to alleviate signs of brachycephalic obstructive airway syndrome in dogs. *Journal of the American Veterinary Medical Association* 253: 1158–1163.

Zang, M., Chen, K., and Yu, P. (2010). Reconstruction of large tracheal defects in a canine model: lessons learned. *Journal of Reconstructive Microsurgery* 26: 391–399.

41

Surgical Diseases of the Lungs

Eric Monnet

Surgery of the lungs in dogs and cats is mostly due to acquired pulmonary disease. Congenital disease of the lungs is either compatible or incompatible with life (Lopez 2007). The severe anomalies of agenesis or hypoplasia cause death shortly after birth. Hypoplasia of one lung or lung lobe is rarely diagnosed unless chest radiographs are taken or a necropsy performed (Saperstein *et al.* 1976). Congenital tracheoesophageal and bronchoesophageal fistulas are extremely rare in dogs and cats (Basher *et al.* 1991; Johnson 2005).

Surgery of the lungs requires access to the thoracic cavity by thoracotomy or thoracoscopy. Thoracic surgery interferes with pulmonary and cardiac function, so the surgeon must possess a thorough understanding of pulmonary and cardiac physiology. It also requires appropriate monitoring of the patient to document and treat those changes.

Cyst, bullae, and bleb

Cystic and bullous lesions in the lungs are characterized by a thin-walled cavity within the lung parenchyma (Anderson 1987; Nelson & Sellon 2005; Lopez 2007). Cysts can be filled with fluid or air and are covered by respiratory epithelium (Aron & Kornegay 1983; Nelson & Sellon 2005). Pulmonary cysts are most commonly associated with trauma (Aron & Kornegay 1983). Blunt trauma to the chest with pulmonary contusion seems to be the most common cause of pulmonary cysts in dogs and cats (Aron & Kornegay 1983). Younger animals appear to be more at risk for the development of a cyst after trauma. If an infection is present, the cyst will

become a pneumatocele or an abscess with destruction of the respiratory epithelium. Pneumatoceles can also result from pneumonia (Nelson & Sellon 2005).

Lung bullae and blebs (pseudocysts) are similar to cysts, but have no epithelial lining (Berzon *et al.* 1979; Kramek *et al.* 1985; Kramek & Caywood 1987; Nelson & Sellon 2005). Bullae and blebs are described as large blisters with a fibrous wall. Bullae are large air spaces that develop within the lung parenchyma, whereas blebs are small accumulations of air between the visceral pleura and the lung parenchyma (Figure 41.1) (Anderson 1987). These cavities develop from traumatic rupture and coalescence of alveoli, and are frequently secondary to obstructive lung disease (Kramek *et al.* 1985; Kramek & Caywood 1987; Lipscomb *et al.* 2003; Lopez 2007).

Bullae and cysts show similar complications of infection, abscessation, rupture causing pneumothorax, and

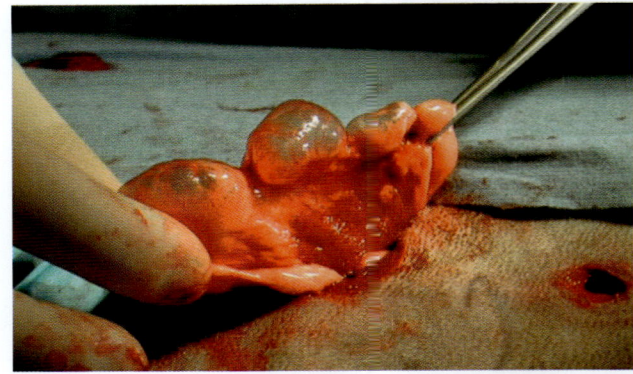

Figure 41.1 Bullae in the periphery of a cranial lung lobe in a dog.

---

local compression of lung tissue leading to dyspnea, exercise intolerance, and abdominal respiration (Nelson & Sellon 2005). Auscultation may reveal decreased ventilatory sounds on the affected side and increased heart sounds on the contralateral side (displaced heart due to a space-occupying cyst).

Spontaneous idiopathic pneumothorax warrants close examination of radiographs detailing the lung profile and parenchyma for bleb, bullae, or cyst formation (Puerto *et al.* 2002; Lipscomb *et al.* 2003). Computed tomography (CT) has been recommended for the diagnosis of bullae in dogs with spontaneous pneumothorax (Puerto *et al.* 2002; Au *et al.* 2006). Atelectasis of the lobe containing the ruptured cavity occurs and may obscure identification of underlying cysts.

Conservative support of spontaneous pneumothorax by continuous chest drainage should be tried for 2–3 days before partial or complete lobectomy (Puerto *et al.* 2002). Many cases respond to this therapy, but the recurrence rate is high (Puerto *et al.* 2002). Lung lobectomy is the treatment of choice for spontaneous pneumothorax in dogs. Thoracoscopy has been used to evaluate visceral surfaces for additional cysts and locate the ruptured cavity (Brissot *et al.* 2003). It can be difficult to accomplish a thorough evaluation of the entire surface of the lungs with the endoscope. Mechanical pleurodesis can be attempted at the time of surgery to induce complete pleural adhesion and reduce the risk of recurrence. Successful production of complete adhesion for control of the disease is uncommon in dogs (Jerram *et al.* 1999). It should not be the primary treatment for spontaneous pneumothorax in dogs.

Bronchoesophageal fistulas

Congenital tracheoesophageal and bronchoesophageal fistulas are extremely rare in dogs and cats (Basher *et al.* 1991; Johnson 2005). Bronchoesophageal fistulas can result from foreign bodies that become wedged into the esophagus. Pressure necrosis can induce the formation of a fistula between the esophagus and the lung parenchyma or an airway. Saliva and food can then access the airway of a lung lobe and induce pneumonia. Dogs with a bronchoesophageal fistula are often presented for weight loss, elevated temperature, and coughing associated with eating. Thoracic radiography with water-soluble iodine is the best diagnostic tool (Figure 41.2). Flexible endoscopy of the esophagus is also a valid diagnostic technique to visualize the location and size of the fistula (Figure 41.3).

The only treatment is surgical lung lobectomy and closure of the fistula. An intercostal thoracotomy is indicated because it allows better exposure of the esophagus. After identification of the affected lung lobe, a lung

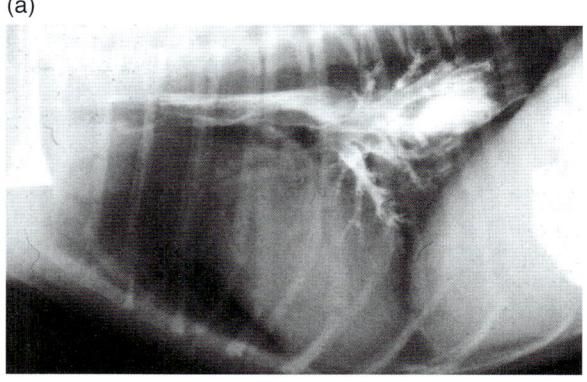

(a)

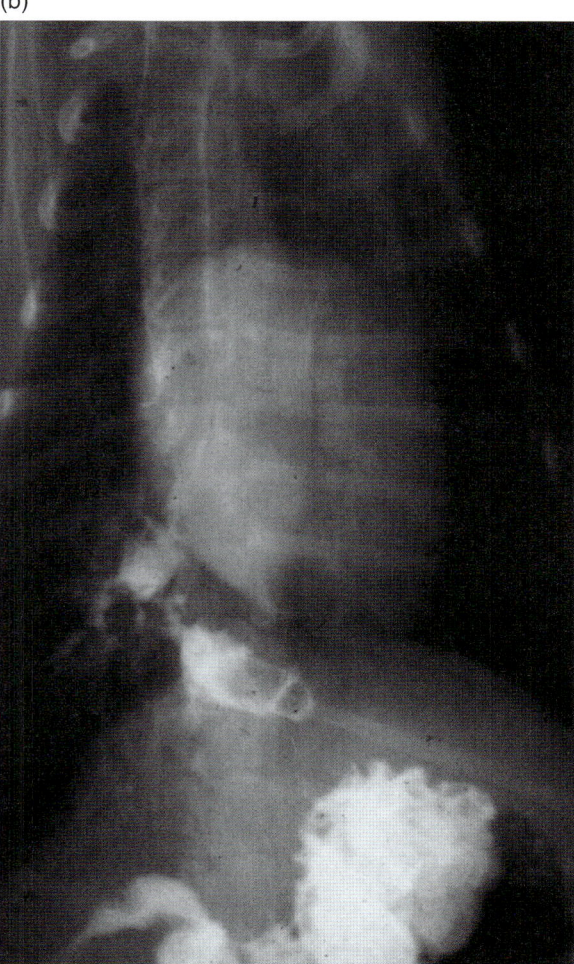

(b)

Figure 41.2 (a) Lateral and (b) ventrodorsal radiographs with water-soluble iodine demonstrating a bronchoesophageal fistula in a caudal lobe.

lobectomy is performed. The fistula is then resected from the esophagus (Figure 41.4). The edges of the esophagus are débrided and closed with two simple continuous sutures using monofilament absorbable suture material.

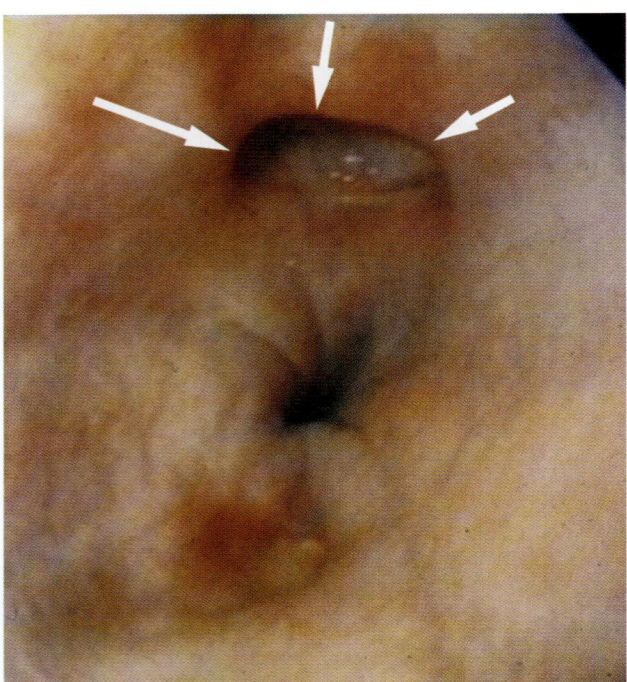

Figure 41.3 Endoscopy of the esophagus. The bronchoesophageal fistula (white arrows) is visible in the distal part of the esophagus.

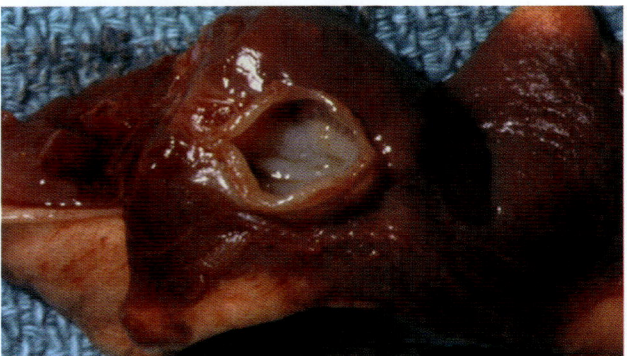

Figure 41.4 The lung lobe with the bronchoesophageal fistula.

Consolidated lung lobe and abscess

A consolidated lung lobe results most commonly from pneumonia. The pneumonia is usually secondary to a foreign body, bacterial or fungal infection, or parasites (Murphy *et al.* 1997a). Lung abscesses are more common in cats than in dogs, although they are relatively uncommon in both. Thoracic penetrating wounds, vascular obstruction, and neoplastic tissue with a necrotic center can also present as an abscess in the lung parenchyma (Nelson & Sellon 2005). Lung abscesses are commonly associated with pyothorax in dogs and cats because the abscess has ruptured into the pleural space at the time of diagnosis (Rooney & Monnet 2002;

Waddell *et al.* 2002). A consolidated lung lobe induces a low *V/Q* mismatch and significant desaturation of the arterial blood, which will interfere with the activity level of the patient.

Barbed seeds or hulls (grass awns) and other small bodies inhaled into the bronchi resist dislodgment by coughing and work their way along the small air passages (Arnoczky & O'Neill 1979). A plant awn frequently breaks into parenchymal tissue and causes a septic focus that develops into an abscess. Awns may migrate some distance, leaving lung abscesses, pyothorax, and draining tracts in their wake. Small rocks, nuts, or other dense objects that gain entrance into the bronchial tree may obstruct or act like a one-way valve at a small bronchus. The foreign body will be encapsulated in dense fibrous tissue surrounding an abscess. It can also create a fistulous tract. The part of the involved lobe with the foreign body usually becomes atelectatic and secondarily septic.

History

This condition is manifested as a chronic debilitating disease with various degrees of respiratory distress and persistent low-grade fever.

Diagnosis

In a study by Murphy *et al.* (1997b), the mean age of presentation of 59 dogs treated with lung lobectomy for pneumonia was 5.0 ± 2.8 years. Anemia of a chronic disorder may be present. Lung abscess involves part of a lobe and it may be thick or thin walled, or may rupture into the airway or pleural space, but rarely erodes a blood vessel. Ventilatory sounds range from moist rales and friction rub to no sounds over the mass. Muffled sounds are due to pleural effusion. If pleural effusion is present, a chest drain to relieve the respiratory distress may be necessary. Severe leukocytosis with a degenerative left shift is present on blood work.

If a foreign body has been inhaled, vague and intermittent signs of respiratory disease may be noted. Initial inhalation of the foreign body causes severe dry coughing, followed by periods without clinical signs and periods of low-grade respiratory infection with a moist cough and fever. A temporary response to antibiotic therapy is common.

Chest radiography aids in locating the involved region. The pleural space may have to be lavaged and drained before a definite radiographic diagnosis can be made. An abscess has the density of water, unless it has ruptured and drained. In the latter case, air contrast may be seen in the abscessed cavity if it connects with the respiratory system. A consolidated lung lobe may or may not be present as an alveolar pattern with an air

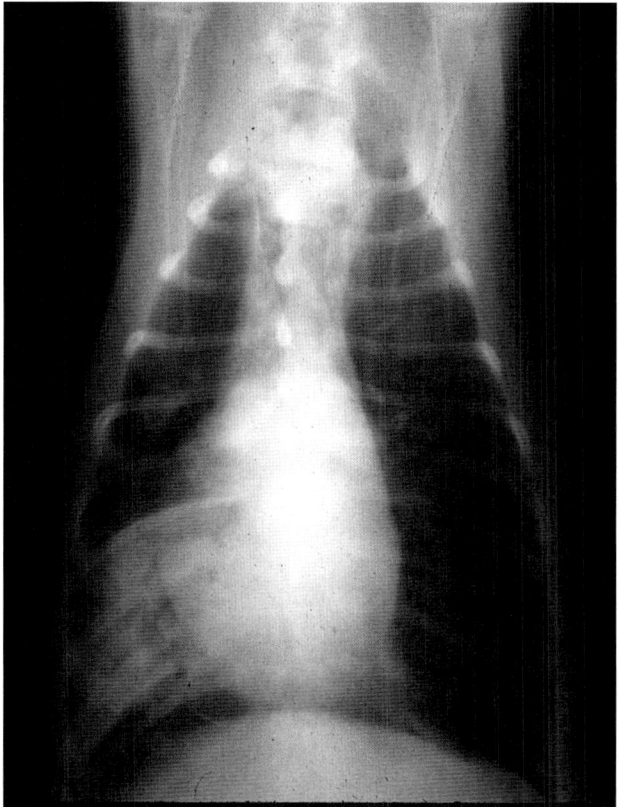

Figure 41.5 Thoracic radiograph of a dog with an abscess in the right caudal lung lobe.

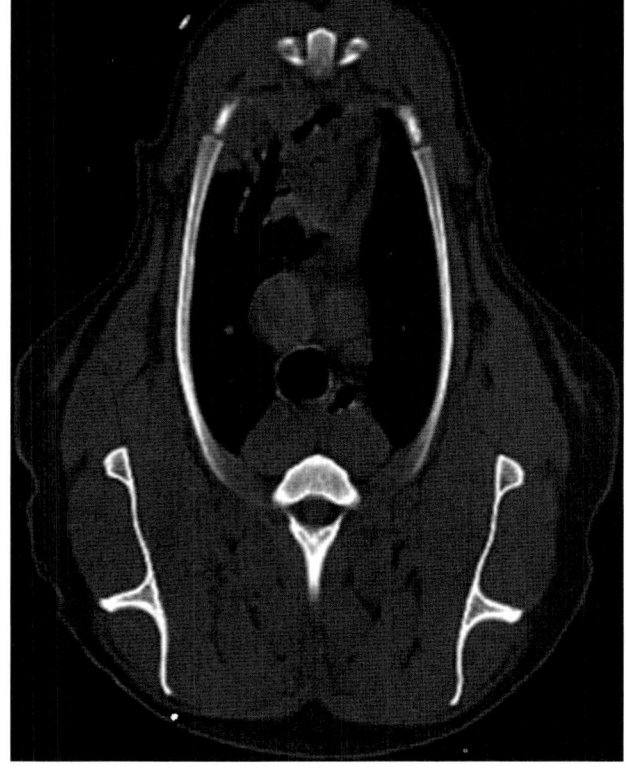

Figure 41.6 Computed tomography scan of a dog with a foreign body in its left cranial lung lobe.

bronchogram generalized to the entire lobe (Figure 41.5). CT can also be used to identify a foreign body in a lung lobe or help further localize the lesion (Figure 41.6).

If a foreign body is present in the lower airway, radiographic examination may show an area of increased lung density compatible with local atelectasis, bronchopneumonia, abscess with a thick fibrous capsule, or granuloma. Radiopaque bodies are easily seen, whereas radiolucent bodies are difficult to outline when located deep in the bronchial system. Exudation coming from a single main bronchus during bronchoscopy is supportive of a local infection, with a high index of suspicion for a foreign body.

Medical approach

Medical management should be optimized before surgical intervention is begun. Bronchoalveolar lavage should be used to collect fluid from the diseased lung and a culture and sensitivity performed. The most commonly isolated bacteria in dogs with pneumonia are *Escherichia coli*, *Klebsiella pneumoniae*, *Staphylococcus*, *Streptococcus*, *Pseudomonas*, and *Fusobacterium* (Murphy *et al.* 1997b; Nelson & Sellon 2005). In cats, *Nocardia*

and *Corynebacterium* were present (Nelson & Sellon 2005). Appropriate antibiotics are given for at least 2–3 weeks (Murphy *et al.* 1997a; Nelson & Sellon 2005). If a pleural effusion is present, a thoracostomy tube might be indicated if the amount of effusion is interfering with lung ventilation and expansion. Pleural lavage is actively pursued if a pyothorax is present. If the condition is not improving within a week of appropriate medical treatment or if the condition of the patient is deteriorating, surgery is then indicated to remove the diseased lung.

Surgical approach

An aggressive approach to surgical exploration is frequently beneficial because it decreases recovery time by removing the initiating cause. Patients are prepared so that exposure of both hemithoraces is possible. A sternotomy is the method of choice because it allows evaluation of both sides of the thoracic cavity with its organs. Adhesions of lung lobes to the lateral wall are possible, but not necessarily very common. These can be dissected free by careful digital pressure and sharp dissection without significant lung damage (except in well-organized lesions).

Usually adhesions are not present along the sternum because the mediastinum prevents their formation.

The involved lung lobe is located, and a partial or complete lobectomy is performed. If several lobes are involved the entire diseased parenchyma should be removed. Sheets of fibrin covering lung surfaces are undesirable and should be removed because they can harbor bacteria. Decortication is indicated if chronic restrictive pleuritis is present preventing lung reexpansion. If only one lung lobe requires decortication, a lung lobectomy is preferred. Decortication is a difficult surgical procedure that results in lesions of the lung parenchyma and induction of air leakage. Chest drains are placed, and the thoracic cavity is closed.

Bacterial pneumonia in dogs as a cause of a consolidated lung lobe seems to have a higher mortality rate than an abscess due to a foreign body or fungal infection (Murphy et al. 1997b). The mortality rate was 20% in a study of 59 cases and it correlated with the amount of lung parenchyma removed (Murphy et al. 1997b). If one lung lobe was removed the mortality rate was 14%, whereas it was 60% if three lobes were resected. No more than 50% of the lung parenchyma can be removed at the time of surgery. Of the dogs that survived the surgery, 54% had resolution of their pneumonia (Murphy et al. 1997b). The dogs that resolved their pneumonia had a median survival time of 96 months, while the dogs that did not had a median survival time of 10 months after surgery.

Bronchiectasis

Bronchiectasis is a localized or diffuse destructive lung disease that results in severe dilatation of large airways with accumulation of secretions. Proteolytic enzymes and cytokines produced by inflammatory cells induce severe lysis of the muscular and elastic support of the airway. The inflamed bronchial walls lose collagen and elastin elements, and a granulomatous reaction develops. Bronchiectasis can be associated with primary ciliary dyskinesia as a result of chronic respiratory disease (Hawkins et al. 2003; Johnson 2005). It is the most devastating complication of chronic bronchitis. If the lesion is localized to a portion of the wall of a bronchi it is sacculated, whereas if it affects the entire wall of the bronchi it is cylindrical. Bronchiectasis in young animals can be assumed to be congenital. Dilated and sacculated bronchi develop and retain secretions, resulting in recurring infections (Johnson 2005). Bronchiectasis manifests grossly as a prominent lump in the lungs. It induces atelectasis of the surrounding alveoli because it is obstructing the airway and compressing alveoli (Lopez 2007).

Patients with bronchiectasis have a chronic history of cough with frequent bouts of pneumonia. Moist crackles can be heard on auscultation. Loud bronchial sounds can be present if severe dilatation of a bronchus is present. Nasal discharge can also occur if a pneumonia is present. Recurrent fever with signs of respiratory infection, anorexia, and debilitation with exercise intolerance are present in these patients (Hawkins et al. 2003). American cocker spaniels and miniature poodles were 7 and 14 times more at risk than other breeds to be presented for bronchiectasis (Hawkins et al. 2003). The right cranial lung lobe was the most commonly affected lobe in a retrospective study of 316 cases (Hawkins et al. 2003).

Thoracic radiography shows signs of atelectasis, consolidation, and fibrosis of bronchi. Dilated bronchi can also be seen, although radiography is fairly insensitive to these changes. Cylindrical dilation is more common than sacculated bronchiectasis (Hawkins et al. 2003). CT or bronchoscopy is more helpful for the diagnosis. Contrast bronchography is needed to outline the bronchi for positive diagnosis. Bronchoscopy is the most reliable diagnostic technique. Loss of circular shape of the bronchi, sacculation or dilatation of the bronchi, hyperemia of the mucosa, and large amounts of secretions are commonly seen during bronchoscopy. Bronchoalveolar lavage typically shows a suppurative inflammation with neutrophils and monocytes. Culture for aerobic and anaerobic bacteria is indicated (Hawkins et al. 2003; Johnson 2005).

Lobectomy of the affected lobes is recommended in patients with one or two involved lobes. Removal of affected lobes eliminates the initiating foci for recurrent infection. Continuous monitoring of remaining lobes and intense medical management of respiratory infection are mandatory to prevent recurrence. Prognosis is guarded. Median survival of dogs treated for bronchiectasis is 16 months (Hawkins et al. 2003).

Lung laceration

Blunt or penetrating trauma to the thoracic cavity can induce lung laceration (Hankins et al. 1977; Spackman & Caywood 1987; Shahar et al. 1997). Dogs or cats with lung laceration are usually presented with a pneumothorax. Since the trauma is the cause of the laceration, lung contusions are present and aggravate the clinical presentation of the patient. Lung lacerations are usually small and resolve on their own or with the aid of chest drainage to control the accumulation of air and blood in the chest. Rupture of the visceral pleura of the lung by blunt trauma is commonly associated with rib fractures. Ends of fractured ribs lacerate the parenchyma and bronchi as they are depressed medially by the impact. Lung lacerations not associated with rib fractures have been noted. Lateral compression of the chest wall with a closed glottis causing a rapid increase in airway pressure has been suggested as a cause of explosive rupture. The rapid decrease in these pressures immediately after chest compression may result in additional shearing tears.

Radiographic evidence of fractured ribs, increased lung density (contusion, edema), and free air and fluid in the thorax aids in identifying lung lobe lacerations. Air and fluid are quickly dispersed to both sides of the thorax in most trauma cases.

Medical treatment

Medical treatment is the treatment of choice for patients with traumatic pneumothorax and lung laceration due to blunt trauma or penetrating wounds. The patient needs to be stabilized before any surgery can be started. Usually lung contusions aggravate gas exchange. Chest tubes can be placed with heavy sedation and local analgesia if the pneumothorax is interfering with ventilation. If the pneumothorax does not resolve in 3–4 days, surgery is then indicated to treat pneumothorax. If a wound is present, it should be explored and débrided as soon as the patient is stabilized. If the thoracic wall is not intact, it should be repaired so as to be able to establish negative pressure in the pleural space. Minimal suture material and foreign material should be used to repair the chest wall because the wound is contaminated.

Surgical approach

If the pneumothorax resulting from a lung laceration does not resolve in 3–4 days, a median sternotomy should be performed to enable inspection of the entire thoracic cavity and individual lung lobes. Flooding the chest with saline during positive-pressure ventilation locates air leaks. Some lacerations may not leak continuously. Maintaining intermittent elevated pressure in the airway is recommended as a way of maximizing the observation of a leak.

Unsealed lacerations are closed in a mattress pattern using absorbable suture (4-0 or 5-0). Contused or edematous lung tissue is friable and tends to tear when sutured. In these cases, suture mounted on Teflon pledgets should be used to provide an adequate seal without tearing the tissue. Deep lacerations into the lung parenchyma may involve large airways that leak profusely. If the lesions are peripheral, a partial lung lobectomy should be performed. If the lesion is close to the hilus of the lung, the airway can be closed with simple interrupted absorbable sutures (4-0 or 5-0). The parenchyma is then closed with mattress sutures as already described.

Chest tubes are placed after surgery and lavage of the pleural space should be performed for 2–3 days. Cytology can be performed on the chest fluid to evaluate for the presence of pyothorax.

Lung lobe torsion

The extent of movement of each lung lobe is limited by the presence of other lung lobes, as well as the surrounding structures. Pulmonary ligaments are thin sheets of pleura that stabilize the caudal lung lobes by creating an attachment of these lobes to the caudal mediastinum. Lung lobe torsion is an uncommon condition that has been reported in dogs and cats (Rawlings *et al.* 1970; Lord *et al.* 1973; Alexander *et al.* 1974; Moses 1980; Johnston *et al.* 1984; Silberstein *et al.* 1991; Hoover *et al.* 1992; Neath *et al.* 2000; White & Corzo-Menendez 2000; Rooney *et al.* 2001; Spranklin *et al.* 2003; Hofeling *et al.* 2004; Choi & Yoon 2006; Murphy & Brisson 2006; Millard *et al.* 2008; Latimer *et al.* 2017). Dogs with deep narrow chests have a higher incidence of lung lobe torsion, and the right cranial and middle lobes are more frequently affected (Lord *et al.* 1973; Johnston *et al.* 1984; Miller & Sherrill 1987; Gelzer *et al.* 1997). However, cats, Yorkshire terriers, and pugs have also been diagnosed with lung lobe torsion (Rooney *et al.* 2001; Choi & Yoon 2006; Murphy & Brisson 2006; Millard *et al.* 2008). Most torsions cause venous and bronchus obstruction, but a portion of the arterial blood flow remains. The lobe becomes severely congested and consolidated as fluid moves into the interstitial tissue and airways. The condition is associated with chronic respiratory disease, chylothorax, trauma, thoracic surgery, and neoplasia (Williams & Duncan 1986; Fossum *et al.* 1993; Kerpsack *et al.* 1994; Neath *et al.* 2000). Recurring lung lobe torsion has been reported in three dogs, with a time interval from the initial torsion of 5–180 days (Johnston *et al.* 1984).

Clinical signs

Although nonspecific, clinical signs are related to local and systemic effects of the consolidated or necrotic lung lobe and accumulation of fluid in the pleural space. Dogs can manifest an acute or chronic presentation. Coughing with hemoptysis is very common in dogs with lung lobe torsion. Pugs are more commonly presented with chronic clinical signs. Patients are depressed, have a cough, and show various degrees of respiratory distress. Anorexia with weight loss and occasional vomiting occurs in long-standing cases (1–3 weeks). Moist rales are heard with muffled respiratory and cardiac sounds due to accumulation of pleural fluid.

Diagnosis

Thoracocentesis produces large amounts of a serosanguineous or chylous fluid (Williams & Duncan 1986; Gelzer *et al.* 1997; Neath *et al.* 2000; Murphy & Brisson 2006). Cytologic study of this fluid reveals significant numbers of erythrocytes and leukocytes but rare evidence of sepsis.

Radiography shows evidence of pleural effusion and lung consolidation. Pleural fluid may have to be drained before the consolidated lung lobe can be seen (Siems *et al.* 1998; Seiler *et al.* 2008). Fluid may remain trapped around the affected lobe after chest drainage. Early in the process, radiographs of the lobe indicate air bronchograms, but this air is absorbed and replaced by fluid within 2–3 days. The lobe may reach an inflated size but is consolidated (Figure 41.7).

The obstructed orifice of the main bronchus supplying the affected lobe can be demonstrated by positive contrast bronchography and bronchoscopy (Moses 1980). The orifice may have ridges of wrinkled mucosa and appear narrow when observed through the bronchoscope (Moses 1980).

Medical therapy

Initial therapy is symptomatic and aimed at stabilization. Respiratory distress is relieved with chest drainage,

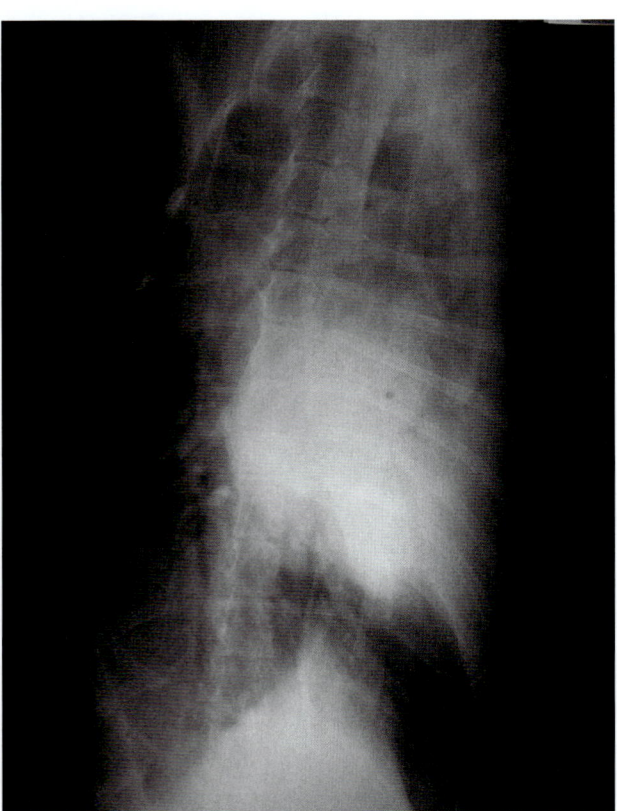

Figure 41.7 Ventrodorsal radiograph of a dog with a lung lobe torsion of the left cranial lung lobe.

oxygen therapy, and medical care of associated respiratory disease. Intravenous fluid therapy is indicated if dehydration is present and is given before surgery in all cases to provide adequate circulating blood volume. Antibiotics are given before surgery. Surgery should be performed as soon as possible.

Surgical approach

A median sternotomy should be used to approach the thoracic cavity because it will allow complete exploration of the thoracic cavity and of all lung lobes. Total lobectomy of the involved lung lobe is the treatment of choice (see later section on lobectomy). Most torsioned lung lobes are congested, friable, and necrotic. They should not be untwisted because it would release inflammatory cytokines and endotoxins.

The lung lobe should remain in the twisted position. Stapling equipment should be used for the lobectomy because it can be performed with the lung in an abnormal position. If stapling equipment is not available, the pedicle of the lobe is clamped with noncrushing forceps before the lobe is untwisted (Lord *et al.* 1973; Teunissen *et al.* 1976). After untwisting the lung lobe, a lung lobectomy can be performed with sutures. Effusion associated with the torsion, even if it is chylous, will resolve within 7 days of surgery (Johnston *et al.* 1984; Kerpsack *et al.* 1994; Neath *et al.* 2000; Murphy & Brisson 2006).

Neoplasia

Primary pulmonary neoplasia is most commonly diagnosed in middle-aged dogs and cats (Ogilvie *et al.* 1989b; McNiel *et al.* 1997). Metastatic pulmonary neoplasia is more common than primary lung neoplasia. Primary lung neoplasia represents 1% of all tumors in dogs (Withrow 2001). Most primary lung tumors are carcinomas from the bronchi. Squamous cell carcinoma is occasionally diagnosed in dogs and cats (McNiel *et al.* 1997; Withrow 2001). Osteosarcoma and other mesenchymal tumors have been diagnosed (Withrow 2001). Primary pulmonary histolytic sarcoma has been described in dogs (Marlowe *et al.* 2018). Papillary (bronchoalveolar in origin) carcinoma represents 76% of lung tumors in dogs, solid (bronchial in origin) carcinomas 10%, mucoepidermal (combination of squamous cell carcinoma and adenocarcinoma) carcinomas 7%, acinar (bronchial in origin) adenocarcinomas 6%, and squamous cell carcinomas 1% (McNiel *et al.* 1997).

Primary lung tumors have high metastatic potential. At the time of diagnosis, multiple lung masses or tumor invasion is present in 37–55% of cases. Bronchial lymph nodes are invaded in 22–25% of cases (Ogilvie *et al.* 1989a,b; McNiel *et al.* 1997). At the time of necropsy, metastasis has been documented in 100% of squamous cell carcinomas, 90% of anaplastic carcinomas, and 50% of carcinomas (Brodey & Craig 1965). Lung tumors metastasize usually to the lymph nodes and lung parenchyma. Metastases have been reported in the pericardium, pleura, heart, pancreas, and adrenal glands (Brodey & Craig 1965). Canine pulmonary lymphomatoid granulomatosis is a rare lymphoid neoplasm with a predilection for pulmonary involvement (Postorino et al. 1989; Berry et al. 1990). It may have a better prognosis than other neoplasms of the lungs.

A solitary mass in a caudal lung lobe is the most common radiologic sign of a primary lung tumor. Cavitation of the mass can be seen if the mass has a necrotic center. Hilar lymph nodes should be evaluated on radiography and CT since they are prognostic indicators (McNiel et al. 1997; Withrow 2001). Fine-needle aspiration of a large peripheral mass can provide a diagnosis in 80% of cases, but the complication rate can be elevated (Teske et al. 1991). Thoracic masses may cause hypertrophic osteopathy (Liptak et al. 2004).

Primary and metastatic neoplasia of the lung is not surgically approached unless it appears as a solitary nodule, diagnostic biopsy is desired, or a salvage procedure is feasible. A lung lobectomy by either thoracotomy or thoracoscopy is recommended.

A mean survival time of 13 months after surgical treatment has been reported (McNiel et al. 1997). Dogs with well-differentiated tumors had a significantly longer median disease-free interval (493 days) than dogs with moderately differentiated tumors (191 days) or poorly differentiated tumors (0 days) (McNiel et al. 1997). Squamous cell carcinoma is associated with a shorter survival time (8 months) than adenocarcinoma (19 months) (McNiel et al. 1997). Dogs with a smaller tumor (<100 mL) survived for 20 months, whereas dogs with a larger tumor (>100 mL) survived for only 8 months (McNiel et al. 1997). Dogs with papillary adenocarcinoma have the longest survival time (495 days) and disease-free interval (365 days) (McNiel et al. 1997). Dogs with other tumor types have a median survival time of 44 days and disease-free interval of 14 days. Dogs with a well-differentiated tumor had a survival time of 790 days and disease-free interval of 493 days. In dogs where the regional lymph nodes are involved, the survival time (26 days) and disease-free interval (6 days) are significantly shorter than in dogs without lymph node involvement (survival time 452 days, disease-free interval 351 days) (McNiel et al. 1997). Biopsy of the hilar lymph nodes is important at the time of surgery. Dogs with a well-differentiated adenocarcinoma less than 4 cm in diameter, no lymph node metastasis, and no pleural effusion have the best prognosis. Half of these patients survived for 1 year (Mehlhaff et al. 1984; Ogilvie et al. 1989b; McNiel et al. 1997). Squamous cell carcinoma seems to have a worse prognosis (50% survival at 8 months) (Mehlhaff et al. 1984; McNiel et al. 1997). Cats have a worse prognosis than dogs because the disease is more advanced at the time of diagnosis (Mehlhaff & Mooney 1985). Primary pulmonary histolytic sarcoma treated surgically (374 days) had a significantly better overall survival than dogs treated medically (131 days) (Marlowe et al. 2018).

Surgery of the lungs

Partial lung lobectomy

Excision of a portion of a lung lobe to remove isolated disease or for diagnostic biopsy is relatively safe. Lesions involving the distal two-thirds or less of a lung lobe can be excised using partial lobectomy. Nonresponsive lung abscesses, cysts or bullae, small tumors, and severe lacerations are treated by this technique.

The affected lobe is approached through an intercostal thoracotomy. If the affected area is near the apex of a lung lobe, a simple wedge or distal lobe amputation is performed. The area of the lung lobe to be removed is identified, and a pair of crushing forceps is placed across the lobe at the resection level (Figure 41.8). If a wedge is taken out, two pairs of forceps are used to outline it. A continuous overlapping hemostatic/pneumostatic suture (3-0 or 4-0 absorbable suture) is placed 4–5 mm proximal to the forceps. The suture is tied at its beginning

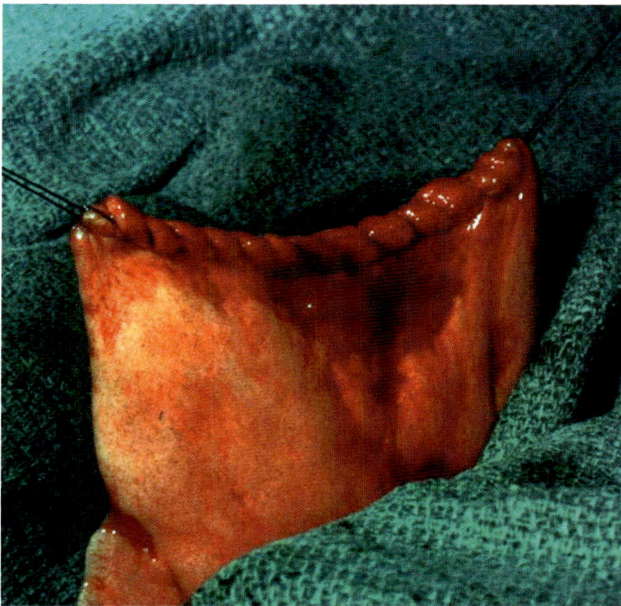

Figure 41.8 Partial lung lobectomy with suture. A continuous mattress suture has been placed followed by a simple continuous mattress suture.

and at its end so that adequate tissue compression is achieved, and a piece (8–10 cm long) is left at each side of the lobe to control the lung. The lung lobe is incised on the proximal side of the forceps, leaving a narrow strip of uninjured lung distal to the compressing suture. The edge of the lung incision is oversewn with a very closely spaced simple continuous pattern of absorbable suture (4-0 or 5-0). The lobe is allowed to drop back into the thoracic cavity, the chest is filled with saline until the incision is covered, the lungs are inflated, and the suture line checked for leaks. Leaks are closed with simple interrupted or cruciate sutures of similar material.

Partial lobectomy in the proximal third of the lobe encounters relatively large bronchi and blood vessels. These are ligated individually with suture ligatures (fixation ligatures) to reduce hemorrhage or air leak, and the lung edge is sutured as previously described.

Mechanical stapling equipment can be used in lieu of suture techniques (Hess *et al.* 1979). The stapler is positioned across the lobe proximal to the lesion, and a double row of fine staples is placed (Figure 41.9). The lobe distal to the staples is cross-clamped to prevent leakage

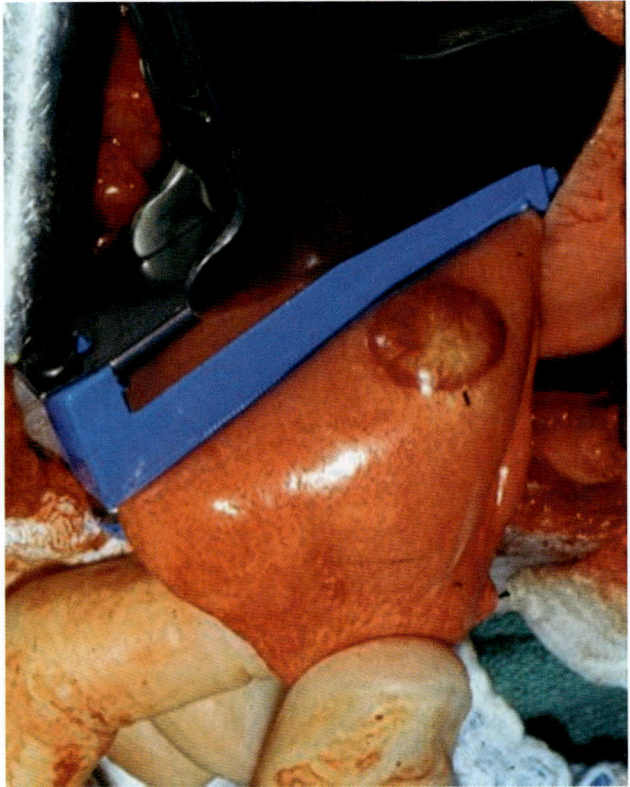

Figure 41.9 Partial lobectomy using stapling equipment. The stapler is placed across the lung lobe proximal to the lesion, and two rows of staples are simultaneously placed to seal the lung edge. The lung lobe distal to the stapler is excised and the stapler removed.

and excised between the clamp and staples. Small air leaks and hemorrhage are occasionally found along the stapled surface because the physical construction of the staples in a "B" configuration allows small vessels and bronchi to remain patent. These leaks are controlled by a few interrupted sutures. This technique is very rapid and is warranted in patients in critical condition. Stapling equipment is too large to use in the thorax of small patients.

Partial lung lobectomy can also be performed with thoracoscopy using staples or thoracoscopically assisted. Specially designed staples (Endo GIA®, United States Surgical Corporation, Norwalk, CT, USA) are used to perform partial lung lobectomy. Endo GIA staples come in three different dimensions: 30, 45, and 60 mm length for the cartridge. Staple lengths are 2.0, 2.5, 3.5, or 4.8 mm when opened. Thoracoscopy with an intercostal approach is preferred (Lansdowne *et al.* 2005); 12 mm cannulas are required to introduce the Endo GIA into the thoracic cavity. Similar to open-chest surgery, the staples have to be placed across the lobe proximal to the lesions. Staple lengths of 2.5 mm are used for partial lung lobectomy. If a thoracoscopic-assisted approach is used, one cannula is placed in an intercostal space to visualize where the lesion to resect is located, and another cannula will then be placed in the intercostal space at the level of the lesion to resect. The tip of the lung lobe will be grasped with an atraumatic grasping forceps through the cannula. The lung lobe will then be partially exteriorized after enlarging the cannula site. The partial lung lobectomy can be performed as during an intercostal thoracotomy. The lung lobe will then be returned to the thoracic cavity.

Complete lung lobectomy

The standard surgical approach is an intercostal thoracotomy over the affected lung area and its hilus or a median sternotomy. The lung lobectomy may be a little more complicated with a median sternotomy, although this approach is more appropriate if several lung lobes have to be removed or an exploration of the pleural space is required. The remaining lung lobes are packed out of the way with moist laparotomy sponges, and the visceral pleura is incised to expose the pulmonary vessels.

The arterial supply to the lobe is approached first to control blood flow to the lobe, preventing congestion and reducing the chance of severe arterial hemorrhage as the hilar dissection is performed. The pulmonary artery supplying the affected lung lobe is dorsal to the left bronchi and ventrolateral to the right bronchi. The pulmonary artery is exposed by sharp and blunt dissection until its circumference is clear of pleura and

(a)

(b)

(c)

(d)

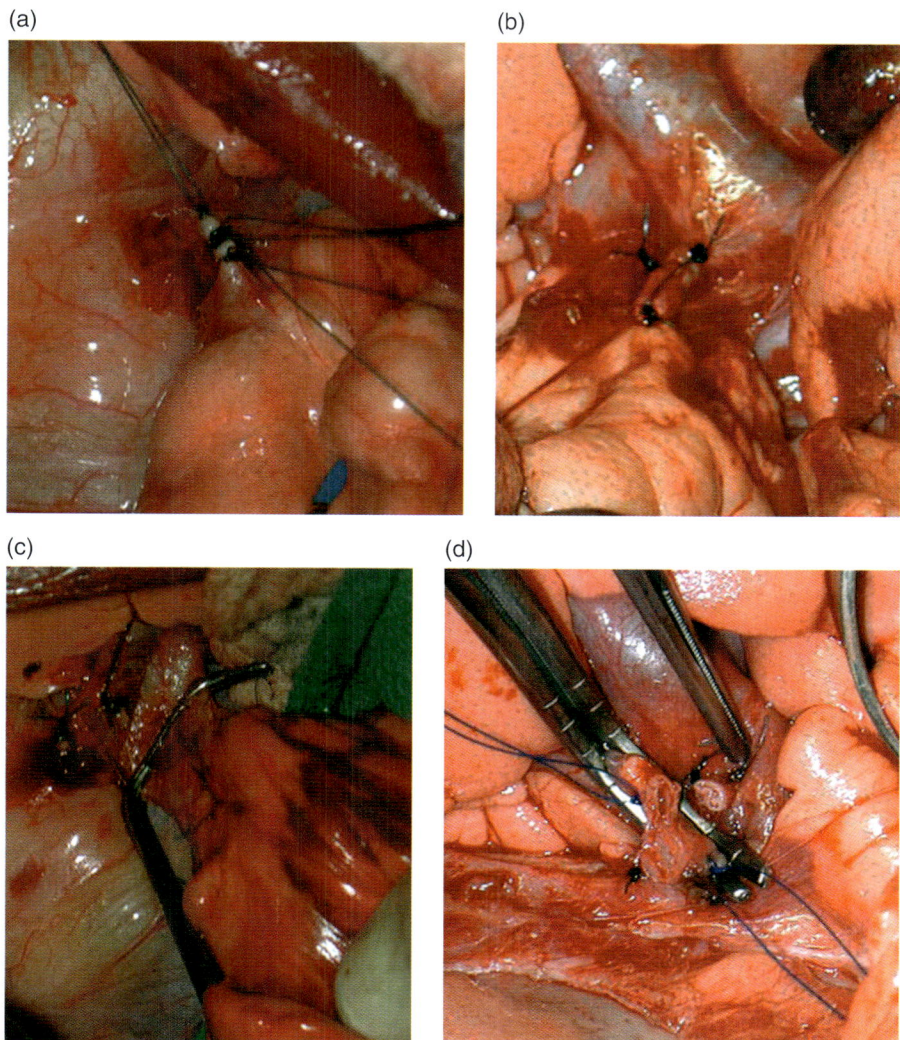

Figure 41.10 (a) The artery and vein supplying the lung lobe are each triple ligated, with the central ligatures being a fixation type. The vessels are transected between the two most distal sutures. (b) The vein is double ligated instead of triple ligated. (c) The clamped bronchus is transected distal to the noncrushing clamp. (d) The transected bronchus is collapsed with a continuous horizontal mattress suture. The end is oversewn with a simple continuous suture pattern.

perivascular tissue (Figure 41.10). Right-angle forceps assist in dissecting the blind side. The artery is then triple ligated with two encircling sutures and one transfixation. A simple ligature of 2-0 or 3-0 suture material (nonabsorbable) is tied at the proximal end of the artery near its branch point, taking care not to encroach on the lumen of the parent vessel. A similar suture is placed distal to the point at which the artery is transected. A transfixing suture is tied 1 mm distal to the proximal suture to prevent its migration. The artery is transected between the two distal sutures.

The lobe is retracted dorsally and the pulmonary vein is approached on the ventral side of the bronchus. Care is taken as the dissection is extended around the

pulmonary vein to prevent laceration of this delicate vessel. Sharp dissection (scissors) combined with gentle blunt dissection with forceps is needed to isolate the vein. The vein is ligated as for the artery. Care should be used to ensure that the venous drainage from other lung lobes in the area is not interfered with by incorporating an adjacent vein in the ligatures. The vein is ligated with two encircling sutures with 3-0 nonabsorbable suture.

The main bronchus supplying the lobe is dissected free of remaining tissue. The bronchus is cross-clamped with two pairs of noncrushing-type forceps proximal and distal to a convenient point for transection close to the lung lobe (Figure 41.10). The bronchus is transected between the forceps, and the lung is removed, providing more room in the chest to complete the operation. The bronchus, near its origin and proximal to the remaining clamp, is sutured with continuous horizontal mattress sutures (2-0 to 3-0 nonabsorbable monofilament suture). These sutures collapse the bronchus as they are tied. A simple continuous suture pattern is used to oversew the mucosa and cartilage on the distal end of the bronchus (3-0 or 4-0 absorbable suture). The bronchial suture line is tested for air leaks by flooding the thorax with warm saline and producing 25–30 cmH$_2$O pressure in the ventilation system. Additional sutures may be placed to close major leaks. Suture hole leaks are closed by suturing surrounding pleura and subpleural tissue over the end of the bronchus and vessel stumps. Complete coverage of the raw tissues exposed during surgery aids in decreasing adhesions, reduces postoperative air leaks, and speeds healing of the exposed stumps.

An alternate technique is mechanical suturing with automatic stapling equipment. Stapling the entire pedicle *in situ* has met with few problems (Scott *et al.* 1976; Hess *et al.* 1979; LaRue *et al.* 1987). A premium TA30 V3 or TA55 (United States Surgical Corporation) is usually used with 3.5 mm staples to occlude vessels and bronchi during lobectomy (Figure 41.11) (Hess *et al.* 1979; LaRue *et al.* 1987). The equipment may be difficult to position in a small thorax. Leakage of air and blood through the B-shaped staples usually seals spontaneously. Sutures are used to stop minor leaks. This technique decreases surgery time, especially when multiple lobes are removed.

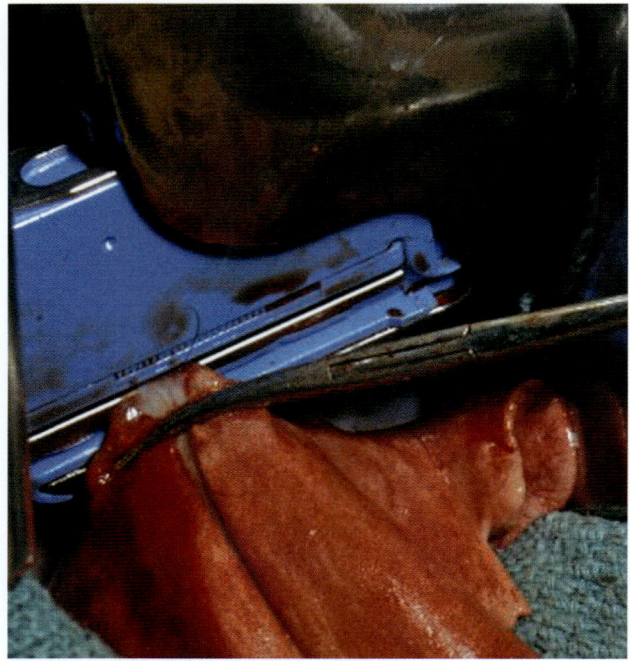

Figure 41.11 Lung lobectomy with staples.

Complete lung lobectomy can be performed with thoracoscopy. The thoracoscopy is performed with an intercostal approach (Lansdowne *et al.* 2005). One-lung ventilation can facilitate the procedure (Kudnig *et al.* 2003, 2004, 2006; Lansdowne *et al.* 2005; Mayhew *et al.* 2019). Different techniques to induce one-lung ventilation have been described (Lansdowne *et al.* 2005; Mayhew *et al.* 2009, 2012, 2019). The technique with an obturator seems to be more appropriate in dogs than using a double lumen endotracheal tube. To introduce the Endo GIA stapler into the thoracic cavity, 12 mm cannulas are used. The staples are placed at the hilus of the lung lobe as during open-chest surgery (Website Chapter 41: Respiratory tract/lung lobectomy thoracoscopy). If a caudal lung lobe is resected, the dorsal ligament has to be dissected first. Endo GIA 60-3.5 is recommended for a lung lobectomy in dogs. The lung lobe is then placed in a retrieving bag to prevent contamination of the thoracic wall with tumor cells. A thoracoscopic-assisted approach can also be used to perform a complete lung lobectomy (Scott *et al.* 2019; Singh *et al.* 2019). It has been shown that thoracoscopy does not affect short- or long-term outcomes when used to perform a lung lobectomy for neoplasia (Mayhew *et al.* 2013; Bleakley *et al.* 2015).

Pneumonectomy

Acute restriction of more than 60% of the pulmonary artery outflow is fatal in dogs because it can induce acute pulmonary hypertension (Tronc *et al.* 1999). This observation correlates well with dogs surviving a 50% total lung loss but dying with a 75% loss (Brugarolas & Takita 1973). Excision of an entire left lung is tolerated if the right lung is healthy because it only represents 42% of the lung mass. Because the right lung is larger than the left, a right pneumonectomy removes more than 50% of the lung and is likely to be fatal. However, if the disease process has induced a slow and progressive reduction in lung function, pneumonectomy of the right side is possible in dogs (Liptak *et al.* 2004). Transient respiratory acidosis has been noted in dogs undergoing pneumonectomy (Brugarolas & Takita 1973). Healthy dogs undergoing staged lobectomies during a 6-month period can survive on the equivalent of one and one-half healthy caudal lung lobes. Lung regeneration can be anticipated in multiple partial lobectomies in an attempt to restore normal lung capacity (Rannels & Rannels 1988). This hyperplastic response increases alveolar, bronchiolar, and vascular components. Lung regeneration can be anticipated in multiple partial lobectomies. It may account for gradual improvement in exercise tolerance in these patients (Brugarolas & Takita 1973).

Pneumonectomy is accompanied by secondary changes in the contralateral lung and the myocardium. Accompanying lung regeneration is a decrease in compliance, vital capacity, and perfusion compared with the normal lung. Right ventricular hypertrophy and an increase in pulmonary vascular resistance and residual lung capacity are noted (Lucas *et al.* 1983). The lung remaining after pneumonectomy is more sensitive to positive end-expiratory pressure, as manifested by a greater increase in pulmonary vascular resistance with a given level of positive end-expiratory pressure. This is correlated with a lower cardiac output (Lores *et al.* 1985).

Pneumonectomy is indicated for lesions already described when they have extended to all lobes of one lung while sparing the contralateral lung. The same surgical conditions exist as described for lobectomy (i.e., neoplasia, abscess, trauma), and the same sequence of vessel and bronchus ligation is followed.

Control of the right or left branch of the main pulmonary artery (lobar artery) early in the procedure reduces the chance of major hemorrhage during hilar dissection. The artery is transected and oversewn or ligated, depending on its size. Small arteries (<5 mm diameter) can be double ligated, whereas larger arteries are oversewn or stapled. Before the lobar artery is oversewn, a noncrushing vascular clamp is placed on the lobar artery adjacent to the main pulmonary artery, and a crushing clamp is placed 1 cm distally. The artery is transected between clamps, leaving 5 mm of artery distal to the noncrushing clamp. The cut edge of the proximal segment of the lobar artery is oversewn using a double layer of simple continuous monofilament nonabsorbable suture (4-0 to 5-0) (Figure 41.12). In small dogs and cats, the lobar artery is ligated twice (5 mm apart), and a fixation ligature is juxtapositioned distal to the proximal ligature. The vessel is transected between the two distal sutures. The veins are ligated using the same method in all dogs and cats.

The bronchus is transected using the cut-and-sew technique after the endotracheal tube is advanced into the contralateral bronchus. Monofilament nonabsorbable suture is anchored in the tracheal wall immediately adjacent to the bronchus and used for traction. The bronchus is clamped distal to the amputation site. The first suture line is placed approximately 5–10 mm distal to the carina. Simple interrupted horizontal mattress sutures (3-0 or 4-0 monofilament nonabsorbable suture) are placed full thickness through the bronchus and tied. The bronchus is transected 3 mm distal to the suture line. The ends of the incision may be tapered to obtain a smooth closure and secure seal. The edge of the bronchus is oversewn with a simple continuous suture. The resection and closure should not reduce the size of the other mainstem bronchus.

All ligatures are checked for security, and the endotracheal tube is withdrawn proximal to the carina. The tracheal incision is submerged in saline and examined for

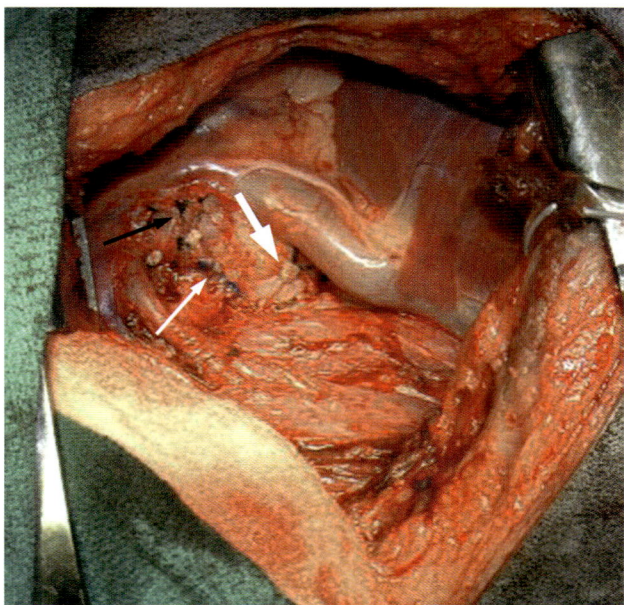

Figure 41.12 Pneumonectomy on the left side. The pulmonary artery has been oversewn (black arrow). One pulmonary vein (large white arrow) and the primary bronchus (small white arrow) were ligated. Other small vessels were also ligated during the dissection.

air leaks while the intratracheal pressure is raised to 20–25 cmH$_2$O. Extra sutures are used as needed to stop air leaks. However, the main bronchus has tracheal-type cartilage rings that resist collapse, and the sutures or staples tend to cut through the bronchus.

References

Alexander, J.W., Hoffer, R.E., and Bolton, G.R. (1974). Torsion of the diaphragmatic lobe of the lung following surgical correction of a patent ductus arteriosus. *Veterinary Medicine, Small Animal Clinician* 69: 595–597.

Anderson, G.I. (1987). Pulmonary cavitary lesions in the dog: a review of seven cases. *Journal of the American Animal Hospital Association* 23: 89–94.

Arnoczky, S.P. and O'Neill, J.A. (1979). Lung lobectomy. *Veterinary Clinics of North America: Small Animal Practice* 9: 219–229.

Aron, D.N. and Kornegay, J.N. (1983). The clinical significance of traumatic lung cysts and associated pulmonary abnormalities in the dog and cat. *Journal of the American Animal Hospital Association* 19: 903–912.

Au, J.J., Weisman, D.L., Stefanacci, J.D., and Palmisano, M.P. (2006). Use of computed tomography for evaluation of lung lesions associated with spontaneous pneumothorax in dogs: 12 cases (1999–2002). *Journal of the American Veterinary Medical Association* 228: 733–737.

Basher, A.W., Hogan, P.M., Hanna, P.E. et al. (1991). Surgical treatment of a congenital bronchoesophageal fistula in a dog. *Journal of the American Veterinary Medical Association* 199: 479–482.

Berry, C.R., Moore, P.F., Thomas, W.P. et al. (1990). Pulmonary lymphomatoid granulomatosis in seven dogs (1976–1987). *Journal of Veterinary Internal Medicine* 4: 157–166.

Berzon, J.L., Rendano, V.T., and Hoffer, R.E. (1979). Recurrent pneumothorax secondary to ruptured pulmonary blebs: a case report. *Journal of the American Animal Hospital Association* 15: 707–711.

Bleakley, S., Duncan, C.G., and Monnet, E. (2015). Thoracoscopic lung lobectomy for primary lung tumors in 13 dogs. *Veterinary Surgery* 44: 1029–1035.

Brissot, H.N., Dupre, G.P., Bouvy, B.M., and Paquet, L. (2003). Thoracoscopic treatment of bullous emphysema in 3 dogs. *Veterinary Surgery* 32: 524–529.

Brodey, R.S. and Craig, P.H. (1965). Primary pulmonary neoplasms in the dog: a review of 29 cases. *Journal of the American Veterinary Medical Association* 147: 1628–1643.

Brugarolas, A. and Takita, H. (1973). Regeneration of the lung in the dog. *Journal of Thoracic and Cardiovascular Surgery* 65: 187–190.

Choi, J. and Yoon, J. (2006). Lung lobe torsion in a Yorkshire terrier. *Journal of Small Animal Practice* 47: 557.

Fossum, T.W., Wellman, M., Relford, R.L., and Slater, M.R. (1993). Eosinophilic pleural or peritoneal effusions in dogs and cats: 14 cases (1986–1992). *Journal of the American Veterinary Medical Association* 202: 1873–1876.

Gelzer, A.R., Downs, M.O., Newell, S.M. et al. (1997). Accessory lung lobe torsion and chylothorax in an Afghan hound. *Journal of the American Animal Hospital Association* 33: 171–176.

Hankins, J.R., McAslan, T.C., Shin, B. et al. (1977). Extensive pulmonary laceration caused by blunt trauma. *Journal of Thoracic and Cardiovascular Surgery* 74: 519–527.

Hawkins, E.C., Basseches, J., Berry, C.R. et al. (2003). Demographic, clinical, and radiographic features of bronchiectasis in dogs: 316 cases (1988–2000). *Journal of the American Veterinary Medical Association* 223: 1628–1635.

Hess, J.L., DeYoung, D.W., and Grier, R.L. (1979). Use of mechanical staples in veterinary thoracic surgery. *Journal of the American Animal Hospital Association* 15: 569–573.

Hofeling, A.D., Jackson, A.H., Alsup, J.C., and O'Keefe, D. (2004). Spontaneous midlobar lung lobe torsion in a 2-year-old Newfoundland. *Journal of the American Animal Hospital Association* 40: 220–223.

Hoover, J.P., Henry, G.A., and Panciera, R.J. (1992). Bronchial cartilage dysplasia with multifocal lobar bullous emphysema and lung torsions in a pup. *Journal of the American Veterinary Medical Association* 201: 599–602.

Jerram, R.M., Fossum, T.W., Berridge, B.R. et al. (1999). The efficacy of mechanical abrasion and talc slurry as methods of pleurodesis in normal dogs. *Veterinary Surgery* 28: 322–332.

Johnson, L.R. (2005). Diseases of the small airways. In: *Textbook of Veterinary Internal Medicine*, 6e (ed. S.J. Ettinger and E.D. Feldman), 1233–1239. St Louis, MO: Elsevier.

Johnston, G.R., Feeney, D.A., O'Brien, T.D. et al. (1984). Recurring lung lobe torsion in three Afghan hounds. *Journal of the American Veterinary Medical Association* 184: 842–845.

Kerpsack, S.J., McLoughlin, M.A., Graves, T.K. et al. (1994). Chylothorax associated with lung lobe torsion and a peritoneopericardial diaphragmatic hernia in a cat. *Journal of the American Animal Hospital Association* 30: 351–354.

Kramek, B.A. and Caywood, D.D. (1987). Pneumothorax. *Veterinary Clinics of North America: Small Animal Practice* 17: 285–300.

Kramek, B.A., Caywood, D.D., and O'Brien, T.D. (1985). Bullous emphysema and recurrent pneumothorax in the dog. *Journal of the American Veterinary Medical Association* 186: 971–974.

Kudnig, S.T., Monnet, E., Riquelme, M. et al. (2003). Effect of one-lung ventilation on oxygen delivery in anesthetized dogs with an open thoracic cavity. *American Journal of Veterinary Research* 64: 443–448.

Kudnig, S.T., Monnet, E., Riquelme, M. et al. (2004). Cardiopulmonary effect of thoracoscopy in anesthetized normal dogs. *Veterinary Anaesthesia and Analgesia* 31: 121–128.

Kudnig, S.T., Monnet, E., Riquelme, M. et al. (2006). Effect of positive end-expiratory pressure on oxygen delivery during one-lung ventilation for thoracoscopy in normal dogs. *Veterinary Surgery* 35: 534–542.

Lansdowne, J.L., Monnet, E., Twedt, D.C., and Dernell, W.S. (2005). Thoracoscopic lung lobectomy for treatment of lung tumors in dogs. *Veterinary Surgery* 34: 530–535.

LaRue, S.M., Withrow, S.J., and Wykes, P.M. (1987). Lung resection using surgical staples in dogs and cats. *Veterinary Surgery* 16: 238–240.

Latimer, C.R., Lux, C.N., Sutton, J.S., and Culp, W.T.N. (2017). Lung lobe torsion in seven juvenile dogs. *Journal of the American Veterinary Medical Association* 251: 1450–1456.

Lipscomb, V.J., Hardie, R.J., and Dubielzig, R.R. (2003). Spontaneous pneumothorax caused by pulmonary blebs and bullae in 12 dogs. *Journal of the American Animal Hospital Association* 39: 435–445.

Liptak, J.M., Monnet, E., Dernell, W.S. et al. (2004). Pneumonectomy: four case studies and a comparative review. *Journal of Small Animal Practice* 45: 441–447.

Lopez, A. (2007). Respiratory system. In: *Pathologic Basis of Veterinary Diseases*, 4e (ed. M.D. McGavin and J.F. Zachary), 463–558. St Louis, MO: Mosby/Elsevier.

Lord, P.F., Greiner, T.P., Greene, R.W., and DeHoff, W.D. (1973). Lung lobe torsion in the dog. *Journal of the American Animal Hospital Association* 9: 473–482.

Lores, M.E., Keagy, B.A., Vassiliades, T. et al. (1985). Cardiovascular effects of positive end-expiratory pressure (PEEP) after pneumonectomy in dogs. *Annals of Thoracic Surgery* 40: 464–468.

Lucas, C.L., Murray, G.F., Wilcox, B.R., and Shallal, J.A. (1983). Effects of pneumonectomy on pulmonary input impedance. *Surgery* 94: 807–816.

Marlowe, K.W., Robat, C.S., Clarke, D.M. et al. (2018). Primary pulmonary histiocytic sarcoma in dogs: a retrospective analysis of 37 cases (2000–2015). *Veterinary and Comparative Oncology* 16: 658–663.

Mayhew, K.N., Mayhew, P.D., Sorrell-Raschi, L., and Brown, D.C. (2009). Thoracoscopic subphrenic pericardectomy using double-lumen endobronchial intubation for alternating one-lung ventilation. *Veterinary Surgery* 38: 961–966.

Mayhew, P.D., Culp, W.T., Pascoe, P.J. et al. (2012). Evaluation of blind thoracoscopic-assisted placement of three double-lumen endobronchial tube designs for one-lung ventilation in dogs. *Veterinary Surgery* 41: 664–670.

Mayhew, P.D., Hunt, G.B., Steffey, M.A. et al. (2013). Evaluation of short-term outcome after lung lobectomy for resection of primary lung tumors via video-assisted thoracoscopic surgery or open thoracotomy in medium- to large-breed dogs. *Journal of the American Veterinary Medical Association* 243: 681–688.

Mayhew, P.D., Steffey, M.A., Fransson, B.A. et al. (2019). Long-term outcome of video-assisted thoracoscopic thoracic duct ligation and pericardectomy in dogs with chylothorax: a multi-institutional study of 39 cases. *Veterinary Surgery* 48: O112–O120.

McNiel, E.A., Ogilvie, G.K., Powers, B.E. et al. (1997). Evaluation of prognostic factors for dogs with primary lung tumors: 67 cases (1985–1992). *Journal of the American Veterinary Medical Association* 211: 1422–1427.

Mehlhaff, C.J. and Mooney, S. (1985). Primary pulmonary neoplasia in the dog and cat. *Veterinary Clinics of North America: Small Animal Practice* 15: 1061–1067.

Mehlhaff, C.J., Leifer, C.E., Patnaik, A.K., and Schwarz, P.D. (1984). Surgical treatment of primary pulmonary neoplasia in 15 dogs. *Journal of the American Animal Hospital Association* 20: 799–803.

Millard, R.P., Myers, J.R., and Novo, R.E. (2008). Spontaneous lung lobe torsion in a cat. *Journal of Veterinary Internal Medicine* 22: 671–673.

Miller, H.G. and Sherrill, A. (1987). Lung lobe torsion: a difficult condition to diagnose. *Veterinary Medicine* 82: 797–798.

Moses, B.L. (1980). Fiberoptic bronchoscopy for diagnosis of lung lobe torsion in a dog. *Journal of the American Veterinary Medical Association* 176: 44–47.

Murphy, K.A. and Brisson, B.A. (2006). Evaluation of lung lobe torsion in pugs: 7 cases (1991–2004). *Journal of the American Veterinary Medical Association* 228: 86–90.

Murphy, S.T., Mathews, K.G., Ellison, G.W., and Bellah, J.R. (1997a). Pulmonary lobectomy in the management of pneumonia in five cats. *Journal of Small Animal Practice* 38: 159–162.

Murphy, S.T., Ellison, G.W., McKiernan, B.C. et al. (1997b). Pulmonary lobectomy in the management of pneumonia in dogs: 59 cases (1972–1994). *Journal of the American Veterinary Medical Association* 210: 235–239.

Neath, P.J., Brockman, D.J., and King, L.G. (2000). Lung lobe torsion in dogs: 22 cases (1981–1999). *Journal of the American Veterinary Medical Association* 217: 1041–1044.

Nelson, O.L. and Sellon, R.K. (2005). Pulmonary parenchymal disease. In: *Textbook of Veterinary Internal Medicine*, 6e (ed. S.J. Ettinger and E.D. Feldman), 1239–1250. St Louis, MO: Elsevier.

Ogilvie, G.K., Haschek, W.M., Withrow, S.J. et al. (1989a). Classification of primary lung tumors in dogs: 210 cases (1975–1985). *Journal of the American Veterinary Medical Association* 195: 106–108.

Ogilvie, G.K., Weigel, R.M., Haschek, W.M. et al. (1989b). Prognostic factors for tumor remission and survival in dogs after surgery for primary lung tumor: 76 cases (1975–1985). *Journal of the American Veterinary Medical Association* 195: 109–112.

Postorino, N.C., Wheeler, S.L., Park, R.D. et al. (1989). A syndrome resembling lymphomatoid granulomatosis in the dog. *Journal of Veterinary Internal Medicine* 3: 15–19.

Puerto, D.A., Brockman, D.J., Lindquist, C., and Drobatz, K. (2002). Surgical and nonsurgical management of and selected risk factors for spontaneous pneumothorax in dogs: 64 cases (1986–1999). *Journal of the American Veterinary Medical Association* 220: 1670–1674.

Rannels, D.E. and Rannels, S.R. (1988). Compensatory growth of the lung following partial pneumonectomy. *Experimental Lung Research* 14: 157–182.

Rawlings, C.A., Lebel, J.L., and Mitchum, G. (1970). Torsion of the left apical and cardiac pulmonary lobes in a dog. *Journal of the American Veterinary Medical Association* 156: 726–733.

Rooney, M.B. and Monnet, E. (2002). Medical and surgical treatment of pyothorax in dogs: 26 cases. *Journal of the American Veterinary Medical Association* 221: 86–92.

Rooney, M.B., Lanz, O., and Monnet, E. (2001). Spontaneous lung lobe torsion in two pugs. *Journal of the American Animal Hospital Association* 37: 128–130.

Saperstein, G., Harris, S., and Leipold, H.W. (1976). Congenital defects in domestic cats. *Feline Practice* 6: 18–43.

Scott, R.N., Faraci, R.P., Hough, A., and Chretien, P.B. (1976). Brochial stump closure techniques following pneumonectomy: a serial comparative study. *Annals of Surgery* 184: 205–211.

Scott, J.E., Singh, A., Case, J.B. et al. (2019). Determination of optimal location for thoracoscopic-assisted pulmonary surgery for lung lobectomy in cats. *American Journal of Veterinary Research* 80: 1050–1054.

Seiler, G., Schwarz, T., Vignoli, M., and Rodriguez, D. (2008). Computed tomographic features of lung lobe torsion. *Veterinary Radiology and Ultrasound* 49: 504–508.

Shahar, R., Shamir, M., and Johnston, D.E. (1997). A technique for management of bite wounds of the thoracic wall in small dogs. *Veterinary Surgery* 26: 45–50.

Siems, J.J., Jakovljevic, S., and Van Alstine, W. (1998). Radiographic diagnosis: lung lobe torsion. *Veterinary Radiology and Ultrasound* 39: 418–420.

Silberstein, A., Mercier, M., Jaafar, M., and Cadore, J.L. (1991). Lung lobe torsion: a rare complication of thoracic surgery in the dog. *Point Vétérinaire* 23 (138): 105–110.

Singh, A., Scott, J., Case, J.B. et al. (2019). Optimization of surgical approach for thoracoscopic-assisted pulmonary surgery in dogs. *Veterinary Surgery* 48: O99–O104.

Spackman, C.J. and Caywood, D.D. (1987). Management of thoracic trauma and chest wall reconstruction. *Veterinary Clinics of North America: Small Animal Practice* 17: 431–447.

Spranklin, D.B., Gulikers, K.P., and Lanz, O.I. (2003). Recurrence of spontaneous lung lobe torsion in a pug. *Journal of the American Animal Hospital Association* 39: 446–451.

Teske, E., Stokhof, A.A., van der Ingh, T.S.G.A.M. et al. (1991). Transthoracic needle aspiration biopsy of the lung in dogs with pulmonic disease. *Journal of the American Animal Hospital Association* 27: 289–294.

Teunissen, G.H., Wolverkamp, W.T., and Goedegebuure, S.A. (1976). Necrosis of a pulmonary lobe in a dog. *Tijdschrift voor Diergeneeskunde* 101: 1129–1133.

Tronc, F., Gregoire, J., Leblanc, P., and Deslauriers, J. (1999). Physiologic consequences of pneumonectomy. Consequences on the pulmonary function. *Chest Surgery Clinics of North America* 9: 459–473, xii–xiii.

Waddell, L.S., Brady, C.A., and Drobatz, K.J. (2002). Risk factors, prognostic indicators, and outcome of pyothorax in cats: 80 cases (1986–1999). *Journal of the American Veterinary Medical Association* 221: 819–824.

White, R.N. and Corzo-Menendez, N. (2000). Concurrent torsion of the right cranial and right middle lung lobes in a whippet. *Journal of Small Animal Practice* 41: 562–565.

Williams, J.H. and Duncan, N.M. (1986). Chylothorax with concurrent right cardiac lung lobe torsion in an Afghan hound. *Journal of the South African Veterinary Association* 57: 35–37.

Withrow, S.J. (2001). Lung cancer. In: *Small Animal Clinical Oncology*, 3e (ed. S.J. Withrow and E.G. MacEwen), 361–370. Philadelphia, PA: WB Saunders.

Section 7

Urinary Tract

42

Pathophysiology of Renal Disease

Cathy Langston and Serge Chalhoub

Renal physiology and its importance in overall body function

Each nephron is a functional unit composed of a glomerulus and its associated renal tubule, and the kidneys are composed of thousands of nephrons. Superficial cortical nephrons have relatively short loops of Henle that only penetrate a short distance into the renal medulla, whereas juxtamedullary nephrons have long loops of Henle that penetrate deep into the inner medulla. It is thought that the latter represents the majority of canine and feline nephron morphology (DiBartola 2012).

The glomerular capillary is a modified capillary bed that acts as a filter of blood plasma. The glomerulus is characterized by invaginations of fenestrated capillary tufts into Bowman's capsule. The capillaries are supplied by an afferent arteriole and drained by an efferent arteriole. The capillary endothelium is surrounded by the glomerular basement membrane, which in turn is covered by the foot processes of the epithelial podocytes. These pseudopodia interdigitate and form filtration slits along the capillary wall. The resultant structure is freely permeable to water and small dissolved solutes, but not to most cells and large proteins (Guyton & Hall 2020).

The main determinants of passage across this filtration barrier are molecular size and charge. Particles with a molecular mass over 60 kDa do not typically pass through the glomerular membrane. Negatively charged particles are retained in the capillaries to a greater extent than neutral or positively charged particles, mainly due to an extensive network of negatively charged glycoproteins on the podocytes and their associated foot processes, the basement membrane, and the capillary endothelium (Brown 1993; Guyton & Hall 2020). The product of the glomerular filtration process is the ultrafiltrate. Mesangial cells are in contact with the basement membrane in areas where there are no foot processes. They are not part of the filtration barrier, but they can contract and affect filtration dynamics and secrete prostaglandins.

The ultrafiltrate flows from Bowman's space into the proximal convoluted tubule in the renal cortex (Figure 42.1). The walls of the proximal convoluted tubule are made up of a singer layer of interdigitated cells that are united by apical tight junctions. The proximal tubule is divided into three functional segments (S1–S3) based on regional differences in function. Sodium moves from the ultrafiltrate across the luminal side of the tubule cells by cotransport or exchange mechanisms, in a process driven by the gradient created by the Na^+/K^+-ATPase pump on the basolateral side of the tubule cells. During passage through the proximal tubule about 60% of the sodium in the ultrafiltrate is reabsorbed, and all of the glucose and amino acids are normally reabsorbed. Bicarbonate is also reabsorbed in this segment. Water is osmotically reabsorbed, which maintains the osmolality of the ultrafiltrate constant and relatively similar to plasma (Anderson 2001; Briggs et al. 2017).

The ultrafiltrate enters the loop of Henle with its characteristic hairpin turn in the outer medulla. The descending segment of the loop does not allow the reabsorption of electrolytes and other molecules, but allows the reabsorption of water. Hence, as the ultrafiltrate reaches the bottom of the loop its osmolality increases, reaching a maximum of approximately 2800 mOsmol/kg in dogs and 3200–4980 mOsmol/kg in cats (DiBartola 2012). As

Small Animal Soft Tissue Surgery, Second Edition. Edited by Eric Monnet.
© 2023 John Wiley & Sons, Inc. Published 2023 by John Wiley & Sons, Inc.
Companion website: www.wiley.com/go/monnet/small

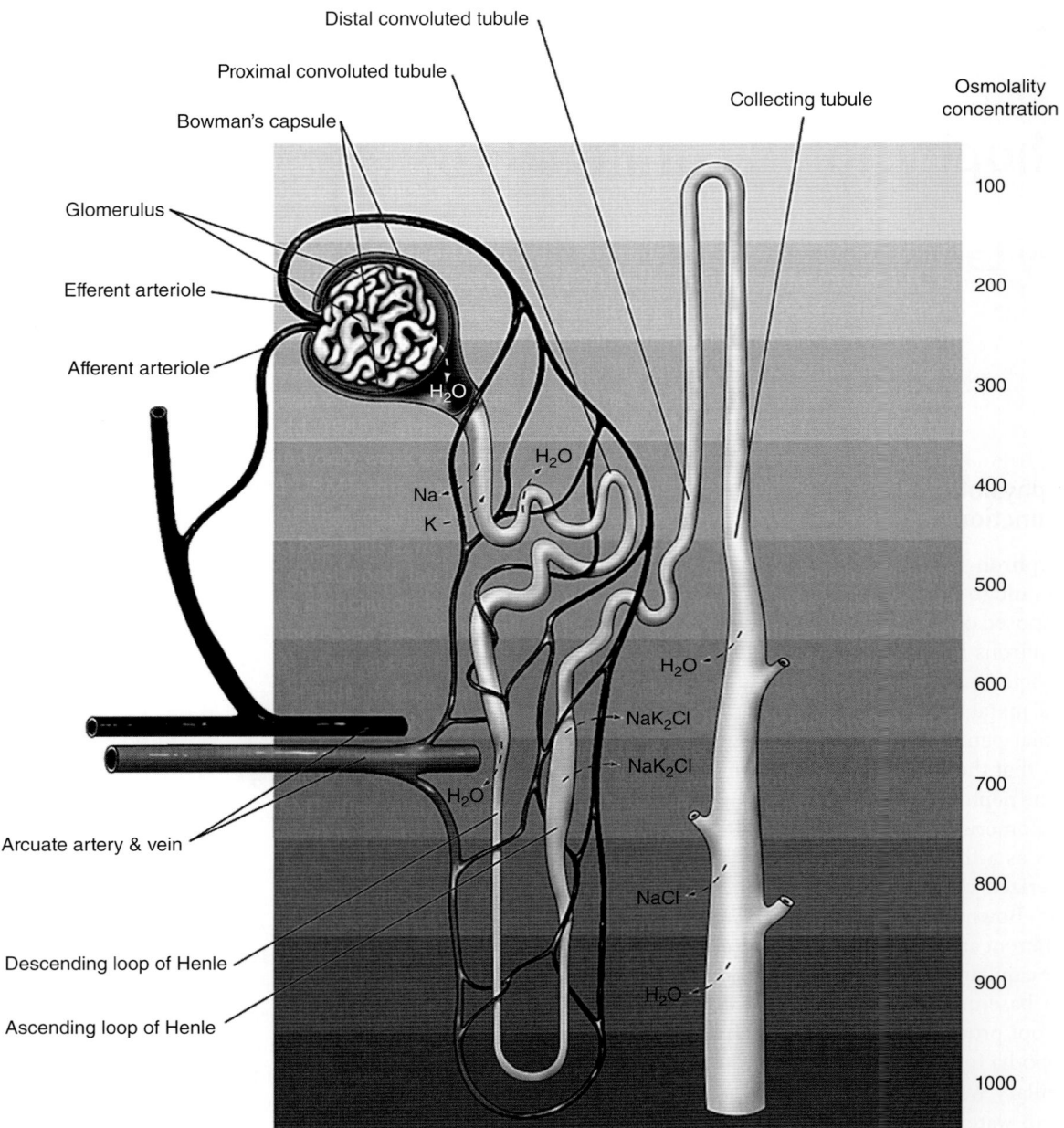

Figure 42.1 Ultrafiltrate created at the glomerulus is the same osmolality as blood. In the proximal tubule, Na+/K+-ATPase pumps on the basolateral side pump sodium into the interstitium. Water is passively reabsorbed in the descending loop of Henle, creating a concentrated ultrafiltrate. A luminal Na+/K+/2Cl– pump in the ascending loop of Henle dilutes the urine, as that segment is impermeable to water. A luminal NaCl pump in the distal tubule further dilutes the ultrafiltrate. In the collecting tubule and duct, antidiuretic hormone (ADH) opens water channels (aquaporins) that allow reabsorption of water, creating a concentrated urine if needed. In the absence of ADH, the urine remains dilute.

the ultrafiltrate reaches the thicker ascending loop, which is impermeable to water, a Na+/K+/2Cl– cotransporter pumps NaCl into the tubular cells. Approximately 30% of the sodium load of the ultrafiltrate is reabsorbed in this manner (Briggs *et al.* 2017). Loop diuretics inhibit this cotransporter. The resultant ultrafiltrate is hyposo-

molar (100 mOsmol/kg) to plasma as it reaches the distal tubule.

The morphologic conformation of the loop of Henle (descending limb from the proximal tubule, connected to the parallel ascending limb by a hairpin turn) is important for the countercurrent multiplier. The multiplier system generates an osmotic gradient due to active NaCl reabsorption across the ascending limb, which creates an osmotic difference between the tubular fluid and the surrounding interstitium, and a low water permeability of the ascending limb that keeps the gradient active. This, combined with a high water permeability of the descending loop, allows water to diffuse into the interstitium by osmosis due to the high NaCl concentration caused by the ascending limb reabsorption, and therefore causes an increase in the osmolality of the descending loop's tubular fluid. The now hypertonic fluid travels to the ascending limb, where water cannot diffuse, but NaCl will be transported out into the interstitium by active transport, thereby reducing the tonicity of the tubular fluid as it reaches the distal tubule, to the point of being hypotonic to plasma. These steps are repeated over and over, thus increasing the osmolality of the tubular fluid of the descending limb (the multiplier effect) (Allon 2017; Guyton & Hall 2020; Verlander et al. 2019).

The distal tubule is the site of a luminal NaCl cotransporter. The initial portion of the distal tubule is relatively impermeable to water. Specialized distal tubular cells that reside in the angle between the efferent and afferent arteriole comprise the macula densa. The macula densa cells detect changes in tubular fluid flow. Along with the renin-secreting juxtaglomerular cells in the afferent arteriole, they form the juxtaglomerular apparatus (Guyton & Hall 2020).

The principal cells of the collecting ducts predominate and are involved in antidiuretic hormone (ADH)-stimulated water reabsorption via aquaporin channels. Water leaves the lumen via the aquaporin channels passively due to the high osmolality of the interstitium, creating a concentrated urine (Guyton & Hall 2020). The intercalated cells are mainly concerned with acid secretion and bicarbonate transport. The distal tubule and cortical collecting ducts are also the main sites of action of aldosterone. It is within these segments that the urine's final composition and concentration will be determined.

Determinants of glomerular filtration rate

Glomerular filtration rate (GFR) is defined as the total filtration rate of both kidneys. The hydrostatic pressure of the glomerular capillary is quantitatively the most important force enhancing filtration and is opposed by the hydrostatic pressure of Bowman's space. The oncotic pressure in the glomerular capillary opposes filtration, whereas the oncotic pressure in Bowman's space is typically negligible.

Although the net filtration pressure of the glomerulus is approximately the same as systemic capillaries (about 15 mmHg), the GFR is much higher than the movement of fluid in systemic capillaries because of the ultrafiltration coefficient (K_f). The K_f depends on the surface area for filtration and the permeability of the capillary to water and molecules, and can change in response to disease, hormones, and neurologic stimulation on mesangial cells (Barrett et al. 2019; Inker et al. 2017; DiBartola 2012; Guyton & Hall 2020).

Changes in the afferent and efferent arterioles can also greatly change GFR. Variations in resistance of these vessels can modify renal blood flow (RBF) and consequently GFR. Local (e.g., prostaglandins), neurologic (e.g., norepinephrine), and humoral (e.g., angiotensin II) substances act on these vessels in various physiologic and pathophysiologic situations (Okusa et al. 2019).

Renal blood flow

The kidneys receive 20–25% of the cardiac output, and the major sites of resistance to blood flow are the afferent and efferent arterioles. The majority of RBF is distributed to the renal cortex (90%), while the remaining blood flow is distributed between the outer medulla (<10%) and inner medulla (2–3%). Disruption of blood flow will primarily affect the medullary regions of the kidneys, which already exist in a state of relative hypoxia (Padanilam 2003; Versteilen et al. 2004; Okusa et al. 2019).

The kidneys have an intrinsic ability to autoregulate blood flow, permitting a relatively constant blood flow despite variations in arterial perfusion pressure. GFR and RBF are maintained when mean arterial pressure ranges between 80 and 180 mmHg (DiBartola 2012).

Acute kidney injury and chronic kidney disease

Acute kidney injury (AKI) is a collection of conditions characterized by an insult to the kidneys that results in an abrupt decline in GFR of variable magnitude, depending on the type of injury, the extent, and the duration, with the resultant accumulation of nitrogenous waste products such as blood urea nitrogen (BUN) and creatinine (Okusa et al. 2019; Ronco et al. 2019; Kerl 2020).

AKI can range from mild increases in creatinine (i.e., >0.3 mg/dL in 48 hours) without overt azotemia to complete lack of function, which results in the significant retention of nitrogenous waste products and lack of fluid balance control, acid–base dysregulation, and electrolyte disturbances. Elevations in serum creatinine above its reference range do not occur until 75% or more of nephrons are no longer functional, highlighting the insensitivity of creatinine as an AKI marker (Polzin 2017). Azotemia is defined by an increase in blood nonprotein nitrogenous compounds such as BUN and creatinine that are normally eliminated by the kidneys. Uremia can be the result of AKI depending on its magnitude, and encompasses the clinical signs associated with loss of nephron function.

Chronic kidney disease (CKD) is defined as structural or functional renal damage that has existed for at least three months and results in a permanent reduction of functional nephrons (DiBartola 2012; Langston 2017a). CKD usually results in a decrease in GFR that is often progressive and may or may not be detectable by routine lab analysis.

Urine output and renal failure

Normal daily urine output (UOP) ranges from 20 to 40 mL/kg in dogs and cats (DiBartola 2012). There are four broad categories of UOP associated with renal failure: anuric (no urine produced), oliguric (UOP less than 1 mL/kg per hour), nonoliguric (UOP 1–2 mL/kg per hour), and polyuric (UOP >2 mL/kg per hour). However, an additional category, relative oliguria, should be considered in which UOP may be 1 mL/kg per hour or more, but does not vary with volume status (i.e., the patient may not be able to excrete the volume of administered fluids even with increased volume administration).

Differentiating acute kidney injury from chronic kidney disease

It may be difficult to differentiate between AKI and CKD. A history of renal disease, irregular kidneys on physical exam or medical imaging, weight loss, anemia, polyuria, polydipsia, and past elevations in renal parameters may be more indicative of CKD and may help in differentiation, but are nonspecific. Cats are also more prone to azotemic CKD than dogs are, whereas dogs are more prone to protein-losing nephropathies. Questioning the owners about the possibility of their pet ingesting drugs or toxins and travel history (e.g., leptospirosis, tick-borne diseases) is important. Kidney size during physical examination may also help, as small kidneys tend to reflect CKD and larger than normal kidneys support AKI. Other physical examination and history findings suggestive of CKD include poor body condition and/or hair coat, weight loss, halitosis (uremic breath), uremic buccal ulcers, heat-seeking behavior, gastrointestinal symptoms such as decreased appetite, anorexia and vomiting, and muscle wasting. On ultrasound, small and irregular kidneys, evidence of infarcts, or renal asymmetry may suggest CKD. The presence of renal pelvic distention, ureteral dilation, or ureteroliths may suggest AKI or an acute obstructive component to preexisting chronic disease. A dilated renal pelvis without evidence of ureteroliths is suggestive of pyelonephritis, although

ureteral obstruction can occur without renal pelvic dilation. AKI can occur in a patient with previously normal renal function, or as an acute deterioration of preexisting renal disease.

BUN and creatinine values are insensitive markers of renal function, for both AKI and CKD. It may take up to five days for these values to increase after a renal insult. Symmetric dimethylarginine (SDMA) is more sensitive than BUN or creatinine at detecting GFR changes in CKD and may also be useful for AKI detection (Hall et al. 2014, 2016; Dahlem et al. 2017). GFR measurement is a more accurate measure of renal function than BUN or creatinine concentrations. Although relatively simple protocols exist for measuring GFR in chronic stable disease, measuring GFR in an AKI setting tends to be impractical in clinical practice. Cystatin C, kidney injury molecule (KIM)-1, and neutrophil gelatinase-associated lipocalin (NGAL) have been investigated as markers of early kidney injury (Bonventre 2007, 2008; Bagshaw & Gibney 2008; Coca et al. 2008; Ferguson et al. 2008; Parikh & Devarajan 2008; Vaidya et al. 2008, 2009; Waikar & Bonventre 2008; Wu & Parikh 2008; Haase et al. 2009; Yerramilli et al. 2016; Bland et al. 2018). KIM-1 in particular may provide a useful in-clinic rapid test to detect AKI.

Acute kidney injury

AKI can be caused by hemodynamic disturbances, intrinsic parenchymal damage, postrenal disorders, or by a combination of these. It is difficult to differentiate the relative contribution of each cause to AKI, as hemodynamic and postrenal disorders can lead to intrinsic damage if left untreated (Devarajan 2006; Okusa et al. 2019; Hingorani et al. 2009; Macedo & Mehta 2009; Chang et al. 2010; Langston 2017b). The classification of AKI has evolved to define it as a syndrome in human medicine (such as cardiorenal, hepatorenal, nephrotoxic, etc.), as it is a major complication of hospitalization and seen frequently in the intensive care unit (ICU) (Ronco et al. 2019). In veterinary medicine, classification of AKI is mostly based on relative anatomic origin.

Hemodynamic acute kidney injury

Hemodynamic causes of AKI include diseases characterized by renal hypoperfusion, but where the basic integrity of the renal parenchymal tissue is preserved. In these cases, GFR is often corrected once renal perfusion is restored in a timely fashion. However, severe or persistent renal hypoperfusion can lead to ischemic intrinsic AKI. Any condition that can cause systemic hypotension will activate arterial and cardiac baroreceptors and initiate a series of neural and humoral responses. These responses include activation of the sympathetic nervous system, with the subsequent release of norepinephrine, release of renin from the juxtaglomerular cells leading to the creation of angiotensin II, and ADH release from the posterior hypothalamus (Badr & Ichikawa 1988; Cowgill & Francey 2005; Macedo & Mehta 2009; Okusa *et al.* 2019). The main effect is to maintain systemic blood pressure, preserve cardiac and cerebral perfusion pressure, divert blood from acutely less important vascular beds such as the splanchnic circulation, stimulate thirst, and promote renal reabsorption of water and sodium.

The kidneys receive a large portion of cardiac output, but the vast majority of that blood is directed to the renal cortex. Blood leaving the efferent arterioles in the cortex enters the vasa recta in the medulla. The characteristic low blood flow of the vasa recta is important in the physiologic function of the countercurrent multiplier system. However, this low flow leaves the medulla in a state of relative hypoxia even in normal circumstances. For instance, the renal cortex has an average partial pressure of oxygen of about 50 mmHg, whereas the outer medulla has a partial pressure of oxygen of only 10–20 mmHg (Brezis & Rosen 1995). Slight changes in blood flow and oxygen can lead to hypoxic damage (Brezis & Rosen 1995; Heyman *et al.* 2008; Hill *et al.* 2008; Le Dorze *et al.* 2009).

The kidneys can maintain GFR and renal perfusion via autoregulation by protective mechanisms that include stretch receptors within afferent arterioles that detect a decrease in pressure, and trigger the relaxation of afferent arteriolar smooth muscle and subsequent vasodilatation. Other protective mechanisms include intrarenal synthesis of prostaglandin E_2, prostacyclin, nitric oxide (NO), kallikrein, and kinins, which promote afferent arteriolar vasodilatation, and angiotensin II, which induces preferential efferent arteriolar vasoconstriction and hence maintains intraglomerular pressure and subsequently GFR (Okusa *et al.* 2019; Kontogiannis & Burns 1998). Some of the major causes of hemodynamic AKI are listed in Table 42.1.

Several classes of drugs commonly used in a surgical setting may impair renal protective adaptive mechanisms and can exacerbate AKI from hypotension. For example, nonsteroidal anti-inflammatory drugs (NSAIDs), including selective cyclooxygenase (COX)-II inhibitors, inhibit renal prostaglandin synthesis. In moderate and severe hypotensive states, this can lead to inadequate afferent arteriolar vasodilatation and subsequent fall in RBF and GFR (Wali & Henrich 2002; Papich 2008). In a similar fashion, animals on angiotensin-converting enzyme (ACE) inhibitors or angiotensin receptor blockers (ARBs) may not be able to compensate adequately for hypotensive episodes during

Table 42.1 Major causes of hemodynamic acute kidney injury.

Intravascular depletion
  Hemorrhage from trauma, surgery, gastrointestinal tract
  Gastrointestinal loss from vomiting, diarrhea
  Blood volume sequestering
  Renal losses by drug-induced or osmotic diuresis, diabetes insipidus, Addison disease
  Increased insensible losses (i.e., panting, fever)
  Third-space losses (i.e., pancreatitis, hypoalbuminemia, liver failure)

Decreased cardiac output
  Myocardial, pericardial, valvular, or conduction diseases
  Pulmonary hypertension
  Pulmonary thromboembolism
  Systemic vasodilatation, disseminated intravascular coagulation, sepsis
  Positive-pressure ventilation
  Secondary to drugs: antihypertensives, afterload reduction, diuretics

Vasoactive mediators
  Hypercalcemia
  Endotoxins
  Radiocontrast agents
  Calcineurin inhibitors
  Angiotensin-converting enzyme (ACE) inhibitors
  Epinephrine, norepinephrine

Pharmacologic causes
  Anesthetic agents that impair renal autoregulation
  Nonsteroidal anti-inflammatory drugs impairing prostaglandin synthesis
  ACE inhibitors or angiotensin receptor blockers

surgical procedures (Engelhardt & Brown 1987; Brown *et al.* 2001; Lefebvre *et al.* 2007). Vasoactive substances, such as contrast agents and epinephrine used as a pressor agent, can induce intense intrarenal vasoconstriction, which leads to AKI (Margulies *et al.* 1990; Solomon 1998; Tepel *et al.* 2000). Renal compensatory mechanisms are overwhelmed during moderate to severe hypotension, and intrinsic AKI may follow.

Intrinsic acute kidney injury

Intrinsic AKI refers to diseases involving the renal parenchymal tissue (Table 42.2). As stated previously, hemodynamic AKI can lead to ischemic AKI if prolonged or severe. Intrinsic AKI can be divided into four anatomic locations: large renal vessel diseases, glomerular diseases, renal tubular injury, and tubulointerstitial diseases. Ischemic or toxic acute tubular injury accounts

Table 42.2 Major causes of intrinsic acute kidney injury.

Large renal vessels (rare)
   Surgical trauma
   Compression
   Thromboembolism
   Vasculitis

Glomerular diseases
   Amyloidosis
   Glomerulonephritis
   Malignant hypertension
   Hypercalcemia
   Radiocontrast agents, drugs
   Hemolytic–uremic syndrome
   Immune-mediated hemolytic anemia and secondary microthrombi
   Disseminated intravascular coagulation
   Hyperviscosity syndromes (erythrocytosis)

Renal tubular injury
   Ischemia caused by renal hypoperfusion
   Exogenous toxins (antibiotics, antineoplastic agents, radiocontrast agents)
   Endogenous toxins (hemoglobin, myoglobin, myeloma light chains, tumor lysis)

Tubulointerstitial diseases
   Allergic interstitial nephritis (antibiotics, nonsteroidal anti-inflammatory drugs)
   Infectious causes (pyelonephritis, leptospirosis)
   Neoplasia
   Systemic lupus erythematosus

for almost 90% of all intrinsic AKI in humans (Ronco et al. 2019; Okusa et al. 2019).

In humans, ischemic acute tubular injury is most often observed in patients who have major surgery, trauma, severe hypovolemia, sepsis, and burns (Gill et al. 2005). Sepsis can induce renal hypoperfusion by creating a combination of systemic vasodilatation and intrarenal vasoconstriction (De Vriese 2003; Schrier & Wang 2004; Langenberg et al. 2005; Bagshaw et al. 2007). In human patients with septic shock, 60-day mortality is 3–5 times greater in those who develop AKI (Ronco et al. 2019). Acute tubular injury from hypoperfusion is most severe in the outer medulla of the kidney, where oxygen tension is normally low and metabolic oxygen demand is normally high.

Some drugs and toxins have the potential to produce direct renal toxicity by causing intrarenal vasoconstriction (radiocontrast agents, NSAIDs), direct tubular toxicity (aminoglycosides, cisplatin, grapes, lilies), tubular dysfunction without necrosis (i.e., aminoglycosides), acute interstitial nephritis (i.e., penicillins), or tubular obstruction (i.e., trimethoprim sulfa) (Dillon 2001). Other drugs that are initially harmless to the kidneys can be metabolized by the kidneys into toxic metabolites (Okusa et al. 2019). Contrast nephropathy usually presents as an acute decline in GFR within 1–2 days of administration, a peak in creatinine level in 3–5 days, and a return to baseline within a week (McCullough 2008). The high proportion of cardiac output delivered to the kidneys makes them particularly vulnerable to toxic damage. In addition to the high delivery of toxins, the kidneys can concentrate certain toxins via the countercurrent system and also by active tubular absorption/secretion.

Drugs that can cause tubulointerstitial AKI such as β-lactam antibiotics (e.g., ampicillin and cephalosporins) can act as haptens and trigger infiltration of inflammatory cells and subsequent allergic reaction, causing an acute interstitial nephritis (Langston 2017a,b). NSAIDs are also reported to cause interstitial nephritis (Dillon 2001). Escherichia coli is the most frequently isolated cause of bacterial pyelonephritis (Barsanti et al. 1994; Norris et al. 2000; Barsanti 2006; Labato 2009). Other infectious causes include leptospirosis, which will trigger tubulointerstitial inflammation and damage (Niwattayakul et al. 2002; Langston & Heuter 2003; Andrade et al. 2008).

Direct kidney injury, as well as localized changes secondary to anoxia, promotes the migration of inflammatory cells into renal tissue. Release of inflammatory cytokines (interleukin-, tumor necrosis factor), chemokines, heat shock proteins, nitric oxide, and reactive oxygen species from damaged cells induces a proinflammatory environment (Misseri et al. 2004). There is also promotion of inflammatory cell adhesion molecules by the injured cells (Devarajan 2006). Hypoxic cells have upregulation of hypoxia inducible factor (HIF) genes and their respective targets, and upregulation of HIF is associated with lethal cellular damage (Furuichi et al. 2009).

Injury and loss of tubular cells by necrosis and apoptosis, can lead to loss of kidney function, tubular obstruction, and a decrease in GFR. Both necrosis, with its associated inflammatory response, and apoptosis occur with AKI. It is not clear why some cells are destined for apoptosis and others for necrosis but this may be related to the duration of ischemia (Allen et al. 1992; Wiegele et al. 1998). During AKI, the basolateral Na^+/K^+-ATPase can be lost, leading to a decrease in sodium reabsorption and increase in fractional sodium excretion (Racusen 2001). This can lead to increased tubuloglomerular feedback and a further drop in GFR.

Postrenal acute kidney injury

Postrenal AKI is caused by acute obstruction of the urinary tract from the ureters to the distal urethra (Table 42.3) (Cowgill & Francey 2005; Langston 2017a,b; Kennedy & White 2022). The type and degree of kidney damage that results from postrenal obstruction depend on numerous factors, including duration of obstruction, whether the obstruction is partial or complete, existing renal disease, species, and function of the contralateral kidney (Wen *et al.* 1999). Acute obstruction causes ureteral peristalsis to increase, and intraluminal ureteral and tubular pressures to rise (Klahr & Morrissey 2002). This induces the production and release of prostaglandin E_2, prostacyclin, and nitric oxide, which cause afferent arteriolar vasodilatation and hence increased RBF. Glomerular capillary hydraulic pressure increases, but the increase in tubular pressure exceeds this increase and GFR declines (Wen *et al.* 1999; Klahr & Morrissey 2002; Fischer *et al.* 2009). The incidence of nephrolithiasis and ureterolithiasis in cats has increased sharply in the past decade, making this a common cause of AKI in this species (Kyles *et al.* 2005; Kennedy & White 2022).

Table 42.3 Major causes of postrenal acute kidney injury.

Ureteral obstructions
  Intraluminal: calculi, blood clots, dried solidified blood, debris, strictures
  Extraluminal: neoplasia, accidental ligation
  Intramural: post-ureterotomy edema, suture reaction, strictures

Trigonal obstructions
  Neoplasia
  Calculi
  Neurologic causes
  Prostatic causes (benign prostatic hyperplasia, carcinoma, prostatitis, cystic prostatitis)

Urethral obstructions
  Calculi
  Neoplasia (urothelial [transitional] cell carcinoma being the most common)
  Stricture
  Debris
  Blood clots

Urinary tract/bladder rupture
  Calculi
  Neoplasia
  Iatrogenic (surgical, bladder expression, catheterization)
  Trauma

Mechanism of acute kidney injury

The main effect of kidney injury from prolonged hemodynamic, intrinsic renal, or postrenal causes is a decrease in GFR (Okusa *et al.* 2019). The decrease in the filtration capacity of the kidney occurs before any damage is visible on histopathology, and even before traditional renal function markers such as SDMA, BUN, and creatinine increase. There are three major proposed mechanisms for the decrease in GFR.

The first mechanism is a drop in filtration pressure within the glomerulus caused by afferent arteriolar vasoconstriction due to endothelial cell injury (Burke *et al.* 1980; Alejandro *et al.* 1995). The resultant reduction in glomerular capillary ultrafiltration coefficient (K_f) and permeability leads to a direct fall in GFR capability. Endothelial cell injury leads to an imbalance of vasoactive substances, with a predominance of vasoconstrictive mediators (Okusa *et al.* 2019). The second mechanism involves tubular back leakage and creates an effective decrease in GFR. In this setting, damaged tubular epithelial cells allow glomerular filtrate to leak back into the renal interstitium and be reabsorbed into the systemic circulation. The main determinant of this mechanism is the depletion of ATP, leading to disruption of tight junctions (Lee *et al.* 2006; Okusa *et al.* 2019). The third mechanism is a result of tubular obstruction such as when sloughed tubular epithelial cells form casts in the tubular lumen (Okusa *et al.* 2019).

Another consequence of AKI is a decrease in the ability of the kidney to concentrate urine. This can be explained by a loss of ADH-responsive aquaporin channels in the collecting ducts (Kwon *et al.* 1999).

Phases of acute kidney injury

AKI can be divided into five phases: insult, initiation, extension, maintenance, and recovery (Bock 1998; Molitoris 2003; Langston 2017a,b). The insult and initiation phases are the periods where the animal is exposed to the damaging insult and parenchymal renal injury is evolving, but not yet established. Acute tubular injury is preventable in this setting. This period can last from a few hours to many days. The end portion of the initiation phase is called the extension phase. This phase is characterized by the kidneys being subject to altered renal perfusion, continued hypoxia, inflammation, and ongoing cellular damage (Cowgill & Francey 2005). During the maintenance phase, parenchymal damage is established and GFR decreases. As a result of ongoing cellular damage, renal cells undergo necrosis or apoptosis. UOP may decrease in this period. The maintenance phase usually lasts about 1–2 weeks, but may be prolonged (Bonventre & Weinberg 2003; Cowgill & Francey 2005).

In the recovery phase, there is repair and regeneration of renal tissue. Renal function may recover completely, partially, or not at all. An increase in urine production during this phase does not correspond necessarily to a meaningful improvement in GFR. The renal injury induces growth factor production, which allows remaining surviving cells to enter the cell cycle, replicate, repopulate, and dedifferentiate into mature epithelial cells. Growth factors involved include insulin-like growth factor-1, epidermal growth factor (EGF), transforming growth factor (TGF), platelet-derived growth factor, fibroblast growth factor, nerve growth factor, hepatocyte growth factor, and vascular endothelial growth factor (Ichimura & Bonventre 2001). These growth factors allow repair, but also favor fibrosis and other negative aspects, leading to progression of renal damage and loss of function. The recovery phase can last weeks to months (Cowgill & Francey 2005).

Anoxia leads to depletion of cellular ATP stores and consequently to disruption of the endothelial cell actin cytoskeleton (Kwon et al. 2002). The endothelial cells become deformed, and this leads to red blood cell sludging and vascular congestion. Hypoxia also leads to dysregulation of intracellular ionic concentrations of Na^+ and Ca^{2+}. These two ions enter the cell because the lack of energy causes defective membrane pumps, and consequently cells swell and burst (Le Dorze et al. 2009).

Role of endothelial cells in acute kidney injury

Endothelial cells play an important role in the development of AKI. Under normal circumstances, intrarenal production of vasodilatory mediators such as prostacyclin and prostaglandin E_2 mediates vasodilatation of afferent arterioles, which decreases renal vascular resistance and maintains RBF. When an initial insult damages the endothelial cells of renal vessels, the damage leads to an inability to regulate local blood flow, cell migration into tissues, and coagulation (Sutton et al. 2002; Molitoris & Sutton 2004). Intrarenal vasoconstriction may occur when there is an imbalance of production of normal vasodilatory substances (nitric oxide) and vasoconstrictive substances (endothelin). Endothelial nitric oxide synthase (eNOS) function is decreased with hypoxic/ischemic renal damage, and inducible nitric oxide synthase (iNOS) activity is increased. This leads to an increase in reactive oxygen species, which can further damage cells (Goligorsky et al. 2002, 2004; Andreoli 2009). Ischemic damage to endothelial cells leads to disruption of actin filaments and loss of cellular integrity (Brady et al. 1996; Racusen 2001). Damaged endothelial cells change their interactions with inflammatory cells, and express more P and E selectins as well as intercellular adhesion molecule (ICAM)-1, the integrins responsible for the attachment of inflammatory cells (Eppihimer et al. 1997; Molitoris & Marrs 1999; Friedewald & Rabb 2004; Singbartl & Ley 2004).

Complications arising from acute kidney injury

AKI will disrupt multiple aspects of renal function, including the kidney's role in maintaining body fluid homeostasis, excretion of Na^+, K^+, water, and the body's waste products, urinary acidification mechanisms, and acid–base buffer mechanisms.

Intravascular volume overload is a consequence of the kidney's inability to regulate sodium and water excretion. This can lead to clinically relevant consequences, ranging from mild hypertension to severe pulmonary edema. Dehydration can occur from excess sodium or water loss (Okusa et al. 2019; Bouchard & Mehta 2009).

Hyperkalemia is a common sequela of AKI and is potentially life-threatening (Alosaif et al. 2005). Mild hyperkalemia (<6.0 mEq/L) is usually asymptomatic, but higher levels will frequently manifest with electrocardiogram (ECG) abnormalities. Life-threatening cardiac abnormalities induced by hyperkalemia include bradycardia, heart block, ventricular tachycardia or fibrillation, and asystole. Hyperkalemia can also lead to hyporeflexia, muscle weakness, and respiratory failure (Mattu et al. 2000; Esposito et al. 2004; Kahloon et al. 2005; DiBartola 2012).

Normal protein metabolism leads to the production of a large quantity of fixed nonvolatile acids that are normally eliminated by the kidneys to preserve acid–base homeostasis. Hyperphosphatemia is a common consequence of AKI and leads to excessive parathyroid hormone secretion, calcium disorders, and tissue mineralization (Finco et al. 1992; Knochel & Agarwal 1996).

Anemia can develop quite rapidly in AKI. It is usually mild to moderate and multifactorial in origin. Causes include lack of secretion of erythropoietin from the kidneys, hemolysis, bleeding, and reduced red blood cell survival time. Bleeding can be a consequence of uremic thrombocytopathia, gastrointestinal ulceration, and vasculitis (Radtke et al. 1979; Eschbach 1989; Cowgill 1992; King et al. 1992; Fishbane & Masani 2005; Weiss & Goodnough 2005).

Cardiac complications include arrhythmias, myocardial infarction, and pulmonary embolism. These abnormalities can be triggered by hypervolemia, acidosis, hyperkalemia, and other metabolic sequelae of AKI (Cowgill & Francey 2005; Okusa et al. 2019).

The inflammatory response in AKI, especially if prolonged, leads to a catabolic state and the patient ends up with net protein breakdown. Nitrogenous waste products accumulate and lead to uremic syndrome (Williams et al. 1991; Druml 1998).

Preventive measures in acute kidney injury

Prevention of AKI involves avoiding or reducing risk factors while attempting to protect the kidneys. Optimization of cardiovascular function and intravascular volume is by far the most important aspect of AKI prevention (Langston 2017a,b). Proper maintenance of blood pressure is essential in avoiding hemodynamic AKI. Timely and effective hemostasis and replacement of any blood loss with proper crystalloids and colloids or blood products will also minimize the development of AKI. Volume depletion is a known risk factor for nephrotoxic AKI caused by radiocontrast agents, aminoglycosides, cisplatin, hemolysis, and other nephrotoxins. The use of proper, established dosages for drugs is essential. Diuretics, NSAIDs, ACE inhibitors, ARBs, and other vasodilator drugs should be used with caution in patients with suspected hypovolemia or renal disease. With preexisting renal disease, it is important to realize that some drugs may not be eliminated in the same manner as if the kidneys were healthy, and that drug dosages should be modified accordingly. The use of pressors in periods of hypotension during surgery should be judicious. Pressors can effectively reduce RBF and promote AKI. Prolonged anesthesia should be avoided as much as possible. Risk factors can be cumulative (Lane *et al.* 1994; Grauer 1996, 1999).

Outcome

The prognosis for recovery from AKI depends on the cause, duration of damage, comorbidity, extent of damage, and the speed at which AKI is diagnosed (Langston *et al.* 1997; Adin & Cowgill 2000; Cowgill & Francey 2005; Anderson *et al.* 2006; Harison *et al.* 2012; Langston 2017a,b). A review of 99 cases of AKI in dogs demonstrated a mortality of nearly 60% from death or euthanasia (Vaden *et al.* 1997). Almost 60% of the surviving dogs developed CKD. Failure to survive was associated with the severity of azotemia, hypocalcemia, anemia, proteinuria, cause (i.e., ethylene glycol), and disseminated intravascular coagulation. In another case series, mortality for dogs with hospital-acquired AKI was 62%. In this study, age and initial urine production were predictors of mortality. Survival from hemodynamic and infectious causes is greater than survival from toxic causes (Behrend *et al.* 1996; Cowgill & Francey 2005). Mortality in cats was approximately 50% in one series, of which half had persistent azotemia (Worwag & Langston 2008).

In a study of hospitalized cats and dogs, patients were monitored for the progression of AKI and changes in creatinine. Dogs and cats with initial creatinine <1.6 mg/dL had ≥1 other creatinine measurement within 2, 3,

and 7 days of hospitalization were included in the study. AKI was defined as increase in creatinine by >0.3 mg/dL. Patients were then placed into levels 0–2, and mortality assessed at 30 and 90 days. Level 0 was defined as an initial creatinine ≤1.6 mg/dL and a change of <0.3 mg/dL. Level 1 was patients with a starting creatinine of ≤1.6 mg/dL and a change of ≥0.3 mg/dL. Level 3 was pets that started with a creatinine of >1.6 mg/dL and had a change of ≥0.3 mg/dL. Dogs placed in level 1 within 2 days were approximately three times more likely to die within 90 days. Dogs placed in level 2 within 2, 3, or 7 days were approximately three times more likely to die within 30 or 90 days. Cats placed in level 2 within 3 or 7 days were approximately three times more likely to die at 30 days and four times more likely to die if placed in this level within 7 days. If placed in level 2 within 2 or 3 days, cats were approximately three times more likely to die within 90 days. Therefore, the study concluded that detecting increasing azotemia, even if still within reference range, predicted mortality in hospitalized patients with AKI (Harison *et al.* 2012).

Chronic kidney disease

CKD is a common problem in veterinary medicine, especially in cats. The prevalence of kidney disease has been estimated to range between 0.5% and 7% in dogs and between 1.6% and 20% in cats. The incidence increases in older animals, and the causes are multifactorial. Tubulointerstitial inflammation and fibrosis are common findings regardless of the inciting cause. Tubulointerstitial disease, far from being merely a result of glomerular damage, plays a prominent role in the progression of CKD (Remuzzi *et al.* 2008). Glomerular damage increases the amount of protein in the ultrafiltrate delivered to the tubule. Most of the protein is reabsorbed by the tubules, which induces damage to the tubular cells and interstitium. Glomerular hypertension or hypoperfusion may damage the associated tubule. As nephron mass decreases, remaining nephrons hypertrophy, but this adaptation can lead to tubulointerstitial disease. Damage leads to transition of epithelial tubular cells into mesenchymal fibroblasts. TGF-β and EGF provide the strongest stimulus for the transition.

Chronic hypoxia is one of the most important contributors to tubulointerstitial fibrosis. Resultant angiotensin production and inhibition of nitric oxide cause vasoconstriction that may worsen the hypoxia. Because the diffusion distance between tubular cells and peritubular capillaries is increased, with tubular atrophy and increased interstitial compartment volume, fibrosis further impairs this relationship, worsening the hypoxia. The remaining tubules become hypermetabolic, further increasing oxygen consumption and worsening the hypoxic environment (Remuzzi *et al.* 2008). While careful attention to modifiable risk factors, such as ensuring adequate hydration and blood pressure during anesthesia to preserve RBF and avoidance of nephrotoxins, will allow many patients with CKD to withstand surgical procedures, it has been our clinical experience that some patients with severe CKD will progress to end-stage disease (frequently oliguric to anuric) after surgical procedures, despite all precautions.

CKD is recognized as a disease entity, but the initiating cause is often unknown. In cats, a current theory is that of mini active kidney injuries. An initial insult to the kidney may lead to maladaptive repair mechanisms to the basement membranes, leaving the kidney open to further damage either by mini active kidney injuries or by a slow sustained injury. This leads to a progressive loss of nephron mass and function, leading to detectable CKD (Cowgill *et al.* 2016).

References

Absosaif, N.Y., Tolba, Y.A., Heap, M. et al. (2005). The outcome of acute renal failure in the intensive care unit according to RIFLE: model application, sensitivity, and predictability. *American Journal of Kidney Diseases* 46: 1038–1048.

Adams, L.G. (2000). Renal failure, chronic. In: *The 5-Minute Veterinary Consult: Canine and Feline*, 2e (ed. L.P. Tilley and F.W.K. Smith Jr.). Baltimore, MD: Lippincott Williams & Wilkins.

Adin, C.A. and Cowgill, L.D. (2000). Treatment and outcome of dogs with leptospirosis: 36 cases (1990–1998). *Journal of the American Veterinary Medical Association* 216: 371–375.

Alejandro, V., Scandling, J.D. Jr., Sibley, R.K. et al. (1995). Mechanisms of filtration failure during postischemic injury of the human kidney. A study of the reperfused renal allograft. *Journal of Clinical Investigation* 95: 820–831.

Allen, J., Winterford, C., Axelsen, R.A., and Gobe, G.C. (1992). Effects of hypoxia on morphological and biochemical characteristics of renal epithelial cell and tubule cultures. *Renal Failure* 14: 453–460.

Allon, M. (2017). Disorders of potassium metabolism. In: *Primer on Kidney Diseases*, 7e (ed. D. Weiner). Philadelphia, PA: WB Saunders.

Anderson, R.J. (2001). Clinical and laboratory diagnosis of acute renal failure. In: *Acute Renal Failure: A Companion to Brenner and Rector's the Kidney* (ed. B.A. Molitoris and W.F. Finn). Philadelphia, PA: WB Saunders.

Anderson, R.B., Aronson, L.R., Drobatz, K.J., and Atilla, A. (2006). Prognostic factors for successful outcome following urethral rupture in dogs and cats. *Journal of the American Animal Hospital Association* 42: 136–146.

Andrade, L., de Francesco, D.E., and Seguro, A.C. (2008). Leptospiral nephropathy. *Seminars in Nephrology* 28: 383–394.

Andreoli, S.P. (2009). Acute kidney injury in children. *Pediatric Nephrology* 24: 253–263.

Badr, K.F. and Ichikawa, I. (1988). Prerenal failure: a deleterious shift from renal compensation to decompensation. *New England Journal of Medicine* 319: 623–629.

Bagshaw, S.M. and Gibney, R.T.N. (2008). Conventional markers of kidney function. *Critical Care Medicine* 36: S152–S158.

Bagshaw, S.M., Langenberg, C., Wan, L. et al. (2007). A systematic review of urinary findings in experimental septic acute renal failure. *Critical Care Medicine* 35: 1592–1598.

Barrett, K.E., Barman, S.M., Yuan, J. et al. (2019). Renal function and micturition. In: *Ganong's Review of Medical Physiology*, 26e (ed. K.E. Barrett, S.M. Barman, J. Yuan and H. Brooks). New York: Lange Medical/McGraw-Hill.

Barsanti, J.A. (2006). Genitourinary infections. In: *Infectious Diseases of the Dog and Cat*, 3e (ed. C.E. Greene). Saunders Elsevier: St. Louis, MO.

Barsanti, J.A., Finco, D.R., and Brown, S.A. (1994). Disease of the lower urinary tract. In: *The Cat: Diseases and Clinical Management*, 2e (ed. R.G. Sherding). New York: Churchill Livingstone.

Behrend, E., Grauer, G.F., Mani, I. et al. (1996). Hospital-acquired acute renal failure in dogs: 29 cases (1983–1992). *Journal of the American Veterinary Medical Association* 208: 537–541.

Bland, K.S., Clark, M.E., Cote, O., and Bienzle, D. (2018). A specific immunoassay for detection of feline kidney injury molecule 1. *Journal of Feline Medicine and Surgery* 21: 1069–1079.

Bock, H.A. (1998). Pathogenesis of acute renal failure: new aspects. *Contributions to Nephrology* 124: 43–55; discussion 55–63.

Bonventre, J.V. (2007). Diagnosis of acute kidney injury: from classic parameters to new biomarkers. *Contributions to Nephrology* 156: 213–219.

Bonventre, J.V. (2008). Kidney injury molecule-1 (KIM-1): a specific and sensitive biomarker of kidney injury. *Scandinavian Journal of Clinical and Laboratory Investigation Supplement* 241: 78–83.

Bonventre, J.V. and Weinberg, J.M. (2003). Recent advances in the pathophysiology of ischemic acute renal failure. *Journal of the American Society of Nephrology* 14: 2199–2210.

Bouchard, J. and Mehta, R.L. (2009). Fluid accumulation and acute kidney injury: consequence or cause. *Current Opinion in Critical Care* 15: 509–513.

Brady, P.A., Alekseev, A.E., Aleksandrova, L.A. et al. (1996). A disrupter of actin microfilaments impairs sulfonylurea-inhibitory gating of cardiac KATP channels. *American Journal of Physiology* 271: H2710–H2716.

Brezis, M.L. and Rosen, S. (1995). Hypoxia of the renal medulla: its implications for disease. *New England Journal of Medicine* 332: 647–655.

Briggs, J.P., Kriz, W., and Schnermann, J.B. (2017). Overview of kidney function and structure. In: *Primer on Kidney Diseases*, 7e (ed. D. Weiner). Philadelphia, PA: Elsevier Saunders.

Brown, S.A. (1993). Determinants of glomerular ultrafiltration in cats. *American Journal of Veterinary Research* 54: 970–975.

Brown, S.A., Brown, C.A., Jacobs, G. et al. (2001). Effects of the angiotensin converting enzyme inhibitor benazepril in cats with induced renal insufficiency. *American Journal of Veterinary Research* 62: 375–383.

Burke, T.J., Cronin, R.E., Duchin, K.L. et al. (1980). Ischemia and tubule obstruction during acute renal failure in dogs: mannitol in protection. *American Journal of Physiology* 238: F305–F314.

Chang, C.H., Lin, C.Y., Tian, Y.C. et al. (2010). Acute kidney injury classification: comparison of AKIN and RIFLE criteria. *Shock* 23: 247–252.

Coca, S.G., Yalavarthy, R., Concato, J., and Parikh, C.R. (2008). Biomarkers for the diagnosis and risk stratification of acute kidney injury: a systematic review. *Kidney International* 73: 1008–1016.

Cowgill, L.D. (1992). Pathophysiology and management of anemia in chronic progressive renal failure. *Seminars in Veterinary Medicine and Surgery (Small Animal)* 7: 175–182.

Cowgill, L.D. and Francey, T. (2005). Acute uremia. In: *Textbook of Veterinary Internal Medicine*, 6e (ed. S.J. Ettinger and E.C. Feldman). Philadelphia, PA: Elsevier Saunders.

Cowgill, L.D., Polzin, D.J., Elliott, J. et al. (2016). Is progressive chronic kidney disease a slow acute kidney injury? *Veterinary Clinics: Small Animal Practice* 46: 995–1013.

Dahlem, D.P., Neiger, R., Schweighauser, A. et al. (2017). Plasma symmetric dimethylarginine concentration in dogs with acute kidney injury and chronic kidney disease. *Journal of Veterinary Internal Medicine* 31: 799–804.

De Vriese, A.S. (2003). Prevention and treatment of acute renal failure in sepsis. *Journal of the American Society of Nephrology* 14: 792–805.

Devarajan, P. (2006). Update on mechanisms of ischemic acute kidney injury. *Journal of the American Society of Nephrology* 17: 1503–1520.

DiBartola, S.P. (2012). Applied renal physiology. In: *Fluid, Electrolyte, and Acid–Base Disorders in Small Animal Practice*, 4e (ed. S.P. DiBartola). St Louis, MO: Saunders Elsevier.

Dillon, J.J. (2001). Nephrotoxicity from antibacterial, antifungal, and antiviral drugs. In: *Acute Renal Failure: A Companion to Brenner and Rector's the Kidney* (ed. B.A. Molitoris and W.F. Finn). Philadelphia, PA: WB Saunders.

Druml, W. (1998). Protein metabolism in acute renal failure. *Mineral and Electrolyte Metabolism* 24: 47–54.

Engelhardt, J.A. and Brown, S.A. (1987). Drug-related nephropathies. Part II. Commonly used drugs. *Compendium on Continuing Education for the Practicing Veterinarian* 9: 281–288.

Eppihimer, M.J., Russell, J., Anderson, D.C. et al. (1997). Modulation of P-selectin expression in the postischemic intestinal microvasculature. *American Journal of Physiology* 273: G1326–G1332.

Eschbach, J.W. (1989). The anemia of chronic renal failure: pathophysiology and the effects of recombinant erythropoietin. *Kidney International* 35: 134–148.

Esposito, C., Bellotti, N., Fasoli, G. et al. (2004). Hyperkalemia-induced ECG abnormalities in patients with reduced renal function. *Clinical Nephrology* 62: 465–468.

Ferguson, M.A., Vaidya, V.S., and Bonventre, J.V. (2008). Biomarkers of nephrotoxic acute kidney injury. *Toxicology* 245: 182–193.

Finco, D.R., Brown, S.A., Crowell, W.A. et al. (1992). Effects of dietary phosphorus and protein in dogs with chronic renal failure. *American Journal of Veterinary Research* 53: 2264–2271.

Fischer, J.R., Lane, I.F., and Stokes, J.E. (2009). Acute postrenal azotemia: etiology, clinicopathology, and pathophysiology. *Compendium on Continuing Education for the Practicing Veterinarian* 31: 520–529.

Fishbane, S. and Masani, N. (2005). Anemia in chronic kidney disease. In: *Chronic Kidney Disease, Dialysis, and Transplantation*, 2e (ed. B.J.G. Pereira, M.H. Sayegh and P. Blake). Philadelphia, PA: Elsevier Saunders.

Friedewald, J.J. and Rabb, H. (2004). Inflammatory cells in ischemic acute renal failure. *Kidney International* 66: 486–491.

Furuichi, K., Kaneko, S., and Wada, T. (2009). Chemokine/chemokine receptor-mediated inflammation regulates pathologic changes from acute kidney injury to chronic kidney disease. *Clinical and Experimental Nephrology* 13: 9–14.

Gill, N., Nally, J.V. Jr., and Fatica, R.A. (2005). Renal failure secondary to acute tubular necrosis: epidemiology, diagnosis, and management. *Chest* 128: 2847–2863.

Goligorsky, M.S., Brodsky, S.V., and Noiri, E. (2002). Nitric oxide in acute renal failure: NOS versus NOS. *Kidney International* 61: 855–861.

Goligorsky, M.S., Brodsky, S.V., and Noiri, E. (2004). NO bioavailability, endothelial dysfunction, and acute renal failure: new insights into pathophysiology. *Seminars in Nephrology* 24: 316–323.

Grauer, G.F. (1996). Prevention of acute renal failure. *Veterinary Clinics of North America. Small Animal Practice* 26: 1447–1459.

Grauer, G.F. (1999). Prevention of hospital-acquired acute renal failure. *Veterinary Forum* 46–53.

Guyton, A.C. and Hall, J.C. (2020). The urinary system: functional anatomy and urine formation by the kidneys. In: *Textbook of Medical Physiology*. Philadelphia, PA: Elsevier Saunders.

Haase, M., Bellomo, R., Devarajan, P. et al. (2009). Accuracy of neutrophil gelatinase-associated lipocalin (NGAL) in diagnosis and prognosis in acute kidney injury: a systematic review and meta-analysis. *American Journal of Kidney Diseases* 54: 1012–1024.

Hall, J.A., Yerramilli, M., Obare, E. et al. (2014). Comparison of serum concentrations of symmetric dimethylarginine and creatinine as kidney function biomarkers in cats with chronic kidney disease. *Journal of Veterinary Internal Medicine* 28: 1676–1683.

Hall, J.A., Yerramilli, M., Obare, E. et al. (2016). Serum concentrations of symmetric dimethylarginine and creatinine in dogs with naturally occurring chronic kidney disease. *Journal of Veterinary Internal Medicine* 30: 794–802.

Harison, E., Langston, C.E., Palma, D., and Lamb, K. (2012). Acute azotemia as a predictor of mortality in dogs and cats. *Journal of Veterinary Internal Medicine* 26: 1093–1098.

Heyman, S.N., Rosen, S., and Rosenberger, C. (2008). Renal parenchymal hypoxia, hypoxia adaptation, and the pathogenesis of radiocontrast nephropathy. *Clinical Journal of the American Society of Nephrology* 3: 288–296.

Hill, P., Shukla, D., Tran, M.G.B. et al. (2008). Inhibition of hypoxia inducible factor hydroxylases protects against renal ischemia-reperfusion injury. *Journal of the American Society of Nephrology* 19: 39–46.

Hingorani, S., Molitoris, B.A., and Himmelfarb, J. (2009). Ironing out the pathogenesis of acute kidney injury. *American Journal of Kidney Diseases* 53: 569–571.

Ichimura, T. and Bonventre, J.V. (2001). Growth factors, signaling, and renal injury and repair. In: *Acute Renal Failure: A Companion to Brenner and Rector's the Kidney* (ed. B.A. Molitoris and W.F. Finn). Philadelphia, PA: WB Saunders.

Inker, L.A., Levey, A.J., Gilbert, S.J. et al. (2017). Assessment of kidney function in acute and chronic settings. In: *Primer on Kidney Diseases*, 7e (ed. D. Weiner). Philadelphia, PA: Elsevier Saunders.

Kahloon, M.U., Aslam, A.K., Aslam, A.F. et al. (2005). Hyperkalemia induced failure of atrial and ventricular pacemaker capture. *International Journal of Cardiology* 105: 224–226.

Kennedy, J.A. and White, J.A. (2022). Feline ureteral obstruction: a case-control study of risk factors (2016–2019). *Journal of Feline Medicine and Surgery* 24: 298–303.

Kerl, M. (2020). Acute kidney injury. In: *Cote's Clinical Veterinary Adviser Dogs and Cats*, 4e (ed. L.A. Cohn and E. Cote). St. Louis, MO: Elsevier.

King, L.G., Giger, U., Diserens, D., and Nagode, L.A. (1992). Anemia of chronic renal failure in dogs. *Journal of Veterinary Internal Medicine* 6: 264–270.

Klahr, S. and Morrissey, J. (2002). Obstructive nephropathy and renal fibrosis. *American Journal of Physiology* 283: F861–F875.

Knochel, J.P. and Agarwal, R. (1996). Hypophosphatemia and hyperphosphatemia. In: *Brenner and Rector's the Kidney*, 5e (ed. B.M. Brenner). Philadelphia, PA: WB Saunders.

Kontogiannis, J.B. and Burns, K.D. (1998). Role of AT1 angiotensin II receptors in renal ischemic injury. *American Journal of Physiology* 274: F79–F90.

Kwon, T.-H., Frokiaer, J., Fernandez-Llama, P. et al. (1999). Reduced abundance of aquaporins in rats with bilateral ischemia-induced acute renal failure: prevention by α-MSH. *American Journal of Physiology* 277: 413–427.

Kwon, O., Phillips, C.L., and Molitoris, B.A. (2002). Ischemia induces alterations in actin filaments in renal vascular smooth muscle cells. *American Journal of Physiology* 282: F1012–F1019.

Kyles, A.E., Hardie, E.M., Wooden, B.G. et al. (2005). Clinical, clinicopathologic, radiographic, and ultrasonographic abnormalities in cats with ureteral calculi: 163 cases (1984–2002). *Journal of the American Veterinary Medical Association* 226: 932–936.

Labato, M.A. (2009). Uncomplicated urinary tract infection. In: *Kirk's Current Veterinary Therapy XIV* (ed. J.D. Bonagura and D.C. Twedt). St. Louis, MO: Saunders Elsevier.

Lane, I.F., Grauer, G.F., and Fettman, M.J. (1994). Acute renal failure. Part I. Risk factors, prevention, and strategies for protection. *Compendium on Continuing Education for the Practicing Veterinarian* 16: 15–18, 20–23, 26–29.

Langenberg, C., Bellomo, R., May, C. et al. (2005). Renal blood flow in sepsis. *Critical Care* 9: R363–R374.

Langston, C.E. (2017a). Chronic kidney disease. In: *Textbook of Veterinary Internal Medicine*, 11e (ed. S.J. Ettinger, E.C. Feldman and E. Cote). St. Louis, MO: Elsevier.

Langston, C.E. (2017b). Acute kidney injury. In: *Textbook of Veterinary Internal Medicine*, 11e (ed. S.J. Ettinger, E.C. Feldman and E. Cote). St. Louis, MO: Elsevier.

Langston, C.E. and Heuter, K.J. (2003). Leptospirosis: a re-emerging zoonotic disease. *Veterinary Clinics of North America. Small Animal Practice* 33: 791–807.

Langston, C.E., Cowgill, L.D., and Spano, J.A. (1997). Applications and outcome of hemodialysis in cats: a review of 29 cases. *Journal of Veterinary Internal Medicine* 11: 348–355.

Le Dorze, M., Legrand, M., Payen, D., and Ince, C. (2009). The role of the microcirculation in acute kidney injury. *Current Opinion in Critical Care* 15: 503–508.

Lee, D.B., Huang, E., and Ward, H.J. (2006). Tight junction biology and kidney dysfunction. *American Journal of Physiology* 290: F20–F34.

Lefebvre, H.P., Brown, S.A., Chetboul, V. et al. (2007). Angiotensin-converting enzyme inhibitors in veterinary medicine. *Current Pharmaceutical Design* 13: 1347–1361.

Macedo, E. and Mehta, R.L. (2009). Prerenal failure: from old concepts to new paradigms. *Current Opinion in Critical Care* 15: 467–473.

Margulies, K.B., McKinley, L.J., Cavero, P.G., and Burnett, J.C.J. (1990). Induction and prevention of radiocontrast-induced nephropathy in dogs with heart failure. *Kidney International* 38: 1101–1108.

Mattu, A., Brady, W.J., and Robinson, D.A. (2000). Electrocardiographic manifestations of hyperkalemia. *American Journal of Emergency Medicine* 18: 721–729.

McCullough, P.A. (2008). Acute kidney injury with iodinated contrast. *Critical Care Medicine* 36: S204–S211.

Misseri, R., Rink, R.C., Meldrum, D.R., and Meldrum, K.K. (2004). Inflammatory mediators and growth factors in obstructive renal injury. *Journal of Surgical Research* 119: 149–159.

Molitoris, B.A. (2003). Transitioning to therapy in ischemic acute renal failure. *Journal of the American Society of Nephrology* 14: 265–267.

Molitoris, B.A. and Marrs, J. (1999). The role of cell adhesion molecules in ischemic acute renal failure. *American Journal of Medicine* 106: 583–592.

Molitoris, B.A. and Sutton, T.A. (2004). Endothelial injury and dysfunction: role in the extension phase of acute renal failure. *Kidney International* 66: 496–499.

Niwattayakul, K., Homvijitkul, J., Niwattayakul, S. et al. (2002). Hypotension, renal failure, and pulmonary complications in leptospirosis. *Renal Failure* 24: 297–305.

Norris, C.R., Williams, B.J., Ling, G.V. et al. (2000). Recurrent and persistent urinary tract infections in dogs: 383 cases (1969–1995). *Journal of the American Animal Hospital Association* 36: 484–492.

Okusa, M.D., Portilla, D.T., Maarten, W. et al. (2019). Pathophysiology of acute kidney injury. In: *Brenner and Rector's the Kidney*, 11e (ed. G. Chertrow, V. Luyckx, P. Marsden, et al.). Philadelphia, PA: Elsevier Saunders.

Padanilam, B.J. (2003). Cell death induced by acute renal injury: a perspective on the contributions of apoptosis and necrosis. *American Journal of Physiology* 284: F608–F627.

Papich, M.G. (2008). An update on nonsteroidal anti-inflammatory drugs (NSAIDs) in small animals. *Veterinary Clinics of North America. Small Animal Practice* 38: 1243–1266.

Parikh, C.R. and Devarajan, P. (2008). New biomarkers of acute kidney injury. *Critical Care Medicine* 36: S159–S165.

Polzin, D.J. (2017). Chronic kidney disease. In: *Textbook of Veterinary Internal Medicine*, 8e (ed. E. Cote, S. Ettinger and E.C. Feldman). St. Louis, MO: Elsevier Saunders.

Racusen, L.C. (2001). The morphologic basis of acute renal failure. In: *Acute Renal Failure: A Companion to Brenner & Rector's the Kidney* (ed. B.A. Molitoris and W.F. Finn). Philadelphia, PA: WB Saunders.

Radtke, H.W., Claussner, A., Erbes, P.M. et al. (1979). Serum erythropoietin concentration in chronic renal failure: relationship to degree of anemia and excretory renal function. *Blood* 54: 877–884.

Remuzzi, G., Perico, N., and De Broe, M.E. (2008). Tubulointerstitial diseases. In: *Brenner and Rector the Kidney*, 8e (ed. B.M. Brenner). Philadelphia, PA: Saunders Elsevier.

Ronco, C., Bellomo, R., and Kellum, J.A. (2019). Acute kidney injury. *Lancet* 394: 1949–1964.

Schrier, R.W. and Wang, W. (2004). Acute renal failure and sepsis. *New England Journal of Medicine* 351: 159–169.

Singbartl, K. and Ley, K. (2004). Leukocyte recruitment and acute renal failure. *Journal of Molecular Medicine* 82: 91–101.

Solomon, R. (1998). Contrast-medium-induced acute renal failure. *Kidney International* 53: 230–242.

Sutton, T.A., Fisher, C.J., and Molitoris, B.A. (2002). Microvascular endothelial injury and dysfunction during ischemic acute renal failure. *Kidney International* 62: 1539–1549.

Tepel, M., van der Giet, M., Schwarzfeld, C. et al. (2000). Prevention of radiographic-contrast-induced reductions in renal function by acetylcysteine. *New England Journal of Medicine* 343: 180–184.

Vaden, S.L., Levine, J., and Breitschwerd, E.B. (1997). A retrospective case control of acute renal failure in 99 dogs. *Journal of Veterinary Internal Medicine* 11: 58–64.

Vaidya, V.S., Ferguson, M.A., and Bonventre, J.V. (2008). Biomarkers of acute kidney injury. *Annual Review of Pharmacology and Toxicology* 48: 463–493.

Vaidya, V.S., Ford, G.M., Waikar, S.S. et al. (2009). A rapid urine test for early detection of kidney injury. *Kidney International* 76: 108–114.

Verlander, J.W., Clapp, W.L., Taal, M.W. et al. (2019). Anatomy of the kidney. In: *Brenner and Rector's the Kidney*, 11e (ed. G. Chertrow, V. Luyckx, P. Marsden, et al.). Philadelphia, PA: Elsevier Saunders.

Versteilen, A.M.G., Di Maggio, F., Leemreis, J.R. et al. (2004). Molecular mechanism of acute renal failure following ischemia/reperfusion. *International Journal of Artificial Organs* 27: 1019–1029.

Waikar, S.S. and Bonventre, J.V. (2008). Biomarkers for the diagnosis of acute kidney injury. *Nephron. Clinical Practice* 109: c192–c197.

Wali, R.K. and Henrich, W.L. (2002). Recent developments in toxic nephropathy. *Current Opinion in Nephrology and Hypertension* 11: 155–163.

Weiss, G. and Goodnough, L.T. (2005). Anemia of chronic disease. *New England Journal of Medicine* 352: 1011–1023.

Wen, J.G., Frokiaer, J., and Jorgensen, T.M. (1999). Obstructive nephropathy: an update of the experimental research. *Urological Research* 27: 29–39.

Wiegele, G., Brandis, M., and Zimmerhackl, L.B. (1998). Apoptosis and necrosis during ischaemia in renal tubular cells (LLC-PK1 and MDCK). *Nephrology, Dialysis, Transplantation* 13: 1158–1167.

Williams, B., Hattersley, J., Layward, E., and Walls, J. (1991). Metabolic acidosis and skeletal muscle adaptation to low protein diets in chronic uremia. *Kidney International* 40: 779–786.

Worwag, S. and Langston, C.E. (2008). Feline acute intrinsic renal failure: 32 cats (1997–2004). *Journal of the American Veterinary Medical Association* 232: 728–732.

Wu, I. and Parikh, C.R. (2008). Screening for kidney diseases: older measures versus novel biomarkers. *Clinical Journal of the American Society of Nephrology* 3: 1895–1901.

Yerramilli, M., Farace, G., Quinn, J., and Yerramilli, M. (2016). Kidney disease and the nexus of chronic kidney disease and acute kidney injury: the role of novel biomarkers as early and accurate diagnostics. *Veterinary Clinics: Small Animal Practice* 46: 961–993.

43

Upper Urinary Tract Obstruction

Eric Monnet

The presence of uroliths in the renal pelvis may or may not result in clinical problems. Nephroliths can cause obstruction of urine flow, may be associated with pyelonephritis (which can make infection difficult to treat), or can result in progressive enlargement of the kidney and deterioration of renal function. However, nephroliths can remain in the kidney for long periods without causing clinical problems (Ross et al. 1999, 2007). The presence of uroliths in the ureter can result in complete or partial ureteral obstruction.

Pathophysiology of upper urinary tract stones

The physiologic response to upper urinary tract obstruction is extremely complex and depends on the species, the age of the animal, the degree of obstruction, the length of time the obstruction has existed, and whether the obstruction is unilateral or bilateral (Wen et al. 1998, 1999, 2000). After complete unilateral ureteral obstruction, both renal blood flow and ureteral pressure increase for 1–1.5 hours on the affected side. The blood flow then begins to decline, while ureteral pressure continues to increase. After 5 hours, renal blood flow decreases further and ureteral pressure decreases. Ureteral pressure is near normal by 24 hours after obstruction. Renal blood flow continues to decrease and by 2 weeks after obstruction is 20% of normal in conscious dogs (Vaughan et al. 1970a,b; Gulmi et al. 1995; Lanzone et al. 1995; Bhangdia et al. 2003). Glomerular filtration rate (GFR) increases in the affected kidney initially, but then decreases (Wen et al. 1998, 1999, 2000, 2008). The GFR in the contralateral kidney increases.

After relief of complete unilateral ureteral obstruction in dogs, return of GFR ranges from nearly normal after 4 days of obstruction to 46% of normal after 2 weeks (Wen et al. 1998, 1999, 2000). Return of concentrating ability can occur if obstruction is less than 1 week, but is permanently impaired after 4 weeks of obstruction (Wen et al. 1998, 1999, 2000). Interestingly, destruction of the obstructed kidney occurs more quickly and return of function occurs more slowly if the contralateral kidney is present and functioning (Wen et al. 1998, 1999, 2000). In contrast to the rapid irreversibility of renal function in complete obstruction, partial obstruction results in less severe destruction and more return of function after relief of obstruction. In one model using dogs, total GFR was normal after 4 weeks of partial obstruction.

In the ureter, obstruction leads to hydroureter and thickening of the smooth muscle layer. Thickening is due to muscular hypertrophy, not hyperplasia, and the muscle is gradually replaced by fibrous tissue (Chuang et al. 1995, 1998, 2001). Over 90% of the muscle layer is fibrous tissue by 42 days after obstruction in the rat, but the exact time this takes in dogs and cats is not known.

Patient evaluation

Physical examination findings

Clinical findings reported in dogs with upper urinary tract obstruction include hematuria, abdominal pain, vomiting, anorexia, depression or lethargy, and emaciation. Abdominal pain was common in dogs with calculi (Hardie & Kyles 2004). The most common clinical signs reported in cats with ureteral obstruction are nonspecific, such as reduced appetite, lethargy, and weight loss (Kyles et al. 2005a,b). Clinical signs may also be referable to uremia, such as vomiting, polyuria, and polydipsia, or directly to ureteral obstruction, such as stranguria, pollakiuria, hematuria, and abdominal pain (Kyles *et al.* 2005a,b).

Clinicopathologic evaluation

A complete blood count, chemistry profile, urinalysis, and urine culture should be performed. The blood urea nitrogen (BUN) and creatinine concentrations depend on the hydration status of the patient, kidney function, presence and extent of ureteral obstruction, and function of the contralateral kidney. In one study of 163 cats with ureteral calculi, 83% of cats had a BUN or creatinine concentration above the reference range and 33% were markedly azotemic (creatinine >10 mg/dL; reference range 1.1–2.2 mg/dL) (Kyles *et al.* 2005a,b). Of cats with unilateral calculi, 76% were azotemic compared with 96% of cats with bilateral calculi. In addition, hyperphosphatemia was observed in 54%, hyperkalemia in 35%, and anemia in 48% of cats with ureteral calculi (Kyles *et al.* 2005a,b). Urine should be evaluated for the presence of crystalluria, hematuria, and urinary tract infection.

Imaging

Most uroliths of the upper urinary tract are diagnosed using abdominal radiography and ultrasonography. When urolithiasis is diagnosed, the entire urinary tract should be evaluated for calculi (Kyles *et al.* 2005a).

Plain radiography

Plain abdominal radiography allows evaluation of renal size and shape; radiolucent and small radiopaque calculi and moderate-to-severe hydroureter may not be seen on plain abdominal radiography.

Contrast study

Intravenous excretory urography may aid in visualization of the dilated ureter and renal pelvis proximal to the site of obstruction, but contrast excretion is often poor due to ureteral obstruction and opacification of the ureter is frequently inadequate. Dopamine at a low dose can improve the diagnostic quality of an excretory urogram in the presence of renal disease (Choi *et al.* 2001). Percutaneous antegrade pyelography provides good visualization of the renal pelvis and ureter, and has been used to determine if obstruction is present, with 100% sensitivity and specificity in cats (Adin *et al.* 2003). It facilitated diagnosis of radiodense and nonradiodense ureteral lesions. Under ultrasound guidance, a needle is placed through the greater curvature of the kidney into the renal pelvis. Urine is withdrawn until the renal pelvis

is reduced in size by half and a volume of aqueous iodinated contrast material equal to half the urine volume removed is infused into the pelvis of the kidney under ultrasound guidance. Care should be exercised, as the dilated renal pelvis protrudes beyond the renal parenchyma and inadvertent needle penetration of this portion of the pelvis can result in persistent urine leakage. If contrast solution is leaking in the renal parenchyma or in the perirenal tissue, then interpretation of the antegrade pyelogram is difficult.

Ultrasound

Ureteral calculi can be imaged with abdominal ultrasonography. In one study in cats, the sensitivity of survey radiography alone for the diagnosis of ureteral calculi was 81%, the sensitivity of ultrasonography alone was 77%, and the sensitivity of a combination of survey radiography and ultrasonography was 90% (Kyles *et al.* 2005a,b). In cats, ultrasound has been associated with 100% sensitivity and 33% specificity for the diagnosis of obstruction of the ureter (Adin *et al.* 2003). Abdominal ultrasound is particularly useful for the evaluation of ureteral and renal pelvic dilation secondary to obstruction. Dilatation of the ureter, renal pelvis, or both was observed ultrasonographically in 92% of cats with ureteral calculi (Kyles *et al.* 2005b). The renal resistive index of the kidney may be helpful in separating obstructive from nonobstructive disease (Rivers *et al.* 1996, 1997; Choi *et al.* 2003; Lee *et al.* 2006; Novellas *et al.* 2007, 2010). The resistive index can be affected by factors other than renal disease (Novellas *et al.* 2008a,b).

Computed tomography

Helical computed tomographic (CT) excretory urography is the modality of choice for imaging urolithiasis in many human hospitals. In cats, the sensitivity of CT and ultrasonography for the diagnosis of ureteral dilation is similar, but CT is superior in the determination of the number and position of ureteral calculi (Rozear & Tidwell 2003; Hardie & Kyles 2004). CT seems to be superior to ultrasound to determine the number and location of ureteral stones in cats (Testault *et al.* 2021).

Renal scintigraphy

Renal scintigraphy has been used clinically to evaluate the obstructed kidney and ureter. Technetium-99m diethylenetriamine pentaacetic acid (DTPA) scintigraphy can be used to measure the GFR of individual kidneys (Krawiec *et al.* 1988; Moe & Heiene 1995; Kampa *et al.* 2003; Hecht *et al.* 2006, 2010). Total GFR in a normal dog should be between 2.53 and 5.41 mL/min/kg. Measurement of GFR is operator dependent (Kampa *et al.* 2003). The GFR in the obstructed kidney will be reduced and scintigraphy cannot predict the GFR after relief of the obstruction. Measurement of the GFR of the contralateral kidney may assist in the decision to perform a nephrectomy on the obstructed kidney. Addition of diuretics can increase the accuracy of the diagnosis of ureteral obstruction by scintigraphy (Hecht *et al.* 2006, 2010). Kidney function can be evaluated in the presence of ureteral obstruction with magnetic resonance imaging with intravenous injection of DTPA (Wen *et al.* 2000, 2008).

Management of nephroliths

Medical management

In dogs, struvite nephroliths can be successfully dissolved. An appropriate antibiotic is administered in patients with urinary tract infection determined from culture and sensitivity. A prescription diet is fed, with restricted protein content and low levels of phosphate and magnesium. Average dissolution time varies from 6 weeks (without infection) to 3 months (with urinary tract infection). Calcium oxalate stones are usually difficult to dissolve.

Extracorporeal shock-wave lithotripsy, using both dry and waterbath techniques, has been used to fragment nephroliths in the dog (Block *et al.* 1996; Adams & Senior 1999). Several treatments may be required. Lithotripsy is not currently recommended for cats because the cat kidney is more sensitive to shock wave–induced injury (Adams & Senior 1999).

Surgical management

In general, surgery should aim to preserve the kidney. Nephrectomy should only be performed in cases of severe hydronephrosis with minimal remaining renal parenchyma. Surgical removal of nephroliths is indicated in patients with obstruction of the renal pelvis, uncontrolled infection, or deterioration of renal function. In the dog and cat, the undilated renal pelvis is completely surrounded by renal parenchyma.

Nephrotomy

Nephrotomy is indicated for removal of calculi where dilatation of the renal pelvis and proximal ureter does not extend beyond the kidney parenchyma and pyelolithotomy is not feasible. For nephrotomy, the kidney is mobilized and the renal artery (or arteries) is temporarily occluded with vascular clamps or a tourniquet. An incision is made though the renal capsule along the convex surface of the kidney and the parenchyma is bluntly dissected to the renal pelvis. The incision length should

be limited to that needed to retrieve the calculi. After calculi removal, the pelvis, calyces, and proximal ureter are flushed. For closure, the nephrotomy incision is apposed with digital pressure and the capsule sutured with a continuous suture pattern or mattress sutures. A technique without suture has been reported (Gahring *et al.* 1977). Bisection nephrotomy has been reported and it temporarily reduces renal function in the operated kidney by 30–50% (Gahring *et al.* 1977; Bolliger *et al.* 2005; King *et al.* 2006). However, Stone *et al.* (2002) reported that neither bisection nephrotomy nor intersegmental nephrotomy adversely affected GFR. Intersegmental nephrotomy is performed along the division between the parenchyma supplied by the dorsal and ventral branches of the renal artery. Four weeks after surgery the GFR was increased by 176% in both groups (Stone *et al.* 2002). In normal kidneys, nephrotomy does not induce a reduction of GFR (Bolliger *et al.* 2005; King *et al.* 2006). It is also feasible to insert a rigid endoscope and grasping instruments or baskets through a limited nephrotomy to retrieve nephroliths.

Pyelolithotomy

Pyelolithotomy can be performed to remove a nephrolith that has caused dilatation of the renal pelvis and proximal ureter beyond the renal parenchyma (Greenwood & Rawlings 1981). Usually this procedure is performed when the renal pelvis has some dilatation and the stones have migrated from the renal calyces to the renal pelvis. The kidney is mobilized from its peritoneal attachments and rotated medially to expose its dorsal surface and the renal pelvis. After placing two stay sutures on the renal pelvis and proximal ureter, the dilated renal pelvis and proximal ureter are incised longitudinally. The calculus is removed and the renal pelvis flushed. The incision is closed in a continuous pattern with 5-0 or 6-0 absorbable suture material. Pyelolithotomy removes the need for vascular occlusion and results in reduced blood loss.

Nephrectomy

Nephrectomy should be considered the last option and is reserved for cases where there is no kidney function remaining or there is end-stage hydronephrosis with severe infection and when the other kidney is able to support the patient (Gookin *et al.* 1996). Therefore a study of kidney function with GFR evaluation is preferable before a nephrectomy is considered.

The kidney is dissected from its peritoneal attachment. The renal arteries and veins are dissected, and it is not unusual to identify more than one renal artery to the kidney. The renal arteries are triple ligated first with

3-0 monofilament nonabsorbable suture. Two encircling sutures are placed first, then a transfixing suture is placed between the two encircling sutures. The renal arteries are transected, leaving one encircling suture and the transfixing suture in the patient. The veins are double ligated with encircling sutures with the same suture material. The ureter is identified, ligated, and transected near where it enters the bladder. After transection of the ureter close to the bladder, traction is placed on the kidney to pull the ureter through the retroperitoneal space. The site is then inspected for bleeding.

Management of ureteroliths

Medical management

Cats and dogs with ureteroliths are usually treated medically, initially with fluid diuresis alone or in combination with diuretic drug therapy (e.g., mannitol), which may result in ureterolith passage. Patients are closely monitored to determine if the ureterolith has passed and the obstruction resolved. Glucagon increases GFR (which results in diuresis), exhibits a spasmolytic effect on the ureteral smooth muscle, and may facilitate the passage of ureteroliths. Prazosin, an α-adrenergic receptor antagonist, and amitriptyline can cause ureteral smooth muscle relaxation, which may facilitate the passage of ureteroliths. Studies demonstrating the efficacy of glucagon, prazosin, or amitriptyline in dogs and cats with ureterolithiasis are lacking.

Extracorporeal shock-wave lithotripsy has been used to fragment ureteroliths in the dog (Bailey & Burk 1995; Block *et al.* 1996; Adams & Senior 1999), but is not currently recommended for cats.

Severe azotemia should be treated with hemodialysis, if available, or drainage of urine via a nephrostomy tube placed in the pelvis of the obstructed kidney. Nephrostomy tubes can be placed percutaneously under ultrasound guidance (Kyles *et al.* 2005b; Berent 2011). Nephrostomy tube placement requires that the renal pelvis is dilated and may not be possible in animals with acute obstruction. Nephrostomy tube placement has the additional advantage of allowing evaluation of the remaining function in the obstructed kidney. Pyelogram can also be performed with a nephrostomy tube.

Surgical management

Surgical removal of ureteral calculi is indicated when a ureter is partially or completely obstructed, as indicated by hydronephrosis and hydroureter proximal to the calculus, and immobility of the ureteral calculus determined by repeated radiographic or ultrasonographic examinations. Initial attempts should be made to retropulse the urinary calculi in the renal pelvis, as it is

often safer and simpler to perform a pyelolithotomy than a ureterotomy. A ventral cystotomy is performed and a catheter is advanced retrograde into the ureter. If the ureteral calculi are not movable, then they can be removed by ureterotomy or, when located in the distal ureter, by ureteroneocystostomy. In cats, it has been recommended that ureteral calculi in the proximal third of the ureter be removed by ureterotomy, whereas ureteral calculi in the distal two-thirds of the ureter can be managed by partial ureterectomy and ureteroneocystostomy (Kyles *et al.* 2005b).

Ureterotomy

Ureterotomy can be performed at any level of the ureter. Ureteral calculi may be directly observed or palpated. Ureteral dilation tends to begin proximally and extend distally, so that the dilated ureter may not extend all the way to the level of the calculus. If a calculus cannot be identified, a cystotomy should be performed and the ureter should be catheterized from the bladder. A longitudinal or a transverse incision is made with a scalpel blade in the dilated ureter proximal to the ureteral calculi. Transverse incision seems to be associated with less complication than longitudinal incision in human patients with ureteral stones (Douglas *et al.* 2003). Normally the calculus is readily removed, but occasionally it becomes embedded in the ureteral wall (Osborne & Polzin 1986). If the calculus is embedded in the wall, a resection anastomosis is required to remove the stone. After the calculus is removed, the ureter is flushed with warm saline and a catheter or, in cats, a length of suture material is passed proximally into the renal pelvis and distally into the bladder to assure that no additional calculi remain. The ureterotomy incision is closed with 5-0 to 8-0 monofilament suture material in a simple continuous suture pattern using a full-thickness bite to ensure a watertight seal. A stent can be placed in the ureter during the closure to help divert urine to prevent urine leakage and stenosis.

Ureteroneocystostomy

Ureteroneocystostomy involves implantation of the middle to distal ureter into the bladder after resection of distal ureteral lesions (Waldron *et al.* 1987; Kochin *et al.* 1993; Gregory *et al.* 1996). Surgical techniques for ureteroneocystostomy can be divided into intravesical or extravesical techniques (see Chapter 47). Intravesical techniques, such as the mucosal apposition technique, are performed from within the bladder lumen and require a cystotomy for access, in contrast with extravesical techniques such as the modified Lich–Gregoir technique (see Chapter 47). The mucosal apposition technique works well in dogs, but the modified Lich–Gregoir technique is preferred in cats, particularly when there is minimal preexisting ureteral dilatation, as it is associated with a reduced degree of postoperative swelling and ureteral obstruction (Kochin *et al.* 1993; Gregory *et al.* 1996). It should be noted that in both dogs and cats, postoperative hydroureter and hydronephrosis can occur in many patients due to partial ureteral obstruction after surgery; this has been reported in up to 50% of patients after ureteral reimplantation (Holt *et al.* 1982; Waldron *et al.* 1987; Holt & Moore 1995). Ureteral implantation with an extravesical technique has been used to treat 12 cats with stones in one or both ureter (Lorange & Monnet 2020). Treatment was successful in 11 of the 12 cats, and in the long term the creatinine concentration was 2 mg/dL. Four years after surgery the survival rate was 80%.

Ureteroureterostomy

Ureteroureterostomy is the technique utilized to reappose the ureter after ureteral resection. The procedure is technically more difficult than ureteroneocystostomy and is associated with a high incidence of postoperative ureteral obstruction (Adin & Scansen 2011; Zaid *et al.* 2011). Hence ureteroureterostomy is normally performed only when the proximal end of the ureter cannot be implanted into the bladder directly.

Renal descensus and psoas cystopexy

Tension on the ureteroneocystostomy or ureteroureterostomy should be avoided. Tension can be reduced by performing renal descensus and psoas cystopexy (Stone & Barsanti 1992). Renal descensus involves dissecting the kidney from its peritoneal attachments so that it remains attached by the renal vessels, repositioning the kidney more caudally and performing a nephropexy to attach the kidney to the body wall. Psoas cystopexy involves pulling the apex of the bladder cranially and laterally toward the kidney and suturing the bladder to the psoas muscle dorsally. With the combination of a psoas cystopexy and repositioning of the kidney caudally, a ureteroneocystostomy can be performed with the proximal third of the ureter. An alternative technique for reducing the tension on the anastomosis is nephrocystopexy. This involves dissecting the kidney from its retroperitoneal attachments, repositioning it caudally, pulling the bladder forward, and suturing the kidney directly to the bladder.

Boari tube

If the ureter is too short to reach the bladder, a Boari tube can be created from the bladder to be able to perform a ureteroneocystostomy without tension (Aronson *et al.* 2018). A Boari tube can also be combined with a psoas cystopexy to reduce tension.

Urinary diversion

Urine can be diverted after ureterotomy or ureteroureterostomy by placement of a ureteral stent or nephrostomy tube (Nwadike *et al.* 2000; Kyles *et al.* 2005b; Berent 2011; Palm & Culp 2016; Wormser *et al.* 2016; Culp *et al.* 2016). In cats, nephrostomy tubes are associated with a high complication rate, with problems of poor drainage, tube dislodgment, and urine leakage. Ureterotomy incisions in cats can heal satisfactorily without urine drainage via a nephrostomy tube. Ureteral stents can be used in cats during a ureterotomy or a ureteroneocystostomy. It seems to help reduce azotemia faster after ureterotomy (Culp *et al.* 2016). However, it is also associated with a high rate of complications (Wormser *et al.* 2016; Culp *et al.* 2016). A subcutaneous urinary bypass system can also be implanted to correct obstruction of ureter in dogs and cats. The different options for urinary diversion in dogs and cats are presented in Chapter 50. The subcutaneous urinary bypass systems are associated with long-term complications, mostly related to infection and obstruction of the bypass system (Kopecny *et al.* 2019; Dirrig *et al.* 2020; Kulendra *et al.* 2021; Deprey *et al.* 2021).

Complications after surgery of the ureter

Surgery of the ureter is associated with a high incidence of uroabdomen because of leakage of urine from incision in the ureter. In series of 101 cats, uroabdomen occurred in 16% of cases that survived the surgery (Kyles *et al.* 2005b). Leakage occurred in 16% of the cats following a ureterotomy and 15% of the cats in which a ureterocystostomy was performed (Kyles *et al.* 2005b). Placement of a drain during the abdominal surgery helps palliate the clinical signs. Although nephrostomy tube use has been advocated to prevent uroabdomen, 25% of the cases that had a nephrostomy tube placed had a uroabdomen compared with 12% of cats that did not have one placed (Kyles *et al.* 2005b). Ureteral obstruction is the second most common complication: 5% after ureterotomy and 11% after neoureterocystostomy in cats treated for ureteral calculi (Kyles *et al.* 2005b).

Stricture formation is another reported complication of ureterotomy, though the incidence is not known in cats or dogs (Lechevallier *et al.* 2008). Previous ureteral surgery was the most common cause of stricture formation in 10 cats (Zaid *et al.* 2011).

References

Adams, L.G. and Senior, D.F. (1999). Electrohydraulic and extracorporeal shock-wave lithotripsy. *Veterinary Clinics of North America: Small Animal Practice* 29: 293–302, xv.

Adin, C.A. and Scansen, B.A. (2011). Complications of upper urinary tract surgery in companion animals. *Veterinary Clinics of North America: Small Animal Practice* 41: 869–888.

Adin, C.A., Herrgesell, E.J., Nyland, T.G. et al. (2003). Antegrade pyelography for suspected ureteral obstruction in cats: 11 cases (1995–2001). *Journal of the American Veterinary Medical Association* 222: 1576–1581.

Aronson, L.R., Cleroux, A., and Wormser, C. (2018). Use of a modified Boari flap for the treatment of a proximal ureteral obstruction in a cat. *Veterinary Surgery* 47: 578–585.

Bailey, G. and Burk, R.L. (1995). Dry extracorporeal shock wave lithotripsy for treatment of ureterolithiasis and nephrolithiasis in a dog. *Journal of the American Veterinary Medical Association* 207: 592–595.

Berent, A. (2011). Ureteral obstructions in dogs and cats: a review of traditional and new interventional diagnostic and therapeutic options. *Journal of Veterinary Emergency and Critical Care* 21: 86–103.

Bhangdia, D.K., Gulmi, F.A., Chou, S.Y. et al. (2003). Alterations of renal hemodynamics in unilateral ureteral obstruction mediated by activation of endothelin receptor subtypes. *Journal of Urology* 170: 2057–2062.

Block, G., Adams, L.G., Widmer, W.R., and Lingeman, J.E. (1996). Use of extracorporeal shock wave lithotripsy for treatment of nephrolithiasis and ureterolithiasis in five dogs. *Journal of the American Veterinary Medical Association* 208: 531–536.

Bolliger, C., Walshaw, R., Kruger, J.M. et al. (2005). Evaluation of the effects of nephrotomy on renal function in clinically normal cats. *American Journal of Veterinary Research* 66: 1400–1407.

Choi, J., Lee, H., Chang, D. et al. (2001). Effect of dopamine on excretory urographic image quality and the prevention of contrast-induced nephropathy in dogs. *Journal of Veterinary Medical Science* 63: 383–388.

Choi, H., Won, S., Chung, W. et al. (2003). Effect of intravenous mannitol upon the resistive index in complete unilateral renal obstruction in dogs. *Journal of Veterinary Internal Medicine* 17: 158–162.

Chuang, Y.H., Chuang, W.L., Huang, S.P. et al. (1995). The temporal relationship between the severity of hydroureter and the dynamic changes of obstructed ureters in a rat model. *British Journal of Urology* 76: 303–310.

Chuang, Y.H., Chuang, W.L., Liu, K.M. et al. (1998). Tissue damage and regeneration of ureteric smooth muscle in rats with obstructive uropathy. *British Journal of Urology* 82: 261–266.

Chuang, Y.H., Chuang, W.L., and Huang, C.H. (2001). Myocyte apoptosis in the pathogenesis of ureteral damage in rats with obstructive uropathy. *Urology* 58: 463–470.

Culp, W.T., Palm, C.A., Hsueh, C. et al. (2016). Outcome in cats with benign ureteral obstructions treated by means of ureteral stenting versus ureterotomy. *Journal of the American Veterinary Medical Association* 249: 1292–1300.

Deprey, J., Baldinger, A., Livet, V. et al. (2021). Risk factors and clinical relevance of positive urine cultures in cats with subcutaneous ureteral bypass. *BMC Veterinary Research* 17: 199.

Dirrig, H., Lamb, C.R., Kulendra, N., and Halfacree, Z. (2020). Diagnostic imaging observations in cats treated with the subcutaneous ureteral bypass system. *Journal of Small Animal Practice* 61: 24–31.

Douglas, L.L., Wedderburn, K., Rattray, C.A., and Cadogan, C.M. (2003). Transverse ureterotomy in open ureterolithotomy. *West Indian Medical Journal* 52: 140–144.

Gahring, D.R., Crowe, D.T. Jr., Powers, T.E. et al. (1977). Comparative renal function studies of nephrotomy closure with and without sutures in dogs. *Journal of the American Veterinary Medical Association* 171: 537–541.

Gookin, J.L., Stone, E.A., Spaulding, K.A., and Berry, C.R. (1996). Unilateral nephrectomy in dogs with renal disease: 30 cases (1985–1994). *Journal of the American Veterinary Medical Association* 208: 2020–2025.

Greenwood, K.M. and Rawlings, C.A. (1981). Removal of canine renal calculi by pyelolithotomy. *Veterinary Surgery* 22: 12–21.

Gregory, C.R., Lirtzman, R.A., Kochin, E.J. et al. (1996). A mucosal apposition technique for ureteroneocystostomy after renal transplantation in cats. *Veterinary Surgery* 25: 13–17.

Gulmi, F.A., Matthews, G.J., Marion, D. et al. (1995). Volume expansion enhances the recovery of renal function and prolongs the diuresis and natriuresis after release of bilateral ureteral obstruction: a possible role for atrial natriuretic peptide. *Journal of Urology* 153: 1276–1283.

Hardie, E.M. and Kyles, A.E. (2004). Management of ureteral obstruction. *Veterinary Clinics of North America: Small Animal Practice* 34: 989–1010.

Hecht, S., Daniel, G.B., and Mitchell, S.K. (2006). Diuretic renal scintigraphy in normal dogs. *Veterinary Radiology and Ultrasound* 47: 602–608.

Hecht, S., Lawson, S.M., Lane, I.F. et al. (2010). (99m) Tc-DTPA diuretic renal scintigraphy in dogs with nephroureterolithiasis. *Canadian Veterinary Journal* 51: 1360–1366.

Holt, P.E. and Moore, A.H. (1995). Canine ureteral ectopia: an analysis of 175 cases and comparison of surgical treatments. *Veterinary Record* 136: 345–349.

Holt, P.E., Gibbs, C., and Pearson, H. (1982). Canine ectopic ureter: a review of twenty-nine cases. *Journal of Small Animal Practice* 23: 195–198.

Kampa, N., Bostrom, I., Lord, P. et al. (2003). Day-to-day variability in glomerular filtration rate in normal dogs by scintigraphic technique. *Journal of Veterinary Medicine. A, Physiology, Pathology, Clinical Medicine* 50: 37–41.

King, M.D., Waldron, D.R., Barber, D.L. et al. (2006). Effect of nephrotomy on renal function and morphology in normal cats. *Veterinary Surgery* 35: 749–758.

Kochin, E.J., Gregory, C.R., Wisner, E. et al. (1993). Evaluation of a method of ureteroneocystostomy in cats. *Journal of the American Veterinary Medical Association* 202: 257–260.

Kopecny, L., Palm, C.A., Drobatz, K.J. et al. (2019). Risk factors for positive urine cultures in cats with subcutaneous ureteral bypass and ureteral stents (2010–2016). *Journal of Veterinary Internal Medicine* 33: 178–183.

Krawiec, D.R., Twardock, A.R., Badertscher, R.R. II et al. (1988). Use of Tc-diethylenetriaminepentaacetic acid for assessment of renal function in dogs with suspected renal disease. *Journal of the American Veterinary Medical Association* 192: 1077–1079.

Kulendra, N.J., Borgeat, K., Syme, H. et al. (2021). Survival and complications in cats treated with subcutaneous ureteral bypass. *Journal of Small Animal Practice* 62: 4–11.

Kyles, A.E., Hardie, E.M., Wooden, B.G. et al. (2005a). Clinical, clinicopathologic, radiographic, and ultrasonographic abnormalities in cats with ureteral calculi: 163 cases (1984–2002). *Journal of the American Veterinary Medical Association* 226: 932–936.

Kyles, A.E., Hardie, E.M., Wooden, B.G. et al. (2005b). Management and outcome of cats with ureteral calculi: 153 cases (1984–2002). *Journal of the American Veterinary Medical Association* 226: 937–944.

Lanzone, J.A., Gulmi, F.A., Chou, S.Y. et al. (1995). Renal hemodynamics in acute unilateral ureteral obstruction: contribution of endothelium-derived relaxing factor. *Journal of Urology* 153: 2055–2059.

Lechevallier, E., Traxer, O., and Saussine, C. (2008). Open surgery for upper urinary tract stones. *Progrès en Urologie* 18: 952–954.

Lee, J.I., Kim, M.J., Park, C.S., and Kim, M.C. (2006). Influence of ascorbic acid on BUN, creatinine, resistive index in canine renal ischemia-reperfusion injury. *Journal of Veterinary Science* 7: 79–81.

Lorange, M. and Monnet, E. (2020). Postoperative outcomes of 12 cats with ureteral obstruction treated with ureteroneocystostomy. *Veterinary Surgery* 49: 1418–1427.

Moe, L. and Heiene, R. (1995). Estimation of glomerular filtration rate in dogs with 99M-Tc-DTPA and iohexol. *Research in Veterinary Science* 58: 138–143.

Novellas, R., Espada, Y., and Ruiz de Gopegui, R. (2007). Doppler ultrasonographic estimation of renal and ocular resistive and pulsatility indices in normal dogs and cats. *Veterinary Radiology and Ultrasound* 48: 69–73.

Novellas, R., Riuz de Gopegui, R., and Espada, Y. (2008a). Determination of renal vascular resistance in dogs with diabetes mellitus and hyperadrenocorticism. *Veterinary Record* 163: 592–596.

Novellas, R., Ruiz de Gopegui, R., and Espada, Y. (2008b). Increased renal vascular resistance in dogs with hepatic disease. *Veterinary Journal (London)* 178: 257–262.

Novellas, R., de Gopegui, R., and Espada, Y. (2010). Assessment of renal vascular resistance and blood pressure in dogs and cats with renal disease. *Veterinary Record* 166: 618–623.

Nwadike, B.S., Wilson, L.P., and Stone, E.A. (2000). Use of bilateral temporary nephrostomy catheters for emergency treatment of bilateral ureter transection in a cat. *Journal of the American Veterinary Medical Association* 217: 1862–1865.

Osborne, C.A. and Polzin, D.J. (1986). Nonsurgical management of canine obstructive urolithopathy. *Veterinary Clinics of North America: Small Animal Practice* 16: 333–347.

Palm, C.A. and Culp, W.T. (2016). Nephroureteral obstructions: the use of stents and ureteral bypass systems for renal decompression. *Veterinary Clinics of North America: Small Animal Practice* 46: 1183–1192.

Rivers, B.J., Walter, P.A., Letourneau, J.G. et al. (1996). Estimation of arcuate artery resistive index as a diagnostic tool for aminoglycoside induced acute renal failure in dogs. *American Journal of Veterinary Research* 57: 1536–1544.

Rivers, B.J., Walter, P.A., Letourneau, J.G. et al. (1997). Duplex Doppler estimation of resistive index in arcuate arteries of sedated, normal female dogs: implications for use in the diagnosis of renal failure. *Journal of the American Animal Hospital Association* 33: 69–76.

Ross, S.J., Osborne, C.A., Lulich, J.P. et al. (1999). Canine and feline nephrolithiasis: epidemiology, detection, and management. *Veterinary Clinics of North America: Small Animal Practice* 29: 231–250.

Ross, S.J., Osborne, C.A., Lekcharoensuk, C. et al. (2007). A case–control study of the effects of nephrolithiasis in cats with chronic kidney disease. *Journal of the American Veterinary Medical Association* 230: 1854–1859.

Rozear, L. and Tidwell, A.S. (2003). Evaluation of the ureter and ureterovesicular junction using helical computed tomographic excretory urography in healthy dogs. *Veterinary Radiology and Ultrasound* 44: 155–164.

Stone, E.A. and Barsanti, J.A. (1992). Surgical therapy for urinary tract trauma. In: *Urologic Surgery of the Dog and Cat*, 189–196. Philadelphia, PA: Lea & Febiger.

Stone, E.A., Robertson, J.L., and Metcalf, M.R. (2002). The effect of nephrotomy on renal function and morphology in dogs. *Veterinary Surgery* 31: 391–397.

Testault, I., Gatel, L., and Vanel, M. (2021). Comparison of nonenhanced computed tomography and ultrasonography for detection of ureteral calculi in cats: a prospective study. *Journal of Veterinary Internal Medicine* 35: 2241–2248.

Vaughan, E.D. Jr., Sorenson, E.J., and Gillenwater, J.Y. (1970a). The renal hemodynamic response to chronic unilateral complete ureteral occlusion. *Investigative Urology* 8: 78–90.

Vaughan, E.D. Jr., Sweet, R.C., and Gillenwater, J.Y. (1970b). Peripheral renin and blood pressure changes following complete unilateral ureteral occlusion. *Journal of Urology* 104: 89–92.

Waldron, D.R., Hedlund, C.S., Pechman, R.D. et al. (1987). Ureteroneocystostomy: a comparison of the submucosal tunnel and transverse pull through techniques. *Journal of the American Animal Hospital Association* 23: 285–290.

Wen, J.G., Chen, Y., Frøkiaer, J. et al. (1998). Experimental partial unilateral ureter obstruction. I. Pressure flow relationship in a rat model with mild and severe acute ureter obstruction. *Journal of Urology* 160: 1567–1571.

Wen, J.G., Frøkiaer, J., Jorgensen, T.M., and Djurhuus, J.C. (1999). Obstructive nephropathy: an update of the experimental research. *Urological Research* 27: 29–39.

Wen, J.G., Chen, Y., Ringgaard, S. et al. (2000). Evaluation of renal function in normal and hydronephrotic kidneys in rats using gadolinium diethylenetetramine-pentaacetic acid enhanced dynamic magnetic resonance imaging. *Journal of Urology* 163: 1264–1270.

Wen, J.G., Pedersen, M., Dissing, T.H. et al. (2008). Evaluation of complete and partially obstructed kidneys using Gd-DTPA enhanced dynamic MRI in adolescent swine. *European Journal of Pediatric Surgery* 18: 322–327.

Wormser, C., Clarke, D.L., and Aronson, L.R. (2016). Outcomes of ureteral surgery and ureteral stenting in cats: 117 cases (2006–2014). *Journal of the American Veterinary Medical Association* 248: 518–525.

Zaid, M.S., Berent, A.C., Weisse, C., and Caceres, A. (2011). Feline ureteral strictures: 10 cases (2007–2009). *Journal of Veterinary Internal Medicine* 25: 222–229.

44

Urolithiasis of the Lower Urinary Tract

Eric Monnet

The presence of urinary calculi in the bladder and urethra is fairly common in dogs and cats (Thumchai *et al.* 1996; Ling *et al.* 1998a,b,c,d; Franti *et al.* 1999). It requires medical and surgical attention. Animals can be presented with an acute and complete obstruction or a chronic partial obstruction. Acute lower urinary tract obstruction represents a medical emergency with electrolyte abnormalities. The diagnosis and localization of the stones require physical examination and imaging.

Patient evaluation

Physical examination findings

The presence of calculi in the urinary bladder can result in hematuria, inappropriate urination, stranguria, or pollakiuria. Palpation of the caudal abdomen allows an assessment of bladder size, firmness, and pain. Occasionally calculi may be palpated. Animals with urinary calculi are frequently asymptomatic (Langston *et al.* 2008).

The presence of urethral calculi can result in complete or partial urethral obstruction. Urethral calculi are more frequently diagnosed in male dogs and cats compared with female dogs and cats. In the male dog, the most common site for urethral calculi to lodge is just proximal to the os penis, though they can lodge in any portion of the urethra. In the male cat, the most common site for urethral calculi is the junction of the intrapelvic and penile urethra. Urethral calculi can result in clinical signs of urethral obstruction, including stranguria, pollakiuria, and a distended urinary bladder. The patient develops postrenal uremia and hyperkalemia, resulting in progressive depression and vomiting. Urethral obstruction can result in urinary bladder rupture.

Clinicopathologic evaluation

Evaluation of patients with lower urinary tract calculi should include a complete blood count, chemistry panel, urinalysis, urine sediment examination, and urine culture. Urethral obstruction results in fluid, electrolyte, and acid–base imbalances, typically a hyperkalemic metabolic acidosis. Hyperkalemia can result in bradycardia, absent or flattened P waves, prolonged PR interval, widened QRS complexes, and spiked T waves on electrocardiographic examination.

Imaging

In patients with lower urinary tract calculi, the entire urinary tract should be evaluated. Calcium oxalate, struvite, calcium phosphate, and silica uroliths are generally radiopaque and can usually be seen on plain radiography. Urate and cystine uroliths are not normally visible on plain radiographs and require contrast radiography (positive contrast cystography, double contrast cystography, positive contrast urethrography) or ultrasonography (Feeney *et al.* 1999; Langston *et al.* 2008).

Medical management: dietary modification and antibiotic therapy

Medical treatment is indicated when there is no urinary obstruction (Lulich *et al.* 2009a; Westropp *et al.* 2010; Wisener *et al.* 2010). The goal of medical treatment is to modify the environment (alter pH), treat the infection if present, and modify excretion of certain substances (Kruger & Osborne 1986; Lulich *et al.* 1998, 1999a, 2009a; Bartges *et al.* 1999; Kruger *et al.* 1999; Osborne *et al.* 1999a,b,d; Westropp *et al.* 2010; Wisener *et al.* 2010).

Small Animal Soft Tissue Surgery, Second Edition. Edited by Eric Monnet.
© 2023 John Wiley & Sons, Inc. Published 2023 by John Wiley & Sons, Inc.
Companion website: www.wiley.com/go/monnet/small

Struvite, urate, and cystine uroliths can be medically dissolved. Dissolution requires that the urolith be bathed in undersaturated urine, including calculi present in the urinary bladder or urethroliths flushed back into the bladder. Determining the type of urolith should preferably be based on quantitative urolith analysis.

Small uroliths may be obtained via catheter-assisted retrieval (Lulich & Osborne 1992). The technique is usually performed to obtain calculi for analysis, and can be accomplished without anesthesia if the patient will tolerate urethral catheterization. After the urethral catheter is placed, the bladder is distended with sterile saline solution, agitated, and urine aspirated.

If medical treatment is failing or not appropriate, then the urinary stones should be removed by either a nonsurgical or a surgical approach. The technique with the least amount of morbidity should be used. When stones are present in the urethra it is important to make every effort to retropulse the stones into the bladder. Therefore a cystotomy is performed, which typically carries less morbidity than a urethrotomy or a urethrostomy.

Nonsurgical approach for removal of calculi in the lower urinary tract

Voiding hydropropulsion

Small cystic calculi can be removed by inducing voiding while the dog is positioned vertically so that the calculi are present in the trigone area and are passed with the voided urine (Lulich *et al.* 1993, 1999b). The procedure is usually performed under general anesthesia. The bladder is filled via cystoscopy or urethral catheterization, the dog is positioned vertically, and the bladder agitated to allow the calculi to settle into the trigone. The bladder is slowly manually compressed to raise intravesicular pressure and initiate a detrusor contraction. Digital pressure is maintained until voiding is complete. The bladder is refilled and the procedure repeated until there are no calculi in the voided urine.

Cystoscopic retrieval

Cystic calculi can be retrieved during cystoscopy using stone baskets. The basket is usually placed through the working channel of the scope, allowing the stone to be grasped within the basket. The cystoscope and basket are slowly withdrawn through the urethra.

Laser lithotripsy

The laser energy of the holmium:YAG laser is absorbed in less than 0.5 mm of fluid, making it safe for urologic procedures (Davidson *et al.* 2004; Adams *et al.* 2008; Lulich *et al.* 2009b). Larger cystic calculi can be fragmented using a holmium:YAG laser placed through the operating channel of a rigid or flexible endoscope. The fragments can be removed by basket retrieval or voiding hydropropulsion. Complete removal of uroliths was reported in 79% (52 of 66) of dogs with cystic calculi using laser lithotripsy (Lulich *et al.* 2009b). A success rate of 83% and 100% has been reported in male and female dogs with uroliths in the bladder or the urethra (Adams *et al.* 2008). Laser time ranged from 2 to 328 minutes, and 37% of the dogs had 2–5 stones. Total procedure time was longer for stones in the bladder than stones in the urethra. Fragments of stones were removed with a basket grasper. In 6 dogs a second anesthesia was necessary 3–5 days after the first procedure to remove fragments that were left in the bladder at the time of fragmentation.

Electrohydraulic lithotripsy

With electrohydraulic lithotripsy, the electrode is passed through an endoscope allowing hydraulic shock waves generated within the bladder to fragment the urolith. Complete removal of uroliths was reported in only 19% (5 of 26) of dogs with cystic calculi using electrohydraulic lithotripsy (Defarges & Dunn 2008).

Extracorporeal shock-wave lithotripsy

With extracorporeal shock-wave lithotripsy (ESWL), the urolith is fragmented using shock waves generated outside the body (Adams *et al.* 2005; Lulich *et al.* 2009a). ESWL is best suited to the upper urinary tract, where uroliths are fixed in position, rather than the bladder, where they tend to move out of the focal spot (Block *et al.* 1996). Complete removal of uroliths in a single session of ESWL was reported in 57% (8 of 14) of dogs with cystic calculi (Adams *et al.* 2005). This procedure is more efficient in dogs than in cats (Adams *et al.* 2005).

Cystoscopy with laser or electrohydraulic lithotripsy

Urethral calculi can be successfully removed during cystoscopy using laser or electrohydraulic lithotripsy (Defarges & Dunn 2008; Lulich *et al.* 2009b).

Surgical removal of calculi in the lower urinary tract

Following removal of calculi in the lower urinary tract, imaging studies should be taken to determine if stones have been inadvertently missed, particularly in patients with multiple uroliths. Incomplete urolith removal has been reported in up to 20% of dogs following cystolithotomy (Grant *et al.* 2010).

Retrograde urohydropulsion

Retrograde urohydropulsion is performed in male dogs or cats to push the calculi into the bladder, relieving any urethral obstruction and allowing the calculi to be retrieved via a cystotomy (Osborne *et al.* 1999c). First the patient has to be placed under general anesthesia. A urethral catheter is passed to the level of the obstruction (note that the catheter must be large in order to withstand the mechanical forces of the procedure). A mixture of saline and water-soluble lubricant is used to dilate and lubricate the urethra. An assistant directly presses on the intrapelvic urethra via the rectum while the operator flushes sterile saline into the urethral catheter, providing an increased pressure of saline within the urethra distal to the calculus. The assistant releases the urethra while the operator continues to flush, hopefully pushing the calculus retrograde up the urethra. Care should be taken not to overdistend the bladder during the procedure. Plain or contrast radiography may be needed to determine if all urethral calculi have been successfully pushed into the bladder. The catheter advanced in the urethra should be left in place until the bladder is opened to retrieve the stones. If the catheter is removed prematurely, the stones may migrate back into the urethra during the procedure.

Cystotomy with laparotomy

Cystotomy is the traditional technique for removal of cystic calculi. Cystotomy can be performed via a short caudal midline laparotomy (Website Chapter 44: Urinary surgery/cystotomy). A catheter is placed in the urethra before surgery and is connected to an extension set to facilitate access underneath the surgical drapes by the nurses during surgery. For male dogs, the prepuce is flushed with dilute betadine in order for it to be within the surgical field. After exposure of the bladder in the caudal abdomen, it is isolated from the rest of the abdomen with laparotomy sponges. A ventral cystotomy is recommended as it provides better access to the trigone and proximal urethra, and is associated with a similar risk of adhesions or leakage as a dorsal incision (Crowe 1986; Desch & Wagner 1986). After placing stay sutures at the apex and the trigone area, the bladder is opened by a blade at the apex. The incision is extended with Metzenbaum scissors toward the trigone, staying on the ventral midline. Stones are usually removed with a small sterile spoon. Forceps can also be used to grab larger stones. After removal of the stones, the urethra is flushed retrogradely with the catheter placed before surgery. The catheter is flushed with sterile saline while it is removed from the urethra. It is important to place sterile laparotomy sponges around the bladder to catch the stones while the urethra is being flushed. The urethra is then flushed normogradely with a catheter placed from the trigone.

Prior to closure of the bladder, it is important to collect a biopsy of the bladder mucosa for aerobic/anaerobic culture. It has been shown that cultures of the bladder mucosa combined with stones yield better results than cultures of urine only (Gatoria *et al.* 2006).

The bladder is closed with a simple apposition one-layer closure, using absorbable monofilament suture material (Website Chapter 44: Urinary surgery/cystotomy closure) (Radasch *et al.* 1990). The monofilament suture can be placed full thickness and be exposed in the lumen of the bladder. In an experiment in rats, polyglytone 6211 and glycomer 631 have been shown to be the desirable suture for urinary surgery because of their tensile strength and fast rate of resorption in urine (Karabulut *et al.* 2010). It has also been shown that rapidly absorbed monofilament absorbable suture is desirable for closure of the urinary bladder because it does not increase the risk of urolithiasis around the suture (Morris *et al.* 1986; Edlich *et al.* 1987; Hanke *et al.* 1994; Biondo-Simões *et al.* 1998). Monofilament absorbable sutures lose their strength in urine infected with *Proteus* faster than catgut does (Greenberg *et al.* 2004). However, since their rate of degradation with hydrolysis is more predictable than the rate of degradation of catgut, monofilament absorbable sutures are still recommended in the presence of infection (Edlich *et al.* 1987).

Transvesicular percutaneous cystolithotomy

After a midline incision, the apex of the bladder is localized and exteriorized. A screw-in cannula is then introduced into the apex of the bladder. A rigid 30° cystoscope is introduced into the bladder and a basket forceps is used to retrieve stones in the bladder and the urethra. Results have been reported on 23 dogs and 4 cats (Runge *et al.* 2011). Patient weight was between 1.8 and 42.6 kg. The number of uroliths retrieved ranged from 1 to more than 35 and the median size was 4.5 mm. The procedure time was 50–80 minutes.

Laparoscopy-assisted cystotomy

A laparoscopy-assisted technique has been used to perform a cystotomy to remove bladder stones (Website Chapter 44: Laparoscopic-assisted cystotomy) (Rawlings *et al.* 2003; Pinel *et al.* 2013). As for the laparotomy technique, a catheter is placed in the urethra before surgery. The catheter is connected to a sterile fluid bag. After insufflation of the abdominal cavity with carbon dioxide, a cannula is placed caudal to the umbilicus to introduce the camera. After inspection of the abdominal cavity, the apex of the bladder is localized. The bladder is gently distended with saline. Another cannula is placed midline at the level of the apex of the bladder. A grasping forceps is then introduced to pull the apex of the bladder against the abdominal wall. The hole of the cannula with the grasping forceps is enlarged to expose the wall of the bladder, which also deflates the abdominal cavity. The wall of the bladder is then pexied temporarily to the abdominal wall to prevent urine leakage into the abdomen. A 5 mm cannula is placed in the apex of the bladder and the endoscope is introduced to visualize the stones. With the catheter in the urethra, a flow of saline is created from the catheter up the cannula to evacuate the small stones. To increase the flow of saline the sterile bag of saline can be pressurized and suction applied to the cannula. Larger stones that do not fit in the cannula are removed with grasping forceps placed next to the cannula. After removal of all the stones, the catheter in the urethra is retrieved slowly while the endoscope is advanced in the urethra to ensure that no stones are left behind. Obviously in male dogs the endoscope will not go beyond the ischiatic arch. The cannula in the bladder is removed and the bladder is closed routinely. The temporary cystopexy is removed and the abdomen is closed routinely.

Urethrotomy

The main indication for urethrotomy is to remove urethral calculi in male dogs that cannot be retropulsed into the bladder (Smeak 2000). Urethrotomy can also be performed to remove a mass in the urethra (Haine et al. 2020). The most common site for urethral calculi to lodge in male dogs is just proximal to the os penis. Calculi in this site can be removed using a prescrotal urethrotomy. After midline incision the retractor preputial muscle is retracted laterally to visualize the urethra (Figure 44.1). The urethra is then incised with a no. 11 blade over the stones or just distal to them (Figure 44.2). It is important to remain on midline during the incision, because the ischiocavernosus

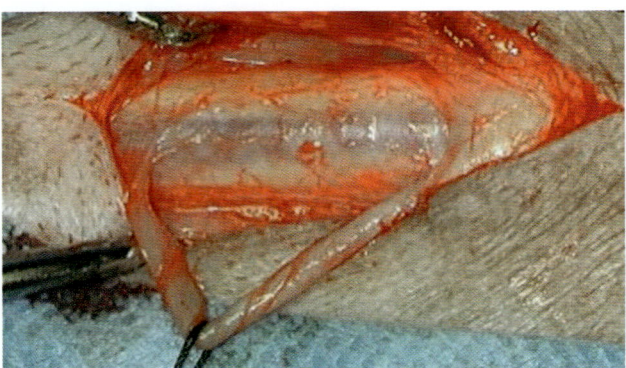

Figure 44.1 Urethrotomy: the retractor penile muscle has been retracted laterally. The urethra is exposed.

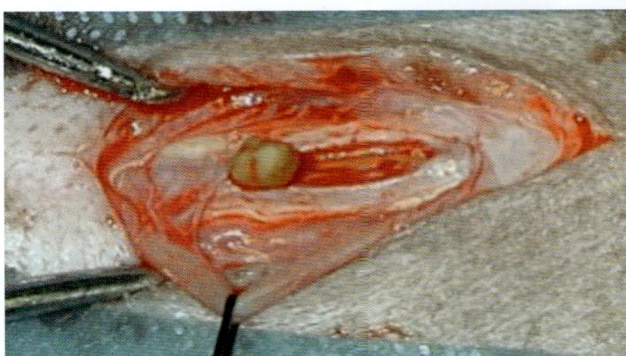

Figure 44.2 Urethrotomy: the urethra is opened over the stones.

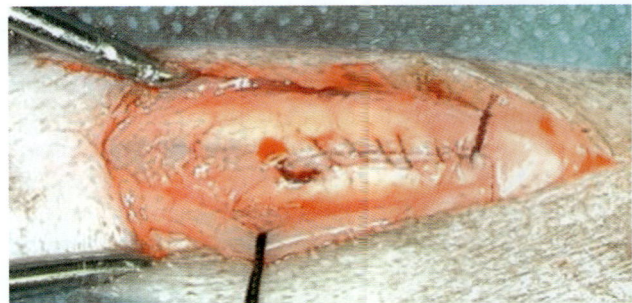

Figure 44.3 Urethrotomy: the urethra is closed with 5-0 monofilament absorbable suture with a simple continuous pattern.

tissue is present on each side of the urethra. If the ischiocavernosus tissue is traumatized, it will bleed profusely during surgery and may create a hematoma after surgery. The stone is removed and a urinary catheter is placed normograde and retrograde to ensure the urethra is patent. The urethrotomy is then closed with 5-0 monofilament absorbable suture in a simple continuous pattern (Figure 44.3). The urethrotomy can be left to heal by secondary intention, although bleeding from the incision is expected for a few days (Weber et al. 1985).

Less frequently, calculi lodge at the ischial arch because the urethra remains wide past the ischiatic arch in dogs. These can be removed via a perineal urethrotomy (Banerjee 1968; Reimer et al. 2004). Surgical closure of the urethrotomy should be performed.

Following a urethrotomy, hematuria is expected for 4–5 days after surgery. This is the most common complication after urethrotomy (Waldron et al. 1985; Weber et al. 1985). The risk of stenosis is limited with a longitudinal incision that has been sutured with apposition of the mucosa.

Urethrostomy

Urethrostomy is performed in patients that repeatedly (Carb & Yoshioka 1982) form calculi despite appropriate medical management to reduce the likelihood of urethral obstruction (Blake 1968; Wilson & Harrison 1971;

Smith 1987, 2002; Bradley 1989; Smeak *et al.* 1990; Bilbrey *et al.* 1991; Smeak 2000; Baines *et al.* 2001; Bernarde & Viguier 2004; Bass *et al.* 2005; Phillips & Holt 2006). A urethrostomy can also be performed after penile amputation for trauma or neoplasia (Burrow *et al.* 2011; Bolfer *et al.* 2015)

In the male dog, urethrostomy can be performed in five locations: antepubic, perineal, scrotal, transpelvic, and prescrotal (Carb & Yoshioka 1982; Bradley 1989; Bilbrey *et al.* 1991; Chiaramonte *et al.* 2022; Taylor & Smeak 2021). The scrotal location is preferred, as the urethra is relatively superficial and wide, there is less hemorrhage, and the dog rapidly adapts to urinating through the stoma. Perineal, antepubic, subpubic, and transpubic urethrostomies are the options available in cats (Blake 1968; Bone 1969; Mendham 1970; Wilson & Harrison 1971; Ellison & Lewis 1989; Bernarde & Viguier 2004; Bass *et al.* 2005).

Scrotal urethrostomy

Scrotal urethrostomy is the most common urethrostomy procedure in the male dog because the urethra is wide until the level of the ischiatic arch. Therefore stones that migrate into the urethra should be expelled easily with a scrotal urethrostomy (Bilbrey *et al.* 1991; Newton & Smeak 1996; Smeak 2000).

Scrotal urethrostomy is not indicated if the level of obstruction is more proximal. The scrotal urethra is approached by an incision around the base of the scrotum (castrated dogs) or via a castration and scrotal ablation (intact dogs). After exposure of the urethra, the urethra is opened with a no. 11 blade. It is important to keep the incision on the midline, because the ischiocavernosus muscles are present on each side and will bleed profusely if incised during the procedure. The stoma should be around 2–3 cm long. The urethrostomy can be completed with either simple interrupted sutures or two continuous suture patterns (Newton & Smeak 1996). It is important to achieve accurate mucosa to skin apposition without tension on the stoma. Usually, 4-0 absorbable suture material is used to perform the urethrostomy (Figure 44.4). The most common complication is hemorrhage from the surgical site for a few days after surgery; stricture formation is uncommon (Newton & Smeak 1996). It is important to prevent self-mutilation since it will increase the risk of stricture formation. Sedation might be required to reduce the incidence of hemorrhage after surgery.

Perineal urethrostomy in dogs

Perineal urethrostomy is performed in a similar manner, except in a deeper location of the urethra. Tension-relieving sutures between the tunic of the penis and the

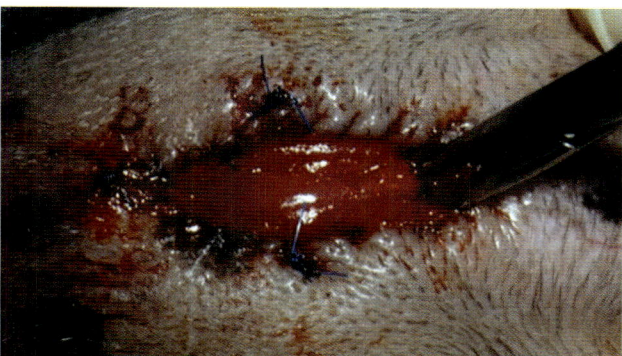

Figure 44.4 Scrotal urethrostomy in a dog. A clamp has been introduced in the urethra in the caudal part of the urethrostomy to show the width of the urethra at the level of the ischiatic arch.

subcutaneous tissue are recommended. This procedure is rarely performed in dogs because it may result in severe urine scalding. Scrotal urethrostomy is more appropriate for a male dog.

Perineal urethrostomy in cats

Perineal urethrostomy is indicated in cats that experience multiple episodes of urethral obstruction despite appropriate medical management. The technique is performed using an elliptical incision around the penis and scrotum (Figure 44.5) (Website Chapter 44: Urinary surgery/perineal urethrostomy cat) (Carbone 1967; Blake 1968; Bone 1969; Osborne *et al.* 1996; Smith 2002; Agrodnia *et al.* 2004). The penis is freed from its attachments to the pubis by elevating the paired ischiocavernosus muscles from the pelvis (Figure 44.6). Once this is completed, it is possible to place a finger between the floor of the pelvic canal and the penis. No dissection should occur dorsal to the penis to preserve the innervation to the bladder. Dissection continues cranially to the level of the bulbourethral glands, which can be difficult to see in castrated male cats (Figure 44.7). A catheter is placed in the urethra and the urethra incised distally. The urethral incision is extended to the level of the bulbourethral glands, which represent the distal end of the wider intrapelvic urethra (Figure 44.8) (Phillips & Holt 2006). A single simple interrupted suture is placed between the tunic of the penis proximally and the subcutaneous tissue at the dorsal end of the incision to reduce tension on the anastomosis. Four simple interrupted sutures (4-0 to 5-0 nonabsorbable suture material) are preplaced to form the proximal end of the stoma. These sutures should be placed from the urethral mucosa to the skin. These sutures are tightened to check the apposition of mucosa and skin and then tied. The urethral mucosa and skin are then sutured for a further 1–1.5 cm distally (Figure 44.9). A simple interrupted or simple

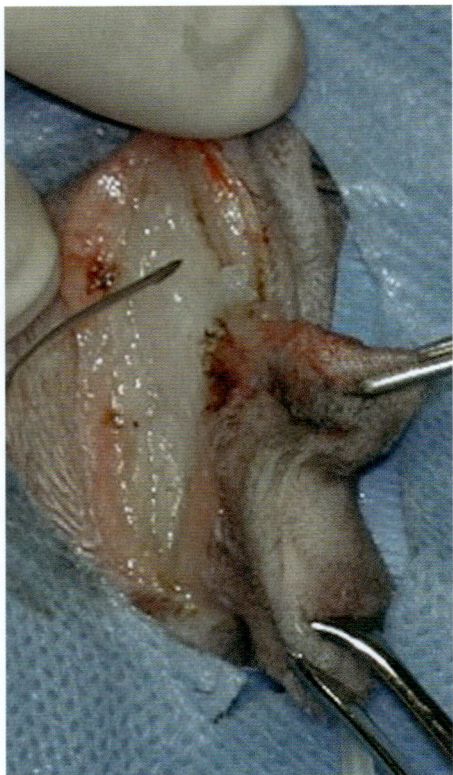

Figure 44.5 Elliptical incision at the base of the prepuce and scrotum.

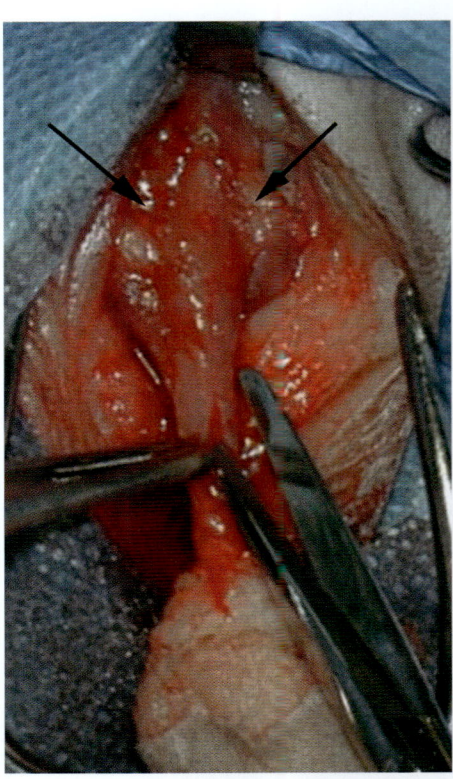

Figure 44.7 The dissection is carried forward until the bulbourethral glands can be seen (black arrows). They are usually striated. They can be atrophied in a castrated male.

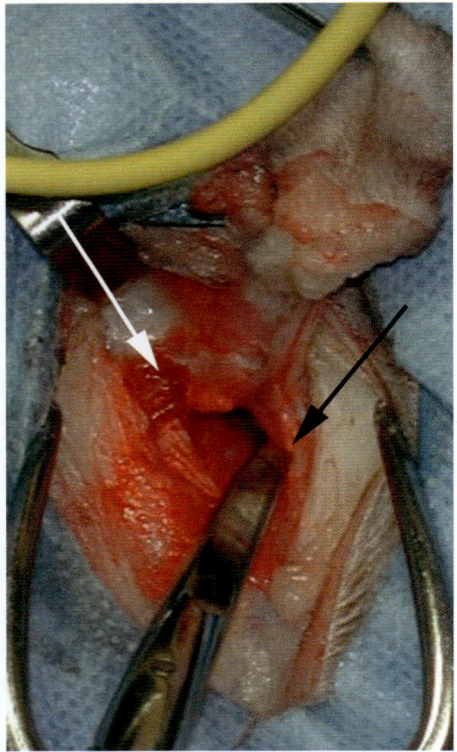

Figure 44.6 The ischiocavernosus muscles are detached from the ischium with Mayo scissors. The muscle on the left side has been already detached (white arrow), while the one on the right (black arrow) is about to be detached with the Mayo scissors.

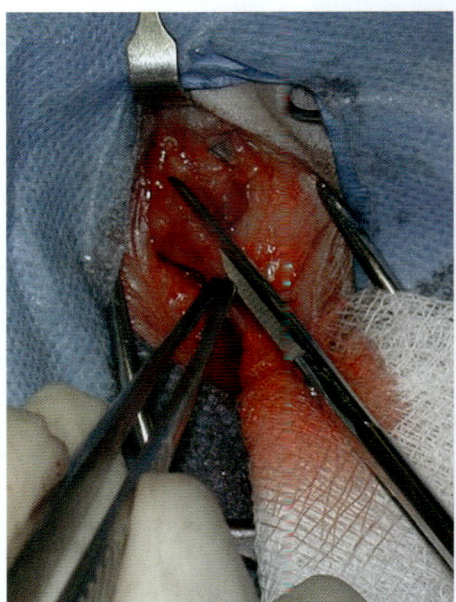

Figure 44.8 The urethra is opened with a pair of Metzenbaum scissors up to the level of the bulbourethral glands.

continuous suture pattern can be used (Figure 44.10) (Agrodnia *et al.* 2004). The penis is ligated distal to the stoma and transected and the remaining skin incision closed. After surgery, an Elizabethan collar is placed to prevent self-mutilation.

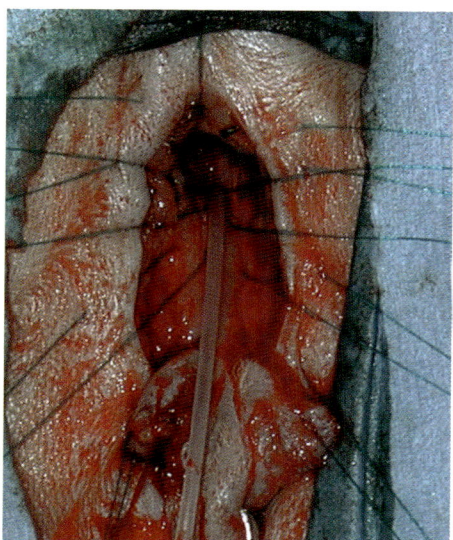

Figure 44.9 Sutures are preplaced between the uroepithelium of the urethra and the skin. It is important to achieve good apposition of the skin with the urethra.

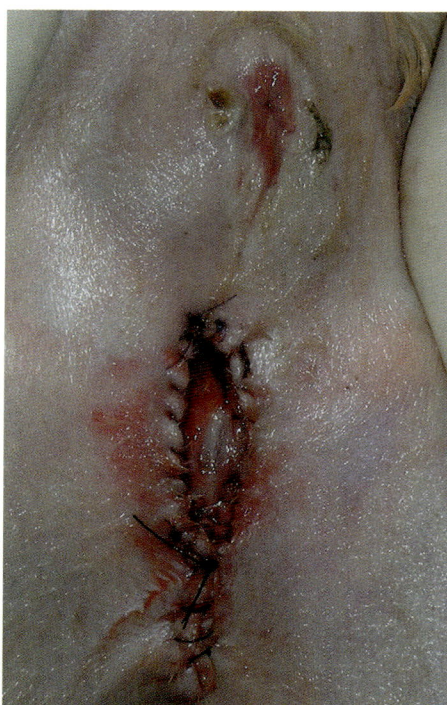

Figure 44.10 The perineal urethrostomy has been completed with a continuous suture in the ventral part.

The most common immediate complication is incisional hemorrhage; the site should not be disturbed unless the cat is unable to urinate. Other complications include stricture formation, urinary tract infection, subcutaneous urine leakage, urinary incontinence, and perineal hernia (Carbone 1965; Sackman *et al.* 1991; Osborne *et al.* 1996; Agrodnia *et al.* 2004; Bass *et al.* 2005; Ruda & Heiene 2012; Slunsky *et al.* 2018; Slunsky

et al. 2019; Segal *et al.* 2020; Nye *et al.* 2020). A high incidence of bacterial cystitis has been reported after perineal urethrostomy in male cats (Osborne *et al.* 1991, 1996; Griffin & Gregory 1992). Preservation of the urethral branches of the pudendal nerve during surgery is important for the preservation of continence after surgery (Gregory 1984; Gregory *et al.* 1984; Griffin *et al.* 1989). However, it has been shown that the degree of dissection around the urethra does not seem to affect the urethral pressure profile in cats (Sackman *et al.* 1991). Stricture formation is the most common complication and is usually caused by failure to extend the incision cranial to the bulbourethral gland or by failing to prevent the cat self-traumatizing the site (Phillips & Holt 2006; Segal *et al.* 2020). The urethrostomy can be successfully revised in most cats with strictures (Phillips & Holt 2006). If revision is not possible, then transpubic or subpubic urethrostomy is recommended (Ellison & Lewis 1989; Bernarde & Viguier 2004). Subcutaneous urine leakage is usually the result of poor mucosal to skin apposition or trauma to the stoma. Perineal hernia and urinary incontinence are rare and reflect excessive intrapelvic dissection.

Prepubic urethrostomy

Prepubic or antepubic urethrostomy is performed in both male and female cats and dogs with irreparable obstruction of the intrapelvic urethra (McCully 1955; Mendham 1970; Carb & Yoshioka 1982; Baines *et al.* 2001). In the male dog, a technique of creating the urethrostomy opening in the prepuce has been described after penile amputation (Pavletic & O'Bell 2007).

A standard approach to the caudal abdomen is made. The maximum length of normal urethra should be maintained: in the female, the urethra should be transected close to the vagina, whereas in the male dog it should be transected distal to the prostate. It is important that the location of the urethrostomy opening be chosen to create a gentle arc with the urethra and prevent kinking at the bladder neck. The exact position depends on the length of the remaining urethra and the conformation of the animal. The urethra is exteriorized lateral to the abdominal incision and two simple interrupted sutures placed between the adventitia of the urethra and the linea alba to reduce tension on the stoma. The exteriorized urethra is spatulated and a stoma created with simple interrupted sutures. The abdominal incision is closed routinely.

Prepubic urethrostomy is associated with significant complications, but is a viable salvage procedure (Mendham 1970; McLaren 1988; Bradley 1989; Baines *et al.* 2001). Postoperative urinary obstruction can occur due to strictures associated with the urethrostomy opening, kinking of the urethra, or inappropriate choice of urethrostomy site. Animals are prone to urinary tract infections and should be periodically tested and appropriately treated. Urinary incontinence can occur, but is uncommon. Urine scalding of the skin is uncommon, even in cats with pendulous inguinal skin folds. In a retrospective study on 16 cats, 7 developed urine scalding or skin necrosis and 6 had urinary incontinence; 6 cats were euthanized between 6 and 84 months because of urinary incontinence (3 cats), skin necrosis (2 cats), and urinary tract infection (1 cat) (Baines *et al.* 2001).

Subpubic urethrostomy

A subpubic urethrostomy has been reported in cats as a salvage procedure for stricture after perineal urethrostomy (Ellison & Lewis 1989). The surgical procedure is similar to antepubic urethrostomy. To increase the length of the urethra, an osteotomy of the pubis is performed, exteriorizing a longer segment of urethra. Increasing the length of the urethra should reduce the risk of incontinence.

Transpelvic urethrostomy

Transpelvic urethrostomy has been proposed as an alternative procedure in cats to rescue failure of a perineal urethrostomy, and instead of a perineal urethrostomy if the distal urethra is strictured. It has also been performed in female dog with a vestibulovaginal stricture (Chiaramonte *et al.* 2022). The surgery is started like a perineal urethrostomy but extended more cranially along the urethra. The caudal part of the pubis and ischium are removed to allow ventral mobilization of the distal urethra. The distal urethra is sutured to the skin in a similar manner to a perineal urethrostomy. In a study of 11 cats with chronic lower urinary tract obstruction, 10 had a successful outcome between 9 and 42 months of follow-up. One cat developed a lower urinary tract infection 6 months after surgery, and one cat had transient urinary incontinence (Bernarde & Viguier 2004).

References

Adams, L.G., Williams, J.C. Jr., McAteer, J.A. et al. (2005). in vitro evaluation of canine and feline calcium oxalate urolith fragility via shock wave lithotripsy. *American Journal of Veterinary Research* 66: 1651–1654.

Adams, L.G., Berent, A.C., Moore, G.E., and Bagley, D.H. (2008). Use of laser lithotripsy for fragmentation of uroliths in dogs: 73 cases (2005–2006). *Journal of the American Veterinary Medical Association* 232: 1680–1687.

Agrodnia, M.D., Hauptman, J.G., Stanley, B.J., and Walshaw, R. (2004). A simple continuous pattern using absorbable suture for perineal urethrostomy in the cat: 18 cases (2000–2002). *Journal of the American Animal Hospital Association* 40: 479–483.

Baines, S.J., Rennie, S., and White, R.S. (2001). Prepubic urethrostomy: a long-term study in 16 cats. *Veterinary Surgery* 30: 107–113.

Banerjee, B.J. (1968). Perineal urethrotomy in acute urinary retention of dogs. *Indian Veterinary Journal* 45: 256–262.

Bartges, J.W., Osborne, C.A., Lulich, J.P. et al. (1999). Canine urate urolithiasis. Etiopathogenesis, diagnosis, and management. *Veterinary Clinics of North America: Small Animal Practice* 29: 161–191, xii–xiii.

Bass, M., Howard, J., Gerber, B., and Messmer, M. (2005). Retrospective study of indications for and outcome of perineal urethrostomy in cats. *Journal of Small Animal Practice* 46: 227–231.

Bernarde, A. and Viguier, E. (2004). Transpelvic urethrostomy in 11 cats using an ischial ostectomy. *Veterinary Surgery* 33: 246–252.

Bilbrey, S.A., Birchard, S.J., and Smeak, D.D. (1991). Scrotal urethrostomy: a retrospective review of 38 dogs (1973 through 1988). *Journal of the American Animal Hospital Association* 27: 560–564.

Biondo-Simões, M.L.P., Collaço, L.M., Veronese, C. et al. (1998). Behavior of chromic catgut and polyglecaprone 25 sutures in the urinary bladder of rats, with special reference to stone formation. *Acta Cirurgica Brasileira* 13: 26–28.

Blake, J.A. (1968). Perineal urethrostomy in cats. *Journal of the American Veterinary Medical Association* 152: 1499–1506.

Block, G., Adams, L.G., Widmer, W.R., and Lingeman, J.E. (1996). Use of extracorporeal shock wave lithotripsy for treatment of nephrolithiasis and ureterolithiasis in five dogs. *Journal of the American Veterinary Medical Association* 208: 531–536.

Bolfer, L., Schmit, J.M., McNeill, A.L. et al. (2015). Penile amputation and scrotal urethrostomy followed by chemotherapy in a dog with penile hemangiosarcoma. *Journal of the American Animal Hospital Association* 51: 25–30.

Bone, W.J. (1969). Perineal urethrostomy in the male cat. *Veterinary Medicine, Small Animal Clinician* 64: 518–520.

Bradley, R.L. (1989). Prepubic urethrostomy. An acceptable urinary diversion technique. *Problems in Veterinary Medicine* 1: 120–127.

Burrow, R.D., Gregory, S.P., Giejda, A.A., and White, R.N. (2011). Penile amputation and scrotal urethrostomy in 18 dogs. *Veterinary Record* 169: 657–665.

Carb, A. and Yoshioka, M.M. (1982). Antepubic urethrostomy in the dog. *Journal of the American Animal Hospital Association* 18: 290–294.

Carbone, M.G. (1965). Perineal urethrostomy in the male cat: a report on twenty cases. *Journal of the American Veterinary Medical Association* 146: 843–853.

Carbone, M.G. (1967). A modified technique for perineal urethrostomy in the male cat. *Journal of the American Veterinary Medical Association* 151: 301–305.

Chiaramonte, A., Anglin, E., Takacs, J.D. et al. (2022). Transpelvic urethrostomy in a female dog with congenital vestibulovaginal and urethral stenosis: a case report. *Veterinary Surgery* 51: 706–712.

Crowe, D.T. (1986). Ventral versus dorsal cystotomy: an experimental investigation. *Journal of the American Animal Hospital Association* 22: 382–386.

Davidson, E.B., Ritchey, J.W., Higbee, R.D. et al. (2004). Laser lithotripsy for treatment of canine uroliths. *Veterinary Surgery* 33: 56–61.

Defarges, A. and Dunn, M. (2008). Use of electrohydraulic lithotripsy in 28 dogs with bladder and urethral calculi. *Journal of Veterinary Internal Medicine* 22: 1267–1273.

Desch, J.P. and Wagner, S.D. (1986). Urinary bladder incisions in dogs: comparison of ventral and dorsal. *Veterinary Surgery* 15: 153–155.

Edlich, R.F., Rodeheaver, G.T., and Thacker, J.G. (1987). Considerations in the choice of sutures for wound closure of the genitourinary tract. *Journal of Urology* 137: 373–379.

Ellison, G. and Lewis, D.B.F. (1989). Subpubic urethrostomy to salvage a failed perineal urethrostomy in a cat. *Compendium on Continuing Education for the Practicing Veterinarian* 11: 946–951.

Feeney, D.A., Weichselbaum, R.C., Jessen, C.R., and Osborne, C.A. (1999). Imaging canine urocystoliths: detection and prediction of mineral content. *Veterinary Clinics of North America: Small Animal Practice* 29: 59–72.

Franti, C.E., Ling, G.V., Ruby, A.L., and Johnson, D.L. (1999). Urolithiasis in dogs. V: regional comparisons of breed, age, sex, anatomic location, and mineral type of calculus. *American Journal of Veterinary Research* 60: 29–42.

Gatoria, I.S., Saini, N.S., Rai, T.S., and Dwivedi, P.N. (2006). Comparison of three techniques for the diagnosis of urinary tract infections in dogs with urolithiasis. *Journal of Small Animal Practice* 47: 727–732.

Grant, D.C., Harper, T.A., and Werre, S.R. (2010). Frequency of incomplete urolith removal, complications, and diagnostic imaging following cystotomy for removal of uroliths from the lower urinary tract in dogs: 128 cases (1994–2006). *Journal of the American Veterinary Medical Association* 236: 763–766.

Greenberg, C.B., Davidson, E.B., Bellmer, D.D. et al. (2004). Evaluation of the tensile strengths of four monofilament absorbable suture materials after immersion in canine urine with or without bacteria. *American Journal of Veterinary Research* 65: 847–853.

Gregory, C.R. (1984). Electromyographic and urethral pressure profilometry. Clinical application in male cats. *Veterinary Clinics of North America: Small Animal Practice* 14: 567–574.

Gregory, C.R., Holliday, T.A., Vasseur, P.B. et al. (1984). Electromyographic and urethral pressure profilometry: assessment of urethral function before and after perineal urethrostomy in cats. *American Journal of Veterinary Research* 45: 2062–2065.

Griffin, D.W. and Gregory, C.R. (1992). Prevalence of bacterial urinary tract infection after perineal urethrostomy in cats. *Journal of the American Veterinary Medical Association* 200: 681–684.

Griffin, D.W., Gregory, C.R., and Kitchell, R.L. (1989). Preservation of striated muscle urethral sphincter function with use of a surgical technique for perineal urethrostomy in cats. *Journal of the American Veterinary Medical Association* 194: 1057–1060.

Haine, D.L., Miller, R., and Barnes, D. (2020). Prescrotal urethrotomy for urethroscopic ablation of a hemorrhagic urethral mucosal mass. *Canadian Veterinary Journal* 61: 1299–1302.

Hanke, P.R., Timm, P., Falk, G., and Kramer, W. (1994). Behavior of different suture materials in the urinary bladder of the rabbit with special reference to wound healing, epithelization and crystallization. *Urologia Internationalis* 52: 26–33.

Karabulut, R., Sonmez, K., Turkyilmaz, Z. et al. (2010). An in vitro and in vivo evaluation of tensile strength and durability of seven suture materials in various pH and different conditions: an experimental study in rats. *Indian Journal of Surgery* 72: 386–390.

Kruger, J.M. and Osborne, C.A. (1986). Etiopathogenesis of uric acid and ammonium urate uroliths in non-Dalmatian dogs. *Veterinary Clinics of North America: Small Animal Practice* 16: 87–126.

Kruger, J.M., Osborne, C.A., and Lulich, J.P. (1999). Canine calcium phosphate uroliths: etiopathogenesis, diagnosis, and management. *Veterinary Clinics of North America: Small Animal Practice* 29: 141–159.

Langston, C., Gisselman, K., Palma, D., and McCue, J. (2008). Diagnosis of urolithiasis. *Compendium on Continuing Education for the Practicing Veterinarian* 30: 447–450, 452–454; quiz 455.

Ling, G.V., Franti, C.E., Johnson, D.L., and Ruby, A.L. (1998a). Urolithiasis in dogs. III: prevalence of urinary tract infection and interrelations of infection, age, sex, and mineral composition. *American Journal of Veterinary Research* 59: 643–649.

Ling, G.V., Franti, C.E., Johnson, D.L., and Ruby, A.L. (1998b). Urolithiasis in dogs. IV: survey of interrelations among breed, mineral composition, and anatomic location of calculi, and presence of urinary tract infection. *American Journal of Veterinary Research* 59: 650–660.

Ling, G.V., Franti, C.E., Ruby, A.L., and Johnson, D.L. (1998c). Urolithiasis in dogs. II: breed prevalence, and interrelations of breed, sex, age, and mineral composition. *American Journal of Veterinary Research* 59: 630–642.

Ling, G.V., Franti, C.E., Ruby, A.L. et al. (1998d). Urolithiasis in dogs. I: mineral prevalence and interrelations of mineral composition, age, and sex. *American Journal of Veterinary Research* 59: 624–629.

Lulich, J.P. and Osborne, C.A. (1992). Catheter-assisted retrieval of urocystoliths from dogs and cats. *Journal of the American Veterinary Medical Association* 201: 111–113.

Lulich, J.P., Osborne, C.A., Carlson, M. et al. (1993). Nonsurgical removal of urocystoliths in dogs and cats by voiding urohydropropulsion. *Journal of the American Veterinary Medical Association* 203: 660–663.

Lulich, J.P., Osborne, C.A., Thumchai, R. et al. (1998). Management of canine calcium oxalate urolith recurrence. *Compendium on Continuing Education for the Practicing Veterinarian* 20: 178–180.

Lulich, J.P., Osborne, C.A., Lekcharoensuk, C. et al. (1999a). Canine calcium oxalate urolithiasis: case-based applications of therapeutic principles. *Veterinary Clinics of North America: Small Animal Practice* 29: 123–139.

Lulich, J.P., Osborne, C.A., Sanderson, S.L. et al. (1999b). Voiding urohydropropulsion. Lessons from 5 years of experience. *Veterinary Clinics of North America: Small Animal Practice* 29: 283–291, xiv.

Lulich, J.P., Adams, L.G., Grant, D. et al. (2009a). Changing paradigms in the treatment of uroliths by lithotripsy. *Veterinary Clinics of North America: Small Animal Practice* 39: 143–160.

Lulich, J.P., Osborne, C.A., Albasan, H. et al. (2009b). Efficacy and safety of laser lithotripsy in fragmentation of urocystoliths and urethroliths for removal in dogs. *Journal of the American Veterinary Medical Association* 234: 1279–1285.

McCully, R.M. (1955). Antepubic urethrostomy for the relief of recurrent urethral obstruction in the male cat. *Journal of the American Veterinary Medical Association* 126: 173–179.

McLaren, I.G. (1988). Prepubic urethrostomy involving transplantation of the prepuce in the cat. *Veterinary Record* 122: 363.

Mendham, J.H. (1970). A description and evaluation of antepubic urethrostomy in the male cat. *Journal of Small Animal Practice* 11: 709–721.

Morris, M.C., Baquero, A., Redovan, E. et al. (1986). Urolithiasis on absorbable and non-absorbable suture materials in the rabbit bladder. *Journal of Urology* 135: 602–603.

Newton, J.D. and Smeak, D.D. (1996). Simple continuous closure of canine scrotal urethrostomy: results in 20 cases. *Journal of the American Animal Hospital Association* 32: 531–534.

Nye, A.K., Luther, J.K., Mann, F.A. et al. (2020). Retrospective multicentric study comparing durations of surgery and anesthesia and likelihoods of short- and long-term complications between cats positioned in sternal or dorsal recumbency for perineal urethrostomy. *Journal of the American Veterinary Medical Association* 257: 176–182.

Osborne, C.A., Caywood, D.D., Johnston, G.R. et al. (1991). Perineal urethrostomy versus dietary management in prevention of recurrent lower urinary tract disease. *Journal of Small Animal Practice* 32: 296–305.

Osborne, C.A., Caywood, D.D., Johnston, G.R. et al. (1996). Feline perineal urethrostomy: a potential cause of feline lower urinary tract disease. *Veterinary Clinics of North America: Small Animal Practice* 26: 535–549.

Osborne, C.A., Jacob, F., Lulich, J.P. et al. (1999a). Canine silica urolithiasis. Risk factors, detection, treatment, and prevention. *Veterinary Clinics of North America: Small Animal Practice* 29: 213–230, xiii.

Osborne, C.A., Lulich, J.P., Polzin, D.J. et al. (1999b). Medical dissolution and prevention of canine struvite urolithiasis: twenty years of experience. *Veterinary Clinics of North America: Small Animal Practice* 29: 73–111.

Osborne, C.A., Lulich, J.P., and Polzin, D.J. (1999c). Canine retrograde urohydropropulsion: lessons from 25 years of experience. *Veterinary Clinics of North America: Small Animal Practice* 29: 267–281.

Osborne, C.A., Sanderson, S.L., Lulich, J.P. et al. (1999d). Canine cystine urolithiasis: cause, detection, treatment, and prevention. *Veterinary Clinics of North America: Small Animal Practice* 29: 193–211.

Pavletic, M.M. and O'Bell, S.A. (2007). Subtotal penile amputation and preputial urethrostomy in a dog. *Journal of the American Veterinary Medical Association* 230: 375–377.

Phillips, H. and Holt, D.E. (2006). Surgical revision of the urethral stoma following perineal urethrostomy in 11 cats: (1998–2004). *Journal of the American Animal Hospital Association* 42: 218–222.

Pinel, C.B., Monnet, E., and Reems, M.R. (2013). Laparoscopic-assisted cystotomy for urolith removal in dogs and cats – 23 cases. *Canadian Veterinary Journal* 54: 36–41.

Radasch, R.M., Merkley, D.F., Wilson, J.W., and Barstad, R.D. (1990). Cystotomy closure: a comparison of the strength of appositional and inverting suture patterns. *Veterinary Surgery* 19: 283–288.

Rawlings, C.A., Mahaffey, M.B., Barsanti, J.A., and Canalis, C. (2003). Use of laparoscopic-assisted cystoscopy for removal of urinary calculi in dogs. *Journal of the American Veterinary Medical Association* 222: 759–761.

Reimer, S.B., Kyles, A.E., Schulz, K.S. et al. (2004). Unusual urethral calculi in two male dogs. *Journal of the American Animal Hospital Association* 40: 157–161.

Ruda, L. and Heiene, R. (2012). Short- and long-term outcome after perineal urethrostomy in 86 cats with feline lower urinary tract disease. *Journal of Small Animal Practice* 53: 693–698.

Runge, J.J., Berent, A.C., Mayhew, P.D., and Weisse, C. (2011). Transvesicular percutaneous cystolithotomy for the retrieval of cystic and urethral calculi in dogs and cats: 27 cases (2006–2008). *Journal of the American Veterinary Medical Association* 239: 344–349.

Sackman, J.E., Sims, M.H., and Krahwinkel, D.J. (1991). Urodynamic evaluation of lower urinary tract function in cats after perineal urethrostomy with minimal and extensive dissection. *Veterinary Surgery* 20: 55–60.

Segal, U., Shani, J., Zemer, O., and Joseph, R. (2020). Evaluation of urethral orifice cross-section dimensions following perineal urethrostomy in male cats. *Journal of Small Animal Practice* 61: 475–479.

Slunsky, P., Brunnberg, M., Lodersted, S., and Brunnberg, L. (2018). Effect of intraoperative positioning on the diameter of the vertebral canal in cats during perineal urethrostomy (cadaveric study). *Journal of Feline Medicine and Surgery* 20: 38–44.

Slunsky, P., Brunnberg, M., Loderstedt, S. et al. (2019). Effect of intraoperative positioning on postoperative neurological status in cats after perineal urethrostomy. *Journal of Feline Medicine and Surgery* 21: 931–937.

Smeak, D.D. (2000). Urethrotomy and urethrostomy in the dog. *Clinical Techniques in Small Animal Practice* 15: 25–34.

Smeak, D.D., Fingeroth, J.M., and Bojrab, M.J. (1990). Scrotal urethrostomy. In: *Current Techniques in Small Animal Surgery*, 3e (ed. M.J. Bojrab), 381–385. Philadelphia, PA: Lea & Febiger.

Smith, C.W. (1987). Perineal urethrostomy in the cat: technique, indications and complications. *Modern Veterinary Practice* 68: 153–157.

Smith, C.W. (2002). Perineal urethrostomy. *Veterinary Clinics of North America: Small Animal Practice* 32: 917–925, vii.

Taylor, C.J. and Smeak, D.D. (2021). Perineal urethrostomy in male dogs – technique description, short- and long-term results. *Canadian Veterinary Journal* 62: 1315–1322.

Thumchai, R., Lulich, J.P., Osborne, C.A. et al. (1996). Epizootiologic evaluation of urolithiasis in cats: 3,498 cases (1982–1992). *Journal of the American Veterinary Medical Association* 208: 547–551.

Waldron, D.R., Hedlund, C.S., Tangner, C.H. et al. (1985). The canine urethra: a comparison of first and second intention healing. *Veterinary Surgery* 14: 213–217.

Weber, W.J., Boothe, H.W., Brassard, J.A., and Hobson, H.P. (1985). Comparison of the healing of prescrotal urethrotomy incisions in the dog: sutured versus nonsutured. *American Journal of Veterinary Research* 46: 1309–1315.

Westropp, J.L., Ruby, A.L., Campbell S.J., and Ling, G.V. (2010). Canine and feline urolithiasis: pathophysiology, epidemiology, and management. In: *Mechanisms of Disease in Small Animal Surgery*, 3e (ed. M.J. Bojrab and E. Monnet), 387–392. Jackson, WY: Teton New Media.

Wilson, G.P. III and Harrison, J.W. (1971). Perineal urethrostomy in cats. *Journal of the American Veterinary Medical Association* 159: 1789–1793.

Wisener, L.V., Pearl, D.L., Houston, D.M. et al. (2010). Risk factors for the incidence of calcium oxalate uroliths or magnesium ammonium phosphate uroliths for dogs in Ontario, Canada, from 1998 to 2006. *American Journal of Veterinary Research* 71: 1045–1054.

45

Ureteral Ectopia and Urinary Incontinence

Philipp D. Mayhew and Allyson Berent

Urinary incontinence (UI) is defined as the inability to retain voluntary control over urination. It is a common presenting clinical sign in dogs and occurs with less frequency in cats. The etiopathogenesis of the condition is varied, but can be broadly divided into neurogenic causes, nonneurogenic anatomic defects, or functional compromise. In some cases, functional abnormalities are predisposed to by anatomic alterations. An example of this would be urethral sphincter mechanism incompetence (USMI), which is often associated with a short urethra and intrapelvic bladder in dogs (Adams & DiBartola 1983; Mahaffey et al. 1984; Holt 1985c; Power et al. 1998) and vaginal aplasia and severe urethral hypoplasia in cats (Holt & Gibbs 1992; Holt & Thrusfield 1993).

Overall, ectopic ureters (EU) and USMI made up 82% of the diagnosed cases of UI in dogs in one study (Holt 1990a). The most common causes of incontinence in juvenile dogs are EU and congenital sphincter mechanism incontinence (Holt 1990a; Forsee et al. 2013). In young cats EU and urethral hypoplasia are most common (Holt 1990a). In adult dogs USMI, prostatic disease, urogenital neoplasia, and neurogenic causes are most common, whereas neurogenic incontinence followed by a variety of urethral and bladder conditions is the most common cause of acquired incontinence in adult cats (Holt 1990a; Lonc et al. 2020).

Companion animals that are incontinent pets are very frustrating for owners to live with, and the condition is a common cause of euthanasia due to the severity of environmental contamination that is caused. A methodical approach to diagnosis and treatment is required, as often multiple conditions can coexist in the same patient. In most cases a combination of careful clinical history,

physical examination, laboratory testing, and imaging is required. Treatment of UI can be frustrating, with some common disease processes, such as USMI and ureteral ectopia, being associated with relatively high treatment failure rates after both medical and surgical management (Holt 1985b, 1990b; McLaughlin & Miller 1991; Massat et al. 1993; Holt & Hotson-Moore 1995; Muir et al. 1994; Aaron et al. 1996; Scott et al. 2002; White 2001; Rawlings et al. 2001; Barth et al. 2005; Holt et al. 2005; Mayhew et al. 2006; Berent et al. 2008, 2012; Noel et al. 2017). However, even in the most challenging cases, if a willingness to pursue multimodality therapy exists, many patients can be cured, or significantly improved, with treatment and in recent years better outcomes have been documented in some studies.

Anatomic considerations

Anatomic structures relevant to incontinence include the ureters, bladder, urethra, and prostate gland. The ureters are retroperitoneal in location, arising from the renal hilus and passing in a sometimes convoluted fashion to enter the dorsal aspect of the bladder. Prior to entry they make a characteristic J-shaped turn cranially, which can sometimes be detected using contrast imaging studies (Mason et al. 1990). The ureterovesicular opening is normally horseshoe shaped and can be seen best during cystoscopic examination (Cannizzo et al. 2003; Samii et al. 2004; Berent 2016). These openings are usually visible in normal dogs during open surgery, but in cats they can be challenging to visualize and magnification is usually required. The ureters receive their blood supply from a cranial and caudal

Small Animal Soft Tissue Surgery, Second Edition. Edited by Eric Monnet.
© 2023 John Wiley & Sons, Inc. Published 2023 by John Wiley & Sons, Inc.
Companion website: www.wiley.com/go/monnet/small

source. Cranially branches of the renal artery supply the ureteral artery, which courses alongside the ureter, and anastomose with branches from the prostatic and vaginal arteries caudally.

The bladder is usually located within the peritoneal cavity in dogs (Evans & Christensen 1993), although intrapelvic bladders have been recognized in clinically normal dogs (Mahaffey et al. 1984). In cats the bladder is located more cranially and is always located within the abdominal cavity. The urethra in feline patients is consequently longer than its canine counterpart (Dyce et al. 2002). The bladder has two principal functions, firstly as a storage organ for urine, and secondly as the muscular force behind the voiding phase of micturition mediated by the detrusor muscle. The detrusor muscle of the bladder wall is made up of three layers of muscle, outer and inner longitudinal layers, and a thick middle circular layer. Smooth muscle cells in the bladder wall are attached to each other by "tight junctions" (Sharp & Wheeler 2005). Membrane depolarization leads to a well-coordinated wave of contraction across the detrusor. Chronic distension can disrupt the tight junctions and lead a loss of coordinated bladder contraction. The bladder receives its blood supply from the cranial and caudal vesical arteries originating from the internal iliac artery.

The urethra extends from the bladder trigone to the vestibule (or end of the penis in males) and plays a very significant role in most causes of UT. The wall of the urethra is also made up of an inner and outer longitudinal and a middle circular layer of smooth muscle, which turns to striated muscle in the distal urethra. Blood supply is from the vaginal and external and internal pudendal arteries. The prostate gland completely encircles the male canine urethra from the bladder neck to the post-prostatic membranous urethra. It is mostly retroperitoneal (Evans & Christensen 1993) and is anchored along with the urethra and bladder by lateral umbilical ligaments, within which courses the neurovascular supply. The prostate gland enlarges continuously in dogs throughout life under the influence of testosterone, and 95% of 9-year-old dogs have evidence of benign prostatic hyperplasia (Berry et al. 1986). The prostatic artery arises from the internal pudendal artery and approaches the gland from the dorsal aspect. The prostate gland can become pathologically enlarged due to hyperplasia or neoplasia. It is unusual, but primary prostatic disease of any type can be associated with UI in dogs, possibly due to mechanical interference with the urethral sphincter mechanism (Holt 1990a). In cats, because of the elongated urethra, there is a relatively longer preprostatic urethra. The prostate gland only partially encircles the urethra in cats, being absent ventrally (Dyce et al. 2002). Age-related benign prostatic hyperplasia in cats is not a frequently encountered phenomenon as it is in dogs, and prostatic disease has only very rarely been implicated as a cause of UI in cats (Lonc et al. 2020).

The nervous supply of the urethra and bladder has great relevance to UI, as many cases are neurogenic in origin. The bladder receives sympathetic, parasympathetic, and somatic innervation. The sympathetic innervation through the hypogastric nerve originates from spinal segments L1–L4/5 in dogs. Its principal function is to cause contraction of urethral smooth muscle, mediated through α-adrenergic receptors, and relaxation of the detrusor muscle, mediated through β-adrenergic receptors. Sympathetic tone predominates during the storage phase of micturition. Parasympathetic innervation is through the pelvic nerve, originating from spinal segments S1–S3. Parasympathetic stimulation causes contraction of the bladder detrusor muscle and relaxation of the urethral sphincter mechanism. Detrusor contraction is stimulated by stretch receptors within the wall of the bladder that sense overdistension, leading to stimulation of parasympathetic fibers that initiate the voiding phase. The somatic innervation is through the pudendal nerve, originating from spinal segments S1–S3, and provides voluntary innervation to the external urethral sphincter. During bladder filling the pudendal nerve maintains the tonic contracted state of the external sphincter. During the voiding phase, and under voluntary control, inhibition of pudendal innervation causes relaxation of the striated muscle and allows free passage of urine.

Physiology of continence

The urethral sphincter mechanism constitutes the primary mechanism for retention of continence by providing resistance to outflow during the storage phase of micturition. Continence occurs when the resting urethral pressure exceeds the intravesical pressure in the bladder. The term "urethral sphincter" has been used frequently, although it should not be thought of as a discrete anatomic structure but as a tubular area of high tension rather than a solitary point of high pressure (Stolzenburg et al. 2006). The sphincter mechanism is contributed to by smooth and striated muscle along with the fibroelastic tissues of the urethral wall. Pressure profilometry studies have demonstrated that certain areas of the urethra contribute greater amounts of resting urethral tone during the storage phase of urination and that males and females have different anatomic configurations of these structures (Awad & Downie 1976).

In normal female dogs it is considered that smooth muscle provides the greatest contribution to resting urethral tone (Awad & Downie 1976) and detailed anatomic studies have shown that the majority of urethral smooth muscle in normal female dogs resides in the trigone and proximal urethral segments, as a continuation of the middle layer of detrusor smooth muscle (Cullen *et al.* 1981; Stolzenburg *et al.* 2002). This coincides with urodynamic observations that static urethral pressure is maximal in the proximal urethra in clinically normal female dogs under conditions of fluid flow (Cass & Hinman 1968). The clinical observation that the α-adrenergic agents provide the most effective therapeutic effect in female dogs with USMI, coupled with the knowledge that most α-adrenergic receptors are located on smooth muscle, provides further evidence for this hypothesis. The striated muscle component of the urethral wall, which is under somatic innervation, is located more distally and the fibrovascular components are distributed throughout the length of the urethra (Awad & Downie 1976). It should be noted, however, that urodynamic and morphometric variables have been shown to be significantly affected by age and the stage of the estrus cycle (Noel *et al.* 2017). In male dogs striated muscle comprises more than 50% of the urethral wall caudal to the body of the prostate gland, and this area has often been termed the "external urethral sphincter mechanism"(Gookin *et al.* 1996; Cullen *et al.* 1981). However, it has been estimated that approximately 85% of the overall continence mechanism or urethral wall tension is composed of the urethral smooth muscle and nonneural components (fibroelastic components) in the proximal urethra (Awad & Downie 1976).

In male dogs the location of the urethral sphincter mechanism is more controversial (Stolzenburg *et al.* 2006). It has been suggested based on anatomic studies that the primary area of smooth muscle responsible for maintenance of continence appears to be in the bladder neck (Cullen *et al.* 1981). However, in urodynamic studies of male dogs little increase in closure pressure was found until the mid-prostatic urethra (Awad & Downie 1976). It is generally agreed that the striated muscle component of the prostatic and postprostatic urethra in male dogs contributes more substantially to resting urethral tone than it does in females (Awad & Downie 1976).

Cats appear to have anatomically and functionally different sphincter mechanisms compared to dogs and so assumptions for one species should not be extrapolated to the other (Cullen *et al.* 1983a,b). They too have a predominance of smooth muscle in the vesicle neck and proximal urethra, but with a greater longitudinal component than in dogs (Cullen *et al.* 1983a; Frenier *et al.* 1992). The smooth muscle sphincter is better developed than in the dog, with approximately twice the relative volume of circular smooth muscle in the feline urethra compared to the canine. They also have a striated external urethral sphincter mechanism in the mid to distal urethra that is relatively similar in volume to that of dogs, although there may not be a completely encircling striated sphincter muscle in the prostatic region in cats (Cullen *et al.* 1983b). The resting urethral tone of the feline sphincter mechanism may rely more heavily on the fibroelastic components and the narrow diameter of the male urethra compared to the dog (Cullen *et al.* 1983b; Gregory 1984).

Pathophysiology of urinary incontinence

Urethral sphincter mechanism incontinence

The most common cause of UI in dogs is USMI, which has sometimes been termed "hormone-responsive incontinence" or "postspaying" incontinence in female dogs. This condition is seen in a congenital form as well as an acquired form in male and female dogs, as well as female cats, although the incidence in females is much greater than in males (Holt 1985a, 1990a; Holt & Gibbs 1992; Holt & Thrusfield 1993; Aaron *et al.* 1996; Scott *et al.* 2002; Angioletti *et al.* 2004; Reichler *et al.* 2006). It does not appear to have been reported in male cats. The condition can be seen in all breeds of dogs, although certain breeds such as the Old English sheepdog, Rottweiler, Dobermann, Weimaraner, Irish setter, and boxer are overrepresented (Arnold *et al.* 1989; Holt & Thrusfield 1993). The German shepherd and dachshund were found to be underrepresented (Arnold *et al.* 1989). Larger-breed dogs have been found to be particularly at risk (Holt & Thrusfield 1993; Aaron *et al.* 1996; Byron *et al.* 2017). Dogs >20 kg (31%) are more likely to develop USMI than those under 20 kg (9.3%) (Arnold *et al.* 1989).

A number of different pathologic factors have been investigated with regard to USMI, although it remains an incompletely understood condition. The introduction of urethral pressure profilometry (UPP) in studies of incontinent dogs first elucidated the role of decreased urethral tone in the etiopathogenesis of USMI. Studies were able to show that maximal urethral pressure (MUP) and maximal urethral closure pressure (MUCP) were decreased when populations of continent dogs were compared to their incontinent counterparts (Rosin & Barsanti 1981; Richter & Ling 1985; Holt 1988). Response to α-adrenergic stimulation provides further evidence that a decrease in urethral tone plays a principal role in the pathogenesis of the disease (Rosin & Ross 1981; White & Pomeroy 1989; Richter & Ling 1985). The factors that might lead to this loss of tone have been the subject of much investigation.

The role of hormonal factors has been investigated due to the observation that a large number of animals develop symptoms of USMI after neutering. This is true for male and female dogs (Aaron *et al.* 1996; Arnold *et al.* 1989; Power *et al.* 1998; Thrusfield *et al.* 1998; Angioletti *et al.* 2004). Approximately 5–20% of spayed female dogs are affected with USMI and incontinence occurs within three years of surgery in approximately 75% of cases (Holt 1985a; Arnold *et al.* 1989; Holt & Thrusfield 1993; Angioletti *et al.* 2004). Conversely, much smaller incidences of USMI have been reported in unspayed populations, with only 10 of 5315 dogs affected in one study (Holt & Thrusfield 1993). An epidemiologic study has proved an association between spaying and incontinence, with spayed females being 4.9 times more likely to develop incontinence compared to their unspayed counterparts (Thrusfield 1985), although a more recent systematic review found only weak evidence for the association of spaying and USMI; this may have been partially due to the paucity of high-quality studies directly evaluating the hypothesis (Beauvais *et al.* 2012). The timing of spaying has been questioned lately and there is some weak evidence for an association between early spaying (<3 months) and an increased risk of USMI developing (Beauvais *et al.* 2012). Age appears to be important, particularly for larger breeds of dogs anticipated to weigh >25 kg, where delaying spaying to the end of the first year of life resulted in a lower incidence of USMI post spaying (Byron *et al.* 2017). No significant differences in the incidence of USMI after ovariectomy (OVE) versus ovariohysterectomy (OVH) have been reported in several studies that have investigated this possibility (Okkens *et al.* 1997; Arnold *et al.* 1989; Van Goethem *et al.* 2006; Corriveau *et al.* 2017). The role of estrogens in the pathogenesis of USMI has been investigated, but remain somewhat uncertain. It is known that estrogen therapy is essential to the development of continence in young animals and a significant number of juvenile female dogs with UI will spontaneously improve after the first estrus (Holt 1985a). It is also known that MUCP decreases significantly in the year after ovariectomy (Reichler *et al.* 2004). This apparently beneficial effect of estrogens on the urethral sphincter mechanism has been investigated, and is related to estrogen-induced increase in expression of α-2 adrenergic receptors on urethral smooth muscle and their sensitivity to α-adrenergic agents (Creed 1983; Miodrag *et al.* 1988). After removal of the ovaries, it has been hypothesized that the loss of endogenous estrogen could cause a decrease in urethral tone. Unfortunately, this is likely to be too simplistic an explanation and does not consider all the factors involved. Firstly, studies have shown that levels of endogenous estrogens are no different in incontinent spayed female dogs compared to those in entire dogs in anestrus (Richter & Ling 1985). Secondly,

response to treatment with exogenous estrogen administration has yielded mixed therapeutic responses, with a significant proportion of dogs not responding to treatment in some studies (Adams & DiBartola 1983; Holt 1985a; Arnold *et al.* 1989; Mandigers & Nell 2001). In male dogs with USMI, an even poorer response to exogenous estrogen therapy has been reported (Aaron *et al.* 1996).

Recently the role of follicle-stimulating hormone (FSH) and luteinizing hormone (LH) in the incontinent female dog has been investigated. After ovariectomy the negative feedback mechanism on the production of FSH and LH is interrupted, leading to large increases in their plasma levels (Olson *et al.* 1992; Concannon 1993). In one study plasma levels rose rapidly in the first 3 weeks, fell again until 10 weeks, but then started to increase again until they reached a steady-state level at about 42 weeks postoperatively. Steady-state levels were 14–17 times greater than they had been preovariectomy (Reichler *et al.* 2004). A causal relationship for the role of elevated FSH and LH was hypothesized by the observation that some incontinent dogs become continent after administration of a GnRH analog (Reichler *et al.* 2006), which reduces the elevations in FSH and LH levels that develop after OHE/OVE. However, in this study no relationship existed between the elevations in LH/FSH and MUCP, so it was hypothesized that despite there being a beneficial effect of GnRH analog treatment in some dogs, the effect may occur independent of measurable increases in urethral tone (Reichler *et al.* 2004).

Anatomic factors have long been implicated in the development of USMI in dogs. Anatomic texts state that the normal canine bladder is intra-abdominal (Evans & Christensen 1983), although some observers have noted that intrapelvic bladder location can be seen in dogs with no apparent associated morbidity (Adams & DiBartola 1983; Mahaffey *et al.* 1984; Holt 1985c). However, bladder location has been shown to be highly significant (Holt 1985c). In a study of 57 incontinent and 42 continent bitches, an intrapelvic bladder neck location was found to be present in 54 of 57 incontinent and only 7 of 42 continent dogs (Holt 1985c). This effect has also been shown to be independent of degree of bladder filling (Holt 1985c). In summary, it can be stated that whilst not pathognomonic of USMI, there appears to be a strong association between intrapelvic bladder location and USMI. Shortened urethral length was also found to be strongly associated with incontinence in the same study. In another study, vaginal position was related to continence using retrograde vaginourethrograms (Gregory *et al.* 1999). In this study, the location of the cranial vagina was found to be intrabdominal in 25 of 30 continent bitches and only 11 of 30 incontinent bitches, a difference found to be statistically significant (Gregory *et al.* 1999). The significance of the anatomic location of the lower urogenital tract has been hypothesized to be related to the influence of intra-abdominal pressure on the urethral sphincter mechanism. It is suggested that in animals with intra-abdominal bladder necks, increases in intra-abdominal pressure are transmitted to the bladder neck and proximal urethra as well as the bladder, whereas in animals with intrapelvic bladder necks the pressure is only exerted on the bladder. In the absence of good urethral tone, UI could therefore result (Holt 1985c). This theory has formed the basis of many surgical procedures that attempt to move the bladder neck/proximal urethra into the abdomen, such as colposuspension and vas deferentopexy (Holt 1985b; Weber *et al.* 1997; Rawlings *et al.* 2001).

In male dogs, studies using contrast urethrocystograms have also shown that an intrapelvic bladder predisposes to USMI, although short urethral length was not found to be a significant factor, unlike in female dogs (Power *et al.* 1998). The authors of this study suggested that bladder location is related to prostate size and that castrated dogs, which generally have smaller prostate glands, may be more likely to have intrapelvic bladders and therefore be incontinent (Power *et al.* 1998). Castration was shown to be a risk factor for incontinence (Power *et al.* 1998). Other studies have shown a close temporal relationship to castration with most dogs that become incontinent, doing so within a median of one month after castration (Aaron *et al.* 1996).

In cats, USMI is much less common and reported cases are mostly congenital (Holt & Gibbs 1992; Holt 1985b). There are some very significant differences between the pathologic findings in cats compared to dogs. Clinically, animals appear to have severe incontinence, with prolific urine staining from a younger age than those with ectopic ureters (Holt 1992). Most cats have severe concurrent anatomic abnormalities of the lower urinary tract, with marked hypoplasia of the urethra being seen in most cases (Holt 1992). Vaginal aplasia was present in eight of nine cats in one study. The uterine horns in these cases were found to enter the dorsal aspect of the bladder (in six of seven cases there was communication between the uterine horns and bladder lumina) (Holt 1992).

Ectopic ureters

Ectopic ureters develop due to a defect in the embryologic development of the metanephric duct, which becomes the ureter later in development. This results in an abnormal location of the termination of the ureteral orifice(s) (Owen 1973a,b). In humans a different set of developmental changes occurs, resulting in the duplication of parts of the excretory mechanism. Over 80% of people with EU have duplex kidneys in which separate anterior and posterior segments are drained by two different duct systems, although both do not usually develop normally (Albers *et al.* 1995). Although this has been reported in a dog and a cat, it appears to be extremely rare (O'Handley *et al.* 1979; Ghantous & Crawford 2006).

In normal animals the ureteral orifices are seen characteristically as horseshoe-shaped slits in the dorsolateral aspects of the bladder trigone. They are seen on cystoscopic examination as jets of urine entering the bladder during the passage of ureteral peristaltic waves. A significant female sex predilection for EU occurs in dogs, with almost 90% of affected dogs being female in one large study (Holt & Hotson-Moore 1995). In cats 43% of cases reported were female (Holt 1992). EUs have been found to be more common in certain breeds of dogs, including Labrador retrievers, golden retrievers, fox terriers, Siberian huskies, Newfoundlands, bulldogs, and poodles (Hayes 1984; Holt & Hotson-Moore 1995).

Two general subtypes of EU occur: intra- and extramural. In animals with intramural EU, normal entry into the dorsal trigone area will occur, but either no opening into the bladder lumen exists (most commonly) or else an opening into the bladder is present along with openings into the urethra or vagina more distally. In these cases, the ureter continues as an intramural tunnel and terminates in one or more openings within the urethra or vagina. In recent studies using cystoscopy, the frequency of multiple openings appears to be greater than previously thought, with one study reporting more than one ureteral opening in 32% of cases (Cannizzo *et al.* 2003). Earlier studies may have underestimated the occurrence of this abnormality (Holt & Hotson-Moore 1995). Ureteral troughs are extensions of the normal ureteral opening within the wall of the urethral mucosa. They also are increasingly recognized and were found to be present in 72% of dogs in one study using cystoscopy (Cannizzo *et al.* 2003). In one large study, 92% of EUs emptied into the urethra and the remaining 8% entered the vagina in dogs (Holt & Hotson-Moore 1995). The frequency in cats is similar, with 90% of EUs terminating in the urethra and the remaining 10% in the vagina in another study (Holt 1992). In dogs, extramural ureteral ectopia, where the ureter completely bypasses the bladder to enter at a location more distal, appears to be exceedingly rare, with none of 175 cases in one report having this anomaly (Holt & Hotson-Moore 1995), although canine cases have been reported (Singer 1959; Lapish 1985; Mason *et al.* 1990; Lane & Lappin 1995; Mouatt & Watt 2001; Fox *et al.* 2016). It should be noted that misdiagnosis of extramural EU is commonplace when only traditional contrast radiography is employed for diagnosis (Mason *et al.* 1990). The occurrence of extramural EUs in cats appears to be more common, with many cases bypassing the bladder completely (Holt 1992). Other pathologic processes affecting the urinary tract are frequently encountered in dogs with EU and include renal dysplasia, hydronephrosis, hydroureter, hypoplastic bladder, vestibular follicle formation, hymenal remnants, persistent paramesonephric remnants, vestibulovaginal stenosis, vaginal septum, dual vagina, and ureterocele (McLoughlin *et al.* 1989; Holt *et al.* 1982; Holt & Hotson-Moore 1995; Lamb & Gregory 1998; Cannizzo *et al.* 2003; Samii *et al.* 2004).

The presence of hydroureter and hydronephrosis is very common in patients with EU. In one study 42% of dogs had hydroureter and 19% had both hydroureter and hydronephrosis (Holt & Hotson-Moore 1995). It is thought that some degree of functional ureteral obstruction exists due to the presence of the long intramural ureteral tunnel acting as a flap-like valve that becomes intermittently obstructed during periods of increased urethral pressure (McLoughlin & Chew 2000). It is also possible that abnormal ureteral peristalsis or intermittent bacterial infection may play a role in dilatation of the renal pelvis and ureters (Holt & Hotson-Moore 1995). Urinary tract infection (UTI) is particularly common in dogs and cats with EU, being present in 64–79% of cases (Stone & Mason 1990; McLaughlin & Miller 1991; Mayhew *et al.* 2006). Screening for and treatment of UTIs prior to surgical intervention are essential in all cases. More recently the presence of congenital distal ureteral orifice stenosis in association with intramural ureteral ectopia, and sometimes other urinary tract disorders, has also been increasingly recognized as a component of the disease complex (Meler *et al.* 2018).

The presence of decreased bladder storage capacity has been hypothesized to be present in some dogs with EU as a developmental response to urine chronically bypassing the bladder, thereby reducing residual volume during the storage phase of micturition (Lane & Lappin 1995). Subjective radiographic evidence of this abnormality has been documented in dogs with ectopic ureters (Mason *et al.* 1990). In these cases, bladders were radiographically small, sometimes tubular, and intrapelvic in location (Mason *et al.* 1990). Further evidence for the occurrence of this abnormality comes from cystometrographic studies that have shown reduced urinary bladder capacity and poor bladder accommodation in 44% of dogs with EUs (Lane & Lappin 1995; Lane *et al.* 1995). Little information is available on the potential treatment of this condition, although some anecdotal evidence supports the use of anticholinergic agents such as oxybutynin (Lane & Lappin 1995).

UI in patients with EU is not purely related to urine bypassing the urethral sphincter mechanism at the proximal urethra. A significant proportion of animals whose EUs are surgically treated remain incontinent. It has been hypothesized that many animals suffer from other concurrent abnormalities that predispose to UI, principally USMI. Other explanations for persistent UI include poor surgical technique (Stone & Mason 1990), recanalization of the ureteral tunnel (Holt & Hotson-Moore 1995), and decreased bladder capacity (Lane & Lappin 1995). Evidence from UPP lends support to the theory that USMI may be present in cases with EU, as MUPs were significantly lower in dogs with EU compared to healthy controls (Koie *et al.* 2000). Another study documented that 6 of 9 dogs with EU had abnormal urethral pressure profiles, consistent with urethral sphincter mechanism incompetence (Lane *et al.* 1995). Those that remained incontinent after surgical correction had significantly lower MUPs, MUCPs, and functional profile areas, compared to those who became continent postoperatively. It was suggested that dogs with a urethral closure pressure less than $19\,cmH_2O$ may have an increased risk of postoperative incontinence. Care needs to be taken in interpretation of these data, as the clinical utility of UPP has been questioned by some (Lose 2001) and clinical recommendations should be made with care based on these results, as dogs with abnormal urethral profiles can still ultimately become continent. It has been hypothesized that the much longer functional length of the male dog urethra may confer greater resting urethral pressure in dogs, making retrograde passage of urine into the bladder more likely, thereby maintaining continence (Holt & Hotson-Moore 1995; McLoughlin & Chew 2000). It has also been suggested that for the same reason EUs may be a more frequent asymptomatic finding in male dogs (McLoughlin & Chew 2000).

Rarely, ureteroceles can occur in dogs and cats with EU and can be associated with UI (McLoughlin *et al.* 1989; Lautzenhiser & Bjorling 2002; Sutherland-Smith *et al.* 2004; Eisele *et al.* 2005; Tattershall & Welsh 2006; Rogatko *et al.* 2019). Ureteroceles are caused by congenital abnormalities that result in cystic dilatations of the distal ureters. The exact mechanism by which they form has not yet been fully elucidated (McLoughlin *et al.* 1989). Ureteroceles can be orthotopic where the ureterovesicular junction is located in the normal location at the bladder trigone. Orthotopic ureteroceles are often asymptomatic or associated with signs related to an obstructive disorder, such as dysuria, hematuria, and pain. Ectopic ureteroceles often are associated with other anomalies such as renal dysplasia or duplex kidney (McLoughlin *et al.* 1989), and are more commonly associated with UI, as the ureteral opening can be in the urethra or another location distal to the urethral sphincter mechanism.

Neurogenic incontinence

Neurogenic incontinence is common after spinal cord injury and less common in animals with brain lesions. Broadly, two forms of incontinence are seen, depending on whether the spinal cord lesion is upper motor neuron (UMN) or lower motor neuron (LMN). With lesions cranial to L4 (UMN) urethral tone becomes excessive. The consequence is that the bladder fills and, because of urethral sphincter mechanism spasticity and an inability to contract the detrusor muscle, the bladder fails to empty until the intravesicular pressure overcomes the elevated resting urethral tone. This results in overflow incontinence. In these situations, bladder size should always be assessed, as a full bladder in the presence of overflow incontinence is typical of a UMN bladder. In these cases, the bladder must be periodically evacuated by manual expression or catheterization until function returns, otherwise detrusor muscle atony can result, which may cause long-term detrusor dysfunction. After about a month there is usually a return of reflexive detrusor function that may allow emptying to occur.

In LMN lesions there is loss of tone within the urethral sphincter mechanism and an inability to contract the detrusor muscle due to loss of parasympathetic innervation from the pelvic nerves. In these cases constant dribbling occurs due to a loss of the normal urethral resting tone. The most common causes of LMN disease in dogs are degenerative lumbosacral stenosis and trauma. In cats the most common cause is low lumbar and/or pelvic trauma after motor vehicle accidents. Affected cats may have complete paralysis of the lower urogenital tract as well as the rectum (Holt 1985b).

Treatment for neurogenic causes of UI relies on treatment of the underlying neurologic disease. Until normal function hopefully returns, supportive care in these cases must be instituted to avoid further morbidity such as urine scalding and ascending UTI. Readers are referred to other sources for a more complete description of the medical and surgical management of neurogenic causes of UI (Sharp & Wheeler 2005).

Miscellaneous causes of urinary incontinence

Several other, less common causes of incontinence occur in dogs and cats. Prostatic disease has occasionally been implicated as a possible cause of UI in dogs, although this is uncommon. In some cases, prostatic hemorrhage may be confused by owners as evidence of true UI. However, it is hypothesized that prostatic disease can interfere with the functioning of the urethral sphincter

mechanism (Holt 1990a). Some evidence for the role of primary prostatic disease in rare cases of UI comes from a urodynamic study of nine dogs that had abnormally low MUCP and MUP, although in this report none of the dogs was clinically incontinent (Basinger et al. 1989). A more common reason for prostatic disease to be related to UI is as a complication of prostatic surgery. Total prostatectomy in dogs with prostatic disease resulted in postoperative UI in 17 of 18 cases in two studies (Basinger et al. 1989; Hardie et al. 1990), although interestingly continence is maintained in most dogs without prostatic disease (Basinger et al. 1989). A more recent study demonstrated a lower incidence of 35% permanent incontinence post prostatectomy, possibly related to earlier diagnosis and a tendency toward smaller lesions being operated earlier (Bennett et al. 2018). Incontinence occurs due to removal of part of the prostatic urethra that is the area of highest urethral tone in the male canine urethra (Awad & Downie 1976). This hypothesis has been further confirmed by urodynamic studies that demonstrate decreased urethral tone post prostatectomy (Basinger et al. 1989). Less invasive prostatic procedures such as marsupialization or omentalization result in UI much less frequently (Hardie et al. 1990). Prostatic omentalization for treatment of prostatic abscesses did not result in any long-term cases of UI in one study (White & Williams 1995).

Ureterovaginal fistulae are an acquired form of ureteral ectopia that usually occurs as an iatrogenic lesion caused during ovariohysterectomy. It has rarely been reported in both cats and dogs, and usually results in symptoms of UI in the weeks after surgery. It is generally due to a connection being established between the vaginal vault and one or both ureters when they are erroneously ligated in combination during the procedure (Allen & Webbon 1980; MacCoy et al. 1988; Day et al. 1993; Lamb 1994). Treatment of this condition necessitates surgery to reposition the ureteral opening(s) into the trigone of the bladder, usually by neoureterocystostomy.

Detrusor instability, sometimes also termed reflex dyssynergia, detrusor-urethral dyssynergia, or detrusor-striated sphincter dyssynergia, is a complex condition that is common in people, but remains poorly characterized in animals. It has been reported by several authors principally in dogs (Holt 1990a; Gookin & Bunch 1996; Diaz Espineira et al. 1998). Detrusor instability is a functional anomaly where contraction of the detrusor muscle and relaxation of the striated external urethral sphincter component do not occur in a coordinated fashion during the voiding phase of micturition, and is characterized by pollakiuria, urgency, and incontinence. It can be primary or occur secondary to other conditions such as UTI or bladder neoplasia (Holt 1990a). Two forms are generally recognized: excessive sympathetic tone leading to contraction of the smooth muscle (sympathetic dyssynergia) and excessive somatic innervation causing excessive striated external sphincter tone (somatic dyssynergia). The sympathetic form of the condition appears to be more common (Diaz Espineira *et al.* 1998). Diagnosis of this condition relies on concurrent measurements of bladder pressure and urine flow rates (Gookin & Bunch 1996). Clinically, animals have signs similar to partial or complete urethral obstruction that include passing small spurts of urine, followed by an inability to void, although UI can also be associated with the condition in some cases. Diagnosis requires the use of simultaneous cystometrographic and UPP and has been infrequently reported (Gookin & Bunch 1996).

Bladder, urethral, and vaginal mass lesions associated with inflammatory or neoplastic disease can be occasional causes of UI in dogs and this is presumably due to interference with the normal functioning of the urethral sphincter mechanism. In animals with primary bladder wall tumors, interference with function of the detrusor muscle may be the cause (Holt 1990a). One study found that 9% of dogs presenting for bladder or urethral neoplasia presented with UI (Norris *et al.* 1992). In these cases, treatment of the underlying lesion is critical, but can be challenging in many cases. Readers are referred to other sources for a more complete discussion of the management of lower urogenital tract neoplasia.

Animals with intersex presentations can also present with UI. A variety of combinations of intersex lesions exist and not all will result in UI. Incontinence may occur secondary to USMI or to the anatomical abnormalities presented. The most common intersex abnormality associated with UI is the male-like arrangement, where a vagina and uterine horns are present in a dog with male-appearing external genitalia. In these dogs the vagina may be continuous with the urethra, leading to retrograde vaginal filling and pooling during urination. Urine can then be passed out between urination episodes (Holt 1990a).

Pervious urachus occurs when the normal regression of the umbilical ligament fails to occur and a patent channel is retained through which urine can pass out at the umbilicus. This is a very rare anomaly and can be confirmed by contrast radiography. Simple treatment by excision of the urachal stalk will resolve the UI.

History, clinical signs, and physical examination

A careful clinical history can help to discern the various underlying causes for UI, although few findings are pathognomonic for one particular disease. Most dogs

and cats with congenital USMI will have a history of never having been continent as young puppies, and in many cases owners will not consider the clinical signs abnormal until the time they expect them to be housebroken. Most cases of USMI are, however, not congenital and UI appears within three years of neutering in approximately 75% of cases (Holt 1985a; Arnold *et al.* 1989). There is also a relationship between neutering and USMI in male dogs, with the majority of cases developing UI within a month of castration (Aaron *et al.* 1996). In cats with USMI, the incontinence has been described as "copious" and earlier in onset compared to cats with ureteral ectopia (Holt & Gibbs 1992). The most common clinical sign associated with canine ureteral ectopia is also intermittent or continuous UI since birth or since current ownership (Holt & Gibbs 1992; Stone & Mason 1990; McLaughlin & Miller 1991; Holt & Hotson-Moore 1995), although adult-onset UI can also occur. Stranguria secondary to an enlarged nonpatent ectopic ureter or concurrent UTIs has also been reported (Smith *et al.* 1980). Patients with USMI and EU will often retain the ability to urinate normally and might only experience incontinence during periods of increased intra-abdominal pressure, such as when they are recumbent, excited, or barking (Holt 1985a). Male dogs with EU may retain continence more readily than females, possibly due to the long length of their urethra offering greater resistance to urine outflow, or due to the possibility that urine may travel retrograde into the bladder because of the high resistance in the prostatic urethra (Steffey & Brockman 2004). Some patients with EU may only present with recurrent UTIs as a symptom and maintain their continence.

Dogs with detrusor instability may produce bursts of urine flow, but often have an inability to produce a continuous stream. Some may show signs of complete urethral obstruction and persistent severe stranguria. Incontinence can occur, but is not always documented in these cases (Gookin & Bunch 1996; Diaz Espineira *et al.* 1998).

On physical examination most dogs and cats presenting with UI will have evident staining around the vulva or prepuce and will lick frequently at the site. Many will have an obvious urine odor emanating from the area. Most patients with EU or USMI will have few other noticeable clinical signs. Animals with neurogenic incontinence may have other clinical signs referable to the neurologic system, such as paresis, paralysis, pain, or fecal incontinence. Dogs and cats with intersex abnormalities may have atypical external genitalia and those with a pervious urachus have urine emanating from the umbilicus and/or urine scalding and associated dermatitis at the site.

Diagnostic imaging

A multitude of imaging modalities have been used for the investigation of UI in dogs. Over the last 20 years an evolution has occurred in our knowledge of the capabilities of different modalities, resulting in newer modalities replacing older ones. In many cases, imaging modalities are now combined with therapeutic treatments such as cystoscopic-guided interventions, and these have revolutionized the treatment of some causes of UI.

Plain and contrast radiographic techniques

Plain radiography can provide some nonspecific information in the investigation of UI. A rough estimate of renal size can be obtained, along with the possible presence of any radiopaque uroliths. Bladder location may be confirmed, although if the bladder is empty and collapsed it may be more difficult to visualize clearly. Spinal/pelvic trauma can often be visualized on plain radiography.

A variety of contrast radiographic techniques have been used, principally for the diagnosis of anatomic urogenital tract defects. These include intravenous urography (IVU), positive or negative contrast cystography, and retrograde urethrography or vaginourethrography. IVU was the gold standard imaging modality for many years for diagnosis of EU (Alexander 1993); however, it has now been largely superseded by the use of intraoperative fluoroscopy and cystoscopy. When an IVU is performed, intravenous injection of a renally excreted iodine-based contrast media is used. Sequential radiographs are taken precontrast and at 5, 10, and 15 minutes postcontrast, or at 5-minute intervals until the distal ureters are opacified (Lamb & Gregory 1998; Mantis *et al.* 2008). Images can also be obtained via fluoroscopy during the IVU procedure (Samii *et al.* 2004).

Diagnosis of EU is usually based on the loss of the normal J-shaped turn that the distal ureters take prior to entering the bladder. Alteration of the J-shaped angle to a straight line is considered highly suggestive of EU by some, even when the exact site of termination is not seen (Mason *et al.* 1990). However, others have questioned the significance of this finding and have found that no association exists between the shape of the ureterovesicular junction and the surgical diagnosis of EU (Cannizzo *et al.* 2003). In this study only 32% of dogs received a double-contrast cystogram (Cannizzo *et al.* 2003). In many cases IVU is performed in combination with a negative contrast pneumocystogram, as this has been shown to better delineate the vesicoureteral junctions, which can be obscured by positive contrast that accumulates within the bladder (Mason *et al.* 1990). However, in another study IVU only diagnosed 12 of 17

dogs with ectopic ureters and the authors felt that concurrent use of cystograms was not helpful in these cases (Samii *et al.* 2004). There are several other disadvantages of IVU for the diagnosis of EU. It can be difficult to discern extramural from intramural passage of the EU and misdiagnosis of extramural EU that were found to be intramural at surgery occurred in 7 of 18 dogs in one study (Mason *et al.* 1990). There is often superimposition of pelvic bones over the area, which can obscure visualization, and in dogs with multiple ureteral openings urine can appear to flow into the bladder through proximal openings, leading to misdiagnosis of some intramural EUs with multiple openings. More recent studies have compared IVU to ultrasonography, cystography, and helical computed tomography (CT). Ultrasonography was found to give a more accurate determination of the site of ureteral termination in the bladder in cases with normal ureteral anatomy (Lamb & Gregory 1998).

Retrograde vaginourethrography is performed by placing a foley catheter into the vagina of female animals, securing it in place just caudal to the urethral orifice (Holt *et al.* 1982; Mantis *et al.* 2008). Retrograde urethrography is performed by placing a urinary catheter into the penile urethra of male patients and injecting a diluted iodinated contrast agent retrograde up the urethra (Mantis *et al.* 2008). An iodinated contrast agent is injected into the catheter. Retrograde studies can be used to diagnose EU and ureterovaginal fistulae, as well as some of the associated pathologies of USMI such as intrapelvic bladder location and short urethra (Leveille 1998). Vestibulovaginal stenosis may be diagnosed using retrograde vaginourethography. The theoretical advantage of a retrograde study is that when the bladder is filled up with contrast agent there should be a greater chance of shunting contrast up the EUs, thus better delineating the position of the ureterovesicular junctions. A number of studies have found the specificity of retrograde studies to be relatively low, however (Samii *et al.* 2004; Mantis *et al.* 2008), and EU was diagnosed in only 47% of dogs with the disease in one study using this modality (Samii *et al.* 2004). The authors found that unless hydroureter was present in dogs, retrograde filling of the ureter, required to diagnosis their ectopic nature, did not occur, leading to false-negative results (Samii *et al.* 2004).

Ultrasonography

Ultrasonographic evaluation of the urinary tract allows important evaluation of both the upper and lower urinary tracts. The kidneys should always be imaged for evidence of hydronephrosis, pyelonephritis, or other abnormalities. Ureteral distension secondary to EU can usually be detected ultrasonographically. Ultrasonography has been described as an excellent diagnostic imaging tool for diagnosis of ureteral ectopia, when performed by experienced operators. The ureterovesicular junctions are visualized as small convex structures on the dorsal aspect of the bladder mucosa (Douglass 1993; Lamb & Gregory 1998). They will be visible in most normal dogs, although in cases with completely intrapelvic bladders it may be impossible to image this area adequately (Lamb 1994). The hallmark ultrasonographic sign of ureteral ectopia is the absence of ureteral urine jets entering the bladder as a series of small echogenic foci streaming periodically from the ureterovesicular junction. This, in combination with visualization of the ureter passing caudal to the bladder trigone, confirms the diagnosis of EU (Lamb & Gregory 1998).

In a retrospective study comparing contrast radiographic methods to ultrasonography for the diagnosis of EU, ultrasound was found to have higher sensitivity, specificity, and accuracy compared to retrograde urethrography and retrograde urethrovaginography (Mantis et al. 2008). The results must be interpreted with caution, as ultrasonographic diagnosis is always heavily influenced by operator experience with the technique. It is also important to remember that dogs with multiple fenestrations may appear to have urine entering the bladder, despite more distal openings being present concurrently. The principal difficulty with ultrasonography for imaging of EU is determination of the side of the lesion, which can be challenging (Mantis et al. 2008). Dogs with USMI may have few ultrasonographic abnormalities, although a pelvic bladder may be detectable. Ureteroceles and space-occupying lesions of the upper and lower tracts should be visible ultrasonographically.

Cystoscopy

The use of cystoscopy has been increasingly reported for the diagnosis of many lower urinary tract abnormalities and is now considered a standard diagnostic test in the investigation of UI in many institutions. In female dogs cystoscopy is usually performed using a rigid sheathed 1.9 mm or 2.7 mm telescope (Canizzo et al. 2001; Berent 2016) in female dogs/cats, or a 2.7 mm flexible fiberoptic ureteroscope in male dogs (Berent et al. 2008). Sterile saline is used for irrigation through the side ports to maintain bladder and urethral distension. Guidewires, catheter, biopsy instruments, or laser fibers can be placed through the working channels of the sheath if interventions are to be performed concurrently (Canizzo et al. 2001, 2003; Samii et al. 2004; Berent et al. 2008, 2016). Rigid endoscopes offer superior image quality to their flexible counterparts, but in male dogs flexible uroendoscopes must be used for cystoscopy due to the

anatomy of the male urethra. Uroendoscopes with outer diameters from 2.5 to 3.1 mm can be used for male dogs weighing over 8 kg (Canizzo et al. 2001; Berent et al. 2008). In most cases instruments will not easily pass through the small working channel (3.2 Fr) of these small scopes (Canizzo et al. 2001). However, passage of a laser fiber during cystoscopic-guided laser ablation of male canine ectopic ureters has been reported using a 7.5 Fr (2.5 mm) flexible ureteroscope (Berent et al. 2008). Even smaller uroendoscopes are manufactured that can be used in female and even male cats (1.9 mm and 1 mm outer diameter, respectively) (Canizzo et al. 2001). However, as the diameter of these endoscopes decreases, so do the image quality and their durability.

A wide variety of urinary disorders can be diagnosed using cystourethroscopy and vestibulovaginoscopy and it gives a thorough evaluation of the entire lower urinary tract. Recent studies using cystoscopy for the diagnosis of EUs has revealed the high levels of concurrent lower urinary tract abnormalities that might be overlooked with traditional contrast radiography and ultrasound (Samii et al. 2004; Cannizzo et al. 2003). In addition, most authors believe that characterization of the ureterovesicular junction is better using cystoscopy and better recognition of anomalies such as ureteral troughs and multiple ureteral openings occurs (Samii et al. 2004; Cannizzo et al. 2003). Recently in one study cystoscopy was able to diagnose EUs in 24 of 25 dogs affected with the condition (Cannizzo et al. 2003). In another study cystoscopy had 100% sensitivity and 75% specificity in a population of 24 dogs suspected of having EU (Samii et al. 2004). Cystoscopy has also been used for diagnosis and treatment of associated disorders such as persistent paramesonephric remnants (Burdick et al. 2014), ureteroceles (Rogatko et al. 2019), and congenital distal ureteral orifice stenosis (Meler et al. 2018). The main drawbacks of cystoscopy are that only the lower urinary tract can be visualized and so another form of imaging such as ultrasonography, retrograde ureteropyelography (during cystoscopy), or IVU needs to be used in combination with this modality in cases where upper tract abnormalities are suspected.

Cystoscopy is currently considered the diagnostic procedure of choice in the authors' practice, as the opportunity exists for concurrent diagnosis and treatment of EUs during a single intervention (see the discussion of cystoscopic-guided laser ablation). This does require a high degree of technical skill and specialized equipment, but has gained much greater popularity in recent years and is available in many centers. Cystourethroscopy is also used to assess urethral length and bladder size, for the determination of short urethral syndrome or hypoplastic bladders. During a cystoscopy the vestibule and vagina should be routinely and carefully evaluated for a persistent paramesonephric remnant (seen in over 90% of dogs with EU in one study) (Cannizzo *et al.* 2003; Burdick *et al.* 2014), a vaginal septum/dual vagina, or a vestibulovaginal stenosis.

Computed tomography

Contrast-enhanced computed tomography (CECT) has recently been reported for imaging the lower urinary tract of dogs (Barthez *et al.* 1998; Rozear & Tidwell 2003; Cannizzo *et al.* 2003; Berent *et al.* 2008; Fox *et al.* 2016; Schwarz *et al.* 2021). The advantages of CECT for diagnosis of EU include the fact that the course of each ureter can be traced individually without superimposition of structures, as is seen with other contrast radiographic techniques. Additionally, good information on the morphology of the upper urinary tract can be gleaned (Samii *et al.* 2004). Several recent studies have evaluated CECT specifically for the diagnosis of EU in dogs (Samii *et al.* 2004; Fox *et al.* 2016). A correct diagnosis of EU was possible in 16 of 17 and 10 of 10 dogs in these studies (Samii *et al.* 2004; Fox *et al.* 2016). The authors suggested that advantages of CECT include the fact that it is a more rapid imaging study compared to some other techniques and that it is largely operator independent, thus removing some of the experience-related variability in results obtained with techniques such as ultrasonography and cystoscopy (Samii *et al.* 2004). Clear differentiation of intramural versus extramural location is also possible with CECT. This should be done with concurrent pneumocystography. More recently, a slight advantage of four-dimensional CECT over traditional CECT has been demonstrated (Schwarz *et al.* 2021).

Urethral pressure profilometry

The urethral pressure profile gives a graphic representation of the pressure within the urethra during the resting phase. A variety of methods have been used to measure the UPP, including perfusion and microtransducer methods (Gregory 1994; Gookin *et al.* 1996). Standard measurements include the MUP, which is the highest pressure within the urethral profile; the MUCP, which is the difference between the MUP and the intravesicular pressure; and the functional profile length (FPL), which is the length of the urethra over which the urethral pressure exceeds the intravesicular pressure.

UPP can be a very useful diagnostic tool in the evaluation of a variety of causes of UI in dogs and has also been investigated in cats (Gregory & Willits 1986; Frenier *et al.* 1992). It is particularly helpful in the diagnosis of USMI. Multiple studies have shown that urethral tone is reduced in incontinent male and female dogs with USMI compared to their continent counterparts (Richter & Ling 1985; Holt 1988). In a large population of continent and incontinent female dogs, Holt found that the incontinent population had significantly lower MUCP compared to the continent dogs. In addition to these findings, UPPs have also been used to assess response to various medical and surgical treatments for incontinent patients. The therapeutic benefit of the α-adrenergic drug phenylpropanolamine was demonstrated in both male and female dogs using UPPs in one study (Richter & Ling 1985). In this study MUCPs were shown to be significantly lower than normal in incontinent dogs pretreatment, but returned to within the normal range posttreatment. Clinically, most animals showed a clinical improvement that mirrored the improvement in MUCP (Richter & Ling 1985). The therapeutic effect of colposuspension has also been evaluated using UPP, with somewhat conflicting results (Gregory & Holt 1994; Rawlings *et al.* 2000). One study (Gregory & Holt 1994) demonstrated increases in MUCP and FPL postoperatively, whereas another demonstrated decreases in MUCP but increases in leak point pressures (Rawlings *et al.* 2000). The authors hypothesized that these somewhat conflicting results may have been due to differences in UPP technique as well as anesthetic protocols (Rawlings *et al.* 2000).

The use of UPP has not, however, gained widespread clinical use due to the technical difficulty in obtaining repeatable results between patients. There are many different extrinsic factors that can affect the results (Gregory & Holt 1994; Gookin *et al.* 1996), including differing sedation and technique protocols. Generally it is considered that due to this inherent variability, investigators need to establish standardized techniques and reference ranges for their own laboratories in order to use this technique for assessment of clinical cases (Gookin *et al.* 1996).

References

Aaron, A., Eggleton, K., Power, C. et al. (1996). Urethral sphincter mechanism incompetence in male dogs: a retrospective analysis of 54 cases. *Veterinary Record* 139: 542–546.

Adams, W.M. and DiBartola, S.P. (1983). Radiographic and clinical features of pelvic bladder in the dog. *Journal of the American Veterinary Medical Association* 182: 1212–1217.

Albers, P., Foster, R.S., Bihrle, R. et al. (1995). Ectopic ureters and ureteroceles in adults. *Urology* 45: 870–875.

Alexander, L.G. (1993). Ectopic ureter and ureterocele. In: *Disease Mechanisms in Small Animal Surgery*, 2e (ed. M.J. Bojrab), 515–519. Philadelphia, PA: Lippincott Williams & Wilkins.

Allen, W.E. and Webbon, P.M. (1980). Two cases of urinary incontinence associated with acquired vagino-ureteral fistula. *Journal of Small Animal Practice* 21: 367–371.

Angioletti, A., De Francesco, I., Vergottini, M. et al. (2004). Urinary incontinence after spaying in the bitch: incidence and oestrogen therapy. *Veterinary Research Communications* 28: 153–155.

Arnold, S., Arnold, P., Hubler, M. et al. (1989). Urinary incontinence in spayed bitches: prevalence and breed predisposition. *Schweizer Archiv für Tierheilkunde* 131: 259–263.

Awad, S.A. and Downie, J.W. (1976). Relative contributions of smooth and striated muscles to the canine urethral pressure profile. *British Journal of Urology* 48: 347–354.

Barth, A., Reichler, I.M., Hubler, M. et al. (2005). Evaluation of long-term effects of endoscopic injection of collagen into the urethral submucosa for treatment of urethral sphincter incompetence in female dogs: 40 cases (1993-2000). *Journal of the American Veterinary Medical Association* 226: 73–76.

Barthez, P.Y., Begon, D., and Delisle, F. (1998). Effect of contrast medium dose and image acquisition timing on ureteral opacification in the normal dog as assessed by computed tomography. *Veterinary Radiology & Ultrasound* 39: 524–527.

Basinger, R.R., Rawlings, C.A., Barsanti, J.A. et al. (1989). Urodynamic alterations associated with clinical prostatic diseases and prostatic surgery in 23 dogs. *Journal of the American Animal Hospital Association* 25: 385–392.

Beauvais, W., Cardwell, J.M., and Brodbelt, D.C. (2012). The effect of neutering on the risk or urinary incontinence in bitches – a systematic review. *Journal of Small Animal Practice* 53: 198–204.

Bennett, T.C., Matz, B.M., Henderson, R.A. et al. (2018). Total prostatectomy as a treatment for prostatic carcinoma in 25 dogs. *Veterinary Surgery* 47: 367–377.

Berent, A.C. (2016). Advances in urinary tract endoscopy. *Veterinary Clinics of North America. Small Animal Practice* 46: 113–135.

Berent, A.C., Mayhew, P.D., and Porat-Mosenco, Y. (2008). Use of cystoscopic-guided laser ablation for treatment of intramural ureteral ectopia in male dogs: four cases (2006-7). *Journal of the American Veterinary Medical Association* 232: 1026–1034.

Berent, A.C., Weisse, C., Mayhew, P.D. et al. (2012). Evaluation of cystoscopic-guided laser ablation of intramural ectopic ureters in female dogs. *Journal of the American Veterinary Medical Association* 240: 716–725.

Berry, S.J., Coffey, D.S., and Ewing, L.L. (1986). Effects of aging on prostate growth in beagles. *American Journal of Physiology* 250: R1039–R1046.

Burdick, S., Berent, A.C., Weisse, C. et al. (2014). Endoscopic-guided laser ablation of vestibulovaginal septal remnants in dogs: 36 cases (2007≠2011). *Journal of the American Veterinary Medical Association* 244: 944–949.

Byron, J.K., Taylor, K.H., Phillips, G.S. et al. (2017). Urethral sphincter mechanism incompetence in 163 neutered female dogs: diagnosis, treatment, and relationship of weight and age at neuter to development of disease. *Journal of Veterinary Internal Medicine* 31: 442–448.

Canizzo, K.L., McLoughlin, M.A., Chew, D.J. et al. (2001). Uroendoscopy. *Veterinary Clinics of North America. Small Animal Practice* 31: 789–807.

Cannizzo, K.L., McLoughlin, M.A., Mattoon, J.S. et al. (2003). Evaluation of transurethral cystoscopy and excretory urography for diagnosis of ectopic ureters in female dogs: 25 cases (1992–2000). *Journal of the American Veterinary Medical Association* 223: 475–481.

Cass, A.S. and Hinman, F. (1968). Constant urethral flow in female dog. I. Normal vesical and urethral pressures and effect of muscle relaxant. *Journal of Urology* 99: 442–446.

Concannon, P.W. (1993). Biology of gonadotrophin secretion in adult and prepubertal female dogs. *Journal of Reproduction and Fertility* 47 (Suppl): 3–27.

Corriveau, K.M., Giuffrida, M.A., Mayhew, P.D. et al. (2017). Outcome of laparoscopic ovariectomy and laparoscopic-assisted ovario-hysterectomy in dogs: 278 cases (2003–2013). *Journal of the American Veterinary Medical Association* 251: 443–450.

Creed, K.E. (1983). Effect of hormones on urethral sensitivity to phenylephrine in normal and incontinent dogs. *Research in Veterinary Science* 34: 177–181.

Cullen, W.C., Fletcher, T.F., and Bradley, W.E. (1981). Histology of the canine urethra II. Morphometry of the male pelvic urethra. *Anatomical Record* 199: 187–195.

Cullen, W.C., Fletcher, T.F., and Bradley, W.E. (1983a). Morphometry of the female feline urethra. *Journal of Urology* 129: 190–192.

Cullen, W.C., Fletcher, T.F., and Bradley, W.E. (1983b). Morphometry of the male feline pelvic urethra. *Journal of Urology* 129: 186–189.

Day, D.G., Bailey, M.Q., Evans, K.L. et al. (1993). Postoperative evaluation of renal function after surgical correction of a uretero-vaginal fistula in a cat. *Journal of the American Veterinary Medical Association* 202: 104–106.

Diaz Espineira, M.M., Viehoff, F.W., and Nickel, R.F. (1998). Idiopathic detrusor-urethral dyssynergia in dogs: a retrospective analysis of 22 cases. *Journal of Small Animal Practice* 39: 264–270.

Douglass, J.P. (1993). Bladder wall mass effect caused by the intramural portion of the canine ureter. *Veterinary Radiology & Ultrasound* 34: 107.

Dyce, K.M., Sack, W.O., and Wensing, C.J.G. (2002). The pelvis and reproductive organs of the carnivores. In: *Textbook of Veterinary Anatomy*, 3e (ed. K.M. Dyce, W.O. Sack and C.J.C. Wensing), 435–453. Philadelphia, PA: WB Saunders.

Eisele, J.G., Jackson, J., and Hager, D. (2005). Ectopic ureterocele in a cat. *Journal of the American Animal Hospital Association* 41: 332–335.

Evans, H.E. and Christensen, G.C. (1993). The urogenital system. In: *Miller's Anatomy of the Dog*, 3e (ed. H.E. Evans), 494–559. Philadelphia, PA: WB Saunders.

Forsee, K.M., Davis, G.J., Mouat, E.E. et al. (2013). Evaluation of the prevalence of urinary incontinence in spayed female dogs: 566 cases (2003–2008). *Journal of the American Veterinary Medical Association* 14: 959–962.

Fox, A.J., Sharma, A., and Secrest, S.A. (2016). Computed tomographic excretory urography features of intramural ectopic ureters in 10 dogs. *Journal of Small Animal Practice* 57: 210–213.

Frenier, S.L., Knowlen, G.G., Speth, R.C. et al. (1992). Urethral pressure response to a-adrenergic agonist and antagonist drugs in anesthetized healthy male cats. *American Journal of Veterinary Research* 53: 1161–1165.

Ghantous, S.N. and Crawford, J. (2006). Double ureters with ureteral ectopia in a domestic short-haired cat. *Journal of the American Animal Hospital Association* 42: 462–466.

Gookin, J.L. and Bunch, S.E. (1996). Detrusor-striated sphincter dyssynergia in a dog. *Journal of Veterinary Internal Medicine* 10: 339–344.

Gookin, J.L., Stone, E.A., and Sharp, N.J. (1996). Urinary incontinence in dogs and cats. Part I. Urethral pressure profilometry. *Compendium on Continuing Education for the Practicing Veterinarian* 18: 407–417.

Gregory, C.R. (1984). Electromyographic and urethral pressure profilometry: clinical application in male cats. *Veterinary Clinics of North America. Small Animal Practice* 14: 567–574.

Gregory, C.R. (1994). Developments in the understanding of the pathophysiology of urethral sphincter mechanism incompetence in the bitch. *British Veterinary Journal* 150: 135–150.

Gregory, S.P. and Holt, P.E. (1994). The immediate effect of colposuspension on resting and stressed urethral pressure profiles in anesthetized incontinent bitches. *Veterinary Surgery* 23: 330–340.

Gregory, C.R. and Willits, N.H. (1986). Electromyographic and urethral pressure evaluations: assessment of urethral function in female and ovariohysterectomized female cats. *American Journal of Veterinary Research* 47: 1472–1475.

Gregory, S.P., Holt, P.E., Parkinson, T.J. et al. (1999). Vaginal position and length in the bitch: relationship to spaying and urinarty incontinence. *Journal of Small Animal Practice* 40: 180–184.

Hardie, E.M., Stone, E.A., Spaulding, K.A. et al. (1990). Subtotal canine prostatectomy with the neodymium:yttrium-aluminum-garnet laser. *Veterinary Surgery* 19: 348–355.

Hayes, H.M.J. (1984). Breed associations of canine ectopic ureter: a study of 217 female cases. *Journal of Small Animal Practice* 25: 501–504.

Holt, P.E. (1985a). Urinary incontinence in the bitch due to sphincter mechanism incompetence: prevalence in referred dogs and retrospective analysis of sixty cases. *Journal of Small Animal Practice* 26: 181–190.

Holt, P.E. (1985b). Urinary incontinence in the bitch due to sphincter mechanism incompetence: surgical treatment. *Journal of Small Animal Practice* 26: 237–246.

Holt, P.E. (1985c). Importance of urethral length, bladder neck position and vestibulovaginal stenosis in sphincter mechanism incompetence in the incontinent bitch. *Research in Veterinary Science* 39: 364–372.

Holt, P.E. (1988). "Simultaneous" urethral pressure profilometry: comparisons between continent and incontinent bitches. *Journal of Small Animal Practice* 29: 761–769.

Holt, P.E. (1990a). Urinary incontinence in dogs and cats. *Veterinary Record* 127: 347–350.

Holt, P.E. (1990b). Long-term evaluation of colposuspension in the treatment of urinary incontinence due to incompetence of the urethral sphincter mechanism in the bitch. *Veterinary Record* 127: 537–542.

Holt, P.E. (1993). Surgical management of congenital urethral sphincter mechanism incompetence in eight female cats and a bitch. *Veterinary Surgery* 22: 98–104.

Holt, P.E. and Gibbs, C. (1992). Congenital urinary incontinence in cats: a review of 19 cases. *Veterinary Record* 130: 437–442.

Holt, P.E. and Hotson-Moore, A. (1995). Canine ureteral ectopia: an analysis of 175 cases and comparison of surgical treatments. *Veterinary Record* 136: 345–349.

Holt, P.E. and Thrusfield, M.V. (1993). Association in bitches between breed, size, neutering and docking, and acquired urinary incontinence due to incompetence of the urethral sphincter mechanism. *Veterinary Record* 133: 177–180.

Holt, P.E., Gibbs, C., and Pearson, H. (1982). Canine ectopic ureter – a review of twenty-nine cases. *Journal of Small Animal Practice* 23: 195–208.

Holt, P.E., Coe, R.J., and Hotson Moore, A. (2005). Prostatopexy as a treatment for urethral sphincter mechanism incompetence in male dogs. *Journal of Small Animal Practice* 46: 567–570.

Koie, H., Yamaya, Y., and Sakai, T. (2000). Four cases of lowered urethral pressure in canine ectopic ureter. *Journal of Veterinary Medical Science* 62: 1221–1222.

Lamb, C.R. (1994). Acquired ureterovaginal fistula secondary to ovariohysterectomy in a dog: diagnosis using ultrasound-guided nephropyelocentesis and antegrade ureterography. *Veterinary Radiology and Ultrasound* 35: 201–203.

Lamb, C.R. and Gregory, S.P. (1998). Ultrasonographic findings in 14 dogs with ectopic ureter. *Veterinary Radiology & Ultrasound* 39: 218–223.

Lane, I.F. and Lappin, M.R. (1995). Urinary incontinence and congenital urogenital anomalies in small animals. In: *Current Veterinary Therapy XII* (ed. J. Bonagura and R.W. Kirk), 1022–1026. Philadelphia, PA: WB Saunders.

Lane, I.F., Lappin, M.R., and Seim, H.B. (1995). Evaluation of results of preoperative urodynamic measurements in nine dogs with ectopic ureters. *Journal of the American Veterinary Medical Association* 206: 1348–1357.

Lapish, J.P. (1985). Hydronephrosis, hydroureter, and hydrometra associated with ectopic ureter in a bitch. *Journal of Small Animal Practice* 26: 613–617.

Lautzenhiser, S.J. and Bjorling, D.E. (2002). Urinary incontinence in a dog with an ectopic ureterocele. *Journal of the American Animal Hospital Association* 38: 29–32.

Léveillé, R. (1998). Ultrasonography of urinary bladder disorders. Veterinary Clinics of North America. *Small Anim Practice* 28: 799–821.

Lonc, K.M., Kaneene, J.B., Carneiro, P.A.M. et al. (2020). Retrospective analysis of diagnoses and outcomes of 45 cats with micturition disorders presenting as urinary incontinence. *Journal of Veterinary Internal Medicine* 34: 216–226.

Lose, G. (2001). Urethral pressure measurement: problems and clinical value. *Scandinavian Journal of Urology and Nephrology. Supplementum* 207: 61–66.

MacCoy, M.D., Ogilvie, G., Burke, T. et al. (1988). Post-ovariohysterectomy ureterovaginal fistula in a dog. *Journal of the American Animal Hospital Association* 24: 469–471.

Mahaffey, M.B., Barsanti, J.A., Barber, D.L. et al. (1984). Pelvic bladder in dogs without urinary incontinence. *Journal of the American Veterinary Medical Association* 184: 1477–1479.

Mandigers, P.J.J. and Nell, T. (2001). Treatment of bitches with acquired urinary incontinence with oestriol. *Veterinary Record* 149: 764–767.

Mantis, P., Brockman, D., Whatmough, C. et al. (2008). Sensitivity, specificity and accuracy of diagnostic imaging methods for the diagnosis of ectopic ureters in the dog. *European Journal of Companion Animal Practice* 18: 21–27.

Mason, L.K., Stone, E.A., Biery, D.N. et al. (1990). Surgery of ectopic ureters: pre- and postoperative radiographic morphology. *Journal of the American Animal Hospital Association* 26: 73–79.

Massat, B.J., Gregory, C.R., Ling, G.V. et al. (1993). Cystourethropexy to correct refractory urinary incontinence due to urethral sphincter mechanism incompetence. *Veterinary Surgery* 22: 260–269.

Mayhew, P.D., Lee, K.C.L., Gregory, S.P. et al. (2006). Comparison of two surgical techniques for management of intramural ureteral ectopia in dogs: 36 cases (1994-2004). *Journal of the American Veterinary Medical Association* 229: 389–393.

McLaughlin, R. and Miller, C.W. (1991). Urinary incontinence after surgical repair of ureteral ectopia in dogs. *Veterinary Surgery* 20: 100–103.

McLoughlin, M.A. and Chew, D.J. (2000). Diagnosis and surgical management of ectopic ureters. *Clinical Techniques in Small Animal Practice* 15: 17–24.

McLoughlin, M.A., Hauptman, J.G., and Spaulding, K. (1989). Canine ureteroceles: a case report and literature review. *Journal of the American Animal Hospital Association* 25: 699–706.

Meler, E., Berent, A.C., Weisse, C. et al. (2018). Treatment of congenital distal ureteral orifice stenosis by endoscopic laser ablation in dogs: 16 cases (2010-2014). *Journal of the American Veterinary Medical Association* 253: 452–462.

Miodrag, A., Castleden, C.M., and Vallance, T.R. (1988). Sex hormones and the female urinary tract. *Drugs* 36: 491–504.

Mouatt, J.G. and Watt, P.R. (2001). Ectopic ureter repair and colposuspension in seven bitches. *Australian Veterinary Practitioner* 31 (4): 160–167.

Muir, P., Goldsmid, S.E., and Bellenger, C.R. (1994). Management of urinary incontinence in five bitches with incompetence of the urethral sphincter mechanism by colposuspension and a modified sling urethroplasty. *Veterinary Record* 134: 38–41.

Noel, S.M., Claeys, S., and Hamaide, A.J. (2017). Surgical management of ectopic ureters in dogs: clinical outcome and prognostic factors for long-term continence. *Veterinary Surgery* 46: 631–641.

Norris, A.M., Laing, E.J., Valli, V.E. et al. (1992). Canine bladder and urethral tumors: a retrospective study of 115 cases (1980-1985). *Journal of Veterinary Internal Medicine* 6: 145–153.

O'Handley, P., Carrig, C.B., and Walshaw, R. (1979). Renal and ureteral duplication in a dog. *Journal of the American Veterinary Medical Association* 174: 484–487.

Okkens, A.C., Kooistra, H.S., and Nickel, R.F. (1997). Comparison of long-term effects of ovariectomy versus ovariohysterectomy in bitches. *Journal of Reproduction and Fertility* 51 (Suppl): 227–231.

Olson, P.N., Mulnix, J.A., and Nett, T.M. (1992). Concentrations of luteinizing hormone and follicle-stimulating hormone in the serum of sexually intact and neutered dogs. *American Journal of Veterinary Research* 53: 762–766.

Owen, R.R. (1973a). Canine ureteral ectopia – a review. 1. Embryology and aetiology. *Journal of Small Animal Practice* 14: 407–417.

Owen, R.R. (1973b). Canine ureteral ectopia – a review. 2. Incidence, diagnosis and treatment. *Journal of Small Animal Practice* 14: 419–427.

Power, S.C., Eggleton, K.E., Aaron, A.J. et al. (1998). Urethral sphincter mechanism incompetence in the male dog: importance of bladder neck position, proximal urethral length and castration. *Journal of Small Animal Practice* 39: 69–72.

Rawlings, C.A., Mahaffey, M.B., Chernosky, A. et al. (2000). Immediate urodynamic and anatomic response to colposuspension in female beagles. *American Journal of Veterinary Research* 61: 1353–1357.

Rawlings, C.A., Barsanti, J.A., Mahaffey, M.B. et al. (2001). Evaluation of colposuspension for treatment of incontinence in spayed female dogs. *Journal of the American Veterinary Medical Association* 219: 770–775.

Reichler, I.M., Pfeiffer, E., Piche, A. et al. (2004). Changes in plasma gonadotropin concentrations and urethral closure pressure in the bitch during the 12 months following ovariectomy. *Theriogenology* 62: 1391–1402.

Reichler, I.M., Jochle, W., Piche, C.A. et al. (2006). Effect of a long acting GnRH analogue or placebo on plasma LH/FSH, urethral pressure profiles and clinical signs of urinary incontinence due to sphincter mechanism incontinence in bitches. *Theriogenology* 66: 1227–1236.

Richter, K.P. and Ling, G.V. (1985). Clinical response and urethral pressure profile changes after phenylpropanolamine in dogs with primary sphincter incompetence. *Journal of the American Veterinary Medical Association* 187: 605–611.

Rogatko, C.P., Berent, A.C., Adams, L.G. et al. (2019). Endoscopic laser-ablation for the treatment of orthotopic and ectopic ureteroceles in dogs: 13 cases (2008–2017). *Journal of Veterinary Internal Medicine* 33: 670–679.

Rosin, A.H. and Barsanti, J.A. (1981). Diagnosis of urinary incontinence in dogs: role of the urethral pressure profile. *Journal of the American Veterinary Medical Association* 187: 605–611.

Rosin, A.H. and Ross, L. (1981). Diagnosis and pharmacological management of disorders of urinary incontinence in the dog. *Compendium on Continuing Education for the Practicing Veterinarian* 3: 601–610.

Rozear, L.M. and Tidwell, A.S. (2003). Evaluation of the ureter and ureterovesicular junction using helical computed tomographic excretory urography in healthy dogs. *Veterinary Radiology & Ultrasound* 44: 155–164.

Samii, V.F., McLoughlin, M.A., Mattoon, J.S. et al. (2004). Digital fluoroscopic excretory urography, digital fluoroscopic urethrography, helical computed tomography, and cystoscopy in 24 dogs with suspected ureteral ectopia. *Journal of Veterinary Internal Medicine* 18: 271–281.

Schwarz, T., Bommer, N., Parys, M. et al. (2021). Four-dimensional CT excretory urography is an accurate technique for diagnosis of canine ureteral ectopia. *Veterinary Radiology & Ultrasound* 62: 190–198.

Scott, L., Leedy, M., Bernay, F. et al. (2002). Evaluation of phenylpropanolamine in the treatment of urethral sphincter mechanism incompetence in the bitch. *Journal of Small Animal Practice* 43: 493–496.

Sharp, N.J.H. and Wheeler, S.J. (2005) Postoperative care. In: *Small Animal Spinal Disorders*, 2e (ed. S. NJH and S.J. Wheeler), 339–362. Philadelphia, PA: Elsevier Mosby.

Singer, A. (1959). Surgical correction of congenital incontinence in a pup – a case report. *Journal of the American Veterinary Medical Association* 134: 646.

Smith, C.W., Stowater, J.L., and Knellex, S.K. (1980). Bilateral ectopic ureter in a male dog with urinary incontinence. *Journal of the American Veterinary Medical Association* 177: 1022–1024.

Steffey, M.A. and Brockman, D.J. (2004). Congenital ectopic ureters in a continent male dog and cat. *Journal of the American Veterinary Medical Association* 224: 1607–1610.

Stolzenburg, J.U., Dorschnera, W., Postenjak, M. et al. (2002). Sphincteric musculature of female canine urethra in comparison to woman including 3D reconstruction. *Cells, Tissues, Organs* 170: 151–161.

Stolzenburg, J.U., Neuhaus, J., Liatsikos, E.N. et al. (2006). Histomorphology of canine urethral sphincter systems, including three-dimensional reconstruction and magnetic resonance imaging. *Urology* 67: 624–630.

Stone, E., A. and Mason, L.K. (1990). Surgery of ectopic ureters: types, method of correction and post-operative results. *Journal of the American Animal Hospital Association* 26: 81–88.

Sutherland-Smith, J., Jerram, R.M., Walker, A.M. et al. (2004). Ectopic ureters and ureteroceles in dogs; presentation, cause and diagnosis. *Compendium on Continuing Education for the Practicing Veterinarian* 26: 303–310.

Tattershall, J.A. and Welsh, E. (2006). Ectopic ureterocele in a male dog: a case report and review of the surgical management. *Journal of the American Animal Hospital Association* 42: 395–400.

Thrusfield, M.V. (1985). Association between urinary incontinence and spaying in bitches. *Veterinary Record* 116: 695.

Thrusfield, M.V., Holt, P.E., and Muirhead, R.H. (1998). Acquired urinary incontinence in bitches: its incidence and relationship to neutering practices. *Journal of Small Animal Practice* 39: 559–566.

Van Goethem, B., Schaeffers-Okkens, A., and Kirpensteijn, J. (2006). Making a rational choice between ovariectomy and ovariohysterectomy in the dog: a discussion of the benefits of either technique. *Veterinary Surgery* 35: 136–143.

Weber, U.T., Arnold, A., Hubler, M. et al. (1997). Surgical treatment of male dogs with urinary incontinence due to urethral sphincter mechanism incompetence. *Veterinary Surgery* 26: 51–56.

White, R.N. (2001). Urethropexy for the management of urethral sphincter mechanism incompetence in the bitch. *Journal of Small Animal Practice* 42: 481–486.

White, R.A.S. and Pomeroy, C.J. (1989). Phenylpropanolamine: an a-adrenergic agent for the management of urinary incontinence in the bitch associated with urethral sphincter mechanism incompetence. *Veterinary Record* 125: 478–480.

White, R.A.S. and Williams, J.M. (1995). Intracapsular prostatic omentalization: a new technique for management of prostatic abscesses in dogs. *Veterinary Surgery* 24: 390–395.

46

Treatment Strategies for Urethral Sphincter Mechanism Incompetence

Philipp D. Mayhew and Allyson Berent

Medical management

A large proportion of urethral sphincter mechanism incompetence (USMI) patients will respond to medical management and many dogs with ureteral ectopia complicated by USMI may require adjunctive medical management to become continent after ectopic ureteral repair.

The most frequently used class of drugs is the α-adrenergic agents, including phenylpropanolamine (PPA) (1.5 mg/kg orally [p.o.] every [q] 8 h) and pseudoephedrine (0.2–0.4 mg/kg p.o. q 8–12 h) (Lane & Westropp 2009). These drugs increase urethral tone by stimulating urethral smooth muscle. Urodynamic studies have shown that phenylpropanolamine increases maximal urethral pressure and maximal urethral closure pressure (Richter & Ling 1985). Clinical reports have demonstrated their effectiveness *in vivo*, with response rates in female incontinent dogs of 70–90% (Richter & Ling 1985; White & Pomeroy 1989; Scott *et al.* 2002). Occasional reports document that some dogs can become refractory to PPA over time (White & Pomeroy 1989; Bacon *et al.* 2002). A sustained-release formula of PPA that is combined with diphenylpyraline hydrochloride has been described for treatment of female dogs that either lacked response or became refractory to the traditional immediate-release preparation of oral PPA (Bacon *et al.* 2002). Of 11 dogs treated with this preparation, 6 were continent at follow-up (Bacon *et al.* 2002). Possible side effects of PPA include anxiety, restlessness, tachycardia, and hypertension, but these are rarely serious. Response to PPA in male dogs appears to be less predictable. In one study only 5 of 16 (31%) male dogs were continent after treatment, with 2 further dogs showing some improvement (Aaron *et al.* 1996). Another study reported that 7 of 8 male dogs became continent after PPA therapy (Richter & Ling 1985). Little information exists on the effectiveness of PPA in feline USMI (Barsanti & Downey 1984).

Estrogen therapy has also been investigated as a treatment for USMI due the known association between spaying (and therefore loss of endogenous estrogen production) and USMI. Estrogens are known to upregulate both the expression and sensitivity of α-adrenergic receptors (Creed 1983; Miodrag *et al.* 1988). A synergistic effect between estrogens and α-adrenergic agents may exist due to this mechanism of action and this can allow dose reductions over time (Lane & Westropp 2009). Several estrogen preparations have been used, including diethylstilbestrol (0.1–1 mg/dog p.o. q24h for 5–7 days, then weekly as needed), stilbestrol (0.04–0.06 mg/dog p.o. q 24h for 7 days, reduced weekly to 0.01–0.02 mg/dog/day), and estriol (0.5–1 mg/dog p.o. q24h for 5–7 days, then q2–3 days as needed). Estrogen therapy has received mixed reviews in the literature as to its efficacy, with some studies suggesting a poor response to therapy (Adams & DiBartola 1983; Holt 1985), while others suggest that correctly tailored therapy might yield very favorable responses (Angioletti *et al.* 2004). Care must be taken in interpretation of these results that analyze responses in very different study populations. The most comprehensive study of 129 female dogs that were newly diagnosed with urinary incontinence showed a 61% continence rate at 42 days post treatment, with a further 22% showing improvement

Small Animal Soft Tissue Surgery, Second Edition. Edited by Eric Monnet.
© 2023 John Wiley & Sons, Inc. Published 2023 by John Wiley & Sons, Inc.
Companion website: www.wiley.com/go/monnet/small

(Mandigers & Nell 2001). Side effects seen in this study included swollen vulva, swollen teats, and/or attractiveness to males in 12/129 cases, although these effects were short term in all but one dog. Other potential side effects of estrogen therapy include bone marrow suppression, although this appears to be an uncommon problem when appropriate dosing regimens are followed (Mandigers & Nell. 2001; Lane & Westropp 2009). Overall it is considered that α-adrenergic agents are more effective in the treatment of USMI in female dogs compared to estrogens. Male dogs generally have a poor response to treatment with estrogens; none of eight dogs treated in one study became continent (Aaron *et al.* 1996) and their use in males is generally discouraged (Lane & Westropp 2009). The use of testosterone in male dogs has also been tried, with uniformly poor results (Aaron *et al.* 1996), though the use of methyltestosterone (0.5 mg/kg p.o. per day) or testosterone cypionate (2.2 mg/kg intramuscularly [i.m.] q30 days) has been used with some success (A. Berent, personal communication). Little information is available concerning the use of estrogens in cats, although their use has been discouraged by some authors (Lane & Westropp 2009).

Recently the use of GnRH analogs (leuprolide acetate) for the treatment of USMI in female spayed dogs has been reported (Reichler *et al.* 2006a,b). It was hypothesized that the rapid rise in plasma follicle-stimulating hormone (FSH) and luteinizing hormone (LH) that occurs after spaying may be involved in the pathogenesis of USMI in female dogs. It was shown that leuprolide acetate therapy resulted in a significant decrease in FSH and LH levels after treatment; however, this change did not correlate with changes in the urethral pressure profile (UPP) that would have suggested a direct link between GnRH treatment and urethral tone (Reichler *et al.* 2006a; Barth *et al.* 2005). Nevertheless, significant response to therapy was noted with leuprolide acetate, with dogs demonstrating a 71% decrease in episodes of incontinence. Efficacy was not as great as for PPA, which was administered at the start of the trial and resulted in a 91% decrease in incontinent episodes (Reichler *et al.* 2006b). In the absence of evidence for a GnRH direct effect on urethral tone, the authors hypothesized that the effect may be mediated through an increased fluid-holding capacity of the bladder, which was shown to be increased by cystometric studies (Reichler *et al.* 2006a; Barth *et al.* 2005).

Medical management for detrusor instability/detrusor dyssynergia can be challenging, as the underlying abnormalities are not always the same between cases. Detrusor hyperactivity should be carefully distinguished from reflex dyssynergia, as one is of excessive elimination and one is typically of urine retention.

If incontinence occurs with an empty bladder, it is typically due to abnormal detrusor contractions during the storage phase, and so anticholinergic drugs have been proposed to treat this. Oxybutynin (0.5–1.25 mg total dose for small dogs and cats, 2.5–3.75 mg total dose for larger dogs) is the most commonly used drug and can be used in combination with α-adrenergic agents (Lane & Westropp 2009). If signs mimic functional obstruction, more typical of reflex dyssynergia, and if physical obstruction has been ruled out, sympathetic or somatic dyssynergia may be present (Gookin & Bunch 1996; Diaz Espineira *et al.* 1998). In these cases specific drug therapy to reduce smooth muscle tone (prazosin, phenoxybenzamine) or striated external sphincter tone (dantrolene, diazepam) should be attempted. One should never use an α-adrenergic agonist in cases where stranguria and urine retention are present. If it is clinically indistinguishable which part of the sphincter is most affected, it is usually recommended to start a therapeutic trial of a sympatholytic drug first (Diaz Espineira *et al.* 1998).

Surgical management

A variety of surgical procedures have been described for treatment of USMI in dogs when medical treatment failures occur. Currently a variety of "open" surgical options exist for the treatment of USMI in male and female dogs and female cats, as well as the minimally invasive option of submucosal collagen injection, which aims to increase resistance to urine outflow. Open surgical options are primarily aimed at either (i) relocating the bladder neck and proximal urethra into the abdomen to expose the bladder neck and proximal urethra to increases in intraabdominal pressure; or (ii) to increase the resistance to urine outflow in the urethra by direct pressure or constriction. In male dogs a higher proportion of USMI cases may require surgery due to the documented poor response to medical management in this sex (Aaron *et al.* 1996). In cats, due to the different pathophysiology and anatomy of USMI, different techniques are applicable. In this species only one surgical technique has been reported in greater than single-case reports. In this technique, bladder neck reconstruction was performed, with the aim of lengthening the shortened urethra that is present in most cats with USMI (Holt & Gibbs 1992).

Surgical techniques in female dogs

Colposuspension

This is the most common technique described for the treatment of USMI in female dogs (Rawlings *et al.* 2000; Gregory & Holt 1994). Two studies, one in experimental dogs (Rawlings *et al.* 2000) and one in clinically incontinent bitches (Gregory & Holt 1994), evaluated the urodynamic effects of colposuspension in female dogs. In experimental beagles colposuspension was found to increase leak point pressures, and move the bladder and urethra cranially, although maximum urethral closure pressure (MUCP) was decreased (Rawlings *et al.* 2000). In clinically affected dogs there were significant increases in both functional profile length (FPL) and MUCP (Gregory & Holt 1994). Both studies supported the hypothesis that colposuspension may restore continence by increasing pressure transmission to the proximal urethra and bladder neck. Colposuspension was first reported by Holt in 1985 and of the 33 dogs treated, 55% were cured of incontinence and another 36 were improved, with only 3/33 nonresponders in a mean follow-up period of one year (Holt 1985). In a larger follow-up study of 150 dogs, Holt reported similar results, with a cure rate of 53% and a further 37% improved. Only 9% failed to respond to surgery in a mean follow-up time of 2.8 years. Nine dogs in this study that initially responded relapsed 6 weeks to 15 months after surgery (Holt 1990). Others have found similar short-term results after colposuspension, but much higher rates of relapse after surgery. One study reported a cure rate of 55% two months after surgery, with a further 36% improved. However, this improvement rate was not sustained and only 3 of 22 dogs (14%) were completely continent one year after surgery without medications. When colposuspension and medical management were combined, 81% of dogs were considered either completely continent or greatly improved, however (Rawlings *et al.* 2001). Colposuspension has also been used in combination with neoureterostomy or ureteroneocystostomy for treatment of dogs with ureteral ectopia to attempt to decrease the incidence of persistent postoperative incontinence (Mouatt & Watt 2001; Noel *et al.* 2017). This technique was successful in 5 of 7 dogs treated (Mouatt & Watt 2001).

Technique

Prior to surgery a urethral catheter is placed (Holt & Stone 1997; Rawlings *et al.* 2000; Rawlings 2002; McLoughlin & Chew 2009). Routine aseptic preparation of the entire abdomen extending caudally to the vulva is performed. A caudal midline celiotomy is performed that extends from the umbilicus to the pubis. Fat and other connective tissue are dissected from the rectus abdominal insertions and prepubic tendon. The urethra and uterus or uterine body remnant are identified. Ovariohysterectomy or ovariectomy can be performed at this point if the dog is intact. A stay suture is placed at the apex or ventral surface of the bladder to provide cranial traction. As the bladder is moved cranially, the uterine body and vagina will also tend to move in a cranial direction. Once the cranial urethra has been moved far enough cranially so that it is beyond the pubic brim, small windows are dissected in the tissues lateral to the urethra to expose the vagina dorsally. Sutures are placed in a mattress pattern by first passing lengths of 2-0 nonabsorbable suture through the prepubic tendon, being careful to remain medial to the caudal superficial epigastric vessels on either side. Two to three sutures are passed on either side, through the lateral aspect of the muscular wall of the vagina and then back through the prepubic tendon on the same side. They should be all preplaced before tying. A subjective estimate of suture tightness must be made as the sutures are being tied to ensure that a therapeutic effect occurs, but conversely that urethral obstruction does not result. A small finger or the blunt end of a forceps can be placed between the urethra and body wall prior to definitive closure to ensure that the risk of postoperative urethral obstruction is minimal.

Postoperative care and complications

A urethral catheter is usually placed for 1–3 days postoperatively. Dysuria was the most common complication and occurred in 6% of cases in one study, but can usually be managed with urethral catheterization and anti-inflammatory medication (Holt 1990). If complete urethral obstruction occurs, which is rare, suture removal or replacement must be performed. The principle long-term complication of colposuspension is recurrence of urinary incontinence (Holt 1990; Rawlings *et al.* 2001).

Urethropexy and cystourethropexy

The aims of the urethropexy techniques are similar to that of colposuspension, in that the bladder and proximal urethra are moved cranially into an intra-abdominal position to allow intra-abdominal pressure to be exerted on the proximal urethra and trigone area (Massat *et al.* 1993; White 2001; McLoughlin & Chew 2009). The technical difference is that sutures are placed through the lateral wall of the urethra itself rather than by creating a vaginal sling around the urethra, as is the case with colposuspension. In addition to repositioning, however, an additional mechanism of action may be a direct effect of increasing urethral resistance at the level where the sutures are applied (White 2001). The authors of one large study of 100 dogs undergoing urethropexy found that there was an appreciable "kink" on postoperative retrograde vaginourethrograms and that there was a palpable increase in pressure during postoperative passage of a urethral catheter in many dogs (White 2001).

However, these subjective observations have not been substantiated with urodynamic studies demonstrating the effect of urethropexy techniques on the urethral sphincter mechanism postoperatively. Care should be taken when interpreting the clinical efficacy of these procedures, as different studies used somewhat differing techniques of urethropexy. The original study of 10 female dogs with USMI treated by cystourethropexy showed that only 2 of 10 dogs were continent postoperatively without medications (Massat *et al.* 1993). With medical management this figure increased to only 4 of 10 dogs and several cases demonstrated recurrence of urinary incontinence after initially being continent (Massat *et al.* 1993). Nevertheless, in a much larger study of 100 dogs performed by White, the continence rates postoperatively were better and found to be similar to those for colposuspension (White 2001). In this study 56% of dogs were cured by surgery, but the postoperative complication rate was high at 21%; 83% were found to have significant improvement in their continence rates. However, cure rates were found to decrease over time with this procedure also, and at >3 years postoperatively only 48% of dogs were considered to still have an "excellent" outcome.

Technique

The patient is positioned in dorsal recumbency and the entire abdomen is aseptically prepared for surgery (Massat *et al.* 1993; White 2001; McLoughlin & Chew 2009). A ventral midline celiotomy is performed extending to the pubic brim. A stay suture is placed in the bladder apex and is used to put cranial traction on the bladder and urethra. The margins of the rectus abdominis sheath are cleared of fat so that they can be clearly visualized. In the original technique reported by Massat, sutures of 2-0 monofilament nonabsorbable suture (polypropylene is usually used) were passed through the rectus sheath and into the lateral most aspects of the urethra on both sides. Each suture was left untied until the end. Up to 6–10 horizontal mattress sutures were placed on each side of the urethra (Massat *et al.* 1993). In White's technique a suture of 2-0 or 0 polypropylene was passed through the prepubic tendon and then passed transversely through the muscular layers of the urethra, being careful not to enter the lumen. Once placed through the urethra the suture was passed caudal to the opposite prepubic tendon. A second suture was then placed through the urethral wall approximately 3–5 mm cranial to the first (White 2001). Once both sutures were placed, they were tied and the remainder of the celiotomy incision was closed routinely.

Postoperative care and complications

Careful monitoring of postoperative urination is essential. Postoperative complications in one study occurred in 21% of dogs and included increased frequency of micturition in 14 cases, dysuria in 6 cases, and anuria in 3 cases (White 2001). These 3 anuric cases required a second surgery to release the overly tight sutures in order to allow them to urinate again (White 2001). The other major complication is recurrence of urinary incontinence postoperatively, as already discussed (Massat *et al.* 1993; White 2001).

Urethral sling procedures

Several procedures that involve the creation of a sling around the proximal to mid-urethra have been reported that aim to increase resistance to urine outflow without necessarily changing the position of the bladder or urethra (Bushby & Hankes 1980; Muir *et al.* 1994; Nickel *et al.* 1998; McLoughlin & Chew 2009; Claeys *et al.* 2010; Hamon *et al.* 2019). These techniques have in some cases been performed in combination with colposuspension.

Technique

A technique reported by Muir involves the creation of a sling from two rectangular, seromuscular pedicle flaps that are elevated from the ventral bladder trigone area (Muir *et al.* 1994; Bushby & Hankes 1980; Nickel *et al.* 1998; McLoughlin & Chew 2009). The two flaps, approximately 2–2.5 cm long, are caudally based and are passed around the bladder neck and sutured together dorsally. Each flap should be 4–10 mm wide, depending on the size of the dog (Muir *et al.* 1994). The resultant defect in the ventral trigonal area is then closed primarily with simple interrupted sutures. This modified sling urethroplasty was reported in 5 dogs and performed concurrently with colposuspension, but was not found to offer an advantage compared to colposuspension alone, as only 2 of 5 dogs were continent postoperatively (Muir *et al.* 1994). A further case using this technique was reported and resulted in initial cure, followed by a recurrence of urinary incontinence at six weeks (Bushby & Hankes 1980).

Another modification of the sling technique reported the use of a polyester ribbon. From a ventral midline approach, the adductor muscles were dissected away from the midline until the obturator foramina could be identified. The ribbon was passed through the obturator foramina, around the urethra, and secured ventral to the pelvis with a titanium clip. This technique was designed principally for use in large-breed dogs and its use in conjunction with colposuspension or in isolation was evaluated (Nickel *et al.* 1998). A modification of this technique is less invasive and performed through an episiotomy approach (Claeys *et al.* 2010). A polypropylene tape is passed using a transobturator inside-out approach, which was adapted from a technique used in women. Short-term results of this technique were promising, but long-term outcomes showed significant recurrence of urinary incontinence. with only 40% of incontinent dogs remaining continent at a median follow-up of 85 months (range 28–95 months). However, with the addition of medical management in addition to the sling procedure, approximately 80% of dogs were able to retain continence (Hamon *et al.* 2019). Complications of the surgical procedure included an iatrogenic urethral tear in one dog (Claeys *et al.* 2010).

Postoperative care and complications

Principal complications of the sling procedures include dysuria postoperatively and persistent postoperative incontinence. In the study by Muir, 3 of 5 dogs had an increase in frequency of urination in the days postoperatively, which resolved (Muir *et al.* 1994). The urethral sling created using polyester ribbon resulted in a postoperative continence rate of 50%. Dogs that underwent the sling and colposuspension did not have a higher continence rate than those that underwent colposuspension alone (Nickel *et al.* 1998). Additionally, 2 of 13 dogs that had the ribbons placed developed fistulas associated with the ribbons postoperatively, which only healed after ribbon removal (Nickel *et al.* 1998)

Surgical techniques in male dogs

Vas deferentopexy

This technique is aimed at reproducing the effects of colposuspension in male dogs by using traction on the vas deferens of castrated males to pull the bladder neck and proximal urethra into a more cranial location (Weber *et al.* 1997; Salomon *et al.* 2002). If not already neutered, dogs must be castrated prior to undergoing vas deferentopexy. The procedure has been described using an "open" and laparoscopic technique. Other authors have voiced concerns that because the tissues of the vas deferens contain receptors for androgens and estrogens, castration might lead to weakening of the deferent ducts over time, with resulting recurrence of clinical signs (Holt *et al.* 2005).

Technique

Dogs are placed in dorsal recumbency and the entire abdomen is aseptically prepared for celiotomy (Weber *et al.* 1997). If the dog is not already castrated, this procedure is performed first prior to celiotomy using a standard castration technique. A standard ventral caudal celiotomy is performed, extending from the umbilicus to the pubis. The vas deferens is slowly withdrawn from each inguinal canal and pulled in a cranial direction to pull the urethra cranially. Both deferent ducts are pulled at a 60° angle to midline and at the point where the duct meets the abdominal wall the deferentopexy is performed. A 4–5 mm incision perpendicular to the celiotomy in the rectus sheath is created and the ends of each duct are pulled through. After removal of the abdominal retractor, traction is placed on the ducts such that the prostate gland is seen to move approximately 1 cm cranially. The ducts are then sutured to the body wall with 2-0 polydioxanone. In the original technique a polydioxanone band was also sutured down to the ducts to prevent their future displacement.

A laparoscopic-assisted deferentopexy has also been described in a dog (Salomon *et al.* 2002). A three-port technique was used and the distal ends of the vas deferens were coagulated and cut and then pulled cranially. The ducts were sutured to the rectus sheath using a similar technique as for the "open" version described earlier. The ducts were secured to the rectus sheath through two small percutaneous skin incisions over the anticipated locations of the pexy sites. However, the dog described did not respond to therapy and only became continent with the addition of PPA (Salomon *et al.* 2002).

Postoperative care and complications

This technique was performed in 7 dogs, 5 of which had intrapelvic bladders preoperatively. The bladders of all dogs were located intra-abdominally postoperatively (Weber *et al.* 1997). Clinically 3 of 7 dogs were continent after surgery and a further 3 were improved but only continent with medical therapy. One dog remained incontinent long term (Weber *et al.* 1997). No other major complications were recorded.

Prostatopexy

This technique for use in male dogs also aims to move the bladder neck and proximal urethra into an intra-abdominal position (Holt *et al.* 2005). It was hypothesized that it may have advantages over vas deferentopexy as castration is not necessary for this technique. Avoidance of castration may be beneficial, as it is known that there is an association between castration and USMI in male dogs (Aaron *et al.* 1996; Power *et al.* 1998; Holt *et al.* 2005).

Technique

Dogs are placed in dorsal recumbency and the entire abdomen is aseptically prepared for celiotomy

(Holt *et al.* 2005). A standard ventral caudal celiotomy is performed, extending from the cranial margin of the prepuce to the pubis. Cranial traction is applied to the bladder until the cranial end of the prostate gland can be visualized. Two sutures of nonabsorbable monofilament suture were passed through the prepubic tendon and through the ventral and caudal prostatic capsule approximately 1 cm from the urethra on either side. The sutures were all preplaced prior to tightening and care was taken not to overtighten the sutures, thereby overcompressing the urethra.

Postoperative care and complications

Postoperatively only 1 of 9 dogs was cured by the surgery, although 4 more were significantly improved (Holt *et al.* 2005). Postoperative retrograde urethrocystograms showed that the bladder was positioned intra-abdominally in all dogs. There were no other major complications reported. It appears that male dogs do not respond as well as females to currently available surgical therapies for the treatment of USMI.

Surgical techniques in female cats

Bladder neck reconstruction

Cats with USMI may have a somewhat different pathophysiology from the disease process that occurs in female dogs and response to medical management has not been well documented, although it is suggested to be poor (Holt 1993; Lane & Westropp 2009). Severe anatomic abnormalities of the feline lower urogenital tract usually accompany the condition and include severe urethral and vaginal hypoplasia, with bladder hypoplasia occurring less commonly (Holt & Gibbs 1992; Holt 1993). Due to these abnormalities, many of the techniques described in dogs that are designed to move the bladder neck and proximal urethra intra-abdominally, such as colposuspension or urethropexy, are not applicable.

Technique

The essential goal of these techniques was to create a new tubular urethra in cats that lacked such a structure (Holt 1993). Both techniques described are performed through a standard ventral midline celiotomy, with the cat in dorsal recumbency. In the first technique the caudoventral bladder is excised cranially to the extent of the ureterovesicular junctions. Only enough bladder is left dorsally to create a tubular urethra that can house a 4 Fr urinary catheter. Once excised, the tubular area of bladder that remains is sutured together to create a new tubular "urethra." The second variation of the technique aims to preserve as much bladder volume as possible. In this technique a ventral cystotomy is performed back to the level of the ureterovesicular junctions. Two ventral triangular bladder flaps are then created, by incising from the caudal tip of the cystotomy incision cranially in a craniolateral direction to the level of the ureterovesicular junctions. The defect is then primarily sutured to create the urethral tube caudally of similar dimensions to the first technique. However, closure then continues around the cut margin of the two elevated flaps cranially, resulting in no loss of bladder volume. Although only small numbers of cats have been treated with these two procedures, the authors suggested that cats with bladder hypoplasia might be better treated using the flap reconstruction technique, whereas cats with normal-sized bladders may be adequately treated with the bladder neck resection technique (Holt 1993). This technique can also be used in dogs, although it has been reported in only one dog to date (Holt 1993).

Postoperative care and complications

Bladder neck reconstruction has been reported to have significant success in a report of 8 cats. Of 8 cats treated with two different modifications of the technique, 3 cats became completely continent, while 4 other cats were significantly improved. One was lost to follow-up (Holt 1993). Dysuria was seen in 1 of 8 cats in the study, and 2 cats developed recurrent cystitis that responded to medical management after surgery.

Injectable bulking agents

Urethral bulking agents are used in dogs that failed medical management of USMI, or cannot tolerate the side effects of medications such as PPA and diethylstilbestrol (DES). Periurethral submucosal injections of various agents have been used, including polytetrafluoroethylene (PTFE), collagen, hydroxyapatite, dextranomer/hyaluronic acid copolymer, and cross-linked gelatin (Barth *et al.* 2005; Luttman *et al.* 2019; Chen *et al.* 2020). This has been reported mainly for use in female dogs with USMI. If concurrent ectopic ureters exist, it is recommended that the ureteral ectopia be treated prior to treatment with bulking agents. Initial reports showed a control rate of 53% for incontinence treated with one of two series of injections. The rate of continence increased to 75% when PPA was used in combination (Arnold 1997). Nearly 10% of dogs with USMI are not helped by the collagen and drug therapy. Using submucosal collagen, a more recent study demonstrated success in 68% of 40 dogs, with a mean duration of effect of 17 months (Barth *et al.* 2005). With the addition of PPA the continence rate improved to nearly 85%. Other materials like hydroxyapatite (Coaptite®, Boston Scientific, Marlborough, MA, USA), ethylene vinyl alcohol copolymer suspended in dimethyl sulfoxide (DMSO; Tegress®, Bard, Murray Hill, NJ, USA), and extracellular matrix derived from porcine urinary bladder (ACell Vet®, Columbia, MD, USA) have been used, but have not been as beneficial as collagen (Contigen®, Bard), in the authors' experience. In a recent study collagen injection was compared to the use of dextranomer/hyaluronic acid copolymer (Luttman *et al.* 2019). In this study, dogs undergoing collagen injection experienced both increased levels of continence post procedure as well as duration of effect (Luttman *et al.* 2019). Cross-linked gelatin was used in a recent study of 15 dogs with USMI and continence was achieved in 87% of dogs after one injection and 100% of dogs after two injections, with a mean duration of continence of 11.1 months (Chen *et al.* 2020).

Technique

Injections are performed via cystoscopic guidance into the periurethral tissue submucosa (Arnold 1997; Barth *et al.* 2005; Byron *et al.* 2009; Luttman *et al.* 2019; Chen *et al.* 2020). A routine cystoscopy should be performed prior to considering a collagen injection to rule out other anatomic anomalies such as proximal ureteral ectopia. Once the ureteral openings are identified in their normal locations, the bladder is filled to about 66–75% capacity, so that the urethra remains open and stretched. The cystoscope is then pulled into the urethra, and within the proximal 2–3 cm, where the urethra is at its narrowest (the lumen of the mucosa is starting to meet), the collagen should be injected. The material is provided in a syringe, and a long, flexible 5 Fr collagen injection needle is required. The needle is typically 20 gauge and has a Huber metallic tip. The needle should be primed with the collagen and carefully placed in the working channel of the cystoscope, being careful to not damage the metallic tip. Due to the 5 Fr size of the needle, the appropriate-sized cystoscope should be used (>2.7 mm rigid). Once the ideal location is identified in the urethra, the needle is exteriorized from the proximal tip of the cystoscope through the working channel. It is very important to try to stay parallel to the urethral lumen, and this often requires utilizing the 30° cystoscope angle to turn the cystoscope in an appropriate orientation. Once the needle is nearly parallel with the mucosal lumen, the tip of the needle is gently pierced through the urethral mucosa, remaining fairly superficial so that the muscularis is not entered. Once the bevel of the needle is under the tissue, the cystoscope should remain very stable and an assistant should start injecting the material 0.1 mL at a time. Care must be taken not to advance the needle into the muscularis, which usually results in no bleb forming. Within 0.2 mL a bleb of blanching tissue should be seen moving into the urethral lumen from under the urethral mucosa. If this does not occur, the needle is likely too deep and should be backed out before a second attempt is made. It should be remembered during injection that the entire syringe contains only 2.5 mL. It is typically recommended to make 3–4 blebs at the 2, 6, and 10 o'clock positions. The goal is to have all of the blebs meet in the lumen of the urethra so that it appears almost closed (Figure 46.1). It is the authors' impression that injecting two rows of collagen improves the continence rate and longevity, and does not increase the complication rate. It is not unusual to have a small amount of bleeding after removing the needle, but this will resolve within a few minutes.

Postoperative care and complications

An initial success rate of 68% in 40 dogs after six months has been reported, although the long-term outcome continence rate was only 28% (at the time of death or the end of the study). Continence was reported to last a mean of 17 months (ranging from 1 to 64 months) (Barth *et al.* 2005). The authors have tried different types of bulking agents, such as hydroxyapatite, and have not found a benefit when compared to bovine collagen (Contigen). This technique is much more effective in dogs with USMI alone; in situations of anatomic anomalies, such as short/wide urethras, and intrapelvic bladders the results are less favorable. The main complications reported are urinary obstruction after collagen injection, which is very rare and typically short-lived. A urinary catheter for 1–2 days is all that is typically required. One should never inject collagen in the face of an active urinary tract infection, so a negative urine culture should always be obtained prior to this procedure. The authors typically treat the patient with three days of antibiotics and pain analgesics (tramadol or a nonsteroidal anti-inflammatory agent) as needed after the procedure. Most patients can be discharged the same day as the procedure.

Hydraulic occluders

The use of an artificial urethral sphincter (AUS) for refractory incontinence has been performed since the early 1970s in human medicine. The placement of an AUS, using a hydraulic occluder (HO), was first reported in four dogs in 2009 (Rose *et al.* 2009) and has since been reported in a larger cohort of dogs (Currao *et al.* 2013; Reeves *et al.* 2013; Gomes *et al.* 2018) These devices are inflatable silicon occluders that come in various sizes. They are placed around the proximal urethra and are

(a)

(b)

(c)

(d)

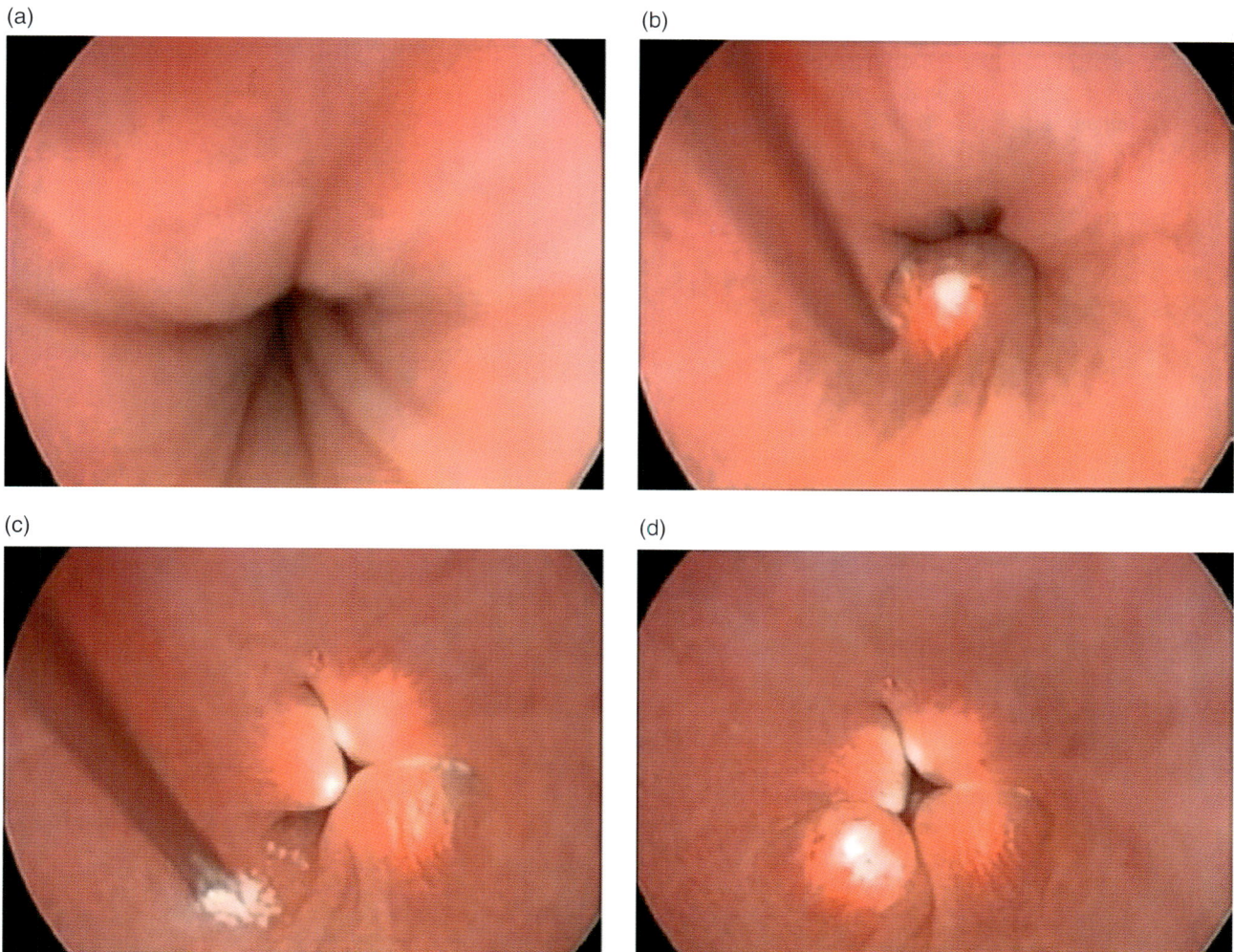

Figure 46.1 Urethral collagen injection in a female dog using rigid cystoscopy. (a) Anatomically normal proximal urethral lumen prior to collagen injection. (b) The collagen needle inserted under the mucosa of the periurethral tissue, creating a bleb of collagen material (white blanched bulge). (c) Three collagen blebs created that are opposing each other in the urethra lumen. The needle is about to be inserted for a fourth and final bleb at the 7 o'clock position. (d) The final result after four blebs have been created in the periurethral tissue.

attached to a subcutaneously placed vascular access port (VAP). In humans an adjustable pump device is used. The use of a custom-designed veterinary device was tested urodynamically in six canine cadavers (Adin *et al.* 2004). Inflation of the device to 25% and 50% resulted in an increase in the maximal urethral closure pressure and cystourethral leak point pressure. Four client-owned animals with acquired USMI were then evaluated over 20–30 months. All four dogs were 100% continent at the end of the study. Three of the four dogs required percutaneous filling of the VAP with saline to improve continence after surgery. One dog was continent without any inflation. One dog developed wound drainage at the port site and required port removal (Rose *et al.* 2009).

In recent clinical studies, most dogs were improved postoperatively, with median continence scores increasing from 3.5/10 preoperatively to 9/10 postoperatively in one study (Gomes *et al.* 2018) and from 3.3/10 to 10/10 in a second study (Currao *et al.* 2013). Most of the dogs in these studies were dogs that failed surgical or endoscopic treatment of their ectopic ureters and were persistently incontinent despite surgery, laser ablation, medications, and collagen injections. The most common complications of hydraulic occluder placement included urethral obstruction, dysuria, cystitis, urine retention, hematuria, and pain when urinating (Currao *et al.* 2013; Reeves *et al.* 2013; Gomes *et al.* 2018).

Procedure

Through a ventral midline celiotomy extending from the umbilicus to the pubis, the bladder is retracted cranially using an apical stay suture (Adin 2009). The vaginal/cervical remnant is then retracted cranially using Allis tissue forceps. The proximal urethra is isolated using blunt dissection and the peri-urethral adipose tissue is gently removed. In an area approximately 2 cm caudal to the bladder neck, the urethra is dissected from the peri-urethral tissue and a circumferential window is made of approximately 1 cm around the urethra ventral to the vagina, using a pair of small Mixter forceps. A 0.25 in. Penrose drain is used to measure a urethral circumference using a sterile marker and ruler. Based on this measurement (in millimeters), an HO size is chosen. Typically, the measurement in millimeters is divided by 2, with the resultant number corresponding to the size of HO chosen. The HO device comes in the following increments: HO-6, 8, 10, 12, 14, 16. The most common size used in dogs <20 kg is 10 and in dogs >20 kg is 12 or 14. The ring of the HO should site around the urethra without any compression. An area lateral to the umbilicus under the skin on the right side of the incision is dissected to the level of the mammary glands. A hemostat is used to puncture a small hole into the abdomen from this pocket and the end of the actuating tubing is pulled through the body wall. Before placement of the HO, the blue boot that secures the VAP is placed on the actuating tubing and then the silicon device is primed with sterile saline (0.9% NaCl). All air is flushed out of the ring and the actuating tubing using a long 18-gauge venous sampling catheter. Once all of the air is removed, and the lumen is filled with saline, the VAP is filled with saline so that all air is ejected. The port and actuating tubing are then connected, making this an air-free system. The blue boot is then secured to the junction of the actuating tubing of the HO and the VAP. The HO is leak tested by infusing the system with sterile saline to ensure there are no leaks.

A length of 2-0 prolene suture material is then placed through one set of eyelets on the HO. The Mixter forceps are used to tunnel under the urethral dissection and the suture material is secured in the forceps as the HO is gently pulled through dorsal to the urethra. Once secured in this dissection, the suture is passed through the opposite eyelets and secured, creating a silicon ring around the urethra (Figures 46.2 and 46.3). Care must be taken to ensure that the ureters are not entrapped by the HO. It is therefore vital to know the ectopic nature of the ureteral openings prior to considering this procedure. In cases of ectopic ureter, the ureteral openings must be repositioned into the bladder trigone prior to this technique being employed to avoid possible ureteral obstruction.

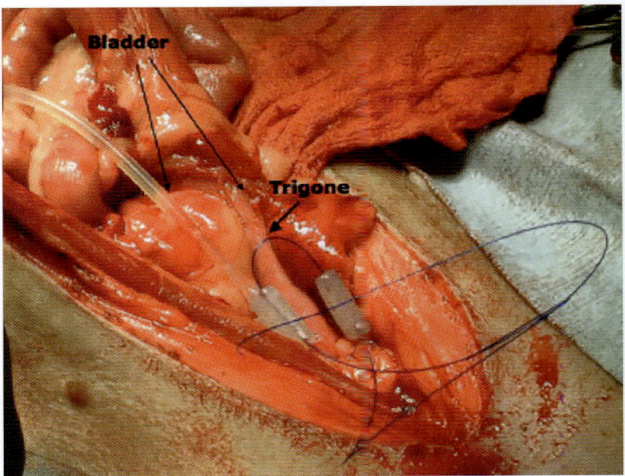

Figure 46.2 Surgical image of a female dog during the placement of a hydraulic occlusion device. The occluder ring is passed around the urethra and permanent suture material (prolene) is passed through the islets to create a ring. This ring is placed at least 1–2 cm caudal to the bladder trigone.

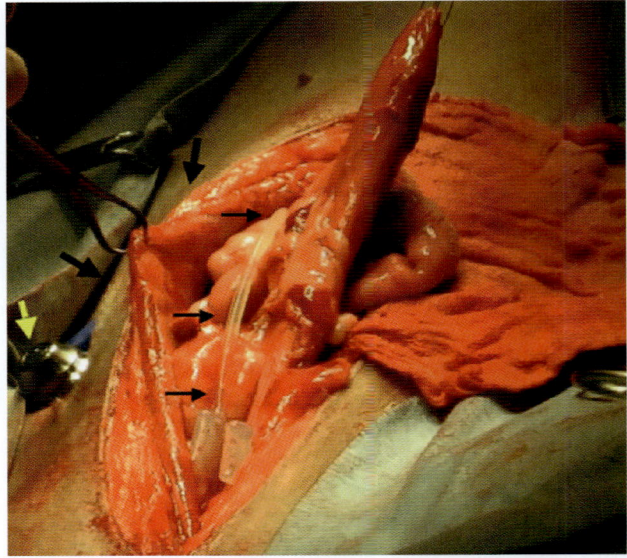

Figure 46.3 Surgical image of a female dog during the placement of a hydraulic occlusion device (cranial is to the top left and caudal to the bottom right). The hydraulic occluder is around the urethra just caudal to the trigone. The actuating tube (black arrows) is passed through the body wall and a pocket is created under the skin for the access port (yellow arrow).

The VAP is then secured to the body wall using 3-0 prolene suture material. The authors typically recommend suturing the port to the dermis rather than the subcutaneous tissue, as it is more secure long term and easier to manipulate in the future.

Postoperative care and complications

Patients are treated with tramadol for pain and two weeks of broad-spectrum antibiotics. This procedure should not be performed if there is any evidence of a urinary tract infection and a negative urine culture should be obtained prior to surgery. Care should be taken to ensure that the patient does not lick the incision, as if the port gets infected than this could be devastating. Typically, no saline is infused into the system at the time of surgery and six weeks is allowed for healing and revascularization of the urethra. After six weeks the system can be inflated. The authors typically perform a urethroscopy to measure the volume it takes to close the HO by 25%, 50%, 75%, and 100%. This relationship is typically not very linear, and the volumes are very small (increments often of 0.05–0.1 mL). Approximately 33% of patients are continent without any inflation and with the presence of the empty HO (Currao *et al.* 2013). If the patient remains incontinent at six weeks, the HO is typically inflated by 25%. This can then be percutaneously adjusted in the future without the need for future anesthesia. It is important to remember that only a Huber needle (22 gauge) should be used for the injection of sterile saline.

References

Aaron, A., Eggleton, K., Power, C., and Holt, P.E. (1996). Urethral sphincter mechanism incompetence in male dogs: a retrospective analysis of 54 cases. *Veterinary Record* 139: 542–546.

Adams, W.M. and DiBartola, S.P. (1983). Radiographic and clinical features of pelvic bladder in the dog. *Journal of the American Veterinary Medical Association* 182: 1212–1217.

Adin, C.A., Farese, J.P., Cross, A.R. et al. (2004). Urodynamic effects of a percutaneously controlled static hydraulic urethral sphincter in canine cadavers. *American Journal of Veterinary Research* 65: 283–288.

Adin, C.A. (2009). Hydraulic occluders for sphincter mechanism incompetence. In: *Proceedings of the American College of Veterinary Surgeons Annual Symposium, October 2009*, 643–647. Washington DC: American College of Veterinary Surgeons.

Angioletti, A., De Francessco, I., Vergottini, M. et al. (2004). Urinary incontinence after spaying in the bitch: incidence and oestrogen therapy. *Veterinary Research Communications* 28: 153–155.

Arnold, S. (1997). [Urinary incontinence in castrated bitches. 2. Diagnosis and treatment]. *Schweiz Arch Tierheilkd* 139: 319–324.

Bacon, N.J., Oni, O., and White, R.A.S. (2002). Treatment of urethral sphincter mechanism incompetence in 11 bitches with a sustained-release formulation of phenylpropanolamine hydrochloride. *Veterinary Record* 151: 373–376.

Barsanti, J.A. and Downey, R. (1984). Urinary incontinence in cats. *Journal of the American Animal Hospital Association* 20: 979–982.

Barth, A., Reichler, I.M., Hubler, M. et al. (2005). Evaluation of long-term effects of endoscopic injection of collagen into the urethral submucosa for treatment of urethral sphincter incompetence in female dogs: 40 cases (1993-2000). *Journal of the American Veterinary Medical Association* 226: 73–76.

Bushby, P.A. and Hankes, G.H. (1980). Sling urethroplasty for the correction of urethral dilatation and urinary incontinence. *Journal of the American Animal Hospital Association* 16: 115–118.

Byron, J.K., Chew, D.J., and McLoughlin, M.A. (2009). Urinary incontinence: treatment with injectable bulking agents. In: *Current Veterinary Therapy XIV* (ed. J.D. Bonagura and D.C. Twedt), 960–964. St. Louis, MO: Saunders Elsevier.

Chen, H., Shipov, A., and Segev, G. (2020). Evaluation of cross-linked gelatin as a bulking agent for the management of urinary sphincter mechanism incompetence in female dogs. *Journal of Veterinary Internal Medicine* 34: 1914–1919.

Claeys, S., de Leval, J., and Hamaide, A. (2010). Transobturator vaginal tape inside out for treatment of urethral sphincter mechanism incompetence: preliminary results in 7 female dogs. *Veterinary Surgery* 39: 969–979.

Creed, K.E. (1983). Effect of hormones on urethral sensitivity to phenylephrine in normal and incontinent dogs. *Research in Veterinary Science* 34: 177–181.

Currao, R.L., Berent, A.C., Weisse, C. et al. (2013). Use of a percutaneously controlled urethral hydraulic occluder for treatment of refractory urinary incontinence in 18 female dogs. *Veterinary Surgery* 42: 440–447.

Diaz Espineira, M.M., Viehoff, F.W., and Nickel, R.F. (1998). Idiopathic detrusor-urethral dyssynergia in dogs: a retrospective analysis of 22 cases. *Journal of Small Animal Practice* 39: 264–270.

Gomes, C., Doran, I., Friend, E. et al. (2018). Long-term outcome of female dogs treated with static hydraulic urethral sphincter for urethral sphincter mechanism incompetence. *Journal of the American Animal Hospital Association* 54: 276–284.

Gookin, J.L. and Bunch, S.E. (1996). Detrusor-striated sphincter dyssynergia in a dog. *Journal of Veterinary Internal Medicine* 10: 339–344.

Gregory, S.P. and Holt, P.E. (1994). The immediate effect of colposuspension on resting and stressed urethral pressure profiles in anesthetized incontinent bitches. *Veterinary Surgery* 23: 330–340.

Hamon, M., Hamaide, A.J., Noel, S.M. et al. (2019). Long-term outcome of the transobturator vaginal tape inside out for treatment of urethral sphincter mechanism incompetence in female dogs. *Veterinary Surgery* 48: 29–34.

Holt, P.E. (1985). Urinary incontinence in the bitch due to sphincter mechanism incompetence: surgical treatment. *Journal of Small Animal Practice* 26: 237–246.

Holt, P.E. (1990). Long-term evaluation of colposuspension in the treatment of urinary incontinence due to incompetence of the urethral sphincter mechanism in the bitch. *Veterinary Record* 127: 537–542.

Holt, P.E. (1993). Surgical management of congenital urethral sphincter mechanism incompetence in eight female cats and a bitch. *Veterinary Surgery* 22: 98–104.

Holt, P.E., Coe, R.J., and Hotson Moore, A. (2005). Prostatopexy as a treatment for urethral sphincter mechanism incompetence in male dogs. *Journal of Small Animal Practice* 46: 567–570.

Holt, P.E. and Gibbs, C. (1992). Congenital urinary incontinence in cats: a review of 19 cases. *Veterinary Record* 130: 437–442.

Holt, P.E. and Stone, E.A. (1997). Colposuspension for urinary incontinence. In: *Current Techniques in Small Animal Surgery*, 4e (ed. M.J. Bojrab), 455–459. Baltimore, MD: Williams and Wilkins.

Lane, I.F. and Westropp, J.L. (2009). Urinary incontinence and micturition disorders: pharmacologic management. In: *Current Veterinary Therapy XIV* (ed. J.D. Bonagura and D.C. Twedt), 955–959. St. Louis, MO: Saunders Elsevier.

Luttman, K., Merle, R., and Nickel, R. (2019). Retrospective analysis after endoscopic urethral injections of glutaraldehyde-cross-linked-collagen or dextranomer/hyaluronic acid copolymer in bitches with urinary incontinence. *Journal of Small Animal Practice* 60: 96–101.

Mandigers, P.J.J. and Nell, T. (2001). Treatment of bitches with acquired urinary incontinence with oestriol. *Veterinary Record* 149: 764–767.

Massat, B.J., Gregory, C.R., Ling, G.V. et al. (1993). Cystourethropexy to correct refractory urinary incontinence due to urethral sphincter mechanism incompetence. *Veterinary Surgery* 22: 260–269.

McLoughlin, M.A. and Chew, D.J. (2009). Surgical treatment of urethral sphincter mechanism incompetence in female dogs. *Compendium on Continuing Education for Practicing Veterinarians* 31 (8): 360–373.

Miodrag, A., Castleden, C.M., and Vallance, T.R. (1988). Sex hormones and the female urinary tract. *Drugs* 36: 491–504.

Mouatt, J.G. and Watt, P.R. (2001). Ectopic ureter repair and colposuspension in seven bitches. *Australian Veterinary Practitioner* 31 (4): 160–167.

Muir, P., Goldsmid, S.E., and Bellenger, C.R. (1994). Management of urinary incontinence in five bitches with incompetence of the urethral sphincter mechanism by colposuspension and a modified sling urethroplasty. *Veterinary Record* 134: 38–41.

Nickel, R.F., Wiegand, U., and Van den Brom, W.E. (1998). Evaluation of a transpelvic sling procedure with and without colposuspension for treatment of female dogs with refractory urethral sphincter mechanism incompetence. *Veterinary Surgery* 27: 94–104.

Noel, S.M., Claeys, S., and Hamaide, A.J. (2017). Surgical management of ectopic ureters in dogs: clinical outcome and prognostic factors for long-term continence. *Veterinary Surgery* 46: 631–641.

Power, S.C., Eggleton, K.E., Aaron, A.J. et al. (1998). Urethral sphincter mechanism incompetence in the male dog: importance of bladder neck position, proximal urethral length and castration. *Journal of Small Animal Practice* 39: 69–72.

Rawlings, C.A. (2002). Colposuspension as a treatment for urinary incontinence in spayed dogs. *Journal of the American Animal Hospital Association* 38: 107–110.

Rawlings, C.A., Barsanti, J.A., Mahaffey, M.B. et al. (2001). Evaluation of colposuspension for treatment of incontinence in spayed female dogs. *Journal of the American Veterinary Medical Association* 219: 770–775.

Rawlings, C.A., Mahaffey, M.B., Chernosky, A. et al. (2000). Immediate urodynamic and anatomic response to colposuspension in female beagles. *American Journal of Veterinary Research* 61: 1353–1357.

Reeves, L., Adin, C., McLoughlin, M. et al. (2013). Outcome after placement of an artificial urethral sphincter in 27 dogs. *Veterinary Surgery* 42: 12–18.

Reichler, I.M., Barth, A., Piche, C.A. et al. (2006a). Urodynamic parameters and plasma LF/FSH in spayed beagle bitches before and 8 weeks after GnRH depot analogue treatment. *Theriogenology* 66: 2127–2136.

Reichler, I.M., Jochle, W., Piche, C.A. et al. (2006b). Effect of a long acting GnRH analogue or placebo on plasma LH/FSH, urethral pressure profiles and clinical signs of urinary incontinence due to sphincter mechanism incontinence in bitches. *Theriogenology* 66: 1227–1236.

Richter, K.P. and Ling, G.V. (1985). Clinical response and urethral pressure profile changes after phenylpropanolamine in dogs with primary sphincter incompetence. *Journal of the American Veterinary Medical Association* 187: 605–611.

Rose, S.A., Adin, C.A., Ellison, G.W. et al. (2009). Long-term efficacy of a percutaneously adjustable hydraulic urethral sphincter for treatment of urinary incontinence in four dogs. *Veterinary Surgery* 38: 747–753.

Salomon, J.F., Cotard, J.P., and Viguier, E. (2002). Management of urethral sphincter mechanism incompetence in a male dog with laparoscopic-guided deferentopexy. *Journal of Small Animal Practice* 43: 501–505.

Scott, L., Leedy, M., Bernay, F. et al. (2002). Evaluation of phenylpropanolamine in the treatment of urethral sphincter mechanism incompetence in the bitch. *Journal of Small Animal Practice* 43: 493–496.

Weber, U.T., Arnold, A., Hubler, M. et al. (1997). Surgical treatment of male dogs with urinary incontinence due to urethral sphincter mechanism incompetence. *Veterinary Surgery* 26: 51–56.

White, R.A.S. and Pomeroy, C.J. (1989). Phenylpropanolamine: an a-adrenergic agent for the management of urinary incontinence in the bitch associated with urethral sphincter mechanism incompetence. *Veterinary Record* 125: 478–480.

White, R.N. (2001). Urethropexy for the management of urethral sphincter mechanism incompetence in the bitch. *Journal of Small Animal Practice* 42: 481–486.

47

Treatment Strategies for Ureteral Ectopia

Philipp D. Mayhew and Allyson Berent

The principal treatment modality for ureteral ectopia is surgery. While medical management of potential concurrent urethral sphincter mechanism incompetence (USMI) could result in improvement of clinical signs with the use of ∝-adrenergic agents and/or estrogen therapy, surgical management to correct the underlying anatomic defect is still warranted to limit the incidence of urinary tract infections (UTIs). Chronic pyelonephritis can cause significant morbidity and patients with ureteral ectopia often have significant vesico-ureteral reflux resulting in pyelonephritis. Additionally, ongoing or worsening hydroureter and/or hydronephrosis is undesirable and a return to normal dimensions of these structures after surgery or laser ablation has been documented in at least some cases (Mason *et al.* 1990; Berent *et al.* 2008).

A variety of surgical procedures have been advocated for treatment of ureteral ectopia and they can be broadly divided into removal of the ectopic ureter along with the affected kidney (ureteronephrectomy), reimplantation of the ureter into the bladder wall, or creation of a new opening into the bladder. In addition, some have advocated treatment with concurrent colposuspension at the time of ectopic ureter treatment in an attempt to reduce the incidence of persistent postoperative incontinence (Mouatt & Watt 2001; Noel *et al.* 2017). Recently, cystoscopic-assisted laser ablation of intramural ureteral ectopia has been reported as a minimally invasive alternative to open surgical treatment in male and female dogs (McCarthy 2006; Berent *et al.* 2008, 2012; Smith *et al.* 2009).

Careful selection of surgical technique depends on a complete understanding of the pathology present in each individual case. UTI should be ruled out prior to any intervention, as UTIs are reported to be present in 64–79% of dogs preoperatively (Stone & Mason 1990; McLaughlin & Miller 1991; Cannizzo *et al.* 2003; Mayhew *et al.* 2006; Noel *et al.* 2017). In feline cases preoperative UTI has been reported to be present in 36% of cases (Holt & Gibbs 1992). A urine sample should be collected via cystocentesis from all patients and urine culture and antibiotic sensitivity testing should be performed. If a UTI is diagnosed, treatment with the appropriate antibiotic should be instituted for 4–6 weeks, as concurrent pyelonephritis is common. Reculture at least a week following cessation of antibiotics should be performed to rule out the presence of an ongoing or resistant UTI.

Imaging should be used to rule out the presence of concurrent pathology. Assessment of renal function is essential, as severe renal damage may necessitate ureteronephrectomy rather than primary ureteral ectopia repair. Ultrasonography can be used to diagnose severe hydronephrosis/hydroureter. In cases where little residual renal parenchyma remains, a judgment must be made as to whether the kidney will retain any filtration capacity postoperatively (Lamb & Gregory 1998). Ultrasonography can also be suggestive of pyelonephritis if echogenic material is visualized within the renal pelvis (Lamb & Gregory 1998). However, the sensitivity of ultrasound for diagnosis of experimentally induced pyelonephritis in one study was only 82% (Neuwirth *et al.* 1993).

Small Animal Soft Tissue Surgery, Second Edition. Edited by Eric Monnet.
Companion website: www.wiley.com/go/monnet/small

Chronic medically unresponsive pyelonephritis may be another indication for ureteronephrectomy in patients with ureteral ectopia. In many cases where hydrone-phrosis is present but some renal parenchyma remains, an objective assessment of the glomerular filtration of that kidney is warranted. Renal scintigraphy using the radioisotope technetium 99mdiethylenetriamine pen-taacetic acid (99mTc-DTPA) is the method of choice to measure glomerular filtration rate (GFR) in these cases (Kerl & Cook 2005) and has been shown to be clinically useful when deciding whether to perform ureterone-phrectomy (Gookin et al. 1996). This is the only method for single kidney GFR assessment and is a rapid nonin-vasive technique that does not require urine collection, unlike most other methods of GFR measurement. The disadvantages of this technique are principally logistic, in that it requires specialized materials and radiation safety precautions must be taken (Kerl & Cook 2005). Excretory urography is a poor method for assessing kidney function as it is heavily affected by the type of contrast medium used, dose, speed of injection, renal blood flow, state of hydration, rate of urine flow, and radiographic technique used (Feeney et al. 1982; Gookin et al. 1996). In patients with bilateral ureteral ectopia, ureteronephrectomy can be performed if one kidney is no longer functioning, but great care must be taken to assess renal function in the contralateral prior to surgery.

In the majority of cases irreversible kidney damage is not present and the choice of surgical technique will depend on the morphologic nature of ectopia and the associated abnormalities of the upper and lower urinary tract. Avoidance of ureteronephrectomy is recom-mended whenever possible.

Creation of a new opening of the ureter in the bladder

The most common surgical treatment for intramural ureteral ectopia is creation of a new stoma from the intramural ureter into the bladder, with or without trig-onal reconstruction. In both cases the ectopic ureter is approached via a ventral midline celiotomy and ventral longitudinal cystotomy and urethrotomy. Two general techniques have been described.

Creation of a new stoma with ligation of the distal ureter

The point of entry of the ureter into the trigone needs to be localized from the mucosal aspect of the bladder. This may be obvious in some cases, but in others the intramu-ral ureteral tunnel can be seen better when light pressure is placed on the urethra distally, resulting in urine

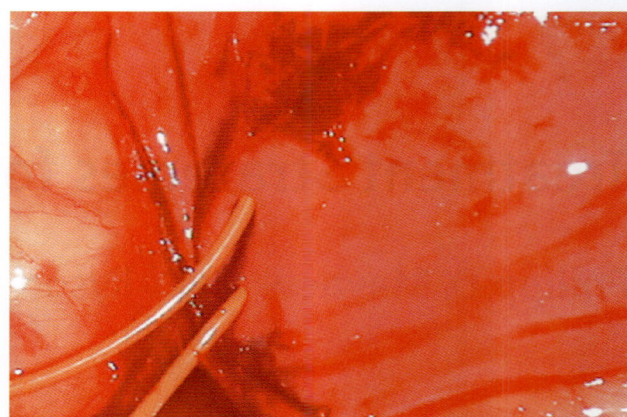

Figure 47.1 The distal openings of both ectopic ureters located within the urethra in this dog have been catheterized using a red rubber catheter. This allows their location within the bladder wall to be palpated more easily.

pooling and distension of the ureteral tunnel. It is also sometimes possible to identify the distal opening of an intramurally tunneling ureter if a partial urethrotomy is performed. Red rubber catheters can then be passed ret-rograde up from the distal orifice (Figure 47.1). Once the point of entry into the trigone has been established, the bladder mucosa and the ectopic ureteral wall are incised parallel to the longitudinal axis of the ureter at the level of the bladder trigone. It can at this point be helpful to pass a red rubber catheter retrograde up the ureter while suturing the new stoma. The edges of the ureteral incision are sutured to the bladder mucosa to create a new ureteral stoma using a fine (4-0 to 5-0) syn-thetic absorbable monofilament suture material in a simple interrupted pattern. The distal ureteral segment is then catheterized with a red rubber catheter via the new ureteral stoma, to facilitate double ligation of the distal ectopic ureteral segment with a synthetic absorb-able suture material. This ensures that no further flow can occur through the distal ureteral tunnel.

Creation of a new stoma with urethral-trigonal reconstruction

In common with the previous technique, a new stoma is created from the ureter into the bladder trigone region. At that point, instead of simple ligation, the distal seg-ment of the ectopic ureteral tunnel is catheterized in an antegrade fashion using the largest sized red rubber catheter that will fit down the tunnel (some ectopic ureteral tunnels are very substantial in diameter). In some cases, the catheter will be seen to exit the distal ureteral opening if it opens into the proximal urethra (Figure 47.2). However, in some cases the distal ureteral tunnel will open more distally within the pelvic canal, in

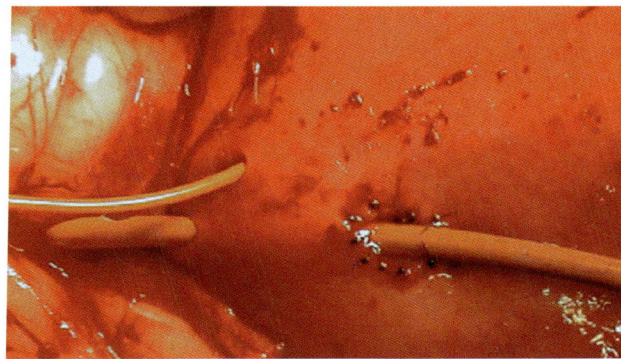

Figure 47.2 After creation of the new stoma has been completed on one side, the distal ectopic ureteral tunnel can be catheterized prior to resection of the intramural tunnel.

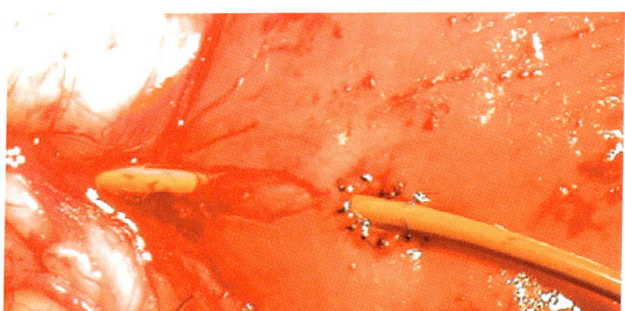

Figure 47.3 An incision has been made over the intramural tunnel prior to its isolation and resection.

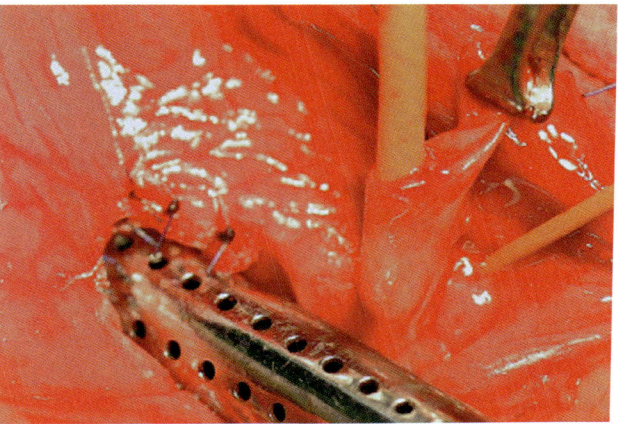

Figure 47.4 In this dog a large dilated intramural tunnel has been dissected out prior to its complete resection. The end of the Poole suction tip is located within the ureter at the site of the new stoma.

which case the catheter will not be seen to emerge from the tunnel. An incision should be made over the distal aspect of the tunnel (Figure 47.3). Fine Metzenbaum scissors should be used to dissect the ureteral tunnel from the surrounding urethra, being careful to disrupt the smooth muscle of the urethral wall as little as possible. In some cases the urethral tunnel may be completely dissected and removed (Figure 47.4). In other cases where the ureter tunnels into the pelvic cavity and dissection to the end of the tunnel is impossible, a pubic symphysiotomy can be performed or the distal end of the ureteral tunnel can be ligated at the most distal point possible, with the remaining segment of ureteral tunnel left in place. After as much as possible of the ureteral tunnel has been dissected out, the urethral wall is reapposed using 4-0 to 5-0 synthetic absorbable monofilament sutures in a simple interrupted or continuous pattern. During suturing profuse hemorrhage will occur, which is usually alleviated once suturing is complete (McLoughlin & Chew 2000).

For both techniques the cystotomy and urethrotomy are closed using a fine (3-0 to 4-0) synthetic absorbable suture material in a simple interrupted or continuous

appositional pattern. The celiotomy incision is thereafter closed routinely. It has been theorized that urethral-trigonal reconstruction might result in reduced postoperative incontinence due to realignment of muscle fibers within the proximal urethral sphincter mechanism (McLoughlin & Chew 2000; McLoughlin & Bjorling 2003). Others have not found that urethral-trigonal reconstruction improved postoperative persistent incontinence rates (Mayhew et al. 2006). In a retrospective study comparing the results of the distal ureteral ligation technique and the urethral-trigonal reconstruction technique in 36 dogs, postoperative incontinence persisted in 71% of the reconstruction group, whereas only 50% of the ligation animals remained incontinent, although these results were not statistically different between groups. Superiority of the reconstruction technique could not be shown and it was hypothesized that removal of the distal ureteral segment could even cause greater disruption to the urethral sphincter mechanism than leaving the ureteral tunnel in situ (Mayhew et al. 2006). One potential advantage of the reconstruction technique is avoidance of recanalization, which has rarely been reported in dogs after simple distal ureteral tunnel ligation (Holt & Hotson-Moore 1995). The incidence of postoperative urinary tract infection could also be affected by leaving a blind-ended distal ureteral tunnel within the urethral wall, although no difference was found in the incidence of postoperative urinary tract infection between the two techniques (Mayhew et al. 2006). It seems, therefore, that in dogs where pubic symphysiotomy would be necessary to resect the very distal segment of the distal ureteral tunnel, this procedure is unwarranted. Three dogs that underwent the procedure remained at least somewhat incontinent postoperatively (Mayhew *et al.* 2006). Most authors now agree that pubic symphysiotomy for distal tunnel resection is probably not warranted, although studies to confirm this hypothesis are lacking (McLoughlin & Chew 2000; Mayhew *et al.* 2006).

Reimplantation of the ureter

This technique is generally indicated to treat extramural ectopic ureters, which are exceedingly rare in dogs and somewhat more common in cats. A ventral midline celiotomy is performed extending caudally all the way to the pubis. Exploration of the peritoneal cavity and close examination of the ureters and their entrance point into the bladder should be performed. It is suspected that many cases of extramural ectopic ureters are misdiagnosed based on preoperative imaging and so confirmation of this anomaly at surgery should always be made (Mason *et al.* 1990; Stone & Mason 1990). In general, the distal end of the affected ureter should be identified and ligated as close to its termination as possible. The ligating suture is left slightly long and care is taken not to twist the ureter during manipulation, which can compromise its blood supply. Several techniques of ureteral reimplantation have been described in both dogs and cats.

Canine reimplantation of the ureter

In dogs a submucosal tunnel technique and a transverse pull-through technique have been described (Waldron *et al.* 1987). For both techniques a ventral cystotomy is performed and stay sutures are placed at the apex of the bladder as well as on both sides of the longitudinal incision to allow good visualization. A location is chosen for the new stoma in the dorsal bladder wall somewhere from the bladder apex to the trigone. A small incision is made in the bladder mucosa and a small oval area of the bladder mucosa is resected corresponding to the anticipated diameter of the distal ureter. For the submucosal tunnel technique, a short oblique submucosal tunnel is created using small mosquito forceps. The long end of the ureteral ligating suture is then used to pull the ureter through into the bladder. The distal end of the ureter is resected back to healthy tissue. The ureter is cut at an oblique angle or a small longitudinal incision is made in the ureteral tip to spatulate the opening. The margins of the ureteral mucosa are then sutured to the surrounding bladder mucosa with 4–6 simple interrupted sutures using fine (5-0 to 6-0) monofilament absorbable suture material (McLoughlin & Chew 2000). The transverse pull-through technique is similar, although no submucosal tunnel is established and the distal ureter is pulled through the bladder wall transversely. However, in a study comparing the two techniques, the pull-through

technique was associated with greater fibrosis at the implantation site and more severe ureteral and renal pelvic distension in the postoperative period (Waldron *et al.* 1987). It should be noted that in both dogs and cats, postoperative hydroureter and hydronephrosis can occur in many patients due to partial ureteral obstruction after surgery, and this has been reported in up to 50% of patients after ureteral reimplantation (Holt *et al.* 1982; Holt & Hotson-Moore 1995; Waldron *et al.* 1987; Mehl *et al.* 2005). Contributing to this may be the loss of normal ureteral peristalsis that occurs after ureteral transection for up to 3 weeks in dogs (Caine & Hermann 1970), or some degree of postoperative ureteral stricturing. Other evidence for partial ureteral obstruction in dogs that undergo ureteral reimplantation has been shown by renal scintigraphy studies that have demonstrated partial ureteral obstruction persisting for 1–2 weeks after ureteroneocystostomy in dogs when measured by 99mTc-DTPA renal scintigraphy (Barthez *et al.* 2000).

Feline reimplantation of the ureter

In cats considerable attention has been given to the subject of ureteroneocystostomy due to the role this procedure plays in feline renal transplantation. Cats are particularly susceptible to ureteral obstruction after reimplantation due to the tiny dimensions of the ureters in this species, the distal feline ureter measuring only 0.4 mm in diameter. Meticulous surgical technique and the use of an operating microscope are considered essential when this microsurgical technique is performed. The same care should be taken when ureteroneocystostomy is performed for treatment of extramural ectopic ureter in cats, which, although a rare disease, occurs with greater frequency compared to dogs (Holt & Hotson-Moore 1992). However, when a ureter is ectopic its diameter is significantly larger than normal, making the reimplantation easier.

The first preimplantation technique described in cats was a simple "drop-in" technique, where the ureter was passed through a small incision in the bladder wall and the distal tip of the ureter was secured to the bladder mucosa with a single suture from the bladder serosa to the adventitia of the ureter (Gregory *et al.* 1992, 1996; Kochin *et al.* 1993). Unfortunately, this technique was not successful due to a very high rate of granulation tissue formation around the stoma site with subsequent obstruction of urine flow (Gregory *et al.* 1992, 1996). An intravesicular technique was then developed that allowed mucosal apposition of the ureteral margin and was not associated with a significant incidence of postoperative ureteral obstruction (Gregory *et al.* 1996). With this technique the distal ureter is drawn transversely through a small incision in the bladder wall. The distal 0.75–1 cm of the ureter is cleared of periureteral fat. The distal tip is resected back to fresh ureteral tissue and then a longitudinal incision 3–5 mm long is made in the distal ureter to achieve spatulation of the distal end. Sutures of 8-0 nylon are placed full thickness through the ureteral wall and into the bladder mucosa, and tied in a simple interrupted appositional fashion. Sutures were placed initially at the extremities of the cut edge of the ureter to fan out the distal ureter as much as possible. It was thought that minimizing the exposure of the periureteral tissues to urine minimized the inflammatory response, thereby reducing granulation tissue formation and subsequent urinary obstruction (Gregory *et al.* 1996). Also a monofilament absorbable suture might reduce the risk of granulation tissue formation.

More recently, extravesicular techniques have been described for reimplantation of ureter in cats and may have some advantages over the intravesicular mucosal appositional technique described by Gregory (Figure 47.5). In this technique a partial-thickness incision through muscularis and submucosa is made and the mucosa of the bladder is exposed. The distal end of the ureter is spatulated and an incision of corresponding length is made in the caudal aspect of the exposed bladder mucosa. Two full-thickness simple interrupted sutures of 7-0 or 8-0 nylon are placed at opposing cranial and caudal margins of the spatulated tip of the ureter and corresponding bladder mucosa. A 4-0 polypropylene stent is then placed into the lumen of the ureter to ensure patency during further suturing, but it must be removed before the last suture is placed. Sutures are then placed

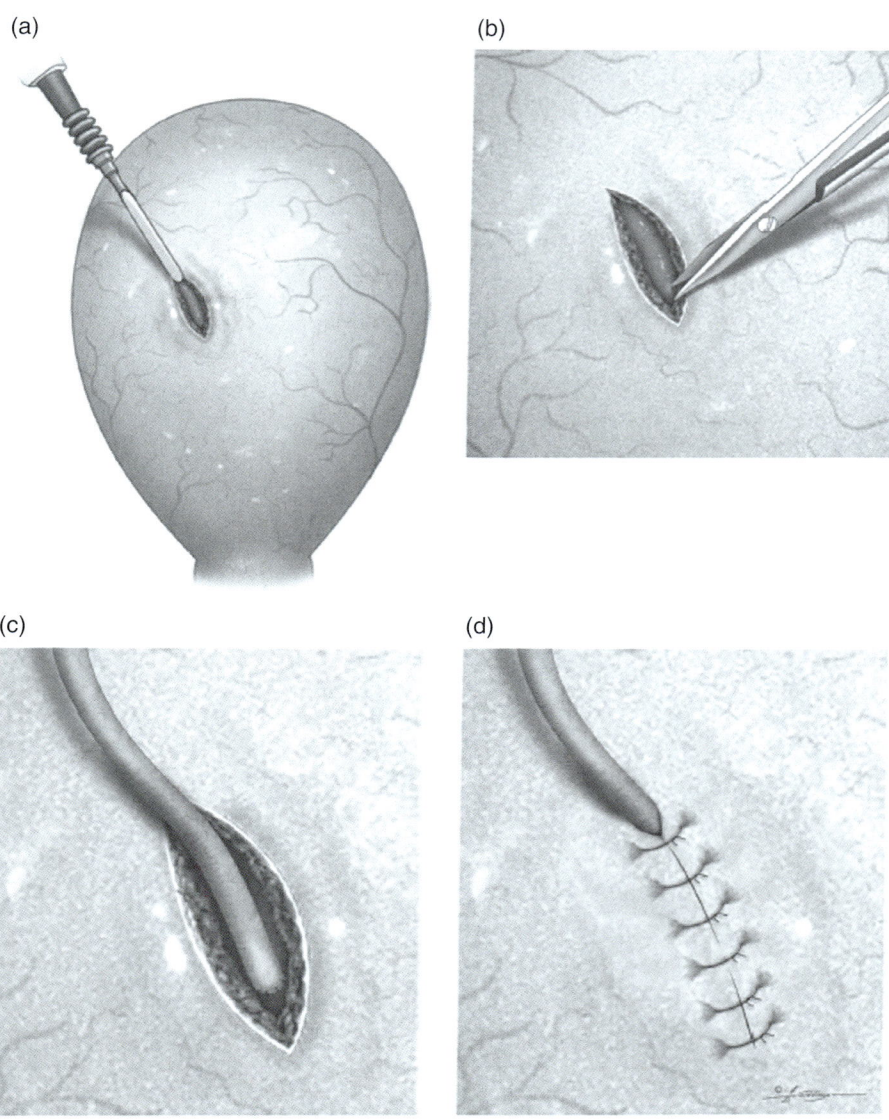

(a)

(b)

(c)

(d)

Figure 47.5 (a–d) Extravesicular technique for reimplantation of a ureter. © D. Giddings.

between the ureteral wall and the bladder mucosa between the two previously placed sutures to complete the circumferential apposition of ureteral to bladder walls. Finally, simple interrupted sutures of 4-0 polydioxanone are placed across the seromuscular layers of the bladder around the stoma site on the serosal side to complete the closure. A variation of this extravesicular technique is to place two simple continuous suture lines of 8-0 nylon between the ureteral and bladder mucosal layers instead of simple interrupted sutures. These two variations of the extravesicular technique were compared to the classical intravesicular mucosal apposition technique described by Gregory in a recent prospective study involving contralaterally nephrectomized cats (Mehl *et al.* 2005). The authors found that cats undergoing extravesicular simple interrupted suturing had lower elevation in serum creatinine in the week postoperatively compared to the other two groups. The extravesicular technique also resulted in less renal pelvic dilatation compared to the intravesicular technique. The authors concluded that although some ureteral dilatation is to be expected after preimplantation in cats, most likely due to transient obstruction to flow, the extravesicular technique sutured with a simple interrupted pattern is most likely the reimplantation technique of choice in cats (Mehl *et al.* 2005).

Ureteronephrectomy

Even though early reports advocated ureteronephrectomy as a good treatment for ureteral ectopia (Owen 1973), removal of the affected kidney and ureter should only be performed in dogs and cats where one kidney is so severely damaged that no significant renal function remains and in cases where function in the contralateral kidney is judged to be normal or adequate. Techniques used to assess function of individual kidney function include ultrasonography and renal scintigraphy and have already been discussed.

Technique

A routine ventral midline celiotomy is performed and the abdominal cavity is fully explored (McLoughlin & Chew 2000; Fossum 2007). The affected kidney is dissected out from its retroperitoneal attachments and reflected medially. The vascular pedicle should be exposed and the renal artery, vein, and ureter identified. The renal artery and vein are double ligated using 2-0 to 3-0 silk ligatures and the most distal ligature is usually transfixed to avoid slippage. After sectioning of the vascular pedicles, the kidney should be completely dissected free with only the ureteral attachment left intact. The ureter is then dissected out of its retroperitoneal bed

all the way down to the bladder. It is ligated at its most distal point as it enters the bladder with two encircling ligatures of a monofilament absorbable suture material. It has been suggested that the distal ureteral intramural tunnel (in cases of intramural ureteral ectopia) should be dissected out of the trigonal and urethral mucosa through a cystotomy incision after the ureteronephrectomy is complete, to avoid ongoing incontinence postoperatively (McLoughlin & Chew 2000). Objective data demonstrating the importance of this have not been published to the authors' knowledge.

Ureteronephrectomy in dogs with ureteral ectopia is associated with few complications when performed correctly (Lapish 1985; Stone & Mason 1990; McLaughlin & Miller 1991; Holt & Hotson-Moore 1995; Gookin *et al.* 1996). Reported complications postoperatively include postoperative oliguria, acute renal failure, blood loss requiring blood transfusion, and pancreatitis (Gookin *et al.* 1996). In a large group of dogs in which the results of ureteronephrectomy were compared to other procedures for the treatment of ureteral ectopia, no obvious improvement in the incidence of postoperative incontinence was seen compared to other procedures, with 40% of dogs remaining at least partially incontinent after surgery (Holt & Hotson-Moore 1995). In this study ureteronephrectomy was, however, associated with a lower complication rate compared to ureteral transplantation (Holt & Hotson-Moore 1995). These results must be interpreted with caution, as the study was not randomized and so results are almost certainly biased by the clinical choices made by the attending clinicians. The reason some dogs undergoing ureteronephrectomy remain incontinent are likely to include unrecognized contralateral ectopia, concurrent USMI, or other urinary tract abnormalities leading to incontinence.

Cystoscopic-guided laser ablation of ectopic ureters

All dogs with intramural ureteral ectopia can be considered candidates for this minimally invasive procedure. The procedure is performed with the use of fluoroscopy, cystoscopy, and a diode or holmium:YAG laser. It can be performed on an outpatient basis at the time of cystoscopic diagnosis, necessitating only one anesthetic episode for both diagnosis and treatment. This procedure can be performed in both dogs and cats with intramural ureteral ectopia and has been described in small case series previously (Berent *et al.* 2008, 2012; Smith *et al.* 2009).

Procedure

The patient is placed in dorsal recumbency and a rigid cystoscope is advanced into the vestibule and urethral orifice in a retrograde fashion by use of manual irrigation with saline (0.9% NaCl) solution. Each ureterovesicular junction (UVJ) is carefully evaluated and the ectopic ureters are identified and their location confirmed. Care should be taken to evaluate for multiple fenestrations, trigonal location, and other anatomic anomalies. A portable C-arm fluoroscopy unit is used to perform retrograde contrast ureteropyelography to confirm the presence of an intramural ectopic tract, as well as to document ureteral and renal pelvis diameter (Figure 47.6). A 0.025–0.035 angled, hydrophilic-tip guidewire is advanced up the ureter through the working channel of the cystoscope, under fluoroscopic and cystoscopic guidance. A 4 or 5 French, open-ended ureteral catheter is advanced over the guidewire into the distal portion of the ureter through the ureteral orifice. A retrograde ureteropyelogram is performed using 5 mL of iodinated nonionic contrast material (240 mg/mL), diluted 50:50 with sterile saline, by injecting retrograde up the ureteral catheter to identify the ureteral path through the urethral wall and determine the anatomic features of the ureter and renal pelvis (Figure 47.6). Then 5–10 mL/kg (4.54 mL/lb) of this mixture is injected into the urethra through the cystoscope for a retrograde cystourethrogram, allowing for a combination cystourethrouretropyelogram. This permits evaluation of the bladder trigone in relation to the ureteral orifice and the transition of the ureter from intra- to extramural (Figure 47.6). Once an intramural ureteral tract is

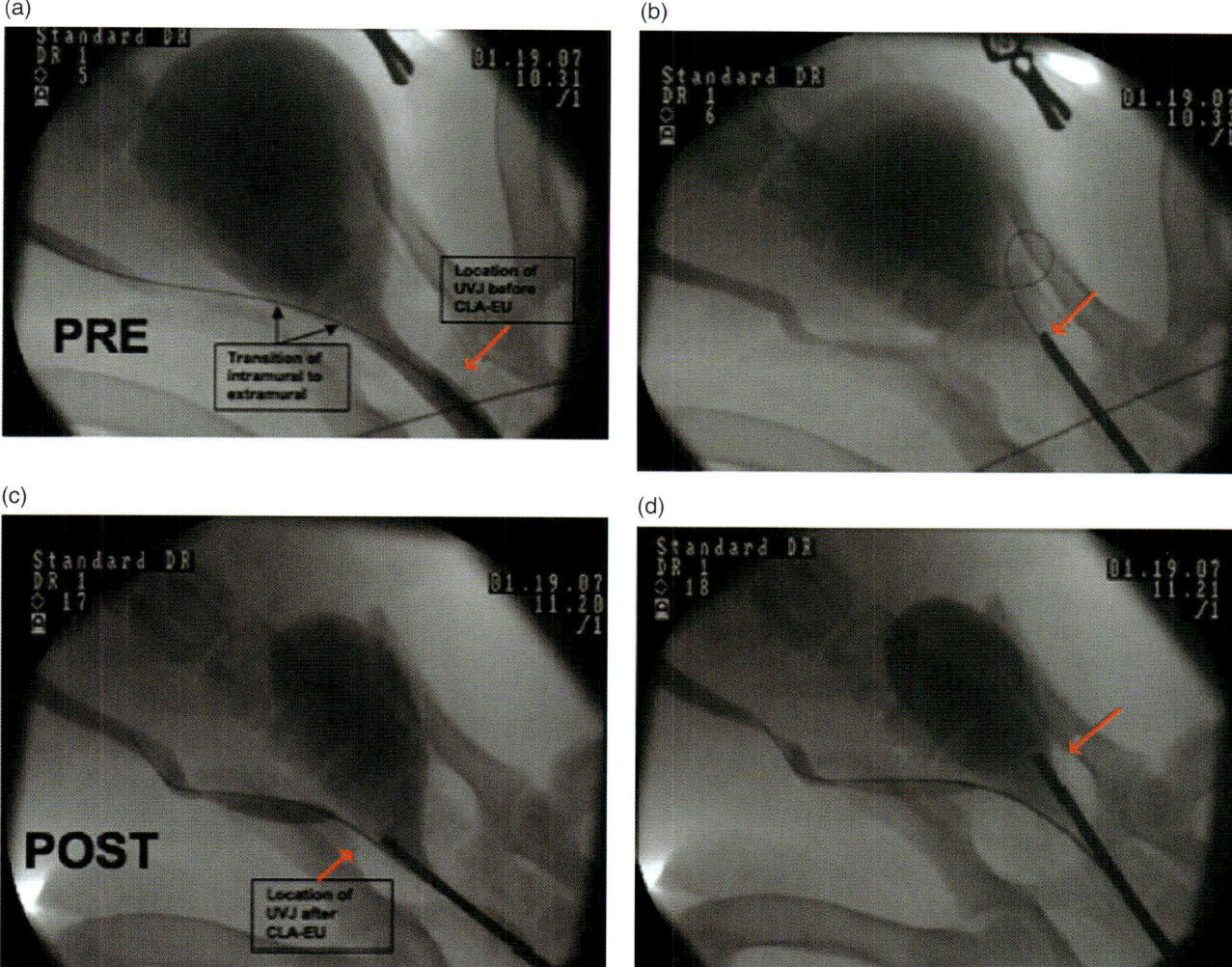

Figure 47.6 Fluoroscopic images of a female dog before and after cystoscopic-guided laser ablation of ectopic ureters. (a) A cystourethrogram and retrograde ureteropyelogram (of the right ureter) are performed simultaneously to confirm intramural travel of the ectopic ureter. A rigid cystoscopy (red arrow) is at the opening of the ectopic ureter prior to laser ablation. A guidewire (black arrows) is up the ureter documenting the ureteral path and protecting the ureter during laser ablation. (b) The left ureteral orifice location prior to laser ablation (red arrow). (c) The location of the new ureteral opening (red arrow; right side) inside the urinary bladder after the procedure. (d) The location of the new ureteral opening (red arrow; left side) inside the urinary bladder after the procedure.

confirmed, the cystoscope is removed over the wire–catheter combination, and they are secured to the drape using a hemostat. The cystoscope is then reinserted into the urethra, next to the wire–catheter combination and the laser fiber (600 μm diode or 400 μm holmium:yttrium aluminum, garnet) is inserted into the working channel of the cystoscope and directed into the ureteral orifice. The cystoscope is directed toward the urethral lumen to angle the laser fiber's tip toward the medial wall of the ureter, avoiding the lateral wall and ureteral catheter (Figure 47.7). The medial ureteral wall is then carefully cut in a continuous manner by use of the diode laser at 16–25 W or a pulsed manner by use of the hol:YAG laser (10–20 Hz, 0.5–1.0 J at a pulse width of 700 ms). When the neo-ureteral orifice is seen within the bladder lumen, cranial to the trigone, or the ureter appears to be diverging from its path alongside the urethra or bladder lumen, suggesting the potential transition from its intramural to its extramural course, a cystourethrogram is performed to confirm that the new UVJ is within the bladder lumen (Figure 47.6). This procedure is repeated on the contralateral side for patients with bilateral ectopia.

A retrograde contrast urethrocystogram and ureteropyelogram are performed in each dog after the cystoscopic-guided laser ablation (CLA) procedure to ensure that there is no extravasation of contrast medium and to document the new location of the ureteral orifice relative to the bladder trigone both cystoscopically and fluoroscopically (Figure 47.6).

The procedure in male dogs has also been reported and is also done via cystoscopy (Berent et al. 2008). This is done with a flexible cystoscope and a 200 μm hol:YAG laser fiber. A few male dogs have also had this procedure performed via percutaneous transurethral needle access to the ischial urethra using fluoroscopic urethral access and serial urethral dilation. The goal is to accommodate a sheath large enough to accept the rigid cystoscope. The procedure can then be performed as described earlier for female dogs. It is important to confirm ureteral ectopia with flexible cystoscopy prior to the transurethral approach being attempted.

Postoperative care and complications

Dogs are administered meloxicam (0.1 mg/kg subcutaneously) upon recovery from the laser procedure, if no chronic kidney disease exists, and the urethra is infused with a bupivacaine (1 mg/kg) solution diluted with an equal volume of sterile saline solution for local transurethral analgesia. Patients are administered 7 days of antibiotics and 2 days of tramadol for pain management after the procedure. In the author's practice a prospective study of 30 female dogs has been completed. For all dogs a cystoscopy was performed at 6–8 weeks after the CLA ureteral ectopia procedure. About 80% of female dogs were continent at >6 months follow-up (~50% with CLA alone, ~60% with additional medications, ~65% with additional collagen injections, and ~80% with the addition of a hydraulic occluder [HO]). The only complication seen was polypoid cystitis seen at the neo-ureteral stoma at 6 weeks during second-look cystoscopy in one dog. Other reported complications include inflammatory reactions at the neo-UVJ or along the laser tract. This is not a common complication noted in this series, of which all dogs were reevaluated postoperatively. In

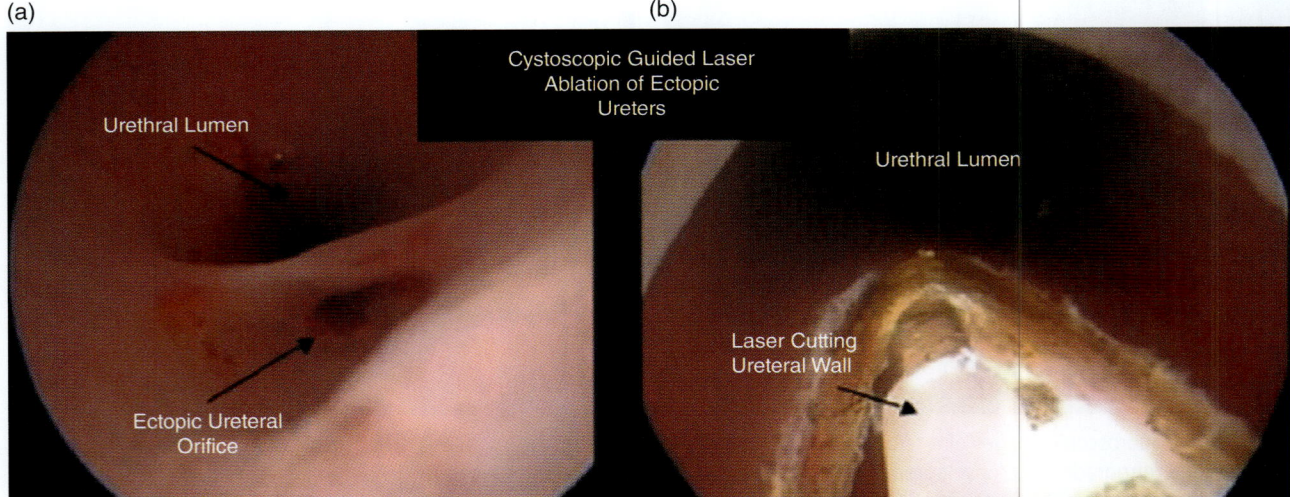

Figure 47.7 Cystoscopy of female dog placed in dorsal recumbency with a left-sided intramural ectopic ureter. (a) Prior to laser ablation. (b) A diode laser is used to cut the medial ureteral wall of the left ureter as it tunnels intramurally inside the urethra. A safety ureteral catheter/guidewire combination is inside the ureteral lumen to protect the lateral wall of the ureteral lumen.

most facilities performing this procedure the use of fluoroscopy is not routine. Care should be taken without fluoroscopy to confirm the intramural nature of these defects. The procedure in male dogs resulted in continence in 100% of cases reported (Berent *et al.* 2008).

This technique is fast, effective, and minimally invasive, avoiding celiotomy, cystotomy, urethrotomy, and ureterotomy. To date this procedure has been performed in both male and female dogs and female cats with success. In female cats you need to use a 1.9 mm rigid cystoscope and a small laser fiber is necessary to fit through the working channel. The CLA ureteral ectopia procedure is safe and appears to be similarly effective to the traditional surgical techniques previously reported, although no randomized study exists to compare the postoperative incontinence rates between procedures. This procedure has been associated with few complications and can be considered at the time of the diagnosis of ectopic ureters. This procedure avoids invasive surgery and if resolution of continence is not seen postoperatively, other more invasive procedures described can be performed subsequently.

Prognosis for ureteral ectopia in dogs and cats

The prognosis for dogs with ureteral ectopia remains guarded, principally due to the high level of persistent postoperative incontinence associated with the disease regardless of treatment modality selected. No surgical or minimally invasive technique has been shown to be superior to any other with regard to postoperative incontinence. No prospective randomized studies exist comparing different approaches to the treatment of ureteral ectopia. The reported outcomes of the different techniques are summarized in Table 47.1. Postoperative incontinence rates for the various "open" surgical techniques vary from 42% to 78% (Holt *et al.* 1982; Stone & Mason 1990; Holt & Hotson-Moore 1995; Noel *et al.* 2017). The CLA technique has a reported postoperative incontinence rate of 53–68% in female dogs (Smith *et al.* 2009; Berent *et al.* 2012). In one study of 32 female dogs, 47% of dogs were completely continent after CLA alone. When the subpopulation of dogs that were not completely continent received additional medical management and/or other interventions (urethral bulking agents or HO placement), the continence rate increased to 77% at a median follow-up of 2.7 years (range 12–62 months). The success has been found after open surgical repair where in combination with medical or interventional management, at a median of 46 months postoperatively, 74% of dogs were considered continent (Noel *et al.* 2017). In 4 male dogs treated with the CLA

technique, a superior outcome was achieved when compared to the female dogs, with 4/4 dogs being continent postoperatively in a median follow-up time of 18 months without any medical management (Berent *et al.* 2008). The prognosis in cats appears to be somewhat better than in dogs. In one report summarizing the outcome for 23 cats, 16 of 18 surgically treated cats that survived the procedure were continent postoperatively (Holt & Gibbs 1992).

Prognostic indicators for a successful outcome after ureteral ectopia surgery have been investigated by several authors. Siberian huskies were shown to have a higher rate of postoperative incontinence in one study (McLaughlin & Miller 1991). Female sex and proximal urethral location of the ectopic ureteral opening were associated with a higher risk of postoperative incontinence in another study (Wiegand *et al.* 1996). The presence of hydroureter and/or hydronephrosis was associated with a decreased risk (Wiegand *et al.* 1996). Urethral pressure profilometry has been shown to be helpful in predicting outcome after surgery in dogs with ureteral ectopia (Lane *et al.* 1995). Preoperative maximal urethral closure pressure (MUCP), functional profile length (FPL), and functional profile area (FPA) were significantly higher in dogs that were continent postoperatively (Lane *et al.* 1995). It was suggested that in dogs with preoperative MUCP >19 cm H_2O and FPA >168 cm H_2O, postoperative continence could have been predicted in 89% of cases. Factors that have been evaluated but were not shown to have a significant effect on postoperative outcome include whether the ectopic ureters are unilateral or bilateral, bladder position (intrapelvic versus intra-abdominal), urethral length, age at the time of surgery, bodyweight, presence of a UTI, or surgical technique (McLaughlin & Miller 1991; Holt & Hotson-Moore 1995; Wiegand *et al.* 1996; Noel *et al.* 2017). Risk factors for successful outcome in cats after surgery for ureteral ectopia have not been evaluated.

In patients with persistent postoperative incontinence, medical management is usually instituted and has been shown to improve postoperative continence rates in most studies (Table 47.1). The α-adrenergic drug propanolamine is most commonly used and has been shown to improve outcome in many studies in dogs that were nonresponsive or only partially responsive to surgery (McLaughlin & Miller 1991; Holt & Hotson-Moore 1995; Mayhew *et al.* 2006). In addition to medical management, endoscopically placed submucosal injections of collagen into the urethral wall have been advocated for persistent postoperative incontinence in dogs with ureteral ectopia, as they have for dogs with USMI (McLoughlin & Chew 2000). However, it has been suggested that response rates to submucosal collagen

Table 47.1 Review of the literature.

Study authors	No. of patients treated	No. of females	No. of males	Treatment modality	% PO incontinence – surgery alone	% PO incontinence – surgery + medication	% PO incontinence – surgery + medication + other	Follow-up time
Stone & Mason (1990)	17 dogs	17	1	Neoureterostomy with distal ureteral ligation	53%	N/A	N/A	Mean 2.4 years
McLaughlin & Miller (1991)	14 dogs	N/A	N/A	Neoureterostomy with distal ureteral ligation	50%	N/A	N/A	2–82 months (median 27 months)
	4 dogs	N/A	N/A	Ureteroneocystostomy	75%	N/A	N/A	
Holt & Hotson-Moore (1995)	49 dogs	N/A	N/A	Ureteroneocystostomy	50%	N/A	N/A	1 month to 15 years (median >2 years)
	44 dogs	N/A	N/A	Neoureterostomy with distal ureteral ligation	32%	N/A	N/A	
	36 dogs	N/A	N/A	Ureteronephrectomy	40%	N/A	N/A	
Lane et al. (1995)	9 dogs	9	0	Neoureterostomy (n = 5), Ureteroneocystostomy (n = 2), Ureteronephrectomy (n = 1)	78%	56%	N/A	>6 months
Mayhew et al. (2006)	21 dogs	17	4	Neoureterostomy with urethral-trigonal reconstruction	71%	43%	N/A	Mean 51 months (range 5–118 months)
	15 dogs	13	2	Neoureterostomy with distal ureteral ligation	50%	43%	N/A	Mean 50 months (range 9–109 months)
Noel et al. (2017)	47 dogs	36	11	Neoureterostomy (n = 50), ureteroneocystostomy (n = 9), ureteronephrectomy (n = 7)	N/A	N/A	74%	Mean of 46 months (range 4–148 months)
Berent et al. (2008)	4 dogs	0	4	CLA	0%	0%	0%	Median 18 months (range 15–20 months)
Smith et al. (2009)	16 dogs 1 cat	17	0	CLA	68%	35%	N/A	N/A
Berent et al. (2012)	32 dogs	32	0	CLA	47%	N/A	77%[a]	Median 2.7 years (range 12–62 months)

CLA, cystoscopic-guided laser ablation; N/A, not available.
[a] Includes the use of a surgically positioned hydraulic occluder.

injection in dogs with ureteral ectopia may be lower than in dogs that only have USMI (Berent, personal communication). Further surgical interventions have been used to increase the chance of postoperative continence in dogs where the traditional surgical approaches have not been successful. Colposuspension has been used concurrently with neoureterostomy to treat female dogs with ureteral ectopia (Mouatt & Watt 2001; Noel et al. 2017). In one study 7 dogs that underwent both procedures had a postoperative long-term continence rate of 71% (Mouatt & Watt 2001) and in another postoperative continence was achieved in 74% of cases (Noel et al. 2017). The use of HOs has also been advocated for use in dogs that have not responded to traditional surgical or CLA repair. In one study 10 of 18 dogs had an HO placed after failed surgical reimplantation or CLA for ectopic ureter repair (Currao et al. 2013) and another study documented the use of an HO in 6 dogs that had failed to become continent after primary treatment of ureteral ectopia (Reeves et al. 2013). There did not seem to be any difference between dogs that had ureteral ectopia with USMI or USMI alone with regard to continence outcomes in those that had an HO placed (Currao et al. 2013).

Persistent UTI is another postoperative issue that can cause ongoing morbidity. In one study episodes of postoperative UTI were recorded in 15% of dogs undergoing neoureterostomy with trigonal reconstruction and 29% of dogs undergoing neoureterostomy with distal ureteral ligation (Mayhew et al. 2006). In this study 66% of dogs were diagnosed with a UTI prior to surgery and so an apparent decrease in the incidence of UTIs may have occurred postoperatively.

References

Barthez, P.Y., Smeak, D.D., Wisner, E.R. et al. (2000). Ureteral obstruction after ureteroneocystostomy in dogs assessed by technetium TC 99m diethylenetriamine pentaacetic acid scintigraphy. *Veterinary Surgery* 29: 499–506.

Berent, A.C., Mayhew, P.D., and Porat-Mosenco, Y. (2008). Use of cystoscopic-guided laser ablation for treatment of intramural ureteral ectopia in male dogs: four cases (2006-7). *Journal of the American Veterinary Medical Association* 232: 1026–1034.

Berent, A.C., Weisse, C., Mayhew, P.D. et al. (2012). Evaluation of cystoscopic-guided laser ablation of intramural ectopic ureters in female dogs. *Journal of the American Veterinary Medical Association* 240: 716–725.

Caine, M. and Hermann, G. (1970). The return of peristalsis in the anastomosed ureter. *British Journal of Urology* 42: 164–170.

Cannizzo, K.L., McLoughlin, M.A., Mattoon, J.S. et al. (2003). Evaluation of transurethral cystoscopy and excretory urography for diagnosis of ectopic ureters in female dogs: 25 cases (1992–2000). *Journal of the American Veterinary Medical Association* 223: 475–481.

Currao, R.L., Berent, A.C., Weisse, C. et al. (2013). Use of a percutaneously controlled urethral hydraulic occluder for treatment of

refractory urinary incontinence in 18 female dogs. *Veterinary Surgery* 42: 440–447.

Feeney, D.A., Barber, D.L., and Osborne, C.A. (1982). The functional aspects of the nephrogram in excretory urography: a review. *Veterinary Radiology* 23: 42–45.

Fossum, T.W. (2007). Surgery of the kidney and ureter. In: *Small Animal Surgery*, 3e (ed. T.W. Fossum), 635–662. St. Louis, MO: Mosby Elsevier.

Gookin, J.L., Stone, E.A., Spaulding, K.A. et al. (1996). Unilateral nephrectomy in dogs with renal disease: 30 cases (1985–1994). *Journal of the American Veterinary Medical Association* 208: 2020–2026.

Gregory, C.R., Gourley, I.M., Kochin, E.J. et al. (1992). Renal transplantation for treatment of end-stage renal failure in cats. *Journal of the American Veterinary Medicine Association* 201: 285–291.

Gregory, C.R., Lirtzman, R.A., Kochin, E.J. et al. (1996). A mucosal apposition technique for ureteroneocysostomy after renal transplantation in cats. *Veterinary Surgery* 25: 13–17.

Holt, P.E. and Gibbs, C. (1992). Congenital urinary incontinence in cats: a review of 19 cases. *Veterinary Record* 130: 437–442.

Holt, P.E. and Hotson-Moore, A. (1995). Canine ureteral ectopia: an analysis of 175 cases and comparison of surgical treatments. *Veterinary Record* 136: 345–349.

Holt, P.E., Gibbs, C., and Pearson, H. (1982). Canine ectopic ureter – a review of twenty-nine cases. *Journal of Small Animal Practice* 23: 195–208.

Kerl, M.E. and Cook, C.R. (2005). Glomerular filtration rate and renal scintigraphy. *Clinical Techniques in Small Animal Practice* 20: 31–38.

Kochin, E.J., Gregory, C.R., Wisner, E. et al. (1993). Evaluation of a method of ureteroneocystostomy in cats. *Journal of the American Veterinary Medical Association* 202: 257–260.

Lamb, C.R. and Gregory, S.P. (1998). Ultrasonographic findings in 14 dogs with ectopic ureter. *Veterinary Radiology & Ultrasound* 39: 218–223.

Lane, I.F., Lappin, M.R., and Seim, H.B. (1995). Evaluation of results of preoperative urodynamic measurements in nine dogs with ectopic ureters. *Journal of the American Veterinary Medical Association* 206: 1348–1357.

Lapish, J.P. (1985). Hydronephrosis, hydroureter, and hydrometra associated with ectopic ureter in a bitch. *Journal of Small Animal Practice* 26: 613–617.

Mason, L.K., Stone, E.A., Biery, D.N. et al. (1990). Surgery of ectopic ureters: pre- and postoperative radiographic morphology. *Journal of the American Animal Hospital Association* 26: 73–79.

Mayhew, P.D., Lee, K.C.L., Gregory, S.P. et al. (2006). Comparison of two surgical techniques for management of intramural ureteral ectopia in dogs: 36 cases (1994–2004). *Journal of the American Veterinary Medical Association* 229: 389–393.

McCarthy, T.C. (2006). Transurethral cystoscopy and diode laser incision to correct an ectopic ureter. *Veterinary Medicine* 101 (9): 558–559.

McLaughlin, R. and Miller, C.W. (1991). Urinary incontinence after surgical repair of ureteral ectopia in dogs. *Veterinary Surgery* 20: 100–103.

McLoughlin, M.A. and Bjorling, D.E. (2003). Ureters. In: *Textbook of Small Animal Surgery*, 3e (ed. D. Slatter), 1619–1628. Philadelphia, PA: Saunders.

McLoughlin, M.A. and Chew, D.J. (2000). Diagnosis and surgical management of ectopic ureters. *Clinical Techniques in Small Animal Practice* 15: 17–24.

Mehl, M.L., Kyles, A.E., Pollard, R. et al. (2005). Comparison of 3 techniques for ureteroneocystostomy in cats. *Veterinary Surgery* 34: 114–119.

Mouatt, J.G. and Watt, P.R. (2001). Ectopic ureter repair and colposuspension in seven bitches. *Australian Veterinary Practitioner* 31 (4): 160–167.

Neuwirth, L., Mahaffey, M., Cromwell, W. et al. (1993). Comparison of excretory urography and ultrasonography for detection of experimentally induced pyelonephritis in dogs. *American Journal of Veterinary Research* 54: 660–669.

Noel, S.M., Claeys, S., and Hamaide, A.J. (2017). Surgical management of ectopic ureters in dogs: clinical outcome and prognostic factors for long-term continence. *Veterinary Surgery* 46: 631–641.

Owen, R.R. (1973). Canine ureteral ectopia – a review. 2. Incidence, diagnosis and treatment. *Journal of Small Animal Practice* 14: 419–427.

Reeves, L., Adin, C., McLoughlin, M. et al. (2013). Outcome after placement of an artificial urethral sphincter in 27 dogs. *Veterinary Surgery* 42: 12–18.

Smith, A.L., Radlinsky, M.A., Rawlings, C. (2009). The use of cystoscopic-guided laser ablation for the treatment of intramural ureteral ectopia: a retrospective evaluation. In: *Proceedings of the American College of Veterinary Surgeons Annual Symposium 2009*, 48. Washington, DC: American College of Veterinary Surgeons.

Stone, E.A. and Mason, L.K. (1990). Surgery of ectopic ureters: types, method of correction and post-operative results. *Journal of the American Animal Hospital Association* 26: 81–88.

Waldron, D.R., Hedlund, C.S., Pechman, R.D. et al. (1987). Ureteroneocystostomy: a comparison of the submucosal tunnel and transverse pull through techniques. *Journal of the American Animal Hospital Association* 23: 285–290.

Wiegand, U., Nickel, R.F., and Van Den Brom, W.E. (1996). Zur prognose bei der behandlung von ektopischen ureteren beim hund. *Kleintierpraxis* 41: 157–167.

48

Neoplasia of the Urinary Tract

Ramesh K. Sivacolundhu and Stephen J. Withrow

Renal Neoplasia

Incidence

Primary renal tumors in dogs are uncommon and secondary/metastatic neoplasia is more common (Burgess & DeRegis 2019; Bryan et al. 2006). Renal tumors comprise 1.6–2.5% and 0.3–1.7% of reported tumors in cats and dogs, respectively (Burgess & DeRegis 2019; Crow 1985). When diagnosed, they usually occur in middle-aged to older dogs, with a mean of 7–9 years of age (Bryan et al. 2006; Baskin & De Paoli 1977). No breed predisposition has been shown in dogs. There is a breed disposition for renal lymphosarcoma in Siamese or Oriental cats, with males being more commonly affected (Gabor et al. 1998). The male to female ratio for canine renal carcinoma has been reported as 1.6:1 to 1.8:1 (Lucke & Kelly 1976; Klein et al. 1988). Nephroblastomas usually occur in young dogs and cats, but have been diagnosed in middle-aged and older dogs also (Klein et al. 1988; Baskin & De Paoli 1977; Bryan et al. 2006; Crow 1985). Secondary metastatic lesions to the kidneys may occur (Hahn et al. 1997), although they are not usually clinically evident until the disease is advanced (Crow 1985). Renal tumors are more common in cats than in dogs, presumably due to lymphoma occurring more commonly in this species (Crow 1985; Wycislo & Piech 2019).

Pathology and biological behavior

Primary renal tumors are usually malignant (Crow 1985; Baskin & De Paoli 1977). They may arise from renal epithelium (carcinomas), mesenchymal tissue (sarcomas), or embryonal tissue of mixed origin (nephroblastomas) (Bryan et al. 2006). The majority of primary renal tumors in dogs are renal carcinomas (Bryan et al. 2006). There are four subtypes: clear cell, chromophobe, papillary, and multilocular cystic (Burgess & DeRegis 2019). Tumors of the renal pelvis are rare and usually arise from transitional epithelial cells (Crow 1985). Renal sarcoma (including hemangiosarcoma, undifferentiated sarcoma, leiomyosarcoma, spindle cell sarcoma, fibromyosarcoma, and malignant fibrous histiocytoma) and nephroblastoma occur far less commonly, with reports describing 60–85% of primary renal cancer cases as epithelial, 11–34% as mesenchymal, and 4–6% as mixed (Klein et al. 1988; Bryan et al. 2006). Bilateral renal involvement has been reported in 4–32.4% of cases (Bryan et al. 2006; Klein et al. 1988). It is unclear whether renal lymphoma represents primary or multicentric disease and it is often considered separately from the more common solid tumors (Bryan et al. 2006). A case of canine lymphoma confined to the kidney with no other organ involvement has been reported (Baskin & De Paoli 1977).

Renal tumors have a moderate to high metastatic rate, with 16–34% having clinically detectable metastases at the time of diagnosis. There will be metastases detectable in the late stage of disease in 70–75% of cases (Burgess & DeRegis 2019). They metastasize readily, primarily via the hematogenous route (Baskin & De Paoli 1977; Crow 1985; Bryan et al. 2006). Pulmonary metastases are most often reported (Lucke & Kelly 1976). Other sites of metastases include lymph nodes, liver, bone, serosal surfaces, ipsilateral adrenal gland, contralateral kidney, other abdominal organs, brain, heart, and skin (Klein *et al*. 1988; Bryan *et al*. 2006; Locke & Barber 2006). Small satellite tumors within the kidney may occur (Lucke & Kelly 1976).

Apart from having metastatic potential, renal carcinomas may be locally aggressive. Most carcinomas are contained within the tumor capsule, but local invasion has been reported to the ureter, lumbar musculature, and adrenal gland (Lucke & Kelly 1976; Baskin & De Paoli 1977; Crow 1985). Intravenous extension and growth to include the renal veins and caudal vena cava can occur (Crow 1985; Lucke & Kelly 1976).

Nephroblastoma is a tumor of embryonic tissue. The tumor arises from neoplastic transformation during nephrogenesis or from nephrogenic nests that persist postnatally (Burgess & DeRegis 2019). Although nephroblastomas may follow a clinically benign course, they have been reported to reach a large size rapidly and cause emaciation, dehydration, and death (Baskin & De Paoli 1977; Crow 1985). They also have metastatic potential (Figure 48.1) (Klein *et al*. 1988; Seaman & Patton 2003; Gasser *et al*. 2003). Paraneoplastic syndromes have been reported rarely in association with primary renal tumors, including polycythemia, hypercalcemia, and hypertrophic osteopathy (Crow 1985; Chiang *et al*. 2007; Grillo *et al*. 2007).

A heritable syndrome of multiple renal cystadenocarcinomas with nodular dermatofibrosis has been reported in German shepherd dogs (Lium & Moe 1985; Klein *et al*. 1988; Moe & Lium 1997). Dogs present with firm, spherical to oval nodules of dense collagen measuring 2–5 mm in diameter, usually found subcutaneously on the limbs and head. The nodules are often very difficult

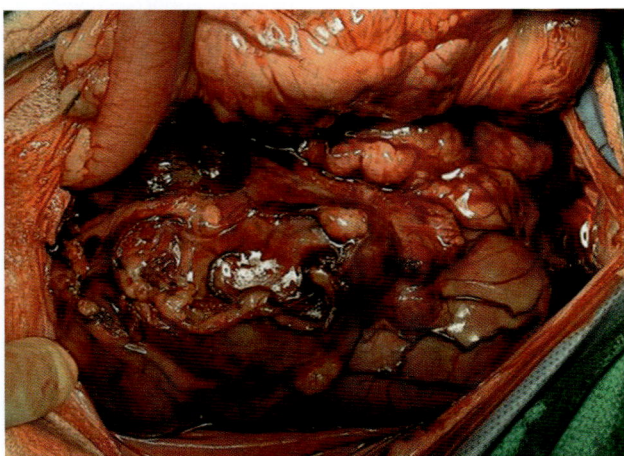

Figure 48.1 Nonresectable nephroblastoma of the right kidney in a 9-month-old dog occupying the majority of the abdominal cavity. Metastases were found at necropsy in the liver, multiple lymph nodes, and lungs.

to see. The kidneys will have multifocal lesions of solid and cystic tumors, and cysts without visible tumor tissue. Cysts range from being barely visible to over 25 cm in diameter. Both kidneys are always affected to varying degrees. Renal changes progress over years. Metastases occur in 47% of dogs to sternal lymph nodes, liver, lungs, and other abdominal lymph nodes, pleura, peritoneum, spleen, and bronchial lymph nodes. The uterus often has lesions diagnosed as leiomyomas on histology. Affected dogs should not be used for breeding (Moe & Lium 1997). The disease is probably associated with an autosomal-dominant mode of inheritance (Burgess & DeRegis 2019).

Renal hemangioma is the most common benign renal tumor in dogs (Baskin & De Paoli 1977; Mott *et al*. 1996). A diagnosis of renal adenoma is controversial as it is difficult to determine biological behavior from histologic criteria alone (Crow 1985).

In cats the most common renal tumor is lymphoma. Renal involvement is most often associated with alimentary or multicentric forms of lymphoma (Crow 1985). Of the primary renal tumors in cats, carcinomas are the most common (tubular and tubulopapillary), followed by transitional cell carcinomas. Nephroblastoma, hemangiosarcoma, and adenoma have also been reported (Henry *et al*. 1999).

Clinical signs

Clinical signs in dogs with renal tumors may be nonspecific and include inappetence or anorexia, lethargy, weakness, cachexia, polyuria/polydipsia, pyrexia, vomiting, and abdominal pain (Burgess & DeRegis 2019; Lucke & Kelly 1976; Bryan *et al*. 2006; Baskin & De Paoli 1977; Locke & Barber 2006). Cases may occasionally present with abdominal distension or shock (Locke & Barber 2006; Moe & Lium 1997). Gross or microscopic hematuria is common and may be intermittent or continuous (Moe & Lium 1997; Mott *et al*. 1996; Bryan *et al*. 2006; Locke & Barber 2006). An abdominal mass may be palpable in advanced cases (Burgess & DeRegis 2019). Rarely animals may present with a paraneoplastic polycythemia syndrome (Burgess & DeRegis 2019).

In cases of hereditary multifocal renal cystadenocarcinomas and nodular dermatofibrosis in German shepherd dogs, skin lesions are always present. Nonspecific clinical signs as already described become more pronounced with time (Moe & Lium 1997).

Clinical signs of cats with primary renal tumors are similarly nonspecific, those of anorexia, weight loss, and depression being the most common. Lethargy, neurologic signs, hematuria, abdominal pain, and abdominal distension have been reported in fewer cases (Henry *et al*. 1999). Clinical signs in cats with renal lymphoma include weight loss, inappetence, and polyuria/polydipsia (Taylor *et al.* 2009).

Diagnostic evaluation

Diagnosis is often delayed due to a lack of overt clinical signs or partial response to empirical treatment (Crow 1985). Evaluation should include a complete blood count, serum biochemical profile, urinalysis, thoracic radiography, and abdominal imaging.

A complete blood count may reveal evidence of anemia secondary to hematuria, neutrophilia due to a stress response or infection, or thrombocytopenia (Bryan *et al.* 2006). Thrombocytopenia could be secondary to blood loss or a paraneoplastic syndrome. Serum biochemistry abnormalities are often nonspecific and may include hypoproteinemia and azotemia (Bryan *et al.* 2006; Klein *et al.* 1988). Urinalysis will frequently show evidence of hematuria and proteinuria (Crow 1985; Locke & Barber 2006). Bacteriuria or pyuria is infrequent (Klein *et al.* 1988; Bryan *et al.* 2006).

Three-view thoracic radiographs are taken to identify evidence of pulmonary or sternal lymph node metastases, with 7–34% of cases having radiographic evidence of metastases at presentation (Bryan *et al.* 2006; Klein *et al.* 1988; Locke & Barber 2006). Abdominal radiography will usually show evidence of solitary or multifocal renal masses, although an abdominal ultrasound examination will give more detail (Locke & Barber 2006; Bryan *et al.* 2006). An abdominal ultrasound examination of the entire abdomen should be performed to assess the degree of local extension of the mass, evaluate the opposite kidney and lymph nodes, and evaluate all other abdominal organs and intra-abdominal surfaces for evidence of metastases (Bryan *et al.* 2006; Crow 1985). Abdominal computed tomography (CT) may also identify the extent of local disease and/or evidence of intra-abdominal metastatic disease (Crow 1985). If abdominal ultrasound or CT is not available, intravenous pyelography may increase the information elucidated from abdominal radiography (Klein *et al.* 1988; Locke & Barber 2006).

An ultrasound- or CT-guided fine-needle aspirate of lesions may be performed in an attempt to diagnose the primary lesion or confirm suspect metastases. Renal cytology may not be diagnostic, but may give more information to direct further diagnostics (e.g., culture versus biopsy) (Borjesson 2003). It is most rewarding in cases of inflammation, which may be due to infectious or noninfectious causes (Wycislo & Piech 2019). Ultrasound-guided or laparoscopic-assisted needle-core biopsy may allow a diagnosis, but risks of bleeding are increased over fine-needle aspiration. It may be more prudent to go straight to surgery if a solitary renal mass

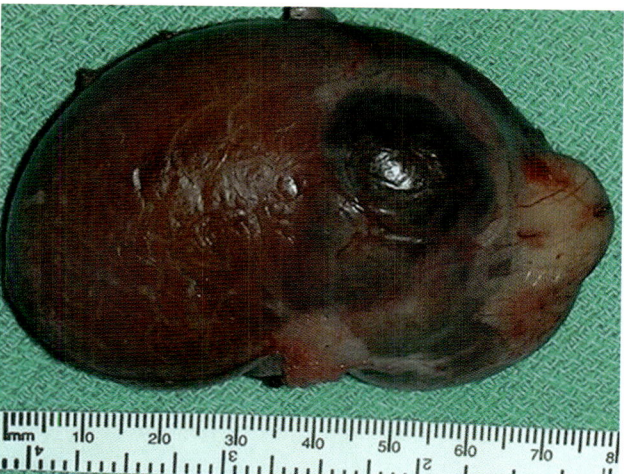

Figure 48.2 Renal hemangiosarcoma in a dog. An ultrasound-guided fine-needle aspirate was not diagnostic on cytology. Definitive diagnosis was made on histology following surgery.

is suspected. If a diagnosis would affect a client's willingness for definitive treatment, then a biopsy is of value. Definitive diagnosis is often made on histopathology following nephrectomy (Figure 48.2) (Bryan *et al.* 2006). If available, nuclear scintigraphy to quantify the glomerular filtration rate of the contralateral kidney may be advisable prior to nephrectomy (Reichle *et al.* 2003).

Diagnostic evaluation in cats should include a complete blood count, biochemical panel, and urinalysis (Henry *et al.* 1999). Affected cats may be anemic, have increases in blood urea nitrogen and/or creatinine, and exhibit hyperkalemia, hypophosphatemia or hyperphosphatemia, hypoglycemia, or hypernatremia. On urinalysis there is often hematuria and/or proteinuria. Three-view thoracic radiography and an abdominal ultrasound examination are warranted for staging purposes (Henry *et al.* 1999). Because of the high incidence of renal lymphoma in cats, fine-needle aspiration of the kidney(s) for cytologic evaluation is warranted (Gabor *et al.* 1998; Taylor *et al.* 2009; Mooney *et al.* 1987). Needle biopsy for histologic evaluation is occasionally required for a diagnosis of renal lymphoma (Mooney *et al.* 1987; Gabor *et al.* 1998; Taylor *et al.* 2009).

Treatment

The treatment for renal neoplasia is nephrectomy and ureterectomy if the disease is unilateral and the remaining kidney is functional (Crow 1985; Klein *et al.* 1988). The tumor is usually contained within the renal capsule, but may invade the renal vein, caudal vena cava, lumbar musculature, or adrenal gland (Crow 1985).

Nephron-sparing surgeries (discussed but rarely employed) include partial nephrectomy or enucleation of the mass (Mott *et al.* 1996). This may be a viable option for dogs with compromised renal function. The aim is to remove a small margin of normal parenchyma with the tumor, preserve adequate renal function, and prevent renal failure. These techniques may be more appropriate for benign tumors, and even centrally located lesions may be removed via a partial nephrectomy (Mott *et al.* 1996).

Radiofrequency ablation of kidney tumors has been reported experimentally in dogs and is used clinically in humans (Ahmed *et al.* 2004; Gervais *et al.* 2005). It is a technique that causes coagulation necrosis of tissue via emission of radiofrequency waves from an electrode inserted directly into the tumor. It is more effective in tumors of smaller diameter, and causes a smaller zone of coagulation necrosis in kidneys compared with liver or subcutaneous tissue. The characteristics of the tumor, including vascularity and electrical conductivity, affect the ablation outcome (Ahmed *et al.* 2004). Radiofrequency ablation is not widely available for clinical use in animals.

There is no proven benefit of chemotherapy for primary renal tumors outside of lymphoma (Crow 1985; Bryan *et al.* 2006). There is, however, a high risk of metastasis, so chemotherapy may have a conceptual role (Bryan *et al.* 2006). Chemotherapeutic agents that have been used for renal carcinomas include doxorubicin-based protocols, cyclophosphamide, 5-fluorouracil, carboplatin, mitoxantrone, paclitaxel, and ifosfamide (Bryan *et al.* 2006; Crow 1985; Locke & Barber 2006). Chemotherapy is indicated for renal lymphoma, although long-term remission is difficult to achieve (Crow 1985). Chemotherapy protocols for renal sarcomas often include doxorubicin, mitoxantrone, or carboplatin (Bryan *et al.* 2006). Chemotherapy for renal hemangiosarcoma usually includes doxorubicin (Locke & Barber 2006). Because of the paucity of cases, there is no evidence to suggest efficacy of chemotherapy against nephroblastoma in dogs. However, it is the standard of care along with surgery and radiation therapy in humans with aggressive forms of the disease (Mehta *et al.* 1991). Chemotherapy agents used for nephroblastoma in dogs include vincristine, actinomycin D, and doxorubicin; vincristine and doxorubicin; and vincristine and cyclophosphamide (Nakayama *et al.* 1984; Frimberger *et al.* 1995; Seaman & Patton 2003).

Prognosis

Primary renal malignancies generally carry a guarded to poor prognosis, especially if they are of mesenchymal origin. Long-term survival is uncommon (Klein *et al.* 1988). All forms of primary renal malignancies are highly metastatic (Bryan *et al.* 2006). An overall metastatic rate of 70–88.9% has been reported for all types of primary renal malignancies, and 32.4% of cases in one study had bilateral involvement (both carcinomas and mesenchymal tumors) (Burgess & DeRegis 2019; Klein *et al.* 1988).

Renal clear cell carcinoma is associated with shorter survival times than other histologic subtypes, with a median survival time of 87 days (Burgess & DeRegis 2019). A metastatic rate of 53.8% has been reported for renal tubular carcinoma. Median survival time for renal carcinomas has been reported as 8 months (Klein *et al.* 1988).

On multivariate analysis, mitotic index was identified as an independent prognostic factor. A mitotic index of >30 has been associated with a median survival time of 187 days, <10 with 1184 days, and 10–30 with a median survival time of 452 days (Edmondson *et al.* 2015).

The prognosis for renal hemangiosarcoma may be better than for the cardiac and splenic forms of the disease. The median survival time for renal hemangiosarcoma was reported as 278 days, with 28% surviving to 1 year. Dogs in that study with a hemoperitoneum had a median survival time of 62 days, compared with 286 days if a hemoperitoneum was not present (Locke & Barber 2006).

The prognosis for nephroblastoma may be slightly better than for both carcinomas and sarcomas (Crow 1985; Klein *et al.* 1988). Even so, nephroblastoma may cause death due to local or metastatic disease (Baskin & De Paoli 1977; Nakayama *et al.* 1984; Klein *et al.* 1988; Frimberger *et al.* 1995; Seaman & Patton 2003).

The prognosis for hereditary multifocal renal cystadenocarcinoma and nodular dermatofibrosis in German shepherd dogs is poor, with severity of clinical signs progressing with age (Moe & Lium 1997).

Ureteral neoplasia

Incidence

Primary ureteral neoplasia is very rare in the dog and has not been reported in the cat (Deschamps *et al.* 2007). Ureteral neoplasia may occur more commonly in association with extension to the ureters from a bladder neoplasm (Hurov *et al.* 1966).

Pathology and biological behavior

The majority of primary ureteral neoplasms are benign (Burton *et al.* 1994; Reichle *et al.* 2003). These include fibropapilloma, fibroepithelial polyp, and leiomyoma (Liska & Patnaik 1977; Hattel *et al.* 1986; Font *et al.* 1993; Reichle *et al.* 2003; Farrell *et al.* 2006). It is unclear if fibroepithelial polyps are truly a benign neoplasm or a chronic inflammatory reaction (Reichle *et al.* 2003). Few malignant primary neoplasms of the ureter have been reported, but include case reports of leiomyosarcoma, transitional cell carcinoma, mast cell tumor, and soft tissue sarcoma (Berzon 1979; Hanika & Rebar 1980; Steffey et al. 2004; Deschamps et al. 2007; Guilherme et al. 2007). Only two of these cases showed evidence of subsequent metastatic disease (Guilherme et al. 2007; Deschamps et al. 2007).

The majority of previously reported benign ureteral masses occurred in the proximal ureter, while the majority of malignant ureteral masses occurred in the distal ureter (Hanika & Rebar 1980; Reichle et al. 2003; Steffey et al. 2004; Deschamps et al. 2007). This is not always the case, with benign masses being reported distally and malignant masses reported in the proximal ureter (Berzon 1979; Reichle et al. 2003; Farrell et al. 2006). The sizes of both benign and malignant ureteral masses vary widely, from 1 cm to over 12 cm in diameter, or they may even occupy the majority of the abdominal cavity (Reichle et al. 2003; Steffey et al. 2004; Farrell et al. 2006; Deschamps et al. 2007; Guilherme et al. 2007).

Clinical signs

Clinical signs may include hematuria, anorexia, lethargy, exercise intolerance, acute abdominal pain, pyrexia, weight loss, vomiting, and an enlarged mass in the cranial abdomen (Berzon 1979; Reichle et al. 2003; Deschamps et al. 2007; Yap et al. 2017). Abdominal pain is usually due to ureteral obstruction, with subsequent hydronephrosis of the ipsilateral kidney resulting in a cranial abdominal mass (Deschamps et al. 2007; Berzon 1979; Farrell et al. 2006).

Diagnostic evaluation

Abdominal radiography and intravenous pyelography may confirm renomegaly and hydronephrosis (Hattel et al. 1986; Reichle et al. 2003). Visualization of abnormalities may be impaired due to a poorly functioning kidney and percutaneous antegrade pyelography may improve results (Reichle et al. 2003). Abdominal ultrasound is often useful in these cases and will generally show hydronephrosis of the affected kidney and some degree of hydroureter proximal to the mass, along with usually identifying the size and location of the ureteral mass (Reichle et al. 2003). Nuclear scintigraphy to quantify glomerular filtration rate may be useful to ensure adequate function of the normal kidney if one is considering nephrectomy and ureterectomy (Reichle et al. 2003).

Treatment

The usual treatment for primary ureteral neoplasia is nephrectomy and ureterectomy (Reichle et al. 2003; Deschamps et al. 2007; Guilherme et al. 2007). One dog was successfully treated for a benign mass via distal ureterectomy and neoureterocystostomy (Reichle et al. 2003).

Prognosis

The prognosis for removal of benign ureteral masses is excellent (Reichle et al. 2003; Burton et al. 1994). The prognosis for removal of malignant ureteral masses is variable. Two dogs with sarcomas showed subsequent evidence of metastatic disease, with survival times of 8 months and 6 months, respectively (Deschamps et al. 2007; Guilherme et al. 2007), and another dog with sarcoma was euthanized 5.5 months after surgery due to progression of a locally recurrent mass (Yap et al. 2017). Three other cases of malignant ureteral tumors (leiomyosarcoma, transitional cell carcinoma, mast cell tumor) did not result in death of the patient for the follow-up times reported (Berzon 1979; Hanika & Rebar 1980; Steffey et al. 2004).

Neoplasia of the urinary bladder and urethra

Incidence

Primary malignancies of the bladder and urethra are rare in dogs and cats, comprising 0.5–1% of all canine cancers, and even less in the cat (Burnie & Weaver 1983; Schwarz et al. 1985; Henry 2003). In dogs, 90% of bladder tumors are malignant (Burgess & DeRegis 2019). Transitional cell carcinoma is the most common cancer of the bladder or urethra in dogs and cats, accounting for 50–75% of all bladder tumors and 75–90% of bladder epithelial tumors (Figures 48.3 and 48.4) (Burgess & DeRegis 2019; Wilson et al. 1979; Burnie & Weaver 1983; Schwarz et al. 1985; Davies & Read 1990; Henry 2003; Wilson et al. 2007). Other epithelial tumors include squamous cell carcinoma, adenocarcinoma, and undifferentiated carcinoma (Burnie & Weaver 1983; Takagi et al. 2005). Nonepithelial tumors of the bladder or urethra include leiomyoma, leiomyosarcoma, hemangioma, hemangiosarcoma, fibroma, fibrosarcoma, rhabdomyosarcoma, myxosarcoma, chondrosarcoma, osteosarcoma, undifferentiated sarcoma, and lymphoma (Tarvin et al. 1978; Wilson et al. 1979; Burnie & Weaver 1983; Swalec et al. 1989; Davies & Read 1990; Moroff et al. 1991; Norris et al. 1992; Struble et al. 1997; Davis & Holt 2003; Olausson et al. 2005; Benigni et al. 2006; Heng et al. 2006; Weisse et al. 2006; Bae et al. 2007). Polypoid cystitis, which may present with a bladder mass or masses, may occur rarely and is not considered a neoplastic disease (Martinez et al. 2003).

Transitional cell carcinoma is usually seen in older dogs with a median age of 11 years, although it may be seen in younger dogs (Knapp et al. 2000a,b; Henry 2003). The median age in cats is 15 years (Wilson et al. 2007).

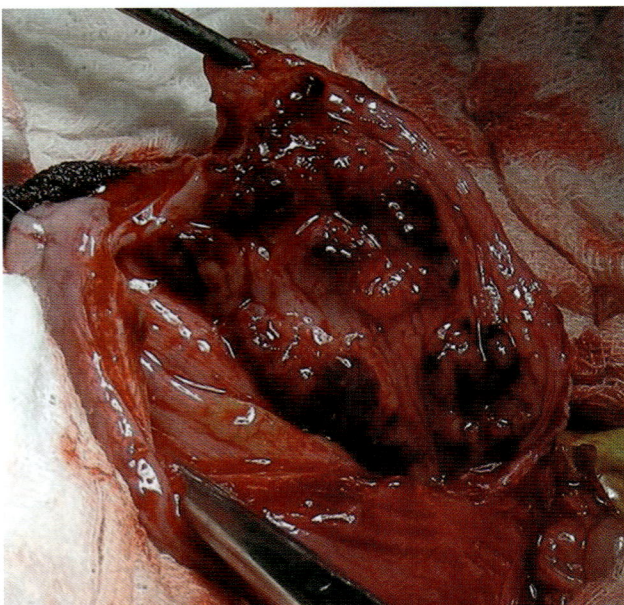

Figure 48.3 High-grade transitional cell carcinoma in a dog. Multifocal lesions occurred throughout the mucosal surfaces of the bladder.

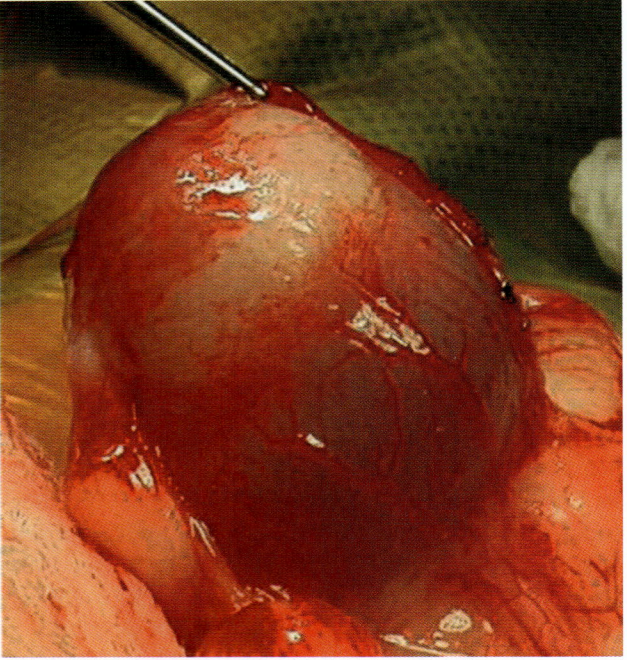

Figure 48.4 High-grade transitional cell carcinoma involving the apex of the bladder in a cat.

It has been reported more commonly in female than in male dogs, with a ratio of 1.7:1–1.95:1 (Norris *et al.* 1992; Knapp *et al.* 2000a,b). Neutered animals of either sex are at four times increased risk compared with intact animals (Burgess & DeRegis 2019). There is a

breed predisposition in Scottish terriers, which are 18 times more likely to be affected than mixed-breed dogs (Knapp *et al.* 2000a,b). Other predisposed breeds include beagles, Shetland sheepdogs, wirehaired fox terriers, West Highland white terriers and other terrier breeds, Eskimo dogs, Samoyeds, keeshonds, collies, Chesapeake Bay retrievers, and schipperkes (Burgess & DeRegis 2019; Knapp *et al.* 2000a,b; Fulkerson & Knapp 2015). In dogs with a high breed-associated risk, the sex predilection is less pronounced (Fulkerson & Knapp 2015).

Polypoid cystitis is reported in dogs, with a mean age of 7.1 years (Martinez *et al.* 2003). No breed predisposition exists and 88% of cases are diagnosed in females (Martinez *et al.* 2003).

Pathology and biological behavior

The majority of canine and feline bladder and urethral tumors are highly malignant, being both locally invasive and having potential for metastatic spread (Wilson *et al.* 1979, 2007; Schwarz *et al.* 1985; Klein *et al.* 1988; Norris *et al.* 1992). Death may be due to local disease or metastases (Norris *et al.* 1992; Wilson *et al.* 2007)

Bladder transitional cell carcinomas of dogs have a multifactorial etiology involving genetic and environmental factors (Glickman *et al.* 2004). The etiology of urethral transitional cell carcinoma is likely similar (Wilson *et al.* 1979). Risk factors include breed, exposure to herbicides, obesity, exposure to older topical insecticides (especially flea and tick dips), dogs living in close proximity to marshes sprayed for mosquito control, and possibly cyclophosphamide administration and female sex (Weller *et al.* 1979; Henry 2003; Glickman *et al.* 1989, 2004; Knapp *et al.* 2000a,b). With regard to the association with insecticides, it is suggested that the "inert" ingredients, comprising over 90% of the product, are the likely carcinogens. Some of those ingredients are lipophilic and stored in fat, possibly accounting for the increased risk of transitional cell carcinoma in obese and female dogs (Glickman *et al.* 1989). Alternatively, the increased risk in females may be due to an increased frequency of urination in male dogs from marking behavior, thereby allowing less contact time for carcinogens in the male urethra (Henry 2003). An increased risk has not been shown with other topical pesticides, such as those containing fipronil or imidacloprid, or with disinfection byproducts in tap water (Raghavan *et al.* 2004; Backer *et al.* 2008). A decreased risk has been associated with regular consumption of yellow or green leafy vegetables at least three times a week. Mechanisms for this are unclear, but may be associated with ingestion of pro- and preformed vitamin A (Raghavan *et al.* 2005).

Transitional cell carcinomas of dogs are usually of an intermediate or high grade on histology (Knapp

Table 48.1 Primary tumor (T).

eTX	Primary tumor cannot be assessed
T0	No evidence of primary tumor
Ta	Noninvasive papillary carcinoma
Tis	Carcinoma in situ: "flat tumor"
T1	Tumor invades subepithelial connective tissue
T2	Tumor invades muscle
T2a	Tumor invades superficial muscle (inner half)
T2b	Tumor invades deep muscle (outer half)
T3	Tumor invades perivesical tissue
T3a	Microscopically
T3b	Macroscopically (extravesical mass)
T4	Tumor invades any of the following: prostate, uterus, vagina, pelvic wall, abdominal wall
T4a	Tumor invades prostate, uterus, vagina
T4b	Tumor invades pelvic wall, abdominal wall

Source: Greene *et al.* (2002).

et al. 2000a,b; Patrick *et al.* 2006). They are often locally advanced at the time of diagnosis. Of affected dogs, 78% are T2 and 20% are T3 (see Table 48.1 for classifications). Transitional cell carcinomas involve the prostate in 29% of male dogs (Fulkerson & Knapp 2015). Tumor grade is associated with survival time (Henry 2003). There are distant metastases in 14–20% of dogs at the time of diagnosis (Fulkerson & Knapp 2015; Knapp *et al.* 2000a,b). The metastatic rate at necropsy is greater than 50% (Fulkerson & Knapp 2015; Henry 2003). Metastases occur most often to lungs, lymph nodes, and liver, but may occur to bone, any abdominal organ, and other distant sites (Henry 2003; Knapp *et al.* 2000a,b). In one study, 9% of dogs with urothelial carcinomas had histologically confirmed skeletal metastases (Charney *et al.* 2017). Death is most often due to progression of local disease and less often to metastases (Knapp *et al.* 2000a,b). The bladder trigone is the most common site for transitional cell carcinomas, frequently leading to partial or complete obstruction of the urinary tract (Knapp *et al.* 2000a,b). In one study, 56% of dogs with primary bladder transitional cell carcinoma had concurrent urethral involvement and 29% of male dogs with the disease had prostatic urethral involvement (Knapp *et al.* 2000a,b). Younger dogs and dogs with larger tumors are at increased risk for metastases (Cannon & Allstadt 2015).

In a study of 65 dogs with transitional cell carcinoma, whole-body CT was conducted at the time of diagnosis. Lung metastases were identified in 35.4%, iliosacral lymphadenomegaly in 47.7%, sternal lymphadenomegaly in 18.5%, and bone metastases in 24.6% of animals (Iwasaki *et al.* 2019).

Feline transitional cell carcinoma is uncommon. Of primary bladder cancers in cats, 60% are transitional cell carcinomas (Burgess & DeRegis 2019). Recurrence is common (Cannon & Allstadt 2015). Cats are more likely to have a mid-body or apical mass in the bladder (Figure 48.4) (Hamlin *et al.* 2019).

Bladder sarcomas are locally invasive and may be associated with widespread metastases (Olausson *et al.* 2005; Bae *et al.* 2007). Osteosarcoma of the bladder has also been reported previously (Woldemeskel 2017). Bladder lymphoma is rare and usually a part of a more extensive disease process (Benigni *et al.* 2006). Bladder tumors in cats are typically locally aggressive and have the ability to metastasize, most often to the lungs and regional lymph nodes (Schwarz *et al.* 1985; Wilson *et al.* 2007). Transitional cell carcinomas are the most common feline bladder cancers, followed by other carcinomas (Schwarz *et al.* 1985).

Paraneoplastic syndromes associated with bladder tumors include hypercalcemia, cancer cachexia, hypertrophic osteopathy, and hyperestrogenism (Norris *et al.* 1992). Polypoid cystitis is rare. It is characterized by inflammation, epithelial proliferation, and development of a polypoid mass or masses without histologic evidence of neoplasia. There is often a history of recurrent urinary tract infection. Polypoid cysts may be an inflammatory and hyperplastic reaction to chronic irritation of the bladder mucosa. It is unclear if they represent preneoplastic lesions (Martinez *et al.* 2003). Polypoid cystitis and transitional cell carcinoma may occur concurrently (Wycislo & Piech 2019).

Clinical signs

The most common clinical signs seen with bladder cancer are those referable to the urinary tract. Urinary tract signs are similar to those associated with urinary tract infections (Fulkerson & Knapp 2015). Norris *et al.* (1992) reported that 84% of cases had dysuria, 50% had hematuria, and 37% had pollakiuria in a series of 115 dogs. Less common clinical signs include incontinence, polyuria/polydipsia, or nonspecific signs such as exercise intolerance, dullness and vomiting, fecal tenesmus, and decreased appetite (Norris *et al.* 1992; Burnie & Weaver 1983; Schwarz *et al.* 1985). Occasionally animals present with dyspnea due to pulmonary metastases, or lameness due to bone metastases or (rarely) hypertrophic osteopathy (Schwarz *et al.* 1985; Norris *et al.* 1992; Brodey 1971). Clinical signs associated with urethral cancer are similar. The most common clinical signs are stranguria, hematuria, and pollakiuria (Tarvin *et al.* 1978; Moroff *et al.* 1991). In a study of infiltrative urethral disease in female dogs, 7 of 41 dogs (17%) presented with total urinary tract obstruction (Moroff *et al.* 1991). In the same study, 16 of 41 dogs (39%) presented with a vaginal discharge (Moroff *et al.* 1991).

Over two-thirds (70%) of animals have some physical abnormality detected on clinical examination, including a urethral mass palpable by digital rectal or vaginal examination, a palpable abdominal mass, prostatomegaly, a distended bladder, or abdominal pain (Norris *et al.* 1992). In another study of 41 female dogs with infiltrative urethral disease, all 41 dogs had a thick, irregularly shaped urethra detected on rectal examination and/or an irregularly shaped urethral papilla on vaginal examination (Moroff *et al.* 1991).

Skin metastases may occur rarely, presenting as erythematous ulcerated or proliferative lesions (Reed *et al.* 2013). Tumor may have spread via direct extension, lymphatic spread, or vascular dissemination. A mechanism of transepidermal spread via urine-scalded skin was also postulated (Reed *et al.* 2013).

Diagnostic evaluation

Bloodwork

Blood should be submitted for a complete blood count and biochemical panel as part of a minimum database. The most common abnormality seen is a neutrophilia. Other abnormalities may include anemia, azotemia, and rarely hypercalcemia (Norris *et al.* 1992).

Urine tests

A urinalysis is often the first screening test used to diagnose bladder cancer and is abnormal in 93% of cases (Norris *et al.* 1992). While urine sediment examination shows evidence of transitional cell carcinoma in 30–40% of cases, the urinalysis may also be indistinguishable from dogs with cystitis, including leukocytes, erythrocytes, and bacteria (Norris *et al.* 1992; Tarvin *et al.* 1978; Henry 2003). Reactive nonneoplastic transitional cells look very similar morphologically to transitional carcinoma cells (Henry 2003). Caution should be exercised when obtaining the urine sample, since tumor seeding may rarely occur following a cystocentesis (Nyland *et al.* 2002).

Early detection of a cancer has the potential to provide more time for appropriate therapy, help delay onset of clinical signs, and improve outcomes associated with a smaller tumor burden (Wiley *et al.* 2019). A qualitative rapid latex agglutination urine dipstick test has been evaluated as a screening test for transitional cell carcinoma. It measures a glycoprotein antigen complex associated with bladder cancer (Borjesson *et al.* 1999). While it is a sensitive test, with reported sensitivities of over 85%, the specificity is relatively low compared with control dogs with other urinary tract disease (Borjesson *et al.* 1999; Henry *et al.* 2003b). False-positive results were seen with significant glucosuria, proteinuria, pyuria, or hematuria (Henry *et al.* 2003b; Borjesson *et al.* 1999). The test is associated with a high negative predictive value, indicating that it is highly unlikely that dogs with a negative result will have bladder cancer (Henry *et al.* 2003b). There is a polymerase chain reaction (PCR) test developed that may be performed on a voided urine sample for the presence of genetic mutation of the *BRAF* gene, which is noted in 80% of dogs with bladder or prostate cancer (Burgess & DeRegis 2019; Mochizuki *et al.* 2015). This is a rapid and highly sensitive test (Wiley *et al.* 2019).

Dogs with transitional cell carcinomas are at high risk for urinary tract infections. The bacteria may become resistant to antibiotics and could possibly enhance tumor progression and diminish treatment response. Periodic urinalyses are indicated (Fulkerson & Knapp 2015). In one study (Budreckis *et al.* 2015), 55% of dogs had a positive urine culture during the treatment course. Prior to the start of chemotherapy, 25% of dogs had a positive culture. Dogs with urethral involvement were more likely to have a positive culture and 43.3% of positive cultures had multiple bacteria present. Risk and complications of urinary tract infections may be greater than the risk of tumor seeding associated with multiple cystocenteses (Budreckis *et al.* 2015).

Cytology

Cytology of bladder masses can be rewarding to help differentiate between cystic lesions, inflammation, and neoplasia (Wycislo & Piech 2019). Fine-needle aspiration with ultrasound guidance yields a diagnosis in 91% of cases (Norris *et al.* 1992). Tumor seeding along the needle tract may occur, resulting in tumor implantation of the ventral abdominal wall (Nyland *et al.* 2002). For this reason, traumatic urethral catheterization is preferred and will yield small samples for histopathologic evaluation in over 80% of cases (Moroff *et al.* 1991; Lamb *et al.* 1996). Ultrasound guidance of the catheter allows accurate placement of the catheter for sample acquisition. However, the small samples may limit the accuracy of the diagnosis (Lamb *et al.* 1996). Biopsies from multiple sites are indicated due to the small sample size and because of the masses being heterogeneous in nature (Henry 2003). A prostatic or urethral wash was reported as diagnostic in 77% of dogs with bladder or urethral cancer (Norris *et al.* 1992). Cytology is not always definitive and a biopsy with histopathology may be required for definitive diagnosis of benign or malignant lesions. Well-differentiated transitional cell carcinoma, with minimal pleomorphism, may be difficult to diagnose cytologically (Wycislo & Piech 2019).

Radiography and computed tomography

Three-view thoracic radiography is routinely performed to assess for the presence of pulmonary metastases or intrathoracic lymphadenopathy (Henry 2003). Most dogs with pulmonary metastases present with an interstitial nodular pattern or a diffuse unstructured interstitial opacity (Walter *et al.* 1984). Other patterns that may be seen include localized (lobar), interstitial or alveolar infiltrates, or normal pulmonary opacity (Walter *et al.* 1984). Evidence of pulmonary metastases is seen in 17% of animals at presentation (Norris *et al.* 1992). Dogs with a diffuse interstitial opacity associated with pulmonary metastases may be difficult to differentiate from those with normal aging changes (Walter *et al.* 1984).

Abdominal radiographs occasionally show evidence of prostatomegaly (12%), sublumbar lymphadenopathy (9%), lumbar vertebral and pelvic bone metastases (8%), or a caudal abdominal mass (6%) (Norris *et al.* 1992). Combining abdominal radiography with a positive or double-contrast retrograde urethrocystogram increases diagnostic ability to 96% for demonstration of a bladder mass (Norris *et al.* 1992). Contrast urography shows a filling defect and/or irregularity or reduced patency in up to 96% of cases (Burgess & DeRegis 2019). Contrast urethrocystography is similarly sensitive for demonstrating primary urethral tumors (Tarvin *et al.* 1978). In another study, contrast urethrocystography was normal in 5 of 9 dogs (55%) with granulomatous urethritis and in 4 of 24 dogs (16%) with epithelial neoplasia (Moroff *et al.* 1991).

CT may be more accurate to evaluate animals for evidence of metastases (Iwasaki *et al.* 2019). Whole-body CT could be helpful in detecting skeletal metastases as a source of bone pain (Charney *et al.* 2017).

Ultrasound

Abdominal ultrasound examination offers the advantages of improved detection of intra-abdominal lesions (compared with radiographs) and the ability to obtain biopsy samples via catheterization under ultrasound guidance. Suspected intra-abdominal metastatic lesions should be subjected to fine-needle aspiration for cytologic assessment (Henry 2003). Transitional carcinoma may appear sonographically similar to other tumors, benign polyps, cystitis, and urethritis (Burgess & DeRegis 2019).

Cystoscopy

Cystoscopy allows direct visualization of the extent of the lesion under magnification and allows procurement of biopsy samples for histopathology (Childress *et al.* 2011; Henry 2003). Brush cytology may be performed in patients too small for a biopsy port in the endoscopic equipment, although diagnostic accuracy is compromised due to similarities in the cytologic appearances of neoplastic and nonneoplastic transitional cells (Henry 2003). In 92 dogs, diagnostic samples were obtained in 96% of female dogs and 65% of male dogs (Childress *et al.* 2011). Alternatively, biopsy specimens may be procured surgically (Henry 2003). Granulomatous urethritis, polypoid cystitis, reactive tissue surrounding calculi, and neoplasms (transitional cell carcinomas or other neoplasms) may all produce mass lesions of the lower urinary tract (Childress *et al.* 2011; Burgess & DeRegis 2019). Additionally, polypoid cystitis and transitional cell carcinoma may occur concurrently (Wycislo & Piech 2019).

Cystoscopy often results in low-grade urethral and bladder mucosal injury. This may result in transient hematuria for 2–3 days. It occasionally may result in stranguria, pollakiuria, and inappropriate urination for 2–5 days. Incontinence in a previously continent bitch is rare and may occur for 3–5 days. Urethral perforation and bladder rupture are rare (Morgan & Forman 2015).

Nuclear scintigraphy

Nuclear scintigraphy may be performed to exclude bone metastases, especially in animals with unexplained lameness; 8% of dogs with transitional cell carcinoma were reported to have bone metastases at the time of diagnosis (Norris *et al.* 1992).

Treatment

Treatment options for bladder cancer include surgery, chemotherapy, and radiation therapy. Selection of treatment options will be influenced by tumor location, expected tumor type, and presence of gross metastases. The majority of bladder tumors are transitional cell carcinomas (Norris *et al.* 1992). It is important to distinguish transitional cell carcinomas from other disease, as the treatment and prognosis may vary considerably (Fulkerson & Knapp 2015).

Surgery

The advisability and extent of surgery depend on tumor location and invasiveness, tumor type, and client expectations (Henry 2003). The goal of surgery may vary from obtaining tissue for diagnosis to attempted removal of affected tissue (Fulkerson & Knapp 2015). If concurrent exposure of the urethra is required, a transpubic approach allows exposure of 95% of the length of the urethra in female dogs (Davies & Read 1990). Surgery is usually considered palliative due to the high metastatic rate. Grossly normal bladder tissue may contain neoplastic or preneoplastic tissue (Henry 2003). Surgical options include partial cystectomy; radical cystectomy and different ureterostomy techniques (to the skin, uterus, or vagina); carbon dioxide laser or electrocautery ablation (debulking) and permanent cystostomy placement; urethral and/or ureteral stenting; and urinary diversion (Ricardo Huppes *et al.* 2017; Delaune *et al.* 2018; Saeki *et al.* 2015; Stone *et al.* 1988; Smith *et al.* 1995; Henry 2003; Liptak *et al.* 2004; Upton *et al.* 2006). Urethral stents may be placed via fluoroscopic guidance in certain cases (Weisse *et al.* 2006). Vaginourethroplasty may be appropriate for resection of mid to distal urethral lesions in female dogs (Davies & Read 1990; White *et al.* 1996).

Partial cystectomy is an option for localized bladder tumors amenable to resection. Precautionary measures must be taken to avoid tumor seeding into surrounding tissues and the abdominal wall. Spread to the abdominal wall is more common in dogs that have had a cystotomy than those that have not. Once detected in the abdominal wall, transitional cell carcinomas grow more aggressively and historically have not responded to medical treatment (Fulkerson & Knapp 2015; Robat *et al.* 2013). Up to 90% of the bladder has been removed successfully in combination with a colonic seromuscular patch, with bladder accommodation occurring over 3 months postoperatively until it was almost normal in size (Pozzi *et al.* 2006). Pollakiuria following partial cystectomy is common due to a decreased capacity for storage, though this generally resolves as the bladder accommodates (Henry 2003). Complete resection of the tumor is uncommon, with only 2 of 102 dogs in one report having complete resections (Knapp *et al.* 2000a,b). Even with complete tumor resection, recurrence of transitional cell carcinoma is likely. This may be due to microscopic neoplasia at the surgical margins or *de novo* tumors due to field carcinogenesis (Knapp *et al.* 2000a,b). Cytoreductive surgery in combination with chemotherapy increases overall survival (Robat *et al.* 2013; Cannon & Allstadt 2015).

Most canine transitional cell carcinomas are trigonal in location. Difficulties in resection occur due to tumor location, frequency of urethral involvement, and metastases being present in 20% or more of dogs at the time of diagnosis (Knapp *et al.* 2000a,b). For management of trigonal masses, surgical options include ablation via laser or electrocautery either surgically or cystoscopically, permanent cystostomy, a urethral stent, urinary diversion, or radical cystectomy (Stone *et al.* 1988; Smith *et al.* 1995; Liptak *et al.* 2004; Upton *et al.* 2006; Weisse *et al.* 2006; Ricardo Huppes *et al.* 2017; Delaune *et al.* 2018).

Laser or electrocautery ablation has been used to palliate signs via an endoscopic or abdominal approach, with or without ultrasound guidance (Liptak *et al.* 2004; Upton *et al.* 2006; Cerf & Lindquist 2012). The goal is to ablate as much tumor as possible without penetrating the serosa of the bladder (Upton *et al.* 2006). Laser ablation is well tolerated with minimal adverse effects. The median survival time for dogs treated with laser ablation and chemotherapy is 299–380 days (Cerf & Lindquist 2012; Upton *et al.* 2006). This is similar to the median survival time for dogs undergoing chemotherapy alone, but resolution of clinical signs is improved with the ablation technique (Upton *et al.* 2006). Urethral involvement was not a prognostic factor and relief is usually provided with one to two treatments (Cerf & Lindquist 2012). Cystoscopic electrocautery ablation is associated with a high complication rate in female dogs. Complications of the technique include iatrogenic urethral perforation, tumor seeding, and urinary tract infection (Liptak *et al.* 2004).

Permanent cystostomy tubes are used palliatively in dogs with stranguria or anuria due to tumors in the trigone or urethra. They are easy to place surgically, usually using an 8 Fr or 12 Fr mushroom-tip or Foley catheter, and are easily managed at home. They cause minimal drainage or irritation and cleaning of the cystostomy site is not routinely required. Four of seven dogs had urinary tract infections after cystostomy tube placement, all of which resolved on antibiotics. The tube is bandaged to the body or placed beneath a stockinette, and owners are instructed to drain the bladder 3–4 times daily. Tubes were managed for up to 148 days (median 106 days) (Smith *et al.* 1995). A low-profile gastrostomy tube has been used as a permanent cystostomy tube. Since the tube lies flush with the skin, it may decrease the likelihood of inadvertent removal (Salinardi *et al.* 2003).

Both balloon-expandable and self-expanding metallic stents have been used for malignant urethral obstructions (Weisse *et al.* 2006). They are a safe and effective palliative option, with the vast majority of dogs being able to urinate after stent placement (McMillan *et al.* 2012; Blackburn *et al.* 2013; Weisse *et al.* 2006). Occasionally the stent may not be able to be placed due to the severity of the obstruction (McMillan *et al.* 2012). Severe incontinence occurs relatively often, in around one-third of cases (Weisse *et al.* 2006; Blackburn *et al.* 2013; McMillan *et al.* 2012). Animals are at risk for urinary tract infections (Blackburn *et al.* 2013). Balloon-expandable coronary stents are available with a smaller delivery system than self-expanding metallic stents, and have been used in the urethra of a cat. Made of stainless steel, they have a high radial force strength and minimal foreshortening during expansion. Their disadvantage is that they will not return to the nominal diameter if they are crushed, and they have poor flexibility (Newman *et al.* 2009). Self-expanding stents are available in longer lengths and are made of nitinol (nickel–titanium alloy), which has excellent biocompatible properties and is less prone to corrosion than is steel (Weisse *et al.* 2006). Stents should be approximately 10% larger than the maximal diameter of the urethra to ensure adequate mucosal apposition, minimize the chance of migration, and decrease trauma to the urethral wall. Stents should not expand to greater than 1.3 times the diameter of the prostatic portion of the urethra or severe mucosal edema may result. Owners must be made aware of the palliative nature of this treatment. Medial survival times reported range from 20 to 78 days (Weisse *et al.* 2006; McMillan *et al.* 2012; Blackburn *et al.* 2013).

Balloon dilatation for treatment of urethral obstruction has resulted in improvement following dilatation in 9 of 12 dogs. The obstruction recurred in 5 dogs 48–296 days later. Three dogs had a second dilatation procedure and all improved for 41–70 days. Complications included hematuria, incontinence, and dysuria. Complications resolved within a few days following treatment (Kim *et al.* 2019).

Radical cystectomy and ureterostomy to different structures constitute an option. Ureters have been anastomosed to the skin, vagina, uterus, or urethra (anastomosis to the colon is associated with an unacceptably high complication rate) (Saeki *et al.* 2015; Ricardo Huppes *et al.* 2017; Delaune *et al.* 2018; Bacon *et al.* 2016). There is a high rate of minor complications including bleeding, edema at the ureterostomy site, and urine scalding. Major complications include ureteral dehiscence, pyelonephritis, oliguria and azotemia, and ureteral obstruction resulting in hydronephrosis (Ricardo Huppes *et al.* 2017; Saeki *et al.* 2015; Delaune *et al.* 2018; Bacon *et al.* 2016). Animals are often managed postoperatively using diapers, which are replaced every 8–12 hours (Ricardo Huppes *et al.* 2017). Major complications associated with ureterocolonic anastomosis were avoided (Ricardo Huppes *et al.* 2017).

Urinary diversion with ureterocolonic anastomosis following total cystectomy was reported in 10 dogs (Stone *et al.* 1988). There was a high incidence of postoperative complications including azotemia in all dogs, hyperchloremic metabolic acidosis in 5 dogs, pyelonephritis in 5 kidneys (2 of which had outflow obstruction), and nausea and vomiting in 3 dogs. This technique is not recommended.

Vaginourethroplasty requires a transpubic approach, which allows exposure of 95% of the length of the urethra in female dogs (Davies & Read 1990). Resection of mid to distal urethral lesions involving up to 50% of the length of the urethra is possible using this technique (Davies & Read 1990; White *et al.* 1996). The technique may be performed for lesions involving up to 85% of the length of the urethra, but urinary incontinence is likely (Davies & Read 1990).

A technique has been described for resection of the entire bladder neck including the trigone and proximal urethra, with preservation of the dorsal neurovascular pedicles (Saulnier-Troff *et al.* 2008). While it is technically challenging, the two dogs treated with this technique regained urinary continence 7 and 17 days postoperatively. One dog was euthanized 8 months later due to a pulmonary metastatic lesion. The other dog had an abdominal wall metastatic lesion identified 6 months later and was euthanized at 580 days due to renal failure.

In cats, transitional cell carcinomas affect the nontrigonal wall in approximately 55% of cases. Surgery is more straightforward and may be more beneficial in these cases (Burgess & DeRegis 2019).

Most polyps associated with polypoid cystitis occur cranioventrally in the bladder wall. Surgical removal of the polyps is the most efficacious treatment (Martinez *et al.* 2003). Concurrent disease such as urinary tract infection and/or urolithiasis should be treated appropriately.

Chemotherapy

Chemotherapy is not curative, but stable disease or even remission may be accomplished. If resistance to a drug develops, other drugs may still be effective (Fulkerson & Knapp 2015). Cytoreductive surgery in combination with chemotherapy increases overall survival (Robat *et al.* 2013).

A number of chemotherapeutic agents have been used for the treatment of canine transitional cell carcinomas, including piroxicam, mitoxantrone, vinblastine, gemcitabine, platinum-based compounds, and combination doxorubicin-based protocols (Fulkerson & Knapp 2015; Helfand *et al.* 1994; Knapp *et al.* 1994, 2000a,b; Henry *et al.* 2003a; Boria *et al.* 2005).

In a series of 34 dogs with unresectable transitional cell carcinoma treated with piroxicam, 2 showed a complete response, 4 showed a partial response, 8 showed stable disease, and 10 showed progressive disease (Knapp *et al.* 1994). In addition, 17% of dogs (6 of 34) had evidence of gastrointestinal irritation, but this resolved on withdrawal of piroxicam and appropriate symptomatic therapy. *In vitro* cytotoxicity assays showed no direct antitumor effects. The protocol was generally well tolerated and 29 of 34 dogs had subjective improvement in quality of life as assessed by their owners. The median survival time for all dogs was 181 days (Knapp *et al.* 1994). Piroxicam is administered at 0.3 mg/kg body weight by mouth once daily (Knapp *et al.* 1994). It is unclear if inhibition of cyclooxygenase (COX) expression is a mechanism by which piroxicam works for this type of neoplasia. The remission rate using the COX-2 selective drug deracoxib or meloxicam is similar to that of piroxicam, but complete remissions are not seen (Burgess & DeRegis 2019; Fulkerson & Knapp 2015). In a series of 18 dogs with transitional cell carcinoma, all 18 tumors stained positive for both COX-1 and COX-2 (Knottenbelt *et al.* 2006). Firocoxib also has efficacy as a single agent (20% partial remission and 33% stable disease) (Knapp *et al.* 2013). It will enhance the activity of cisplatin, but there is a high rate of renal and gastrointestinal toxicoses with cisplatin in these animals (Knapp *et al.* 2013). One-third of dogs treated with piroxicam may have the drug discontinued due to gastrointestinal signs, or azotemia from nephrotoxicity or tumor progression (Allstadt *et al.* 2015). Older dogs had increased risks of adverse gastrointestinal events with piroxicam use, and concurrent use of gastroprotectant medications was not protective (Eichstadt *et al.* 2017).

A long median survival time (of 531 days) was associated with the use of a course of vinblastine followed by piroxicam, which was longer than that seen with the use of both drugs concurrently (medial survival time of 299 days) (Knapp *et al.* 2016). Cisplatin combined with piroxicam has shown a reasonable response rate, with 10 of 14 dogs showing a complete (2 dogs) or partial (8 dogs) response (Knapp *et al.* 2000a,b). The median survival time was 246 days. While gastrointestinal and hematologic toxicities were generally mild, renal toxicity was seen in 10 of 14 dogs, which was unacceptably high (Knapp *et al.* 2000a,b). Another study decreased the dose of cisplatin in combination with piroxicam (Greene *et al.* 2007). This was an attempt to decrease the renal toxicity seen previously. The results showed that the decreased dose had minimal antitumor effects with a high rate of renal and gastrointestinal toxicities (5 of 14 and 8 of 14 dogs, respectively). A different study combined carboplatin with piroxicam, again in an attempt to decrease renal toxicity (Boria *et al.* 2005). Of 29 dogs, 11 showed partial remission, 13 had stable disease, and 5 had progressive disease. Gastrointestinal toxicity was seen in 23 dogs and hematologic toxicity in 11 dogs. The median survival time was 161 days. It was determined that although antitumor activity was enhanced over either drug alone, the frequent toxicity and limited survival benefit (median survival time was no longer than that previously reported for piroxicam alone) did not warrant use of the protocol (Boria *et al.* 2005).

Mitoxantrone is often used with vinblastine and metronomic chlorambucil (Burgess & DeRegis 2019). Mitoxantrone combined with piroxicam has shown some efficacy (Henry *et al.* 2003a). Of 48 treated dogs, 1 showed a complete response, 16 a partial response, 22 had stable disease, and 9 had progressive disease. There was a measurable response in 35.4% of cases and subjective improvement in 75% of cases. The median survival time was 350 days, and gastrointestinal toxicity (18%) and azotemia (10%) were the most common complications (Henry *et al.* 2003a).

A protocol using doxorubicin combined with cyclophosphamide showed some efficacy, with a median survival time reported of 259 days. Of 11 dogs, 1 had life-threatening neutropenia, 7 had mild gastrointestinal signs, and 1 had severe gastrointestinal signs requiring hospitalization (Helfand *et al.* 1994).

Intra-arterial delivery of chemotherapy (carboplatin and meloxicam) is associated with the animal being more likely to have a tumor response and less likely to develop anemia, lethargy, or anorexia. The aim is to increase local concentration of the drugs, decrease systemic effects, and increase tumor response. The impact on long-term outcome and survival has not been determined (Culp *et al.* 2015).

Dogs treated with concurrent cyclophosphamide and furosemide on a metronomic basis had a low (3.6%) incidence of sterile hemorrhagic cystitis. The risk of sterile hemorrhagic cystitis is positively associated with the cumulative dose of cyclophosphamide (Chan *et al.* 2016). Metronomic use of chlorambucil (4 mg/m² orally every 24 hours) and COX-inhibitor drugs are well tolerated and may prolong survival for several months after other treatments have failed (Schrempp *et al.* 2013). Use of toceranib for bladder tumors was associated with a 6.7% partial response rate and 80% stable disease, with a median duration of 128.5 days. There was progression of azotemia in 56% of dogs, so renal function needs to be monitored closely (Gustafson & Biller 2019).

Single-agent vinblastine or single-agent vinorelbine has been used for rescue therapy for dogs with bladder carcinomas (Kaye *et al.* 2015; Arnold *et al.* 2011).

Intravesicular epidermal growth factor (EGF)-anthrax toxin chimera is a new therapeutic strategy for bladder cancer. Cancer cells exposed to the bladder lumen overexpress EGF receptor. Experimentally the toxin chimera triggered apoptosis in exposed bladder cancer cells with exposures as short as 3 minutes. There was a 30% average tumor reduction after a single treatment in dogs that had failed or were not eligible for other treatments (Jack *et al.* 2020).

Radiation therapy

A clear benefit of radiation therapy in the management of bladder tumors has not been shown (Withrow *et al.* 1989; Norris *et al.* 1992; Henry 2003). In a report of

9 dogs treated with surgery and postoperative radiation therapy, 6 had severe complications of incontinence and bladder fibrosis. All 9 cases died of recurrence, complications of radiation therapy, or distant metastases, and there was no improvement in survival over cases treated with surgery alone (Norris *et al.* 1992). In a report of 9 cases of bladder or urethral transitional cell carcinoma treated with debulking and intraoperative radiation with or without postoperative radiation therapy, there were similarly high complication rates with irreversible bladder wall changes. The bladder walls became thickened, fibrotic, and nondistensible by 1–2 months, with resulting incontinence. There was fibrous replacement of muscle and nerve tissue, inflammation, edema, and focal mucosal ulceration. If ureters were included in the intraoperative radiation field, they usually became stenotic and fibrotic, with secondary hydroureter and mild to moderate hydronephrosis (Withrow *et al.* 1989). A report combining six weekly fractions of 5.75 Gy of external beam irradiation with mitoxantrone and piroxicam had minimal side effects, and amelioration of clinical signs in 90% of cases (Poirier *et al.* 2004). Only 2 of 10 cases showed a partial response, and the median survival time was 326 days, which was no different to a previous report using mitoxantrone and piroxicam alone (Henry *et al.* 2003a). Another article further confirmed a high late complication rate of cases receiving definitive radiation of intrapelvic tumors that lived for more than 6 months (Arthur *et al.* 2008).

The use of intensity-modulated radiation therapy may offer hope of increased tumor doses with decreased whole-bladder fibrosis. In 21 dogs with urothelial carcinoma treated with intensity-modulated radiation therapy (54–58 Gy in 20 daily fractions), there was a 60% subjective response rate. The median survival time was 654 days. Acute toxicoses were self-limiting and of low grade. Late grade 3 side effects occurred in 19% of dogs, but this was generally well managed and late in the course of disease (Nolan *et al.* 2012). In a series of 10 dogs treated palliatively with 10 daily doses of 2.7 Gy, there was 7.6% complete response, 53.8% partial response, and 38.5% stable disease. Low-grade acute side effects of radiation occurred in 31% of animals and no late radiation side effects were seen (Choy & Fidel 2016).

Neoadjuvant radiation has been combined with neoadjuvant chemotherapy and adjuvant chemotherapy in 4 dogs. No significant toxicity was seen and all improved clinically (Marconato *et al.* 2012).

Prognosis

Canine transitional cell carcinoma is highly locally invasive at the time of diagnosis and is likely to metastasize. The prognosis is poor, with cure unlikely even with aggressive treatment. Combination protocols using chemotherapy and piroxicam show the most promise in producing tumor responses. Surgery and radiation could be considered in select cases (Henry 2003). In humans, surgery remains the preferred treatment in T1 (tumor invades subepithelial connective tissue) or T2 (tumor invades muscle) bladder tumors in which complete resection is possible (Greene *et al.* 2002). Appropriate treatment for dogs with T3 tumors (tumor invades perivesical tissue), regional metastases, or distant metastases is unknown (Greene *et al.* 2002; Norris *et al.* 1992). The role for surgery and radiation has not been defined (Norris *et al.* 1992). Development of accurate tests for early tumor detection may help diagnose the more treatable T1 and T2 lesions (Henry 2003).

A higher TNM stage is prognostic for survival (Tables 48.1–48.4) (Knapp *et al.* 2000a,b). T1 or T2 tumors were associated with a median survival time of 218 days, compared with 118 days for T3 tumors. Lack of regional node metastases was associated with a median survival time of 234 days compared with 70 days for nodal metastases. Lack of distant metastases was associated with a median survival time of 203 days compared with 105 days with distant metastases. These comparisons all reached statistical significance (Knapp *et al.* 2000a,b). Higher T stage is associated with nodal and distant metastases, male sex, and prostatic involvement. Urethral involvement is associated with the development of metastases. There is a negative association

Table 48.2 Regional nodes (N): regional nodes are those within the true pelvis; all others are distant lymph nodes.

NX	Regional lymph nodes cannot be assessed
N0	No regional lymph node metastasis
N1	Metastasis in a single lymph node, 2 cm or less in greatest dimension
N2	Metastases in a single lymph node, more than 2 cm but not more than 5 cm in greatest dimension; or multiple lymph nodes, none more than 5 cm in greatest dimension
N3	Metastasis in a lymph node, more than 5 cm in greatest dimension

Source: Greene *et al.* (2002).

Table 48.3 Distant metastasis (M).

MX	Distant metastasis cannot be assessed
M0	No distant metastasis
M1	Distant metastasis

Source: Greene *et al.* (2002).

Table 48.4 Stage grouping.

	T	N	M
Stage 0a	Ta	N0	M0
Stage 0is	Tis	N0	M0
Stage I	T1	N0	M0
Stage II	T2a	N0	M0
	T2b	N0	M0
Stage III	T3a	N0	M0
	T3b	N0	M0
Stage IV	T4a	N0	M0
	T4b	N0	M0
	Any T	N1	M0
	Any T	N2	M0
	Any T	N3	M0
	Any T	Any N	M1

Source: Greene *et al.* (2002).

between survival and prostatic involvement. There was a positive association that approached significance between survival and debulking surgery (Knapp *et al.* 2000a,b).

Negative prognostic factors include younger age, trigonal location, partial-thickness excision, and lower frequency of piroxicam administration (daily is better) (Marvel *et al.* 2017; Iwasaki *et al.* 2019). Lymph node or skeletal metastases at the time of diagnosis are a negative prognostic indicator (Allstadt *et al.* 2015; Iwasaki *et al.* 2019). Dogs with prostatic involvement may have shorter survival times (Allstadt *et al.* 2015). Use of whole-body CT at diagnosis may be useful for prognostication (Iwasaki *et al.* 2019). Use of multiple rescue agents is associated with increased survival times (Allstadt *et al.* 2015).

In one study 61% of patients died from causes related to the primary tumor (Burgess & DeRegis 2019), while 60% of cases died due to metastatic disease in another study (Iwasaki *et al.* 2019).

One article found that female dogs survived longer than male dogs (Rocha *et al.* 2000). It was suggested that female dogs have fewer anatomic constraints of the urinary tract, possibly allowing more extensive local tumor progression (Rocha *et al.* 2000).

There is a positive correlation between tumor grade and depth of tumor invasion, tumor grade and presence of metastases, and peritumoral desmoplasia and presence of metastases (Valli *et al.* 1995). Moderate to severe tumor necrosis on histopathology is associated with the presence of fibromyxoid tumor stroma. Fibromyxoid stroma is a strong indicator for invasive growth into muscle and is a poor prognostic factor. This stroma was present in 103 (27%) of 383 cases (de Brot *et al.* 2019).

References

Ahmed, M., Liu, Z., Afzal, K.S. et al. (2004). Radiofrequency ablation: effect of surrounding tissue composition on coagulation necrosis in a canine tumor model. *Radiology* 230: 761–767.

Allstadt, S.D., Rodriguez, C.O. Jr., Boostrom, B. et al. (2015). Randomized phase III trial of piroxicam in combination with mitoxantrone or carboplatin for first-line treatment of urogenital tract transitional cell carcinoma in dogs. *Journal of Veterinary Internal Medicine* 29: 261–267.

Arnold, E.J., Childress, M.O., Fourez, L.M. et al. (2011). Clinical trial of vinblastine in dogs with transitional cell carcinoma of the urinary bladder. *Journal of Veterinary Internal Medicine* 25: 1385–1390.

Arthur, J.J., Kleiter, M.M., Thrall, D.E., and Pruitt, A.F. (2008). Characterization of normal tissue complications in 51 dogs undergoing definitive pelvic region irradiation. *Veterinary Radiology & Ultrasound* 49: 85–89.

Backer, L.C., Coss, A.M., Wolkin, A.F. et al. (2008). Evaluation of associations between lifetime exposure to drinking water disinfection by-products and bladder cancer in dogs. *Journal of the American Veterinary Medical Association* 232: 1663–1668.

Bacon, N., Souza, C.H., and Franz, S. (2016). Total cysto-prostatectomy: technique description and results in 2 dogs. *Canadian Veterinary Journal* 57: 141–146.

Bae, I.H., Kim, Y., Pakhrin, B. et al. (2007). Genitourinary rhabdomyosarcoma with systemic metastasis in a young dog. *Veterinary Pathology* 44: 518–520.

Baskin, G.B. and De Paoli, A. (1977). Primary renal neoplasms of the dog. *Veterinary Pathology* 14: 591–605.

Benigni, L., Lamb, C.R., Corzo-Menendez, N. et al. (2006). Lymphoma affecting the urinary bladder in three dogs and a cat. *Veterinary Radiology & Ultrasound* 47: 592–596.

Berzon, J.L. (1979). Primary leiomyosarcoma of the ureter in a dog. *Journal of the American Veterinary Medical Association* 175: 374–376.

Blackburn, A.L., Berent, A.C., Weisse, C.W., and Brown, D.C. (2013). Evaluation of outcome following urethral stent placement for the treatment of obstructive carcinoma of the urethra in dogs: 42 cases (2004–2008). *Journal of the American Veterinary Medical Association* 242: 59–68.

Boria, P.A., Glickman, N.W., Schmidt, B.R. et al. (2005). Carboplatin and piroxicam therapy in 31 dogs with transitional cell carcinoma of the urinary bladder. *Veterinary and Comparative Oncology* 3: 73–80.

Borjesson, D.L. (2003). Renal cytology. *Veterinary Clinics of North America: Small Animal Practice* 33: 119–134.

Borjesson, D.L., Christopher, M.M., and Ling, G.V. (1999). Detection of canine transitional cell carcinoma using a bladder tumor antigen urine dipstick test. *Veterinary Clinical Pathology* 28: 33–38.

Brodey, R.S. (1971). Hypertrophic osteoarthropathy in the dog: a clinicopathologic survey of 60 cases. *Journal of the American Veterinary Medical Association* 159: 1242–1256.

de Brot, S., Grau-Roma, L., Stirling-Stainsby, C. et al. (2019). A fibromyxoid stromal response is associated with muscle invasion in canine urothelial carcinoma. *Journal of Comparative Pathology* 169: 35–46.

Bryan, J.N., Henry, C.J., Turnquist, S.E. et al. (2006). Primary renal neoplasia of dogs. *Journal of Veterinary Internal Medicine* 20: 1155–1160.

Budreckis, D.M., Byrne, B.A., Pollard, R.E. et al. (2015). Bacterial urinary tract infections associated with transitional cell carcinoma in dogs. *Journal of Veterinary Internal Medicine* 29: 828–833.

Burgess, K.E. and DeRegis, C.J. (2019). Urologic oncology. *Veterinary Clinics of North America: Small Animal Practice* 49: 311–323.

Burnie, A.G. and Weaver, D. (1983). Urinary bladder neoplasia in the dog; a review of seventy cases. *Journal of Small Animal Practice* 24: 129–143.

Burton, C.A., Day, M.J., Hoston-Moore, A., and Holt, P.E. (1994). Ureteric fibroepithelial polyps in two dogs. *Journal of Small Animal Practice* 35: 593–596.

Cannon, C.M. and Allstadt, S.D. (2015). Lower urinary tract cancer. *Veterinary Clinics of North America: Small Animal Practice* 45: 807–824.

Cerf, D.J. and Lindquist, E.C. (2012). Palliative ultrasound-guided endoscopic diode laser ablation of transitional cell carcinomas of the lower urinary tract in dogs. *Journal of the American Veterinary Medical Association* 240: 51–60.

Chan, C.M., Frimberger, A.E., and Moore, A.S. (2016). Incidence of sterile hemorrhagic cystitis in tumor-bearing dogs concurrently treated with oral metronomic cyclophosphamide chemotherapy and furosemide: 55 cases (2009–2015). *Journal of the American Veterinary Medical Association* 249: 1408–1414.

Charney, V.A., Miller, M.A., Heng, H.G. et al. (2017). Skeletal metastasis of canine urothelial carcinoma: pathologic and computed tomographic features. *Veterinary Pathology* 54: 380–386.

Chiang, Y.C., Liu, C.H., Ho, S.Y. et al. (2007). Hypertrophic osteopathy associated with disseminated metastases of renal cell carcinoma in the dog: a case report. *Journal of Veterinary Medical Science* 69: 209–212.

Childress, M.O., Adams, L.G., Ramos-Vara, J.A. et al. (2011). Results of biopsy via transurethral cystoscopy and cystotomy for diagnosis of transitional cell carcinoma of the urinary bladder and urethra in dogs: 92 cases (2003–2008). *Journal of the American Veterinary Medical Association* 239: 350–356.

Choy, K. and Fidel, J. (2016). Tolerability and tumor response of a novel low-dose palliative radiation therapy protocol in dogs with transitional cell carcinoma of the bladder and urethra. *Veterinary Radiology & Ultrasound* 57: 341–351.

Crow, S.E. (1985). Urinary tract neoplasms in dogs and cats. *Compendium on Continuing Education for the Practising Veterinarian* 7: 607–618.

Culp, W.T., Weisse, C., Berent, A.C. et al. (2015). Early tumor response to intraarterial or intravenous administration of carboplatin to treat naturally occurring lower urinary tract carcinoma in dogs. *Journal of Veterinary Internal Medicine* 29: 900–907.

Davies, J.V. and Read, H.M. (1990). Urethral tumors in dogs. *Journal of Small Animal Practice* 31: 131–136.

Davis, G.J. and Holt, D. (2003). Two chondrosarcomas in the urethra of a German shepherd dog. *Journal of Small Animal Practice* 44: 169–171.

Delaune, T., Bernard, F., Matres-Lorenzo, L., and Bernardé, A. (2018). Radical cystectomy and subsequent ureterohysterostomy in a bitch. *Veterinary Surgery* 47: 1106–1111.

Deschamps, J.Y., Roux, F.A., Fantinato, M., and Albaric, O. (2007). Ureteral sarcoma in a dog. *Journal of Small Animal Practice* 48: 699–701.

Edmondson, E.F., Hess, A.M., and Powers, B.E. (2015). Prognostic significance of histologic features in canine renal cell carcinomas: 70 nephrectomies. *Veterinary Pathology* 52: 260–268.

Eichstadt, L.R., Moore, G.E., and Childress, M.O. (2017). Risk factors for treatment-related adverse events in cancer-bearing dogs receiving piroxicam. *Veterinary and Comparative Oncology* 15: 1346–1353.

Farrell, M., Philbey, A.W., and Ramsey, I. (2006). Ureteral fibroepithelial polyp in a dog. *Journal of Small Animal Practice* 47: 409–412.

Font, A., Closa, J.M., and Mascort, J. (1993). Ureteral leiomyoma causing abnormal micturition in a dog. *Journal of the American Animal Hospital Association* 29: 25–27.

Frimberger, A.E., Moore, A.S., and Schelling, S.H. (1995). Treatment of nephroblastoma in a juvenile dog. *Journal of the American Veterinary Medical Association* 207: 596–598.

Fulkerson, C.M. and Knapp, D.W. (2015). Management of transitional cell carcinoma of the urinary bladder in dogs: a review. *Veterinary Journal* 205: 217–225.

Gabor, L.J., Malik, R., and Canfield, P.J. (1998). Clinical and anatomical features of lymphosarcoma in 118 cats. *Australian Veterinary Journal* 76: 725–732.

Gasser, A.M., Bush, W.W., Smith, S., and Walton, R. (2003). Extradural spinal, bone marrow, and renal nephroblastoma. *Journal of the American Animal Hospital Association* 39: 80–85.

Gervais, D.A., McGovern, F.J., Arellano, R.S. et al. (2005). Radiofrequency ablation of renal cell carcinoma: part 1, indications, results, and role in patient management over a 6-year period and ablation of 100 tumors. *American Journal of Roentgenology* 185: 64–71.

Glickman, L.T., Schofer, F.S., McKee, L.J. et al. (1989). Epidemiologic study of insecticide exposures, obesity, and risk of bladder cancer in household dogs. *Journal of Toxicology and Environmental Health* 28: 407–414.

Glickman, L.T., Raghavan, M., Knapp, D.W. et al. (2004). Herbicide exposure and the risk of transitional cell carcinoma of the urinary bladder in Scottish Terriers. *Journal of the American Veterinary Medical Association* 224: 1290–1297.

Greene, F.L., Page, D.L., Fleming, I.D. et al. (ed.) (2002). *Genitourinary Sites*. New York: Springer.

Greene, S.N., Lucroy, M.D., Greenberg, C.B. et al. (2007). Evaluation of cisplatin administered with piroxicam in dogs with transitional cell carcinoma of the urinary bladder. *Journal of the American Veterinary Medical Association* 231: 1056–1060.

Grillo, T.P., Brandao, C.V., Mamprim, M.J. et al. (2007). Hypertrophic osteopathy associated with renal pelvis transitional cell carcinoma in a dog. *Canadian Veterinary Journal* 48: 745–747.

Guilherme, S., Polton, G., Bray, J. et al. (2007). Ureteral spindle cell sarcoma in a dog. *Journal of Small Animal Practice* 48: 702–704.

Gustafson, T.L. and Biller, B. (2019). Use of toceranib phosphate in the treatment of canine bladder tumors: 37 cases. *Journal of the American Animal Hospital Association* 55: 243–248.

Hahn, K.A., McGavin, M.D., and Adams, W.H. (1997). Bilateral renal metastases of nasal chondrosarcoma in a dog. *Veterinary Pathology* 34: 352–355.

Hamlin, A.N., Chadwick, L.E., Fox-Alvarez, S.A., and Hostnik, E.T. (2019). Ultrasound characteristics of feline urinary bladder transitional cell carcinoma are similar to canine urinary bladder transitional cell carcinoma. *Veterinary Radiology & Ultrasound* 60: 552–559.

Hanika, C. and Rebar, A.H. (1980). Ureteral transitional cell carcinoma in the dog. *Veterinary Pathology* 17: 643–646.

Hattel, A.L., Diters, R.W., and Snavely, D.A. (1986). Ureteral fibropapilloma in a dog. *Journal of the American Veterinary Medical Association* 188: 873.

Helfand, S.C., Hamilton, T.A., Hungerford, L.L. et al. (1994). Comparison of three treatments for transitional cell carcinoma of the bladder in the dog. *Journal of the American Animal Hospital Association* 30: 270–275.

Heng, H.G., Lowry, J.E., Boston, S. et al. (2006). Smooth muscle neoplasia of the urinary bladder wall in three dogs. *Veterinary Radiology & Ultrasound* 47: 83–86.

Henry, C.J. (2003). Management of transitional cell carcinoma. *Veterinary Clinics of North America: Small Animal Practice* 33: 597–613.

Henry, C.J., Turnquist, S.E., Smith, A. et al. (1999). Primary renal tumours in cats: 19 cases (1992-1998). *Journal of Feline Medicine and Surgery* 1: 165–170.

Henry, C.J., McCaw, D.L., Turnquist, S.E. et al. (2003a). Clinical evaluation of mitoxantrone and piroxicam in a canine model of human invasive urinary bladder carcinoma. *Clinical Cancer Research* 9: 906–911.

Henry, C.J., Tyler, J.W., McEntee, M.C. et al. (2003b). Evaluation of a bladder tumor antigen test as a screening test for transitional cell carcinoma of the lower urinary tract in dogs. *American Journal of Veterinary Research* 64: 1017–1020.

Hurov, L., Ellett, E.W., and O'Hara, P.J. (1966). Bilateral hydronephrosis resulting from a transitional epithelial carcinoma in a dog. *Journal of the American Veterinary Medical Association* 149: 412–417.

Iwasaki, R., Shimosato, Y., Yoshikawa, R. et al. (2019). Survival analysis in dogs with urinary transitional cell carcinoma that underwent whole-body computed tomography at diagnosis. *Veterinary and Comparative Oncology* 17: 385–393.

Jack, S., Madhivanan, K., Ramadesikan, S. et al. (2020). A novel, safe, fast and efficient treatment for Her2-positive and negative bladder cancer utilizing an EGF-anthrax toxin chimera. *International Journal of Cancer* 146: 449–460.

Kaye, M.E., Thamm, D.H., Weishaar, K., and Lawrence, J.A. (2015). Vinorelbine rescue therapy for dogs with primary urinary bladder carcinoma. *Veterinary and Comparative Oncology* 13: 443–451.

Kim, S., Hosoya, K., Takagi, S., and Okumura, M. (2019). Outcomes following balloon dilation for management of urethral obstruction secondary to urothelial carcinoma in dogs: 12 cases (2010–2015). *Journal of the American Veterinary Medical Association* 255: 330–335.

Klein, M.K., Cockerell, G.L., Harris, C.K. et al. (1988). Canine primary renal neoplasms: a retrospective review of 54 cases. *Journal of the American Animal Hospital Association* 24: 443–452.

Knapp, D.W., Richardson, R.C., Chan, T.C. et al. (1994). Piroxicam therapy in 34 dogs with transitional cell carcinoma of the urinary bladder. *Journal of Veterinary Internal Medicine* 8: 273–278.

Knapp, D.W., Glickman, N.W., DeNicola, D.B. et al. (2000a). Naturally-occurring canine transitional cell carcinoma of the urinary bladder. A relevant model of human invasive bladder cancer. *Urologic Oncology* 5: 47–59.

Knapp, D.W., Glickman, N.W., Widmer, W.R. et al. (2000b). Cisplatin versus cisplatin combined with piroxicam in a canine model of human invasive urinary bladder cancer. *Cancer Chemotherapy and Pharmacology* 46: 221–226.

Knapp, D.W., Henry, C.J., Widmer, W.R. et al. (2013). Randomized trial of cisplatin versus firocoxib versus cisplatin/firocoxib in dogs with transitional cell carcinoma of the urinary bladder. *Journal of Veterinary Internal Medicine* 27: 126–133.

Knapp, D.W., Ruple-Czerniak, A., Ramos-Vara, J.A. et al. (2016). A nonselective cyclooxygenase inhibitor enhances the activity of vinblastine in a naturally-occurring canine model of invasive urothelial carcinoma. *Bladder Cancer* 2: 241–250.

Knottenbelt, C., Mellor, D., Nixon, C. et al. (2006). Cohort study of COX-1 and COX-2 expression in canine rectal and bladder tumours. *Journal of Small Animal Practice* 47: 196–200.

Lamb, C.R., Trower, N.D., and Gregory, S.P. (1996). Ultrasound-guided catheter biopsy of the lower urinary tract: technique and results in 12 dogs. *Journal of Small Animal Practice* 37: 413–416.

Liptak, J.M., Brutscher, S.P., Monnet, E. et al. (2004). Transurethral resection in the management of urethral and prostatic neoplasia in 6 dogs. *Veterinary Surgery* 33: 505–516.

Liska, W.D. and Patnaik, A.K. (1977). Leiomyoma of the ureter of a dog. *Journal of the American Animal Hospital Association* 13: 83–84.

Lium, B. and Moe, L. (1985). Hereditary multifocal renal cystadenocarcinomas and nodular dermatofibrosis in the German shepherd dog: macroscopic and histopathologic changes. *Veterinary Pathology* 22: 447–455.

Locke, J.E. and Barber, L.G. (2006). Comparative aspects and clinical outcomes of canine renal hemangiosarcoma. *Journal of Veterinary Internal Medicine* 20: 962–967.

Lucke, V.M. and Kelly, D.F. (1976). Renal carcinoma in the dog. *Veterinary Pathology* 13: 264–276.

Marconato, L., Nitzl, D.B., Melzer-Ruess, K.J. et al. (2012). Chemotherapy and radiation therapy in 4 dogs with muscle-invasive transitional cell carcinoma of the urinary tract. *Canadian Veterinary Journal* 53: 875–879.

Martinez, I., Mattoon, J.S., Eaton, K.A. et al. (2003). Polypoid cystitis in 17 dogs (1978–2001). *Journal of Veterinary Internal Medicine* 17: 499–509.

Marvel, S.J., Séguin, B., Dailey, D.D., and Thamm, D.H. (2017). Clinical outcome of partial cystectomy for transitional cell carcinoma of the canine bladder. *Veterinary and Comparative Oncology* 15: 1417–1427.

McMillan, S.K., Knapp, D.W., Ramos-Vara, J.A. et al. (2012). Outcome of urethral stent placement for management of urethral obstruction secondary to transitional cell carcinoma in dogs: 19 cases (2007–2010). *Journal of the American Veterinary Medical Association* 241: 1627–1632.

Mehta, M.P., Bastin, K.T., and Wiersma, S.R. (1991). Treatment of Wilms' tumour. Current recommendations. *Drugs* 42: 766–780.

Mochizuki, H., Shapiro, S.G., and Breen, M. (2015). Detection of BRAF mutation in urine DNA as a molecular diagnostic for canine urothelial and prostatic carcinoma. *PLOS ONE* 10: e0144170.

Moe, L. and Lium, B. (1997). Hereditary multifocal renal cystadenocarcinomas and nodular dermatofibrosis in 51 German shepherd dogs. *Journal of Small Animal Practice* 38: 498–505.

Mooney, S.C., Hayes, A.A., Matus, R.E., and MacEwen, E.G. (1987). Renal lymphoma in cats: 28 cases (1977–1984). *Journal of the American Veterinary Medical Association* 191: 1473–1477.

Morgan, M. and Forman, M. (2015). Cystoscopy in dogs and cats. *Veterinary Clinics of North America: Small Animal Practice* 45: 665–701.

Moroff, S.D., Brown, B.A., Matthiesen, D.T., and Scott, R.C. (1991). Infiltrative urethral disease in female dogs: 41 cases (1980–1987). *Journal of the American Veterinary Medical Association* 199: 247–251.

Mott, J.C., McAnulty, J.F., Darien, D.L., and Steinberg, H. (1996). Nephron sparing by partial median nephrectomy for treatment of renal hemangioma in a dog. *Journal of the American Veterinary Medical Association* 208: 1274–1276.

Nakayama, H., Hayashi, T., Takahashi, R., and Fujiwara, K. (1984). Nephroblastoma with liver and lung metastases in an adult dog. *Nippon Juigaku Zasshi* 46: 897–900.

Newman, R.G., Mehler, S.J., Kitchell, B.E., and Beal, M.W. (2009). Use of a balloon-expandable metallic stent to relieve malignant urethral obstruction in a cat. *Journal of the American Veterinary Medical Association* 234: 236–239.

Nolan, M.W., Kogan, L., Griffin, L.R. et al. (2012). Intensity-modulated and image-guided radiation therapy for treatment of genitourinary carcinomas in dogs. *Journal of Veterinary Internal Medicine* 26: 987–995.

Norris, A.M., Laing, E.J., Valli, V.E. et al. (1992). Canine bladder and urethral tumors: a retrospective study of 115 cases (1980–1985). *Journal of Veterinary Internal Medicine* 6: 145–153.

Nyland, T.G., Wallack, S.T., and Wisner, E.R. (2002). Needle-tract implantation following US-guided fine-needle aspiration biopsy of transitional cell carcinoma of the bladder, urethra, and prostate. *Veterinary Radiology & Ultrasound* 43: 50–53.

Olausson, A., Stieger, S.M., Loefgren, S., and Gillingstam, M. (2005). A urinary bladder fibrosarcoma in a young dog. *Veterinary Radiology & Ultrasound* 46: 135–138.

Patrick, D.J., Fitzgerald, S.D., Sesterhenn, I.A. et al. (2006). Classification of canine urinary bladder urothelial tumours based on the World Health Organization/International Society of Urological Pathology consensus classification. *Journal of Comparative Pathology* 135: 190–199.

Poirier, V.J., Forrest, L.J., Adams, W.M., and Vail, D.M. (2004). Piroxicam, mitoxantrone, and coarse fraction radiotherapy for the treatment of transitional cell carcinoma of the bladder in 10 dogs: a pilot study. *Journal of the American Animal Hospital Association* 40: 131–136.

Pozzi, A., Smeak, D.D., and Aper, R. (2006). Colonic seromuscular augmentation cystoplasty following subtotal cystectomy for treatment of bladder necrosis caused by bladder torsion in a dog. *Journal of the American Veterinary Medical Association* 229: 235–239.

Raghavan, M., Knapp, D.W., Dawson, M.H. et al. (2004). Topical flea and tick pesticides and the risk of transitional cell carcinoma of the urinary bladder in Scottish Terriers. *Journal of the American Veterinary Medical Association* 225: 389–394.

Raghavan, M., Knapp, D.W., Bonney, P.L. et al. (2005). Evaluation of the effect of dietary vegetable consumption on reducing risk of transitional cell carcinoma of the urinary bladder in Scottish Terriers. *Journal of the American Veterinary Medical Association* 227: 94–100.

Reed, L.T., Knapp, D.W., and Miller, M.A. (2013). Cutaneous metastasis of transitional cell carcinoma in 12 dogs. *Veterinary Pathology* 50: 676–681.

Reichle, J.K., Peterson, R.A. 2nd, Mahaffey, M.B. et al. (2003). Ureteral fibroepithelial polyps in four dogs. *Veterinary Radiology & Ultrasound* 44: 433–437.

Ricardo Huppes, R., Crivellenti, L.Z., Barboza De Nardi, A. et al. (2017). Radical cystectomy and cutaneous ureterostomy in 4 dogs with trigonal transitional cell carcinoma: description of technique and case series. *Veterinary Surgery* 46: 111–119.

Robat, C., Burton, J., Thamm, D., and Vail, D. (2013). Retrospective evaluation of doxorubicin-piroxicam combination for the treatment of transitional cell carcinoma in dogs. *Journal of Small Animal Practice* 54: 67–74.

Rocha, T.A., Mauldin, G.N., Patnaik, A.K., and Bergman, P.J. (2000). Prognostic factors in dogs with urinary bladder carcinoma. *Journal of Veterinary Internal Medicine* 14: 486–490.

Saeki, K., Fujita, A., Fujita, N. et al. (2015). Total cystectomy and subsequent urinary diversion to the prepuce or vagina in dogs with transitional cell carcinoma of the trigone area: a report of 10 cases (2005–2011). *Canadian Veterinary Journal* 56: 73–80.

Salinardi, B.J., Marks, S.L., Davidson, J.R., and Senior, D.F. (2003). The use of a low-profile cystostomy tube to relieve urethral obstruction in a dog. *Journal of the American Animal Hospital Association* 39: 403–405.

Saulnier-Troff, F.G., Busoni, V., and Hamaide, A. (2008). A technique for resection of invasive tumors involving the trigone area of the bladder in dogs: preliminary results in two dogs. *Veterinary Surgery* 37: 427–437.

Schrempp, D.R., Childress, M.O., Stewart, J.C. et al. (2013). Metronomic administration of chlorambucil for treatment of dogs with urinary bladder transitional cell carcinoma. *Journal of the American Veterinary Medical Association* 242: 1534–1538.

Schwarz, P.D., Greene, R.W., and Patnaik, A.K. (1985). Urinary bladder tumors in the cat: a review of 27 cases. *Journal of the American Animal Hospital Association* 21: 237–245.

Seaman, R.L. and Patton, C.S. (2003). Treatment of renal nephroblastoma in an adult dog. *Journal of the American Animal Hospital Association* 39: 76–79.

Smith, J.D., Stone, E.A., and Gilson, S.D. (1995). Placement of a permanent cystostomy catheter to relieve urine outflow obstruction in dogs with transitional cell carcinoma. *Journal of the American Veterinary Medical Association* 206: 496–499.

Steffey, M., Rassnick, K.M., Porter, B., and Njaa, B.L. (2004). Ureteral mast cell tumor in a dog. *Journal of the American Animal Hospital Association* 40: 82–85.

Stone, E.A., Withrow, S.J., Page, R.L. et al. (1988). Ureterocolonic anastomosis in ten dogs with transitional cell carcinoma. *Veterinary Surgery* 17: 147–153.

Struble, A.L., Lawson, G.W., and Ling, G.V. (1997). Urethral obstruction in a dog: an unusual presentation of T-cell lymphoma. *Journal of the American Animal Hospital Association* 33: 423–426.

Swalec, K.M., Smeak, D.D., and Baker, A.L. (1989). Urethral leiomyoma in a cat. *Journal of the American Veterinary Medical Association* 195: 961–962.

Takagi, S., Kadosawa, T., Ishiguro, T. et al. (2005). Urethral transitional cell carcinoma in a cat. *Journal of Small Animal Practice* 46: 504–506.

Tarvin, G., Patnaik, A., and Greene, R. (1978). Primary urethral tumors in dogs. *Journal of the American Veterinary Medical Association* 172: 931–933.

Taylor, S.S., Goodfellow, M.R., Browne, W.J. et al. (2009). Feline extranodal lymphoma: response to chemotherapy and survival in 110 cats. *Journal of Small Animal Practice* 50: 584–592.

Upton, M.L., Tangner, C.H., and Payton, M.E. (2006). Evaluation of carbon dioxide laser ablation combined with mitoxantrone and piroxicam treatment in dogs with transitional cell carcinoma. *Journal of the American Veterinary Medical Association* 228: 549–552.

Valli, V.E., Norris, A., Jacobs, R.M. et al. (1995). Pathology of canine bladder and urethral cancer and correlation with tumour progression and survival. *Journal of Comparative Pathology* 113: 113–130.

Walter, P.A., Haynes, J.S., Feeney, D.A., and Johnston, G.R. (1984). Radiographic appearance of pulmonary metastases from transitional cell carcinoma of the bladder and urethra of the dog. *Journal of the American Veterinary Medical Association* 185: 411–418.

Weisse, C., Berent, A., Todd, K. et al. (2006). Evaluation of palliative stenting for management of malignant urethral obstructions in dogs. *Journal of the American Veterinary Medical Association* 229: 226–234.

Weller, R.E., Wolf, A.M., and Oyejide, A. (1979). Transitional cell carcinoma of the bladder associated with cyclophosphamide therapy in a dog. *Journal of the American Animal Hospital Association* 15: 733–736.

White, R.N., Davies, J.V., and Gregory, S.P. (1996). Vaginourethroplasty for treatment of urethral obstruction in the bitch. *Veterinary Surgery* 25: 503–510.

Wiley, C., Wise, C.F., and Breen, M. (2019). Novel noninvasive diagnostics. *Veterinary Clinics of North America: Small Animal Practice* 49: 781–791.

Wilson, G.P., Hayes, H.M., and Casey, H.W. (1979). Canine urethral cancer. *Journal of the American Animal Hospital Association* 15: 741–744.

Wilson, H.M., Chun, R., Larson, V.S. et al. (2007). Clinical signs, treatments, and outcome in cats with transitional cell carcinoma of the urinary bladder: 20 cases (1990–2004). *Journal of the American Veterinary Medical Association* 231: 101–106.

Withrow, S.J., Gillette, E.L., Hoopes, P.J., and McChesney, S.L. (1989). Intraoperative irradiation of 16 spontaneously occurring canine neoplasms. *Veterinary Surgery* 18: 7–11.

Woldemeskel, M. (2017). Primary urinary bladder osteosarcoma in a dog. *Journal of Comparative Pathology* 157: 141–144.

Wycislo, K.L. and Piech, T.L. (2019). Urinary tract cytology. *Veterinary Clinics of North America: Small Animal Practice* 49: 247–260.

Yap, F.W., Huizing, X.B., Rasotto, R., and Bowlt-Blacklock, K.L. (2017). Primary ureteral leiomyosarcoma in a dog. *Australian Veterinary Journal* 95: 68–71.

49

Urinary Tract Trauma

Heidi Phillips

Trauma to the urinary tract is not uncommon in veterinary patients and may be the result of blunt trauma, such as motor vehicle injury or a fall; penetrating trauma from bite wounds, ballistic injury, foreign body migration, or other sharp trauma; iatrogenic trauma from surgical procedures, urethral catheterization, or overzealous palpation; trauma related to the presence of obstructive or irritating calculi; or other sources of injury. Additionally, traumatic injury of the urinary tract frequently accompanies injury to the abdomen or pelvis. In studies of traumatized small animals, dogs and cats are frequently victims of motor vehicle injury, often suffering injury to the abdomen or pelvis that may extend to the urinary tract (Kolata & Johnston 1975; Selcer 1982; Streeter *et al.* 2009; Hoffberg *et al.* 2016).

Trauma to the urinary tract can involve the kidneys, ureters, bladder, or urethra and associated urogenital organs such as the prostate. Although the bladder is the most commonly injured organ, concurrent damage to multiple components of the urinary tract as well as other abdominal and thoracic organs, the skeletal system, and skin is possible (Bellah 1999; Aronson 2008). Urologic complications of trauma can be minimized by prompt recognition of urologic damage, sound initial treatment and stabilization, and an accurate and thorough evaluation of the entire urinary tract. This is accomplished through the evaluation and application of historical data and physical examination findings; the results of clinical pathologic testing of blood, urine, and abdominal fluid; abdominal radiographic studies including contrast studies; and advanced diagnostic imaging including abdominal ultrasonography, fluoroscopy, computed tomography

(CT), or magnetic resonance imaging (MRI). Despite the availability of sensitive and accurate diagnostic imaging, abdominal exploratory surgery may be necessary to accurately assess the location and degree of trauma to the urinary tract.

Clinical signs of urinary tract trauma

The clinical signs of urinary tract trauma may range from vague signs such as depressed mentation or vomiting to life-threatening cardiovascular issues (Grimes *et al.* 2018). Signs may be masked by more obvious trauma to other organ systems, or by concurrent illness (Pechman 1982; Bellah 1999; Aronson 2008). Hypovolemic shock and redistribution of body fluids may minimize the presence of abdominal effusion, and injury to the kidneys or ureters may result in the presence of retroperitoneal fluid only. Pain may make palpation of the abdomen or rectum difficult, and injury to other vital organ systems may take priority during stabilization. However, clinical signs that should alert a clinician to the possibility of urinary tract injury include hematuria; anuria; dysuria; abdominal pain; pain, swelling, or bruising in the sublumbar region; ventral abdominal bruising; the presence of abdominal effusion; perineal pain, swelling, or bruising, or other changes in color, texture, or temperature of the perineal skin (Morgan 1982; Pechman 1982; Aumann *et al.* 1998; Bellah 1999; Culp & Silverstein 2015; Grimes *et al.* 2018) (Figure 49.1). The presence of any of the above signs, or bradycardia with electrocardiographic changes suggestive of hyperkalemia, is an indication for radiographic,

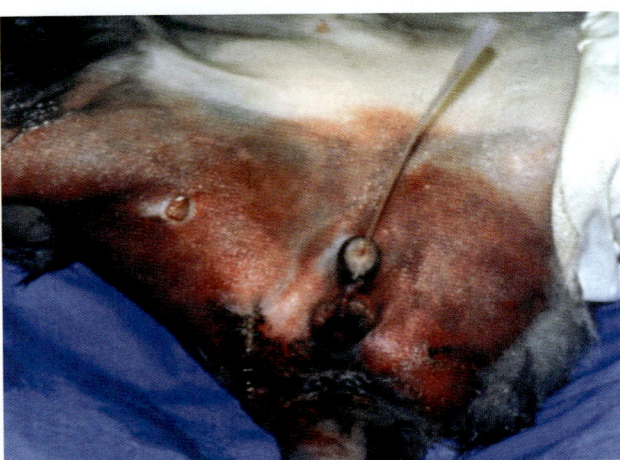

Figure 49.1 Cat having sustained vehicular trauma and disruption of the caudal urethra positioned in dorsal recumbency. Note the significant perineal bruising and discoloration.

ultrasonographic, or CT evaluation of the abdomen and pelvis, and further assessment of the urinary tract with or without intravenous or local infusion of contrast agent (Kleine 1973; Riordan & Schaer 2015).

Initial stabilization

Patients sustaining trauma to the urinary tract frequently experience concurrent trauma to other organ systems (Pechman 1982; Selcer 1982; Culp & Silverstein 2015). Appropriate triage should include prompt attention to immediately life-threatening abnormalities. Patients should be assessed for respiratory, cardiovascular, and neurologic deficiencies, as well as for musculoskeletal and urinary tract injuries. All trauma patients should undergo thoracic radiographic evaluation for signs of rib fracture, pulmonary contusion, or other injury such as diaphragmatic hernia. Although not immediately life-threatening, skin wounds and fractures should also receive appropriate first aid and supportive bandaging following resuscitation and stabilization of the patient.

Depending on time to presentation relative to injury, significant changes in fluid and acid–base balance and electrolytes may be present in the dog or cat with urinary tract trauma and require correction prior to anesthesia and definitive surgical correction (Aronson 2008; Riordan & Schaer 2015). Uroperitoneum or the presence of urine in the retroperitoneal space or perineal tissues may lead to decreased renal excretion of blood urea nitrogen (BUN), creatinine, and potassium, and result in azotemia, electrolyte and acid–base disturbances, depression, and hypovolemic shock. Dehydration may result from decreased fluid intake and excessive fluid losses due to vomiting or third-space accumulation of fluid (Aumann *et al.* 1998; Aronson 2008). The presence of a chemical peritonitis and the osmotic effect of hypertonic urine can lead to marked fluid shifts into the peritoneal cavity. Resuscitative efforts, and the volume and rate of intravenous fluid administration, should be customized to the individual patient's needs. Although potassium-free fluids such as 0.9% sodium chloride are most frequently recommended, the amount of potassium in potassium-deficient isotonic crystalloids is negligible and should not contribute greatly to worsening hyperkalemia in the short term. Additionally, a balanced electrolyte solution may be preferred for its more neutral pH, as compared with the more acidic pH of 0.9% saline. However, intravenous fluids dilute serum potassium levels regardless of which fluid is chosen, and benefit the patient by improving glomerular filtration rate (Stafford & Bartges 2013; Riordan & Schaer 2015).

An electrocardiogram (ECG) should be evaluated in any bradycardic or hyperkalemic patient ($K^+ >5.5$ mEq/L), although cardiac arrhythmias attributable to hyperkalemia are not generally apparent until potassium levels reach or exceed 7.5 mEq/L. Initially in hyperkalemic animals, peaked, narrow T waves are noted on an ECG. As hyperkalemia worsens, bradycardia and prolongation of QRS complexes occur, and the complexes become wide and bizarre. Depressed R waves and depressed ST segments can also occur. Concurrent metabolic acidosis and hypocalcemia secondary to hyperphosphatemia can exacerbate hyperkalemia's effects on the heart and ECG. At potassium concentrations above 7 mEq/L, P waves flatten or become absent, and ultimately atrial standstill, sinoventricular arrhythmias, ventricular flutter and fibrillation, and asystole may occur (Riordan & Schaer 2015).

Immediate therapy to reduce and antagonize serum potassium should be undertaken in patients with significant ECG changes or K^+ concentrations at or exceeding 8 mEq/L. Hyperkalemia increases the resting membrane potential of cells, causing it to approach the depolarization threshold. Administration of calcium gluconate increases the threshold to depolarization and thus modulates the effects of hyperkalemia on the depolarization of cells. Intravenous 10% calcium gluconate should be given at a dose of 0.25–0.5 mL/kg, slowly over 5–10 minutes, to protect the heart from the effects of hyperkalemia. The ECG should continue to be monitored over this time to assess for further development of arrhythmias. In addition to intravenous fluids, other medications may be given to lower serum potassium. Intravenous 25% dextrose solution may be given slowly over 3–5 minutes at a dose of 0.7–1 g/kg, allowing cotransportation of potassium into cells as the dextrose moves intracellularly. Regular insulin (0.1–0.25 units/kg) may also be given to help drive potassium intracellularly, and dextrose is administered concurrently at a dose of 2 g per unit of insulin given. In cases of severe acidosis (pH <7.1) or in patients with excessively low bicarbonate levels (below 10–12 mmol/L), intravenous sodium bicarbonate may be indicated. As sodium bicarbonate treats the metabolic acidosis, it enables hydrogen ions to move extracellularly. This allows potassium to move back into the cells, thereby decreasing serum potassium levels. The dose of sodium bicarbonate is calculated as 0.3 times the base deficit times the body weight in kilograms. One-quarter to one-third of the calculated dose is given slowly intravenously over 15–30 minutes and the patient is then reassessed. A loop diuretic such as furosemide (1–4 mg/kg) or a thiazide diuretic such as hydrochlorothiazide (2–4 mg/kg) can lower potassium levels by increasing urinary potassium excretion, but their use is rarely indicated and must follow rehydration and confirmation of patency of the urinary tract (Riordan & Schaer 2015). Terbutaline is a β-adrenergic receptor agonist that has been shown to induce hypokalemia, and some have recommended its use clinically in the treatment of patients with hyperkalemia (Hall et al. 2010).

Additionally, some severely unstable patients may be unable to tolerate general anesthesia for definitive surgical treatment of urinary tract trauma. Such patients may require placement of a peritoneal dialysis catheter and urethral catheter or percutaneous locking-loop cystostomy tube to divert urine flow from the site of trauma and from the peritoneal cavity (Hoffer & Sclafani 1996; Holmes et al. 2012). Peritoneal dialysis or even hemodialysis may be needed to more completely resolve azotemia as well as fluid, electrolyte, and acid–base imbalances prior to definitive surgery; anesthesia and corrective surgery may then follow adequate resuscitation of the patient (Morgan 1982; Aronson 2008).

An important component of patient care that should not be neglected is pain management. Chemical peritonitis related to uroabdomen, even in the absence of urinary tract infection and abdominal sepsis, is painful. Pure mu agonists such as fentanyl, morphine, or hydromorphone may be used for analgesia in patients with uroabdomen, given as either a constant rate infusion or intermittent injection. Methadone may also be given by intravenous intermittent injection. As these medications are reversible by use of naloxone or partially reversible by use of butorphanol, their effects on the unstable urinary tract trauma patient can be mitigated. Caution should be used in unstable dogs and cats, as opioids can exacerbate hypotension and hypoventilation in shock patients (Stafford & Bartges 2013). Multimodal analgesia combining opioids with other medications such as ketamine, lidocaine, and the use of local anesthesia may achieve high-quality pain control with minimal side effects. Ketamine should be used with caution in patients with uroabdomen, as it is excreted unchanged in the urine and may be resorbed across the peritoneum, resulting in prolonged sedation. Nonsteroidal anti-inflammatory drugs are contraindicated in patients with renal and other urinary tract concerns (Stafford & Bartges 2013).

Clinicopathologic evaluation

A routine complete blood count, serum biochemical screening, and urinalysis should be performed in patients presenting with any abdominal trauma that may affect the urinary tract. A complete blood count may reveal regenerative or nonregenerative anemia, depending on the degree of trauma, time to presentation, and underlying or concurrent abnormalities. Low platelet counts may be due to consumption of platelets in patients with significant hemorrhage. A stress leukogram is possible, or neutrophilia with or without a left shift could be indicative of inflammation or even sepsis in cases of urinary tract infection. Serum biochemical analysis may reveal azotemia and hyperkalemia, hyperphosphatemia, hyponatremia, or hypochloremia. Venous blood gas analysis may demonstrate a metabolic acidosis due to uremia, renal tubular acidosis, or lactic acidosis in hypoperfused patients. Accumulated peritoneal fluid greater than 5–25 mL/kg can usually be obtained by blind closed-needle abdominocentesis, placement of a peritoneal dialysis catheter, or AFAST (abdominal focused assessment with sonography for trauma, triage, and tracking) evaluation of the abdomen followed by ultrasound-guided paracentesis (Heeren et al. 2004; Jandrey 2015). To sample smaller volumes of fluid, diagnostic peritoneal lavage may be necessary, but it dilutes the sample obtained. Undiluted fluid suspected to contain urine should be evaluated for potassium and creatinine levels, and these levels compared with those obtained from peripheral blood. Since potassium is not absorbed across the peritoneal membrane as rapidly as it is excreted into the peritoneal cavity by the disrupted urinary system, potassium levels in the abdominal fluid remain higher than those of the peripheral blood (Stafford & Bartges 2013). Uroperitoneum is suggested by elevation of potassium levels in the abdominal fluid compared with serum in ratios greater than 1.4 : 1 in the dog and 1.9 : 1 in the cat (Schmiedt et al. 2001; Stafford & Bartges 2013). Because relatively small BUN molecules do readily translocate across the peritoneal membrane, assessment of abdominal fluid BUN is not likely to be helpful in diagnosis of uroabdomen. In contrast, the high molecular weight of creatinine molecules permits accurate comparison of abdominal and peripheral values. An abdominal fluid creatinine concentration equal to or greater than twice that of the peripheral blood is highly suggestive of uroperitoneum, with sensitivity of 86% and specificity of 100% (Aumann *et al.* 1998; Wright *et al.* 1999; Heeren *et al.* 2004; Stafford & Bartges 2013). Cytologic evaluation of the abdominal fluid should also be performed to evaluate for signs of sepsis or inflammation, or evidence of damage to other abdominal organs. A nonseptic inflammatory effusion may develop due to chemical peritonitis, or the presence of urinary tract infection may lead to sepsis.

Focused ultrasonography of the canine and feline urinary tracts has been described and can be utilized in cases of suspected urinary tract trauma. As dogs and cats suffering urinary tract trauma may be initially unstable or critically ill, point-of-care sonography can be performed noninvasively to guide the clinician in selecting diagnostic tests and treatment modalities (Cole *et al.* 2021).

Radiographic evaluation of the patient with urinary tract trauma

Plain radiographic films can be helpful in diagnosing urinary tract trauma or in raising the index of suspicion for such trauma, highlighting the need for further imaging. Unfortunately, plain radiography alone is rarely diagnostic for urinary tract injury. To increase diagnostic accuracy, radiographs of the abdomen and pelvis should be taken in two orthogonal planes (Kleine 1973). Radiographic signs that suggest damage to the urinary tract include inability to visualize the kidneys, displacement or asymmetry of one or both kidneys, increased or irregular density in the retroperitoneal space, loss of the lumbar fascial planes, widening of the retroperitoneal space, loss of normal intra-abdominal contrast, or reduced size and displacement or absence of the urinary bladder silhouette (Kleine 1973) (Figure 49.2). The ability to visualize the urinary bladder radiographically does not rule out urinary bladder rupture. Other radiographic signs that should alert the clinician to possible urinary tract injury include fractures of the last three ribs, pelvis, spine, or os penis, or the presence of an abdominal, paracostal, inguinal, or perineal hernia (Pechman 1982) (Figure 49.3).

Radiographic or CT contrast studies can be utilized alone or in combination to evaluate the entire urinary tract and localize any areas of disruption. Uroperitoneum most often develops from trauma to the distal ureters, bladder, or proximal urethra, whereas isolated uroretroperitoneum most often results from focal injury to one or both kidneys or to the proximal ureter without

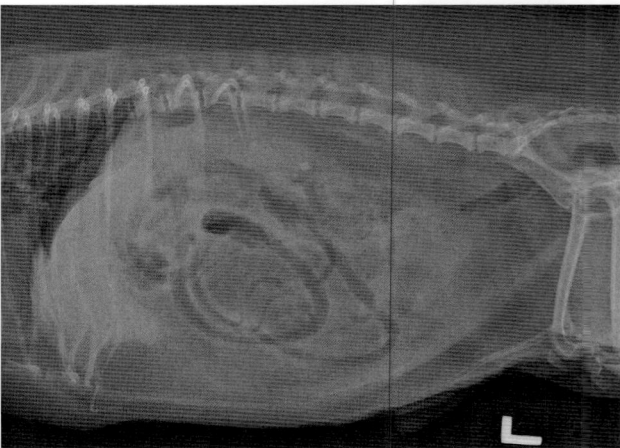

Figure 49.2 Lateral abdominal radiograph of a dog following cystotomy by the primary veterinarian. Dehiscence of the cystotomy incision resulted in uroperitoneum. Note the loss of detail in the peritoneal cavity and absence of the bladder silhouette.

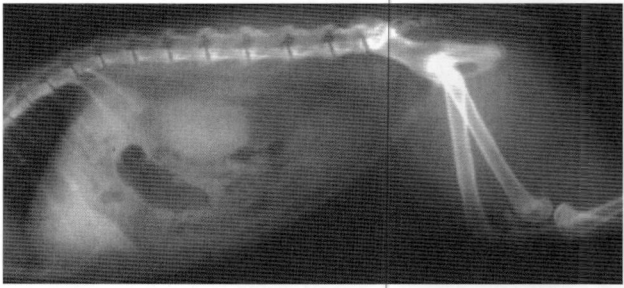

Figure 49.3 Lateral abdominal radiograph of a cat having sustained traumatic disruption of the upper urinary tract. Note widening of the retroperitoneal space and irregular density within the retroperitoneal space.

disruption of the peritoneum (Stafford & Bartges 2013). Suspected injury to the kidneys, ureters, or retroperitoneal space can be evaluated using intravenous pyelography (IVP). However, disruption of the vascular pedicle of the kidneys may sometimes only be detected via renal angiography or CT evaluation. Frequently, IVP allows at least partial examination of the urinary bladder as well, especially the region of the trigone and ureteral orifices. The attending clinician should ensure adequate hydration and correct deficient perfusion as much as possible prior to iodinated contrast studies, as there is an increased risk of renal toxicity when contrast agents are administered intravenously to azotemic, dehydrated animals (Selcer 1982). If the bladder is likely the area of greatest insult and is able to be catheterized via the urethra, a positive-contrast, retrograde, CT cystourethrogram is recommended to yield the most information. A pneumocystogram utilizing carbon dioxide gas may complement a positive-contrast cystogram by highlighting the mucosal surface of the urinary bladder. If the urethra is ruptured or obstructed and urethral catheterization is not possible, a normograde cystourethrogram may be performed under fluoroscopy by percutaneously catheterizing a moderate-sized bladder with an intravenous catheter or temporary locking-loop tube cystostomy. Retrograde or normograde cystourethrograms, and vaginocystourethrograms in females, may be used to evaluate the urethra in addition to the bladder (Kleine 1973; Pechman 1982; Selcer 1982). Finally, CT or MRI with contrast can accurately identify and locate sites of urinary tract disruption anywhere from the kidneys to the urethra (Coburn 2008).

Retroperitoneal hematoma

The retroperitoneum is the actual and potential space located between the ventral parietal peritoneum and the components of the dorsal and lateral abdominal wall, including the quadratus lumborum, psoas muscle groups, transversus abdominis muscles, ribs, spine, and pelvis. Trauma to the retroperitoneal space may occur as an isolated injury, or involve concurrent injury to the kidneys and ureters. Although retroperitoneal hematoma is reported in 12–44% of human victims sustaining blunt abdominal trauma and 5.9–55% of those with penetrating abdominal trauma, there are no reports in the veterinary literature dedicated to retroperitoneal hemorrhage alone (Goins & Rodriguez 1996). This may be because self-limiting retroperitoneal hemorrhage and hematomas are not generally surgical conditions in the veterinary patient and usually respond to conservative management and rest. However, radiographic and ultrasonographic signs of retroperitoneal fluid accumulation should prompt further investigation to determine whether the fluid is hemorrhage, urine, or both, and radiographic contrast studies or advanced diagnostic imaging should be performed to further evaluate the integrity of the urinary tract.

Kidneys

Injuries to the kidneys may include lacerations of the capsule; contusions, fissures, or lacerations to the renal parenchyma; and trauma to the vascular pedicle (Stafford & Bartges 2013). Renal trauma may be confined to one kidney or involve both kidneys and is frequently difficult to diagnose, as clinical signs may be vague and nonspecific (Aronson 2008). A history of trauma, pain on abdominal or lumbar spinal palpation, and gross or microscopic hematuria suggests renal injury (Coburn 2008). In human trauma patients, hematuria is the most common sign indicative of potential renal damage. Although when present it is suggestive of

renal injury, its degree does not correlate well with the severity of injury (Morgan 1982; Miller & McAninch 1996; Aumann et al. 1998; Coccolini et al. 2019). Reports conflict as to whether gross hematuria or microscopic hematuria is an indication for contrast radiographic or advanced imaging studies, but most human trauma centers routinely perform advanced imaging or contrast studies in any traumatized individual with any degree of hematuria. This literature also suggests that hematuria may be cleared by a second or third voiding, or within hours of catheterization (Miller & McAninch 1996; Coburn 2008). Therefore, evaluation of a first voided urine sample or early urinalysis of a catheterized specimen is recommended.

Radiographic signs consistent with kidney trauma in the veterinary patient include an increased or irregular density in the retroperitoneal space, widening of the retroperitoneal space and ventral displacement of the colon, renal asymmetry or displacement, or inability to discern the renal silhouettes (Kleine 1973; Pechman 1982). Renal injury may vary from minor lacerations to complete polar disruption or avulsion of hilar structures, including the vascular pedicle or renal pelvis and proximal ureter (Peters 1996; Coccolini et al. 2019). Although no grading system exists for characterizing renal damage in small animals, the American Association for the Surgery of Trauma classifies renal injuries in people according to the extent and nature of the injury. Grade I injuries include contusions or subcapsular hematomas with an intact renal capsule; grade II injuries are minor parenchymal lacerations extending into the cortex but not medulla; grade III injuries are lacerations of the cortex and medulla that do not extend into the collecting system; grade IV lacerations extend into the collecting system and include damage to main or branching vascular structures with locally contained hemorrhage; and grade V is assigned to multiple or deep lacerations or avulsions involving the cortex, medulla, collecting system, and vessels with associated significant hemorrhage or main-vessel thrombosis (Nash & Carroll 1996; Coccolini et al. 2019).

Point-of-care AFAST or focused urinary ultrasonography can be performed in the acute setting to diagnose renal and retroperitoneal fluid accumulations. Perinephric fluid can be identified using hepatorenal and splenorenal views and, in the trauma patient, may be indicative of renal capsular rupture, trauma to the renal parenchyma with urine leakage, or avulsion of the renal vasculature or proximal ureter (Cole et al. 2021). Uroabdomen or uroretroperitoneum with urinary tract disruption should be considered in any dog or cat with perinephric fluid and a history of recent trauma or surgery. Ultrasonography can be used to serially monitor fluid accumulations, as urine leakage or clinically significant hemorrhage would be expected to increase in volume over serial examinations (Cole *et al.* 2021). IVP, abdominal ultrasound with Doppler color flow assessment, and CT or MRI with contrast could be utilized to determine whether renal injury is present and its severity (Kleine 1973; Nash & Carroll 1996; Coburn 2008). CT angiography and magnetic resonance angiography allow accurate diagnosis of renal vascular injury, because renal nonenhancement using these modalities is thought to be pathognomonic for renal vascular occlusion (Coburn 2008).

Although the need for surgery is dictated by the extent of renal trauma, other factors such as the presence of shock or whether there was blunt or penetrating abdominal trauma causing hematuria may dictate the course of investigation (Morgan 1982; Peters 1996; Coburn 2008). Although accurate and comprehensive imaging is a prerequisite for selection of conservative management of renal trauma, most people with simple renal contusion or subcapsular hematoma, and even some people with simple lacerations, may be successfully managed with rest and observation without high risk of complication (Peters 1996; Coccolini *et al.* 2019). Absolute indications for surgery in people include persistent bleeding represented by an expanding or pulsatile retroperitoneal hematoma, increasing abdominal hemorrhage, or the need for multiple transfusions. Other indications for surgery include urinary extravasation resulting from renal pelvic lacerations or parenchymal lacerations extending to the collection system. Urinomas that subsequently form may be at risk for infection or contribute to chemical peritonitis. Other indications for surgery include suspicion of nonviable tissue or renal arterial or venous thrombosis (Miller & McAninch 1996; Nash & Carroll 1996; Peters 1996; Coburn 2008).

Simple renal capsular lacerations may be closed with fine absorbable suture in a simple continuous or mattress pattern. Generally, parenchymal lacerations extending to the collecting system of veterinary patients do not require separate closure of the collecting system (Morgan 1982; Coburn 2008). The capsular repair may be augmented by suturing of omentum or a transversus abdominis muscle flap over the laceration to offer a more watertight seal (Peters 1996). Parenchymal damage resulting in nonviable tissue confined to a single pole may be resolved by partial nephrectomy (Bellah 1999). The damaged parenchyma is sharply excised and segmental vessels may require individual ligation. The remaining renal capsule is then overseen and the repair can be augmented by omentalization or placement of a muscle flap (Peters 1996; Coburn 2008). If crushing injury or main-vessel thrombosis has occurred or loss of viable parenchyma is not confined to one pole, complete ureteronephrectomy is performed, provided the remaining kidney is thought to be functional (Morgan 1982; Coburn 2008). Because renal arterial branches are end arteries, in patients with vascular damage occlusion or ligation of these segmental vessels results in infarction of the associated parenchyma. However, as a rich network of intravenous renal communication exists, smaller renal veins may be safely ligated if necessary without compromise of venous return (Carroll 1996; Coburn 2008). Care should be taken to avoid ligation of any venous branch draining the ureteral vein, as congestion and loss of the ureter may result (Freedman & Ehrlich 1996).

Although not reported in dogs or cats, in cases of acute vascular pedicle avulsion renal autotransplantation can be considered, but requires microvascular surgical expertise and the use of an operating microscope. If the kidney has been without blood supply for more than 60 minutes, warm ischemic injury will be severe and may negate any benefit to autotransplantation. Intraoperative measures recommended include prevention of hypotension, consideration of mannitol administration to improve perfusion to the autograft, minimal surgical manipulation of the kidney, and rapid cooling by intra-arterial flushing of the autograft kidney with cold phosphate-buffered sucrose solution or iso-osmolar organ storage solution following removal (Novick 1996).

Additionally, although not yet reported, interventional superselective transcatheter arterial embolization techniques could be adapted for exceptional use in selected small animal cases of traumatic persistent renal hemorrhage. Conversely, intravascular stents could be utilized in cases of renal arterial or venous intimal damage, occlusion, or thrombosis.

Finally, rupture of the renal pelvis and avulsion of the proximal ureter from the renal pelvis pose a unique challenge to the veterinary surgeon. Simple rents in the renal pelvis may be closed with fine absorbable suture in an interrupted or simple continuous pattern (Prest & Carroll 1996; Kawashima *et al.* 1997). However, unless significantly dilated, the renal pelvis lies largely within the renal parenchyma and is difficult to visualize. Although not desirable, ureteronephrectomy could be considered for such injuries if the contralateral kidney is functional. Anastomosis of the proximal ureter to the renal pelvis can be performed, but again poor exposure makes the procedure technically difficult. If attempted, excellent proximal and distal exposure and control of the ureteral or renal pelvic remnants should be obtained, with care taken not to damage the ureteral vascular structures. Techniques for ureteral anastomoses are covered in Chapter 55, and the surgeon should adhere to the principles of ureteral surgery, which include gentle tissue handling, accurate mucosal apposition without tension, the use of fine monofilament suture, and, when necessary, spatulation of the ureteral ends to enlarge the ureteral lumen and prevent stricture. To support the repair, divert urine flow, and minimize opportunity for urine leakage and stricture, an ipsilateral nephrostomy tube with or without a ureteral stent could be placed surgically or percutaneously under intraoperative fluoroscopic guidance (Wormser *et al.* 2015). Drainage of the abdomen through the flank using a Jackson–Pratt or other closed-system drain allows accurate monitoring for urine leakage, quantification of intra-abdominal fluid losses, and resolution of peritoneal inflammation (Coburn 1996; Presti & Carroll 1996; Best *et al.* 2005; Streeter *et al.* 2009). Such a drain should be positioned away from the ureteral anastomosis, as direct contact of the drain with the anastomosis may delay healing (Coburn 2008).

Ureters

Ureteral damage in small animal patients is uncommon, accounting for 0.01% of diagnoses of hospitalized patients, but is often related to external trauma (Weisse *et al.* 2002). A retrospective study evaluating ureteral trauma in a small number of dogs and cats and one ferret reported that all noted ureteral injuries were related to blunt abdominal trauma (Weisse *et al.* 2002). Blunt abdominal trauma often results in damage to the proximal ureter, whereas iatrogenic trauma may occur anywhere along the ureter length (Klein & Thorton 1971; Stafford & Bartges 2013). However, laceration, rupture, transection, crushing, or obstruction of ureters may occur with penetrating injury as from bite wounds or from iatrogenic injury at surgery (Payne & Raz 1996; Rosen & McAninch 1996; Bellah 1999) (Figure 49.4). As

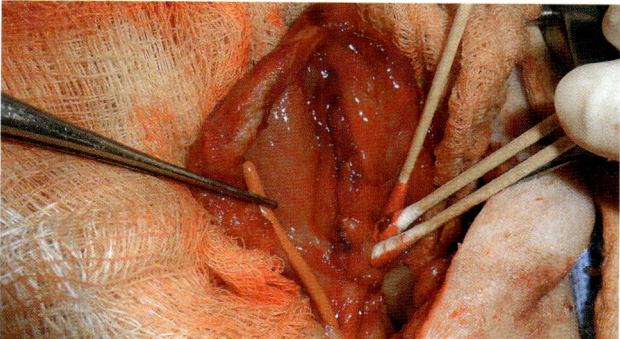

Figure 49.4 Intraoperative photograph taken during exploratory celiotomy following cystotomy performed through two inappropriate incisions. Exploration revealed that one of the cystotomy closures incorporated and traumatized the left ureteral papilla causing ureteral obstruction.

clinical signs of ureteral rupture are frequently nonspecific, and diagnosis often requires a high index of suspicion, patients may become significantly compromised awaiting a diagnosis (Weisse *et al.* 2002; Aronson 2008). Nonspecific clinical signs and physical examination findings in traumatized animals with ureteral injury may include abdominal distension and pain, lethargy, dehydration, weak peripheral pulses, pale mucous membranes, prolonged capillary refill time, tachycardia, vomiting, anorexia, and pyrexia (Morgan 1982; Weisse *et al.* 2002). Only 2 of 10 patients in this study had clinical signs of dysuria, anuria, or hematuria attributable to the urinary tract (Weisse *et al.* 2002). Point-of-care AFAST or focused urinary tract ultrasonography may also be helpful in early diagnosis of dogs and cats with ureteral trauma. Trauma may cause urine leakage, which may be noted as focal or diffuse perinephric or retroperitoneal fluid accumulation. However, trauma may also cause ureteral obstruction by stricture, iatrogenic crushing injury, and blood clots, causing pyelectasia, ureteral dilatation, and unilateral perinephric fluid. Additional diagnostic imaging would be required for more complete and accurate diagnosis (Cole *et al.* 2021).

Radiographic signs of ureteral injury include loss of both retroperitoneal and peritoneal detail, and increased size of or irregular density within the retroperitoneal space (Pechman 1982). Urine and fluid accumulation may be confined to the retroperitoneal space; if disruption of the ventral parietal peritoneum occurs, fluid may spill into the peritoneal cavity, causing uroperitoneum (Aronson 2008). Unilateral ureteral disruption may not result in clinical azotemia and pyelography is generally necessary to diagnose ureteral rupture (Kleine 1973; Kawashima *et al.* 1997; Presti & Carroll 1996; Cole *et al.* 2021). Although the aforementioned study reported that all ureteral ruptures were able to be diagnosed using IVP, contrast CT provides a detailed and accurate assessment of the ureters (Weisse *et al.* 2002). Spiral CT scanners complete initial renal imaging quickly, and a delayed excretory phase of imaging should be requested to permit contrast to pool in the collecting system and opacify the ureter (Coburn 2008). Integrity of the ureters may be confirmed or denied by antegrade pyelography with the aid of percutaneous or intraoperative fluoroscopy (Figure 49.5). At surgery, the bladder may be incised and the ureteral orifices observed for efflux of urine.

For treatment of complications, the ureter can be divided into thirds, having upper, middle, and lower portions. Treatment options for ureteral trauma are contingent on patient stability, function of the contralateral kidney and integrity of the contralateral ureter, concurrent damage to the ipsilateral kidney, location of the injury, and amount of ureteral loss along the length of

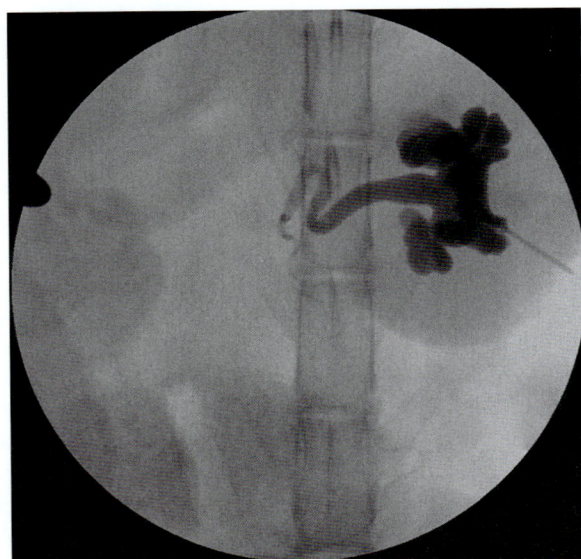

Figure 49.5 Fluoroscopic image taken during antegrade pyelography of the left kidney. Note the renal pelvic dilatation and proximal ureteral dilatation.

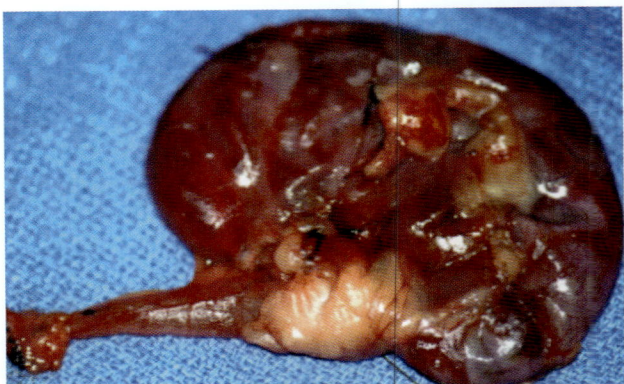

Figure 49.6 Feline kidney and ureter specimen following complete ureteronephrectomy. Severe hydronephrosis had occurred secondary to accidental ligation of the distal ureter.

the damaged ureter (Aronson 2008; Coburn 2008). Iatrogenic crushing of the ureter, as occurs with accidental grasping or ligation during surgery, may not require further treatment once the ureter is released (Bellah 1999). Serial examinations with contrast ureterography reveal that 90% of inappropriately handled or crushed ureters will have a narrowed lumen for about 1 week, but will likely be normal by the 12th week postoperatively. Regarding accidental ligation, a study in dogs showed uniformly excellent results when deligation occurred within 7 days of placing the tie. In contrast, ureters stripped of adventitia experience devascularization, and 50% of these injuries result in persistent stricture (Bellah 1989). Regardless, if there is doubt as to the viability of the ureter, the injured segment should be resected and treated as a laceration or segmental excision, as described shortly (Payne & Raz 1996; Wormser *et al.* 2015). For long-standing ureteral obstruction with severe hydronephrosis, ureteronephrectomy may be required (Figure 49.6).

Surgical options for ureteral rupture, transection, laceration, or stricture include primary repair of lacerations, ureteral spatulated end-to-end anastomosis, ureteral reimplantation, ureteral stenting, or ureteronephrectomy (Morgan 1982; Coburn 1996; Payne & Raz 1996; Peters 1996; Weisse *et al.* 2002). Proximal and middle ureteral disruptions generally require primary repair or ureteral anastomosis, while disruptions of the distal third of the ureter may be treated by excision of the compromised segment and reimplantation of the healthy ureteral end into the bladder via ureteroneocys-

tostomy. Such a direct anastomosis of the lower ureter to the bladder avoids the potential ischemic complications that may occur with a very distal ureteral end-to-end anastomosis (Rosen & McAninch 1996; Coburn 2008). Damage to the middle portion of the ureter may also be treated by reimplantation in exceptional cases, but cranial cystopexy via a psoas hitch and caudal translocation of the kidney by renal descensus may be needed to prevent tension at the anastomosis site (Payne & Raz 1996; Presti & Carroll 1996). Both intravesicular and extravesicular techniques have been described for ureteroneocystostomy (Gregory *et al.* 1996; Hardie *et al.* 2005; Mehl *et al.* 2005).

As in cases of ureteral pelvic disruption or proximal ureteral avulsion, repair of any ureteral injury may benefit from urine diversion and placement of a nephrostomy tube (Coburn 2008). Complications of nephrostomy tube placement include obstruction, infection, and dislodgment with development of uroperitoneum or subcutaneous urine leakage, and placement is often related to surgeon preference. Nephrostomy tubes placed surgically should be secured with a nephropexy to minimize risk of uroperitoneum. Tubes exiting the body should be secured with purse-string and finger-trap sutures in the flank skin with a bandage, and the patient must wear an Elizabethan collar at all times to prevent licking or chewing at the tube and nephrostomy site.

Ureteral repairs performed after trauma in people are often stented, and urologic literature reports that optimal ureteral regeneration requires both urinary diversion and stenting (Bellah 1989; Coburn 2008). In dogs, longitudinal ureteral incisions healed more completely and with less scar tissue when stents were used than when urine was permitted to flow freely. With stenting, ureteral reepithelialization is complete in 4–10 days and regeneration of the mural layers occurs in 4–6 weeks

(Bellah 1989; Coburn 2008). Although other reports indicate that unstented ureterotomies regenerate quickly and completely, most investigators have concluded that diversion of urine complements wound healing (Bellah 1989). Stenting in veterinary patients can be performed with an internal nephroureterostomy or double-pigtail stent, where a loop of stent forms in both the renal pelvis and urinary bladder, preventing dislodgment of the stent. A pigtail or locking-loop nephrostomy tube can be placed concurrently. In a recent study of a small cohort of 12 cats, however, placement of a double-pigtail stent at the time of ureteroneocystostomy had no significant impact on outcome (Lorange & Monnet 2020). Ureteral stents and nephrostomy tubes can be most readily placed percutaneously in patients with renal pelvic dilation of 10 mm or greater using intraoperative fluoroscopy. Ureteral stenting may also be performed surgically by passing the stent retrograde from the ureteral orifice to the renal pelvis, bypassing the site of ureteral injury before or after anastomotic repair. In the former situation, suturing of the ureteral anastomosis may be made easier by suturing over the intraluminal stent (Hoffer & Sclafani 1996; Wormser *et al.* 2015). In one study, end-to-end ureteral anastomosis and double-pigtail ureteral stent placement were successfully used to repair iatrogenic ligation and transection of the ureters of two dogs via an operating microscope (Wormser *et al.* 2015). In another study, treatment by ureteroureterostomy over ureteral stents resulted in life-limiting cystitis and stricture after removal of the stents. Subsequent bilateral subcutaneous ureteral bypass (SUB) procedures led to a successful outcome in this cat and another cat with proximal iatrogenic ureteral trauma (Kulendra *et al.* 2014; Sapora *et al.* 2019). An oversized stent that must be forced into a ureter is likely to cause stricture, whereas undersized stents do not produce stricture. Properly sized and placed ureteral stents cause passive dilatation of the ureter, may minimize the risk for stricture, and provide a conduit for urine on which growth of urothelium can occur (Bellah 1989; Wormser *et al.* 2015). The stent may remain indefinitely, be removed cystoscopically when no longer needed, or be removed surgically in smaller patients or those experiencing complications.

Other factors affecting ureteral healing include methods of suture repair and type of suture utilized. As discussed, a spatulated elliptical anastomosis allows the greatest increase in circumference of the sutured ureterouretestomy, although successful anastomosis can occur without spatulation (Bellah 1989, 1999). Both simple interrupted and simple continuous patterns of anastomosis have been described with success. Although continuous closure takes less time and provides a more watertight seal, its use can promote a purse-string effect on the ureteral lumen. Histologic examination of post-mortem ureteral anastomotic specimens did reveal that continuous sutures produced a smoother pattern of epithelialization, as opposed to the more irregular mucosal healing seen with interrupted suturing of anastomoses (Bellah 1989). Various suture materials have been utilized in ureteral repairs, including polyglycolic acid, polyglactin 910, silk, braided polyester, polypropylene, and nylon. Of these, chromic gut and polypropylene elicited the greatest inflammatory reactions, causing the formation of numerous diverticula and extensive scar tissue. The least fibrosis and greatest internal diameter of ureteral anastomoses were seen with polyglycolic acid. Following complete ureteral transection and repair, normal peristalsis was reported to return from 7–10 days to 3 weeks after anastomosis (Bellah 1989).

In cases of severe loss of ureteral length or when anastomosis cannot occur without undue tension, a Boari bladder flap can be created wherein a full-thickness longitudinal pedicle of bladder is created with its base located at the apex of the bladder (Freedman & Ehrlich 1996; Peters 1996; Presti & Carroll 1996; Aronson *et al.* 2018). The tube is rolled on itself longitudinally and sutured together, the resultant bladder defect is apposed, and the proximal end of the tube is sutured directly to the distal ureteral stump in end-to-end fashion. Although rarely reported in the canine experimental literature, this technique has been shown to result in a higher rate of complications such as urine reflux than the psoas hitch technique (Payne & Raz 1996). However, a modification of the original Boari flap was recently successfully utilized to extend the urinary bladder, replace a segment of mid-distal ureter, and create a site for neoureterocystostomy in a cat with proximal ureteral stricture (Aronson *et al.* 2018). Other complex ureteral reconstruction techniques include transureteroureterostomy, where an end-to-side anastomosis of the damaged ureter to the contralateral ureter is created, and ileal–ureteral replacement (Freedman & Ehrlich 1996; Payne & Raz 1996; Peters 1996; Presti & Carroll 1996). Renal autotransplantation could also be considered to move the kidney furthest caudad in an effort to minimize anastomotic tension involving a severely shortened ureter (Novick 1996). Such techniques should be considered experimental in veterinary patients and accurate information on prognosis is not available at this time.

Urinary bladder

Rupture of the urinary bladder is the most common cause of uroperitoneum and may occur following blunt trauma from motor vehicle accidents or falls, penetrating trauma from fracture fragments or other sharp injury, from overzealous palpation or urethral obstruction, or from poor catheterization techniques (Morgan 1982; Selcer 1982; Aumann *et al.* 1998; Aronson 2008). Bladder rupture is most likely to occur if sudden compression or shear forces at the time of blunt trauma act on a full bladder, and most tears occur at the fundus or apex. Pelvic fracture fragments may penetrate the urinary bladder neck, and in one study 7% of pelvic fractures were associated with bladder rupture. The same study also reported that 15% of patients with pelvic fracture incurred bladder mucosal irregularities and blood clots, and 5% of pelvic fractures were associated with herniation of the bladder caudally through the pelvis or through the abdominal wall (Selcer 1982) (Figure 49.7).

Although the cardinal sign of bladder injury is gross hematuria, a prompt diagnosis of bladder disruption may be difficult to obtain with certainty. In one study of urinary tract trauma associated with pelvic trauma, hematuria was the most frequent sign suggestive of urinary tract trauma and was correlated to actual injury in 61% of dogs. However, gross hematuria is not specific for bladder rupture, and can occur with lesions anywhere in the urinary tract, and also with other bladder injuries including mucosal damage and herniation. In the same report, no clinical signs were observed in 28.5% of bladder ruptures, 40% of mucosal irregularities, and 20% of bladder herniations (Selcer 1982). In another study evaluating uroperitoneum in cats, the bladder was still able to be palpated in 20% of cats with bladder ruptures (Aumann *et al.* 1998). Moreover, it is widely reported that the ability of a patient to urinate or the ability to retrieve urine on urethral catheterization does not rule out bladder injury or rupture. Such findings support the understanding that a prompt diagnosis of urinary tract injury is frequently elusive and requires a

high index of suspicion and specific diagnostics. Other clinical signs or physical examination findings associated with trauma to the bladder include anuria, dysuria, abdominal distension with a fluid wave or pain, pyrexia or hypothermia, bradycardia, and vomiting (Morgan 1982; Aumann *et al.* 1998; Aronson 2008). Severe trauma resulting in bladder rupture leads to uroabdomen, and herniation of the bladder may result in a palpable fluctuant swelling of the body wall, inguinal region, or perineal tissues.

Clinicopathologic findings are as for other types of urinary tract injury, and include azotemia, hyperkalemia, hyperphosphatemia, hyponatremia, hypochloremia, and acid–base disturbances. Abdominal fluid should undergo evaluation for potassium and creatinine values, cytologic abnormalities, and bacterial culture and sensitivity. Organisms isolated from the urinary tract or abdominal fluid in cases of bladder injury include *Enterococcus* spp., *Staphylococcus* spp., *Streptococcus* spp., and *Escherichia coli*, and broad-spectrum antibiotics should be administered empirically to control for and treat infections due to these organisms while culture and sensitivity results are pending (Aumann *et al.* 1998).

Radiographic signs attributable to bladder rupture include loss of detail in the peritoneal cavity and a very small bladder silhouette or absence of the bladder silhouette. Pubic or other pelvic fractures may be noted radiographically, or if bladder herniation has occurred an abnormal soft tissue density may be located in the subcutaneous tissues of the abdominal, inguinal, or perineal regions (Morgan 1982; Selcer 1982). Radiographic contrast studies most likely to aid in the diagnosis of bladder rupture or herniation include positive-contrast retrograde or normograde cystograms (Kleine 1973; Pechman 1982). It is important that the bladder be adequately filled to avoid false-negative studies. To perform a cystogram accurately, the bladder should be emptied via urethral catheterization or temporary locking-loop cystostomy, and a 10–20% water-soluble organic iodide compound injected to fully distend the urinary bladder (Kleine 1973; Pechman 1982). The degree of distension may be sensed by ascertaining difficulty in injecting further, or by observation of distension using fluoroscopy. Following injection, four radiographic views should be obtained: recumbent lateral, ventrodorsal, and two ventrodorsal oblique views. If resistance to filling the urinary bladder is not encountered during injection, a lateral radiograph may be taken to determine whether contrast is leaking into the abdominal cavity. Mucosal abnormalities and other filling defects may be better noted by double-contrast cystography or abdominal ultrasound (Kleine 1973; Morgan 1982). IVP, CT, or

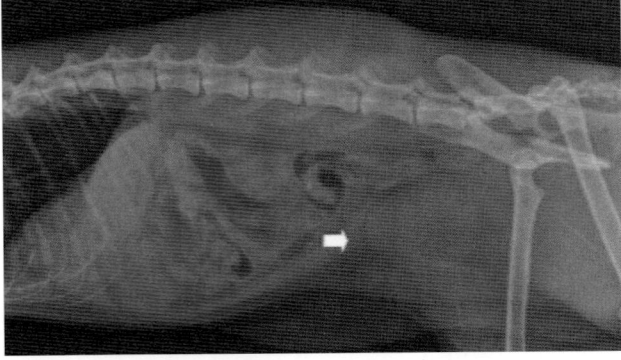

Figure 49.7 Lateral abdominal radiograph of a cat following severe blunt trauma to the abdomen. The prepubic ligament is ruptured, leading to a ventral abdominal wall defect with bladder herniation (white arrow).

MRI evaluation of the urinary tract with contrast may also be helpful in some cases (Peters 1996; Coburn 2008).

Treatment of bladder injury depends on the severity of trauma and the location of injury. Relatively minor trauma to the bladder resulting in mucosal irregularities or blood clot formation is generally amenable to rest and observation (Selcer 1982; Peters 1996; Coburn 2008). Blood clots do not frequently become obstructive due to the presence in the urine of urokinase, which acts as a thrombolytic agent, generally dissolving the clot material over time. A recent case report described the successful management of a urinary bladder blood clot in a cat using tissue plasminogen activator (Young *et al.* 2021). Small tears in the urinary bladder may be managed by an indwelling catheter for 3–5 days. However, complete urinary diversion is difficult to obtain, and most bladder ruptures require definitive surgery to débride and repair the defect (Bellah 1999). Apical and fundic tears may be treated by exploration of the defect, full or partial-thickness débridement of the bladder edges, and suture apposition using a simple interrupted appositional pattern. Ventral midline cystotomy may be necessary to completely assess the scope of bladder trauma or to evaluate for ureteral or urethral defects or avulsion. The cystotomy may also incorporate the ruptured region in some cases, and closure of the cystotomy and defect may occur concurrently. Excision or repair of penetrating pubic fracture fragments may be necessary in cases of fracture-related penetrating injury to prevent ongoing pain and trauma.

Vascularized segments of ileum and colon have been used for enterocystoplasty in people to create a neobladder or augment the remaining urinary bladder following radical resection or tissue loss due to trauma. Augmentation enteroplasty has been used in dogs successfully following severe vehicular trauma (Gonçalves *et al.* 2021). Ureteral dilatation and obstruction, recurrent urinary tract infection, and urinary incontinence were observed in a dog of one report following enterocystoplasty. In humans, hypokalemia, hypochloremia, metabolic acidosis, urinary calculi, diarrhea, and bladder perforation are reported, and dogs should be monitored for these complications as well (Gonçalves *et al.* 2021).

Herniation of the bladder or prostate can occur with traumatic abdominal wall defects, inguinal hernia, and perineal hernia. Depending on the degree of herniation and retroflexion of the bladder and time to presentation and definitive repair, the bladder may undergo ischemic necrosis or even rupture due to vascular compromise. To reduce the urinary bladder in cases of acute herniation, the bladder may be evacuated by blind or ultrasound-guided cystocentesis. The nondistended bladder is then more readily manually reduced through the abdominal, inguinal, or perineal defect. Placement of a urethral catheter helps to keep the bladder deflated and contributes to ongoing reduction of the bladder. Ventral midline abdominal exploration and investigation of bladder damage are indicated in cases of bladder herniation. A partial cystectomy may be necessary when full-thickness ischemic damage has occurred. Repair of the hernia may proceed at that time, or in cases of perineal herniation a cystopexy may be performed and primary hernia repair delayed by 1–3 days to allow some resolution of perineal inflammation and greater visualization at the time of definitive herniorrhaphy (Brissot *et al.* 2004).

Numerous suture materials have been used in the repair of the urinary bladder of small animals, including polyglycolic acid, chromic gut, polyglactin 910, polydioxanone, silk, polypropylene, stainless steel staples, and absorbable staples (Bellah 1989; Greenberg *et al.* 2004). Nonabsorbable and braided suture materials have been shown to be capable of inciting calculus formation in the urinary tract (Bellah 1989; Aronson 2008). Although epithelial cells have been shown to migrate over suture material passed into the lumen of the urinary bladder, some surgeons prefer partial-thickness passage of suture bites, passing through the submucosal holding layer but not through the mucosal layer (Bellah 1989). Epithelial overgrowth of intraluminal suture material may be impeded by physical or chemical qualities of the suture or by infection. Polyglactin 910 may be most appropriate in the presence of urinary tract infection, losing tensile strength less quickly at physiologic and alkaline pH (Bellah 1989). However, polydioxanone has been used successfully in dogs for cystotomy closure, produces minimal tissue reaction, offers more prolonged maintenance of tensile strength, and is the author's choice for cystotomy closure. Additionally, comparison of single- or double-layer appositional patterns with two-layer inverting patterns for cystotomy closure in dogs found more advanced healing in the appositional suture groups (Bellah 1989; Rosen & McAninch 1996). Clinical experience and investigative study in small animals indicate that single-layer appositional closure of the bladder results in functional healing without compromise of luminal volume, and use of a double-layer inverting pattern offers no clear advantage (Thieman-Mankin *et al.* 2012).

A urinary catheter may be placed following bladder repair for 2–5 days to keep the bladder decompressed during healing and to monitor urine output. Wounds of the urinary bladder heal similarly to other compound tissues, typically undergoing a 5-day lag phase of healing, a 14-day fibroblastic phase, and a remodeling period. Compared with other organs, the urinary bladder heals rather quickly, regaining 100% of normal tissue strength by 14–21 days. All cell layers contribute to cell renewal and proliferation to cover mucosal defects in the urinary bladder, and complete reepithelialization of the bladder occurs in 30 days. Regeneration of the bladder following up to 75% partial cystectomy can occur. The bladder remnant undergoes epithelial regeneration, synthesis and remodeling of scar tissue, hypertrophy, and expansion to allow good bladder function to occur within 3 months of partial cystectomy. As much of this renewal process is thought to be dependent on stretching of the bladder remnant, catheter-mediated urine diversion should not continue long term if functional bladder capacity is expected to be achieved (Bellah 1989). However, the owners should expect pollakiuria during this interim period following partial cystectomy. If non-operative management was chosen for a small bladder rupture or laceration, a positive-contrast cystogram is mandatory before catheter removal.

Complications of bladder rupture or injury are few, and intraperitoneal leakage of suture lines is minimized by proper closure. Other rare complications include urinoma, pelvic hematoma, fistulation to the skin, ongoing bladder necrosis, or sepsis from leakage of infected urine (Peters 1996).

Urethra

Partial and complete urethral tears can occur from blunt or penetrating trauma, obstructive urethral calculi, poor catheterization techniques, and iatrogenic trauma during surgeries for sterilization and herniorrhaphy, among others (Pechman 1982; Schulz et al. 1996; Yarrow 1996; Aumann et al. 1998; Aronson 2008; Powers et al. 2010; Flesher et al. 2016; Häußler et al. 2019; Jones et al. 2020). Blunt trauma most commonly results in avulsion of the proximal urethra from the bladder or prostate. Penetrating trauma may result from ballistic missiles or foreign bodies, bite wounds, pubic fractures, fractures of the os penis, or traumatic urethral catheterization (Morgan 1982; Selcer 1982). In one study, 5% of dogs sustaining pelvic fractures had coinciding urethral trauma (Selcer 1982). In addition, pressure necrosis may occur from obstructive calculi or urethral plugs, making urethral rupture more easily induced with even minor trauma. In fact, one study reported that feline lower urinary tract disease was the most common cause of uroperitoneum associated with proximal urethral tears in cats (Aumann et al. 1998). Another study reported trauma from urethral catheterization or calculi to be a common cause of urethral rupture in dogs, second only to vehicular trauma (Anderson et al. 2006). Despite being reported as early as 1996, iatrogenic urethral

trauma related to inadvertent prostatectomy continues to be reported and has been associated most often with the inguinal approach to cryptorchiectomy. The complication has also been reported as a complication of perineal herniorrhaphy and routine prescrotal orchiectomy (Schulz et al. 1996; Yarrow 1996; Powers et al. 2010; Flesher et al. 2016; Häußler et al. 2019; Jones et al. 2020).

Clinical signs and physical examination findings indicative of urethral trauma may be nonspecific as for other areas of the urinary tract (Morgan 1982; Pechman 1982; Anson 1987). Signs specific to the urinary tract can include hematuria, anuria, and dysuria. Proximal urethral rupture and avulsion and prostatic urethral injury may present similar to bladder rupture and cause uroperitoneum (Bellah et al. 1989; Holt 1990; Hay & Rosin 1997). Signs specific to pelvic and penile-urethral injury include painful perineal swelling and changes in character of the perineal skin, ranging from erythema to full-thickness necrosis (Anson 1987; Holt 1989). Ecchymoses may be evident in the perineal and preputial skin, and the distal penis or urethral opening may be traumatized. Clinicopathologic findings are similar to those noted with other urinary tract trauma.

Radiographic signs of urethral injury may include loss of intra-abdominal contrast with proximal urethral rupture, or displacement or absence of the bladder silhouette in cases of urethral avulsion (Kleine 1973; Anson 1987). In one report, changes to the density and appearance of the retroperitoneal space were noted in 60% of dogs with urethral rupture (Selcer 1982). Perineal soft-tissue swelling, the presence of gas lucencies in periurethral soft tissues, or radiopaque obstructive calculi may be noted in some cases of distal urethral disruption (Anson 1987; Holt 1990).

Catheterization of the urethra may occur without incident, may be met with resistance, or may be impossible. If urethral catheterization is possible, some portion of the urethra is likely to be intact, and partial rupture or laceration may have occurred (Meige et al. 2008). A positive-contrast retrograde cystourethrogram is indicated to confirm or deny the integrity of the catheterized urethra, and allows the urethral size, shape, location, and luminal content to be delineated (Kleine 1973; Pechman 1982; Davies et al. 2018). In one recent study, the placement of a radiopaque, hyperattenuating urethral catheter prior to CT evaluation of dogs with multiple pelvic fractures aided in localization of the urethra and surgical planning (Davies et al. 2018). In contrast to nonhyperattenuating catheters, barium sulfate is added to the silicone of a hyperattenuating catheter during the manufacturing process (Mila International, Florence, KY, USA). Percutaneous, normograde, positive-contrast cystography has also been reported (Flesher *et al.* 2016). Following retrograde or percutaneous catheterization with a Mila catheter, red rubber catheter, pediatric Foley catheter, or intravenous catheter in the case of percutaneous normograde cystography, a water-soluble organic iodide contrast agent is given. The contrast agent is diluted to 10–20% iodide, and 10–15 mL of contrast is given to dogs and 5–10 mL to cats (Kleine 1973; Morgan 1982; Pechman 1982; Anson 1987; Flesher *et al.* 2016). A catheter placed retrograde may be slowly withdrawn during injection using fluoroscopic guidance to observe for urethral defects. Alternatively, the full volume may be given into the bladder, and a voiding cystogram performed with bladder expression and serial assessment of radiographs. Pulling the pelvic limbs forward helps to delineate the perineal tissues and allows assessment of the entire urethra. Extravasation of contrast material occurs with both urethral laceration and complete urethral rupture, but in the latter situation contrast generally does not pass the complete tear (Anson 1987).

Management of urethral injuries in dogs and cats depends on the stability of the patient, location and severity of the tear, and presence of concurrent urinary tract or other injury. Minor urethral lacerations in any location may heal spontaneously if appropriate urinary diversion via an indwelling urethral catheter is provided for 7–21 days (Morgan 1982; Anson 1987; Meige *et al.* 2008). In one study of 11 cats with traumatic urethral rupture, placement of an indwelling urethral catheter was accomplished in 10 of 11 cats; however, cystostomy and an "inside to outside" technique were required in 5 cats. Urethral healing was accomplished in all cats, permitting catheter removal in 5–14 days. Very good outcomes were obtained in 8 cats, and 2 cats showed signs of urethral stricture (Meige *et al.* 2008). As placement of a urinary catheter retrograde across a urethral defect or obstruction may be difficult, fluoroscopically guided percutaneous normograde catheterization and retrograde catheterization using the Seldinger technique and a guidewire have been described for male cats and female dogs, respectively (Holmes *et al.* 2012; Robben 2020).

Surgery and urinary diversion is indicated for most partial and complete urethral transections. The surgical approach depends on the location of the urethral tear, and can be based on urethrogram findings. Proximal urethral tears and avulsions can be approached via a ventral midline celiotomy to the pubis. Care should be taken to avoid damage to the neural and vascular supply to the bladder and urethra along the dorsal aspect of each. Ventral midline cystotomy may help to delineate any need for débridement and may help to preserve the ureteral orifices during urethrovesicular anastomosis.

As débridement may leave little tissue available for closure, preservation of the ureteral orifices during closure of the bladder neck can be closely monitored and assured by using stay sutures during closure. A urethral catheter also provides a scaffold on which to suture and, if left in place during healing, a method of urinary diversion (Anson 1987; Hay & Rosin 1997; Cooley *et al.* 1999; Anderson *et al.* 2006).

Complete intrapelvic urethral injuries require pubic osteotomy for adequate exposure; techniques for pelvic symphysiotomy and pubic osteotomy have been described (Layton *et al.* 1987). Precise and anatomic end-to-end anastomosis of the urethra can then proceed unimpeded using a simple interrupted pattern of absorbable suture material (Anson 1987). The use of a urethral catheter as a stent on which to perform urethral anastomosis has been recommended. One report demonstrated that anastomoses sutured over a urethral catheter resulted in fewer strictures than anastomoses performed without a urethral catheter or the use of a catheter without sutured anastomosis (Layton *et al.* 1987). Traumatic pubic fractures may also require repair in conjunction with primary urethral repair (Selcer 1982). Thorough urinary diversion via an indwelling urethral catheter combined with tube cystostomy is recommended. Although Cooley *et al.* (1999) reported no statistical differences in urethral healing when urine diversion was accomplished by indwelling transurethral catheter, cystostomy catheter, or both, it is widely accepted that minimizing urine contact with a site of urethral injury favors urethral healing and decreases the incidence and severity of urethral stricture (Bellah 1989; Coburn 2008). The urethral catheter should be large enough to maintain the size of the lumen, but not so large that it exerts excessive pressure or tension on the anastomotic site. Catheterization for 3–5 days as an adjunct to primary urethral repair has been recommended to allow urothelium to bridge the wound and to prevent urine extravasation (Bellah 1989, 1999). Copious lavage is also recommended and closed-suction abdominal drainage should be considered (Anson 1987).

Complete ruptures of the penile urethra may be treated by primary repair or by scrotal urethrostomy in dogs or perineal urethrostomy in cats (Anson 1987). Prepubic urethrostomy is also an option in female dogs and cats or in cases of more proximal disruption of the male urethra. A recent retrospective study evaluating urethral injuries in dogs and cats concluded that permanent urethrostomy was a viable treatment option for urethral injury (Anderson *et al.* 2006). Additionally, a transpelvic technique for urethrostomy has been described in cats, and was found to preserve urethral length and continence and provide an adequate stoma via an ischial ostectomy (Bernarde & Viguier 2004).

Urethral lacerations associated with fractures of the os penis are a unique category of urethral injury. Most fractures of the os penis may be stabilized concurrently with treatment of a partial urethral injury by indwelling urethral catheterization. If a catheter cannot be passed or in cases of gross displacement of the os penile fragments, the fracture may need to be reduced by direct surgical approach and repair with a plate and screws or stainless steel wire. If the damage to the urethra or os penis is too extensive for primary repair or urethral stenting, proximal permanent urethrostomy should be performed (Anson 1987; Holt 1990).

Inadvertent prostatectomy is also a special problem of urethral injury, as a significant portion of the preprostatic, prostatic, and postprostatic urethra may be lost by inadvertent urethrectomy. Procedures reported for repair of such a urethral defect include cystourethral anastomosis, often over a urethral catheter; urinary bladder retroversion and neourethrocystostomy; and augmentation or patching of the urethral defect with porcine small intestinal submucosa (Schulz et al. 1996; Yarrow 1996; Powers et al. 2010; Flesher et al. 2016; Häußler et al. 2019).

Various suture materials such as polyglycolic acid, polyglactin 910, polydioxanone, and polypropylene have been evaluated for use in the urethra (Layton et al. 1987; Hay & Rosin 1997; Cooley et al. 1999). Although reaction to polypropylene appeared to be the least of all of these suture types, polyglycolic acid, polyglactin 910, and polydioxanone have all been used clinically for urethral anastomosis without suture-related complications (Anson 1987; Bellah 1989). Continuous extraluminal suture patterns have experimentally resulted in the least urethral distortion and reaction, but full-thickness simple interrupted appositional sutures have been used clinically with success.

The most important factors affecting urethral healing are the presence or absence of urine extravasation and urethral continuity (Bellah 1989; Anderson et al. 2006). Leakage of urine, especially infected urine, into the periurethral tissues delays wound healing and exacerbates production of periurethral fibrosis (Anson 1987; Bellah 1989). A urethral wound with any degree of urethral continuity bridged by an intraluminal stent can heal by complete regeneration of urethral mural components without stricture formation (Bellah 1989). In contrast, when there is no continuity between the transected urethral ends, the urethral mucosa retracts into the periurethral tissues, and fibrous tissue proliferation fills the gap between the opposing segments of the urethra, causing an obstructive scar (Anson 1987; Layton et al. 1987; Bellah 1989).

The most common complications following urethral trauma and wound repair are stricture formation and

the development of urethral fistulation (Anson 1987; Bellah 1989, 1999; Peters 1996; Coburn 2008). Factors that favor a successful outcome include accuracy of urethral apposition, adequate hemostasis, achievement of a watertight seal, and elimination of urinary tract infection prior to definitive surgery (Anson 1987; Holt 1990). Although meticulous mucosal apposition of the urethra with fine sutures restores urethral continuity, in most cases of urethral trauma some degree of luminal narrowing will occur over time, and patients should be monitored for recurrence of dysuria (Anson 1987; Layton et al. 1987; Bellah 1989, 1999; Anderson et al. 2006).

References

Anderson, R.B., Aronson, L.R., Drobatz, E.J., and Atilla, A. (2006). Prognostic factors for successful outcome following urethral rupture in dogs and cats. *Journal of the American Animal Hospital Association* 42: 136–146.

Anson, L.W. (1987). Urethra trauma and principles of urethral surgery. *Compendium on Continuing Education for the Practicing Veterinarian* 9: 981–987.

Aronson, L.R. (2008). Urinary tract trauma. *Proceedings of the American Association of Feline Practitioners Fall Conference, September 21–23*. Atlanta, GA: American Association of Feline Practitioners.

Aronson, L.R., Cleroux, A., and Wormser, C. (2018). Use of a modified Boari flap for the treatment of a proximal ureteral obstruction in a cat. *Veterinary Surgery* 47: 577–585.

Aumann, M., Worth, L.T., and Drobatz, K.J. (1998). Uroperitoneum in cats: 26 cases (1986–1995). *Journal of the American Animal Hospital Association* 34: 315–324.

Bellah, J.R. (1989). Wound healing in the urinary tract. *Seminars in Veterinary Medicine and Surgery (Small Animal)* 4: 294–303.

Bellah JR (1999) Diagnosis and management of urinary tract trauma. *Symposium on Soft Tissue Surgery, Palmerston North, Christchurch* (30–31 October). New Zealand.

Bellah, J.R., Spencer, C.P., and Salmeri, K.R. (1989). Hemiprostatic urethral avulsion during cryptorchid orchiectomy in a dog. *Journal of the American Animal Hospital Association* 25: 553–556.

Bernarde, A. and Viguier, E. (2004). Transpelvic urethrostomy in 11 cats using an ischial ostectomy. *Veterinary Surgery* 33: 246–252.

Best, C.D., Petrone, P., Buscarini, M. et al. (2005). Traumatic ureteral injuries: a single institution experience validating the American Association for the Surgery of Trauma Organ Injury Scale grading scale. *Journal of Urology* 173: 1202–1205.

Brissot, H.N., Dupre, G.P., and Bouvy, B.M. (2004). Use of laparotomy in a staged approach for resolution of bilateral or complicated perineal hernia in 41 dogs. *Veterinary Surgery* 33: 412–421.

Carroll, P.R. (1996). Injuries to major abdominal arteries, veins, and renal vasculature. In: *Traumatic and Reconstructive Urology* (ed. J.W. McAninch), 113–125. Philadelphia, PA: WB Saunders.

Coburn, M. (1996). Ureteral injuries from surgical trauma. In: *Traumatic and Reconstructive Urology* (ed. J.W. McAninch), 181–197. Philadelphia, PA: WB Saunders.

Coburn, M. (2008). Genitourinary trauma. In: *Trauma*, 6e (ed. D.V. Feliciano, K.L. Mattox and E.E. Moore), 789–825. New York: McGraw-Hill.

Coccolini, F., Moore, E.E., Kluger, Y. et al. (2019). Kidney and urotrauma: WSES-AAST guidelines. *World Journal of Emergency Surgery* 14: 54.

Cole, L., Humm, K., and Dirrig, H. (2021). Focused ultrasound examination of canine and feline emergency urinary tract disorders. *Veterinary Clinics of North America: Small Animal Practice* 51: 1233–1248.

Cooley, A.J., Waldron, D.R., Smith, M.M. et al. (1999). The effects of indwelling transurethral catheterization and tube cystostomy on urethral anastomoses in dogs. *Journal of the American Animal Hospital Association* 35: 341–347.

Culp WTN, Silverstein DC (2015) Thoracic and abdominal trauma. In: Silverstein DC, Hopper K (eds) Small Animal Critical Care Medicine, 2. Philadelphia, PA: WB Saunders, pp. 728–733.

Davies, D., Marin, S., and Hoey, S.E. (2018). Utility of radiopaque urinary catheter placement before computed tomographic evaluation in two dogs with multiple pelvic fractures. *Veterinary Record Case Reports* 6: e000682. https://doi.org/10.1136-vetreccr-2018-000682.

Flesher, K., Weisse, C., Berent, A., and Lin, R. (2016). Urinary bladder retroversion and neourethrocystostomy for treatment of inadvertent prostatectomy and urethrectomy in a dog. *Journal of the American Veterinary Medical Association* 248: 538–543.

Freedman, A.L. and Ehrlich, R.M. (1996). Ureteral replacement in the reconstruction of the short ureter. In: *Traumatic and Reconstructive Urology* (ed. J.W. McAninch), 249–257. Philadelphia, PA: WB Saunders.

Goins, W.A. and Rodriguez, A. (1996). Retroperitoneal injuries. In: *Complications in Trauma and Critical Care* (ed. K.I. Maull, A. Rodriguez and C.E. Wiles), 442–452. Philadelphia, PA: WB Saunders.

Gonçalves, R., Wade, J., Fransson, B. et al. (2021). Augmentation enterocystoplasty in a polytrauma dog with extensive bladder necrosis. *Veterinary Record Case Reports* 9: 1–7.

Greenberg, C.B., Davidson, E.B., Bellmer, D.D. et al. (2004). Evaluation of the tensile strengths of four monofilament absorbable suture materials after immersion in canine urine with or without bacteria. *American Journal of Veterinary Research* 65: 847–853. https://doi.org/10.2460/ajvr.2004.65.847.

Gregory, C.R., Lirtzman, R.A., Kochin, E.J. et al. (1996). A mucosal apposition technique for ureteroneocystostomy after renal transplantation in cats. *Veterinary Surgery* 25: 13–17.

Grimes, J.A., Fletcher, J.M., and Schmiedt, C.W. (2018). Outcomes in dogs with uroabdomen: 43 cases (2006–2015). *Journal of the American Veterinary Medical Association* 252: 92–97. https://doi.org/10.2460/javma.252.1.92.

Hall, D.J., Rush, J.E., and Rozanski, E.A. (2010). ECG of the month. *Journal of the American Veterinary Medical Association* 236: 299–301.

Hardie, R.J., Schmiedt, C., Phillips, L., and McAnulty, J. (2005). Ureteral papilla implantation as a technique for neoureterocystostomy in cats. *Veterinary Surgery* 34: 393–398.

Häußler, T.C., Thiel, C., Fischer, A. et al. (2019). Inadvertent iatrogenic prostatectomy and urethrectomy in 2 dogs. *Tierärztliche Praxis. Ausgabe K, Kleintiere/Heimtiere* 47: 282–289. https://doi.org/10.1055/a-0948-7713.

Hay, C.W. and Rosin, E. (1997). Repair of an intrapelvic urethral tear in a bitch caused by iatrogenic trauma. *Veterinary Record* 140: 48–49.

Heeren, V., Edwards, L., and Mazzaferro, E.M. (2004). Acute abdomen: diagnosis. *Compendium on Continuing Education for the Practicing Veterinarian* 26: 357–363.

Hoffberg, J.E., Koenigshof, A.M., and Guiot, L.P. (2016). Retrospective evaluation of concurrent intra-abdominal injuries in dogs with traumatic pelvic fractures: 83 cases (2008–2013). *Journal of Veterinary Emergency and Critical Care* 26: 288–294. https://doi.org/10.1111/vec.12430.

Hoffer, E.K. and Sclafani, S.J.A. (1996). Interventional radiology in urologic trauma. In: *Traumatic and Reconstructive Urology* (ed. J.W. McAninch), 157–170. Philadelphia, PA: WB Saunders.

Holmes, E.S., Weisse, C., and Berent, A.C. (2012). Use of fluoroscopically guided percutaneous antegrade urethral catheterization for the treatment of urethral obstruction in male cats: 9 cases (2000–2009). *Journal of the American Veterinary Medical Association* 241: 603–607. https://doi.org/10.2460/javma.241.5.603.

Holt, P.E. (1989). Hindlimb skin loss associated with urethral rupture in two cats. *Journal of Small Animal Practice* 30: 406–409.

Holt, P.E. (1990). Dysuria in the dog. Part 2. Differential diagnosis of dysuria. *In Practice* 12: 147–153.

Jandrey KE (2015) Abdominocentesis and diagnostic peritoneal lavage. In: Silverstein DC, Hopper K (eds) Small Animal Critical Care Medicine, 2. Philadelphia, PA: WB Saunders, pp. 1036–1039.

Jones, S.A., Levy, N.A., and Pitt, K.A. (2020). Iatrogenic urethral trauma during routine prescrotal orchiectomy in a dog. *Topics in Companion Animal Medicine* 40: 100435. https://doi.org/10.1016/j.tcam.2020.100435.

Kawashima, A., Sandler, C.M., Correiere, J.N. et al. (1997). Ureteropelvic junction injuries secondary to blunt abdominal trauma. *Radiology* 205: 487–492.

Klein, L. and Thorton, G. (1971). Radiographic diagnosis of urinary tract trauma. *Journal of the American Animal Hospital Association* 7: 318–327.

Kleine, L.J. (1973). Radiographic diagnosis of urinary tract trauma. *Journal of the American Veterinary Medical Association* 163: 1185.

Kolata, R.J. and Johnston, D.E. (1975). Motor vehicle accidents in urban dogs: a study of 600 cases. *Journal of the American Veterinary Medical Association* 167: 938–941.

Kulendra, E., Kulendra, N., and Halfacree, Z. (2014). Management of bilateral ureteral trauma using ureteral stents and subsequent subcutaneous ureteral bypass devices in a cat. *Journal of Feline Medicine and Surgery* 16: 536–540.

Layton, C.E., Ferguson, H.R., Cook, J.E., and Guffy, M.M. (1987). Intrapelvic urethral anastomosis: a comparison of three techniques. *Veterinary Surgery* 16: 175–182.

Lorange, M. and Monnet, E. (2020). Postoperative outcomes of 12 cats with ureteral obstruction treated with ureteroneocystostomy. *Veterinary Surgery* 49: 1418–1427. http://org.proxy2.library.illinois.edu/10.1111/vsu.13488.

Mehl, M.L., Kyles, A.E., Pollard, R. et al. (2005). Comparison of three techniques for ureteroneocystostomy in cats. *Veterinary Surgery* 34: 114–119.

Meige, F., Sarrau, S., and Autefage, A. (2008). Management of traumatic urethral rupture in 11 cats using primary alignment with a urethral catheter. *Veterinary and Comparative Orthopaedics and Traumatology* 21: 76–84.

Miller, K.S. and McAninch, J.W. (1996). Indications for radiographic assessment in suspected renal trauma. In: *Traumatic and Reconstructive Urology* (ed. J.W. McAninch), 89–94. Philadelphia, PA: WB Saunders.

Morgan, R.V. (1982). Urogenital emergencies. Part I. *Compendium on Continuing Education for the Practicing Veterinarian* 4: 908–915.

Nash, P.A. and Carroll, P.R. (1996). Staging of renal trauma. In: *Traumatic and Reconstructive Urology* (ed. J.W. McAninch), 95–104. Philadelphia, PA: WB Saunders.

Novick, A.C. (1996). Renal autotransplantation: technique and use in the management of the injured kidney and ureter. In: *Traumatic and Reconstructive Urology* (ed. J.W. McAninch), 149–156. Philadelphia, PA: WB Saunders.

Payne, C.K. and Raz, S. (1996). Ureterovaginal and related fistulas. In: *Traumatic and Reconstructive Urology* (ed. J.W. McAninch), 213–249. Philadelphia, PA: WB Saunders.

Pechman, R.D. (1982). Urinary trauma in dogs and cats: a review. *Journal of the American Animal Hospital Association* 18: 33–40.

Peters, P.C. (1996). Urologic trauma. In: *Complications in Trauma and Critical Care* (ed. K.I. Maull, A. Rodriguez and C.E. Wiles), 421–430. Philadelphia, PA: WB Saunders.

Powers, M.Y., Campbell, B.G., and Weisse, C. (2010). Porcine small intestinal submucosa augmentation urethroplasty and balloon dilatation of a urethral stricture secondary to inadvertent prostatectomy in a dog. *Journal of the American Animal Hospital Association* 46: 358–365.

Presti, J.C. and Carroll, P.R. (1996). Ureteral and renal pelvic trauma: diagnosis and management. In: *Traumatic and Reconstructive Urology* (ed. J.W. McAninch), 171–179. Philadelphia, PA: WB Saunders.

Riordan LL, Schaer M (2015) Potassium disorders. In: Silverstein DC, Hopper K (eds) Small Animal Critical Care Medicine, 2. Philadelphia, PA: WB Saunders, pp. 269–273.

Robben, J.H. (2020). A novel insertion technique for urinary catheters in female dogs with the use of a guidewire. *Journal of Veterinary Emergency and Critical Care* 30: 597–600.

Rosen, M.A. and McAninch, J.W. (1996). Wound closures and suture techniques in reconstructive procedures. In: *Traumatic and Reconstructive Urology* (ed. J.W. McAninch), 249–257. Philadelphia, PA: WB Saunders.

Sapora J, Hardie RJ, Evans N (2019) Use of a subcutaneous ureteral bypass device for treatment of bilateral proximal ureteral injury in a 9-month-old cat. Journal of Feline Medicine and Surgery Open Reports 5: 1–6 https://doi.org/10.1177/2055116919831856.

Schmiedt, C., Tobias, K., and Otto, C. (2001). Evaluation of abdominal fluid: peripheral blood creatinine and potassium ratios for diagnosis of uroperitoneum in dogs. *Journal of Veterinary Emergency and Critical Care* 11: 275–280.

Schulz, K.S., Waldron, D.R., Smith, M.M. et al. (1996). Inadvertent prostatectomy as a complication of cryptorchidectomy in four dogs. *Journal of the American Animal Hospital Association* 211–214. https://doi-org.proxy2.library.illinois.edu/10.5326/15473317-32-3-211.

Selcer, B.A. (1982). Urinary tract trauma associated with pelvic trauma. *Journal of the American Animal Hospital Association* 19: 785–793.

Stafford, J.R. and Bartges, J.W. (2013). A clinical review of pathophysiology, diagnosis, and treatment of uroabdomen in the dog and cat. *Journal of Veterinary Emergency and Critical Care* 23: 216–229.

Streeter, E.M., Rozanski, E.A., de Laforcade-Buress, A. et al. (2009). Evaluation of vehicular trauma in dogs: 239 cases (January–December 2001). *Journal of the American Veterinary Medical Association* 235: 405–408.

Thieman-Mankin, K.M., Ellison, G.W., Jeyapaul, C.J. et al. (2012). Comparison of short-term complication rates between dogs and cats undergoing appositional single-layer or inverting double-layer cystotomy closure: 144 cases (1993–2010). *Journal of the American Veterinary Medical Association* 240: 65–68.

Weisse, C., Aronson, L.R., and Drobatz, K. (2002). Traumatic rupture of the ureter: 10 cases. *Journal of the American Animal Hospital Association* 38: 188–192.

Wormser, C., Clarke, D.L., and Aronson, L.R. (2015). End-to-end ureteral anastomosis and double-pigtail ureteral stent placement for treatment of iatrogenic ureteral trauma in two dogs. *Journal of the American Veterinary Medical Association* 247: 92–97.

Wright, K.N., Gompf, R.E., and DeNove, R.C. (1999). Peritoneal effusion in cats: 65 cases (1981–1997). *Journal of the American Veterinary Medical Association* 214: 375–381.

Yarrow, T.G. (1996). Inadvertent prostatectomy as a complication of cryptorchidectomy. *Journal of the American Animal Hospital Association* 32: 376–377. https://doi-org.proxy2.library.illinois.edu/10.5326/15473317-32-5-376.

Young, C.S., Racette, M., and Todd, J.M. (2021). Successful management of urinary bladder blood clot with intravesical tissue plasminogen activator in a cat. *Journal of the American Animal Hospital Association* 38: 128–132.

50

Urinary Diversion Techniques

Maureen Griffin, Allyson Berent, Chick Weisse, and William T.N. Culp

Urinary diversion is typically necessary when an obstruction exists in the urinary collection system. Urinary catheters and stents can be used for various purposes to divert urine through the entire collection system. Most catheters in the urinary system are used for temporary drainage of the renal pelvis, ureter, or urinary bladder. Urinary catheters are classically soft, comfortable, polyurethane-type tubes that have an open lumen. They are also typically multifenestrated. Stents are often more permanent, either looped or expandable to prevent migration, and inserted across a blocked lumen in order to restore patency. Urinary stents can be used in the kidney, ureter, bladder, or urethra for permanent or long-term diversion, particularly when traditional options are considered inappropriate, challenging, or are contraindicated. Stents are most often completely indwelling tubes that can be placed for various purposes, most commonly to bypass a malignant obstruction, stricture, or obstructive stones (i.e., ureterolithiasis). Stents come in different materials (e.g., metal, polyurethane, plastic, rubber), shapes, and sizes.

This chapter discusses the types as well as the placement of various catheters and stents (implants) currently being used in the urinary tract of veterinary patients for urinary diversion. Other surgical procedures for urinary diversion, including ureteral reimplantation and urethrostomy techniques, are discussed in more detail in other chapters.

Kidney

Nephrostomy tubes

The most common reason for stent or catheter placement in the kidney is for drainage of the renal pelvis due to hydronephrosis associated with a renal outflow tract obstruction, typically secondary to a ureteral obstruction. Temporary drainage of the renal pelvis can be accomplished with the placement of a nephrostomy tube, which can be placed surgically or percutaneously using ultrasound and/or fluoroscopic guidance. With the advent of newer and more permanent interventions, like the subcutaneous ureteral bypass (SUB) device or ureteral stenting, temporary nephrostomy tubes are used less frequently. Ureteral obstruction most commonly occurs secondary to ureterolithiasis, trigonal neoplasia obstructing the ureterovesicular junction (UVJ), ureteral strictures/stenosis, accidental ureteral ligation, ureteral trauma, ureteral edema following ureteral surgery, and pyelonephritis. Obstruction can result in life-threatening azotemia, particularly when presenting bilaterally or in animals with concurrent pre-existing renal insufficiency/failure. In cases of ureteral obstruction secondary to a ureterolith, some patients can be managed medically with supportive care until the ureterolith passes, while others may require diversion surgery to avoid permanent damage and/or hemodialysis for stabilization prior to anesthesia and definitive surgery.

Regardless of the cause of ureteral obstruction, the placement of a nephrostomy tube, either surgically or percutaneously, to quickly relieve the obstruction may minimize the morbidity and help determine whether adequate renal function remains to justify more definitive ureteral surgery or a permanent ureteral diversion technique. Nephrostomy tubes may also be helpful after intervention while a surgical site is healing (postureterotomy) or in a patient awaiting future intervention (i.e., ureteral resection anastomosis, ureterotomy, ureteral reimplantation, or ureteral stent/bypass placement). In

Small Animal Soft Tissue Surgery, Second Edition. Edited by Eric Monnet.
© 2023 John Wiley & Sons, Inc. Published 2023 by John Wiley & Sons, Inc.
Companion website: www.wiley.com/go/monnet/small

addition to urinary diversion, these tubes allow the clinician to follow ureteral patency serially with contrast pyeloureterography. If a temporary nephrostomy tube is placed for treatment of obstructive pyonephrosis secondary to ureteral obstruction, an additional procedure is required to permanently relieve or bypass the ureteral obstruction; this differs from placement of a ureteral stent or SUB, which allow for renal pelvis drainage and long-term treatment of the ureteral obstruction in one procedure (Gallagher 2018).

The ideal catheter for this procedure is a locking-loop pigtail catheter (Figure 50.1). Historically, Foley urinary catheters and red rubber catheters have also been used, but they have a tendency to leak, back out, or be inadvertently removed. One study showed complications in 11/24 (46%) cats with ureteral calculi following placement of a nephrostomy Dawson–Mueller (Cook Medical, Bloomington, IN, USA) or Swan–Ganz catheter; the most common complication was uroperitoneum (Kyles *et al.* 2005). A more recent study reported outcomes of 16 cats (18 kidneys) and 4 dogs (4 kidneys) that underwent locking-loop pigtail nephrostomy catheter placement for temporary urine diversion; catheters were placed via laparotomy in 15/22 (68.2%) kidneys and percutaneously in 7/22 (31.8%, including all dogs) kidneys (Berent *et al.* 2012). The catheters remained indwelling for a median of 7 days, and complications occurred in 2/20 (10%) patients, characterized by urine leakage (n = 1) and inadvertent dislodgment (n = 1) (Berent *et al.* 2012). The renal pelvis was successfully decompressed in all cases, and creatinine concentrations improved within 12–72 hours in 16/17 (94.1%) patients (Berent *et al.* 2012). Postprocedure management is important in these patients, as the externalized drainage requires careful management and hospitalization to prevent infection and dislodgment. In humans, nephrostomy tubes are placed for similar reasons but, unlike dogs and cats, tubes can be left in place for months to years given careful maintenance (Lennon *et al.* 1997; Uthappa & Cowan 2005). The risk of infection, discomfort, and inadvertent removal is still possible.

In the authors' experience, if a locking-loop catheter is used, renal pelvic dilatation should be greater than 1 cm in diameter, because the loop of the catheter is 1–1.5 cm in diameter. This allows the locking-loop mechanism (10–15 mm in diameter) to form in the pelvis without backing out. Urine leakage can occur if the entire locking loop is not secured within the renal pelvis. Locking-loop catheter size is most commonly 6 Fr in dogs and 5 Fr in cats (Weisse & Berent 2015). Both percutaneous and surgical nephrostomy tube placement techniques exist, and ultrasound and/or fluoroscopy is required. Because of the nature of the smaller, more mobile kidneys of cats, surgical placement may be more appropriate.

Procedure

Catheter placement is performed using either the modified Seldinger technique or a "one-stab" trocar introduction technique (Dawson–Mueller drainage catheter 5 Fr, locking-loop pigtail catheter 6 Fr) (Figure 50.2).

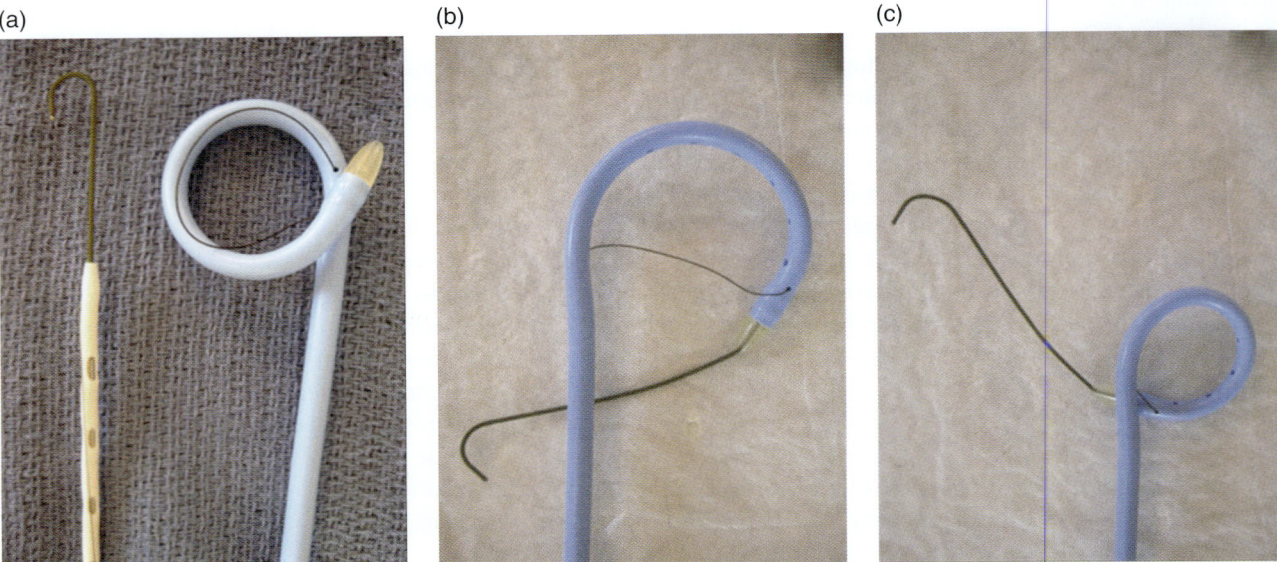

(a) (b) (c)

Figure 50.1 A locking-loop pigtail nephrostomy catheter. (a) A 5 Fr (left) and 6 Fr (right) locking-loop pigtail catheter. The 5 Fr catheter is straightened over its stiff hollow stylette and 0.035 in. guidewire. Notice the loose string of the 6 Fr catheter connecting the distal hole to the most proximal hole. (b) Once the stylette and trocar are removed from the catheter, the pigtail loop can form and the string is tightened. (c) The pigtail is locked in place by the string being completely taut.

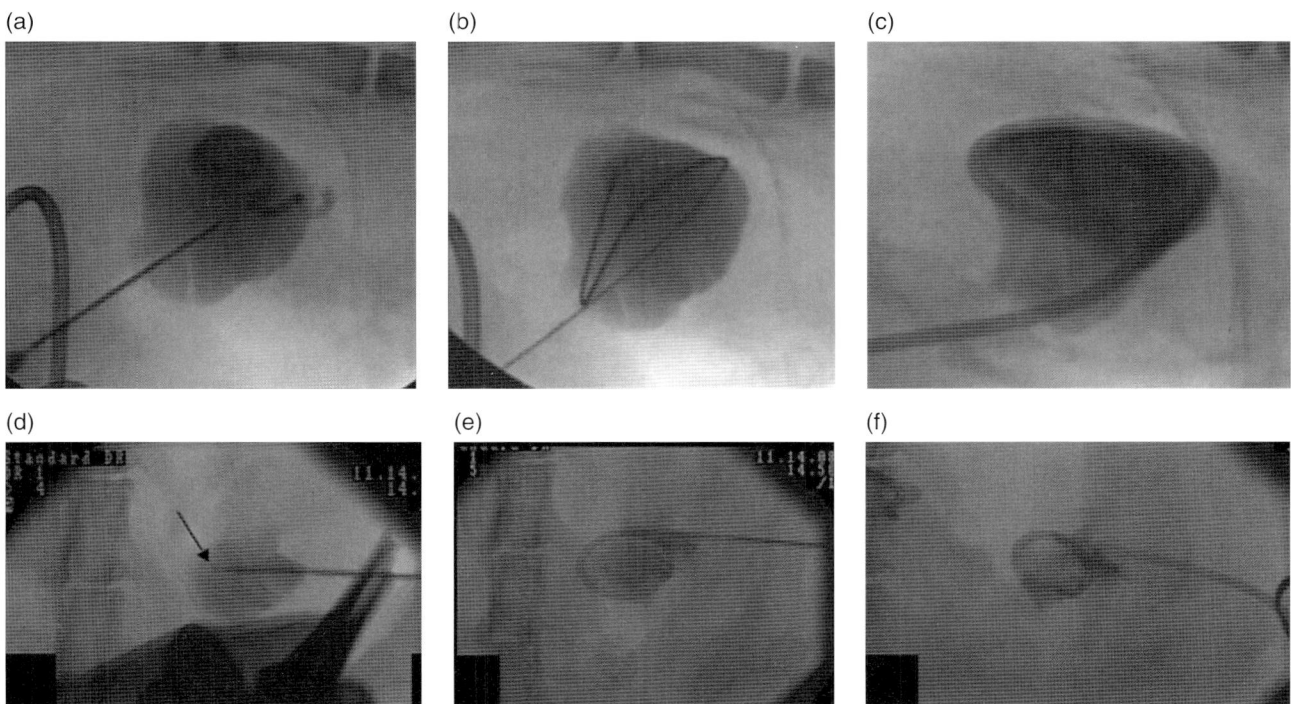

Figure 50.2 The placement of a locking-loop pigtail nephrostomy catheter in two different cats using two different techniques. (a–c) Modified Seldinger technique. (a) Fluoroscopy image of a 22-gauge renal access needle in the renal pelvis after contrast was infused for a pyelogram. (b) A 0.018 in. guidewire is advanced through the needle and coiled inside the renal pelvis. The needle is removed over the wire and the locking-loop pigtail catheter is advanced over the guidewire so that a coil is made inside the renal pelvis. (c) Once the string is pulled, the loop is tightly formed in the renal pelvis to prevent inadvertent removal. (d–f) The one-stab technique. (d) The locking-loop nephrostomy catheter with the sharp trocar (black arrow) being advanced through the greater curvature of the kidney and into the renal pelvis with fluoroscopic guidance. (e) The stiff trocar and stylette are withdrawn as the pigtail catheter is advanced into the dilated renal pelvis. (f) The locking string was pulled so the loop was tightly formed.

Both techniques have been performed successfully in dogs and cats (Berent *et al.* 2009). To aid in performing the modified Seldinger technique, ultrasound guidance is used to perform a pyelocentesis using an over-the-needle catheter or renal access needle. We recommend an 18-gauge needle for dogs and a 22-gauge needle for cats. Once the tip of the catheter is in the renal pelvis, the stylette is removed and an extension set and three-way stopcock are attached to the catheter. Urine is drained and an equal amount of contrast (iohexol 240 mg/mL; Omnipaque™, GE Healthcare, Princeton, NJ, USA) is infused into the renal pelvis to perform a pyelogram and distend the pelvis. The fluoroscopy unit is prealigned over the kidney so that the contrast can be seen as the renal pelvis is filled. Under fluoroscopic guidance, an angle-tipped hydrophilic guidewire (Weasel Wire®, Infiniti Medical, West Hollywood, CA, USA) is advanced through the catheter and coiled (two to three loops if possible) inside the renal pelvis, taking care not to perforate the kidney or ureter. (Note that in the dog, 0.035 in. [0.9 mm] wire fits through the 18-gauge intravenous catheter; in the cat, 0.018 in. [0.46 mm] wire fits through

the 22-gauge catheter.) The catheter is then removed over the wire, and a locking-loop pigtail catheter is advanced over the guidewire through the renal parenchyma and into the renal pelvis. A 5 Fr catheter (Dawson–Mueller drainage catheter) for cats and a 6 Fr catheter (locking-loop drainage catheter, Infiniti Medical) for dogs is passed over the guidewire into the renal pelvis. Once in the renal pelvis, the nephrostomy tube is passed off the hollow trocar and onto the coiled guidewire. When a full loop is present, the locking string is then pulled tight as the guidewire is removed. Contrast infusion through the catheter should show no leakage and confirm that the entire locking loop is situated within the renal pelvis. The catheter is then sutured to the body wall using a purse-string and finger-trap suture pattern and a urine collection system is attached to the catheter for gravity drainage. A secure abdominal bandage is recommended to prevent the tube from being contaminated or accidentally removed.

The one-stab technique is performed using the sharp trocar through the hollow cannula in the locking-loop catheter (Berent *et al.* 2009). A small skin incision is made in the area of the affected kidney. The locking-loop catheter with the sharp trocar left in place can be directly advanced through the body wall, punctured through the greater curvature of the kidney, and into the renal pelvis. The sharp stylette is removed once the catheter is within the renal pelvis, and the catheter is advanced off the hollow trocar until a curl forms within the pelvis. The locking string is subsequently pulled and the locking loop is secured within the renal pelvis. Ultrasound or fluoroscopy can aid in performing this technique. Contrast infusion through the catheter should show no leakage and confirm that the entire locking loop is situated within the renal pelvis. The catheter can be secured to the outside of the body wall as described earlier once the locking mechanism is secured in place.

Both techniques described can also be performed surgically with a standard ventral midline laparotomy approach. Once the catheter is in place, the hub is passed through the body wall using blunt penetration with a hemostat. A nephropexy can then be performed. Both absorbable and nonabsorbable suture material has been used. Surgical bites should include the renal capsule as well as a generous amount of renal parenchyma, with care to avoid penetrating the renal pelvis. We recommend 3-0 suture material for the nephropexy. The catheter can be secured to the outside of the body wall as previously described.

Nephrostomy tube removal

For catheters placed percutaneously, a seal must form to the body wall prior to tube removal, which can take 4 weeks (Mincheff 2007). If the patient is taken to surgery to relieve the obstruction or the obstruction is addressed using other techniques before a seal is formed (e.g., ureteral stenting, shockwave lithotripsy), the tube can either be removed with the site surgically repaired or the tube can be capped and wrapped while left in place for another 2–4 weeks prior to being removed. Fluoroscopy can be used to aid in removal of the nephrostomy tube (Figure 50.3). Using fluoroscopy, the

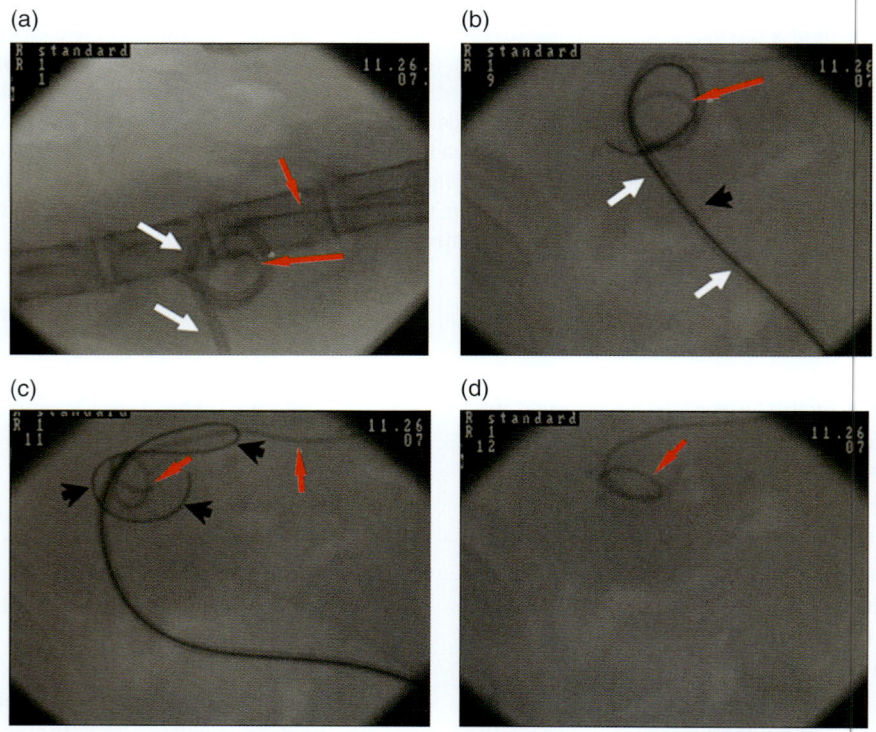

Figure 50.3 Fluoroscopic images during removal of a locking-loop pigtail nephrostomy catheter (white arrows) in a feline patient with a double-pigtail ureteral stent (red arrows). (a) Two catheters are inside the renal pelvis of a feline patient, the locking-loop pigtail nephrostomy catheter (white arrows) and a double-pigtail ureteral stent (red arrows). The stent is placed from the renal pelvis, down the entire ureter, and into the urinary bladder, and remains indwelling. The nephrostomy tube has one loop inside the renal pelvis and is externalized. (b) A guidewire (black arrow) is advanced through the nephrostomy catheter to straighten out the pigtail after the string is unlocked (by cutting the catheter proximally). (c) Once the guidewire (black arrows) is advanced out of the distal end of the nephrostomy catheter, the pigtail straightens out and the catheter is carefully removed through the body wall. Care is taken to avoid entrapping the double-pigtail ureteral stent (red arrows). (d) After the nephrostomy catheter is removed, the double-pigtail ureteral stent remains in place (red arrow) with one loop inside the renal pelvis.

tube is cut approximately 5 cm from the skin and aseptically scrubbed. The string is loosened by cutting the tube. A sterile hydrophilic guidewire is advanced down the tube and curled into the renal pelvis. The tube is then withdrawn over the wire, once the pigtail is straightened out, with gentle traction until it is out of the animal's body and the wire is subsequently removed. The locking string should be removed from the nephrostomy tract. The site can be wrapped for a few hours thereafter to allow the site to close. If a ureteral stent is concurrently in place, fluoroscopy should be used to ensure the pigtails of the stent and nephrostomy tube are not entwined to prevent inadvertent dislodgment of the ureteral stent during nephrostomy tube removal.

Ureter

Ureteral stents

Ureteral stents are classically used in humans to divert urine from the renal pelvis into the urinary bladder, thereby bypassing obstructions secondary to ureterolithiasis, malignant obstructive neoplasia, trauma, or ureteral stenosis/strictures (Zimskind *et al.* 1967; Goldin 1977; Lennon *et al.* 1997; Hubert & Palmer 2005; Uthappa & Cowan 2005; Mustafa 2007). Ureteral stent placement in veterinary patients has been investigated to treat similar conditions (Berent *et al.* 2007, 2011a,b, 2014; Berent 2011; Zaid *et al.* 2011; Lam *et al.* 2012; Wormser *et al.* 2015, 2016; Pavia *et al.* 2018). Multiple goals can be achieved with a ureteral stent:

- To divert urine from the renal pelvis into the urinary bladder to bypass a ureteral obstruction. According to the American College of Veterinary Internal Medicine consensus statement, ureteral stenting or SUB device placement has been recommended to treat cats with obstructive ureteroliths, whereas in dogs ureteral stenting is the recommended procedure (Lulich *et al.* 2016).
- To encourage passive ureteral dilation for ureteral stenosis/strictures, multiple ureteral stones, or future ureteroscopy, which has been documented to occur in over 90% of canine and feline patients (Lennon *et al.* 1997; Berent *et al.* 2007, 2014; Lam *et al.* 2012).
- To decrease surgical tension on the ureter after/during surgery (i.e., resection and anastomosis) and prevent postoperative leakage, stricture formation, and edema-induced obstruction (Kulendra *et al.* 2014b; Manassero *et al.* 2014; Wormser *et al.* 2015, 2016).
- To aid in extracorporeal shockwave lithotripsy for large obstructive ureteroliths or nephroliths that could result in serial ureteral obstructions if the stones do not completely pass down the ureter (Block *et al.* 1996; Lennon *et al.* 1997; Adams & Senior 1999;

Halim 1999; Mustafa 2007; Lulich *et al.* 2009, 2016; Adams 2013).
- To treat obstructive pyonephrosis in dogs (Kuntz *et al.* 2015).

To date, there have been multiple veterinary studies and clinical cases reported in dogs and cats with ureteral stents (Lennon *et al.* 1997; Berent *et al.* 2007, 2011a,b, 2014; Berent 2011; Zaid *et al.* 2011; Lam *et al.* 2012; Nicoli *et al.* 2012; Kulendra *et al.* 2014b; Manassero *et al.* 2014; Kuntz *et al.* 2015; Wormser *et al.* 2015, 2016; Pavia *et al.* 2018). In our experience, success rates in ureteral stent placement are 95% in cats (97% surgically and 20% endoscopically) and 98% in dogs (96% endoscopically, 93% fluoroscopically, and 100% surgically) (Berent *et al.* 2007, 2011a,b, 2014; Berent 2011).

Ureteral stents can be composed of various materials, with the major types incorporating polymeric, metal, and biodegradable compounds (Palm & Culp 2016). The main type of ureteral stent used in both human and veterinary medicine is an indwelling double-pigtail ureteral stent composed of polyurethane material (Figure 50.4). The double-pigtail stent is completely intracorporeal. Typical ureteral stent sizes are ~2 Fr for cats and 3.7, 4.7, or 6 Fr for dogs. The ureteral stent that is preferred by the authors (Vet Stent-Ureter™, Infiniti Medical) is composed of a heat-adaptive polymer and ranges in sizes from 2+ Fr (appropriate for cats, tapered to fit a 0.018 in. guidewire) to 6.0 Fr; the 6.0 Fr stent is specifically designed for dogs with malignant obstructions at the level of the trigone/UVJ and lacks fenestrations at the distal pigtail (whereas other ureteral stents have fenestrations at both pigtails). These ureteral stents are

(a)   (b)

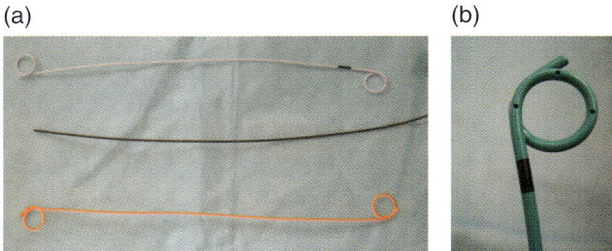

Figure 50.4 A double-pigtail ureteral stent. All are made of polyurethane material. (a) A 2.5 Fr double-pigtail ureteral stent that remains indwelling. The proximal loop remains in the renal pelvis and the distal loop in the urinary bladder. The black tubing is a ureteral dilator and pushing catheter that is used to dilate the feline ureter prior to stent placement, aids in performing a ureteropyelogram, and helps in pushing the ureteral stent over the guidewire when it is straightened out endoscopically so that it can remain indwelling. (b) This is a canine 6 Fr stent that shows the multiple fenestrations at the loop of the stent. Most canine and feline stents are typically multifenestrated.

hydrophilic in nature (to allow placement over the hydrophilic guidewire) and radiopaque.

Procedure

Ureteral stent placement can be performed via minimally invasive or open surgical techniques. Minimally invasive techniques include a percutaneous approach with antegrade stent placement (through the renal pelvis) and the use of cystoscopy with retrograde stent placement. When using cystoscopy, access is obtained in a retrograde manner through the ureteral orifice at the UVJ. In our experience, ureteral stents in dogs are most often placed minimally invasively via cystoscopy (retrograde placement) or a percutaneous technique (antegrade placement). Open surgical techniques for placement of ureteral stents are also possible, and placement can be performed in a retrograde or antegrade fashion. In general, percutaneous ureteral stent placement has only been described for dogs and is not feasible in cats (Berent et al. 2011a; Palm & Culp 2016). Though cystoscopic ureteral stent placement is possible in female cats (20% success), this is much more difficult compared with surgical placement (95% success) (Berent et al. 2014; Kulendra et al. 2014b). In male cats, the narrow nature of the penile urethra typically prevents the use of a standard cystoscope, though newer cystoscopes may provide this option. In general, however, ureteral stents are typically placed via open surgical procedures in cats (Palm & Culp 2016). Surgical stent placement is most common in feline patients and has been highly successful in our experience (95%) (Berent et al. 2007, 2011a, 2014; Berent 2011). This is done via nephrostomy access (antegrade), which is the most effective approach in our experience, cystotomy to access the UVJ (retrograde), or through a ureterotomy incision (antegrade or retrograde). In many cases, the proximal ureter may appear excessively tortuous proximal to the obstructive lesion. Surgical dissection and straightening of the torturous ureter may be necessary to aid in guidewire and stent placement and prevent iatrogenic injury.

Under general anesthesia, the retrograde technique can be performed minimally invasively via cystoscopy with concurrent fluoroscopy (dogs and some female cats) or using an open surgical approach (also with concurrent fluoroscopy) with identification of the UVJ during a cystotomy (Lam et al. 2012; Berent et al. 2014; Kulendra et al. 2014b; Kuntz et al. 2015; Palm & Culp 2016). An angle-tipped hydrophilic guidewire (0.018 in. [0.46 mm] in the cat; 0.025 or 0.035 in. [0.63 or 0.9 mm] in the dog) is advanced into the distal ureter from the UVJ. An open-ended ureteral catheter (dog) or ureteral dilation catheter (cat) is advanced over the wire into the distal ureter and a retrograde ureteropyelogram is

performed. The contrast ureteropyelogram helps to identify any lesions, stones, or other filling defects in the ureter or renal pelvis (Figure 50.5), as well as to outline the path of the ureter for wire passage. Once the ureteropyelogram is performed, the wire is readvanced up the ureter and care is taken to bypass the obstruction without perforating the ureter. If the ureter is penetrated with the guidewire, this hole is small and typically of minimal consequence in our experience, as long as the wire can be readvanced inside the ureteral lumen and past the obstruction to the renal pelvis. This uncommonly occurs in dogs, but may happen more typically in cats. In cases of feline ureteral calculi, the stones are frequently embedded in the mucosa and the surrounding tissue is often very diseased, potentially making the ureter more prone to perforation by the guidewire. The guidewire is coiled inside the renal pelvis and the open-ended ureteral catheter (Figure 50.5) is advanced over the wire, under fluoroscopic guidance, to the level of the renal pelvis. A nephropyelogram can then be performed (through the catheter after removal of the guidewire) to assess for patency of the urinary tract as well as any sites of leakage. The guidewire must then be replaced through the catheter, and the catheter is removed. An indwelling double-pigtail ureteral stent (Vet Stent, Infiniti Medical) is placed over the wire, with one curl remaining in the renal pelvis and the other curl placed in the urinary bladder (Figure 50.5). A pusher catheter can be used over the guidewire, through the endoscope, in order to get the distal loop curled up inside the urinary bladder.

The antegrade technique (Figure 50.6) requires percutaneous or surgical nephrostomy access with a renal access needle or over-the needle catheter (18-gauge dog; 22-gauge cat). In our experience, this is done surgically in cats and percutaneously in dogs. Ultrasound and/or fluoroscopy can aid in identifying the renal pelvis. In general, the location of nephrocentesis should be performed through the center of the greater curvature of the kidney (midway between the cranial and caudal poles and dorsal and ventral axes) toward the UVJ (Palm & Culp 2016). After obtaining access, a ureteropyelogram is performed. Using fluoroscopy, a 0.018 in. hydrophilic guidewire is passed through the catheter into the renal pelvis and down the ureter, guided by the ureteropyelogram, into the urinary bladder, and out the bladder (via cystotomy) or urethra to gain through-and-through access ("flossed"). Once the wire is through and through, the catheter is removed over the guidewire and a ureteral dilator is passed antegrade over the guidewire from the kidney, through the ureter, and into the urinary bladder. The dilator is then removed, and the ureteral stent is placed over the wire. Fluoroscopy should be used to confirm cranial pigtail stent placement within the renal

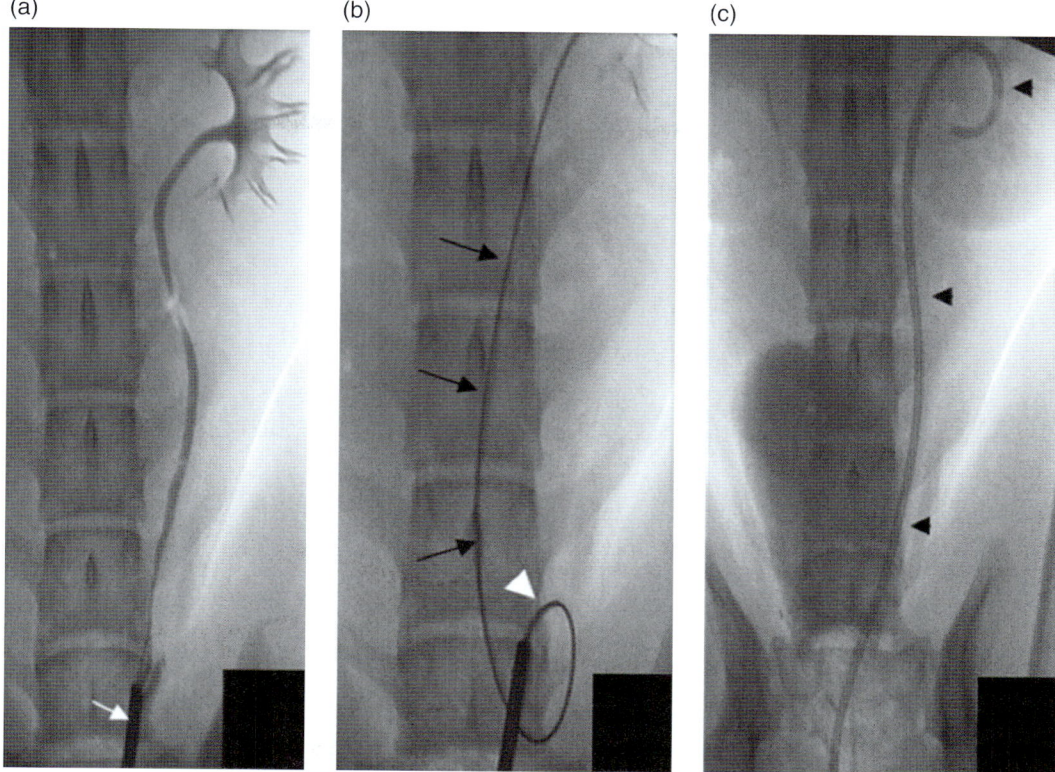

Figure 50.5 Fluoroscopic images of placement of a double-pigtail ureteral stent in a retrograde manner in a female dog using fluoroscopic and cystoscopic guidance. (a) A rigid cystoscope (white arrow) is at the ureterovesicular junction as a guidewire and catheter combination is advanced up the very distal ureter. The wire is removed and the catheter is used for a retrograde ureteropyelogram, seen in this image. (b) The guidewire (black arrows) is advanced up the ureter and into the renal pelvis as the open-ended ureteral catheter (white arrowhead) is advanced over the guidewire. Notice the loop in the distal ureter. This is a common finding in both dogs and cats during endoscopic stent placement. (c) The double-pigtail ureteral stent (black arrowheads) is in place. The proximal loop is curled inside the renal pelvis and the distal loop will be advanced through the cystoscope to form a loop inside the urinary bladder (not shown).

pelvis. The guidewire is then removed, and the caudal stent pigtail is formed in the bladder. This is often the approach for dogs with a trigonal-induced malignant ureteral obstruction when the ureteral orifice cannot be identified cystoscopically, and for small male dogs and male or female cats in which cystoscopy for retrograde ureteral access is not possible. In cases of neoplasia, the wire can be difficult to pass through the tumor (Berent *et al.* 2011b). In cats, antegrade stent placement through the nephrostomy puncture is technically easier than retrograde placement, whereas in dogs this is typically done in a retrograde manner (except in cases of trigonal-induced malignant ureteral obstruction).

Another open surgical technique for ureteral stent placement involves placement of the stent through the ureter following ureterotomy or ureteral resection (Nicoli *et al.* 2012; Kulendra *et al.* 2014b). Stents are typically placed in retrograde fashion in these cases. The guidewire is passed through the ureter, and dilation may be performed prior to stent placement.

Prognosis and complications

Ureteral stent placement is performed noninvasively in a majority of dogs and with surgical assistance in the majority of cats. Ureteral stents should be placed by those experienced with the technique and equipment, as these cases are technically challenging and can become very complicated. The success rates are high, particularly when using the new feline ureteral stent, but the procedure can be very challenging and is not routinely recommended unless the operator has experience with the technique. There is a steep learning curve associated with the procedure, particularly in cats, and the procedure should not be performed without proper understanding of the technique and realization of its potential difficulty. It is important to note that in some cases, ureteral stenting may require concurrent ureterotomy or neoureterocystostomy to complete due to individual case variation and the small diameter of normal cat ureters (0.4 mm) (Kochin *et al.* 1993; Gallagher 2018). A review of the records

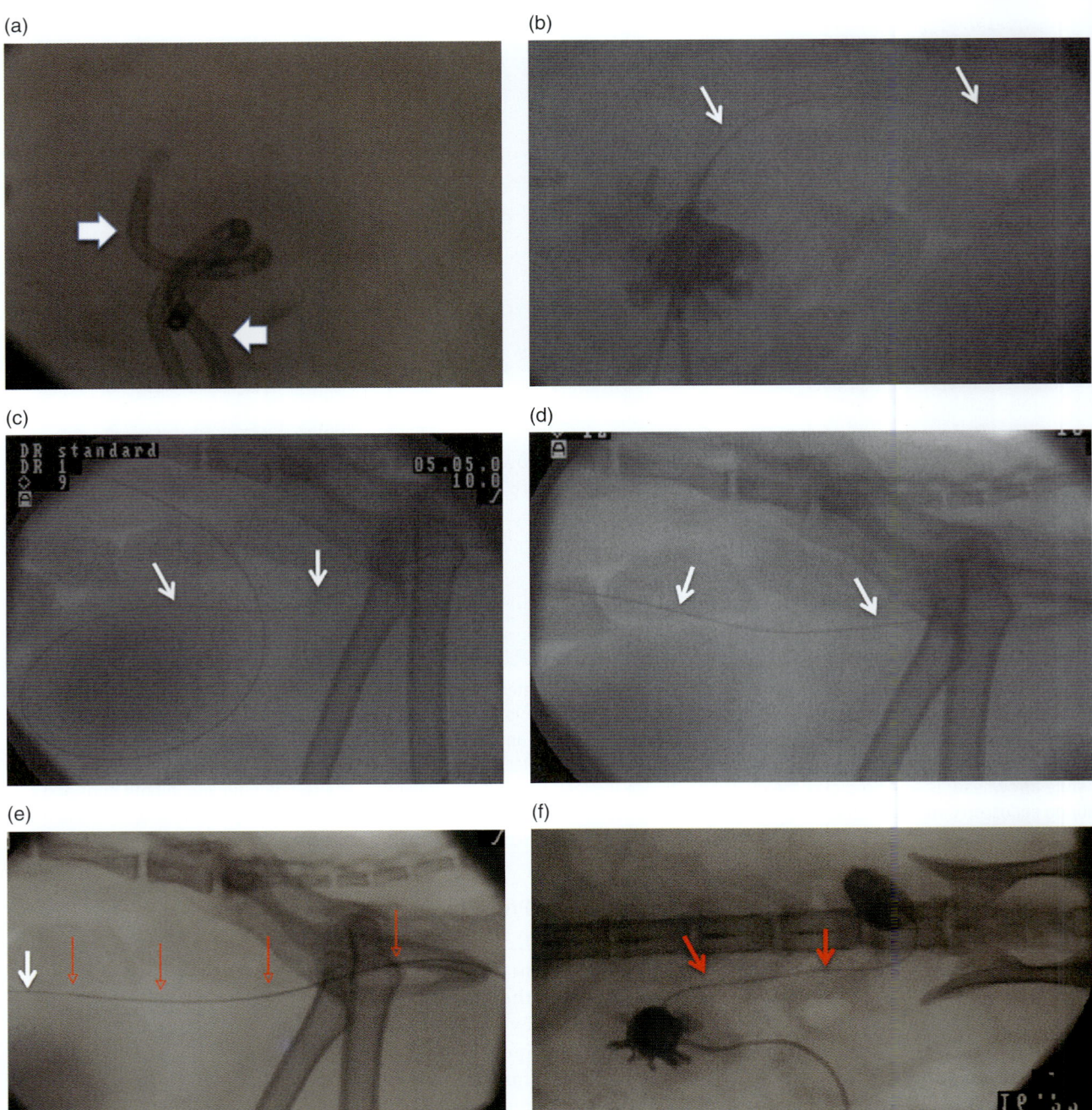

Figure 50.6 Antegrade ureteral stent placement in a male cat. (a) Fluoroscopic image of a cat with bilateral nephrostomy tubes (white arrows) in place. (b) An antegrade pyeloureterogram is performed and a 0.018 in. guidewire (white arrows) is being directed down the ureter past the ureteroliths. (c) The guidewire (white arrows) is advanced from the kidney, down the ureter, and into the urinary bladder and then out of the urethra. (d) The guidewire (white arrows) is pulled straight once through-and-through access is obtained. (e) The ureteral dilator (thin red arrows) is being passed over the guidewire from the urethra and into the ureter. (f) The ureteral stent is in the ureter (red arrows), with one curl in the renal pelvis and the other in the urinary bladder. A nephrostomy tube is inside the renal pelvis and exiting the body wall.

for 84 dogs and 66 cats shows that the success rate for placing the stent was 98% in dogs and 95% in cats. Despite attaining appropriate relief of the ureteral obstruction, studies have documented persistent (though often improved) renal azotemia rates as high as 71% following ureteral stent placement, owing largely to concurrent underlying disease (Berent *et al.* 2014).

Perioperative mortality rates associated with ureteral stent placement in dogs and cats range from 0% to 18%, though the reported procedure-related death rate is very low (Berent *et al.* 2011a,b, 2014; Manassero *et al.* 2014; Kuntz *et al.* 2015; Wormser *et al.* 2016; Deroy *et al.* 2017). Median survival times following ureteral stent placement in dogs and cats range from >415 to 1575 days, though many of these patients died of nonrenal diseases (Berent *et al.* 2014; Manassero *et al.* 2014; Kuntz *et al.* 2015; Wormser *et al.* 2016; Deroy *et al.* 2017; Pavia *et al.* 2018). Long-term survival was not affected by the placement of a stent in the ureter in a series of 117 cats that underwent ureteral surgery or stent placement (Wormser *et al.* 2016). In dogs with malignant ureteral obstructions, a median survival time following stent placement was reported as 57 days in one study, but none died of ureteral-associated disease (Berent *et al.* 2011b). For dogs with benign ureteral obstructions treated with ureteral stents, median follow-up time of 1158 days has been reported, with the majority of dogs (68%) alive at last follow-up, and no dogs died of complications related to the stenting procedure (Kuntz *et al.* 2015).

In humans, it is recommended that stents be removed or exchanged after 3–6 months (Yossepowitch *et al.* 2001; Uthappa & Cowan 2005; Mustafa 2007). However, in veterinary patients, stents are often left in place for multiple years (generally life) and are not typically removed unless they cause a clinical problem. Stent placement may be considered a long-term treatment option for various causes of ureteral obstructions in both dogs and cats, although potential side effects and long-term complications exist (Berent *et al.* 2007, 2011a,b, 2014; Berent 2011; Zaid *et al.* 2011; Nicoli *et al.* 2012; Kulendra *et al.* 2014b; Manassero *et al.* 2014; Kuntz *et al.* 2015; Steinhaus *et al.* 2015; Culp *et al.* 2016; Wormser *et al.* 2016; Deroy *et al.* 2017; Pavia *et al.* 2018). Complications associated with stent placement are most commonly minor in nature, though one study has documented a need for stent removal or exchange in up to 27% of cases (Berent *et al.* 2014).

Possible complications associated with ureteral stent placement include transient or persistent lower urinary tract signs (with dysuria reported in up to 37% of cats long term), infection, urine leakage, stent migration, fracture, encrustation, and obstruction; the rate of these complications is variable across studies (Berent *et al.* 2011b, 2014; Kulendra *et al.* 2014b; Manassero *et al.* 2014; Kuntz *et al.* 2015; Wormser *et al.* 2016). Recurrence of ureteral obstruction has been reported in 22% of cats treated with a ureteral stent or ureteral surgery (Wormser *et al.* 2016). Ureteral stents are associated with encrustation, infection, and chronic pain in human patients (Damiano *et al.* 2002, 2005). Chronic pain can be controlled with α-1 antagonist medications such as alfuzosin or tamsulosin (Damiano *et al.* 2008). Newer stents in cats that are smaller (2+ Fr) and made of a thermoplastic polymer that softens at body temperature are proposed to have a decreased risk of persistent lower urinary tract signs relative to older models, though this remains to be adequately evaluated. With respect to urine leakage, this complication has been documented in animals following ureteral surgery (such as ureterotomy) with concurrent ureteral stent placement as well as in those with ureteral stent placement alone (Berent *et al.* 2014; Wormser *et al.* 2016). Placement of the angle-tipped hydrophilic guidewire can result in ureteral perforation, particularly in cats (<10%). Additionally, because of the small size of the feline ureter, trauma may occur during placement of the stent itself. In an effort to prevent this trauma, care must be taken to advance the stent over the guidewire while holding the ureter securely. The risk of ureteral trauma during stent placement is likely greater when using the older-model pediatric ureteral stents (3 Fr), which are larger and not tapered compared with the currently available feline ureteral stents (2+ and 2.5 Fr). However, in the event of urine leakage following ureteral stent placement, conservative management is often successful and the site of leakage may seal without the requirement for surgery. One study showed that of 8 cats that developed uroperitoneum following ureteral surgery and/or ureteral stent placement, 6 responded to medical management and did not require surgical treatment (Wormser *et al.* 2016). Another study documented uroperitoneum postoperatively in 7/79 feline ureteral stent placements, with 2 of those being associated with a ureterotomy site; 2 of those patients required revision surgery for treatment of the uroperitoneum (Berent *et al.* 2014). If a concurrent ureterotomy is being performed with ureteral stent placement, the authors recommend placing a closed-suction drain in the event there is any leakage to assist with detection of the leakage as well as management.

Subcutaneous ureteral bypass

In human medicine, the SUB device has been used for patients with extensive urinary tract malignancies, ureteral strictures secondary to renal transplantation, or when ureteral stenting or reconstructive surgery fails or is contraindicated (Jurczok *et al.* 2005; Schmidbauer *et al.* 2006; Azhar *et al.* 2010).

The placement of nephrostomy catheters in veterinary medicine has already been described and can result in good outcomes when the appropriate device is used (Berent *et al.* 2009, 2012). The biggest limitation is the externalized drainage, requiring careful management and hospitalization to prevent infection and dislodgment.

The development of an indwelling SUB device (Figure 50.7) using a combination locking-loop nephrostomy catheter and cystostomy catheter was modified from previous reports in human medicine that allowed a nephrostomy tube to remain indwelling long term (median 19 months, range 1 month–10 years) (Jurczok et al. 2005; Schmidbauer et al. 2006). In humans, this device has been shown to reduce complications associated with externalized nephrostomy tubes and improve quality of life (Jurczok et al. 2005; Schmidbauer et al. 2006).

The use of an SUB device has been described in cats and dogs, and its use has increased in veterinary medicine over the past decade (Horowitz et al. 2013; Kulendra et al. 2014a; Johnson et al. 2015; Rossanese & Murgia 2015; Steinhaus et al. 2015; Weisse & Berent 2015; Heilmann et al. 2016; Deroy et al. 2017; Livet et al. 2017; Luca et al. 2017; Berent et al. 2018; Borchert et al. 2018; Cray et al. 2018; Fages et al. 2018; Dirrig et al. 2020). SUB devices allow for bypass of a ureteral obstruction via a nephrostomy tube and cystostomy tube that are connected via a port in the subcutaneous space. Placement of the SUB device does not require manually bypassing (or removing) the ureteral obstruction, and ureteral surgical techniques are not required. This system is designed to be permanent upon placement, and long-term management of these patients is essential. A newer version of the SUB device (SUB 3.0, Norfolk Vet Products, Skokie, IL, USA) consists of a tapered, locking-loop, pigtail catheter in the renal pelvis, a straight, multifenestrated catheter in the urinary bladder, and a "Y-connector" with a piece of actuating tubing connected to a subcutaneous port (Figures 50.7 and 50.8). This has allowed for the mitigation of kinking of the device as it passes through the body wall, as the nephrostomy and cystostomy catheters remain in the abdominal cavity. Two sizes are available for this device for use in cats and small or large dogs. An "X-connector" can also be utilized for bilateral cases to avoid the need for two ports.

Procedure

Placement of an SUB device requires an open surgical approach via a ventral midline laparotomy, and use of fluoroscopy is strongly recommended to ensure appropriate SUB placement. The retroperitoneal fat in the region of the caudal pole of the affected kidney is bluntly dissected away from the renal capsule. A modified Seldinger technique is used for nephrostomy tube placement. An 18-gauge over-the-needle catheter is inserted into the caudal or caudolateral pole of the kidney (midway between the dorsal and ventral axis) into the renal pelvis, and a nephropyelogram is performed. A 0.035 in. J-tip guidewire is passed through the catheter into the renal pelvis, until the J-tip is coiled within the pelvis. The catheter is removed over the wire, and a 6.5 Fr locking-loop nephrostomy catheter is passed over the wire and a hollow cannula into the affected renal pelvis. Once the catheter enters the renal pelvis, the catheter is advanced beyond the end of the cannula and over the guidewire, thereby creating a pigtail within the renal pelvis. A radiopaque marker denotes the last fenestration of the pigtail, and it is important that this entire marker lies within the renal pelvis. The locking string is then pulled taut (not so tight as to create a kink), and the string is clamped with a hemostat just beyond the catheter end to maintain the locking loop. With the aid of fluoroscopy,

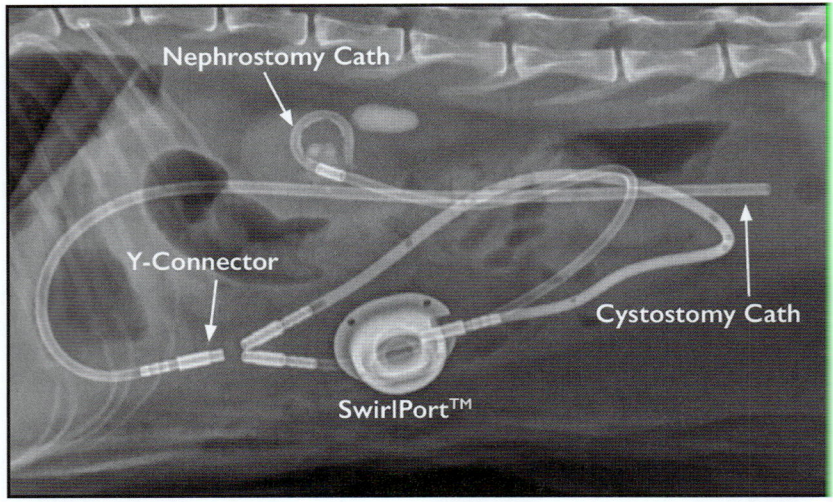

Figure 50.7 The SUB 3.0 system demonstrating the pigtail nephrostomy catheter, straight cystostomy catheter, Y-connector that joins the nephrostomy and cystostomy catheters, and an additional tube that connects to the subcutaneous SwirlPort. Source: Norfolk Veterinary Products, SUB 3.0 brochure.

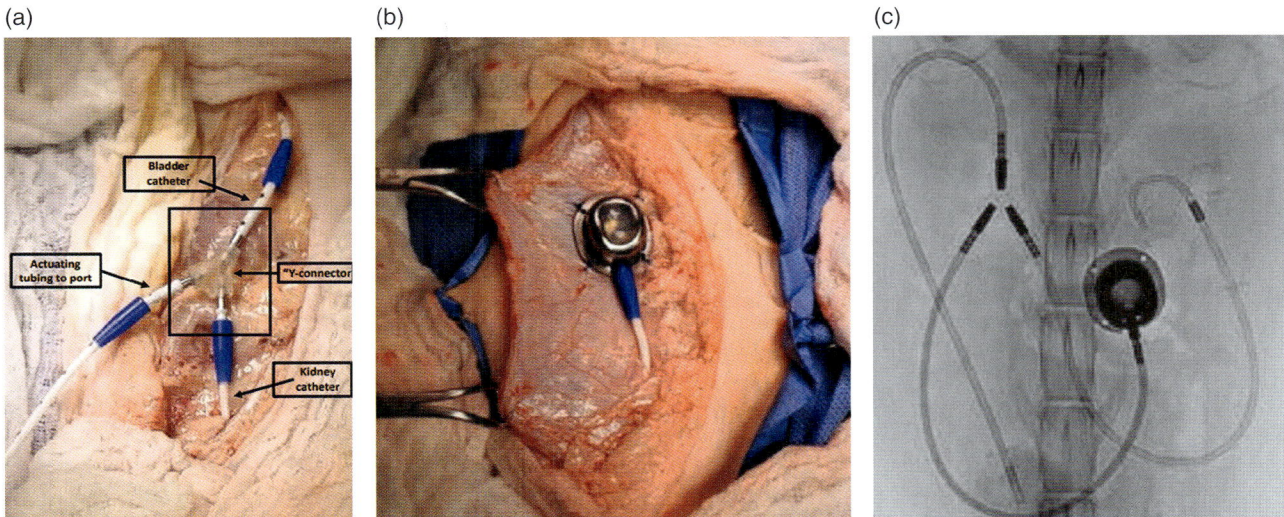

Figure 50.8 A left-sided subcutaneous ureteral bypass (SUB) device in a feline patient. The patient is in dorsal recumbency. (a) The Y-connector connecting the nephrostomy catheter, cystostomy catheter, and actuating tubing. The catheters have been advanced to the final step on the metal barbs, and the blue boots have been preplaced but not yet moved into position over the catheter end and metal barbs of the Y-connector. (b) The access port attached to the catheter (actuating tubing), which is placed subcutaneously. (c) A fluoroscopic image of the SUB in ventrodorsal view, showing the nephrostomy and cystostomy catheters connected to the Y-connector with actuating tubing that connects to the subcutaneous port. Source: Norfolk Veterinary Products, SUB 3.0 surgical guide.

the pelvis is drained and filled with contrast to ensure proper placement. The Dacron cuff is advanced down the catheter to the renal capsule, and sterile cyanoacrylate glue is applied to secure the cuff to the kidney. In patients with a small renal pelvis (less than approximately 8 mm diameter), the nephrostomy catheter can be placed down the proximal ureter rather than within the renal pelvis. With this technique, the locking string should be cut prior to placement so that the catheter does not form a pigtail, and a 0.035 in. angle-tipped hydrophilic guidewire should be used (rather than the J-tip guidewire, with placement through the renal pelvis into the proximal ureter).

Next, a purse-string suture is placed near the apex of the urinary bladder (slightly lateralized) and left loose. The authors prefer to use 3-0 poliglecaprone (Ethicon, Johnson & Johnson, Somerville, NJ, USA) for this suture. A stab incision is then made into the urinary bladder through the purse string. The straight cystostomy catheter is passed over the hollow cannula into the urinary bladder through the stab incision. The purse-string suture is tightened around the catheter and tied. Sterile cyanoacrylate glue is then applied between the cuff and urinary bladder wall. Three simple interrupted sutures of 3-0 poliglecaprone are placed through the Dacron/silicon cuff and full thickness through the urinary bladder. The bladder is then leak tested to ensure that a seal is made.

The skin immediately lateral to the ventral abdominal incision on the ipsilateral side of the affected kidney and nephrostomy tube is dissected off the rectus abdominis muscle and cleared of fat to the level of fascia. The blue boots are preplaced over each catheter end (nephrostomy, cystostomy, and actuating tubing) prior to insertion on the Y-connector. Each catheter end is then advanced onto the barbs of the Y-connector, and the locking string of the nephrostomy catheter is transected once the catheter passes the first rung of the barb (to maintain its tension). Each catheter is then advanced over all rungs of each barb; no string should protrude from the nephrostomy catheter end to prevent leakage. Once the nephrostomy and cystostomy catheters and actuating tubing are connected to the Y-connector as detailed in the instruction manual, the actuating tubing is then passed through the body wall on the side ipsilateral to the ureteral obstruction.

The site of passage of actuating tubing through the body wall should be cranial enough to allow for gentle curvature of each loop without any kink. Once the catheter is in place, a blue boot is placed on the catheter where it will connect to the port, and the catheter is trimmed to an appropriate length. The actuating tubing catheter is then connected to the port with a male adaptor. Once the catheters are secured, the system is leak tested under pressure and patency tested using contrast material to ensure good flow and no leakage or kinking. Only a Huber needle should be used. The port is then secured to the ventrolateral body wall using 3-0 polypropylene via four simple interrupted sutures. The subcutaneous pocket is closed routinely with absorbable suture and any dead space addressed.

Prognosis and complications

There currently exists more outcome data on SUB devices and placement in cats than in dogs. The largest retrospective study documented placement of an SUB device for treatment of 174 obstructed ureters (with benign obstructions) in 134 cats (Berent *et al.* 2018). The SUB device was successfully placed in all 174 cases (Berent *et al.* 2018). Median serum creatinine concentration at admission and discharge was 6.6 and 2.7 mg/dL, respectively (Berent *et al.* 2018). Perioperative mortality occurred in 6.0% of cats; no cats died intraoperatively or due to persistent ureteral obstruction immediately postoperatively (Berent *et al.* 2018). Complications included occlusion of the SUB with blood clots, kinking of the device tubing, leakage of the SUB device, infection, and persistent lower urinary signs (such as dysuria and hematuria) (Berent *et al.* 2018). Mineralization of the catheter was the most common long-term complication (24.2%), with the need for device exchange reaching 12.7%. Device mineralization was statistically associated with a high postoperative serum ionized calcium level (Berent *et al.* 2018). Surgical revision with catheter exchange was required for 9/14 occlusions caused by blood clots and 21/40 occlusions caused by mineralization (12.7% of cases overall); occluded tubes that did not require surgical revision were successfully treated with serial flushing and/or instillation of tissue plasminogen activator for clots (Berent *et al.* 2018). Overall median survival time was 827 days (Borchert *et al.* 2018). New data presented recently showed a dramatic improvement in the rates of mineralization occlusion and chronic infections with serial flushing of the SUB device with tetra sodium-EDTA (tEDTA) (Berent *et al.* 2018; Chik *et al.* 2019). In addition, early data on the SUB 3.0 device support a decreased rate of device kinking with the new design from 15% to 0% (Berent, VIRIES virtual conference 2021).

Decision making

In considering which technique to choose for treatment of ureteral obstruction, veterinary medicine is lacking large, prospective studies comparing outcomes and complication rates for different interventional and surgical procedures in dogs and cats. Therefore, additional information is needed to support broad generalizations regarding preferred treatment modalities, and the optimal treatment modality is likely to be determined by the unique aspects of each clinical case, as well as clinician/institution experience, skill set, and available equipment. However, several retrospective studies have been performed that compare different techniques. For instance, the outcome of cats that underwent ureteral stent placement compared to those that underwent ureterotomy alone for treatment of benign ureteral obstruction has been evaluated (Culp *et al.* 2016). This study demonstrated that cats that underwent ureteral stent placement (n = 26) had greater decreases of creatinine and blood urea nitrogen (BUN) one day postoperatively, and that these cats were more likely to have resolution of azotemia prior to hospital discharge compared to cats that underwent ureterotomy (n = 36) (Culp *et al.* 2016). Furthermore, in general, traditional surgery techniques (ureterotomy, neoureterocystostomy, ureteronephrectomy) for treatment of ureteral obstruction have resulted in relatively high rates of mortality, postoperative complications, recurrent obstruction, and persistent azotemia, such that interventional techniques (ureteral stents and SUBs) are now more commonly performed for treatment of ureteral obstruction in dogs and cats (Kyles *et al.* 2005; Snyder *et al.* 2005; Roberts *et al.* 2011; Culp *et al.* 2016).

One study has shown relatively low perioperative mortality rates and a lower complication rate associated with ureteral surgery compared to ureteral stenting, though inherent bias based on procedure selection in this retrospective study should be noted; the study demonstrates that good outcomes can be obtained with traditional ureteral surgery in cases that are considered good surgical candidates, and when in the hands of surgeons that are experienced with these microsurgical techniques and have the equipment required (such as an operating microscope) to perform these procedures with success (Wormser *et al.* 2016). One study reported an acceptable outcome for 11/12 cats that underwent ureteroneocystostomy for treatment of ureteral obstruction (Lorange & Monnet 2020). Median creatinine concentration was 2.0 mg/dL at a median of 157 days (range 43–1772 days) after ureteroneocystostomy, with no signs of recurrence of obstruction (Lorange & Monnet 2020).

Another retrospective study compared outcomes of cats with ureteral obstruction that underwent ureteral stent or SUB placement (Deroy *et al.* 2017). This study found a lower risk of complications and longer survival time for cats treated with stents compared to SUBs; however, ultimately a prospective study is needed to determine long-term complications and median survival times for these two groups (Deroy *et al.* 2017). In general, SUBs are considered more permanent devices that require open laparotomy for removal or revision (though the need for this is uncommon, especially in cats) as compared to ureteral stents, which can be a temporary or long-term treatment option and also may require exchange or removal. Ureteral stent exchange or removal can be done relatively minimally invasively, and naive placement is typically performed endoscopically in dogs but surgically assisted in cats.

In cases of multiple ureteroliths, bypassing these stones in a cat with a ureteral stent may also be challenging, making the use of an SUB device ideal in many of these patients. In addition, dogs and cats with suspected ureteral strictures may not undergo the expected passive ureteral dilatation around the ureteral stent, and the risk for reobstruction or ureteral stent compression may be greater in these patients; therefore, the authors recommend placement of an SUB device in cats with ureteral strictures (Berent *et al.* 2014). In dogs with ureteral strictures, treatment options include a combination of balloon dilatation of the stricture and ureteral stenting, resection of the ureteral stricture and distal ureter with subsequent ureteroneocystostomy, and SUB device placement. For the subset of cats with ureteral obstructions and circumcaval ureters, the authors also recommend placement of an SUB device rather than a ureteral stent, as there has been a greater rate of reobstruction documented in cats following placement of stents due to the suspected stricture formation associated with circumcaval ureter(s) (Steinhaus *et al.* 2015). Circumcaval ureters are relatively common in cats (14–17% of cats, with a predilection for right ureters in 80%), and this should always be assessed prior to determination of an appropriate treatment technique (Steinhaus *et al.* 2015).

Overall, great care should be taken in choosing the appropriate procedure (interventional or surgical) for each case of ureteral obstruction; most procedures are technically very challenging and should only be performed by clinicians with appropriate experience and equipment. Cats with proximal ureteral strictures, extensive ureteral injury, or trauma associated with urinary calculi in which only a short segment of proximal ureter remains for surgical correction can be challenging cases to address surgically, and successful surgical treatment may involve performing a renal descensus in conjunction with ureteroneocystostomy and cystonephropexy, or the creation of a Boari flap. Additionally, ureteral strictures can be treated by performing a resection of the strictured area and an end to-end anastomosis of the ureter (possibly with placement of a ureteral stent).

With all these surgical techniques, appropriate magnification is essential. Given the technical challenges and risk of complications with these surgical procedures, interventional procedures such as placement of ureteral stents and SUBs have become much more common procedures, with an increasing evidence base for their efficacy and safety in dogs and cats. Ultimately, however, the choice to place a ureteral stent or SUB device or to perform traditional ureteral surgery must be based on the individual case presentation, the experience of the clinician performing the procedure, as well as the availability of equipment.

Postoperative care

Patients treated for ureteral obstruction need to be monitored very carefully long term, as reobstruction is possible, and management of chronic kidney disease is necessary in the majority of patients. This need for monitoring does not depend on the treatment modality chosen, and long-term follow-up schedules are similar regardless of treatment performed. Acutely, feline patients are at a high risk of developing a postobstructive diuresis and potentially fluid overload if fluid balance is not carefully monitored postoperatively. Monitoring fluid inputs and outputs, central venous pressure, body weight, and clinical hydration status is very important. Enteral fluid therapy is often maintained with an esophagostomy feeding tube throughout the entire acute postoperative period. One retrospective study on cats with ureteral obstructions that were treated with ureteral stents or SUBs demonstrated that preoperative serum creatinine, BUN, potassium, and phosphorus concentrations as well as absolute changes in creatinine, BUN, and potassium changes postoperatively relative to preoperatively were positively correlated with duration and/or severity of postobstructive diuresis (Balsa *et al.* 2019). Cats that were anuric preoperatively also had longer durations of postobstructive diuresis (Balsa *et al.* 2019). Regardless of the original azotemia level, with intensive management the majority (91.9%, 34/37) of these patients survived to discharge (Balsa *et al.* 2019). Therefore, care should be taken to maintain appropriate fluid and electrolyte balance in these patients, using enteral hydration (feeding tubes) when possible. Careful monitoring for uroperitoneum and electrolyte imbalances are warranted postoperatively. Abdominal palpation should be discouraged for at least two weeks postoperatively in patients following SUB placement to prevent manipulation of the instrumentation, and intensive palpation should never be performed.

Antibiotic administration should be considered postoperatively and should ideally be based on culture and sensitivity results. Urine from the bladder can be obtained preoperatively via cystocentesis, or urine from the renal pelvis can be obtained at the time of decompression during ureteral stent or SUB device placement. One study showed an incidence of 25% of positive urine cultures postoperatively (and prior to hospital discharge) following ureteral stent or SUB device placement in cats (Kopecny *et al.* 2019). In that study, cats that received antibiotics postoperatively were less likely to have a positive urine culture compared with cats that did not receive antibiotics; type of implant placed and postoperative urethral catheterization were not associated with a positive culture in that study (Kopecny *et al.* 2019). Another study reported a relatively high incidence of urinary tract infection both prior to (33%) and within one month following (31.7%) ureteral stent placement in cats, but these infections were typically able to be cleared in the long term with appropriate antibiotic therapy; use of an externalized catheter following surgery was suspected to be associated with the high postoperative infection rate, but was likely of little clinical consequence long term (Berent *et al.* 2014). These studies also demonstrated the potential for positive urine cultures long term following implant placement, and repeat urine cultures are recommended on a regular basis (such as culture every three months for the first year, then every six months thereafter) (Berent *et al.* 2014; Kopecny *et al.* 2019). For urine collection in patients with an SUB device in place, the authors recommend using the subcutaneous access port. If a cystocentesis is necessary, ultrasound guidance should be used to obtain the urine sample, as avoidance of the SUB device is strongly advised. There does not appear to be significant risk in obtaining urine via cystocentesis for stented patients, though ultrasound guidance may be preferred to avoid damaging or manipulating the stent.

Routine urinary tract ultrasound focusing on renal pelvis diameter, implant location, ureteral diameter, and bladder wall may also be performed to ensure there is no evidence of migration, occlusion, inflammation, or encrustation of the device. In the case of ureteral stents, even if occlusion from urinary debris or crystalline material occurs, appropriate passive dilatation of the ureter around the stent can help prevent reobstruction. This has been appreciated on necropsy, where a guidewire cannot be passed up the lumen of the stent, but the ureter is passively dilated and there is no sign of ureteral obstruction on pyelography or ultrasonography. For patients with SUB devices, flushing of the device through the port to ensure patency is often performed using a 22-gauge Huber needle. The skin over the port is clipped of fur and aseptically prepared. An extension set with a three-way stopcock is used and connected to the Huber needle, with one empty syringe for urine sampling and one syringe filled with sterile saline. The SUB device flush procedure is typically monitored with ultrasound, but can also be monitored with fluoroscopy using contrast material if deemed necessary. Once patency is confirmed, the device can then be infused with 2 mL of tEDTA, while monitoring the renal pelvis with ultrasound, in an effort to chelate

any mineral accumulation and prevent infections. This procedure is highlighted in the instructions for use manual at Norfolk Vet Products, and early data presented recently support this flushing technique as having helped to decrease the rate of device mineralization, occlusion, and infection (Berent *et al.* 2018; Chik *et al.* 2019).

One study assessed for predictors of outcome in cats with ureteral obstruction treated by either ureteral stent or SUB placement, and this showed that these cats had a good overall survival rate, with no parameter determined at presentation associated with survival to discharge (Horowitz *et al.* 2013). In general, however, cats with lower International Renal Interest Society stage chronic kidney disease postprocedure had longer survival times than those with higher stages of chronic kidney disease (Horowitz *et al.* 2013). It is important to consider the underlying disease process and potential chronic kidney disease in these cats, which will require continued long-term management and may be intensive and progressive in nature; however, many of these cats go on to live a relatively long life following treatment for ureteral obstruction.

Bladder

Cystostomy tubes

Cystostomy tubes can be placed permanently to bypass a urethral obstruction or temporarily to avoid bladder distension while a urethral/trigonal lesion is healing. This can be secondary to malignant neoplasia (trigonal, urethral, and prostatic tumors), proliferative/granulomatous urethritis, urethral strictures, urethral tears, reflex dyssynergia, or urethral stones that are difficult to remove surgically. However, with the advent of urethral stents, the use of cystostomy tubes has declined as a method to achieve permanent urinary bypass. Cystostomy tubes can be placed either percutaneously or surgically, and either fluoroscopy or ultrasound can be used to guide placement. Alternative surgical options for bypassing a proximal urethral or trigonal obstruction (such as radical cystectomy and urinary diversion techniques) are discussed elsewhere.

Procedure

With the locking-loop pigtail catheter (Figure 50.9), percutaneous cystostomy tube placement has become a relatively fast and easy technique when necessary. To enable percutaneous placement, the urinary bladder needs to be relatively full. The patient is generally placed in lateral recumbency. Percutaneous placement can be done via either the modified Seldinger technique using

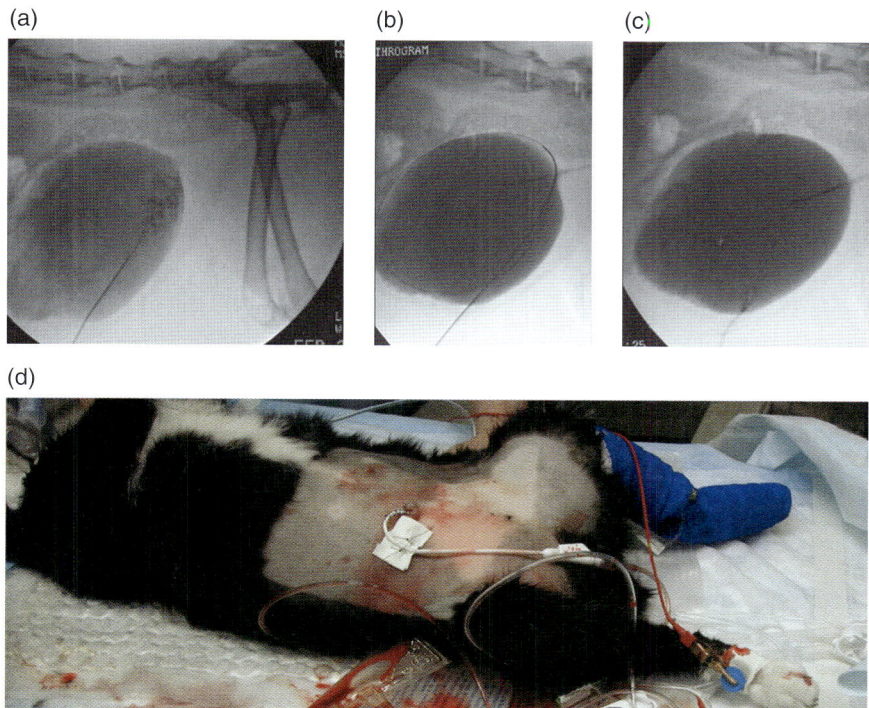

(a)   (b)   (c)

(d)

Figure 50.9 Placement of a percutaneous locking-loop cystostomy tube in a male cat after a urethral tear. (a) An 18-gauge over-the-needle catheter is used to perform a cystocentesis and contrast cystogram under fluoroscopic guidance. (b) A 0.035 in. guidewire is advanced through the catheter and coiled inside the urinary bladder. (c) The 6 Fr locking-loop pigtail catheter is advanced through the body wall, over the guidewire, and into the urinary bladder. The locking string mechanism is pulled tightly to form a secure lock. (d) The catheter is then secured appropriately to the body wall and left to drain.

fluoroscopy or the one-stab technique using ultrasound with or without fluoroscopy. For the modified Seldinger technique, an 18-gauge over-the-needle catheter is advanced into the urinary bladder at the level of the mid-cranial body of the bladder, adjacent to the rectus abdominus or approximately 2 cm lateral to the linea alba, until urine is draining; the catheter should enter the abdomen at a 20–30° angle directed caudally. The stylette is removed and, using an extension set and a three-way stopcock, urine is sampled for culture. Using fluoroscopy, contrast is infused for documentation of the bladder borders. A moistened, 0.035 in. angle-tipped hydrophilic guidewire is advanced though the catheter and into the urinary bladder. The wire is curled within the bladder 2–3 times and visualized with fluoroscopy. Next, the catheter is removed and a locking-loop pigtail catheter (6 or 8 Fr for dogs, 5 or 6 Fr for cats) is advanced over the wire with the hollow cannula still in place. Once the catheter and cannula puncture the bladder wall, the catheter is advanced over the guidewire into the urinary bladder. When the entire pigtail loop of the catheter is well within the urinary bladder, the string is locked and the wire and cannula are removed. The catheter is secured to the body wall using a purse-string suture and finger-trap suture. The catheter should not be pulled so

tightly toward the body wall that it may become dislodged during bladder filling and emptying. A contrast study should be performed through the tube to ensure appropriate placement without leakage. A sterile collection system should then be attached to the catheter, and an abdominal wrap is typically placed to secure the tube to the body wall.

For the one-stab percutaneous technique, a small skin incision is made at the same location, as described earlier. The locking-loop catheter with the sharp trocar left in place can be directly advanced through the body wall and punctured through the bladder. The sharp stylette is then removed once the catheter is within the bladder, and the catheter is advanced off the hollow trocar until a curl forms within the pelvis. The locking string is subsequently pulled and the locking loop is secured within the bladder. Ultrasound or fluoroscopy can aid in performing this technique. Contrast infusion through the catheter should show no leakage and confirm that the entire locking loop is situated within the bladder. The catheter can be secured to the outside of the body wall, as described earlier, once the locking mechanism is secured in place.

An open or laparoscopic-assisted surgical technique for placement of a cystostomy tube allows a cystopexy to be performed concurrently. In addition to a locking-loop pigtail catheter, other tubes, including a latex mushroom-tipped (de Pezzer) catheter, Foley catheter, or low-profile tube, can be placed using an open or laparoscopic-assisted surgical technique (Smith *et al.* 1995; Stiffler *et al.* 2003). Catheter sizes of 8–14 Fr are typically used for surgical cystostomy tube placement (Lipscomb 2018). Foley catheters are recommended for short-term use only due to possible deflation of the balloon with time (Lipscomb 2018). Low-profile silicone gastrostomy tubes can be placed for long-term use; these tubes do not require a bandage to keep the tube secured to the body wall, and a separate tube can be attached to the low-profile tube for drainage (Stiffler *et al.* 2003; Lipscomb 2018).

To place a cystostomy tube surgically, a ventral abdominal laparotomy is performed. A stab incision is first made in the skin paramedian to the abdominal incision at the level of the body of the urinary bladder, adjacent to the proposed cystostomy site, and the distal end of the cystostomy tube is entered into the abdomen through the body wall. A stay suture is placed at the apex of the urinary bladder to assist with manipulation, and the bladder should remain mildly to moderately distended. Using absorbable monofilament suture material, a purse-string suture is placed within the bladder wall on the ventrolateral surface. A stab incision is made into the bladder lumen through the purse string, and the catheter is passed through the stab incision. If a mushroom-tipped catheter is placed, a stylette is needed to stiffen the catheter prior to insertion (and removal) from the urinary bladder. The purse-string suture is tightened around the catheter and tied. Four interrupted sutures (not penetrating the bladder lumen) are then placed in a box pattern between the abdominal wall and bladder wall to create a sutured cystopexy. If a permanent cystopexy is being performed, this suture material is typically nonabsorbable monofilament; if a temporary cystopexy is being performed, this suture material should be absorbable monofilament. The external tube is then secured to the body wall with a purse string and finger-trap pattern and bandage, as already described (with the exception of low-profile tubes). Other surgical techniques that have been described for placement of tube cystostomy include a minimally invasive inguinal approach (dogs and cats) and a laparoscopic percutaneous approach (dogs) (Bray *et al.* 2009; Zhang *et al.* 2010).

Prognosis and complications

The largest retrospective study to date on cystostomy tubes in dogs (n = 37) and cats (n = 39) reported a median duration of tube placement of 11 days; placement times were significantly longer for cases of bladder dysfunction (Beck *et al.* 2007). The underlying disease process resolved and the tube was removed in 42/72 ani-

mals; the remaining animals with follow-up information died or were euthanized with the tube in place (27/72), still had the tube in place at the completion of the study (2/72), or had removal of the tube with persistent clinical signs (1/72) (Beck *et al.* 2007). Cystostomy tubes are commonly associated with secondary infection, with an incidence of 86% in one study (Beck *et al.* 2007). The incidence of other complications, including inadvertent tube removal, eating of the tube by the patient, fistulous tract formation, and mushroom tip breakage during removal, has been reported to be as high as 49% (Beck *et al.* 2007). Thus, cystostomy tube placement is not ideal in circumstances where chemotherapy (for malignant obstructions) or immunosuppressive therapy (for immune-mediated disease/proliferative urethritis) is being used. One study documented leakage and uroperitoneum in three cats following placement of Stamey percutaneous loop cystostomy catheters (Cook Medical, Bloomington, IN, USA) (Hunt *et al.* 2013).

It is important that the tube cystostomy be maintained for an adequate amount of time to allow for adhesions to create a seal between the bladder and body wall to prevent leakage upon tube removal. It is recommended that the tube remain in place for at least 2–4 weeks in nonsurgically placed cystostomy tubes (i.e., those in which a sutured cystopexy was not performed) and 7 days in surgically placed cystostomy tubes (i.e., those with a sutured cystopexy) (Weisse & Berent 2015; Lipscomb 2018). If a tube is removed prematurely, there is a greater risk of uroperitoneum.

Urethra

Urethral catheterization

Urinary diversion in the face of urethral obstruction can be accomplished via standard urethral catheterization. This is a simple and routinely performed procedure in veterinary patients and is primarily used to monitor urine output, establish urine drainage in patients that are recumbent or have mechanical/functional urethral obstructions, allow healing after a urethral tear, or provide urethral patency following urethral or urinary bladder surgery. Unlike urethral stents, these catheters are typically maintained on a temporary basis. Urethral tears are most commonly seen in male cats and occur secondary to iatrogenic trauma while trying to unblock the patient or from vehicular trauma. The management of urethral trauma has been reported using urethral catheterization alone (Meige *et al.* 2008). The most common urethral catheters in use are Foley catheters, which have a balloon tip to prevent the catheter from backing out into the urethra, and red rubber catheters, which are more rigid but, unlike a Foley, do not have a safety mechanism for inadvertent removal. All catheters in the urinary system should be placed with sterile technique. Once placed, they should be secured with suture and connected to sterile urine collection systems.

Procedure

In male dogs, catheters are easily advanced in a retrograde manner up the penile urethra and into the urinary bladder. In female dogs and cats this can be more difficult, requiring digital palpation of the urethral papilla for catheter advancement and sometimes the use of a speculum or cystoscope/vaginoscope to aid in papilla cannulization.

For animals that are either too small (cats and small female dogs) or very difficult (animals that have a urethral tear or malignant obstruction) to easily catheterize retrograde, antegrade access can be attempted (Figure 50.10). This technique can be performed surgically (under general anesthesia) or interventionally (under general anesthesia or heavy sedation) (Holmes *et al.* 2012). When performed surgically, a ventral abdominal approach is used. In addition to normal patient preparation, the vulva or prepuce should be clipped and aseptically prepared. When performing the technique interventionally, the patient is placed in lateral recumbency and an area in the caudolateral abdomen just over the bladder is clipped and aseptically prepared as well as the vulva and prepuce.

A cystocentesis is performed using an 18-gauge over-the-needle catheter directed toward the trigone of the bladder. Urine (5–15 mL) is drained from the bladder and replaced with an equal amount of contrast material diluted 1:1 with sterile saline to identify the proximal urethra. A hydrophilic guidewire (0.035 in.) is advanced into the bladder and aimed toward the bladder trigone under fluoroscopic guidance until it is out of the distal

urethra. When performed surgically, contrast enhancement with the use of fluoroscopy is not necessary. The guidewire is aimed down the urethra and out of the body, gaining through-and-through access. Once the guidewire is outside the urethra, a urinary catheter (open ended; Foley, red rubber, locking-loop catheter, nonlocking pigtail, etc.) is advanced retrograde over the wire through the urethra and into the urinary bladder. This technique is ideal for male cats with urethral tears, as the tear is usually longitudinal in nature and iatrogenically formed in a retrograde manner. Longitudinal urethral tears will usually heal within 5–10 days without surgical intervention, and the catheter should be maintained for that length of time in these patients (Meige *et al.* 2008).

Urethral stents

Urethral stents are most commonly used for the relief of malignant urothelial obstructions in the urethra (Weisse *et al.* 2006; Blackburn 2010; Blackburn *et al.* 2013). Malignant obstructions of the urethra can cause severe discomfort, dysuria, and life-threatening azotemia. More than 80% of animals with transitional cell carcinoma of the urethra and/or prostatic carcinoma experience dysuria and approximately 10% develop complete urinary tract obstruction (Norris *et al.* 1992; Knapp *et al.* 2000). When signs of obstruction occur, more aggressive therapy is indicated. Placement of cystostomy tubes, transurethral resections, and surgical diversionary procedures have been described, but can be associated with an undesirable outcome and high complication rate (Norris *et al.* 1992; Stiffler *et al.* 2003; Liptak *et al.* 2004). Placement of metallic stents using fluoroscopic guidance through a transurethral approach can be a fast, reliable, and safe method to establish urethral patency in both male and female dogs and cats.

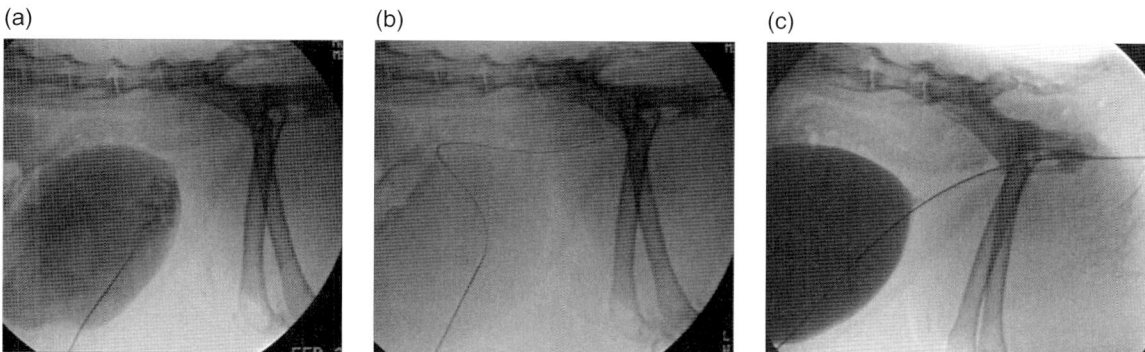

(a)　　　　　(b)　　　　　(c)

Figure 50.10 A male neutered cat with a urethral tear that occurred during catheterization. (a) An 18-gauge over-the-needle catheter is used to perform a cystocentesis, and contrast is injected through the needle to highlight the bladder and proximal urethra during fluoroscopy. (b) A 0.035 in. guidewire is aimed through the catheter, into the bladder, and out through the urethra in an antegrade manner, gaining through-and-through access. (c) An open-ended urethral catheter (5 Fr red rubber catheter) is advanced over the guidewire through the urethra into the urinary bladder and sutured in place at the prepuce.

In our practice, urethral stents have also been placed for benign diseases such as proliferative urethritis, urethral strictures, and reflex dyssynergia when standard medical intervention has failed or surgery is declined or contraindicated. We have also successfully stented cases of extraluminal urethral compression secondary to neoplasia. Urethral stents are usually self-expanding metallic stents (SEMS; Vet Stent-Urethra™, Infiniti Medical) made of laser-cut nitinol, although balloon-expandable metallic stents (Infiniti Medical) made of stainless steel or nitinol have also been used (Figure 50.11). Laser-cut urethral stents are generally not reconstrainable and are associated with minimal foreshortening, thereby allowing precise placement. These stents are placed transurethrally under fluoroscopic guidance using minimally invasive techniques (Figure 50.12).

Procedure

Urethral stent placement is performed under general anesthesia with fluoroscopic guidance. A marker catheter should be placed within a red rubber catheter that is placed within the rectum and descending colon. The prepuce or perineum should be aseptically prepared. Access with a 0.035 in. angled, floppy-tip hydrophilic guidewire is obtained in retrograde fashion in males and retrograde or antegrade fashion in females. Once the wire has been placed, a 7 Fr vascular sheath and dilator are advanced retrograde over the wire into the urinary bladder. A urine sample should be obtained for culture and sensitivity prior to instillation of contrast. The urinary bladder is distended with a 50:50 mixture of sterile saline and contrast (this should be performed through a 4 Fr angiographic catheter in males and the sheath side port in females) (Weisse & Berent 2015). A contrast study should subsequently be performed while withdrawing the catheter or sheath into the distal urethra with maximal distention of the urethra. The length of the urethral obstruction and maximal normal urethral luminal diameter are then determined via extrapolation of the colonic marker catheter. The stent is chosen such that the diameter is equal to or slightly wider than the maximal normal urethral diameter and the length is sufficient to span the obstruction without extending further than 1 cm cranially and caudally. The catheter should then be removed over the guidewire, and the stent delivery system (following flushing with sterile saline) is advanced over the guidewire and placed across the obstruction. Stent delivery is performed carefully under fluoroscopic guidance, and the delivery system is then removed over the wire. An additional contrast cystourethrogram is performed to demonstrate patency of the lower urinary tract. The catheter and sheath are then removed.

Postprocedure care

Most patients are discharged the same day as the urethral stent placement procedure, after demonstrating the ability to urinate. Broad-spectrum antibiotic therapy (7–10 days) may be considered. Pain medication is often not necessary, as the stents do not seem to cause discomfort or dysuria in canine or feline patients, though anti-inflammatory medications can be prescribed if no contraindications exist. Metallic stents remain in place once deployed and are very difficult to remove. It is rare for a tumor to grow through the interstices of the stent, but we have identified cases where the tumor grew behind or in front of the stent and an additional stent may need to be added.

Prognosis and complications

In a retrospective study reviewing urethral stent placement in 42 canine patients with obstructive urethral carcinoma, urethral stenting resulted in adequate relief of the urethral obstruction in 97.5% of dogs (Blackburn et al. 2013). Incontinence of any degree (mild or severe) occurred in 47.4% of females and 78.3% of male dogs; however, only 26.3% of females and 26.1% of males were considered to show severe, or clinically significant, incontinence by their owners (Blackburn et al. 2013). Stranguria was observed in 5.9% of females and 4.3% of males following stent placement (Blackburn et al. 2013). Length, diameter, and location of the stent were not found to be associated with incontinence or stranguria (Blackburn et al. 2013). The median survival time

(a)

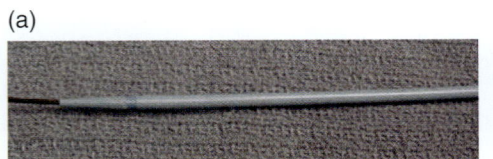

(b)

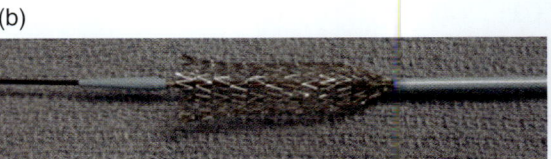

Figure 50.11 Metallic stents used for urethral obstructions. (a) A self-expanding metallic stent is compressed onto a stylette and covered with a sheath to prevent premature deployment. It is advanced over a guidewire and situated in the desired location. (b) The sheath is then deployed off the stylette and the stent opens up to its predetermined diameter and length. Once the stent is fully deployed, the stylette is removed over the wire and the stent remains in place.

(a)

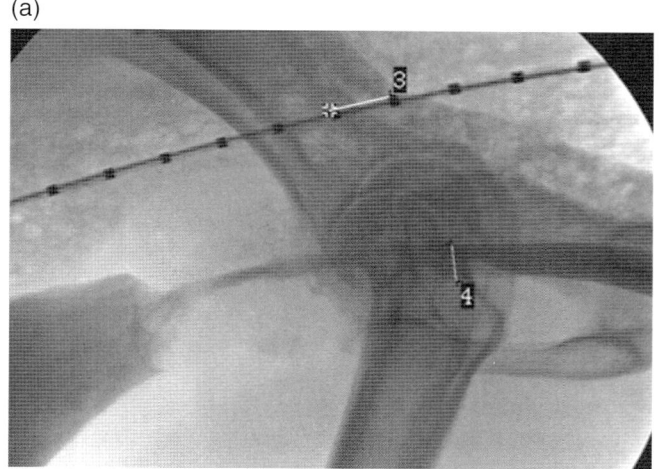

(b)

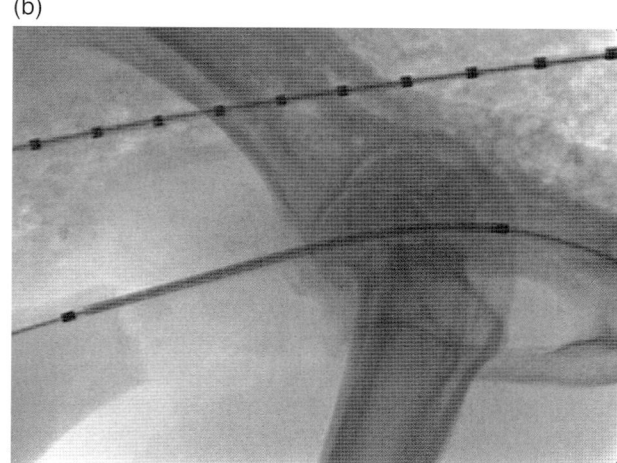

(c)

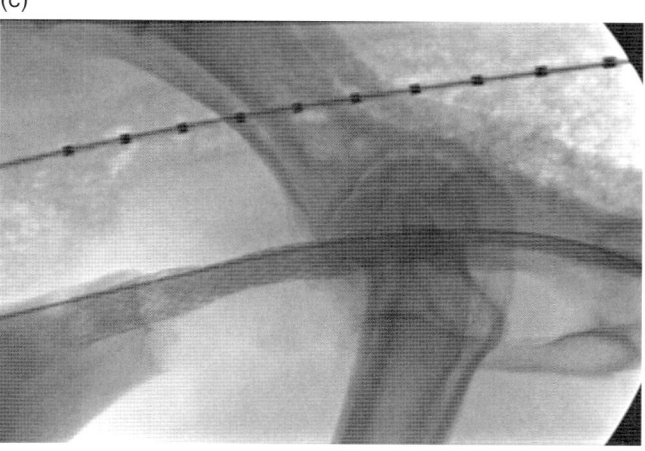

Figure 50.12 Urethral stent placement in an 8-year-old mixed-breed dog with prostatic carcinoma and a urethral obstruction. (a) A marker catheter is placed in the colon in order to adjust for magnification and measure the maximal urethral diameter and obstructive length for appropriate stent size selection. A cysto-urethrogram is performed to measure the widest diameter of the normal urethra to aid in stent sizing. (b) The self-expanding metallic stent is advanced over the guidewire into the urethra and the length of the stent is predetermined to cover approximately 5–10 mm cranial and caudal to the urethral obstruction. (c) The stent is fully deployed. A final urethrogram is performed to confirm urethral patency.

following stent placement was 78 days (Blackburn et al. 2013). The use of prestent nonsteroidal anti-inflammatory drugs and poststent chemotherapy increased the median survival to 251 days (Blackburn 2010; Blackburn et al. 2013).

The most common problem identified following placement of urethral stents is poststent incontinence, and this procedure is not recommended for owners who are not prepared to deal with mild to moderate urinary incontinence. Infection, migration, and stent fracture are rarely seen as major problems with this procedure, particularly if placement is appropriate. Identifying the junction of the bladder trigone and urethra is important to avoid excessive stent inside the urinary bladder and possible stent migration. However, one study documented reobstruction in 4/17 (23.5%) dogs and stent migration in 2/17 (11.8%) dogs following urethral stent placement for obstruction secondary to transitional cell carcinoma (McMillan et al. 2012).

Several reports of urethral stent placement in cats exist to date (Choi et al. 2009; Newman et al. 2009;

Christensen et al. 2010; Hadar et al. 2011; Brace et al. 2014). One retrospective study on 8 cats that underwent urethral stent placement for treatment of nonurolith urethral obstructions found that 4/8 (50%) cats were incontinent postprocedure (with two cats being moderately incontinent and two cats being severely incontinent) (Brace et al. 2014). Similarly to dogs, this procedure should not be recommended for feline owners that are not prepared to deal with urinary incontinence.

References

Adams, L. (2013). Nephroliths and ureteroliths: a new stone age. *New Zealand Veterinary Journal* 61 (4): 212–216.

Adams, L.G. and Senior, D.F. (1999). Electrohydraulic and extracorporeal shock-wave lithotripsy. *Veterinary Clinics of North America. Small Animal Practice* 29 (1): 293–302.

Azhar, R., Hassanain, M., Aljiffry, M. et al. (2010). Successful salvage of kidney allografts threatened by ureteral stricture using pyelovesical bypass. *American Journal of Transplantation* 10 (6): 1414–1419.

Balsa, I.M., Culp, W.T., Palm, C.A. et al. (2019). Factors associated with postobstructive diuresis following decompressive surgery with placement of ureteral stents or subcutaneous ureteral bypass systems for treatment of ureteral obstruction in cats: 37 cases (2010–2014). *Journal of the American Veterinary Medical Association* 254 (8): 944–952.

Beck, A.L., Grierson, J.M., Ogden, D.M. et al. (2007). Outcome of and complications associated with tube cystostomy in dogs and cats: 76 cases (1995–2006). *Journal of the American Veterinary Medical Association* 230 (8): 1184–1189.

Berent, A.C. (2011). Ureteral obstructions in dogs and cats: a review of traditional and new interventional diagnostic and therapeutic options. *Journal of Veterinary Emergency and Critical Care* 21 (2): 86–103.

Berent, A., Weisse, C., Bagley, D., and Casale, P. (2007). Ureteral stenting for benign and malignant disease in dogs and cats. *Veterinary Surgery* 36: E1–E29.

Berent, A., Weisse, C., and Solomon, J. (2009). The use of locking-loop pigtail nephrostomy catheters in dogs and cats. *Veterinary Surgery* 38: E23–E49.

Berent, A., Weisse, C., Letezia, C. et al. (2011a). Ureteral stenting for feline ureteral obstructions: technical and clinical outcomes: 74 ureters (2006–2011). *Journal of Veterinary Internal Medicine* 25 (6): 1052–1062.

Berent, A.C., Weisse, C., Beal, M.W. et al. (2011b). Use of indwelling, double-pigtail stents for treatment of malignant ureteral obstruction in dogs: 12 cases (2006–2009). *Journal of the American Veterinary Medical Association* 238 (8): 1017–1025.

Berent, A.C., Weisse, C.W., Todd, K.L., and Bagley, D.H. (2012). Use of locking-loop pigtail nephrostomy catheters in dogs and cats: 20 cases (2004–2009). *Journal of the American Veterinary Medical Association* 241 (3): 348–357.

Berent, A.C., Weisse, C.W., Todd, K., and Bagley, D.H. (2014). Technical and clinical outcomes of ureteral stenting in cats with benign ureteral obstruction: 69 cases (2006–2010). *Journal of the American Veterinary Medical Association* 244 (5): 559–576.

Berent, A.C., Weisse, C.W., Bagley, D.H., and Lamb, K. (2018). Use of a subcutaneous ureteral bypass device for treatment of benign ureteral obstruction in cats: 174 ureters in 134 cats (2009–2015). *Journal of the American Veterinary Medical Association* 253 (10): 1309–1327.

Blackburn, A. (2010). The use of self expanding urethral stents for the treatment of urothelial carcinoma: 42 dogs. *Journal of Veterinary Internal Medicine* 24: 1577–1583.

Blackburn, A.L., Berent, A.C., Weisse, C.W., and Brown, D.C. (2013). Evaluation of outcome following urethral stent placement for the treatment of obstructive carcinoma of the urethra in dogs: 42 cases (2004–2008). *Journal of the American Veterinary Medical Association* 242 (1): 59–68.

Block, G., Adams, L., Widmer, W., and Lingeman, J. (1996). Use of extracorporeal shock wave lithotripsy for treatment of nephrolithiasis and ureterolithiasis in five dogs. *Journal of the American Veterinary Medical Association* 208 (4): 531–536.

Borchert, C., Berent, A., and Weisse, C. (2018). Subcutaneous ureteral bypass for treatment of bilateral ureteral obstruction in a cat with retroperitoneal paraganglioma. *Journal of the American Veterinary Medical Association* 253 (9): 1169–1176.

Brace, M.A., Weisse, C., and Berent, A. (2014). Preliminary experience with stenting for management of non-urolith urethral obstruction in eight cats. *Veterinary Surgery* 43 (2): 199–208.

Bray, J.P., Doyle, R.S., and Burton, C.A. (2009). Minimally invasive inguinal approach for tube cystostomy. *Veterinary Surgery* 38 (3): 411–416.

Chik, C., Berent, A.C., Weisse, C.W., and Ryder, M. (2019). Therapeutic use of tetrasodium ethylenediaminetetraacetic acid solution for treatment of subcutaneous ureteral bypass device

mineralization in cats. *Journal of Veterinary Internal Medicine* 33 (5): 2124–2132.

Choi, R., Lee, S., and Hyun, C. (2009). Urethral stenting in a cat with refractory obstructive feline lower urinary tract disease. *Journal of Veterinary Medical Science* 71 (9): 1255–1259.

Christensen, N., Culvenor, J., and Langova, V. (2010). Fluoroscopic stent placement for the relief of malignant urethral obstruction in a cat. *Australian Veterinary Journal* 88 (12): 478–482.

Cray, M., Berent, A.C., Weisse, C.W., and Bagley, D. (2018). Treatment of pyonephrosis with a subcutaneous ureteral bypass device in four cats. *Journal of the American Veterinary Medical Association* 252 (6): 744–753.

Culp, W.T., Palm, C.A., Hsueh, C. et al. (2016). Outcome in cats with benign ureteral obstructions treated by means of ureteral stenting versus ureterotomy. *Journal of the American Veterinary Medical Association* 249 (11): 1292–1300.

Damiano, R., Oliva, A., Esposito, C. et al. (2002). Early and late complications of double pigtail ureteral stent. *Urologia Internationalis* 69 (2): 136–140.

Damiano, R., Autorino, R., De Sio, M. et al. (2005). Does the size of ureteral stent impact urinary symptoms and quality of life? A prospective randomized study. *European Urology* 48 (4): 673–678.

Damiano, R., Autorino, R., De Sio, M. et al. (2008). Effect of tamsulosin in preventing ureteral stent-related morbidity: a prospective study. *Journal of Endourology* 22 (4): 651–656.

Deroy, C., Rossetti, D., Ragetly, G. et al. (2017). Comparison between double-pigtail ureteral stents and ureteral bypass devices for treatment of ureterolithiasis in cats. *Journal of the American Veterinary Medical Association* 251 (4): 429–437.

Dirrig, H., Lamb, C., Kulendra, N., and Halfacree, Z. (2020). Diagnostic imaging observations in cats treated with the subcutaneous ureteral bypass system. *Journal of Small Animal Practice* 61 (1): 24–31.

Fages, J., Dunn, M., Specchi, S., and Pey, P. (2018). Ultrasound evaluation of the renal pelvis in cats with ureteral obstruction treated with a subcutaneous ureteral bypass: a retrospective study of 27 cases (2010–2015). *Journal of Feline Medicine and Surgery* 20 (10): 875–883.

Gallagher, A. (2018). Interventional radiology and interventional endoscopy in treatment of nephroureteral disease in the dog and cat. *Veterinary Clinics of North America. Small Animal Practice* 48 (5): 843–862.

Goldin, A.R. (1977). Percutaneous ureteral splinting. *Urology* 10 (2): 165–168.

Hadar, E.N., Morgan, M.J., and De Morgan, O. (2011). Use of a self-expanding metallic stent for the treatment of a urethral stricture in a young cat. *Journal of Feline Medicine and Surgery* 13 (8): 597–601.

Halim, A. (1999). Steinstrasse: a comparison of incidence with and without J stenting and the effect of J stenting on subsequent management. *BJU International* 84 (5): 618–621.

Heilmann, R., Pashmakova, M., Lamb, J.H. et al. (2016). Subcutaneous ureteral bypass devices as a treatment option for bilateral ureteral obstruction in a cat with ureterolithiasis. *Tierärztliche Praxis. Ausgabe K, Kleintiere/Heimtiere* 44 (3): 180–188.

Holmes, E.S., Weisse, C., and Berent, A.C. (2012). Use of fluoroscopically guided percutaneous antegrade urethral catheterization for the treatment of urethral obstruction in male cats: 9 cases (2000–2009). *Journal of the American Veterinary Medical Association* 241 (5): 603–607.

Horowitz, C., Berent, A., Weisse, C. et al. (2013). Predictors of outcome for cats with ureteral obstructions after interventional management using ureteral stents or a subcutaneous ureteral bypass device. *Journal of Feline Medicine and Surgery* 15 (12): 1052–1062.

Hubert, K.C. and Palmer, J.S. (2005). Passive dilation by ureteral stenting before ureteroscopy: eliminating the need for active dilation. *The Journal of Urology* 174 (3): 1079–1080.

Hunt, G.B., Culp, W.T., Epstein, S. et al. (2013). Complications of Stamey percutaneous loop cystostomy catheters in three cats. *Journal of Feline Medicine and Surgery* 15 (6): 503–506.

Johnson, C.M., Culp, W.T., Palm, C.A., and Zacuto, A.C. (2015). Subcutaneous ureteral bypass device for treatment of iatrogenic ureteral ligation in a kitten. *Journal of the American Veterinary Medical Association* 247 (8): 924–931.

Jurczok, A., Loertzer, H., Wagner, S., and Fornara, P. (2005). Subcutaneous nephrovesical and nephrocutaneous bypass. *Gynecologic and Obstetric Investigation* 59 (3): 144–148.

Knapp, D.W., Glickman, N.W., DeNicola, D.B. et al. (2000). Naturally-occurring canine transitional cell carcinoma of the urinary bladder A relevant model of human invasive bladder cancer. *Urologic Oncology: Seminars and Original Investigations* 5 (2): 47–59.

Kochin, E., Gregory, C., Wisner, E. et al. (1993). Evaluation of a method of ureteroneocystostomy in cats. *Journal of the American Veterinary Medical Association* 202 (2): 257–260.

Kopecny, L., Palm, C.A., Drobatz, K.J. et al. (2019). Risk factors for positive urine cultures in cats with subcutaneous ureteral bypass and ureteral stents (2010-2016). *Journal of Veterinary Internal Medicine* 33 (1): 178–183.

Kulendra, E., Kulendra, N., and Halfacree, Z. (2014a). Management of bilateral ureteral trauma using ureteral stents and subsequent subcutaneous ureteral bypass devices in a cat. *Journal of Feline Medicine and Surgery* 16 (6): 536–540.

Kulendra, N.J., Syme, H., Benigni, L., and Halfacree, Z. (2014b). Feline double pigtail ureteric stents for management of ureteric obstruction: short-and long-term follow-up of 26 cats. *Journal of Feline Medicine and Surgery* 16 (12): 985–991.

Kuntz, J.A., Berent, A.C., Weisse, C.W., and Bagley, D.H. (2015). Double pigtail ureteral stenting and renal pelvic lavage for renal-sparing treatment of obstructive pyonephrosis in dogs: 13 cases (2008–2012). *Journal of the American Veterinary Medical Association* 246 (2): 216–225.

Kyles, A.E., Hardie, E.M., Wooden, B.G. et al. (2005). Management and outcome of cats with ureteral calculi: 153 cases (1984–2002). *Journal of the American Veterinary Medical Association* 226 (6): 937–944.

Lam, N.K., Berent, A.C., Weisse, C.W. et al. (2012). Endoscopic placement of ureteral stents for treatment of congenital bilateral ureteral stenosis in a dog. *Journal of the American Veterinary Medical Association* 240 (8): 983–990.

Lennon, G.M., Thornhill, J.A., Grainger, R. et al. (1997). Double pigtail ureteric stent versus percutaneous nephrostomy: effects on stone transit and ureteric motility. *European Urology* 31: 24–29.

Lipscomb, V.J. (2018). Bladder. In: *Veterinary Surgery: Small Animal*, vol. 2 (ed. S. Johnston and K. Tobias), 2219–2233. St. Louis, MO: Elsevier.

Liptak, J.M., Brutscher, S.P., Monnet, E. et al. (2004). Transurethral resection in the management of urethral and prostatic neoplasia in 6 dogs. *Veterinary Surgery* 33 (5): 505–516.

Livet, V., Pillard, P., Goy-Thollot, I. et al. (2017). Placement of subcutaneous ureteral bypasses without fluoroscopic guidance in cats with ureteral obstruction: 19 cases (2014–2016). *Journal of Feline Medicine and Surgery* 19 (10): 1030–1039.

Lorange, M. and Monnet, E. (2020). Postoperative outcomes of 12 cats with ureteral obstruction treated with ureteroneocystostomy. *Veterinary Surgery* 49 (7): 1418–1427.

Luca, G.C., Monteiro, B.P., Dunn, M., and Steagall, P.V. (2017). A retrospective study of anesthesia for subcutaneous ureteral bypass placement in cats: 27 cases. *Journal of Veterinary Medical Science* 79 (6): 992–998.

Lulich, J.P., Adams, L.G., Grant, D., and Osborne, C.A. (2009). Changing paradigms in the treatment of uroliths by lithotripsy. *Veterinary Clinics of North America. Small Animal Practice* 39 (1): 143–160.

Lulich, J.P., Berent, A., Adams, L. et al. (2016). ACVIM small animal consensus recommendations on the treatment and prevention of uroliths in dogs and cats. *Journal of Veterinary Internal Medicine* 30 (5): 1564–1574.

Manassero, M., Decambron, A., Viateau, V. et al. (2014). Indwelling double pigtail ureteral stent combined or not with surgery for feline ureterolithiasis: complications and outcome in 15 cases. *Journal of Feline Medicine and Surgery* 16 (8): 623–630.

McMillan, S.K., Knapp, D.W., Ramos-Vara, J.A. et al. (2012). Outcome of urethral stent placement for management of urethral obstruction secondary to transitional cell carcinoma in dogs: 19 cases (2007–2010). *Journal of the American Veterinary Medical Association* 241 (12): 1627–1632.

Meige, F., Sarrau, S., and Autefage, A. (2008). Management of traumatic urethral rupture in 11 cats using primary alignment with a urethral catheter. *Veterinary and Comparative Orthopaedics and Traumatology* 21 (1): 76–84.

Mincheff, T.V. (2007). Early dislodgement of percutaneous and endoscopic gastrostomy tube. *Journal of the South Carolina Medical Association (1975)* 103 (1): 13–15.

Mustafa, M. (2007). The role of stenting in relieving loin pain following ureteroscopic stone therapy for persisting renal colic with hydronephrosis. *International Urology and Nephrology* 39 (1): 91–94.

Newman, R.G., Mehler, S.J., Kitchell, B.E., and Beal, M.W. (2009). Use of a balloon-expandable metallic stent to relieve malignant urethral obstruction in a cat. *Journal of the American Veterinary Medical Association* 234 (2): 236–239.

Nicoli, S., Morello, E., Martano, M. et al. (2012). Double-J ureteral stenting in nine cats with ureteral obstruction. *Veterinary Journal* 194 (1): 60–65.

Norris, A.M., Laing, E.J., Valli, V.E. et al. (1992). Canine bladder and urethral tumors: a retrospective study of 115 cases (1980–1985). *Journal of Veterinary Internal Medicine* 6 (3): 145–153.

Palm, C.A. and Culp, W.T. (2016). Nephroureteral obstructions: the use of stents and ureteral bypass systems for renal decompression. *Veterinary Clinics of North America. Small Animal Practice* 46 (6): 1183–1192.

Pavia, P.R., Berent, A.C., Weisse, C.W. et al. (2018). Outcome of ureteral stent placement for treatment of benign ureteral obstruction in dogs: 44 cases (2010–2013). *Journal of the American Veterinary Medical Association* 252 (6): 721–731.

Roberts, S.F., Aronson, L.R., and Brown, D.C. (2011). Postoperative mortality in cats after ureterolithotomy. *Veterinary Surgery* 40 (4): 438–443.

Rossanese, M. and Murgia, D. (2015). Management of paraureteral pseudocyst and ureteral avulsion using a subcutaneous ureteral bypass (SUB) system in a cat. *Veterinary Record Case Reports* 3 (1): e000173.

Schmidbauer, J., Kratzik, C., Klingler, H.C. et al. (2006). Nephrovesical subcutaneous ureteric bypass: long-term results in patients with advanced metastatic disease-improvement of renal function and quality of life. *European Urology* 50 (5): 1073–1078; discussion 1078.

Smith, J.D., Stone, E.A., and Gilson, S.D. (1995). Placement of a permanent cystostomy catheter to relieve urine outflow obstruction in dogs with transitional cell carcinoma. *Journal of the American Veterinary Medical Association* 206 (4): 496–499.

Snyder, D., Steffey, M.A., Mehler, S. et al. (2005). Diagnosis and surgical management of ureteral calculi in dogs: 16 cases (1990–2003). *New Zealand Veterinary Journal* 53 (1): 19–25.

Steinhaus, J., Berent, A., Weisse, C. et al. (2015). Clinical presentation and outcome of cats with circumcaval ureters associated with a ureteral obstruction. *Journal of Veterinary Internal Medicine* 29 (1): 63–70.

Stiffler, K.S., Stevenson, M.M., Cornell, K.K. et al. (2003). Clinical use of low-profile cystostomy tubes in four dogs and a cat. *Journal of the American Veterinary Medical Association* 223 (3): 325–329.

Uthappa, M.C. and Cowan, N.C. (2005). Retrograde or antegrade double-pigtail stent placement for malignant ureteric obstruction? *Clinical Radiology* 60 (5): 608–612.

Weisse, C. and Berent, A. (2015). *Veterinary Image-Guided Interventions*. Chichester: Wiley.

Weisse, C., Berent, A., Todd, K. et al. (2006). Evaluation of palliative stenting for management of malignant urethral obstructions in dogs. *Journal of the American Veterinary Medical Association* 229 (2): 226–234.

Wormser, C., Clarke, D.L., and Aronson, L.R. (2015). End-to-end ureteral anastomosis and double-pigtail ureteral stent placement for treatment of iatrogenic ureteral trauma in two dogs. *Journal of the American Veterinary Medical Association* 247 (1): 92–97.

Wormser, C., Clarke, D.L., and Aronson, L.R. (2016). Outcomes of ureteral surgery and ureteral stenting in cats: 117 cases (2006–2014). *Journal of the American Veterinary Medical Association* 248 (5): 518–525.

Yossepowitch, O., Lifshitz, D.A., Dekel, Y. et al. (2001). Predicting the success of retrograde stenting for managing ureteral obstruction. *Journal of Urology* 166 (5): 1746–1749.

Zaid, M.S., Berent, A.C., Weisse, C., and Caceres, A. (2011). Feline ureteral strictures: 10 cases (2007–2009). *Journal of Veterinary Internal Medicine* 25 (2): 222–229.

Zhang, J.-T. Wang, H.-B., Shi, J. et al. (2010). Laparoscopy for percutaneous tube cystostomy in dogs. *Journal of the American Veterinary Medical Association* 236 (9): 975–977.

Zimskind, P.D., Fetter, T.R., and Wilkerson, J.L. (1967). Clinical use of long-term indwelling silicone rubber ureteral splints inserted cystoscopically. *Journal of Urology* 97 (5): 840–844.

51

Idiopathic or Benign Essential Renal Hematuria

Allyson Berent and Chick Weisse

Idiopathic renal hematuria (IRH), or benign essential renal hematuria, is a rare condition of chronic severe unilateral, or less commonly bilateral, renal bleeding. This condition typically results in port wine–colored urine that is not associated with trauma, urolithiasis, neoplasia, or other obvious causes. In humans, it is defined as acute, intermittent, or chronic gross hematuria for which radiologic and hematologic evaluation reveals no source (Bagley & Allen 1990; Tawfiek & Bagley 1998). Other names given to this condition include lateralizing essential hematuria, chronic unilateral hematuria, upper tract hematuria, and benign lateralizing hematuria (Dooley & Pietrow 2004). Although it has been described in the human literature for decades, it is considered a rare condition (Hagen 1963; Copley & Hasbargen 1987; Tawfiek & Bagley 1998; Dooley & Pietrow 2004). The first report in humans was by Wallach et al. (1959), in which a small hemangioma of the kidney causing severe hematuria was described. In veterinary medicine, there have been few cases sporadically reported in the literature. The earliest reports of the condition were in the early 1980s, when Meyer and Senior (1983) described "benign renal bleeding" and Stone et al. (1983) described four dogs with massive hematuria of nontraumatic renal origin.

The anatomic source of hematuria can be broadly divided into conditions arising from either the upper or lower urinary tract. Lower urinary tract disorders causing hematuria are more easily diagnosed with the advent of contemporary imaging such as ultrasound, fluoroscopy, and cystourethroscopy. Causes include bladder or urethral neoplasia (transitional cell carcinoma, prostatic carcinoma), urinary tract infections, urolithiasis,

genitourinary foreign bodies, recent cystocentesis, prostatitis, and vaginitis (Kaufman et al. 1994). These problems are most commonly associated with dysuria, pollakiuria, and potentially genitourinary discharge. Additionally, we have recently seen a case of an intravesicular vascular anomaly causing severe hematuria, without associated dysuria. Upper urinary tract disorders include nephroureterolithiasis, renal or ureteral neoplasia, polycystic kidney disease, telangiectasia (reported in the Pembroke Welsh corgi; Moore & Thornton 1983), glomerulonephritis, pyelonephritis, renal vascular anomalies, and IRH (Stone et al. 1983; Holt et al. 1987; Kaufman et al. 1994). In contrast to humans, massive hematuria from glomerulonephritis is considered very rare in the dog.

In humans, renal vascular abnormalities that rupture, including hemangiomas and abnormal papillary lesions (papillary angiomas) as well as minute venous ruptures, are typically the cause of benign essential renal hematuria (Copley & Hasbargen 1987). Although the long-term course appears to be benign, frequent bouts of hematuria can lead to anemia, ureteral colic during passage of clots, and ureteral/urethral obstructions. In addition, persistent hematuria is distressing to owners. In humans, cystoscopy for evaluation of the ureterovesicular orifice is the diagnostic method of choice. Traditional treatment was unilateral nephrectomy, but this has since changed as nephron preservation is considered necessary. With the advent of contemporary imaging and small ureteroscopes, endourologic treatment via ureteroscopy and electrocautery or laser ablation is now considered the diagnostic and therapeutic choice in human medicine. In 80% of cases, ureteronephroscopy is successful in

Small Animal Soft Tissue Surgery, Second Edition. Edited by Eric Monnet.
© 2023 John Wiley & Sons, Inc. Published 2023 by John Wiley & Sons, Inc.
Companion website: www.wiley.com/go/monnet/small

identifying the lesion in the renal pelvis. Once that is identified, endoscopic-guided therapy is effective in over 90% of patients when a lesion is found (Bagley & Allen 1990; Tawfiek & Bagley 1998; Dooley & Pietrow 2004; Brito *et al.* 2009).

In the veterinary literature this condition is rarely reported. Affected dogs range in age from 2 months to 11 years (Stone *et al.* 1983; Holt *et al.* 1987; Kaufman *et al.* 1994; Mishina *et al.* 1997; Hawthorne *et al.* 1998). Typically this is considered a condition of young dogs, with a majority of the dogs reported under 2 years of age. There does not seem to be a sex predilection. Historically, cases in the veterinary literature were diagnosed before the widespread introduction of cystoscopy, so a diagnosis was made based on normal hematology, serum biochemistry, coagulation profiles, radiography, intravenous pyelography, and exploratory surgery via cystotomy and ureterovesicular junction (UVJ) catheterization. In later reports, ultrasound was performed and showed no lesions (Kaufman *et al.* 1994; Hawthorne *et al.* 1998). Hydronephrosis and hydroureter have also been reported in nearly half of the cases, and this is suspected to be due to the accumulation of blood clots resulting in partial or complete ureteral obstruction (Stone *et al.* 1983; Holt *et al.* 1987). Left-sided lesions appear to be more common (approximately 75%); however, with few cases reported this is hard to discern (Stone *et al.* 1983; Holt *et al.* 1987; Mishina *et al.* 1997; Hawthorne *et al.* 1998). The condition has been reported to occur bilaterally as well (21% of patients) (Stone *et al.* 1983; Holt *et al.* 1987; Kaufman *et al.* 1994; Hawthorne *et al.* 1998). We have identified this condition in an additional 4 cats (2 unilateral and 2 bilateral) and 10 dogs (9 unilateral and 1 bilateral). Nearly two-thirds of these cases that were unilateral were also left-sided. Diagnosis and treatment recommendations are discussed in this chapter. Some novel therapies in veterinary medicine are also considered.

Diagnosis

Diagnosis of IRH has traditionally been one of exclusion in veterinary patients. Dogs or cats can present with chronic, acute, or intermittent severe hematuria. This is sometimes associated with signs of urinary tract disease including dysuria, stranguria, pollakiuria, and pyuria. In rare cases, the severe bleeding can result in blood clot accumulation in the bladder and urethra, resulting in urethral obstruction and dysuria (Hawthorne *et al.* 1998). Although uncommonly identified, a patient with lower urinary tract signs should not have IRH excluded as a possibility. The color of the urine is typically extremely dark ("port wine"). This can

be worse during certain times of the day, and may also be intermittent in nature. Rarely, if a patient is severely anemic, lethargy and exercise intolerance, or syncope, can be seen. There does not seem to be a sex predilection, and most animals will be young in age (from a few weeks to a few years). The oldest reported dog was 11 years (Holt *et al.* 1987). Large-breed dogs have been overrepresented in the literature; however, small-breed dogs and cats have also been diagnosed with the condition. Physical examination in both dogs and cats is typically unremarkable.

Clinicopathologic findings on complete blood count will often reveal a highly regenerative anemia due to blood loss; with chronicity, iron deficiency can ensue and a microcytosis may be documented. Typically, the platelet count is normal but a mild consumptive thrombocytopenia may be seen. On the serum biochemical profile, blood urea nitrogen and creatinine levels are typically normal. Routine urinalysis should be performed, and may be difficult to interpret due to the severe hematuria, making dipstick analysis inaccurate. With the severe degree of hematuria typically seen, evaluation for proteinuria is not diagnostic, as it would be expected to be excessively elevated due to the presence of plasma proteins from the blood in the urine. A urinalysis should also be interpreted during periods when the hematuria has resolved. Typically, the urine specific gravity is normal. A sterile urine sample should always be obtained for culture and sensitivity. A coagulation profile is recommended prior to cystocentesis in an animal with severe hematuria. The urine culture is often negative, and the coagulation profile, including activated partial thromboplastin time (aPTT) and prothrombin time (PT), is typically normal. Von Willebrand factor antigen testing is recommended in all patients, and is also often normal. A platelet function test is recommended when possible, and a buccal mucosal bleeding time should be considered when a platelet function test is not possible. If all these findings are normal, urinary tract imaging is recommended.

It is recommended that abdominal ultrasound should be performed as the first imaging test, which can evaluate for various causes of upper and lower urinary tract bleeding including urolithiasis, neoplasia, and polycystic kidneys. Typically, ultrasonographic findings for IRH are normal, though hydronephrosis and/or hydroureter can be seen secondary to a blood clot(s) or dried solidified blood stones. In our experience, this is a common finding in feline patients with IRH. The inciting lesion is not usually visualized on renal or ureteral ultrasound. Abdominal radiography is also recommended to look for any signs of urolithiasis that can be missed on routine abdominal ultrasound. Evaluation of the entire urinary tract is essential (including the pelvic and penile urethra) to look for urinary stones. Traditionally, an intravenous pyelogram has been recommended; however, we feel that with the newer advanced imaging this is rarely considered helpful. Ideally, computed tomographic angiography (CTA) and/or magnetic resonance angiography (MRA) can be performed to assess the kidney or renal pelvis for subtle vascular lesions, including arteriovenous malformations and aneurysms. While these tests uncommonly reveal abnormal findings, they can be helpful in planning for embolization procedures should they be required in the future. Additionally, these techniques allow the clinician to map out the vasculature to determine options for endovascular treatment.

The next recommended diagnostic test of choice is cystourethroscopy. This technique allows visualization of the entire urethra, prostatic ductules, and vagina. Careful attention should be paid to the UVJ. Because of the typical presence of severe hematuria, it is often necessary to immediately drain the urine from the urinary bladder and then fill with clear sterile saline. For clear identification of the UVJ, a rigid scope (in female dogs) is recommended and should be angled so that the 30° lens is facing the ureteral openings. We typically perform cystoscopy with the patient in dorsal recumbency, and the endoscope is turned so that the angle is down toward the ureters in a dorsal position. Once the UVJ is identified, each ureter should be observed for a few minutes to see at least 2–5 jets of urine from the opening. The bleeding side will typically show a red stream of urine (Figure 51.1). Since it is possible to have bilateral bleeding, careful attention to both orifices is necessary. Additionally, in some canine patients, intermittent bleeding may stop with high fluid flow pressures and so turning off the fluid infusion may be necessary to identify bleeding. If cystoscopy is not an option, than a cystotomy can be performed and each UVJ evaluated carefully for the presence of bleeding. If the side of bleeding cannot be determined, an attempt should be

made to catheterize each UVJ with a soft catheter (in the dog, either a 20-gauge intravenous catheter, 3.5 Fr red rubber catheter, or 4 Fr open-ended ureteral catheter; in the cat, a 25-gauge intravenous catheter ~0.6 mm diameter). Care should be taken when catheterizing the UVJ, particularly in cats, as this process can induce bleeding and edema that can result in temporary ureteral obstruction and misdiagnosis of renal hematuria. The diameter of the feline ureter is 0.4 mm so, if possible, catheterization of the feline UVJ should be avoided and cystoscopy for diagnosis performed in its place.

In patients that have concurrent hydroureter/hydronephrosis secondary to a blood clot, it is important to evaluate both ureters, as the bleeding can still be seen bilaterally. Once the side of the bleeding is documented, various treatment options can be considered. If no bleeding is identified from the UVJ, then careful examination of the entire bladder mucosal surface should be performed to look for a vascular defect or other cause as the source of bleeding. Additionally, if no bleeding is identified, the patient should be evaluated for the presence of a blood clot isolated to the upper urinary tract.

Treatment options

Previously, once a diagnosis of IRH was made based on cystoscopy or ureteral catheterization, aureteronephrectomy was recommended as the treatment of choice. This philosophy has changed over the past few decades in human medicine, and the past few years in veterinary medicine. With the concern that the bleeding is often bilateral, or that the bleeding can become bilateral over time, as well as knowing that the lesion is typically found in the renal pelvis rather than the kidney itself, preservation of renal parenchyma is considered ideal and appropriate. If the bleeding is excessive resulting in life-threatening anemia, then ureteronephrectomy may be the treatment of choice.

Medical treatment

During episodes of severe bleeding, blood transfusions and chronic iron supplementation can be necessary. If a patient receives a packed red blood cell transfusion, there is a significant amount of iron in each unit of blood and supplementation can start approximately one month later. Iron can be given either orally or intramuscularly as ferrous sulfate (10 mg/kg daily) or iron dextrans (10 mg/kg/month in the dog; 50 mg/month in the cat). It is important that iron dextrans are not given intravenously as this could result in severe anaphylaxis.

There have been reports of the use of aminocaproic acid to treat IRH in humans (150 mg/kg divided in four doses per day) (Stefanini *et al.* 1990). There are no

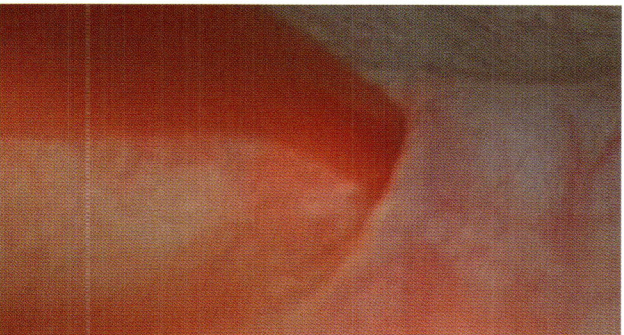

Figure 51.1 Endoscopic image of blood streaming from the left ureteral orifice.

known reports of the use of aminocaproic acid in veterinary medicine. Aminocaproic acid is a derivative and analog of the amino acid lysine, an inhibitor of proteolytic enzymes such as plasmin, which is responsible for fibrinolysis, potentially making this effective in the treatment of bleeding disorders. Side effects that have been reported include gastrointestinal upset, fever, liver disease, and thrombosis.

Minimally invasive surgery

Retrograde ureteronephroscopy and endoscopic coagulation

Retrograde ureteronephroscopy and endoscopic coagulation is the standard for therapy in humans with IRH. This is effective in over 90% of patients when a lesion is identified (Kavoussi *et al.* 1989; Bagley & Allen 1990). Additionally, a phenomenon in humans has been reported where patients in whom no abnormality is found endoscopically will often stop bleeding after the procedure (Bagley & Allen 1990; Tawfiek & Bagley 1998). This is postulated to be due to the increased intraluminal renal pelvic pressure associated with the ureteroscopy and irrigation procedure, resulting in back pressure and inflammation and ultimately in the cessation of bleeding. In about 80% of patients, a lesion can be found in the renal pelvis or renal calyx (Bagley & Allen 1990; Tawfiek & Bagley 1998).

Typically in humans, if a lesion is found and treated, it is expected that the bleeding will stop. In one report, recurrence occurred in approximately 12% of patients a median of 7 months following the procedure (Kavoussi *et al.* 1989). In humans, multiple bleeding lesions or hemangiomas are rarely documented endoscopically, and these are more likely to recur over time. When multiple hemangiomas are identified, the instillation into the renal collection system of topical silver nitrate for chemical cauterization to allow diffuse coagulation to occur has been advocated in certain practices (Bahnson 1987). This is discussed in more detail later.

In veterinary medicine, retrograde ureteronephroscopy for IRH has been performed. This technique is reserved for patients large enough to accept the flexible ureteroscope, which is approximately 8 Fr in diameter. Dogs larger than approximately 18–20 kg can often be accommodated. We have been successful in some smaller dogs with this scope, but it can be challenging. To perform the technique, the patient is placed in dorsal recumbency and a routine cystoscopy is performed. Each ureteral orifice is identified and the side that is bleeding is confirmed. Using both fluoroscopic and endoscopic guidance, an angle-tipped, hydrophilic, 0.9 mm (0.035 in.) guidewire is advanced up the ureter

from the UVJ. It is advanced minimally and followed by a 5 Fr open-ended ureteral catheter. This is guided using fluoroscopy. Once the wire and catheter are in the lumen of the distal ureter, the wire is removed and a retrograde ureteropyelogram is performed using a 1 : 1 mixture of sterile 0.9% saline and iohexol contrast medium (Figure 51.2a). Once the renal pelvis and ureter are highlighted, careful examination for a lesion, mass, or filling defect is recommended. This study is typically normal in patients with IRH. The guidewire is then replaced through the ureteral catheter and advanced up the ureter, without entering the renal pelvis (Figure 51.2b). Care should be taken to avoid irritating the renal pelvis with the tip of the wire, as iatrogenic trauma could mimic a lesion. The cystoscope and catheter are then removed over the guidewire, being careful not to lose guidewire access, and a dual-lumen catheter is carefully advanced over the wire. Typically, a 10 Fr catheter is used. Once this catheter is in the distal ureter, a second guidewire is advanced up this catheter into the ureter, and the catheter is then removed. Alternatively, a dilator is advanced over the wire in order to dilate the ureter sufficiently to accommodate the ureteroscope (Figure 51.2c). The flexible ureteroscope is then advanced over the first guidewire, while the second remains in place as a "safety wire" when diameter permits. The ureteroscope is advanced up the ureter to the renal pelvis with care to avoid ureteral trauma (Figure 51.2d). Very gentle manual irrigation is initiated through the ureteroscope so that the entire ureteral lumen can be visualized. Once in the renal pelvis, careful examination with gentle irrigation of the renal pelvis and each calyx is performed, looking for a potential lesion (Figure 51.2e). When a lesion is identified, irrigation is switched from sterile 0.9% saline to 5% dextrose solution and all the saline is removed via manual suction through the ureteroscope. A 5% dextrose solution is required so that appropriate coagulation can be performed using Bugbee electrocautery via a flexible electrode fiber (Bagley & Allen 1990; Tawfiek & Bagley 1998). Saline will not allow conduction for the electrocautery. The 2–3 Fr electrode fiber is advanced through the working channel of the scope and directed onto the lesion. Settings should begin at approximately 15 W, and can be carefully increased to 20–25 W if necessary. The probe should be directed by the ureteroscope to carefully cauterize the periphery of the lesion and move inward to ablate the entire defect (Figure 51.2f).

Other options for ablation include the holmium:YAG laser (laser lithotriptor) or the Nd:YAG laser (Bagley & Allen 1990; Tawfiek & Bagley 1998; Mugiya *et al.* 2007). For these lasers it is very important to "defocus" the beam so that the fiber is not in direct contact with the

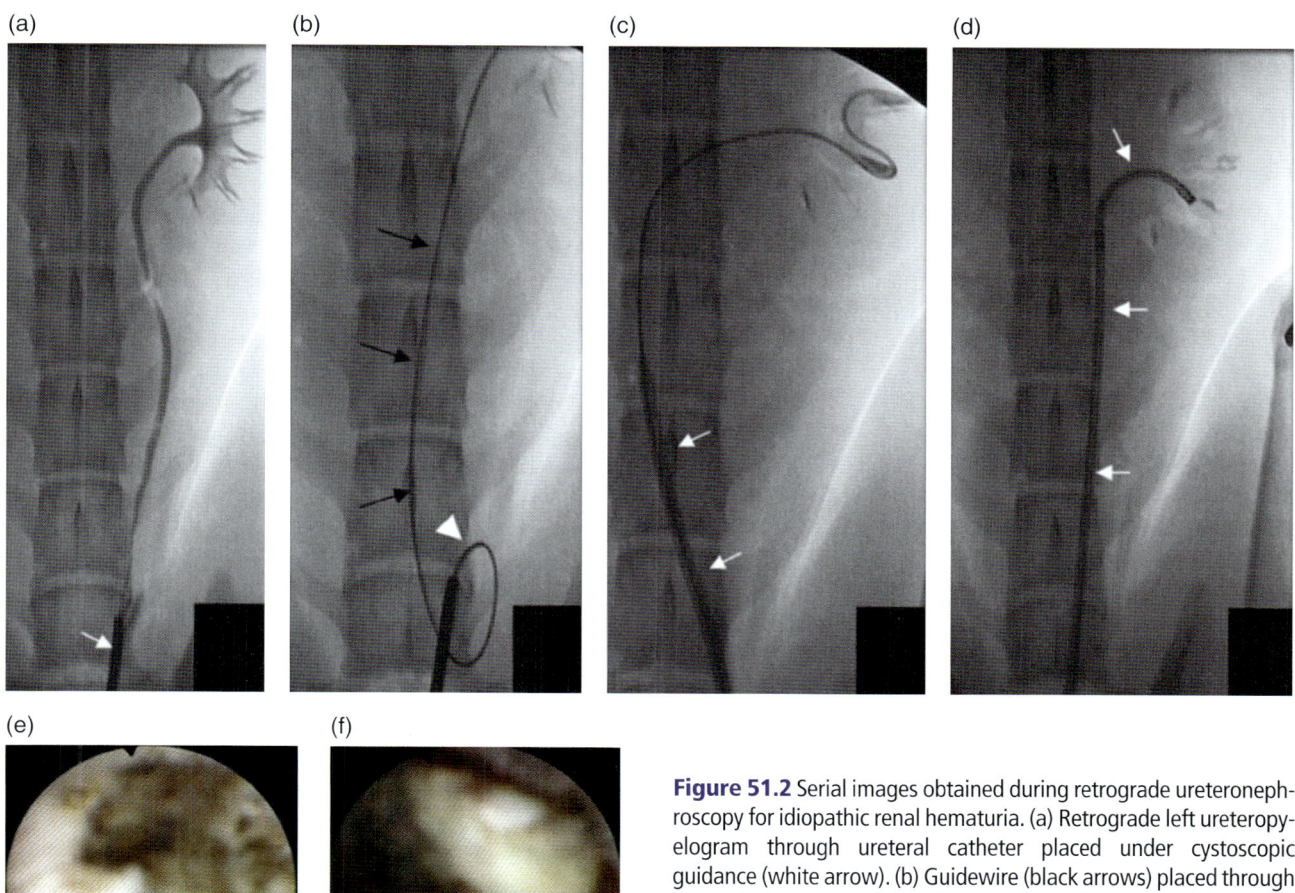

Figure 51.2 Serial images obtained during retrograde ureteronephroscopy for idiopathic renal hematuria. (a) Retrograde left ureteropyelogram through ureteral catheter placed under cystoscopic guidance (white arrow). (b) Guidewire (black arrows) placed through ureteral catheter (arrowhead) and advanced up ureter. (c) Ureteral dilator (white arrows) advanced over guidewire to dilate ureter prior to ureteroscopy. (d) Ureteroscope (white arrows) advanced into renal pelvis. (e) Nephroscopy demonstrating renal pelvis lesion. (f) Nephroscopy and cautery probe (blue) prior to ablation of lesion.

tissue, as it will cut into the renal pelvic mucosa and penetrate into the parenchyma, causing more bleeding. A diode laser is typically not recommended as it is too large in diameter to be easily used through the flexible ureteroscope working channel. In addition, the excessive diameter and stiffness of a diode laser fiber do not allow adequate irrigation and deflection. For ablation with the YAG or diode lasers, 0.9% saline irrigation is typically used. A 5% dextrose solution should not be used for diagnostic nephroscopy, as it will result in red blood cell lysis and obscure the image. It should only be used if electrocautery is the coagulation device chosen during the cautery. Typically, once coagulation is complete, the ureteroscope is removed and the safety wire is advanced into the renal pelvis for placement of an indwelling double-pigtail ureteral stent. The stent will prevent the ureter from becoming obstructed due to procedural-induced edema. The stent can be removed 1–2 weeks after the procedure with simple cystoscopic retrieval.

Transrenalnephroscopy

Another endoscopic option that has been described in a small number of human patients (Gittes & Varady 1981) is transrenalnephroscopy to identify a lesion for cauterization. This technique would be very difficult and unsafe in a canine or feline patient without concurrent hydronephrosis. Traumatic hemorrhage would likely occur during nephrostomy access, obscuring any small lesion from being found.

Sclerotherapy with silver nitrate

Sclerotherapy using silver nitrate irrigation as a coagulating/chemical cauterization agent has been reported for patients diagnosed with IRH (Diamond *et al.* 1981; Bahnson 1987). As already described, once the UVJ is identified via cystoscopy and the bleeding is confirmed at the UVJ, a guidewire and ureteral catheter are advanced up the ureter using endoscopic and fluoroscopic guidance.

Once the catheter is at the ureteropelvic junction, contrast is injected to determine the filling volume of the renal pelvis. Silver nitrate solution (0.25–1.0% solution sterilized) mixed with sterile water or 5% dextrose solution and contrast material is then infused into the renal pelvis based on the predetermined filling volume of the renal pelvis. The solution is left indwelling for 5 minutes and then removed. This technique resulted in the control and resolution of hematuria in four human patients (Diamond *et al.* 1981). If bleeding continues following treatment, repeat infusion has been recommended (Diamond *et al.* 1981).

Sclerotherapy using either silver nitrate or povidone-iodine infusions has also been used successfully in humans to treat another condition known as chyluria (Goel *et al.* 2004; Nandy *et al.* 2004; Sharma *et al.* 2008). In combination these medications may work synergistically, but their use has not been reported in veterinary medicine. Iodine is considered a corrosive agent due to its oxidizing potential and povidone is a thickening and granulating agent. Silver nitrate and povidone-iodine may have chemocauterization effects, resulting in the cessation of bleeding and antisepsis (Kumar *et al.* 2006). In humans, complications identified with silver nitrate include necrotizing ureteritis, bladder wall fibrosis, and hepatic dysfunction (Su *et al.* 2004; Rastinehad *et al.* 2008). There are very few reports on complications with ureteral infusions using povidone-iodine. We have investigated the use of both silver nitrate and povidone-iodine for chemical cauterization

in veterinary patients with IRH, but consider this treatment experimental at present.

Infusion of silver nitrate or povidone-iodine can also be performed in conjunction with a cystotomy and ureteral catheterization to the level of the ureteropelvic junction. This should always be done under fluoroscopic guidance, but is not currently recommended as little is yet known about the effect this will have in veterinary patients. Care should be taken to avoid the silver nitrate from diffusing into the urinary bladder, as bladder fibrosis has been reported in people (Rastinehad *et al.* 2008).

Interventional radiology

A final option that may be considered is selective renal arterial embolization of the branch of the renal artery that is contributing to the bleeding lesion. This has been done in few veterinary patients to date. It is a similar procedure to that described by Mishina *et al.* (1997), but done via angiography in conjunction with cystoscopy. A routine cystoscopy is performed and the side of bleeding is identified and monitored. Using either femoral or carotid arterial access, an angiogram is performed of the distal aorta, documenting the renal arterial anatomy of the affected side (Figure 51.3). Using digital subtraction angiography, each ramus of the ipsilateral renal artery is selectively catheterized. Once the six main branches of the renal arteries are identified (three dorsal and three ventral), catheterization and temporary occlusion of each are attempted. This could be done using an occlusion balloon catheter or an angiographic catheter that is

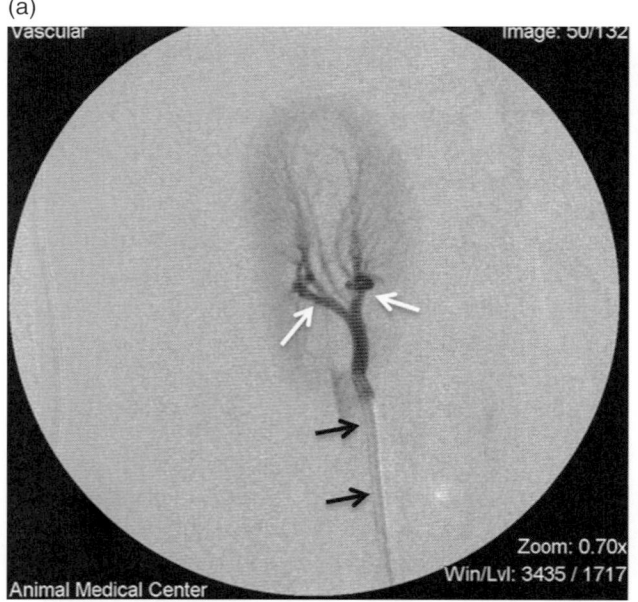
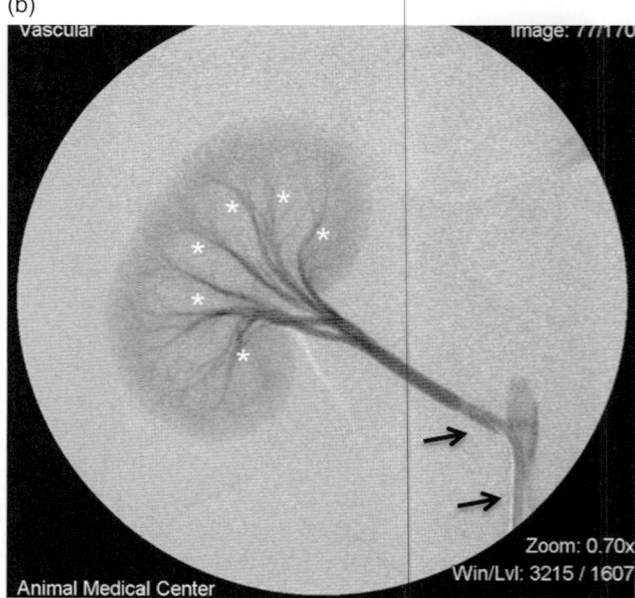

Figure 51.3 Renal angiogram of a dog. (a) The dorsal and ventral distributions of the renal artery (white arrows) are identified. (b) The distribution of the renal artery is also documented on the longitudinal axis of the kidney.

large enough to occlude blood flow. During vascular occlusion, the endoscopist monitors the UVJ for the cessation of bleeding. Once bleeding has stopped, a coil is placed into the appropriate branch of the renal artery through the angiographic catheter and an angiogram performed to confirm embolization. The cystoscope remains in place as the UVJ is monitored further to insure no bleeding recurs once the angiographic catheter is removed. This procedure would ultimately result in only a one-sixth loss of renal blood flow, though collateral circulation could potentially occur. In small dogs or cats, selective occlusion of these six branches can be very difficult and dorsal or ventral occlusion preserving only 50% of the renal tissue may be necessary.

Surgical treatment

Partial ligation of a renal artery

A method of partial occlusion of the renal artery in a dog with IRH has been described (Mishina *et al.* 1997). Following routine laparotomy and cystotomy and identification of bleeding from the left UVJ, blood flow to the left kidney was occluded selectively at the left renal artery. While temporarily occluding the dorsal and ventral ramus of the renal artery, the ureteral catheter was monitored for cessation of bleeding. It was determined that the lesion was being fed by the dorsal ramus of the renal artery and this branch was surgically ligated resulting in resolution of the renal hematuria. This approach can also be performed endovascularly, as described earlier.

Nephrectomy

Similar to humans, ureteronephrectomy on the side of the bleed has traditionally been recommended as the treatment of choice for dogs with IRH. Concerns with this technique include the presence of bilateral hematuria (up to 25% of patients), contralateral hematuria that could develop over time, as well as the risk of chronic renal insufficiency that could develop later in life in a uninephric animal. Since these lesions are typically located in the renal pelvis and not in the renal tissue, if the kidney can be salvaged it is highly recommended.

Conclusion

In summary, IRH is an uncommon disease process in both canine and feline patients. It most commonly occurs in young large-breed dogs and can be seen bilaterally in approximately 20–25% of patients. There is no clear breed or sex predilection. Reports exist of unilateral hematuria progressing over months to years to bilateral hematuria, so avoiding ureteronephrectomy should be considered whenever possible, particularly in young

dogs and cats where future renal function is unknown. Newer, minimally invasive and renoprotective options are currently being investigated in veterinary medicine, including ureteropyeloscopy and electrocauterization, sclerotherapy/chemical cauterization, and selective renal arterial embolization. However, to date no studies regarding efficacy in veterinary medicine have been published. Lesions of the renal pelvis, like hemangiomas, are typically seen during ureteronephroscopy, but can often be missed on histopathology following ureteronephrectomy. For this reason, the disease process is termed benign essential hematuria, rather than IRH, in human medicine.

References

Bagley, D.H. and Allen, J. (1990). Flexible ureteropyeloscopy in the diagnosis of benign essential hematuria. *Journal of Urology* 143: 549–553.

Bahnson, R.R. (1987). Silver nitrate irrigation for hematuria from sickle cell hemoglobinopathy. *Journal of Urology* 137: 1194–1195.

Brito, A.H., Mazzucchi, E., Vicentini, F.C. et al. (2009). Management of chronic unilateral hematuria by ureterorenoscopy. *Journal of Endourology* 23: 1273–1276.

Copley, J.B. and Hasbargen, J.A. (1987). "Idiopathic" hematuria. A prospective evaluation. *Archives of Internal Medicine* 147: 434–437.

Diamond, D.A., Jeffs, R.D., and Marshall, F.F. (1981). Control of prolonged, benign, renal hematuria by silver nitrate instillation. *Urology* 18: 337–341.

Dooley, R. and Pietrow, P.K. (2004). Ureteroscopy of benign hematuria. *Urologic Clinics of North America* 31: 137–143.

Gittes, R.F. and Varady, S. (1981). Nephroscopy in chronic unilateral hematuria. *Journal of Urology* 126: 297–300.

Goel, S., Mandhani, A., Srivastava, A. et al. (2004). Is povidone iodine an alternative to silver nitrate for renal pelvic instillation sclerotherapy in chyluria? *BJU International* 94: 1082–1085.

Hagen, A. (1963). Renal angioma. Four cases of renal angioma of the renal pelvis. *Acta Chirurgica Scandinavica* 126: 657–667.

Hawthorne, J.C., de Haan, J.J., Goring, R.L. et al. (1998). Recurrent urethral obstruction secondary to idiopathic renal hematuria in a puppy. *Journal of the American Animal Hospital Association* 34: 511–514.

Holt, P.E., Lucke, V.M., and Pearson, H. (1987). Idiopathic renal hemorrhage in the dog. *Journal of Small Animal Practice* 28: 253–263.

Kaufman, A.C., Barsanti, J.A., and Selcer, B.A. (1994). Benign essential hematuria in dogs. *Compendium on Continuing Education for the Practicing Veterinarian* 16: 1317–1322.

Kavoussi, L.R., Clayman, R.V., and Basler, J. (1989). Flexible, actively deflectable fiberopticureteronephroscopy. *Journal of Urology* 142: 949–954.

Kumar, B.P., Maddi, A., Ramesh, K.V. et al. (2006). Is povidone-iodine a hemostyptic? A clinical study. *International Journal of Oral and Maxillofacial Surgery* 35: 765–766.

Meyer, D.J. and Senior, D.R. (1983). Hematuria and dysuria. In: *Textbook of Veterinary Internal Medicine* (ed. S.J. Ettinger and E.C. Feldman), 129–133. Philadelphia, PA: WB Saunders.

Mishina, M., Watanage, T., Yugeta, N. et al. (1997). Idiopathic renal hematuria in a dog: the usefulness of a method of partial occlusion of the renal artery. *Journal of Veterinary Medical Science* 59: 293–295.

Moore, F.M. and Thornton, G.W. (1983). Telangiectasia of Pembroke Welsh Corgi dogs. *Veterinary Pathology* 20: 203–208.

Mugiya, S., Ozone, S., Nagata, M. et al. (2007). Ureteroscopic evaluation and laser treatment of chronic unilateral hematuria. *Journal of Urology* 178: 517–520.

Nandy, P., Dwivedi, U.S., Vyas, N. et al. (2004). Povidone iodine and dextrose solution combination sclerotherapy in chyluria. *Urology* 64: 1107–1109.

Rastinehad, A.R., Ost, M.C., Vander Brink, B.A. et al. (2008). Persistent prostatic hematuria. *Nature Clinical Practice Urology* 5: 159–165.

Sharma, G., Chitale, V., Karva, R. et al. (2008). Fluoroscopy guided instillation therapy in chyluria using combination of povidone iodine with contrast agent. Is a single instillation sufficient? *International Brazilian Journal of Urology* 34: 270–275.

Stefanini, M., English, H., and Taylor, A. (1990). Safe and effective prolonged administration of epsilon aminocaproic acid in bleeding from the urinary tract. *Journal of Urology* 143: 559–561.

Stone, E.A., DeNovo, R.C., and Rawlings, C.A. (1983). Massive hematuria of nontraumatic renal origin in dogs. *Journal of the American Veterinary Medical Association* 183: 868–871.

Su, C.M., Lee, Y.C., Wu, W.J. et al. (2004). Acute necrotizing ureteritis with obstructive uropathy following instillation of silver nitrate in chyluria: a case report. *Kaohsiung Journal of Medical Sciences* 20: 512–515.

Tawfiek, E.R. and Bagley, D.H. (1998). Ureteroscopic evaluation and treatment of chronic unilateral hematuria. *Journal of Urology* 160: 700–702.

Wallach, J.B., Sutton, A.P., and Claman, M. (1959). Hemangioma of the kidney. *Journal of Urology* 81: 515–518.

52

Renal Transplant

Chad Schmiedt

Renal transplantation offers a strategy to improve management of animals with chronic kidney disease. Renal transplantation is much more successful and reliable in cats compared to dogs, although chronic complications, primarily related to immunosuppression, continue to occur.

Feline renal transplantation

Timing

The optimal timing of transplantation in cats is unknown. Transplantation in the very early stages of kidney disease exposes stable asymptomatic cats to unnecessary risks associated with anesthesia, surgery, and immunosuppression. This risk is particularly significant in cats with early-stage kidney disease with slow progression. Optimizing medical management of cats with subclinical or minimally clinical kidney disease and evaluating progression over time is a sound strategy prior to transplantation. Conversely, transplantation in cats with end-stage, uremic kidney disease is challenging, because they have a host of metabolic perturbations, are poor anesthetic candidates, and have reduced wound-healing capacity. Cats in IRIS stage 3 chronic kidney disease are reasonable candidates, as they have significant renal disease, have relatively short survival times without intervention, and often remain on reasonable nutritional and metabolic planes. Similarly, some centers also use a serum creatinine concentration of 4 mg/dL as a rough threshold for candidacy for transplantation.

Cats suffering from acute kidney injury or end-stage renal failure should be stabilized prior to transplantation. In cases of moderate kidney disease, stabilization can typically be done in the days prior to transplantation with standard medical therapy to correct dehydration, improve electrolyte imbalances, and administer blood transfusions. In the most severe cases, transplantation centers offering dialysis or renal replacement therapy and transplantation are more suited to receive those cats and facilitate a combined dialysis and transplantation treatment plan. Centers without dialysis may decline cats with significant acute kidney injury or those in end-stage, uremic kidney failure, because the arrangement of logistics surrounding transplantation, including donor cat acquisition and matching and appropriately screening recipients, may take several weeks. Unstable animals with significant kidney dysfunction present major challenges for immediate transplantation.

The nutritional status of preoperative transplantation patients is variable. In some cases, use of feeding tubes is indicated. However, any transcutaneous feeding tube (esophagostomy, gastrostomy, etc.) should be removed prior to immunosuppression, as they are a significant risk for abscess formation after the initiation of immunosuppressive therapy.

Pretransplantation screening

Each transplant center offers specific guidance relative to screening for candidates for renal transplantation. Prior to referring an animal, clinicians should reach out to the center for specific guidance. At a minimum, renal transplant recipients should be free of significant comorbid disease, particularly neoplastic or infectious disease (Adin 2002). Commonly required diagnostic tests are listed in Table 52.1. Some exclusionary criteria may be appropriately managed prior to transplantation; for

Table 52.1 Minimum tests required for renal transplantation in cats.

- Complete blood count
- Biochemical profile
- Urinalysis
- Urine culture
- Urine protein: creatinine ratio
- Thyroid hormone (T4) concentration
- Blood pressure
- Infectious disease testing
  - Toxoplasmosis (IgG and IgM) titers
  - FeLV and FIV tests
  - *Mycoplasma* sp. titers
  - *Bartonella* PCR
- Thoracic radiographs or CT
- Abdominal ultrasound or CT
- Dental evaluation
- Cardiac evaluation with echocardiogram
- Blood type
- Not required at all centers

CT, computed tomography; Ig, immunoglobulin; FeLV, feline leukemia virus; FIV, feline immunodeficiency virus; PCR, polymerase chain reaction.

example, hypertension, hyperthyroidism, and dental disease are exclusionary until they are successfully managed. Following successful management, cats with these conditions can be considered acceptable candidates.

Infectious disease, including urinary tract infections, may be treated and reassessed following the conclusion of therapy. If appropriate, repeat cultures should be performed several weeks following cessation of therapy to verify complete resolution of the infection. Recrudescence of infection following transplantation and immunosuppression may have fatal consequences, so there must be a high confidence of resolution prior to transplantation. A cyclosporine trial may be required to verify complete resolution of infection. For a cyclosporine trial, cats are started on oral cyclosporine (4 mg/kg every 12 h) for 2–4 weeks. Appropriate cyclosporine blood concentrations (300–500 ng/mL at a 12 h trough) are verified or, if the blood concentrations are outside of the appropriate range, the oral dose is adjusted and the trough concentration reevaluated. After initiation of appropriately dosed cyclosporine therapy, diagnostics are repeated to confirm resolution of the infection. Cats with recurrent urinary tract infections, particularly if uroliths are present in the kidney and ureter or there is pyelonephritis, are not candidates for transplantation. Cats with feline immunodeficiency virus (FIV) and feline leukemia virus (FeLV) are not candidates for transplantation.

Immunoglobulin (Ig)G and IgM titers for toxoplasmosis antibodies are required prior to transplantation. Cats that are seropositive and have an active infection may still be candidates if following appropriate therapeutic treatment and will continue on life-long prophylactic clindamycin (25 mg/cat orally [p.o.] every [q]12 h) after transplantation. Trimethoprim-sulfa (15 mg/kg p.o. q12 h) has also been used for those intolerant of clindamycin (Aronson 2016). Seroconversion of seronegative animals has been documented following renal transplantation, so some surgeons prefer to keep all animals on prophylactic clindamycin regardless of preoperative serologic status (Nordquist & Aronson 2008; Aronson 2016; Ludwig *et al.* 2021). For animals who are not on prophylactic therapy and who are seronegative preoperatively, repeating toxoplasmosis titers weeks to months after surgery has been recommended to be sure that seroconversion did not occur following immunosuppression.

Neoplastic disease is a contraindication for transplantation, as cyclosporine will potentiate cancer progression and make treatment challenging. One particular clinical scenario that is frequently a question is a cat with subclinical intestinal thickening noted on pretransplantation screening abdominal imaging. In these animals, obtaining full-thickness intestinal biopsies prior to transplantation is critical to differentiate intestinal lymphoma from inflammatory bowel disease. Cats with intestinal lymphoma are not candidates for transplantation.

Comorbid cardiac disease can be challenging to define, especially with single time-point echocardiographic studies and hypertension in a high percentage of cats with kidney disease. Cats with mild to moderate ventricular wall thickening may still be candidates for transplantation. Ideally, in cats with subclinical ventricular wall thickening, characterization of the progression of cardiac wall changes should be defined 4–6 months after initial diagnosis, particularly when hypertension is present and can be medically controlled. However, that timeline is often not possible in animals with clinically significant kidney disease. Cats with cardiac chamber enlargement are not candidates for renal transplantation.

Cats with a propensity to form stones may be considered for renal transplantation, with a few important caveats. The presence of infection in cats with stones should evoke caution, as the infecting organism may survive in the stones. Repeated negative cultures when not on antibiotics and potentially a cyclosporine trial may help determine if the uroliths are harboring bacteria. One study evaluated renal transplantation in 19 cats with calcium oxalate nephro- or ureteroliths (Aronson *et al.* 2006). Survival time in these cats was 605 days and

5 cats formed calculi in their transplanted kidneys (Aronson *et al.* 2006). Of these 5 cats, 5 died as a result of complications of these nephroliths (Aronson *et al.* 2006).

Cat temperament is a variable that should be also considered prior to transplantation. Owners should be carefully consulted about the demands of daily oral drug administration and frequent veterinary appointments for monitoring. Renal transplantation may not be possible in fractious animals or in animals owned by people without a significant commitment, understanding of the required management, or time available to devote to follow-up care.

Donor cat

Ethics

With current techniques, using a living cat as a kidney donor for a transplantation is an essential aspect of the procedure. The Royal College of Veterinary Surgeons and many in Europe find use of a living renal donor illegal and ethically wrong, as it is viewed as mutilation of a living animal for a medically unnecessary procedure (Royal College of Veterinary Surgeons 2021). Use of "pre-euthanasia" animals is also not endorsed in these countries, as those animals would still be considered living source donors, and, in animals being euthanized for an unrelated condition such as injuries resulting from trauma, prolonging their suffering to arrange for donation is also not appropriate (Royal College of Veterinary Surgeons 2021). Ethically sourced cadavers being euthanized for justifiable animal welfare reasons would be considered acceptable donors (Royal College of Veterinary Surgeons 2021). Successful cadaver donation has not been reported in cats; however, it is not uncommon in humans. Interestingly, because of the long waiting list for transplantation and the benefit of transplantation of even a marginal kidney compared to remaining on dialysis, expanded-criteria donors are becoming more common in human transplantation (Heilman *et al.* 2016). In people, increased consideration is now given to donors with diabetes, cardiac death, hypertension, acute kidney injury (without cortical necrosis), and certain anatomic abnormalities (Heilman *et al.* 2016). Understanding how these preexisting conditions, including cardiac death, influence outcomes in cats will be an important area of research.

In the USA, Asia, and elsewhere, ethical concerns and laws regarding renal donation are not nearly the issue they are in Europe and the practice is accepted by most. Considering the benefits of adoption of these donor animals into supportive and loving homes, and the documented minimal risk of renal donation, the balance is thought to be more positive for the animal. Regardless, the welfare of the renal donor should be a paramount consideration during all aspects of the procedure. One reason so much effort is placed on pre-recipient screening and use of rigorous selection criteria is to optimize the likelihood that the kidney from a donor cat has a reasonable chance to make a positive difference in the life of the recipient.

Donor identification and screening

Cats utilized as renal donors are typically sourced from research colonies, foster or rescue organizations, or humane societies, or they are cats already owned by the owner of the recipient. Screening criteria for the donor serve to maximize the likelihood that the transplanted kidney will optimally serve the recipient and that the donor is medically able to have a normal quality of life following uninephrectomy.

Screening criteria for donor cats are similar to those required for recipients (Adin 2002). Donor cats should be young, healthy animals. While there is not an absolute age limitation, generally donor cats are less than 3 years of age. Donor cats should be the same size or larger than the intended recipient. A complete blood count, biochemical profile, urinalysis, urine culture, urine protein : creatinine, thyroid hormone concentration, toxoplasmosis titers, FeLV/FIV testing, and blood type are required. A baseline blood pressure should also be performed.

Three-dimensional imaging of the donor kidney and renal vasculature has been recommended to ensure normal renal architecture and a single renal artery prior to surgery (Smith *et al.* 2012). Ideal computed tomography (CT) settings were determined to be a 10 second delay post intravenous bolus, two serially acquired helical scans through the renal vasculature to correspond to arterial and venous phases, pitch of 2 (4 mm/s patient translation, 2 mm slice collimation), and 120-K Vp, 160-mA, and 1 second exposure (Smith *et al.* 2012). CT values for normal kidney size and shape have also been reported (Darawiroj & Choisunirachon 2019). The average pre-contrast dimensions of the left kidney included 2.46 ± 0.28 cm (width) $\times 3.52 \pm 0.44$ cm (length) and 2.19 ± 0.31 cm (height), whereas the right kidney was 2.45 ± 0.27 cm (width), 3.54 ± 0.46 cm (length), and 2.05 ± 0.23 cm (height) (Darawiroj & Choisunirachon 2019). The left kidney length : L2 vertebrae length and right kidney length : L2 vertebrae length were 2.29 ± 0.23 and 2.36 ± 0.20, respectively, and the left kidney length : aortic diameter and right kidney length : aortic diameter were 11.72 ± 1.37 and 12.05 ± 1.47, respectively (Darawiroj & Choisunirachon 2019). Normal renal vascular characteristics have also been reported (Caceres *et al.* 2008). Venous multiplicity was observed most frequently on the right vein (45/114 had double right veins) and arterial duplicity was most commonly observed on the left (8/114 kidneys had double left artery) (Caceres *et al.* 2008).

Ultrasound evaluation of the renal architecture and color Doppler evaluation of renal arteries is also possible in screening donor cats. Use of resistive index and contrast-enhanced ultrasound has been described in cats to further assess the renal structure or function, although not specifically in relation to pretransplantation screening (Stock *et al.* 2018; Matos *et al.* 2018; Tipisca *et al.* 2016).

Exclusionary criteria for donors include advanced age, any evidence of renal disease or abnormal renal architecture, infection, hypertension, or any medical condition that could be exacerbated by removal of one kidney. If the donor cat is not already owned by the recipient, it is commonly required that the recipient's family adopt and provide life-long care for that cat.

Outcomes following renal donation

In a study of human kidney donors, and relative to a nondonor population, people who donated kidneys had higher blood pressure, lower glomerular filtration rates, and higher risk for end-stage renal disease and preeclampsia relative to nondonors (O'Keeffe *et al.* 2018). However, the absolute risk for end-stage renal disease remained low at 0.5 events/1000 person-years, and there was no increased risk for other major chronic diseases such as diabetes or psychosocial problems (O'Keeffe *et al.* 2018). Because postdonation health risks will vary with ethnicity, sex, lifestyle, and other factors, the specific risk for chronic complications following renal donation in people is modeled individually for each kidney donor (Matas *et al.* 2017).

In cats, three studies are available to gain insight on outcomes following uninephrectomy for kidney transplantation donation (Lirtzman & Gregory 1995; Danielson *et al.* 2015; Wormser & Aronson 2016). The oldest study evaluated 15 donor cats between two and five years after kidney donation (Lirtzman & Gregory 1995). Of those 15 cats, 2 developed chronic kidney disease. One of those had azotemia, nonregenerative anemia, and proteinuria, and the other was nonazotemic, but had dilute urine and proteinuria (Lirtzman & Gregory 1995). In those 15 cats, immediately post nephrectomy mean serum creatinine increased from 1.36 ± 0.2 to 1.71 ± 0.33 mg/dL (Lirtzman & Gregory 1995).

A second study sought to evaluate the prevalence of kidney failure in a population of 72 donor cats and also measure owner satisfaction with commercially sourced donor cats (Danielson *et al.* 2015). Of those 72 cats, 28 cats had sufficient medical data (serum blood urea nitrogen [BUN] and creatinine, and urine specific gravity) to determine renal function. At the time of the study, cats were a mean of 4.9 years after the nephrectomy, with a mean age of 6.8 years. Of the 28 cats, 5 (17.8%) developed chronic kidney disease; of those, 2 were still alive at the time of the surgery.

Owners of 36 of the 72 cats completed a survey regarding satisfaction with the donor cat as a pet. The response from 83% was that the cats were easily integrated into the house and ~92% were completely satisfied and 8% were mostly satisfied with the donor cat as a pet (Danielson *et al.* 2015).

A final study evaluated outcomes of 141 donor cats, with long-term outcomes available for 99 (Wormser & Aronson 2016). Intraoperative bleeding developed in 2 cats, neither of which required transfusion. Acute postoperative complications developed in 17 cats, including seroma, hematoma, upper respiratory infection, corneal ulceration, and diarrhea. Median follow-up time for the 99 cats was 10 years. At the time of the study, 6 cats with long-term follow-up were identified with urinary tract disease, including 3 with stable chronic kidney disease, 2 with acute kidney injury, and 1 with cystitis (Wormser & Aronson 2016). At follow-up 9 cats were dead, 2 from chronic kidney disease and 4 from ureteral obstruction (Wormser & Aronson 2016). In that study 7% of cats developed renal insufficiency or died from urinary tract disease (Wormser & Aronson 2016). The authors of the study concluded that feline kidney donation had an acceptably low perioperative morbidity and that most cats (84%) had no long-term effects from renal donation (Wormser & Aronson 2016).

Dogs appear to also have a reasonable prognosis following uninephrectomy for kidney donation (Urie *et al.* 2007). In one study, 14 dogs were evaluated up to 2.5 years following kidney donation. Clinically, all dogs in the study were mostly normal after renal donation; one dog was obese, one dogs had dermatitis, and one dog had pyrexia thought to be associated with anxiety. Biochemically, BUN, albumin, total protein, and urine specific gravity did not significantly change following kidney donation, but the serum creatinine concentration did increase significantly from a mean ± standard deviation of 1.22 ± 0.22 to 1.66 ± 0.27 mg/dL. Serum phosphorus decreased significantly after nephrectomy, and hematocrit, red blood cell count, mean corpuscular volume, and mean corpuscular hemoglobin increased significantly. However, all values for all parameters remained within normal limits. All of the harvested kidneys were normal histologically. Four remaining kidneys were biopsied after being the only kidney for an unreported period of time; two were normal and two showed minimal glomerulosclerosis. The remaining kidneys were largest in dogs that were <12 months old at the time of harvest. The authors conclude that canine kidney donors retain normal biochemical parameters following renal donation and that donor age should be considered when selecting a kidney donor (Urie *et al.* 2007).

Pretransplantation medical therapy

Transplant recipients are admitted to the hospital several days prior to surgery. Immunosuppression (modified cyclosporine, 4 mg/kg p.o., q12 h) is started 48 hours prior to surgery. Baseline blood counts, biochemical profile, blood pressure, and so on are obtained. Correction of dehydration and improvement of electrolyte abnormalities should also be performed during this time. Frequently a jugular catheter is placed either the day prior to surgery or the day of surgery to facilitate medication administration and blood sampling postoperatively.

Placement of a transcutaneous feeding tube (esophagostomy, gastrostomy) is a reasonable strategy in the weeks or months prior to transplantation, but it should be removed at least a week prior to immunosuppression. Even with mature stoma sites, once immunosuppression has begun, abscess formation can occur at the stoma site. This can be fatal in an immunocompromised patient.

Anemia is common in cats with chronic kidney disease, and, if indicated, treatment of anemia should be part of optimized pretransplantation medical therapy. Treatment for anemia will depend on the specific patient and timing of transplantation. If a transplantation is in the near future, a packed red blood cell transfusion may be an adequate bridge for the patient and avoids the risk of complications of erythrocyte-stimulating agents (fever, seizures, pure red cell aplasia). However, use of an erythrocyte-stimulating agent, particularly darbepoetin, and iron supplementation may be indicated if transplantation is not planned in the near future (Chalhoub *et al.* 2012).

Surgery

Donor–recipient organization

There are two strategies for timing donor and recipient. In the simultaneous paradigm, donor and recipient are anesthetized at the same time and the donor kidney is harvested while the implantation site is prepared on the recipient's aorta and vena cava. Three surgeons work together: two surgeons work on both the donor and recipient and the third surgeon closes the donor cat after

harvest of the kidney (Aronson 2016). The major advantage to this technique is that it minimizes the time during which the kidney is not receiving blood flow. The disadvantages include the need for two surgical teams and that the allograft is not cooled.

In the delayed paradigm, the donor cat is anesthetized first, and a single surgical team harvests the kidney from the donor, closes the donor, and then implants the kidney into the recipient (Schmiedt *et al.* 2008b). The kidney is flushed with and stored in ice-cold sucrose phosphate solution or a commercially available organ storage solution while the donor cat is closed, the recipient cat is anesthetized, and the implantation site is prepared (McAnulty 1998). The allograft is removed from the storage solution and implanted. The advantages of the delayed technique include being able to perform the transplant with a single surgical team and utilizing cold ischemia to reduce ischemic graft injury during implantation. The disadvantages include extending the duration of the entire procedure.

One experimental study evaluated these two approaches using an autotransplantation model (Csomos *et al.* 2017). In that study, 15 healthy cats were divided into two groups. One group underwent left renal harvest with immediate autotransplantation and right nephrectomy; the second group underwent left renal harvest, sucrose phosphate flushing, and cold storage for a mean duration of 24 minutes. The cats with kidneys that underwent sucrose phosphate flushing and cold storage had a lower peak serum creatinine concentration and returned to reference ranges more quickly compared to the immediate autotransplantation group (Csomos *et al.* 2017). The mean ± standard error of the peak creatinine concentration for the immediate autotransplantation group was 10.7 ± 2.9 mg/dL, which occurred three days after surgery, and for the cold storage group 2.6 ± 0.4 mg/dL, which occurred one day after surgery (Csomos *et al.* 2017).

Another study compared sucrose phosphate solution to heparinized saline for renal flushing in a left kidney autotransplantation model (Katayama *et al.* 2014). In that study each group only had two cats so statistical comparison was not performed, but the cats with kidneys flushed with heparinized saline had higher serum creatinine peaks (5.6 and 5.0 mg/dL) compared to the sucrose phosphate solution cats (2.0 and 1.1 mg/dL). The authors concluded that even with very short ischemia time, cold sucrose phosphate solution will limit ischemia-reperfusion injury (Katayama *et al.* 2014). Therefore, even if a simultaneous transplant paradigm is utilized, flushing with cold sucrose phosphate solution and briefly chilling the kidney may result in improved outcomes.

Renal and ureteral harvest

The left kidney is typically harvested for transplantation because the left renal vein is substantially longer than the right renal vein. The harvest is started by excising the retroperitoneum around the kidney and dissecting the retroperitoneal fat from the kidney. Small amounts of fat can be transplanted with the kidney, particularly around the renal hilus, but too much fat can impair the surgeon's ability to suture the vessels during implantation and transplantation of additional foreign tissue will add to the overall antigenicity of the transplanted kidney. The kidney is dissected until the renal artery and vein and ureter are the only remaining connections. The testicular or ovarian vein typically inserts on the caudal aspect of the left renal vein. The testicular or ovarian vein is ligated and divided near its insertion on the renal vein. The ligatures serve has a marker for the caudal aspect of the renal vein and helps to confirm proper orientation of the vein during the implantation procedure.

During dissection of the kidney, care is taken to avoid excessive traction on the renal vasculature or inadvertent occlusion of the vessels. Rough handling of the vessels will cause vasospasm, which may make implantation more difficult and may add to the ischemic injury to the kidney prior to harvest. Once the kidney is freed from its retroperitoneal attachments, but prior to transection of the vessels, the ureter is dissected from the retroperitoneum. This order of operations gives the kidney and its vasculature a little time to recover from handling prior to removal.

The method of ureteral harvest will depend on how the surgeon plans to implant the allograft ureter. If a ureteral papillae transfer technique is utilized, the entire ureter and a cuff of donor bladder around the papillae must be harvested (Hardie *et al.* 2005; Sutherland *et al.* 2016). If the surgeon plans on implanting the ureter by an intra- or extravesicular mucosal apposition technique, the ureter will be removed entirely but without the ureteral papillae or cuff of donor bladder. For the latter, the harvest is much less complicated. The ureter is dissected from the retroperitoneum; small ureteral vessels are cauterized well away from the ureter to avoid ureteral tissue damage from the cautery; and the ureter is ligated distal to the point of transection and divided. The technique for the papillae harvest and implantation is covered later.

Prior to the renal vessels being clamped and divided, the donor cat is given mannitol (1 g/kg intravenously [i.v.]) over 20 minutes. Prior to the mannitol, some surgeons will also give acepromazine (0.01 mg/kg i.v.), with the theory that it will cause vasodilation of the intraparenchymal renal vasculature and improve perfusion of the mannitol into the kidney. Perioperative antibiotics are not given to the donor until after the kidney is removed, due to concerns about nephrotoxicity of the drugs on the allograft during the ischemic period.

Ideally, the morphology of the renal vasculature would be known prior to surgery. In cats with multiple renal arteries or veins, attempting to anastomose two small renal arteries or veins is not advised. In cats with multiple renal veins, the smaller of the veins may be able to be sacrificed, although there is no published evidence of what size differential is acceptable. Donors with two renal arteries should be avoided unless a Carrel patch technique can be utilized (Budgeon *et al.* 2017).

A Carrel patch technique involves harvesting a cuff of donor aortic wall with the renal artery(s) and is useful when there is a single renal artery with a very early bifurcation, or two renal arteries that exit the aorta in separate locations but very close proximity. For the harvest of a Carrel patch, a Satinsky or similar vascular clamp is used to isolate the desired renal arterial supply, taking care to avoid the contralateral renal arterial supply (Budgeon *et al.* 2017). An ~1 mm patch of aorta is removed with a Beaver mini-blade and Vannas scissors centered over the renal arteries. The defect is closed with 9-0 nylon suture in an overlapping simple continuous pattern (Budgeon *et al.* 2017). Implantation is similar to that described for a simple end-to-side implantation, although the defect in the aortic wall may be slightly larger to accommodate the diameter of the patch. In a series of nine transplantation procedures, a Carrel patch was utilized for cats with or without double renal arteries and no cat had a perioperative vascular complication (Budgeon *et al.* 2017).

Cold flushing and storage technique

Simple *ex vivo* cold storage as already described is routinely successful for 2–3 hours during a transplantation surgery. It has been utilized successfully for up to 7 hours of simple cold storage in clinical feline patients (McAnulty 1998). The recipe for the sucrose phosphate solution is listed in Table 52.2. Typically, the solution is made first thing in the morning on the day of transplantation, put in an intravenous administration bag, and chilled to around 4 °C. Any commercially available organ storage solution approved for kidney storage could be also used, but the sucrose phosphate solution made in-house is the most economical option. UW® Solution (Bridge to Life Ltd., Northbrook, IL, USA) is a common commercially available organ transplant storage solution and has been described for use in cats (McAnulty 1998).

Prior to occlusion and transection of the renal vasculature, a large sterile Mayo bowl is used to create an ice bath. Then 1–2 L of frozen sterile saline is placed in the

Table 52.2 Sucrose phosphate solution for allograft flushing and simple cold storage.

Ingredients	Concentration	g/500 mL
NaH$_2$PO$_4$ (monobasic)	15.5 mmol/L	1.07 g
Na$_2$HPO$_4$ (dibasic)	53.6 mmol/L	3.8 g
Sucrose	140.0 mmol/L	23.9 g
Heparin	1000 IU/L	500 units
Distilled water	–	qs ad 500 mL

qs ad, sufficient quantity to make.

large bowl and broken into small chunks. In our practice, a sterile osteotome is used to break up the frozen saline. A small volume of cold sterile saline is poured over the frozen saline to create a slurry. In the middle of the larger bowl, a smaller sterile bowl is placed and filled with the cold sucrose phosphate solution to create an ice bath. The kidney is harvested and immediately placed in the sucrose phosphate solution for several seconds to achieve immediate surface cooling. The kidney is removed from the solution and placed on a sterile table, and the renal artery and vein are identified. The renal artery is catheterized with an 18- or 20-gauge intravenous catheter, which is attached to the organ storage solution through a fluid administration set. The solution is hung approximately 100 cm above the kidney to achieve an appropriate perfusion pressure. The allograft is flushed until the effluent from the renal vein is clear and the capsular veins have blanched. Periodic gentle pressure on the kidney will help increase venous effluent. The ureter is gently massaged along its length to help the solution move through the ureteral vasculature.

When the flush is complete, the kidney is replaced in the small bowl of sucrose phosphate solution (Figure 52.1). To help insulate the ice bath, surgical towels are placed around the sides of the bowl and the ice bath is covered with sterile surgical drapes until it is needed for implantation.

Vascular anastomosis

The allograft is implanted on the same side from which it was removed from the donor. This is almost always the left side (Figures 52.2 and 52.3). The implantation site is caudal to the native kidneys and cranial to the bladder. Native kidneys are typically biopsied prior to implantation. Rarely, a native kidney may need to be removed to make room for the allograft (renomegaly secondary to polycystic kidney disease) or for a medical reason (chronic obstruction, complete lack of function, etc.).

Historically, a renal artery to external iliac artery end-to-end anastomosis was performed, but resulted in

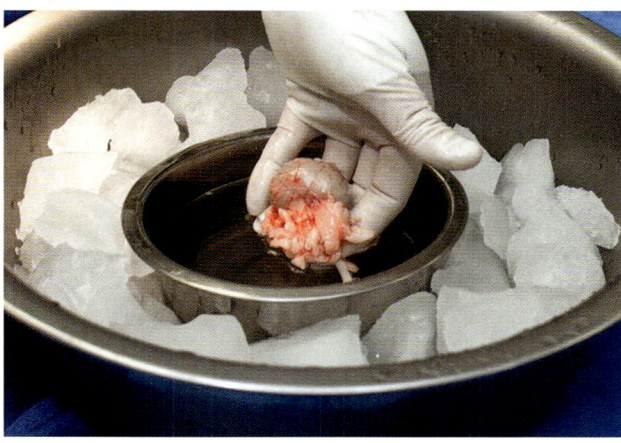

Figure 52.1 A harvested allograft in an ice bath with sucrose phosphate solution. A chilled bath of sucrose phosphate solution is surrounded by a frozen saline slurry. Following harvest, the allograft is flushed with chilled sucrose phosphate solution, then placed in chilled sucrose phosphate solution while the donor is closed and the recipient is prepared for implantation.

ipsilateral hind vascular compromise in some recipients (Gregory *et al*. 1992; Bernsteen *et al*. 1999b). In a study comparing end-to-end versus end-to-side arterial anastomosis techniques, 5/8 of the cats that underwent end-to-end anastomosis developed neuropraxia and lameness in the ipsilateral hindlimb (Bernsteen *et al*. 1999b). The current standard of care is an end-to-side anastomosis of the renal artery to the aorta and the renal vein to the vena cava. Ideally, the anastomosis time should be less than 60 minutes and the implantation is always done with the aid of an operating microscope.

In our practice the venous anastomosis is performed first to minimize the time of aortic occlusion. However, in other practices the aortic anastomosis is performed first (Aronson 2016). For the vein, the vena cava is partially or completely occluded with an aneurysm clamp or other vascular occlusion device, a small defect is made in the wall of the vena cava, and the renal vein is sutured in two simple continuous lines using 7-0 silk or 10-0 polyester fiber suture (Aronson 2016; Schmiedt *et al*. 2008b). The aorta is then occluded with a Cooley vascular clamp or similar and the renal artery is sutured using two simple continuous lines of 9-0 or 8-0 nylon (Aronson 2016; Schmiedt *et al*. 2008b). The venous clamp is removed first and the venous anastomosis is assessed for hemorrhage; the aortic clamp is then removed. There is commonly mild hemorrhage from the needle holes in the vessel walls; this is typically self-limiting. Immediately or shortly after reperfusion the renal artery may experience vasospasm, which is characterized by arterial contraction, blanching of the vessel surface, and poor coloration of the kidney. Topical

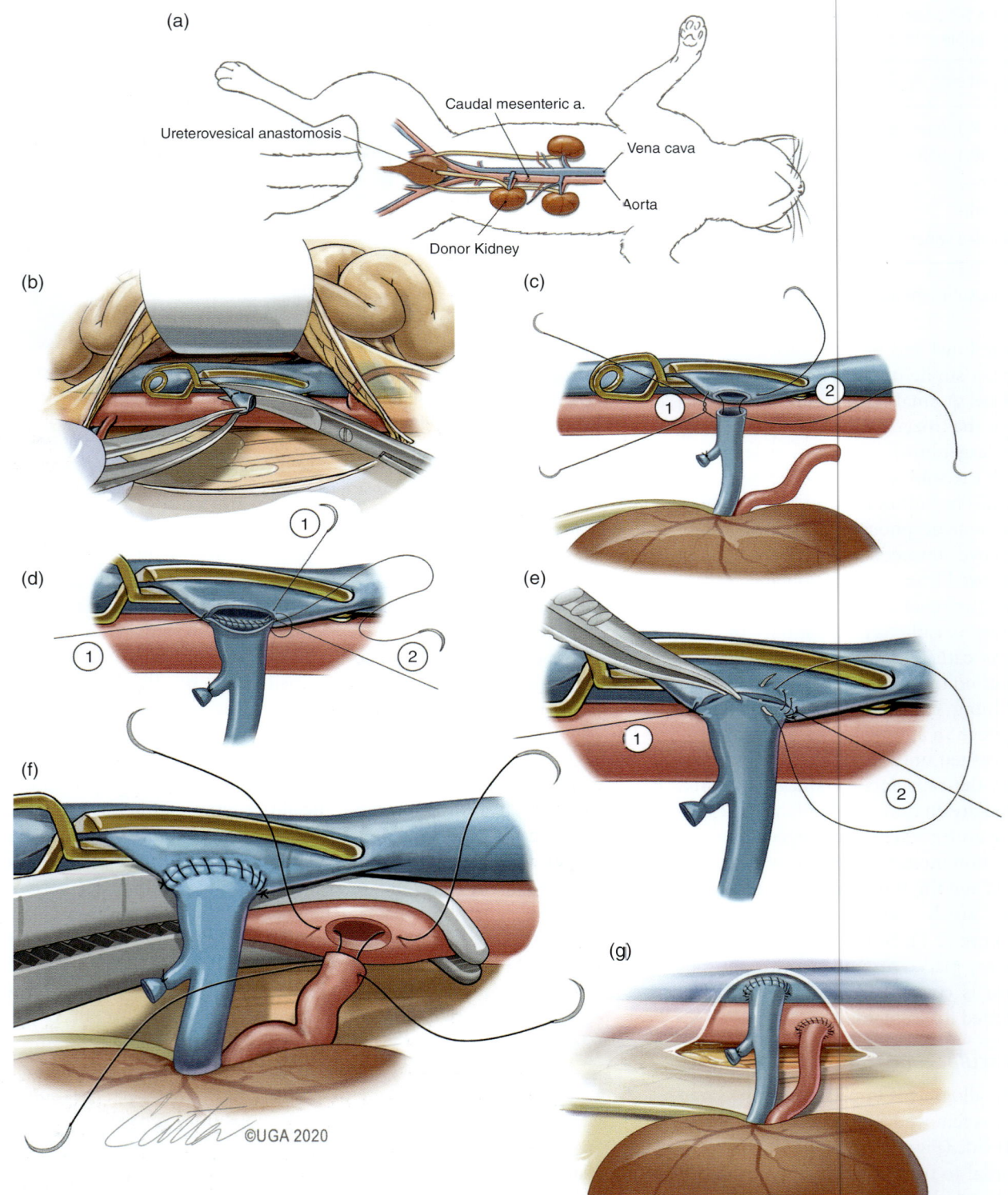

Figure 52.2 Vascular anastomosis technique. (a) The allograft is implanted in the caudal abdomen, typically on the same side from which it was removed from the donor. (b) The implantation technique is begun by partially occluding the caudal vena cava with an aneurysm clamp and creating a vena cavotomy. (c) Two double-armed sutures are tied at the cranial and caudal aspects of the defect in the vena cava, taking care to not cause any twists in the allograft vein. The previously ligated ovarian or testicular vein serves as a marker for the caudal aspect of the allograft vein. (d) The lateral side of the vein is sutured first with a simple continuous pattern through the medial side in an end-to-side technique. (e) The anastomosis is completed by suturing the medial side in a similar pattern. (f) The aorta is then completely occluded using vascular clamps and anastomosed using a similar technique. (g) The venous clamp is released first, followed by the arterial clamp. Illustration by Educational Resources, © University of Georgia.

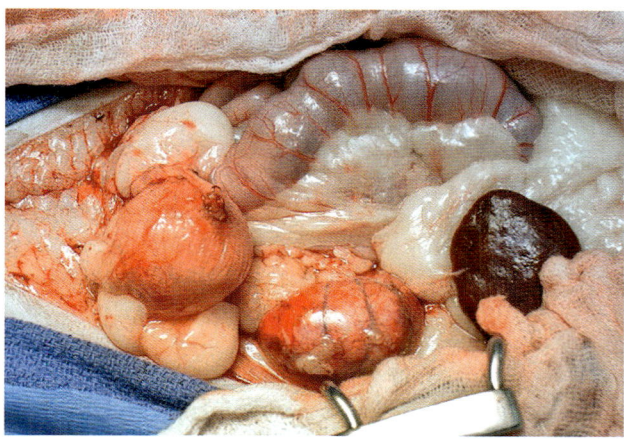

Figure 52.3 A completed transplantation and ureteral implantation. The ureteral papillae transfer technique was used and can be seen inserting on the apex of the bladder.

treatment of the allograft renal artery with chlorpromazine or acepromazine has been suggested as a method to reduce this vasospasm; 1–3 drops of undiluted medication through a 25-gauge needle is applied directly to the surface of the vessel (Schmiedt *et al.* 2008b). In cats without significant intraoperative hemorrhage, a dose of heparin (100 IU/kg i.v.) is given ~60 minutes after removal of the vascular clamps. The cat remains heparinized for 5 days (100 IU/kg heparin subcutaneously [s.c.] q8 h) postoperatively to prevent thrombosis.

Nonsutured methods of vascular anastomosis have been described. Use of nonpenetrating vascular staples has been described for successful anastomosis in research cats, with a significantly shorter anastomosis time compared to sutured anastomosis. Preliminary results of arterial and venous end-to-side vascular coupling devices have also been reported in 6 cats undergoing renal transplantation. In that series, vascular coupling devices significantly reduced anastomosis time to a median time of ~30 minutes (Mickelson *et al.* 2021).

Papillae transfer ureteral implantation

The advantage of the ureteral papilla transfer technique is that it avoids common technical complications of the mucosal apposition technique, including stricture, obstruction by granulation tissue, leakage, and dehiscence (Sutherland *et al.* 2016). The feline ureter is very small (~0.4 mm) and maintaining a patent lumen diameter is technically challenging (Sutherland *et al.* 2016). Harvesting and transplanting the ureter with the normal ureteral opening avoid these technical challenges, as the surgeon sutures the cuff of transplanted donor bladder to the recipient bladder wall. The disadvantages of the ureteral papilla transfer technique include increased harvest time, a more technically demanding harvest, and

potential to injury the contralateral ureter and urethra during the harvest.

During harvest, the ureter is dissected to the trigone of the bladder. Under an operating microscope, the serosal layer of the bladder is sharply excised with scissors to form a small (1–2 mm) cuff around the ureter to be harvested. Extreme caution and anatomic awareness are required not to damage the contralateral ureter or the urethra. The serosal layer is transected until the mucosa bulges through the cut surface. The mucosa is opened laterally and cranially first. Both ureteral papillae are identified and stented with 4-0 monofilament suture, then the medial and caudal aspects of the mucosa cuff are excised. The suture stent is left in the contralateral ureter for most of the closure to insure it is not included in the closure, and a red rubber catheter can be placed in the urethra to aid in identifying its lumen. The bladder is closed in two layers, typically with 8-0 polyglactin 910 followed by 5-0 monofilament absorbable in a simple continuous pattern.

During implantation of a ureter harvested with the papillae, the ureter is wrapped around the recipient bladder. Because the allograft is placed caudal to the native left kidney and much closer to the bladder, when the entire donor ureter and ureteral papilla is preserved there is substantial extra ureteral length. Implanting the ureteral papillae directly into the apex of the bladder without wrapping it around the bladder causes the ureter to bunch up, which can lead to scarring with very sharp angles along its length. To avoid this, the donor ureter is passed dorsal to the bladder, between the urethra and the contralateral (typically right) ureter and over the ventral surface to insert near the bladder apex. This stretches out the ureter and avoids kinks that can result in obstruction. Care is taken at the point where the ureter passes between the contralateral ureter and urethra and abruptly changes direction to move onto the ventral aspect of the bladder, as this is a site of possible occlusion.

A full-thickness defect is made in the apex of the recipient bladder using a 4 mm skin biopsy punch. The location of the ureteral opening is verified with a suture stent and the mucosa of the cuff of the donor bladder is sutured with 8-0 polyglactin 910 in two simple continuous suture lines. The serosa of the cuff is then sutured to the serosa of the recipient bladder with similar suture in a simple interrupted pattern.

A study was reported of 31 feline kidney donors and 30 recipients undergoing ureteral papillae transfers as part of their renal transplantation procedures (Sutherland *et al.* 2016). In the donors, 4 cats developed mild transient increase in serum creatinine postoperatively (range 2.2–3 mg/dL maximum value), but no other complications were noted (Sutherland *et al.* 2016). For the recipient cats, 1 cat had urine leakage diagnosed 3 days after surgery, which resolved without further surgery. Chronically, 5 recipient cats developed retroperitoneal fibrosis and ureteral obstruction. Ureteral obstruction may have resulted from excessive ureteral length in some of these cats (Sutherland *et al.* 2016).

Mucosal apposition ureteral implantation

The mucosal apposition technique for ureteral implantation was described originally as a replacement for the "drop-in" or "modified drop-in" technique, where there was little direct apposition of ureteral mucosa and bladder mucosa (Gregory *et al.* 1996; Kochin *et al.* 1993). The original description of this technique consisted of performing a ventral cystotomy, using a pair of hemostatic forceps to pierce the bladder wall from the inside near the apex and draw the distal ureter into the bladder, everting the bladder mucosa so the interior of the dorsal bladder wall becomes convex, removing a small section of bladder mucosa, and apposing the ureteral mucosa to the defect in the bladder mucosa (Gregory *et al.* 1996). This is known as an intravesical technique, because the ureteroneocystotomy is performed from within the bladder.

This technique was originally reported using 8-0 nylon suture, but other suture can be used as well, including similarly sized polyglactin 910 (Gregory *et al.* 1996; Schmiedt *et al.* 2008b). There is commonly a single ureteral vessel running down the length of the ureter: ligating this vessel at or very near the cut end of the ureter is helpful to maintain an unobstructed field and prevent postoperative hematuria. The distal end of the ureter is cut to remove ureteral tissue damaged when manipulated though the bladder wall with forceps. The periureteral fat can also be removed from the end of the ureter to aid in visualization and definitively identify the ureteral wall. The ureteral lumen is spatulated and a simple interrupted suture is placed at the proximal-most aspect of the spatulation at the "12 o'clock" position. Next, two sutures are placed on the corners of the distal ends of the spatulated ureter. Finally, additional simple interrupted or simple continuous sutures are placed between the three sutures to finish apposing the ureteral and bladder mucosa.

Extravesical strategies have also been described for ureteroneocystotomies in cats (Mehl *et al.* 2005). In one study 15 cats were divided into three groups of 5 cats. One group had an intravesical technique similar to that described earlier, and two groups had extravesical techniques, one group with a single interrupted closure and one group with a simple continuous closure (Mehl *et al.* 2005). In all groups the contralateral kidney was also removed to allow postoperative creatinine to accurately represent the performance of the kidney and operated ureter. In this study, the extravesical simple continuous technique had poor outcomes in several cats and was excluded from analysis. The extravesical simple interrupted and intravesical techniques were compared and the extravesical technique had lower postoperative peak creatinine concentrations compared to the intravesical technique (4.9 ± 3.3 mg/dL extravesical vs. 9.4 ± 2.4 mg/dL intravesical) and more rapid resolution of renal pelvic dilatation. The authors concluded that for cats with normal-sized ureters (i.e., those undergoing kidney transplantation) the extravesical technique seemed to be the best choice (Mehl *et al.* 2005).

Nephropexy

After the vascular anastomosis and ureteral implantation, a nephropexy is performed to prevent torsion of the renal pedicle. The ipsilateral retroperitoneum is elevated from medial to lateral and a pocket is made for the allograft. The retroperitoneum is sutured to the renal capsule in 2–3 locations. The abdomen is lavaged with warm saline.

Prior to closure, 10–15 mL of 1% carboxymethyl cellulose may be instilled into the abdomen to prevent adhesion formation.

Anesthesia considerations

The specific anesthetic strategy will vary for each patient. Whether the transplant will be performed with simultaneous or sequential harvest and implantation techniques may also influence anesthetic decision making.

Donor cats are young, healthy, and have few unique anesthetic considerations. Some centers will avoid perioperative antibiotics until the kidney is removed from the donor to prevent antibiotic renal toxicity during the ischemic period. As mentioned in the section on harvesting, mannitol (1 g/kg i.v.) is given over 20 minutes just prior to harvest, and some surgeons will also give acepromazine (0.01 mg/kg i.v.) prior to the mannitol, based on the theory that acepromazine will vasodilate the intraparenchymal renal vasculature and improve perfusion of the mannitol into the kidney. In our practice, as long as the donor is stable under anesthesia and no contraindication exists, a unit of blood is removed from the donor cat after surgery, but prior to discontinuance of anesthesia. This blood is used as fresh whole blood for the recipient cat.

The recipient cat will present more anesthetic challenges, which will vary directly with the degree of kidney disease and associated comorbidities. Jugular catheters are frequently placed prior to anesthesia to facilitate fluid delivery and blood sampling (Valverde *et al.* 2002).

Arterial catheters are helpful to monitor blood pressures intraoperatively and during recovery. A sterile endotracheal tube is used to minimize airway contamination in immunosuppressed animals. Other routine monitoring devices are critical during the anesthetic event.

In programs that utilized a simultaneous harvest and implantation strategy, the mean anesthetic duration was 4.6 hours ± 27 minutes to 5.2 hours ± 48 minutes (Snell et al. 2015; Valverde et al. 2002). Prolonged anesthesia time has been associated with reduced overall survival time, so minimization of anesthesia time should be a priority (Snell et al. 2015).

Blood products are commonly administered to the recipient before or during the anesthetic event. The most commonly treated intraoperative complications are reported to be hypotension, hypothermia, metabolic acidosis, hypocalcemia, and hypoglycemia (Valverde et al. 2002). The most common complications observed the day after anesthesia include hypertension, hematuria, electrolyte abnormalities, body temperature abnormalities, anemia requiring transfusion, and seizures associated with hypertension (Valverde et al. 2002). No associations were found between survival rate and anesthetic agent or intravenous fluid amount or type, so those decisions should be made based on the characteristics of the specific patient (Valverde et al. 2002). Reversal of μ opioid receptor agonist at the end of anesthesia was associated with better short-term survival, as was a higher hematocrit at the end of anesthesia (Valverde et al. 2002).

Immunosuppression

The standard immunosuppression protocol in cats following renal transplantation is oral, twice-daily cyclosporine and prednisolone. Modified cyclosporine (Neoral®, Novartis, Basel, Switzerland) is microemulsified and is recommended compared to the non-microemulsified cyclosporine (Sandimmune®, Novartis) because of better absorption following oral administration (Colombo & Sartori 2018). Bioavailability of orally administered, microemulsified cyclosporine is reported to be 25–29% in cats (Mehl et al. 2003).

Cyclosporine is started at a dose of 1–4 mg/kg every 12 hours and adjusted to a 12-hour trough concentration of 300–500 ng/mL, erring on the higher side of that range early after transplant and lower on the range as time passes since transplantation (Schmiedt et al. 2008a,b). Cyclosporine is very bitter, so it is frequently administered in gelatin capsules, which are made by the owner immediately prior to administration. Use of gelatin capsules also prevents loss of medication from drool, enables more accurate dosing, and minimizes negative associations between the owner and the cat while medicating.

Absorption of cyclosporine has substantial individual variability, so dosing in renal transplant patients should be based on the individual cat's blood concentrations rather than the oral dose administered (Mehl et al. 2003). This differs from recommendations from dermatologists, who note poor correlation of clinical response in animals with skin disease and trough blood cyclosporine concentration (Schmiedt et al. 2008a,b). Although the clinical standard of care is to evaluate 12-hour trough levels, 2-hour peak concentrations can also be evaluated and have been shown to better correlate with area under the curve compared to 12-hour trough concentrations in cats following oral dosing (Mehl et al. 2003). In cats that have assumed poor absorption based on administration of high doses and persistently low blood concentrations, supplementation of B vitamins may enhance absorption of microemulsified drugs (Francis et al. 2005). Anecdotally, weekly B vitamin supplementation improves cyclosporine blood concentrations after several doses.

Cyclosporine is metabolized by the cytochrome P450 enzyme pathway, so its metabolism can be significantly influenced by other medications that also utilize or influence this pathway (Schmiedt et al. 2008a,b). This has been used clinically in cats where once-daily dosing is desired (McAnulty & Lensmeyer 1999). Ketoconazole, when administered concurrently with cyclosporine at a dose of 10 mg/kg, increased blood cyclosporine concentration 1.8–2.2-fold at 12 and 24 hours after administration (McAnulty & Lensmeyer 1999). This was a result of a reduction in clearance from 2.73 to 1.22 mL/min/kg (McAnulty & Lensmeyer 1999). There are many other drugs with demonstrated interactions with cyclosporine in people, but specifically in cats only a few have been reported. In addition to ketoconazole, itraconazole and clarithromycin have both been shown to reduce cyclosporine clearance and therefore increase levels; there is also preliminary evidence that metoclopramide reduced cyclosporine concentrations in cats (Colombo & Sartori 2018).

Our team has used mycophenolate mofetil (10 mg/kg p.o. q12 h) as part of the immunosuppressive regimen for clinical transplant recipients in two situations. The first is to augment immunosuppression in treatment of an acute rejection reaction. The second is to provide enhanced immunosuppression during the early postoperative period. However, cats on a full dose of mycophenolate and cyclosporine will often have significant gastrointestinal complications (severe anorexia, vomiting, and diarrhea), so the dose of mycophenolate is reduced to 5 mg/kg after 2–3 weeks, then discontinued as the patient stabilizes after the first few months.

Tacrolimus (0.375 mg/kg, p.o. q12 h, adjusted to maintain a blood level of 5–10 ng/mL) has been used to prevent acute rejection in an experimental study of cats following renal transplantation (Kyles *et al.* 2003). In the study, six cats underwent transplantation and received tacrolimus. Of those six, three developed acute active rejection, one cat developed necrotizing vasculitis, and two cats completed the study at day 50 post transplantation (Kyles *et al.* 2003). Tacrolimus-treated cats lived longer than control cats, but given the number of cats with clinical and histopathologic evidence of acute rejection, a substantial proportion may not have had adequate immunosuppression.

Acute complications

Hemorrhage and thrombosis

Thromboembolism can occur systemically or can involve just the allograft (Figure 52.4). If the allograft experiences thrombosis, little can be done to salvage the allograft and it must be removed or replaced. To prevent thromboembolism, a dose of heparin (100 IU/kg) is administered intravenously approximately 60 minutes after release of the vascular clamps. Cats are maintained on heparin (100 IU/kg q8 h s.c.) for 5 days postoperatively, because of the theory that duration of therapy will give sufficient time for endothelial regrowth over the anastomosis site. In cases where cats may be predisposed to ongoing protein loss, for example in cats with underlying glomerulonephritis, continuing on chronic platelet inhibitor therapy (clopidogrel 18.75 mg/cat p.o. q24 h) may be indicated.

When it occurs, hemorrhage typically is noticed in the first 72 hours after surgery and can be severe. Treatment is by discontinuing any clotting inhibitors and treatment

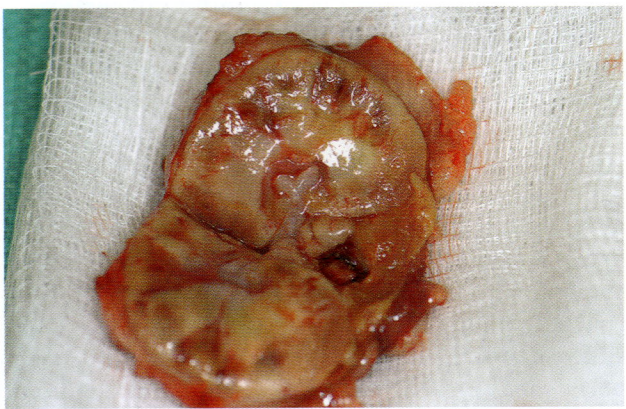

Figure 52.4 A thrombosed renal allograft. The patient had an initial decrease in creatinine immediately following transplantation, but redeveloped azotemia on day 3 following surgery. Ultrasound evaluation demonstrated no blood flow to the allograft. The allograft was removed and replaced with a new allograft.

with fresh whole blood or appropriate blood products. Thrombosis can occur any time after transplantation, but may be more common during the initial healing phase when turbulence and exposed collagen are present at the site of anastomosis. We routinely evaluate blood flow of the allograft with Doppler ultrasound examination on days 1 and 7 postoperatively and as part of the evaluation of any posttransplantation azotemia.

Hypertension

Postoperative hypertension (systolic blood pressure >160–170 mmHg) has been reported in 30–62% of transplant recipients (Schmiedt *et al.* 2008b; Kyles *et al.* 1999; Adin *et al.* 2001). Hypertension has been shown to be a major contributing factor to the development of postoperative neurologic signs, and treatment of hypertension significantly reduced the occurrence of neurologic signs in transplant recipients (Kyles *et al.* 1999). Occurrence of postoperative hypertension can occur regardless of preoperative hypertensive status or preoperative antihypertensive therapy (Adin *et al.* 2001). In one study, reduced time to normal BUN was correlated with occurrence of acute postoperative hypertension (Schmiedt *et al.* 2008b).

The cause for physiologic postoperative hypertension in feline renal transplant recipients is unknown. It has been postulated that hypertension may relate to intrarenal renin production while the graft is not perfused, which is subsequently flushed into systemic circulation on reperfusion, or Goldblatt hypertension secondary to renin production from patchy ischemic areas within the allograft after reperfusion (Schmiedt *et al.* 2010). In experimental cats undergoing renal autotransplantation and with a 30 minute or 3 hour simple cold storage time between harvest and reimplantation, differences were not observed in postreperfusion hemodynamic variables or in circulating renin production, nor was activation of genes for renin, endothelin, or angiotensin-converting enzyme different in kidneys following 2 hours of simple cold or warm ischemia (Schmiedt *et al.* 2010; Schmiedt *et al.* 2009c). However, another study was able to demonstrate a significantly higher level of circulating renin compared to preoperative levels in cats following a 3 hour simple cold storage and renal ischemia (Schmiedt *et al.* 2009b). The role of the renin angiotensin system in acute postoperative hypertension in feline transplant patients remains unclear.

For the first 24–48 hours after transplantation, blood pressure should be monitored every hour. Hypertension is initially treated with hydralazine at a dose of 1–2.5 mg/cat subcutaneously (Kyles *et al.* 1999). If the hypertension does not resolve in 15 minutes, a second dose is given (Kyles *et al.* 1999).

Neurologic signs

Postoperative neurologic signs have been reported in cats following renal transplantation (Kyles *et al.* 1999; Adin *et al.* 2001; Schmiedt *et al.* 2008b; Mathews & Gregory 1997; Gregory *et al.* 1997). Acute neurologic signs occur in the early postoperative period (1 hour to 5 days) and include single or multiple seizure episodes, ataxia, blindness, temporary coma, nonrecoverable coma, and cardiorespiratory arrest (Gregory *et al.* 1997). In an early report on feline transplantation, 37% of perioperative deaths were attributed to the development of seizures or seizure-related complications (Mathews & Gregory 1997). In another study of 61 cats, 9 cats developed neurologic signs (seizures (n = 6) or obtundation and nystagmus (n = 3) (Adin *et al.* 2001). In that study, occurrence of these signs was significantly related to BUN and creatinine concentrations at the time of surgery (Adin *et al.* 2001). However, preoperative BUN and creatinine were not identified as risk factors in another study (Gregory *et al.* 1997). In a third study of 60 cats, postoperative seizures were reported in 2 cats following transplantation (Schmiedt *et al.* 2008b). The first cat had a seizure at 88 hours after transplant, was hypocalcemic, and died of sepsis 8 days postoperatively; the second cat first had a seizure at 10 hours after transplant, was also hypocalcemic, and developed severe pulmonary hypertension secondary to pulmonary thromboembolism (Schmiedt *et al.* 2008b).

The role of serum magnesium as a contributing cause for postoperative neurologic signs in transplant recipients has been evaluated and ionized serum magnesium was found to be commonly reduced in the perioperative period, but no patient was hypomagnesemic when neurologic signs developed, suggesting that hypomagnesemia did not contribute to the onset of neurologic signs (Wooldridge & Gregory 1999).

Importantly, control of postoperative hypertension has been shown to significantly reduce neurologic events, suggesting that hypertensive encephalopathy was a likely cause of the condition in the majority of patients (Kyles *et al.* 1999). In transplant patients, aggressive monitoring and control of hypertension will result in a substantial reduction of postoperative neurologic complications.

Delayed graft function

Delayed graft function is a result of acute ischemic injury to the allograft during the operative period and leads to reduced graft function, increased graft antigenicity, and worse short- and long-term outcomes in humans (Mannon 2018). In people it is defined as acute kidney injury that occurs in the first week after transplant that requires dialysis intervention (Mannon 2018). Identified risk factors in humans, which are also potentially relevant to veterinary transplantation, include increasing donor age, body mass index, and serum creatinine, cold ischemia time, warm ischemia time, and recipient body mass index, previous transplantation, and diabetes (Mannon 2018). Female donors and male recipients are also risk factors in people (Mannon 2018).

Immediate graft function in veterinary transplantation has been defined as a creatinine concentration within normal limits the day after surgery, and it has been suggested that approximately 40% of cats do not have immediate graft function after a renal transplantation (Mehl *et al.* 2006). Delayed graft function has been defined in the veterinary literature as a creatinine over 3 mg/dL at 3 days after surgery without any other identifiable cause of persistent azotemia such as uroperitoneum, graft thrombosis, or ureteral obstruction (Schmiedt *et al.* 2008b). Ischemic injury, particularly warm ischemic injury, which occurs between harvest and implantation is a major contributing cause (Mehl *et al.* 2006). In one study delayed graft function was identified in 5 of 60 cats following renal transplantation, but risk factors specific for cats have not been identified (Schmiedt *et al.* 2008b).

Chronic complications

Neoplasia

Following transplantation, cats have a 6–6.6-fold higher risk of developing posttransplantation malignant neoplasia (PTMN) compared to control cats not receiving transplantation (Schmiedt *et al.* 2009a; Wormser *et al.* 2016). This increased risk of neoplasia is likely due to chronic immunosuppression coupled with chronic antigenic stimulation from the allograft.

Cyclosporine is known to induce cancer progression by several different mechanisms (London *et al.* 1995). Cyclosporine inhibits immune surveillance of abnormal cells by inducing apoptosis of activated T cells, potentiates infection by cancer-causing viruses, and induces cancer progression by a cell-autonomous mechanism (Hojo *et al.* 1999; Durham *et al.* 2014; Andre *et al.* 2004; Gregory *et al.* 1991). Additionally, cyclosporine inhibits cellular ability to repair damaged DNA, triggers the production of transforming growth factor (TGF)-β that may promote cancer progression, and inhibits the apoptosis of abnormal, potentially neoplastic cells (Andre *et al.* 2004).

In one study of 111 cats that received renal transplantation, 25 (22.5%) developed PTMN; 14 of those cases were lymphoma, and the time to occurrence of lymphoma was 617 days from transplantation (Wormser et al. 2016; Durham et al. 2014). Another study documented 9 cases of PTMN in 95 cats following renal transplantation; these occurred a mean of 9 months after transplantation, and 4 of these 9 cats developed lymphoma (Wooldridge et al. 2002). A third study documented 11 cases of PTMN in 45 cats, with 4 of the 11 cases developing lymphoma (Schmiedt et al. 2009a). In that study, time to occurrence was 1020 days for all tumors, and 454 days for cats that developed lymphoma (Schmiedt et al. 2009a).

While many types of malignant neoplasia have been reported, lymphoma is the most common, representing 36–56% of cats with PTMN (Wooldridge et al. 2002; Schmiedt et al. 2009a; Wormser et al. 2016; Durham et al. 2014). One study specifically evaluated cats with posttransplantation lymphoma (Durham et al. 2014). That study evaluated 14 cats that developed lymphoma out of a total of 25 cats with PTMN. Following a diagnosis of lymphoma, the median survival time was 2 days. Of the 7 cats with samples available for evaluation, 5 had multiple organ involvement including lymphoma in the allograft and native kidneys (Durham et al. 2014). All cats had mid- to high-grade diffuse, large B-cell lymphoma (Durham et al. 2014).

Although survival time after diagnosis of neoplasia is very short, cats that develop malignant neoplasia following transplantation do not have significantly different survival times from transplantation compared to cats without malignant neoplasia. In one study cats with PTMN had a median survival time of 646 days, whereas cats without PTMN had a median survival time of 728 days (Wormser et al. 2016). Another study documented a median survival time of 1146 days in cats that did not develop PTMN compared to 1020 days for cats that did develop PTMN (Schmiedt et al. 2009a).

That said, successful treatment of these patients is very challenging and the survival time after diagnosis of PTMN is extremely short, reported to be 2–15 days (Schmiedt et al. 2009a; Wormser et al. 2016). Treatment of these cases is made particularly challenging because of the fundamental role immunosuppression frequently plays in the pathogenesis, coupled with the fundamental need for immunosuppression to prevent allograft rejection.

Diabetes

Posttransplantation diabetes mellitus is a well-recognized complication following renal transplantation in humans and is associated with poor graft function and reduced patient survival (Sezer et al. 2006; Seifi et al. 2009). In people risk factors for developing diabetes following renal transplantation include older age, smoking, increased body mass index, hypertension, pretransplan-

tation insulin secretion abnormalities, and hypertriglyceridemia (Seifi et al. 2009; Sezer et al. 2006). Steroid, cyclosporine, and tacrolimus administration, especially at higher doses, are also known risk factors; steroids predispose for diabetes by causing insulin resistance and tacrolimus and cyclosporine predispose for diabetes because they reducing insulin secretion (van Hooff et al. 2004; Montori et al. 2002).

In cats, posttransplant diabetes mellitus has been reported to occur in approximately 14% of transplant recipients (Case et al. 2007). This incidence in cats after transplantation is 5.45 times higher than control cats with chronic kidney disease that did not have a kidney transplant, and cats that developed posttransplantation diabetes mellitus had a mortality rate 2.38 times higher than cats that underwent transplantation and did not get diabetes (Case et al. 2007). The mean time to diagnosis following renal transplantation was 287 days (31 days–10.7 years) (Case et al. 2007). In cats specific risk factors have not been identified, but in the study cited age, sex, body weight, and percentage change in body weight were not found to be risk factors in the 26 of 187 cats that developed diabetes.

In addition to optimizing diet and supplementing insulin, treatment of posttransplantation diabetes should also involve removing or minimizing steroids from the immunosuppressive regimen and optimizing the dose of cyclosporine to a 12-hour trough blood concentration between 300 and 500 ng/mL. Monitoring of all cats following transplantation should include monitoring for evidence of hyperglycemia and glucosuria.

Infection

Infection is a common complication following renal transplantation, with rates ranging between 28% and 37% (Schmiedt et al. 2008b; Kadar et al. 2005). In one study of 169 cats, 43 cats developed 47 infections a median of 2.5 months after transplantation (Kadar et al. 2005). In that study bacterial infections represented over half of the infections, followed by viral, fungal, and protozoal (Kadar et al. 2005). In another study of 60 cats that underwent kidney transplantation, 22 cats developed 26 infections at some point after surgery, with the median days to infection reported as 40.5 days (Schmiedt et al. 2008b). Just less than half of those infections occurred prior to discharge from the hospital (upper airway infection, i.v. catheter sepsis, incisional infection, and septic peritonitis) (Schmiedt et al. 2008b). Infections occurring after discharge include urinary tract infections (cystitis, pyelonephritis), oral abscessation, viral (herpesvirus, FeLV), fungal dermatitis, local or disseminated mycobacteriosis, nocardiosis, toxoplasmosis, cryptococcosis, and giardiasis (Schmiedt et al. 2008b;

Kadar *et al.* 2005; Griffin *et al.* 2003; Bernsteen *et al.* 1999a; Nordquist & Aronson 2008; Lo *et al.* 2012; Phillips *et al.* 2015; Ludwig *et al.* 2021).

Generally speaking, infections should be treated aggressively and for a longer duration than one would normally in a nonimmunosuppressed animal. Prolonged, repeated, or life-long treatments may be required to manage some infections.

Toxoplasmosis has been a challenging pathogen for immunosuppressed cats (Nordquist & Aronson 2008; Bernsteen *et al.* 1999a; Ludwig *et al.* 2021). As part of the screening process prior to transplantation, *Toxoplasma* IgM and IgG antibody titers are obtained in all cats. Cats with active infection are not candidates for transplantation, but cats that are seropositive, without evidence of an active infection, may still undergo transplantation. Those cats are prophylactically treated with clindamycin (25 mg/cat p.o. q12 h) for life (Aronson 2016; Ludwig *et al.* 2021). Trimethoprim-sulfa (15 mg/kg p.o. q12 h) has also been reported for use in cats that do not tolerate clindamycin (Aronson 2016). Some cats that were seronegative prior to transplantation have become seropositive within 3 months posttransplantation, so some surgeons recommend prophylactically treating all cats with clindamycin or retesting for IgM and IgG antibody titers several months after transplant and regularly thereafter (Aronson 2016; Ludwig *et al.* 2021). Successful renal transplantation has been performed on seropositive cats, provided life-long prophylactic treatment is provided (Ludwig *et al.* 2021).

Acute rejection

In case series of cats receiving a kidney transplant, 13–18% of cats are reported to experience rejection reactions (Mathews & Gregory 1997; Schmiedt *et al.* 2008a,b). An acute rejection reaction can develop at any time following renal transplantation, regardless of the time since transplantation. One study reported a median time to occurrence of acute rejection as 64 days (range 21–251) (Schmiedt *et al.* 2008a,b).

Cats in the early phases of acute rejection may be asymptomatic. As the rejection reaction progresses, cats may become ill, lose their appetite, vomit, and may become polyuric and polydipsic or progress to oliguria. Cats experiencing a rejection reaction may have malaise, a fever, have an enlarged and painful allograft, be azotemic, and have an inflammatory leukogram. These cats will also frequently also have a low 12-hour cyclosporine trough blood concentration, although those data are frequently not known until well after their initial presentation.

In a study of research cats that underwent renal transplantation and received no immunosuppressive medica-

tion postoperatively, 5 of 9 cats reached the study's endpoint of creatinine >7 mg/dL on days 8, 18, 18, 22, and 31. These cats had normal appetites at endpoint, and 4 of the 5 had a normal physical examination, but did have a mean weight loss of 10%. On physical examination 1 of the 5 was depressed. Of the 9 cats, 3 reached the endpoint of >20% of body weight loss after experiencing inappetence for 2–5 days on days 16, 25, and 34. The final cat was found dead on day 24, but had a normal physical examination and appetite prior and no abnormalities other than allograft rejection at necropsy examination. The conclusions of the study were that the median time to clinical rejection as defined by creatinine greater than 7 mg/dL and a loss of >20% of body weight was approximately 22 days (range 8–34) after surgery, and cats may have minimal to no clinical signs while experiencing an acute rejection reaction.

Another study evaluated allograft rejection in cats that were treated with cyclosporine and prednisolone for 14 days and then had their immunosuppressive medication discontinued (Halling *et al.* 2004). All cats had a normal contralateral native kidney for the duration of the study. Complete rejection was defined as lack of blood flow to the allograft as determined by renal ultrasound examination, and this occurred between days 21 and 26 in all cats, or 7–12 days after discontinuance of immunosuppression (Halling *et al.* 2004). During the rejection period all cats have significantly elevated rectal temperatures, but no significant changes in oxidative stress markers including serum creatinine, plasma or urinary creatol, or plasma thiobarbiturate reactive substances (Halling *et al.* 2004). Plasma lactate concentrations were significantly reduced from the preoperative to postoperative time points, as well as from postoperative to rejection time points (Halling *et al.* 2004).

Specific initiators of an acute rejection reaction may be elucidated in a particular patient's history. Cyclosporine absorption may change in a particular cat secondary to dietary lipid concentrations, ineffective administration of medication, or for another unknown reason. We have seen rejection reactions after boarding or after a person unfamiliar with the cat's medication routine takes over care of the animal. Clinically, cyclosporine blood levels commonly change without known cause and that is a critical reason to recheck blood levels frequently, especially in the months following transplantation. Cats with allografts that have been previously injured with ischemic injury in surgery or had a previous rejection reaction may have an increased likelihood of repeated rejection reactions. This is illustrated by reduced postoperative renal function and prolonged surgical time being identified as risk factors for acute rejection in cats (Schmiedt *et al.* 2008a,b).

Clinicians should have a high degree of suspicion for a rejection reaction for a recent-onset azotemia in a renal transplant recipient, particularly in a cat that has a fever. Other causes of azotemia common in transplantation recipients should be ruled out, including dehydration from some other cause like infection, postrenal obstruction from a ureteral stone or stricture, cyclosporine toxicity, and neoplasia. During a rejection reaction abdominal ultrasound examination typically demonstrates an enlarged, hyperechoic allograft with loss of corticomedullary demarcation (Schmiedt et al. 2008a). Hyperechoic changes may also include the ureter and perirenal fat. Peritoneal, or at least perirenal, effusion may be present. Significant increases in graft volume and cross-sectional area have been reported in cats experiencing acute rejection (Schmiedt et al. 2008a,b). The diagnostic utility of resistive index calculations has not been demonstrated in cats undergoing an acute rejection reaction (Schmiedt et al. 2008a,b).

Biopsy of the renal allograft maybe performed, and clinical features of acute or active rejection have been described in cats (De Cock et al. 2004). Distinct differences exist between pathologic lesions observed in cats experiencing a rejection reaction and the well-developed criteria used to score and describe acute rejection in people (De Cock et al. 2004). However, clinically biopsy is infrequently performed because of the cost, invasiveness, longer turnaround times, and lack of pathologists experienced in accurately interpreting feline renal transplant biopsies.

Treatment of rejection reactions involves intravenous doses of immunosuppressive medications, fluid diuresis, correction of electrolyte abnormalities, and other nonspecific symptomatic care. Broad-spectrum antibiotic therapy is often initiated on presentation until a urine culture can guide further care. Intravenous steroids are administered at a 2–4 mg/kg/day prednisone-equivalent dose. Intravenous cyclosporine (4 mg/kg q12 h) should be administered. If intravenous cyclosporine is not available, the oral dose of cyclosporine should be increased relative to what the cat had been receiving, at least dosing at 4 mg/kg every 12 hours. Mycophenolate mofetil (10 mg/kg i.v. q12 h) has been described as a useful immunosuppressive drug in cats (Bacek & Macintire 2011). This drug has been used as a third immunosuppressive drug in cats experiencing a significant rejection reaction or one that may not rapidly respond to immunosuppressive doses of steroids and cyclosporine. Enhanced immunosuppressive treatment and fluid diuresis continue until the creatinine reaches a plateau, at which time the cat can be weaned onto oral immunosuppressive medications. Following a rejection reaction, cats are typically treated with higher doses of steroids and cyclosporine, which are then gradually reduced over several months.

Prognosis for cats with acute rejection is good if the process is caught early and treated rapidly. In one study, 6 of 8 animals identified with acute rejection recovered and had a median survival time of 401 days after diagnosis (range 0–1056 days) (Schmiedt et al. 2008b). For animals with advanced rejection or longer-standing rejection, prognosis is more guarded. Following a single rejection episode cats may be more likely to have repeated episodes, as the allograft will typically become more antigenic with repeated injury.

In people, a different form of rejection, called chronic rejection, describes allografts with an ongoing, low level of immune reaction, an absence of acute inflammation, and no evidence of calcineurin toxicity (Hassaneir & Augustine 2020). Histologically, this type of rejection is characterized by interstitial fibrosis and tubular atrophy, and there is a gradual loss of function of the allograft. The loss of function and associated fibrosis have been historically called chronic allograft nephropathy. Lesions consistent with chronic rejection were observed in 45/77 (69%) of renal biopsy specimens in one survey of feline renal allograft biopsies (De Cock et al. 2004). Little else is known about the functional impact or significance of chronic rejection in individual feline transplant recipients or how those lesions impact the overall population of transplant recipients.

Retroperitoneal fibrosis

Retroperitoneal fibrosis has been reported in cats following renal transplantation (Wormser et al. 2013; Aronson 2002; Byer et al. 2022). The condition is characterized by the formation of fibroinflammatory tissue within the retroperitoneum, which may or may not have an obvious predisposing cause like pyelonephritis, a recent rejection reaction, or another inflammatory event (Wormser et al. 2013). In these patients, azotemia occurs as a result of ureteral obstruction. Diagnosis is often made in azotemic transplant recipients by ultrasound evidence of pyelectasia and hydronephrosis without evidence of another cause like ureteroliths and failure to find the transplanted ureter (Wormser et al. 2013). In a reported series of 138 renal transplant patients, 29 (21%) developed retroperitoneal fibrosis a median 62 days after transplantation (range 4–730 days) (Wormser et al. 2013). In that study, successful treatment with abdominal exploration and ureterolysis was performed in 25 cats (22%) (Wormser et al. 2013), while 6 cats developed recurrence 8–343 days following the first surgery and received a second ureterolysis (Wormser et al. 2013).

Another more recent student described clinically significant retroperitoneal fibrosis in 6 of 81 cats, or 7% of recipients. In this series, all affected cats had at least one subtherapeutic cyclosporine blood level postoperatively and developed clinical signs between 39 and 210 days postoperatively (Byer *et al.* 2022). The cats were taken for revision surgery; 2 died within 5 days of revision, 2 developed recurrences around 1.5 months after surgery, 1 survived long term, and 1 was lost to follow-up (Byer *et al.* 2022).

The cause of retroperitoneal fibrosis in cats is unknown and most likely multifactorial (Wormser *et al.* 2013). Suboptimal immunosuppression may play a role in its pathogenesis (Byer *et al.* 2022).

Ureteral stricture or obstruction

Ureteral obstruction or stricture is an important cause of postoperative azotemia in feline transplant recipients (Figure 52.5). Ureteral stricture or obstruction may or may not be related to retroperitoneal fibrosis or uretero-liths. Stricture may occur at the cystoneoureterostomy site or at any site where there is a bend in the ureter.

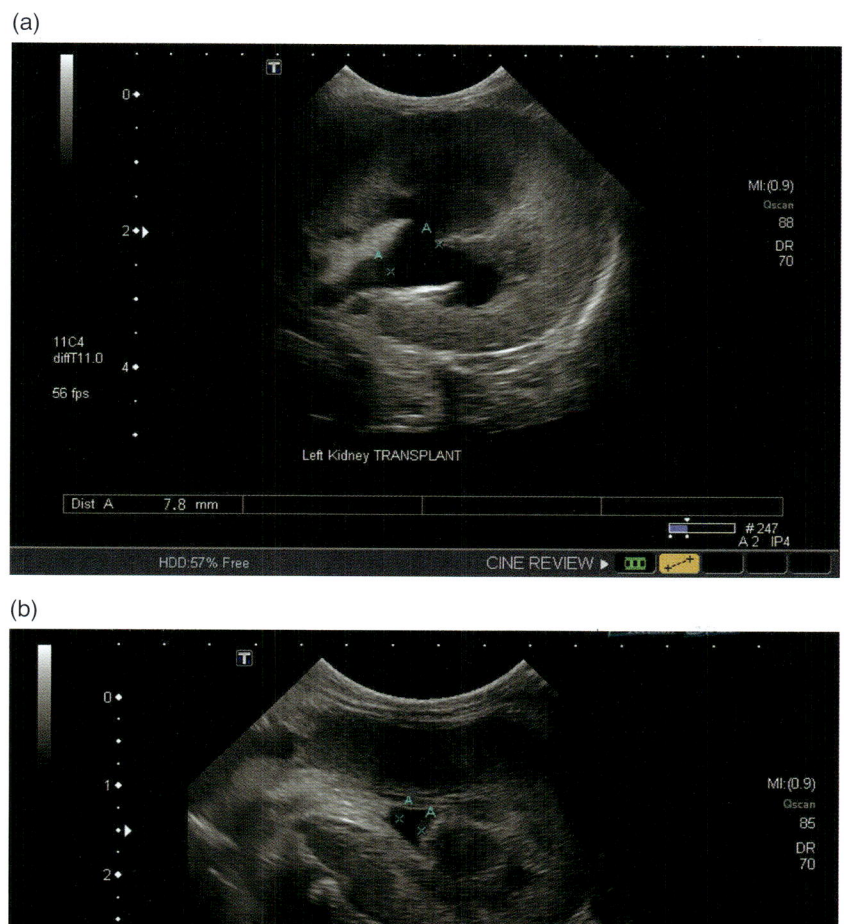

Figure 52.5 (a) Hydronephrosis following renal transplantation secondary to distal ureteral obstruction. The cat became increasingly azotemic approximately 3 weeks after renal transplantation. There was also evidence of hydroureter and a distal ureteral obstruction at the junction of the transplanted ureter and bladder. (b) A ureteroneocystostomy was performed and the hydronephrosis resolved within 1 week.

Stricture at the cystoneoureterostomy site may occur in the days or weeks after transplantation. When using the ureteral papillae transfer technique, wrapping the ureter around the bladder helps to reduce the incidence of ureteral kinking or scarring, but this still may occur, particularly as the ureter travels between the contralateral ureter and the urethra and changes direction to course more cranially. Because of the increased risk of infection with immunosuppression, ureteral obstruction should be addressed with native tissues whenever possible, and chronic use of palliative bypass devices like subcutaneous ureteral bypass devices or ureteral stents should be avoided whenever possible.

Anemia

Frequently, transplant recipients are anemic preoperatively secondary to chronic kidney disease. Acute anemia after transplantation is likely due to blood loss from surgery in the face of preexisting chronic anemia. A higher hematocrit postoperatively has been associated with an improved short-term survival rate and administration of blood products perioperatively is common (Snell *et al.* 2015).

Chronically, anemia related to chronic kidney disease typically begins to resolve in the weeks to a month after transplantation (Aronson *et al.* 2003; Mishina *et al.* 1996). Erythropoietin levels and erythrocyte indices have been evaluated in 14 cats following renal transplantation (Aronson *et al.* 2003). Anemia resolved in most cats 3–49 days after surgery (Aronson *et al.* 2003). Erythropoietin concentrations were reported to be low before transplantation and were variable postoperatively; iron was low before and after surgery (Aronson *et al.* 2003). The authors suggest that low iron may be responsible if anemia is not resolving after transplantation, and cats with poor graft function, including those that have had episodes of acute rejection, did have prolonged recovery from anemia (Aronson *et al.* 2003).

Calcineurin inhibitor nephrotoxicity

Calcineurin inhibitor toxicity can occur in the acute or chronic setting, and in current feline transplantation is almost always due to cyclosporine administration. Acute cyclosporine toxicity results in mild to moderate increases in creatinine, typically in cats with high concentrations of cyclosporine (>800 ng/mL). Cyclosporine causes constriction of the afferent arteriole secondary to impairment of endothelial cell function, resulting in reduced prostaglandin and nitric oxide production and increased thromboxane and endothelin production (Farouk & Rein 2020). Acute cyclosporine toxicity is reversible with reduction of the administered dose or temporary discontinuance to allow for reduction in blood levels. In people, risk factors for acute calcineurin inhibitor toxicity include volume depletion, diuretic use, older donor age, and concomitant use of a nonsteroidal anti-inflammatory drug or a drug that inhibits the cytochrome P450 system (Farouk & Rein 2020).

Chronic calcineurin inhibitor toxicity is ubiquitous in human transplant recipients and is a major cause of reduced allograft function over time (Farouk & Rein 2020). Histologically, lesions associated with chronic calcineurin inhibitor toxicity are very similar to lesions observed with chronic allograft nephropathy, and are thought to be a result of repeated vascular injury with allograft hypoxia by the mechanisms already described, as well as direct tubular injury (Farouk & Rein 2020). Based on the presence of tubular isometric vacuolation lesions, chronic cyclosporine toxicity was reported in 33 of 65 renal biopsy specimens from cats after renal transplants (De Cock *et al.* 2004). Little is known about the clinical consequence or typical course of chronic cyclosporine toxicity in cats.

Miscellaneous complications

Allograft rupture has been reported in a cat after renal transplantation (Palm *et al.* 2010). The cat presented for acute abdominal discomfort that progressed to hemoabdomen several days after hospitalization. At presentation the allograft was enlarged, and was found to be ruptured during a surgical abdominal exploration after hemoabdomen was diagnosed. A necropsy revealed severe chronic active lymphoplasmacytic tubulointerstitial nephritis and a *Pseudomonas* infection in the renal pelvis.

Renal pedicle torsion is observed in the acute postoperative period and was seen with more frequency in earlier reports of feline transplantation (Mathews & Gregory 1997). Developing a secure retroperitoneal pocket for the allograft and suturing the retroperitoneum to the renal capsule at the poles and renal body helps to reduce the risk of this complication (Figure 52.6).

Congestive heart failure was described in 7 of 60 cats following renal transplantation and prior to discharge from the hospital (Schmiedt *et al.* 2008b). Median time to occurrence was 3 days from surgery. Cats that experienced congestive heart failure more commonly had ages between 1 and 5 years, had a heart murmur preoperatively, had reduced graft function postoperatively, and received postoperative blood or hetastarch infusions. All cats should be screened preoperatively for evidence of heart disease. While preoperative congestive heart failure is a contraindication for renal transplantation, the amount of acceptable subclinical heart disease for a transplant recipient is unknown. In our practice, if there is evidence of atrial enlargement cats are not candidates for transplantation; however, mild to moderate thickening

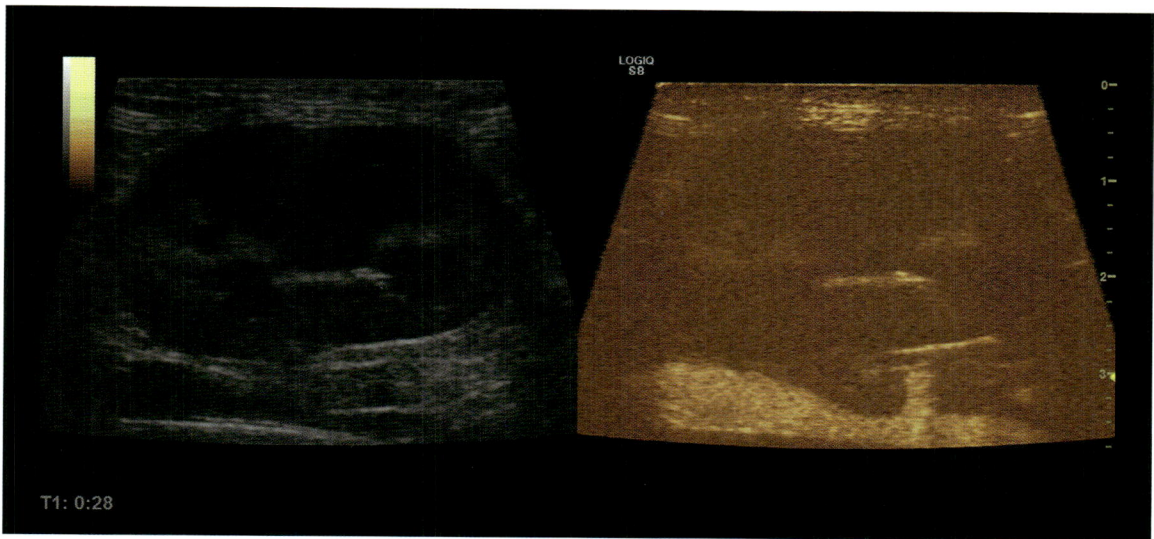

Figure 52.6 Contrast ultrasound imaging demonstrating blood flow in the aorta and proximal allograft artery of a transplanted kidney approximately 2 weeks after transplantation. The cat had become acutely azotemic approximately 1 week after discharge from the hospital. Possible diagnoses are torsion of the allograft pedicle or thromboembolism. On repeat ultrasound examinations blood flow returned to the graft, but significant functional impairment remained.

of the myocardium is acceptable. Often understanding the etiology of the myocardial thickening (hypertension vs. hypertrophic cardiomyopathy) and the rate of progression of cardiac abnormalities is not possible in a single preoperative screening examination, and multiple exams spaced by 4–6 months are not possible given the progression of kidney disease.

Survival

Reported long-term survival times are summarized in Table 52.3. Generally, acute survival has improved over time, with 80%+ of cats currently surviving the first month after surgery, but long-term survival times have remained relatively stable, with around 40% of cats alive 3 years after transplantation (Schmiedt *et al.* 2008b; Snell *et al.* 2015; Adin *et al.* 2001). Median survival time is generally around 2 years, but if only cats that survived the immediate postoperative period are considered, survival times are closer to 3 years, with 45% 3-year survival (Schmiedt *et al.* 2008b).

The human literature separates graft survival and patient survival. Often in the feline transplantation field these two items are connected. In people, other reasons for chronic graft loss include diabetes, hypertension, nonadherence to immunosuppressive therapy, hyperlipidemia, recurrence of primary kidney disease, and immunosuppressive medication toxicity (Hassanein & Augustine 2020). Many of the chronic deaths in cats are related to the effects of chronic immunosuppression, including developing cancer, complications of diabetes, or infection.

Historically, short-term survival was challenged by problems of renal pedicle torsion, seizures or other central nervous system signs, hemorrhage, or thromboembolism (Mathews & Gregory 1997). While hemorrhage and thromboembolism can still be problematic in the postoperative period, renal pedicle torsion and seizures are not common with the evolution of transplantation technique. Risk factors for survival to discharge from the hospital or survival to 30 days have been evaluated in two studies (Schmiedt *et al.* 2008b; Snell *et al.* 2015). Preoperatively, increased BUN and creatinine concentrations and left ventricular wall thickness were identified as risk factors for survival to discharge (Schmiedt *et al.* 2008b). Intraoperatively hypotension was identified as a risk factor, and postoperatively increased creatinine was identified in the same study (Schmiedt *et al.* 2008b). Another study, which evaluated 30-day survival, identified administration of a μ-opioid receptor antagonist during anesthesia recovery as a significant risk factor for survival to 30 days, and failed to confirm the risk factors already identified (Snell *et al.* 2015).

Recipient age has been a repeated finding in three studies as negatively associated with overall survival time (Adin *et al.* 2001; Schmiedt *et al.* 2008b; Snell *et al.* 2015). One study reported a median survival time of 1423 days for animals less than 5 years of age, whereas cats between 5 and 10 years of age had a median survival time of 613 days, and cats over 10 had a median survival time of 150 days (Schmiedt *et al.* 2008b). Another study reported that cats over 12 years of age had a reduced median survival time compared to cats under 12 years

Table 52.3 Survival following renal transplantation.

Reference	Year	No. of cats	Transplant center	% survival at discharge	% survival at 6 months	% survival at 3 years	Median survival (days)	Other
Mathews & Gregory (1997)	1997	66	University of California, Davis	71				28/47 cats with follow-up died median of 12 months. 18/47 cats alive median 22 months
Adin et al. (2001)	2001	61	University of California, Davis		59	41		Age influenced survival
Schmiedt et al. (2008a,b)	2008	60	University of Wisconsin—Madison	77.5	65	40	613	Age, weight, and blood pressure influenced survival
Snell et al. (2015)	2015	94	University of Pennsylvania		78	41	653	84% survived 30 days, age and anesthesia time influenced survival

(Snell *et al.* 2015). A third study documented that cats aged 10–14 years had an increased risk of death, particularly in the first 6 months after surgery, compared to cats aged 0–4 and 5–9 years (Adin *et al.* 2001). Other identified risk factors for overall survival include anesthesia time, weight, and blood pressure (Snell *et al.* 2015; Schmiedt *et al.* 2008b).

Canine renal transplantation

Although used for decades in renal transplantation research, clinical canine renal transplantation is done much less commonly and outcomes are substantially worse than feline renal transplants, for several reasons. Dogs frequently have kidney disease with a glomerular component and are more commonly proteinuric. While cats can also have proteinuric kidney disease, it is more common and frequently more severe in dogs. In part because of this, and because ongoing protein loss from the remaining native kidneys continues to be a concern after surgery, dogs have a greater problem with thromboembolic disease postoperatively compared to cats. Dogs are harder to immunosuppress than cats; their response to cyclosporine alone is often insufficient to prevent rejection, so they require a significantly more robust immunosuppressive regimen, which leaves them also more likely to develop opportunistic infections. Cost of surgery and ongoing cost of drugs are much higher in large dogs compared to cats. A medium to large dog may require $700–900/month of immunosuppressive medication, whereas ongoing costs in a cat are typically $100–150/month. Finally, although not evaluated specifically, the genetic diversity inherent in the vastly different dog breeds must contribute in some way to allograft tolerance or lack thereof. Further, dogs have more blood types and size considerations compared to cats. Logistically, canine donors are not identified and records maintained, while many centers have feline donors available.

Experimentally, a variety of immunosuppression regimens have been evaluated, with little translatable clinical success. Among other immunosuppressive drugs or strategies, donor transfusions, cyclosporine, azathioprine, leflunomide or its derivatives, mycophenolate mofetil, tacrolimus, fractionated bone marrow, antilymphocyte serum, and splenic transplantation have been evaluated experimentally in dogs (Finco *et al.* 1987; Lirtzman *et al.* 1996; Platz *et al.* 1991; Jin *et al.* 2002; Gregory *et al.* 1988a,b; Ochiai *et al.* 1987; Hartner *et al.* 1991; Ayala-Garcia *et al.* 2010).

Microemulsified cyclosporine combined with MNA 715, which is a malononitrilamide and in a class of low molecular weight immunosuppressive agents that are derivatives of leflunomide's primary metabolite, was evaluated in 8 mismatched mongrel dogs (Kyles *et al.* 2002). Of these dogs 4 lived to the study end at 100 days and the other dogs died of intussusception (2), infection (1), and acute rejection (1). These dogs did significantly better than dogs just treated with cyclosporine, which experienced a 50% rate of acute rejection and more mononuclear cell inflammation (Kyles *et al.* 2002). Another experimental study evaluated cyclosporine (20 mg/kg/day), azathioprine (5 mg/kg every other day), and prednisone (1 mg/kg/day) (Bernsteen *et al.* 2003). In that study 2/4 dogs survived to the 100-day study terminus; 1 dog developed an intussusception; and 1 dog developed a severe upper respiratory infection (Bernsteen *et al.* 2003).

Capecitabine, a pyrimidine antimetabolite 5-fluorouracil pro-drug, was evaluated with cyclosporine, ketoconazole, and prednisolone in matched and mismatched beagle dogs (Schmiedt *et al.* 2006; Milovancev *et al.* 2007). The results of those studies were promising because in most dogs good allograft function was maintained over time. However, clinically significant, sometimes fatal, neurologic and ocular toxicity developed in many of the dogs (Milovancev *et al.* 2007; Schmiedt *et al.* 2006; Zarfoss *et al.* 2007). Screening for activity of dihydropyrimidine dehydrogenase, which is a major metabolic enzyme in 5-flourouracil metabolism, prior to initiation of capecitabine therapy may identify animals more likely to have a toxic reaction (Saba *et al.* 2013).

The first reported clinical cases of dogs receiving a kidney transplant were in 1987, where outcomes of 4 dogs were reported with survival times of 0, 12, 38, and 170 days (Gregory *et al.* 1987). Dogs were maintained on cyclosporine and prednisone and died of terminal shock of unknown etiology, chronic infection, or acute rejection (Gregory *et al.* 1987). A second case series described results in 15 dogs administered cyclosporine, azathioprine, and prednisolone (Gregory *et al.* 2006). Of these dogs, 9 died within the first month, of which 5 died of complications from thromboembolism (Gregory *et al.* 2006). The remaining 6 dogs survived over 4 weeks, but bacterial infection was common, suggesting that the immunosuppression was excessive (Gregory *et al.* 2006).

Rabbit anti-dog thymocyte serum as part of the immunosuppressive regimen was described in a number of experimental models and in case series of 15 dogs (Mathews *et al.* 1993, 1994, 2000). In the clinical cases, rabbit anti-dog thymocyte serum was given with cyclosporine, azathioprine, and prednisone. The median survival time of that study was 8 months; 3 dogs died of rejection and 6 dogs died of infection; 2 dogs had a torsion of the renal pedicle, 1 developed fibrocartilaginous emboli, and 1 developed neoplasia (Mathews *et al.* 2000). All animals that were discharged developed some form of infection in the nasal cavity, skin, or urinary tract (Mathews *et al.* 2000).

More recently, 26 clinical cases of renal transplantation were reported with a median survival time of 24 days (Hopper *et al.* 2012). In that study, all dogs received microemulsified cyclosporine and some were treated with azathioprine (2–3 mg/kg every other day) or leflunomide (4–6 mg/kg once a day) (Hopper *et al.* 2012). While 7 dogs in that study lived over a year, the perioperative mortality was significant, with 8 dogs dying of thromboembolic disease (Hopper *et al.* 2012). Increasing age was associated with an increased risk of death (Hopper *et al.* 2012).

Despite decades of research, renal transplantation in dogs remains an unsolved clinical problem. Few centers offer transplantation and much, if not all, of the clinical research has stalled. New immunosuppressive drugs or therapies are needed that offer affordable and effective immunosuppression without overly predisposing recipients to opportunistic infections. Further work also needs to be done to understand peritransplantation coagulopathies, why these occur more commonly in dogs, and what can be done to prevent their occurrence.

References

Adin, C.A. (2002). Screening criteria for feline renal transplant recipients and donors. *Clinical Techniques in Small Animal Practice* 17: 184–189.

Adin, C.A., Gregory, C.R., Kyles, A.E., and Cowgill, L. (2001). Diagnostic predictors of complications and survival after renal transplantation in cats. *Veterinary Surgery* 30: 515–521.

Andre, N., Roquelaure, B., and Conrath, J. (2004). Molecular effects of cyclosporine and oncogenesis: a new model. *Medical Hypotheses* 63: 647–652.

Aronson, L.R. (2002). Retroperitoneal fibrosis in four cats following renal transplantation. *Journal of the American Veterinary Medical Association* 221: 984–9, 975.

Aronson, L.R. (2016). Update on the current status of kidney transplantation for chronic kidney disease in animals. *Veterinary Clinics of North America: Small Animal Practice* 46: 1193–1218.

Aronson, L.R., Preston, A., Bhalerao, D.P. et al. (2003). Evaluation of erythropoiesis and changes in serum erythropoietin concentration in cats after renal transplantation. *American Journal of Veterinary Research* 64: 1248–1254.

Aronson, L.R., Kyles, A.E., Preston, A. et al. (2006). Renal transplantation in cats with calcium oxalate urolithiasis: 19 cases (1997–2004). *Journal of the American Veterinary Medical Association* 228: 743–749.

Ayala-Garcia, M.A., Soel, J.M., Diaz, E. et al. (2010). Induction of tolerance in renal transplantation using splenic transplantation: experimental study in a canine model. *Transplantation Proceedings* 42: 376–380.

Bacek, L.M. and Macintire, D.K. (2011). Treatment of primary immune-mediated hemolytic anemia with mycophenolate mofetil in two cats. *Journal of Veterinary Emergency and Critical Care* 21: 45–49.

Bernsteen, L., Gregory, C.R., Aronson, L.R. et al. (1999a). Acute toxoplasmosis following renal transplantation in three cats and a dog.

Journal of the American Veterinary Medical Association 215: 1123–1126.

Bernsteen, L., Gregory, C.R., Pollard, R.E. et al. (1999b). Comparison of two surgical techniques for renal transplantation in cats. *Veterinary Surgery* 28: 417–420.

Bernsteen, L., Gregory, C.R., Kyles, A.E. et al. (2003). Microemulsified cyclosporine-based immunosuppression for the prevention of acute renal allograft rejection in unrelated dogs: preliminary experimental study. *Veterinary Surgery* 32: 213–219.

Budgeon, C., Hardie, R.J., and McAnulty, J.F. (2017). A Carrel patch technique for renal transplantation in cats. *Veterinary Surgery* 46: 1139–1144.

Byer, B.J., Hardie, R.J., and McAnulty, J.F. (2022). Retroperitoneal fibrosis as a postoperative complication following renal transplantation in cats. *Journal of Feline Medicine and Surgery* 24: 304–310.

Caceres, A.V., Zwingenberger, A.L., Aronson, L.R., and Mai, W. (2008). Characterization of normal feline renal vascular anatomy with dual-phase CT angiography. *Veterinary Radiology & Ultrasound* 49: 350–356.

Case, J.B., Kyles, A.E., Nelson, R.W. et al. (2007). Incidence of and risk factors for diabetes mellitus in cats that have undergone renal transplantation: 187 cases (1986–2005). *Journal of the American Veterinary Medical Association* 230: 880–884.

Chalhoub, S., Langston, C.E., and Farrelly, J. (2012). The use of darbepoetin to stimulate erythropoiesis in anemia of chronic kidney disease in cats: 25 cases. *Journal of Veterinary Internal Medicine* 26: 363–369.

Colombo, S. and Sartori, R. (2018). Ciclosporin and the cat: current understanding and review of clinical use. *Journal of Feline Medicine and Surgery* 20: 244–255.

Csomos, R.A., Hardie, R.J., Schmiedt, C.W. et al. (2017). Effect of cold storage on immediate graft function in an experimental model of renal transplantation in cats. *American Journal of Veterinary Research* 78: 330–339.

Danielson, K.C., Hardie, R.J., and McAnulty, J.F. (2015). Outcome of donor cats after unilateral nephrectomy as part of a clinical kidney transplant program. *Veterinary Surgery* 44: 914–919.

Darawiroj, D. and Choisunirachon, N. (2019). Morphological assessment of cat kidneys using computed tomography. *Anatomia, Histologia, Embryologia* 48: 358–365.

De Cock, H.E., Kyles, A.E., Griffey, S.M. et al. (2004). Histopathologic findings and classification of feline renal transplants. *Veterinary Pathology* 41: 244–256.

Durham, A.C., Mariano, A.D., Holmes, E.S., and Aronson, L. (2014). Characterization of post transplantation lymphoma in feline renal transplant recipients. *Journal of Comparative Pathology* 150: 162–168.

Farouk, S.S. and Rein, J.L. (2020). The many faces of calcineurin inhibitor toxicity—what the FK? *Advances in Chronic Kidney Disease* 27: 56–66.

Finco, D.R., Rawlings, C.A., Crowell, W.A. et al. (1987). Efficacy of azathioprine versus cyclosporine on kidney graft survival in transfused and nontransfused unmatched mongrel dogs. *Journal of Veterinary Internal Medicine* 1: 61–66.

Francis, M.F., Cristea, M., and Winnik, F.M. (2005). Exploiting the vitamin B12 pathway to enhance oral drug delivery via polymeric micelles. *Biomacromolecules* 6: 2462–2467.

Gregory, C.R., Gourley, I.M., Taylor, N.J. et al. (1987). Preliminary results of clinical renal allograft transplantation in the dog and cat. *Journal of Veterinary Internal Medicine* 1: 53–60.

Gregory, C.R., Gourley, I.M., Cain, G.R. et al. (1988a). Effects of combination cyclosporine/mizoribine immunosuppression on canine renal allograft recipients. *Transplantation* 45: 856–859.

Gregory, C.R., Gourley, I.M., Haskins, S.C. et al. (1988b). Effects of mizoribine on canine renal allograft recipients. *American Journal of Veterinary Research* 49: 305–311.

Gregory, C.R., Madewell, B.R., Griffey, S.M., and Torten, M. (1991). Feline leukemia virus-associated lymphosarcoma following renal transplantation in a cat. *Transplantation* 52: 1097–1099.

Gregory, C.R., Gourley, I.M., Kochin, E.J., and Broaddus, T.W. (1992). Renal transplantation for treatment of end-stage renal failure in cats. *Journal of the American Veterinary Medical Association* 201: 285–291.

Gregory, C.R., Lirtzman, R.A., Kochin, E.J. et al. (1996). A mucosal apposition technique for ureteroneocystostomy after renal transplantation in cats. *Veterinary Surgery* 25: 13–17.

Gregory, C.R., Mathews, K.G., Aronson, L.R. et al. (1997). Central nervous system disorders after renal transplantation in cats. *Veterinary Surgery* 26: 386–392.

Gregory, C.R., Kyles, A.E., Bernsteen, L., and Mehl, M. (2006). Results of clinical renal transplantation in 15 dogs using triple drug immunosuppressive therapy. *Veterinary Surgery* 35: 105–112.

Griffin, A., Newton, A.L., Aronson, L.R. et al. (2003). Disseminated *Mycobacterium avium* complex infection following renal transplantation in a cat. *Journal of the American Veterinary Medical Association* 222: 1097–1101, 1077–78.

Halling, K.B., Ellison, G.W., Armstrong, D. et al. (2004). Evaluation of oxidative stress markers for the early diagnosis of allograft rejection in feline renal allotransplant recipients with normal renal function. *Canadian Veterinary Journal* 45: 831–837.

Hardie, R.J., Schmiedt, C., Phillips, L., and McAnulty, J. (2005). Ureteral papilla implantation as a technique for neoureterocystostomy in cats. *Veterinary Surgery* 34: 393–398.

Hartner, W.C., Markees, T.G., De Fazio, S.R. et al. (1991). The effect of antilymphocyte serum, fractionated donor bone marrow, and cyclosporine on renal allograft survival in mongrel dogs. *Transplantation* 52: 784–789.

Hassanein, M. and Augustine, J.J. (2020). Chronic kidney transplant rejection. In: *StatPearls*. Treasure Island, FL: StatPearls Publishing https://www.ncbi.nlm.nih.gov/books/NBK549762.

Heilman, R.L., Mathur, A., Smith, M.L. et al. (2016). Increasing the use of kidneys from unconventional and high-risk deceased donors. *American Journal of Transplantation* 16: 3086–3092.

Hojo, M., Morimoto, T., Maluccio, M. et al. (1999). Cyclosporine induces cancer progression by a cell-autonomous mechanism. *Nature* 397: 530–534.

van Hooff, J.P., Christiaans, M.H., and van Duijnhoven, E.M. (2004). Evaluating mechanisms of post-transplant diabetes mellitus. *Nephrology, Dialysis, Transplantation* 19 (Suppl 6): vi8–vi12.

Hopper, K., Mehl, M.L., Kass, P.H. et al. (2012). Outcome after renal transplantation in 26 dogs. *Veterinary Surgery* 41: 316–327.

Jin, M.B., Nakayama, M., Ogata, T. et al. (2002). A novel leflunomide derivative, FK778, for immunosuppression after kidney transplantation in dogs. *Surgery* 132: 72–79.

Kadar, E., Sykes, J.E., Kass, P.H. et al. (2005). Evaluation of the prevalence of infections in cats after renal transplantation: 169 cases (1987–2003). *Journal of the American Veterinary Medical Association* 227: 948–953.

Katayama, M., Okamura, Y., Shimamura, S. et al. (2014). Influence of phosphate-buffered sucrose solution on early graft function in feline renal autotransplantation. *Research in Veterinary Science* 97: 409–411.

Kochin, E.J., Gregory, C.R., Wisner, E. et al. (1993). Evaluation of a method of ureteroneocystostomy in cats. *Journal of the American Veterinary Medical Association* 202: 257–260.

Kyles, A.E., Gregory, C.R., Wooldridge, J.D. et al. (1999). Management of hypertension controls postoperative neurologic disorders after renal transplantation in cats. *Veterinary Surgery* 28: 436–441.

Kyles, A.E., Gregory, C.R., Griffey, S.M. et al. (2002). An evaluation of combined immunosuppression with MNA 715 and microemulsified cyclosporine on renal allograft rejection in mismatched mongrel dogs. *Veterinary Surgery* 31: 358–366.

Kyles, A.E., Gregory, C.R., Craigmill, A.L. et al. (2003). Pharmacokinetics of tacrolimus after multidose oral administration and efficacy in the prevention of allograft rejection in cats with renal transplants. *American Journal of Veterinary Research* 64: 926–934.

Lirtzman, R.A. and Gregory, C.R. (1995). Long-term renal and hematologic effects of uninephrectomy in healthy feline kidney donors. *Journal of the American Veterinary Medical Association* 207: 1044–1047.

Lirtzman, R.A., Gregory, C.R., Levitski, R.E. et al. (1996). Combined immunosuppression with leflunomide and cyclosporine prevents MLR-mismatched renal allograft rejection in a mongrel canine model. *Transplantation Proceedings* 28: 945–947.

Lo, A.J., Goldschmidt, M.H., and Aronson, L.R. (2012). Osteomyelitis of the coxofemoral joint due to *Mycobacterium* species in a feline renal transplant recipient. *Journal of Feline Medicine and Surgery* 14: 919–923.

London, N.J., Farmery, S.M., Will, E.J. et al. (1995). Risk of neoplasia in renal transplant patients. *Lancet* 346: 403–406.

Ludwig, H.C., Schlicksup, M.D., Beale, L.M., and Aronson, L.R. (2021). *Toxoplasma gondii* infection in feline renal transplant recipients: 24 cases (1998–2018). *Journal of the American Veterinary Medical Association* 258: 870–876.

Mannon, R.B. (2018). Delayed graft function: the AKI of kidney transplantation. *Nephron* 140: 94–98.

Matas, A.J., Hays, R.E., and Ibrahim, H.N. (2017). Long-term non-end-stage renal disease risks after living kidney donation. *American Journal of Transplantation* 17: 893–900.

Mathews, K.G. and Gregory, C.R. (1997). Renal transplants in cats: 66 cases (1987–1996). *Journal of the American Veterinary Medical Association* 211: 1432–1436.

Mathews, K.A., Gallivan, G.J., and Mallard, B.A. (1993). Clinical, biochemical, and hematologic evaluation of normal dogs after administration of rabbit anti-dog thymocyte serum. *Veterinary Surgery* 22: 213–220.

Mathews, K.A., Holmberg, D.L., Johnston, K. et al. (1994). Renal allograft survival in outbred mongrel dogs using rabbit anti-dog thymocyte serum in combination with immunosuppressive drug therapy with or without donor bone marrow. *Veterinary Surgery* 23: 347–357.

Mathews, K.A., Holmberg, D.L., and Miller, C.W. (2000). Kidney transplantation in dogs with naturally occurring end-stage renal disease. *Journal of the American Animal Hospital Association* 36: 294–301.

Matos, I., Azevedo, P., and Carreira, L.M. (2018). Pilot study to evaluate the potential use of the renal resistive index as a preliminary diagnostic tool for chronic kidney disease in cats. *Journal of Feline Medicine and Surgery* 20: 940–947.

McAnulty, J.F. (1998). Hypothermic storage of feline kidneys for transplantation: successful ex vivo storage up to 7 hours. *Veterinary Surgery* 27: 312–320.

McAnulty, J.F. and Lensmeyer, G.L. (1999). The effects of ketoconazole on the pharmacokinetics of cyclosporine A in cats. *Veterinary Surgery* 28: 448–455.

Mehl, M.L., Kyles, A.E., Craigmill, A.L. et al. (2003). Disposition of cyclosporine after intravenous and multi-dose oral administration in cats. *Journal of Veterinary Pharmacology and Therapeutics* 26: 349–354.

Mehl, M.L., Kyles, A.E., Pollard, R. et al. (2005). Comparison of 3 techniques for ureteroneocystostomy in cats. *Veterinary Surgery* 34: 114–119.

Mehl, M.L., Kyles, A.E., Reimer, S.B. et al. (2006). Evaluation of the effects of ischemic injury and ureteral obstruction on delayed graft function in cats after renal autotransplantation. *Veterinary Surgery* 35: 341–346.

Mickelson, M.A., Hardie, R.J., Hespel, A.M., and Dreyfus, J. (2021). Evaluation of a microvascular anastomotic coupler for end-to-side arterial and venous anastomosis for feline renal transplantation. *Veterinary Surgery* 50: 213–222.

Milovancev, M., Schmiedt, C.W., Bentley, E. et al. (2007). Use of capecitabine to prevent acute renal allograft rejection in dog erythrocyte antigen-mismatched mongrel dogs. *Veterinary Surgery* 36: 10–20.

Mishina, M., Watanabe, T., Maeda, H. et al. (1996). Renal transplantation in cats with chronic renal failure. *Journal of Veterinary Medical Science* 58: 655–658.

Montori, V.M., Basu, A., Erwin, P.J. et al. (2002). Posttransplantation diabetes: a systematic review of the literature. *Diabetes Care* 25: 583–592.

Nordquist, B.C. and Aronson, L.R. (2008). Pyogranulomatous cystitis associated with *Toxoplasma gondii* infection in a cat after renal transplantation. *Journal of the American Veterinary Medical Association* 232: 1010–1012.

Ochiai, T., Nagata, M., Nakajima, K. et al. (1987). Studies of the effects of FK506 on renal allografting in the beagle dog. *Transplantation* 44: 729–733.

O'Keeffe, L.M., Ramond, A., Oliver-Williams, C. et al. (2018). Mid- and long-term health risks in living kidney donors: a systematic review and meta-analysis. *Annals of Internal Medicine* 168: 276–284.

Palm, C.A., Aronson, L.R., and Mayhew, P.D. (2010). Feline renal allograft rupture. *Journal of Feline Medicine and Surgery* 12: 330–333.

Phillips, H., Occhipinti, L.L., and Aronson, L.R. (2015). Septicemia and infection due to ESBL-producing *K. pneumoniae* following feline renal allograft transplantation. *Journal of the American Animal Hospital Association* 51: 119–129.

Platz, K.P., Sollinger, H.W., Hullett, D.A. et al. (1991). RS-61443—a new, potent immunosuppressive agent. *Transplantation* 51: 27–31.

Royal College of Veterinary Surgeons (2021). 27. Miscellaneous procedures: legal and ethical considerations. https://www.rcvs.org.uk/setting-standards/advice-and-guidance/code-of-professional-conduct-for-veterinary-surgeons/supporting-guidance/miscellaneous (accessed September 1, 2022).

Saba, C.F., Schmiedt, C.W., Freeman, K.G., and Edwards, G.L. (2013). Indirect assessment of dihydropyrimidine dehydrogenase activity in cats. *Veterinary and Comparative Oncology* 11: 265–271.

Schmiedt, C.W., Penzo, C., Schwab, M. et al. (2006). Use of capecitabine after renal allograft transplantation in dog erythrocyte antigen-matched dogs. *Veterinary Surgery* 35: 113–124.

Schmiedt, C.W., Delaney, F.A., and McAnulty, J.F. (2008a). Ultrasonographic determination of resistive index and graft size for evaluating clinical feline renal allografts. *Veterinary Radiology & Ultrasound* 49: 73–80.

Schmiedt, C.W., Holzman, G., Schwarz, T., and McAnulty, J.F. (2008b). Survival, complications, and analysis of risk factors after renal transplantation in cats. *Veterinary Surgery* 37: 683–695.

Schmiedt, C.W., Grimes, J.A., Holzman, G., and McAnulty, J.F. (2009a). Incidence and risk factors for development of malignant neoplasia after feline renal transplantation and cyclosporine-based immunosuppression. *Veterinary and Comparative Oncology* 7: 45–53.

Schmiedt, C.W., Hurley, K.A., Tong, X. et al. (2009b). Measurement of plasma renin concentration in cats by use of a fluorescence resonance energy transfer peptide substrate of renin. *American Journal of Veterinary Research* 70: 1315–1322.

Schmiedt, C.W., Mercurio, A.D., Glassman, M.M. et al. (2009c). Effects of renal autograft ischemia and reperfusion associated with renal transplantation on arterial blood pressure variables in clinically normal cats. *American Journal of Veterinary Research* 70: 1426–1432.

Schmiedt, C.W., Mercurio, A., Vandenplas, M. et al. (2010). Effects of renal autograft ischemic storage and reperfusion on intraoperative hemodynamic patterns and plasma renin concentrations in clinically normal cats undergoing renal autotransplantation and contralateral nephrectomy. *American Journal of Veterinary Research* 71: 1220–1227.

Seifi, S., Rahbar, M., Lessan-Pezeshki, M. et al. (2009). Posttransplant diabetes mellitus: incidence and risk factors. *Transplantation Proceedings* 41: 2811–2813.

Sezer, S., Bilgic, A., Uyar, M. et al. (2006). Risk factors for development of posttransplant diabetes mellitus in renal transplant recipients. *Transplantation Proceedings* 38: 529–532.

Smith, D., Chudgar, A., Daly, B., and Cooper, M. (2012). Evaluation of potential renal transplant recipients with computed tomography angiography. *Archives of Surgery* 147: 1114–1122.

Snell, W., Aronson, L., Phillips, H. et al. (2015). Influence of anesthetic variables on short-term and overall survival rates in cats undergoing renal transplantation surgery. *Journal of the American Veterinary Medical Association* 247: 267–277.

Stock, E., Paepe, D., Daminet, S. et al. (2018). Contrast-enhanced ultrasound examination for the assessment of renal perfusion in cats with chronic kidney disease. *Journal of Veterinary Internal Medicine* 32: 260–266.

Sutherland, B.J., McAnulty, J.F., and Hardie, R.J. (2016). Ureteral papilla implantation as a technique for neoureterocystostomy in cats undergoing renal transplantation: 30 cases. *Veterinary Surgery* 45: 443–449.

Tipisca, V., Murino, C., Cortese, L. et al. (2016). Resistive index for kidney evaluation in normal and diseased cats. *Journal of Feline Medicine and Surgery* 18: 471–476.

Urie, B.K., Tillson, D.M., Smith, C.M. et al. (2007). Evaluation of clinical status, renal function, and hematopoietic variables after unilateral nephrectomy in canine kidney donors. *Journal of the American Veterinary Medical Association* 230: 1653–1656.

Valverde, C.R., Gregory, C.R., and Ilkiw, J.E. (2002). Anesthetic management in feline renal transplantation. *Veterinary Anaesthesia and Analgesia* 29: 117–125.

Wooldridge, J.D. and Gregory, C.R. (1999). Ionized and total serum magnesium concentrations in feline renal transplant recipients. *Veterinary Surgery* 28: 31–37.

Wooldridge, J.D., Gregory, C.R., Mathews, K.G. et al. (2002). The prevalence of malignant neoplasia in feline renal-transplant recipients. *Veterinary Surgery* 31: 94–97.

Wormser, C. and Aronson, L.R. (2016). Perioperative morbidity and long-term outcome of unilateral nephrectomy in feline kidney donors: 141 cases (1998–2013). *Journal of the American Veterinary Medical Association* 248: 275–281.

Wormser, C., Phillips, H., and Aronson, L.R. (2013). Retroperitoneal fibrosis in feline renal transplant recipients: 29 cases (1998–2011). *Journal of the American Veterinary Medical Association* 243: 1580–1585.

Wormser, C., Mariano, A., Holmes, E.S. et al. (2016). Post-transplant malignant neoplasia associated with cyclosporine-based immunotherapy: prevalence, risk factors and survival in feline renal transplant recipients. *Veterinary and Comparative Oncology* 14: e126–e134.

Zarfoss, M., Bentley, E., Milovancev, M. et al. (2007). Histopathologic evidence of capecitabine corneal toxicity in dogs. *Veterinary Pathology* 44: 700–702.

Section 8

Reproductive Tract

53

Pyometra

Natali Krekeler and Fiona Hollinshead

Pyometra is an acute or chronic suppurative infection with accumulation of pus in the uterine lumen in predominantly middle-aged to aged bitches. Up to 24% of intact bitches develop pyometra before 10 years of age (Egenvall *et al.* 2001).

Pathophysiology

Originally, cystic endometrial hyperplasia (CEH) and pyometra were defined as one disease entity. It was believed that the condition of CEH arose first and therefore predisposed the uterus to secondary bacterial infection, which resulted in pyometra. More recently, it has been proposed that the two conditions be distinguished as (i) cystic endometrial hyperplasia–mucometra complex and (ii) endometritis–pyometra complex. Although both diseases bear many similarities with each other and can be found as subsequent events, the conditions have the potential to derive *de novo* (De Bosschere *et al.* 2001). Any stimulus in a progesterone-influenced uterus can lead to CEH and therefore the presence of CEH in pyometra could merely be the result of a uterine reaction to the bacterial infection (Figure 53.1). Another condition that grossly resembles CEH but is highly organized, often localized, and histologically similar to placentation sites has been proposed to be named "pseudo-placentational endometrial hyperplasia" (Schlafer & Gifford 2008).

The pathogenesis of pyometra is not thoroughly understood. It is currently believed that pyometra results from the interaction of *Escherichia coli* (*E. coli*) with the progesterone-influenced canine uterus. Research is focusing on the variation in bacterial pathogenicity in combination with uterine pathology and potentially impaired host immune function.

Predisposing factors

Many factors, such as the influence of age, ovarian hormones, breed, parity, and treatment with exogenous hormones, have been shown to play a role in the development of the disease. Pyometra has initially been described as a condition of older, ovary-intact bitches that still undergo estrous cycles. The mean age is between 7 and 8.5 years, although a range from 4 months to 18 years has been reported. A breed predisposition has been reported for the golden retriever, Cavalier King Charles spaniel, miniature schnauzer, Irish terrier, rough Saint Bernard, Leonberger, Airedale terrier, rough collie, and Rottweiler. Other breeds, such as dachshunds and fox terriers, were underrepresented (Egenvall *et al.* 2001).

Pyometra is believed to be facilitated by the unique canine estrous cycle, during which an estrogen phase is followed by a relatively long progesterone-dominated phase (diestrus). The length of the diestrus phase in a nonpregnant bitch is not significantly shorter than that of a pregnant bitch, suggesting that a luteolytic mechanism, as present in other domestic species, is missing in the dog (Concannon *et al.* 1989; Hoffmann *et al.* 2004). Studies show that the overwhelming proportion of affected bitches present within 2–12 weeks of their last heat (Børresen 1979; Blendinger & Bostedt 1991). Under the influence of progesterone, uterine leukocyte inhibition and myometrial contractions are decreased, which supports bacterial growth (Borel *et al.* 1999). The progesterone influence in diestrus results in uterine stromal

Small Animal Soft Tissue Surgery, Second Edition. Edited by Eric Monnet.
© 2023 John Wiley & Sons, Inc. Published 2023 by John Wiley & Sons, Inc.
Companion website: www.wiley.com/go/monnet/small

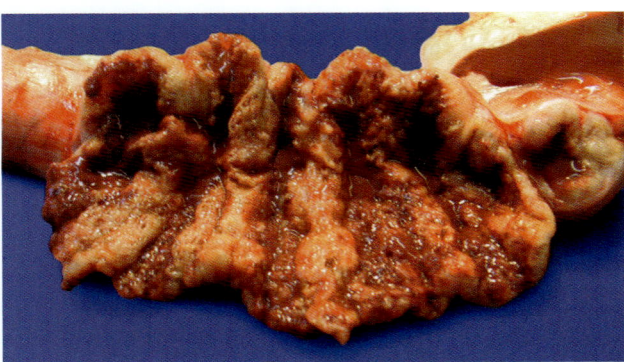

Figure 53.1 An opened uterine horn from a bitch with pyometra. Note the degree of cystic endometrial change in the uterine wall. Although both cystic endometrial hyperplasia (CEH) and pyometra bear many similarities to each other, the conditions have the potential to derive *de novo*. Any stimulus in a progesterone-influenced uterus can lead to CEH and therefore the presence of CEH in pyometra could merely be the result of a uterine reaction to the bacterial infection.

and glandular epithelial proliferation and increased glandular secretion (Lee *et al.* 2006). These effects are cumulative. Therefore, the risk of uterine disease increases with each estrous cycle (Sugiura *et al.* 2004).

Although there is no evidence of abnormal ovarian hormone concentrations in the pathogenesis of pyometra, it has been shown that progesterone is necessary to initiate a CEH reaction and estrogen potentiates the effect (Chen *et al.* 2001; Noakes *et al.* 2001). Exogenous administration, especially of estradiol early in diestrus ("mismating shot"), can be linked to an increased risk of developing the disease.

The role of E. coli

In diestrus, the most common time for the diagnosis of pyometra, the uterus of healthy bitches has been found to be free of cultivable bacterial growth (Watts *et al.* 1996). Uropathogenic *E. coli* is the most commonly isolated pathogen from canine uteri with pyometra (>90% of cases) (Fransson *et al.* 1997; Chen *et al.* 2003). Other, mostly vaginal commensals have sometimes been reported (e.g., *Streptococcus canis*, *Staphylococcus aureus*, *Proteus* spp., *Klebsiella* spp.). *E. coli* can also be found in the intestine of dogs, where it is not pathogenic (Wådas *et al.* 1996; Chen *et al.* 2003). However, *E. coli* possess specific uropathogenic virulence factors (UVF) that augment pathogenicity in the urinary and genital tracts (Lloyd *et al.* 2007). Biochemical fingerprinting has shown that the same bacterial strains isolated from the uterus in bitches affected by pyometra and urinary tract infections are also found in the feces of these dogs (Wådas *et al.* 1996). Therefore, *E. coli* isolates in bitches with pyometra are thought to be derived from normal

bacterial flora in the intestine and are not specific "infectious strains" spread between animals. The urinary tract and the vagina are thought to function as bacterial reservoirs and bacteria ascend into the uterus during estrus while the cervix is relaxed.

UVFs of *E. coli* include fimbrial adhesins, toxins, host defense avoidance mechanisms (capsule or somatic-specific antigen), and a number of iron-acquisition systems (Johnson 1991). Since attachment to the mucosal surface is a critical first step in facilitating microbial persistence and starting the "cross-talk" with the host that triggers the inflammatory response, research has focused on adhesins. The UVFs best known for their involvement in adhesion of *E. coli* to the urinary epithelium are type-1, P, and S pili. They have all been found in *E. coli* isolated from canine pyometra (Chen *et al.* 2003). FimH, the mannose-binding lectin of type-1 pili, has been demonstrated to facilitate bacterial binding to the canine endometrial epithelium (Krekeler *et al.* 2012). However, in a pyometra disease model it has been shown that the disease could only be induced reliably if *E. coli* were inoculated into the uterus during diestrus. Inoculation in estrus or anestrus did not result in pyometra (Arora *et al.* 2006). This suggests that the bitch's immune response differs during different stages of the estrous cycle.

The role of the host's immune response

Data on changes in immune response during different stages of the estrous cycle in the bitch are very limited. No significant difference was observed between prostaglandin gene expression in anestrus and diestrus uteri. Uteri with pyometra did show an increase in cyclooxygenase (COX)-2, *PGFS*, and *mPGES-1* gene transcription, believed to be the result of an *E. coli*-stimulated endotoxin release (Silva *et al.* 2009). A reduced proliferative response of peripheral blood monocytes to an *E. coli* pyometra strain was observed in diestrus compared with other stages of the cycle (Sugiura *et al.* 2004). Mucin-1 is part of the epithelial cell glycocalyx and has been shown to be increased in estrus and decreased in diestrus. Furthermore, it is negatively correlated to *E. coli* binding to epithelial cells (Ishiguro *et al.* 2007).

The role of the bitch's immune response has been emphasized by the diagnosis of endometritis in the bitch. It was widely believed that endometritis did not exist in the canine species and that a bacterial infection would always result in pyometra. However, more recent studies have shown that bacteria could be isolated from subfertile bitches without showing the hallmarks of pyometra. Interestingly, the mean age of these bitches was lower than those with pyometra (Fontaine *et al.* 2009). This suggests that bitches might contain bacteria in the form of subclinical endometritis for quite some time before some unknown factors allow bacterial proliferation and subsequent pyometra. This is concurrent with the finding that *E. coli* can undergo biofilm formation (Fiamengo *et al.* 2020), which may allow them to persist in the uterus for a prolonged period of time before causing disease at an opportune time, for example when increased uterine pathologies or a compromised host immune defense occurs. The biofilm state would also explain the inability to culture bacteria in diestrus. The presence of bacteria that are not cultivable by traditional methods has also been demonstrated in a microbiome study, as bacterial richness in diestrus was comparable to anestrus and estrus (Lyman *et al.* 2019).

Pyometra in cats

Pyometra in cats is believed to have a similar pathophysiology as in dogs. However, due to the characteristics of the feline estrous cycle, the presentation differs. Being induced ovulators, cats, unlike dogs, usually have repeated estrous cycles if ovulation does not occur through mating or artificial induction. However, cats can also undergo spontaneous ovulation (Lawler *et al.* 1993), which leads on to a progesterone-dominated diestrus phase or pseudopregnancy for approximately 40 days, which predisposes them to the development of CEH and subsequent pyometra. Therefore, cats with pyometra present most often 2–5 weeks after estrous in which they have either undergone mating and induced ovulation or a spontaneous ovulation. Interestingly, corpora lutea are only present in about half of the cases of pyometra. As in dogs, CEH can often be observed in cats at time of hysterectomy. Oriental purebred cats have a higher incidence of pyometra than other breeds, which correlates with an increased spontaneous ovulation rate in those cats (Hagman *et al.* 2014).

Clinical signs

The degree of systemic illness depends largely on the integrity of the cervix. In a "closed-cervix" pyometra, dogs presented are commonly systemically ill because of the endotoxemia resulting from the build-up and subsequent resorption of *E. coli* toxins in the uterine lumen. Bacteremia can also occur. In an "open-cervix" pyometra, a bloody, purulent vulvar discharge might be the only clinical sign. However, systemic clinical signs are often observed concurrently or in cases of closed-cervix pyometra. Systemic clinical signs secondary to pyometra are associated with renal and hepatic dysfunction, anemia, heart arrhythmias, and/or hypoglycemia. Pyrexia is not always present in cases of pyometra.

Prerenal azotemia, with elevated serum blood urea nitrogen (BUN) and creatinine levels, can be observed due to poor renal perfusion as a result of shock or dehydration. The commonly observed polyuria is due to tubular insensitivity to antidiuretic hormone caused by *E. coli* endotoxins. This results in reduced tubular concentrating ability. Polydipsia is a compensatory effect of the polyuria. The observed proteinuria is attributed to a significant glomerulopathy, a result of immune-complex deposition. Membranoproliferative glomerulonephritis has commonly been associated with pyometra, but recent studies dispute this and attribute the histologic changes purely to glomerular sclerosis of aging dogs (Heiene *et al.* 2007). Especially polyuria and polydipsia are usually reversed quite quickly after surgical or medical treatment of the disease. However, proteinuria seems to be a valuable prognostic indicator for postsurgical progression to renal failure.

Hypoalbuminemia and hypercholesterolemia can be observed and are attributed to an acute-phase reaction. Hepatocellular damage can lead to a mild to moderate increase in serum level of the liver enzymes alanine aminotransferase and, particularly, alkaline phosphatase, which is commonly elevated.

Nonregenerative, mostly normocytic, and normochromic anemia can result from suppressed erythropoiesis caused by chronic inflammation and bacterial toxins. Serum iron levels are low and iron is sequestered by myeloid macrophages, presumably to limit the iron availability for iron-dependent bacteria such as *E. coli*. Leukocytosis, which is commonly present, results in an increased myeloid to erythroid ratio in the bone marrow. Leucopenia seems to be a good prognostic indicator for the development of peritonitis (Jitpean *et al.* 2014). Myeloid proliferation as well as extramedullary myelopoiesis in spleen, lymph nodes, and liver are features of the condition.

Cardiac arrhythmias and myocardial injury can occur due to endotoxins, shock, or electrolyte imbalances.

Diagnosis

Signalment

- Commonly middle-aged to old intact bitches (>6 years), but age at presentation can range from as early as 4 months to more than 16 years.
- Present within 8–12 weeks of their last estrus.
- Breed predisposition.
- Treatment with exogenous estrogens for misalliance or long-term, high-dose use of progestogens.
- Nulliparous bitches have a higher incidence.

- Spayed bitches may present with a "stump" pyometra if they concurrently have ovarian remnant syndrome or have received exogenous hormone therapy.

History

The most important historical finding is to establish the time that has elapsed since the last estrus, and if the administration of exogenous progesterones or estrogens has occurred. Owners' observation of polydipsia, polyuria, apathy, anorexia, vomiting, abdominal distension, and/or vaginal discharge should be noted.

Clinical examination

Pyrexia is sometimes present, although hypothermia, attributed to endotoxemia, has also been observed in some bitches. Mucous membranes can be pale or in cases of severe septic shock show petechial hemorrhages. Hemopurulent vaginal discharge may or may not be present depending on the patency of the cervix. Assessment of uterine distension by abdominal palpation should be undertaken very carefully, as the enlarged pus-filled uterus can be friable and prone to rupture.

Clinical signs are not definitive, and therefore pyometra should be suspected in any ovary-intact bitch presenting 4–12 weeks after having been in heat with any of the following signs: vaginal discharge, depression, polydipsia, polyuria, vomiting, and/or pyrexia.

Laboratory findings

An elevated white blood cell count (average 37×10^9/L) is typical for pyometra (70% of cases) and is mainly due to a neutrophilia with a left shift. Toxic change is often observed. However, in some cases the white cell count can be lower than the reference range due to the pooling of neutrophils in the uterus. Hypergammaglobulinemia, hypoalbuminemia, hypercholesterolemia, and elevation in C-reactive protein can be found frequently in pyometra cases. Increase in serum levels of liver enzymes (alanine aminotransferase and alkaline phosphatase), BUN, and creatinine can be attributed to the consequences of sepsis and/or dehydration. Severe vomiting or diarrhea can result in electrolyte imbalances. In general, laboratory abnormalities tend to be more severe in animals with a closed-cervix pyometra.

Urinalysis may be performed by ultrasound-guided cystocentesis and might reveal isosthenuria, bacteriuria, glucosuria, and/or proteinuria. Urine should be collected via guided cystocentesis to exclude the risk of uterine puncture and subsequent peritoneal contamination with uterine contents. A midstream urine sample can be used for culture and sensitivity, as the causative agent is often also located in the bladder. However, a bacterial culture and especially sensitivity are best performed on a sample taken from the cranial vagina using a long-guarded swab, such as the swabs used in mares for obtaining uterine cytologic samples. However, antibiotic treatment should commence immediately on the assumption that *E. coli* is the most likely isolate.

Cytologic examination of either the vulval discharge or a vaginal swab will reveal degenerate neutrophils and phagocytosed bacteria.

Brucella canis can be the causal bacterial agent for pyometra, so performing a serologic assay such as a rapid slide agglutination test to screen for the presence of *B. canis* is recommended.

Serum levels of the hormone progesterone in most cases of pyometra will be >2 ng/mL. However, some bitches present in anestrus with a chronic pyometra. This is important to confirm before initiating medical therapy (see later).

Diagnostic imaging and vaginoscopy

Ultrasonography is the method of choice for the diagnosis of pyometra. The tubular uterine horns appear distended and filled with heterogenic fluid (Figure 53.2). The uterine wall is commonly thickened and shows irregular edges with small hypoechoic areas, which are consistent with cystic changes of the uterine glands (Figure 53.3). However, if the uterus is severely distended with fluid, the uterine wall can appear thinned.

Abdominal radiographs can be taken to confirm uterine distension (Figure 53.4). Fetal skeletal ossification is only visible after day 45 following the luteinizing hormone (LH) peak. Prior to that, a distinction between uterine distension as a result of pyometra or pregnancy is not possible.

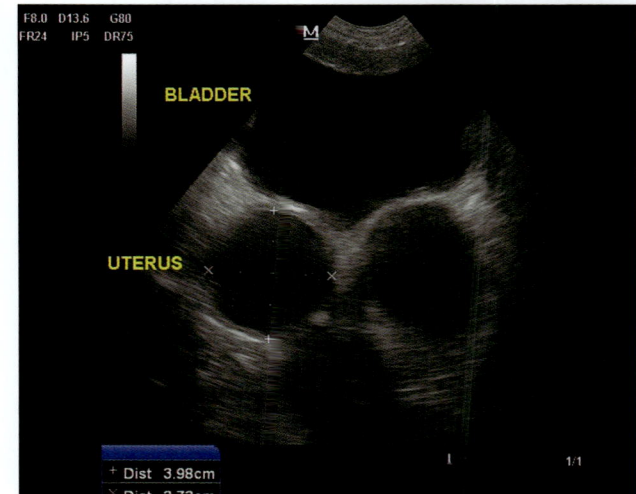

Figure 53.2 Ultrasonographic image of the caudal abdomen of a bitch with loops of fluid-filled uterine horns in pyometra. Source: Courtesy of Dr. Michelle Kutzler, Oregon State University, USA.

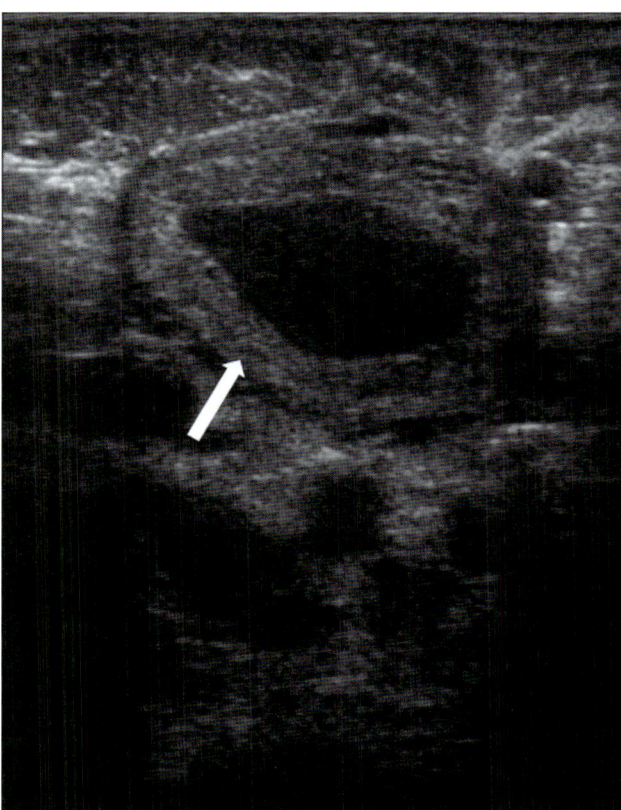

Figure 53.3 Ultrasonographic image of the caudal abdomen of a bitch with pyometra. Note the fluid-filled uterus and thickened uterine wall with evidence of cystic changes (arrow).

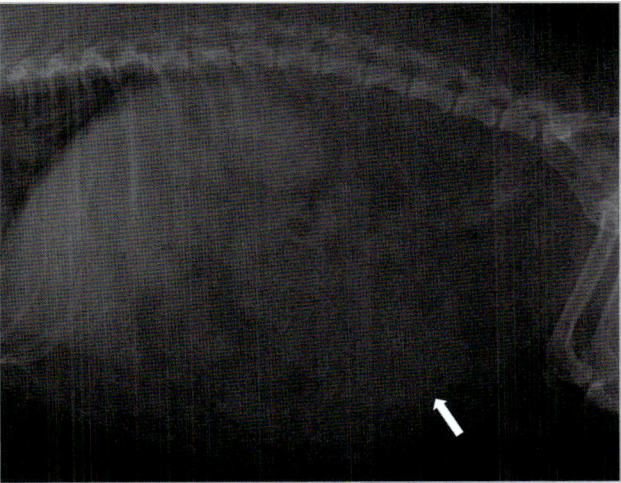

Figure 53.4 Lateral abdominal radiographic image. Note the fluid-filled uterus (arrow). Source: Courtesy of Melbourne Veterinary Hospital, Victoria, Australia.

Performing vaginoscopy and a urinalysis is indicated in dogs with purulent vulval discharge but without apparent uterine enlargement and/or systemic clinical signs. Determination of the anatomic origin of the purulent discharge will help to differentiate between pyometra, vaginitis, and cystitis.

Differential diagnosis

See Table 53.1.

Uterine enlargement

- Mucometra, hemometra, hydrometra (not associated with systemic clinical signs and neutrophilia).
- Pregnancy (can be excluded by ultrasonography 25 days after the LH peak or by radiography 42 days after the LH peak).
- Metritis, retained fetal membrane (typically within first days postpartum).

Systemic clinical signs

- Polyuria and polydipsia.
- Diabetes mellitus.
- Hyperadrenocorticism.
- Renal disease.
- Diabetes insipidus (not usually associated with leukocytosis).

Purulent vulvar discharge

- Vaginitis (primary/congenital or secondary/acquired).
- Perivulval dermatitis.

Treatment

Pyometra in the bitch can be treated either surgically or medically and, in some cases, treatment with a combination of both therapies can be effective. Historically, pyometra has most commonly been treated by ovariohysterectomy (OVH). However, with the recent development of new pharmacologic agents and treatment protocols, canine pyometra can be successfully treated medically with appropriate case selection. Initial medical treatment to initiate cervical opening and drainage of pus, in patients presenting with a closed pyometra prior to surgery, can be beneficial to facilitate stabilization of systemic derangements associated with endotoxemia, bacteremia, and sepsis. This can reduce the morbidity and mortality that can be associated with anesthesia and immediate surgical treatment. Bitches left untreated can die, but even with treatment the mortality rate of bitches affected by pyometra is 4% (Verstegen *et al.* 2008).

Indications for surgical treatment or medical therapy

Indications for surgical treatment of pyometra include bitches without significant reproductive value or not intended for future breeding, emergency presentations

Table 53.1 Most common characteristics in canine pyometra.

Clinical presentation		Comments
Signalment	Nulliparous, diestral bitches >6 years	Also in young dogs; exogenous hormones and breed predisposition
Clinical signs	Vaginal discharge, lethargy, anorexia, polyuria, polydipsia, vomiting	
Laboratory findings		
White blood cells	WBC >35 × 109/L Neutrophilia with left shift/toxic change	Normal leukocyte count and leukopenia possible
Red blood cells	Packed cell volume <35	Dehydration can mask anemia
Serum biochemistry	Hyperproteinemia, hyperglobulinemia, elevated ALP, ALT, BUN	ALP elevation in 50–75% of cases
Urinalysis	Proteinuria, bacteriuria	Proteinuria is a prognostic indicator for post-treatment renal failure
Progesterone concentration	>2–4 ng/mL	Can be <2 ng/mL in open-cervix pyometra
Diagnostic imaging		
Ultrasonography	Thick-walled tubular uterus filled with hypoechoic/heterogenic fluid	
Radiography	Fluid-dense tubular structure	Pregnancy can only be detected more than 42 days post LH peak

ALP, alkaline phosphatase; ALT, alanine aminotransferase; BUN, blood urea nitrogen; LH, luteinizing hormone; WBC, white blood cell count.

such as uterine rupture or torsion concurrent with pyometra, and older bitches (>4 years), especially those with significant cystic and degenerative endometrial changes detected on ultrasound. Additionally, bitches that are refractory, bitches that have been treated medically previously, or chronic cases that do not readily respond to medical treatment are also candidates for OVH. Historically, closed pyometra was an indication for surgical management. However, uterine rupture is a very rare event and many cases of closed pyometra are successfully managed with careful medical therapy aimed at opening the cervix. Medical treatment is only recommended for young, genetically valuable breeding bitches (<4 years old) that are not azotemic or systemically unwell.

Medical management of pyometra

The primary objectives of medical management of canine pyometra are to (i) remove the effects of progesterone by inducing luteolysis or preventing progesterone from binding to its receptors; (ii) promote the emptying/drainage of the pus-filled uterus by inducing cervical relaxation and myometrial contractions; and (iii) inhibit further proliferation of bacteria and their release of endotoxins through the use of broad-spectrum antibiotics.

Ecbolic and luteolytic therapy

Repeated doses of prostaglandin $PGF_{2\alpha}$ result in luteolysis of the canine corpus luteum. The resultant reduction in progesterone concentrations promotes cervical relaxation and reduction in uterine secretions. $PGF_{2\alpha}$ also stimulates myometrial contractions, which facilitate drainage of pus from the uterus. There are two forms of $PGF_{2\alpha}$: its natural form (dinoprosttromethamine) and synthetic derivatives (e.g., cloprostenol). Natural $PGF_{2\alpha}$ induces greater myometrial contractions and therefore faster evacuation of pus from the uterus compared with synthetic $PGF_{2\alpha}$. However, cloprostenol has been associated with fewer side effects and requires fewer injections due to its longer half-life. Different dose rates apply to each of the different forms of $PGF_{2\alpha}$. Use of high doses of $PGF_{2\alpha}$ in the past has been associated with a number of detrimental side effects, including hypersalivation, vomiting, diarrhea, pyrexia, and panting. In rare cases, uterine rupture (especially if the cervix is closed), shock, and death can potentially occur. $PGF_{2\alpha}$ has a very small therapeutic index, so use of low doses and administration by an intramuscular or subcutaneous route are imperative. Recently developed treatment regimens, involving low doses of natural forms of $PGF_{2\alpha}$ with small incremental dosage increases, have been used very successfully in the bitch with minimal or no

Table 53.2 Dosages of commonly used luteolytic, antiluteotrophic, and antiprogestogenic drugs for the medical treatment of canine pyometra.

Drug	Dosage	Protocol	Action
PGF2a			
Dinoprosttromethamine	10 μg/kg s.c.	Five times on day 1	Luteolysis
	25 μg/kg s.c.	Five times on day 2	Myometrial contractions
	50 μg/kg s.c.	Five times daily on days 3–7[a]	Cervical opening
Cloprostenol	1 μg/kg s.c.	Once daily	
Dopamine agonists			
Cabergoline	5 μg/kg p.o.	Once daily for 7 days	Antiprolactin, antiluteotrophic
Bromocriptine	10–25 μg/kg p.o.	Three times daily for 7 days	
Antiprogestin			
Aglepristone	10 mg/kg s.c.	Days 1, 2, and 8	Progesterone receptor antagonist
PGE1			
Misoprostol	10 μg/kg p.o.	Days 1, 2, and 3	Cervical opening
	200 μg (<20 kg) intravaginally		
	400 μg (>20 kg) intravaginally		

p.o., orally; s.c., subcutaneously.

[a] Depending on response to treatment.

side effects. The recommended treatment protocol (Table 53.2) for pyometra with dinoprosttromethamine (Lutalyse®, Zoetis, Parsippany, NJ, USA) is to start with 10 μg/kg subcutaneously 3–5 times on the first day, then 25 μg/kg subcutaneously 3–5 times on the second day, and then 50 μg/kg subcutaneously 3–5 times daily until resolution (Verstegen *et al.* 2008). Doses greater than 50 μg/kg should not often be required. Side effects at these low doses are rare, and if they occur it is usually within 20–30 minutes after administration and they do not last longer than 30 minutes.

Side effects are usually only seen at the start of treatment, as bitches tend to develop tolerance to $PGF_{2\alpha}$ if it is started at these low doses and slowly increased in a tapered manner. There is some variation in tolerance to $PGF_{2\alpha}$ between individuals, with some bitches tolerating more rapid dose increases than others.

It is recommended not to feed the patient or administer oral antibiotics prior to treatment in case vomiting occurs. The recommended dose for the synthetic form of $PGF_{2\alpha}$ (cloprostenol) is 1 μg/kg subcutaneously once a day. This is commonly used with other pharmacologic agents. Greater side effects and prolonged resolution are often seen with this single-dose regimen of synthetic $PGF_{2\alpha}$. In many countries the use of $PGF_{2\alpha}$ in dogs is off-label, and consent from the owner before treatment is required.

Dopamine agonists can also be used for the treatment of pyometra in the bitch. Dopamine agonists are ergot-derived alkaloid compounds that have antiprolactin activity. They can therefore be used from 25 days after ovulation when prolactin is present to treat pyometra through an antiluteotrophic activity. There are two commonly used dopamine agonists: cabergoline and bromocriptine. Cabergoline is associated with few to no side effects and involves once-daily administration compared with bromocriptine, which requires administration 2–3 times a day and is associated with a number of side effects, including vomiting, anorexia, depression, and some behavioral changes.

Dopamine agonists are commonly used in combination with $PGF_{2\alpha}$ as together they potentiate the luteolytic effect, resulting in more rapid luteolysis, a faster subsequent drop in progesterone concentration, and cervical opening within 24–48 hours. The recommended dose for cabergoline is 5 μg/kg orally each 24 hours for 7 days, and for bromocriptine is 10–25 μg/kg orally three times a day for 7 days when used in combination with natural or synthetic $PGF_{2\alpha}$ (Table 53.2).

Progesterone receptor antagonists or "antiprogestins" are synthetic steroids that reversibly bind to progesterone receptors with a greater affinity than natural progesterone, resulting in decreased progesterone activity and reduction of bacteria adhering to the surface of the endometrium (Galac *et al.* 2000; Arnold *et al.* 2006). The progesterone receptor antagonists include aglepristone (Alizin®, Virbac, Carros, France) and mifepristone. Aglepristone has minimal or no side effects and has been used very effectively to treat closed pyometra, as it causes cervical opening with no or minimal uterine contractions. It is best used in combination with $PGF_{2\alpha}$ to potentiate luteolysis and stimulate uterine contractions. Initiation of aglepristone treatment 24–48 hours prior to $PGF_{2\alpha}$ treatment may also reduce the risk of uterine rupture in a closed pyometra. Aglepristone can be used alone to treat pyometra, but is more effective when used in combination with $PGF_{2\alpha}$ (Gobello *et al.* 2003; Fieni 2006) or misoprostol, which is a synthetic PGE1 analog that also facilitates cervical opening. The recommended dose of aglepristone is 10 mg/kg subcutaneously on days 1, 2, and 8. An additional injection of aglepristone can be given on day 14 or 15 after the onset of treatment if resolution of the pyometra has not occurred. Bitches that present with poor liver and kidney function should not be medically treated with aglepristone.

Antimicrobial treatment

The most commonly isolated pathogen from canine uteri with pyometra is *E. coli*. Therefore, initiation of empirical treatment pending culture and sensitivity results with a broad-spectrum antibiotic such as ampicillin (22 mg/kg orally [p.o.] three times daily), amoxicillin, and clavulanic acid (12.5–25 mg/kg p.o. 2–3 times daily), or cefazolin (22 mg/kg intravenously [i.v.] or intramuscularly [i.m.] three times daily) is indicated. Broad-spectrum antibiotic therapy should be initiated immediately. A culture and sensitivity on either the vaginal discharge or, preferably, a sample of uterine fluid is important, as infections with antibiotic-resistant organisms or pathogens such as *Pseudomonas* can occur. Antibiotic treatment should be continued for 10–14 days after resolution of the pyometra (see the following assessment parameters).

Assessing response to therapy

There are a number of parameters that should be measured and assessed throughout the medical management of a bitch with pyometra that indicate the response to treatment and determine when luteolytic treatment can cease or surgical treatment needs to be implemented. After initiation of medical therapy, a clinical improvement is usually seen within 48 hours. Resolution of all clinical signs should occur within 7–10 days.

Monitoring of vaginal discharge is important. A significant increase in the volume of purulent uterine discharge is usually seen within 24 hours of treatment. The nature of the vaginal discharge will gradually change, from purulent to serosanguineous and eventually serous. Complete emptying of the uterus is typically achieved after 5–7 days of medical treatment. $PGF_{2\alpha}$ treatment should be continued for as long as a vaginal discharge is present. On vaginal cytology the number of neutrophils present will decrease over the course of treatment and a minimal number should be detected after 7 days. Most pyometra cases present with a leukocytosis characterized by a neutrophilia with a left shift and the presence of toxic neutrophils. After 10–15 days of medical therapy most leukograms will return to normal.

Ultrasound is the most important tool in evaluating the efficacy of treatment. A significant reduction in the size of the uterine lumen should be seen 3–5 days after the onset of medical therapy. Initially daily ultrasound assessments are recommended to assess response to therapy. When uterine dimensions have returned to normal and there is no fluid present in the uterus, luteolytic treatment can be ceased. Reduction in uterine wall size and often a reduction in the degree of CEH are detected on ultrasound after removal of progesterone and bacterial infection. In refractory cases when the uterine lumen has not reduced in size after 3–5 days of treatment, OVH is recommended. Treatment for longer than 7–10 days can increase the risk of secondary complications such as disseminated intravascular coagulation (DIC).

Measurement of serum progesterone to determine the effectiveness of luteolysis after treatment with $PGF_{2\alpha}$ can be carried out at 48 hours and again at 5–7 days after onset of treatment (with progesterone concentrations <2 ng/mL). In refractory cases, checking serum progesterone levels for incomplete luteolysis is advised. Progesterone receptor antagonists displace endogenous progesterone, thus elevating systemic levels. Therefore, using serum progesterone concentrations to assess luteolysis must be interpreted with caution. Serum progesterone concentration 3 weeks after initiation of aglepristone treatment should be below 2 ng/mL. Monitoring for DIC is important in chronic cases of pyometra.

Prognosis after medical treatment

Following medical treatment, the prognosis for future fertility is positive (average 86% in bitches and 95% in queens) if appropriate case selection for medical treatment has been performed; that is young, healthy bitches. The likelihood of recurrence of pyometra depends on a number of factors, including the age and parity of the bitch, the degree of CEH changes and preexisting uterine pathology. Pregnancy rates after treatment are variable (50–90%) (Verstegen *et al.* 2008) as is the risk of reoccurrence of pyometra at the subsequent heat (10–80%) (Blendinger 2007). However, the probability of a bitch previously treated for pyometra developing pyometra or becoming pregnant at a subsequent heat is the same as the probability for a naive bitch of the same age, breed, and parity (Verstegen *et al.* 2008). Bitches that do not respond to medical therapy within 5 days have a poor prognosis with regard to fertility and an increased likelihood of pyometra developing at their next heat.

Management after medical treatment of pyometra

Uterine regeneration after treatment of pyometra is important for the fertility of the bitch at her next estrus. Prolongation of the anestrus period with an androgen receptor agonist such as mibolerone (for dose, see manufacturer's recommendation) starting 1 month after the cessation of treatment of the pyometra for a period of 2–3 months may be beneficial, especially in bitches known to have a short inter-estrous interval (<4–6 months). Exogenous progestogen administration is contraindicated. It is important that the bitch is mated or inseminated on the first estrus following treatment of a pyometra and bred on each subsequent heat until the desired number of puppies has been achieved, depending on the general health of the bitch. The bitch should then be spayed before her next heat to prevent recurrence of the disease. It is important that the bitch becomes pregnant at her subsequent estrous cycle, and therefore use of high-quality semen and timed insemination with extenders containing antibiotics are indicated. Use of frozen-thawed semen is not advised in these cases. Close monitoring with vaginal cytology (presence of neutrophils during estrus) and ultrasound (intraluminal uterine fluid during diestrus) to detect recurrence of pyometra in these cases is important.

Surgical treatment for pyometra

The primary aim of surgical treatment for pyometra is to remove the pus-filled uterus, both ovaries, and the entire cervix. The same surgical technique as for elective OVH is used for treating pyometra. However, there are a number of additional considerations when carrying out an OVH on a bitch with pyometra.

Preoperative considerations

Evaluation of the patient's hematologic, metabolic (acidosis), renal (urine output), cardiac (arrhythmia), and hydration status should be immediately carried out and continually monitored before, during, and after surgery. Correction of hydration and electrolyte and acid–base derangements is imperative prior to anesthesia and surgery. Dehydration and hypotension should be corrected with crystalloid intravenous fluid therapy prior to surgery and continued for the duration of surgery and postoperatively. Hypertonic saline (4 mg/kg of 7.5% saline) with colloids (10–20 mL/kg every [q]12–24 hours) may be required for cases presenting with hypovolemic and endotoxic shock. Furthermore, these endotoxic patients may also require corticosteroids (prednisolone sodium succinate 30–60 mg/kg i.v.). Many pyometra cases may present with not only shock but also both prerenal and renal azotemia. Ionotropic support in the form of a continuous-rate infusion of low-dose dopamine (1–5 µg/kg/min) or dobutamine (1–20 µg/kg/min) along with intensive fluid therapy may be required before and during surgery in these cases. Patients with poor renal function often also present with hypokalemia. Care should be taken to correct this electrolyte abnormality with potassium supplementation.

Administration of antiarrhythmic drugs, diuretics, and glucose may also be required. Oxygen therapy should be provided to all patients presenting in shock and ventilatory support may be required for animals with pulmonary compromise. Intravenous broad-spectrum antibiotics effective against *E. coli* (see earlier discussion) should be given after intravenous fluids have been initiated and prior to surgery. If the patient presents in a critical condition, stabilization with medical therapy may only be possible for a few hours prior to surgery. In less critical patients, initiation of medical luteolytic treatment to dilate the cervix and facilitate drainage of pus from the uterus (see the medical therapy section) may hasten systemic stabilization and reduce the anesthetic and surgical risk (uterine rupture and leakage through the oviducts during surgery).

There are a number of anesthetic protocols that can be used for a pyometra patient. Emergency cases requiring surgery present with depression, dehydration, hypotension, and sometimes hypovolemic shock. These cases require intensive monitoring during and after surgery and have additional anesthetic considerations. Preoxygenation therapy is important in facilitating perfusion.

Surgical considerations and technique

The bitch is placed in dorsal recumbency and the entire ventral abdomen is clipped and prepared for aseptic surgery. A ventral midline incision is made 2–3 cm caudal to the xiphoid and extending down to the pubis. It is important to examine the abdominal cavity for any pus and evidence of peritonitis. The presence of a tear in the uterus and pus in the abdominal cavity is a poor prognostic indicator for survival. Careful and minimal handling is required, as the friable and distended uterus can readily rupture and/or pus can leak through the oviducts into the peritoneal cavity.

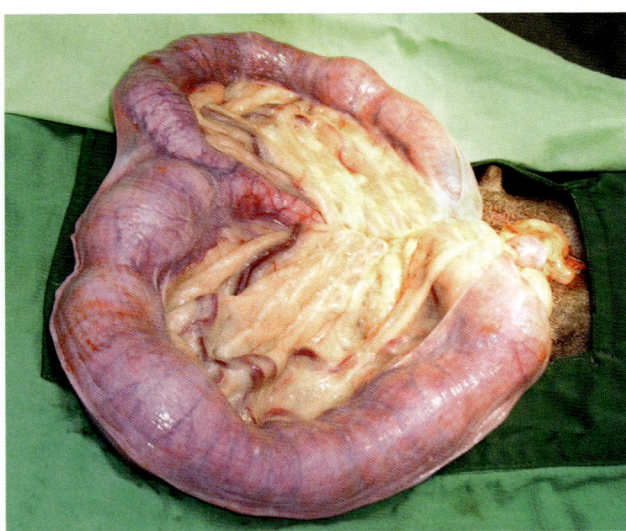

Figure 53.5 Intraoperative image of an enlarged, fluid-filled uterus in a bitch with pyometra.

Therefore, careful exteriorization by lifting the uterus out of the abdominal cavity with minimal pressure or tension is required (Figure 53.5). A spay hook is contraindicated, as is correcting any torsions that may be present. To help prevent pus leaking or spilling into the abdominal cavity, the use of saline-soaked laparotomy sponges is important.

Removal of the uterus, both ovaries, and the entire cervix is required. Clamps and ligation are carried out in the same manner as for OVH. The pedicles should be ligated with an absorbable monofilament suture material such as 2-0 polydioxanone or polyglyconate. After removal of the uterus, lavage of the abdominal cavity, and in particular the stump, with warmed isotonic saline is recommended. A sample of fluid from the uterus can be obtained after its removal from the abdominal cavity for culture and sensitivity testing. The incision should be routinely closed unless peritonitis is present and placement of a drainage system is required. We do not recommend placement of an indwelling catheter for daily lavage in management of canine pyometra as has been previously reported.

More recently laparoscopic-assisted OVH has been described for a carefully selected subset of surgical patients. It has been recommended for open or closed cervix pyometra in systemically stable patients with only moderately distended uterine horns (<5 cm) and no existing uterine perforation. Three- and one-portal approaches have been reported (Adamovich-Rippe *et al.* 2013).

Postoperative care, complications, and prognosis

Intensive postoperative monitoring 24–48 hours after surgery for signs of shock, sepsis, dehydration, electrolyte/acid–base derangements, hypoglycemia, hypoproteinemia, and anemia is essential. Postoperative management involves systemic support with intravenous fluids for a minimum of 24 hours and until the patient is eating and drinking. Pain should be managed with opioids such as morphine (0.1–0.2 mg/kg i.v. q4–6 h) or buprenorphine (0.0 mg/kg subcutaneously [s.c.] q8 h). Hematologic and immunologic parameters usually return to normal 7 days after OVH. Oral antibiotic therapy based on culture and sensitivity results should be ongoing for 7–10 days after surgery.

Postoperative complications include peritonitis, septicemia, endotoxemia, anorexia, anemia, pyrexia, vomiting, renal insufficiency, and hepatic disease, but these usually resolve within two weeks. Stump pyometra should not occur if the entire cervix and both ovaries are completely removed.

The prognosis after surgical treatment of pyometra is generally very good, with reported survival rates between 83% and 100%. Reported complications include peritonitis, urinary tract infection, wound infection, uveitis, and cardiac arrhythmia. It has been reported that the indicator of leucopenia, followed by fever/hypothermia, depression, and pale mucous membranes, was associated with peritonitis and prolonged hospitalization. The renal status of the patient before and after surgery is also an indicator for prognosis. Measurement of protein in the urine is therefore an important prognostic indicator, and monitoring of protein excretion patterns in bitches with compromised renal function postoperatively is advised. Other factors influencing prognosis include the nature of the pyometra (closed vs. open), severity of the metabolic derangements, dehydration status, presence of uterine rupture, and presence of other concurrent disease.

Possible alternative endoscopic treatment of canine pyometra

Techniques have been described to treat both closed and open pyometra with a noninvasive transcervical endoscopic cervical catheterization technique. That involves flushing the uterus with warm sterile saline containing $PGF_{2\alpha}$ in combination with oral antibiotics. This treatment is repeated two days later if uterine fluid is detected on ultrasound. Promising results were initially reported, with resolution of pyometras within 3–5 days (Verstegen *et al.* 2008), but there has been limited information published since these initial reports.

References

Adamovich-Rippe, K.N., Mayhew, P.D., Runge, J.J. et al. (2013). Evaluation of laparoscopic-assisted ovariohysterectomy for treatment of canine pyometra. *Veterinary Surgery* 2013 42 (5): 572–578.

Arnold, S., Hubler, M., and Reichler, I. (2006). Canine pyometra: new approaches to an old disease. *Proceedings of the World Small Animal Veterinary Association Conference*, Prague, Czech Republic.

Arora, N., Sandford, J., Browning, G.F. et al. (2006). A model for cystic endometrial hyperplasia/pyometra complex in the bitch. *Theriogenology* 66: 1530–1536.

Blendinger, K. (2007). Success rate of conservative treatment of canine pyometra and fertility: which is the treatment of choice? *Proceedings of the 56th SCIVAC Congress*, Rimini, Italy.

Blendinger, K. and Bostedt, H. (1991). The age and stage of estrus in bitches with pyometra. Statistical inquiry and interpretive study of the understanding of variability. *Tierarztliche Praxis* 19: 307–310.

Borel, I.M., Freire, S.M., Rivera, E. et al. (1999). Modulation of the immune response by progesteroneinduced lymphocyte factors. *Scandinavian Journal of Immunology* 49: 244–250.

Børresen, B. (1979). Pyometra in the dog. I. A pathophysiological investigation. II. Anamnestic, clinical and reproductive aspects. *Nordisk Veterinaermedicin* 31: 251–257.

Chen, Y.M., Wright, P.J., and Lee, C.S. (2001). A model for the study of cystic endometrial hyperplasia in bitches. *Journal of Reproduction and Fertility* 57 (Suppl): 407–414.

Chen, Y.M., Wright, P.J., Lee, C.S., and Browning, G.F. (2003). Uropathogenic virulence factors in isolates of *Escherichia coli* from clinical cases of canine pyometra and feces of healthy bitches. *Veterinary Microbiology* 94: 57–69.

Concannon, P.W., McCann, J.P., and Temple, M. (1989). Biology and endocrinology of ovulation, pregnancy and parturition in the dog. *Journal of Reproduction and Fertility* 39 (Suppl): 3–25.

De Bosschere, H., Ducatelle, R., Vermeirsch, H. et al. (2001). Cystic endometrial hyperplasia–pyometra complex in the bitch: should the two entities be disconnected? *Theriogenology* 55: 1509–1519.

Egenvall, A., Hagman, R., Bonnett, B.N. et al. (2001). Breed risk of pyometra in insured dogs in Sweden. *Journal of Veterinary Internal Medicine* 15: 530–538.

Fiamengo, T.E., Runcan, E.E., Premanandan, C. et al. (2020). Evaluation of biofilm production by *Escherichia coli* isolated from clinical cases of canine pyometra. *Topics in Companion Animal Medicine* 39: 100429.

Fieni, F. (2006). Clinical evaluation of the use of aglepristone, with or without cloprostenol, to treat cystic endometrial hyperplasia–pyometra complex in bitches. *Theriogenology* 66: 1550–1556.

Fontaine, E., Levy, X., Grellet, A. et al. (2009). Diagnosis of endometritis in the bitch: a new approach. *Reproduction in Domestic Animals* 44 (Suppl 2): 196–199.

Fransson, B., Lagerstedt, A.S., Hellmen, E., and Jonsson, P. (1997). Bacteriological findings, blood chemistry profile and plasma endotoxin levels in bitches with pyometra or other uterine diseases. *Zentralblatt fur Veterinarmedizin Reihe A* 44: 417–426.

Galac, S., Kooistra, H.S., Butinar, J. et al. (2000). Termination of midgestation pregnancy in bitches with aglepristone, a progesterone receptor antagonist. *Theriogenology* 53: 941–950.

Gobello, C., Castex, G., Klima, L. et al. (2003). A study of two protocols combining aglepristone and cloprostenol to treat open cervix pyometra in the bitch. *Theriogenology* 60: 901–908.

Hagman, R., Holst, B.S., Möller, L., and Egenvall, A. (2014). Incidence of pyometra in Swedish insured cats. *Theriogenology* 82 (1): 114–120.

Heiene, R., Kristiansen, V., Teige, J., and Jansen, J.H. (2007). Renal histomorphology in dogs with pyometra and control dogs, and longterm clinical outcome with respect to signs of kidney disease. *Acta Veterinaria Scandinavica* 49: 13.

Hoffmann, B., Busges, F., Engel, E. et al. (2004). Regulation of corpus luteum-function in the bitch. *Reproduction in Domestic Animals* 39: 232–240.

Ishiguro, K., Baba, E., Torii, R. et al. (2007). Reduction of mucin-1 gene expression associated with increased *Escherichia coli* adherence in the canine uterus in the early stage of dioestrus. *Veterinary Journal (London)* 173: 325–332.

Jitpean, S., Ström-Holst, B., Emanuelson, U. et al. (2014). Outcome of pyometra in female dogs and predictors of peritonitis and prolonged postoperative hospitalization in surgically treated cases. *BMC Veterinary Research* 10 (1): 1–2.

Johnson, J.R. (1991). Virulence factors in *Escherichia coli* urinary tract infection. *Clinical Microbiology Reviews* 4: 80–128.

Krekeler, N., Marenda, M.S., Browning, G.F. et al. (2012). Uropathogenic virulence factor Fim H facilitates binding of uteropathogenic *Escherichia coli* to canine endometrium. *Comparative Immunology, Microbiology and Infectious Diseases* 35: 461–467.

Lawler, D.F., Johnston, S.D., Hegstad, R.L. et al. (1993). Ovulation without cervical stimulation in domestic cats. *Journal of Reproduction and Fertility. Supplement* 47: 57–61.

Lee, K., Jeong, J., Tsai, M.J. et al. (2006). Molecular mechanisms involved in progesterone receptor regulation of uterine function. *Journal of Steroid Biochemistry and Molecular Biology* 102: 41–50.

Lloyd, A.L., Rasko, D.A., and Mobley, H.L. (2007). Defining genomic islands and uropathogen-specific genes in uropathogenic *Escherichia coli*. *Journal of Bacteriology* 189: 3532–3546.

Lyman, C.C., Holyoak, G.R., Meinkoth, K. et al. (2019). Canine endometrial and vaginal microbiomes reveal distinct and complex ecosystems. *PLOS ONE* 14 (1): e0210157.

Noakes, D.E., Dhaliwal, G.K., and England, G.C. (2001). Cystic endometrial hyperplasia/pyometra in dogs: a review of the causes and pathogenesis. *Journal of Reproduction and Fertility. Supplement* 57: 395–406.

Schlafer, D.H. and Gifford, A.T. (2008). Cystic endometrial hyperplasia, pseudo-placentational endometrial hyperplasia, and other cystic conditions of the canine and feline uterus. *Theriogenology* 70 (3): 349–358.

Silva, E., Leitao, S., Ferreira-Dias, G. et al. (2009). Prostaglandin synthesis genes are differentially transcripted in normal and pyometra endometria of bitches. *Reproduction in Domestic Animals* 44 (Suppl 2): 200–203.

Sugiura, K., Nishikawa, M., Ishiguro, K. et al. (2004). Effect of ovarian hormones on periodical changes in immune resistance associated with estrous cycle in the beagle bitch. *Immunobiology* 209: 619–627.

Verstegen, J., Dhaliwal, G., and Verstegen-Onclin, K. (2008). Mucometra, cystic endometrial hyperplasia, and pyometra in the bitch: advances in treatment and assessment of future reproductive success. *Theriogenology* 70: 364–374.

Wådas, B., Kuhn, I., Lagerstedt, A.S., and Jonsson, P. (1996). Biochemical phenotypes of *Escherichia coli* in dogs: comparison of isolates isolated from bitches suffering from pyometra and urinary tract infection with isolates from faeces of healthy dogs. *Veterinary Microbiology* 52: 293–300.

Watts, J.R., Wright, P.J., and Whithear, K.C. (1996). Uterine, cervical and vaginal microflora of the normal bitch throughout the reproductive cycle. *Journal of Small Animal Practice* 37: 54–60.

54

Cesarean Section

Wendy Baltzer

The most common indication for cesarean section is to relieve dystocia in the bitch or queen. Among insured Swedish intact female dogs, the incidence of dystocia is approximately 2%, and 60–80% of dogs with dystocia will undergo cesarean section as part of their treatment (Darvelid & Linde-Forsberg 1994; Bergstrom *et al.* 2006; Munnich & Kuchenmeister 2009). However, up to 32% of cesarean sections performed are elective procedures based upon breed, fetal size compared to pelvic canal diameter, previous dystocia, and owner convenience (Ryan & Wagner 2006a,b; Munnich & Kuchenmeister 2009). While the procedure and perioperative care may be similar, puppy mortality is 12.7–19.6% for emergency procedures and only 3.6% for an elective cesarean (Moon-Massat 2003; Schmidt *et al.* 2021). There is also an increased risk of death for the dam with an emergency cesarean (Moon *et al.* 2000). Determination of when to perform a cesarean is vital to a successful outcome for both the neonates and the dam, as are adequate preparation and management of the patients, whether the procedure is elective or emergent.

Indications for an elective cesarean section

While no standard indicators have been identified in small animals for the performance of an elective cesarean section, in humans planned cesarean is performed in cases of fetal malposition, multiple fetuses, or fetal abnormality; or if maternal compromise occurs (cardiac disease, diabetes, preeclampsia, hypertension, placenta previa or abruption, infectious disease such as acquired immunodeficiency syndrome, toxoplasmosis, or syphilis) (Gregory *et al.* 2002; Wilmink *et al.* 2010). While exceedingly rare in humans, uterine rupture can occur if a uterine scar is present, including a scar from a previous cesarean (Gregory *et al.* 2002).

In small animals, indications for an elective cesarean may include brachycephalic breed (particularly bulldogs due to fetopelvic disproportion), previous uterine inertia in large-breed dogs, diabetes mellitus, gestational diabetes, maternal cardiac condition or other maternal compromise, and in the fetus, oversize, anatomic abnormalities, or death (Munnich & Kuchenmeister 2009; Ryan & Wagner 2006b). Some practitioners advocate elective cesarean for dams 6 years of age or older, litter sizes of two or fewer, litter sizes of eight or more, or when an owner lives in an area with limited access to emergency veterinary services (Smith 2007). In Labrador retrievers, the risk for requiring a cesarean is not influenced by weight and size of litter, parity, whelping season, or maternal inbreeding coefficient. What increases the risk may be reduced dam weight when the largest puppy has increased body weight (0.66 kg), number of malpositioned fetuses, and quality of uterine contractions (uterine inertia) (Dorf *et al.* 2018).

Elective cesarean performed prior to full term in humans results in greater neonatal morbidity and mortality; therefore, accurate determination of gestational age is vital (Wilmink *et al.* 2010). In dogs, the placenta is unlikely to be able to meet the nutritional needs of the fetus for more than two days beyond the due date, and intrauterine death can result if cesarean section is delayed (Lopate 2008). Canine gestation can vary from 57 to 72 days, with most lasting 63 ± 1 days after the preovulatory luteinizing hormone (LH) surge (Feldman & Nelson 2004). Because of this wide variability in gestational length, mating dates cannot be used to predict an

Small Animal Soft Tissue Surgery, Second Edition. Edited by Eric Monnet.
© 2023 John Wiley & Sons, Inc. Published 2023 by John Wiley & Sons, Inc.
Companion website: www.wiley.com/go/monnet/small

optimal elective cesarean date. Ideally, the date of the LH and preovulatory progesterone surge is known, because the progesterone concentrations were measured during the breeding process (Concannon *et al.* 1975). A rise in serum progesterone above 1.5 ng/mL and at least twice the baseline level taken before breeding has a 90% accuracy of predicting the parturition date within two days (Kutzler *et al.* 2003a). Planned cesarean can be safely performed 63 days following the LH surge (Smith 2007). Most commonly, the serum progesterone level is determined and should drop to less than 2 ng/mL within 24 hours of parturition (Concannon *et al.* 1975). Commercial kits for detection of serum progesterone levels may not be accurate to levels as low as 3 ng/mL or less, and should be used with caution. In conjunction with the decrease in serum progesterone within one day of parturition, there is an increase in serum C-reactive protein (1.2 ± 0.19 mg/dL) to slightly above the reference range (0–1.07 mg/dL) (Rota *et al.* 2019).

Another method used to estimate the reduction in progesterone is the resulting drop in the dam's body temperature to below 37.8 °C (100 °F), and this method of predicting parturition within 24 hours has been deemed a reliable method in practice (Biddle & Macintire 2000; Davidson 2001; Ryan & Wagner 2006b).

Ultrasound as a prediction method

Ultrasound can be used to predict the date of parturition. If the pregnancy is suspected to be less than 20 days and the dam is less than 10 kg in body weight, the inner chorionic cavity diameter is measured in millimeters (mm) and entered into the following equation (Luvoni & Grioni 2000; Kutzler *et al.* 2003b):

$$Days\ prior\ to\ parturition = (mm - 68.68)/1.53$$

For dogs weighing between 11 and 40 kg and less than 20 days pregnant, the inner chorionic cavity diameter is entered into the following equation:

$$Days\ prior\ to\ parturition = (mm - 82.13)/1.8$$

For dogs weighing up to 10 kg and more than 20 days pregnant, the biparietal diameter is determined and entered into the following equation:

$$Days\ prior\ to\ parturition = (mm - 25.11)/0.61$$

For dogs between 11 and 40 kg, the equation is as follows:

$$Days\ prior\ to\ parturition = (mm - 29.18)/0.7$$

When measuring the gestational sacs using ultrasound, two transverse plane images, at 90° to each other, should be averaged for these calculations. In addition, at least two different fetal structures should be measured and averaged (Luvoni & Grioni 2000; Son *et al.* 2001; Kutzler *et al.* 2003b; Luvoni & Beccaglia 2006). For toy and giant breeds, the formula for biparietal diameter can be used on day 30 of the suspected gestation length; however, for toy breeds, 1 day is added for the gestational length and 2 days are subtracted for giant breeds (>40 kg) (Kutzler *et al.* 2003b). These formulas have claimed to be accurate within 2 days of parturition in up to 88% of cases when using the inner chorionic cavity measurement or biparietal diameter measurement (Son *et al.* 2001; Beccaglia & Luvoni 2006; Luvoni & Beccaglia 2006; Lopate 2008). Litter size has not been shown to affect fetal size or rate of growth related to determination of parturition date in most cases; however, singletons and very large litters may affect calculation of parturition date in some cases (Kutzler *et al.* 2003b; Lopate 2008). In Drever bitches, each additional pup in the litter more than the average litter size (6.8 ± 2.1) decreased gestation by 0.25 days and each pup less than the average litter size increased gestation by 0.25 days (Gavrilovic *et al.* 2008). In English bulldogs, the number of pups in the litter did not affect gestation or calculations of biparietal diameter (distance between the parietal bones on skull of rostral-most fetuses), and this calculation significantly increased (>3 cm) from 48 to 6 hours of delivery (de Freitas *et al.* 2021). In this same breed, inner chorionic cavity diameter, measured by taking two measurements at 90° to each other using two-dimensional ultrasound close to the trophoblastic reaction, predicted delivery within +/− 1 day (de Freitas *et al.* 2021).

Radiography as a prediction method

Radiography has been advocated for predicting the timing of parturition in dogs. For example, the first evidence of mineralization of the fetal skull occurs between 43 and 46 days. Visualization of the scapula, humerus, and femur usually occurs between 46 and 51 days, while radiographically identifiable pelves and ribs occur between 53 and 59 days, with the coccygeal vertebrae, fibula, and distal extremities the last to be seen between 55 and 64 days of gestation (Rendano *et al.* 1984; Toal *et al.* 1986; Lopate 2008). Radiographs have also been used to detect fetal distress (flexion or balling of the fetus or hyperextension of the hindlimbs) and fetal death (bones of skull overriding, gas within the uterus or fetus confirmed in two views), which indicate the need for a cesarean. However, once these signs develop on radiography, most fetuses have already died up to 24 hours prior (Rendano 1983). Consequently, many veterinarians regard radiography as a poor modality to assess fetal viability (Wykes 2003; Feldman & Nelson 2004; Root-Kustritz 2005).

Foam stability test as a development prediction method

The foam stability test has been advocated to determine whether fetal lung development is sufficient for birth. Using ultrasound guidance, 1 mL of amniotic fluid is obtained and mixed in a glass tube with 1 mL of 100% ethanol and shaken vigorously for 15 seconds. If bubbles form and remain present for at least 15 minutes at the fluid–air interface, adequate fetal surfactant is present in the lungs, and female fetuses are at least 62 days' gestation and the males 63 days'. More than one fetus must be tested or at least one male, since females produce surfactant 1 day earlier than males (Ruaux 2010).

Tocodynamometer as a prediction method

Commercial services are available (Veterinary Perinatal Specialties Inc., Wheat Ridge, CO, USA) that supply the owner with a tocodynamometer, a recorder to store uterine contraction history, a modem to transfer the history to a perinatal service, and a Doppler ultrasound to monitor fetal heart rates. The service monitors the recordings and sends interpretations to the referring veterinarian. Stillbirth rates may be decreased using these monitoring services, especially for older dogs or dogs with a prior history of dystocia (Davidson 2001; Jutkowitz 2005).

Indications for an emergency cesarean section

Breeds considered to have a higher incidence of dystocia include English bulldogs, pugs, Boston terriers, French bulldogs, boxers, shih tzu, Yorkshire terriers, and Labrador retrievers (Smith 2007). The most common reasons for dystocia in the boxer have been cited as primary uterine inertia in 60% of cases and fetal malpresentation in 26% (Linde-Forsberg & Persson 2007). Maternal factors contributing to dystocia include pelvic canal narrowing due to previous fracture, vaginal tumors or strictures, and maternal stress (Eneroth *et al.* 1999). Fetopelvic disproportion has been documented in the Scottish terrier and Boston terrier breeds, with Scottish terriers at increased risk of dystocia with a dorsoventrally flattened pelvic canal. Boston terriers are at increased risk with a dorsoventrally flattened pelvic canal and large fetuses with large heads. Miniature and small breeds of dogs accounted for 59.4% of dystocias in one recent report (Munnich & Kuchenmeister 2009). Radiographic assessment of brachycephalic and Scottish and Boston terriers is recommended if dystocia is suspected.

Primary uterine inertia or disorganized uterine contractions can be a familial cause of dystocia and can result in fetal death from placental separation. Primary uterine inertia may be due to small litter size, large litter size, hypocalcemia, uterine torsion, or low serum oxytocin concentration (Wallace 1994). Secondary uterine inertia is the failure of the uterus to respond to oxytocin and is usually the result of uterine exhaustion due to large litter size or prolonged attempts to deliver a large fetus, but hypocalcemia may also play a role (Smith 2007). Determination of serum ionized calcium levels is warranted if secondary uterine inertia is suspected (no response to oxytocin administration and absent straining on pressure to the vagina in the pelvic canal) and radiography or ultrasound has ruled out a large fetus and fetal malposition. Serum ionized calcium must be measured, because total calcium levels are an insensitive measure of calcium homeostasis (Drobatz & Casey 2000; Kudnig & Mama 2000).

Fetal malposition occurs when the fetus enters the uterine body in the transverse position, two fetuses enter the uterine body simultaneously, or the fetus enters posterior with the hindlimbs flexed forward at the hips (breech). Normal presentations for dogs and cats include head and forelimbs first, as well as hindlimbs first (Darvelid & Linde-Forsberg 1994; Barber 2003).

A diagnosis of dystocia may be made if fetal malposition is present, 72 days have passed since breeding, the dam has been abdominally straining for 1 hour continuously without producing any puppies, green or black vaginal discharge is present prior to producing any puppies, fetuses are dead at birth, there has been more than 3 hours since the last puppy was produced and radiography indicates that more are present, or the dam is distressed, dehydrated, or depressed (Darvelid & Linde-Forsberg 1994; Wallace 1994; Smith 2007).

An emergency cesarean section is indicated as soon as possible if there are indications of fetal distress, including reduced fetal heart rate measured with ultrasound. A fetal heart rate of less than 150 bpm indicates severe distress, heart rates between 150 and 170 bpm indicate moderate to severe distress, while heart rates greater than 180 bpm are normal. Uterine contractions can reduce fetal heart rate; therefore repeated measurement at least 30–60 seconds apart is recommended to determine if fetal distress is present (Traas 2008a,b). Dystocia lasting longer than 4.5–6 hours is associated with increased fetal death; therefore, cesarean section is warranted once the dam has been stabilized (Darvelid & Linde-Forsberg 1994; Ekstrand & Linde-Forsberg 1994; Gaudet 1985).

Preoperative considerations

Physical examination and bloodwork

Whether undergoing an elective or emergency cesarean, the dam should have comprehensive bloodwork performed, including ionized calcium, glucose, hematocrit, total protein, blood urea nitrogen, creatinine, sodium, potassium, chloride, and white blood cell count at a minimum. Maternal blood volume increases by approximately 40% and the resulting hemodilution causes a relative anemia, with hematocrit as low as 30–35%, and lowered blood urea nitrogen and creatinine (Kaneko et al. 1993; Seymour 1999; Pascoe & Moon 2001). If the hematocrit, creatinine, and blood urea nitrogen are normal or elevated, dehydration should be suspected as a possible cause. The heart rate of the dam will remain elevated throughout labor and is not an indicator of dystocia or hemodynamic status (Lucio et al. 2009). Because of the increased blood volume and decreased peripheral vascular resistance, cardiac work is increased to maintain the higher cardiac output that is needed (Seymour 1999; Ryan & Wagner 2006b). In addition, baroreceptor response to hemorrhage or hypotension is compromised during pregnancy, so that maternal risk of death secondary to these complications is increased (Brooks & Keil 1994).

Cardiac decompensation or failure can occur in pregnant dogs that were previously stable, and therefore a thorough physical examination of the dam is vital (Seymour 1999). Hyperglycemia may occur due to progesterone-mediated insulin resistance and can also result in enlarged fetuses. Hypoglycemia may develop if the dam has been in labor for a prolonged period of time or has a very large litter, and may be treated with intravenous dextrose.

Preparation of the patient

Intravenous fluid therapy and correction of electrolyte and acid–base imbalances should begin prior to induction of anesthesia. Intravenous fluid therapy with a balanced solution such as lactated Ringer solution warmed to body temperature prevents a drop in uterine blood flow and can be administered at 10 mL/kg if not dehydrated, 20 mL/kg if mildly dehydrated, and 30 mL/kg if severely dehydrated in a bolus (Kudnig & Mama 2000; Ryan & Wagner 2006b). Thereafter, fluids can be given at 10–20 mL/kg/h during anesthesia. Colloids such as hetastarch or blood products can be administered in cases of refractory hypotension (Ryan & Wagner 2006b).

Because oxygen consumption increases with pregnancy and functional residual lung capacity is decreased, hypoxemia of the dam and fetuses is not uncommon, unless the dam is preoxygenated with a mask giving 3–5 L/min of 100% oxygen prior to induction of anesthesia (Jutkowitz 2005; Ryan & Wagner 2006b). $PaCO_2$ is decreased to 30–33 mmHg during pregnancy due to increased minute ventilation and increased sensitivity of the respiratory center to carbon dioxide (Greene 1995). This means that hyperventilation can worsen hypocapnia during maternal stress or anesthetic induction, resulting in decreased oxygen transfer to the fetuses through the Bohr effect as well as decreased uterine blood flow (Greene 1995; Moon-Massat 2003). There should be as little stress as possible placed on the dam prior to anesthesia. Once anesthetized, careful ventilation and monitoring of $PaCO_2$ should be carried out during the procedure.

Minimizing anesthetic time

In order to minimize anesthetic time, it is recommended that the abdomen be clipped and an initial scrub performed prior to induction of anesthesia. Premedication of the dam can have adverse effects on the fetuses, so use of short-acting drugs that can be antagonized is recommended (Ryan & Wagner 2006a). Opioids can be administered as a premedicant along with atropine (0.01 mg/kg intravenously [i.v.] or 0.02 mg/kg subcutaneously [s.c.]) to provide analgesia but minimize bradycardia in the fetus and dam. The opioids hydromorphone, morphine, and oxymorphone are used as premedicants because they can be antagonized in the neonate with naloxone (Moon-Massat 2003; Ryan & Wagner 2006a). Glycopyrrolate is not recommended since very little will cross the placental barrier to prevent bradycardia in the fetuses (Ryan & Wagner 2006a). Benzodiazepines can be used intravenously immediately prior to induction and can be reversed in the fetuses with flumazenil (0.1 mg/kg i.v.) (Ryan & Wagner 2006a). Because of their significant adverse effects on the fetuses and/or dam, acepromazine, ketamine, and α_2-adrenoceptor agonists (xylazine, medetomidine) are not recommended for cesarean section (Moon et al. 2000; Moon-Massat & Erb 2002).

The risk of regurgitation is increased in the dam during general anesthesia due to decreased lower esophageal tone and increased intra-abdominal pressure. Esophagitis can result from the increased acidity of the gastric contents, another side effect of pregnancy, and premedication with metoclopramide (0.2–0.4 mg/kg i.v. or intramuscularly [i.m.]) has been recommended by some veterinarians (Seymour 1999). The incidence of pneumonia following cesarean section is unknown, although 5 of 9 cases of maternal mortality had evidence of pneumonia in one canine study (Pascoe & Moon 2001).

Anesthetic considerations

Induction and maintenance of anesthesia must be tailored to each patient; however, decreased puppy vigor has been associated with the use of thiobarbiturates, ketamine, and inhalant anesthetics. Inhalant anesthetics such as isoflurane or halothane are minimally metabolized, but must be exhaled to eliminate the drug; therefore, their excessive use should be avoided or the puppies may have to be intubated and ventilated in order to resolve inhalant anesthetic-induced apnea at birth (Moon-Massat & Erb 2002). In addition, the minimum alveolar concentration required in the dam is reduced by 25% for halothane and 40% for isoflurane in humans and sheep, so judicious use is especially important during a cesarean section (Palahniuk & Shnider 1974; Gin & Chan 1994). Sevoflurane has not been associated with reduced puppy vigor (Gendler *et al.* 2007). Propofol induction followed by maintenance with isoflurane inhalant is a commonly used method of anesthesia for cesarean section (Moon *et al.* 2000; Ryan & Wagner 2006a); however, evidence suggests that alfaxalone as an induction agent may increase puppy vigor within the first 60 minutes following cesarean birth (Doebeli *et al.* 2013). Both propofol and alfaxalone induction of the dam for emergency cesarean result in similar puppy survival, but puppy Apgar scores were higher in the alfaxalone group (Doebeli *et al.* 2013). Following induction, 15–20 minutes under general anesthesia with intravenous fluid support should occur prior to delivery of the neonates to allow drug metabolism by the dam to occur and reduce depression in the neonates (Short & Bufalari 1999). In cases of severe maternal compromise or maternal cardiac disease, etomidate (1–2 mg/kg i.v.) is used for induction of general anesthesia, and can be used with midazolam to reduce any excitatory side effect (Robertson 1992; Pablo & Bailey 1999).

Surgical procedure

The ventral abdomen is clipped and a preliminary scrub performed prior to induction of general anesthesia. Care is taken not to traumatize the nipples during preparation. Positioning of the dam in dorsal recumbency does not cause aortocaval hypotension in dogs <30 kg (Probst & Webb 1983; Probst *et al.* 1987); however, in larger dogs the table may be tilted 10–15° to one side to remove pressure from the caudal vena cava (Gilson 2015). The dog's head is kept no lower than the abdomen to prevent increased pressure on the diaphragm from the uterus and fetuses. After the dog is induced, the final surgical scrub is performed and a ventral midline incision made from 1–2 cm cranial to the umbilicus to 1 cm cranial to the pubis. The incision can be extended if needed to exteriorize the uterus. The incision through the subcutaneous tissue is performed with care to prevent incising the mammary glands. The incision into the linea alba is also performed with care, as it is stretched thin and directly overlying the uterus in most animals. The uterus is then identified and each horn gently exteriorized. The uterus and especially the uterine body are packed off with saline-moistened laparotomy sponges.

An incision is made into the body of the uterus parallel to the incision made in the abdominal wall (Figure 54.1). The fetuses are milked through the incision and the fetal sac removed from the fetus's head (Figure 54.2). The umbilicus is double clamped, then transected between the clamps and the puppy quickly transferred to personnel for resuscitation. The umbilicus is left clamped and at least 1 cm long on the fetus to facilitate umbilical injections or blood draws. An incision can be made in each uterine horn with very large litters in order to expedite removal of the fetuses; however, care must be taken to ensure that a placenta is not transected. The uterine body and pelvic canal are thoroughly inspected for any remaining fetuses. Each fetal membrane must be removed or ruptured to allow passage of the next fetus down to the uterine incision (Traas 2008a,b). There are some surgeons who leave the placenta in place if it is firmly adhered to the uterus, fearing excessive hemorrhage or placental fragment retention with traction on the placenta, while others slowly and gently massage the uterus and remove all fetal membranes prior to closure (Gilson 2003; Traas 2008b). If the cervix is not open, the fetal membranes must be entirely removed (Traas 2008b).

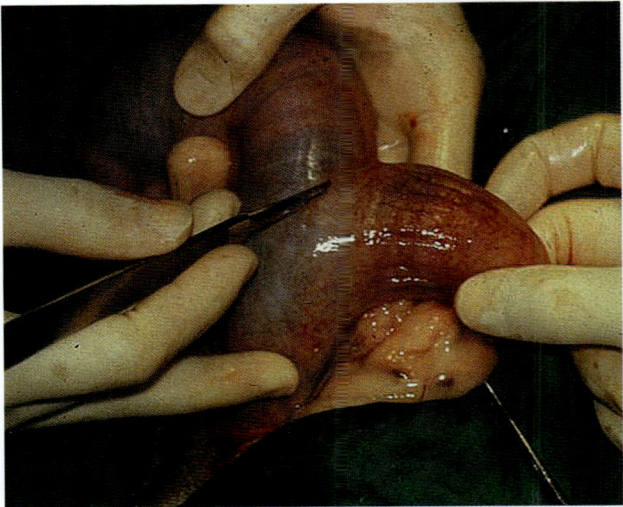

Figure 54.1 An incision is made with a scalpel blade into the uterine body, with care being taken not to incise a fetus that may be located directly below the incision.

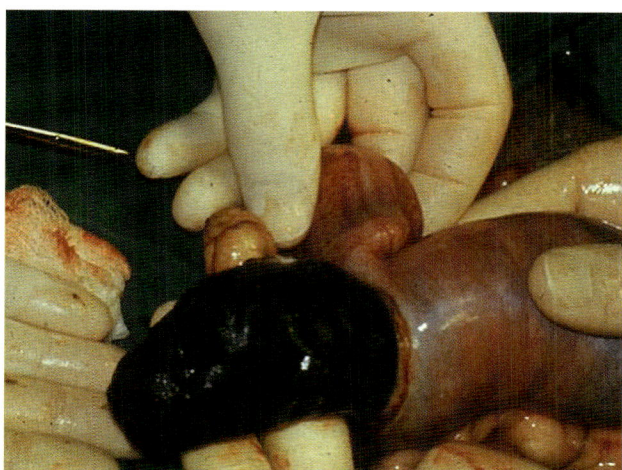

Figure 54.2 The fetuses are milked to the incision with gentle pressure on the uterus cranial to the fetus. Once the fetal head is exteriorized, the fetal membranes are removed.

Hysterotomy closure is most commonly performed in two layers, with a simple continuous layer first, and care taken that sutures are not entering the lumen or penetrating the mucosa. The second layer is an inverting pattern such as a Cushing. The suture of choice is 3-0 or 4-0 monofilament synthetic absorbable for both layers (Figure 54.3). The surgeon's gloves and instruments are changed, and the abdomen is lavaged (warm lactated Ringer solution, 100–200 mL/kg) and closed (Gilson 2003). Care is taken to ensure generous bites in the linea alba, which has been stretched and thinned by the weight of the gravid uterus. Apposition of the abdominal musculature and linea alba should be done with monofilament synthetic absorbable suture in either a simple interrupted or continuous pattern. Closure of the skin should be performed with a simple continuous intradermal pattern using monofilament synthetic absorbable suture. No skin sutures or staples are placed, as the neonates could become entangled in them. The skin should be cleaned of all antiseptics prior to exposure to the neonates (Hedlund 2007). Oxytocin can be administered after the hysterotomy incision has been closed to facilitate expulsion of fetal membranes and placenta, reduce uterine hemorrhage, and stimulate uterine involution (Traas 2008b). Dosages of 2 IU/kg or a maximum of 20 IU of oxytocin, subcutaneously or intramuscularly, can be administered (Gilson 2003; Ryan & Wagner 2006b). Survival of the fetuses at birth is reportedly 92% with cesarean section and 80% survival one week following surgery (Moon & Erb 1998; Moon-Massat & Erb 2002).

An alternative surgical procedure to hysterotomy is *en bloc* ovariohysterectomy, in which the uterine body and arteries and the ovarian pedicles are clamped. The uterus is then removed with the fetuses so that the support staff can remove the fetuses and revive them. This procedure is effective for cases where infectious material may be present in the uterus, the fetuses are dead, or the dam is in a critical condition. Surgery must be as brief as possible. Survival of fetuses was found to be 75% for puppies and 42% for cats with this method (Robbins & Mullen 1994). It is vital, if live fetuses are present, that the time from placement of the first clamp on any vessels to extraction of the fetuses is less than 60 seconds (Hedlund 2007). There can be more postoperative complications and a longer hospital stay for the dam using *en bloc* ovariohysterectomy compared with hysterotomy cesarean (Gaudet 1985; Robbins & Mullen 1994).

The incidence of infection in the uterus following cesarean section is low, with only 1 of 21 dogs having a positive uterine culture in one study (Olson & Mather 1978). The most likely organisms to cause infection are *Escherichia coli* and *Staphylococcus* spp., which can be prevented in most cases with perioperative intravenous antibiotics such as a first- or second-generation cephalosporin (Ryan & Wagner 2006b). Perioperative antibiotics and culture and sensitivity of uterine contents are indicated if necrosis is present (fetal death, uterine torsion), uterine infection is suspected, or a break in asepsis has occurred (Ryan & Wagner 2006b). Transmission of *Staphylococcus pseudointermedius* from the milk of the dam to the puppies resulting in fatal sepsis has recently been reported in a Boston terrier following an elective cesarean section (Zakosek Pipan et al. 2019). S. pseudointermedius is considered a commensal colonizer, but has been associated with pyoderma and neonatal puppy death (Bannoehr & Guardabassi 2012; Zakosek Pipan et al. 2019).

Postoperative analgesia

Local infiltration of anesthetics at the surgical incision in the dam is useful, and often lidocaine (2 mg/kg) or bupivacaine (2 mg/kg in combination with lidocaine) is administered following closure of the skin incision.

The most common method of systemic analgesia utilizes opioids, given orally, transdermally, or via injection (Ryan & Wagner 2006b). If respiratory or behavioral depression occurs in the neonate, naloxone (1 drop of 0.4 mg/mL) under the tongue of the puppy or kitten can reverse these effects and can be titrated to effect (Mathews 2005). The opioid can be combined with a nonsteroidal anti-inflammatory drug (NSAID) to lower the dose of opioid required and reduce sedation in the dam; however, small amounts may be transferred to the neonate in the milk. NSAIDs could theoretically damage neonatal renal development, although no definitive research has been performed to determine if this actually occurs.

(a)   (b)   (c)

(d)

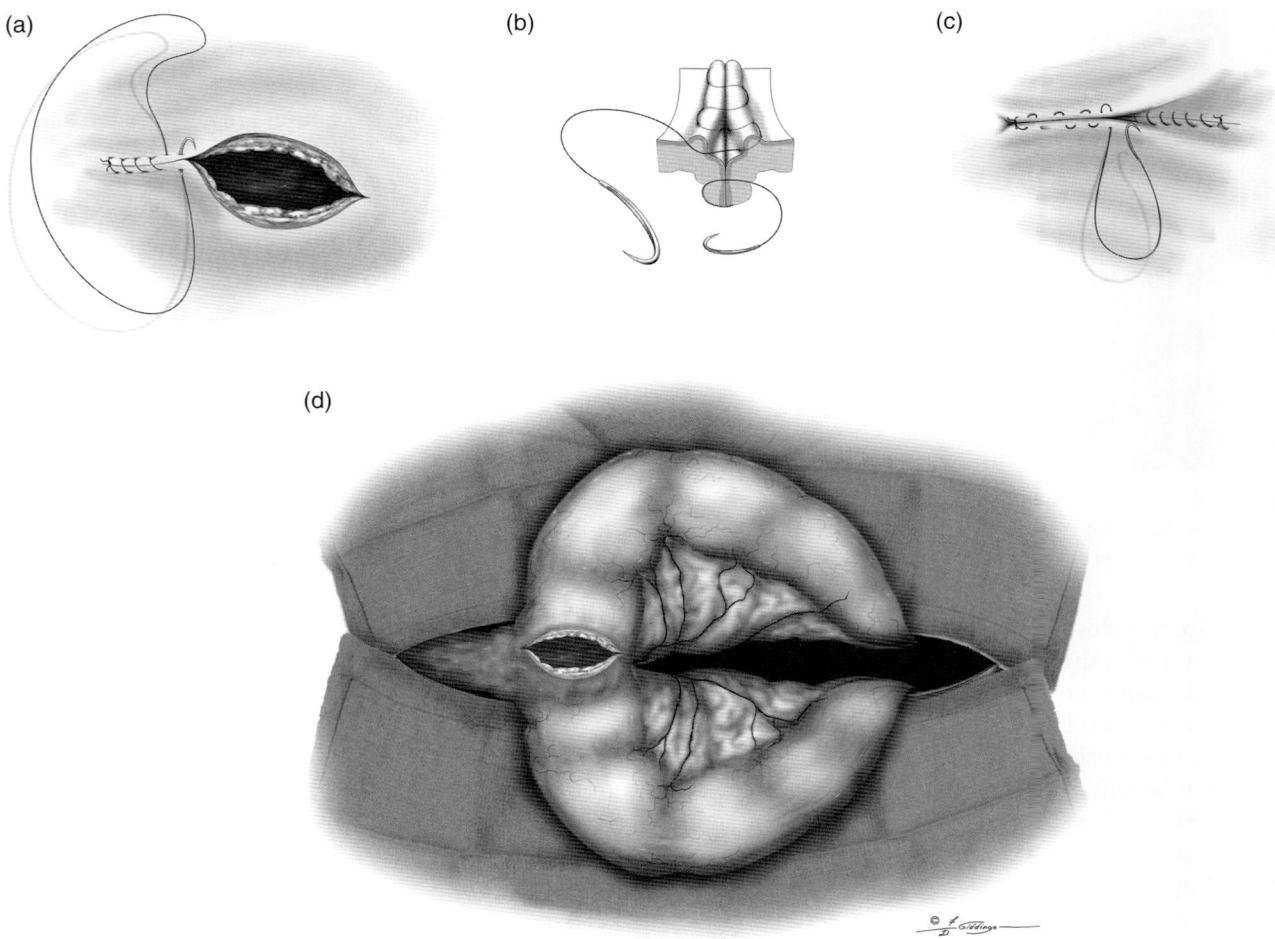

Figure 54.3 The hysterotomy incision (d) is closed with monofilament absorbable suture in a simple continuous pattern (a) for the first layer, with care taken to ensure that no sutures penetrate the mucosa of the uterus and enter the lumen. The second layer is an inverting pattern such as a Cushing (b, c). The suture of choice is 3-0 or 4-0 absorbable, synthetic monofilament for both layers. Source: © D. Giddings.

A single dose of a cyclooxygenase (COX)-2 selective NSAID, such as meloxicam, following cesarean section has been advocated (Mathews 2005). Bitches given a loading dose of 4 mg/kg day 1 then 2 mg/kg every 12 hours orally for 2–5 days of carprofen following cesarean section transmitted low quantities into the milk (<700 ng/mL). Puppies drinking the milk received 1/10 the dose an adult dog would receive at 2 mg/kg every 12 hours; however, mastitis increases the concentration of carprofen in milk by approximately twofold, to 1300 ng/mL (Ferrari *et al.* 2022). The low dose received by the puppies and lack of clinical signs of renal disease 6 months following birth may warrant its use postoperatively following cesarean section, but further research determining renal function in puppies is needed (Ferrari *et al.* 2022).

Care must be taken to ensure that the dam does not become hypothermic and that she responds to her neonates once awake, cleaning and stimulating them, as well as allowing them to nurse.

Neonatal care

The neonates are often depressed due to hypoxia and anesthetics that were administered to the dam. The neonate must be warmed and the membranes cleared from the oropharynx and nasal passages with a bulb syringe. If the neonate is not effectively breathing or vocalizing, oxygen may be administered via a mask (Davidson 2014). Inhalant anesthetics such as isoflurane are minimally metabolized and must be eliminated by respiration in the neonate (Jutkowitz 2005). Rubbing the neonate with a warm towel for 30 seconds over the right and left lateral thorax will warm it as well as stimulate respiration (Figure 54.4) (Traas 2008a). For the first three days of life, neonates have a tactile respiratory reflex when the umbilical and genital areas are stimulated. Therefore, rubbing these areas with a towel can stimulate respiration (Fox 1964). If opioids were administered to the dam, they can be reversed in the neonate with naloxone (0.25 mg/kg or one drop equaling 1–5 µg of 0.4 mg/mL

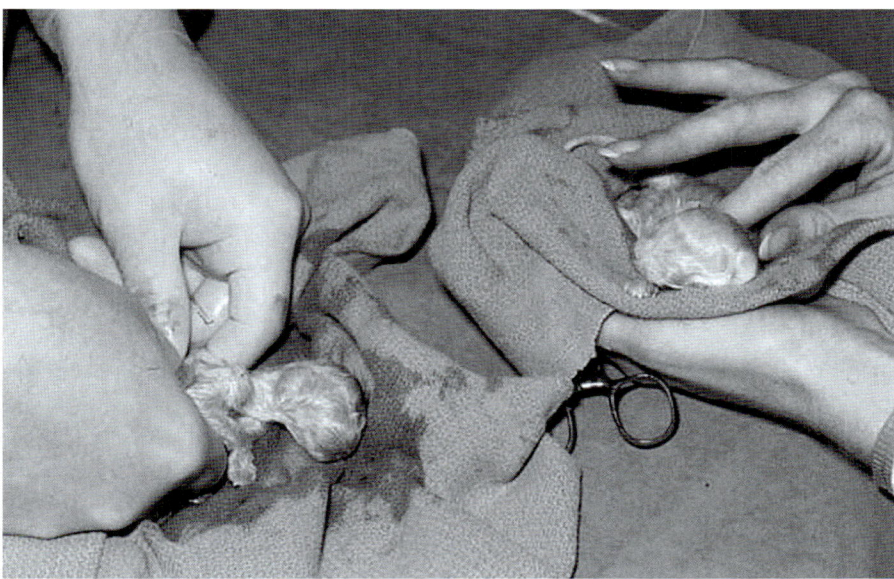

Figure 54.4 Resuscitation of the neonate involves vigorous rubbing of the right and left lateral thorax. The umbilical and perineal areas are also rubbed gently to stimulate a respiratory reflex.

sublingually [s.l.], i.m., or s.c.) (Ryan & Wagner 2006a,b; Traas 2008a). If the neonate does not begin breathing or remains bradycardic, intubation of the trachea with a small endotracheal tube or tomcat catheter is performed to administer oxygen to reverse the hypoxemia. Once the puppy or kitten begins breathing regularly, supplemental oxygen can be administered with a mask or by placing the neonate in an oxygen cage (Ryan & Wagner 2006b). Expansion of the neonate's lungs can be attempted with a tight-fitting mask placed over the face and pressure slowly increased over a 3 second period to 20 cmH$_2$O until the chest wall expands. Alternatively, a cuffed endotracheal tube can be placed and the patient ventilated up to a pressure of 30–60 cmH$_2$O until the chest wall has expanded (Moon *et al.* 2001).

Ventilatory support can be continued with breaths of no greater than 10 cmH$_2$O at 30 breaths per minute (Traas 2008a). The acupuncture point called Renzhong (or Jen Chung) has been used to stimulate ventilation in the neonate, although this technique has not been substantiated (Rattan 1999; Skarda 1999; Davidson 2014). A 25-gauge needle is placed into the base of the nasal philtrum until bone is touched and then the needle is turned to stimulate spontaneous breathing (Traas 2008a). Doxapram has been used to stimulate respiration in neonates in veterinary medicine in the past; however, its use is controversial. Doxapram may cause decreased cerebral blood flow in newborns and worsen obtundation in the neonate (Roll & Horsch 2004). It is considered a central nervous system stimulant and has a short duration of action to stimulate respiratory rate and volume

(Ryan & Wagner 2006b). Doxapram may be ineffective if the neonate is hypoxic (Moon *et al.* 2000). In addition, it may not improve hypoxemia, since it also increases oxygen consumption and the work of respiration (Ryan & Wagner 2006b). In neonates that are not hypoxic, but rather apneic or breathing with shallow gasping respirations, doxapram may improve ventilation if given at a dose of 1–5 mg sublingually, subcutaneously, or intravenously (Ryan & Wagner 2006b; Traas 2008a).

Recurrence of narcosis can occur since the duration of action of naloxone is shorter than that of many opioids; therefore, a second dose of naloxone may be required. If benzodiazepines were administered to the dam, these should be antagonized in the neonate with flumazenil (0.1 mg/kg i.v. or through the umbilicus) (Figure 54.5) (Ryan & Wagner 2006b).

In cases of severe bradycardia (refractory to intubation and ventilatory support) or cardiac arrest, chest compressions can be performed at a rate of one to two per second, with pauses for ventilation. All neonates must have intubation and ventilatory support for cardiopulmonary resuscitation. If cardiac arrest has occurred, epinephrine is administered via the umbilical vein or an intraosseous catheter placed in the proximal femur or other suitable site. The dose of epinephrine is 0.1–0.3 mg/kg either intravenously or intraosseously, followed by cardiac compressions so that the drug can reach the myocardium. Atropine is not effective in neonatal puppies and kittens and therefore is not recommended to resuscitate newborns (McMichael & Dhupa 2000). If the neonate fails to respond and breathe

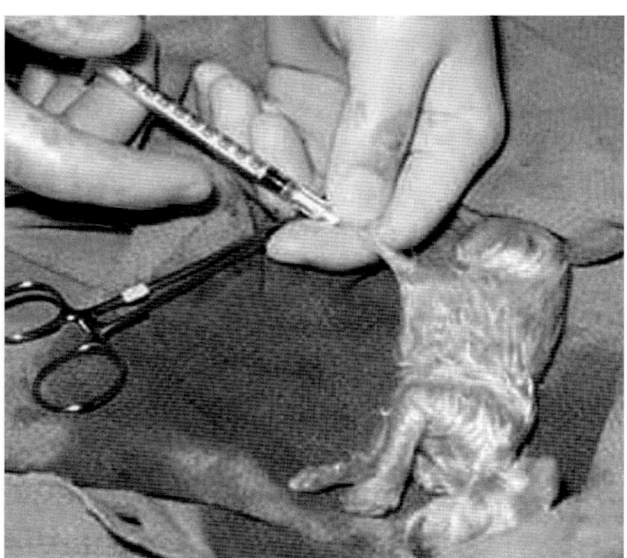

Figure 54.5 Administration of naloxone or flumazenil or intravenous fluids through the umbilical vein is used as an emergency method of intravenous access in the neonate.

spontaneously and continues with bradycardia for greater than 15 minutes, sodium bicarbonate can be administered. The sodium bicarbonate (8.4%) is diluted 1:2 with normal saline and administered intravenously (umbilical vein or intraosseous catheter) at a dose of 0.5–1.0 mL/kg (prior to dilution) (Traas 2008a).

Intravenous fluids and dextrose can be administered following a prolonged resuscitation process in the neonate, such as 10% dextrose at a dose of 2–4 mL/kg slowly intravenously or intraosseously. Hypoglycemia is diagnosed if blood glucose falls below 30–40 mg/dL (Davidson 2014). A neonate can be easily fluid overloaded due to its inability to concentrate or dilute its urine, so judicious use of fluids is recommended (60–180 mL/kg daily) (Grundy 2006).

Once the neonate has begun vocalizing and moving spontaneously, it can be placed in an incubator at 50–60% relative humidity with oxygen supplementation. The temperature should be 32.2 °C (90 °F) to prevent hypothermia. If no incubator is available, the neonates can be placed on a warm air blanket or warm water bottles covered with towels (Traas 2008a,b). Once the dam is stable and alert, the neonates may be placed with her, with some authors recommending bathing the neonates in amniotic fluid to increase acceptance by the mother (Abitbol & Inglis 1997). All neonates should receive a complete physical examination and be inspected for congenital defects including atresia ani, hypospadias, cleft palate, and umbilical hernia.

Neonatal blood lactate concentrations are similar at birth whether born vaginally or via cesarean section; however, neonates have a greater chance of survival if blood lactate rapidly declines in the first 24 hours following birth. In addition, non-survivor neonates were more likely to have higher blood lactate levels (>5.0 mmol/L) in conjunction with lower Apgar score (<3) than surviving neonates (Castagnetti et al. 2017).

Complications and prognosis

Maternal mortality rates following cesarean section are 1% (Moon & Erb 1998). Performance of an ovariohysterectomy at the time of cesarean section (whether by owner request or because of decreased uterine viability) does not decease lactation subsequently (Robbins & Mullen 1994; Tobias 2010). Repeat cesarean surgeries in dogs are associated with a high rate of uterine body and horn adhesions, which can complicate exteriorization of the uterus at the repeat cesarean (Choppillil 2019). There is also the rarer occurrence of perimetrial cyst formation; however, this did not prevent subsequent pregnancy. As with primary cesarean sections, prognosis was improved with elective versus emergency procedures (Choppillil 2019).

Complications following cesarean section can include hemorrhage, hypovolemia, and hypotension. If the dam appears to be having a prolonged recovery, monitoring for these complications should be performed including hematocrit, total protein, systemic blood pressure, and heart rate. Intravenous fluids and supportive care can be continued as well as administration of blood products. However, continued hemorrhage may have to be treated with ovariohysterectomy. The incidence of hemorrhage associated with dystocia is 6.7% and following cesarean without ovariohysterectomy is 23%, as recently reported (Doodnaught et al. 2020). Reduction in the incidence of postpartum hemorrhage following cesarean has been achieved in humans by administration of oxytocin and tranexamic acid, and these medications have been reported previously in cases of hemorrhage following cesarean in a dog (Simonazzi et al. 2016; Doodnaught et al. 2020). In the dog, 1 unit oxytocin was administered intramuscularly postoperatively and tranexamic acid at 10 mg/kg intravenously every 8 hours for 24 hours, with the recommendation that dogs remain hospitalized for 24 hours postoperatively for serial systemic blood pressure and hematocrit measurements (Doodnaught et al. 2020).

Uterine, urinary, or gastrointestinal tract trauma can occur during cesarean section and owners should be informed prior to consent to the surgery. Later, postoperative complications can include endometritis, mastitis, wound infection, wound dehiscence, and peritonitis (Gilson 2003).

Survival rates for neonates born via cesarean section are 92% at birth, 87% at 2 hours of age, and 80% at 7 days of age (Moon & Erb 1998), but that number drops with emergency cesareans when 19.6% of puppies are born dead (Schmidt *et al.* 2021). Neonatal mortality was associated with puppy lodgment in the pelvic canal or length of anesthesia >80 minutes. Reduction of time between induction and surgery start time (<30 minutes) and expedient cesarean if obstructive dystocia is present are recommended (Schmidt *et al.* 2021). More than 50% of dystocia cases caused by uterine inertia require repeated dosing with oxytocin and/or denaverine; therefore, repeat treatment is warranted, but if no response occurs cesarean section should be considered (Munnich & Kuchenmeister 2009). More frequent lower doses of oxytocin (0.25–0.5 IU/dog) have been advocated in the medical management of dystocia, with some success. However, following two doses of oxytocin 15–30 minutes apart without success, one should consider cesarean section (Munnich & Kuchenmeister 2009). Vitality of the neonate can be sustained and a successful outcome achieved with cesarean section if surgery is timed correctly (not waiting too long to choose surgery) and appropriate perioperative and surgical procedures are performed (Linde-Forsberg & Eneroth 1998; Munnich & Kuchenmeister 2009). The number of stillbirths was higher with increasing duration of the expulsion stage. The duration of expulsion in litters with normal puppies (without hypoxia) was 5.5 hours, whereas it was 10 hours for litters with dead/hypoxic puppies regardless of the method of management chosen for treatment of the dystocia, including cesarean section (Munnich & Kuchenmeister 2009). Improvement in neonate survival can be achieved, among other methods, by decreasing the number of emergency cesarean sections and not using methoxyflurane or xylazine for the anesthesia (Moon *et al.* 2000). Proper management of the dam and neonates is of vital importance for a positive outcome for all of them, and this means having well-trained staff and surgeons with equipment in place at the time of surgery.

References

Abitbol, M.L. and Inglis, S.R. (1997). Role of amniotic fluid in newborn acceptance and bonding in canines. *Journal of Maternal-Fetal Medicine* 6: 49–52.

Bannoehr, J. and Guardabassi, L. (2012). Staphylococcus pseudointermedius in the dog: taxonomy, diagnostics, ecology, epidemiology and pathogenicity. *Veterinary Dermatology* 23: 253–266.

Barber, J. (2003). Parturition and dystocia. In: *Small Animal Theriogenology* (ed. M.V. Root-Kustritz), 241–279. Burlington, VT: Butterworth-Heinemann.

Beccaglia, M. and Luvoni, G.C. (2006). Comparison of the accuracy of two ultrasonographic measurements in predicting the parturition date in the bitch. *Journal of Small Animal Practice* 47: 670–673.

Bergstrom, A., Nodtvedt, A., Lagerstedt, A.S. et al. (2006). Incidence and breed predilection for dystocia and risk factors for cesarean section in a Swedish population of insured dogs. *Veterinary Surgery* 35: 786–791.

Biddle, D. and Macintire, D.K. (2000). Obstetrical emergencies. *Clinical Techniques in Small Animal Practice* 15: 88–93.

Brooks, V.L. and Keil, L.C. (1994). Hemorrhage decreases arterial pressure sooner in pregnant compared with nonpregnant dogs: role of baroreflex. *American Journal of Physiology* 266: H1610–H1619.

Castagnetti, C., Cunto, M., Bini, C. et al. (2017). Time-dependent changes and prognostic value of lactatemia during the first 24 hours of life in brachicephalic newborn dogs. *Theriogenology* 94: 100–104.

Choppillil, J. (2019). Outcome and complications of repeat cesarean deliveries in dogs. *Pharma Innovation Journal* 8: 456–459.

Concannon, P.W., Hansel, W., and Visek, W.J. (1975). The ovarian cycle of the bitch: plasma estrogen, LH and progesterone. *Biology of Reproduction* 13: 112–121.

Darvelid, A.W. and Linde-Forsberg, C. (1994). Dystocia in the bitch: a retrospective study of 182 cases. *Journal of Small Animal Practice* 35: 402–407.

Davidson, A.P. (2001). Uterine and fetal monitoring in the bitch. *Veterinary Clinics of North America: Small Animal Practice* 31: 305–313.

Davidson, A.P. (2014). *Veterinary Clinics of North America: Small Animal Practice* 44: 199–204.

Doebeli, A., Michel, E., Bettschart, R. et al. (2013). Apgar score after induction of anesthesia for canine cesarean section with alfaxalone versus propofol. *Theriogenology* 80: 850–854.

Dolf, G., Gaillard, C., Russenberger, J. et al. (2018). Factors contributing to the decision to perform cesarean section in Labrador retrievers. *BMC Veterinary Research* 14: 57.

Doodnaught, G.M., O'Toole, E., and Pang, D.S.J. (2020). Management of severe peripartum hemmorrhage following cesarean section in a dog. *Canadian Veterinary Journal* 61: 589–594.

Drobatz, K.J. and Casey, K.K. (2000). Eclampsia in dogs: 31 cases (1995–1998). *Journal of the American Veterinary Medical Association* 217: 216–219.

Ekstrand, C. and Linde-Forsberg, C. (1994). Dystocia in the cat: a retrospective study of 155 cases. *Journal of Small Animal Practice* 35: 459–464.

Eneroth, A., Linde-Forsberg, C., Uhlhorn, M. et al. (1999). Radiographic pelvimetry for assessment of dystocia in bitches: a clinical study in two terrier breeds. *Journal of Small Animal Practice* 40: 257–264.

Feldman, E.C. and Nelson, R.W. (2004). Breeding, pregnancy and parturition. In: *Canine and Feline Endocrinology and Reproduction*, 3e, 775–806. St Louis, MO: WB Saunders.

Ferrari, D., Lundgren, S., Holmberg, J. et al. (2022). Concentration of carprofen in the milk of lactating bitches after cesarean section and during inflammatory conditions. *Theriogenology* 181: 59–68.

Fox, M.W. (1964). The ontogeny of behavior and neurologic responses in the dog. *Journal of Animal Behavior* 12: 301–310.

de Freitas, L.A., Costa, P.P.C., Waller, S.B. et al. (2021). Breed-specific ecobiometry and ultrasound factors predictive of fetal maturity in healthy English Bulldog bitches subjected to elective cesarean section. *Research, Society and Development* 10 (10): e555101019091.

Gaudet, D.A. (1985). Retrospective study of 128 cases of canine dystocia. *Journal of the American Animal Hospital Association* 21: 813–818.

Gavrilovic, B.B., Andersson, K., and Linde-Forsberg, C. (2008). Reproductive patterns in the domestic dog: a retrospective study of the Drever breed. *Theriogenology* 70: 783–794.

Gendler, A., Brourman, J.D., and Graf, K.E. (2007). Canine dystocia: medical and surgical management. *Compendium on Continuing Education for the Practicing Veterinarian* 29: 551–562.

Gilson, S.D. (2003). Cesarean section. In: *Textbook of Small Animal Surgery*, 3e (ed. D. Slatter), 1517–1520. Philadelphia, PA: WB Saunders.

Gilson, S.D. (2015). Cesarean section. In: *Small Animal Surgical Emergencies* (ed. L.R. Aronson), 391–396. Chichester: Wiley.

Gin, T. and Chan, M.T. (1994). Decreased minimum alveolar concentration of isofluorane in pregnant humans. *Anesthesiology* 81: 829–832.

Greene, S.A. (1995). Anesthetic considerations for surgery of the reproductive system. *Seminars in Veterinary Medicine and Surgery (Small Animal)* 10: 2–7.

Gregory, K.D., Korst, L.M., Gornbein, J.A. et al. (2002). Using administrative data to identify indications for elective primary cesarean delivery. *Health Services Research* 37: 1387–1401.

Grundy, S.A. (2006). Clinically relevant physiology of the neonate. *Veterinary Clinics of North America: Small Animal Practice* 36: 443–459.

Hedlund, C.S. (2007). Surgery of the reproductive and genital systems. In: *Small Animal Surgery*, 3e (ed. T.W. Fossum), 702–744. St Louis, MO: Mosby Elsevier.

Jutkowitz, L.A. (2005). Reproductive emergencies. *Veterinary Clinics of North America: Small Animal Practice* 35: 397–420.

Kaneko, M., Nakayama, H., Igarashi, N. et al. (1993). Relationship between the number of fetuses and the blood constituents of beagles in late pregnancy. *Journal of Veterinary Medical Science* 55: 681–682.

Kudnig, S.T. and Mama, K. (2000). Perioperative fluid therapy. *Journal of the American Veterinary Medical Association* 221: 1112–1121.

Kutzler, M.A., Mohammed, H.O., Lamb, S.V. et al. (2003a). Accuracy of canine parturition date prediction from the initial rise in preovulatory progesterone concentration. *Theriogenology* 60: 1187–1196.

Kutzler, M.A., Yeager, A.E., Mohammed, H.O. et al. (2003b). Accuracy of canine parturition date prediction using fetal measurements obtained by ultrasonography. *Theriogenology* 60: 1309–1317.

Linde-Forsberg, C. and Eneroth, A. (1998). Parturition. In: *Manual of Small Animal Reproduction and Neonatology* (ed. G.M. Simpson, G.C.W. England and M.J. Harvey), 127–142. Gloucester, British Small Animal Veterinary Association.

Linde-Forsberg, C. and Persson, G. (2007). A survey of dystocia in the boxer breed. *Acta Veterinaria Scandinavica* 49: 8.

Lopate, C. (2008). Estimation of gestational age and assessment of canine and feline maturation using radiology and ultrasonography: a review. *Theriogenology* 70: 397–402.

Lucio, C.F., Silva, L.C.G., Rodrigues, J.A. et al. (2009). Peripartum haemodynamic status of bitches with normal birth or dystocia. *Reproduction in Domestic Animals* 44: 133–136.

Luvoni, G.C. and Beccaglia, M. (2006). The prediction of parturition date in canine pregnancy. *Reproduction in Domestic Animals* 41: 27–32.

Luvoni, G.C. and Grioni, A. (2000). Determination of gestational age in medium and small size bitches using ultrasonographic fetal measurements. *Journal of Small Animal Practice* 41: 292–294.

Mathews, K.A. (2005). Analgesia for the pregnant, lactating and neonatal to pediatric cat and dog. *Journal of Veterinary Emergency and Critical Care* 15: 273–284.

McMichael, M.A. and Dhupa, N. (2000). Pediatric critical care medicine: specific syndromes. *Compendium on Continuing Education for the Practicing Veterinarian* 22: 353–358.

Moon, P.F. and Erb, H.N. (1998). Perioperative management and mortality rates of dogs undergoing cesarean section in the United States and Canada. *Journal of the American Veterinary Medical Association* 213: 365–369.

Moon, G.J., Erb, H.N., Ludders, J.W. et al. (2000). Perioperative risk factors for puppies delivered by cesarean section in the United States and Canada. *Journal of the American Animal Hospital Association* 36: 359–368.

Moon, G.J., Massat, B.J., and Pascoe, P.J. (2001). Neonatal critical care. *Veterinary Clinics of North America: Small Animal Practice* 31: 343–367.

Moon-Massat, P.F. (2003). Cesarean section. In: *Textbook of Small Animal Surgery*, 3e (ed. D. Slatter), 2597–2602. Philadelphia, PA: WB Saunders.

Moon-Massat, P.F. and Erb, H.N. (2002). Perioperative factors associated with puppy vigor after delivery by cesarean section. *Journal of the American Animal Hospital Association* 38: 90–96.

Munnich, A. and Kuchenmeister, U. (2009). Dystocia in numbers. Evidence-based parameters for intervention in the dog: causes for dystocia and treatment recommendations. *Reproduction in Domestic Animals* 44 (Suppl 2): 141–147.

Olson, P.N. and Mather, E.C. (1978). Canine vaginal and uterine bacterial flora. *Journal of the American Veterinary Medical Association* 172: 708–711.

Pablo, L.S. and Bailey, J.E. (1999). Etomidate and telazol. *Veterinary Clinics of North America: Small Animal Practice* 29: 779–792.

Palahniuk, R.J. and Shnider, S.M. (1974). Maternal and fetal cardiovascular and acid–base changes during halothane and isoflurane anesthesia in the pregnant ewe. *Anesthesiology* 41: 462–472.

Pascoe, P.J. and Moon, P.F. (2001). Periparturient and neonatal anesthesia. *Veterinary Clinics of North America: Small Animal Practice* 31: 315–340.

Probst, C.W. and Webb, A.I. (1983). Postural influence on systemic blood pressure, gas exchange and acid/base status in the term-pregnant bitch during general anesthesia. *American Journal of Veterinary Research* 44: 1963–1965.

Probst, C.W., Broadstone, R.V., and Evans, A.T. (1987). Postural influence on systemic blood pressure in large full-term pregnant bitches during general anesthesia. *Veterinary Surgery* 16: 471–473.

Rattan, J.C. (1999). Acupuncture resuscitation techniques questioned. *Journal of the American Veterinary Medical Association* 214: 616–618.

Rendano, V.T. (1983). Radiographic evaluation of fetal development in the bitch and fetal death in the bitch and queen. In: *Current Veterinary Therapy* (ed. R.W. Kirk), 947–952. Philadelphia, PA: WB Saunders.

Rendano, V.T., Lein, D.H., and Concannon, P.W. (1984). Radiographic evaluation of prenatal development in the Beagle: correlation with time of breeding, LH release, and parturition. *Veterinary Radiology* 25: 132–141.

Robbins, M.A. and Mullen, H.S. (1994). En bloc ovariohysterectomy as a treatment for dystocia in dogs and cats. *Veterinary Surgery* 23: 48–52.

Robertson, S. (1992). Advantages of etomidate: use as an anesthetic agent. *Veterinary Clinics of North America: Small Animal Practice* 22: 277–280.

Roll, C. and Horsch, S. (2004). Effects of doxapram on cerebral blood flow velocity in preterm infants. *Neuropediatrics* 35: 126–129.

Root-Kustritz, M.V. (2005). Pregnancy diagnosis and abnormalities of pregnancy in the dog. *Theriogenology* 64: 755–765.

Rota, A., Milani, C., Contiero, B. et al. (2019). Evaluation of serum C-reactive protein concentration as a marker of impending parturition and correlation with progesterone profile in peripartum bitches. *Animal Reproduction Science* 204: 111–116.

Ruaux, C.G. (2010). The respiratory system. In: *Small Animal Pediatrics: The First 12 Months of Life* (ed. M.E. Peterson and M. Kutzler), 328–339. St Louis, MO: Elsevier.

Ryan, S.D. and Wagner, A.E. (2006a). Cesarean section in dogs: anesthetic management. *Compendium on Continuing Education for the Practicing Veterinarian* 28: 44–54.

Ryan, S.D. and Wagner, A.E. (2006b). Cesarean section in dogs: physiology and perioperative considerations. *Compendium on Continuing Education for the Practicing Veterinarian* 28: 34–43.

Schmidt, K., Feng, C., Wu, T., and Duke-Novakovski, T. (2021). Influence of maternal, anesthetic, and surgical factors on neonatal survival after emergency cesarean section in 78 dogs: a retrospective study (2002–2020). *Canadian Veterinary Journal* 62: 961–968.

Seymour, C. (1999). Cesarean section. In: *BSAVA Manual of Small Animal Anesthesia and Analgesia* (ed. C. Seymour and R. Gleed), 217–222. Gloucester: British Small Animal Veterinary Association.

Short, C.E. and Bufalari, A. (1999). Propofol anesthesia. *Veterinary Clinics of North America: Small Animal Practice* 29: 747–788.

Simonazzi, G., Bisulli, M., Saccone, G. et al. (2016). Tranexamic acid for preventing postpartum blood loss after cesarean delivery: a systematic review and meta-analysis of randomized controlled trials. *Acta Obstetricia et Gynecologica Scandinavica* 95: 28–37.

Skarda, R.T. (1999). Anesthesia case of the month: dystocia, cesarean section and acupuncture resuscitation of newborn kittens. *Journal of the American Veterinary Medical Association* 214: 37–39.

Smith, F.O. (2007). Challenges in small animal parturition: timing elective and emergency cesarean sections. *Theriogenology* 68: 348–353.

Son, C., Jeong, K., Kim, J. et al. (2001). Establishment of the prediction table of parturition day with ultrasonography in small pet dogs. *Journal of Veterinary Medical Science* 63: 715–721.

Toal, R.L., Walker, M.A., and Henry, G.A. (1986). A comparison of real-time ultrasound, palpation, and radiography in pregnancy detection and litter size determination in the bitch. *Veterinary Radiology* 27: 102–108.

Tobias, K.M. (2010). Cesarean section. In: *Manual of Small Animal Soft Tissue Surgery*, 255–259. Ames, IA: Wiley Blackwell.

Traas, A.M. (2008a). Resuscitation of canine and feline neonates. *Theriogenology* 70: 343–348.

Traas, A.M. (2008b). Surgical management of canine and feline dystocia. *Theriogenology* 70: 337–342.

Wallace, M.S. (1994). Management of parturition and problems of the periparturient period of dogs and cats. *Seminars in Veterinary Medicine and Surgery (Small Animal)* 9: 28–37.

Wilmink, F.A., Hukkelhoven, C.W., Lunshof, S. et al. (2010). Neonatal outcome following elective cesarean section beyond 37 weeks of gestation: a 7-year retrospective analysis of a national registry. *American Journal of Obstetrics and Gynecology* 202: 250.e1–250.e8.

Wykes, P.M. (2003). Normal and abnormal parturition. In: *Textbook of Small Animal Surgery*, 3e (ed. D. Slatter), 1510–1517. Philadelphia, PA: WB Saunders.

Zakosek Pipan, M., Svara, T., Zdovc, I. et al. (2019). *Staphylococcus pseudointermedius* septicemia in puppies after elective cesarean section: confirmed transmission via dam's milk. *BMC Veterinary Research* 14: 41.

55

Congenital Vaginal Defects

Fran Smith

Normal sexual development begins early in gestation, although gonadal sex of the developing fetus is initially undifferentiated and morphologically indistinguishable until after day 30 of gestation (Pretzer 2008). Errors in the establishment of chromosomal, gonadal, or phenotypic sex may result in congenital vaginal defects (Lyle 2007). Thus, abnormalities in the development of the urogenital sinus may result in varying malformations of the vagina and vestibule, such as persistent hymen and septal remnants.

Vaginal defects

Development

Vertical bands of tissue can be located at the vestibulovaginal junction or anywhere within the vagina. A persistent hymen or annular stricture is a transverse vertical band that can result when the caudal aspect of the paramesonephric ducts fails to fuse or cannulate with the urogenital sinus. An elongated vertical vaginal band, a vaginal septum, or rarely a duplication of the vagina is a longitudinal vertical band that can result when the paramesonephric ducts fail to unite or fuse with each other, leaving a medial partition.

Vertical bands of tissue are commonly identified at the vestibulovaginal junction in otherwise normal bitches, and in bitches with other congenital developmental abnormalities. These vertical bands are very common in bitches with ectopic ureters.

Clinical signs

Vertical vaginal bands are commonly associated with bitches that refuse copulation. These bitches may avoid the male, behave aggressively, and, if forced to allow intromission, exhibit signs of pain (Soderberg 1986). Clinical signs other than mating difficulties have not been clearly demonstrated. Chronic urinary tract infections, chronic vaginal discharge, vaginitis, urine pooling, and chronic cystitis have been associated with congenital vaginal defects (Hammel & Bjorling 2002). No direct cause and effect between congenital vaginal anomalies and the above clinical signs have been clearly defined (Lane & Lappin 1995). There is a report of a young Labrador retriever bitch with hematic-like vaginal discharge caused by a congenital abnormality of the muscular layer of the vagina complicated by hemato-pyocolpos. The case was resolved by ovariohysterectomy and partial vaginectomy with vaginoplasty (Alonge et al. 2015)

Diagnosis

Diagnostic techniques used to evaluate the vagina and vestibulovaginal junction include digital examination, rigid or flexible endoscopy, and positive-contrast radiography. Digital examination in either the awake or sedated patient allows the identification of either a central vertical band or of two openings in the vaginal vault. Vertical vaginal bands are the most commonly encountered defect. The vaginal septum was digitally palpable in 11 of 15 bitches in one study (Root et al. 1995). Bitches with an annular or circumferential opening of the vestibulovaginal junction may present challenges during digital examination. The combination of sedation and estrus may facilitate digital examination in some bitches.

If the opening between the vestibule and the cranial vaginal vault does not allow penetration of the finger during digital examination, consider a diagnosis of annular constriction or vestibulovaginal stenosis. While differences in the expanse of the vaginal vault will occur because of the tremendous range in size of bitches, the vagina should be large enough to allow passage of the fetus during delivery.

The author uses a rigid sigmoidoscope (Welch Allyn 36019, Welch Allyn, Skaneateles Falls, NY, USA) with a disposable sigmoidoscope speculum (Welch Allyn Kleenscope) and rectal insufflators (Welch Allyn 30200) as a first choice to visualize the vaginal vault (Figure 55.1). For very tight annular strictures, a rigid endoscope used for transcervical insemination (Karl Storz, Tuttlingen, Germany) is very effective (Figure 55.2) (McCarthy 2006). Other rigid or flexible endoscopes are very effective in visualizing the vestibule, vestibulovaginal junction, and cranial vagina. Equipment choices can be based on availability and capital expense. Videovaginoscopy allows documentation of any abnormality found and can aid in planning any surgical treatment that is indicated (Burdick *et al.* 2014).

Positive-contrast retrograde vaginoscopy can be used to identify the extent of a stricture. Positive-contrast vaginography in a group of 12 bitches was successful in identifying the vaginal septum. This technique is particularly effective in investigating the extent of an elongated vertical band prior to considering surgical repair (Figure 55.3). Surgical repair should not be considered for any bitch that does not demonstrate clinical signs. In the case of a bitch that is important to a breeding program, the combination of artificial insemination followed by cesarean section at term can result in a superior outcome than with attempted resection of the vaginal septa.

Treatment

Correction of many congenital vaginal defects will require episiotomy to facilitate surgical correction (Wykes & Olson 1993; Tobias 1995; McLouglin 2003; Sicard & Fingland 2006). Episiotomy requires a general surgery pack, Gelpi or Weitlaner retractors, and a sterile Foley or other sterile urinary catheter. The procedure may be performed under local, epidural, or general anesthesia. The bitch should be positioned in ventral recumbency with the rear end elevated (Trendelenburg position) (McLouglin 2003; Sicard & Fingland 2006). It is very important that the surgical table be well padded to prevent inadvertent injury to the femoral nerves while performing the resection. Place a purse-string suture in the anus and secure the tail upright and toward the head. The patient is surgically clipped and prepared from dorsal to the anus to below the vulvar commissure. The entire perianal area should be prepared. The vestibule and vagina are flushed with a dilute antiseptic solution. The bladder is catheterized to remove urine and facilitate identification of the urethra. Drape both sides of the vulvar clefts and the dorsal commissure of the vulva. Insert a finger in the vestibule and identify the caudodorsal aspect of the vaginal canal. This point represents the dorsal extent of the incision. Make a median skin incision from the caudodorsal aspect of the vaginal canal to the dorsal aspect of the vulvar cleft (Figure 55.4). Using Metzenbaum or Mayo scissors, continue the incision in the same plane, incising the muscular layer and the mucosa. Apply the retractor to visualize the vaginal defect.

A thin septal band can often be removed using biopsy forceps. The band can be grasped with forceps along its base and separated from the attachment along the vestibulovaginal junction (Figure 55.5). The tissue remnant for the opposite surface is then removed. Sutures may or may not be required. Thicker septa will need to be removed by a direct surgical approach, typically requiring an episiotomy.

If a vaginal band is present, place a curved instrument cranial to the band and retract the band caudally. Transect the band at the dorsal and ventral attachments. Close the mucosal defects using small absorbable suture in a continuous suture pattern. To correct an annular constriction, circumferentially excise thin membranes at the mucosal attachment. If submucosal fibrous tissue is present, it should be carefully dissected and excised. The

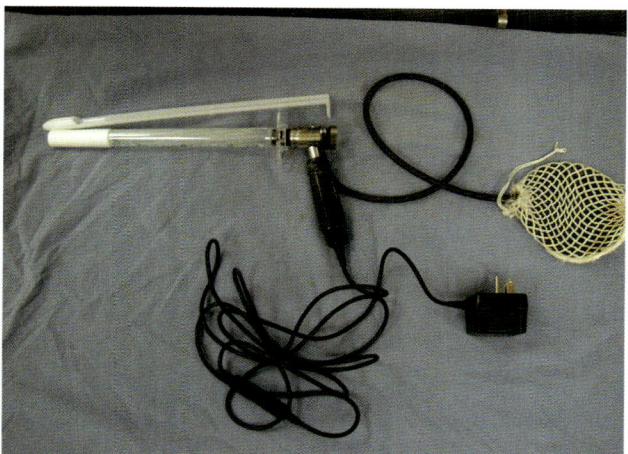

Figure 55.1 Welch Allyn sigmoidoscope with insufflator used to visualize congenital defects of the vulva and vagina.

(a)

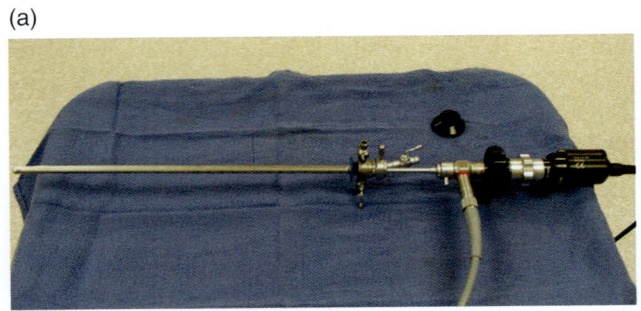

(b)

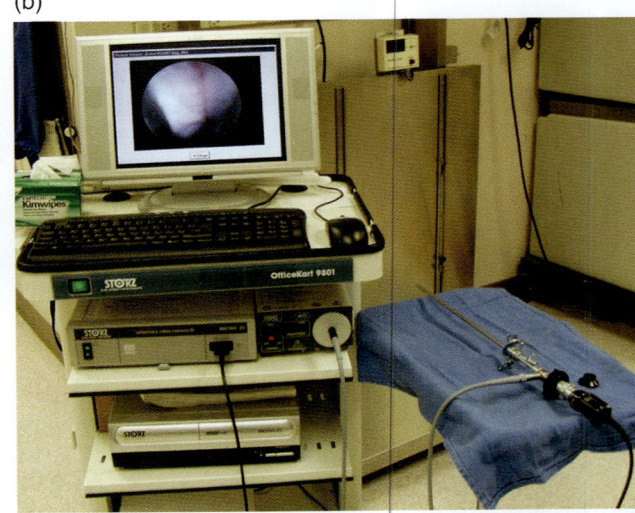

Figure 55.2 (a) Endoscopy unit that includes a rigid-fiber endoscope. (b) Light source, computer, camera, and video screen with recording capabilities.

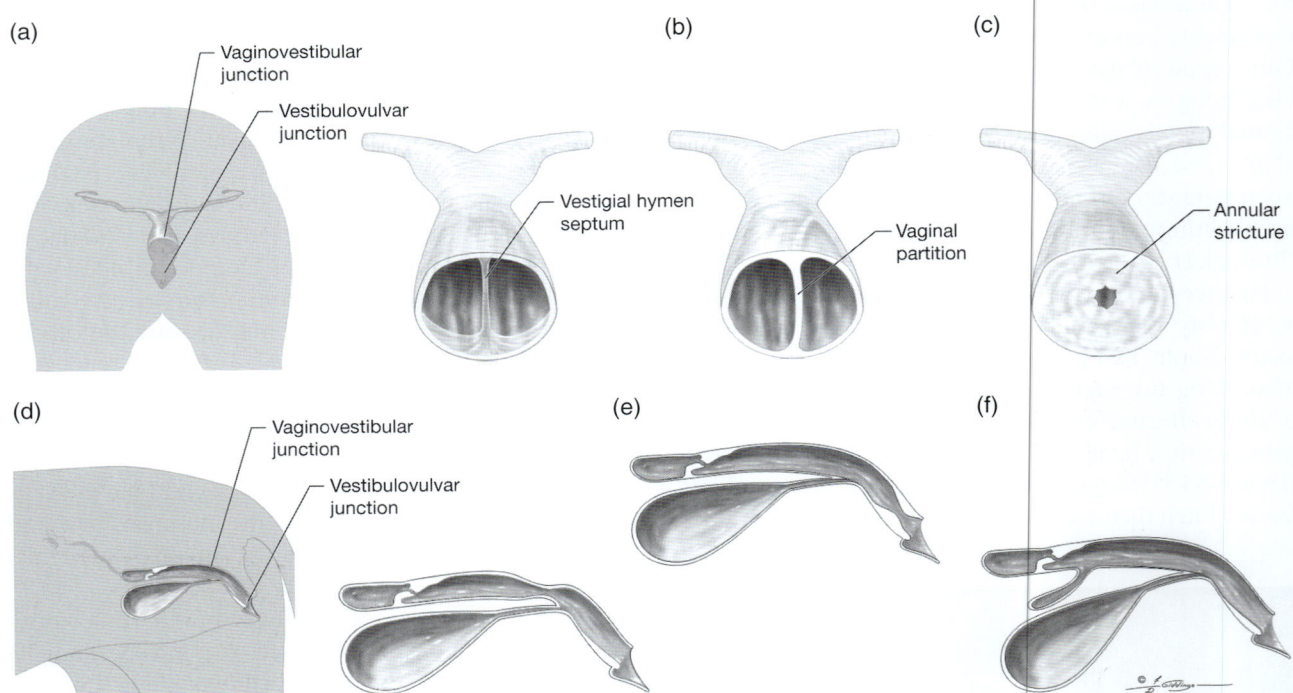

Figure 55.3 Different types and locations of congenital vaginal defects in the bitch, demonstrating the variability of the defects. (a) Normal anatomy of the caudal reproductive tract. (b) Incomplete fusion of the paramesonephric ducts resulting in incomplete partitioning of the vagina. (c) Annular stricture at the vaginovestibular orifice. (d) Stenosis of vaginovestibular junction. (e) Stenosis at the vestibulovulvar junction. (f) Secondary vaginal pouch. © D. Giddings.

mucosal defect is closed with small absorbable suture in either a simple interrupted or simple continuous pattern.

Complete resection of an annular stricture at the vestibulovaginal junction is difficult and time-consuming (Kyles *et al.* 1996). In certain cases, a narrowed region of the vagina can be enlarged by using a vestibulovaginoplasty procedure. Short hypoplastic segments of the vagina may be corrected by extending the vaginal incision beyond the affected area and closing the vaginal defect in a "T" fashion, or by rotation of a vestibular mucosal flap with the base located at the vestibulovaginal junction. The flap is placed where the defect was created by extending the vaginal incision (Figure 55.6). Following excision of the septa or completion of the

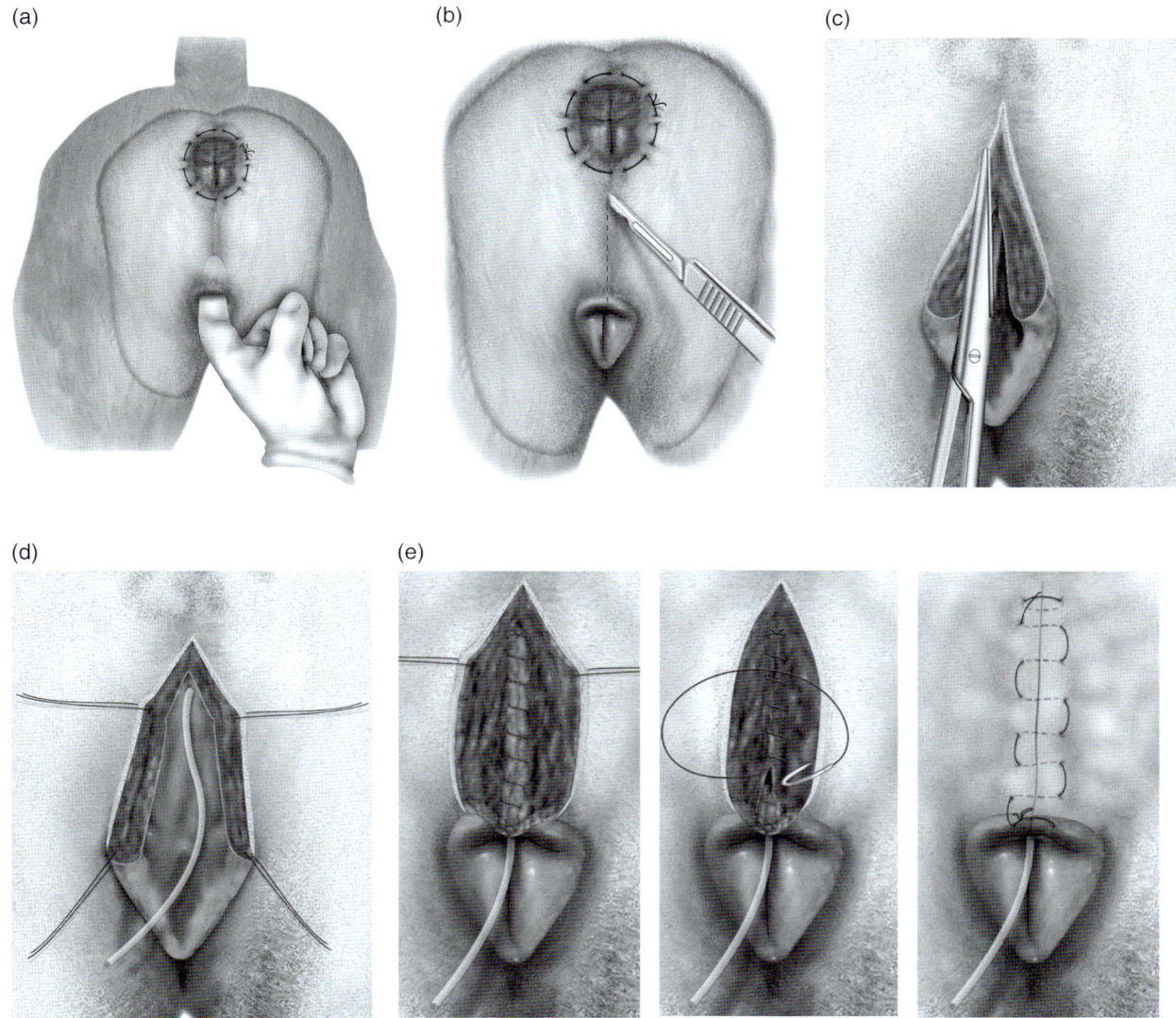

Figure 55.4 (a–e) Surgical technique for an episiotomy in a bitch. © D. Giddings.

correction, the episiotomy is closed in three layers. First, the mucosal layer is closed by apposing the edges with 3-0 absorbable suture in a continuous pattern with knots exposed to the lumen. Second, the muscular layer and the subcutaneous tissue are closed simultaneously using absorbable suture in a simple continuous pattern. Third, the skin is closed separately using small suture material in either a continuous or simple interrupted pattern. Following closure, remove the urethral catheter and the purse-string suture from the anus.

Strictures that are located more cranially may not be amenable to correction via episiotomy. These defects may require more extensive surgery involving an abdominal approach and potential pubic osteotomy. Surgery of this magnitude must be carefully considered

by the clinician and with counseling of the owner. If the purpose of the surgery is to facilitate reproduction, artificial insemination and cesarean section are likely a safer and more cost-effective alternative.

In rare occasions, vaginectomy is undertaken. This procedure may be performed after failed surgery of the vestibulovaginal junction, with very cranial strictures, or for confirmed urine pooling after removal of a septal band. A midline abdominal incision is required, followed by a complete ovariohysterectomy and then isolation of the vagina from its peritoneal support. The vaginal branches of the urogenital arteries and veins are ligated and the vagina is transfixed just cranial to the urethral tubercle. It is important to avoid damage to the vascular and nerve supply to the urethra and bladder.

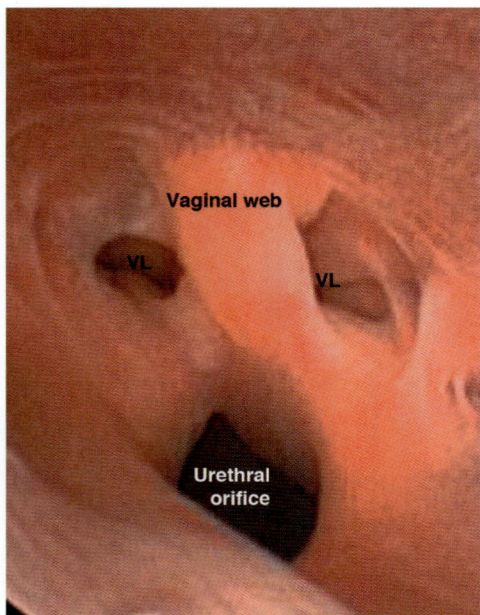

Figure 55.5 A vaginal septum in a spayed female dog as visualized through an endoscope. VL, vaginal lumen.

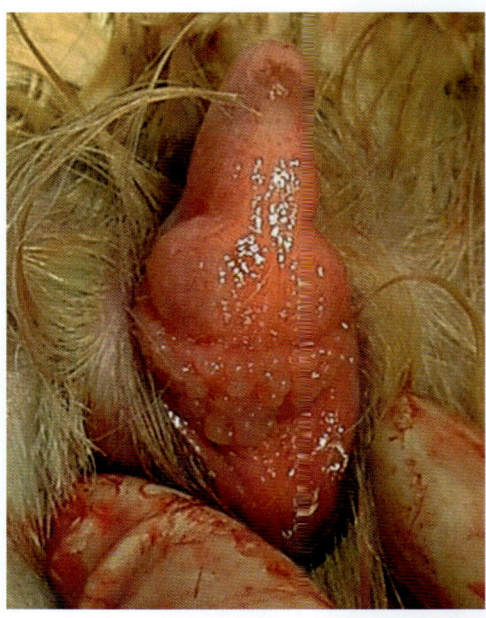

Figure 55.7 Severe clitoral hypertrophy in a Kerry blue terrier bitch with XX sex reversal.

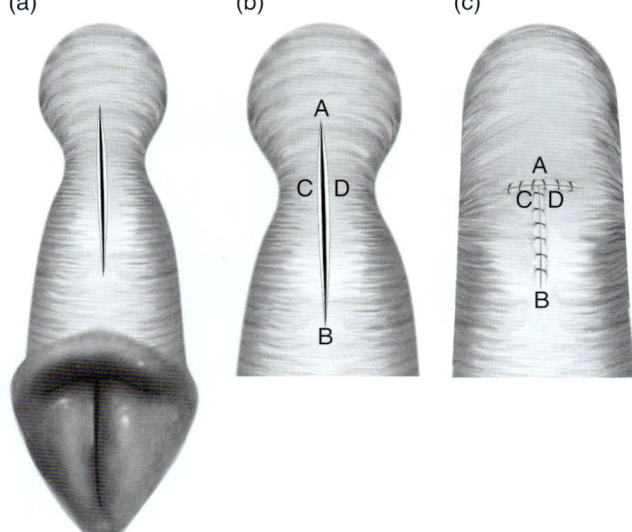

Figure 55.6 Surgical technique used for the correction of segmental vaginal stenosis. (a) A longitudinal incision is made beyond the limit of the stenosis. (b, c) The incision is then closed in a transverse fashion. © D. Giddings.

Endoscopic-guided laser ablation of vestibulovaginal septal remnants has been described in dogs. The vaginal membrane involved was transected using an endoscopic-guided laser with a holmium:yttrium-aluminum-garnet and diode laser. This procedure was safe, effective, and minimally invasive in 36 cases (Burdick *et al.* 2014).

Clitoral hypertrophy

Clitoral hypertrophy may occur in the bitch either as a congenital or an acquired problem (Figure 55.7). Acquired causes of clitoral hypertrophy include exogenous administration of androgenic substances and hyperadrenocorticism. The bitch that presents with congenital clitoral hypertrophy is typically afflicted with disorders of sexual differentiation. These bitches usually have disorders of gonadal sex (gonadal sex does not agree with chromosomal sex) and are frequently categorized as XX sex reversal. The condition is most common in the American cocker spaniel, English cocker spaniel, beagle, Weimaraner, Kerry blue terrier, and pug. The mode of inheritance in most breeds is uncertain. In the American cocker spaniel it is inherited as an autosomal recessive trait.

Treatment of clitoral hypertrophy is reserved for bitches with significant clinical signs, including chronic vaginitis, chronic vestibulitis, and secondary urinary tract infection. The treatment is surgical and includes an episiotomy for exposure of the clitoris and clitoral fossa. The urethra is catheterized and clitoris is dissected from its attachment and the surrounding mucosa. Significant hemorrhage may be encountered, particularly in animals with XX sex reversal. Control hemorrhage as indicated. The edges of the mucosa are aligned and closed with absorbable suture, eliminating the clitoral fossa. The episiotomy is closed in a routine manner.

References

Alonge, S., Romussi, S., Grieco, V., and Luvoni, G.C. (2015). Congenital abnormality of the vagina complicated by haemato-pyocolpos in a 1-year labrador retriever. *Reproduction in Domestic Animals* 50 (3): 514–516.

Burdick, S., Berent, A., Weisse, C., and Langston, C. (2014). Endoscopic-guided laser ablation of vestibulovaginal septal remnant in dogs: 36 cases (2007–2011). *Journal of the American Veterinary Medical Association* 244 (8): 944–949.

Hammel, S.P. and Bjorling, D.E. (2002). Results of vulvoplasty for treatment of recessed vulva in dogs. *Journal of the American Animal Hospital Association* 38: 79–83.

Kyles, A.E., Vaden, S., Hardie, E.M., and Stone, E.A. (1996). Vestibulovaginal stenosis in dogs: 18 cases (1987–1995). *Journal of the American Veterinary Medical Association* 209: 1889–1893.

Lane, I.F. and Lappin, M.R. (1995). Urinary incontinence and congenital urogenital anomalies in small animals. In: *Current Veterinary Therapy XII* (ed. J.D. Bonagura and R.W. Kirk), 1022–1026. St Louis, MO: WB Saunders.

Lyle, S.K. (2007). Disorder of sexual development in the dog and cat. *Theriogenology* 68: 338–343.

McCarthy, T. (2006). Otheroscopies. In: *Veterinary Endoscopy for the Small Animal Practitioner* (ed. T. McCarthy), 426–427. Elsevier Saunders: St Louis, MO.

McLouglin, M.A. (2003). Surgical techniques of the reproductive tracts. In: *Proceedings of the Society for Theriogenology*, 202–203. Columbus, OH: Society for Theriogenology.

Pretzer, S.D. (2008). Canine embryonic and fetal development: a review. *Theriogenology* 70: 300–303.

Root, M.V., Johnston, S.D., and Johnston, G.R. (1995). Vaginal septa in dogs: 15 cases (1983–1992). *Journal of the American Veterinary Medical Association* 206: 56–58.

Sicard, G.K. and Fingland, R.B. (2006). Surgery of the vagina and vulva. In: *Saunders Manual of Small Animal Practice*, 3e (ed. S.J. Birchard and R.G. Sherding), 1009–1010. Saunders Elsevier: St Louis, MO.

Soderberg, S.F. (1986). Vaginal disorders. *Veterinary Clinics of North America Small Animal Practice* 16: 543–559.

Tobias, K.M. (1995). Surgical correction of congenital anomalies of the reproductive tract. *Seminars in Veterinary Medicine and Surgery (Small Animal)* 10: 13–20.

Wykes, P.M. and Olson, P.V. (1993). Vaginal vestibule and vulva. In: *Textbook of Small Animal Surgery*, 2e (ed. D.H. Slatter), 1308–1311. Philadelphia, PA: WB Saunders.

56

Ovariectomy and Ovariohysterectomy

Thomas J. Smith and Bernard Séguin

There are numerous indications to neuter a female dog or cat. These include eliminating pregnancy, the nuisance of proestrus (or spotting) in dogs, undesirable behaviors during estrus, decreasing the incidence of neoplasia, cystic endometrial hyperplasia, and pyometra. Neutering early in life has been shown to significantly decrease the risk of developing mammary tumors in dogs and cats.

In dogs, the relative risk of developing mammary gland tumors later in life is 0.5% if the ovariohysterectomy (OVH) is performed before the first estrus, 8% if the OVH is performed between the first and second estrus, and 26% if the OVH is performed between second estrus and 2.5 years of age (Schneider *et al.* 1969). However, if the OVH is performed within two years of developing mammary tumors in dogs, the tumor is more likely to have benign behavior and OVH at this time prolongs survival (Sorenmo *et al.* 2000; Chang *et al.* 2005, 2009). In cats, there is a 91% reduction in risk of developing mammary carcinoma if the neuter is performed before 6 months of age and an 86% reduction compared with intact females if the neuter is performed before 1 year of age (Overley *et al.* 2005).

Effects of age of patient at time of neutering

The effects of age at time of neutering have been investigated in several studies. In dogs, neutering when an animal is growing leads to delayed closure of the growth plates of the radius and ulna such that these bones end up being longer. This effect is greatest in dogs neutered at an early age (7 weeks of age in the study). Neutered dogs also show immature vulvar development and increased activity levels (Salmeri *et al.* 1991a,b). Another study concluded that early gonadectomy (<24 weeks of age) in dogs increases the risk of contracting an infectious disease (Howe *et al.* 2001).

It has also been shown that early gonadectomy (<5.5 months old vs. >5.5 months old) can lead to an increased rate of cystitis and urinary incontinence among female dogs (Spain *et al.* 2004a). The risk of urinary incontinence was greatest for dogs spayed before 3 months old. Early gonadectomy can also lead to an increased incidence of hip dysplasia, noise phobia, and sexual behavior. Conversely, early-age gonadectomy leads to a decreased incidence of separation anxiety, escape behavior, inappropriate elimination when frightened, and relinquishment for any reason. Therefore it has been recommended to delay gonadectomy until at least 3 months of age and ideally until after 4–5 months old. Neutering does not affect food intake, weight gain, and back-fat depth (Salmeri *et al.* 1991b) and indeed early-age gonadectomy can lead to a decreased incidence of obesity (Spain *et al.* 2004a).

Intact cats weigh less, have less fat, and have earlier closure of the growth plates. Intact cats also display more aggression toward other cats, are less affectionate, and have greater development of their secondary sex characteristics (Stubbs *et al.* 1996) Early gonadectomy (<5.5 months old vs. >5.5 months old) in female cats is safe and does not lead to serious problems (Howe *et al.* 2000; Spain *et al.* 2004b). Early gonadectomy can

Small Animal Soft Tissue Surgery, Second Edition. Edited by Eric Monnet.
© 2023 John Wiley & Sons, Inc. Published 2023 by John Wiley & Sons, Inc.
Companion website: www.wiley.com/go/monnet/small

lead to increased shyness and decreased incidence of asthma, gingivitis, and hyperactivity (Spain *et al.* 2004b).

In conclusion, early gonadectomy is safe to perform in dogs and cats, but in female dogs it may be prudent to wait until the animal is at least 3 months old or even older. However, it is best to perform the procedure before the first estrus in female dogs and 6 months of age in cats to reduce the risk of mammary tumors.

Ovariohysterectomy versus ovariectomy

Making a rational choice between ovariectomy (OVE) and OVH in the dog can be challenging. From the perspective of surgically related complications, the risks of hemorrhage, vaginal bleeding, inadvertent ligation of the ureter, and formation of stump granulomas are less likely when performing OVE than OVH (van Goethem *et al.* 2006). Regarding ovarian remnant syndrome, OVE may allow incisions to be made more cranially, allowing better visualization of the ovary and hence less chance of leaving ovarian remnants. Long-term complications including urinary sphincter mechanism incontinence and weight gain are similar in both OVE and OVH. Development of endometritis, pyometra, and stump pyometra seems more common in dogs that had OVH. Okkens *et al.* (1981a,b) reported a 35% incidence of stump pyometra in dogs after OVH, while none of the dogs that received OVE had endometritis or pyometra. Stump pyometras were associated with an ovarian remnant. A potential disadvantage of OVE is that since the uterus is not removed, the potential for uterine tumors to develop exists, where it does not exist in OVH because the entire uterus is removed. However, it is estimated that the risk of developing a benign or malignant uterine tumor in dogs is 0.03% and 0.003%, respectively (van Goethem *et al.* 2006). In one study, incisions were shorter for OVE than OVH, but there was no difference in pain scores between the two groups and the surgical time was not significantly different either (Peeters & Kirpensteijn 2011).

Surgical techniques

Canine ovariohysterectomy and ovariectomy

Canine midline ovariohysterectomy

The dog is placed in dorsal recumbency. The length of the ventral midline abdominal incision is based on the size of the animal (Stone 2003). The distance between the umbilicus and the pubis is divided into thirds. The incision is initially made in the cranial third, because the ovaries are more difficult to exteriorize than the uterine body. However, the length of the incision should be sufficient to visualize the intra-abdominal structures and safely perform the procedure.

The right or left uterine horn is located by means of an index finger, or spay hook. The spleen and other organs are avoided. Once the uterine horn is exteriorized, it is followed cranially until the ovary is found. A clamp is placed on the proper ligament of the ovary and is used to retract the ovary while the suspensory ligament is stretched or broken with the index finger to better exteriorize the ovary (Hill & Smeak 2010). A window is made in the meso-ovarium, avoiding any vessels within it, immediately caudal to the ovarian vessels. The ovarian pedicle is triple clamped, and the pedicle severed between the clamp closest to the ovary and the middle clamp. The clamp most distant to the ovary is removed so that the pedicle ligature can be placed in the groove that is formed from the crushed tissue. Both authors highly recommend that a second ligature is placed for additional hemostasis should the first ligature fail. In addition, two ligatures are still considered to be the standard of care for this procedure.

The pedicle is grasped with small hemostats or thumb forceps, the remaining clamp is removed, and the pedicle is inspected for bleeding. The pedicle is gently replaced into the abdomen and visually inspected. As the tension on the pedicle is released, it is possible that hemorrhage may occur. The procedure is repeated on the other side.

The right and left broad ligaments are severed or torn. Sutures or electrocoagulation can be used to control bleeding. The uterine horns are pulled up, out of the abdominal cavity and caudally until the uterine body comes into sight. The incision may be lengthened to adequately expose the cervix. Three clamps are placed on the uterine body just cranial to the cervix. The uterine body is severed between the most cranial and middle clamps. In a large dog, the uterine arteries are individually ligated caudal to the most caudal clamp. The caudal clamp is removed, and the uterus is ligated in the groove that is formed from the crushed tissue. If the arteries were not ligated individually, a second ligature is placed on the uterine body. The uterine pedicle is grasped with a small hemostat above the clamp, the clamp is removed, and the pedicle is inspected for bleeding. The pedicle is gently replaced into the abdomen and the hemostat is removed.

A simple minimally invasive technique for OVE has been recently described relying on the creation of two midline portals, one cranial and one caudal, and with the aid of a 30 cm Hauptner shaft biopsy forceps, but without laparoscopy (Pukacz *et al.* 2009).

Canine flank ovariohysterectomy or ovariectomy

A flank approach has been described for OVE or OVH in dogs (Dorn 1975; McGrath *et al.* 2004). A grid approach is performed in either the right or left flank depending on the surgeon's preferences.

Canine laparoscopic ovariohysterectomy and ovariectomy

Laparoscopic OVE or OVH has been described with one, two, or three portals (Website Chapter 56: Reproductive tract/female reproductive tract/laparoscopic ovariectomy) (Austin *et al.* 2003; van Goethem *et al.* 2003; Davidson *et al.* 2004; Devitt *et al.* 2005; van Nimwegen *et al.* 2005; Mayhew & Brown 2007; Van Nimwegen & Kirpensteijn 2007a; Gower & Mayhew 2008; Culp *et al.* 2009; Dupré *et al.* 2009). In the one-portal technique, a working telescope is used to introduce one instrument into the working channel. The working telescope is 10 mm in diameter and therefore a 10 mm portal is used. Because the working channel is small, only 5 mm instruments can be used, which may prolong surgical time (Dupré *et al.* 2009). In the two- and three-portal procedures, one portal is placed caudal to the umbilicus to introduce the 5 mm endoscope with the camera. The other portals are placed either cranial to the umbilicus in the two-portal procedure or on either side of the camera portal. Usually one portal is 10 or 12 mm in diameter, which allows the utilization of larger vessel sealant devices. The larger device provides more effective hemostasis of the ovarian pedicle, which is particularly interesting in large-breed dogs or obese dogs with the ovarian pedicle covered with adipose tissue. In the one- and two-portal procedures, a percutaneous suture is used to stabilize the ovary against the abdominal wall under minimal tension to visualize the ovarian pedicle. Suture, vascular clip, harmonic scalpel, laser, electrocoagulation, and vessel sealant device can be used to provide adequate hemostasis (van Goethem *et al.* 2003; Devitt *et al.* 2005; van Nimwegen *et al.* 2005; Mayhew & Brown 2007; Van Nimwegen & Kirpensteijn 2007a; Dupré *et al.* 2009). OVH is either performed completely with laparoscopy or laparoscopically assisted while both ovarian pedicles are ligated with laparoscopy, but then both uterine horns are exteriorized through a portal that was initially placed at the level of the cervix. Then the uterine body is ligated as described during a regular OVH with an open approach. The laparoscopically assisted technique seems to be most commonly used to perform OVH because it eliminates the need to control the uterine body inside the abdominal cavity with sutures.

After insufflation of the abdominal cavity with CO_2 to a pressure of less than 15 mmHg, the patient, initially in dorsal recumbency, is tilted on one side to help visualize and ligate the ovarian pedicle on the nondependent side. The patient will then be tilted onto the other side to ligate the other ovarian pedicle. During a laparoscopic OVE the ovaries are retrieved through one portal. Usually ovaries of dogs weighing less than 30 kg can be retrieved through a 10–12 mm portal. If the ovaries are too large, the hole of the portal will have to be enlarged just enough to extract the ovary.

A number of studies have recently investigated the efficacy and variations of laparoscopic techniques. Hancock *et al.* (2005) and Devitt *et al.* (2005) have reported less pain associated with harmonic scalpel-assisted laparoscopy and laparoscopic OVH compared with open laparotomy in dogs, respectively. Mayhew and Brown (2007) reported that the use of a novel 5 mm bipolar vessel sealant device significantly shortened surgical time and provided excellent hemostasis during laparoscopic-assisted OVH. Dupré *et al.* (2009) reported on surgical times and perioperative complication rates of single-port and two-port laparoscopic OVE in dogs using a bipolar vessel shear-divider device. They concluded that single-port laparoscopic OVE using the device is feasible, safe, and does not significantly increase total surgical time in comparison with a two-portal approach. In another study, bipolar electrocautery was found to decrease laparoscopic OVE time and laparoscopic intraoperative hemorrhage, and facilitated exteriorization of the ovaries compared with the use of monopolar electrocautery (van Goethem *et al.* 2003). Case *et al.* (2011) showed that the level of pain in the one- and two-portal procedures was not significantly different and that surgical time was significantly prolonged with the one-portal procedure.

Canine ovariectomy by natural orifice transluminal endoscopic surgery

Freeman *et al.* (2009) studied 10 healthy female dogs that had OVE performed using an electrocautery snare via a gastrotomy that was subsequently closed with a prototype T-fastener. The mean operative time was 154 minutes and no animals died. In a single dog, incomplete ovary excision resulted in the need to convert to an open procedure.

Feline ovariectomy and ovariohysterectomy

Currently, the midline celiotomy or left flank approach is most commonly performed (Howard 2006). Selection of either technique is often made due to personal choice and previous training. Indications for flank spays include excessive mammary gland development due to lactation or mammary gland hyperplasia, lactating animals, ability to observe wounds at a distance in shelter cats, and reduced potential for evisceration (McGrath *et al.* 2004). Contraindications to a flank approach include breeds that are known to change their coat color following fur clipping such as oriental breeds (Gorelick 1974), gravid uterus, pyometra, obesity, and any suspicion of concurrent abdominal disease necessitating exploratory laparotomy (Pearson 1973; Dorn 1975; Dorn & Swift 1977; Janssens & Hanssens 1991; Salmeri *et al.* 1991a,b; McGrath *et al.* 2004). A recent clinical study reported that postoperative pain scores between cats having either flank or midline OVH were similar, but there was significantly more wound tenderness following the flank approach (Grint *et al.* 2006). Feline laparoscopic OVE (Van Nimwegen & Kirpensteijn 2007b) has been described as a feasible procedure. The relative benefits and potential cost of this procedure may not be advantageous when compared with flank OVE.

Feline midline ovariohysterectomy

OVH in the cat via a midline approach is similar in principle to that in the dog, with the exception that the feline incision is made in the central third (from umbilicus to pubis) instead of the cranial third as it is in the dog (Stone 2003). The suspensory ligament often does not need to be torn to allow exteriorization of the ovary. The cervix is closer to the level of the urinary bladder trigone in cats than in dogs, and therefore when ligating the uterine body in cats it is recommended to remain distant from the cervix to avoid entrapment of the ureters. When reflecting the uterus caudally out of the abdominal cavity, the ureter on the side of the bladder that the uterus is passing can be caught if ligatures are placed too close to the cervix. On completion of the OVH, the incisions in the abdominal wall and skin are closed in a routine fashion.

Feline flank ovariohysterectomy

A flank approach has been described for OVE or OVH in cats (Krzaczynski 1974; Coe *et al.* 2006). The cat is traditionally placed in right lateral recumbency and the pelvic limbs held in extension using ropes or sandbags. After making an incision in the left flank at a point located two finger widths behind the last rib and one finger width below the transverse process, the uterus is easily identified lying ventral to the sublumbar fat and adjacent or dorsal to the bladder (Feathers 1974; Hogues 1991; McGrath *et al.* 2004; Burrow *et al.* 2006; Coe *et al.* 2006; Grint *et al.* 2006). OVH is then performed as already described.

Several potential complications have been reported while using the flank approach, including the possibility that the entire uterine body may be difficult to remove, a dropped ovarian pedicle may be difficult to recover, and it may be difficult to expose the opposite ovary and uterine bifurcation (Ghanawat & Mantri 1996; Fingland 1998; Hedlund 2002; Stone 2003; Howard 2006).

Feline laparoscopic ovariectomy

Laparoscopic OVE has been described in 14 cats in which laser and bipolar electrocoagulation were compared (Van Nimwegen & Kirpensteijn 2007b). A midline three-portal technique is used as described for the dog (van Nimwegen *et al.* 2005). A Hasson technique was used for the placement of the first cannula. The ovary is grasped and lifted upward using the self-retaining grasping forceps through the cranial port. During bipolar electrocoagulation the proper ligament, suspensory ligament, and ovarian pedicle are coagulated using a 3 mm diameter bipolar electrocoagulation forceps and cut using endoscopic scissors. During laser OVE, major blood vessels of the ovarian pedicle are coagulated using the bipolar electrocoagulation forceps. The ovary is resected by sequentially cutting the proper ligament, pedicle, and suspensory ligament using the laser fiber in contact mode with 10 W continuous wave laser power. Iatrogenic hemorrhage is controlled using the bipolar electrocoagulation forceps. After complete resection, the ovary is removed from the abdomen through the caudal port, after removal of the trocar sheath. After reinsertion of the caudal trocar, the same procedure is performed for the right ovary. After removal of the instruments, each port is closed with a cruciate suture with 4-0 monofilament absorbable material. Subcutaneous tissues and skin are closed in routine fashion.

Complications

Despite being routine, OVH in the dog has been reported as having the highest complication rate of all elective procedures in North America (Pollari & Bonnett 1996; Pollari *et al.* 1996; Bradley *et al.* 2000). Numerous potential complications are associated with elective OVH (Bradley *et al.* 2000). The frequency of complications following OVH has been reported to be 12.2–31.5% (Berzon 1979; Pollari & Bonnett 1996; Pollari *et al.* 1996; Coolman *et al.* 1999). Minor complications occurring during surgery or within the first postoperative week are most common (Berzon 1979; Pollari & Bonnett 1996; Pollari *et al.* 1996; Coolman *et al.* 1999). Examples include reversible anesthetic complications, intraoperative bleeding, postoperative pyrexia, patient-inflicted incisional trauma, seroma, suture infection, and delayed healing (Joshua 1965; Dorn & Swift 1977; Berzon 1979; Pollari & Bonnett 1996; Pollari *et al.* 1996; Coolman *et al.* 1999). Less common major complications include anesthetic death, severe hemorrhage/exsanguination, hydroureter/hydronephrosis, stump pyometra, recurrent estrus from residual ovarian tissue (ovarian remnant syndrome), ovarian or uterine stump granulomas, draining fistulous tracts, vaginoperitoneal or vaginoureteral fistula, adhesion formation, retained surgical sponges, bowel obstruction, and tetanus (Joshua 1965; Furneaux *et al.* 1973; Pearson 1973; Dorn & Swift 1977; Berzon 1979; Allen & Webbon 1980; Kunin & Terry 1980; Pearson & Gibbs 1980; Rubin *et al.* 1983; De Baerdemaecker 1984; Spackman *et al.* 1984; MacCoy *et al.* 1988; Banks *et al.* 1991; Muir *et al.* 1993; Bagley *et al.* 1994; Lamb 1994; McEvoy 1994; Pollari & Bonnett 1996; Pollari *et al.* 1996; Smith & Davies 1996; Coolman *et al.* 1999; Ganssbauer *et al.* 2000).

Hemorrhage is reported as the most common complication in dogs weighing more than 25 kg (79%) (Berzon 1979) and the most common cause of death following routine OVH (Pearson 1973). Vaginal bleeding has also been reported as a complication after OVH. Vaginal bleeding is believed to be caused by the use of nonabsorbable multifilament ligatures around the uterine body, which can lead to erosion through the uterine vessels, resulting in intermittent vaginal bleeding (van Goethem *et al.* 2006).

Ovarian remnant syndrome is caused by incomplete removal of ovarian tissue and has been reported in both the dog and cat. Clinical signs include proestrus, estrus, and pseudopregnancy, and arguably stump pyometra. Several causes have been suggested for ovarian remnant syndrome, including dropping of ovarian tissue, improper clamp placement, and a small surgical incision (Wallace 1989). Less than half of the cases in one study were operated on by new graduates (Miller 1995). It is more common to inadvertently leave ovarian tissue on the right side than on the left (Wallace 1991; Ball *et al.* 2010). Some cases may be due to the presence of an accessory ovary or ovarian tissue that has extended into the ligament of the ovary, a situation that has been reported in cats but not dogs (McEntee 1990). Treatment of this condition involves exploratory laparotomy and removal of the suspected area of ovarian remnants. Removal of the remnants during estrus or diestrus is recommended, because enlarged ovarian structures (follicles or corpora lutea) make the remnants more easily identifiable.

Uterine stump pyometra, abscess, and granuloma are complications associated with the remaining uterine body. Uterine stump abscess is characterized by inflammation and bacterial infection of the portion of the uterine body that is not removed during OVH (Nelson & Feldman 1986). The term "stump pyometra" refers to a uterine stump abscess that is associated with cystic endometrial hyperplasia secondary to the activity of endogenous (from ovarian tissue remnants) or exogenous progestogens. Uterine stump abscesses are uncommon in dogs and cats (Feldman & Nelson 2004). Uterine stump inflammation and granuloma can be caused by ligatures of nonabsorbable suture material, poor aseptic technique, or excessive residual devitalized uterine body.

Fistulas are usually an indication of a foreign body reaction. These may occur typically in response to the presence of a retained surgical sponge (Frank & Stanley 2009) or are associated with nonabsorbent suture material, typically multifilament sutures (Grassi *et al.* 1994). Fistulous tracts associated with use of multifilament sutures originate most often in the ovarian pedicle (Pearson 1973).

Accidental ligation of a ureter, causing hydronephrosis or atrophy of the kidney (Joshua 1965; Turner 1972; Smith 1974; Okkens *et al.* 1981a,b; Kyles *et al.* 1996; Mehl & Kyles 2003) is prevented by careful identification of uterine horns and body before ligation of the uterine body. Granulation formation may involve the ureter, leading to partial or complete obstruction (Kanazono *et al.* 2009). Relief of unilateral complete obstruction after 4 days resulted in nearly complete return of renal function in one dog (Kanazono *et al.* 2009). Relief of obstruction after 14 days resulted in 46% recovery of glomerular filtration rate and tubular function by 4 months, whereas relief of obstruction after 40 days resulted in little recovery of renal function (Vaughan & Gillenwater 1971; Vaughan *et al.* 1973; Fink *et al.* 1980; Kanazono *et al.* 2009).

Urinary incontinence after OVH can be caused by adhesions or granulomas of the uterine stump that interfere with urinary bladder sphincter function (Pearson & Gibbs 1980; Okkens *et al.* 1981a,b). A common ligature around the vagina and ureter may produce vaginoureteral fistulization and urinary incontinence (Pearson & Gibbs 1980; MacCoy *et al.* 1988). However, the most common cause of urinary incontinence in spayed dogs is urethral sphincter mechanism incompetence. This condition is present in 0.2–0.3% of intact female dogs and 3–20% of spayed dogs (van Goethem *et al.* 2006). It is hypothesized that this condition has an underlying hormonal cause.

Inactivity and increased food intake contribute to weight gain. In particular, gonadectomy adversely affects the ability to regulate food intake and thus predisposes these animals to obesity (Salmeri *et al.* 1991a,b; van Goethem *et al.* 2006). This can lead to body weight gain of 26–38% following OVH (Dorn & Swift 1977; van Goethem *et al.* 2006). In one study, it was observed that 21.4% of all dogs were overweight and that spayed females were twice as likely to be obese compared with intact female dogs (Edney & Smith 1986). This is in contrast to the results of another study where gonadectomy did not influence food intake, weight gain, or back-fat depth (Salmeri *et al.* 1991a,b).

Intestinal pathology has been associated with OVH in dogs and cats, mostly because of entrapment and adhesions (Joshua 1965; Muir *et al.* 1991; Pollari & Bonnett 1996; Pollari *et al.* 1996; Smith & Davies 1996; Coolman *et al.* 1999; Swift 2009).

References

Allen, W.E. and Webbon, P.M. (1980). Two cases of urinary incontinence in cats associated with acquired vagino-ureteral fistula. *Journal of Small Animal Practice* 21: 367–371.

Austin, B., Lanz, O.I., Hamilton, S.M. et al. (2003). Laparoscopic ovariohysterectomy in nine dogs. *Journal of the American Animal Hospital Association* 39: 391–396.

Bagley, R.S., Dougherty, S.A., and Randolph, J.F. (1994). Tetanus subsequent to ovariohysterectomy in a dog. *Progress in Veterinary Neurology* 5: 63–65.

Ball, R.J., Birchard, S.J., May, L.R. et al. (2010). Ovarian remnant syndrome in dogs and cats: 21 cases (2000–2007). *Journal of the American Veterinary Medical Association* 236: 548–553.

Banks, S.E., Fleming, I.R., and Browning, T.N. (1991). Urinary incontinence in a bitch caused by vaginoureteral fistulation. *Veterinary Record* 128: 108.

Berzon, J.L. (1979). Complications of elective ovariohysterectomies in the dog and cat at a teaching institution: clinical review of 853 cases. *Veterinary Surgery* 8: 89–91.

Bradley, K.J., Billet, J.-P., and Barr, F.J. (2000). Dysuria resulting from an encapsulated haematoma in a recently spayed bitch. *Journal of Small Animal Practice* 41: 465–467.

Burrow, R., Wawra, E., Pinchbeck, G. et al. (2006). Prospective evaluation of postoperative pain in cats undergoing ovariohysterectomy by midline or flank approach. *Veterinary Record* 158: 657–660.

Case, J.B., Marvel, S.J., Boscan, P., and Monnet, E.L. (2011). Surgical time and severity of postoperative pain in dogs undergoing laparoscopic ovariectomy with one, two, or three instrument cannulas. *Journal of the American Veterinary Medical Association* 239: 203–208.

Chang, S.C., Chang, C.C., Chang, T.J., and Wong, M.L. (2005). Prognostic factors associated with survival two years after surgery in dogs with malignant mammary tumors: 79 cases (1998–2002). *Journal of the American Veterinary Medical Association* 227: 1625–1629.

Chang, C.C., Tsai, M.H., Liao, J.W. et al. (2009). Evaluation of hormone receptor expression for use in predicting survival of female dogs with malignant mammary gland tumors. *Journal of the American Veterinary Medical Association* 235: 391–396.

Coe, R.J., Grint, N.J., Tivers, M.S. et al. (2006). Feline ovariohysterectomy: comparison of flank and midline surgical approaches. Surgical technique and owner satisfaction. *Veterinary Record* 159: 309–313.

Coolman, B.R., Marretta, S.M., Dudley, M.B., and Averill, S. (1999). Partial colonic obstruction following ovariohysterectomy: a report of three cases. *Journal of the American Animal Hospital Association* 35: 169–172.

Culp, W.T.N., Mayhew, P.D., and Brown, D.C. (2009). The effect of laparoscopic versus open ovariectomy on postsurgical activity in small dogs. *Veterinary Surgery* 38: 811–817.

Davidson, E.B., Moll, H.D., and Payton, M.E. (2004). Comparison of laparoscopic ovariohysterectomy and ovariohysterectomy in dogs. *Veterinary Surgery* 33: 62–69.

De Baerdemaecker, G.C. (1984). Post spaying vaginal discharge in a bitch caused by acquired vaginoureteral fistula. *Veterinary Record* 115: 62.

Devitt, C.M., Cox, R.E., and Hailey, J.J. (2005). Duration, complication, stress, and pain of open ovariohysterectomy versus a simple method of laparoscopic-assisted ovariohysterectomy in dogs. *Journal of the American Veterinary Medical Association* 227: 921–927.

Dorn, A.S. (1975). Ovariohysterectomy by the flank approach. *Veterinary Medicine, Small Animal Clinician* 70: 569–573.

Dorn, A.S. and Swift, R.A. (1977). Complications of canine ovariohysterectomy. *Journal of the American Animal Hospital Association* 13: 720–724.

Dupré, G., Fiorbianco, V., Skalicky, M. et al. (2009). Laparoscopic ovariectomy in dogs: comparison between single portal and two-portal access. *Veterinary Surgery* 38: 818–824.

Edney, A.T. and Smith, P.M. (1986). Study of obesity in dogs visiting veterinary practices in the United Kingdom. *Veterinary Record* 118: 391–396.

Feathers, D.J. (1974). Locating site of incision for flank approach to feline ovariohysterectomy. *Veterinary Medicine, Small Animal Clinician* 69: 1069.

Feldman, E.C. and Nelson, R.W. (2004). Cystic endometrial hyperplasia/pyometra complex. In: *Canine and Feline Endocrinology and Reproduction*, 3e, 852–867. St Louis, MO: WB Saunders.

Fingland, R.B. (1998). Ovariohysterectomy. In: *Current Techniques in Small Animal Surgery*, 4e (ed. M.J. Bojrab), 489–496. Baltimore, MD: Williams & Wilkins.

Fink, R.L., Caridis, D.T., Chmiel, R., and Ryan, G. (1980). Renal impairment and its reversibility following variable periods of complete ureteral obstruction. *Australian and New Zealand Journal of Surgery* 50: 77–83.

Frank, J.D. and Stanley, B.J. (2009). Enterocutaneous fistula in a dog secondary to an intraperitoneal gauze foreign body. *Journal of the American Animal Hospital Association* 45: 84–88.

Freeman, L.J., Rahmani, E.Y., Sherman, S. et al. (2009). Oopherectomy by natural orifice transluminal endoscopic surgery: feasibility study in dogs. *Gastrointestinal Endoscopy* 69: 1321–1332.

Furneaux, R.W., Baysen, B.G., and Mero, K.N. (1973). Complications of ovariohysterectomies. *Canadian Veterinary Journal* 14: 98–99.

Ganssbauer, B., Kramer, S., Mayer-Lindbergen, A., and Nolte, I. (2000). Tetanus following ovariohysterectomy in a dog. *Tierärztliche Praxis* 28: 225–229.

Ghanawat, H.G. and Mantri, M.B. (1996). Comparative study of various approaches for ovariohysterectomy in cats. *Indian Veterinary Journal* 73: 987–988.

Gorelick, J. (1974). Discoloration of exotic cat's hair following flank ovariohystrectomy. *Veterinary Medicine, Small Animal Clinician* 69: 943.

Gower, S. and Mayhew, P.D. (2008). Canine laparoscopic and laparoscopic-assisted ovariohysterectomy and ovariectomy. *Compendium on Continuing Education for the Practicing Veterinarian* 30: 430–440.

Grassi, F., Romagnoli, S., Camillo, F. et al. (1994). Iatrogenic enterovaginal fistula following hysterectomy. *Journal of Small Animal Practice* 35: 32–34.

Grint, N.J., Murison, P.J., Coe, R.J., and Waterman Pearson, A.E. (2006). Assessment of the influence of surgical technique on postoperative pain and wound tenderness in cats following ovariohysterectomy. *Journal of Feline Medicine and Surgery* 8: 15–21.

Hancock, R.B., Lanz, O.I., Waldron, D.R. et al. (2005). Comparison of postoperative pain after ovariohysterectomy by harmonic scalpel-assisted laparoscopy compared with median celiotomy and ligation in dogs. *Veterinary Surgery* 34: 273–282.

Hedlund, C.S. (2002). Surgery of the reproductive and genital systems. In: *Small Animal Surgery*, 2e (ed. T.W. Fossum, C.S. Hedlund, D.A. Hulse, et al.), 616–618. St Louis, MO: Mosby.

Hill, L.N. and Smeak, D.D. (2010). Suspensory ligament rupture technique during ovariohysterectomy in small animals. *Compendium on Continuing Education for the Practicing Veterinarian* 32: E1–E8.

Hogues, M. (1991). Comparative study of various approaches to feline ovariohysterectomy. *Indian Journal of Veterinary Surgery* 12: 29–30.

Howard, S. (2006). Ovariohysterectomy in cats. *Veterinary Record* 159: 464.

Howe, L.M., Slater, M.R., Boothe, H.W. et al. (2000). Long-term outcome of gonadectomy performed at an early age or traditional age in cats. *Journal of the American Veterinary Medical Association* 217: 1661–1665.

Howe, L.M., Slater, M.R., Boothe, H.W. et al. (2001). Long-term outcome of gonadectomy performed at an early age or traditional age in dogs. *Journal of the American Veterinary Medical Association* 218: 217–221.

Janssens, L.A. and Hanssens, G.H. (1991). Bilateral flank ovariectomy in the dog: surgical technique and sequelae in 72 animals. *Journal of Small Animal Practice* 32: 249–252.

Joshua, J.O. (1965). The spaying of bitches. *Veterinary Record* 77: 642–647.

Kanazono, S., Aikawa, T., and Yoshigae, Y. (2009). Unilateral hydronephrosis and partial ureteral obstruction by entrapment in a granuloma in a spayed dog. *Journal of the American Animal Hospital Association* 45: 301–304.

Krzaczynski, J. (1974). The flank approach to feline ovariohysterectomy (an alternate technique). *Veterinary Medicine, Small Animal Clinician* 69: 572–574.

Kunin, S. and Terry, M. (1980). A complication following ovariohysterectomy in a dog. *Veterinary Medicine, Small Animal Clinician* 75: 1000–1001.

Kyles, A.E., Douglass, J.P., and Rottman, J.B. (1996). Pyelonephritis following inadvertent excision of the ureter during ovariohysterectomy in a bitch. *Veterinary Record* 139: 471–472.

Lamb, C.R. (1994). Acquired ureterovaginal fistula secondary to ovariohysterectomy in a dog: diagnosis using ultrasound-guided nephropyelocentesis and antegrade ureterography. *Veterinary Radiology and Ultrasound* 35: 201–203.

MacCoy, D.M., Ogilvie, G., Burke, T., and Parker, A. (1988). Postovariohysterectomy ureterovaginal fistula in a dog. *Journal of the American Animal Hospital Association* 24: 469–471.

Mayhew, P.D. and Brown, D.C. (2007). Comparison of three techniques for ovarian pedicle hemostasis during laparoscopic-assisted ovariohysterectomy. *Veterinary Surgery* 36: 541–547.

McEntee, K. (ed.) (1990). *Reproductive Pathology of Domestic Mammals*. New York: Academic Press.

McEvoy, F.J. (1994). Iatrogenic renal obstruction in a dog. *Veterinary Record* 135: 457–458.

McGrath, H., Hardie, R.J., and Davis, E. (2004). Lateral flank approach for ovariohysterectomy in small animals. *Compendium on Continuing Education for the Practicing Veterinarian* 26: 922–931.

Mehl, M.L. and Kyles, A.E. (2003). Ureteroureterostomy after proximal ureteric injury during an ovariohysterectomy in a dog. *Veterinary Record* 153: 469–470.

Miller, D.M. (1995). Ovarian remnant syndrome in dogs and cats: 46 cases (1988–1992). *Journal of Veterinary Diagnostic Investigation* 7: 572–574.

Muir, P., Goldsmid, S.E., and Bellenger, C.R. (1991). Megacolon in a cat following ovariohysterectomy. *Veterinary Record* 129: 512–513.

Muir, P., Goldsmid, S.E., Simpson, D.J., and Bellenger, C.R. (1993). Incisional swelling following celiotomy in cats. *Veterinary Record* 132: 189–190.

Nelson, R.W. and Feldman, E.C. (1986). Pyometra. *Veterinary Clinics of North America: Small Animal Practice* 16: 561–576.

Okkens, A.C., Dieleman, S.J., and van de Gaag, I. (1981a). Urological complications following ovariohysterectomy in dogs. *Tijdschrift voor Diergeneeskunde* 106: 1189–119 .

Okkens, A.C., Dieleman, S.J., and van de Gaag, I. (1981b) []. Gynaecological complications following ovariohysterectomy in dogs, due to: (1) partial removal of the ovaries, (2) inflammation of the uterocervical stump]. *Tijdschrift voor Diergeneeskunde* 106: 1142–1158.

Overley, B., Shofer, F.S., Goldschmidt, M.H. et al. (2005). Association between ovariohysterectomy and feline mammary carcinoma. *Journal of Veterinary Internal Medicine* 19: 560–563.

Pearson, H. (1973). The complications of ovariohysterectomy in the bitch. *Journal of Small Animal Practice* 14: 257–266.

Pearson, H. and Gibbs, C.A. (1980). Urinary incontinence in the dog due to accidental vagino-ureteral fistulation during hysterectomy. *Journal of Small Animal Practice* 21: 287–291.

Peeters, M.E. and Kirpensteijn, J. (2011). Comparison of surgical variables and short-term postoperative complications in healthy dogs undergoing ovariohysterectomy or ovariectomy. *Journal of the American Veterinary Medical Association* 238: 189–194.

Pollari, F.L. and Bonnett, B.N. (1996). Evaluation of postoperative complications following elective surgeries of dogs and cats at private practices using computer records. *Canadian Veterinary Journal* 37: 672–678.

Pollari, F.L., Bonnett, B.N., Bamsey, S.C et al. (1996). Postoperative complications of elective surgeries in dogs and cats determined by examining electronic and paper medical record. *Journal of the American Veterinary Medical Association* 208: 1882–1886.

Pukacz, M., Kienzle, B., and Braun, J. (2009). Simple, minimally invasive technique for ovariohysterectomy in the dog. *Veterinary Record* 165: 688–690.

Rubin, S., Faulkner, R.T., and Ward, G.. (1983). Tetanus following ovariohysterectomy in a dog: a case report and review. *Journal of the American Animal Hospital Association* 19: 293–298.

Salmeri, K.R., Bloomberg, M.S., Scruggs, S.L., and Shille, V. (1991a). Gonadectomy in immature dogs: effects on skeletal, physical, and behavioral development. *Journal of the American Veterinary Medical Association* 198: 1193–1203

Salmeri, K.R., Olson, P.N., and Bloomberg, M.S. (1991b). Elective gonadectomy in dogs: a review. *Journal of the American Veterinary Medical Association* 198: 1183–1192

Schneider, R., Dorn, C.R., and Taylor, D.O.N. (1969). Factors influencing canine mammary cancer development and postsurgical survival. *Journal of the National Cancer Institute* 43: 1249–1261.

Smith, K.W. (1974). Female genital system. In: *Canine Surgery* (ed. J. Archibald), 272. Santa Barbara, CA: American Veterinary Publications.

Smith, M.C. and Davies, N.L. (1996). Constipation following ovariohysterectomy in a cat. *Veterinary Record* 138: 163.

Sorenmo, K.U., Shofer, F.S., and Goldschmidt, M.H. (2000). Effect of spaying and timing of spaying on survival of dogs with mammary carcinoma. *Journal of Veterinary Internal Medicine* 14: 266–270.

Spackman, C.J.A., Caywood, D.D., Johnston, G.R. et al. (1984). Granulomas of the uterine and ovarian stumps: a case report. *Journal of the American Animal Hospital Association* 20: 449–453.

Spain, C.V., Scarlett, J.M., and Houpt, K.A. (2004a). Long-term risks and benefits of early-age gonadectomy in dogs. *Journal of the American Veterinary Medical Association* 224: 380–387.

Spain, C.V., Scarlett, J.M., and Houpt, K.A. (2004b). Long-term risks and benefits of early-age gonadectomy in cats. *Journal of the American Veterinary Medical Association* 224: 372–379.

Stone, E.A. (2003). Ovary and uterus. In: *Textbook of Small Animal Surgery*, 3e (ed. D. Slatter), 1487–1502. Philadelphia, PA: WB Saunders.

Stubbs, W.P., Bloomberg, M.S., Scruggs, S.L. et al. (1996). Effects of prepubertal gonadectomy on physical and behavioral development in cats. *Journal of the American Veterinary Medical Association* 209: 1864–1871.

Swift, I. (2009). Ultrasonographic features of intestinal entrapment in dogs. *Veterinary Radiology and Ultrasound* 50: 205–207.

Turner, T. (1972). An unusual case of hydronephrosis in a spayed Alsatian bitch. *Veterinary Record* 91: 588–590.

Van Goethem, B.E.B.J., Rosenveldt, K.W., and Kirpensteijn, J. (2003). Monopolar versus bipolar electrocoagulation in canine laparoscopic ovariectomy: a nonrandomized, prospective, clinical trial. *Veterinary Surgery* 32: 464–470.

Van Goethem, B.E.B.J., Schaefers-Okkens, A., and Kirpensteijn, J. (2006). Making a rational choice between ovariectomy and ovariohysterectomy in the dog: a discussion of the benefits of either technique. *Veterinary Surgery* 35: 136–143.

Van Nimwegen, S.A. and Kirpensteijn, J. (2007a). Comparison of Nd:YAG surgical laser and Remorgida bipolar electrosurgery forceps for canine laparoscopic ovariectomy. *Veterinary Surgery* 36: 533–540.

Van Nimwegen, S.A. and Kirpensteijn, J. (2007b). Laparoscopic ovariectomy in cats: comparison of laser and bipolar electrocoagulation. *Journal of Feline Medicine and Surgery* 9: 397–403.

Van Nimwegen, S.A., Van Swol, C.F., and Kirpensteijn, J. (2005). Neodymium:yttrium aluminum garnet surgical laser versus bipolar electrocoagulation for laparoscopic ovariectomy in dogs. *Veterinary Surgery* 34: 353–357.

Vaughan, E.D. Jr. and Gillenwater, J.Y. (1971). Recovery following complete chronic unilateral obstruction: functional, radiographic, and pathological alterations. *Journal of Urology* 106: 27–35.

Vaughan, E.D. Jr., Sweet, R.E., and Gillenwater, J.Y. (1973). Unilateral ureteral occlusion: pattern of nephron repair and compensatory response. *Journal of Urology* 109: 979–982.

Wallace, M.S. (1989). Estrus after ovariohysterectomy. Diagnosis of the ovarian remnant syndrome in the bitch and queen. *Proceedings of the Society for Theriogenology*, 316–319.

Wallace, M.S. (1991). The ovarian remnant syndrome in the bitch and queen. *Veterinary Clinics of North America: Small Animal Practice* 21: 501–507.

57

Scrotal and Testicular Trauma and Neoplasia

Fran Smith

Scrotum

Lesions of the scrotum and the scrotal contents are uncommon except for traumatic events (Larsen & Smith 1986). The scrotum normally contains the testes, epididymides, and spermatic cords. Clinical problems involving the scrotum typically present as the presence of fluid in the scrotum, pain and discomfort with or without discoloration of the scrotum, and changes in size, shape, or consistency of the scrotal contents. Scrotal dermatitis may accompany any of these signs. Pyoderma, dermatophytes, keratinization defects, immune-mediated skin disease, and food allergy can result in scrotal lesions. The client's complaint may be that the dog is reluctant to sit or is repeatedly licking his scrotum.

Lacerations and penetrating wounds

Lacerations of the scrotum caused by bite wounds, bullets, and automobiles should be considered contaminated wounds. When the tunica vaginalis has been open for less than 24 hours and the damage is not severe, the cavity can be flushed with a sterile solution containing antibiotics (Larsen & Smith 1986). The tunica parietalis should be sutured and the scrotal wall repaired. For older injuries, treat the exposed tissues as an open wound. The goal of all treatment of scrotal wounds is to minimize inflammation.

In human patients suffering penetrating scrotal injuries, 40% underwent immediate surgical intervention, whereas 60% underwent scrotal ultrasound. Of the patients that underwent scrotal ultrasound, 80% were found to have testicular injuries upon scrotal exploration. Among the patients with negative ultrasound

(122 patients), 14 were managed conservatively and 8 underwent exploration; all 8 were negative for testicular injury. Scrotal ultrasound sensitivity and specificity in this group were 100% and 84.6%, respectively (Churukanti *et al.* 2016).

Penetrating wounds that go through the tunica vaginalis visceralis and tunica albuginea should only be closed at the tunica vaginalis parietalis and skin level. This limited closure minimizes swelling and the resultant pressure necrosis. Adhesions between the visceral and parietal layers of the tunica vaginalis may occur after repair of a penetrating wound. If the tunica albuginea has been ruptured and testicular tissue has bulged through the ruptured area, the testis should be removed. Systemic antibiotics should be administered in all cases of scrotal trauma.

A case of scrotal mutilation in a young golden retriever beginning at 4–5 months of age was diagnosed in this dog secondary to bilateral sperm granuloma. Evaluation of the history, physical examination, and laboratory findings indicated that a bilateral congenital abnormality was the likely cause. The dog was treated by castration and scrotal ablation (Althouse *et al.* 1993).

Hernia

A scrotal hernia can cause acute onset of severe pain and swelling. The hernia allows abdominal contents to extend through the inguinal canal and migrate into the vaginal process next to the spermatic cord. Strangulation of the abdominal contents of the hernia is a surgical emergency. Severe damage to the scrotal wall and testes often requires surgical removal of the affected tissue. Ultrasound is a valuable tool in identification of a scrotal hernia.

Small Animal Soft Tissue Surgery, Second Edition. Edited by Eric Monnet.
© 2023 John Wiley & Sons, Inc. Published 2023 by John Wiley & Sons, Inc.
Companion website: www.wiley.com/go/monnet/small

Dermatitis

Scrotal skin is thinner than most of the skin on the body and is readily irritated. Chemical irritation, extremes of heat and cold, insect bites, drug eruption from agents such as diethylcarbamazine, and trauma from activity through brush or rough terrain may result in rapid progression from a minor scrape to a lesion resembling pyotraumatic dermatitis (Figure 57.1) (Graves 2006). The affected area rapidly becomes firm, thickened, warm to the touch, and exquisitely painful. Treatment must be aggressive to avoid thermal injury to the testicles. Topical therapy is usually successful and includes corticosteroids, antihistamines, and judicious use of tranquilizers. In refractory cases, surgery to remove the scrotal lesion may be necessary.

Tumors

Any tumor that affects the skin may be found on the scrotum. The most commonly diagnosed scrotal tumor is the mast cell tumor, which accounted for 88% of all scrotal tumors in one study and 75% in another (Veiga *et al.* 2009; Taylor 2010). Other tumors reported are melanoma, histiocytoma, hemangioma, neurofibroma, papilloma, sebaceous adenoma, fibroma, fibrosarcoma, squamous cell carcinoma, and apocrine gland tumor. Risk factors and etiology of scrotal tumors are undefined. These tumors are generally visible and palpable. The presenting complaint is often licking of the scrotum or a nonhealing lesion on the scrotum.

Careful physical examination is warranted for any dog with a scrotal tumor to identify any other cutaneous lesion. Fine-needle aspirates may be obtained and histopathology should be performed to establish tumor type and stage the disease (Taylor 2010). A typical surgical work-up should be performed including complete blood count, chemistry panel, urinalysis, and possibly thoracic radiography. Benign tumors may be removed locally and do not require castration and scrotal ablation. Malignant tumors and especially mast cell tumors require castration and scrotal ablation to avoid metastatic disease. Prognosis for benign tumors is excellent.

Testes

The testes are positioned obliquely within the scrotum with the long axis oriented dorsocaudally. The testes are covered with peritoneum originating from within the abdomen. The outer layer is the parietal vaginal tunic. The inner layer of the visceral vaginal tunic is continuous with the parietal peritoneum of the abdomen (McLouglin 2003). The tunica albuginea, a dense white capsule, covers the testis. Within the tunica albuginea are superficial branches of the testicular artery and vein. The testes and epididymides are attached to the parietal vaginal tunic by the caudal ligaments of the epididymides. Partial indirect stabilization of the testes is provided by the spermatic cords and vaginal tunics. Arterial supply to the testes originates from the aorta at the level of the fourth lumbar vertebra. The testicular veins follow the arterial pattern but from the pampiniform plexus in the spermatic cord, which serves an important function in temperature regulation of the testes.

Testicular function is regulated by gonadotropins and depends on precise thermoregulation. Scrotal temperature is maintained below core body temperature through a combination of spermatic cord vascular supply, cremaster muscle function, and the structure of the scrotum. The scrotum should contain two freely movable testicles of similar size and shape (Graves 2006). Size of testicles is correlated with breed of dog and especially with adult body weight. There is tremendous variability in testicular size even between dogs of the same breed. An enlarged painful testicle is consistent with inflammation, varicocele, neoplasia, granuloma, spermatocele, or torsion. An enlarged nonpainful testicle is most often seen with neoplasia (Graves 2006). One small testicle in the presence of one normal testicle suggests a degenerative process (Figure 57.2).

Trauma

Testicles are not commonly traumatized in dogs and cats due to their mobile nature within the scrotum. Clinical signs usually indicate pain and swelling of the affected testicle, with possible hindlimb lameness. In more severe cases scrotal swelling and bruising may be seen. Severe blunt trauma may result in local hemorrhage and rupture of the tunica albuginea. Diagnosis of testicular trauma is by careful physical examination. Rupture of

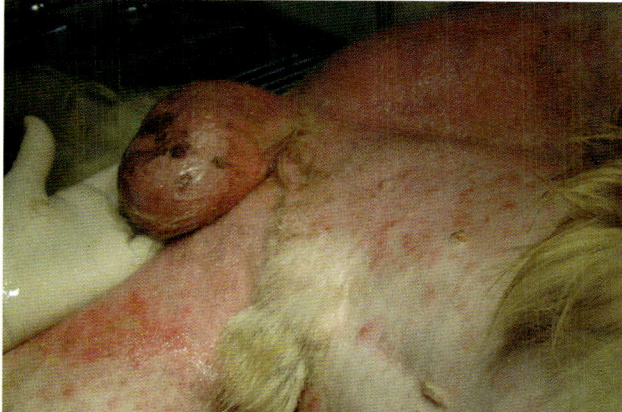

Figure 57.1 Severe scrotal dermatitis in a golden retriever with atopy and a scrotal contact scald from a floor cleaning disinfectant.

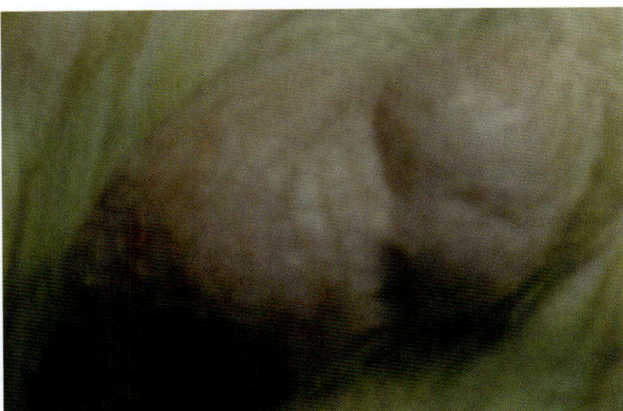

Figure 57.2 Testicular asymmetry in a dog with unilateral testicular atrophy.

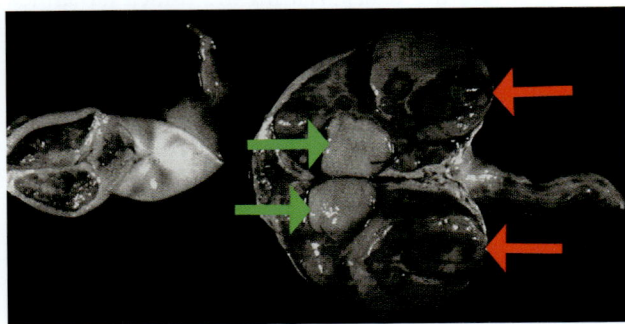

Figure 57.3 A hemisectioned testis shows the difference in gross appearance between an interstitial cell tumor (red arrows) and a functional seminoma (green arrows).

Table 57.1 Breeds at increased risk for testicular tumor development.

All testicular tumors	Sertoli cell tumors
Siberian husky	West Highland white terrier
Norwegian elkhound	Weimaraner
Afghan hound	Airedale
Shetland sheepdog	Pekingese
Fox terrier	
	Interstitial cell tumors
Seminomas	Bull terrier
Keeshond	Dalmatian
Great Dane	Old English sheepdog
Old English sheepdog	
Samoyed	
Scottish terrier	
Bulldog	

the tunica albuginea may be difficult to detect because of local swelling. Local hypothermia, swelling, loss of sensation, and blue discoloration are indicators of irreversible damage due to ischemia (Boothe 2006). Severe testicular trauma may require unilateral or bilateral castration. Castration should be delayed until the testicular damage is completely evaluated.

Tumors

Incidence and risk factors

Testicular tumors are the second most common tumor in the male dog, with an incidence of 7–16% (Boothe 2006; Veiga *et al.* 2009). More than 40% of the dogs diagnosed with testicular tumors have multiple tumor types at the time of diagnosis (Figure 57.3) (Taylor 2010). The incidence of testicular tumors increases with age, with a mean of 10 years of age at the time of diagnosis. The etiology of testicular tumors is unclear. Risk factors for development of testicular tumors include increasing age, breed (Table 57.1), environmental elements, and cryptorchidism. German shepherd working dogs serving in Vietnam had an increased incidence of testicular tumors compared with German shepherd dogs in the USA, implicating environmental factors as a contributor to the increased incidence (Taylor 2010).

Cryptorchidism is a significant risk factor for the development of Sertoli cell tumors and seminomas, increasing the risk by 8.8 and 16 times, respectively, compared with the incidence in scrotal testicles (Taylor 2010). The long-term exposure to core body temperature results in degeneration of the germinal epithelium of the testicle and spermatogenesis ceases, although hormonal function continues (Boothe 2006). The risk of testicular neoplasia is 13.6 times greater in cryptorchid dogs and the scrotal testicle shows the same type of testicular tumor in 40% of dogs (Graves 2006). In the retained abdominal testicle, the remaining Sertoli cells may undergo neoplastic changes, resulting in Sertoli cell tumors. Intermediate temperature in the inguinal area may stimulate spermatogenic cell neoplasia, and a higher incidence of inguinal seminomas is observed in dogs with inguinal cryptorchidism.

Clinical signs and paraneoplastic syndromes

Testicular tumors arise from three different cell types (Figure 57.4). Sertoli cell tumors arise from the sustentacular cell of the seminiferous tubules. Sertoli cell tumors can produce estrogen and estrogen-associated illness and clinical signs (Table 57.2). Hormone production is more likely in cryptorchid testicles. Dogs with Sertoli cell tumors may present for feminization, haircoat changes, or acute abdominal distress if testicular torsion is present (McEntee 2002; Graves 2006). Estrogen toxicity is a serious complication of Sertoli cell tumors,

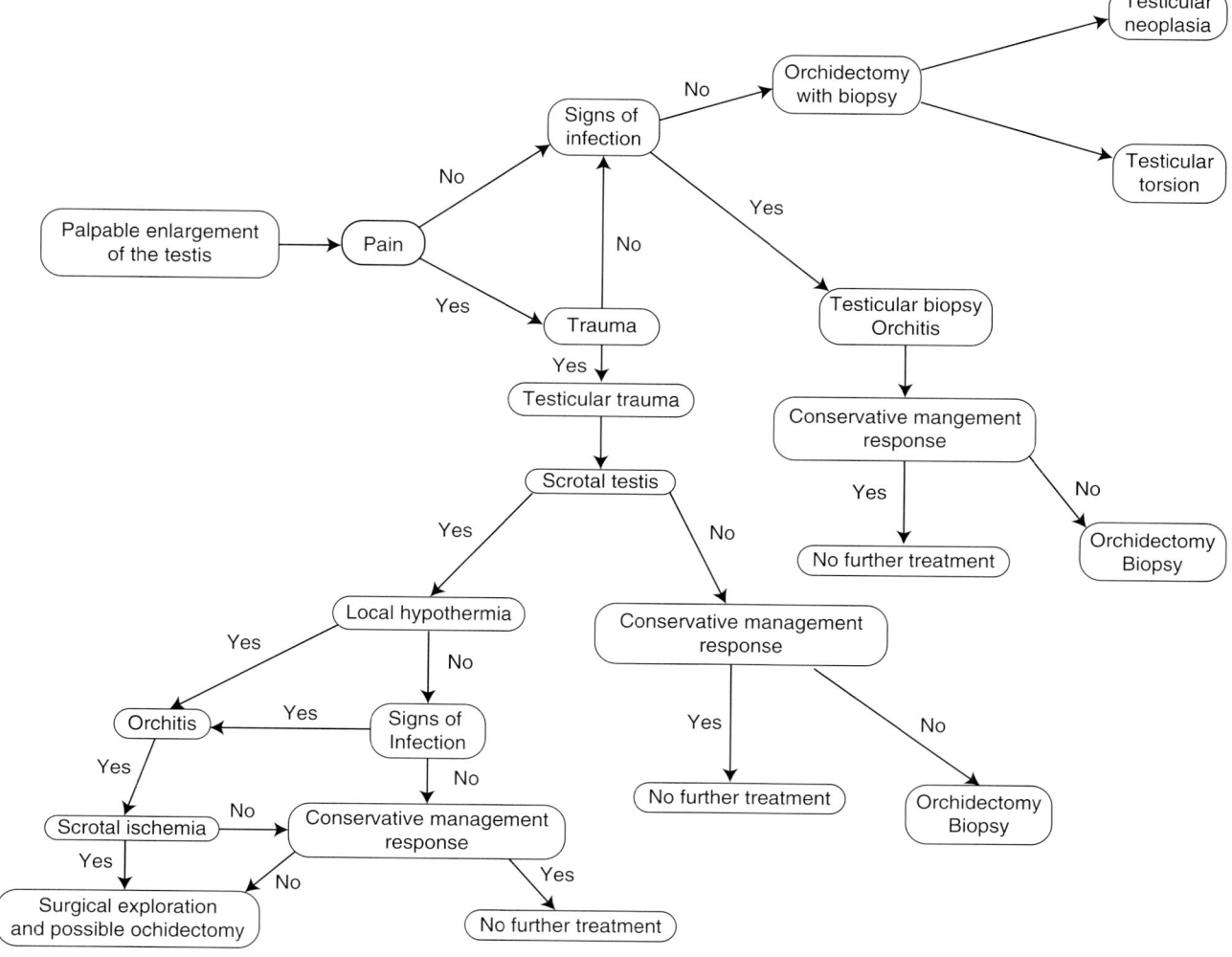

Figure 57.4 A clinical summary of canine testicular tumors that includes the signalment, diagnostic procedures, treatment, and prognosis for each tumor type. Source: M.C. McEntee 2002 / with permission of Elsevier.

Table 57.2 A clinical summary of canine testicular tumors that includes clinical presentation, diagnostic procedures, treatment, and prognosis.

Clinical presentation

Majority of dogs are asymptomatic and a testicular mass is detected on physical examination. There may be contralateral atrophy in dogs with functional testicular tumors

Signs of feminization syndrome most commonly seen with Sertoli cell tumors, including gynecomastia, galactorrhea, attraction of males, symmetric alopecia, pendulous prepuce, change in semen quality, and signs of bone marrow suppression

Dogs with interstitial cell tumors and increased testosterone may present with perineal hernia, tail gland and perianal gland hyperplasia, and adenomas

Diagnostics

Physical examination and palpation of the testicles

Ultrasound examination of the testicles and abdomen

Complete bloodwork

Treatment

Orchidectomy is the treatment of choice

Cisplatin chemotherapy for metastatic Sertoli cell tumors or seminomas. Limited information available

Radiation therapy effective in treatment of metastatic seminomas based on small series of cases

Prognosis

Majority of dogs are cured with surgery alone

Guarded prognosis for dogs with hyperestrogenism and bone marrow failure. Treatment should include supportive measures such as antibiotic therapy and blood products with as few as 20% of the patients making a full recovery from the myelosuppression (Taylor 2010).

Interstitial cell tumors may produce testosterone. The excessive testosterone produced by the interstitial cell tumor may contribute to an increased incidence of perineal hernia, perianal gland tumors, and prostatic hyperplasia.

Diagnosis

Diagnosis of testicular tumors includes physical examination, imaging, and laboratory evaluation. A rectal examination should be performed. A complete blood count and full chemistry panel should be performed to rule out myelosuppression. Ultrasonography should be performed on the abdomen of cryptorchid patients and on the scrotal testicle of all patients (McEntee 2002). Color Doppler ultrasonography may be helpful in differentiating testicular neoplasms from nonneoplastic findings in the testicle. Vascular signals in neoplasms were significantly intensified around and inside solid tumors versus inflammatory and degenerative lesions of the testicle (Bigliardi et al. 2019). Testicular biopsy or fine-needle aspiration may be considered to differentiate inflammatory causes of testicular enlargement from neoplasia.

Metastases

Metastatic disease may occur in 9–14% of Sertoli cell tumors, in less than 10% of seminomas, and very rarely with interstitial cell tumors that are considered benign. Metastasis may affect the regional lymph nodes, liver, brain, kidney, spleen, adrenal gland, and pancreas. There is a single report of a seminoma in a Great Pyrenees with metastases to the skin (Spugnini et al. 2000). Malignant Leydig cell tumors in dogs are very rare. Kudo et al. reported two cases in dogs with malignant Leydig cell (interstitial cell) tumors with cutaneous metastases. One dog had cutaneous metastases to the corner of the mouth; the other had multiple cutaneous masses in the dorsal neck region, the thoracic back region, and the right hindlimb. The tumors were positive for inhibin-alpha and melanin-A. Mitotic indexes were very high (Kudo et al. 2019).

Treatment

Castration is the treatment of choice for all testicular tumors (Dhaliwal et al. 1999). In the case of a valuable breeding dog, unilateral castration of the obviously affected testicle may be performed (McEntee 2002). Many of these dogs will have testicular tumors affecting the remaining testicle, which may influence future fertility. Dogs with estrogen toxicity will require supportive care including antibiotics, fluid therapy, and blood products.

Orchidectomy on scrotal testicles may be performed using either an open or closed technique (Tobias 1995; Boothe 1996, 2006). For the closed technique, the dog is placed in dorsal recumbency and the prescrotal area is surgically prepared. One of the testicles is pushed cranially into the prescrotal area. An incision is made through the skin overlying the testis. The incision is continued through the subcutaneous tissue and spermatic fascia to expose the parietal vaginal tunic. The testicle is exteriorized and freed from the scrotal attachment by incising the spermatic fascia and scrotal ligament close to the testes. Fat and fascia are reflected using a gauze sponge to allow exteriorization of the testis and spermatic cord. The intact spermatic cord is double ligated using transfixation ligatures of absorbable suture. The spermatic cord and cremaster muscle are transected distal to the ligatures and returned to the inguinal region. The subcutaneous tissue is closed routinely using absorbable suture in either a continuous or interrupted pattern. A subcuticular pattern may be used to align the skin. Skin sutures are optional.

In the open method, the parietal vaginal tunic is incised, exposing the spermatic cord. The spermatic cord is double ligated with absorbable sutures using transfixation ligatures. Alternatively, the parietal vaginal tunic is incised over the testis. The spermatic cord is double ligated using transfixation ligature of absorbable material. The parietal vaginal tunic and cremaster muscle are ligated using a transfixation ligature. The spermatic cord and cremaster muscle are transected and returned to the inguinal area. Routine closure of the subcutaneous tissue with absorbable suture and subcuticular or skin sutures completes the procedure.

References

Althouse, G.C., Evans, E., and Hopkins, S.M. (1993). Episodic scrotal mutilation with concurrent bilateral sperm granuloma in a dog. *Journal of the American Veterinary Medical Association* 202 (5): 776–778.

Bigliardi, E., Denti, L., DeCesaris, V. et al. (2019). Colour Doppler ultrasound imaging of blood flows variations in neoplastic and non-neoplastic testicular lesions in dogs. *Reproduction in Domestic Animals* 54 (1): 63–71.

Boothe, H.W. (1996). Testes and epididymides. In: *Textbook of Small Animal Surgery*, 2e (ed. D. Slatter), 1325–1331. Philadelphia, PA: WB Saunders.

Boothe, H.W. (2006). Surgery of the testes and scrotum. In: *Saunders Manual of Small Animal Practice*, 3e (ed. S.J. Birchard and R.G. Sherding), 969–970. St Louis, MO: Saunders Elsevier.

Churukanti, G., Kim, A., Rich, D. et al. (2016). Role of ultrasonography for testicular injuries in penetrating scrotal trauma. *Urology* 95: 208–212.

Dhaliwal, R.S., Kitchell, B.E., Knight, B.L. et al. (1999). Treatment of aggressive testicular tumors in four dogs. *Journal of the American Animal Hospital Association* 35: 311–318.

Graves, T.K. (2006). Diseases of the testes and scrotum. In: *Saunders Manual of Small Animal Practice*, 3e (ed. S.J. Birchard and R.G. Sherding), 963–968. St Louis, MO: Saunders Elsevier.

Kudo, T., Kamiie, J., Aihara, N. et al. (2019). Malignant Leydig cell tumor in dogs: two cases and a review of the literature. *Journal of Veterinary Diagnostic Investigation* 31 (4): 557–561.

Larsen, R.E. and Smith, F.O. (1986). Lesions of the scrotum and scrotal structures. In: *Small Animal Reproduction and Infertility* (ed. T.J. Burke), 237–244. Philadelphia, PA: Lea & Febiger.

McEntee, M.C. (2002). Reproductive oncology. *Clinical Techniques in Small Animal Practice* 17: 133–149.

McLouglin, M.A. (2003). Surgical techniques of the reproductive tracts. In: *Proceedings of the Society for Theriogenology*, vol. 2003, 206–208.

Spugnini, E.P., Bartolazzi, A., and Ruslander, D. (2000). Seminoma with cutaneous metastases in a dog. *Journal of the American Animal Hospital Association* 36: 253–256.

Taylor, K.H. (2010). Male reproductive tumors. In: *Cancer Management in Small Animal Practice* (ed. C.J. Henry and M.L. Higginbotham), 282–286. Saunders Elsevier: Maryland Heights, MO.

Tobias, K.M. (1995). Surgical correction of congenital anomalies of the reproductive tract. *Seminars in Veterinary Medicine and Surgery (Small Animal)* 10: 13–20.

Veiga, G.A.L., D'Oliveira, K.S., Brito, K.D. et al. (2009). Retrospective study of tumors at the genital tract of dogs presented at the veterinary hospital of Unisa during the period of February 2000 to December 2008. In: *Proceedings of the 34th World Small Animal Veterinary Association Congress 2009*. Sao Paulo, Brazil.

58

Prostatic Disease

Michelle Kutzler

Prostatic disease in dogs may be noninfectious and non-neoplastic or may be infectious or neoplastic. Accurate diagnosis requires understanding of clinical signs and interpretation of diagnostic tests. Prostatomegaly due to any cause may be an asymptomatic incidental finding, or it may cause tenesmus because of mechanical interference with defecation. Prostatomegaly in a castrated dog should immediately prompt a search for prostatic neoplasia or the possibility of a remaining cryptorchid testicle(s). German shepherds and Doberman pinschers have a higher reported incidence of all prostatic diseases (Krawiec & Heflin 1992). Prostate disease is extremely rare in cats.

Noninfectious, nonneoplastic prostate diseases

Causes of noninfectious, nonneoplastic prostate disease include benign prostatic hyperplasia (BPH), intraparenchymal prostatic cysts, paraprostatic cysts, prostatic calculi, squamous metaplasia, and persistent Müllerian duct syndrome (PMDS).

Benign prostatic hyperplasia

BPH is the most common cause of prostatomegaly in intact male dogs. The prostate gland is symmetrically enlarged due to an androgen-mediated, age-related increase in the number of acinar basal cells in both the stromal and glandular elements of the prostate (McNeal 1984; Leav *et al.* 2001). BPH is histologically apparent in up to 16% of intact male dogs by 2 years of age. By 5 years of age, 50% of intact male dogs will have evidence of BPH. By 9 years of age, the prevalence has increased to 95%.

BPH often causes no clinical signs. In one study reporting on prostatic disease in 177 dogs, nearly half of the histologically confirmed cases of BPH had no clinical signs (Krawiec & Heflin 1992). Physical examination findings typically include a symmetric, nonpainful enlarged prostate in an otherwise healthy sexually intact adult male dog. After 4 years of age, intraparenchymal prostatic cyst formation may accompany BPH because of hyperplastic obstruction of parenchymal ducts causing accumulation of prostatic secretions (see next section for further information). If intraparenchymal prostatic cysts accompany BPH, the prostate may be asymmetrically enlarged depending on the size and location of the cysts. The prevalence of intraparenchymal prostatic cyst formation in intact male dogs with no clinical evidence of urologic problems is 14% (Hastak *et al.* 1982; Black *et al.* 1998). However, intraparenchymal prostatic cyst formation may predispose the prostate to bacterial infection.

When clinical signs are present in cases of BPH, they usually include sanguineous urethral (preputial) discharge and/or hematuria, since prostatic fluid normally refluxes into the urinary tract between ejaculations. In a 14-year retrospective study on canine prostatic disease, urethral bleeding was the only presenting sign observed in 23% of cases and of these cases, 95% were BPH. Blood loss can be associated with sexual arousal. Blood loss from the prostate resulting in blood dripping from the urethra/prepuce is not reported commonly as a clinical sign of BPH in the dog, although urethral discharge and hematuria are (Krawiec & Heflin 1992). The source of blood may be dilated veins coursing over the enlarged, adenomatous gland; these veins are readily visible during

Small Animal Soft Tissue Surgery, Second Edition. Edited by Eric Monnet.
© 2023 John Wiley & Sons, Inc. Published 2023 by John Wiley & Sons, Inc.
Companion website: www.wiley.com/go/monnet/small

cystoscopy. One study reported greatly increased vascularity of the prostatic parenchyma with many grossly visible dilated veins (Huggins & Clark 1940). In stud dogs used for breeding, there may also be evidence of hemospermia and/or infertility.

Tenesmus is observed less commonly because as the prostate enlarges, it falls cranioventrally into the abdomen so as not to put pressure on the rectum or colon. Although widely described as a clinical sign associated with prostatic disease, constipation and tenesmus are only presenting signs when the prostate is morbidly enlarged and/or adhered within the pelvic cavity. In one report, constipation developed following calcification of an enlarged, cystic prostate (Akpavie & Sullivan 1986). Signs of tenesmus are more commonly associated with infectious or neoplastic causes of prostate enlargement, which cause adhesions between the prostate capsule and the pelvic wall preventing the prostate from falling cranioventrally as it enlarges.

Unlike the situation in men, BPH rarely causes stranguria or urine retention in dogs. BPH in humans originates from the transition zone, a specific inner region of the prostate, where its growth can impinge the urethra (McNeal 1978). In contrast, canine hyperplasia is a diffuse process that develops from the peripheral terminal glands and expands away from the urethra. When symptoms of stranguria or urine retention occur in dogs, they are inevitably associated with neoplastic invasion into the urethral and/or bladder.

Intraparenchymal prostatic cysts

Intraparenchymal prostatic cysts are most often observed within the prostatic parenchyma of aging dogs (>4 years) and are often associated with BPH. Occasionally these intraparenchymal prostatic cysts may reach several centimeters in diameter. Some dogs with BPH have small (in millimeters) cystic changes within the prostate. The finding of a large (in centimeters) intraparenchymal cyst is often associated with BPH. Intraparenchymal cysts may predispose the prostate to bacterial infection (bacterial prostatitis and prostatic abscess), but often they are merely an incidental finding during prostate ultrasonography. In a study including 85 adult, intact male dogs examined for medical problems unrelated to the urinary tract or prostate gland, the prevalence of intraparenchymal prostatic cysts was 14% (Ruel *et al.* 1998). Although an incidental finding, 42% of the dogs with intraparenchymal prostatic cysts cultured positive for bacteria (Black *et al.* 1998).

Intraparenchymal prostatic cysts are filled with prostatic fluid, the production of which depends on androgens. As a result, any treatment (surgical or medical) that reduces prostatic exposure to androgens will result

in cyst shrinkage and elimination in most cases not complicated by neoplasia (Berry *et al.* 1986). Percutaneous fine-needle aspiration of intraparenchymal prostatic cysts for diagnostic or treatment purposes has resulted in serious iatrogenic bacterial infections (e.g., acute prostatitis, peritonitis) even when sterile techniques were used. For this reason, other methods should be considered first before sticking a needle into the prostate.

Paraprostatic cysts

Paraprostatic cysts are uncommon, large cysts resulting from dilated embryonic Müllerian duct remnants (Feeney *et al.* 1985). Paraprostatic cysts vary in size, shape, and location. Most paraprostatic cysts are located cranial or dorsal to the prostate or the trigone of the urinary bladder (Stowater & Lamb 1989) and are outside of the prostatic parenchyma, but are attached to it by a stalk (Stowater & Lamb 1989). They may extend cranially, displacing the bladder, or caudally, into the pelvic canal (Stowater & Lamb 1989). The major differential consideration for the paraprostatic cyst is pyometra of the uterine masculinus, which appears sonographically as multiple, convoluted, tubular cavitations (Johnston *et al.* 1991).

Although paraprostatic cysts can become extremely large, they are not usually associated with other prostatic pathology. Paraprostatic cysts are typically not clinically discernible until their size is sufficient to impinge on the colon or urethra (Stowater & Lamb 1989), or if secondary infection occurs (iatrogenic or ascending) and an abscess develops (Stowater & Lamb 1989). Physical examination findings may include a large mid to caudal abdominal mass in an otherwise healthy male dog. Paraprostatic cysts are often asymptomatic, but clinical signs may be associated with mechanical interference with abdominal viscera. For paraprostatic cysts, complete surgical excision with castration is recommended. When the cyst is not amenable to complete surgical excision, omentalization is recommended. For a valuable stud dog, pharmacologic management with percutaneous fine-needle drainage may be an alternative treatment, albeit temporary.

Prostatic calculi

Prostatic calculi are rare in dogs (Feeney *et al.* 1985). Prostatic calculi, generally composed of calcium phosphate or carbonate, form secondary to chronic inflammation along the urethra or in periurethral areas and are located in cyst-like cavitations.

Squamous metaplasia of the prostate

Squamous metaplasia of the prostatic columnar epithelium occurs in response to hyperestrogenism. Metaplasia causes symmetric enlargement of the gland and diminished flow of prostatic fluid through the ducts. Squamous metaplasia of the prostate is most associated with estrogen-secreting testicular neoplasia, but exogenous estrogen can also cause it. Testicular tumors are common in dogs over 10 years of age.

Squamous metaplasia of the prostate may be asymptomatic or may cause symptoms like BPH. Physical examination findings with squamous metaplasia of the prostate may include a symmetric, nonpainful prostate, a testicular mass with atrophy of the contralateral testis, and other findings caused by hyperestrogenism (alopecia, pigmentation, gynecomastia, pendulous prepuce, and scrotum). There may be other clinical and laboratory signs of hyperestrogenism.

Dogs with squamous metaplasia should be treated promptly by removing the source of estrogen before additional sequelae of estrogen toxicity develop. In dogs with benign estrogen-secreting testicular tumors, castration is the treatment of choice. Additional therapy to treat bone marrow suppression caused by hyperestrogenism may be required.

Persistent Müllerian duct syndrome

PMDS is an autosomal recessive trait in miniature schnauzers and bassett hounds, with expression limited to dogs with an XY chromosome constitution that are also homozygous for these recessive genes. PMDS has also been reported in Persian cats, domestic short hair (DSH) cats, and domestic long hair (DLH) cats. This syndrome results from the failure of Müllerian-inhibiting activity (mutation in the gene for the macrophage migration inhibitory factor [MIF] receptor) with normal synthesis of testosterone during development. As a result, Müllerian-derived structures (uterine tubes, uterus, cervix, and cranial vagina) are retained.

Approximately 50% of animals affected with PMDS are either unilaterally or bilaterally cryptorchid, but otherwise appear to be normal males externally. Affected males with scrotal testes are fertile. Male and female offspring as well as parents and siblings of affected males are carriers of the trait.

Internally, retained testes are attached to the cranial ends of a normal uterus (uterus masculinus), with an epididymis associated with each testis. The vas deferens are present within the myometrium. The cranial portions of the vagina and prostate are often present. A pyometra of the uterine masculinus can occur secondary to infection without hormonal influence and appears as multiple, convoluted, tubular cavitations (Johnston *et al.* 1991). Externally, normal male animals may go unnoticed until they develop pyometra or a urinary tract infection (or dysuria) or prostatic infection. Squamous

metaplasia of the prostate has been reported in animals affected with PMDS and concurrent Sertoli cell tumors.

Definitive diagnosis is made by histologic examination of the internal genitalia and gonads as well as cytogenetic determination of an XY karyotype. When removing the uterus, it is important to remove as much of the vagina as possible. Small-diameter communications between the cranial vagina and prostatic urethra are a source of ascending infection into the uterus.

Infectious prostate diseases

Causes of infectious prostate disease include prostatitis and abscesses. Inflammation of the prostate is almost always the consequence of an infection. Bacterial prostatitis can be either acute or chronic, with the latter being the most common clinical presentation. Acute prostatitis may develop into a prostatic abscess.

Chronic bacterial prostatitis

Chronic bacterial prostatitis (CBP) is the second most common prostate disorder in intact male dogs after BPH. CBP has been estimated to be a primary or a complicating factor in 20–74% of all prostatic diseases in adult male dogs. An increased risk for CBP has been reported in bouvier de Flandres, Scottish terriers, Bernese mountain dogs, German pointers and Doberman pinschers (Krawiec & Heflin 1992).

CBP results when bacteria from the urinary tract ascend into the hyperplastic prostate. Hypersecretory and cystic degenerative changes that occur with BPH create ideal conditions for bacterial overgrowth. Disturbances in the normal defense mechanisms (urine flow during micturition, urethral high-pressure zone, bactericidal effects of prostatic fluid, and local immunoglobulin [Ig]A production) predispose to CBP. The causative organisms are usually those that are common in the urinary tract: *Escherichia coli* (most common), *Pseudomonas*, *Proteus*, *Staphylococcus*, and *Streptococcus*. CBP can occasionally be caused by *Brucella canis*, a potential zoonotic pathogen, via a hematogenous route.

CBP is usually occult in the early stages such that this condition often goes undiagnosed for months to years. The prostate is typically symmetrically enlarged and nonpainful. Infertility, hemospermia, or pyospermia may be present. However, signs of systemic illness are unlikely in dogs with CBP. Clinical signs associated with CBP include recurrent urinary tract infection, hematuria, and purulent or sanguineous urethral discharge. Recurrent urinary tract infection caused by the same pathogen is a hallmark of CBP, because the pathogen persists within the prostate during antimicrobial therapy for the bacteriuria. Although the urine can be sterilized and the symptoms controlled during therapy, discontinuation of treatment leads to reinfection of the urine and recurrence of clinical signs (Meares 1982). Constant or intermittent dripping of sanguineous or purulent exudate from the penis, independent of urination, is another common finding associated with CBP attributed to an increased secretory rate of prostatic fluid induced by infection (Barsanti & Finco 1980). This is attributed to the increased secretory rate of prostatic fluid caused by inflammation (Barsanti & Finco 1980).

Diagnosis is based upon ultrasonographic findings consistent with CBP and more than 10^4 bacteria of a single species per milliliter of seminal plasma. CBP is almost always associated with BPH and, as such, CBP is difficult to treat successfully. Because of the difficulty in treatment, it is much more important to localize the source of infection when CBP is suspected. CBP should be considered whenever recurrent urinary tract infection occurs in the male dog.

Acute bacterial prostatitis

Acute bacterial prostatitis is an uncommon occurrence in dogs and when it does occur, it is primarily in younger (usually intact) male dogs. Acute bacterial prostatitis can occur as the only disease in a particular prostate gland, or it may occur concomitantly with a paraprostatic cyst (etiology for a prostatic abscess) or prostatic neoplasia. The route of infection in cases of acute bacterial prostatitis is usually ascending through the urethra. However, hematogenous spread or spread from the kidneys, bladder, testes, or epididymides is also possible. Causative organisms are similar to those reported for CBP.

Acute bacterial prostatitis is manifested by severe acute abdominal pain. Acute bacterial prostatitis does not cause prostatic enlargement. However, constipation and tenesmus are still sequelae secondary to avoidance of pain induced by defecation. Over 70% of dogs with acute prostatitis have signs of systemic illness. Clinical signs include fever, tachycardia, dehydration, depression, anorexia, vomiting, weakness, hematuria, gait abnormalities, tense abdomen, prostatic pain on rectal exam, and neutrophilia with a left shift. If left untreated, acute bacterial prostatitis can extend through the capsule into the abdomen, resulting in peritonitis (Lattimer 1994).

Prostatic abscess

Prostatic abscess occurs rarely in the dog. It is a severe disorder involving infection of the prostate gland, resulting in the production of pocket(s) of suppurative material and destruction of glandular tissue. Prostatic abscesses may develop as a sequela to squamous meta-

plasia of the prostate gland (Barsanti & Finco 1980), prostatitis, and prostatic neoplasia. Intraparenchymal prostatic cysts that develop concurrently with BPH and chronic prostatitis are frequently misdiagnosed as prostatic abscesses, and these two conditions can be differentiated on the basis of clinical signs. Clinical signs associated with prostatic abscesses are like those of acute bacterial prostatitis. An asymmetrically enlarged prostate may be palpated on rectal exam or an abdominal mass can be palpated abdominally if the prostate is severely enlarged. Symptoms arise from compression or displacement of adjacent structures, prostatic pain, or systemic illness. Symptoms include fever, depression, anorexia, vomiting, caudal abdominal pain, dysuria, tenesmus, and gait abnormalities. As with acute prostatitis, patients with a prostatic abscess often have neutrophilia with a left shift and can present in septic shock. Additionally, hemorrhagic or purulent urethral/preputial discharge may be present. In contrast to prostatic abscess, there is no evidence of pain or systemic involvement in cases of intraparenchymal prostatic cysts that develop concurrently with BPH, and chronic prostatitis and this condition can be treated simply by removal of available androgens to the prostate (either surgically or medically).

Neoplastic prostate diseases

Prostate tumors occur almost exclusively in dogs, with few sporadic cases reported in cats. While there has been no breed predilection reported, middle- to large-breed dogs are more commonly affected. The mean age at diagnosis in dogs is 8.5–11.2 years and prostate tumors are rarely reported prior to 6 years of age (Schrank & Romagnoli 2020). Prostate carcinomas can occur in intact and castrated dogs. However, prostate carcinomas are very rare in intact dogs and are the most common prostate disorder in castrated dogs (Leav *et al.* 2001; Schrank & Romagnoli 2020). Castration at any age has not shown a sparing effect on developing prostatic carcinoma (Obradovich *et al.* 1987); however, the influence of early-age castration (<8 weeks of age) has not been evaluated.

Although urinary transitional cell carcinomas often metastasize into the prostate from the bladder, adenocarcinomas are the most frequent prostate neoplasm in dogs. Primary and metastatic squamous cell carcinomas, urothelial carcinomas, undifferentiated carcinomas, and leiomyosarcomas have also been reported in the prostate of dogs (Johnston *et al.* 1991). However, benign neoplasms of the canine prostate have not been reported.

Prostatic adenocarcinomas arise from the glandular or ductal epithelial cells within the prostate, which are different from men and indicate that separate susceptibility factors promote hyperplastic and neoplastic development in dogs (Leav *et al.* 2001). More than half of the canine prostate carcinomas exhibited intratumoral heterogeneity (Cornell *et al.* 2000). Prostate adenocarcinomas show features of glandular differentiation, including typical variation in acinar size, shape, and spacing, with acini lined by cells with a cuboidal or columnar appearance containing enlarged nuclei and prominent nucleoli (Cornell *et al.* 2000).

In dogs, prostate adenocarcinomas are locally invasive and highly malignant. Initially, prostatic adenocarcinomas grow into the urethra, causing urethral obstruction, followed by invasion into or putting external pressure on the colon, causing bloody stools and tenesmus. The metastatic rate for prostate tumors is 85–100%. The most common sites for metastasis include lungs (50%), iliac and sublumbar lymph node (30%), and bone (15–45%). The pelvis and lumbosacral spine are the most common sites of bony metastasis.

Clinical signs of canine prostate carcinoma referable to the urinary tract (e.g., hematuria, stranguria, incontinence) are seen in 62% of dogs. Constipation and tenesmus occur in 30% of cases secondary to avoidance of pain induced by defecation. Prostatic enlargement tends to be asymmetric, firm, nonmobile (firmly adhered to pelvic canal), and painful on palpation. In intact dogs, prostatic carcinoma is not always associated with prostatomegaly. However, in castrated dogs, prostatomegaly is highly associated with prostatic carcinoma.

Clinical signs of canine prostate carcinoma referable to involvement of the musculoskeletal system or spinal cord are seen in 36% of cases (Cornell *et al.* 2000) and this is the most common reason to observe stiffness or weakness of the rear legs in association with prostate disease (Barsanti & Finco 1980). Of dogs with prostatic adenocarcinoma, 40% had concomitant locomotor problems. Signs of systemic disease (e.g., weight loss, anorexia) are reported in 42% of dogs (Cornell *et al.* 2000). Gross metastases were present in 80% of dogs with prostate carcinoma, with lymph nodes, lung, and bone being the most frequent sites (Cornell *et al.* 2000). Skeletal metastases were observed in 22% of cases (with the predominance in the axial skeleton) (Cornell *et al.* 2000).

Tumor location often precludes early diagnosis. Most tumors are consequently locally advanced and have metastasized (70–80%) at the time of diagnosis, with a median survival of 30 days without treatment (Cornell *et al.* 2000). Finding neoplastic cells on cytologic examination of prostatic fluid is diagnostically important, but not finding neoplastic cells does not eliminate the possibility of neoplasia. In men, prostatic intraepithelial neoplasia (PIN) is the most likely precursor of some prostate cancers, with foci of high-grade PIN present in 85% of men with prostate cancer. However, studies have disagreed on the frequency of PIN in cases of canine prostate carcinoma (Cornell *et al.* 2000; Waters *et al.* 1997). In addition, PIN has been reported in the prostate glands of older dogs with and without carcinoma (Waters *et al.* 1997).

Diagnosis

Clinical signs of prostatic disease

Most prostatic diseases are associated with prostatomegaly. Clinical signs associated with prostatic disease are variable, depending on the degree of prostatomegaly and the specific disorder. Prostatic size is correlated with body weight and age (Berry *et al.* 1986) as well as breed (O'Shea 1962). The beagle prostate increases in size for at least six years whether it is normal or hyperplastic. Prostatic enlargement is common in intact male dogs more than 5 years old. Scottish terriers are reported to have prostates that are four times larger than those from other breeds of similar weights and ages (O'Shea 1962).

Most common clinical signs associated with prostatic disease include urethral discharge, hematuria, and tenesmus. Urethral discharge can be clear, purulent, or hemorrhagic. The sources of prostatic hemorrhage are dilated prostatic veins and/or increased vascularity within the prostatic parenchyma associated with hyperplasia, infection, or neoplasia (Huggins & Clark 1940). Although widely described as a clinical sign associated with prostatic disease, tenesmus is only present when the prostate is morbidly enlarged. In one report, constipation developed following mineralization of a grossly enlarged paraprostatic cyst (Akpavie & Sullivan 1986). Additional clinical signs associated with prostatic disease include fever, cachexia, abnormal hindlimb gait, and caudal abdominal pain. In addition to history and clinical signs, diagnosis of prostatic diseases is based upon examination by means of palpation, imaging, prostatic fluid, and histology.

In addition to history and clinical signs, diagnosis of prostatic diseases is based on examination by means of palpation, imaging, prostatic fluid, and histology.

Palpation of the testes and prostate gland

In intact male dogs, the scrotum should be palpated to confirm the presence of two scrotal testicles as well as to rule out the presence of a testicular tumor. A cursory examination of the prostate can be performed by simultaneous rectal and abdominal palpation. Rectal palpation permits examination of only the dorsal or dorsocaudal aspect of the prostate (Hastak *et al.* 1982).

Simultaneous rectal and abdominal palpation not only allows for the cranial aspects of the prostate to be examined, but also facilitates better palpation per rectum because the prostate can be pushed into or near the pelvic canal, which is especially important in large-breed dogs (Barsanti & Finco 1980).

The prostate should be evaluated for size, symmetry, surface contour, consistency, mobility, and pain. The normal prostate is bilobed, symmetric, smooth, movable, and nonpainful. When symmetric, nonpainful prostatomegaly is an incidental physical exam finding in an otherwise normal, healthy, older, intact male dog, a tentative diagnosis of BPH is justified. Ultrasound would be confirmatory, but there is usually no urgency. Rectal palpation of the prostate is a simple method commonly used to evaluate prostate size, but the clinician should be aware that this method is limited to only the dorsal or dorsal-caudal aspects of enlarged prostates (Hastak et al. 1982).

Prostate imaging

Radiographically, the prostate gland is of soft tissue opacity and its identification is influenced by the differential subject opacity of surrounding tissues. It is normally intrapelvic and may, therefore, be difficult to see radiographically. In addition, ascites and emaciation may alter the radiographic contrast and therefore make it difficult to identify the prostate gland on survey radiographs (Johnston et al. 1991). However, generalized enlargement of the prostate gland produces cranial and possibly dorsal displacement of the urinary bladder. The size, location, and contour of the prostate may be evaluated by radiographically in lateral and dorsoventral survey views. A normal-sized prostate displaces neither the colon nor the bladder from their normal position. BPH, paraprostatic cysts, prostatic abscesses, and squamous metaplasia may displace the colon dorsally. But enlargement of the sublumbar (iliac) lymph nodes causes ventral displacement of the colon. Paraprostatic cysts may also cause displacement of the urinary bladder.

Radiographic diagnosis of prostatomegaly is made when the ventrodorsal and craniocaudal prostate gland dimensions exceed 70% of the pubic–promontory distance (distance between the cranial aspect of the pubic bone and the sacral promontory) on lateral survey radiographs (Feeney et al. 1987a) or exceeding 50% of the width of the pelvic inlet on a ventrodorsal radiograph. However, the exact dimensions of the prostate cannot always be accurately determined on abdominal radiographs due to superposition of osseous structures, and may be further impaired by lack of abdominal serosal detail due to lack of fat, abdominal effusion, or focal peritonitis associated with prostatitis (Lattimer 1994). In addition, radiographic magnification may yield erroneous results. The guidelines for diagnosing prostatomegaly from pubic–promontory distance are useful for clinical practice, but remain imprecise and subjective and do not consider the effect of age.

Paraprostatic cysts appear as a mid- or caudal-abdominal, soft tissue mass. On survey radiographs alone, they may be difficult to differentiate from the urinary bladder or may appear as a "second" bladder-like structure. In some cases of paraprostatic cysts, calcified walls have been reported. However, mineralization of the prostatic parenchyma may indicate present or past inflammation or neoplasia, with the latter being the most common (Bradbury et al. 2009). Prostatic mineralization has been shown to be highly predictive of neoplasia in neutered male dogs, but less reliable in intact male dogs. Overt osteodestructive processes or other evidence of bone metastasis in pelvic bones or mid and cranial lumbar vertebral bodies may also be evident radiographically with prostatic neoplasia.

Distention retrograde contrast urethrocystography (DRCU) has been described as a method for determining prostatic integrity. In a normal prostate or with BPH, no or minimal positive contrast will be identified in the prostatic parenchyma near the urethra (urethroprostatic reflux) (Feeney et al. 1984). However, larger volumes of contrast material accumulating within the prostatic parenchyma (intraprostatic reflux; sometimes referred to as parenchymal-positive contrast "blushes") have been reported to occur with all types of prostate diseases and can occur in normal dogs as well (Barsanti & Finco 1980; Feeney et al. 1984). Irregularity or an undulant pattern to the prostatic urethral surface has been associated with noninflammatory nonneoplastic prostatic disease, inflammatory nonneoplastic disease, as well as prostatic adenocarcinoma or urethral transitional cell carcinoma. Narrowing of the prostatic urethral diameter during DRCU has been reported to occur in association with prostatic abscesses and neoplasia (Feeney et al. 1987a). However, since prostatic urethral diameter varies in normal dogs with the degree of bladder distension, changes in prostatic diameter must be interpreted cautiously (relative to the measurement of maximal urethral diameter). DRCU can be helpful in differentiating the urinary bladder from a paraprostatic cyst if ultrasonography is not available. In addition, the absence of positive results on contrast studies does not rule out the present of prostatic disease (Feeney et al. 1987b). Based on the author's experience, ultrasonography is a better method for imaging prostatic integrity compared to DRCU in most instances.

Transabdominal ultrasonography is the best imaging modality for evaluation of the prostate because it is a safe, noninvasive method that allows for precise measurements to be taken as well as allowing evaluation of the prostatic parenchyma. When findings of imaging techniques were compared within the same patients, ultrasonographic assessment of both the prostate symmetry and contour was more sensitive for a diagnosis than survey radiography, and equally sensitive to distension retrograde urethrocystography (Feeney *et al.* 1987a,b). Ultrasonography has been shown to be a useful technique for evaluation of the response to drug-induced prostatic involution in dogs (Cartee *et al.* 1990).

The dog can be imaged in dorsal, dorsal oblique, or lateral recumbency. Because the hair coat is thin in the suprapubic area, clipping is usually not necessary. However, hair may be clipped from the ventral abdomen between the cranial aspect of the prepuce and pubic bone from the midline to the inguinal fold to facilitate imaging. Alcohol and/or coupling gel is applied to the skin to improve contact. A 5 or 7.5 MHz real-time convex or sector transducer is recommended because of its $\geq 90°$ field of view and ability for the transducer head to follow the body contour of the caudal abdomen better than that of a linear array transducer. To image the prostate, the transducer is placed against the ventral abdominal wall cranial to the pubis. If the prostate remains within the pelvic canal, a finger can be inserted into the rectum to displace the prostate gland cranially.

The prostate should be imaged in both sagittal (longitudinal) and transverse planes to ensure that all areas of the prostate are seen. The true sagittal plane can be confirmed by observing the hypoechoic urethral tract. Since most prostatic diseases are associated with prostatomegaly, the prostate should be carefully measured. Prostate dimensions are measured on both the

sagittal and transverse planes (Ruel *et al.* 1998). In a study of 100 healthy intact male dogs, maximum predicted values of prostate size were found to vary by age, breed of dog, and body weight (O'Shea 1962; Berry *et al.* 1986; Ruel *et al.* 1998). Formulas for calculating the maximum prostatic dimension in a normal intact dog are shown in Table 58.1. In the author's experience, normal prostatic height on sagittal plane for a dog castrated before 1 year of age is about 1 cm.

The ultrasonographic appearance of a prostate from a normal intact dog should have a uniform background echogenicity that is referred to as homogeneous, with a fine to medium texture and moderately hyperechoic, similar to that of the spleen (Figure 58.1) (Feeney

Table 58.1 Canine prostate measurement formulas.

$$L = (0.055 \times BW) + (0.143 \times A) + 3.31$$
$$W = (0.047 \times BW) + (0.089 \times A) + 3.4$$
$$H_{sag} = (0.046 \times BW) + (0.06 \times A) + 2.68$$
$$H_{tr} = (0.044 \times BW) + (0.083 \times A) + 2.25$$
$$V = (0.867 \times BW) + (1.885 \times A) + 15.88$$

Using 100 clinically normal intact sexually mature dogs, multiple regression analyses were used to establish formulas for calculating the maximal predictive value of prostate length (L, cm), width (W, cm), height (H_{sag}, height on sagittal image, cm; H_{tr}, height on transverse image, cm), and volume (V, cm³), based on body weight (BW, kg) and age (A, years). Source: Data from Ruel *et al.* (1998).

(a)

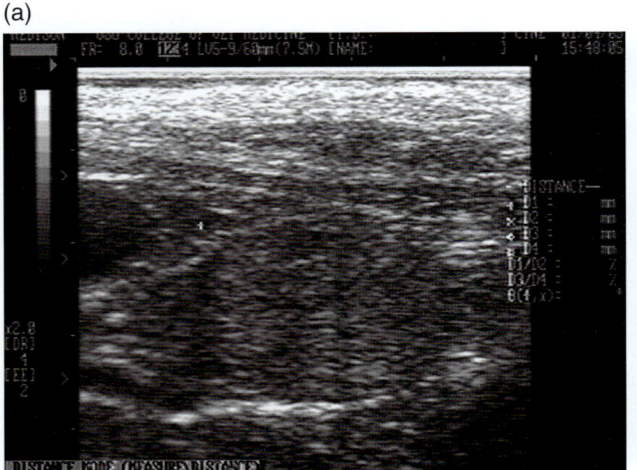

(b)

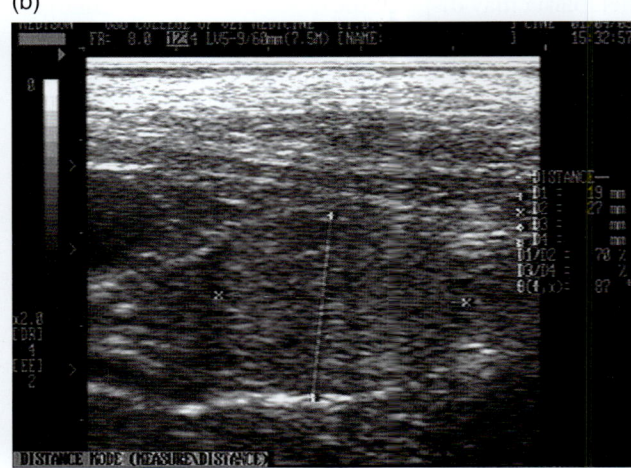

Figure 58.1 Sagittal ultrasonographic image of a normal prostate from an intact dog (a) without and (b) with measuring calipers. The prostate is ovoid with a smooth margin and the parenchyma has a homogeneous echotexture of medium echogenicity.

et al. 1985). The echogenicity within the prostate should be assessed for focal, multifocal, or diffuse changes in echotexture. The ultrasonographic appearance of canine prostatic diseases is summarized in Table 58.2 (Bradbury *et al.* 2009).

Transrectal ultrasonography is commonly performed in humans for prostatic imaging. Transrectal ultrasonography in dogs allows for tumor measurements, including urethral penetration of the tumor (identification of abnormal tissue within the urethral lumen) and tumor extension into the urinary tract (Culp *et al.* 2019). Transrectal ultrasonography is superior to transabdominal ultrasonography for imaging prostate tumors in dogs and is comparable to results obtained from magnetic resonance imaging (MRI) (Culp *et al.* 2019).

Both computed tomography (CT) and MRI are excellent methods for prostatic imaging as well as imaging of adjacent structures where metastasis may be a concern. CT can be helpful for surgical or radiation treatment planning. In humans, MRI serves as an accurate modality for assessing prostatic volume, provided that serial measurements are correlated with the weight of an excised prostate.

However, there is little information in the veterinary literature of the usefulness for diagnosing prostatic disease in the dog. Both are expensive procedures to perform in dogs, these technologies are not widely available in referral practices, and both require immobilization of the dog with general anesthesia. Bone scintigraphy may also be helpful in imaging osseous metastatic lesions before they could be identified by radiography (Lee-Parritz & Lamb 1988).

Prostatic fluid analysis

Cytology and culture of prostatic tissue and/or fluid are the next diagnostic steps. Prostatic fluid should be assessed by cytologic evaluation and quantitative bacterial culture in any dog suspected to have prostate disease.

Prostatic fluid may be obtained by ejaculation (collection of the third fraction), prostatic wash, or percutaneous fine-needle aspiration, where the former is the preferred method of collection, especially in cases of

Table 58.2 Ultrasonographic appearance of several canine prostatic diseases.

Disease	Shape	Echotexture
Benign prostatic hyperplasia (BPH)	Symmetric prostatomegaly with smooth margins; large intraparenchymal cyst formation may result in some degree of asymmetry	Homogeneous echotexture of normal to slightly increased echogenicity; the central hilar echo may be absent and small anechoic fluid-filled cavities (1–100 mm) may be present within the parenchyma
Chronic prostatitis[a]	Symmetric prostatomegaly with smooth margins; large intraparenchymal cysts from concurrent BPH may result in some degree of asymmetry	May be indistinguishable from BPH; homogeneous to heterogeneous mixed echotexture of normal to slightly increased echogenicity to coarsely hyperechoic due to irregular hyperechoic foci; may have regions of dystrophic mineralization resulting from fibrosis and chronic inflammation that may be indistinguishable from neoplasia
Acute prostatitis[a]	Symmetric normal-sized prostate with smooth margins	Heterogeneous mixed echotexture of coarsely hyperechoic and hypoechoic parenchyma; hypoechoic areas result from edema and small fluid-filled cavities
Prostatic abscess[a]	Symmetric prostatomegaly with smooth margins to asymmetric irregularly shaped, depending upon the size of the abscess	Heterogeneous mixed echotexture of coarsely hyperechoic and hypoechoic parenchyma with one or more large anechoic to hypoechoic fluid-filled cavities
Neoplasia[a,b,c]	Asymmetric irregularly shaped prostatomegaly with capsular disruption and extension into adjacent tissues	Heterogeneous mixed echotexture of focal hypoechoic areas with poorly defined and coalescing mineralized hyperechoic foci with acoustic shadowing; anechoic cavities from intraparenchymal cysts may also be present
Paraprostatic cyst	Very large (>15 cm), well circumscribed, ovoid	Anechoic or hypoechoic fluid adjacent to the prostate; may be appear like the urinary bladder and may contain single or multiple, thin hyperechoic septa, may be mineralized

[a] Iliac and sublumbar lymph nodes may be enlarged.
[b] Irregular contour of caudal lumbar vertebral bodies and large lymph nodes may be present.
[c] Urethra and bladder neck may have an irregular margin.

suspected bacterial infection and concomitant cystitis. In a study comparing these methods, paired urethral and ejaculate specimens were found to agree with specimens collected by needle aspiration in 80% of cases. However, if the prostatic lesion does not communicate with the urethra, the results of the first two methods may be misleading (Huggins & Clark 1940; Barsanti & Finco 1980; Barsanti et al. 1980; Bell et al. 1995; Powe et al. 2004; Root Kustritz 2006). Prostatic fine-needle aspiration or biopsy is an effective method of obtaining cells for cytology and culture and tissue for histopathology. In one study, complications associated with fine-needle aspiration or punch biopsy included hematuria for fewer than four days and periprostatic hemorrhage (Barsanti et al. 1980). In another report, a sterile intraparenchymal prostatic cyst was aspirated and developed into a prostatic abscess seven days later. Prostatic biopsies are not recommended if bacterial prostatitis is suspected, unless neoplasia is also suspected or if the existence of CBP cannot be confirmed by other tests (Barsanti & Finco 1980). Needle aspiration is contraindicated in patients with acute prostatitis or prostatic abscesses, since large numbers of bacteria may be seeded along the needle tract.

Prostatic fluid should be assessed by cytologic evaluation and quantitative bacterial culture in any dog suspected to have prostate disease. Prostatic fluid can be collected "aseptically" via ejaculation, if care is taken to change collection containers after first and second fractions are collected and the tip of the penis does not touch the collection vessel. Increased numbers of squamous epithelial cells typically are found in prostatic wash and ejaculate samples from dogs with prostatic squamous metaplasia. In one study, the presence of squamous epithelial cells and Gram-positive cocci bacteria in conjunction with the absence of neutrophils was indicative that contamination occurred during ejaculated prostatic fluid collection (Barsanti et al. 1980). Low numbers of neutrophils (<5 per high-power field) can normally be found in voided urine and in an ejaculate (Barsanti & Finco 1980). Prostatic inflammation and infection are well correlated with the appearance of macrophages in prostatic fluid (Barsanti et al. 1983). However, the severity of inflammatory infiltrate (septic suppurative inflammation) is not always correlated to the type or number of bacteria present. Bacteria may be seen within neutrophils.

Cytologic evaluation of prostatic fluid from dogs with BPH reveals many erythrocytes and epithelial dysplasia (Kawakami et al. 1995). Most inflammatory cells (>80%), if present, are mononuclear cells (lymphocytes and plasmocytes) (Mahapokai et al. 2001). This contrasts with bacterial prostatitis or prostatic abscess, in which the cytologic evaluation of prostatic fluid reveals degenerative neutrophils. Extreme care must be taken if performing a fine-needle aspirate with a presumptive diagnosis of a bacterial prostatitis or prostatic abscess, because of the potential to cause septic peritonitis. Fine-needle aspiration of a paraprostatic cyst yields a fluid (not urine) that is clear and yellow to turbid and brown (Barsanti & Finco 1980). This fluid will be obtained on aspiration unless the cyst is secondarily infected.

In addition to fine-needle aspirate, prostatic fluid can be collected from dogs with prostatic neoplasia via prostatic wash or by collecting the third fraction of the ejaculate. However, if the lesion does not communicate with the urethra, results may be misleading. The appearance of neoplastic cells on prostatic fluid cytologic examination is diagnostically significant, but not finding neoplastic cells does not eliminate the possibility of neoplasia.

Prostatic fluid bacterial culture results should be negative. Positive culture results indicate concomitant bacterial prostatitis or abscess, and/or urinary tract infection, and/or contamination of the ejaculate with preputial organisms (Barsanti et al. 1983). If positive, generally large numbers of a single bacterial species are isolated. Common bacterial causes of prostatitis and abscessation are E. coli, Staphylococcus spp., Streptococcus spp., Proteus spp., Pseudomonas spp., and B. canis. In rare cases, prostatitis can result from nonbacterial organisms (e.g., Blastomyces, Pythium) that cause systemic disease. It is of interest to note that urine bacterial culture results are well correlated with prostatic fluid culture results, such that a cystocentesis would be a safer alternative to a fine-needle aspirate of the prostate if prostatic fluid could not be collected by ejaculation or prostatic wash (Barsanti et al. 1983).

In striking contrast to humans, the prostatic fluid pH in dogs with prostatitis (6.3) is similar to dogs without infection (6.25) (Barsanti et al. 1983). Serum and seminal acid phosphatase concentrations do not differ between normal dogs and dogs with prostatic disorders.

Histopathology

Although definitive diagnosis of BPH or squamous metaplasia requires histopathologic confirmation, it is difficult to justify a prostatic biopsy when the results of less invasive methods strongly support the diagnosis of BPH and the absence of more sinister prostatic diseases (Barsanti et al. 1980; Krawiec & Heflin 1992). However, histopathologic evaluation is essential for tumor diagnosis.

Adenocarcinoma is the most frequent histologic type of prostatic neoplasia, although more than half exhibit intratumoral heterogeneity (Cornell et al. 2000). Histologic features of prostatic carcinoma include variation in glandular acinar size, shape, and spacing, with acinar cells containing enlarged nuclei and prominent nucleoli (Cornell *et al.* 2000). PIN, a common precursor prostatic neoplasia in humans, has been reported in the prostates of older dogs with and without neoplasia (Waters & Bostwick 1997). In cases of canine prostatic neoplasia, the occurrence of PIN is too variable to be clinically useful, occurring in between 7% (Cornell *et al.* 2000) and 66% (Waters *et al.* 1997) of cases of dogs with prostatic neoplasia. Tumor markers frequently used in human medicine, such as prostate-specific antigen and prostatic acid phosphatase, are not useful in diagnosing prostatic neoplasia in the dog (Bell *et al.* 1995; Gobello *et al.* 2002; Oliveira *et al.* 2006; Goodman *et al.* 2011).

Urinalysis

If a cystocentesis is performed, care should be taken to avoid the prostate during urine collection. Regardless of the method of urine collection, inflammatory sediment is usually present on urinalysis. Macroscopic or microscopic hematuria may be found. Urine bacterial culture results were well correlated with evidence of prostatic infection (Barsanti *et al.* 1983). Results of bacterial culture of fluid collected after prostatic massage are not interpretable if there is concurrent urinary tract infection.

Hematology

Serum biochemistry profiles are generally unremarkable. A complete blood count should be performed in all dogs with suspected squamous metaplasia to assess for possible bone marrow suppression from hyperestrogenism.

Treatment

Castration

Most types of prostate disease, with the exception of neoplasia and paraprostatic cysts, can be prevented or cured by neutering male dogs (Obradovich *et al.* 1987; Freitag *et al.* 2007). Routine castration is the most effective method for reducing prostatic size and activity, since dihydrotestosterone is required to maintain prostatic function. However, healthy intact dogs with BPH or intraparenchymal prostatic cysts, showing no clinical signs, do not necessarily require treatment and can have treatment delayed until clinical signs occur. It is important to note that BPH and intraparenchymal prostatic cysts increase the risk for an ascending bacterial prostatic infection by urethral flora.

Surgical castration

The prostate begins to involute soon after castration and is significantly smaller within 7–10 days (Barsanti &

Finco 1980). Clinical signs attributable to nonneoplastic prostate diseases are typically completely resolved within 4 weeks after castration. Prostate secretion decreases to a minimal amount within 30 days, whereas size continues to decrease for 60–90 days. On the cellular level, the acinar epithelial cells become small and the acini eventually collapse (Barsanti & Finco 1980). Castration is recommended as the primary treatment for BPH and as an ancillary treatment in intraparenchymal prostatic cysts, bacterial prostatitis (chronic and acute), and prostatic abscesses. Because of diminished prostatic fluid production, intraparenchymal prostatic cysts decrease in size and resolve completely after castration. In dogs with experimentally induced *E. coli* bacterial prostatitis, castration resolved the infection within 4.2 weeks compared to 9.5 weeks in intact dogs.

Medical (nonsurgical) castration

Although surgical castration is superior to medical treatments for reducing prostatic size, medical (nonsurgical) management is an alternative for owners who decline surgery because of the value of their dog as a stud, or in cases in which other disorders put the animal at great anesthetic or surgical risk. By a variety of mechanisms, these drugs have anti-androgenic effects that are effective in reducing prostatic size, but will eventually wane after treatment is discontinued because the source of androgen (testes) still exists.

Finasteride (5α-reductase inhibitor), deslorelin acetate (decreases testosterone concentration), flutamide (androgen receptor blocker), and delmadinone acetate (decreases testosterone concentration) are all effective for the control of BPH in dogs (Cartee *et al.* 1990; Coffey & Walsh 1990; Laroque *et al.* 1994; Kawakami *et al.* 1995; Lange *et al.* 2001; Shibata *et al.* 2001; Albouy *et al.* 2008).

Antimicrobials

Intermittent tissue concentrations of bactericidal antimicrobials that are 4–8 times the minimum inhibitory concentration are usually sufficient for a clinical cure of prostatic bacterial infections, excluding prostatic abscessation that also requires drainage. However, cure of prostatic infections is difficult because most antimicrobial agents useful against the prostatitis organisms diffuse poorly into prostatic fluids. If there is no specific secretory or active transport mechanism, the ability of an antibiotic to cross any membrane depends upon the pKa of the drug, its lipid solubility, and the degree of protein binding. Only the nonionized forms can cross epithelial membranes (Barsanti & Finco 1980).

Chloramphenicol reaches levels in canine prostatic fluid that are about 60% of the levels in canine plasma

(Meares 1982). In comparison, doxycycline and tetracycline reach levels in canine prostatic fluid that are less than 20% of that in plasma. Drugs such as ampicillin, penicillin, and cephalothin with low lipid solubility cannot cross lipid membranes.

Basic drugs, such as trimethoprim-sulfonamide, macrolides, or fluoroquinolones, will readily diffuse from the more alkaline blood (pH 7.4) to the more acidic prostatic fluid (pH <7.0) (Baumueller *et al.* 1977; Meares 1982; Barsanti *et al.* 1983). Unlike enrofloxacin, ciprofloxacin has poorer penetration of prostatic tissue and is not the preferred fluoroquinolone for the treatment of prostatic bacterial infections (Dorfman *et al.* 1995).

Antibiotics should be continued for at least 4–6 weeks, regardless of the earlier disappearance of clinical signs. Prostatic fluid should be recultured 3–7 days after discontinuation of the antibiotics. Acute bacterial prostatitis should be treated with an appropriate antibiotic, as determined by a culture and sensitivity, as the prostatic blood barrier is disrupted in most cases of ABP so that most antibiotics will penetrate the capsule. If left untreated, bacterial prostatitis can extend through the capsule into the abdomen, resulting in peritonitis (Lattimer 1994).

Prostatic drainage

Ultrasound-guided fine-needle drainage of intraparenchymal prostatic cysts, paraprostatic cysts, or prostatic abscesses should be done in conjunction with other treatment modalities (e.g., castration, antimicrobial therapy, omentalization), as drainage alone may be inadequate. Percutaneous ultrasound-guided drainage followed by alcoholization of the cavity is reported to be an effective method for resolving prostatic abscesses (Boland *et al.* 2003). However, owners need to be aware that treatment of intraparenchymal prostatic cysts or paraprostatic cysts by percutaneous drainage alone will likely require reaspiration.

Paraprostatic cyst or abscess excision with omentalization

The recommended treatment for paraprostatic cysts causing symptoms of prostate disease is surgical removal with castration (Head & Francis 2002). When the paraprostatic cyst or abscess is not amenable to complete surgical excision, drainage, or digital exploration of the gland through bilateral capsulectomy, débridement with resection of the majority of the cyst/abscess wall and packing the residual cyst/abscess cavity with omentum (intracapsular omentalization) are recommended (Figures 58.2 and 58.3) (White & Williams 1995; White 2000).

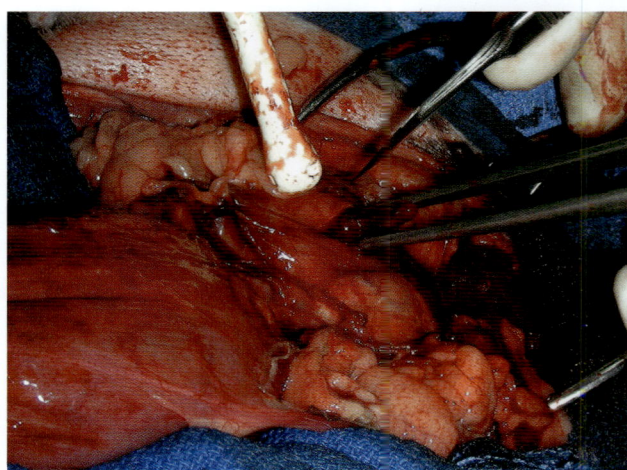

Figure 58.2 A prostatic abscess is opened with a blade. The entire abscess is flushed with saline and all the septa present in the abscess are broken down with digital palpation.

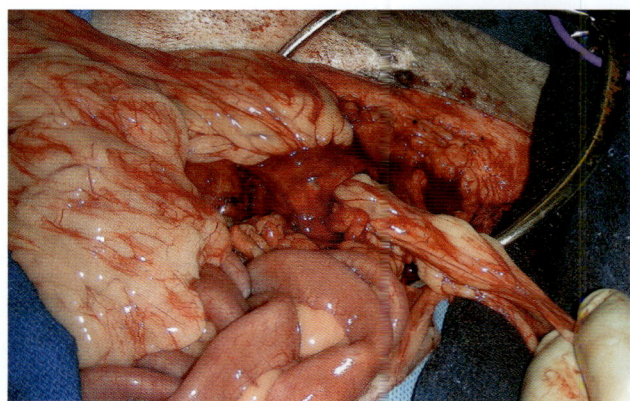

Figure 58.3 The omentum has been introduced into the prostate. It passes dorsal to the urethra since the abscess was bilateral. An abdominal drain was placed at the end of surgery.

Intracapsular omentalization has an up to 20% incidence of postoperative urinary incontinence (temporary or permanent) (Del Magno *et al.* 2021). Other reported postoperative complications include urinary retention, dysuria, urethral tear, oliguric kidney injury, cardiac arrhythmia, and persisting urinary tract obstruction (Del Magno *et al.* 2021). Minor complications (n = 10) consisted of temporary urinary incontinence (n = 2) and permanent urinary incontinence n = 5).

Prostatectomy

Both complete and subtotal/partial prostate removal in dogs with neoplasia have been previously described.

Complete prostatectomy

Complete prostatectomies are difficult to perform and require careful dissection of the prostate to avoid damaging the urethra and minimize neurovascular damage to the bladder. Intraoperative identification of the neurovascular supply to the gland is essential to avoid avascular necrosis or neurogenic incontinence associated with surgery. Complete prostatectomy is associated with a high complication rate, such that most surgeons do not recommend the procedure (Rawlings *et al.* 1994, 1997; Goldsmid & Bellenger 1991; Robertson & Bojrab 1984). The overall median survival time following complete prostatectomy is 231 days (range 24–1255 days), with one- and two-year survival rate of 32% and 12%, respectively (Bennett *et al.* 2018). Advances in surgical modalities may result in fewer complications following prostatectomy. In one study, a robot-assisted radical prostatectomy was performed in a 6-year-old neutered male Bernese mountain dog using a daVinci Si Surgical System through a transperitoneal approach (Schlake *et al.* 2020). An interfascial nerve-sparing approach was used to preserve the neurovascular bundles. Although there was no postoperative urinary incontinence with this method, peritoneal carcinomatosis 43 days after surgery resulted in the dog being euthanized (Schlake *et al.* 2020). Regardless of method used or if used in combination with adjunct therapies, case selection for total prostatectomy plays a significant role in postoperative outcomes (Bennett *et al.* 2018).

Subtotal or partial prostatectomy with intraoperative adjunctive therapy

Advantages of a subtotal resection compared with complete prostatectomy include reduced operative time and preservation of the vas deferens in breeding animals. Subtotal or partial prostatectomy with neodymium: yttrium-aluminum-garnet (Nd: YAG) laser dissection to remove focal prostatic neoplastic lesions had a median survival of 183 days (range 91–239 days). Nd-YAG laser energy creates well-defined areas of coagulative necrosis, with little tissue charring and without development of postoperative incontinence. It is important to use low power (1–2 W) with long exposure (400–1500 seconds), as higher power (35–60 W) with shorter exposure (1–2 seconds) laser ablation in canine prostates has been associated with intraoperative death, incontinence, and recurrent urinary tract and prostatic infections (L'Eplattenier *et al.* 2006).

Intraoperative orthovoltage radiotherapy (radiation therapy to surgically exposed prostate tumors) has also been used as an intraoperative adjunctive therapy for treating prostate tumors. The reported survival time following intraoperative orthovoltage radiotherapy was 41–750 days, with survival time primarily dependent upon the degree to which the tumor had metastases prior to treatment (Turrel 1987).

Intraoperative photodynamic therapy (PDT) has been used as a treatment option for prostatic carcinoma (Dobson et al. 2018). Researchers have demonstrated the biological responses of the prostate and adjacent vital structures to meso-tetra-(m-hydroxyphenyl) chlorin (mTHPC) or aluminum disulfonated phthalocyanine (AlS2Pc). Other workers using the photosensitizer photofrin found that interstitial PDT in the canine prostate produced modest volumes of tissue necrosis, which varied in relation to the amount of hemorrhage, which was unpredictable. Intraoperative PDT using a halogen broad-band lamp after local administration of 5-aminolevulinic acid in six dogs with prostatic adenocarcinoma resulted in a median survival time of 41 days (range 10–68 days) (L'Eplattenier *et al.* 2008).

Adjunctive prostatic neoplasia treatments

Definitive-intent, intensity-modulated radiotherapy has been used in dogs to treat prostate tumor, with the total prescribed radiation dose ranging from 48 to 54 Gy (median 50 Gy), delivered as daily doses of 2.5–2.8 Gy (Walz *et al.* 2020). Diarrhea was the most common toxicity observed (Walz *et al.* 2020). Following definitive-intent, intensity-modulated radiotherapy, the median event-free survival was 220 days and median overall survival was 563 days (Walz *et al.* 2020). External beam radiation therapy to the pelvis is also used in veterinary medicine to treat malignancies of the prostate, bladder, perineal area, and regional (medial iliac) lymph nodes. However, daily treatments (Monday–Friday) of external beam radiation therapy (43–54 Gy in 2.7–3.3 Gy fractions for 19–28 days) are reported to have limited success, with the complication of colitis developing in 56% of cases (Bell *et al.* 1991; Anderson *et al.* 2002). Survival following treatment ranged from 209 to 934 days (Anderson *et al.* 2002). Radiation potentiators (e.g., cisplatin) used in conjunction with external beam radiation reportedly increase survival times (Anderson *et al.* 2002).

Fluoroscopy-guided prostatic artery catheterization followed by radioembolization (RE) with Yttrium-90 microspheres (dose escalation from 60 to 200 Gy per prostate hemigland) has been shown in dogs to induce a significant dose-dependent decrease (25–60%) in prostate size by 40 days, with no radiographic or no gross changes in the rectum, urethra, penis, or bladder (Mouli *et al.* 2021). Histology revealed RE-induced changes in the treated prostatic tissues of the highest-dose group, with gland atrophy and focal necrosis, but no extraprostatic RE-related histologic findings were observed (Mouli *et al.* 2021).

More than 90% of canine prostate carcinomas express cyclooxygenase 1 and 2 (Sorenmo *et al.* 2004; L'Eplattenier *et al.* 2007). Treatment of dogs with piroxicam, a selective cyclooxygenase-2 inhibitor, has been used successfully in the reduction of several canine carcinomas. Of the dogs treated with piroxicam (0.3 mg/kg orally every 24–48 h), 75% had a reduction in invasive transitional cell carcinoma volume that was strongly associated with the induction of apoptosis. In dogs with prostate carcinoma, piroxicam treatment alone resulted in prolonged survival compared to untreated dogs (7 vs. 0.7 months, respectively) and also improved clinical signs associated with stranguria and tenesmus (Sorenmo *et al.* 2004). Combining cisplatin therapy (60 mg/m^2 intravenously every 21 days) with piroxicam therapy resulted in complete or partial tumor remission in 71% of dogs, compared to no tumor remission with cisplatin therapy alone. Other nonsteroid anti-inflammatory drugs (e.g., meloxicam, firocoxib, carprofen) have been used in combination with other chemotherapeutics (e.g., carboplatin, mitoxantrone, toceranib phosphate, cyclophosphamide, chlorambucil, lomustine) with varying degrees of tumor regression and improvement in clinical signs (Ravicini *et al.* 2018; Pan *et al.* 2016).

The chemotherapeutic paclitaxel has been used in human medicine for the treatment of recurrent or inoperable tumors (Boon 2002). Paclitaxel works by arresting the cell cycle in the G0/G1 and G2/M phases, thereby suppressing indiscriminate proliferation of tumor cells (Zhang *et al.* 2014). Oral administration of paclitaxel (5–12.5 mg/kg) was well tolerated in dogs with prostate cancer, with adverse effects limited to mild neutropenia (Chae *et al.* 2020). Clinical responses included reduction in mass size and improvement of symptoms, but disease progression resulted in euthanasia of all dogs (Chae *et al.* 2020).

Similar to the veterinary melanoma vaccine (Oncept®, Merial, Duluth, GA, USA), immunotherapy with prostate cancer vaccines may soon be available for dogs. Several prostate cancer vaccines – such as the personalized dendritic cell vaccine sipuleucel-T (Provenge®, Dendreon Pharmaceuticals, Seal Beach, CA, USA) or the recombinant viral prostate cancer vaccine PSA-TRICOM (Prostvac®-VF, Bavarian Nordic, Hellurup, Denmark) – have been used in human clinical trials with varying degrees of success (Thomas & Prendergast 2016). However, vaccine immunotherapy is not yet a standard treatment for men, due to the tumor environment's complex interaction between the immune system and malignant cells (Mitsogiannis *et al.* 2022).

Palliative care should be considered in animals with metastatic disease and those with advanced localized disease not amenable to definitive therapy. The efficacy of palliative treatments has not been established conclusively. Palliative radiotherapy may provide short-term relief from urinary obstruction or other clinical signs resulting from local disease. Permanent cystostomy tube placement may provide relief from urinary obstruction. Placement of a stent in the urethra can palliate some of the clinical signs related to urinary obstruction (Weisse 2006; Blackburn 2010). Although there is no evidence that canine prostatic neoplasia is androgen dependent, castration is recommended, since BPH can occur concurrently and may contribute to clinical signs associated with prostatomegaly. Systemic treatment with chemotherapy, nonsteroidal anti-inflammatories, or paclitaxel may provide some additional relief.

Prognosis

The prognosis and outcome of prostatic disease depend upon the condition. For BPH with or without intraparenchymal prostatic cysts, the prognosis is excellent. Dogs not showing clinical signs may remain symptoms free for months to years. Castration is curative of clinical signs of BPH and intraparenchymal prostatic cysts will decrease in size. Castration of juvenile dogs prevents BPH, intraparenchymal prostatic cysts, and testicular tumors.

The prognosis is fair for prostatitis in general. Acute prostatitis is generally more amenable to cure than chronic prostatitis, but systemic illness makes it a more urgent and potentially life-threatening disease than chronic prostatitis. Prostatic fluid and urine should be collected for culture and cytology two weeks after completion of antibiotics, and again four weeks later. Infection generally will not recur if finasteride is continued or if castration is performed.

Prostatic abscess formation is a possible sequela of acute prostatitis. The prognosis is guarded to poor for prostatic abscess. Morbidity can be high with surgical intervention, with reported mortality rates of 24–51% within the first year following therapy.

With rare exceptions, the prognosis for animals with prostatic tumors is poor; advanced disease at the time of diagnosis is the major causative factor for this poor prognosis. Due to the severity of clinical disease (advanced local and distant metastasis), most dogs with clinical signs caused by prostate tumors are euthanized within one month of diagnosis.

Animals treated with a single 30 Gy dose of intraoperative radiation have shown a median survival of four months; animals treated with conventional external beam radiotherapy (57 Gy) have shown a median survival of seven months (Turrel 1987). Dogs receiving piroxicam therapy had a median survival of seven months, compared to a median survival of less than one month in those not receiving such therapy.

References

Akpavie, S.O. and Sullivan, M. (1986). Constipation associated with calcified cystic enlargement of the prostate in a dog. *Veterinary Record* 118: 694–695.

Albouy, M., Sanquer, A., Maynard, L., and Eun, H.M. (2008). Efficacies of osaterone and delmadinone in the treatment of benign prostatic hyperplasia in dogs. *Veterinary Record* 163: 179–183.

Anderson, C.R., McNiel, E.A., Gillette, E.L. et al. (2002). Late complications of pelvic irradiation in 16 dogs. *Veterinary Radiology and Ultrasound* 43: 187–192.

Barsanti, J.A. and Finco, D.R. (1980). Canine bacterial prostatitis. *Veterinary Clinics of North America. Small Animal Practice* 9: 679–700.

Barsanti, J.A., Prasse, K.W., Crowell, W.A. et al. (1983). Evaluation of various techniques for diagnosis of chronic bacterial prostatitis in the dog. *Journal of the American Veterinary Medical Association* 183: 219–224.

Barsanti, J.A., Shotts, E.B. Jr., Prasse, K., and Crowell, W. (1980). Evaluation of diagnostic techniques for canine prostatic diseases. *Journal of the American Veterinary Medical Association* 177: 160–163.

Baumueller, A., Kjaer, T.B., and Madsen, P.O. (1977). Prostatic tissue and secretion concentrations of rosamicin and erythromycin: experimental studies in the dog. *Investigative Urology* 15: 158–160.

Bell, F.W., Klausner, J.S., Hayden, D.W. et al. (1991). Clinical and pathologic features of prostatic adenocarcinoma in sexually intact and castrated dogs: 31 cases (1970–1987). *Journal of the American Veterinary Medical Association* 199: 1623–1630.

Bell, F.W., Klausner, J.S., Hayden, D.W. et al. (1995). Evaluation of serum and seminal plasma markers in the diagnosis of canine prostatic disorders. *Journal of Veterinary Internal Medicine* 9: 149–153.

Bennett, T.C., Matz, B.M., Henderson, R.A. et al. (2018). Total prostatectomy as a treatment for prostatic carcinoma in 25 dogs. *Veterinary Surgery* 47: 367–377.

Berry, S.J., Coffey, D.S., and Ewing, L.L. (1986). Effects of aging on prostate growth in beagles. *American Journal of Physiology* 250: R1039–R1046.

Black, G.M., Ling, G.V., Nyland, T.G., and Baker, T. (1998). Prevalence of prostatic cysts in adult, large-breed dogs. *Journal of the American Animal Hospital Association* 34: 177–180.

Blackburn, A. (2010). The use of self expanding urethral stents for the treatment of urothelial carcinoma: 42 dogs [abstract]. *Journal of Veterinary Internal Medicine* 24: 1577–1583.

Boland, L.E., Hardie, R.J., Gregory, S.P., and Lamb, C.R. (2003). Ultrasound-guided percutaneous drainage as the primary treatment for prostatic abscesses and cysts in dogs. *Journal of the American Animal Hospital Association* 39: 151–159.

van der Boon, J. (2002). New drug slows prostate-cancer progression. *Lancet Oncology* 3: 201.

Bradbury, C.A., Westropp, J.L., and Pollard, R.E. (2009). Relationship between prostatomegaly, prostatic mineralization, and cytologic diagnosis. *Veterinary Radiology and Ultrasound* 50: 167–171.

Cartee, R.E., Rumph, P.F., Kenter, D.C. et al. (1990). Evaluation of drug-induced prostatic involution in dogs by transabdominal B-mode ultrasonography. *American Journal of Veterinary Research* 51: 1773–1778.

Chae, H.K., Yang, J.I., An, J.H. et al. (2020). Use of oral paclitaxel for the treatment of bladder tumors in dogs. *Journal of Veterinary Medical Science* 82: 527–530.

Coffey, D.S. and Walsh, P.C. (1990). Clinical and experimental studies of benign prostatic hyperplasia. *Urologic Clinics of North America* 17: 461–475.

Cornell, K.K., Bostwick, D.G., Cooley, D.M. et al. (2000). Clinical and pathologic aspects of spontaneous canine prostate carcinoma: a retrospective analysis of 76 cases. *Prostate* 45: 173–183.

Culp, W.T.N., Johnson, E.G., Giuffrida, M.A. et al. (2019). Use of transrectal ultrasonography for assessment of the size and location of prostatic carcinoma in dogs. *American Journal of Veterinary Research* 80: 1012–1019.

Del Magno, S., Pisani, G., Dondi, F. et al. (2021). Surgical treatment and outcome of sterile prostatic cysts in dogs. *Veterinary Surgery* 50: 1009–1016.

Dobson, J., de Queiroz, G.F., and Golding, J.P. (2018). Photodynamic therapy and diagnosis: principles and comparative aspects. *Veterinary Journal* 233: 8–18.

Dorfman, M., Barsanti, J., and Budsberg, S.C. (1995). Enrofloxacin concentrations in dogs with normal prostates and dogs with chronic bacterial prostatitis. *American Journal of Veterinary Research* 56: 386–390.

Feeney, D.A., Johnston, G.R., and Klausner, J.S. (1985). Two-dimensional, gray-scale ultrasonography: applications in canine prostatic disease. *Veterinary Clinics of North America. Small Animal Practice* 15: 1159–1176.

Feeney, D.A., Johnston, G.R., Klausner, J.S. et al. (1987a). Canine prostatic disease: comparison of radiographic appearance with morphologic and microbiologic findings: 30 cases (1981–1985). *Journal of the American Veterinary Medical Association* 190: 1018–1026.

Feeney, D.A., Johnston, G.R., Klausner, J.S. et al. (1987b). Canine prostatic disease: comparison of ultrasonographic appearance with morphologic and microbiologic findings: 30 cases (1981–1985). *Journal of the American Veterinary Medical Association* 190: 1027–1034.

Feeney, D.A., Johnston, G.R., Osborne, C.A., and Tomlinson, M.J. (1984). Maximum distention retrograde urethrocystography in healthy male dogs: occurrence and radiographic appearance of urethroprostatic reflux. *American Journal of Veterinary Research* 45: 948–952.

Freitag, T., Jerram, R.M., Walker, A.M. et al. (2007). Surgical management of common canine prostatic conditions. *Compendium on Continuing Education for the Practicing Veterinarian* 29: 656–658, 660, 662–663.

Gobello, C., Castex, G., and Corrada, Y. (2002). Serum and seminal markers in the diagnosis of disorders of the genital tract of the dog: a mini review. *Theriogenology* 57: 1285–1291.

Goldsmid, S.E. and Bellenger, C.R. (1991). Urinary incontinence after prostatectomy in dogs. *Veterinary Surgery* 20: 253–256.

Goodman, L.A., Jarrett, C.L., Krunkosky, T.M. et al. (2011). 5-Lipoxygenase expression in benign and malignant canine prostate tissues. *Veterinary and Comparative Oncology* 9: 149–157.

Hastak, S.M., Gammmelgaard, J., and Holm, H.H. (1982). Transrectal ultrasonic volume determination of the prostate: a preoperative and postoperative study. *Journal of Urology* 127: 1115–1118.

Head, L.L. and Francis, D.A. (2002). Mineralized paraprostatic cyst as a potential contributing factor in the development of perineal hernias in a dog. *Journal of the American Veterinary Medical Association* 221: 533–535.

Huggins, C. and Clark, P.J. (1940). Quantitative studies of prostatic secretion. II. The effect of castration and/or estrogen injection on the normal and the hyperplastic prostate glands of dogs. *Journal of Experimental Medicine* 72: 747–762.

Johnston, G.R., Feeney, D.A., Rivers, B., and Walter, P.A. (1991). Diagnostic imaging of the male canine reproductive organs. *Veterinary Clinics of North America. Small Animal Practice* 21: 553–589.

Kawakami, E., Tsutsui, T., Shimizu, M. et al. (1995). Comparison of the effects of chloradinone acetate pellet implantation and orchidectomy on benign prostatic hypertrophy in the dog. *International Journal of Andrology* 18: 248–255.

Krawiec, D.R. and Heflin, D. (1992). Study of prostatic diseases in dogs: 177 cases (1981–1986). *Journal of the American Veterinary Medical Association* 200: 1119–1122.

Lange, K., Cordes, E.K., Hopper, H.O., and Günzel-Apel, A.R. (2001). Determination of concentration of sex steroids in blood plasma and semen of male dogs treated with delmadinone acetate or finasteride. *Journal of Reproduction and Fertility. Supplement* 57: 83–91.

Laroque, P.A., Prahalada, S., Gordon, L.R. et al. (1994). Effects of chronic oral administration of a selective 5 alpha-reductase inhibitor, finasteride, on the dog prostate. *Prostate* 24: 93–100.

Lattimer, J.C. (1994). The prostate gland. In: *Textbook of Veterinary Diagnostic Radiology*, 2e (ed. D.E. Thrall), 479. Philadelphia, PA: WB Saunders.

Leav, I., Schelling, K.H., Adams, J.Y. et al. (2001). Role of canine basal cells in postnatal prostatic development, induction of hyperplasia, and sex hormone-stimulated growth, and the ductal origin of carcinoma. *Prostate* 48: 210–224.

Lee-Parritz, D.E. and Lamb, C.R. (1988). Prostatic adenocarcinoma with osseous metastases in a dog. *Journal of the American Veterinary Medical Association* 192: 1569–1572.

L'Eplattenier, H.F., Klem, B., Teske, E. et al. (2008). Preliminary results of intraoperative photodynamic therapy with 5-aminolevulinic acid in dogs with prostate carcinoma. *Veterinary Journal (London)* 178: 202–207.

L'Eplattenier, H.F., Lai, C.L., van den Ham, R. et al. (2007). Regulation of COX-2 expression in canine prostate carcinoma: increased COX-2 expression is not related to inflammation. *Journal of Veterinary Internal Medicine* 21: 776–782.

L'Eplattenier, H.F., van Nimwegen, S.A., van Sluijs, F.J., and Kirpensteijn, J. (2006). Partial prostatectomy using Nd: YAG laser for management of canine prostate carcinoma. *Veterinary Surgery* 35: 406–411.

Mahapokai, W., van den Ingh, T.S., van Mil, F. et al. (2001). Immune response in hormonally induced prostatic hyperplasia in the dog. *Veterinary Immunology and Immunopathology* 78: 297–303.

McNeal, J.E. (1978). Origin and evolution of benign prostatic enlargement. *Investigative Urology* 15: 340–345.

McNeal, J.E. (1984). Anatomy of the prostate and morphogenesis of BPH. *Progress in Clinical and Biological Research* 145: 27–53.

Meares, E.M. Jr. (1982). Prostatitis: review of pharmacokinetics and therapy. *Reviews of Infectious Diseases* 4: 475–483.

Mitsogiannis, I., Tzelves, L., Dellis, A. et al. (2022). Prostate cancer immunotherapy. *Expert Opinion on Biological Therapy* 22: 577–590.

Mouli, S.K., Raiter, S., Harris, K. et al. (2021). Yttrium-90 radioembolization to the prostate gland: proof of concept in a canine model and clinical translation. *Journal of Vascular and Interventional Radiology* 32: 1103–1112.e12.

Obradovich, J., Walshaw, R., and Goullaud, E. (1987). The influence of castration on the development of prostatic carcinoma in the dog. *Journal of Veterinary Internal Medicine* 1: 183–187.

Oliveira, K.S., Araújo, E.G., Menezes, L.B. et al. (2006). CYR61, a cellular proliferation marker in dogs with prostatic disease. *Theriogenology* 66: 1618–1620.

O'Shea, J.D. (1962). Studies on the canine prostate gland. I. Factors influencing its size and weight. *Journal of Comparative Pathology* 72: 321–331.

Pan, X., Tsimbas, K., Kurzman, I.D., and Vail, D.M. (2016). Safety evaluation of combination CCNU and continuous toceranib phosphate (Palladia(®)) in tumour-bearing dogs: a phase I dose-finding study. *Veterinary Comparative Oncology* 14: 202–209.

Powe, J.R., Canfiel, P.J., and Martin, P.A. (2004). Evaluation of the cytologic diagnosis of canine prostatic disorders. *Veterinary Clinical Pathology* 33: 150–154.

Ravicini, S., Baines, S.J., Taylor, A. et al. (2018). Outcome and prognostic factors in medically treated canine prostatic carcinomas: a multi-institutional study. *Veterinary Comparative Oncology* 16: 450–458.

Rawlings, C.A., Crowell, W.A., Barsanti, J.A., and Oliver, J.E. Jr. (1994). Intracapsular subtotal prostatectomy in normal dogs: use of an ultrasonic surgical aspirator. *Veterinary Surgery* 23: 182–189.

Rawlings, C.A., Mahaffey, M.B., Barsanti, J.A. et al. (1997). Use of partial prostatectomy for treatment of prostatic abscesses and cysts in dogs. *Journal of the American Veterinary Medical Association* 211: 868–871.

Robertson, J.J. and Bojrab, M.J. (1984). Subtotal intracapsular prostatectomy: results in normal dogs. *Veterinary Surgery* 13: 6–10.

Root Kustritz, M.V. (2006). Collection of tissue and culture samples from the canine reproductive tract. *Theriogenology* 66: 567–574.

Ruel, Y., Barthez, P.Y., Mailles, A., and Begon, D. (1998). Ultrasonographic evaluation of the prostate in healthy intact dogs. *Veterinary Radiology and Ultrasound* 39: 212–216.

Schlake, A., Dell'Oglio, P., Devriendt, N. et al. (2020). First robot-assisted radical prostatectomy in a client-owned Bernese mountain dog with prostatic adenocarcinoma. *Veterinary Surgery* 49: 1458–1466.

Schrank, M. and Romagnoli, S. (2020). Prostatic neoplasia in the intact and castrated dog: how dangerous is castration? *Animals* 10: 85.

Shibata, Y., Fukabori, Y., Ito, K. et al. (2001). Comparison of histological compositions and apoptosis in canine spontaneous benign prostatic hyperplasia treated with androgen suppressive agents chlormadinone acetate and finasteride. *Journal of Urology* 165: 289–293.

Sorenmo, K.U., Goldschmidt, M.H., Shofer, F.S. et al. (2004). Evaluation of cyclooxygenase-1 and cyclooxygenase-2 expression and the effect of cyclooxygenase inhibitors in canine prostatic carcinoma. *Veterinary and Comparative Oncology* 2: 13–23.

Stowater, J.L. and Lamb, C.R. (1989). Ultrasonographic features of paraprostatic cysts in nine dogs. *Veterinary Radiology* 30: 232–239.

Thomas, S. and Prendergast, G.C. (2016). Cancer vaccines: a brief overview. *Methods in Molecular Biology* 1403: 755–761.

Turrel, J.M. (1987). Intraoperative radiotherapy of carcinoma of the prostate gland in ten dogs. *Journal of the American Veterinary Medical Association* 190: 48–52.

Walz, J.Z., Desai, N., Van Asselt, N. et al. (2020). Definitive-intent intensity-modulated radiation therapy for treatment of canine prostatic carcinoma: a multi-institutional retrospective study. *Veterinary Comparative Oncology* 18: 381–388.

Waters, D.J. and Bostwick, D.G. (1997). Prostate intraepithelial neoplasia occurs spontaneously in the canine prostate. *Journal of Urology* 157: 713–716.

Waters, D.J., Hayden, D.W., Bell, F.W. et al. (1997). Prostatic intraepithelial neoplasia in dogs with spontaneous prostate cancer. *Prostate* 30: 92–97.

Weisse, C. (2006). Evaluation of palliative stenting for management of malignant urethral obstructions in dogs. *Journal of the American Veterinary Medical Association* 229: 226–234.

White, R.A. (2000). Prostatic surgery in the dog. *Clinical Techniques in Small Animal Practice* 15: 46–51.

White, R.A. and Williams, R.A. (1995). Intracapsular prostatic omentalization: a new technique for management of prostatic abscesses in dogs. *Veterinary Surgery* 24: 390–395.

Zhang, D., Yang, R., Wang, S., and Dong, Z. (2014). Paclitaxel: new uses for an old drug. *Drug Design, Development and Therapy* 8: 279–284.

59

Cryptorchidism

Carlos Gradil and Robert McCarthy

Cryptorchidism is the most common congenital defect of the testes in dogs, with a reported incidence ranging from 1.2% to 10% (Sojka 1980; Kawakami *et al.* 1984; Turba & Willer 1988; Ruble & Hird 1993; Khan *et al.* 2018). Retained testes can be unilateral or bilateral, but most commonly cryptorchidism is a unilateral condition, with the right testicle being most frequently retained (Dunn 1968; Reif *et al.* 1979; Wallace & Cox 1980; Crane 1990). Cryptorchidism is found more frequently in small breeds compared with large-breed dogs, and within a breed the risk of cryptorchidism is higher in the smaller counterparts. A very high prevalence has been reported within certain highly inbred lines (Table 59.1) (Pullig 1953; Priester *et al.* 1970; Cox *et al.* 1978). In the cat, the incidence of cryptorchidism ranges from 0.37% to 3.8%, with an increased risk in Persian cats (Henderson 1951; Millis *et al.* 1992; Richardson & Mullen 1993).

Causes

Canine cryptorchidism is heritable and transmitted as a sex-limited autosomal recessive trait (Burke & Reynolds 1993). Because the gene(s) responsible for testicular descent are autosomal, cryptorchidism can be carried by both females and males. Inguinal hernia, umbilical hernia, hip dysplasia, patellar luxation, and penile and preputial defects are all reported with increased frequency in cryptorchid male dogs (Hayes *et al.* 1985). Cryptorchidism is presumed to be heritable in cats and a polygenic mode of inheritance has been suggested (Herron & Stern 1980).

Nonhereditary causes of cryptorchidism have not been described in dogs or cats, but in humans may be related to any process that alters intra-abdominal pressure. Examples include umbilical infection with concurrent peritonitis or trauma to the inguinal canal with subsequent inflammation or adhesions (Romagnoli 1991).

Normal development

Normal testicular descent is complete by about day 10 after birth in normal dogs and prior to birth in cats (Hoskins & Taboada 1992). In a newborn puppy or kitten, the testes are small and soft and can move between scrotum and inguinal canal, especially when the pup is stressed or frightened (Howard & Bjorling 1989; Romagnoli 1991). Testicular descent is regulated by both androgenic and nonandrogenic factors, and is mediated by the gubernaculums, a gelatinous tissue of mesenchymal origin. Testicular descent takes place in two phases:

- *Phase I: intra-abdominal migration.* The embryonic testes develop caudal to the kidney. From this location, the testes are pulled caudally by the gubernacula that connect the caudal pole of the testis to the inguinal canal. The testes descend from their intra-abdominal position to the inguinal area under the influence of insulin-like growth factor 3. This process can be inhibited by 17ß-estradiol in the mouse embryonic Leydig cell (Nef *et al.* 2000).
- *Phase II: inguinal–scrotal phase.* Regression of the gubernacula is induced by androgens, and

Table 59.1 Risk of cryptorchidism by breed.

Breeds at increased risk (in decreasing order)
Toy poodle
Pomeranian
Yorkshire terrier
Miniature dachshund
Cairn terrier
Chihuahua
Maltese
Boxer
Pekingese
English bulldog
Old English sheepdog
Miniature poodle
Miniature schnauzer
Shetland sheepdog
Siberian husky
Standard poodle

Breeds at decreased risk
Mongrel
Beagle
Labrador retriever
Golden retriever
Saint Bernard
Great Dane
English setter

Source: Johnston, S.D., Root Kustritz, M.V., and Olsen, P.N.S. (2001). Disorders of the canine testes and epididymides. In: *Canine and Feline Theriogenology*, 312–332. Philadelphia, PA: WB Saunders (Table 18.1, p. 314).

abdominal pressure pushes the testes through the inguinal canal. Prenatal antiandrogen-treated mice have maldescended testes in an inguinal position (Nef *et al.* 2000).

Abnormal development

The pathogenesis of abnormal testicular descent is not well understood. Smaller breeds and smaller counterparts within a breed (i.e., toy vs. standard poodles) are generally at increased risk for cryptorchidism. Thus, abnormal testicular descent may simply be related to physical size and/or rate of growth of the testes, epididymides, and gubernacula. Breakdown of the cranial suspensory ligament is an essential component of normal testicular migration, and failure of breakdown to occur may prevent outgrowth of the gubernacula and subsequent testicular descent.

Although postulated, insufficiency of the hypothalamic–pituitary–testicular axis and its production of gonadotropin-releasing hormone (GnRH), luteinizing hormone (LH), and testosterone form an unlikely cause of cryptorchidism in dogs. This is based on the inconsistent response to treatment of cryptorchidism with exogenous gonadotropic hormones.

Testes must be scrotal and thus 4–5 °C cooler than core body temperature to produce normal sperm. Therefore, a bilaterally cryptorchid male does not produce normal sperm and is sterile. A unilaterally cryptorchid animal can produce sperm of variable semen quality, including oligospermia and azoospermia. Unilateral cryptorchids can impregnate a female in estrus. Both unilateral and bilateral cryptorchid dogs produce testosterone (Matheuws & Comhaire 1989; Kawakami *et al.* 1995), so most will show sexual desire and can achieve erection (Badinand *et al.* 1972). The lack of significant differences between testosterone levels in intact male dogs and unilaterally cryptorchid dogs can probably be explained in part by a compensatory increase in testosterone production in the intact contralateral testicle (Heilkenbrinker 1986).

Clinical signs

In general, cryptorchidism in dogs causes no clinical signs unless complicated by neoplasia or spermatic cord torsion. The risk of neoplasia in a retained testis has been reported to be 9–14 times higher than in a scrotal testis, with Sertoli cell tumors and seminomas predominating (Pendergrass & Hays 1975; Hayes *et al.* 1985). Sertoli cell tumors are frequently associated with signs of feminization such as symmetric alopecia and gynecomastia, while other neoplasms such as seminomas rarely cause any clinical signs other than the presence of a palpable mass. Testicles retained within the abdomen are more mobile than those within the scrotum and are therefore more susceptible to spermatic cord torsion. Typical clinical signs include acute abdominal pain and collapse. In one study, over 90% of torsions of the spermatic cord involved a retained testis (Pearson & Kelly 1975).

In cryptorchid cats, testes produce testosterone, and the cats show typical secondary sex characteristics of urine marking, aggressive behavior, and urine odor. In a cryptorchid cat, an examination of the penis for the presence of spines is an excellent diagnostic technique because penile spines are testosterone dependent, becoming atrophied after six weeks of castration.

Diagnosis

Diagnosis of cryptorchidism is generally straightforward in puppies and kittens and is determined by history and palpation of the scrotal and inguinal region. It is recommended to wait until about 6 months of age before declaring a dog cryptorchid, as this is when the inguinal ring finally closes (Johnston *et al.* 2001). A definitive diagnosis of cryptorchidism should not be made in cats under 7–8 months of age (Sojka 1980). In adult animals with an unknown history, diagnosis and localization of an undescended testicle can be more challenging.

Monorchidism (aplasia of one testis) has not been diagnosed in the dog. Therefore, if only one scrotal testis is evident, the other testis is retained. Retained testes are smaller, and abdominally retained testes typically weigh less than inguinal testes. Testicles in the extrainguinal region are generally palpable, but those in the intrainguinal region or abdominal cavity are not palpable unless they are neoplastic. Differentiation of bilaterally cryptorchid dogs from castrated male dogs may be done by rectal palpation of the prostate, which is often enlarged in intact males. Inguinal lymph nodes and fat may be easily confused for small inguinal testes. In a study in cats, palpation to locate the retained testicle was successful only 48% of the time (Richardson & Mullen 1993).

Laboratory assessment

Laboratory assessment can be useful in the diagnosis of cryptorchidism in both dogs and cats. Measurement of anti-Mullerian hormone (AMH) and inhibin-B for canine and feline is the gold standard. Basal levels of LH and testosterone are unreliable in differentiation of normal dogs from dogs with one or both testicles retained; consequently, hormone challenge testing is required. In general, a serum testosterone level of greater than 1 ng/mL after treatment with either GnRH (Purswell & Wilcke 1993) or LH (human chorionic gonadotropin, hCG) indicates the presence of at least one testicle (Table 59.2). Samples from prepubertal males may produce false negatives for testosterone.

Table 59.2 Gonadotropin-releasing hormone (GnRH) and human chorionic gonadotropin (hCG) stimulation protocol.

GnRH

Dose: 2 μg/kg intramuscularly

At 0 and 2 h post injection, draw blood into a polymer gel-free tube. Allow blood adequate time to clot prior to centrifugation to avoid fibrin formation. After centrifugation, transfer the serum into a vial suitable for shipping or frozen storage

hCG

Dose: 250 IU subcutaneously

For T measurement, process sample as above

Ultrasonography may be attempted for diagnosis and localization of a retained testicle, but the decreased size and large number of possible locations make it difficult to visualize. A helpful characteristic is the mediastinum testis that appears as an echogenic linear structure in the center of the echogenically homogeneous testis.

Medical treatment

Medical treatment has been shown to have variable success in dogs with cryptorchidism. The most common medical treatment, not including acupuncture and herbal medicine, is the use of drugs providing LH activity, such as hCG. As an alternative, administration of GnRH can induce an increase in endogenous LH (Feldman & Nelson 1996). Most of the studies reporting the success of hormonal treatment are based on clinical case reports that lack control animals. Interestingly, the predisposition to neoplasia remains whether the testis is retained or not. Therefore, medical treatment should not be recommended, as this is a heritable disease, and castration should be considered.

Surgical treatment

The treatment of choice for cryptorchidism in both dogs and cats is bilateral castration. Even if the condition is unilateral, both the descended and undescended testicles should be removed to prevent hereditary transmission of this defect. Alternatively, if an owner prefers to preserve the dog's gonadal hormones, then a vasectomy can be performed on the descended testicle. The surgical approach for removal of the retained testis depends on its location.

Extrainguinal testis

A testis located outside the inguinal canal is generally easily palpable and can often be removed by pushing it caudally to a prescrotal position, where it can be excised routinely. Alternately, an incision can be made directly over it. Either an open (incision through the tunica albuginea) or closed (tunic left intact) surgical technique of castration is appropriate once the testicle is exposed.

Inguinal testis

A testis trapped within the inguinal canal is common in dogs and especially common in cats. The testis cannot be palpated externally and is not visible within the abdominal cavity. A testis located in this area requires incision directly over the inguinal canal. Meticulous dissection is necessary, with close attention paid to hemostasis, as the testis must be carefully distinguished from inguinal fat and lymph node. Once the testis and associated structures are exposed, removal is routine.

Intra-abdominal testis

An abdominal testis may be located anywhere along the path of abdominal migration (i.e., from the caudal pole of the kidney to the inguinal canal). Traditionally, abdominally retained testicles have been removed through a combined ventral median and parapreputial abdominal skin incision in dogs and through a caudal ventral midline incision in cats (Boothe 1993). Bilateral retained testes are often located caudal to the kidney, while a unilateral retained testis is more commonly located in the caudal abdomen lateral to the bladder.

The key to finding a retained abdominal testis is first to identify the ductus deferens at the prostate, then to follow the ductus to the retained testis. Following this rule will avoid reported complications such as inadvertent prostatectomy, ureteral damage, urethral transection, and lymph node excision. Use of small laparotomy incisions and a spay hook to retrieve retained testicles has been recommended (Kirby 1980), but potential complications are unacceptable, and this technique is not advocated (Bellah *et al.* 1989; Millis *et al.* 1992; Schultz *et al.* 1996). Adequate exposure is critical when performing this surgery.

An inguinal approach adapted from equine surgery has been described for use in both dogs and cats (Steckel 2011). In this procedure an incision is made over the inguinal ring and the undescended testicle is located for removal by identification and opening of the vaginal process. Traction on the testicular adnexa is used to deliver the testicle through the inguinal canal, where it is removed extracorporeally. This approach may be somewhat less invasive than using the traditional midline and parapreputial incision, but the anatomic features are somewhat unfamiliar to most small animal surgeons.

Laparoscopic cryptorchidectomy

Laparoscopic cryptorchidectomy is a quick, efficient, and minimally invasive technique that provides excellent visualization of all involved structures. Minimally invasive surgery has become commonplace in human surgery, and owners are coming to expect the same level of treatment for their pets. The advantages are the same in animals as they are in humans. Recovery is hastened, allowing outpatient surgery where previously recovery would take days or weeks. Additionally, a reduction in perioperative pain is a major benefit for all patients (Miller *et al.* 2004; Lhermette & Sobel 2008).

To perform laparoscopic cryptorchidectomy, the patient is first placed in a head-down (Trendelenburg) position and a urinary catheter placed. The Trendelenburg position shifts the abdominal viscera forward to improve exposure, while the urinary catheter evacuates the urinary bladder during the procedure. The abdomen is distended to a pressure of 10–15 mmHg using either a Verress needle or Hasson technique. The optical port is placed just caudal to the umbilicus and the caudal abdominal region is explored. If the retained testicle is not easily visualized, the inguinal ring should be examined closely to see if the ductus deferens and testicular vasculature extend into the inguinal canal. If they do, the laparoscopic procedure is abandoned and converted into routine open surgery for retrieval of an inguinal testis.

Once an intra-abdominal testicle has been located, two additional instrument ports are placed under direct visualization, one on each side just lateral to the rectus abdominis muscle about halfway from the umbilicus to the pubis (Figure 59.1). A grasping instrument is passed through the instrument port on the affected side to grasp and stabilize the testicle away from abdominal viscera.

Ligation of the testicular vasculature and associated structures is accomplished by stainless steel clips (Endoclip™, Medline Industries, Northfield, IL, USA), pre-tied suture loop (Surgitie Ligating Loop™, Covidien, Dublin, Ireland), or a vessel-sealant device (Force Triad™, Covidien) passed through the opposite instrument port. The instrument port on the affected side is then enlarged slightly, and the testicle is removed.

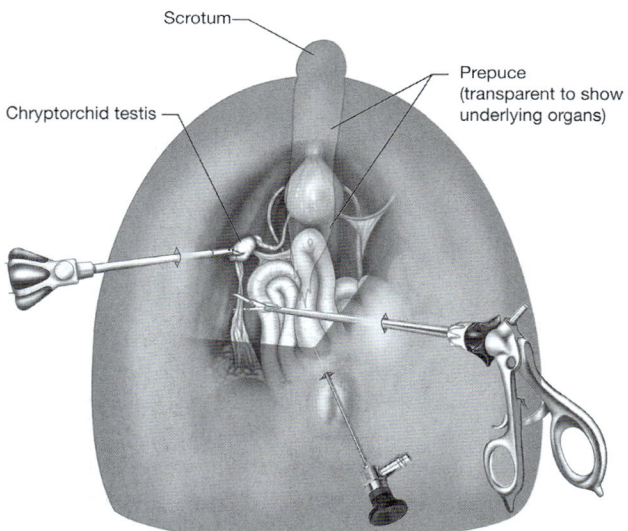

Figure 59.1 Laparoscopic cryptorchidectomy. The entire surgery is performed in the abdomen under laparoscopy. A grasper (instrument port 1) is used to hold the testicle, while a vessel-sealant device (instrument port 2) is used to ligate the vascular pedicle and the ductus deferens. Instrument port 1 is enlarged slightly so that the testicle can be retrieved from the abdomen. © D. Giddings.

A second technique with only two cannulas is possible. Two cannulas are placed on midline. A grasping instrument is passed through the instrument portal and the intra-abdominal testicle is pulled against the abdominal wall. The intra-abdominal testicle is transfixed with a heavy suture passed through the abdominal wall. After the intra-abdominal testicle has been stabilized, ligation of the testicular vasculature and associated structures is accomplished as already described. The instrument portal is then enlarged slightly, and the testicle is removed.

A single-incision laparoscopic procedure can be accomplished by using a multiple-access (SILS™, Medtronic) laparoscopic port (Runge *et al.* 2014). In this situation the telescope, grasping instrument, and ligation tool are all passed through multiple openings in a single low-profile, malleable port. The cryptorchid testicle is then retrieved through the single-port incision.

Laparoscopic-assisted technique

An alternate "laparoscopic-assisted" technique can also be employed. In this technique the retained testicle is identified as previously, but an instrument port is created only on the affected side. The testicle is grasped, brought against the body wall, and then exteriorized by enlarging the instrument port. Ligation of vascular and associated structures is accomplished extracorporeally and the ligated stump is returned to the abdomen.

Potential complications after any laparoscopic technique include cardiovascular and pulmonary changes associated with carbon dioxide pneumoperitoneum, trocar injuries to abdominal viscera or major vessels, subcutaneous emphysema, visceral herniation, and wound infection or hematoma formation at the trocar entry sites. The differences in complications associated with laparoscopic-assisted cryptorchidectomy compared with open cryptorchidectomy have not been investigated. In humans, various laparoscopic procedures are associated with substantially fewer complications than the corresponding open procedures. Results of studies in humans indicate that decreased use of analgesics, decreased duration of hospitalization, and faster return to work are associated with use of laparoscopic procedures compared with similar open procedures (Anderson *et al.* 2003; Klinger *et al.* 2003; Rassweiler *et al.* 2003). Comparable findings are likely in animals with minimally invasive procedures.

References

Anderson, B., Hallen, M., Leveau, P. et al. (2003). Laparoscopic extraperitoneal inguinal hernia repair versus open mesh repair: a prospective randomized controlled trial. *Surgery* 133: 464–472.

Badinand, F., Szumowki, P., and Breton, A. (1972). Etude morphobiologique et biochimique du sperme du chien cryptorchide. *Recueil de médecine vétérinaire* 148: 655–688.

Bellah, J.R., Spencer, C.P., and Salmeri, K.R. (1989). Hemiprostatic urethral avulsion during cryptorchid orchiectomy in a dog. *Journal of the American Animal Hospital Association* 25: 553–556.

Boothe, H.W. (1993). Testes and epididymides. In: *Textbook of Small Animal Surgery*, 2e (ed. D. Slatter and E.A. Stone), 1325–1326. Philadelphia, PA: WB Saunders.

Burke, T.J. and Reynolds, H.A. (1993). The testes. In: *Disease Mechanisms in Small Animal Surgery*, 2e (ed. M.J. Bojrab), 546–547. Philadelphia, PA: Lea & Febiger.

Cox, V.S., Wallace, L.J., and Jensen, C.R. (1978). An anatomic and genetic study of canine cryptorchidism. *Teratology* 18: 233–240.

Crane, S.W. (1990). Orchiectomy of retained and descended testes in the dog and cat. In: *Current Techniques in Small Animal Surgery*, 3e (ed. M.J. Bojrab), 416–422. Philadelphia, PA: Lea & Febiger.

Dunn, M.L. (1968). Cryptorchidism in dogs: a clinical survey. *Journal of the American Animal Hospital Association* 4: 180–182.

Feldman, E.C. and Nelson, R.W. (1996). Disorders of the testes and epididymides. In: *Canine and Feline Endocrinology and Reproduction*, 697–710. Philadelphia, PA: WB Saunders.

Hayes, H.M., Wilson, G.P., and Pendergrass, T.W. (1985). Canine cryptorchidism and subsequent testicular neoplasia: case–control study with epidemiologic update. *Teratology* 32: 51–56.

Heilkenbrinker, T. (1986). Untersuchungen über die Auswirkungen einseitiger Kastration und abdominaler Hodenreposition auf inkretorische und exkretorische Funktionen der skrotalen Keimdrüse beim Hund. PhD thesis, School of Veterinary Medicine, Hanover.

Henderson, W. (1951). Cryptorchidism in the adult cat. *North American Veterinarian* 32: 634–636.

Herron, M.A. and Stern, B. (1980). Prognosis and management of feline infertility. In: *Current Veterinary Therapy VII* (ed. R.W. Kirk), 1231–1236. Philadelphia, PA: WB Saunders.

Hoskins, J.D. and Taboada, J. (1992). Congenital defects of the dog. *Compendium on Continuing Education for the Practicing Veterinarian* 14: 873–897.

Howard, P.E. and Bjorling, D.E. (1989). The intersexual animal: associated problems. *Problems in Veterinary Medicine* 1: 74–84.

Johnston, S.D., Root Kustritz, M.V., and Olson, P.N.S. (2001). Disorders of the canine testes and epididymides. In: *Canine and Feline Theriogenology*, 312–332. Philadelphia, PA: WB Saunders.

Kawakami, E., Tsutsui, T., and Yamada, Y. (1984). Cryptorchism in the dog: occurrence of cryptorchidism and semen quality in the cryptorchid dog. *Japanese Journal of Veterinary Sciences* 46: 303–308.

Kawakami, E., Tsutsui, T., and Saito, S. (1995). Changes in peripheral plasma luteinizing hormone and testosterone concentrations and semen quality in normal and cryptorchid dogs during sexual maturation. *Laboratory Animal Science* 45: 258–263.

Khan, F.A., Gartley, C.J., and Khanam, A. (2018). Canine cryptorchidism: an update. *Reproduction in Domestic Animals* 53: 1263–1270.

Kirby, F.D. (1980). A technique for castrating the cryptorchid dog or cat. *Veterinary Medicine (London)* 75: 632.

Klinger, H.C., Remzi, M., and Janetschek, G. (2003). Benefits of laparoscopic renal surgery are more pronounced in patients with high body mass index. *European Urology* 43: 522–527.

Lhermette, P. and Sobel, D. (2008). *BSAVA Manual of Canine and Feline Endoscopy and Endosurgery*. Gloucester: British Small Animal Veterinary Association, p. viii.

Matheuws, D. and Comhaire, F.H. (1989). Concentrations of oestradiol and testosterone in peripheral and spermatic venous blood of dogs with unilateral cryptorchidism. *Domestic Animal Endocrinology* 6: 203–209.

Miller, N.A., Van Lue, S.J., and Rawlings, C.A. (2004). Use of laparoscopic assisted cryptorchidectomy in dogs and cats. *Journal of the American Veterinary Medical Association* 224: 875–878.

Millis, D.L., Hauptman, J.G., and Johnson, C.A. (1992). Cryptorchidism and monorchidism in cats: 25 cases (1980–1989). *Journal of the American Veterinary Medical Association* 200: 1128–1130.

Nef, S., Shipman, T., and Parada, L.F. (2000). A molecular basis for estrogen-induced cryptorchidism. *Developmental Biology* 224: 354–361.

Pearson, H. and Kelly, D.F. (1975). Testicular torsion in the dog: a review of 13 cases. *Veterinary Record* 97: 200–204.

Pendergrass, T.W. and Hays, H.M. (1975). Cryptorchidism and related defects in dogs: epidemiologic comparisons with man. *Teratology* 12: 51–56.

Priester, W.A., Glass, A.G., and Waggoner, N.S. (1970). Congenital defects in domesticated animals: general consideration. *American Journal of Veterinary Research* 31: 1871–1879.

Pullig, T. (1953). Cryptorchidism in cocker spaniels. *Journal of Heredity* 44: 250.

Purswell, B.J. and Wilcke, J.R. (1993). Response to gonadotrophin-releasing hormone by the intact male dog: serum testosterone, luteinizing hormone and follicle-stimulating hormone. *Journal of Fertility Supplement* 47: 335–341.

Rassweiler, J., Seemann, O., Schulze, M. et al. (2003). Laparoscopic versus open radical prostatectomy: a comparative study at a single institution. *Journal of Urology* 169: 1689–1693.

Reif, J.S., Maguire, T.J., Kenney, R.M. et al. (1979). A cohort study of canine testicular neoplasia. *Journal of the American Veterinary Medical Association* 175: 719–723.

Richardson, E.F. and Mullen, H. (1993). Cryptorchidism in cats. *Compendium on Continuing Education for the Practicing Veterinarian* I5: 1342–1369.

Romagnoli, S.E. (1991). Canine cryptorchidism. *Veterinary Clinics of North America. Small Animal Practice* 21: 533–544.

Ruble, R.P. and Hird, D.W. (1993). Congenital abnormalities in immature dogs from a pet store: 253 cases (1987–1988). *Journal of the American Veterinary Medical Association* 202: 633–636.

Runge, J.J., Mayhew, P.D., Case, J.B. et al. (2014). Single-port laparoscopic cryptorchidectomy in dogs and cats: 25 cases (2009–2014). *Journal of the American Veterinary Medical Association* 245: 1258–1265.

Schultz, K.S., Waldron, D.R., Smith, M.M. et al. (1996). Inadvertent prostatectomy as a complication of cryptorchidectomy in four dogs. *Journal of the American Animal Hospital Association* 32: 211–214.

Sojka, N.J. (1980). The male reproductive system. In: *Current Therapy in Theriogenology* (ed. D.W. Morrow), 865–869. Philadelphia, PA: WB Saunders.

Steckel, R.R. (2011). Use of an inguinal approach adapted from equine surgery for cryptorchidectomy in dogs and cats: 26 cases (1999–2010). *Journal of the American Veterinary Medical Association* 239: 1098–1103.

Turba, E. and Willer, S. (1988). The population genetics of cryptorchidism in German boxers. *Monash Veterinary* 43: 316–319.

Wallace, L.J. and Cox, V.S. (1980). Canine cryptorchidism. In: *Current Veterinary Therapy VII: Small Animal Practice* (ed. R.W. Kirk), 1244–1246. Philadelphia, PA: WB Saunders.

60

Paraphimosis

Michelle Kutzler

Paraphimosis is an inability to completely withdraw the penis into the prepuce (Somerville & Anderson 2001). It is the opposite of phimosis, which is the inability to extrude the penis from the prepuce (see Chapter 62). Paraphimosis occurs 14 times more frequently than phimosis (Kustritz & Olson 1999). It is most seen in young intact male dogs, but has also been reported in castrated male dogs. Paraphimosis is rare in cats. Although a clear breed predisposition has not been established, boxers and poodles are overrepresented in case reports.

Causes

Paraphimosis may occur secondary to (i) a hypoplastic prepuce (congenital or acquired from early-age castration); (ii) trauma (e.g., os penis fracture); (iii) a relatively small or stenotic preputial orifice; (iv) diphallia (duplicated penis) (Laube *et al.* 2017); (v) constriction of preputial hair around the penis (Hart & Peterson 1971); (vi) ineffective preputial musculature that cannot effectively retract the penis into the prepuce (Chaffee & Knecht 1975); (vii) hypospadias (Lee 1976); (viii) neurologic deficits in dogs with posterior paresis (e.g., intervertebral disk disease [IVDD], spinal tumors) or in cats following castration (Swalec & Smeak 1989); (ix) balanoposthitis; (x) large penile tumor (e.g., transmissible venereal tumor; Figure 60.1); (xi) priapism (see Chapter 61); or (xii) as an idiopathic event (Ndiritu 1979; Root-Kustritz 2001). About 30% of paraphimosis cases are idiopathic.

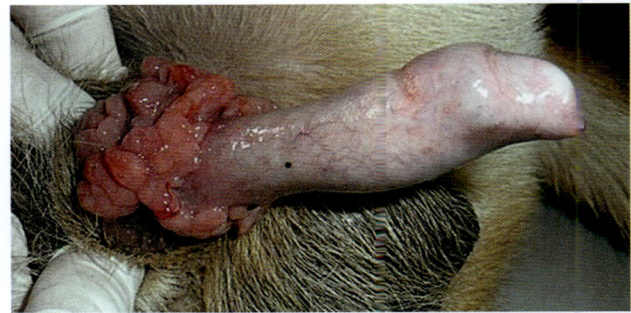

Figure 60.1 Paraphimosis occurred following examination of this dog's penis and prepuce secondary to an owner complaint of intermittent hemorrhagic preputial discharge. A large transmissible venereal tumor (TVT) was present at the base of the penis. The paraphimosis resolved quickly with the application of a topical lubricant to penile mucosa near the preputial opening and gently sliding the prepuce over the swollen glans of the penis. The dog was neutered and the TVT regressed spontaneously over 4 weeks.

Diagnosis

Clinicians can make a diagnosis of paraphimosis by visual inspection of the penis protruding from the prepuce. The entire length of the penis should be examined to determine if any other urogenital abnormalities exist. The prepuce should also be examined. The cranial preputial muscles (paired muscles originating from the cutaneous trunci) normally draw the prepuce cranially about 1 cm in front of the tip of the penis. If the prepuce is too short (hypoplastic), then the prepuce may end at the tip of the penis or be shorter than the penis, allowing the tip of the penis to remain continuously exposed. The penile mucosa may be erythematous, dry, inflamed, congested, edematous, ischemic, and painful, which may lead to self-mutilation (Somerville & Anderson 2001). Chronic protrusion of the penis may lead to excoriation and subsequent cornification of the mucosa. If there is evidence or history of trauma and/or concurrent stranguria, radiographs should be taken of the penis to identify concomitant os penis fracture.

Treatment

The goal of any paraphimosis treatment is to replace the penis in the prepuce as soon as possible before tissue compromise and to prevent recurrence (Kustritz & Olson 1999). Clinicians can reduce penile size (edema and inflammation) using cold compression bandages, massage with topical hyperosmotic solutions, and systemic anti-inflammatory therapy (Root-Kustritz 2001). Urination should be closely monitored. If in doubt about urethral patency and/or bladder integrity, a urinary catheter should be placed. Prior to attempting manual replacement of the penis, the hair around the preputial opening should be shaved or plucked and copious amounts of lubricant should be applied to the penile mucosa (Figure 60.2). In addition, general or regional anesthesia will reduce preputial muscle contraction, facilitating replacing the penis into the prepuce. If digital pressure on the penis is not sufficient to facilitate replacement within the prepuce, a preputiotomy can be performed. If a preputiotomy is performed, the tissues should be carefully closed to the original state. Castration is often performed in conjunction with surgical correction of paraphimosis to prevent recurrence, but castration alone is not successful in correcting paraphimosis.

If the penis can be returned to the prepuce but does not remain in the prepuce, several surgical techniques can be performed (Olsen & Salwei 2001). Surgical repair or reconstruction of abnormalities requires a thorough understanding of normal anatomy and basic reconstruction principles. These techniques include purse-string suture at the preputial orifice; preputial orifice narrowing; preputial lengthening (preputioplasty); cranial preputial advancement (Papazoglou 2001; Yiapanis et al. 2021); preputial muscle myorraphy; and phallopexy. In some cases, preputial advancement in combination with tissue grafting (Massari et al. 2018) and/or with phallopexy (Wasik & Wallace 2014) is needed. Phallopexy (the author's preferred method for penile retention) is a technique of creating a permanent adhesion between the dorsal surface of the penis and the

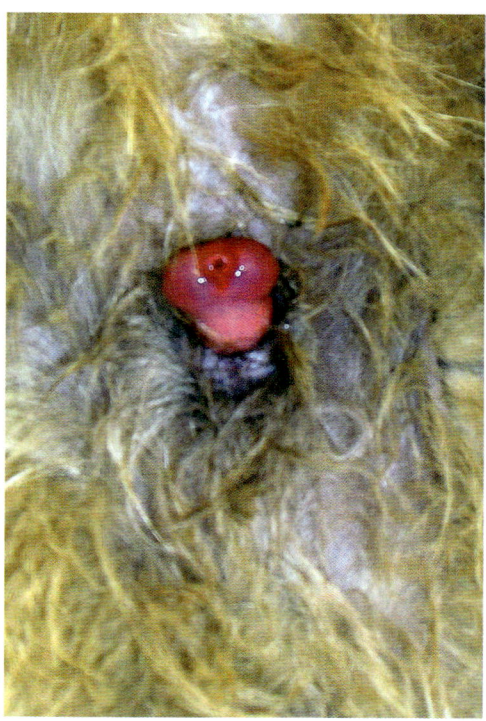

Figure 60.2 Following semen collection for an infertility evaluation, this male developed a paraphimosis secondary to inversion of the prepuce during detumescence (natural resolution of erection and penile retraction). This was resolved quickly with the application of a topical lubricant to penile mucosa near the preputial opening and gently sliding the prepuce over the swollen glans of the penis.

preputial mucosa (Somerville & Anderson 2001). Phallopexy should be performed on the dorsal surface of the penile shaft to avoid the urethra and the looser preputial tissues present on the ventral side (Figure 60.3). During this procedure, care must be taken to avoid incising into the underlying cavernous tissue (Somerville & Anderson 2001). Urine pooling and balanoposthitis may result if this procedure is performed too far caudally in the prepuce (Somerville & Anderson 2001). The penile tip should be retained inside the preputial orifice by 5–10 mm when the penis is in the nonerect state (Proescholdt et al. 1977).

If the penis has been severely damaged or despite all the previous techniques cannot be returned to the prepuce, penile amputation with concurrent urethrostomy should be performed (Pavletic & O'Bell 2007). A complete or subtotal penile amputation can be performed, depending upon the extent of the injury. To perform a complete penile amputation, the prepuce is reflected caudally following excision of the suspensory structures and ligation of the preputial blood supply. The dorsal and deep arteries of the penis, both branches of the

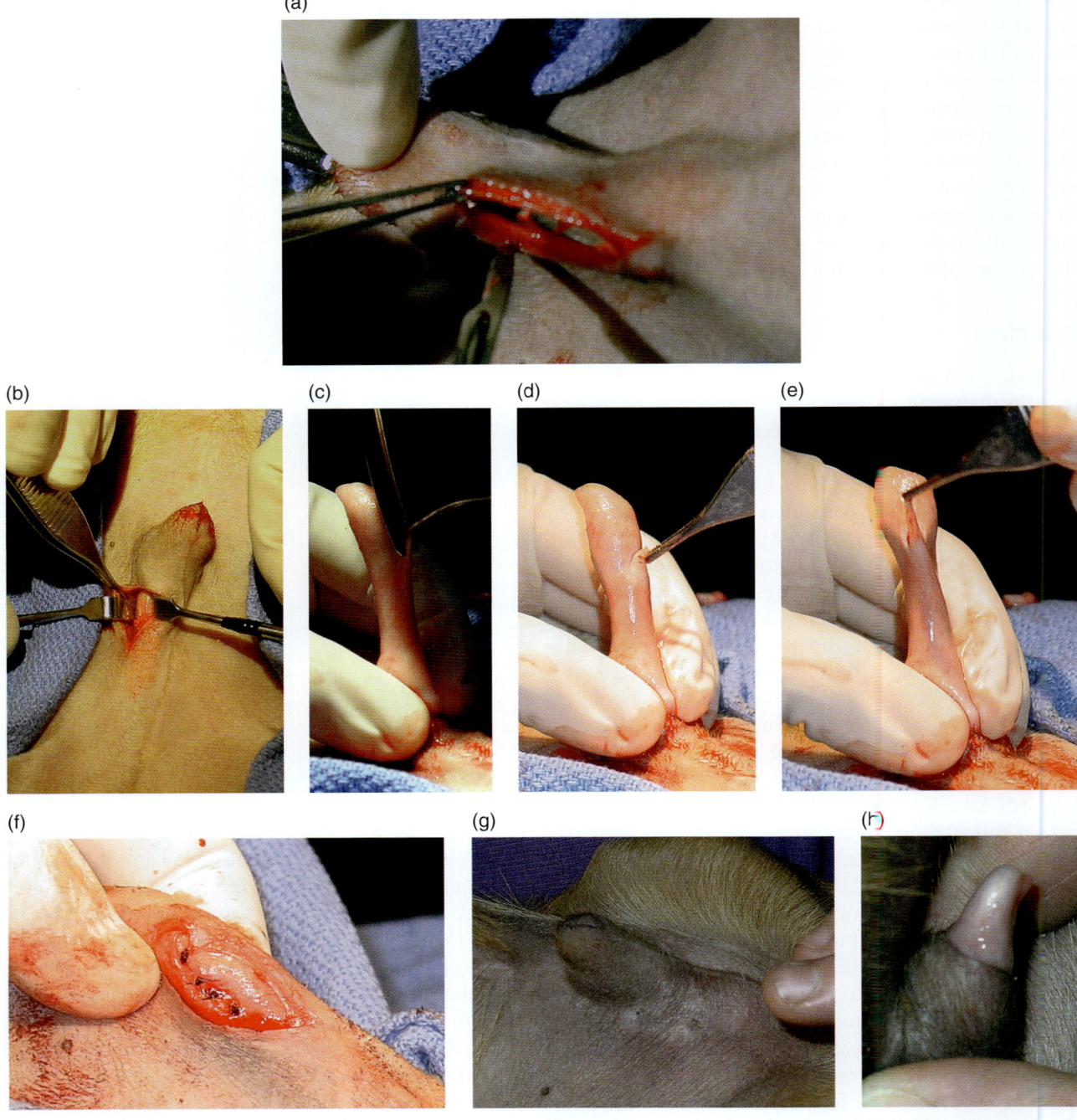

Figure 60.3 Phallopexy is a technique of creating a permanent adhesion between the dorsal surface of the penis and the preputial mucosa. (a) An incision is made through the dorsolateral aspect of the middle of the prepuce into the preputial cavity. (b) The penis is visualized and then exteriorized through the incision. (c) Phallopexy should be performed on the dorsal surface of the penile shaft to avoid the urethra and the looser preputial tissues present on the ventral side. (d) During this procedure, care must be taken to avoid incising into the underlying cavernous tissue. (e) A strip of penile mucosa approximately 2 mm wide by 20 mm long is removed. (f) An opposing strip of preputial mucosa is removed from the dorsal surface and the exposed mucosal edges are sutured (4-0 polydioxanone [PDS] interrupted sutures were used here). (g) Two weeks following the phallopexy surgery, the skin incision has healed completely. (h) Only the penile tip can be expressed out of the prepuce with the phallopexy in place.

perineal artery, are ligated when the penis is amputated from the ischial attachments (Wilson 1975). A segment of the urethra should be retained to perform a scrotal urethrostomy.

A midline preputiotomy incision can be used to expose the penile shaft and the amputation performed caudal to the preputial fornix (Pavletic & O'Bell 2007). A release incision cranial to the prepuce can be used to facilitate caudal displacement of the preputial mucosa, which facilitates urethral anastomosis to this structure. The terminal portion of the urethra is anastomosed to the preputial mucosa, which allows the dog to urinate through the preputial orifice. Unlike a perineal urethrostomy, preputial urethrostomy eliminates the potential for local skin irritation during urination. Preputial urethrostomy is also easier to perform in those dogs in which penile amputation is required adjacent to the preputial fornix.

Prognosis

The prognosis is good to guarded for resolution of paraphimosis, depending on the severity and duration of clinical signs. It is important to inform the owner that erection and ejaculation may be impaired following long-standing paraphimosis (Kustritz & Olson 1999). Balanoposthitis secondary to phimosis may occur following surgical retention of the penis within the preputial cavity. Urethral stricture formation and recurrent urinary tract infections may result following penile amputation.

References

Chaffee, V.W. and Knecht, C.D. (1975). Canine paraphimosis: sequel to inefficient preputial muscles. *Veterinary Medicine, Small Animal Clinician* 70: 1418–1420.

Hart, B.L. and Peterson, D.M. (1971). Penile hair rings in male cats may prevent mating. *Laboratory Animal Science* 21: 422.

Kustritz, M.V. and Olson, P.N. (1999). Theriogenology question of the month. Priapism or paraphimosis. *Journal of the American Veterinary Medical Association* 214 (10): 1483–1484.

Laube, R., Cook, A., and Winkler, K. (2017). Diphallia in a mixed-breed puppy: case report. *Journal of the American Animal Hospital Association* 53: 281–284.

Lee, J. (1976). Paraphimosis in a pseudohermaphrodite dog. *Veterinary Medicine, Small Animal Clinician* 71 (8): 1076–1077.

Massari, F., Montinaro, V., Buracco, P., and Romanelli, G. (2018). Combined caudal-superficial-epigastric axial pattern flap and full-thickness buccal mucosa graft for single-stage preputial reconstruction in six dogs. *Journal of Small Animal Practice* 59: 415–421.

Ndiritu, C.G. (1979). Lesions of the canine penis and prepuce. *Modern Veterinary Practice* 60 (9): 712–715.

Olsen, D. and Salwei, R. (2001). Surgical correction of a congenital preputial and penile deformity in a dog. *Journal of the American Animal Hospital Association* 37 (2): 187–192.

Papazoglou, L.G. (2001). Idiopathic chronic penile protrusion in the dog: a report of six cases. *Journal of Small Animal Practice* 42 (10): 510–513.

Pavletic, M.M. and O'Bell, S.A. (2007). Subtotal penile amputation and preputial urethrostomy in a dog. *Journal of the American Veterinary Medical Association* 230 (3): 375–377.

Proescholdt, T.A., DeYoung, D.W., and Evans, L.E. (1977). Preputial reconstruction for phimosis and infantile penis. *Journal of the American Animal Hospital Association* 13: 725–727.

Root-Kustritz, M.V. (2001). Disorders of the canine penis. *Veterinary Clinics of North America: Small Animal Practice* 31 (2): 247–258. vi.

Somerville, M.E. and Anderson, S.M. (2001). Phallopexy for treatment of paraphimosis in the dog. *Journal of the American Animal Hospital Association* 37 (4): 397–400.

Swalec, K.M. and Smeak, D.D. (1989). Priapism after castration in a cat. *Journal of the American Veterinary Medical Association* 195: 963–964.

Yiapanis, C., Atamna, R., Gan El, M. et al. (2021). Cranial translation of the elevated prepuce in dogs before and after two modifications: A cadaveric study. *Veterinary Surgery* 50: 1463–1471.

Wasik, S.M. and Wallace, A.M. (2014). Combined preputial advancement and phallopexy as a revision technique for treating paraphimosis in a dog. *Australian Veterinary Journal* 92: 433–436.

Wilson, G.P. (1975). Surgery of the male reproductive tract. *Veterinary Clinics of North America* 5: 537–550.

61

Priapism

Michelle Kutzler

Priapism is an uncommon disorder in male cats and dogs. It is characterized by a persistent penile erection that lasts for more than one hour, resulting in pain and dysuria. The term comes from the Greek god Priapus, who had a disproportionately large and permanent erection.

Normal anatomy and physiology of erection

The penis is attached to the ischial arch by the crura and ischiocavernous muscles. The penis consists of the root, body, and glans. The root is not externally visible. The body of the penis is made up of cavernous tissue. The dog has two separate corpora cavernosa with a complete septum and a corpus spongiosum similar to humans, making the dog model particularly useful in erectile dysfunction studies (Dong *et al*. 2011). The distal corpus cavernosum is ossified (os penis) and extends distally from just behind the bulb to the tip of the glans (Beach 1984). There is a ventral groove within the os penis to accommodate the penile urethra, the proximal end of which is a common site of urethral obstruction with urinary calculus (Herron 1972).

The glans penis of the dog is divided into two principal parts: the pars longa glandis and bulbus glandis. Applying pressure behind the bulbus glandis results in contraction of the ischiourethralis muscle, which inserts on a fibrous ring encircling the common trunk of the left and right dorsal veins of the penis (Hart & Kitchell 1966). Contraction of the ischiourethralis muscle occludes the dorsal vein, resulting in engorgement of the cavernous tissues within the penis. Transection of the ischiourethralis muscle prevents canine erection, including partial penile erection of the bulbus glandis (Hart 1972). Detumescence requires relaxation of these smooth muscle fibers, which allows drainage through the pudendal veins (Vali & Bookstein 1987).

The blood supply to the corpus spongiosum penis is by the deep and dorsal penile arteries (Figure 61.1). Erection occurs when there is an increase in cavernosal arterial blood flow coupled with a decrease venous outflow from the corpora via the dorsal penile vein, resulting in sinusoidal relaxation and filling of the corpora cavernosa (Lue *et al*. 1984a, 1985a; Carati *et al*. 1988). The inferior epigastric artery can serve as a donor vessel to increase blood flow to the corpus cavernosa when flow has been reduced to the dorsal penile artery (Floth *et al*. 1991). In the dog, the rapid engorgement of the bulb is also dependent upon dilatation of helicine arteries in the erectile tissue (Hart 1974a,b). The circumflex vein drains into the deep dorsal vein and provides additional drainage to the distal two thirds of the cavernous bodies (Breza *et al*. 1990). Minor cavernous vein leakage in the presence of normal arterial flow has minimal effect on the development of erection (Aboseif *et al*. 1990). The spinal nuclei for control of erection are located in the intermediolateral gray matter at the S1–S3 and T12–L3 in dogs (Lue *et al*. 1984b). The sacral nuclei axons fuse to form the pelvic nerve (nervus erigens), whose visceral parasympathetic efferent fibers (cavernous nerves) are located on the lateral aspect of the urethra (Langley & Anderson 1895; Lue *et al*. 1984b). The cavernous nerves penetrate the tunica albuginea of the corpora cavernosa alone and enter with the deep

Small Animal Soft Tissue Surgery, Second Edition. Edited by Eric Monnet.
© 2023 John Wiley & Sons, Inc. Published 2023 by John Wiley & Sons, Inc.
Companion website: www.wiley.com/go/monnet/small

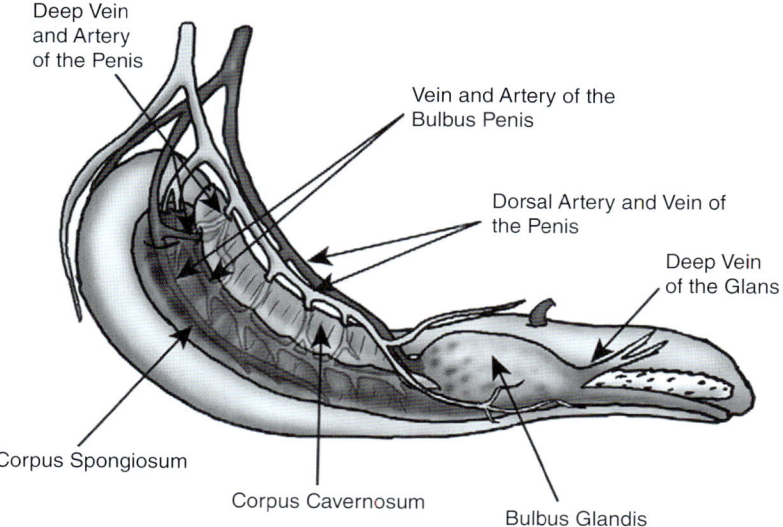

Figure 61.1 Anatomy and vascular supply of the canine penis. Source: Lavely, J.A. (2009) / with permission of Elsevier.

penile artery and cavernous vein (Lue *et al.* 1984b). These nerves can be easily damaged during urogenital surgery. Erection can be induced via electrostimulation of the cavernous nerves along the posterolateral aspect of the prostate in intact and castrated males (Müller *et al.* 1988; Floth *et al.* 1991).

Etiology

Priapism is generally not initiated by sexual stimuli and results from disturbances in the normal regulatory mechanisms that initiate and maintain penile flaccidity. Priapism is most likely to develop secondary to trauma during mating or during castration (Wilson 1975). Other causes of priapism can be categorized as either high flow (nonischemic) or low flow (ischemic) (Rochat 2001; Lavely 2009).

High-flow priapism

High-flow priapism results from the development of arteriovenous fistulas or a persistent increase in blood flow from a neuro-arterial disturbance (Pohl *et al.* 1986). Arteriovenous fistulas are reported infrequently dogs and cats. Occasionally, arteriovenous fistulas develop on the prepuce (Trower *et al.* 1997). Clinically, a preputial arteriovenous fistula presents as a network of large tortuous pulsating blood vessels that enlarge gradually over several months (Trower *et al.* 1997). However, an experimentally produced arteriovenous fistula between the inferior epigastric artery and deep dorsal vein does not have any significant impact on cardiac output, nor does it lead to priapism (Godziachvili & Saba 1997).

Persistent pelvic nerve stimulation results in a persistent increase in penile blood flow. Persistent pelvic nerve stimulation can result from inflammation from a genitourinary infection, multifocal distemper-associated myelitis lesions, or constipation (Wilson 1975; Orima *et al.* 1989; Swalec & Smeak 1989; Guilford *et al.* 1990; Gunn-Moore *et al.* 1995). Lumbar stenosis (L7–S1) and spinal cord injuries in association with medullar compression can also result in stimulation of the erection center or the pelvic nerves (Payan-Carreira *et al.* 2013).

Intracavernous administration of vasodilatory drugs (e.g., 2–10 mg papaverine-HCl) decreases arterial resistance and increases venous resistance (Bjorling 1984; Lue *et al.* 1986b; Breza *et al.* 1990; Floth *et al.* 1991; Godziachvili & Saba 1997). Sporadic cases of iatrogenic acepromazine-induced priapism have been reported in both intact dogs and cats. In addition, there is one report of a dog that received trazodone that developed a priapism (Murphy *et al.* 2017). Some antipsychotic medications used for humans inadvertently consumed by pets can also result in a priapism.

Low-flow priapism

Low-flow priapism is associated with a poorer prognosis as the damage from the ischemia is more severe (Pohl *et al.* 1986; Spycher & Hauri 1986). In low-flow priapism, the danger is not in the priapism itself, but in the reduction of oxygen and an elevation of carbon dioxide partial pressure. This partial pressure change results from the associated vascular stasis in the corpus cavernosum and spongiosum. The combination of spongiosum and partial pressure change results in sickling of erythrocytes and trabecular edema formation that occlude the venous outflow (Hashmat *et al.* 1981). Decreased venous outflow can result from occlusive thromboembolic lesions secondary to systemic disease (e.g., hemoglobinopathy) or compressive masses (e.g., penile metastasis from urogenital tumors or abscess within the pelvic cavity) that impair blood drainage from the penis (Wilson 1975; Rogers *et al.* 2002; Lavely 2009; Martins-Bessa *et al.* 2010).

Presentation

The persistently erect penis may be within the prepuce (partial erection) or the prepuce may be behind the bulbus glandis (full erection). An important differential when presented with a priapism case is paraphimosis (see Chapter 60). In priapism the penis will be firm, whereas in paraphimosis the penis will be flaccid (Figure 61.2). The penile mucosa may be dry, inflamed, excoriated, and is often dark red to purple in color secondary to blood congestion. The male frequently licks the penis because it is painful and self-mutilation may occur. If neglected, the penis will become necrotic. In the event of urethral obstruction, stranguria may be present, which can progress to uremia secondary to cystorrhexis if left untreated.

Diagnosis

Other than direct examination, the diagnosis can be made using ultrasound and radiography. B-mode ultrasonography of the perineum and the entire penile shaft can be used to verify engorgement of the corpus

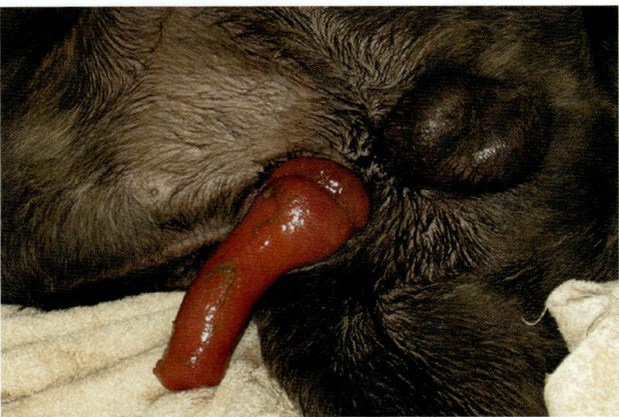

Figure 61.2 Paraphimosis in an 11-month-old mastiff. The penis is markedly swollen and cannot be replaced into the prepuce. Source: Lavely, J.A. (2009) / with permission of Elsevier.

(a)

(b)

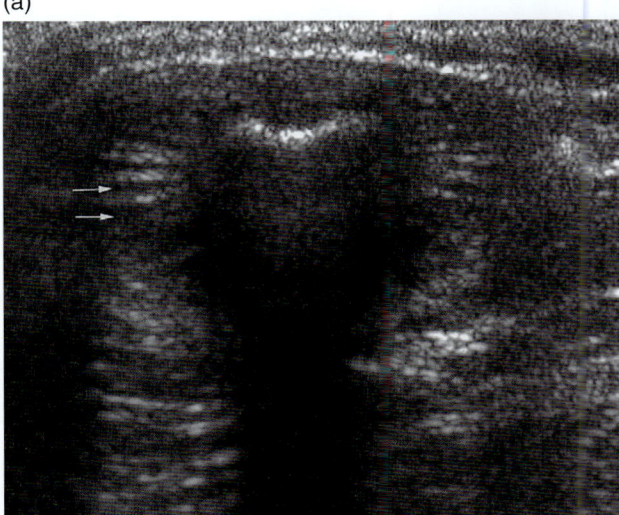

Figure 61.3 (a) Transverse ultrasound image of the priapism illustrated in Figure 61.2. Note the engorged vessels in the corpus cavernosum indicated by the arrows. (b) Transverse ultrasound image of a normal nonerect canine penis for the purposes of comparison. Source: Lavely, J.A. (2009) / with permission of Elsevier.

cavernosum and spongiosum (Figure 61.3) as well as to rule out etiologic factors (e.g., neoplasia) (Goericke-Pesch *et al.* 2013). Local and regional penile blood flow can be determined using color-flow Doppler ultrasonography (Breza *et al.* 1990). Doppler ultrasonography can also be used to diagnose an arterial to cavernosum fistula.

Penile angiography (cavernosography) can be used to show patency (or the lack thereof) of the corpus cavernosum and spongiosum (Shokeir *et al.* 2004). Cavernosography can be used to identify thromboemboli or masses resulting in decreased venous outflow and the extent of venous outflow impairment, as well as for diagnosing arteriovenous communication (Ninomiya *et al.* 1984; Root-Kustritz & Olson 1999). Characteristic angiographic findings of arteriovenous fistulas include premature venous filling, absence of the normal capillary phase, and reduced distal arterial flow (Hosgood 1989). The procedure consists of an intracavernous infusion of heparinized saline using a 19–21-gauge butterfly catheter, followed by infusion of 60% Hypaque™ meglumine contrast medium (GE Healthcare, Chicago, IL, USA) to opacify abnormally draining veins (Stief *et al.* 1988).

Treatment

Priapism is an emergency condition requiring aggressive acute treatment to induce detumescence. The goal of therapy is to restore normal circulation within the penile erectile tissues, as well as to preserve the penis from severe injury, desiccation, ischemia, necrosis, and urethral obstruction (Van Harreveld & Gaughan 1999; Johnston *et al.* 2001). Regardless of the primary cause, priapism if prolonged leads to irreversible thrombosis and fibrosis of the erectile tissues and main venous outflow tracts of the penis. Histologically, severe cavernosal congestion develops with large hemoglobin crystals and organizing fibrin thrombi (Swalec & Smeak 1989; Foster *et al.* 1999).

Medical treatment with oral pseudoephedrine (1.72 mg/kg) twice daily until resolution has successfully induced detumescence in one dog (Lavely 2009). Following unsuccessful medical treatment with ephedrine and terbutaline, treatment with gabapentin successfully resolved a priapism in one cat (Lavely 2014). In addition, intravenous benztropine mesylate (0.015 mg/kg), an anticholinergic and anti-histaminergic drug, has been used successfully in horses to induce detumescence, but must be administered within 6 hours after the onset of priapism when venous drainage in the cavernous spaces is still preserved (Hart 1974b; Wilson *et al.* 1991). In humans, some success has been reported using gonadotropin-releasing hormones, anti-androgens, hydroxyurea, and phosphodiesterase-5 inhibitors (Lavely 2014).

If pharmacologic reversal has failed, then venous outflow should be increased via drainage and flushing of the cavernous tissues with heparinized saline (0.9% NaCl) solution in combination with intracavernosal infusion of phenylephrine (Hart 1974b; Bjorling 1984; Lue

et al. 1986a; Sidi 1988; Godziachvili & Saba 1997; Moon *et al.* 1999; Rochat 2001). Phenylephrine diluted in saline (100–500 μg/mL) can be injected at a rate of 1–3 μg/kg with continuous cardiovascular monitoring (Lavely 2014). Better success rates have been reported when cavernosal flushing is administered shortly after the onset of priapism (Van Harreveld & Gaughan 1999). However, the penis may be irreparably damaged at time of initial presentation, necessitating amputation and urethrostomy (Burrow *et al.* 2011). In this case, conservative methods of treatment failed to achieve detumescence. Decompression through surgical methods such as the tunica albuginea incision, which includes an incision of the bulbus glandis as well as the pars longa glandis (Orima *et al.* 1989), is usually successful without permanent damage provided the treatment is done within 12 hours of the onset of the situation (Kalsi *et al.* 2002).

Conservative treatment consists of various combinations of cold-water compresses, topical hypertonic solutions, penile lubrication, anti-inflammatories, broad-spectrum antibiotics, and diuretics (Gunn-Moore *et al.* 1995). Unfortunately, conservative treatment is usually not successful. Since the fully erect penis cannot be manually reduced into the prepuce because it is too large and long, it becomes congested, dry, and eventually necrotic. Surgery can be performed to enlarge the diameter of the preputial opening to facilitate return of the penis within the prepuce (see Chapter 62). However, penile retraction into the preputial cavity does not in itself treat the priapism and the penis will eventually undergo necrosis. If this occurs, penile amputation with urethrostomy and castration may need to be performed (Burrow *et al.* 2011).

Conservative surgical treatment for arteriovenous fistulas involves ligating the proximal supplying vessels to reduce blood flow through the fistula (Trower *et al.* 1997). The prognosis for dogs with arteriovenous fistulas depends on the size and site of the fistula and the degree of cardiovascular failure at the time of diagnosis (Hosgood 1989).

References

Aboseif, S.R., Wetterauer, U., Breza, J. et al. (1990). The effect of venous incompetence and arterial insufficiency on erectile function: an animal model. *Journal of Urology* 144: 790–793.

Beach, F.A. (1984). Hormonal modulation of genital reflexes in male and masculinized female dogs. *Behavioral Neuroscience* 98: 325–332.

Bjorling, D.E. (1984). Traumatic injuries of the urogenital system. *Veterinary Clinics of North America: Small Animal Practice* 14: 61–76.

Breza, J., Aboseif, S.R., Lue, T.F. et al. (1990). Cavernous vein arterialization for vasculogenic impotence. *Urology* 35: 513–518.

Burrow, R.D., Gregory, S.P., Giejda, A.A., and White, R.N. (2011). Penile amputation and scrotal urethrostomy in 18 dogs. *Veterinary Record* 169: 657.

Carati, C.J., Creed, K.E., and Keogh, E.J. (1988). Vascular changes during penile erection in the dog. *Journal of Physiology* 400: 75–88.

Dong, Q., Deng, S., Wang, R., and Yuan, J. (2011). in vitro and in vivo animal models in priapism research. *Journal of Sexual Medicine* 8: 347–359.

Floth, A., Paick, J.S., Suh, J.K. et al. (1991). Hemodynamics of revascularization of the corpora cavernosa in an animal model. *Urology Research* 19: 281–284.

Foster, S.F., Hunt, G.B., and Malik, R. (1999). Congenital urethral anomaly in a kitten. *Journal of Feline Medicine and Surgery* 1: 61–64.

Godziachvili, V. and Saba, A. (1997). Arteriovenous fistula combined with basal external penile compression: a new cure for male impotence. *American Surgery* 63 (8): 704–709.

Goericke-Pesch, S., Hölscher, C., Failing, K., and Wehrend, A. (2013). Functional anatomy and ultrasound examination of the canine penis. *Theriogenology* 80: 24–33.

Guilford, W.G., Shaw, D.P., O'Brien, D.P. et al. (1990). Fecal incontinence, urinary incontinence, and priapism associated with multifocal distemper encephalomyelitis in a dog. *Journal of the American Veterinary Medical Association* 197: 90–92.

Gunn-Moore, D.A., Brown, P.J., Holt, P.E. et al. (1995). Priapism in seven cats. *Journal of Small Animal Practice* 36: 262–266.

Hart, B.L. (1972). The action of extrinsic muscles during copulation in the male dog. *Anatomical Record* 173: 1–6.

Hart, B.L. (1974a). Physiology of sexual function. *Veterinary Clinics of North America* 4: 557–571.

Hart, B.L. (1974b). Gonadal androgen and sociosexual behavior of male mammals: a comparative analysis. *Psychological Bulletin* 81: 383–400.

Hart, B.J. and Kitchell, R.L. (1966). Penile erection and contraction of penile muscles in the spinal and intact dog. *American Journal of Physiology* 210: 257–262.

Hashmat, A.L., Macchia, R.J., and Waterhouse, K. (1981). Treatment of priapism by corporoglans shunt. A report on 20 cases. *Journal of Urology* 125: A234.

Herron, M.A. (1972). The effect of prepubertal castration on the penile urethra of the cat. *Journal of the American Veterinary Medical Association* 160: 208–211.

Hosgood, G. (1989). Arteriovenous fistulas: pathophysiology, diagnosis and treatment. *Compendium on Continuing Education for the Practicing Veterinarian* 11: 625–636.

Johnston, S.D., Root-Kustritz, M.V., and Olson, P.N.S. (2001). Disorders of the canine penis and prepuce. In: *Canine and Feline Theriogenology*, 356–367. Philadelphia, PA: WB Saunders Company.

Kalsi, J.S., Arya, M., Minhas, S. et al. (2002). Priapism: a medical emergency. *Hospital Medicine* 63: 224–225.

Langley, J. and Anderson, H.K. (1895). The innervation of the pelvic and adjoining viscera: part II, the bladder; part III, the external generative organs; part IV, the internal generative organs; part V, position of the nerve cells on the course of efferent nerve fibres. *Journal of Physiology* 19: 71–139.

Lavely, J.A. (2009). Priapism in dogs. *Topics in Companion Animal Medicine* 24: 49–54.

Lavely, J.A. (2014). Priapism in dogs. In: *Kirk's Current Veterinary Therapy XV*, ch. 73. St. Louis, MO: Elsevier.

Lue, T.F., Takamura, T., Umraiya, M. et al (1984a). Hemodynamics of canine corpora cavernosa during erection. *Urology* 24: 347–352.

Lue, T.F., Zeineh, S.J., Schmidt, R.A. et al. 1984b). Neuroanatomy of penile erection: its relevance to iatrogenic impotence. *Journal of Urology* 131: 273–280.

Lue, T.F., Hellstrom, W.J.G., McAninch, J.N. et al. (1986a). Priapism: a refined approach to diagnosis and treatment. *Journal of Urology* 136: 104–108.

Lue, T.F., Hricak, H., Schmidt, R.A. et al. (1986b). Functional evaluation of penile veins by cavernosography in papaverine-induced erection. *Journal of Urology* 135: 479–482.

Martins-Bessa, A., Santos, T., Machado, J. et al. (2010). Priapism secondary to perineal abscess in a dog—a case report. *Reproduction in Domestic Animals* 45: 558–563.

Moon, D.G., Lee, D.S., and Kim, J.J. 1999). Altered contractile response of penis under hypoxia with metabolic acidosis. *International Journal of Impotence Research* 11: 265–271.

Müller, S.C., Hsieh, J.T., Lue, T. et al. (1988). Castration and erection. *European Urology* 15: 118–124.

Murphy, L.A., Barletta, M., Graham, L.F. et al. (2017). Effects of acepromazine and trazodone on anesthetic induction dose of propofol and cardiovascular variables in dogs undergoing general anesthesia for orthopedic surgery. *Journal of the American Veterinary Medical Association* 250: 408–416.

Ninomiya, H., Fukase, T., and Nakamura, T. (1984). Scanning electron microscopy of celluloid replicas of the penile spines of the domestic cat. *Experimental Animals* 33: 525–528.

Orima, H., Tsuitsui, T., Waki, T. et al. (1989). Surgical treatment of priapism observed in a dog and a cat. *Nippon Juigaku Zasshi* 51: 1227–1229.

Payan-Carreira, R., Colaço, B., Rocha, C. et al. (2013). Priapism associated with lumbar stenosis in a dog. *Reproduction in Domestic Animals* 48: e58–e64.

Pohl, J., Pott, B., and Kleinhans, G. (1986). Priapism: a three phase concept of management according to aetiology and prognosis. *British Journal of Urology* 58: 113–118.

Rochat, M.C. (2001). Priapism: a review. *Theriogenology* 56: 713–722.

Rogers, L., Lopez, A., and Gillis, A. (2002). Priapism secondary to penile metastasis in a dog. *Canadian Veterinary Journal* 43: 547–549.

Root-Kustritz, M.V. and Olson, P.N. (1999). Priapism or paraphimosis. *Journal of the American Veterinary Medical Association* 214: 1483–1484.

Shokeir, A.A., Osman, Y., El-Azab, M. et al. (2004). Tunica albuginea acellular matrix graft for treatment of Peyronie's disease. *Scandinavian Journal of Urology and Nephrology* 38: 499–503.

Sidi, A.A. (1988). Vasoactive intracavernous pharmacotherapy. *Urologic Clinics of North America* 15: 95–101.

Spycher, M.A. and Hauri, D. (1986). The ultrastructure of the erectile tissue in priapism. *Journal of Urology* 135: 142–147.

Stief, C.G., Diederichs, W., Benard, F. et al. (1988). The diagnosis of venogenic impotence: dynamic or pharmacologic cavernosometry? *Journal of Urology* 140: 1561–1563.

Swalec, K.M. and Smeak, D.D. (1989). Priapism after castration in a cat. *Journal of the American Veterinary Medical Association* 195: 963–964.

Trower, N.D., White, R.N., and Lamb, C.R. (1997). Arteriovenous fistula involving the prepuce of a dog. *Journal of Small Animal Practice* 38: 455–458.

Valji, K. and Bookstein, J.J. (1987). The veno-occlusive mechanism of the canine corpus cavernosum: angiographic and pharmacologic studies. *Journal of Urology* 138: 1467–1470.

Van Harreveld, P.D. and Gaughan, E.M. (1999). Partial phallectomy to treat priapism in a horse. *Australian Veterinary Journal* 77: 167–169.

Wilson, G.P. (1975). Surgery of the male reproductive tract. *Veterinary Clinics of North America* 5: 537–550.

Wilson, D.V., Nickels, F.A., and Williams, M.A. (1991). Pharmacologic treatment of priapism in two horses. *Journal of the American Veterinary Medical Association* 199: 1183–1184.

62

Phimosis

Dietrich Volkmann

Phimosis is the inability of the penis to extend beyond the preputial orifice. The condition is rare and can have a number of developmental and acquired causes (Ndiritu 1979).

Causes

In anatomically normal dogs, the tip of the penis and hence the urethral opening are positioned at or just outside the preputial opening during urination. Urine does not therefore accumulate inside the preputial cavity before flowing out (Proescholdt et al. 1977). Developmental disorders that lead to phimosis include a smaller than appropriate preputial opening, an inherently small or short penis (penile hypoplasia, micropenis, infantile penis), or persistence of tissue bands that connect the penis to the preputial mucosa (Biewenga 1974; Jacobs & Baughman 1977; Proescholdt et al. 1977; Sarierler & Kara 1998; Olsen & Salwei 2001; Bouzalas et al. 2009). Acquired conditions may result in fibrosis and stenosis of the preputial opening as a consequence of trauma (bite wounds, excessive licking, suckling activity by littermates, grooming by the dam) or infection (balanoposthitis) (Smith & Gourley 1990; Staub et al. 2006).

Balanoposthitis may also be secondary to an inherently narrow preputial opening that causes the accumulation of urine inside the preputial cavity, leading to urine scalding and eventually infection due to overgrowth of resident bacteria (Biewenga 1974; Saporito 2008). Balanoposthitis may also cause ulceration of the preputial and penile mucosae. If it is allowed to persist for long enough, the irritated and denuded surfaces of the penis and preputial mucosa may form adhesions, rendering the penis immobile within the preputial cavity (Saporito 2008). Phimosis may also be the consequence of an excessively thick penis, as may be seen in cases of neoplasia (see Chapter 70).

Presentation

Most cases of phimosis due to a congenital cause manifest in juvenile or young adult dogs. Owners report that their dogs lick their prepuces excessively, dribble urine from their preputial orifices after urination, suffer from an offensive preputial discharge, or have a fluid-distended prepuce. The same presenting clinical signs may be noted in older dogs that suffer from an acquired form of phimosis. The diagnosis is often obvious once attempts are made to extend the penis for examination:

- The preputial orifice may be too tight to allow extension of the penis.
- The penis may be too small (thin and short) to be extended through the preputial orifice.
- The penis may be adhered to the preputial mucosa.
- A scar or partially healed wound may be present at or near the preputial orifice.
- A penile tumor may be palpable through the preputial skin.

In cases where urine is voided into the preputial cavity, a secondary balanoposthitis may be evident as inflammation (reddening, swelling, and ulceration) of the tissues at the preputial opening. In extreme cases, fluid (usually retained urine) may be palpable inside the preputial cavity. Phimosis will obviously prevent the extension of the erect penis, thus preventing normal copulation.

Small Animal Soft Tissue Surgery, Second Edition. Edited by Eric Monnet.
© 2023 John Wiley & Sons, Inc. Published 2023 by John Wiley & Sons, Inc.
Companion website: www.wiley.com/go/monnet/small

Diagnosis

Other than by direct examination, the diagnosis can be made using contrast radiography or ultrasonography. Contrast radiography is accomplished by filling the preputial cavity with saline and then taking radiographs of the penis and prepuce (Sarierler & Kara 1998). Ultrasonographic examination can largely achieve the same results as contrast radiography. Ultrasonography will allow the detection of adhesions between the penis and preputial mucosa that were not detected by palpation through the preputial skin. When present, any accumulated fluid inside the prepuce may be aspirated to verify that it is urine, or to submit it for bacterial culture and sensitivity testing in cases that suffer from significant balanoposthitis and require antimicrobial therapy in addition to corrective surgery. The approach to the diagnosis of intrapreputial tumors is discussed in Chapter 70.

Treatment

All reported cases of phimosis required surgical correction. In its simplest form, corrective surgery involves the widening of an excessively narrow preputial opening (Papazoglou & Kazakos 2002). A longitudinal, full-thickness incision of 10–15 mm is made through the dorsal aspect of the preputial ring. In extreme cases, it may be necessary to excise a full-thickness V-shaped wedge at the same location. The placement of the incision at the ventral aspect of the preputial opening is considered ill-advised, as it may result in the persistent exposure of the tip of the penis. The raw edges of the incision are then closed by suturing the preputial mucosal edge to the skin edge, resulting in a V-shaped suture line (Figure 62.1). The suture pattern can be simple interrupted or simple continuous with nonabsorbable suture materials.

In cases where adhesions are present between the penis and the preputial mucosa, the preputial cavity must be exposed through a mid-ventral longitudinal incision that allows access to the adhesions, which are then freed by blunt and sharp dissection (Saporito 2008). Once separated, the defects in the penile and preputial mucosa should be closed using absorbable suture material. Leaving the defects open is likely to result in the formation of new adhesions and recurrence of the problem.

In cases of phimosis due to penile hypoplasia, the prepuce can be shortened so that the tip of the shorter than normal penis comes to be positioned closer to the preputial orifice (Proescholdt *et al.* 1977; Papazoglou & Kazakos 2002). This will result in improved voiding of urine with less urine retention inside the prepuce, which is inciting the balanoposthitis. A section of the prepuce is removed by making two transverse incisions through the preputial skin and the full circumference of the preputial mucosa (Figure 62.2). In order to allow smooth

(a)

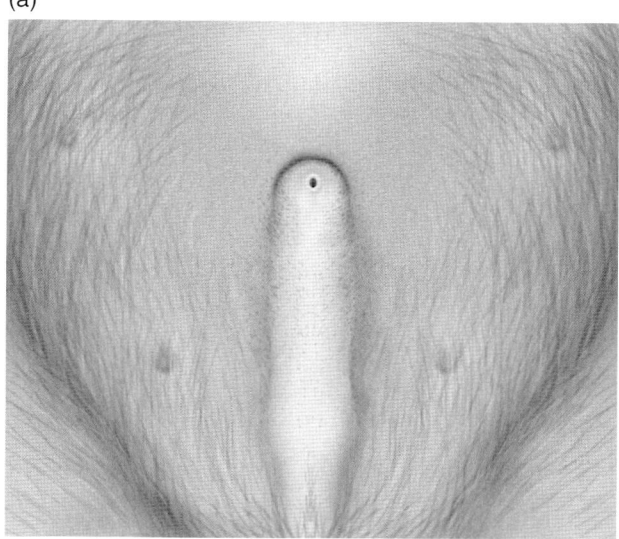

(b)

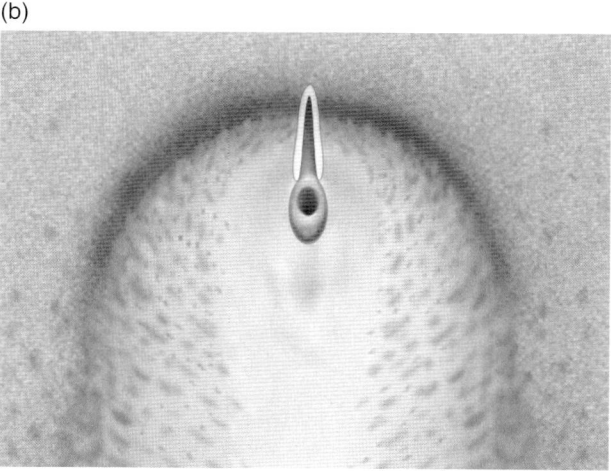

(c)

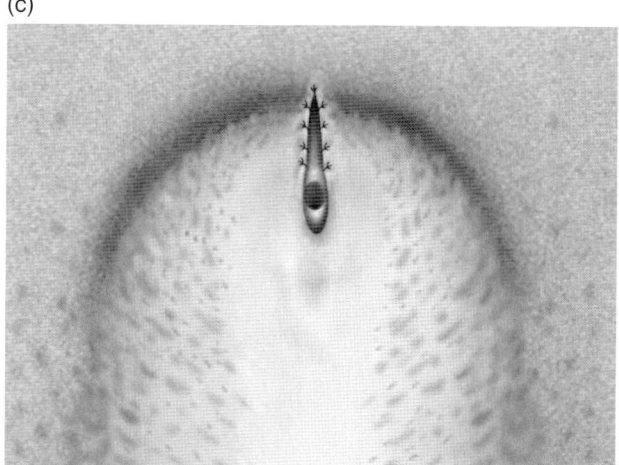

Figure 62.1 (a) Widening the preputial orifice. (b) A full-thickness longitudinal incision or wedge-shaped excision is made through the dorsal aspect of the narrow preputial opening. (c) Skin and mucosal edges are sutured together to create a wider opening. © D. Giddings.

(a)

(b)

(c)

(d)

(e)

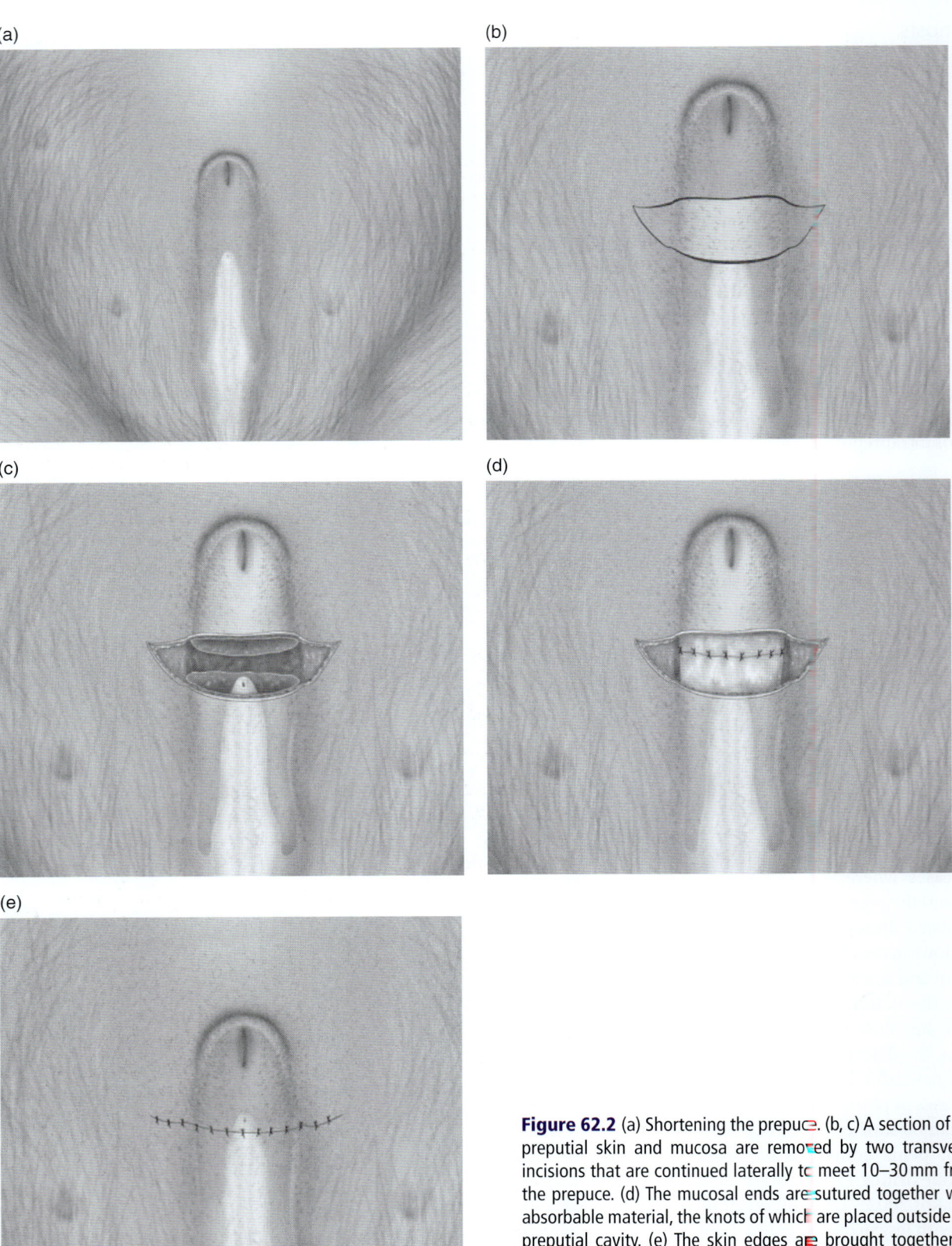

Figure 62.2 (a) Shortening the prepuce. (b, c) A section of the preputial skin and mucosa are removed by two transverse incisions that are continued laterally to meet 10–30 mm from the prepuce. (d) The mucosal ends are sutured together with absorbable material, the knots of which are placed outside the preputial cavity. (e) The skin edges are brought together by simple interrupted sutures of nonabsorbable material. The knots of the mucosal sutures therefore become buried between the two layers of the original incision. © D. Giddings.

closure of the defect, the skin incisions are continued laterally to meet approximately 10–30 mm on either side of the prepuce. The isolated skin and tubular section of the preputial mucosa are then freed from the deeper tissues and removed. The cranial and caudal free edges of the preputial mucosa are sutured together with absorbable suture material, placing the knots outside the preputial lumen (they become buried between the mucosa and overlying skin once the latter has been closed). The cranial and caudal skin edges are sutured together with nonabsorbable suture material in a simple interrupted pattern.

Supportive care for cases that have undergone preputial surgery varies according to the extent of the intervention or the severity of tissue compromise prior to surgery. All dogs undergoing preputial surgery should be fitted with an Elizabethan collar to prevent licking of the surgical site. Pain management should be provided through the administration of systemic anti-inflammatory agents or analgesics to hasten wound healing and reduce self-trauma to the surgical site. When significant infection of the preputial cavity was present prior to surgery, a course of broad-spectrum antimicrobial therapy is indicated until the wounds are completely healed. In chronic cases, the choice of antimicrobial agent should be based on the results of bacterial culture and antimicrobial sensitivity testing.

The prognosis for virtually all phimosis cases that have been subjected to appropriate corrective surgery is good to excellent. Formation of adhesions between the penis and preputial mucosa or the development of preputial stenosis secondary to fibrosis could occur but has not been reported. While no specific mode of inheritance has been discovered or proposed for the congenital malformations associated with phimosis, several authors suggest that affected dogs should not be used for breeding.

References

Biewenga, W.J. (1974). Schijnbare incontinentia urinae bijeen pup. *Tijdschrift voor Diergeneeskunde* 99: 841–843.

Bouzalas, I.G., Papazoglou, L.G., Flouraki, E. et al. (2009). Correction of a preputial fusion abnormality and stenotic preputial opening in a dog. *Australian Veterinary Practitioner* 39: 144–146.

Jacobs, D. and Baughman, G.L. (1977). Preputial defect in a puppy. *Modern Veterinary Practice* 58: 522–523.

Ndiritu, C.G. (1979). Lesions of the canine penis and prepuce. *Modern Veterinary Practice* 60: 712–715.

Olsen, D. and Salwei, R. (2001). Surgical correction of a congenital preputial and penile deformity in a dog. *Journal of the American Animal Hospital Association* 37: 187–192.

Papazoglou, L.G. and Kazakos, G.M. (2002). Surgical conditions of the canine penis and prepuce. *Compendium on Continuing Education for the Practicing Veterinarian* 24: 204–218.

Proescholdt, T.A., DeYoung, D.W., and Evans, L.E. (1977). Preputial reconstruction for phimosis and infantile penis. *Journal of the American Animal Hospital Association* 13: 725–727.

Saporito, K. (2008). A challenging case: phimosis in a young adult dog. *Veterinary Medicine (London)* 103: 22–26.

Sarierler, M. and Kara, M.E. (1998). Congenital stenosis of the preputial orifice in a dog. *Veterinary Record* 143: 201.

Smith, M.M. and Gourley, I.M. (1990). Preputial reconstruction in a dog. *Journal of the American Veterinary Medical Association* 196: 1493–1496.

Staub, A.K., Kramer, M., and Thiel, C. (2006). Traumatische phimose als ursache für harnabsatzbeschwerden bei einem terrier-mix-welpen: diagnostik und therapie. *Praktische Tierarzt* 87: 526–529.

63

Penile and Preputial Trauma and Neoplasia

Dawna Voelkl

A wide range of acquired conditions affect the canine penis and prepuce. Trauma and neoplasia are the most common causes of disruption of the normal anatomic architecture of the prepuce and penis and often compromise urinary and reproductive function.

Trauma to the prepuce and penis

Injury to the prepuce and penis is usually the consequence of sharp trauma, as may occur during hunting, blunt-force trauma as in vehicular accidents, dog fights, gunshots, or breeding (Johnston *et al.* 2001). The degree of trauma varies widely, from superficial lacerations of the prepuce to penile amputation. The need for surgical intervention is largely dictated by the existence of, or potential for, urethral obstruction and, more rarely, by the presence of extensive hemorrhage.

Lacerations of the prepuce and penis

While lacerations of the external prepuce are readily apparent, injuries to the penis may be less obvious, with the only presenting clinical sign being serosanguineous to sanguineous preputial discharge. Small volumes of blood may drip slowly and continuously from the preputial orifice or large amounts may be released intermittently as the preputial cavity fills and overflows. Hemorrhage from a lacerated penis may be exacerbated by penile erection, particularly when wounds are deep and penetrate the cavernous spaces.

Management of lacerations to the prepuce and penis is determined by the depth, extent, and nature of the defect, the volume of hemorrhage, involvement of the os penis, and compromise of the urethra. Superficial lacerations

of the external prepuce are repaired as for any skin wound; however, full-thickness lacerations generally require a two-layer closure, beginning with closure of the preputial mucosal defect using 3-0 absorbable suture material.

Minor injuries to the penis that produce little hemorrhage, for example punctures, are managed as open wounds, treated with topical antimicrobial ointments, and allowed to heal by second intention. Surgical débridement, ligation of compromised vasculature, and a double-layer closure of the tunica albuginea and penile mucosa using absorbable suture must be performed for lacerations demonstrating significant hemorrhage (Johnston & Archibald 1984). Postoperative care includes administration of systemic antimicrobials and anti-inflammatory medications, application of topical antibiotic ointments, and prevention of sexual excitement and penile erection through isolation and/or sedation. In cases where urethral integrity is known to have been, or is suspected to be, compromised, placement of an indwelling urinary catheter for the first several days following repair may deter stricture formation. If the laceration has significantly compromised the urethral orifice, a urinary catheter should be placed and reconstruction undertaken by suturing urethral to penile mucosa at the glans using 5-0 absorbable suture material (Johnston & Archibald 1984). In some cases, the ability to achieve normal penile erection and breed by natural service may be compromised following healing due to disruption of normal architecture or damage to the penile innervation (Figure 63.1). Deep lacerations to the glans penis involving the urethra may be treated with

---

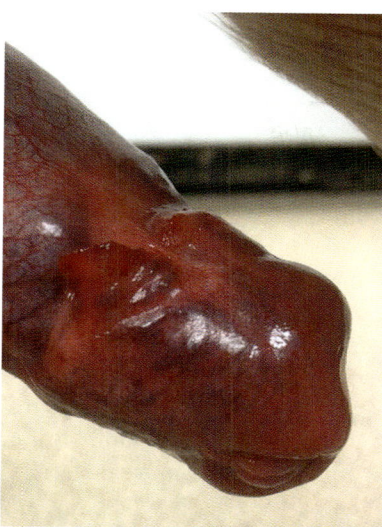

Figure 63.1 Penile laceration permitted to heal by second intention in a middle-aged proven pointer dog. The dog appeared to lack sensation to the glans penis and was no longer capable of natural mating.

partial penile amputation and prescrotal urethrostomy (Esposito *et al.* 2021).

Traumatic truncation and amputation of the penis

Traumatic penile truncation or amputation has been reported in the dog (Brown 1979; Park *et al.* 2007). In cases of loss of a portion of the glans penis distal to the os, preservation of the remaining penis may be attempted. The wound may be approached through extrusion of the remaining penis through the external preputial orifice or, if the penis has been truncated to such a degree as to prohibit extrusion achieving adequate exposure, the wound may be approached through a ventral midline preputiotomy. The injury site is cleaned and débrided, and a new urethral opening fashioned through apposition of the urethral mucosa to the penile mucosa using 5-0 absorbable suture material, with an indwelling urinary catheter employed as a guide (Johnston & Archibald 1984). In cases where a large portion of the penis has been lost or where the os penis is exposed, partial penile amputation with preputial urethrostomy or complete penile amputation with scrotal or perineal urethrostomy is indicated. The most practical and definitive treatment for complete traumatic amputation is use of the tunica albuginea to close defects in the corpus cavernosum penis and performance of a scrotal or perineal urethrostomy, depending on the site of trauma, although successful surgical reattachment of an amputated penis has been reported in a dog injured while hunting wild boar. Reattachment of the penis was

accomplished through anastomosis of the urethra, corpus cavernosum penis and urethra, and the dorsal veins of the penis (Park *et al.* 2007).

Fracture of the os penis

Dogs suffering from fracture of the os penis may be presented following acute trauma with concurrent laceration of the penis, penile deviation, sanguineous preputial discharge, and/or dysuria. Alternatively, chronic fractures of the os penis may result in clinical presentations of hematuria and/or dysuria months to years after a traumatic episode or apparently spontaneously, in the absence of a known history of trauma (Stead 1972; Elkins *et al.* 1990; Kelly & Clark 1995). Urinary obstruction is associated with displaced bony fragments acutely and callus formation resulting from healed fractures in chronic cases.

While clinical signs of hematuria and/or dysuria in the presence of penile deviation, crepitus, and pain on palpation of the penis are suggestive of a fracture of the os penis, radiography confirms the diagnosis. Placement of a urinary catheter prior to radiography or performance of retrograde contrast urethrography is useful in evaluating the degree of urethral canal impingement, particularly in cases of chronic fracture and callus formation.

The approach to treatment of fractures of the os penis depends on the duration of the fracture, presence and severity of concurrent soft tissue damage, and degree of compromise of urethral integrity. Fractures of the os penis are most often simple and transverse; however, comminuted fractures are possible (Johnston & Archibald 1984). In young dogs, fracture with displacement may occur between ossification centers (Petrelli *et al.* 2020). Simple acute fractures may be managed conservatively via closed reduction and placement of an indwelling urinary catheter to impart stability during healing. The catheter is positioned proximal to the fracture site and left in place for 5–7 days, during which time systemic antimicrobial and anti-inflammatory medications are administered. Temporary perineal urethrotomy may be performed if maintenance of urethral patency is problematic following catheter withdrawal (Johnston & Archibald 1984).

In acute cases in which concurrent disruption of the urethra is suspected and/or the fracture is comminuted or moderately displaced, more extensive interventions may be required. Urethral catheterization is performed, with urethrotomy used to confirm placement of the catheter, and surgical repair of the fracture is pursued. Fractures of the os penis may be reduced openly and stabilized through internal fixation using a titanium or stainless steel finger plate (Stead 1972; Kelly & Clark 1995). Under general anesthesia, the penis is extruded from the external preputial orifice, cleaned, and a tourniquet is temporarily applied proximal to the os. The penile mucosa and tunica albuginea are incised along the lateral aspect of the penis in the area of the os. Following reduction of the fracture, the finger plate is positioned along the lateral aspect of the dorsal portion of the os penis in order to avoid the urethra, which courses in the ventral groove of the bone. The incision is then closed in two layers, the tunica albuginea and penile mucosa, using 3-0 absorbable suture in a simple continuous pattern. Urinary catheterization is maintained for several days postoperatively, as is broad-spectrum antimicrobial coverage (Stead 1972).

Progressive dysuria with or without attendant hematuria is the hallmark of urinary outflow compromise secondary to callus formation in healed fractures of the os penis. Thus chronic fracture of the os penis must always be considered when other more common causes of dysuria, such as urinary calculi, have been excluded. Radiography is the diagnostic modality of choice and may reveal exostoses or masses of soft tissue opacity consistent with an organized hematoma. Contrast retrograde urethrography is useful for determining the degree of urethral obstruction in the area of the lesion.

Surgical remediation of urinary obstruction due to exostoses and organized hematomas secondary to chronic fractures of the os penis may be accomplished through resection of the lateral wall of the urethral groove of the os penis along with callus removal (partial ostectomy), complete removal of the os penis (total ostectomy), or penile amputation and urethrostomy, depending on the size and location of the offending lesion. Partial ostectomy is approached either directly with the penis extruded from the external preputial orifice or through a ventral midline preputiotomy incision. Access to the caudal aspect of the os penis is improved with employment of the latter approach (Hayes *et al.* 1994). Following urethral catheterization, skin and preputial mucosal incisions are made beginning 2 cm caudal to the preputial orifice and extending to 1 cm beyond the caudal end of the os penis. The penis is then delivered through the preputiotomy incision. A temporary tourniquet may be placed on the penis proximal to the surgical site or the dorsal vessels of the penis may be occluded for 10-minute intervals using clamps or ligatures (Stead 1972; Johnston & Archibald 1984). A ventral approach to the os penis is then undertaken via incisions in the penile mucosa, the tunica albuginea, and the erectile tissue of the pars longa glandis and bulbus glandis. At the caudal extent of the incision, the retractor penis muscle is reflected. The urethra is then dissected from the ventral groove of the os penis and one lateral

wall of the groove is freed from surrounding erectile tissue. The urinary catheter is removed and using rongeurs the lateral wall of the groove is removed. Rongeurs are also used to reduce the size of exostoses and to perform a wedge ostectomy to correct deviations of the penis caused by loss of normal architecture of the os. Vascular occlusion is released, the surgical area is assessed for sites of hemorrhage, and ligation is performed as indicated. In order to facilitate identification of the urethra during closure, the urinary catheter may be reinserted. The tunica albuginea is closed using 3-0 absorbable suture in a simple interrupted pattern, the penile mucosa is closed similarly with a simple continuous suture, and the skin of the preputiotomy incision closed using nonabsorbable suture material (Johnston & Archibald 1984).

Highly comminuted fractures of the os penis or recalcitrant urethral obstruction in acute or chronic cases may necessitate penile amputation and urethrostomy. Penile amputation is generally favored over total ostectomy of the os penis, as removal of the os penis in its entirety is technically challenging, may precipitate profuse hemorrhage, and may injure the urethra, resulting in stricture formation and urinary obstruction (Johnston & Archibald 1984). Often penile amputation must be performed just caudal to or at the level of the preputial fornix. Traditionally, scrotal or perineal urethrostomy has been performed in conjunction with radical penile resection. However, a technique for subtotal penile amputation caudal to the fornix has been described, with anastomosis of the urethral mucosa to a caudally translocated preputial orifice creating a preputial urethrostomy. Potential advantages to this procedure over scrotal or perineal urethrostomy include reduction in urine scalding and in the risk for development of ascending urinary tract infection (Pavletic & O'Bell 2007).

Injury to the proximal penis

Injury to the corpus cavernosum and musculature of the proximal penis may result from blunt-force trauma, particularly when exerted in a caudal to cranial direction, as well as nonphysiologic bending of the penis or forced uncoupling during copulation. Clinical signs may include pain referable to the pelvic and/or caudal vertebral regions, stiff hindlimb gait, pain on palpation of the penis proximal to the os, and systemic manifestations such as anorexia and lethargy. Abnormalities of urination may or may not be present. Radiography and retrograde contrast urethrography are useful for ruling out fractures of the os penis and urethral obstruction secondary to calculi or mass impingement, respectively. While ultrasonography of the proximal penis and perineal regions may be used, magnetic resonance imaging of the pelvic cavity and urogenital system is a highly sensitive method for identifying otherwise occult lesions, including hematomas of the proximal corpus cavernosum and musculature of the penile crura. Treatment of hemorrhage in the proximal penis in the absence of lacerations, fractures of the os penis, or other visible trauma is generally nonsurgical and conservative, with provision of cage rest, analgesia, and anti-inflammatory medications. Prognosis for life is very good; however, insufficient clinical data have been gathered to allow evaluation of future breeding soundness in affected dogs (Hicks *et al.* 2007).

Neoplasia of the prepuce and penis

Neoplasia of the prepuce and penis is relatively rare in the dog. Broadly, neoplasia can be divided into tumors affecting the soft tissues of the penis and prepuce and those associated with the os penis.

Neoplasia of the soft tissues

The skin and subcutaneous tissues of the external prepuce may be affected by neoplasia associated with the integument in other body regions. Reported preputial neoplasms include mast cell tumor, papilloma, carcinoma, and glomangioma (Johnston *et al.* 2001; Galofaro *et al.* 2006). The transmissible venereal tumor (TVT) may also affect the prepuce in addition to the penis.

In some cases, tumor resection with adequate margins results in extensive loss of preputial integument. Penile amputation with scrotal urethrostomy has traditionally been performed. However, alternative approaches have been described, including multiple-stage repair utilizing a caudal superficial epigastric artery axial pattern flap and a single procedure using a buccal mucosa graft to reconstruct the preputial mucosa in addition to the aforementioned flap (Castro *et al.* 2017; Massari *et al.* 2018). Successful reconstruction and return to function of the prepuce require catering for contracture, lest paraphimosis may result (Massari *et al.* 2018).

Most reported penile tumors have been documented to be primary; however, metastasis to the penis from remote sites is possible. Lymphosarcoma, hemangiosarcoma, squamous cell carcinoma, and extramedullary plasmacytoma have been identified as primary tumors of the penis proper, with TVT affecting the penile mucosa primarily (Patnaik *et al.* 1988; Michels *et al.* 2001; Agrawal *et al.* 2004; Marolf *et al.* 2006; Gorenstein *et al.* 2016). Chondrosarcoma of the penile urethra has also been reported (Davis & Holt 2003).

Unifying clinical signs of penile neoplasia include stranguria and hematuria progressing to dysuria over weeks to months, urinary bladder distension, abdominal pain, and enlargement of the preputial cavity (Figure 63.2). Penile prolapse was reported to occur in association with lymphosarcoma of the penis in one dog. Passage of a urinary catheter is usually readily accomplished. Plain radiography in addition to retrograde contrast urethrography is useful both to localize the mass lesion and to determine the degree of impingement on the urethra. Thoracic and abdominal radiographs should also be obtained to evaluate whether distant metastases are present prior to pursuing treatment for the penile neoplasm. Depending on the location, extent, and invasiveness of the penile mass, partial or complete penile amputation and urethrostomy may be performed.

Metastasis of neoplasms to the penis is rare but reported (Figure 63.3). However, a case of "malignant priapism" in which metastasis of an undifferentiated car-

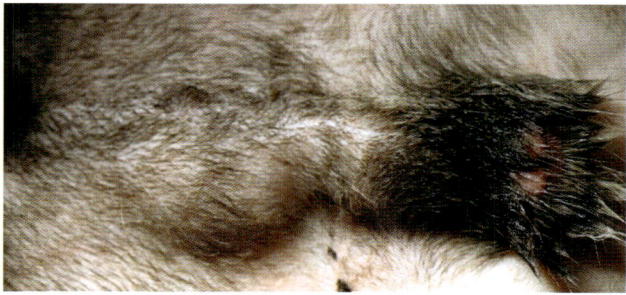

Figure 63.2 Enlarged preputial cavity of a 13-year-old male castrated mixed-breed dog discovered incidentally during routine physical examination.

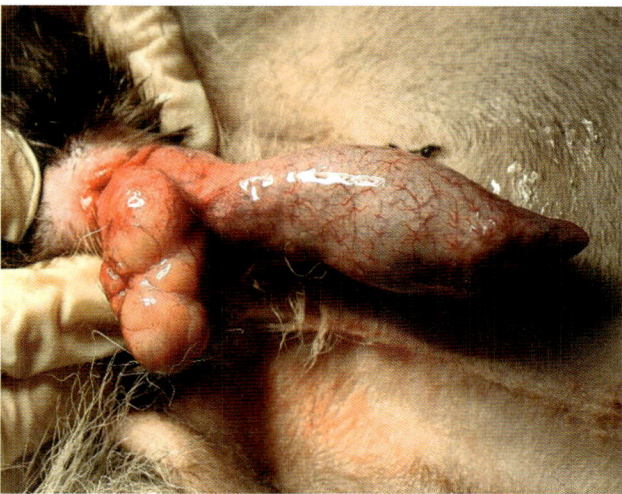

Figure 63.3 Same dog as in Figure 63.1. Penile neoplasm, suspected to be a secondary metastasis of a neuroendocrine tumor associated with the adrenal gland. Presumptive diagnosis was based on cytologic evaluation of a fine-needle aspirate from the mass. Penile amputation with urethrostomy was recommended.

cinoma originating in the urinary bladder or prostate colonized penile vasculature resulting in recalcitrant priapism has been reported (Rogers *et al.* 2002).

TVT is the most common neoplasm affecting the canine preputial and penile mucosa and occurs worldwide, particularly in tropical climates (Ndiritu 1979). Exfoliation and transfer of neoplastic cells during sexual contact form the primary, and highly efficient, mode of transmission. Because the tumor involves primarily mucosal surfaces, stranguria and dysuria are not typically included in the clinical history, unless the urethral orifice is occluded. Instead, intermittent to continuous serosanguineous to purulent preputial discharge, preputial swelling, genital licking, and urinary tract infection are more commonly reported. Presumptive diagnosis is based on appearance of the lesions, which may begin as small, firm nodules and progress to pedunculated, cauliflower-like masses that may ulcerate and bleed. Definitive diagnosis is confirmed based on cytologic evaluation of impression smears, swab samples, and/or fine-needle aspirates. Immunohistochemical analysis allows differentiation of TVT from other round cell tumors (Mozos *et al.* 1996). TVT demonstrates a relatively low rate of metastasis, 17% or less (Rogers *et al.* 1998), and up to 19% of affected animals undergo spontaneous remission (Nayak *et al.* 1987).

Surgical resection of TVT with wide margins is recommended, followed by adjunctive chemotherapy or radiation, as recurrence rates following exclusively surgical remediation may reach 44%. For cases in which there is recurrence, metastasis, or the tumor is not resectable, chemotherapy or radiation therapy is recommended. Single- and multiple-drug protocols have been employed. Monotherapy using vincristine (0.025 mg/kg intravenously once weekly until regression) has been widely utilized. In one study, a median of 5 treatments were required to induce tumor regression; however, up to 16 treatments were necessary to induce complete remission in some cases. Poor response was associated with increased patient age, relatively large tumor volume, and provision of therapy during "hot and rainy" months (Scarpelli *et al.* 2010). Multidrug therapy using a combination of vincristine, cyclophosphamide, and methotrexate administered at weekly intervals has also been demonstrated to be efficacious in inducing regression of localized but nonresectable TVT (Brown *et al.* 1980).

Idiopathic mucosal penile squamous papillomas are solitary, pedunculated, pink, cauliflower-like masses arising from the penile mucosa. These lesions may approach 8 cm in diameter and ulcerate, yet are often completely inapparent. Enlargement of the preputial cavity, genital licking, and intermittent sanguineous preputial discharge that may be misinterpreted as hematuria constitute the most common presenting concerns. Treatment is surgical resection, often via a ventral midline preputiotomy, as the masses are often located on the most caudal extent of the free portion of the penis. The etiology of idiopathic mucosal penile squamous papillomas has been hypothesized to be a reaction to trauma, as no viral antigen has been detected and no evidence of malignant transformation is apparent (Cornegliani *et al.* 2007).

Neoplasia associated with the os penis

Neoplasia of the os penis must be considered as a differential diagnosis for urinary obstruction associated with a mass lesion in the area of the penile bone. Neoplasms reported to affect the os penis include ossifying fibroma, benign mesenchymal tumors, chondrosarcoma, osteosarcoma, and osteochondrosarcoma (Bleier *et al.* 2003; Mirkovic *et al.* 2004; Root Kustritz & Fick 2007; Peppler *et al.* 2009; Webb *et al.* 2009). Hemangiosarcoma associated with the os penis has also been reported (Bolfer *et al.* 2015; Fry *et al.* 2014). Nonneoplastic bone hyperplasia as well as osteomyelitis precipitating hyperostosis may present similarly to neoplasms of the os penis (Maeta *et al.* 2021; Silveira *et al.* 2020). Clinical signs are referable to impingement on the urethra by a mass lesion and include stranguria, dysuria, anuria, hematuria, distension of the urinary bladder, and abdominal pain. Signs of systemic illness may also be apparent, including anorexia, vomiting, and lethargy. Clinicopathologic abnormalities may include postrenal azotemia and uremia. A mass may be palpable in association with the os penis.

Diagnosis is initiated through visualization of the mass by radiography or computed tomography. The os penis may be eroded and evidence of osteolysis present. Thoracic and abdominal radiography should be performed to determine the presence of metastases. Cytologic evaluation of a fine-needle aspirate or excisional biopsy at surgery characterizes the neoplasm. Retrograde urethrography with contrast is performed in order to evaluate the degree of urethral obstruction prior to surgical intervention. Partial or complete penile amputation allows mass removal and urethrostomy provides definitive treatment for urethral obstruction. However, surgical intervention will not be curative if metastases are present at the time of surgery.

References

Agrawal, D.K., Chauhan, R.S., Singh, S.P. et al. (2004). Lymphoma in a male crossbred dog around the bulbar gland of the penis. *Journal of Immunology and Immunopathology* 6: 72–73.

Bleier, T., Lewitschek, H.P., and Reinacher, M. (2003). Canine osteosarcoma of the penile bone. *Journal of Veterinary Medicine A, Physiology, Pathology, Clinical Medicine* 50: 397–398.

Bolfer, L., Schmit, J.M., McNeill, A.L. et al. (2015). Penile amputation and scrotal urethrostomy followed by chemotherapy in a dog with penile hemangiosarcoma. *Journal of the American Animal Hospital Association* 51: 25–30.

Brown, B.G. (1979). Urethroplasty for traumatic loss of the penis: a case report. *Auburn Veterinarian* 36: 22–23.

Brown, N.O., Calvert, C., and MacEwen, E.G. (1980). Chemotherapeutic management of transmissible venereal tumors in 30 dogs. *Journal of the American Veterinary Medical Association* 176: 983–986.

Castro, J.L.C., Huppes, R.R., Sprada, A.G. et al. (2017). Axial pattern flap from the caudal epigastric artery for the correction of surgical defects created by resection of tumors or traumas in cats and dogs: 16 cases (2012–2015). *Journal of Agricultural Science* 9: 170–174.

Cornegliani, L., Vercelli, A., and Abramo, F. (2007). Idiopathic mucosal penile squamous papillomas in dogs. *Veterinary Dermatology* 18: 439–443.

Davis, G.J. and Holt, D. (2003). Two chondrosarcomas in the urethra of a German shepherd dog. *Journal of Small Animal Practice* 44: 169–171.

Elkins, A.D., Pechman, R., Kearney, M.T., and Herron, M. (1990). Urinary obstruction resulting from a mass in the caudal os penis of a dog. *Journal of the American Animal Hospital Association* 26: 133–135.

Esposito, F., Cinti, F., Minci, S., and Pisani, G. (2021). Successful treatment and long-term outcome of a traumatic urethral laceration in a 3-week-old puppy. *Veterinary Record Case Reports* 9: e80.

Fry, J.K., Burney, D., Hottinger, H. et al. (2014). Pollakiuria and stranguria in a Labrador retriever with penile HSA. *Journal of the American Hospital Association* 50: 141–147.

Galofaro, V., Rapisarda, G., Ferrara, G., and Iannelli, N. (2006). Glomangioma in the prepuce of a dog. *Reproduction in Domestic Animals* 41: 568–570.

Gorenstein, T.G., Jark, P.C., Feliciano, M.A.R. et al. (2016). Extramedullary plasmacytoma in the penile bone of a dog: case report. *Brazilian Journal of Veterinary and Animal Sciences* 68: 292–298.

Hayes, A.G., Pavletic, M.M., Schwartz, A., and Boudrieau, R.J. (1994). A preputial splitting technique for surgery of the canine penis. *Journal of the American Animal Hospital Association* 30: 291–295.

Hicks, D.G., Bagley, R.S., Gavin, P.R. et al. (2007). Imaging diagnosis: corpus cavernosum, ischiocavernosus, and bulbospongiosus muscle injury in a dog. *Veterinary Radiology and Ultrasound* 48: 239–242.

Johnston, E.J. and Archibald, J. (1984). Male genital system. In: *Canine and Feline Surgery* (ed. J. Archibald and E.J. Catcott), 293–320. Santa Barbara, CA: American Veterinary Publications.

Johnston, S.D., Root Kustritz, M.V., and Olson, P.N.S. (ed.) (2001). *Canine and Feline Theriogenology*. Philadelphia, PA: WB Saunders.

Kelly, S.E. and Clark, W.T. (1995). Surgical repair of fracture of the os penis in dog. *Journal of Small Animal Practice* 36: 507–509.

Maeta, N., Miyama, T.S., Kutara, K. et al. (2021). Dysuria associated with non-neoplastic bone hyperplasia of the os penis a a pug dog. *Veterinary Sciences* 8: 6–12.

Marolf, A., Specht, A., Thompson, M., and Castleman, W. (2006). Imaging diagnosis: penile hemangiosarcoma. *Veterinary Radiology and Ultrasound* 47: 474–475.

Massari, F., Montinaro, V., Buracco, P., and Romanelli, G. (2018). Combined caudal-superficial-epigastric axial pattern flap and full-thickness buccal mucosa graft for single stage preputial reconstruction in six dogs. *Journal of Small Animal Practice* 59: 415–421.

Michels, G.M., Knapp, D.W., David, M. et al. (2001). Penile prolapse and urethral obstruction secondary to lymphosarcoma of the penis in a dog. *Journal of the American Animal Hospital Association* 37: 474–477.

Mirkovic, T.K., Shmon, C.L., and Allen, A.L. (2004). Urinary obstruction secondary to an ossifying fibroma of the os penis in a dog. *Journal of the American Animal Hospital Association* 40: 152–156.

Mozos, E., Méndez, A., Gómez-Villamandos, J.C. et al. (1996). Immunohistochemical characterization of canine transmissible venereal tumor. *Veterinary Pathology* 33: 257–263.

Nayak, N.C., Nandi, S.N., and Bhownik, N.K. (1987). Canine transmissible venereal tumour (CTVT) with a note on metastasis. *Indian Veterinary Journal* 64: 252–253.

Ndiritu, C.G. (1979). Lesions of the canine penis and prepuce. *Modern Veterinary Practice* 60: 712–715.

Park, J., Cho, K., Han, T. et al. (2007). Replantation of a traumatically amputated penis in a dog. *Journal of Veterinary Clinics* 24: 627–630.

Patnaik, A.K., Matthiesen, D.T., and Zawie, D.A. (1988). Two cases of canine penile neoplasm: squamous cell carcinoma and mesenchymal chondrosarcoma. *Journal of the American Animal Hospital Association* 24: 403–406.

Pavletic, M.M. and O'Bell, S.A. (2007). Subtotal penile amputation and preputial urethrostomy in a dog. *Journal of the American Veterinary Medical Association* 230: 375–377.

Peppler, C., Weissert, D., Kappe, E. et al. (2009). Osteosarcoma of the penile bone (os penis) in a dog. *Australian Veterinary Journal* 87: 52–55.

Petrelli, A., Longo, M., Willems, A., and Liuti, T. (2020). Medical management of a penile fracture with presumed pyelonephritis in a juvenile dog. *Veterinary Record Case Reports* 8: e001176.

Rogers, K.S., Walker, M.A., and Dillon, H.B. (1998). Transmissible venereal tumor: a retrospective study of 29 cases. *Journal of the American Animal Hospital Association* 34: 463–470.

Rogers, L., López, A., and Gillis, A. (2002). Priapism secondary to penile metastasis in a dog. *Canadian Veterinary Journal* 43: 547–549.

Root Kustritz, M.V. and Fick, J.L. (2007). Theriogenology question of the month. Neoplasia of the os penis. *Journal of the American Veterinary Medical Association* 230: 197–198.

Scarpelli, K.C., Valladão, M.L., and Metze, K. (2010). Predictive factors for the regression of canine transmissible venereal tumor during vincristine therapy. *Veterinary Journal (London)* 183: 362–363.

Silveira, B.C., Ribeiro, A.P., Lourenco, L.D. et al. (2020). Chronic osteomyelitis in a canine penile bone: case report. *Brazilian Journal of Veterinary and Animal Sciences* 72: 317–322.

Stead, A.C. (1972). Fracture of the os penis in the dog: two case reports. *Journal of Small Animal Practice* 13: 19–22.

Webb, J.A., Liptak, J.M., Hewitt, S.A., and Vince, A.R. (2009). Multilobular osteochondrosarcoma of the os penis in a dog. *Canadian Veterinary Journal-Revue vétérinaire Canadienne* 50: 81–84.

Section 9

Endocrine

64

Primary Hyperparathyroidism

Nicholas J. Bacon

Historically, primary hyperparathyroidism has been defined as the presence of increased parathyroid hormone (PTH) concentration or PTH in the reference range, in the face of increased ionized serum calcium, in the absence of azotemia, and with one or two enlarged parathyroid glands visualized on ultrasonography or at surgery (Feldman *et al.* 2005; Gear *et al.* 2005; Rasor *et al.* 2007).

Anatomy

The parathyroid glands in dogs and cats are tan-colored ovoid structures closely associated with each thyroid gland. The external parathyroid is cranially located, sitting on the ventral aspect of the thyroid capsule (Hullinger 1993), sometimes even a few millimeters from the capsule in loose fascia. The internal parathyroid is more caudally located, often two-thirds of the distance toward the caudal pole. It can be within the thyroid parenchyma, but is also occasionally found protruding through the parenchyma on the dorsal surface, especially when enlarged. Ultrasound of enlarged glands normally shows them to be located in either the cranial or caudal pole, although in 10% of dogs the gland is present in the mid-body of the thyroid (Wisner *et al.* 1997). A normal parathyroid is approximately 1 mm thick and 5 mm long (Flanders 1993). Dogs and cats have four parathyroid glands and ectopic parathyroid tissue is rare. Embryologically, the glands arise from the third and fourth pharyngeal pouches and remain associated with the thyroid glands. Theoretically, parathyroid tissue can migrate anywhere within the neck down to the heart base and reportedly ectopic parathyroid tissue is present in 35–50% of cats and 6–100% of dogs (Nicholas & Swingle 1925; Reed *et al.* 1928) and this tissue occasionally has become neoplastic (Kishi *et al.* 2014; Erickson *et al.* 2021).

The majority of the blood supply to the thyroid and parathyroid glands comes from the cranial thyroid artery, a branch of the carotid artery (Hullinger 1993). The caudal thyroid artery is a branch of the brachiocephalic artery and is present in most dogs, but this artery is absent in cats (Nicholas & Swingle 1925). The venous drainage of the thyroid and parathyroid is similar to that of the arterial supply, by way of the cranial and caudal thyroid veins. The cranial vein drains into the internal jugular vein, and the caudal vein enters the brachycephalic vein. Lymphatic drainage is by way of the cranial and caudal deep cervical lymph nodes. Efferent lymphatics reach the venous system by way of the right lymphatic duct and left tracheal duct (Hullinger 1993; Radlinsky 2007).

Physiology

PTH release is controlled by calcium receptors on the chief cells in the parathyroid glands in response to hypocalcemia. PTH has a short half-life (3–5 minutes) in serum and so a steady rate of secretion is necessary to maintain serum PTH concentrations (Schenck *et al.* 2006). Natural variations in PTH concentration occur in healthy dogs. Aging is associated with increased concentrations of plasma PTH in dogs (Aguilera-Tejero *et al.* 1998), and a diurnal rhythm in PTH secretion has been identified in dogs, with an early morning peak in PTH observed (López *et al.* 2005).

Small Animal Soft Tissue Surgery, Second Edition. Edited by Eric Monnet.
© 2023 John Wiley & Sons, Inc. Published 2023 by John Wiley & Sons, Inc.
Companion website: www.wiley.com/go/monnet/small

PTH elevates plasma calcium concentration directly by mobilizing calcium from the bone and increasing urinary phosphate excretion (Ganong 2001), and indirectly through its actions on the intestine mediated through vitamin D_3 (Sutton & Dirks 1986). Serum calcium exists in three fractions: protein bound (40%), complexed to phosphate, citrate, sulfate, lactate, or bicarbonate (10%), and ionized. Ionized calcium (iCa) comprises approximately 50% of serum total calcium and is the most biologically active fraction. It is fluctuations in iCa that directly affect PTH release (Forman & Lorenzo 1991; Ganong 2001).

Almost all (99%) of total body calcium is stored with phosphorus in the bone and PTH mobilizes calcium rapidly from the bone by acting on osteoblasts, and then in a sustained fashion through action on osteocytes. The action of PTH on osteoblasts causes release of osteoclast-stimulating factor, resulting in a rapid degradation of bone by osteoclasts and subsequent increase in serum calcium and phosphorus. PTH also increases differentiation of macrophage precursors into more osteoclasts (Bonczynski 2007). The more sustained osteocyte activity is again in direct response to PTH and it results in calcium and phosphorus being released from the bone matrix crystals hydroxyapatite and calcium phosphate. The action of PTH on osteocytes is potentiated synergistically by 1,25-dihydroxy-vitamin D_3 (Reeve & Zanelli 1986; Sutton & Dirks 1986; Flanders 1993).

Vitamin D exists in two forms: cholecalciferol (vitamin D_3) in animals, and ergocalciferol (vitamin D_2) predominantly in plants. Cholecalciferol can be produced in the skin of most mammals from the activation of the provitamin 7-dehydrocholesterol by ultraviolet light, although dogs and cats can synthesize less cholecalciferol in the skin than many other mammals (Gross et al. 2000; Mellanby et al. 2005; Schenck et al. 2006). Dietary vitamin D is transported to the liver and metabolized to 25-hydroxyvitamin D_3 (cholecalciferol) by the liver. PTH then potentiates hydroxylation of 25-hydroxyvitamin D_3 in the kidneys to 1,25-dihydroxyvitamin D_3 (calcitriol). Calcitriol is the most active metabolite and causes a 100-fold increase in bone calcium resorption, enhances intestinal calcium and phosphorus absorption threefold compared with cholecalciferol, and increases calcium resorption in the kidney (Gross et al. 2000; Flanders 2003). Hydroxylation of cholecalciferol to calcitriol is inhibited by hypercalcemia, hyperphosphatemia, excess calcitriol, and absence of PTH (Flanders 2003).

The increase in calcium absorption across the small intestinal mucosa is affected by a combination of actions, mediated by vitamin D_3: increased permeability of cell membranes to calcium, production of intracellular calcium-binding proteins in the enterocytes of the duodenum and jejunum, and increased activity of a membrane-bound calcium/magnesium pump that transports calcium out of the cell and into the blood (Sutton & Dirks 1986; Flanders 1993).

PTH directly increases serum calcium concentration by increasing the rate of calcium reabsorption in the distal renal tubules. PTH has no effect on the proximal tubules, where calcium is reabsorbed by diffusion. However, PTH does inhibit reabsorption of phosphorus in the proximal renal tubules, leading to increased phosphorus excretion (Morrow & Volmer 2002; Flanders 2003; Schenck et al. 2006).

Calcitonin antagonizes PTH and is secreted by the C cells of the thyroid gland in response to hypercalcemia. It reduces plasma calcium concentration by reducing its absorption from the bone by inhibiting osteoclasts (Ganong 2001; Schenck et al. 2006). Calcitonin will also inhibit renal phosphorus reabsorption and increase calcium reabsorption (Flanders 2003). PTH synthesis and secretion are also inhibited in the face of elevated serum calcium by a negative feedback loop to the parathyroid glands.

History and clinical signs

Primary hyperparathyroidism is rare, comprising 0.5% cases referred to one large academic institution (Blois et al. 2011). Dogs with primary hyperparathyroidism have a median age of 9.3 years (Gear et al. 2005) and a mean age of 11.8 years (Feldman & Nelson 2004; Feldman et al. 2005; Ham et al. 2009), although a recent paper of 100 dogs with parathyroid carcinoma had an older median age of 11 years (Erickson et al. 2021). Mean body weight is 18–22.2 kg (Feldman et al. 2005; Ham et al. 2009). Reportedly Labrador retrievers, golden retrievers, and German shepherd dogs are at increased risk (Feldman et al. 2005), but other papers have found mixed breeds to be more affected (Erickson et al. 2021) and a familial predisposition in keeshonden has been described (DeVries et al. 1993), with this breed comprising 19–40% of affected animals in several studies (Feldman et al. 2005; Goldstein et al. 2007; Rasor et al. 2007). Primary hyperparathyroidism is an autosomal-dominant, genetically transmitted disease in keeshonden, although the gene mutations responsible have yet to be identified (Goldstein et al. 2007; Skelly & Franklin 2007). In one study, 14% were German shepherd dogs and 14% keeshonden, the latter being closely related dogs (Gear et al. 2005). No sex predisposition is seen (Feldman et al. 2005; Gear et al. 2005; Erickson et al. 2021).

All clinical signs associated with primary hyperparathyroidism are related to the hypercalcemia secondary to the elevation in PTH. With an increasing number of "wellness" examinations being performed in an ever-aging population of pets, asymptomatic hypercalcemic patients are being diagnosed more commonly and reportedly 21–42% of cases are incidental findings (Feldman *et al.* 2005; Gear *et al.* 2005; Rasor *et al.* 2007; Ham *et al.* 2009). Sometimes years can pass between the onset of clinical signs or the diagnosis of hypercalcemia and treatment (Sawyer *et al.* 2012; Guttin *et al.* 2015).

If the animal is symptomatic, clinical signs are normally vague and nonspecific (Wisner *et al.* 1997), the majority of cases having an insidious onset (Gear *et al.* 2005). Polyuria and polydipsia are well-recognized clinical signs, the former caused by hypercalcemia reducing expression of aquaporin-2 (a vasopressin-regulated water channel) in the renal collecting ducts (Earm *et al.* 1998). Lethargy, weakness, vomiting, diarrhea, inappetence, weight loss, tremors, and stiffness are common (Berger & Feldman 1987; Gear *et al.* 2005), and in up to 50% of dogs, signs consistent with urolithiasis or urinary tract infections had been observed for days or months (DeVries *et al.* 1993; Feldman *et al.* 2005; Gear *et al.* 2005). Occasionally dogs present with pathologic fractures, presumably due to osteolysis from chronically elevated PTH, but with earlier detection this is becoming increasingly rare (Gear *et al.* 2005).

The masses themselves are typically less than 10 mm in diameter and thus symptoms due to the physical presence of the mass in the neck are rare (Berger & Feldman 1987; DeVries *et al.* 1993; Feldman *et al.* 1997; Sawyer *et al.* 2012). In fact, 71% of dogs with primary hyperparathyroidism have no obvious abnormalities observed on clinical examination (Feldman *et al.* 2005).

Information about the animal's diet should be part of the history, as calcium can be increased if the animal is on calcium supplements, calcium-rich phosphate binders, or vitamin D supplements (Bonczynski 2007). Some commercial dog foods have also been found to contain vitamin D concentrations over 100 times higher than that stated on the manufacturer's data sheet (Mellanby *et al.* 2005).

Primary hyperparathyroidism is rare in cats, with few cases described to date. It is associated with a mean age of 13.3 years, mean weight of 4.9 kg, and 62.5% are domestic shorthair cats. Clinical signs are reportedly lethargy (56%), anorexia (53%), vomiting (41%), weight loss (31%), polyuria (19%), polydipsia (16%), and diarrhea (9%). Unlike dogs, a mass or thyroid slip was palpable on the ventral neck in 37.5% cases, with the masses ranging from 2 to 20 mm in diameter (Kallet *et al.* 1991; Marquez *et al.* 1995; den Hertog *et al.* 1997; Reimer *et al.* 2005; Garrett *et al.* 2007; Sellon *et al.* 2009; Singh *et al.* 2018).

Diagnosis

Hematology

In most cases this is unremarkable. Mild anemia and mild polycythemia are seen only rarely (Feldman *et al.* 2005; Gear *et al.* 2005).

Serum chemistry

An elevation in iCa concentration is the most sensitive means of detecting hypercalcemia. One recent study defined hypercalcemia as iCa above 1.33 mmol/L (reference range 1.13–1.33 mmol/L) (Messinger *et al.* 2009), and in dogs with primary hyperparathyroidism the reported range is 1.48–2.55 mmol/L, with a median of 1.89 mmol/L (Gear *et al.* 2005; Ham *et al.* 2009) and a mean of 1.67–1.71 mmol/L (Feldman *et al.* 2005; Ham *et al.* 2009). An elevated reading should always be validated by a second sample and it has been suggested that sampling should be at least 30 days apart (Feldman *et al.* 2005). Most routine serum chemistry profiles report total calcium, which also includes protein-bound and complexed forms (Messinger *et al.* 2009). Total calcium and iCa may be poorly correlated in a patient. Equations using the dog's serum albumin to "correct" total protein to more accurately estimate iCa have proven inaccurate (Meuten *et al.* 1982a; Finco 1983; Messinger *et al.* 2009).

Hypergammaglobulinemia secondary to inflammatory conditions will also affect total calcium (LeBlanc *et al.* 2008). The calcium ion binds to the increased number of negatively charged globulins, resulting in an increased total calcium concentration but an iCa concentration within the reference range (Stockham & Scott 2002). A monoclonal β-gammopathy in association with primary hyperparathyroidism and hypercalcemia has also been reported, which decreased following the removal of a parathyroid adenoma (Benchekroun *et al.* 2009).

A diagnosis of hypercalcemia using total calcium is made if the concentration is 12 mg/dL or more (reference range 9.9–11.4 mg/dL) (Feldman *et al.* 2005). Total calcium elevation is often 2.97–5.83 mmol/L, median 3.47 mmol/L (Gear *et al.* 2005), or 12.1–23.4 mg/dL, mean 14.5 mg/dL; 48% of dogs had calcium greater than 14 mg/dL (Feldman *et al.* 2005).

Primary hyperparathyroidism comprises only 13% of cases of ionized hypercalcemia, with 58% being neoplasia (predominantly lymphoma and various carcinomas) and 17% being chronic or acute renal failure (Messinger *et al.* 2009). A recent review of the malignancy-associated causes comprised lymphoma (38%), unknown (22%), anal sac carcinoma (12%), other carcinomas (10%), bone neoplasia (7%), sarcoma (5%), multiple myeloma

(3%), leukemia (2%), and thymoma (1%). Dogs presenting with *ionized* hypercalcemia that is moderate to severe (>1.5 mmol/L) are significantly more likely to have primary hyperparathyroidism, malignancy-associated hypercalcemia, or hypervitaminosis D (Coady *et al.* 2019). In studies with *total* serum calcium, dogs with primary hyperparathyroidism had significantly lower concentrations than dogs with neoplasia (Kruger *et al.* 1996), but dogs with primary hyperparathyroidism, lymphoma, and anal sac adenocarcinoma had higher serum total calcium than dogs with chronic renal failure or vitamin D toxicosis (Feldman *et al.* 2005).

Serum inorganic phosphorus should be evaluated, as an elevation in both calcium and phosphorus is suggestive of renal failure or vitamin D toxicosis (Feldman *et al.* 2005). However, in primary hyperparathyroidism, phosphate concentration is more likely to be normal or decreased (Gear *et al.* 2005). A concomitant hypophosphatemia is seen in up to 65% of cases, with 98% of dogs being below the lower half of the reference limit (Feldman *et al.* 2005). Alkaline phosphatase is increased in 48–50% of dogs, urea is elevated in 37–47%, creatinine is elevated in 3–36%, and cholesterol elevated in 41% (DeVries *et al.* 1993; Feldman *et al.* 2005; Gear *et al.* 2005). These values must be taken in the context that some dogs were pretreated with glucocorticoids or were subsequently diagnosed with hyperadrenocorticism.

Cats presenting with *ionized* hypercalcemia that is moderate to severe (>1.6 mmol/L) are significantly more likely to have malignancy-associated hypercalcemia or idiopathic hypercalcemia (Coady *et al.* 2019).

Urinalysis

The mean urine specific gravity is 1.012 (range 1.006–1.017) (DeVries *et al.* 1993) and is significantly more dilute than in "normal" control dogs. Urine culture can be positive in 29% of dogs, often in association with cystic calculi (Feldman *et al.* 2005).

Parathyroid hormone assays

Intact PTH concentration is best determined using the two-site immunoradiometric assay, which has been validated for use in dogs (Torrance & Nachreiner 1989a,b). The test typically takes several days before results are available and a "point-of-care" assay has recently been described in dogs (Ham *et al.* 2009), although this is expensive and currently poorly available to veterinary patients. However, accurate results are available 10–20 minutes after blood sampling (Ham *et al.* 2009).

The upper limit of the PTH reference range is 13–17 pmol/L (Feldman *et al.* 2005; Ham *et al.* 2009). In order to diagnose primary hyperparathyroidism in the face of hypercalcemia, one study required PTH to be in the upper half of the reference range or higher (Messinger *et al.* 2009), although in one study of 210 dogs, 73% had a serum PTH concentration within the reference range (Feldman *et al.* 2005). In this study mean PTH concentration was 11.3 pmol/L (range 2.3–121 pmol/L). In one study of 29 dogs with primary hyperparathyroidism, PTH values ranged from 57 to 680 pg/mL (median 167.5 pg/mL). No correlation could be detected between PTH and total or ionized calcium (Gear *et al.* 2005). If ionized calcium is high and the phosphate is low, renal secondary hyperparathyroidism cannot be ruled out (Feldman 2000). Elevated PTH has also been identified in up to 92–95% dogs with hyperadrenocorticism, but these cases are not hypercalcemic (Ramsey 2001; Ramsey *et al.* 2005; Tebb *et al.* 2005). The term "adrenal secondary hyperparathyroidism" has been suggested for these dogs (Ramsey *et al.* 2005).

Feldman *et al.* (1997) investigated whether comparing the level of intact PTH from each jugular vein could be used to accurately localize the primary parathyroid tumor. In only 8% of dogs was the serum PTH from the jugular vein ipsilateral to the parathyroid tumor greater than that from the contralateral vein. In 92% the concentrations were similar and not helpful in localizing abnormal parathyroid tissue. A more recent study using a "point-of-care" analyzer in dogs with unilateral disease found that PTH concentration on the affected side was much higher than that on the unaffected side in only 43% of dogs (Ham *et al.* 2009), again suggesting that this was not a useful differentiating test.

The reference range for PTH in cats is lower than that for dogs at 0–4 pmol/L (Reimer *et al.* 2005). In one study of 26 cats with hyperparathyroidism, 77% had a PTH above the reference range, and 23% were within the normal reference range. PTH had a median value of 9.7 pmol/L (interquartile range 3.8–17.0) (Singh *et al.* 2018)

Diagnostic imaging
Ultrasound

Since most hyperfunctioning parathyroid tissue occurs in the normal location of the parathyroid glands, cervical ultrasound is economical and readily available, and so is commonly the first line of imaging modality. It detected a parathyroid nodule in 100% dogs in one study (Feldman *et al.* 1997, 2005; Erickson *et al.* 2021). Normal parathyroid glands in healthy dogs range from 2 to 4.6 mm in diameter when imaged ultrasonographically, with a strong positive correlation between diameter and body weight (Wisner *et al.* 1997; Wisner & Nyland 1998; Reusch *et al.* 2000; Benchekroun *et al.* 2009). Ultrasound can detect nodules >2.1 mm diameter. In a study of 23 normal dogs, the largest parathyroid gland measured

3 mm in dogs weighing less than 10 kg, 3.5 mm in dogs weighing 10–19 kg, 4 mm in dogs weighing 20–29 kg, and 4.6 mm in dogs weighing over 30 kg. Two to four glands are normally visible, with all four glands normally visible in dogs over 30 kg (Reusch et al. 2000; Liles et al. 2010). Multiple structures as well as ultrasound artifacts can be misinterpreted as parathyroid tissue including cysts, follicular adenomas, thyroid lobules, and lymphoid tissue. In one study on 10 cadavers, of 35 structures presumed to be parathyroid glands on ultrasound, only 26 (74% positive predictive values) were parathyroid tissue when all glands were examined histologically (Liles et al. 2010). Ultrasound examination is normally performed with a 10 MHz sector scanning transducer or a 7.5–10 MHz linear array transducer, and abnormal parathyroid tissue is typically round or oval and anechoic or hypoechoic compared with surrounding thyroid parenchyma (Wisner & Nyland 1998) (Figure 64.1). They are typically well-defined structures and this becomes more apparent with increasing size. In a study of 142 parathyroid masses, the median greatest diameter was 6 mm (range 3–23 mm) (Feldman et al. 2005) and neoplastic lesions (median diameter 5.5–8 mm, range 2–25 mm) typically are significantly larger than hyperplastic glands (median 2 mm, range 2–6 mm), regardless of whether the hyperplasia is primary or secondary (Wisner et al. 1997; Sawyer et al. 2012; Erickson et al. 2021), although it is not advisable to use ultrasonographic findings alone to differentiate hyperplasia from neoplasia as there is much overlap between groups (Secrest & Grimes 2019). In 70–100% of dogs, a solitary parathyroid nodule is identified, with up to 13–25% of dogs having two abnormally large glands and less than 5% having three or more nodules (Feldman et al. 2005; Gear et al. 2005; Rasor et al. 2007; Ham et al. 2009; Burkhardt et al. 2021; Erickson et al. 2021).

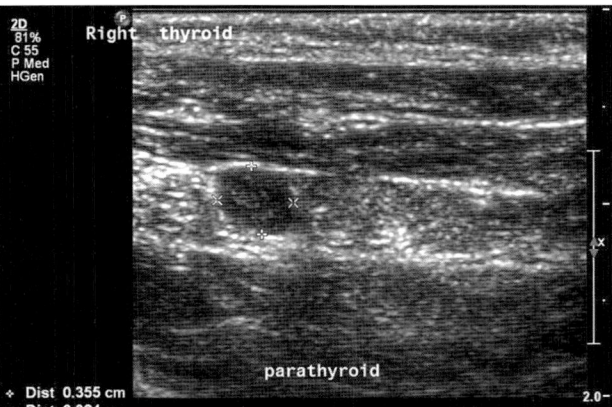

Figure 64.1 Ultrasound image showing oval hypoechoic parathyroid gland at the cranial end of the thyroid gland.

The side identified correlates to surgical findings in up to 72–93% of dogs (Gear et al. 2005; Burkhardt et al. 2021). However, ultrasonography is operator dependent and the skill of the individual performing the examination is a major factor in the value of this test (Feldman et al. 1997).

Up to 47% of dogs in one study had concurrent renal abnormalities on ultrasound, including renal calculi, hyperechogenic cortices, and pyelectasia (Gear et al. 2005). The only consistent abnormality identified during abdominal radiography and ultrasonography in 210 dogs was cystic calculi in 24% (Feldman et al. 2005).

Parathyroid masses can be up to 12 mm in diameter in cats (Reimer et al. 2005), but ultrasound examination of feline parathyroids is more difficult and therefore unreliable. In one study 92% of cats had at least one mass, nodule, or enlargement associated with the thyroid or parathyroid glands (Singh et al. 2018), but in another study 0–6 hypoechoic nodules per thyroid were identified in cat cadavers, and 0–3 nodules in the thyroids of clinically healthy cats, neither of which is consistent with the known normal anatomy of cats. This caused the authors to conclude that parathyroids may not be ultrasonographically observable in healthy cats, or may be indistinguishable from thyroid tissue. A normal reference range for feline parathyroid size in healthy cats as determined by ultrasound is therefore unknown (Woods et al. 2017).

Nuclear medicine

A dog has been diagnosed with primary hyperparathyroidism following a thyroid technetium scan that demonstrated a defect in the posterior pole of the left thyroid, subsequently confirmed by surgery (van Vonderen et al. 2003).

Double-phase parathyroid scintigraphy using ^{99m}Tc-sestamibi has shown to be successful in humans for preoperative localization of hyperfunctioning parathyroid tissue with high accuracy (sensitivity >90%), reliability, and an 82% true-positive rate (Gotway et al. 2002; Elaraj et al. 2010), but it has proven to be disappointing in dogs. Parathyroid scintigraphy correctly identified the presence and location of hyperfunctioning parathyroid tissue in only one of six dogs with a parathyroid adenoma, with many false negative results (Matwichuk et al. 2000).

Magnetic resonance imaging

In humans, magnetic resonance imaging (MRI) is used in patients with persistent or recurrent hyperparathyroidism, in whom it has been shown to be effective in locating remaining abnormal parathyroid tissue, especially in the area of the trachea, esophagus, and cranial mediastinum. A 90% accuracy has been reported in detection of parathyroid adenomas in the human neck as small as 0.5 cm prior to neck exploration (Hamilton et al. 1988). In instances in which no neck lesion is identified or an ectopic parathyroid gland is suspected, electrocardiogram (ECG)-gated axial images of the mediastinum can be effective (Johnson et al. 2007). In most cases, abnormal parathyroid tissue demonstrates isointense to low signal intensity relative to muscle on T1-weighted images, with increased signal intensity typically present on T2-weighted images. Intense contrast enhancement is frequently observed (Gotway et al. 2001).

There is a case report of a functional metastatic parathyroid adenocarcinoma being identified preoperatively by MRI in the mediastinum of a dog, which was persistently hypercalcemic despite two previous neck surgeries with all detectable parathyroid tissue removed. The MRI appearance was heterogeneous enhancement, with numerous low-signal intensity foci within the tissue. The mass was heterogeneously enhanced following intravenous gadolinium contrast administration (Kishi et al. 2014).

The role of MRI in veterinary patients has yet to be further elucidated, in part due limited spatial resolution in cats and most dogs (Taeymans et al. 2008).

Computed tomography

Computed tomography (CT) has been used in humans both to identify abnormally intensely enhancing parathyroid glands with 46–87% sensitivity, and to describe space-occupying masses and invasion of vital vasculature in mediastinal masses (Gotway et al. 2002; Yoon et al. 2004).

In healthy dogs with normal parathyroids, the mean size is $4.2 \times 2.5 \times 2.9$ mm, but they are not reliably identifiable. When they are visible, the CT dimensions appear larger than would be expected, suggesting that visibility on CT does not imply parathyroid disease (Lautscam et al. 2020). A report of four dogs undergoing CT identified nodules 3–50 mm in diameter (Erickson et al. 2021).

The CT findings in three cats have been described and a mass was found in the area of thyroid/parathyroid in all cases (Singh et al. 2018).

Differential diagnosis

Some of the disorders associated with hypercalcemia include lymphoma (Meuten et al. 1982a; Weir et al. 1986; Kubota et al. 2002), apocrine gland adenocarcinoma of the anal sac (Meuten et al. 1982b; Hobson et al. 2006), hypervitaminosis D (Gunther et al. 1988; Mellanby et al. 2005), acute and chronic renal failure, multiple

myeloma, thymoma (Foley et al. 2000), melanoma (Pressler et al. 2002), hypoadrenocorticism (Willard et al. 1982), mycosis (Dow et al. 1986), and idiopathic hypercalcemia of cats (Midkiff et al. 2000).

Hypercalcemia of malignancy: parathyroid hormone-related protein

Dogs with neoplasms, especially lymphoma, apocrine gland adenocarcinoma of the anal sac, or multiple myeloma, comprise 58% of dogs with ionized hypercalcemia (Messinger et al. 2009) and are typically hypercalcemic due to the synthesis and secretion of parathyroid hormone-related protein (PTHrP) by the tumor. This has polypeptide segments that are homologous to native PTH and that cause hypercalcemia by increasing bone resorption and the renal tubular reabsorption of calcium (Rosol & Capen 1988; Strewler 2000).

PTHrP is measured by an immunoradiometric two-site assay and in normal healthy dogs lies within the reference range (0.3–1.0 pmol/L). Dogs with hypercalcemia due to lymphoma have an elevated PTHrP (median 5.05 pmol/L, range 0.5–16.0 pmol/L) and PTH below the reference range in most but not all cases (Mellanby et al. 2006). This is presumably due to suppression of PTH secretion by the negative feedback effects of high concentrations of calcium and PTHrP (Motellón et al. 2000). A similar relationship between ionized calcium, PTHrP, and PTH was seen in hypercalcemic dogs with adenocarcinoma of the apocrine gland of the anal sac.

PTHrP in seven hypercalcemic dogs with parathyroid adenoma was within the reference range. PTHrP in two hypercalcemic dogs with parathyroid carcinoma was greater than the reference range in both cases, at 1.8 and 8.1 pmol/L, all nine dogs also having the expected elevations in PTH (Mellanby et al. 2006).

Such elevations in both PTH and PTHrP in hypercalcemic dogs are rare. Other possibilities include a dog with primary hyperparathyroidism also having an additional malignancy secreting PTHrP. An association between primary hyperparathyroidism and a secondary malignancy is well recognized in people and has occasionally been described in dogs and cats, including a dog with simultaneous primary hyperparathyroidism and multiple myeloma (Strodel et al. 1988; Hutcheson et al. 1995; Walker et al. 2000; Sztukowski et al. 2021). Another possibility is the rare example of a tumor producing both PTH and PTHrP (Uchimura et al. 2002). Malignancies growing within the bone marrow and metastasis of solid tumors to the skeleton are other possible causes.

When measured in 12 cats with hyperparathyroidism, PTHrP was 0.0 pmol/L in all cases (Singh et al. 2018).

Multiple endocrine neoplasia syndrome

A patient with hyperplasia or neoplasia in two or more endocrine glands simultaneously is rare, but is occasionally seen with parathyroid tumors. Only two of the four recognized multiple endocrine neoplasia (MEN) patterns involve the parathyroid gland. MEN type 1 (MEN 1) consists of tumors of the parathyroid gland, pancreatic islets, anterior pituitary gland, and less commonly adrenal cortical tumors. This has been rarely reported in dogs. MEN type 2 (specifically MEN 2A) consists of medullary thyroid carcinoma, unilateral or bilateral pheochromocytoma, and a parathyroid tumor. Parathyroid adenoma, bilateral pheochromocytoma, and medullary thyroid carcinoma has been described in a Rottweiler (Soler Arias *et al.* 2016) and one study found that 3% of dogs with parathyroid carcinoma had MEN 2 syndrome (Erickson *et al.* 2021). In this study 18% of dogs were also found to have adrenal abnormalities on abdominal ultrasonography, which might have underestimated the number of pheochromocytoma, adrenal cortical tumors, and pituitary tumors in this population.

MEN type 1 has been described in a cat (Reimer *et al.* 2005).

Hypoadrenocorticism

Hypercalcemia is seen in 18–30% of dogs with hypoadrenocorticism (Peterson *et al.* 1996; Adler *et al.* 2007). Furthermore, it is an important differential diagnosis for hypercalcemia, as it is the cause in 5–25% of hypercalcemic dogs (Elliott *et al.* 1991; Messinger *et al.* 2009). In a recent study of eight dogs with hypoadrenocorticism, four of five dogs with ionized hypercalcemia had a PTH concentration within the reference range (Gow *et al.* 2009) and it was concluded that hypercalcemia associated with spontaneous hypoadrenocorticism is independent of PTH. The exact pathogenesis of the hypercalcemia is not clear. Possibilities include decreased glomerular filtration, increased tubular calcium reabsorption, excessive intestinal absorption of calcium, and increased bone resorption (Walser *et al.* 1963; Hahn *et al.* 1981; Walker & Davies 1981).

Hypervitaminosis D

The parathyroid glands in healthy dogs are relatively inactive, possibly the result of the relatively large amount of vitamin D in commercial dog food (Kallfelz & Dzanis 1989) and cases of hypercalcemia through dietary oversupplementation have been reported (Mellanby *et al.* 2005). Hypervitaminosis D as a cause of ionized hypercalcemia is rare, comprising only 3% of dogs (Messinger *et al.* 2009), but is most commonly seen secondary to ingestion of either rodenticides containing cholecalciferol or anti-psoriatic ointments that contain vitamin D analogues. Hypervitaminosis D has been reported following treatment of hypoparathyroidism.

Renal failure

Chronic renal failure is commonly associated with hyperparathyroidism through parathyroid gland hyperplasia (Flanders 2003). Increased serum phosphorus concentration, decreased 1,25-dihydroxyvitamin D_3 concentration (because of fewer functional nephrons to hydroxylate cholecalciferol to calcitriol), greater skeletal resistance to the calcemic effects of PTH, and elevation of the serum calcium "set point" for inhibition of PTH are all possible explanations for parathyroid hypersecretion (Feinfeld & Sherwood 1988; Flanders 2003). Most dogs and cats with renal failure have a normal or low concentration of serum calcium, but 10–20% of dogs have mild to moderate hypercalcemia (Feldman 1995) and they comprise 17% of dogs with ionized hypercalcemia (Messinger *et al.* 2009). The exact reason some chronic renal failure patients with secondary hyperparathyroidism become hypercalcemic is not known (Coburn & Slatopolsky 1986). The reason most cats and dogs are normocalcemic or hypocalcemic in the face of hyperparathyroidism may be due to low 1,25-dihydroxyvitamin D_3 decreasing intestinal calcium absorption, the calcemic effect of PTH on bone, a reduction in functional renal tubule cells to reabsorb calcium, and hyperphosphatemia (Feinfeld & Sherwood 1988; Flanders 2003).

The prevalence of hyperparathyroidism in cats with azotemic chronic kidney disease is as high as 84% (Barber & Elliott 1998), and the PTH of those that subsequently develop azotemia is significantly higher than those that remain nonazotemic; that is, renal secondary hyperparathyroidism can precede azotemia. This occurs even in the absence of hyperphosphatemia and hypocalcemia (Finch *et al.* 2012).

Up to 77% of hyperthyroid cats have elevated PTH concentrations (Barber & Elliott 1996), and this can result in calcification of soft tissues, including the kidney, which may cause progression of chronic kidney disease. Dietary phosphate restriction, which decreases PTH concentration, has been shown to prolong the survival of cats with chronic kidney disease (Barber & Elliott 1996; Elliott *et al.* 2000).

Granulomatous/inflammatory

This was the final diagnosis in 4% of dogs with ionized hypercalcemia (Messinger *et al.* 2009). It is believed to be due to extrarenal synthesis of calcitriol (1,25-dihydroxyvitamin D_3) by activated macrophages (Sharma 2000; Mellanby *et al.* 2006; LeBlanc *et al.* 2008).

Removal of the granulomatous or inflammatory process tends to result in rapid normocalcemia (LeBlanc et al. 2008). In one study of 38 dogs with blastomycosis, only 5% had ionized hypercalcemia and 95% were normocalcemic. When total calcium is measured, 2.5–6.4% of dogs are hypercalcemic (Legendre et al. 1981; Crews et al. 2007).

Surgical therapy

Exploratory surgery with parathyroidectomy in dogs with primary hyperparathyroidism serves as both a diagnostic test and definitive therapy (Wisner et al. 1997). Surgical exploration of the neck is warranted in a hypercalcemic dog with inappropriate levels of PTH and the absence of PTHrP, even with normal cervical ultrasound findings, as occasionally enlarged glands are identified at surgery that had not been detected by preoperative ultrasound (Ham et al. 2009). Surgery should be advocated to reduce the risk of urolithiasis and urinary tract infection (DeVries et al. 1993), as well as improving the clinical signs seen with hypercalcemia such as polydipsia, polyuria, weakness, and decreased appetite (Feldman et al. 2005). Surgical time is reduced by accurate preoperative planning to localize the abnormal gland(s) and morbidity is reduced by familiarity with the local anatomy and an appropriate postoperative plan. With appropriate treatment the prognosis can be excellent (Berger & Feldman 1987).

Preoperative considerations: hypercalcemia

Preoperative treatment of hypercalcemia is contentious and there are no published standards (Bonczynski 2007). Recommendations exist in patients with serum calcium levels greater than 14 mg/dL, or if calcium-associated neurologic or cardiac signs exist, or if azotemia is present. If these conditions are present, then intravenous fluid therapy should be started 12–24 hours before surgery, ideally with 0.9% saline. During diuresis, care is taken not to overhydrate the patient and packed cell volume, total protein, weight, and respiratory rate are monitored twice daily. If hypercalcemia persists despite rehydration and diuresis, renal calcium excretion can be encouraged with furosemide at 2–4 mg/kg every 8–12 hours (Vasilopulos 2003; Schenck et al. 2006).

Calcitonin is effective for rapidly reducing serum calcium concentrations (Flanders 2003). Isolated case examples of its use to treat hypercalcemia exist in veterinary medicine; hypervitaminosis D has been treated with salmon calcitonin at a dose of 4.5 units/kg subcutaneously every 8 hours in a dog (Dougherty et al. 1990), and 4 units/kg intramuscularly was used successfully in a cat (Peterson et al. 1991).

Bisphosphonates are used as standard of care in human oncology to treat hypercalcemia of malignancy (Fan 2007). Their main mechanism of action is inhibition of bone resorption by reduction of osteoclast activities and induction of osteoclast apoptosis (programmed cell death) (Body 1998), thereby reducing serum calcium levels. However, bisphosphonates do not affect the increased renal tubular reabsorption seen with elevations in PTH and PTHrP (Rizzoli et al. 1992; Chisholm et al. 1996), and so dogs with primary hyperparathyroidism or with hypercalcemia and great elevations in PTHrP may respond less favorably to bisphosphonate therapy (Walls et al. 1994). The use of bisphosphonates to reduce serum calcium concentrations in tumor-bearing dogs and cats is poorly documented (Fan 2007). Published work has mostly concerned animals with hypercalcemia secondary to excessive PTHrP (not PTH) treated with intravenous saline diuresis and diuretics (Kadar et al. 2004; Fan et al. 2005; Hostutler et al. 2005). One study showed that clodronate could reduce hypercalcemia following experimental vitamin D toxicosis in dogs (Ulutas et al. 2006).

To prevent acute hypocalcemia after surgery, some authors have also recommended supplementing dogs preoperatively with vitamin D if total calcium is 14 mg/dL or higher, for example with dihydrotachysterol and calcium gluconate (Feldman 2005), with alfacalcidol (0.05 μg/kg) the day before surgery with or without calcium gluconate (Gear et al. 2005), or with calcitriol (20 ng/kg per day orally starting 1–2 days before surgery) (Ham et al. 2009). However, this preoperative treatment has not been shown to prevent hypocalcemia after surgery.

Surgical technique

Following a wide ventral neck clip, the patient is positioned in dorsal recumbency with the neck outstretched and a sandbag placed beneath it for further extension. The forelimbs are pulled caudally and tied in place. A ventral midline skin incision is made from the level of the larynx cranially midway to the manubrium caudally. The sphincter colli muscles are incised to expose the longitudinal fibers of the paired sternohyoideus muscles (Radlinsky 2007). Dissection is continued through the midline of sternohyoideus and sternothyroideus. The thyroid glands lie in the peritracheal fascia medial to the thyrohyoideus muscle. Locally, the recurrent laryngeal nerve and carotid sheath (containing the vagus nerve and carotid artery and vein) should be identified. Each parathyroid–thyroid complex is inspected separately. If necessary, a blunt-ended Gelpi retractor can be placed between the cranial trachea and neck muscles to help expose each thyroid. Preoperative ultrasound will guide the surgeon toward one side or the other, but it is imperative that every parathyroid is gently palpated to ensure there is only one abnormal gland. Normal parathyroid tissue is soft and pale tan in color. When diseased, it becomes firmer, typically spherical, and often stands proud from the thyroid tissue. This is important, as in some cases the abnormalities are subtle and parathyroid glands can be mistaken grossly for thyroid nodular disease. Any abnormal parathyroid tissue should be different to the touch, however (Liles *et al.* 2010). Parathyroid adenoma is usually a solitary disease, and if more than one gland is enlarged and firm, then hyperplasia should be suspected. When a dog has two parathyroid nodules, they can be either bilateral or ipsilateral (Rasor *et al.* 2007).

The abnormal parathyroid gland is removed through a combination of sharp and blunt dissection. Iris scissors, fine dissecting scissors, or bipolar cautery should be used to make a hole in the capsule between the parathyroid and thyroid gland (Figure 64.2), and then blunt dissection is used to "roll" the gland out of the thyroid bed. Hemorrhage is typically minimal and easily controlled with cautery. If the parathyroid mass is clearly adherent to the thyroid parenchyma, then a partial thyroidectomy is indicated. This is most easily achieved by an encircling monofilament absorbable ligature at the thyroid gland mid-body, or within palpably normal parenchyma away from the parathyroid nodule. Care should be taken to ensure that residual thyroid tissue has a visible blood supply. If in doubt (and the contralateral thyroid–parathyroid complex is normal), then a unilateral thyroidectomy is warranted.

Surgical decision making involving a firm solitary parathyroid adenoma is straightforward. The primary parathyroid mass may be small, but if one gland has a palpably firmer texture compared with its partners, the decision can be made to remove it. Problems arise during surgery when several glands appear enlarged or when no gland appears enlarged and none is noticeably firmer. All four glands may become enlarged due to renal secondary hyperparathyroidism and removal of one to three glands may decrease serum calcium levels sufficiently to ameliorate clinical signs (Flanders 2003). Parathyroid gland hyperplasia can present with one to four enlarged glands, with the other glands atrophied and unable to be found. In these dogs, all large parathyroid glands should be removed. Naturally, if all four are resected, the patient will likely need lifelong medical supplementation with vitamin D with or without dietary calcium, and so removal of three may be sufficient to reduce the hypercalcemia (Flanders 2003).

If no gland appears asymmetrically enlarged or firm, possibilities include the following:

- Explore the entire cervical region, among the loose peritracheal fascia, for evidence of ectopic parathyroid tissue. There has been one report of a mediastinal ectopic adenocarcinoma (Patnaik *et al.* 1978) and a metastatic parathyroid carcinoma has been removed from a similar location (Figure 64.3) (Kishi *et al.* 2014).
- Parathyroid hyperplasia is affecting all parathyroid glands symmetrically and there is no normal parathyroid tissue to use as a reference (Flanders 2003).

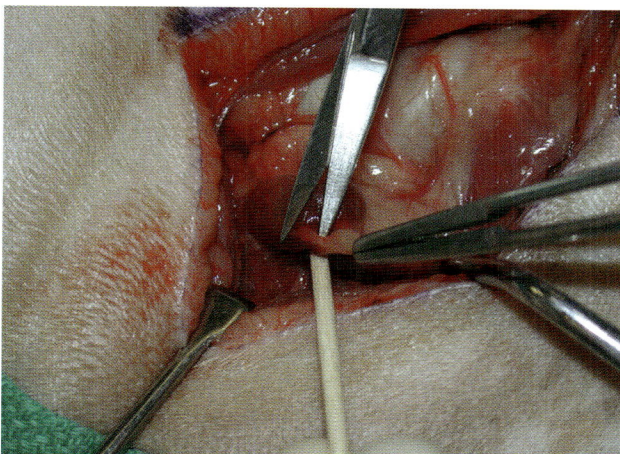

Figure 64.2 Following a ventral neck approach, a left-sided parathyroid adenoma is removed from the surface of the thyroid gland using sharp dissection with iris scissors.

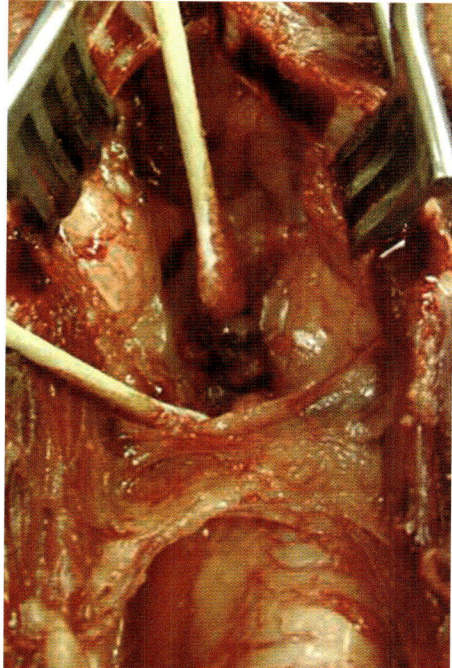

Figure 64.3 Parathyroid adenoma removed from the cranial mediastinum after median sternotomy.

One parathyroid gland (the largest or most prominent) can be removed for histologic evaluation to rule out hyperplasia. If present and the dog is still hypercalcemic, the surgeon should consider second surgery, a percutaneous ablation technique, or long-term medical therapy. If hyperplasia is not demonstrated, it is possible that a functional ectopic tumor exists.

- Consider performing MRI postoperatively from the tongue base to the heart base to look for evidence of ectopic parathyroid tissue (see the previous section on imaging).
- In patients with ionized hypercalcemia and PTH concentration within the reference range, consider atypical hypoadrenocorticism (Gow et al. 2009) and perform a basal cortisol assay or adrenocorticotropic hormone (ACTH) stimulation test.

Closure of the wound is in three layers: the divided muscle, the subcutaneous tissue, and skin. Use of a drain is not routinely recommended.

Recently a minimally invasive approach adopted from human surgery has been described in canine cadavers and a limited number of clinical canine cases. A 15 mm midline approach is made just caudal to the cricoid cartilage of the larynx and blunt suction dissectors and fine elevators used to allow ingress of a 5 mm 30° rigid endoscope. The parathyroid nodule is then removed by a combination of electrocautery and blunt and sharp dissection. Further work is required to determine the benefits of minimally invasive video-assisted parathyroidectomy (MIVAP) on a larger number of patients (Sumner et al. 2022).

Postoperative care

The greatest postoperative concern, reportedly occurring in 8–63% dogs (Berger & Feldman 1987; Ham et al. 2009; Burkhardt et al. 2021), is hypocalcemia due to chronic suppression of the remaining parathyroid glands through negative feedback from the hypersecretory tumor. Aggressive calcium uptake by bone in the postoperative period has also been suggested as a possible etiology in humans (Headley 1998). The suppressed glands require 2–3 weeks to begin secreting PTH (Flanders 2003). The parathyroid glands optimize their response to falling calcium levels by a phenomenon called hysteresis, a mechanism that allows the glands to increase PTH secretion in response to decreasing postoperative plasma calcium concentrations, even though still exposed to hypercalcemia (Conlin et al. 1989; Domingo et al. 2007). However, atrophied glands cannot compensate for the rapid fall in calcium after parathyroidectomy and hypocalcemia can result. Clinical signs of hypocalcemia include seizures, muscle twitching, face

rubbing, lethargy, and anorexia. Seizures and muscle twitching are due to neuronal hyperexcitability caused by sodium leaking into the neuron. The nerve cell membrane becomes more permeable to sodium in the face of low calcium concentrations and the altered membrane potential can result in spontaneous nerve depolarizations and muscle twitching.

After parathyroidectomy, total or ionized calcium drops rapidly for the first 24–48 hours and then begins to plateau, often normalizing within 1–7 days, with a median of 36 hours (Gear et al. 2005; Ham et al. 2009). Preoperative total calcium concentrations were significantly higher (median 4.2 mmol/L) in dogs that became hypocalcemic after surgery compared with dogs that remained normocalcemic (median 3.4 mmol/L) in one study (Gear et al. 2005), and this was confirmed in a larger group of 54 dogs with a moderate correlation between ionized calcium concentration before surgery and hypocalcemia afterward (Dear et al. 2017). Dogs with a preoperative serum ionized calcium concentration ≥1.75 mEq/L reportedly have 7.5 times greater odds of becoming hypocalcemic postoperatively (Burkhardt et al. 2021). Other studies have shown no correlation between preoperative ionized calcium and postoperative ionized calcium nadirs, or preoperative PTH concentrations between hypocalcemic and nonhypocalcemic populations (Arbaugh et al. 2012; Milovancev & Schmiedt 2013). Some authors have also concluded that preoperative ionized calcium concentration has a positive association with postoperative ionized calcium concentrations (Armstrong et al. 2018).

When faced with an acute onset of severe clinical signs, intravenous calcium gluconate (0.5 mL/kg of a 10% solution over 60 minutes) should be administered as a bolus and supported by a constant-rate infusion until vitamin D supplementation is at therapeutic levels (Schenck et al. 2006; Bonczynski 2007; Ham et al. 2009). An algorithm for treatment of postoperative hypocalcemia is shown in Figure 64.4. Vitamin D supplementation with or without calcium supplementation may be continued from a few weeks to indefinitely. Vitamin D supplementation should be tapered down two weeks after surgery while monitoring iCa.

Efforts to minimize postoperative hypocalcemia include supplementing dogs preoperatively with vitamin D (dihydrotachysterol or alfacalcidol), although this treatment has not been shown to be effective in preventing hypocalcemia. Also it is important for the other parathyroid gland to be exposed to a normal calcium level to encourage PTH production. Therefore supplementation before normocalcemia has been reached may slow down the response from the remaining glands.

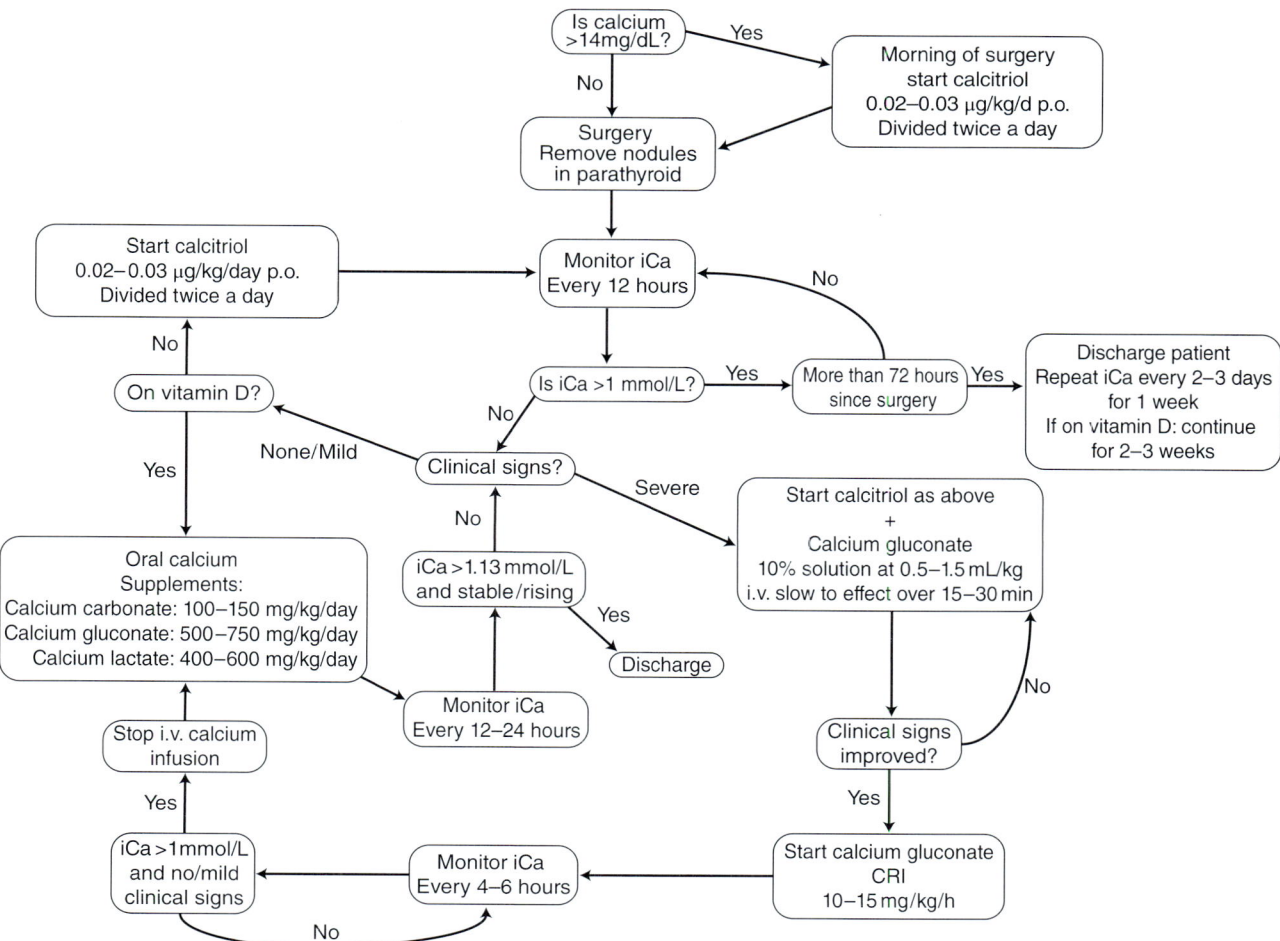

Figure 64.4 Algorithm for preoperative and postoperative management of calcium levels in primary hyperparathyroidism. CRI, continuous-rate infusion; iCA, ionized calcium; i.v., intravenously; p.o., orally.

Dihydrotachysterol has a long onset of action (3–5 days) and alfacalcidol is a hydroxylated vitamin D analogue with a shorter half-life (1–3 days). It has the advantage of reaching therapeutic levels quickly and is also eliminated from the body faster, allowing for tighter control of calcium (Gear *et al.* 2005). In one study where seven dogs did not resolve their hypercalcemia within seven days of surgery, five of them were prophylactically receiving calcium supplementation preoperatively (Erickson *et al.* 2021).

One study examined the benefit of pretreatment with calcitriol prior to parathyroidectomy. Starting on the day of surgery 55 dogs were treated prophylactically (mean dose 23 ng/kg/day, range 6–52 ng/kg/day), and 23 dogs received no calcitriol. It was found that calcitriol did not slow down the acute drop in calcium postoperatively and did not identify any protective effect of calcitriol administration in preventing postoperative hypocalcemia (Armstrong *et al.* 2018).

In cats, the only reported postoperative complication was respiratory distress occurring in 9.4%, presumed to be due to damage to the recurrent laryngeal nerve during neck dissection. Clinical signs of hypocalcemia were not observed in any cat (Singh *et al.* 2018), although 34% became hypocalcemic at a median of 36 hours postoperatively. Preoperative ionized calcium was not associated with the lowest postoperative ionized calcium, hypocalcemia during hospitalization or at discharge, or hypercalcemia at discharge. In this study 19% remained hypercalcemic for the duration of hospitalization.

Histopathology

In dogs with primary hyperparathyroidism, solitary adenoma is seen in approximately 74–90% of dogs, adenomatous hyperplasia in 5–24%, and carcinoma in 4–20% (DeVries *et al.* 1993; Feldman 1995; Wisner *et al.* 1997; Gear *et al.* 2005; Ham *et al.* 2009), although in recent studies a higher prevalence of 15–25% of parathyroid nodules has been reported as parathyroid carcinoma (Armstrong *et al.* 2018; Secrest & Grimes 2019).

Parathyroid adenoma and hyperplasia are difficult to distinguish with hematoxylin and eosin staining (Feldman 1995; Feldman & Nelson 1996) and diagnosis is often based on size alone. Adenoma is arbitrarily defined as an encapsulated nodule with a diameter of at least 5 mm, and hyperplasia as a diffuse form affecting all glands or a (multi)nodular lesion with nodules less than 5 mm in diameter in one or more glands with the unaffected glands atrophied (DeVries *et al.* 1993). This leads to some disagreement between pathologists when classifying benign parathyroid disease. In one recent study three pathologists disagreed on the classification of 35% of submitted parathyroid glands (Ham *et al.* 2009). It has even been suggested that there may not be a true distinction between parathyroid adenoma and nodular hyperplasia, because there is no functional difference between them and they simply represent a continuum of morphologic structures (van Vonderen *et al.* 2003). It is argued that since the success of surgery is dictated by the removal of all abnormal parathyroid tissue and a return to normocalcemia, the relevance of classifying which of the two benign "cured" processes is responsible may be academic (Ham *et al.* 2009).

Parathyroid carcinoma is rare, with 12 academic institutions over a 10-year period only identifying 100 cases (Erickson *et al.* 2021). Parathyroid carcinoma usually affects a single gland and is diagnosed histologically if there is capsular or vascular invasion by the abnormal parathyroid tissue, the presence of mitotic figures within the parenchymal cells, or fibrous trabeculae on histopathology (Schantz & Castleman 1972). The median nodule diameter is 5 mm (range 64–85 mm) with capsular invasion (84%), nuclear atypia (84%), or fibrous trabeculae (62%) commonly seen. Extracapsular invasion (29%), vascular invasion (15%), and necrosis (14%) are less commonly seen and mitotic count is typically very low, with most carcinomas being considered low grade (Sawyer *et al.* 2012; Erickson *et al.* 2021).

In 32 cats, parathyroid adenoma was diagnosed in 62.5%, parathyroid carcinoma in 22%, parathyroid hyperplasia in 9.4%, and parathyroid cystadenoma in 6.3% (Singh *et al.* 2018).

Nonsurgical therapy

Percutaneous ultrasound-guided ethanol ablation

A reduced-cost, low level of invasiveness and short duration of anesthesia may make an ethanol ablation procedure the preferred choice in some patients. The cost is estimated to be one-third of the cost for surgical parathyroidectomy (Guttin *et al.* 2015).

Dogs are anesthetized and under ultrasound guidance a 25- or 27-gauge, 1.5 in. needle is inserted into the affected parathyroid gland. Ethanol (95%) is injected until the entire gland is infiltrated and a change in echogenicity of the whole nodule is identified ultrasonographically (Long *et al.* 1999; Rasor *et al.* 2007). It has also been described injecting an equivalent volume of ethanol as the mass (product of maximum length, width, height), with volumes ranging from 0.02 to 2 mL given (Guttin *et al.* 2015). Total calcium and iCa are measured immediately and then every 12 hours for 3 days (Gear *et al.* 2005).

In the original report, 7 of 8 dogs (88%) were successfully treated with a single treatment (Long *et al.* 1999). More recently, 12 of 15 dogs (80%) were treated successfully with a single procedure, with hypercalcemia resolving in 1–4 days; 1 dog responded to a second treatment and 2 dogs failed to respond to a second treatment (Rasor *et al.* 2007). In a later study, 2 of 5 dogs showed a partial response with a reduction in blood calcium, although it remained above the reference range. The other 3 dogs failed to respond. This was attributed to attempts to ablate glands 5 mm or less in diameter, or to operator inexperience (Gear *et al.* 2005). The most recent study reports 27 treatments in 24 dogs with hypercalcemia resolving after 85% procedures, with the interval between treatment and resolution being 12 hours–3 weeks. Of those that resolved, 96% did so within 72 hours and 23% subsequently became hypocalcemic. Complications occurred in 11% dogs, but 89% of patients had long-term normocalcemia (Guttin *et al.* 2015).

Periprocedural or postprocedural adverse effects are rare, and treatment failures are often attributed to misidentification of parathyroid nodules, injection failure, or injection of nodules that are not actively secreting PTH.

Percutaneous ultrasound-guided heat ablation

Patients are anesthetized and placed on a cautery ground pad. Ultrasound locates the abnormal parathyroid gland and is then used to direct an 18- or 20-gauge over-the-needle intravenous catheter into the gland. The catheter sleeve acts as an insulator for the surrounding normal soft tissues. Radiofrequency energy is applied at 10–20 W until the tissue becomes hyperechoic (typically at least 90 seconds), redirecting the needle if necessary to ablate the entire gland (Pollard *et al.* 2001; Rasor *et al.* 2007) and causing cell death by thermal necrosis (Long *et al.* 1999). Blood flow disperses the high temperature, which tends to reduce the trauma to the surrounding tissues. Dogs with small nodules (<2–3 mm) are poor candidates for heat ablation, as needle insertion and manipulation can be difficult. Conversely, when the cross-sectional area of the nodule is greater than 0.35 mm², these patients seem to have a higher rate of local recurrence. Surgery is therefore advisable with very large or small nodules (Bucy et al. 2016).

In the original report, 8 of 9 dogs (89%) were successfully treated (Pollard et al. 2001). In another study, 43 of 48 dogs (90%) responded to a single treatment, with hypercalcemia resolving in 1–6 days, but mean time to resolution was significantly longer than following parathyroidectomy or ethanol ablation. In that study 1 dog resolved after a second treatment and 4 dogs failed treatment and remained hypercalcemic (Rasor et al. 2007). A recent study of 8 dogs described uneventful ablation in a single procedure in all cases with a rapid decrease in serum calcium to normal by 48–72 hours (Leal et al. 2018), with 3 dogs becoming hypocalcemic, but only 1 clinically affected. No long-term complications or relapses were seen. A larger study reported only 22/32 (69%) dogs having a successful radiofrequency ablation, with those that were unsuccessful developing recurrent hypercalcemic postoperatively a median of 5 months later (range 2–25 months) (Bucy et al. 2016).

There is no significant difference between the success rate for parathyroidectomy and heat ablation, but there is a significant difference between the success rate for parathyroidectomy and ethanol ablation (Rasor et al. 2007). The disadvantage of both the ethanol and heat ablation techniques is the lack of tissue for histopathologic examination. Other than hypocalcemia, complications arise in a small number of dogs due to leakage of ethanol or extension of thermal necrosis from the parathyroid gland into the surrounding tissues, causing damage to structures such as the recurrent laryngeal nerve and vagosympathetic trunk (Long et al. 1999). Following percutaneous techniques, dysphonia/change in bark is reported in 8% of dogs, a cough in 4%, and Horner's syndrome in 1% (Long et al. 1999; Pollard et al. 2001; Rasor et al. 2007).

Recurrent/persistent hypercalcemia

Persistent hypercalcemia can be seen due to multiglandular disease, ectopic parathyroid glands, incomplete excision of autonomously functioning parathyroid tissue, or malignant disease with residual functional metastasis (Feldman 2005). In one study, surgical failure was attributed to lack of parathyroid tissue being detected on histopathology (Rasor et al. 2007).

Recurrent hypercalcemia following parathyroidectomy can be seen in 4–17% of cases from a few months to years after surgery. In these reported cases it is caused by a second parathyroid adenoma or hyperplasia

(Feldman 2005; Gear et al. 2005; Rasor et al. 2007; Ham et al. 2009).

Relapse of hypercalcemia has also been reported in 2–28% of dogs following ultrasound-guided heat ablation treatment (Rasor et al. 2007; Bucy et al. 2016) and in 8–13% of dogs following ultrasound-guided ethanol ablation treatment (Long et al. 1999; Guttin et al. 2015).

Prognosis

All patients should be examined 14 days postoperatively for suture removal and calcium measurement. It is prudent to recheck calcium at three-month intervals thereafter, or more frequently if clinical signs suggestive of hypercalcemia arise.

Surgical excision alone is the most widely performed treatment for primary hyperparathyroidism and a cure rate of 94% is reported if all autonomously functioning parathyroid tissue is removed (Rasor et al. 2007). A greater than 50% decrease in serum PTH concentration by 30–45 minutes after parathyroidectomy can be used to confirm the removal of hyperfunctional tissue (Ham et al. 2009). What defines the success of parathyroidectomy should be return to a normal calcium level, and not necessarily a normal PTH level. In people, up to 33% of patients will have a normal calcium but elevated PTH after parathyroidectomy, and this is attributed to the existence of a new PTH set point (Dolev et al. 2008).

Although a malignancy, parathyroid carcinoma appears to behave in a low-grade fashion, with thoracic metastases seen in only 1% of patients at presentation and subsequent metastasis rare, with the prescapular lymph node, lung, kidney, and bladder suspected or confirmed in 5% of dogs (Erickson et al. 2021). The prognosis after resection of parathyroid carcinoma is reportedly good, with a median survival time of 614–735 days reported, and recurrence of hypercalcemia reported in <1% of cases following tumor excision and no dog demonstrating local recurrence of the primary tumor (Sawyer et al. 2012; Erickson et al. 2021).

Of note is the often-witnessed phenomenon of asymptomatic dogs doing exceptionally well after surgery and improving in attitude and mobility, especially when the hypercalcemia was diagnosed incidentally. Many symptoms of hypercalcemia such as muscular weakness and lethargy are attributed to old age in many dogs, yet the atrophic changes to the muscle are reversible with successful treatment of the primary disease (Feldman 1989), and it is only then that owners become aware how affected their animals had been. Similar functional musculoskeletal improvements are witnessed in asymptomatic people following treatment of primary hyperparathyroidism, where a significant improvement in bone density is seen in the lumbar spine and femoral neck compared with untreated patients (Steward *et al.* 2008).

In one study 37% of dogs developed renal failure postoperatively, and these dogs had significantly higher preoperative total calcium concentrations (median 4.0 mmol/L) compared with those with normal renal function (median 3.3 mmol/L) (Gear *et al.* 2005).

Prognosis in cats is good if all autonomously secreting tissue is removed, with a median survival time of 1109 days, not associated with preoperative ionized calcium, hypocalcemia at discharge, hypercalcemia at discharge, or diagnosis of carcinoma (Singh *et al.* 2018).

References

Adler, J.A., Drobatz, K.J., and Hess, R.S. (2007). Abnormalities of serum electrolyte concentrations in dogs with hypoadrenocorticism. *Journal of Veterinary Internal Medicine* 21: 1168–1173.

Aguilera-Tejero, E., Sanchez, J., Estepa, J.C. et al. (1998). Mineral metabolism in healthy geriatric dogs. *Research in Veterinary Science* 64: 191–194.

Arbaugh, M., Smeak, D., and Monnet, E. (2012). Evaluation of preoperative serum concentrations of ionized calcium and parathyroid hormone as predictors of hypocalcemia following parathyroidectomy in dogs with primary hyperparathyroidism: 17 cases (2001–2009). *Journal of the Veterinary Medical Association* 241: 233–236.

Armstrong, A.J., Hauptman, J.G., Stanley, B.J. et al. (2018). Effect of prophylactic calcitriol administration on serum ionized calcium concentrations after parathyroidectomy: 78 cases (2005–2015). *Journal of Veterinary Internal Medicine* 32 (1): 99–106.

Barber, P.J. and Elliott, J. (1996). Study of calcium homeostasis in feline hyperthyroidism. *Journal of Small Animal Practice* 37: 575–582.

Barber, P.J. and Elliott, J. (1998). Feline chronic renal failure: calcium homeostasis in 80 cases diagnosed between 1992 and 1995. *Journal of Small Animal Practice* 39: 108–116.

Benchekroun, G., Desmyter, A., Hidalgo, A. et al. (2009). Primary hyperparathyroidism and monoclonal gammopathy in a dog. *Journal of Veterinary Internal Medicine* 23: 211–214.

Berger, B. and Feldman, E.C. (1987). Primary hyperparathyroidism in dogs: 21 cases (1976–1986). *Journal of the American Veterinary Medical Association* 191: 350–356.

Blois, S.L., Dickie, E., Kruth, S.A., and Allen, D.G. (2011). Multiple endocrine disease in dogs: 35 cases (1996–2009). *Journal of the American Veterinary Medical Association* 238: 1616–1621.

Body, J.J. (1998). Bisphosphonates. *European Journal of Cancer* 34: 263–269.

Bonczynski, J. (2007). Primary hyperparathyroidism in dogs and cats. *Clinical Techniques in Small Animal Practice* 22: 70–74.

Bucy, D., Pollard, R., and Nelson, R. (2016). Analysis of factors affecting outcome of ultrasound-guided radiofrequency heat ablation for treatment of primary hyperparathyroidism in dogs. *Veterinary Radiology and Ultrasound* 58 (1): 83–89.

Burkhardt, S.J., Sumner, J.P., and Mann, S. (2021). Ambidirectional cohort study on the agreement of ultrasonography and surgery in the identification of parathyroid pathology, and predictors of postoperative hypocalcemia in 47 dogs undergoing parathyroidectomy due to primary hyperparathyroidism. *Veterinary Surgery* 50: 1379–1388.

Chisholm, M.A., Mulloy, A.L., and Taylor, A.T. (1996). Acute management of cancer-related hypercalcemia. *Annals of Pharmacotherapy* 30: 507–513.

Coady, M., Fletcher, D.J., and Goggs, R. (2019). Severity of ionized hypercalcemia and hypocalcemia is associated with etiology in dogs and cats. *Frontiers in Veterinary Science* 6: 276.

Coburn, J.W. and Slatopolsky, E. (1986). Vitamin D, parathyroid hormone, and renal osteodystrophy. In: *The Kidney*, 3e (ed. E.M. Brenner and F.C. Rector), 1657–1729. Philadelphia, PA: WB Saunders.

Conlin, P.R., Fajtova, V.T., Mortensen, R.M. et al. (1989). Hysteresis in the relationship between serum ionized calcium and intact parathyroid hormone during recovery from induced hyper and hypocalcemia in normal humans. *Journal of Clinical Endocrinology and Metabolism* 69: 593–599.

Crews, L.J., Sharkey, L.C., Feeney, D.A. et al. (2007). Evaluation of total and ionized calcium status in dogs with blastomycosis: 38 cases (1997–2006). *Journal of the American Veterinary Medical Association* 231: 1545–1549.

Dear, J.D., Kass, P.H., Della Maggiore, A.M., and Feldman, E.C. (2017). Association of hypercalcemia before treatment with hypocalcemia after treatment in dogs with primary hyperparathyroidism. *Journal of Veterinary Internal Medicine* 31: 349–354.

DeVries, S.E., Feldman, E.C., Nelson, R.W., and Kennedy, P.C. (1993). Primary parathyroid gland hyperplasia in dogs: six cases (1982–1991). *Journal of the American Veterinary Medical Association* 202: 1132–1136.

Dolev, Y., Black, M.J., Hier, M.P. et al. (2008). Defining success of parathyroidectomy in hyperparathyroidism. *Otolaryngology Head and Neck Surgery* 139 (2 Suppl 1): 36.

Domingo, V., Lopez, I., Mendoza, F.J. et al. (2007). Circadian variation of the Ca²⁺ PTH curve during hypercalcaemia in dogs. *Journal of Veterinary Medicine A Physiology, Pathology, Clinical Medicine* 54: 545–548.

Dougherty, S.A., Center, S.A., and Dzanis, D.A. (1990). Salmon calcitonin as adjunct treatment for vitamin D toxicosis in a dog. *Journal of the American Veterinary Medical Association* 196: 1269–1272.

Dow, S.W., Legendre, A.M., Stiff, M., and Greene, C. (1986). Hypercalcemia associated with blastomycosis in dogs. *Journal of the American Veterinary Medical Association* 188: 706–709.

Earm, J.H., Christensen, B.M., Frøkiaer, J. et al. (1998). Decreased aquaporin-2 expression and apical plasma membrane delivery in kidney collecting ducts of polyuric hypercalcemic rats. *Journal of the American Society of Nephrology* 9: 2181–2193.

Elaraj, D.M., Sippel, R.S., Lindsay, S. et al. (2010). Are additional localization studies and referral indicated for patients with primary hyperparathyroidism who have negative sestamibi scan results? *Archives of Surgery* 2010 145: 578–581.

Elliott, J., Dobson, J.M., Dunn, J.K. et al. (1991). Hypercalcemia in the dog: a preliminary study of 40 cases. *Journal of Small Animal Practice* 32: 564–571.

Elliott, J., Rawlings, J.M., Markwell, P.J., and Barber, P.J. (2000). Survival of cats with naturally occurring chronic renal failure: effect of dietary management. *Journal of Small Animal Practice* 41: 235–242.

Erickson, A.K., Regier, P.J., Watt, M.M. et al. (2021). Incidence, survival time, and surgical treatment of parathyroid carcinomas in dogs: 100 cases (2010–2019). *Journal of the American Veterinary Medical Association* 259 (11): 1309–1317.

Fan, T.M. (2007). The role of bisphosphonates in the management of patients that have cancer. *Veterinary Clinics of North America: Small Animal Practice* 37: 1091–1110 vi.

Fan, T.M., de Lorimier, L.-P., Charney, S.C., and Hintermeister, J.G. (2005). Evaluation of intravenous pamidronate administration in 33 cancer-bearing dogs with primary or secondary bone involvement. *Journal of Veterinary Internal Medicine* 19: 74–80.

Feinfeld, D.A. and Sherwood, L.M. (1988). Parathyroid hormone and 1,25(OH)$_2$D$_3$ in chronic renal failure. *Kidney International* 33: 1049–1058.

Feldman, E.C. (1989). Canine primary hyperparathyroidism. In: *Current Veterinary Therapy X: Small Animal Practice* (ed. R.W. Kirk and J.D. Bonagura), 985. Philadelphia, PA: WB Saunders.

Feldman, E.C. (1995). Disorders of the parathyroid glands. In: *Textbook of Veterinary Internal Medicine*, 4e (ed. S.J. Ettinger and E.C. Feldman), 1437–1465. Philadelphia, PA: WB Saunders.

Feldman, E.C. (2000). Disorders of the parathyroid glands. In: *Textbook of Veterinary Internal Medicine*, 5e (ed. S.J. Ettinger and E.C. Feldman), 1379–1400. Philadelphia, PA: WB Saunders.

Feldman, E.C. (2005). Disorders of the parathyroid glands. In: *Textbook of Veterinary Internal Medicine*, 6e (ed. S.J. Ettinger and E.C. Feldman), 1508–1535. Philadelphia, PA: WB Saunders.

Feldman, E.C. and Nelson, R.W. (1996). Hypercalcemia and primary hyperparathyroidism. In: *Canine and Feline Endocrinology and Reproduction*, 2e, 455–493. Philadelphia, PA: WB Saunders.

Feldman, E.C. and Nelson, R.W. (2004). Hypercalcemia and primary hyperparathyroidism. In: *Canine and Feline Endocrinology and Reproduction*, 3e, 660–711. WB Saunders: St Louis, MO.

Feldman, E.C., Wisner, E.R., Nelson, R.W. et al. (1997). Comparison of results of hormonal analysis of samples obtained from selected venous sites versus cervical ultrasonography for localizing parathyroid masses in dogs. *Journal of the American Veterinary Medical Association* 211: 54–56.

Feldman, E.C., Hoar, B., Pollard, R., and Nelson, R.W. (2005). Pretreatment clinical and laboratory findings in dogs with primary hyperparathyroidism: 210 cases (1987–2004). *Journal of the American Veterinary Medical Association* 227: 756–761.

Finch, N.C., Syme, H.M., and Elliott, J. (2012). Parathyroid hormone concentration in geriatric cats with various degrees of renal function. *Journal of the American Veterinary Medical Association* 241: 1326–1335.

Finco, D.R. (1983). Interpretations of serum calcium concentrations in the dog. *Compendium of Continuing Education for the Small Animal Practitioner* 5: 778–787.

Flanders, J.A. (1993). Parathyroid glands. In: *Disease Mechanisms in Small Animal Surgery*, 2e (ed. M.J. Bojrab, D.D. Smeak and M.S. Bloomberg), 583–588. Philadelphia, PA: Lippincott, Williams & Wilkins.

Flanders, J.A. (2003). Parathyroid gland. In: *Textbook of Small Animal Surgery*, 3e (ed. D. Slatter), 1711–1723. Philadelphia, PA: Saunders.

Foley, P., Shaw, D., Runyon, C. et al. (2000). Serum parathyroid hormone-related protein concentration in a dog with a thymoma and persistent hypercalcemia. *Canadian Veterinary Journal* 41: 867–870.

Forman, D.T. and Lorenzo, L. (1991). Ionized calcium: its significance and clinical usefulness. *Annals of Clinical and Laboratory Science* 21: 297–304.

Ganong, W.F. (2001). Hormonal control of calcium metabolism and physiology of bone. In: *Review of Medical Physiology*, 20e, 369–382. New York: Lange Medical Books.

Garrett, L.D., Craig, C.L., Szladovits, B., and Chun, R. (2007). Evaluation of buffy coat smears for circulating mast cells in healthy cats and ill cats without mast cell tumor-related disease. *Journal of the American Veterinary Medical Association* 231: 1685–1687.

Gear, R.N., Neiger, R., Skelly, B.J., and Herrtage, M.E. (2005). Primary hyperparathyroidism in 29 dogs: diagnosis, treatment,

outcome and associated renal failure. *Journal of Small Animal Practice* 46: 10–16.

Goldstein, R.E., Atwater, D.Z., Cazolli, D.M. et al. (2007). Inheritance, mode of inheritance, and candidate genes for primary hyperparathyroidism in Keeshonden. *Journal of Veterinary Internal Medicine* 21: 199–203.

Gotway, M.B., Reddy, G.P., Webb, W.R. et al. (2001). Comparison between MR imaging and ^{99m}Tc MIBI scintigraphy in the evaluation of recurrent of persistent hyperparathyroidism. *Radiology* 218: 783–790.

Gotway, M.B., Leung, J.W.T., Gooding, G.A. et al. (2002). Hyperfunctioning parathyroid tissue: spectrum of appearances on noninvasive imaging. *American Journal of Roentgenology* 179: 495–502.

Gow, A.G., Gow, D.J., Bell, R. et al. (2009). Calcium metabolism in eight dogs with hypoadrenocorticism. *Journal of Small Animal Practice* 50: 426–430.

Gross, C., Wedekind, J.E. et al. (2000). Nutrients. In: *Small Animal Clinical Nutrition* (ed. M.S. Hand, C.D. Thatcher, R.L. Remillard and P. Roudebush), 84–86. Mark Morris Institute: Topeka, KS.

Gunther, R., Felice, L.J., Nelson, R.K., and Franson, A.M. (1988). Toxicity of a vitamin D$_3$ rodenticide to dogs. *Journal of the American Veterinary Medical Association* 193: 211–214.

Guttin, T., Know, V.W., and Diroff, J.S. (2015). Outcomes for dogs with primary hyperparathyroidism following treatment with percutaneous ultrasound-guided ethanol ablation of presumed functional parathyroid nodules: 27 cases (2008–2011). *Journal of the American Veterinary Medical Association* 24: 771–777.

Hahn, T.J., Halstead, L.R., and Baran, D.T. (1981). Effects off short term glucocorticoid administration on intestinal calcium absorption and circulating vitamin D metabolite concentrations in man. *Journal of Clinical Endocrinology and Metabolism* 52: 111–115.

Ham, K., Greenfield, C.L., Barger, A. et al. (2009). Validation of a rapid parathyroid hormone assay and intraoperative measurement of parathyroid hormone in dogs with benign naturally occurring primary hyperparathyroidism. *Veterinary Surgery* 38: 122–132.

Hamilton, R., Greenberg, B.M., Gefter, W. et al. (1988). Successful localization of parathyroid adenomas by magnetic resonance imaging. *American Journal of Surgery* 155: 370–373.

Headley, C.M. (1998). Hungry bone syndrome following parathyroidectomy. *ANNA Journal* 25 (3): 283–289.

den Hertog, E., Goossens, M.M., van der Linde-Sipman, J.S., and Kooistra, H.S. (1997). Primary hyperparathyroidism in two cats. *Veterinary Quarterly* 19: 81–84.

Hobson, H.P., Brown, M.R., and Rogers, K.S. (2006). Surgery of metastatic anal sac adenocarcinoma in five dogs. *Veterinary Surgery* 35: 267–270.

Hostutler, R.A., Chew, D.J., Jaeger, J.Q. et al. (2005). Uses and effectiveness of pamidronate disodium for treatment of dogs and cats with hypercalcemia. *Journal of Veterinary Internal Medicine* 19: 29–33.

Hullinger, G.A. (1993). The endocrine system. In: *Miller's Anatomy of the Dog*, 3e (ed. H.E. Evans), 559–585. Philadelphia, PA: WB Saunders.

Hutchesson, A.C., Bundred, N.J., and Ratcliffe, W.A. (1995). Survival in hypercalcaemic patients with cancer and co-existing primary hyperparathyroidism. *Postgraduate Medical Journal* 71 (831): 28–31.

Johnson, N.A., Tublin, M.E., and Ogilvie, J.B. (2007). Parathyroid imaging: technique and role in the preoperative evaluation of primary hyperparathyroidism. *American Journal of Roentgenology* 188: 1706–1715.

Kadar, E., Rush, J.E., Wetmore, L., and Chan, D.L. (2004). Electrolyte disturbances and cardiac arrhythmias in a dog following pamidronate, calcitonin, and furosemide administration for hypercalcemia of malignancy. *Journal of the American Animal Hospital Association* 40: 75–81.

Kallet, A.J., Richter, K.P., Feldman, E.C., and Brum, D.E. (1991). Primary hyperparathyroidism in cats: seven cases (1984–1989). *Journal of the American Veterinary Medical Association* 199: 1767–1771.

Kallfelz, F.A. and Dzanis, D.A. (1989). Overnutrition: an epidemic problem in pet animal practice? *Veterinary Clinics of North America. Small Animal Practice* 19: 433–446.

Kishi, E.N., Holmes, S.P., Abbott, J.R., and Bacon, N.J. (2014). Functional metastatic parathyroid adenocarcinoma in a dog. *Canadian Veterinary Journal* 55: 383–388.

Kruger, J.M., Osborne, C.A., Nachreiner, R.F., and Refsal, K.R. (1996). Hypercalcemia and renal failure. Etiology, pathophysiology, diagnosis, and treatment. *Veterinary Clinics of North America. Small Animal Practice* 26: 1417–1445.

Kubota, A., Kano, R., Mizuno, T. et al. (2002). Parathyroid hormone-related protein (PTHrp) produced by dog lymphoma cells. *Journal of Veterinary Medical Science* 64: 835–837.

Lautscam, E., von Klopman, C., Schaub, S. et al. (2020). CT iaging features of the normal parathyroid gland in the dog. *Tierarztliche Praxis Ausgabe K Kleintiere/Heimtiere* 48 (5): 313–320.

Leal, R.O., Pascual, L.F., and Hernandez, J. (2018). The use of percutaneous ultrasound-guided radiofrequency heat ablation for the treatment of primary hyperparathyroidism in eight dogs: outcome and complications. *Veterinary Sciences* 5: 91.

LeBlanc, C.J., Echandi, R.L., Moore, R.R. et al. (2008). Hypercalcemia associated with gastric pythiosis in a dog. *Veterinary Clinical Pathology* 37: 115–120.

Legendre, A.M., Walker, M., Buyukmihci, N., and Stevens, R. (1981). Canine blastomycosis: a review of 47 clinical cases. *Journal of the American Veterinary Medical Association* 178: 1163–1168.

Liles, S.R., Linder, K.E., Cain, B., and Pease, A.P. (2010). Ultrasonography of histologically normal parathyroid gland and thyroid lobules in normocalcemic dogs. *Veterinary Radiology and Ultrasound* 51: 447–452.

Long, C.D., Goldstein, R.E., Hornof, W.J. et al. (1999). Percutaneous ultrasound-guided chemical parathyroid ablation for treatment of primary hyperparathyroidism in dogs. *Journal of the American Veterinary Medical Association* 215: 217–221.

López, I., Aguilera-Tejero, E., Estepa, J.C. et al. (2005). Diurnal variations in the plasma concentration of parathyroid hormone in dogs. *Veterinary Record* 157: 344–347.

Marquez, G.A., Klausner, J.S., and Osborne, C.A. (1995). Calcium oxalate urolithiasis in a cat with a functional parathyroid adenocarcinoma. *Journal of the American Veterinary Medical Association* 206: 817–819.

Matwichuk, C.L., Taylor, S.M., Daniel, G.B. et al. (2000). Double-phase parathyroid scintigraphy in dogs using technetium-99M-sesta-mibi. *Veterinary Radiology and Ultrasound* 41: 461–469.

Mellanby, R.J., Mee, A.P., Berry, J.L., and Herrtage, M.E. (2005). Hypercalcaemia in two dogs caused by excessive dietary supplementation of vitamin D. *Journal of Small Animal Practice* 46: 334–338.

Mellanby, R.J., Craig, R., Evans, H., and Herrtage, M.E. (2006). Plasma concentrations of parathyroid hormone-related protein in dogs with potential disorders of calcium metabolism. *Veterinary Record* 159: 833–838.

Messinger, J.S., Windham, W.R., and Ward, C.R. (2009). Ionized hypercalcemia in dogs: a retrospective study of 109 cases (1998–2003). *Journal of Veterinary Internal Medicine* 23: 514–519.

Meuten, D.J., Chew, D.J., Capen, C.C., and Kociba, G.J. (1982a). Relationship of serum total calcium to albumin and total protein in dogs. *Journal of the American Veterinary Medical Association* 180: 63–67.

Meuten, D.J., Capen, C.C., Kociba, G.J., and Cooper, B.J. (1982b). Hypercalcemia of malignancy: hypercalcemia associated with an adenocarcinoma of the apocrine glands of the anal sac. *American Journal of Pathology* 108: 366–370.

Midkiff, A.M., Chew, D.J., Randolph, J.F. et al. (2000). Idiopathic hypercalcemia in cats. *Journal of Veterinary Internal Medicine* 14: 619–626.

Milovancev, M. and Schmiedt, C.W. (2013). Preoperative factors associated with postoperative hypocalcemia in dogs with primary hyperparathyroidism that underwent parathyroidectomy: 62 cases (2004–2009). *Journal of the American Veterinary Medical Association* 242: 507–515.

Morrow, C.K. and Volmer, P.A. (2002). Hypercalcemia, hyperphosphatemia and soft tissue mineralization. *Compendium on Continuing Education for the Practicing Veterinarian* 24: 380–388.

Motellón, J.L., Javort Jiménez, F., de Miguel, E. et al. (2000). Parathyroid hormone-related protein, parathyroid hormone, and vitamin D in hypercalcemia of malignancy. *Clínica Chimica Acta* 290: 189–197.

Nicholas, J.S. and Swingle, W.W. (1925). An experimental and morphological study of the parathyroid glands of the cat. *American Journal of Anatomy* 34: 469.

Patnaik, A.K., MacEwen, E.G., Erlandson, R.A. et al. (1978). Mediastinal parathyroid adenocarcinoma in a dog. *Veterinary Pathology* 15: 55–63.

Peterson, E.N., Kirby, R., Sommer, M., and Bovee, K.C. (1991). Cholecalciferol rodenticide intoxication in a cat. *Journal of the American Veterinary Medical Association* 199: 904–906.

Peterson, M.E., Kintzer, P.P., and Kass, P.H. (1996). Pretreatment clinical and laboratory findings in dogs with hypoadrenocorticism: 225 cases (1979–1993). *Journal of the American Veterinary Medical Association* 208: 85–91.

Pollard, R.E., Long, C.D., Nelson, R.W. et al. (2001). Percutaneous ultrasonographically guided radiofrequency heat ablation for treatment of primary hyperparathyroidism in dogs. *Journal of the American Veterinary Medical Association* 218: 1106–1110.

Pressler, B.M., Rotstein, D.S., Law, J.M. et al. (2002). Hypercalcemia and high parathyroid hormone-related protein concentration associated with malignant melanoma in a dog. *Journal of the American Veterinary Medical Association* 221 (263–265): 240.

Radlinsky, M.G. (2007). Thyroid surgery in dogs and cats. *Veterinary Clinics of North America. Small Animal Practice* 37: 789–798. viii.

Ramsey, I.K. (2001). Increased parathyroid hormone concentrations in dogs with hyperadrenocorticism. *19th Annual American College of Veterinary Internal Medicine Forum*, Denver, CO.

Ramsey, I.K., Tebb, A., Harris, E. et al. (2005). Hyperparathyroidism in dogs with hyperadrenocorticism. *Journal of Small Animal Practice* 46: 531–536.

Rasor, L., Pollard, R., and Feldman, E.C. (2007). Retrospective evaluation of three treatment methods for primary hyperparathyroidism in dogs. *Journal of the American Animal Hospital Association* 43: 70–77.

Reed, C.I., Lackey, R.W., and Payte, J.I. (1928). Observations on parathyroidectomized dogs, with particular attention to the regional incidence of tetany, and to the blood mineral changes in this condition. *American Journal of Physiology* 84: 176–188.

Reeve, J. and Zanelli, J.M. (1986). Parathyroid hormone and bone. *Clinical Science* 71: 231–238.

Reimer, S.B., Pelosi, A., Frank, J.D. et al. (2005). Multiple endocrine neoplasia type I in a cat. *Journal of the American Veterinary Medical Association* 227: 101–104.

Reusch, C.E., Tomsa, K., Zimmer, C. et al. (2000). Ultrasonography of the parathyroid glands as an aid in differentiation of acute and chronic renal failure in dogs. *Journal of the American Veterinary Medical Association* 217: 1849–1852.

Rizzoli, R., Caverzasio, J., Bauss, F., and Bonjour, J.P. (1992). Inhibition of bone resorption by the bisphosphonate Bm-21.0955 is not associated with an alteration of the renal handling of calcium in rats infused with parathyroid hormone-related protein. *Bone* 13: 321–325.

Rosol, T.J. and Capen, C.C. (1988). Inhibition of in vitro bone resorption by a parathyroid hormone receptor antagonist in the canine adenocarcinoma model of humoral hypercalcemia of malignancy. *Endocrinology* 122: 2098–2102.

Sawyer, E.S., Northrup, N.C., Schmiedt, C.W. et al. (2012). Outcome of 19 dogs with parathyroid carcinoma after surgical excision. *Veterinary and Comparative Oncology* 10 (1): 57–64.

Schantz, A. and Castleman, B. (1972). Parathyroid carcinoma: a study of 70 cases. *Cancer* 31: 600–605.

Schenck, P.A., Chew, D.J., Nagode, L.A. et al. (2006). Disorders of calcium: hypercalcemia and hypocalcemia. In: *Fluid, Electrolyte and Acid–Base Disorders in Small Animal Practice*, 3e (ed. S.P. DiBartola), 122–194. St Louis, MO: WB Saunders.

Secrest, S. and Grimes, J. (2019). Ultrasonographic size of the canine parathyroid gland may not correlate with histopathology. *Veterinary Radiology and Ultrasound* 60: 729–733.

Sellon, R.K., Fidel, J., Houston, R., and Gavin, P.R. (2009). Linear-accelerator-based modified radiosurgical treatment of pituitary tumors in cats: 11 cases (1997–2008). *Journal of Veterinary Internal Medicine* 23: 1038–1044.

Sharma, O.P. (2000). Hypercalcemia in granulomatous disorders: a clinical review. *Current Opinion in Pulmonary Medicine* 6: 442–447.

Singh, A., Giuffrida, M.A., Thomson, C.B. et al. (2018). Perioperative characteristics, histological diagnosis, and outcome in cats undergoing surgical treatment of primary hyperparathyroidism. *Veterinary Surgery* 48: 367–374.

Skelly, B.J. and Franklin, R.J. (2007). Mutations in genes causing human familial isolated hyperparathyroidism do not account for hyperparathyroidism in keeshond dogs. *Veterinary Journal* 174: 652–654.

Soler Arias, E.A., Castillo, V.A., Trigo, R.H., and Caneda Aristarain, M.E. (2016). Multiple endocrine neoplasia similar to human subtype 2A in a dog: medullary thyroid carcinoma, bilateral pheochromocytoma and parathyroid adenoma. *Open Veterinary Journal* 6 (3): 165–171.

Steward, D.L., Bhatki, A.M., and Falciglia, M. (2008). The effects of surgery for primary hyperparathyroidism. *Otolaryngology Head and Neck Surgery* 139 (2 Suppl 1): 46.

Stockham, S.L. and Scott, M.A. (2002). *Fundamentals of Veterinary Clinical Pathology*. Ames, IA: Iowa State Press.

Strewler, G.J. (2000). The parathyroid hormone-related protein. *Endocrinology and Metabolism Clinics of North America* 29: 629–645.

Strodel, W.E., Thompson, N.W., Eckhauser, F.E., and Knol, J.A. (1988). Malignancy and concomitant primary hyperparathyroidism. *Journal of Surgical Oncology* 37 (1): 10–12.

Sumner, J.P., Espinheira Gomes, F.N.C.M., and Flanders, J.A. (2022). Minimally invasive video-assisted parathyroidectomy in dogs: technique description and feasibility study. *Veterinary Surgery* 51 (Suppl 1): O167–O173.

Sutton, R.A. and Dirks, J.H. (1986). Calcium and magnesium: renal handling and disorders of metabolism. In: *The Kidney*, 3e (ed. B.M. Brenner and F.C. Rector), 551–617. Philadelphia, PA: WB Saunders.

Sztukowski, K., Gin, T., Neel, J., and Lunn, K. (2021). Simultaneous primary hyperparathyroidism and multiple myeloma in a dog with hypercalcaemia. *Veterinary Record Case Reports* 9: e198.

Taeymans, O., Dennis, R., and Saunders, J.H. (2008). Magnetic resonance imaging of the normal canine thyroid gland. *Veterinary Radiology and Ultrasound* 49: 238–242.

Tebb, A.J., Arteaga, A., Evans, H., and Ramsey, I.K. (2005). Canine hyperadrenocorticism: effects of trilostane on parathyroid hormone, calcium and phosphate concentrations. *Journal of Small Animal Practice* 46: 537–542.

Torrance, A.G. and Nachreiner, R. (1989a). Human-parathormone assay for use in dogs: validation, sample handling studies, and parathyroid function testing. *American Journal of Veterinary Research* 50: 1123–1127.

Torrance, A.G. and Nachreiner, R. (1989b). Intact parathyroid hormone assay and total calcium concentration in the diagnosis of disorders of calcium metabolism in dogs. *Journal of Veterinary Internal Medicine* 3: 86–89.

Uchimura, K., Mokuno, T., Nagasaka, K. et al. (2002). Lung cancer associated with hypercalcemia induced by concurrently elevated parathyroid hormone and parathyroid hormone-related protein levels. *Metabolism: Clinical and Experimental* 51: 871–875.

Ulutas, B., Voyvoda, H., Pasa, S., and Alingan, M.K. (2006). Clodronate treatment of vitamin D-induced hypercalcemia in dogs. *Journal of Veterinary Emergency and Critical Care* 16: 141–145.

Vasilopulos, R.J. (2003). Humoral hypercalcemia of malignancy: diagnosis and treatment. *Compendium on Continuing Education for the Practicing Veterinarian* 25: 129–136.

van Vonderen, I.K., Kooistra, H.S., Peeters, M.E. et al. (2003). Parathyroid hormone immunohistochemistry in dogs with primary and secondary hyperparathyroidism: the question of adenoma and primary hyperplasia. *Journal of Comparative Pathology* 129: 61–69.

Walker, D.A. and Davies, M. (1981). Addison's disease presenting as a hypercalcemic crisis in a patient with idiopathic hypoparathyroidism. *Clinical Endocrinology* 14: 419–423.

Walker, M.C., Jones, B.R., Guildford, W.G. et al. (2000). Multiple endocrine neoplasia type 1 in a crossbred dog. *Journal of Small Animal Practice* 41: 67–70.

Walls, J., Ratcliffe, W.A., Howell, A., and Bundred, N.J. (1994). Response to intravenous bisphosphonate therapy in hypercalcaemic patients with and without bone metastases: the role of parathyroid hormone-related protein. *British Journal of Cancer* 70: 169–172.

Walser, M., Robinson, B.H., and Duckett, J.W. Jr. (1963). The hypercalcemia of adrenal insufficiency. *Journal of Clinical Investigation* 42: 456–465.

Weir, E.C., Norrdin, R.W., Barthold, S.W. et al. (1986). Primary hyperparathyroidism in a dog: biochemical, bone histomorphometric, and pathologic findings. *Journal of the American Veterinary Medical Association* 189: 1471–1474.

Willard, M.D., Schall, W.D., McCaw, D.E., and Nachreiner, R.F. (1982). Canine hypoadrenocorticism: report of 37 cases and review of 39 previously reported cases. *Journal of the American Veterinary Medical Association* 180: 59–62.

Wisner, E.R. and Nyland, T.G. (1998). Ultrasonography of the thyroid and parathyroid glands. *Veterinary Clinics of North America: Small Animal Practice* 28: 973–978.

Wisner, E.R., Penninck, D., Biller, D.S. et al. (1997). High-resolution parathyroid sonography. *Veterinary Radiology and Ultrasound* 38: 462–466.

Woods, S.J., Palm, C., Sheley, M. et al. (2017). Ultrasonography does not consistently detect parathyroid glands in healthy cats. *Veterinary Radiology and Ultrasound* 58: 737–743.

Yoon, J., Feeney, D.F., Cronk, D.E. et al. (2004). Computed tomographic evaluation of canine and feline mediastinal masses in 14 patients. *Veterinary Radiology and Ultrasound* 45: 542–546.

65

Feline Hyperthyroidism

Marie-Pauline Maurin and Carmel T. Mooney

Hyperthyroidism (thyrotoxicosis) is a multisystemic disorder resulting from excess production of the active thyroid hormones triiodothyronine (T_3) and/or thyroxine (T_4) from an abnormally functioning thyroid gland. Feline hyperthyroidism was first described over four decades ago (Holzworth *et al*. 1980; Peterson 1979). Since that time, its prevalence has increased dramatically. It is now recognized as the most common endocrine disorder affecting cats. It has an apparent prevalence of just over 8% in primary care practices in England, making it a disease of some significance in the general cat population (Stephens *et al*. 2014). Improved awareness, easier availability of testing methods, and aging of the cat population may have contributed to the increasing prevalence of feline hyperthyroidism, although they are unlikely to be the sole cause.

Pathogenesis and etiology

The most common pathologic abnormality associated with hyperthyroidism in cats is benign adenomatous hyperplasia (adenoma), accounting for >98% of cases. The majority (>60%) of cats have bilateral lobe involvement, whereas unilateral lobe involvement is less common (approximately 30% of cases) (Peterson & Broome 2015). Asymmetric thyroid lobe enlargement predominates in bilateral cases and in unilateral cases atrophy of the contralateral lobe is expected. A small number of cats (<4%) may have involvement of ectopic thyroid tissue (primarily mediastinal or less likely lingual), either in association with cervical thyroid lobe involvement or occasionally alone.

Functional thyroid carcinoma is a rare (<2%) cause of hyperthyroidism in cats (Peterson & Broome 2015). Given the high prevalence of benign thyroid disease, it may be difficult to differentiate thyroid carcinoma alone from concurrence of benign and malignant disease. Indeed, there is some evidence that malignant transformation can occur in hyperthyroid cats. The prevalence of suspected thyroid carcinoma (characterized by severe hyperthyroidism, and large, multifocal, intrathoracic masses refractory to medical management) increases from 0.4% in cats medically managed for ≤1 year to approximately 20% in those managed for >4–6 years (Peterson *et al*. 2016a).

The underlying etiology of feline hyperthyroidism is unclear and there can be difficulty in dissociating cause from effect in diseased animals. It has been likened to human toxic nodular goiter, for several reasons. Pathologically, affected thyroid tissue in cats contains single or multiple nodules of autonomous tissue that continue to grow when transplanted into nude mice and when cultured in thyroid-stimulating hormone (TSH)-free media (Peterson 2014). However, unlike in the human disease, common or unifying gene mutations have not been identified.

Several risk factors, apart from advancing age, have been associated with an increased risk of developing hyperthyroidism. These most notably include living indoors, using cat litter, and feeding canned foods (especially pop-top cans) of particular flavors such as fish, liver, or giblet (McLean *et al*. 2017; Kohler *et al*. 2016). Because of this dietary association, a potential role for

---

Small Animal Soft Tissue Surgery, Second Edition. Edited by Eric Monnet.
© 2023 John Wiley & Sons, Inc. Published 2023 by John Wiley & Sons, Inc.
Companion website: www.wiley.com/go/monnet/small

iodine has long been speculated. Cats may be exposed to other goitrogenic compounds or thyroid disruptors through their food and environment, including isoflavones, selenium, bisphenol-A, and polybrominated diphenyl ethers, which could contribute to the development of thyroid adenomatous lesions (van Hoek *et al.* 2015; Jones *et al.* 2019). However, none of these factors has been confirmed to induce hyperthyroidism. There is a long-established decreased risk of hyperthyroidism in Siamese and Himalayan breeds and more recently Tonkinese, Abyssinian, British shorthair, Burmese, and Persian breeds have been identified as at decreased risk. Longhaired non-purebreeds may be at increased risk (Crossley *et al.* 2017). Gender and neutering status do not appear to be important (Stephens *et al.* 2014).

Feline hyperthyroidism is likely a multifactorial disease where genetics and other factors may play a role. However, as a single cause has not been identified, prevention is not currently possible.

Signalment

Hyperthyroid cats are usually middle-aged to older, with an average age at onset of 12–13 years. Less than 10% of cats are younger than 10 years and hyperthyroidism has not been convincingly diagnosed in cats below 6 years. No sex predilection has been identified.

Clinical features

Excess thyroid hormones have an impact on every organ system and the majority of hyperthyroid cats present with a variety of clinical signs, although occasionally one predominates. There is usually an insidious onset and as the majority of cats remain clinically well, signs may be present for many months before owners seek veterinary attention. The severity of the clinical signs therefore varies from mild to severe depending on disease duration, the ability of the cat to cope with thyroid hormone excess, and/or the presence or absence of comorbidities (Peterson *et al.* 1983; Broussard *et al.* 1995).

The most commonly reported signs include weight loss despite a normal to increased appetite, unkempt haircoat, polyuria/polydipsia, tachycardia, hyperactivity/nervousness, and intermittent gastrointestinal signs (diarrhea and vomiting) (Thoday & Mooney 1992; Bucknell 2000). The overall increase of metabolic rate results in mild to severe weight loss that can progress to muscle weakness and wastage, leading to cachexia if left untreated (Peterson *et al.* 2016b). The direct and indirect effects of thyroid hormones on cardiac muscle generally result in a reversible hypertrophic cardiomyopathy (Weichselbaum *et al.* 2005). Cardiovascular signs include tachycardia and development of a cardiac murmur, with

their prevalence increasing with the severity of the hyperthyroidism (Watson *et al.* 2018).

Occasionally hyperthyroid cats are presented as depressed and anorexic rather than hyperactive and polyphagic. These cats often have significant concurrent diseases such as chronic kidney disease, or the hyperthyroidism has progressed and irreversible cardiac damage has led to congestive cardiac failure.

Demonstration of goiter is important for diagnosing hyperthyroidism. Each thyroid lobe is located just below the cricoid cartilage on the either side of the trachea. The classic method of palpation requires restraining the animal in a sitting position, holding the front limbs, and gently extending the neck while palpating on either side of the trachea and sweeping slowly downward from the larynx to the manubrium. Alternatively, cervical palpation can be attempted from behind the cat, sweeping down the trachea as the cat's head is turned to each side. Clinician preference dictates the technique used, although the former is considered to have better repeatability. Palpation of a mobile subcutaneous mass, nodule, or "blip" that slips under the fingertips determines the presence of a goiter (Norsworthy *et al.* 2002a; Paepe *et al.* 2008; Boretti *et al.* 2009; Mooney & Peterson 2012). However, with such a subjective diagnostic test, sensitivity and specificity may vary with clinician experience (Paepe *et al.* 2008; Lovelace 2009). Goiter may be palpable in cats that do not have hyperthyroidism, and such cases require reevaluation at regular intervals.

Undoubtedly cats are currently being diagnosed with hyperthyroidism before clinical signs are apparent or their owners realize that they are ill. Investigation for hyperthyroidism should be prompted if there is any discernible loss of weight or decrease in muscle mass, as this appears to be lost before body condition score is affected (Peterson *et al.* 2016a). The development of a cardiac murmur or identification of goiter is also an important indicator. Unfortunately the prevalence and size of goiter are related to the severity of disease. In previous studies of highly symptomatic cats, >90% had palpable thyroid gland enlargement (Thoday & Mooney 1992; Norsworthy *et al.* 2002b). Currently, palpable goiter is identified in 80% of affected cats (Wehner *et al.* 2019), and the majority are small and <5 mm. The absence of goiter should therefore not be used to rule out a diagnosis of hyperthyroidism.

Supportive diagnostic tests

Hematology

Hematologic changes in hyperthyroid cats are generally mild and clinically insignificant but include mild erythrocytosis and a stress leukogram with mature neutrophilia, lymphopenia, and eosinopenia (Broussard *et al.* 1995; Peterson *et al.* 1983; Thoday & Mooney 1992).

Biochemistry

A mild to marked increase in one or more liver enzyme activities – alanine aminotransferase (ALT), aspartate aminotransferase (AST), alkaline phosphatase (ALP), and lactate hydrogenase (LDH) – is most commonly observed (Mooney 2002). The severity reflects the increase in total T4 concentrations. The increased liver enzyme activities are not associated with parenchymal abnormalities or hepatic dysfunction function (Berent *et al.* 2007) and decline to within reference intervals with successful treatment of the hyperthyroidism. However, concurrent hepatic disease should be investigated if there are marked elevations of liver enzyme activities in association with a mild elevation of serum total T4 concentration (Mooney & Peterson 2012).

Hyperthyroidism and chronic kidney disease are common conditions in older cats, and it is not surprising that a proportion (2–10%) of hyperthyroid cats present with concurrent azotemia (Williams *et al.* 2010b; Peterson *et al.* 2018). Increased thyroid hormone concentrations have hemodynamic effects with consequences on kidney function, notably by increasing glomerular filtration rate (GFR). Loss of muscle mass is also associated with decreased creatinine concentrations. Kidney disease may therefore be masked in hyperthyroid cats (Vaske *et al.* 2016).

Abnormalities in calcium and phosphate homeostasis are common in hyperthyroid cats. Hyperphosphatemia in the absence of azotemia occurs in approximately 40% and mild ionized hypocalcemia in up to 50% of cases (Williams *et al.* 2012, 2013). In association with these changes, parathyroid hormone (PTH) concentrations are increased in approximately 75% of hyperthyroid cats. The pathophysiologic mechanisms are largely unknown. Nevertheless, the fact that hyperparathyroidism exists in the face of low ionized calcium concentrations may play some role in the potential development of hypoparathyroidism post bilateral thyroidectomy.

Other biochemical changes include mild hyperglycemia, reflecting a stress response (Mooney & Peterson 2012). Fructosamine concentration is significantly lower in hyperthyroid than in healthy cats, reflecting increased protein turnover (Graham *et al.* 1999; Crenshaw *et al.* 1996). This should be factored in when monitoring diabetic cats with concurrent hyperthyroidism. Hypokalemia, with associated clinical signs, is an unusual feature of hyperthyroidism.

Urinalysis is useful for eliminating other relevant differential diagnoses such as diabetes mellitus. Urine specific gravity is variable in hyperthyroidism, ranging from dilute to concentrated. Mild proteinuria may be present as a consequence of hypertension, hyperfiltration, or altered tubular function. Concurrent urinary tract infections with associated clinical signs are unusual in hyperthyroid cats. Hyperthyroid cats have a low (<5%) prevalence of subclinical bacteriuria that is not different from cats of a similar age and sex (Peterson *et al.* 2020b). Routine urine culture is therefore not recommended for hyperthyroid cats.

Cardiac imaging (radiographs, ultrasound, electrocardiography)

Thoracic radiography, cardiac ultrasonography, and electrocardiography (ECG) may provide evidence for hypertrophic cardiomyopathy (cardiomegaly, sinus tachycardia, and increased R-wave amplitude in lead II, left ventricular caudal wall hypertrophy, and hypertrophy of the interventricular septum) in hyperthyroid cats. However, they are rarely indicated unless there are clinical signs of congestive cardiac failure present.

Thyroid imaging

Cervical ultrasonography can provide information on the dimensions and volume of the thyroid lobes. In hyperthyroid cats affected thyroid lobes are generally uniformly enlarged and less echogenic than healthy thyroid tissue. Cystic changes within the thyroid parenchyma can also be identified (Barberet *et al.* 2010; Miller *et al.* 2017). Thyroid ultrasonography is heavily reliant on good operator skills and provides no information on function.

Computed tomography (CT) can also be used to determine the size and volume of affected thyroid tissue (Drost *et al.* 2006). This imaging modality is becoming more accessible and can easily be performed in cats that are not or only mildly sedated (Bush *et al.* 2017). As with ultrasonography, no information on thyroid function is provided.

Definitive diagnostic tests

The diagnosis of hyperthyroidism is confirmed by demonstration of increased thyroidal radioisotope uptake or increased circulating concentrations of the thyroid hormones.

Thyroid scintigraphy

There is increased thyroidal uptake of radioactive iodine (^{123}I or ^{131}I) and technetium-99m as pertechnetate (99mTcO4$^-$) in hyperthyroid cats. The latter isotope is usually preferred as it is widely available, relatively inexpensive, has a rapid uptake (imaging procedures can start within 20 minutes of administration), gives a low radiation dose, and provides superior image quality. Percentage thyroid uptake, thyroid-to-background ratio, or thyroid-to-salivary uptake can be measured after injection. Whatever parameter is used, increased values are found in almost all hyperthyroid cats and are strongly correlated with circulating thyroid hormone concentrations. The thyroid-to-salivary ratio is often preferred as the most accurate measurement, although quantitative thyroid uptake provides more information on functional volume and metabolic activity and is therefore most useful for assessing radioactive iodine treatment dose (Peterson *et al.* 2016c).

Although scintigraphy provides the most sensitive and specific test for diagnosing hyperthyroidism, it requires access to sophisticated equipment that is beyond the reach of most veterinary practices.

Thyroid scintigraphy also provides information on unilateral versus bilateral thyroid lobe involvement, potential location of affected ectopic thyroid tissue, and existence of multifocal lesions. It is therefore particularly useful when there is no palpable thyroid lobe enlargement, when thyroid carcinoma is suspected, or where bilateral thyroidectomy has previously been carried out (Peterson & Broome 2015).

Thyroid hormone concentrations

Measurement of circulating total T_4 is considered the most appropriate first-line diagnostic test for hyperthyroidism in cats. Methods for its measurement are widely available and relatively cheap and special sample handling is not required. It is a highly specific diagnostic test; false-positive results are rare, if they occur at all. Values are above the reference interval in >90% of hyperthyroid cats; typical reference intervals range from approximately 15 to 50–60 nmol/L. Values may remain within the reference interval (usually within the upper third to half) in early disease, and represent 20–40% of cats classified as having mild disease (Peterson *et al.* 2015). Reference interval values in hyperthyroidism may also be due to the suppressive effect of severe concurrent nonthyroidal illness (NTI). Diagnosing hyperthyroidism in such cases is not difficult, as total T_4 concentrations are expected to be suppressed to within the lower half or below the reference interval in euthyroid cats with significant NTI (Peterson *et al.* 2020a). If a reference interval value is found, and the cat is considered to have mild hyperthyroidism, retesting after 3–6 weeks is recommended, at which point serum total T_4 concentrations may have increased into the thyrotoxic range.

Measurement of circulating free T_4 concentration is a more sensitive diagnostic test. Increased concentrations are found in >95% of hyperthyroid cats, with <15% of mildly affected cases maintaining reference interval values (Peterson *et al.* 2015). However, this test lacks diagnostic specificity, with approximately 15% of euthyroid cats with NTI having increased values (Peterson *et al.* 2020a). Free T_4 concentrations are only accurately measured using equilibrium dialysis, a technique that is confined to specialist laboratories; special sample handling is required.

Measurement of circulating canine TSH (cTSH) can provide some diagnostic information. However, the assay used has a relatively high limit of detection such that suppressed values cannot be accurately measured. Undetectable cTSH concentrations (typically defined as <0.03 ng/mL) are found in 98% of hyperthyroid cats (Peterson *et al.* 2015). Yet approximately 30% of cats with NTI also have undetectable concentrations, rendering it a poorly specific diagnostic test. Nevertheless, the combination of a high reference interval total T_4, increased free T_4, and undetectable cTSH concentration is consistent with hyperthyroidism. On the other hand, a high reference interval total T_4 and detectable cTSH concentration make hyperthyroidism less likely.

Treatment

Different treatment methods of feline hyperthyroidism exist, each with advantages and disadvantages (Peterson 2020). There are two curative treatments: administration of radioactive iodine and surgical thyroidectomy. Temporary inhibition of thyroid hormone synthesis by administration of antithyroid drugs or iodine-restricted diets can be useful as a sole treatment, prior to surgical thyroidectomy, and while awaiting radioactive iodine treatment. Overall, the preferred option is radioactive iodine administration, although treatment should be tailored to each individual cat.

Young cats without concurrent disease should be directed to a curative treatment with either surgery or radioiodine whenever possible. In older cats or those with concurrent diseases, long-term medical management may be more appropriate. Cats with mild disease may temporarily respond to dietary management. Cats with severe clinical signs and/or large thyroid tumors should be directed to a curative therapy as soon as possible, because they are likely to be resistant to medical management. Facilities and skilled surgeon availability, and cat compliance in accepting the treatment, are also considerations. A systematic approach taking into account all factors is therefore crucial to guide the decision as to the most appropriate treatment in individual cats.

Medical management

Methimazole and its pro drug, carbimazole, have a reliable effect on suppressing thyroid hormone production. Carbimazole is rapidly converted to methimazole after oral absorption, with 5 mg approximating 3 mg methimazole. Methimazole is concentrated within the thyroid gland and inhibits the synthesis of thyroid hormones by inhibiting oxidation of iodide, organification of iodide, and coupling of iodothyronines to form T_4 and T_3. Methimazole is licensed for cats as both tablet (1.25 mg, 2.5 mg, and 5 mg) and liquid (5 mg/mL) preparations. Carbimazole is licensed for cats as a controlled-release tablet formulation (10 mg and 15 mg). Conventional carbimazole is available for human use. Methimazole and carbimazole can also be reformulated for transdermal application to the nonhaired pinna of the ear, and this may be of particular benefit in fractious cats or those that vomit.

The starting dose for methimazole is 1.25–5 mg/cat administered every 12 hours, depending on the severity of the hyperthyroidism. Using the total dose administered once daily is feasible, but attainment of euthyroidism is less reliable and takes longer. The starting dose for controlled-release carbimazole is 15 mg/cat every 24 hours. In mild cases, a lower starting dose of 10 mg/cat is recommended. Higher doses of methimazole/carbimazole are required when transdermal preparations are used because of reduced bioavailability (Hill *et al.* 2011).

Euthyroidism should be achieved within approximately 1 week after starting treatment. Cats should be reassessed after 10 days if receiving controlled-release carbimazole tablets or 3 weeks if receiving methimazole. Once euthyroidism has been restored, the dose of medication is decreased, aiming for the lowest dose possible that maintains a serum total T_4 concentration within the lower half of the reference interval and free T_4 concentration within the reference interval. Rechecks are recommended every 3–6 months or earlier if clinically indicated.

Mild clinical side effects occur in approximately 10–25% of cats and are observed mainly during the first 4–8 weeks of treatment. The most common clinical signs include anorexia, vomiting, and lethargy. They are not dose dependent and should spontaneously resolve despite continuation of the medication. Such gastrointestinal side effects may be less frequent in cats treated with transdermal methimazole (Sartor *et al.* 2004). Other side effects such as self-induced excoriation of the face/neck and lymphadenopathy are rarely reported (Niessen *et al.* 2007; Peterson *et al.* 1988). Hemolytic anemia, neutropenia, thrombocytopenia, and hepatopathy, while all serious and potentially life-threatening, are rare (<5% of cases).

Drug withdrawal and an alternate treatment for hyperthyroidism are required for these more serious adverse effects.

Surgical treatment

Surgical anatomy

The feline thyroid gland is divided into two lobes located just below the cricoid cartilage on either side of the trachea. An isthmus of tissue may connect the two lobes but, unlike in humans, this is nonfunctional. The right lobe is located slightly more cranial than the left. Each lobe is encapsulated and includes an external (cranial) and internal (caudal) parathyroid gland. The latter are removed during thyroidectomy as they cannot be visualized during surgery. The cranial thyroid artery arising from the common carotid artery on each side provides the major blood supply to each lobe. The artery enters the cranial pole and branches off to the parathyroid gland before entering thyroid tissue. Arising from the brachycephalic trunk, a caudal thyroid artery can be present in some cats. The cranial and caudal thyroid veins provide venous drainage, branched from the internal jugular vein. The recurrent laryngeal nerve travels dorsally and medially to the right thyroid lobe. The right common carotid artery and the right vagosympathetic trunk are located medially to this lobe. The left lobe is in close proximity to the esophagus dorsally, the caudal laryngeal nerve dorso-medially, and the left common carotid laterally, although slightly more separated because of the position of the esophagus.

Indications

Surgical thyroidectomy is an effective and curative treatment option for feline hyperthyroidism. It is considered a treatment of choice when radioactive iodine is unavailable. It is ideally suited for unilateral cases, avoiding postoperative complications such as hypothyroidism and hypoparathyroidism. However, just over 60% of hyperthyroid cats have bilateral involvement and this is often asymmetric (Peterson & Broome 2015). In many of these cases distinction between a small hyperfunctional lobe and an atrophic lobe can be challenging. Scintigraphy prior to surgery is ideal for optimal surgical planning. In its absence, the risk benefit of routine bilateral thyroidectomy must be carefully evaluated and discussed with the owners. The external parathyroid glands should be identified and preserved with their vascularization, avoiding postoperative hypoparathyroidism. While this may not be considered as important during unilateral compared with bilateral thyroidectomy, some unilateral cases may develop recurrent hyperthyroidism involving the contralateral lobe, thereby requiring repeat surgery.

Preoperative stabilization

Preoperative control of thyroid hormone production with antithyroid drugs is necessary to decrease the risk of cardiac and metabolic complications associated with anesthetizing hyperthyroid cats. B-blockers (propranolol/atenolol) can also be used pre- and intraoperatively to control tachycardia and supraventricular tachyarrhythmias in cats where medical treatment cannot be tolerated or where such arrhythmias develop under anesthesia.

Anesthetic management

If the hyperthyroidism is controlled preoperatively, a range of anesthetic protocols can be safely used. However, anticholinergic agents and drugs that stimulate or potentiate adrenergic activity capable of inducing tachycardia and arrythmias should be avoided. For these reasons, acepromazine combined with an opioid is preferred for premedication. Propofol is usually used for induction and the anesthesia should be maintained with isoflurane or sevoflurane.

Minimizing the anesthetic time is important, while it is crucial to continuously monitor the blood pressure, oxygen saturation, electrocardiogram, and temperature. Hyperthyroid cats may have reduced body fat, increasing the risk of hypothermia. Intraoperative analgesia can be provided using a constant-rate infusion of fentanyl (Naan *et al.* 2006). Postoperative analgesia using buprenorphine is acceptable if the surgery was routine.

Thyroid storm is a life-threatening exaggerated clinical response to a sudden increase in thyroid hormone concentrations, recognized in humans as a potential adverse effect of surgical handling of thyroid tissue. It is not a well-recognized syndrome in cats.

Surgical techniques

Magnification is recommended for meticulous dissection of the thyroid lobes. Bipolar electrocautery is also advised for precise and effective hemostasis. Cotton buds are useful for delicate dissection of the parathyroid gland.

The cat is placed in dorsal recumbency with the neck extended and slightly elevated using a small sandbag or a rolled towel and the front limbs are retracted caudally. A ventral midline approach is used from the larynx to the manubrium. The sternohyoid and sternothyroid muscles are separated along the midline and retracted laterally, allowing visualization of the thyroid lobes and the external parathyroid glands (Figure 65.1). The paratracheal fascia lateral to the proximal trachea can be bluntly dissected using cotton buds. The recurrent laryngeal nerve and carotid sheath should be identified and preserved. If

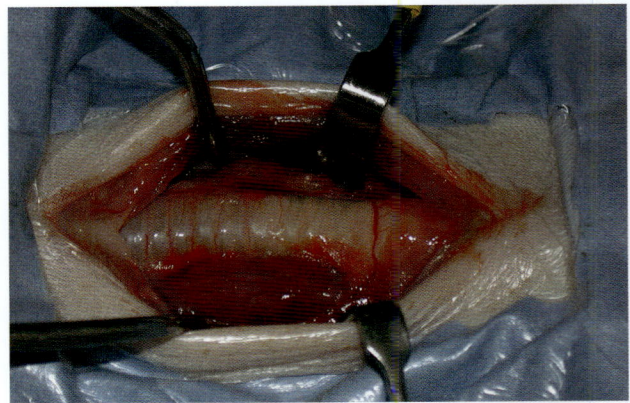

Figure 65.1 Appearance of bilateral thyroid lobe enlargement at the time of surgery. The external parathyroid glands are easily visualized as small spherical pale glands at the cranial pole of each thyroid lobe.

no preoperative scintigraphy has been performed, inspection of both thyroid lobes is required. Adenomatous thyroid tissue is usually darker red or brown. In unilateral cases, the contralateral lobe can be atrophied, pale, thin, and difficult to visualize. If the opposite lobe does not look atrophic, it should at least be biopsied as it is likely affected (Padgett 2002; Sisserer 2014). Routine closure of the neck muscles and skin is performed.

Two main techniques exist called extracapsular and intracapsular thyroidectomy. For each technique, a modified version has been developed.

The extracapsular technique involves removing the entire thyroid lobe with its capsule and both parathyroid glands (internal and external) after ligation of the cranial and caudal thyroid arteries. This technique carries an unacceptably high risk of postoperative hypocalcemia. The modified extracapsular technique differs by preserving the cranial thyroid artery supply to the external parathyroid gland. This is best achieved by using bipolar cautery instead of a ligature, allowing minimal dissection around the parathyroid tissue and therefore better preservation of the blood supply (Welches *et al.* 1989; Flanders *et al.* 1987; Flanders 1999).

The intracapsular technique involves a dorsal incision of the thyroid capsule and peeling away of the thyroid tissue, leaving the entire capsule *in situ* (Figure 65.2). This technique allows preservation of the blood supply to the external parathyroid gland. However, it carries a high risk of recurrence by leaving thyroid tissue adherent to the capsule, which can subsequently regrow. This technique is also time consuming. The modified version of the intracapsular technique includes removal of almost the entirety of the capsule, leaving the external parathyroid gland and its associated vasculature intact, decreasing the risk of recurrence (Figure 65.3).

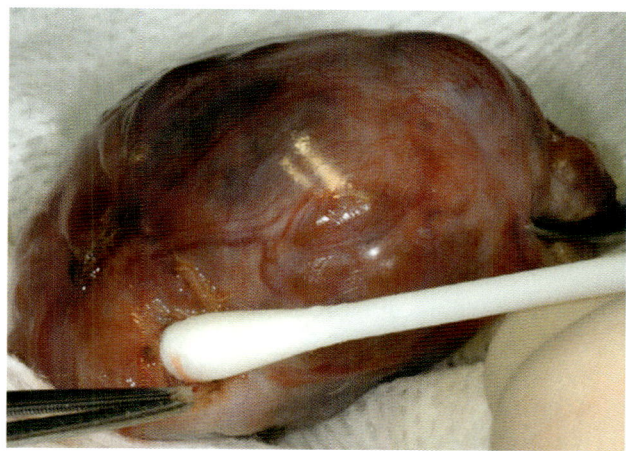

Figure 65.2 Modified intracapsular thyroidectomy. Intraoperative view: a moistened cotton-tipped swab is used in the dissection of the parathyroid gland.

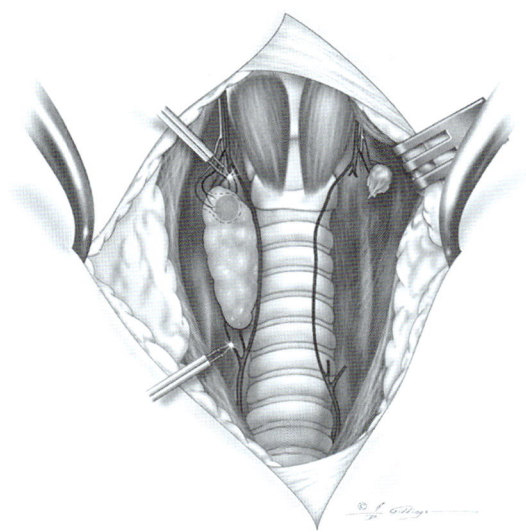

Figure 65.3 The appearance of the tissues remaining following a modified intracapsular thyroidectomy. © D. Giddings.

For bilateral cases, there is no significant difference in the rate of postoperative hypocalcemia or recurrence between the two modified techniques (Welches *et al*. 1989). Because of the increased risk of hemorrhage obscuring the surgical field during the dissection and prolonged time for performing the modified intracapsular technique, the modified extracapsular technique is often preferred. The choice of technique is not as crucial for unilateral disease, as only one parathyroid gland is necessary to maintain calcium homeostasis. However, a cautious approach is recommended based on the possibility of recurrence developing on the contralateral side.

To decrease the risk of postoperative hypocalcemia, a staged approach with a 3–4-week delay between each

unilateral thyroidectomy has been reported (Flanders *et al*. 1987). However, this has limited benefit and two anesthetic procedures are required.

Irrespective of technique used, if blood supply to the external parathyroid gland is compromised, a technique of local auto-transplantation can be performed. The parathyroid tissue is placed within a recipient bed in one of the sternohyoid muscles by bluntly dissecting it parallel to the muscle fibers. The myotomy is closed with a simple continuous suture to secure the gland within its recess. This allows revascularization within 1–2 weeks and potentially decreases the duration and severity of postoperative hypocalcemia, at least in some cases. However, it may also contribute to seeding of diseased thyroid tissue (Padgett *et al*. 1998).

Postoperative complications

The main postoperative complication is hypocalcemia. While reported in up to 82% of cats depending on the surgical technique, it only occurs in 6% of cases when the operation is carried out by an experienced surgeon (Birchard 2006; Flanders *et al*. 1987; Naan *et al*. 2006; Welches *et al*. 1989). This complication usually occurs if the parathyroid glands are inadvertently injured or removed during bilateral thyroidectomy. Postoperative hypocalcemia usually occurs within 1–5 days of surgery. Clinical signs include anorexia, vocalization, irritability, muscle twitching, tetany, and generalized convulsions (Mooney & Peterson 2012).

If a bilateral thyroidectomy is performed, the cat should be monitored for clinical signs and serum total, or ionized calcium concentration, should be assessed at least once daily for 1–5 days after surgery. Mild, transient, and clinically silent hypocalcemia can be observed without the need for supplementation. However, more severe hypocalcemia with associated clinical signs should be immediately treated with intravenous 10% calcium gluconate at a dose of 0.5–1.5 mL/kg infused slowly over at least 20 minutes, ensuring careful evaluation for bradycardia either by auscultation or continuous ECG monitoring. Subsequently a dose of 6.5–10 mL/kg can be infused over 24 hours as oral supplementation with calcium (equivalent to 25–50 mg/kg/day elemental calcium) and calcitriol/alfacalcidol (20–30 ng/kg/day) commences. Subcutaneous calcium solutions should not be administered, even if diluted, because of the risk of sterile abscess formation and skin sloughing (Mooney & Peterson 2012).

It is difficult to predict how long it will take for parathyroid function to recover and it can take days, weeks, or months. Recovery is related to reversible parathyroid damage or activation of accessory parathyroid tissue. Calcium homeostasis may also be provided by mechanisms other than PTH (Flanders *et al*. 1991).

Recurrence of hyperthyroidism is relatively uncommon, ranging from 0% to 22% of cases depending on the technique used (Flanders 1999). It can occur after unilateral thyroidectomy, but is also possible even after bilateral parathyroidectomy. After unilateral thyroidectomy, a second surgery may be considered. However, repeat surgery after previous bilateral thyroidectomy is contraindicated, as it carries a higher risk of life-threatening complications (Mooney & Peterson 2012). In general, cats with ectopic thyroid tissue or multifocal tissue involvement have a higher risk of recurrence. Medical therapy or radioactive iodine may be more appropriate treatment options in these cases.

Other complications are directly related to the surgeon's skills and can be avoided with careful dissection. They are a result of iatrogenic damage to the important surrounding structures, which could cause hemorrhage, laryngeal edema, Horner's syndrome, laryngeal paralysis, and voice change (Naan *et al.* 2006).

Radioactive iodine treatment

Administration of radioactive iodine (^{131}I) is the treatment of choice for feline hyperthyroidism. It is a simple curative treatment that is becoming increasingly available in many (but not all) countries. Radioactive iodine can be administered intravenously, orally, or subcutaneously, with the latter preferred because of minimal side effects, safer administration, and only requiring light sedation. The radioisotope ^{131}I emits both γ-rays and β-particles. The β-particles cause 80% of the tissue damage, but only travel a short distance (1–2 mm). It is therefore locally destructive to the abnormal thyroid tissue wherein it is concentrated, but spares adjacent atrophic thyroid and parathyroid tissue, and other important cervical structures.

The goal of therapy is to resolve hyperthyroidism without causing hypothyroidism. Thyroid hormone concentrations usually normalize within days to a few weeks after administration. Various methods have been used to assess and determine the most appropriate dose of ^{131}I for effective treatment while minimizing exposure to handling personnel. The dose can be determined using tracers or a scoring system, or a predetermined fixed dose is used (Turrel *et al.* 1984; Théon *et al.* 1994; Peterson & Becker 1995; Meric & Rubin 1990). The scoring system method, including the severity of the clinical thyrotoxicosis, elevation in circulating total T_4 concentration, and estimated size of the goiter by palpation, is currently a popular and easily implemented method. Over 90% of cats become euthyroid after one treatment, but hypothyroidism is a possibility (Peterson & Becker 1995; Fernandez *et al.* 2019). Fixed-dose regimes can result in under- or overtreatment of a significant number of hyperthyroid cats. Given the earlier diagnosis and milder form of the disease seen today, fixed low doses (74 MBq) are as successful (>95% of cases) in treating hyperthyroidism as standard doses (148 MBq), while at the same time decreasing the risk of subclinical and clinical hypothyroidism (Lucy *et al.* 2017). An algorithm incorporating a score for thyroid hormone concentrations and thyroid volume and percent technetium uptake as assessed by thyroid scintigraphy, providing an individualized dose for each cat, appears most successful (>95% of cases) in treating hyperthyroid cats while minimizing persistence of hyperthyroidism and development of hypothyroidism (Peterson & Rishniw 2021). Cats with severe hyperthyroidism, extreme elevations in thyroid hormone concentrations, and very large goiters are less likely to respond to radioactive iodine. This is particularly true for cats that have been medically managed for several years (Peterson *et al.* 2016a).

The prognosis following radioiodine treatment is excellent. The median survival times (MST) reported are up to four years (Peterson & Becker 1995; Milner *et al.* 2006). Hyperthyroid cats treated by radioactive iodine generally die from other conditions developing with age, such as kidney disease or malignancy.

Other treatments

Other methods for feline hyperthyroidism treatment have been described. Percutaneous ultrasound-guided single or staged injections of ethanol into affected thyroid tissue have been reported (Goldstein *et al.* 2001; Wells *et al.* 2001). However, numerous complications related to this treatment occur, including dysphonia, Horner's syndrome, gagging, and laryngeal paralysis. Percutaneous ultrasound-guided radiofrequency heat ablation showed similar complications, with recurrence of hyperthyroidism in all treated cats (Mallery *et al.* 2003). These treatments are therefore no longer recommended.

For cats with concurrent NTI or with serious adverse effects to methimazole, or where owners are unable to medicate and if surgery or radioactive iodine is not considered a feasible option, nutritional management with an iodine-restricted diet can be considered. Severely restricted iodine diets have been commercially available for some time (i.e., Hill's Prescription Diet y/d). Unfortunately, the efficacy of these diets remains limited. Undoubtedly, when they are used almost all cats demonstrate a reduction of thyroid hormone concentrations. However, time to euthyroidism can be prolonged, a variable percentage of cats return to a euthyroid state, and in those that do improvement of clinical signs is limited, suggesting periods of hyperthyroidism interspersed with euthyroidism (Gilman 2019; Grossi *et al.* 2019). Such diets are likely to be most successful in cats with mild hyperthyroidism. Cats chronically managed with an iodine-restricted diet should be frequently monitored (every six months) and more frequently if clinical signs dictate. There are many limitations to this alternative treatment. It is not a diet designed for many illnesses cats may concurrently have, such as allergic dermatitis or inflammatory bowel disease. Additionally, cats must not have any access to other sources of food containing iodine (Gilman 2019). This can be a particular challenge in multicat households or in those with outdoor access.

Complications of treatment: kidney disease and hypothyroidism

It is well recognized that hyperthyroidism is associated with increased GFR and decreased creatinine concentrations and is capable of masking or improving preexisting chronic kidney disease. A decline in GFR is generally apparent within one month of treatment of hyperthyroidism and remains stable for approximately six months (Boag *et al.* 2007).

Hyperthyroid cats with evidence of preexisting kidney disease based on increased creatinine concentration and inappropriately dilute urine will exhibit a decline in kidney function once hyperthyroidism is treated. They are often considered to have a poor prognosis with a predicted median survival of approximately six months, and this is likely reflective of the stage of kidney disease that develops (Milner *et al.* 2006; Williams *et al.* 2010a). The implications of worsening kidney function regarding survival should be discussed with owners prior to selection of their preferred treatment option for hyperthyroidism.

Cats without evidence of preexisting kidney disease may show evidence of such disease once hyperthyroidism is successfully managed. The prevalence by which it develops varies widely, from just over 10% to approaching 50% of cases. However, this is modulated by the treatment used for the hyperthyroidism, and whether or not subclinical or overt hypothyroidism develops.

Predicting in which cats azotemia will develop is difficult. Assessment of GFR is considered reasonable, while urine specific gravity is variably predictable. Measurement of serum symmetric dimethylarginine (SDMA) concentration helps predict impending azotemia with high diagnostic specificity but poor sensitivity in some but not all studies, and is not recommended in isolation (Peterson *et al.* 2018; Buresova *et al.* 2019; DeMonaco *et al.* 2020; Yu *et al.* 2020). Predicting the possible unmasking of chronic kidney disease is perhaps not crucial, as survival of cats that develop azotemia is no different than for those cats that do not develop azotemia after treatment of hyperthyroidism (Williams *et al.* 2010a). However, the prevalence of azotemia increases and survival decreases in those cats that develop hypothyroidism after treatment (Williams *et al.* 2010b).

As with emerging kidney disease, the prevalence of hypothyroidism varies depending on the treatment used for the hyperthyroidism. Additionally, azotemia can be affected by development of both overt and subclinical hypothyroidism. Overt hypothyroidism is usually defined by decreased thyroid hormone concentrations together with an elevated cTSH concentration. Subclinical disease is defined as reference interval thyroid hormone concentrations together with an elevated cTSH concentration, although it is recognized that some of these cats may be clearly hypothyroid when assessed by thyroid scintigraphy (Peterson *et al.* 2017). The development of hypothyroidism is least likely with dietary followed by medical management (Williams *et al.* 2010b; Vaske *et al.* 2016). It can occur after surgical thyroidectomy, but is dependent on whether bilateral thyroidectomy is carried out and the technique used (Covey *et al.* 2019). Its likelihood increases with radioactive iodine therapy, particularly if relatively high doses are used (Lucy *et al.* 2017). In many cases, the development of hypothyroidism is temporary and if azotemia does not develop, continued monitoring is recommended to ascertain if this is the case. However, if subclinical or overt hypothyroidism and azotemia develop, improved kidney function and better survival are possible by decreasing the dose of medical management or by providing L-thyroxine supplementation (Williams *et al.* 2014; Peterson *et al.* 2017).

Conclusion

Feline hyperthyroidism is a common disease of older cats of unknown etiology. It can be successfully cured by thyroidectomy or radioactive iodine therapy. Medical management is noncurative. Even though it treats hyperthyroidism, it does not prevent continuous growth of the thyroid gland and potential development of thyroid carcinoma.

References

Barberet, V., Baeumlin, Y., Taeymans, O. et al. (2010). Pre- and post-treatment ultrasonography of the thyroid gland in hyperthyroid cats. *Veterinary Radiology & Ultrasound* 51: 324–330.

Berent, A.C., Drobatz, K.J., Ziemer, L. et al. (2007). Liver function in cats with hyperthyroidism before and after 131I therapy. *Journal of Veterinary Internal Medicine* 21: 1217–1223.

Birchard, S.J. (2006). Thyroidectomy in the cat. *Clinical Techniques in Small Animal Practice* 21: 29–33.

Boag, A.K., Neiger, R., Slater, L. et al. (2007). Changes in the glomerular filtration rate of 27 cats with hyperthyroidism after treatment with radioactive iodine. *Veterinary Record* 161: 711–715.

Boretti, F.S., Sieber-Ruckstuhl, N.S., Gerber, B. et al. (2009). Thyroid enlargement and its relationship to clinicopathological parameters and T(4) status in suspected hyperthyroid cats. *Journal of Feline Medicine and Surgery* 11: 286–292.

Broussard, J.D., Peterson, M.E., and Fox, P.R. (1995). Changes in clinical and laboratory findings in cats with hyperthyroidism from 1983 to 1993. *Journal of the American Veterinary Medical Association* 206: 302–305.

Bucknell, D.G. (2000). Feline hyperthyroidism: spectrum of clinical presentations and response to carbimazole therapy. *Australian Veterinary Journal* 78: 462–465.

Buresova, E., Stock, E., Paepe, D. et al. (2019). Assessment of symmetric dimethylarginine as a biomarker of renal function in hyperthyroid cats treated with radioiodine. *Journal of Veterinary Internal Medicine* 33: 516–522.

Bush, J.L., Nemanic, S., Gordon, J., and Bobe, G. (2017). Computed tomographic characteristics of the thyroid glands in eight hyperthyroid cats pre- and postmethimazole treatment compared with seven euthyroid cats. *Veterinary Radiology & Ultrasound* 58: 176–185.

Covey, H.L., Chang, Y.M., Elliott, J., and Syme, H.M. (2019). Changes in thyroid and renal function after bilateral thyroidectomy in cats. *Journal of Veterinary Internal Medicine* 33: 508–515.

Crenshaw, K.L., Peterson, M.E., Heeb, L.A. et al. (1996). Serum fructosamine concentration as an index of glycemia in cats with diabetes mellitus and stress hyperglycemia. *Journal of Veterinary Internal Medicine* 10: 360–364.

Crossley, V.J., Debnath, A., Chang, Y.M. et al. (2017). Breed, coat color, and hair length as risk factors for hyperthyroidism in cats. *Journal of Veterinary Internal Medicine* 31: 1028–1034.

DeMonaco, S.M., Panciera, D.L., Morre, W.A. et al. (2020). Symmetric dimethylarginine in hyperthyroid cats before and after treatment with radioactive iodine. *Journal of Feline Medicine and Surgery* 22: 531–538.

Drost, W.T., Mattoon, J.S., and Weisbrode, S.E. (2006). Use of helical computed tomography for measurement of thyroid glands in clinically normal cats. *American Journal of Veterinary Research* 67: 467–471.

Fernandez, Y., Puig, J., Powell, R., and Seth, M. (2019). Prevalence of iatrogenic hypothyroidism in hyperthyroid cats treated with radioiodine using an individualised scoring system. *Journal of Feline Medicine and Surgery* 21: 1149–1156.

Flanders, J.A. (1999). Surgical options for the treatment of hyperthyroidism in the cat. *Journal of Feline Medicine and Surgery* 1: 127–134.

Flanders, J.A., Harvey, H.J., and Erb, H.N. (1987). Feline thyroidectomy. A comparison of postoperative hypocalcemia associated with three different surgical techniques. *Veterinary Surgery* 16: 362–366.

Flanders, J.A., Neth, S., Erb, H.N., and Kallfelz, F.A. (1991). Functional analysis of ectopic parathyroid activity in cats. *American Journal of Veterinary Research* 52: 1336–1340.

Gilman, O. (2019). Can iodine-restricted diets normalise serum total thyroxine (TT4) and subsequently improve clinical signs in cats with hyperthyroidism? *Veterinary Evidence* 4: 1–8.

Goldstein, R.E., Long, C., Swift, N.C. et al. (2001). Percutaneous ethanol injection for treatment of unilateral hyperplastic thyroid nodules in cats. *Journal of the American Veterinary Medical Association* 218: 1298–1302.

Graham, P.A., Mooney, C.T., and Murray, M. (1999). Serum fructosamine concentrations in hyperthyroid cats. *Research in Veterinary Science* 67: 171–175.

Grossi, G., Zoia, A., Palagiano, P. et al. (2019). Iodine-restricted food versus pharmacological therapy in the management of feline hyperthyroidism: a controlled trial in 34 cats. *Open Veterinary Journal* 9: 196–204.

Hill, K.E., Gieseg, M.A., Kingsbury, D. et al. (2011). The efficacy and safety of a novel lipophilic formulation of methimazole for the once daily transdermal treatment of cats with hyperthyroidism. *Journal of Veterinary Internal Medicine* 25: 1357–1365.

van Hoek, I., Hesta, M., and Biourge, V. (2015). A critical review of food-associated factors proposed in the etiology of feline hyperthyroidism. *Journal of Feline Medicine and Surgery* 17: 837–847.

Holzworth, J., Theran, P., Carpenter, J.L. et al. (1980). Hyperthyroidism in the cat: ten cases. *Journal of the American Veterinary Medical Association* 176: 345–353.

Jones, B., Engdahl, J.N., and Weiss, J. (2019). Are persistent organic pollutants important in the etiology of feline hyperthyroidism? A review. *Acta Veterinaria Scandinavica* 61: 45.

Kohler, I., Ballhausen, B.D., Stockhaus, C. et al. (2016). Prevalence of and risk factors for feline hyperthyroidism among a clinic population in southern Germany. *Tierarztl Prax Ausg K Kleintiere Heimtiere* 44: 149–157.

Lovelace, K. (2009). Comparing thyroid palpation techniques. *Journal of Feline Medicine and Surgery* 11: 525–526.

Lucy, J.M., Peterson, M.E., Randolph, J.F. et al. (2017). Efficacy of low-dose (2 millicurie) versus standard-dose (4 millicurie) radioiodine treatment for cats with mild-to-moderate hyperthyroidism. *Journal of Veterinary Internal Medicine* 31: 326–334.

Mallery, K.F., Pollard, R.E., Nelson, R.W. et al. (2003). Percutaneous ultrasound-guided radiofrequency heat ablation for treatment of hyperthyroidism in cats. *Journal of the American Veterinary Medical Association* 223: 1602–1607.

McLean, J.L., Lobetti, R.G., Mooney, C.T. et al. (2017). Prevalence of and risk factors for feline hyperthyroidism in South Africa. *Journal of Feline Medicine and Surgery* 19: 1103–1109.

Meric, S.M. and Rubin, S.I. (1990). Serum thyroxine concentrations following fixed-dose radioactive iodine treatment in hyperthyroid cats: 62 cases (1986–1989). *Journal of the American Veterinary Medical Association* 197: 621–623.

Miller, M.L., Peterson, M.E., Randolph, J.F. et al. (2017). Thyroid cysts in cats: a retrospective study of 40 cases. *Journal of Veterinary Internal Medicine* 31: 723–729.

Milner, R.J., Channell, C.D., Levy, J.K., and Schaer, M. (2006). Survival times for cats with hyperthyroidism treated with iodine 131, methimazole, or both: 167 cases (1996–2003). *Journal of the American Veterinary Medical Association* 228: 559–563.

Mooney, C.T. (2002). Pathogenesis of feline hyperthyroidism. *Journal of Feline Medicine and Surgery* 4: 167–169.

Mooney, C.T. and Peterson, M.E. (2012). *Manual of Canine and Feline Endocrinology*. Gloucester: BSAVA.

Naan, E.C., Kirpensteijn, J., Kooistra, H.S., and Peeters, M.E. (2006). Results of thyroidectomy in 101 cats with hyperthyroidism. *Veterinary Surgery* 35: 287–293.

Niessen, S.J., Voyce, M.J., de Villiers, L. et al. (2007). Generalised lymphadenomegaly associated with methimazole treatment in a hyperthyroid cat. *Journal of Small Animal Practice* 48: 165–168.

Norsworthy, G.D., Adams, V.J., McElhaney, M.R., and Milios, J.A. (2002a). Palpable thyroid and parathyroid nodules in asymptomatic cats. *Journal of Feline Medicine and Surgery* 4: 145–151.

Norsworthy, G.D., Adams, V.J., McElhaney, M.R., and Milios, J.A. (2002b). Relationship between semi-quantitative thyroid palpation and total thyroxine concentration in cats with and without hyperthyroidism. *Journal of Feline Medicine and Surgery* 4: 139–143.

Padgett, S. (2002). Feline thyroid surgery. *Veterinary Clinics of North America: Small Animal Practice* 32: 851–859, vi.

Padgett, S.L., Tobias, K.M., Leathers, C.W., and Wardrop, K.J. (1998). Efficacy of parathyroid gland autotransplantation in maintaining serum calcium concentrations after bilateral thyroparathyroidectomy in cats. *Journal of the American Animal Hospital Association* 34: 219–224.

Paepe, D., Smets, P., van Hoek, I. et al. (2008). Within- and between-examiner agreement for two thyroid palpation techniques in healthy and hyperthyroid cats. *Journal of Feline Medicine and Surgery* 10: 558–565.

Peterson, M.E. (2014). Animal models of disease: feline hyperthyroidism: an animal model for toxic nodular goiter. *Journal of Endocrinology* 223: T97–T114.

Peterson, M.E. (2020). Hyperthyroidism in cats: considering the impact of treatment modality on quality of life for cats and their owners. *Veterinary Clinics of North America: Small Animal Practice* 50: 1065–1084.

Peterson, J.J.G. and Andrews, L.K. (1979). Spontaneous hyperthyroidism in the cat. *Scientific Proceedings of the American College of Veterinary Internal Medicine, Seattle*, 108.

Peterson, M.E. and Becker, D.V. (1995). Radioiodine treatment of 524 cats with hyperthyroidism. *Journal of the American Veterinary Medical Association* 207: 1422–1428.

Peterson, M.E. and Broome, M.R. (2015). Thyroid scintigraphy findings in 2096 cats with hyperthyroidism. *Veterinary Radiology & Ultrasound* 56: 84–95.

Peterson, M.E. and Rishniw, M. (2021). A dosing algorithm for individualized radioiodine treatment of cats with hyperthyroidism. *Journal of Veterinary Internal Medicine* 35: 2140–2151.

Peterson, M.E., Kintzer, P.P., Cavanagh, P.G. et al. (1983). Feline hyperthyroidism: pretreatment clinical and laboratory evaluation of 131 cases. *Journal of the American Veterinary Medical Association* 183: 103–110.

Peterson, M.E., Kintzer, P.P., and Hurvitz, A.I. (1988). Methimazole treatment of 262 cats with hyperthyroidism. *Journal of Veterinary Internal Medicine* 2: 150–157.

Peterson, M.E., Guterl, J.N., Nichols, R., and Rishniw, M. (2015). Evaluation of serum thyroid-stimulating hormone concentration as a diagnostic test for hyperthyroidism in cats. *Journal of Veterinary Internal Medicine* 29: 1327–1334.

Peterson, M.E., Broome, M.R., and Rishniw, M. (2016a). Prevalence and degree of thyroid pathology in hyperthyroid cats increases with disease duration: a cross-sectional analysis of 2096 cats referred for radioiodine therapy. *Journal of Feline Medicine and Surgery* 18: 92–103.

Peterson, M.E., Castellano, C.A., and Rishniw, M. (2016b). Evaluation of body weight, body condition, and muscle condition in cats with hyperthyroidism. *Journal of Veterinary Internal Medicine* 30: 1780–1789.

Peterson, M.E., Guterl, J.N., Rishniw, M., and Broome, M.R. (2016c). Evaluation of quantitative thyroid scintigraphy for diagnosis and staging of disease severity in cats with hyperthyroidism: comparison of the percent thyroidal uptake of pertechnetate to thyroid-to-salivary ratio and thyroid-to-background ratios. *Veterinary Radiology & Ultrasound* 57: 427–440.

Peterson, M.E., Nichols, R., and Rishniw, M. (2017). Serum thyroxine and thyroid-stimulating hormone concentration in hyperthyroid cats that develop azotaemia after radioiodine therapy. *Journal of Small Animal Practice* 58: 519–530.

Peterson, M.E., Varela, F.V., Rishniw, M., and Polzin, D.J. (2018). Evaluation of serum symmetric dimethylarginine concentration as a marker for masked chronic kidney disease in cats with hyperthyroidism. *Journal of Veterinary Internal Medicine* 32: 295–304.

Peterson, M.E., Davignon, D.L., Shaw, N. et al. (2020a). Serum thyroxine and thyrotropin concentrations decrease with severity of nonthyroidal illness in cats and predict 30-day survival outcome. *Journal of Veterinary Internal Medicine* 34: 2276–2286.

Peterson, M.E., Li, A., Soboroff, P. et al. (2020b). Hyperthyroidism is not a risk factor for subclinical bacteriuria in cats: a prospective cohort study. *Journal of Veterinary Internal Medicine* 34: 1157–1165.

Sartor, L.L., Trepanier, L.A., Kroll, M.M. et al. (2004). Efficacy and safety of transdermal methimazole in the treatment of cats with hyperthyroidism. *Journal of Veterinary Internal Medicine* 18: 651–655.

Sissener, T. (2014). *Feline Soft Tissue and General Surgery*. Philadelphia, PA: Elsevier.

Stephens, M.J., O'Neill, D.G., Church, D.B. et al. (2014). Feline hyperthyroidism reported in primary-care veterinary practices in England: prevalence, associated factors and spatial distribution. *Veterinary Record* 175: 458.

Théon, A.P., Van Vechten, M.K., and Feldman, E. (1994). Prospective randomized comparison of intravenous versus subcutaneous administration of radioiodine for treatment of hyperthyroidism in cats. *American Journal of Veterinary Research* 55: 1734–1738.

Thoday, K.L. and Mooney, C.T. (1992). Historical, clinical and laboratory features of 126 hyperthyroid cats. *Veterinary Record* 131: 257–264.

Turrel, J.M., Feldman, E.C., Hays, M., and Hornof, W.J. (1984). Radioactive iodine therapy in cats with hyperthyroidism. *Journal of the American Veterinary Medical Association* 184: 554–559.

Vaske, H.H., Schermerhorn, T., and Grauer, G.F. (2016). Effects of feline hyperthyroidism on kidney function: a review. *Journal of Feline Medicine and Surgery* 18: 55–59.

Watson, N., Murray, J.K., Fonfara, S., and Hibbert, A. (2018). Clinicopathological features and comorbidities of cats with mild, moderate or severe hyperthyroidism: a radioiodine referral population. *Journal of Feline Medicine and Surgery* 20: 1130–1137.

Wehner, A., Koehler, I., Ramspott, S., and Hartmann, K. (2019). Relationship between total thyroxine, thyroid palpation and a clinical index in hyperthyroid and healthy cats and cats with other diseases. *Journal of Feline Medicine and Surgery* 21: 741–749.

Weichselbaum, R.C., Feeney, D.A., and Jessen, C.R. (2005). Relationship between selected echocardiographic variables before and after radioiodine treatment in 91 hyperthyroid cats. *Veterinary Radiology & Ultrasound* 46: 506–513.

Welches, C.D., Scavelli, T.D., Matthiesen, D.T., and Peterson, M.E. (1989). Occurrence of problems after three techniques of bilateral thyroidectomy in cats. *Veterinary Surgery* 18: 392–396.

Wells, A.L., Long, C.D., Hornof, W.J. et al. (2001). Use of percutaneous ethanol injection for treatment of bilateral hyperplastic thyroid nodules in cats. *Journal of the American Veterinary Medical Association* 218: 1293–1297.

Williams, T.L., Elliott, J., and Syme, H.M. (2010a). Association of iatrogenic hypothyroidism with azotemia and reduced survival time in cats treated for hyperthyroidism. *Journal of Veterinary Internal Medicine* 24: 1086–1092.

Williams, T.L., Peak, K.J., Brodbelt, D. et al. (2010b). Survival and the development of azotemia after treatment of hyperthyroid cats. *Journal of Veterinary Internal Medicine* 24: 863–869.

Williams, T.L., Elliott, J., and Syme, H.M. (2012). Calcium and phosphate homeostasis in hyperthyroid cats: associations with development of azotaemia and survival time. *Journal of Small Animal Practice* 53: 561–571.

Williams, T.L., Elliott, J., Berry, J., and Syme, H.M. (2013). Investigation of the pathophysiological mechanism for altered calcium homeostasis in hyperthyroid cats. *Journal of Small Animal Practice* 54: 367–373.

Williams, T.L., Elliott, J., and Syme, H.M (2014). Effect on renal function of restoration of euthyroidism n hyperthyroid cats with iatrogenic hypothyroidism. *Journal of Veterinary Internal Medicine* 28: 1251–1255.

Yu, L., Lacorcia, L., Finch, S., and Johnstone T. (2020). Assessment of serum symmetric dimethylarginine and creatinine concentrations in hyperthyroid cats before and after a fixed dose of orally administered radioiodine. *Journal of Veterinary Internal Medicine* 34: 1423–1431.

66

Canine Thyroid Neoplasia

Deanna R. Worley

Thyroid cancer is considered a common canine cancer, typically with a slow disease progression, and affecting mostly the older dog population. Of all the reported cancers in the dog population, thyroid cancer comprises 1.1% of tumors (Wucherer & Wilke 2010). Thyroid tumors are the most common endocrine tumor occurring in dogs (Barber 2007). Of all canine thyroid masses, 90% are either thyroid carcinoma or thyroid adenocarcinoma, and the majority of affected dogs present between 10 and 15 years of age (Wucherer & Wilke 2010). Of 1722 dogs prospectively studied for diagnosis of multiple distinct malignancies at a single oncology service, the diagnosis of thyroid carcinoma along with malignant melanoma and mast cell tumors were overrepresented (Rebhun & Thamm 2010). Furthermore, 33% of the dogs diagnosed with a thyroid tumor in that study were found to have additional distinct malignancies, which suggests a need for thorough staging for any dog presenting with a thyroid tumor (Rebhun & Thamm 2010). The more commonly affected breeds of dogs include golden retrievers, Labrador retrievers, and beagles in one cohort of 156 dogs having unilateral thyroidectomy (Reagan et al. 2019). Siberian huskies might be overrepresented, but thyroid tumors can affect any breed of dog (Wucherer & Wilke 2010). The majority of thyroid tumors present as unilateral in the bilobed thyroid gland (Reagan et al. 2019).

Clinical features

Most commonly a thyroid tumor is diagnosed following palpation of a cervical mass that is either discrete and mobile or fixed in the region of the normal thyroid gland, which is not normally palpable. Either or both lobes of the thyroid gland can be affected. Ectopic thyroid tumors can occur on the midline from the sublingual space to the base of the heart.

Common clinical signs include a palpable tumor, and varying symptoms due to increasing size and compressive or invasive mass effect of the tumor resulting in coughing, dysphagia, dyspnea, or dysphonia/laryngeal paralysis. Horner's syndrome may rarely be seen if the tumor mass also involves the preganglionic segment or sympathetic trunk. In one study of 156 dogs having unilateral thyroid lobectomy, the inciting clinical sign was owner palpation and discovery of a ventral cervical mass in over 50% of the dogs, whereas in 25% of the dogs the tumor was discovered during a physical examination (Reagan et al. 2019). Further, 5% of dogs presented with respiratory changes, and laryngeal paralysis was noted in 10 of the 156 dogs (6.4%) (Reagan et al. 2019). Among reported clinical signs in another contemporary cohort of 73 dogs receiving thyroidectomy for tumors having gross vascular invasion, a mass was noted in 80% of dogs, coughing in 6%, dysphonia in 6%, vomiting in 4%, dysphagia in 3%, and 19% of dogs did not have any clinical signs (Latifi et al. 2021). In another multi-institutional cohort of dogs having functional thyroid tumors causing hyperthyroidism, the more commonly reported clinical signs were polyuria/polydipsia and weight loss, with less frequently polyphagia, alopecia, and panting (Frederick et al. 2020).

Thyrotoxic crisis or thyroid storm is a rare life-threatening crisis that may occur with functional thyroid tumors and/or following tumor manipulation, resulting in excess circulation of thyroid hormone causing acute hypertension, tachyarrhythmias, hyperthermia, central nervous system dysfunction, gastrointestinal dysfunction, and even multiorgan dysfunction (Merkle *et al.* 2021; Lee *et al.* 2017). This should be considered when preparing an anesthetic protocol for dogs with thyroid tumors (Merkle *et al.* 2021; Lee *et al.* 2017).

Diagnostic procedures

Physical examination

The most important criteria for assessment of thyroid tumor resectability are determining tumor discreteness and mobility via digital palpation. Mobility is defined as movement ≥1 cm in all planes (Tuohy *et al.* 2012). For larger thyroid masses or for dogs resistant to deep cervical palpation, the aid of sedation or anesthesia may be necessary for thorough palpation and to allow for relaxed musculature. Preoperative laryngeal function assessment is also critical for determining tumor involvement of the recurrent laryngeal nerve, and should be paired with an immediate postoperative laryngeal assessment upon extubation, especially following thyroidectomy for ascertaining potential iatrogenic disruption of the paired nerves. Thorough palpation of the entire cervical region and hyoid apparatus is also warranted for potential ectopic thyroid tumors. In the multi-institutional retrospective study of 156 dogs having a unilateral thyroid lobectomy, the majority of thyroid masses were assessed as being mobile, with 15 of 156 dogs having documentation of a fixed thyroid tumor (Reagan *et al.* 2019). Surprisingly a preoperative laryngeal function exam was documented in just 2 dogs in that study, but was likely performed in most dogs (Reagan *et al.* 2019). Tumor size and volume have been described as historical prognostic indicators. In the same study, the maximal single-dimension measurement recorded in 133 of 156 dogs ranged from 1 cm to over 18 cm, with a mean measurement of 4.4 cm; 30 tumors measured at or over 7 cm in diameter (Reagan *et al.* 2019). Of note is that even when thyroid tumors palpate as freely movable, gross vascular invasion may be present (Latifi *et al.* 2021).

Thyroid function

The majority of canine thyroid tumors are nonfunctional. In the cohort of 156 dogs presenting for unilateral thyroidectomy, 5% of dogs presented with elevated serum thyroid hormone measurements, and 10% of dogs presented with clinical signs associated with hyperthyroidism (Reagan *et al.* 2019). In the same study, a prior diagnosis of hyperthyroidism was made in about 10% of dogs, hypothyroidism in 7%, and hyperparathyroidism in 2%; 5 additional dogs (3.2%) had hyperadreno-

corticism, hypoadrenocorticism, hyperadrenocorticism with hyperparathyroidism, or hyperadrenocorticism with hypothyroidism (Reagan *et al.* 2019). Of 50 dogs with thyroid tumors with gross vascular invasion, the preoperative measurements of total T4 (measuring both free and bound serum thyroxine) levels were increased in 9 dogs, decreased in 6 dogs, and normal in the remaining 35 dogs (Latifi *et al.* 2021).

Blood typing

Routine blood typing is done at the discretion of the surgeon for discrete mobile thyroid tumors. For thyroid tumors with gross vascular invasion and/or for fixed primary tumors, it is encouraged.

Echocardiography and electrocardiography

Cardiac evaluation should be considered, particularly for dogs that have functional thyroid tumors causing hyperthyroidism.

Radiographs of the chest

Metastatic-view thoracic radiographs are indicated as a minimum for tumor staging of thyroid tumors for the presence of pulmonary metastasis. Up to 40% of dogs have been reported to have metastasis at presentation.

Ultrasound of the neck

Ventral cervical ultrasound aids in assessing the origin of cervical masses, if there are any gross tumor-associated vascular thrombi, and the size of regional cervical lymph nodes, which are often not palpable. Ultrasound also aids in precise aspiration of structures for cytology. The utility of cervical ultrasound is operator dependent and it is not as sensitive as contrast-enhanced cervical computed tomography (CT) imaging.

Computed tomography of the neck

Contrast-enhanced CT imaging from the base of the tongue to the heart base is a sensitive tool for assessing thyroid tumor, ectopic thyroid tumors, gross vascular invasion, and for any regional lymphadenopathy. Especially for fixed thyroid tumors and for ectopic tumors, the inclusion of an angiogram may further delineate the tumor and tumor involvement with the surrounding anatomy. Another advantage of CT imaging is the option to perform pre-contrast pulmonary imaging, as CT imaging of the lungs is more sensitive at detecting metastatic lesions and smaller metastatic lesions than thoracic radiography. Indirect CT lymphography may also be considered for determining which of the regional lymph nodes might be at risk for metastasis.

Thyroid tumors may be discovered incidentally during routine CT imaging of the head and neck. In one study of 4000 dogs having a CT scan for any reason and including the cervical region, 34 dogs were found to have incidental thyroid lesions, with the majority of lesions being thyroid carcinomas (Bertolini *et al.* 2017).

In the case series of 73 dogs having thyroidectomy with gross vascular invasion, all dogs had preoperative contrast-enhanced cervical CT imaging, with the median maximal tumor length range of 2–12 cm and the median length being 5 cm (Latifi *et al.* 2021).

Radionuclide scan

Thyroid scintigraphy, either with sodium pertechnetate ($^{99m}TcO_4$) or radioiodine (^{123}I), is used to assess if a patient is a good candidate for radioiodine (^{131}I) treatment of the thyroid tumor, for identification of ectopic thyroid tissue, and for identification of metastatic thyroid tissue (van den Berg *et al.* 2020). Radioiodine, both the lower-energy ^{123}I and ^{131}I, is actively trapped in the thyroid gland and incorporated into thyroid hormone, which is mediated by the sodium iodide symporter and represents actual uptake, whereas pertechnetate is not organified or incorporated into thyroid hormone but represents the trapping mechanism (van den Berg *et al.* 2020; Turrel *et al.* 2006; Lyssens *et al.* 2021). Thyroid scintigraphy is accomplished either via planar imaging or with a SPECT camera (single-photon emission computed tomography). SPECT imaging captures multiple 2D images that can be reconstructed to provided 3D imaging and a more sensitive study (van den Berg *et al.* 2020). Whereas planar imaging is limited for assessing thyroid tissue, SPECT imaging has increased sensitivity for also detecting pulmonary metastasis, especially when compared to thoracic radiographs; the sensitivity compared to thoracic CT imaging is unknown (van den Berg *et al.* 2020).

Cytology

Cytologic aspiration of a thyroid tumor is often rewarding in obtaining a pretreatment diagnosis of at least an epithelial or neuroendocrine tumor. In one study, 106 canine unilateral thyroid tumors were fine-needle aspirated, with only 13 tumor cytologies being either nondiagnostic or not representative of the tumor (Reagan *et al.* 2019). In another study of 60 dogs having thyroid tumor fine-needle aspirates, cytologic diagnoses were noted as thyroid carcinoma (48%), neuroendocrine (30%), undifferentiated carcinoma (5%), and nondiagnostic in only 17% of dogs (Latifi *et al.* 2021).

Treatment

Dogs with discrete mobile thyroid tumors, whether unilateral or bilateral, are amenable for surgical treatment and surgery provides the opportunity for the longest patient survival of all modalities. Select ectopic basihyoid and other ectopic thyroid tumors also benefit from surgical resection. With other treatment modalities being available, there is limited enthusiasm for and great caution over resection of thyroid tumors that are clearly fixed and/or invasive to the trachea or esophagus.

Surgical excision

A ventral cervical exploratory surgery can be pursued for discrete mobile thyroid tumors, bypassing other imaging modalities such as cervical ultrasonography or CT, and with the disadvantage of not knowing if any gross vascular invasion is present, if there are any aberrant vascular patterns, or the stage of regional lymph nodes without performing an additional deeper surgical dissection.

Patients are placed in dorsal recumbency, with a towel under the neck for support and elevation, for the ventral midline cervical exploratory. Meticulous dissection and judicious hemostasis are encouraged, along with identification of normal structures, particularly the recurrent laryngeal nerves and the esophagus, which can be deceptive in appearance. The recurrent laryngeal nerve should be treated gently and with avoidance of any electrocautery dose. An attempt should be made to resect gross tumor thrombi *en bloc* with the thyroid tumor, and thyroid tumors are resected marginally. Due to tumor-associated angiogenesis, the vascular pattern may likely appear as numerous and abnormal. The jugular vein or carotid artery could be entrapped by the tumor and even the recurrent laryngeal nerve, with a need for sacrifice while ideally preserving the contralateral laryngeal nerve. A cuff of skeletal muscle is resected *en bloc* for any thyroid tumors focally fixed to the strap muscles. Various tools aid with hemostasis in the neck, including monopolar electrocautery, bipolar electrocautery, cotton-tipped applicators, hemoclips, and vessel-sealant devices. Use of a vessel-sealant device may enable a shorter operation time when performing thyroidectomies (Lorange *et al.* 2019).

Staging lymphadenectomy and sentinel lymph node mapping are generally considered as elective for this disease, yet a recent case series highlights a different perspective. Of 22 dogs having thyroidectomy for thyroid tumors, all had extirpation performed of at least an ipsilateral medial retropharyngeal lymph node, and in some dogs also of any enlarged deep cervical or superficial cervical lymph nodes if present and variable contralateral nodes (Skinner *et al.* 2021). Lymph node metastasis was found in 10 of the 22 dogs, highlighting a potential need for improved lymph node staging in dogs with thyroid carcinoma (Skinner *et al.* 2021).

Of 156 dogs having unilateral thyroidectomy, residual macroscopic disease was left in 7% of dogs, gross vascular invasion was found in 35% and lymph node metastasis in 7% (Reagan et al. 2019). Perioperative complications occurred in 20% of dogs, with surgical hemorrhage being the most common (8% of the 156 dogs) and most receiving blood transfusions (Reagan et al. 2019). Postoperative complications occurred in 13%, with aspiration pneumonia being the most common (3% of the 156 dogs) and with 2 of the dogs having bilateral laryngeal paralysis (Reagan et al. 2019). Other reported postoperative complications included hematochezia, Horner's syndrome, hemorrhage, hyperthermia, hypothyroidism, transient vestibular disease, laryngeal paralysis, respiratory arrest, and death (Reagan et al. 2019). Less than 3% of dogs did not survive the hospitalization prior to discharge (Reagan et al. 2019). Factors associated with the complication rate included whether the thyroid tumor was palpated as fixed and an increasing number of days of hospitalization (Reagan et al. 2019). Factors found not to be associated with complication rate included tumor size, malignancy of the thyroid mass, concurrent endocrinopathy, anesthetic time, and presence of gross vascular invasion (Reagan et al. 2019).

Of 73 dogs with thyroid tumors with gross vascular invasion, gross vascular invasion was discovered unexpectedly intraoperatively in 85% of dogs, while preoperative contrast-enhanced CT imaging detected gross vascular invasion in 45% of the dogs (Latifi et al. 2021). In that same population of dogs, 26% had thyroid tumors invading the soft tissues of muscle and the esophagus, with three dogs receiving partial esophagectomy (Latifi et al. 2021). There were limited complications following thyroidectomy with *en bloc* resection of the gross vascular tumor thrombi; two dogs required transfusions for intraoperative bleeding, one dog sustained a small esophageal perforation, and two dogs died postoperatively prior to hospital dismissal (Latifi et al. 2021). Aspiration pneumonia occurred in 4% of cases (Latifi et al. 2021). Of the dogs having elective lymph node resections, metastasis was found in over 40%, with an unclear impact on overall patient survival (Latifi et al. 2021).

A surgical sequela of removing both thyroid lobes is hypocalcemia if none of the parathyroid glands can be preserved, and also hypothyroidism. Of 15 dogs with mobile discrete bilateral thyroid tumors, parathyroid glands could not be salvaged in 9 dogs, and a single parathyroid gland was reimplanted in 4 dogs and preserved in 2 dogs during thyroidectomy (Tuohy et al. 2012). In the same study, 11 dogs experienced transient hypocalcemia, with 7 dogs having no preserved parathyroid tissue, 3 parathyroid glands were reimplanted, and 1 was

preserved (Tuohy et al. 2012). Many dogs required lifelong calcitriol supplementation and most required thyroid hormone supplementation (Tuohy et al. 2012). The median survival time for this population of dogs was three years, with some dogs having gross vascular invasion and varying tumor sizes (Tuohy et al. 2012).

Another surgical sequela may be hypothyroidism if resecting a hormonally active tumor. In a cohort of 27 dogs having thyroidectomy for functional thyroid tumors, permanent thyroid hormone supplementation was required for 9 unilateral thyroid tumor resections and all 5 of the bilateral thyroid tumor resections, while temporary thyroid hormone supplementation was required for 6 unilateral thyroid tumor resections (Frederick et al. 2020). Median survival time for this cohort of dogs was three years (Frederick et al. 2020). Similar results are found in another case series of dogs with functional thyroid tumors (Scharf et al. 2020).

Ectopic thyroid tumor lesions if present may need to be removed from the thorax via median sternotomy or thoracoscopy, or from the hyoid apparatus via partial hyoidectomy if ectopic lesions develop outside of the cervical space. In a case series of five dogs receiving partial hyoid apparatus resection for ectopic thyroid tumors, all dogs were able to drink and eat within a day following surgery, which also included partial resection of the tongue root (Milovancev et al. 2014). Intraoperatively, hyoid apparatus-stabilizing sutures were placed, with unclear effectiveness. Two dogs had mild transient inspiratory stridor or inspiratory stertor, which did not require treatment, and one dog was noted to have a persistent change in bark without exercise intolerance or respiratory problems (Milovancev et al. 2014). Surgery was well tolerated by these dogs (Milovancev et al. 2014).

External beam radiation therapy

Radiation therapy can be administered in a palliative-intent protocol for nonresectable thyroid carcinomas. In a contemporary cohort of 20 dogs treated with hypofractionated radiation therapy, and with most dogs having distant metastasis, the median survival time was 170 days (Tsimbas et al. 2019). Following radiation therapy of a thyroid tumor, hypothyroidism may develop regardless of the radiation protocol used and with a median time to diagnosis of six months following therapy (Amores-Fuster et al. 2017). However, there is a historically reported low incidence of radiation-induced hypothyroidism and hypoparathyroidism (Brearley et al. 1999; Theon et al. 2000).

Stereotactic body radiation therapy (SBRT) has also been described for thyroid tumors. In a case series of 23 dogs receiving SBRT for thyroid tumors, 70% of dogs had clinical signs of tumor compression due to tumor size, with signs of coughing, dysphagia, and dyspnea, and with visualized laryngeal paralysis in 33% of the dogs (Lee *et al.* 2020). The majority of dogs had bilateral and or ectopic basihyoid tumors, and 70% of all the dogs were classified as having nonresectable tumors (Lee *et al.* 2020). These dogs had larger tumors (median longest tumor diameter 16.6 cm) and represented a cohort of more advanced disease, with 57% having stage III disease and 44% stage IV disease (Lee *et al.* 2020). Of the dogs presenting with clinical signs, improvement was seen in 80% with a median time of 16 days (Lee *et al.* 2020). The overall tumor response rate (complete and partial responses) was 70% (Lee *et al.* 2020). Median progression-free survival was 315 days and median survival time was 362 days for this population of dogs with advanced disease and with a low radiation toxicity profile (Lee *et al.* 2020). Three of the four euthyroid dogs developed hypothyroidism and required permanent supplementation (Lee *et al.* 2020).

[131]I radiation therapy

Radioiodine is used for treatment of fixed or metastatic thyroid tumors with active iodine pumps in the neoplastic tissue. Being a radioactive therapeutic, its use is limited to facilities able to accommodate radioactive isotopes, prolonged housing of radioactive patients and radioactive biologic waste, proximity to a cyclotron, and adherence to radiation safety protocols and regulations. Dogs being treated may need to be isolated for several days or weeks, as the half-life of ^{131}I is 8.1 days.

Of 39 dogs receiving treatment of ^{131}I for fixed invasive thyroid tumors, including ectopic sites and with 7 dogs having metastasis, adverse events occurred in 3 dogs, with all 3 developing bone marrow suppression with secondary sequelae resulting in death 1–4 months after injection (Turrel *et al.* 2006). Transient posttreatment hypothyroidism was noted in other dogs, requiring tapered supplementation (Turrel *et al.* 2006). [131]I was noted to prolong the overall survival time in this cohort of dogs with nonresectable thyroid tumors, with a median survival time greater than two years and without any survival advantage for dogs having resection of residual disease (Turrel *et al.* 2006). In a different cohort of 20 dogs receiving radioiodine for sublingual ectopic thyroid tumors, either as sole therapy (with 5 of the dogs having metastatic disease) or following surgical resection, the median survival times did not significantly vary (347 days versus 976 days) (Broome *et al.* 2014). In another cohort of five dogs having treatment of ^{131}I for functional nonresectable ectopic thyroid tumors with clinical signs of hyperthyroidism, bone marrow suppression occurred in one dog and signs of hyperthyroidism resolved in all (Lyssens *et al.* 2021). Four dogs became

euthyroid after treatment and one developed hypothyroidism requiring supplementation (Lyssens *et al.* 2021). There was a measurable decrease in tumor size in all five dogs and an overall median survival time of two years (Lyssens *et al.* 2021).

Chemotherapy

The potential survival benefit of chemotherapy for dogs with thyroid carcinoma is still unknown for both macroscopic and microscopic disease (Sheppard-Olivares *et al.* 2020; Tuohy *et al.* 2012; Reagan *et al.* 2019). In one of the largest studies to date evaluating toceranib phosphate for treatment of measurable thyroid tumors in 42 dogs, clinical benefit (either complete response, partial response, or stable disease) was documented for the majority of treated dogs, whether for treatment-naive thyroid tumors or for thyroid tumors previously treated, though there were no differences in progression-free interval or in overall survival times between groups (Sheppard-Olivares *et al.* 2020). Historically reported sole-therapy and adjuvant chemotherapy protocols also include carboplatin, doxorubicin, cyclophosphamide, and other agents, again with unclear benefit to overall survival.

Long-term monitoring

Follow-up monitoring is advised every three months for the next year and a half, with a taper to every six months thereafter. Monitoring should include assessments for local disease recurrence, whether there is any regional lymphatic metastasis, hormone assessment, and checking for development of any distant metastatic disease.

Prognosis

Following marginal excision of thyroid lobe tumors, the local recurrence rate is low. In a cohort of 73 dogs having gross vascular invasion and thyroidectomy, the local tumor recurrence rate was suspected to be 10%, with a median time to recurrence of 238 days following surgery (Latifi *et al.* 2021). Distant metastasis was reported in 12% of dogs at a median of 375 days post surgery (Latifi *et al.* 2021). The median overall survival time was 621 days for these dogs, with 82.5% of dogs alive at one year following surgery (Latifi *et al.* 2021). These dogs had excellent or good outcomes even with gross vascular invasion.

In a cohort of 156 dogs having unilateral thyroidectomy, local recurrence was suspected to occur in 12% of dogs and metastatic disease developed in 8% (Reagan *et al.* 2019). The overall median survival time was 911 days (Reagan *et al.* 2019). In that study, a higher mitotic index and larger maximal tumor diameter size were significantly associated with shorter progression-free interval, and the higher mitotic index was associated with decreased survival times (Reagan *et al.* 2019). Historically and recently, the median survival time has been reported at over 3 years following surgery for mobile discrete tumors, versus 6–12 months for fixed invasive tumors (Klein *et al.* 1995; Carver *et al.* 1995; Scharf *et al.* 2020).

Typically, metastasis progresses to regional lymph nodes and lung, but also rarely to atypical sites such as the spinal canal and pelvic region, kidneys, liver, spleen, and bones (Reagan *et al.* 2019; Latifi *et al.* 2021; Lee *et al.* 2020).

References

Amores-Fuster, I., Cripps, P., and Blackwood, L. (2017). Post-radiotherapy hypothyroidism in dogs treated for thyroid carcinomas. *Veterinary and Comparative Oncology* 15: 247–251.

Barber, L.G. (2007). Thyroid tumors in dogs and cats. *Veterinary Clinics of North America. Small Animal Practice* 37: 755–773. vii.

Bertolini, G., Drigo, M., Angeloni, L., and Caldin, M. (2017). Incidental and nonincidental canine thyroid tumors assessed by multidetector row computed tomography: a single-centre cross sectional study in 4520 dogs. *Veterinary Radiology and Ultrasound* 58: 304–314.

Brearley, M.J., Hayes, A.M., and Murphy, S. (1999). Hypofractionated radiation therapy for invasive thyroid carcinoma in dogs: a retrospective analysis of survival. *Journal of Small Animal Practice* 40: 206–210.

Broome, M.R., Peterson, M.E., and Walker, J.R. (2014). Clinical features and treatment outcomes of 41 dogs with sublingual ectopic thyroid neoplasia. *Journal of Veterinary Internal Medicine* 28: 1560–1568.

Carver, J.R., Kapatkin, A., and Patnaik, A.K. (1995). A comparison of medullary thyroid carcinoma and thyroid adenocarcinoma in dogs: a retrospective study of 38 cases. *Veterinary Surgery* 24: 315–319.

Frederick, A.N., Pardo, A.D., Schmiedt, C.W. et al. (2020). Outcomes for dogs with functional thyroid tumors treated by surgical excision alone. *Journal of the American Veterinary Medical Association* 256: 444–448.

Klein, M.K., Powers, B.E., Withrow, S.J. et al. (1995). Treatment of thyroid carcinoma in dogs by surgical resection alone: 20 cases (1981–1989). *Journal of the American Veterinary Medical Association* 206: 1007–1009.

Latifi, M., Skinner, O.T., Spoldi, E. et al. (2021). Outcome and postoperative complications in 73 dogs with thyroid carcinoma with gross vascular invasion managed with thyroidectomy. *Veterinary and Comparative Oncology* 19: 685–696.

Lee, A., Shin, C.W., Son, W.G. et al. (2017). Anesthesia case of the month. *Journal of the American Veterinary Medical Association* 250: 1379–1385.

Lee, B.I., LaRue, S.M., Seguin, B. et al. (2020). Safety and efficacy of stereotactic body radiation therapy (SBRT) for the treatment of canine thyroid carcinoma. *Veterinary and Comparative Oncology* 18: 843–853.

Lorange, M., De Arburn Parent, R., Huneault, L. et al. (2019). Use of a vessel-sealing device versus conventional hemostatic techniques in dogs undergoing thyroidectomy because of suspected thyroid carcinoma. *Journal of the American Veterinary Medical Association* 254: 1186–1191.

Lyssens, A., van den Berg, M.F., Peremans, K. et al. (2021). 131 treatment in dogs with hyperthyroidism caused by a non-resectable ectopic thyroid tumour: 5 cases (2008–2019). *Journal of Small Animal Practice* 62: 137–144.

Merkle, J.E., Boudreaux, B., Langohr, I. et al. (2021). Thyroid storm in a dog secondary to thyroid carcinoma. *Journal of Veterinary Emergency and Critical Care* 31: 428–431.

Milovancev, M., Wilson, D.M., Monnet, E., and Seguin, B. (2014). Partial resection of the hyoid apparatus during surgical treatment of ectopic thyroid carcinomas in dogs: 5 cases (2011–2013). *Journal of the American Veterinary Medical Association* 244: 1319–1324.

Reagan, J.K., Selmic, L.E., Fallon, C. et al. (2019). Complications and outcomes associated with unilateral thyroidectomy in dogs with naturally occurring thyroid tumors: 156 cases (2003–2015). *Journal of the American Veterinary Medical Association* 255: 926–932.

Rebhun, R.B. and Thamm, D.H. (2010). Multiple distinct malignancies in dogs: 53 cases. *Journal of the American Animal Hospital Association* 46: 20–30.

Scharf, V.F., Oblak, M.L., Hoffman, K. et al. (2020). Clinical features and outcome of functional thyroid tumours in 70 dogs. *Journal of Small Animal Practice* 61: 504–511.

Sheppard-Olivares, S., Bello, N.M., Wood, E. et al. (2020). Toceranib phosphate in the treatment of canine thyroid carcinoma: 42 cases (2009–2018). *Veterinary and Comparative Oncology* 18: 519–527.

Skinner, O.T., Souza, C.H.M., and Kim, D.Y. (2021). Metastasis to ipsilateral medial retropharyngeal and deep cervical lymph nodes in 22 dogs with thyroid carcinoma. *Veterinary Surgery* 50: 150–157.

Theon, A.P., Marks, S.L., Feldman, E.S. and Griffey, S. (2000). Prognostic factors and patterns of treatment failure in dogs with unresectable differentiated thyroid carcinomas treated with megavoltage irradiation. *Journal of the American Veterinary Medical Association* 216: 1775–1779.

Tsimbas, K., Turek, M., Christensen, N. et al. (2019). Short survival time following palliative-intent hypofractionated radiotherapy for non-resectable canine thyroid carcinoma: a retrospective analysis of 20 dogs. *Veterinary Radiology and Ultrasound* 60: 93–99.

Tuohy, J.L., Worley, D.R., and Withrow, S. (2012). Outcome following simultaneous bilateral thyroid lobectomy for treatment of thyroid gland carcinoma in dogs: 15 cases (1994–2010). *Journal of the American Veterinary Medical Association* 241: 95–103.

Turrel, J.M., McEntee, M.C., Burke, B.F., and Page, R.L. (2006). Sodium iodide I-131 treatment of dogs with nonresectable thyroid tumors: 39 cases (1990–2003). *Journal of the American Veterinary Medical Association* 229: 542–548.

van den Berg, M.F., Daminet, S., Stock, E. et al. (2020). Planar and single-photon emission computed tomography imaging in dogs with thyroid tumors: 68 cases. *Journal of Veterinary Internal Medicine* 34: 2651–2659.

Wucherer, K.L. and Wilke, V. (2010). Thyroid cancer in dogs: an update based on 638 cases (1995–2005). *Journal of the American Animal Hospital Association* 46: 249–254.

67

Canine and Feline Insulinoma

Floryne O. Buishand and Jolle Kirpensteijn

Insulin-secreting tumors, more commonly known as insulinomas, originate from endocrine β cells in the islets of Langerhans in the pancreas. Insulinoma is uncommon in dogs and rare in cats. Irrespective of its medical rarity, many cases of insulinoma have been described in the dog. The first canine insulinoma was reported in 1935 by Slye and Wells, followed by more than 400 dogs with insulinoma in the last three decades. In contrast, only nine cases of feline insulinoma have been reported (O'Brien *et al.* 1990; Kraje 2003; Greene & Bright 2008; Schaub & Wigger 2013; Cervone *et al.* 2019; Gifford *et al.* 2020). Therefore this chapter mainly focuses on canine insulinoma.

Pathology

Insulinoma is the most common pancreatic endocrine tumor in the dog. Immunohistochemically, neoplastic β cells in dogs and humans have been shown to produce a variety of hormones in addition to insulin. These hormones include glucagon, somatostatin, gastrin, serotonin, growth hormone, and pancreatic polypeptide (Heitz *et al.* 1982; Hawkins *et al.* 1987; O'Brien *et al.* 1987; Robben *et al.* 2002; Fernandez *et al.* 2009; Madarame *et al.* 2009). Although multiple hormones have been demonstrated immunohistochemically in insulinoma, the occurrence of mixed clinical syndromes is rare and therefore insulinomas are named after insulin, the hormone that is principally secreted, and the most common clinical sign, hyperinsulinemia-induced hypoglycemia.

In 90% of cases, primary canine insulinoma are solitary tumors and their diameter is usually smaller than 2.5 cm (Steiner & Bruyette 1996; Feldman & Nelson 2004).

Most insulinomas are located in the left or right pancreatic lobe, rather than in the pancreatic body (Mehlhaff *et al.* 1985; Tryfonidou *et al.* 1998; Tobin *et al.* 1999). Multiple primary tumors are present in 10–14% of cases and although very rare, diffuse tumor growth in the pancreas can be observed.

In 1969, Capen and Martin stated that 60% of insulinomas are carcinomas and 40% are adenomas. According to these authors, hyperinsulinism was more commonly diagnosed in dogs with β-cell carcinomas than in dogs with β-cell adenomas. Yet in a more recent study, insulinomas in 35 dogs were all classified as adenocarcinomas (Mehlhaff *et al.* 1985). Although there is still some controversy in the literature concerning the benign or malignant nature of β-cell tumors in the dog, in general canine insulinomas are considered to be malignant in more than 95% of cases, because even though they may lack histologic criteria of malignancy, they almost always tend to metastasize (Leifer *et al.* 1986; Caywood *et al.* 1988; Buishand *et al.* 2010). In 40–50% of dogs, macroscopically visible insulinoma metastases are already present at surgery, primarily in regional lymph nodes (i.e., duodenal, hepatic, splenic, and greater mesenteric) and/or the liver (Figure 67.1) (Mehlhaff *et al.* 1985; Leifer *et al.* 1986; Tryfonidou *et al.* 1998). Other metastatic sites include duodenum, mesentery, omentum, spleen, kidney, heart, and spinal cord. Pulmonary metastases seem rare. Clinical staging of insulinoma is performed in accordance with the World Health Organization's TNM (tumor, node, metastasis) system (Table 67.1) (Owen 1980).

Dogs with insulinoma are divided into one of three clinical stages based on extent of neoplasia: T1N0M0

Small Animal Soft Tissue Surgery, Second Edition. Edited by Eric Monnet.
© 2023 John Wiley & Sons, Inc. Published 2023 by John Wiley & Sons, Inc.
Companion website: www.wiley.com/go/monnet/small

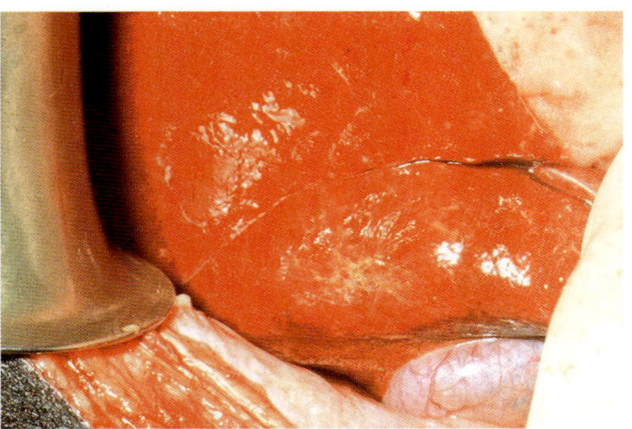

Figure 67.1 A large insulinoma metastasis in the liver of a dog.

Table 67.1 TNM classification for canine insulinoma.

T Primary tumor
  T0: No evidence of tumor
  T1: Tumor present
N Regional lymph nodes
  N0: No regional lymph nodes involved
  N1: Regional lymph nodes involved
M Distant metastasis
  M0: No evidence of distant metastasis
  M1: Distant metastasis present

(clinical stage I), T1N1M0 (clinical stage II), and T0N0M1, T1N0M1, or T1N1M1 (clinical stage III).

Pathophysiology

Insulinomas hypersecrete insulin, producing an increased insulin concentration in the blood. The elevated insulin levels inhibit glycogenolysis and gluconeogenesis and thereby suppress glucose secretion by hepatocytes. Moreover, the high insulin levels stimulate glucose uptake by muscle and adipose tissue. In normal β cells, insulin secretion is tightly regulated by the blood glucose concentration. In contrast to most other cells, the entrance of glucose into β-cells via facilitative glucose transporters (GLUTs) is insulin independent. With increasing blood glucose concentrations, insulin secretion gradually increases, eventually reaching a plateau level. Conversely, when blood glucose concentrations decrease, insulin secretion is inhibited.

Neoplastic β-cells are less sensitive to the negative feedback of low blood glucose concentrations. Therefore insulinomas secrete inappropriately high amounts of insulin despite declining blood glucose concentrations, resulting in a profound hypoglycemia (Feldman & Nelson 2004).

The clinical signs of hyperinsulinemia-induced hypoglycemia are due to activation of the autonomic nervous system and the lack of an energy substrate available to the central nervous system. The latter is called neuroglycopenia and results in neurologic signs, since nervous tissue can use only glucose for its energy supply and diffusion of glucose across the blood–brain barrier as well as cerebral oxidation are severely impaired in a situation of low blood glucose concentration. Activation of the autonomic nervous system involves both neuronally released transmitters and catecholamines released by the adrenal medulla.

Signalment

Insulinomas are most frequently diagnosed in middle-sized to large-breed dogs. Although a real breed predilection has not been established German shepherds, Irish setters, boxers, golden retrievers, poodles, fox terriers, collies, and Labrador retrievers appear most frequently affected. Insulinomas are also reported to occur in smaller breeds such as West Highland white terriers. There is no sex predisposition for the disease (Mehlhaff *et al.* 1985; Leifer *et al.* 1986; Caywood *et al.* 1988). Based on 214 dogs from eight reports, the mean age of dogs with insulinoma at the time of diagnosis is 9.1 years (range 3–15 years) (Mehlhaff *et al.* 1985; Tryfonidou *et al.* 1998; Tobin *et al.* 1999; Moore *et al.* 2002; Bryson *et al.* 2007; Fernandez *et al.* 2009; Madarame *et al.* 2009; Buishand *et al.* 2010).

Clinical signs

Common clinical signs of dogs with insulinoma are due to neuroglycopenia and include seizures, collapse, generalized weakness, posterior paresis, lethargy, ataxia, and exercise intolerance. Hypoglycemia-induced stimulation of the autonomic nervous system may result in muscle tremors, nervousness, and hunger (Table 67.2).

Clinical signs of canine insulinoma often occur intermittently. In the initial stages hypoglycemic episodes are preceded by fasting, exercise, excitement, or stress, because those situations lead to increased glucose utilization. Paradoxically, an episode might also follow directly after a meal, because the neoplastic β cells respond excessively to the postprandial rise in blood glucose concentration, indicating some sensitivity to the glucose feedback loop.

At first hypoglycemic attacks occur at widely spaced intervals, but as the disease progresses they will succeed each other at shorter intervals and will become more severe. The severity of clinical signs depends on the glucose nadir: convulsions and loss of consciousness often

Table 67.2 Clinical signs reported in 197 dogs.

	Number of dogs	Percentage of dogs
Collapse	94	48
Seizures	83	42
Generalized weakness	63	33
Exercise intolerance	30	15
Ataxia	29	15
Paresis posterior	20	10
Tremors	19	10
Disorientation	14	7
Lethargy	11	6
Shaking	11	6
Polyphagia	10	5
Hysteria	8	4
Polyuria and polydipsia	8	4
Focal facial seizures	6	3
Status epilepticus	4	2
Anxiousness	3	2
Inappetence	3	2
Asymptomatic	2	1

occur when blood glucose concentration is below 50 mg/dL (<2.8 mmol/L). The rate of decrease in the blood glucose concentration and the duration of hypoglycemia also determine the severity of the clinical signs. For example, a blood glucose concentration that gradually declines to 36 mg/dL (2 mmol/L) over an extended period is less likely to result in clinical signs of hypoglycemia compared with a blood glucose concentration of 36 mg/dL that develops rapidly over a few hours. Between hypoglycemic attacks, affected dogs usually do not have clinical signs.

Prolonged and severe episodes of hypoglycemia may eventually induce laminar cortical necrosis in the cerebrum, leading to coma and death (Capen & Martin 1969). The mean duration of clinical signs prior to diagnosis is 3.6 months (range 1 day–3.5 years) (Mehlhaff et al. 1985; Tryfonidou et al. 1998; Tobin et al. 1999).

Physical examination

Physical examination findings are usually unremarkable in dogs with insulinoma. Weight gain can be found in some dogs due to the anabolic effects of insulin. Weakness, epileptic seizures, and changes in mentation or behavior were the most common clinical signs in a multicentric study of 116 canine insulinoma cases, with one-third of the dogs showing an abnormal neurologic examination (Ryan et al. 2021). In rare cases dogs may show peripheral neuropathy, characterized by proprioception deficits, poor spinal reflexes, poor muscle tone, and muscle atrophy (Van Ham et al. 1997; Moore et al. 2002). The exact etiology of this peripheral neuropathy is not known. Because similarities exist between tumor and nervous tissue antigens, insulinoma-associated peripheral polyneuropathy is most likely caused by an immune response against peripheral nerves (Van Ham et al. 1997). Dogs have been reported to recover from peripheral polyneuropathy after surgical removal of the insulinoma.

Clinical pathology

Routine complete blood count in dogs with insulinoma is usually within normal limits. A consistent abnormality in biochemistry profiles is hypoglycemia. Sometimes a blood glucose concentration within the reference interval is found, because the blood glucose concentration can significantly fluctuate during the course of a day. In these cases, fasting samples and repeated testing may be necessary to confirm hypoglycemia.

Additional abnormalities that have been reported in dogs with insulinoma include mildly increased plasma levels of albumin, alkaline phosphatase, alanine transaminase, bile acids, amylase, and lipase, as well as mildly decreased plasma urea and creatinine concentrations and hypoglobulinemia. However, these findings are nonspecific and do not have diagnostic value (Lester et al. 1999; Tobin et al. 1999; Fernandez et al. 2009).

Differential diagnoses

In the elderly dog, common differential diagnoses of hypoglycemia include laboratory error, insulinoma, hypoadrenocorticism, hepatic insufficiency, portosystemic shunting, sepsis, and nonpancreatic neoplasia. Nonpancreatic tumors associated with hypoglycemia include hepatocellular carcinoma, hepatoma, leiomyosarcoma, metastatic mammary carcinoma, primary pulmonary carcinoma, adrenocortical carcinoma, and leukemia. In the past, several mechanisms were suggested to explain the hypoglycemia due to nonpancreatic tumors such as deranged tumor metabolism with excessive utilization of glucose. Now there is convincing evidence that incompletely processed insulin-like growth factors cause the hypoglycemia (Boari et al. 1995; Zini et al. 2007).

Delayed separation of blood cells and plasma during sample processing is also a common differential diagnosis of hypoglycemia. The glucose concentration in whole blood may decrease by 10 mg/dL/h (0.56 mmol/L/h) because erythrocytes and leukocytes continue to utilize glucose. It is advisable to collect blood for glucose measurement in a sodium fluoride-coated tube, because sodium fluoride inhibits glucose metabolism by blood cells.

Less common differential diagnoses are neonatal and juvenile hypoglycemia, pregnancy toxemia, and hunting dog hypoglycemia. Sporadically, hypoglycemia is the result of glycogen storage disease, growth hormone deficiency, glucagon deficiency, severe polycythemia, renal failure, cardiac failure, or nesidioblastosis. Finally, hypoglycemia might also be iatrogenic, induced by drugs like insulin and sulfonylurea (Rogers & Luttgen 1985; Fernandez *et al.* 2009; Polansky *et al.* 2018).

Diagnosis

Glycemia and insulin levels

A blood glucose concentration below 50 mg/dL (2.8 mmol/L) is often accompanied by clinical signs, but values just below the lower limit of the reference range may not be. Hence the presumptive diagnosis of canine insulinoma is not defined by hypoglycemia alone, but is commonly based on signalment and history, combined with the fulfillment of Whipple's triad (Whipple & Frantz 1935): presence of clinical signs, hypoglycemia, and relief of clinical signs after glucose administration or feeding.

To demonstrate hypoglycemia it may be necessary to fast the dog. Fasting for 24 hours is in most cases sufficient to reveal hypoglycemia; if not, fasting is prolonged for up to 72 hours (Leifer *et al.* 1986). Fasting should be supervised by hourly evaluation of blood glucose concentration, since in dogs with insulinoma blood glucose levels decrease before symptoms occur, possibly triggering sudden and severe symptoms (Rogers & Luttgen 1985; Fernandez *et al.* 2009).

While Whipple's triad fits any cause of hypoglycemia, the next step in the diagnostic work-up (Table 67.3) is to exclude differential diagnoses. The plasma insulin concentration should be determined. Two commonly used insulin assays are a chemiluminescent immunoassay and a competitive enzyme-linked immunosorbent assay (Madarame *et al.* 2009). In cases of insulinoma, circulating insulin concentrations are typically within the reference range (10–170 pmol/L or 2–21 µU/mL) or higher, despite hypoglycemia (Fernandez *et al.* 2009). The simultaneous occurrence of blood glucose below 62.5 mg/dlL(<3.5 mmol/L) and plasma insulin above 70 pmol/L (>10 µU/mL) is diagnostic for insulinoma. Plasma insulin concentrations greater than the high end of the reference interval have been reported in 56–83% of dogs with insulinoma (Fernandez *et al.* 2009). Several explanations have been suggested for the occurrence of insulinoma with plasma insulin concentrations within the reference interval:

Table 67.3 Diagnostic work-up for canine insulinoma.

Step 1	Confirmation of hypoglycemia and fulfillment of Whipple's triad
Step 2	Excluding differential diagnoses
	Blood analysis
	Hematocrit
	Na$^+$, K$^+$, Ca^{2+}
	ACTH stimulation test
	Alkaline phosphatase, bile acids, ammonia
	Urea, creatinine
	Lipase
	Abdominal ultrasound
Step 3	Determination of plasma insulin concentration during hypoglycemia
Step 4	Preoperative insulinoma staging computed tomography scan

- Insulinoma may episodically secrete insulin in short bursts, which causes wide fluctuations in plasma insulin levels.
- Insulinoma may secrete abnormal insulin, which is rapidly broken down.
- Insulinoma may secrete excessive amounts of proinsulin instead of insulin.
- Circulating insulin-like growth factors may contribute to hypoglycemia (Madarame *et al.* 2009).

Regardless of the underlying mechanism, the plasma insulin concentration should be suppressed when blood glucose levels drop below 62.5 mg dL (3.5 mmol/L) and the absence of this response indicates inappropriate secretion of insulin.

To improve the diagnostic value of glucose and insulin measurements, insulin-to-glucose ratios, such as the amended insulin-to-glucose ratio (AIGR), have been determined in the past. However because AIGR lacks specificity and reference intervals vary between laboratories, these ratios are generally considered of little additional diagnostic value. Likewise, provocation tests such as the intravenous glucose tolerance test and glucagon tolerance test do not have enough additional value to justify their routine use. Moreover the use of these tests in human and veterinary medicine is discouraged, because thee tests can be dangerous since they can induce hypoglycemic episodes (Rogers & Luttgen 1985; Leifer *et al.* 1986; Steiner & Bruyette 1996).

Imaging modalities

Diagnostic imaging techniques like transabdominal ultrasonography, computed tomography (CT), single-photon emission computed tomography (SPECT),

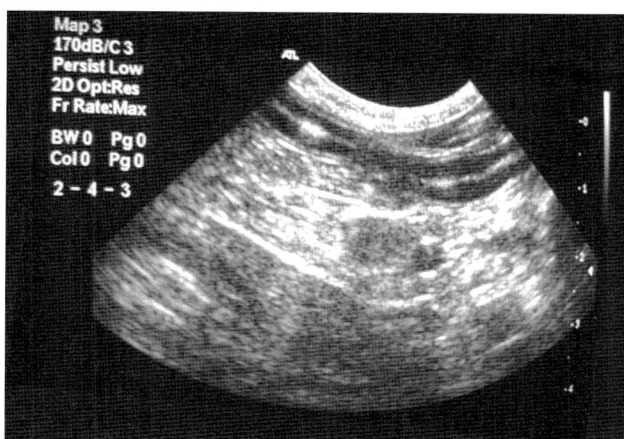

Figure 67.2 Ultrasound is believed to have low sensitivity in detecting canine insulinoma. A hypoechoic mass lesion is present on this ultrasonographic image.

somatostatin receptor scintigraphy, and magnetic resonance imaging (MRI) can be of great help in the identification and preoperative staging of insulinoma.

Radiography of the abdomen does not contribute to a diagnosis of insulinoma because of the small size of the tumors and border effacement from the surrounding soft tissues of the cranial abdomen. Ultrasound was found to have low sensitivity in detecting canine insulinoma (Robben *et al.* 2005); only 5 of 14 primary insulinomas were correctly identified by ultrasound, and no lymph node metastases were detected by ultrasound (Figure 67.2). Similar results were obtained using SPECT. A small case series has recently investigated the potential of MRI to detect insulinomas in dogs (Walczak *et al.* 2019). In all four dogs, the insulinomas displayed a high-intensity signal on T2-weighted fat-saturated images, and the tumors were primarily isointense to normal pancreatic tissue on post-contrast T2-weighted fat-saturated images.

Conventional pre- and post-contrast CT has proved to be a more sensitive method than ultrasonography, correctly identifying 10 of 14 primary tumors and 2 of 5 lymph node metastases. However, conventional pre- and post-contrast CT was not found to be a very specific method, because it also identified many false-positive lesions. More recently, dual- and triple-phase contrast-enhanced CT (CECT) techniques have been developed and the use of dynamic CECT for the presurgical localization of insulinoma in dogs has been reported (Iseri *et al.* 2007; Mai & Caceres 2008; Buishand *et al.* 2018). Using CECT, after an intravenous injection of contrast medium, CT images are acquired during the arterial, portal, and delayed venous phases. A recent case series of 27 dogs with insulinoma demonstrated that CECT had a high sensitivity (96%) in detecting canine

insulinoma. Detection of lymph node metastases with CECT scans had a sensitivity of 67% and detection of liver metastases had a sensitivity of 75% (Figure 67.3). Despite the high sensitivity in detecting the primary tumors, CECT scans predicted the correct location of insulinomas within the pancreas in only 52% of cases. There was no specific post-contrast phase in which insulinomas could be visualized best, but major location errors mainly occurred in single- or double-phase CECT scans compared to triple-phase CECT scans (Buishand *et al.* 2018). A small single-center study of 35 dogs suggested that hyperattenuation of insulinomas in the arterial phase is the predominant feature, and that hypoattenuation or isoattenuation is much less common. In this study 33 of 35 nodules were identified. Pancreatic insulinoma location at surgery matched that described on the CT images in 17 of 19 cases where location was described in the surgical report (Coss *et al.* 2021).

Despite advancements in preoperative diagnostic imaging modalities, exploratory laparotomy remains the most reliable method of detecting primary and metastatic insulinoma. Careful inspection and palpation of the pancreas and adjacent structures, with or without the use of intravenous methylene blue infusion (3 mg/kg, administered over 30–40 min, for intraoperative staining), reveals most primary and metastatic insulinomas (Figure 67.4). Since intravenous methylene blue has been found to induce fatal hemolytic anemia or acute renal failure, its use is not routinely recommended (Steiner & Bruyette 1996). When intraoperative inspection and palpation are unsuccessful in detecting the tumor, intraoperative ultrasound can be used to visualize both the primary insulinoma as well as possible liver metastases. Definitive diagnosis is obtained by histologic examination of tumor samples.

Treatment

Insulinoma therapy can be divided into medical management and surgical treatment. Surgery is considered the treatment of choice because it has been associated with the longest survival times (Caywood *et al.* 1988; Tobin *et al.* 1999; Polton *et al.* 2007); however, most dogs are also treated with medical management at some point in the disease course, for example preoperative stabilization, postoperative treatment of residual disease, or cases in which surgery is not performed.

Medical therapy
Emergency treatment

An acute hypoglycemic crisis typically occurs after exercise, excitement, or eating; immediately after surgery in dogs with inoperable neoplasia; or as a result of inadvertently

(a)

(b)

(c)

(d)

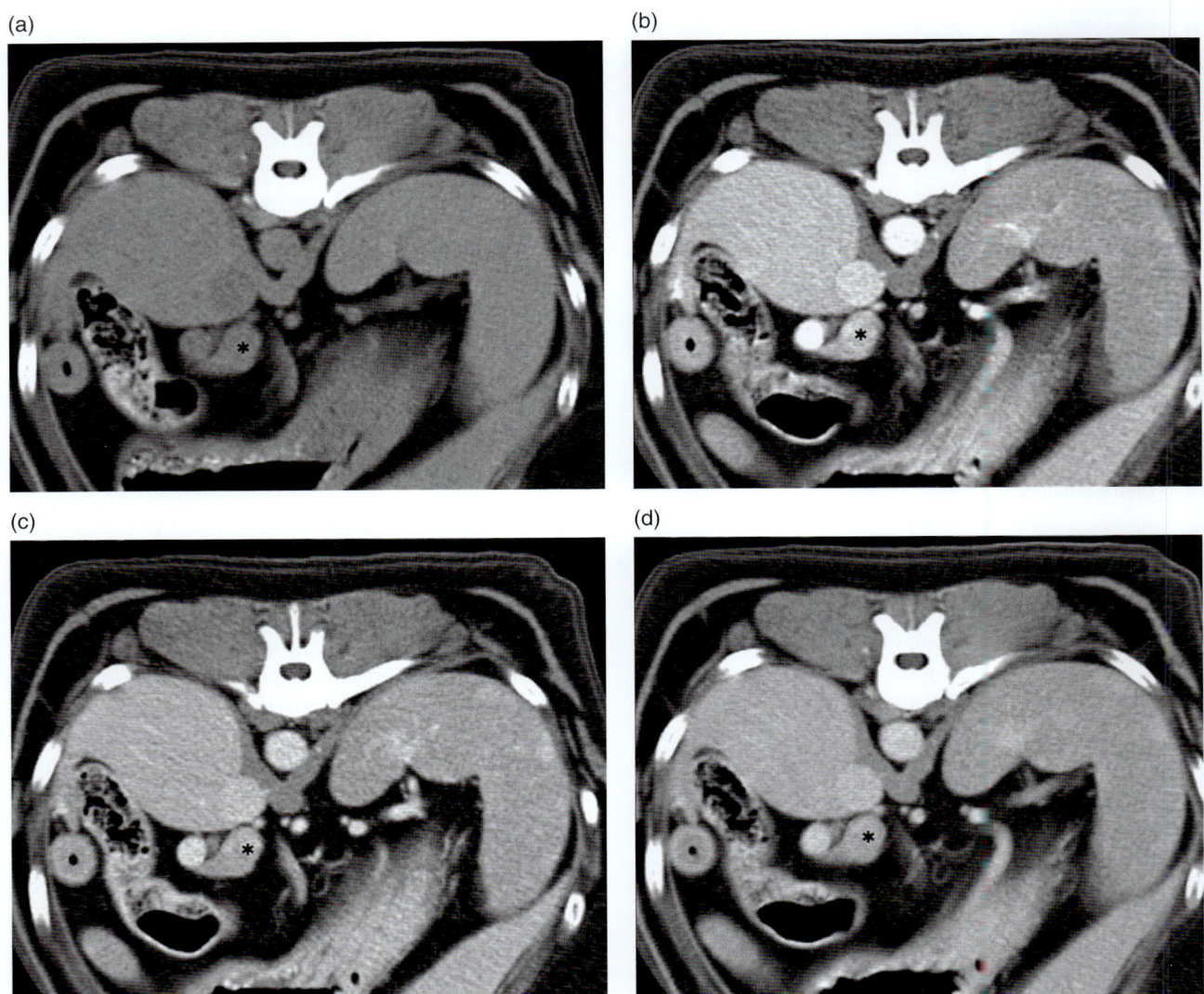

Figure 67.3 Transverse triple-phase contrast-enhanced computed tomography (CECT) in a dog with metastatic insulinoma lymphade-nopathy (asterisk). The metastatic lymph node is homogenously iso-attenuating on pre-contrast images (a) and all post-contrast phases – arterial (b), portal (c), and delayed venous (d) – demonstrate hyperattenuation.

aggressive intravenous dextrose administration result-ing in a massive release of insulin from insulinoma and rebound hypoglycemia. Dogs with acute and severe sei-zures should be treated immediately (Table 67.4), since the shorter the period of hypoglycemia, the lower the risk of irreversible brain damage (Feldman & Nelson 2004; Rijnberk & Kooistra 2010).

Long-term treatment

Dogs with insulinoma should be fed 4–6 small meals a day of a high-protein, high-fat, and high-complex car-bohydrate diet. This type of diet decreases postprandial hyperglycemia, thereby preventing a marked insulin surge. Restricting exercise to brief walks on a leash might

also help to reduce clinical hypoglycemia (Capen & Martin 1969). In some dogs this approach is sufficient to control insulin-induced hypoglycemia. If clinical signs persist, despite frequent feedings and restricted exercise, additional medication should be initiated.

Diazoxide is the preferred drug for treatment of insulinoma-induced hypoglycemia. Diazoxide raises blood glucose concentrations mainly through direct inhibition of pancreatic insulin release, but also through stimulation of hepatic gluconeogenesis and glycogenoly-sis and inhibition of glucose uptake by tissues (Leifer et al. 1986; Caywood et al. 1988; Tobin et al. 1999). It is recommended to start with an oral dose of 5 mg/kg twice daily. If hypoglycemic symptoms persist, the initial dose

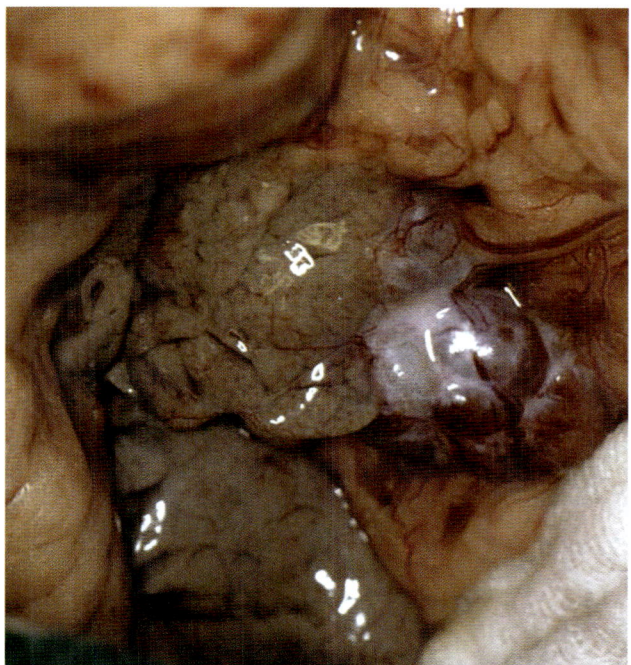

Figure 67.4 The use of intravenous methylene blue infusion reveals most primary and metastatic insulinomas, but it should be used with care.

can be gradually increased to 30 mg/kg twice daily (Steiner & Bruyette 1996). Possible side effects of diazoxide treatment are anorexia, vomiting, and ptyalism. These side effects may be prevented by dividing the daily dose and by administering diazoxide with food. The use of diazoxide is contraindicated in patients with liver, kidney, or heart failure (Elie & Zebre 1995; Steiner & Bruyette 1996).

An alternative to diazoxide therapy is glucocorticoid therapy. Glucocorticoids, such as prednisolone, antagonize the effects of insulin at the cellular level and increase gluconeogenesis (Rijnberk & Kooistra 2010). The recommended initial dose of prednisolone is 0.25 mg/kg orally twice daily, which can be increased to 2.0–3.0 mg/kg twice daily (Steiner & Bruyette 1996).

However, dosages greater than 1.1 mg/kg orally twice daily are considered immunosuppressive, and the use of high dosages of glucocorticoids often gives rise to clinical signs of iatrogenic Cushing syndrome (Elie & Zebre 1995).

In addition to the commonly used drugs already described, treatment with somatostatin (analogs, streptozocin, and toceranib phosphate) has been described (Simpson *et al.* 1995; Robben *et al.* 1997, 2006; Moore *et al.* 2002; Flesner *et al.* 2019). Octreotide is a somatostatin analog that binds to the somatostatin receptors on β cells, thereby inhibiting the synthesis and secretion of insulin. There have been conflicting reports

Table 67.4 Emergency treatment for hypoglycemic seizures caused by insulinoma.

Seizures at home

Step 1	Rub glucose syrup on patient's gum. Do not pour syrup into the patient's mouth, since it is easily aspirated by a seizuring patient
Step 2a	Once patient is sternal, feed a small meal
Step 2b	If seizures do not decrease within 1–2 min, administer diazepam, if available, rectally (1 mg/kg), and continue rubbing glucose syrup on patient's gum
Step 3	Call the veterinarian

Seizures in hospital

Step 1	Small dog: administer 6–12 mL of 20% glucose, or 2.5–5 mL of 50% glucose, intravenously (i.v.) slowly over 5–10 min Large dog: administer 20–35 mlLof 20% glucose, or 8–15 mL of 50% glucose, i.v. slowly over 5–10 min
Step 2	Once patient is sternal, feed a small meal
Step 3	Initiate long-term medical therapy

Intractable seizures in hospital

Step 1	Start a continuous rate infusion of 2.5–5% glucose at 1.5–2 times maintenance rate
Step 2	Add dexamethasone 0.5–1 mg/kg to i.v. fluids and administer over 6 h; if necessary, repeat every 12–24 h
Step 3	Start with a 50 ng/kg bolus of glucagon, followed by a continuous-rate infusion at an initial rate of 5–10 ng/kg per min
Step 4	Diazepam (1 mg/kg) or propofol (2–6 mg/kg) can be given to effect if the patient is still seizuring after normalization of the blood glucose concentration
Step 5	If above fails, anesthetize patient with pentobarbital for 4–8 h while continuing above therapy; consider surgical excision of insulinoma

on the effectiveness of octreotide therapy in dogs with insulinoma. Several reports show that both somatostatin and octreotide significantly decrease plasma insulin concentrations and reduce the clinical signs of hypoglycemia (Lohtrop 1989; Meleo 1990; Robben *et al.* 1997). However, in a study conducted by Simpson *et al.* (1995), octreotide treatment did not lead to any improvement in clinical signs or blood glucose and insulin concentrations. These contradictory results may be explained by the variable expression of somatostatin receptors on neoplastic β cells. Another explanation for treatment failures in dogs with insulinoma could be the relatively short (3–4 h) suppressive effect of octreotide on plasma insulin concentration in dogs. Furthermore, some dogs become refractory to octreotide treatment (Lohtrop 1989). The most recent study on the use of octreotide (Robben *et al.* 2006) demonstrated that a single subcutaneous dose of 50 µg produced consistent suppression of plasma insulin concentrations and a corresponding increase in blood glucose concentrations in 12 dogs with insulinoma. Octreotide administration at this dosage was not associated with side effects, and therefore further studies on the effectiveness of slow-release octreotide preparations in long-term treatment of dogs with insulinoma are warranted.

Streptozocin is a nitrosourea compound that selectively destroys pancreatic β cells. Streptozocin is extremely nephrotoxic, and therefore induction of diuresis is mandatory to ameliorate its toxic renal effects. A successful treatment protocol includes a 0.9% NaCl diuresis (18 mL/kg per hour intravenously) for seven hours. Three hours after initiating the diuresis, streptozocin (500 mg/m²) is administered over a two-hour period. An antiemetic should be administered immediately before or after streptozocin therapy. Streptozocin treatment is repeated every three weeks until there is evidence of tumor progression, recurrence of hypoglycemia, or development of streptozocin-induced toxicosis. Common side effects of streptozocin therapy include vomiting, diabetes mellitus, and renal failure (Moore *et al.* 2002).

Glucagon is a readily available treatment for insulin-induced hypoglycemia and one study concluded that glucagon therapy in insulinomas is an effective treatment to manage hypoglycemia. The median glucagon constant-rate infusion dose was significantly higher for the nonsurvivors than for survivors. No other correlation was found between any of the independent variables evaluated when comparing blood glucose trends, length of hospitalization, and outcome (Harris *et al.* 2020).

Finally, a recent case study described the use of tyrosine kinase inhibitor toceranib phosphate in a dog with stage III insulinoma. After partial pancreatectomy, the dog had long-term glycemic control with survival over 24 months while receiving prednisone 0.63 mg/kg orally once daily and toceranib phosphate 2.5 mg/kg orally every other day (Flesner *et al.* 2019). In one small study, the use of toceranib combined with palliative treatment in dogs with suspect metastatic or recurrent insulinoma increased survival time (median 399 days, range 125–476 days) compared to a control group (median 67 days, range 23–387 days; *P* = 0.04), while the treatment group had a higher incidence of grade 1–2 gastrointestinal toxicity (Alonso-Miguel *et al.* 2021).

Surgical therapy
Preoperative considerations and anesthesia

Dry food should be withheld 12 hours before surgery. Canned food can be fed until 6 hours before surgery. If dogs are clinically hypoglycemic, easily digestible liquid food preparations should be given until 1–2 hours before surgery. If clinical signs occur in this immediate preoperative period, the animal should be administered glucose solution intravenously (1–5 mL of 50% dextrose administered over 10 min), because it is important to stabilize blood glucose concentration before surgery.

During anesthesia, dogs should receive a continuous intravenous infusion of a balanced electrolyte solution containing 2.5–5.0% dextrose. Since some anesthetics increase blood glucose concentration, administering intravenous glucose solutions without monitoring blood glucose can lead to hyperglycemia, stimulating the insulinoma to secrete even more insulin. Additionally, manipulation of the tumor during surgery can trigger increased insulin secretion, leading to a more profound hypoglycemia. To prevent this vicious circle, it is important to regularly monitor blood glucose concentration during surgery and to modify the rate of the intravenous glucose solution according to the measured blood glucose levels. Glucose infusion is normally stopped as soon as the primary tumor is removed, which often suddenly lowers plasma insulin concentrations and stimulates a rise in blood glucose concentration. Normoglycemia is typically restored or hyperglycemia is induced within minutes after insulinoma resection. Continuous glucose monitoring (every 10 min post resection) is required.

Surgical techniques

Depending on pancreatic localization, an insulinoma can be removed by local enucleation or partial pancreatectomy (Figures 67.4–67.6). Partial pancreatectomy is the preferred method, because it results in longer survival times than local enucleation (Mehlhaff *et al.* 1985). Therefore, local enucleation should only be considered if the insulinoma is located in the body of the pancreas, or in the most proximal portions (i.e., close to the corpus) of the right and left lobes, in which case extreme caution should be taken to prevent damage to the ductal system and the pancreaticoduodenal arteries that are located near or in the pancreatic tissue (Steiner & Bruyette 1996). With any technique, it is important to evaluate the entire pancreas to assess for the presence of multiple nodules.

Partial pancreatectomy is commonly performed using either the suture–fracture technique or the dissection–ligation technique. The suture–fracture technique is easier to perform than the dissection–ligation technique and has no obvious disadvantages (Allen *et al.* 1989). After incising the mesoduodenum or omentum on each side of the pancreas, nonabsorbable sutures are passed around the pancreas, just proximal to the pancreatic mass. The ligature is tightened, allowing it to crush through the

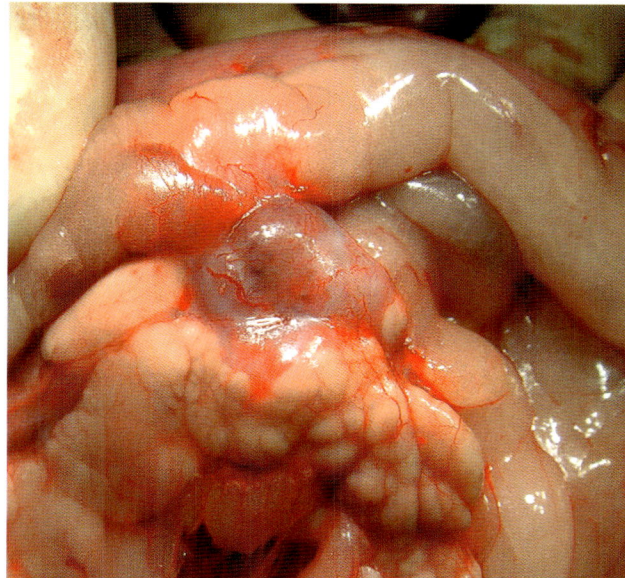

Figure 67.5 Intraoperative view of an insulinoma: note the difference in color between the tumor and the normal pancreas.

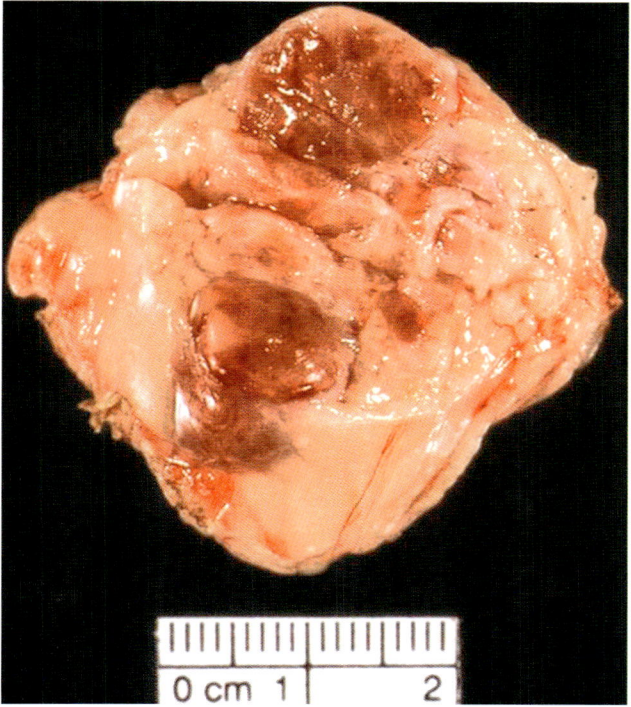

Figure 67.6 View of a postoperatively transected insulinoma.

(a)

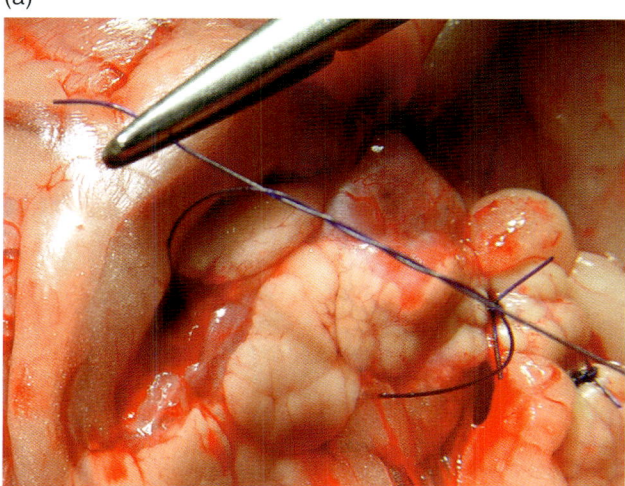

(b)

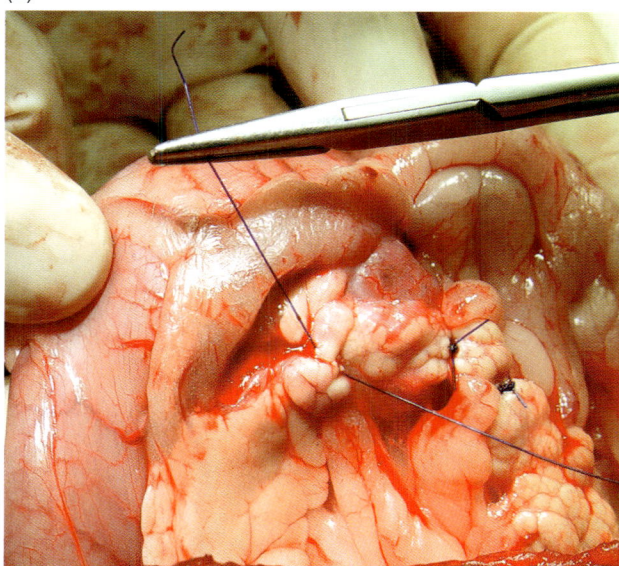

Figure 67.7 (a) During the suture–fracture technique, the ligature is tightened, (b) allowing it to crush through the pancreatic parenchyma, thereby ligating vessels and ducts.

pancreatic parenchyma, thereby ligating vessels and ducts (Figure 67.7). Hereafter, the pancreatic tissue distal to the ligature is excised. Using the dissection–ligation technique, the pancreatic capsule is incised and bluntly dissected down to the pancreatic duct and vessels. The duct and vessels are individually ligated, using double ligatures, and then transected between the two ligatures.

More recently, vessel-sealant devices have been developed. These systems provide safe and quick hemostasis, sealing blood vessels up to 7 mm in diameter and tissue bundles without dissection or isolation (Belli *et al.* 2003). The use of a bipolar vessel-sealant device for partial pancreatectomy in dogs with insulinoma was safe and effective, decreased surgery duration, and improved surgical performance in lesions with difficult access compared with the suture–fracture technique (Wouters *et al.* 2011). No clinical signs associated with pancreatitis were observed in any of the dogs (Figure 67.8). Alternatively, a stapling device can be used to remove the pancreatic part that contains the insulinoma (Figure 67.9).

(a) (b)

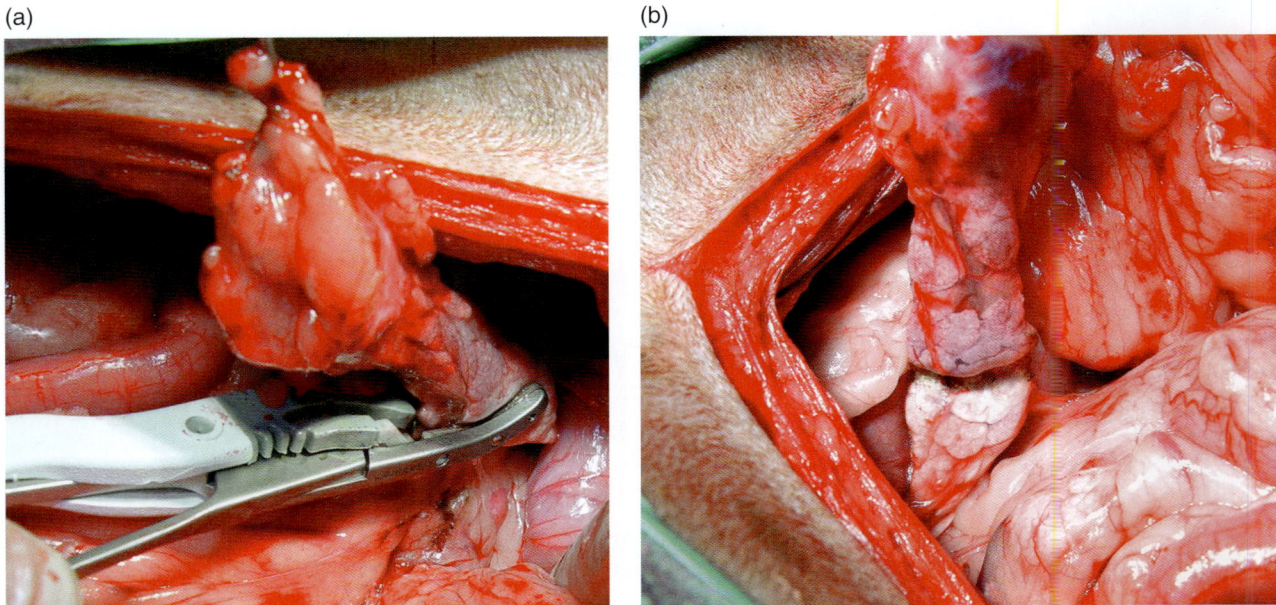

Figure 67.8 A vessel-sealing device (a) allows rapid resection of the tumor and (b) causes minimal side effects while ensuring that there is no leakage.

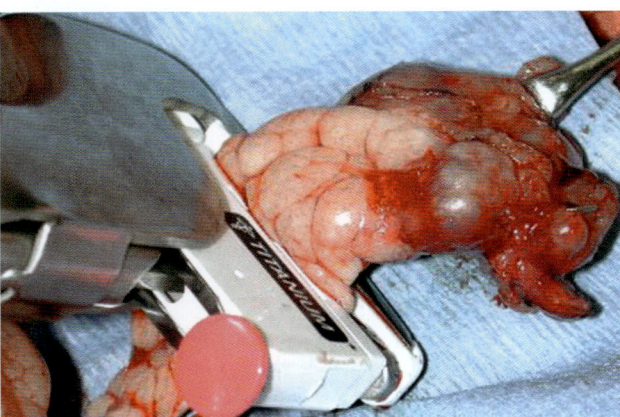

Figure 67.9 A stapling device is used to remove a pancreatic insulinoma.

Up until now, the literature has only reported the use of laparoscopic resection of a single canine insulinoma (Mcclaran *et al.* 2017). In human medicine, several recent large case series and comparative studies on the short- and long-term outcomes of laparoscopic pancreatectomy have demonstrated clear advantages over the open approach. Extrapolating this to veterinary medicine, the authors expect that the role of laparoscopic resection of canine insulinomas will significantly extend in the coming decade. Laparoscopic partial pancreatectomy can be used in cases with isolated pancreatic insulinomas located in the distal two-thirds of either the right or left pancreatic lobe. Open surgery will remain

the preferred technique in cases in which pancreatic tumors have extensive metastases to abdominal lymph nodes or the liver. However, selected abdominal lymph nodes are accessible using a laparoscopic technique (Buishand *et al.* 2015).

Segmental pancreatectomy that leaves the distal portion of a lobe is not indicated. For instance, it is tempting to remove a tumor located in the middle of either pancreatic leg *en bloc* with the surrounding pancreatic tissue, but leave the most distal part of the pancreas in place. This part of the pancreas may still have an adequate blood supply, but often has no ductal structure that leads to the duodenum, leading to local pancreatitis or sterile pancreatic abscesses. If pancreatic abscesses occur after partial pancreatectomy, they are treated by repeated ultrasound-guided aspiration and flushing with sterile solutions instead of reoperation. Based on our experience, most abscesses will resolve in this manner.

The presence of metastatic disease is evaluated in two ways: (i) gross inspection of common target organs including lymph nodes (duodenal, hepatic, splenic, greater mesenteric) and liver; and (ii) on the basis of the blood glucose concentrations after the glucose infusion has stopped. All macroscopically enlarged lymph nodes should be excised and submitted for histologic examination. Enlarged lymph nodes do not always contain tumor cells, but can also be enlarged because of inflammation associated with the tumor or other causes. In the case of liver metastases, debulking of the metastasis is warranted to decrease tumor mass and to increase the effects of medical therapy after surgery. Partial hepatectomy is performed on all affected liver lobes. We have been photocoagulating small multiple metastases with a neodymium:yttrium aluminum garnet (Nd:YAG) surgical laser. No data are available to document the efficacy of this technique.

After surgery, dogs should be closely monitored and adequately treated in case of postoperative complications. The most common complications of insulinoma surgery are acute pancreatitis, persistent hypoglycemia, and diabetes mellitus. Inappetence and vomiting occurred in 27.3% and 24.2%, respectively, of 33 dogs that underwent surgery for insulinoma. Risk factors for postoperative vomiting were longer duration of clinical signs before surgery, higher preoperative total protein concentration, and lack of liver metastasis. No significant risk factors for inappetence or survival were identified (Hixon et al. 2019).

If hyperglycemia develops after surgery, insulin might be required to lower the blood glucose level until the suppressed β cells are producing their normal insulin. In the case of persistent very low blood glucose (<50 mg/dL, <2.8 mmol/L), medical therapy using diazoxide should be initiated. In addition, these dogs might also need a glucose infusion after surgery to stabilize their blood glucose concentration. In the presence of subnormal to normal postoperative blood glucose concentrations, dogs receive frequent meals of dry food. The authors recommend initiating diazoxide therapy only when clinical signs of hypoglycemia reoccur. Once a dog is eating properly and is able to maintain normal blood glucose levels, diazoxide therapy is discontinued.

Prognosis

Canine insulinoma has a guarded prognosis because metastasis, tumor regrowth, and return of clinical signs are almost inevitable. The prognosis for dogs treated with surgery combined with medical treatment is significantly better than the prognosis for dogs receiving medical treatment alone (Polton et al. 2007). Reported median disease-free interval and median survival time (MST) of dogs that underwent partial pancreatectomy were 12 months (range 0–55 months) and 14 months (range 0–51 months), respectively (Leifer et al. 1986; Dunn et al. 1992; Tryfonidou et al. 1998; Tobin et al. 1999; Polton et al. 2007; Del Busto et al. 2020). In contrast, the MST of 21 dogs treated medically was only 4 months (range 0–18 months) (Tobin et al. 1999; Polton et al. 2007; Ryan et al. 2021). Other prognostic factors include TNM stage, age, and postoperative blood glucose concentrations. In the study of Caywood et al.

(1988), dogs with clinical stage I insulinoma had a median disease-free interval of 14 months, significantly longer than the disease-free interval of dogs with clinical stage II and III insulinoma, these dogs remaining normoglycemic for a median of only 1 month. Furthermore, dogs with clinical stage I and II insulinoma had a significantly longer MST (18 months) than dogs with clinical stage III insulinoma (<6 months) (Caywood et al. 1988). In contrast to the latter study, a more recent study by Buishand et al. (2010) did not demonstrate a significant difference in the disease-free interval between dogs with insulinoma confined to the pancreas and dogs with metastatic disease. This study demonstrated that disease in dogs with clinical stage III insulinoma remained subclinical for a significantly shorter period after surgery than in dogs with clinical stage I and II insulinoma. Furthermore, it was found that the Ki67 index can act as a biomarker of canine insulinoma that can be used to predict clinical outcome (Buishand et al. 2010, 2014). Young dogs have a worse prognosis than older dogs. Dogs that are hyperglycemic, or normoglycemic immediately postoperatively, survive significantly longer than dogs with hypoglycemia postoperatively (Tryfonidou et al. 1998). In a study of 49 dogs with surgically treated insulinoma, 80% of dogs had immediate resolution of hypoglycemia and 20% remained persistently hypoglycemic postoperatively. The MST for all dogs was 561 days. The MST for dogs that had resolution of hypoglycemia was 746 days. Of those that had resolution of hypoglycemia, 44% experienced recurrence of hypoglycemia by 2 years postoperatively. Pathologic stage was a predictor of persistent postoperative hypoglycemia, which, in turn, was a predictor of survival time (Cleland et al. 2021).

Feline insulinoma

Insulinoma is rare in cats. Nine cats, ranging in age from 12 to 17 years, have been reported to have insulinoma (O'Brien et al. 1990; Kraje 2003; Greene & Bright 2008; Schaub & Wigger 2013; Cervone et al. 2019; Gifford et al. 2020). There are few data to establish a sex or breed predilection, but it is remarkable that of the nine reported cases, seven cats were castrated males and three insulinomas were found in Siamese cats. Clinical signs of feline insulinoma are similar to those of canine insulinoma, including seizures, weakness, disorientation, and muscle fasciculations. Presumptive diagnosis is based on demonstration of hypoglycemia with concomitant normal to increased plasma insulin concentration. Surgical excision of the insulinoma and metastases, if needed, followed by prednisone treatment (0.5 mg/kg orally twice daily), is the treatment of choice. To our knowledge, there are no reports on the use of diazoxide, streptozocin, or octreotide in cats with insulinoma. In two cats clinical signs did not reoccur for at least 32 months after surgery, but in the other cats the disease-free interval ranged from 5 days to 18 months. Necropsy was only performed on the cat surviving for 18 months and this revealed metastases to the pancreatic lymph nodes and the liver. It is suspected that the long-term prognosis for insulinoma in the cat is poor, because of the high likelihood of metastatic disease (O'Brien *et al.* 1990; Kraje 2003; Greene & Bright 2008).

References

Allen, S.W., Cornelius, L.M., and Mahaffey, E.A. (1989). A comparison of two methods of partial pancreatectomy in the dog. *Veterinary Surgery* 18: 274–278.

Alonso-Miguel, D., García-San José, P., González Sanz, S. et al. (2021). Evaluation of palliative therapy, alone or in combination with toceranib phosphate, in dogs diagnosed with metastatic or recurrent beta-cell neoplasia. *New Zealand Veterinary Journal* 69 (4): 234–239.

Belli, G., Fantini, C., Ciciliano, F. et al. (2003). Pancreaticoduodenectomy in portal hypertension: use of the Ligasure. *Journal of Hepato-Biliary-Pancreatic Surgery* 10: 215–217.

Boari, A., Barreca, A., Bestetti, G.E. et al. (1995). Hypoglycemia in a dog with a leiomyoma of the gastric wall producing an insulin-like growth factor II-like peptide. *European Journal of Endocrinology* 132: 744–750.

Bryson, E.R., Snead, E.C., McMillan, C. et al. (2007). Insulinoma in a dog with pre-existing insulin-dependent diabetes mellitus. *Journal of the American Animal Hospital Association* 43: 65–69.

Buishand, F.O., Kik, M., and Kirpensteijn, J. (2010). Evaluation of clinicopathological criteria and the Ki67 index as prognostic indicators in canine insulinoma. *Veterinary Journal* 185: 62–67.

Buishand, F.O., Visser, J., Kik, M. et al. (2014). Evaluation of prognostic indicators using validated canine insulinoma tissue microarrays. *Veterinary Journal* 201: 57–63.

Buishand, F.O., Nimwegen, S.A., and Kirpensteijn, J. (2015). Laparoscopic surgery of the pancreas. In: *Small Animal Laparoscopy and Thoracoscopy* (ed. B.A. Fransson and P.D. Mayhew), 167–178. Wiley Blackwell: Hoboken, NJ.

Buishand, F.O., Vilaplana Grosso, F.R., Kirpensteijn, J. et al. (2018). Utility of contrast-enhanced computed tomography in the evaluation of canine insulinoma location. *Veterinary Quarterly* 38: 53–62.

Capen, C.C. and Martin, S.L. (1969). Hyperinsulinism in dogs with neoplasia of the pancreatic islets: a clinical, pathologic, and ultrastructural study. *Veterinary Pathology* 6: 309–341.

Caywood, D.D., Klausner, J.S., O'Leary, T.P. et al. (1988). Pancreatic insulin-secreting neoplasms: clinical, diagnostic, and prognostic features in 73 dogs. *Journal of the American Animal Hospital Association* 24: 577–584.

Cervone, M., Harel, M., Ségard-Weisse, E., and Krafft, E. (2019). Use of contrast-enhanced ultrasonography for the detection of a feline insulinoma. *Journal of Feline Medicine and Surgery Open Reports* 5: 2055116919876140.

Cleland, N.T., Morton, J., and Delisser, P.J. (2021). Outcome after surgical management of canine insulinoma in 49 cases. *Veterinary and Comparative Oncology* 19 (3): 428–441.

Coss, P., Gilman, O., Warren-Smith, C., and Major, A.C. (2021). The appearance of canine insulinoma on dual phase computed tomographic angiography. *Journal of Small Animal Practice* 62 (7): 540–546.

Del Busto, I., German, A.J., Treggiari, E. et al. (2020). Incidence of postoperative complications and outcome of 48 dogs undergoing surgical management of insulinoma. *Journal of Veterinary Internal Medicine* 34 (3): 1135–1143.

Dunn, J.K., Heath, M.K., Herrtage, M.E. et al. (1992). Diagnosis of insulinoma in the dog: a study of 11 cases. *Journal of Small Animal Practice* 33: 514–520.

Elie, M.S. and Zebre, C.A. (1995). Insulinoma in dogs, cats, and ferrets. *Compendium on Continuing Education for the Practicing Veterinarian* 17: 51–59.

Feldman, E.C. and Nelson, R.W. (2004). *Canine and Feline Endocrinology and Reproduction*, 3e, 616–644. St. Louis, MO: WB Saunders.

Fernandez, N.J., Barton, J., and Spotswood, T. (2009). Hypoglycemia in a dog. *Canadian Veterinary Journal* 50: 423–426.

Flesner, B.K., Fletcher, J.M., Smithee, T. et al. (2019). Long-term survival and glycemic control with toceranib phosphate and prednisone for a metastatic canine insulinoma. *Journal of the American Hospital Association* 55: e55105.

Gifford, C.H., Morris, A.P., Kenney, K.J., and Estep, J.S. (2020). Diagnosis of insulinoma in a Maine Coon cat. *Journal of Feline Medicine and Surgery Open Reports* 6: 2055116919894782.

Greene, S.N. and Bright, R.M. (2008). Insulinoma in a cat. *Journal of Small Animal Practice* 49: 38–40.

Harris, M.E., Weatherton, L., and Bloch, C.P. (2020). Glucagon therapy in canines with an insulinoma: a retrospective descriptive study of 11 dogs. *Canadian Veterinary Journal* 61 (7): 737–742.

Hawkins, K.L., Summers, B.A., Kuhajda, F.P. et al. (1987). Immunocytochemistry of normal pancreatic islets and spontaneous islet cell tumors in dogs. *Veterinary Pathology* 24: 170–179.

Heitz, P.U., Kasper, M., Polak, J.M. et al. (1982). Pancreatic endocrine tumors: immunocytochemical analysis of 125 tumors. *Human Pathology* 13: 263–271.

Hixon, L.P., Grimes, J.A., Wallace, M.L., and Schmiedt, C.W. (2019). Risk factors for gastrointestinal upset and evaluation of outcome following surgical resection of canine pancreatic β-cell tumors. *Canadian Veterinary Journal* 60 (12): 1312–1318.

Iseri, T., Yamada, K., Chijiwa, K. et al. (2007). Dynamic computed tomography of the pancreas in normal dogs and in a dog with pancreatic insulinoma. *Veterinary Radiology and Ultrasound* 48: 328–331.

Kraje, A.C. (2003). Hypoglycemia and irreversible neurologic complications in a cat with insulinoma. *Journal of the American Veterinary Medical Association* 233: 812–814.

Leifer, C.E., Peterson, M.E., and Matus, R.E. (1986). Insulin-secreting tumor: diagnosis and medical and surgical treatment in 55 dogs. *Journal of the American Veterinary Medical Association* 181: 60–64.

Lester, N.V., Newell, S.M., Hill, R.C. et al. (1999). Scintigraphic diagnosis of insulinoma in a dog. *Veterinary Radiology and Ultrasound* 40: 174–178.

Lohtrop, C.D. (1989). Medical treatment of neuroendocrine tumors of the gastroenteropancreatic system with somatostatin. In: *Current Veterinary Therapy X* (ed. R.W. Kirk), 1020–1024. Philadelphia, PA: WB Saunders.

Madarame, H., Kayanuma, H., Shida, T. et al. (2009). Retrospective study of canine insulinomas: eight cases (2005–2008). *Journal of Veterinary Medical Science* 71: 905–911.

Mai, W. and Caceres, A.V. (2008). Dual-phase computed tomographic angiography in three dogs with pancreatic insulinoma. *Veterinary Radiology and Ultrasound* 49: 141–148.

Mcclaran, J.K., Pavia, P., Fischetti, A.J. et al. (2017). Laparoscopic resection of a pancreatic β cell tumor in a dog. *Journal of the American Animal Hospital Association* 53: 338–345.

Mehlhaff, C.J., Peterson, M.E., Patnaik, A.K. et al. (1985). Insulin-producing islet cell neoplasms: surgical considerations and general management in 35 dogs. *Journal of the American Animal Hospital Association* 21: 607–612.

Meleo, K. (1990). Management of insulinoma patient with refractory hypoglycemia. *Problems in Veterinary Medicine* 2: 602–609.

Moore, A.S., Nelson, R.W., Henry, C.J. et al. (2002). Streptozocin for treatment of pancreatic islet cell tumors in dogs: 17 cases (1989–1999). *Journal of the American Veterinary Medical Association* 221: 811–818.

O'Brien, T.D., Hayden, D.W., O'Leary, T.P. et al. (1987). Canine pancreatic endocrine tumors: immunohistochemical analysis of hormone content and amyloid. *Veterinary Pathology* 24: 308–314.

O'Brien, T.D., Norton, F., Turner, T.M. et al. (1990). Pancreatic endocrine tumor in a cat: clinical, pathological and immunohistochemical evaluation. *Journal of the American Animal Hospital Association* 26: 453–457.

Owen, L.N. (1980). *TNM Classification of Tumours in Domestic Animals*. Geneva: World Health Organization.

Polansky, B.J., Martinez, S.A., and Calkley, M.D. (2018). Resolution of hyperinsulinemic hypoglycemia following partial pancreatectomy in a dog with nesidioblastosis. *Journal of the American Veterinary Medical Association* 253: 893–896.

Polton, G.A., White, R.N., Brearly, M.J. et al. (2007). Improved survival in a retrospective cohort of 28 dogs with insulinoma. *Journal of Small Animal Practice* 48: 151–156.

Rijnberk, A. and Kooistra, H.S. (2010). *Clinical Endocrinology of Dogs and Cats*, 2e. Hannover: Schluttersche.

Robben, J.H., Visser-Wisselaar, H.A., Rutteman, G.R. et al. (1997). in vitro and in vivo detection of functional somatostatin receptors in canine insulinomas. *Journal of Nuclear Medicine* 38: 1036–1042.

Robben, J.H., Van Garderen, E., Mol, J.A. et al. (2002). Locally produced growth hormone in canine insulinomas. *Molecular and Cellular Endocrinology* 197: 187–195.

Robben, J.H., Pollak, Y.W., Kirpensteijn, J. et al. (2005). Comparison of ultrasonography, computed tomography, and single-photon emission computed tomography for detection and localization of canine insulinoma. *Journal of Veterinary Internal Medicine* 19: 15–22.

Robben, J.H., Van den Brom, W.E., Mol, J.A. et al. (2006). Effect of octreotide on plasma concentrations of glucose, insulin, glucagon, growth hormone, and cortisol in healthy dogs and dogs with insulinoma. *Research in Veterinary Science* 80: 25–32.

Rogers, A.S. and Luttgen, P.J. (1985). Hyperinsulinism. *Compendium on Continuing Education for the Practicing Veterinarian* 7: 829–840.

Ryan, D., Pérez-Accino, J., Gonçalves, R. et al. (2021). Clinical findings, neurological manifestations and survival of dogs with insulinoma: 116 cases (2009–2020). *Journal of Small Animal Practice* 62 (7): 531–539.

Schaub, S. and Wigger, A. (2013). Ultrasound-aided diagnosis of an insulinoma in a cat. *Tierärztliche Praxis. Ausgabe K, Kleintiere/Heimtiere* 41: 338–342.

Simpson, K.W., Stepien, R.L., Elwood, C.M. et al. (1995). Evaluation of the long-acting somatostatin analog octreotide in the management of insulinoma in three dogs. *Journal of Small Animal Practice* 36: 161–165.

Slye, M. and Wells, H.G. (1935). Tumor of islet tissue with hyperinsulinism in a dog. *Archives of Pathology* 19: 537–542.

Steiner, J.M. and Bruyette, D.S. (1996). Canine insulinoma. *Compendium on Continuing Education for the Practicing Veterinarian* 18: 13–23.

Tobin, R.L., Nelson, R.W., Lucroy, M.D. et al. (1999). Outcome of surgical versus medical treatment of dogs with beta cell neoplasia: 39 cases (1990–1997). *Journal of the American Animal Hospital Association* 215: 226–230.

Tryfonidou, M.A., Kirpensteijn, J., and Robben, J.H. (1998). A retrospective evaluation of 51 dogs with insulinoma. *Veterinary Quarterly* 20: S114–S115.

Van Ham, L., Braund, K.G., Roels, S. et al. (1997). Treatment of a dog with an insulinoma-related peripheral polyneuropathy with corticosteroids. *Veterinary Record* 141: 98–100.

Walczak, R., Paek, M., Uzzle, M. et al. (2019). Canine insulinomas appear hyperintense on MRI T2-weighted images and isointense on T1-weighted images. *Veterinary Radiology & Ultrasound* 60: 330–337.

Whipple, A.O. and Frantz, V.K. (1935). Adenoma of islet cells with hyperinsulinism. *Annals of Surgery* 101: 1299–1335.

Wouters, E.G.H., Buishand, F.O., Kik, M. et al. (2011). Use of a bipolar vessel-sealing device in resection of canine insulinoma. *Journal of Small Animal Practice* 52: 139–145.

Zini, E., Glaus, T.M., Minuto, F. et al. (2007). Paraneoplastic hypoglycemia due to an insulin-like growth factor type-II secreting hepatocellular carcinoma in a dog. *Journal of Veterinary Internal Medicine* 21: 193–195.

68

Adrenal Tumors

Pierre Amsellem, Michael Schaer, and James P. Farese

Primary adrenal tumors constitute a small percentage of tumors reported in dogs and cats. They represent 1–2% of all tumors in dogs and 0.2% of all tumors in cats (Myers 1997). Over a 20-year period at the University of California–Davis, 195 (41%) of 472 neoplastic adrenal lesions were reported as adrenocortical tumors (ATs), 151 (32%) were pheochromocytomas, and 126 (27%) were metastatic lesions. In cats, 6 (30%) were adrenocortical tumors, 2 (10%) were pheochromocytoma, and 12 (60%) were metastatic lesions. Lymphoma was the most common cancer to spread to the adrenal glands in both species (Lunn & Page 2013; Labelle & De Cock 2005). More than 50% of pheochromocytomas are considered malignant (Lunn & Page 2013; Gilson *et al.* 1994b; Kyles *et al.* 2003; Von Dehn *et al.* 1995). Approximately 30–50% of pheochromocytomas invade adjacent vasculature and approximately 20–30% have been reported to metastasize. Approximately half of adrenocortical tumors are malignant, 10–20% invade adjacent vasculature, and reported metastasis rates range from 0% to 50% (Hunt *et al.* 1992; Johnston 1977; Kintzer & Peterson 1994).

Improved diagnostic imaging has led to an improved ability to diagnose adrenal tumors, and many of these are accidentally discovered during routine abdominal ultrasound for nonspecific ailments. These adrenal masses ("incidentalomas") pose a major diagnostic challenge for the clinician (Grumbach *et al.* 2003; Young 2007). The majority of adrenocortical tumors are functional, with clinical signs reflecting the type of hormone being produced by the neoplasm. The differential diagnosis includes adrenocortical adenoma, adrenocortical adenocarcinoma, pheochromocytoma, aldosteronoma,

and various combinations of coexisting disorders. Figure 68.1 illustrates the general approach to a newly identified adrenal mass. Adrenocortical nodular hyperplasia is sometimes confused with adrenocortical tumors, but hyperplasia is always bilateral and pituitary dependent. The prognosis for adrenal tumors depends on the extent of disease and whether benign or malignant, invasion of surrounding tissues, and presence of metastatic disease.

Adrenocortical adenocarcinoma, adrenal adenoma, adrenocortical adenomatous hyperplasia

History and physical findings

Each of these conditions can cause clinical signs of Cushing's disease because of their ability to produce cortisol and/or intermediary products of steroid metabolism such as androstenedione, progesterone, or 17-hydroxyprogesterone. The most common historical and physical examination findings are polydipsia, polyuria, pendulous abdomen, hepatomegaly (in dogs with hepatic glycogen accumulation), panting, and various skin changes such as alopecia, hyperpigmentation, calcinosis cutis, epidermal atrophy, or easy bruising (Reusch & Feldman 1991). Many of these signs can vary from clinically inapparent to grossly overt, depending on whether the tumor is secreting hormones and which particular products are entering the bloodstream. In cats, hypercortisolism can cause extremely friable skin. Additional findings can include hypertension, lethargy, weakness, pulmonary calcification and/or thrombus formation, dilute urine, and proteinuria. Clinical signs

Small Animal Soft Tissue Surgery, Second Edition. Edited by Eric Monnet.
© 2023 John Wiley & Sons, Inc. Published 2023 by John Wiley & Sons, Inc.
Companion website: www.wiley.com/go/monnet/small

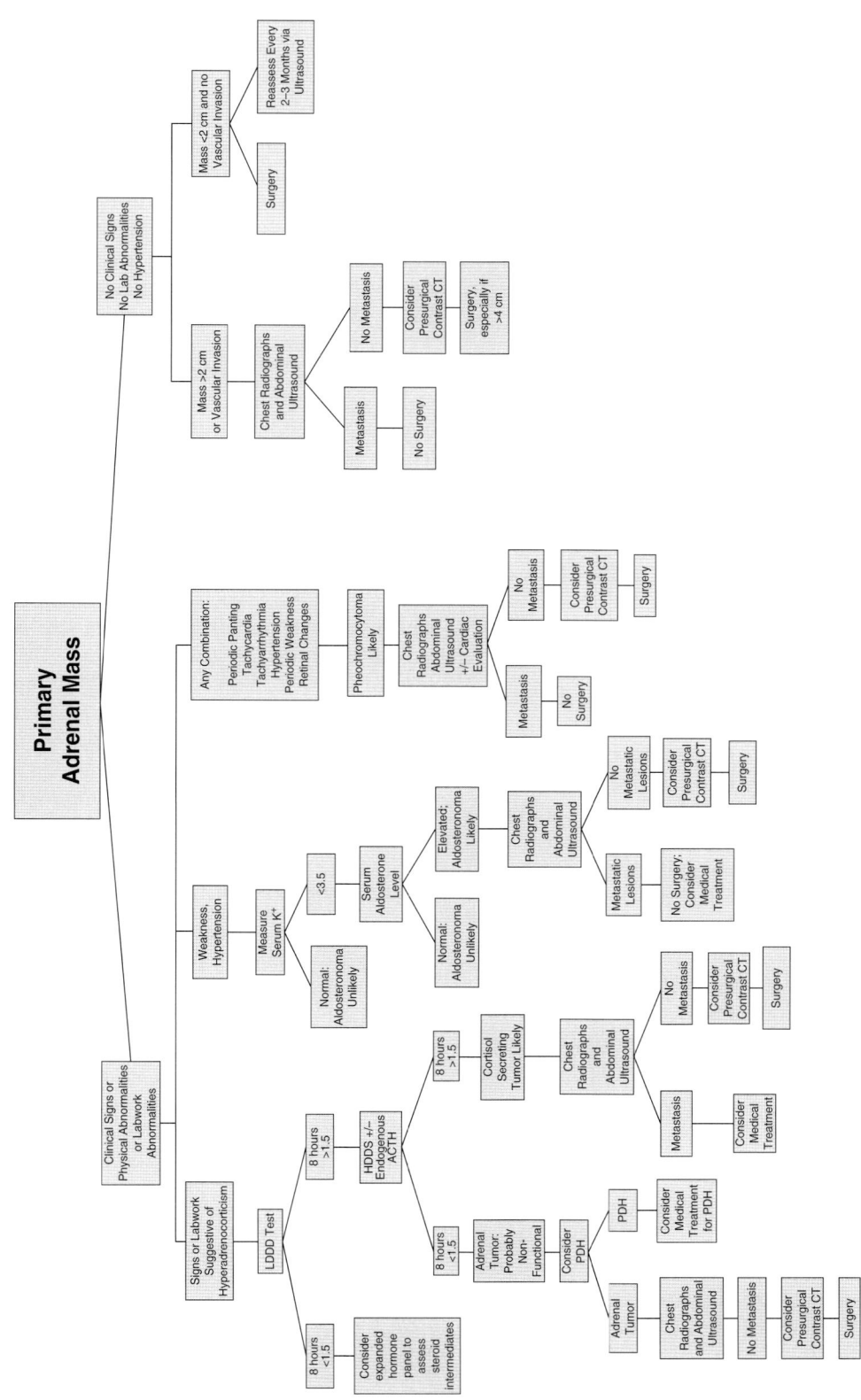

Figure 68.1 Algorithm showing the clinical approach to primary adrenal tumors.

related to excessive sex hormones have also been reported (Millard *et al.* 2009; Syme *et al.* 2001). None of these signs can be used to distinguish one etiology from the other. Various infections can occur because of the immunologic impairment cause by hypercortisolism, the most frequent involving the skin and the urinary tract. If the tumor is a large adenocarcinoma (greater than 5 cm), it can sometimes be detected on abdominal palpation. A malignant tumor can also invade the caudal vena cava and cause abdominal ascites (Kyles *et al.* 2003). More rarely it can invade the spinal canal and cause cord dysfunction.

Adrenocortical tumors in dogs can sometimes have a spontaneous hemorrhage, or it can bleed following accidental blunt abdominal trauma (Evans *et al.* 1991) or from excessive localizing pressure during abdominal ultrasound examination. The clinical signs are dramatic and are characterized as a clinically stable patient that suddenly vomits, becomes weak in all four legs, and finally collapses. Clinical signs are typical of hypovolemia, including weakness, mental dullness, tachycardia, increased respiratory rate, weak pulses, pale mucous membranes, and decreased body temperature. Abdominal pain is sometimes present.

General laboratory test results

Functional adrenocortical adenocarcinoma, adrenal adenoma, and adrenocortical adenomatous hyperplasia cannot be distinguished with routine laboratory tests. All will give findings typical of Cushing's disease, with various combinations and degrees of abnormalities involving elevated liver enzymes (serum alkaline phosphatase, alanine aminotransferase), serum lipids, eosinopenia, lymphopenia, and thrombocytosis., The total bilirubin is usually normal, but it can be elevated with steroid hepatopathy. The fasting and postfeeding serum bile acids can also be elevated from steroid hepatopathy. The urine concentration will range from hyposthenuria to normal; it can even simulate diabetes insipidus. Urinalysis should always be followed by urinate bacterial culture to screen for the presence of urinary tract infection, because of the patient's altered immune status from hypercortisolism (Feldman & Nelson 2004).

Endocrinological test results

The endocrinologic evaluation of an adrenocortical mass can be confusing, because of the wide variations in test results that can occur. The most commonly used tests include ACTH stimulation, low-dose dexamethasone suppression (LDDS), and high-dose dexamethasone sup-

pression (HDDS) tests (Reusch & Feldman 1991). The following discussion will characterize the adrenal tumor and adrenocortical adenomatous hyperplasia features with each of these tests. Note that adrenocortical adenomatous hyperplasia will give the same test results as pituitary-dependent hyperplasia (PDH).

ACTH stimulation test

The ACTH stimulation test results can range from low to elevated with adrenocortical tumors (AT). This broad range depends on the numbers of ACTH receptor sites on the surface of the target tissue and the degree of tumor autonomy. Adrenal neoplasia commonly shows an elevated response to ACTH similar to PDH. As a result of these response variations, the ACTH stimulation test is unable to distinguish between AT and PDH. There are some dogs with both functional adrenal tumors and PDH that will show normal cortisol secretion during the ACTH stimulation test. There are others that produce increased amounts of steroid intermediates such as androstenedione, progesterone, and 17-hydroxyprogesterone, which will require special laboratories to make these determinations (Norman *et al.* 1999; Syme *et al.* 2001), but caution should be exercised with some interpretations because some nonadrenal tumors can increase these steroid intermediates (Behrend *et al.* 2005a). It is therefore prudent to freeze extra serum from the ACTH stimulation test in case there is a need to do these intermediate steroid determinations for the "atypical Cushing's" patient.

Cats show a variable, wide-ranging result with ACTH stimulation, therefore making it undependable.

Low-dose dexamethasone suppression test

The normal dog will show adrenocortical suppression (<1.7 μg/dL) eight hours after receiving 0.01 mg/kg of dexamethasone intravenously, whereas patients with PDH and functional AT will not suppress to this degree after eight hours. There are rare exceptions to this characterization that will require additional diagnostic tests. If the Cushing's patient shows cortisol suppression (>50%) after four hours but then goes on to increase to a value >1.7 μg/dL, PDH will be the diagnosis, because functional adrenocortical tumors will not suppress beyond the slightest change because of physiologic fluctuations. Therefore, the LDDS will only diagnose hypercortisolism and sometimes distinguish PDH from AT if the four-hour cortisol sample is suppressed by more than 50% from the baseline value.

The LDDS (0.01 mg/kg) test gives undependable results in the cat. Results in the cat are much more reliable at a larger dose of 0.1 mg/kg.

High-dose dexamethasone suppression test

This test is still being used in dogs and cats to help distinguish AT from PDH, although its inconsistent results have made it an unpopular test for humans. Under ideal circumstances, the patient with PDH will show serum cortisol suppression by 50% or more from the baseline. However, caution with interpreting this test is recommended, because up to 25% of dogs with PDH will not suppress (Feldman 1983). Furthermore, there might even be dogs with AT that will suppress with this test, although this is rare. Therefore, the HDDS cannot reliably be the sole criterion for making a diagnosis of an adrenal tumor in dogs and cats (Galac *et al.* 2019).

Plasma ACTH

The functional adrenal tumor will hypersecrete cortisol, which in turn will decrease ACTH production by the anterior pituitary gland because of negative feedback inhibition. This differs from PDH, which overrides the negative feedback mechanism, allowing elevated amounts of ACTH release from the anterior pituitary despite the presence of hypercortisolemia. Therefore, the dog with a functional adrenal tumor will have a plasma ACTH level of less than 40 pg/mL, with many being <10 pg/mL or less (Feldman 1981; Pineiro *et al.* 2009). Values of 45 pg/mL or greater typify PDH.

The diagnostic accuracy of this test in the cat remains to be shown.

Imaging

Abdominal radiographs are not as sensitive as computerized tomography (CT) and magnetic resonance imaging (MRI) techniques. Radiography can detect adrenal masses that exceed 5 cm in diameter or smaller masses if they are mineralized (Penninck *et al.* 1988). Adrenocortical tumors measuring <4 cm in diameter can be benign or malignant, while those that are ≥4 cm in diameter are typically malignant. A left-sided adrenal tumor can be seen just cranial to the left kidney, whereas the right-sided neoplasm is located just medial to the cranial pole of the right kidney. Some 50% of adrenocortical masses will calcify, but this will not distinguish between benign and malignant tumors. Pheochromocytomas rarely are mineralized. Any animal with a suspect adrenal mass should have thoracic radiographs performed to evaluate for pulmonary metastasis.

As mentioned, spontaneous peri-adrenal hemorrhage can occur. Acute peri-adrenal bleeding may show a loss of detail and an increased soft tissue density in the retroperitoneal space on plain film radiography. This abnormality is readily detected with more advanced diagnostic imaging.

Abdominal ultrasonography is a valuable aid for diagnosing adrenal gland tumors (Figure 68.2). In general, adrenal tumors tend to be abnormally enlarged and rounded. They are usually solitary, but on rare occasions bilateral adrenal tumors can occur. They can be of the same functional type or they can be completely different from each other. There is no diagnostic imaging test that can distinguish between a glucocorticoid-secreting adrenocortical tumor, an adrenomedullary tumor (pheochromocytoma), and an aldosteronoma. Each of these tumors has a similar shape and size and all three can invade the caudal vena cava. Any adrenal tumor that exceeds 2 cm in diameter should be suspicious as a possible malignant neoplasm. A functional glucocorticoid-secreting tumor should cause contralateral adrenal gland atrophy because of negative feedback inhibition on ACTH secretion, but often the atrophy is not detectable on imaging (Hoerauf & Reusch 1999).

An adrenal mass less than 2 cm in diameter in an asymptomatic dog and cat can be a benign lesion, or it can be a nonfunctional tumor with either benign or malignant behavior. These lesions should be closely monitored for any change in size or infiltrative behavior; in such cases surgery might be strongly indicated.

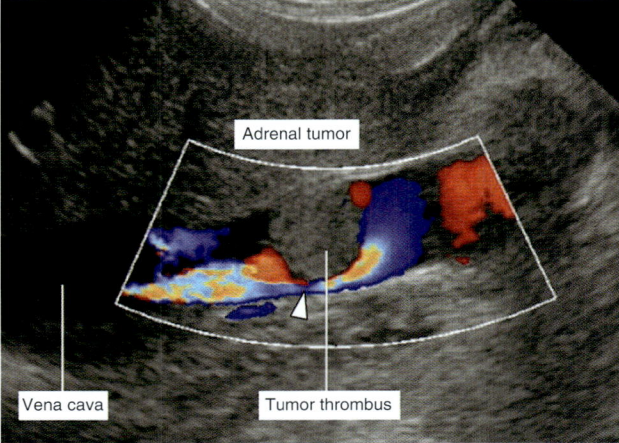

Figure 68.2 Ultrasonographic image of an adrenal tumor thrombus within the vena cava. Note the pattern of blood flow (arrowhead) depicted by color Doppler around the thrombus.

The use of CT scans has greatly facilitated the detection of adrenal tumors. CT also provides the examiner the opportunity to evaluate the vena cava for tumor invasion (Figure 68.3). It has a reported sensitivity and specificity of 80% and 90%, respectively (Kyles *et al.* 2003). Adrenal tumors discovered in the absence of clinical signs (i.e., found as incidental findings) and lacking obvious malignant behavior have been termed incidentalomas. CT-guided fine-needle aspiration biopsy is not typically recommended, because it rarely makes an accurate distinction between benign and malignant disease and can be dangerous (Quayle *et al.* 2007). Small incidentalomas should be closely monitored via periodic ultrasounds for any change in size or infiltrative behavior (Figure 68.1). CT is also used for surgical planning and assessment of renal and vascular involvement. This topic will be discussed further in the surgical section.

MRI of normal canine adrenal glands has been described in the literature (Llabres-Diaz & Dennis 2003). MRI should provide very detailed information regarding the anatomic location of the adrenal tumor, any vascular involvement, as well as any evidence of regional metastasis. This procedure may be helpful to the oncologic surgeon who has to plan a surgical strategy for tumor resection. MRI use is dictated by cost restriction, availability, and the clinical signs of the patient.

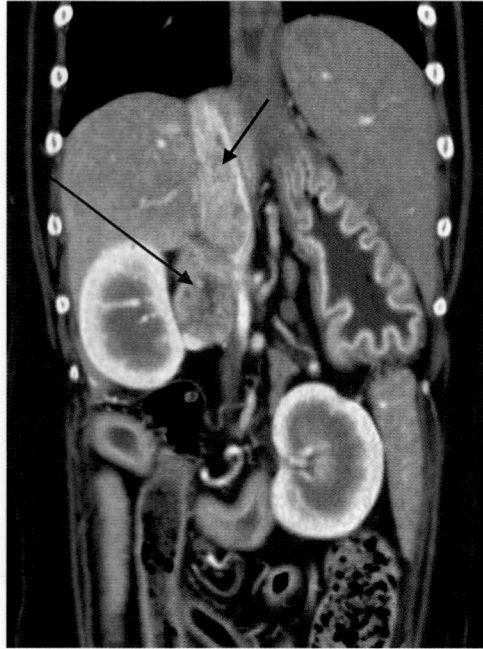

Figure 68.3 Coronal computed tomography image of a right-sided adrenal mass (blue arrow) with a caval thrombus (black arrow).

Preoperative preparation

Because hypercortisolism is a catabolic condition, all dogs and cats should have a thorough preoperative medical evaluation in order to detect any coexisting infections, especially those involving the skin and urinary tract. A complete urinalysis should be done, and any evidence of pyuria and bacteriuria should prompt submission of the sample for bacterial culture and sensitivity. All underlying infections should be treated and brought under control prior to surgery. A serum biochemistry evaluation, complete blood count, and thoracic radiograph should also be done preoperatively. Coexisting lung pathology such as pulmonary calcification or pulmonary thrombosis will strongly accentuate the anesthetic risk for the patient. Neither of these pulmonary disorders is amenable to treatment. CT and MRI techniques will further define the anatomic borders of the tumor and its tendency to invade nearby structures. Any borderline hyperglycemia >150–200 mg/dL should be followed up at a later date in order to detect and treat diabetes mellitus.

The patient's blood pressure should also be evaluated. Any systolic value that repeatedly exceeds 160 mmHg should be considered as hypertension. For dogs, a calcium channel blocker such as amlodipine (0.12–0.2 mg/kg body weight once daily) and angiotensin-converting enzyme (ACE) inhibitors such as enalapril (0.1–0.5 mg/kg body weight orally [p.o.] twice daily) are commonly used. Treatments for hypertension will vary according to the clinician's experience and preference; however, most surgeons recommend a 1–2-week course of phenoxybenzamine (PBZ; 0.5 mg/kg p.o. every 12 hours) for hypertensive dogs (Herrera *et al.* 2008; Kyles *et al.* 2003). Hypertensive cats are best treated with amlodipine (0.06–0.1 mg body weight p.o. once daily). Because hypercortisolism can predispose the patient to hypercoagulation, a serum antithrombin 3 globulin determination and a thromboelastogram may be helpful to evaluate the patient's potential for thrombosis-caused complications.

Patient management during and after surgery

Surgical removal of a cortisol-producing adrenal tumor can leave the patient with life-threatening hypocortisolemia during the surgical and postoperative phases. This is avoided by providing glucocorticoid drugs during and after surgery. A recommended method involves administering dexamethasone at a dose of 0.05–0.1 mg/kg body weight (Feldman & Nelson 2004; Kyles *et al.* 2003). It should be noted that dexamethasone does not interfere with the measurement of endogenous cortisol levels. This dose is given at the end of surgery and then usually every 12 hours that day. On the first postoperative day, a repeat ACTH stimulation test should be done before any glucocorticoid is given, in order to determine whether adrenalectomy has corrected the hypercortisolemia (if present preoperatively) and to assess for the presence of functional metastatic tumors. A low post-stimulation cortisol value can indicate the absence of functional tumor cells, although metastasis with non-functional tumor cells is still possible. A high poststimulation cortisol level is indicative of either incorrect diagnosis of the source of the excess cortisol or metastatic disease. If the serum cortisol concentration is low postoperatively, dexamethasone can then be given subcutaneously every 12 hours until the patient can receive oral replacement therapy. Once this occurs, prednisone can be given at a replacement dose of 0.25–0.5 mg/kg once or twice daily. This dose can then be slowly reduced over the ensuing 4–6 weeks. An ACTH stimulation test should be done within a week after the prednisone is discontinued in order to access the patient's adrenocortical reserve.

Postoperative mineralocorticoid drug treatment is required in dogs that undergo bilateral adrenalectomy for bilateral adrenal tumors. The postoperative management of those dogs was reported to be uncomplicated in a series of nine dogs with bilateral adrenal tumors (Oblak *et al.* 2016). Intraoperative and postoperative mineralocorticoid drug treatment is necessary in a small number of dogs with a solitary cortisol-secreting adrenal tumor. In most cases the contralateral adrenal gland will be able to produce ample amounts of aldosterone in order to maintain normal serum sodium and potassium concentrations. If hyponatremia and hyperkalemia do occur postoperatively, replacement hormone treatment can begin with either deoxycorticosterone pivalate (2 mg/kg body weight subcutaneously [s.c.] approximately once every 21–30 days) or oral fludrocortisone acetate tablets (starting at 0.02 mg/kg divided twice daily).

Prophylaxis against thromboembolism has been recommended with heparin treatment (Feldman & Nelson 2004). Heparin can be administered as a single agent at a dose ranging from 35 to 220 units/kg intravenously. This broad range of dosage represents the different methodologies and therapeutic philosophies of various veterinary authors. One method combining the techniques of Feldman, Nelson, Garvey, and Smiley calls for the intraoperative administration of plasma (as a source of antithrombin 3 globulin) containing heparin at dose of 35 units/kg body weight. This is followed postoperatively with heparin administered for two doses 12 hours apart at a subcutaneous dose of 35 units/kg body weight, and then tapered to 10 units/kg body weight given subcutaneously every 12 hours for the next 2–3 days. On the fifth postoperative day, hetastarch (10–20 mL/kg body weight over a period of 6 hours) is given as a single dose, with the thought that it will reduce the potential for thromboembolism for a period of days. This latter recommendation with hetastarch is not consistently recommended in the literature.

Intraoperative antibiotics are administered routinely, but antimicrobial drugs are not continued postoperatively unless there is a documented infection, the most common being urinary tract infections that should have been detected preoperatively. If an indwelling urinary catheter is used during the intraoperative and immediate postoperative periods, the catheter tip or the patient's urine should be submitted to the laboratory for bacterial culture and sensitivity in order to detect any secondary nosocomial infection.

Acute pancreatitis has been observed in some dogs in the immediate postoperative period. This potentially life-threatening disorder might occur as a result of intraoperative hypotension causing ischemic injury to the pancreas, microthromboemboli to the pancreas, or as a result of intraoperative injury to the pancreas during surgical retraction. Any vomiting that occurs during the immediate postoperative period should call for the recommended therapeutic actions for managing this condition, such as continued intravenous fluids, restriction of food and water, and analgesic drugs as deemed appropriate. The postoperative glucocorticoid treatments should be continued despite the presence of acute pancreatitis, especially in light of the fact that the patient might not have enough endogenous glucocorticoids to meet the bodily demands during this stressful complication.

All insulin-dependent diabetics should continue to receive their insulin requirements. Failure to do so can result in diabetic ketoacidosis, hyperosmolar nonketotic diabetes, and predisposition to infection. This especially applies to the cat with a functional adrenocortical tumor, because most cats with hypercortisolism also have insulin-dependent diabetes. The clinician should closely monitor the blood glucose postoperatively, because the decline in elevated blood cortisol levels might reverse any insulin resistance that might have occurred preoperatively.

Dogs that develop metastatic adrenocortical carcinoma might benefit from mitotane treatment. Mitotane is an adrenocorticolytic drug that has been used to treat humans with adrenocortical carcinoma (Luton *et al.* 1990). One of the studies using this drug in dogs with adrenocortical carcinoma showing signs of hypercorticism have shown a good response to treatment (Kintzer & Peterson 1994; Van Sluijs *et al.* 1995). Most of the 32 dogs in Kinzer's study were shown to require 2–20 times the normal maintenance dose of 50 mg/kg per week, with 19 dogs developing signs of drug toxicosis and three developing signs of glucocorticoid and mineralocorticoid deficiencies.

Adrenal medullary tumor (pheochromocytoma)

Pheochromocytoma is a rare tumor in dogs and even more rare in the cat (Henry *et al.* 1993; Patnaik *et al.* 1990). It is frequently undiagnosed because of its rare occurrence, it might not be endocrinologically active, and some are benign lesions that might not cause any clinical signs in the patient. Pheochromocytoma is usually a solitary tumor, but it can occur bilaterally as well. It can even coexist with an adrenocortical tumor. To make matters even more confusing for the clinician, it can also coexist with PDH (Lunn & Page 2013; Feldman & Nelson 2004; Von Dehn *et al.* 1995). Pheochromocytomas are usually slow-growing tumors that can range in size from less than 0.5 cm in diameter to more than 10 cm in diameter. Some 50% are benign and approximately 50% are malignant. They are usually diagnosed if they are endocrinologically active, with their hypersecretion of catecholamine hormones, norepinephrine, and/or epinephrine, or if they assume malignant behavior and metastasize to other areas of the body or invade the posterior vena cava.

History and physical findings

The benign and endocrinologically silent pheochromocytoma might be an incidental finding (adrenal incidentaloma) during the medical evaluation for some other condition. Those that hypersecrete catecholamines can cause abnormalities that are characteristic to those hormones (Barthez *et al.* 1997; Bouayad *et al.* 1987; Gilson *et al.* 1994b). Some of the signs attributed to hyperepinephrinemia include panting, anxiety, restlessness, palpably strong heart beats, warm and reddened skin (due to flushing), and sometimes collapse and muscular weakness. The latter sign can be due to cardiac tachyarrhythmias. Polydipsia and polyuria can also be present. Refractory hypertension is the main sign associated with increased secretion of catecholamines, and it might have a fluctuating tendency that parallels the tumor's production of norepinephrine and epinephrine (Herrera *et al.* 2008). If the tumor invades the posterior vena cava, ascites might be apparent. The owner's history might describe the panting, anxiety, pacing, strong heart beats against the dog's chest wall, and skin flushing as episodic occurrences because of the tumor's intermittent secretory pattern. The physical examination findings can range from normal to those signs associated with increased catecholamine secretion. Cardiac tachyarrhythmias may or may not be present at the time of the examination.

Several blood pressure determinations should be done on dogs and cats with suspect pheochromocytomas. This can be done by direct intra-arterial measurements or indirectly using the oscillometric and Doppler methods. Although there are various values for defining hypertension in the veterinary literature, it is generally agreed that a systolic pressure exceeding 160 mmHg and a diastolic reading exceeding 100 mmHg constitute the acceptable reference points. More details regarding hypertension classification in dogs and cats are found in the American College of Veterinary Internal Medicine consensus statement (Acierno *et al.* 2018).

The tests should be repeated in the suspect adrenal medullary tumor patient because of the episodic secretory nature of catecholamine-secreting tumors, which will cause variable results. Because there are several different causes (chronic renal disease, hyperadrenocorticism) of hypertension in the dog and cat that may or may not coexist with a pheochromocytoma, a thorough medical work-up along with detailed imaging studies are essential in order to accurately evaluate each individual patient. The clinician should also be aware that only 50% of pheochromocytomas are found to have clinical evidence of hypertension (Lunn & Page 2013; Bouayad *et al.* 1987; Von Dehn *et al.* 1995).

Abnormal laboratory tests

There are no consistent abnormalities on the hemogram or the serum biochemistry panel with pheochromocytoma. The blood glucose can be elevated due to the increased glycogenolysis and gluconeogenesis that can occur from the increased epinephrine secretion. In most cases, the elevation is not high enough to be classified as clinical diabetes mellitus. Proteinuria can be caused by the effects of hypertension on the kidney and renal insufficiency can be a sequel to chronic hypertension.

Diagnostic imaging

Abdominal radiographs will be abnormal if an adrenal tumor invades and completely obstructs the lumen of the vena cava and causes ascites. Tumors less than 3 cm in diameter are rarely visible on plain radiographs, and those that are detected are notably larger than 5 cm and rarely calcify. Thoracic radiographs can show any cardiomegaly that has resulted from the excess cardiac workload associated with elevated circulating catecholamine blood levels.

Abdominal ultrasound plays a key role in the diagnosis of adrenal tumors; however, this technique cannot specifically distinguish adrenocortical from adrenal medullary tumors. Generally speaking, a dog showing no clinical signs of hyperadrenocorticism with unilateral adrenomegaly and a normal-sized contralateral adrenal gland should be suspicious for a pheochromocytoma or a nonfunctional adrenocortical tumor. Functional adrenocortical tumors can cause contralateral adrenal atrophy caused by negative feedback inhibition on corticotrophin-releasing hormone and ACTH, although this is not always evident ultrasonographically. A skilled ultrasonographer can demonstrate tumor infiltration into the vena cava when present, and into nearby blood vessels such as the phrenicoabdominal artery and vein.

CT and MRI are very accurate and noninvasive methods for imaging pheochromocytomas and adrenocortical tumors. The detail provided by these techniques is very helpful in preoperative planning and for establishing the tumor's anatomic relationship with nearby blood vessels and organs, for example invasion into the ipsilateral kidney or renal vasculature.

Metaiodobenzylguanidine (MIBG) is a structural analog of guanethidine derivative with a molecular structure similar to norepinephrine. Labeling it with iodine 131 allows the chromaffin tissue of the adrenal medullary tumor to be imaged with a gamma camera (Feldman & Nelson 2004). Although this technique has been used more commonly in humans, it has only been used occasionally in the dog. While the test can sometimes distinguish the pheochromocytoma from an adrenocortical tumor in humans, the accuracy and availability of CT and MRI techniques minimize the usefulness of the MIBG study as a routine diagnostic test.

Serum and urine catecholamine levels

In humans, there is available technology to routinely determine plasma and urine epinephrine and norepinephrine concentrations. Additional tests can be done to measure the urine metabolites including metanephrine, normetanephrine, and vanillylmandelic acid. These same tests are not readily available in veterinary medicine because of technological and economic factors. There is one report using urinary catecholamine and metanephrine to creatinine ratios for helping to make the diagnosis of pheochromocytoma in the dog (Kook et al. 2007). Since the first edition of this textbook, new methodologies for detection of catecholamine urinary metabolites have become available in the dog. One study (Quante et al. 2010) concluded that dogs with high urinary concentrations of normetanephrine (four times normal) are highly suggestive of pheochromocytoma. Another study (Gostelow et al. 2013) showed that plasma-free normetanephrine and metanephrine concentrations have excellent sensitivity and specificity for the diagnosis of pheochromocytoma in dogs.

Preoperative preparation and intraoperative monitoring

Surgery should be postponed until the dog's blood pressure is brought under control. This is optimally done with PBZ given orally at home. PBZ is an alpha-adrenergic antagonist that irreversibly binds to both α-1 and α-2 adrenergic receptors and blocks the α-adrenergic response to circulating epinephrine and norepinephrine. Herrera et al. (2008) have reported a much improved survival in dogs that were treated with PBZ at a dosage of 1–2 mg/kg per day for approximately 20 days preoperatively. The median dosage was 0.6 mg/kg (range 0.1–2.5 mg/kg) every 12 hours. PBZ is used to reverse vasoconstriction and hypovolemia before surgery and to control fluctuations of blood pressure and heart rate during anesthesia. Once the blood pressure is stable, surgery can be scheduled. Barrera et al. (2013), in a later study, did not find any protective effect from PBZ. However, this study only had six dogs with pheochromocytomas treated with PBZ. At this point, the authors continue to pretreat dogs with suspected pheochromocytoma with PBZ, which is given last on the night before surgery. It is strongly recommended that strict anesthetic monitoring be done during and after surgery. An intra-arterial catheter should be placed to allow for accurate blood pressure monitoring. Another intra-arterial catheter can be used for frequent arterial blood gas determinations intraoperatively. Because of the anticipated blood pressure and heart rate swings that can occur with surgical manipulation of the tumor, the anesthesiologist should be ready to administer certain critical drugs such as the α-adrenergic-blocking injectable drug phentolamine (0.1 mg/kg intravenously [i.v.]) and the catecholamine drug dopamine (2–5 μg/kg/min i.v.) under the appropriate circumstances.

Tachyarrhythmias pose a definite intraoperative threat to the patient. Therefore, constant electrocardiographic monitoring is essential during the intraoperative and immediate postoperative stages. Antiarrhythmic drugs such as lidocaine should be readily available for treating ventricular tachycardia. For other severe tachyarrhythmias β-blocking drugs might be needed, but in humans it is essential to treat with α-blockers before administering the β-blocker in order to avoid life-threatening hypertension. This same guideline might also be applicable to the dog, although experience is limited.

Postoperative monitoring

If the tumor is completely resected, the postoperative cardiac rhythm and blood pressure recordings should normalize. Persistent hypertension can reflect residual tumor in the patient, either from incomplete tumor removal or from functional metastatic lesions. Diagnostic efforts should search for other causes of hypertension such as chronic renal disease or hyperadrenocorticism. Cardiac monitoring should be done for 24–48 hours after surgery. Tachyarrhythmias can occur from residual functional tumor tissue or from metastatic disease. A complete cardiac assessment should be done in order to rule out cardiac disease that may or may not be due to the increased blood levels of epinephrine and norepinephrine.

Aldosteronoma

An aldosteronoma is a neoplasm of the zona glomerulosa of the adrenal cortex. There is a higher incidence of this syndrome in the cat compared to the dog. A functional tumor will produce and secrete supraphysiologic amounts of aldosterone that will cause hyperaldosteronism and clinical signs related to the increased mineralocorticoid hormone production. There is one case report of an adrenocortical tumor in the dog that produced excessive amounts of deoxycorticosterone (Reine *et al.* 1999) and another that produced excessive amounts of corticosterone and aldosterone (Behrend *et al.* 2005b). The veterinary literature is scant on publications describing this syndrome in the dog, but there have been several reported involvements in the cat (Ash *et al.* 2005; DeClue *et al.* 2005; Flood *et al.* 1999; Kooistra 2006; Moore *et al.* 2000; Shiel & Mooney 2007). Similar clinical signs caused by this syndrome can also occur with idiopathic hyperplasia of the zona glomerulosa involving one or both adrenal glands (Kooistra 2006). Aldosteronoma in the cat has an approximately even distribution for being either an adenoma or an adenocarcinoma.

History and physical findings

The clinical signs are due to excessive amounts of aldosterone production. The main action of aldosterone occurs at the distal convoluted renal tubule, where it promotes sodium absorption and potassium excretion. The sodium retention affects total body sodium levels, while the serum concentration is usually maintained between normal and high normal. The sodium retention may also cause hypertension, which can induce retinal hemorrhage and blindness. The excessive potassium excretion will cause hypokalemia and an enormous loss of total body potassium stores. Hypokalemia with serum values <3.0 mEq/L will have adverse effects on the skeletal and cardiac muscles. Clinically this will cause severe skeletal muscle weakness. It can also cause rhabdomyolysis and abnormalities in cardiac excitation and conduction.

Feline hyperaldosteronism may result from either an adrenocortical tumor or bilateral adrenocortical hyperplasia (Kooistra 2006). The main clinical signs in the cat are skeletal muscle weakness (including ventral cervical flexion) and hypertension (systolic >180 mmHg). The latter can cause retinal hemorrhage and detached retina. Chronic hypertension can also have adverse effects on the heart and kidneys. It is important to look for other causes of hypertension in the older cat, especially chronic renal insufficiency and hyperthyroidism. Polydipsia and polyuria can also occur from hypokalemia, because the low potassium concentration can impair the action of antidiuretic hormone (ADH, vasopressin) at the distal renal tubule and collecting duct. It can also impair ADH release from the posterior pituitary gland (Shiel & Mooney 2007). Hypokalemia can also affect the hypertonic medullary interstitial gradient by interfering with solute accumulation (DiBartola & DeMorais 2006).

Abnormal laboratory tests

Resting plasma aldosterone concentrations are frequently markedly elevated when the cause is an adrenocortical tumor. However, they might be normal or only slightly elevated with adrenocortical hyperplasia, which might then be further defined with certain adrenal dynamic tests such as plasma renin activity determination and the ratio of plasma aldosterone to plasma renin activity ratio (Javadi *et al.* 2005; Kooistra 2006). These tests are restricted to those laboratories that can measure plasma renin concentrations. The serum sodium is usually normal despite the increased in total body sodium. The hypokalemia can decrease to dangerously low levels (<3.0 mEq/L). This can potentially cause a metabolic alkalosis because of the direct effects of aldosterone on the distal renal tubular H^+-ATPase pumps of the cortical and medullary collecting tubules, as well as hypokalemia-associated transcellular shifting and hydrogen ion secretion. Hypokalemia also promotes increased bicarbonate ion absorption in the proximal renal tubule, which will further exacerbate the metabolic alkalosis. The associated metabolic alkalosis has been reported more frequently in humans compared to dogs and cats; there is only one case report describing it in a dog (Reine *et al.* 1999). A more specific diagnosis of hyperaldosteronism using the plasma aldosterone/renin ratio has been described by Javadi *et al.* (2006).

Because severe hypokalemic myopathy can cause severe rhabdomyolysis, the serum creatine kinase concentration can be markedly elevated. Myoglobinemia can subsequently occur and can be renal tubulotoxic, thereby compromising renal function. The blood urea nitrogen (BUN) and serum creatinine concentrations can elevate from the myoglobinuria, but the hypertension can also cause renal pathology through the loss of renal arteriolar autoregulation. This can cause elevated intraglomerular capillary pressure and progressive renal damage. Hypertension can then occur from both renal failure and the hyperaldosteronism.

Diagnostic imaging

In primary hyperaldosteronism, abdominal ultrasound and advanced imaging such as CT and MRI are used to detect an adrenocortical tumor. As with other adrenal tumors that have malignant potential, thoracic radiographs should always be done to assess for possible pulmonary metastatic lesions.

Preoperative preparation

The patient should have a complete medical evaluation preoperatively. This should include a complete blood count, serum chemistry panel, blood gas measurement, electrocardiogram, thoracic radiography, and blood pressure determinations. The hypokalemia can be treated with slowly administered intravenous potassium chloride solution diluted in lactated Ringer's solution. The usual therapeutic recommendation is 0.5 mEq/kg/h; however, in situations where the serum potassium is <2.5 mEq/L, a larger dose ranging from 1.0 to 1.5 mEq/kg/h might have to be given along with simultaneous electrocardiographic monitoring. Spironolactone can be given orally at a dose of 2–4 mg/kg/day. This drug will block the effects of aldosterone at the renal distal tubule. Oral potassium supplementation using potassium gluconate can be used at a dose of 2 mEq/4.5 kg of body weight twice daily. Blood pressure readings that exceed 180 mmHg should be treated with a calcium channel blocker such as amlodipine (cat: 0.625 mg–0.125 mg orally once daily; dog: 0.125–0.2 mg/kg once daily). Skeletal muscle weakness caused by the hypokalemia can be profound. This can even involve the muscles of respiration, which can cause impaired ventilation and subsequent hypercarbia. It is therefore prudent to delay surgery until the hypokalemia is corrected and any other accompanying abnormalities are resolved, thus making the patient less of an anesthetic risk.

Intraoperative and postoperative medical management

The anesthetist should monitor the breathing quality, PCO_2 concentration, and electrocardiogram very closely. Blood gases (including blood pH) and serum potassium concentration should also be closely monitored. Although most anesthesiologists refrain from adding potassium to the intravenous fluids during most surgeries, intraoperative potassium supplementation might be required during surgery if the patient becomes hypokalemic. Any swings in blood pressure should be corrected with appropriate pressor or antipressor drugs.

Postoperative evaluation should entail monitoring the serum potassium concentration, electrocardiogram, and arterial blood pressure. The serum potassium level can become elevated as a result of hypoaldosteronism caused by negative feedback inhibition on normal aldosterone production cause by the preoperative hyperaldosteronism. This will hopefully self-correct over the ensuing days after surgery, but elevated serum potassium levels exceeding 7.0 mEq/L should be treated with furosemide (1–2 mg/kg body weight, p.o., s.c., i.v., or intramuscularly), which acts as a kaliuretic agent. Any hypotension should prompt an immediate assessment for postoperative hemorrhage.

Surgical considerations

The caudal vena cava can be divided into prerenal, renal, prehepatic, hepatic, and posthepatic following the normal flow of blood (Harder *et al.* 2002). In the dog, the venous drainage of the adrenal glands is through the short adrenal veins into the phrenicoabdominal veins and then into the caudal vena cava (Bezuidenhout 2013). However, drainage of the left adrenal vein into the left renal vein has also been described (Hullinger 1993). This anatomic particularity may explain why, in rare cases, left adrenal tumor thrombi extend into the left renal vein rather than the vena cava (Chiti *et al.* 2021). The right adrenal capsule may be continuous with the tunica externa of the vena cava.

Dogs with hyperadrenocorticism may be at higher risk of surgical wound infection. Prophylactic antibiotics are thus used intraoperatively.

Operative planning

As previously stated, in addition to abdominal ultrasound (Figure 68.2), contrast-enhanced CT is ideal for surgical planning (Figure 68.3) (Schultz *et al.* 2009). Contrast-enhanced CT has a high sensitivity and specificity to detect caval invasion/thrombosis (Schultz *et al.* 2009), but false positives are possible (Kyles *et al.* 2003), especially if contrast filling of the caudal vena cava is inadequate. To improve the quality of contrast filling of the caudal vena cava, iodinated contrast could be injected via a hindlimb catheter into the saphenous vein or the caudal vena cava. This can be administered as a bolus or as a slow infusion (Dr. David Reese, University of Florida, personal communication). In humans, to reduce the risk of catecholamine release in patients with suspected pheochromocytoma, it has been recommended to premedicate patients with phenoxybenzamine or to use nonionic iodinated contrast material (Hunter *et al.* 1994). Catecholamine release has not been documented after contrast injection in dogs (Rosenstein 2000). As a precaution, it may be prudent to use nonionic iodinated contrast material in dogs with adrenal masses. Slice thickness through the adrenals and vasculature should be 1–2 mm to allow visualization of the thin phrenicoabdominal veins (Schultz *et al.* 2009).

CT will help stage the disease and determine tumor resectability. Large masses that invade the paraspinal musculature (Rosenstein 2000) or the spinal column (Platt *et al.* 1998) are usually deemed nonresectable. Vascular or renal capsule invasion does not preclude resectability. Large or extensive tumor thrombi can be extracted and are not usually criteria for nonresectability (Kyles *et al.* 2003). Ipsilateral nephrectomy can be performed if there is local invasion, assuming the opposite kidney is functional. If a nephrectomy is likely based on CT changes (invasion of parenchyma or renal vasculature), the glomerular filtration rate can be measured preoperatively using scintigraphy to assess the function of each kidney preoperatively (Krawiec *et al.* 1988). Contrast CT results in an excretory urogram, which provides a crude, less reliable evaluation of renal function. The final decision on resectability and need for nephrectomy is often made at surgery. Finally, in the coming years, as is the case in humans, the contrast-enhanced CT appearance of adrenal masses may give us an idea of the histopathologic diagnosis (Schultz *et al.* 2009).

Surgical approaches

Both midline celiotomy and lateral flank approaches are utilized and the decision is largely based on surgeon preference. Surgical preparation should include the caudal thorax, should a sternotomy be required for access to the posthepatic vena cava. A midline approach allows for complete abdominal exploratory and evaluation of both adrenal glands (Figure 68.4). A Balfour retractor is used. Variably sized malleable retractors and moistened laparotomy sponges should be on hand. The pancreas is protected throughout the procedure, as it is very near the surgery site.

For a left adrenalectomy, the descending colon is retracted to the right. For a right adrenalectomy, the proximal duodenum is retracted toward the left side to access the retroperitoneum, the hepatorenal ligament is severed, and the liver is retracted cranially using moistened laparotomy sponges and malleable retractors. The vena cava may be retracted medially using a malleable retractor. Alternatively, a vessel loop may be placed

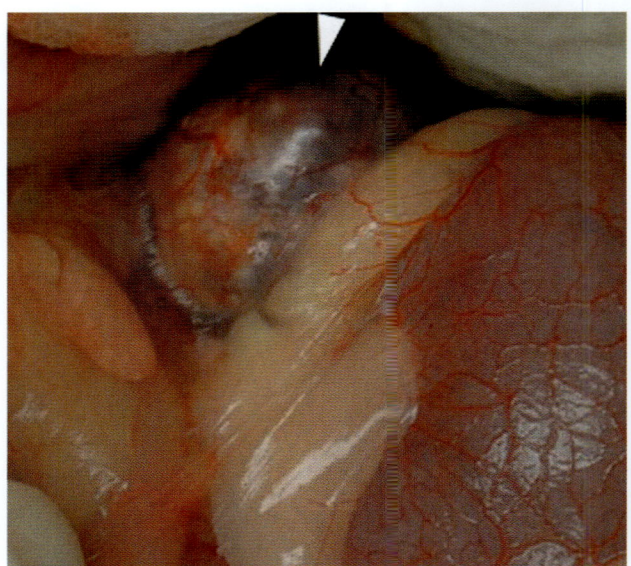

Figure 68.4 Intraoperative photograph of a right-sided pheochromocytoma invading the vena cava via the phrenicoabdominal vein. Note the tumor thrombus visible through the wall of the vein (white arrow). The right kidney (bottom left) is being digitally retracted by the surgeon. Photograph taken via a midline celiotomy approach.

around the vena cava to provide slight traction on the vessel and help with dissection.

The retroperitoneal space is entered and the mass separated from the surrounding tissues using a combination of sharp and blunt dissection and electrocautery. Use of vessel sealer or bipolar cautery can be useful to isolate some very vascular pheochromocytomas. In most cases, the renal vein and the renal capsule can be separated from the mass using blunt dissection and cotton-tip applicators. Right-angle forceps may also be useful in the blunt separation of the mass from the vena cava. Vascular clips are used to ligate the phrenicoabdominal vein on both sides of the adrenal mass. Additional abdominal lesions (e.g., regional lymph nodes, liver, etc.) should be biopsied before closure. Over 50% of dogs with adrenal tumors have additional lesions (e.g., regenerative liver nodule), but the gross appearance should not dictate an intraoperative decision of euthanasia, as in one study only 9% of the biopsies indicated metastases (Schwartz *et al.* 2008). The abdominal wall is usually closed using nonabsorbable suture material to reduce the risk of dehiscence in an animal with hyperadrenocorticism and delayed healing.

A retroperitoneal approach has been described for adrenalectomy (Johnston 1977; Van Sluijs *et al.* 1995). The approach can be performed for either a right or a left adrenalectomy. The animal is placed in lateral recumbency and a skin incision is made caudal to the last rib ventral to the epaxial muscles. The abdominal muscles are separated following the direction of their fibers until the retroperitoneum is entered. This approach does not allow evaluation of the other abdominal structures (e.g., liver) or of the contralateral adrenal gland, so it is recommended that advanced imaging such as CT be performed first for proper staging. This approach was initially believed to reduce the risk of postoperative pancreatitis (Johnston 1977), but this has not proven to be true in a more recent study (Van Sluijs et al. 1995). This technique should be reserved for small adrenal masses without vascular invasion.

Laparoscopic transabdominal adrenalectomy has been reported for small to medium-sized (<5 cm) right- or left-sided adrenocortical carcinoma and pheochromocytomas without vascular invasion (Figure 68.5) (Jimenez Pelaez et al. 2008; Pitt et al. 2016; Mayhew et al. 2014). This is usually performed in lateral oblique recumbency. This approach allows partial exploratory of the abdominal organs and good visualization of the retroperitoneal structures. When comparing open and laparoscopic approaches, laparoscopic adrenalectomy was faster (median surgical time of 90 vs. 120 minutes) than open surgery (Mayhew et al. 2014). However, rupture of the tumor capsule during dissection seemed to occur more frequently in dogs treated laparoscopically (particularly with right-sided tumors) than with open surgery (Mayhew et al. 2014). In another laparoscopic adrenalectomy case series, the tumor fragmented after capsular rupture in two dogs and intracapsular "piecemeal" excision was then recommended (Jimenez Pelaez et al. 2008). This approach may increase the risk of local recurrence.

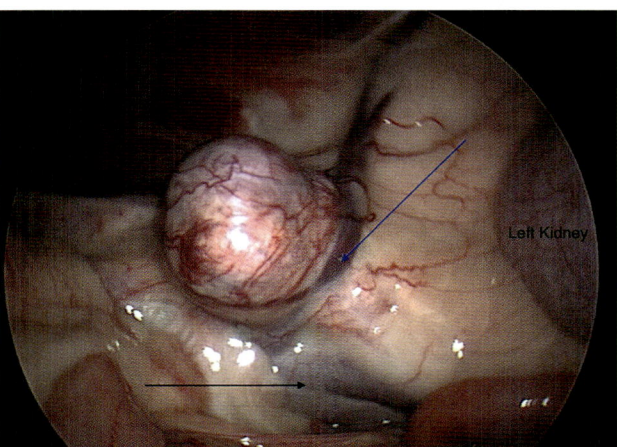

Figure 68.5 Intraoperative laparoscopic view of a left adrenal tumor. The phrenicoabdominal vein (blue arrow) and the vena cava (black arrow) are visible. Source: Courtesy of Dr. Philipp Mayhew.

Positioning the dog in sternal recumbency with the pelvis and thorax elevated and without support under the abdomen to allow ventral displacement of the abdominal organs has also been recommended (Naan et al. 2013). Because of improved visualization, sternal positioning was associated with shorter duration of surgery compared to lateral oblique recumbency for dogs with cortical adrenal tumors (Naan et al. 2013).

In the hands of the most experienced laparoscopic surgeons, dogs with adrenal pheochromocytoma without vascular invasion may also be good candidates for laparoscopic adrenalectomy (Pitt et al. 2016). In any case, when performing laparoscopic adrenalectomy, one should be ready to convert to an open approach, should significant hemorrhage occur.

Adrenal tumors with vascular invasion

Macroscopic vascular invasion due to a tumor thrombus or a blood thrombus has been reported in approximately 25% of reviewed cases (Kyles et al. 2003; Schwartz et al. 2008) and may occur in 10–20% of canine adrenocortical tumors and 30–50% of dogs with pheochromocytoma (Kyles et al. 2003). Tumor thrombi associated with adrenal tumors have been reported in the phrenicoabdominal veins, renal vein, and caudal vena cava (Anderson et al. 2001; Kyles et al. 2003; Schwartz et al. 2008; Chiti et al. 2021). Caval invasion has been described with both left- and right-sided adrenal masses (Kyles et al. 2003). The route of invasion into the vena cava is most commonly via the phrenicoabdominal vein (Kyles et al. 2003; Schultz et al. 2009), although direct caval wall invasion has been reported (Kyles et al. 2003; Lipscomb 2019). Vascular thrombi associated with adrenal tumors have been classified into three groups (Kyles et al. 2003): (1) phrenicoabdominal vein only; (2) involvement of the prehepatic vena cava with or without the phrenicoabdominal vein; and (3) involvement of the intrahepatic and/or posthepatic vena cava.

Prior to thrombectomy, the goal of tumoral dissection is usually to isolate the adrenal mass, so that it remains attached to the caudal vena cava only by a stalk (phrenicoabdominal vein with endoluminal thrombus). For left-sided tumors, after the adrenal mass is isolated, it can be passed underneath the mesentery so that the mass is on the same side as the vena cava. This facilitates exposure prior to venotomy (Knight et al. 2019).

For group 1 cases, the phrenicoabdominal vein is ligated as close as possible to the vena cava and removed en bloc with the mass (Figure 68.6) (Gilson et al. 1994a). For group 2 cases, Rumel tourniquets are placed on either side of the thrombus (Figure 68.7). For right-sided tumors, tourniquets may only be necessary around the vena cava, one cranial to the renal veins and one caudal

(a)

(b)

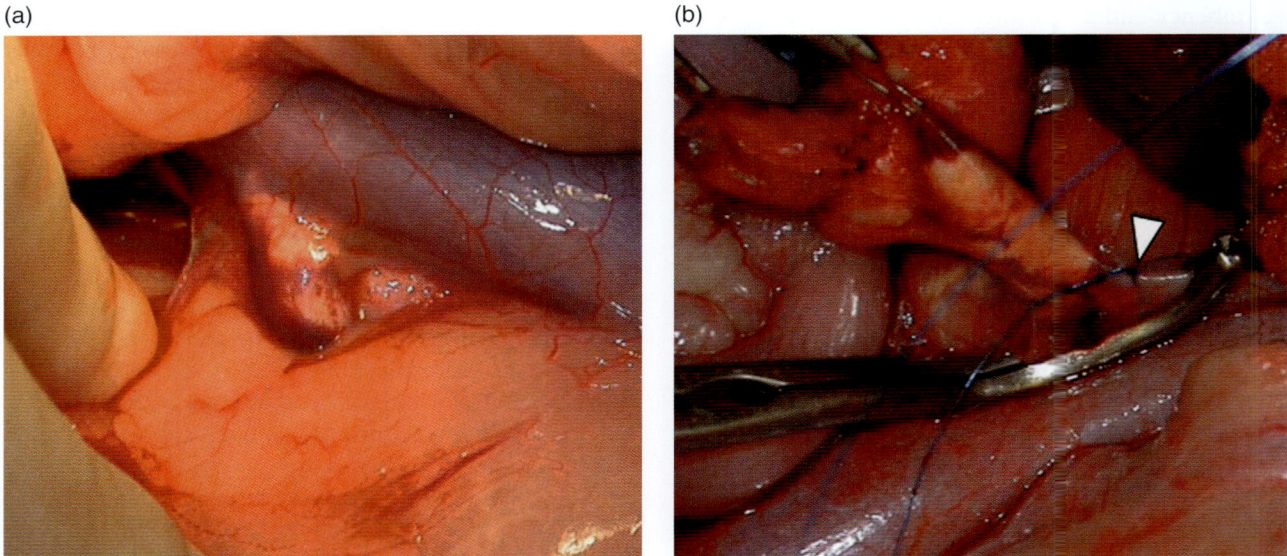

Figure 68.6 (a) Right-sided pheochromocytoma with invasion into the right phrenicoabdominal vein. (b) Satinsky forceps has been placed to isolate the planned venotomy site where the phrenicoabdominal vein enters the vena cava. Arrowhead indicates where 5-0 prolene suture has been preplaced at the cranial aspect of the anticipated venotomy site. The venotomy site is closed with a simple continuous closure.

(a)

(b)

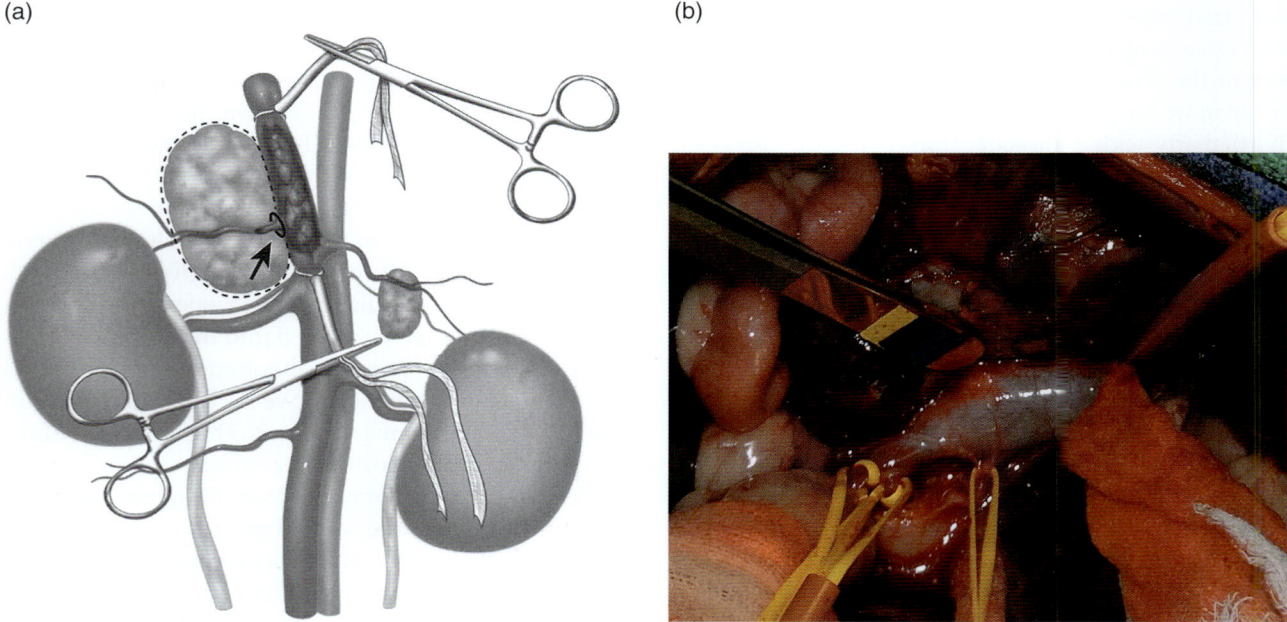

Figure 68.7 (a) Illustration from a ventral abdominal perspective depicting the placement of Rumel tourniquets for inflow occlusion and the dissection plane around the adrenal mass (dotted line) prior to venotomy for left-sided pheochromocytoma. © D. Giddings. (b) Tourniquets have been preplaced around the vena cava, both renal veins and the phrenicoabdominal vein from the contralateral side. Source: Courtesy of Dr. Eric Monnet.

to the liver. For left-sided tumors the anatomic location of the renal veins requires that individual Rumel tourniquets be placed on the vena cava (cranially and caudally) as well as the right and left renal veins. Alternatively, the caudal vena cava and the left renal vein may be occluded together with a single tourniquet. If the thrombus is small and can be included safely within a Satinsky forceps (Figures 68.8 and 68.9), the venotomy site may be isolated in like fashion, leaving the Rumel tourniquets loose during venotomy and repair of the caval defect.

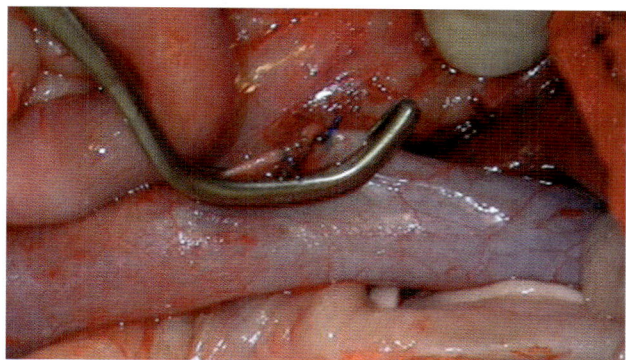

Figure 68.8 The tumor thrombus was included in the Satinsky clamp before opening the vena cava. The venotomy site was closed with a simple continuous closure.

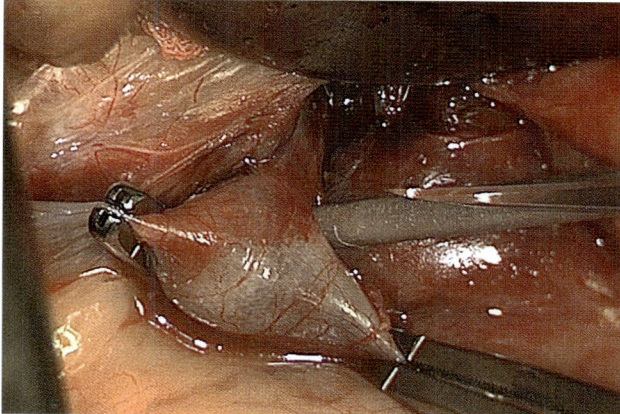

Figure 68.10 A Satinsky clamp has been placed and a no. 15 blade is used to start the venotomy. Source: Courtesy of Dr. Eric Monnet.

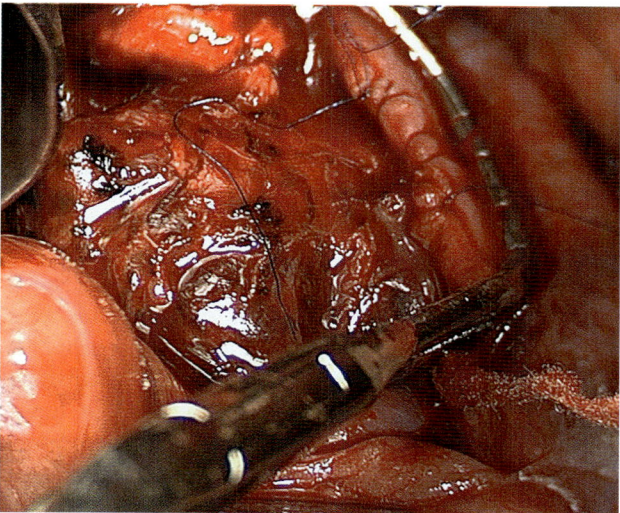

Figure 68.9 A Satinsky clamp has been placed instead of tourniquets for the removal of a tumor thrombus. Source: Courtesy of Dr. Eric Monnet.

Thus, in this scenario the Rumels are only in place in the event of bleeding complications associated with use of the Satinsky forceps.

For caval venotomy, stay sutures can be placed cranial and caudal to the planned venotomy. An incision is made with a no. 15 blade at the junction between the phrenicoabdominal vein and the caudal vena cava (Figure 68.10). The venotomy is extended 360° around the thrombus using fine scissors to separate the phrenicoabdominal vein from the caudal vena cava. The caval incision may need to be extended craniad to extract a large-diameter thrombus in one piece. However, care should be taken to minimize the size of the caval incision to allow for more rapid closure of the venotomy and to leave room for a prehepatic cranial tourniquet to be placed before the porta hepatis (Lipscomb 2019). The

thrombus is typically not adherent to the caval wall and is usually successfully extracted with gentle traction on the adrenal mass. This is performed with one hand, while the other hand or that of an assistant milks the thrombus out of the vena cava (Gilson *et al.* 1994a). The venotomy is closed using 5-0 or 6-0 polypropylene in a simple continuous pattern (Figure 68.9) and this closure is usually performed while the Rumel tourniquets are occluding blood flow. To speed up the suturing, the stay sutures previously placed in the vena cava can be pretied and used to suture the defect in the vein. The caudal tourniquet is released first to fill the vein, before tying the last knot to evacuate any air from the vein and thereby reduce the risk of air embolism (Gilson et al. 1994a). Alternatively, to minimize venous occlusion time, a Satinsky clamp can be placed over the venotomy site so that the tourniquet can be released sooner. The venotomy is then repaired as described over the clamp.

Safe prehepatic caval occlusion times have not been evaluated in dogs. In normal dogs, acute ligation of the prehepatic vena cava cranial to the phrenicoabdominal vein has been associated with a 50–80% mortality rate within 24 hours as a result of decreased venous return and shock (Nesbit & Wear 1961; Whittenberger & Huggins 1940). Similarly, safe renal vein occlusion times have not been clearly evaluated, but as little as 15 minutes of renal vein occlusion leads to tissue hypoxia and local acidosis protein degeneration in the tubular epithelial cells (Darewicz *et al.* 1976). At our institutions, we have arbitrarily limited occlusion time of both the caudal vena cava and the renal veins to 8 minutes in our clinical cases. However, caval occlusion times of up to 25 minutes have been reported in a dog that survived an adrenalectomy (Knight *et al.* 2019). Another less invasive option for adrenal tumors reported in dogs with a small

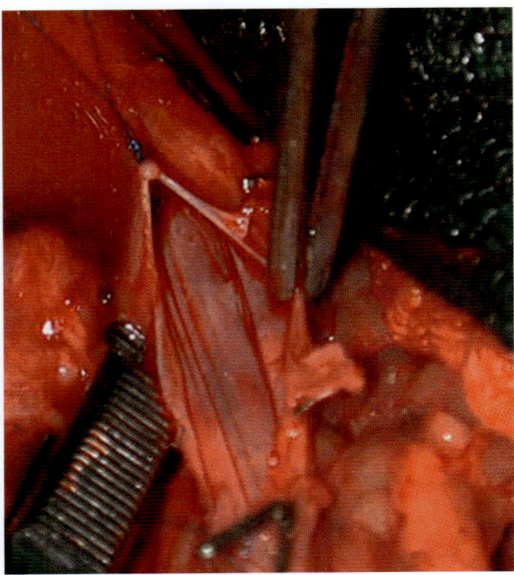

Figure 68.11 A long venotomy has been performed to remove a tumor thrombus extending cranial to the liver. Source: Courtesy of Dr. Eric Monnet.

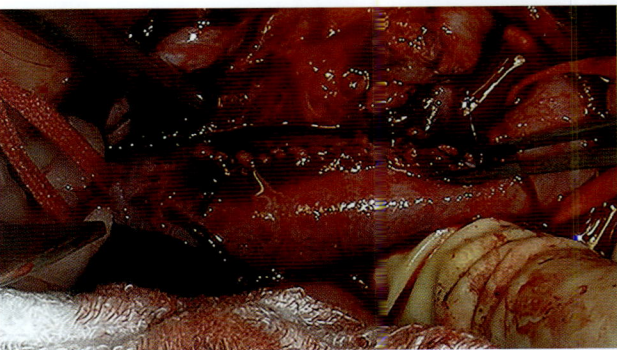

Figure 68.12 A long venotomy has been closed with a simple continuous suture pattern with 6-0 monofilament polypropylene. A simple continuous suture pattern was started at each end of the venotomy and met in the middle. The caudal tourniquet was realized before completing the closure of the venotomy to remove air in the vena cava. Source: Courtesy of Dr. Eric Monnet.

caval thrombus is phrenicoabdominal venotomy to retrieve the caval thrombus prior to phrenicoabdominal vein ligation (Mayhew *et al.* 2018).

Finally, for group 2 tumors there is *en bloc* excision of the adrenal mass with the portion of prehepatic vena cava that contains a thrombus (Louvet *et al.* 2005). There is experimental evidence, however, that progressive complete caval occlusion will be asymptomatic and result in the development of collateral vessels caudal to the occlusion (Peacock *et al.* 2003). Venograms and necropsy showed multiple collaterals extending from the renal capsular vessels, the vena cava, and the iliac veins to the lumbar, vertebral, and azygous veins (Peacock *et al.* 2003). The use of a caval gradual occlusion device has not been evaluated in dogs with adrenal tumors. In dogs with adrenal masses, caval occlusion is often partial and the reduction in caval blood flow as assessed subjectively is only mild to moderate, thus the capacity of the collateral circulation may not be sufficient to accommodate *en bloc* caval resection.

Massive tumor thrombi (group 3 tumors) can sometimes extend cranially into the hepatic or posthepatic vena cava (Figure 68.11). In such cases, placement of the Rumel tourniquet can either be done prehepatically and only partially tightened around the tumor thrombus that is removed (Kyles *et al.* 2003), or posthepatically beyond the cranial extent of the thrombus via extension of the abdominal incision into a caudal sternotomy (Gilson *et al.* 1994a; Lipscomb 2019). In the latter scenario, the surgeon must also be prepared to perform Pringle's

maneuver to reduce back-bleeding from the hepatic veins (Kirkali & Obek 2008; Lipscomb 2019). Because some tumor thrombi have a fragile stalk connection to the main portion of the mass, the latter approach may be a safer way to ensure complete thrombectomy and prevention of fragmentation and subsequent embolism of the thrombus. Though uncommon, partial occlusion of the vena cava around massive tumor thrombi prehepatically can result in dislodgment and fatal embolism of tumor thrombi fragments to the heart and/or lungs. With posthepatic vena cava occlusion, venous return will be significantly decreased and hypotension may ensue. In one study, 8 minutes of total posthepatic caval occlusion resulted in a 62% decrease in systolic blood pressure, but rapid hemodynamic recovery ensued after release of the occlusion (Hunt *et al.* 1992). The venotomy is closed with a simple continuous suture pattern with 5-0 or 6-0 polypropolene suture. The caudal tourniquet is released first to fill the vein, before tying the last knot to evacuate any air from the vein and thereby reduce the risk of air embolism (Figure 68.12).

Finally, renal venotomy has been reported in five dogs with left-sided adrenal tumors and renal vein tumor thrombosis (Chiti *et al.* 2021). This technique may avoid the need for nephrectomy in select cases of renal venal tumor thrombosis.

Histopathology results

Cortical tumors

When distant metastases, capsular invasion or vascular invasion is evident on imaging or at surgery, or when a certain threshold tumor size is reached adrenocortical tumors are classified as carcinomas (Labelle & De Cock 2005).

However, the fact that the tumor invades local vasculature has not been correlated with the risk of systemic metastasis. Histopathology is always required to differentiate adenomas from carcinomas; nevertheless, even with a tissue sample it may be difficult to have a definitive diagnosis. In one study, pathologists associated tumor size over 2 cm, microscopic capsular invasion, and a trabecular growth pattern with carcinomas (Labelle & De Cock 2005). Immunohistochemical staining for the proliferation marker Ki67 can also be used in difficult cases to differentiate adenomas from carcinomas (Labelle & De Cock 2005). There is no grading system available to correlate histopathology findings and risk of metastases for adrenal carcinomas.

Medullary tumors

Most pheochromocytomas are usually easily distinguished from adrenocortical tumors. However, there is some overlap and poorly differentiated pheochromocytomas can be mistaken for cortical tumors. In difficult cases, histochemistry using chromogranin A stain can be used, as pheochromocytomas usually stain positive for chromogranin A. Pheochromocytomas have also been differentiated into benign or malignant using the degree of pleomorphism, mitotic index, and presence of capsular and/or lymphatic invasion (Capen 2002). However, there are no clear-cut histopathologic criteria or grading system in place for pheochromocytoma. Thus, tumor behavior (large size, presence of metastasis, presence of a tumor thrombus, etc.) is often used to determine malignancy (Gilson *et al.* 1994b) (Figure 68.8).

Prognosis

A high perioperative mortality rate (as high as 60%) was initially reported for adrenal surgery (Scavelli *et al.* 1986); however, in that study many cases were euthanized at surgery because of suspected metastatic lesions that were not confirmed histologically (Scavelli *et al.* 1986). In one study in dogs with adrenal tumors, the incidence of macroscopic lesions involving other organs was high (53%), but histologic confirmation of metastases in those dogs was very low (9%) (Barthez *et al.* 1997). Consequently, euthanasia is not recommended based on identification of gross lesions alone at the time of surgery. A recent study of dogs with adrenal tumors without vascular invasion and less then 3 cm in diameter had a perioperative mortality rate of 3% in 33 dogs undergoing open adrenalectomy (Cavalcanti *et al.* 2020). This suggests that early detection and surgical treatment may further decrease operative mortality. More recent studies showed a perioperative mortality of approximately 20% and that the presence of a tumor

thrombus did not seem to affect survival (Kyles *et al.* 2003; Schwartz *et al.* 2008).

For pheochromocytomas, the use of phenoxybenzamine preoperatively has reduced mortality from 48% to 13% (Herrera *et al.* 2008). Further reduction in perioperative mortality is likely possible if CT is used routinely for surgical planning, Rumel tourniquets are placed around the major vessels early in the course of dissection, blood products are readily available, and all physiologic parameters are adequately monitored and controlled. Histologically, confirmed metastases have been reported in 14% of surgical cases of adrenocortical tumors (Anderson *et al.* 2001; Kyles *et al.* 2003). Reported sites of metastases include lungs, peritoneum, liver, kidney, ovary, and mesenteric lymph node (Anderson *et al.* 2001; Labelle & De Cock 2005). Histologically confirmed metastases have been reported in 36% of cases in a study that included both surgical and necropsy cases (Gilson *et al.* 1994b). Sites of metastases for pheochromocytoma include local lymph nodes, liver, spleen, kidney, lungs, bone, peritoneum, heart, pancreas, spinal canal, and jejunum (Barthez *et al.* 1997; Gilson *et al.* 1994b).

In recent studies, mean survival time is approximately two years after adrenalectomy for a cortical or a medullary tumor, suggesting that animals that survive through the perioperative period typically achieve long-term survival (Anderson *et al.* 2001; Schwartz *et al.* 2008). This in turn would suggest either a low frequency or a slow growth of metastases in animals with adrenal tumors. There are reports of long-term survival (up to 30 months) without clinical signs after visceral metastases from an adrenal carcinoma were identified at surgery (Kyles *et al.* 2003; Barthez *et al.* 1997). Follow-up ultrasonography and thoracic radiographs are recommended every three months after successful resection of an adrenal malignancy.

References

Acierno, M.J., Brown, S., Coleman, A.E. et al. (2018). ACVIM consensus statement: guidelines for the identification, evaluation, and management of systemic hypertension in dogs and cats. *Journal of Veterinary Internal Medicine* 32: 1803–1822.

Anderson, C.R., Birchard, S.J., Powers, B.E. et al. (2001). Surgical treatment of adrenocortical tumors: 21 cases (1990–1996). *Journal of the American Animal Hospital Association* 37: 93–97.

Ash, R.A., Harvey, A.M., and Tasker, S. (2005). Primary hyperaldosteronism in the cat: a series of 13 cases. *Journal of Feline Medicine and Surgery* 7: 173–182.

Barrera, J.S., Bernard, F., Ehrhart, E. et al. (2013). Evaluation of risk factors for outcome associated with adrenal gland tumors with or without invasion of the caudal vena cava and treated via adrenalectomy in dogs: 86 cases (1993–2009). *Journal of the American Veterinary Medical Association* 242: 1715–1721.

Barthez, P.Y., Marks, S.L., Woo, J. et al. (1997). Pheochromocytoma in dogs: 61 cases (1984–1995). *Journal of Veterinary Internal Medicine* 11: 272–278.

Behrend, E.N., Kemppainen, R.J., Boozer, A.L. et al. (2005a). Serum 17-alpha-hydroxyprogesterone and corticosterone concentrations in dogs with nonadrenal neoplasia and dogs with suspected hyperadrenocorticism. *Journal of the American Veterinary Medical Association* 227: 1762–1767.

Behrend, E.N., Weigand, C.M., Whitley, E.M. et al. (2005b). Corticosterone- and aldosterone-secreting adrenocortical tumor in a dog. *Journal of the American Veterinary Medical Association* 226: 1662–1666.

Bezuidenhout, A.J. (2013). Veins. In: *Miller's Anatomy of the Dog* (ed. H.E. Evans and A. De Lahunta), 682–716. St. Louis, MO: Elsevier Saunders.

Bouayad, H., Feeney, D.A., Caywood, D.D., and Hayden, D.W. (1987). Pheochromocytoma in dogs: 13 cases (1980–1985). *Journal of the American Veterinary Medical Association* 191: 1610–1615.

Capen, C.C. (2002). Tumor of the endocrine glands. In: *Tumors in Domestic Animals*, 4e (ed. D.J. Meuten), 607–696. Ames, IA: Blackwell.

Cavalcanti, J.V.J., Skinner, O.T., Mayhew, P.D. et al. (2020). Outcome in dogs undergoing adrenalectomy for small adrenal gland tumours without vascular invasion. *Veterinary and Comparative Oncology* 18: 599–606.

Chiti, L.E., Mayhew, P.D., and Massari, F. (2021). Renal venotomy for thrombectomy and kidney preservation in dogs with adrenal tumors and renal vein invasion. *Veterinary Surgery* 50: 872–879.

Darewicz, J., Cylwik, B., and Gruszecki, W. (1976). Effects of clamping the renal vein in dogs on certain biochemical and histopathological changes. *International Urology and Nephrology* 8: 271–276.

Declue, A.E., Breshears, L.A., Pardo, I.D. et al. (2005). Hyperaldosteronism and hyperprogesteronism in a cat with an adrenal cortical carcinoma. *Journal of Veterinary Internal Medicine* 19: 355–358.

Dibartola, S.P. and Demorais, G.A. (2006). Disorders of potassium: hypokalemia and hyperkalemia. In: *Fluid, Electrolyte and Acid-Base Disorders in Small Animal Practice* (ed. S.P. Dibartola), 91–121. St. Louis, MO: Saunders Elsevier.

Evans, K., Hosgood, G., Boon, G.D., and Kowalewich, N. (1991). Hemoperitoneum secondary to traumatic rupture of an adrenal tumor in a dog. *Journal of the American Veterinary Medical Association* 198: 278–280.

Feldman, E.C. (1981). Effect of functional adrenocortical tumors on plasma cortisol and corticotropin concentrations in dogs. *Journal of the American Veterinary Medical Association* 178: 823–826.

Feldman, E.C. (1983). Distinguishing dogs with functioning adrenocortical tumors from dogs with pituitary-dependent hyperadrenocorticism. *Journal of the American Veterinary Medical Association* 183: 195–200.

Feldman, E.C. and Nelson, R.W. (2004). The adrenal gland. In: *Canine and Feline Endocrinology and Reproduction*, 251–484. St. Louis, MO: Saunders Elsevier.

Flood, S.M., Randolph, J.F., Gelzer, A.R., and Refsal, K. (1999). Primary hyperaldosteronism in two cats. *Journal of the American Animal Hospital Association* 35: 411–416.

Galac, S., Rosenberg, D., and Pey, P. (2019). Cushing's syndrome (hypercortisolism). In: *Feline Endocrinology* (ed. E. Feldman, F. Fracassi and M. Peterson), 452–484. Milan: Edra.

Gilson, S.D., Withrow, S.J., and Orton, E.C. (1994a). Surgical treatment of pheochromocytoma: technique, complications, and results in six dogs. *Veterinary Surgery* 23: 195–200.

Gilson, S.D., Withrow, S.J., Wheeler, S.L., and Twedt, D.C. (1994b). Pheochromocytoma in 50 dogs. *Journal of Veterinary Internal Medicine* 8: 228–232.

Gostelow, R., Bridger, N., and Syme, H.M. (2013). Plasma-free metanephrine and free normetanephrine measurement for the diagnosis of pheochromocytoma in dogs. *Journal of Veterinary Internal Medicine* 27: 83–90.

Grumbach, M.M., Biller, B.M., Braunstein, G.D. et al. (2003). Management of the clinically inapparent adrenal mass ("incidentaloma"). *Annals of Internal Medicine* 138: 424–429.

Harder, M.A., Fowler, D., Pharr, J.W. et al. (2002). Segmental aplasia of the caudal vena cava in a dog. *Canadian Veterinary Journal* 43: 365–368.

Henry, C.J., Brewer, W.G. Jr., Montgomery R.D. et al. (1993). Clinical vignette. Adrenal pheochromocytoma. *Journal of Veterinary Internal Medicine* 7: 199–201.

Herrera, M.A., Mehl, M.L., Kass, P.H. et al. (2008). Predictive factors and the effect of phenoxybenzamine on outcome in dogs undergoing adrenalectomy for pheochromocytoma. *Journal of Veterinary Internal Medicine* 22: 1333–1339.

Hoerauf, A. and Reusch, C. (1999). Ultrasonographic characteristics of both adrenal glands in 15 dogs with functional adrenocortical tumors. *Journal of the American Animal Hospital Association* 35: 193–199.

Hullinger, R.L. (1993). The endocrine system. In: *Miller's Anatomy of the Dog*, 4e (ed. H.E. Evans and A. De Lahunta), 559–585. St. Louis, MO: Elsevier Saunders.

Hunt, G.B., Malik, R., Bellenger, C.R., and Pearson, M.R. (1992). A new technique for surgery of the caudal vena cava in dogs using partial venous inflow occlusion. *Research in Veterinary Science* 52: 378–381.

Hunter, T.B., Dye, J., and Duval, J.F. (1994). Selective use of low-osmolality contrast agents for i.v. urography and CT: safety and effect on cost. *American Journal of Roentgenology* 163: 965–968.

Javadi, S., Djajadiningrat-Laanen, S.C., Kooistra, H.S. et al. (2005). Primary hyperaldosteronism, a mediator of progressive renal disease in cats. *Domestic Animal Endocrinology* 28: 85–104.

Javadi, S., Galac, S., Boer, P. et al. (2006). Aldosterone-to renin cortisol-to-adrencorticotropic hormone ratios in healthy dogs and dogs with primary hypoadrenocorticism. *Journal of Veterinary Internal Medicine* 20: 556–561.

Jimenez Pelaez, M., Bouvy, B.M., and Dupre, G.P. (2008). Laparoscopic adrenalectomy for treatment of unilateral adrenocortical carcinomas: technique, complications, and results in seven dogs. *Veterinary Surgery* 37: 444–453.

Johnston, E.J. (1977). Adrenalectomy via retroperitoneal approach in dogs. *Journal of the American Veterinary Medical Association* 170: 1092–1095.

Kintzer, P.P. and Peterson, M.E. (1994). Mitotane treatment of 32 dogs with cortisol-secreting adrenocortical neoplasms. *Journal of the American Veterinary Medical Association* 205: 54–61.

Kirkali, Z. and Obek, C. (2008). Advanced tumors: tumor thrombus. In: *Renal Cell Cancer. Diagnosis and Therapy* (ed. J. De La Rosette, C.N. Sternberg and H. Van Poppel), 250–264. London: Springer.

Knight, R.C., Lamb, C.R., Brockman, D.J. and Lipscomb, V.J. (2019). Variations in surgical technique for adrenalectomy with caudal vena cava venotomy in 19 dogs. *Veterinary Surgery* 48: 751–759.

Kooistra, H.A. (2006). Hyperaldosteronism in cats. In: *World Small Animal Veterinary Association World Congress, 2006*, 318–319. https://www.vin.com/apputil/content/defaultadv1.aspx?id=3859002&pid=11223&.

Kook, P.H., Boretti, F.S., Hersberger, M. et al. (2007). Urinary catecholamine and metanephrine to creatinine ratios in healthy dogs at home and in a hospital environment and in 2 dogs with pheochromocytoma. *Journal of Veterinary Internal Medicine* 21: 388–393.

Krawiec, D.R., Twardock, A.R., Badertscher, R.R. 2nd et al. (1988). Use of 99mTc diethylenetriaminepentaacetic acid for assessment of renal function in dogs with suspected renal disease. *Journal of the American Veterinary Medical Association* 192: 1077–1080.

Kyles, A.E., Feldman, E.C., De Cock, H.E. et al. (2003). Surgical management of adrenal gland tumors with and without associated tumor thrombi in dogs: 40 cases (1994–2001). *Journal of the American Veterinary Medical Association* 223: 654–662.

Labelle, P. and De Cock, H.E. (2005). Metastatic tumors to the adrenal glands in domestic animals. *Veterinary Pathology* 42: 52–58.

Lipscomb, V.J. (2019). Surgical management of an adrenal gland tumor that had extended into the thoracic portion of the caudal vena cava in a dog. *Journal of the American Veterinary Medical Association* 254: 1309–1315.

Llabres-Diaz, F.J. and Dennis, R. (2003). Magnetic resonance imaging of the presumed normal canine adrenal glands. *Veterinary Radiology & Ultrasound* 44: 5–19.

Louvet, A., Lazard, P., and Denis, B. (2005). Phaeochromocytoma treated by en bloc resection including the suprarenal caudal vena cava in a dog. *Journal of Small Animal Practice* 46: 591–596.

Lunn, K.F. and Page, R.L. (2013). Tumors of the endocrine system. In: *Small Animal Clinical Oncology*, 4e (ed. S.J. Withrow and D.M. Vail), 504–531. St. Louis, MO: Saunders-Elsevier.

Luton, J.P., Cerdas, S., Billaud, L. et al. (1990). Clinical features of adrenocortical carcinoma, prognostic factors, and the effect of mitotane therapy. *New England Journal of Medicine* 322: 1195–1201.

Mayhew, P.D., Culp, W.T., Hunt, G.B. et al. (2014). Comparison of perioperative morbidity and mortality rates in dogs with noninvasive adrenocortical masses undergoing laparoscopic versus open adrenalectomy. *Journal of the American Veterinary Medical Association* 245: 1028–1035.

Mayhew, P.D., Culp, W.T.N., Balsa, I.M., and Zwingenberger, A.L. (2018). Phrenicoabdominal venotomy for tumor thrombectomy in dogs with adrenal neoplasia and suspected vena caval invasion. *Veterinary Surgery* 47: 227–235.

Millard, R.P., Pickens, E.H., and Wells, K.L. (2009). Excessive production of sex hormones in a cat with an adrenocortical tumor. *Journal of the American Veterinary Medical Association* 234: 505–508.

Moore, L.E., Biller, D.S., and Smith, T.A. (2000). Use of abdominal ultrasonography in the diagnosis of primary hyperaldosteronism in a cat. *Journal of the American Veterinary Medical Association* 217: 213–215.

Myers, N.C. (1997). Adrenal incidentalomas. Diagnostic workup of the incidentally discovered adrenal mass. *Veterinary Clinics of North America. Small Animal Practice* 27: 381–399.

Naan, E.C., Kirpensteijn, J., Dupre, G.P. et al. (2013). Innovative approach to laparoscopic adrenalectomy for treatment of unilateral adrenal gland tumors in dogs. *Veterinary Surgery* 42: 710–715.

Nesbit, R.M. and Wear, J.B. (1961). Ligation of inferior vena cava above renal veins. *Annals of Surgery* 154 (Supplement): 332–344.

Norman, E.J., Thompson, H., and Mooney, C.T. (1999). Dynamic adrenal function testing in eight dogs with hyperadrenocorticism associated with adrenocortical neoplasia. *Veterinary Record* 144: 551–554.

Oblak, M.L., Bacon, N.J., and Covey, J.L. (2016). Perioperative management and outcome of bilateral adrenalectomy in 9 dogs. *Veterinary Surgery* 45: 790–797.

Patnaik, A.K., Erlandson, R.A., Lieberman, P.H. et al. (1990). Extra-adrenal pheochromocytoma (paraganglioma) in a cat. *Journal of the American Veterinary Medical Association* 197: 104–106.

Peacock, J.T., Fossum, T.W., Bahr, A.M. et al. (2003). Evaluation of gradual occlusion of the caudal vena cava in clinically normal dogs. *American Journal of Veterinary Research* 64: 1347–1353.

Penninck, D.G., Feldman, E.C., and Nyland, T.G. (1988). Radiographic features of canine hyperadrenocorticism caused by autonomously functioning adrenocortical tumors: 23 cases (1978–1986). *Journal of the American Veterinary Medical Association* 192: 1604–1608.

Pineiro, M.I., Benchekroun, G., De Fornel-Thibaud, P., and Maurey-Guenec, C. (2009). Accuracy of an adrenocorticotrophic hormone (ACTH) immunoluminometric assay for differentiating ACTH-dependent from ACTH-independent hyperadrenocorticism in dogs. *Journal of Veterinary Internal Medicine* 23: 850–855.

Pitt, K.A., Mayhew, P.D., Steffey, M.A. et al. (2016). Laparoscopic adrenalectomy for removal of unilateral noninvasive pheochromocytomas in 10 dogs. *Veterinary Surgery* 45: O70–O76.

Platt, S.R., Sheppard, B.J., Graham, J. et al. (1998). Pheochromocytoma in the vertebral canal of two dogs. *Journal of the American Animal Hospital Association* 34: 365–371.

Quante, S., Boretti, F.S., Kook, P.H. et al. (2010). Urinary catecholamine and metanephrine to creatinine ratios in dogs with hyperadrenocorticism or pheochromocytoma, and in healthy dogs. *Journal of Veterinary Internal Medicine* 24: 1093–1097.

Quayle, F.J., Spitler, J.A., Pierce, R.A. et al. (2007). Needle biopsy of incidentally discovered adrenal masses is rarely informative and potentially hazardous. *Surgery* 142: 497–502.

Reine, N.J., Hohenhaus, A.E., Peterson, M.E., and Patnaik, A.K. (1999). Deoxycorticosterone-secreting adrenocortical carcinoma in a dog. *Journal of Veterinary Internal Medicine* 13: 386–390.

Reusch, C.E. and Feldman, E.C. (1991). Canine hyperadrenocorticism due to adrenocortical neoplasia. Pretreatment evaluation of 41 dogs. *Journal of Veterinary Internal Medicine* 5: 3–10.

Rosenstein, D.S. (2000). Diagnostic imaging in canine pheochromocytoma. *Veterinary Radiology & Ultrasound* 41: 499–506.

Scavelli, T.D., Peterson, M.E., and Matthiesen, D.T. (1986). Results of surgical treatment for hyperadrenocorticism caused by adrenocortical neoplasia in the dog: 25 cases (1980-1984). *Journal of the American Veterinary Medical Association* 189: 1360–1364.

Schultz, R.M., Wisner, E.R., Johnson, E.G., and Macleod, J.S. (2009). Contrast-enhanced computed tomography as a preoperative indicator of vascular invasion from adrenal masses in dogs. *Veterinary Radiology & Ultrasound* 50: 625–629.

Schwartz, P., Kovak, J.R., Koprowski, A. et al. (2008). Evaluation of prognostic factors in the surgical treatment of adrenal gland tumors in dogs: 41 cases (1999-2005). *Journal of the American Veterinary Medical Association* 232: 77–84.

Shiel, R. and Mooney, C.T. (2007). Diagnosis and management of primary hyperaldosteronism in cats. *In Practice* 29: 194–201.

Syme, H.M., Scott-Moncrieff, J.C., Treadwell, N.G. et al. (2001). Hyperadrenocorticism associated with excessive sex hormone production by an adrenocortical tumor in two dogs. *Journal of the American Veterinary Medical Association* 219: 1725–1728.

Van Sluijs, F.J., Sjollema, B.E., Voorhout, G. et al. (1995). Results of adrenalectomy in 36 dogs with hyperadrenocorticism caused by adreno-cortical tumour. *Veterinary Quarterly* 17: 113–116.

Von Dehn, B.J., Nelson, R.W., Feldman, E.C., and Griffey, S.M. (1995). Pheochromocytoma and hyperadrenocorticism in dogs: six cases (1982–1992). *Journal of the American Veterinary Medical Association* 207: 322–324.

Whittenberger, J.L. and Huggins, C. (1940). Ligation of the inferior vena cava. *Archives of Surgery* 41: 133–1343.

Young, W.F. Jr. (2007). Clinical practice. The incidentally discovered adrenal mass. *New England Journal of Medicine* 356: 601–610.

Section 10

Ear Surgery

69

Anatomy of the Ear

Jamie R. Bellah

In dogs and cats, the ears provide structure and receptors that support the functions of hearing and balance. The temporal bone houses most of the vestibulocochlear organ, which is composed of three parts that are anatomically and functionally distinct: the external ear, the middle ear, and the internal ear.

Pinna

The anatomy of the ear is quite similar in general for all dog breeds, but the appearance and shape of the pinna vary, providing the unique appearance characteristic to many breeds. In dogs, the pinna is erect or pendulous to varying degrees. The appearance of feline ears is also quite similar, with less variation in the shape of the pinna. Noted exceptions are the Scottish Fold breed, which has a rostroventral directed fold at the distal aspect of the auricle (Hudson & Hamilton 1993), and the American Curl breed, which has pinnal apices that curl back (Njaa *et al.* 2012). A small, thin pouch is present at the caudolateral margin and is termed the cutaneous marginal pouch, a structure that has no known function (Kumar 2005). The purpose of the pinna is to collect and localize sound waves for transmission to the tympanum and its mobility allows localization of the sound source (Evans 1993a; Njaa *et al.* 2012).

The auricular cartilage forms the major portion of the ear structural support and has two sections (Figure 69.1). The scapha is the flat cartilage that supports the major portion of the pinna, and the concha is the tubular-shaped cartilage that forms the vertical and horizontal ear canals. The most distal aspect of the scapha is the apex and the helix comprises the medial and lateral borders of the scapha. The prominent antihelix is a transversely oriented fold that is located at the concave base of the auricular cartilage and separates the distal pinna from the vertical ear canal, which continues proximally and becomes the distal portion of the horizontal ear canal. Vessels and nerves coursing along the outer concave surface penetrate the cartilage of the pinna toward the inner convex surface through multiple small perforations. Ridges on the inner surface of the concha are formed by folds in the cartilage where intrinsic auricular muscles are attached (Hudson & Hamilton 1993). The most proximal portion of the auricular cartilage overlaps the annular cartilage (a ring or cylinder of cartilage that supports most of the length of the horizontal ear canal). The annular cartilage overlaps the external acoustic meatus, which is the osseous extension of the skull and the lateral aspect of the tympanic cavity. Fibrous tissue connections occur between these intersecting segments of the ear canal. These junctions provide some flexibility to the canal, but also provide regions predisposed to canal rupture or drainage in traumatic events and when para-auricular abscessation occurs (Tobias & Morris 2005).

The pinna has a broad margin that is covered by tightly adhered skin on its concave surface and a lesser, more mobile skin on the convex surface (Heine 2004). Hair follicles are much more numerous on the convex surface of the pinna. Both sides contain apocrine sweat glands and sebaceous glands (Njaa *et al.* 2012). Some breeds (i.e., poodles and cocker spaniels) may have more hair within the ear canal (hirsute).

Small Animal Soft Tissue Surgery, Second Edition. Edited by Eric Monnet.
© 2023 John Wiley & Sons, Inc. Published 2023 by John Wiley & Sons, Inc.
Companion website: www.wiley.com/go/monnet/small

The external ear has both extrinsic and intrinsic auricular muscles that connect ear canal cartilages to the head or that provide interconnections as already described. Numerous auricular muscles attach to the pinna at rostroauricular and caudoauricular locations and in one ventroauricular location (Heine 2004). The scutiform cartilage is L-shaped and directly adjacent to the auricular cartilage rostromedially, and since rostral auricular muscles are attached to it is still considered a portion of the external ear (Bacon 2012). The scutiform cartilage is sometimes excised (partially or completely) in resection or ablative procedures.

External ear canal

The opening of the external ear canal is dorsolateral in location (Figure 69.1). It is bordered by the tragus cartilage laterally and the antihelix (a transverse ridge) medially. The antitragus is a cartilage structure (with lateral and medial processes) and is separated from the tragus by the intertragic incisure. The intertragic incisure is the landmark for guidance of an otoscope or otoendoscope to examine the ear canal (Njaa *et al.* 2012). The tragohelicine incisure (pretragic incisure) is located at the rostral aspect of the tragus and separates the tragus from the lateral crus of the helix. The medial crus of the helix is located ventral and rostral to the tragohelicine incisure. These incisures are the surgical landmarks for the vertical ear canal incisions during lateral ear resection. As the

proximal portion of the auricular cartilage becomes funnel shaped it forms the vertical ear canal, and then deviates medially to become the horizontal ear canal. A ridge of cartilage, dorsal and medial within the canal, is an anatomic demarcation of the vertical and horizontal ear canals. Elevating this ridge by upward traction on the pinna facilitates examination of the horizontal canal (Njaa *et al.* 2012; Radlinsky 2016). The annular cartilage, a separate band of cartilage, fits within the conchal tube and has fibrous attachments to the osseous external meatus (Njaa *et al.* 2012). The horizontal ear canal extends to the external acoustic meatus (Figure 69.2). The terminal portion of the horizontal canal is therefore surrounded by bone where it is not pliable and cannot be dilated during otoscopy (Radlinsky 2016). The zygomatic arch of the temporal bone is a close neighbor to the dorsorostral margin of the external acoustic meatus (Njaa *et al.* 2012). This zygomatic bony structure varies between dog breeds, resulting in a deeper location of the acoustic meatus in breeds such as pit bulls and other broad-headed breeds. The depth and more acute access angles may interfere with scope insertion for myringotomy procedures (Njaa *et al.* 2012). The dorsal aspect of the parotid salivary gland lies over the lateral wall of the vertical ear canal.

Hair is present in the external ear canal in most dogs and the concentration of follicles decreases from distal to proximal locations. Most hair follicles are simple; however, the cocker spaniel breed is characterized by

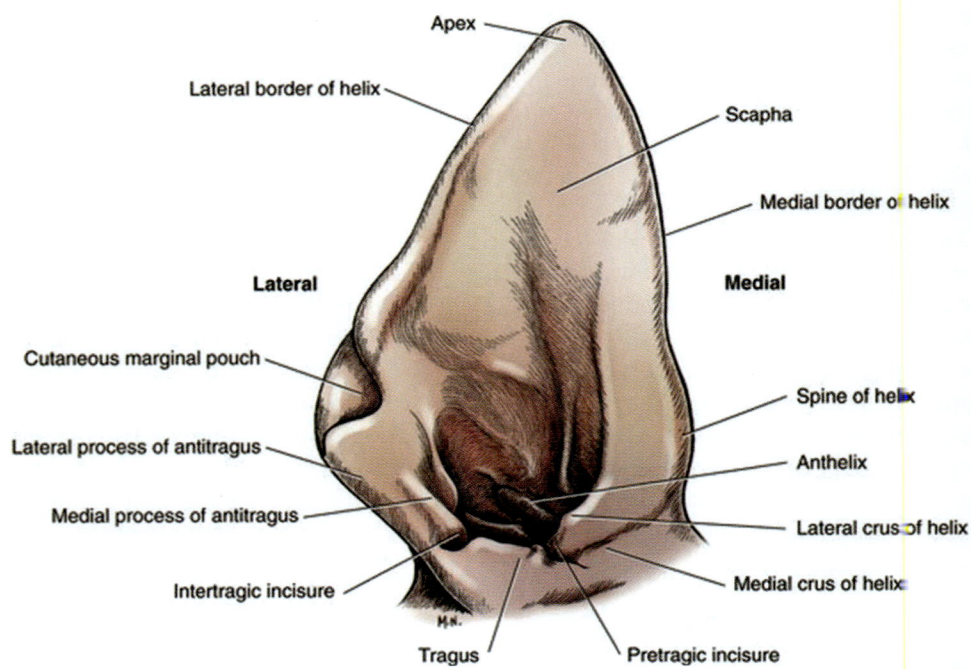

Figure 69.1 Right external ear of the dog. L, lateral; M, medial. Source: Cole LK (2009) / with permission of The Ohio State University.

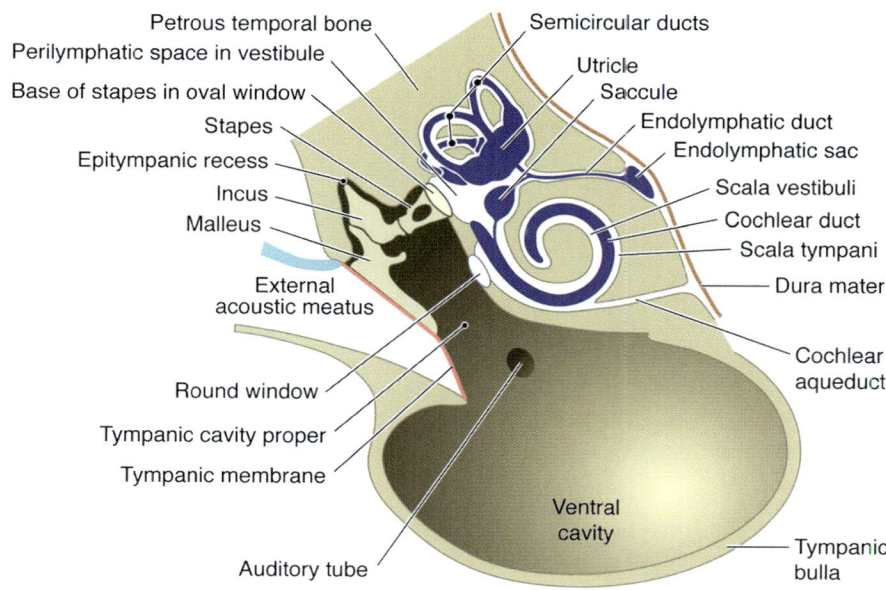

Figure 69.2 Schematic drawing of the inner ear, middle ear, and external acoustic meatus of the dog. Source: Cole LK (2009) / with permission of The Ohio State University.

excessive numbers of compound hair follicles (Stout-Graham *et al*. 1990). The histology of the ear canal, including the presence of sebaceous and apocrine tubular glands, and the self-cleaning function of the external ear, where stratum corneum keratinocytes transport from the tympanic membrane toward the external auditory canal in a radial direction (a process called epithelial migration), have been well described (Cole 2009; Njaa *et al*. 2012). The sebaceous glands are more superficial, whereas the ceruminous glands are located deeper in the dermis. Ceruminous glands (modified apocrine glands) are more concentrated in the proximal portions of the ear canal, with ducts opening into hair follicles or directly to the canal surface. Cerumen is composed of secretions from sebaceous and ceruminous glands and desquamated keratinized squamous epithelial cells, and forms an emulsion that coats the ear canal (Njaa *et al*. 2012). Long-haired breeds tend to have more glandular tissue than short-haired breeds (Cole 2009). The pH of ear canal epithelium in normal dogs is 4.6–7.2. Cerumen from ears with otitis externa has a greater concentration of cerumen gland constituents, creating a more acidic medium that may be less supportive of bacterial growth. Dogs with acute and chronic otitis externa have a pH ranging from 5.2 to 7.2 and 6.0 to 7.4, respectively (Cole 2009). The dermal layer of the external ear canal, made up of collagen and elastic fibers, is separated from the cartilaginous layer by subcutaneous tissue (Njaa *et al*. 2012). The tympanic membrane is the medial termination of the external ear canal. The normal

Table 69.1 Most common flora of the external ear canal in the dog.

Normal flora	Flora in otitis externa
Staphylococcus	*Staphylococcus (pseudo)intermedius*
Bacillus sp.	*Pseudomonas aeruginosa*
Escherichia coli	*Proteus* sp.
Corynebacterium sp.	*Beta-streptococcus*
Streptococci	*Corynebacterium* sp.
Micrococcus sp.	*Enterococcus* sp.
Pseudomonas sp. (rare)	*Escherichia coli*
Proteus sp. (rare)	Yeast (common)
Yeast	

Source: Adapted from Cole 2009.

bacterial flora of the external ear canal of the dog and bacteria commonly found in otitis externa are listed in Table 69.1.

Middle ear

The tympanic cavity is an air-filled structure that contains three auditory ossicles and associated muscles and ligaments. The tympanic membrane is the lateral boundary of the middle ear (Figures 69.2 and 69.3). The tympanum is positioned at a 45° angle to the axis of the horizontal ear canal (Figures 69.4 and 69.5).

The outer surface of the tympanum is stratified squamous epithelium (derived from ectoderm of the

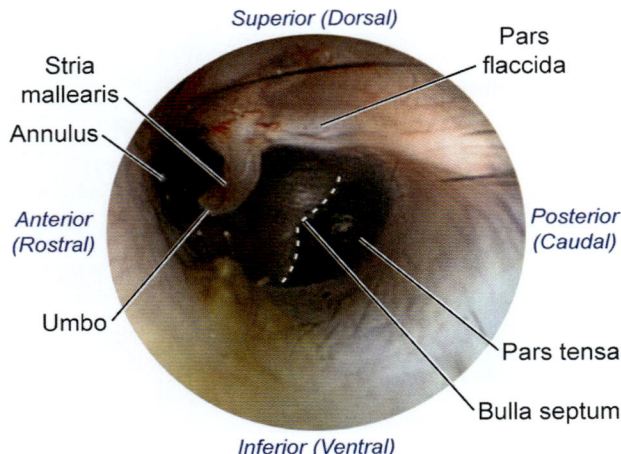

Figure 69.3 Left tympanic membrane of the dog. Source: Cole LK (2009) / with permission of The Ohio State University.

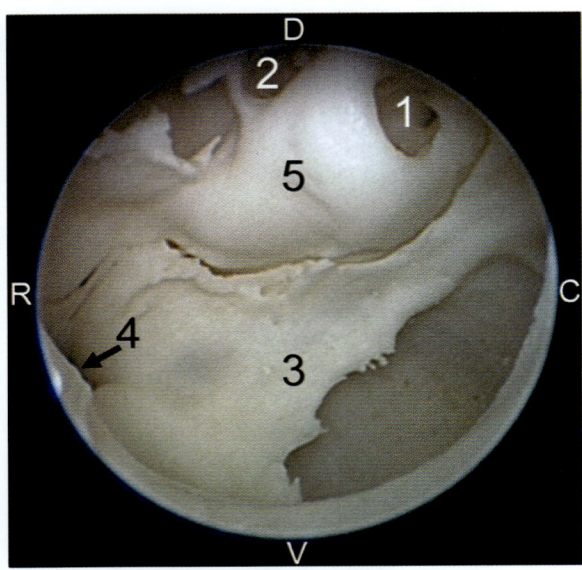

Figure 69.4 View of the left middle ear of a dog skeleton, with the tympanic membrane removed. 1, cochlear (round) window; 2, vestibular (oval) window; 3, bulla septum; 4, Eustachian tube; 5, promontory; C, caudal; D, dorsal; R, rostral; V = ventral. Source: Cole LK (2009) / with permission of The Ohio State University.

first pharyngeal groove) and continuous with the external ear canal. The central layer of the tympanum is fibrous connective tissue that is from the pharyngeal wall. The inner epithelial layer originates from the pharyngeal pouch (Evans 1993b). The tympanic membrane (which appears concave otoscopically) is divided into two sections: the upper and flatter pars flaccida and the lower, thinner, and larger pars tensa. The two sections are similar histologically (Njaa et al. 2012). A bulging pars flaccida indicates a primary secretory

otitis media where mucous fills the middle ear cavity, presumably secondary to auditory tube dysfunction in King Charles spaniels (Stern-Bertholtz et al. 2003). The manubrium of the malleus attaches to the medial surface of the pars tensa and its outline seen externally is called the stria mallearis. The stria mallearis is hook or C shaped in the dog, and straight in the cat (Njaa et al. 2012). The umbo is the point where the tympanum appears most depressed and is located opposite the distal aspect of the manubrium. Although not confirmed in dogs, the umbo is believed to be the germination center of the eardrum in humans (Tinling & Chole 2006; Cole 2009).

In dogs, the tympanic membrane regenerates by day 14, with complete healing in 3–5 weeks (Njaa et al. 2012; Steiss et al. 1992). The tympanic cavity is an air-filled structure that has three regions: the epitympanic recess, the tympanic cavity proper, and the ventral cavity. In metacephalic dogs the middle ear cavity volume has been determined to be 1.5 mL, increasing in nonlinear fashion by body weight (Defalque et al. 2005). The head of the malleus and the incus occupy most of the epitympanic recess, while the tympanic cavity proper is next to the tympanum. The malleus, incus and stapes (acting as a piston) transmit and amplify pressure wave–induced air vibrations from the tympanum to produce fluid pressure waves within inner ear structures (Njaa et al. 2012). The ability to detect sound is explained by the "lever ratio," a ratio between the length of the manubrium of the malleus and the long process of the incus. The greater the lever ratio, the grater the ability to hear faint audible sounds (Hudson & Hamilton 1993). Muscles that originate in the tympanic bulla and attach to the auditory ossicles, the tensor tympani muscle that inserts on the malleus and the larger stapedius muscle that inserts on the stapes, protect the middle ear from loud, repetitive noise by contracting (Sims 1988). The chorda tympani, a small branch of the facial nerve, passes beneath the base of the muscular process of the malleolus. This location is medial and close to the pars flaccida. The chorda tympani exits the middle ear and merges with the lingual band of the mandibular nerve. The nerve can be damaged in this location, resulting in impairment of taste (Njaa et al. 2012).

The ventral cavity is the largest region of the tympanic bulla. In dogs the ventral cavity is one chamber, but in cats the tympanic bulla is divided into dorsolateral and ventromedial compartments by an incomplete bony septum (Hudson & Hamilton 1993). At the caudodorsal aspect of this septum, an opening near the cochlear window allows communication between the two compartments (Hudson & Hamilton 1993). Small tympanic bone spicules and bone crests have been identified to be

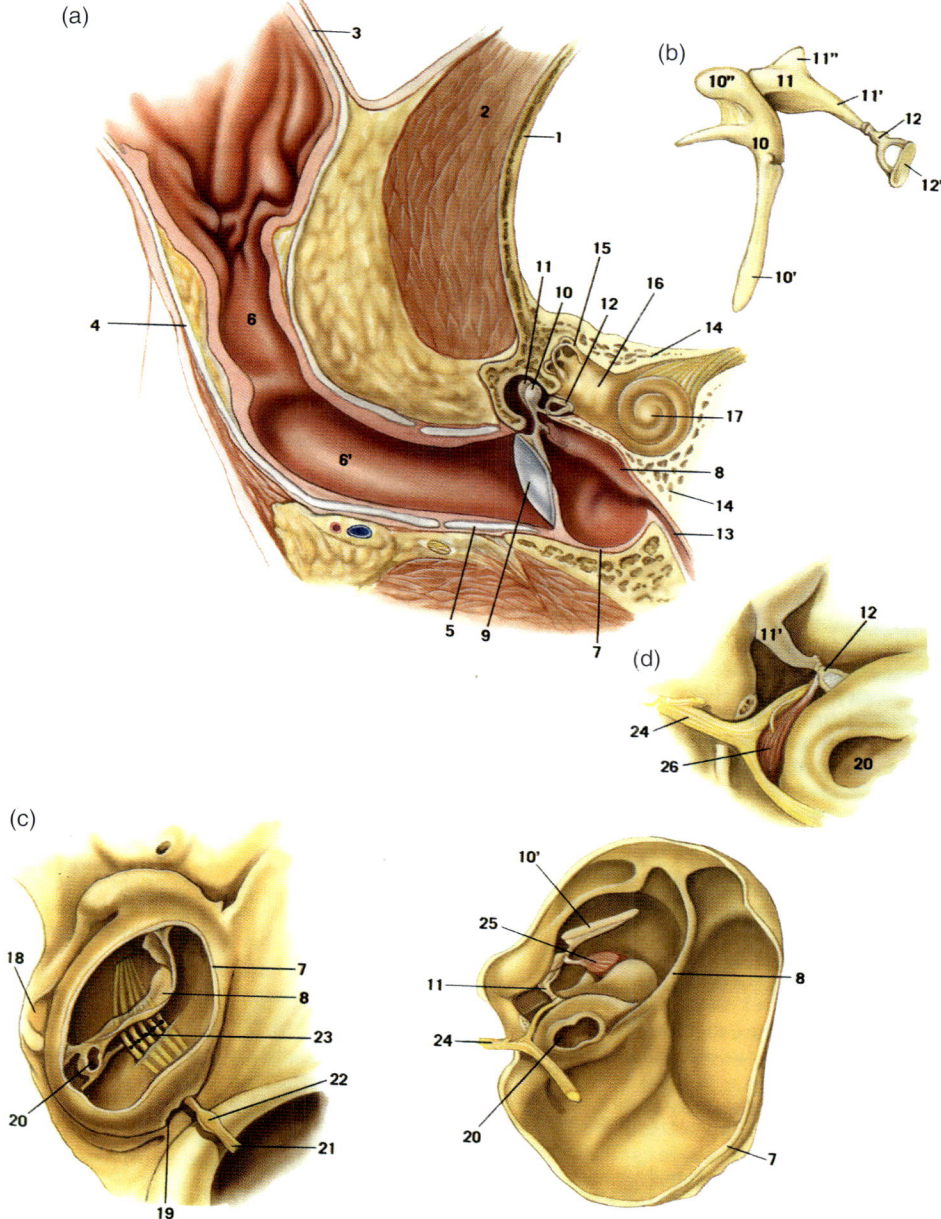

Figure 69.5 Feline aural anatomy. (a) Schematic illustration of structures of the right ear, transverse section through the external ear canal, cranial view. (b) Articulation of the left middle ear ossicles, caudal view. (c) Schematic illustration of sympathetic nerves through the middle ear cavity, ventral tympanic bulla removed, ventral view. (d) Enlargement of structures of middle ear cavity, ventral bulla removed, ventral view in slight rostral rotation to see additional middle ear structures. 1, skull; 2, musculus temporalis; 3–6′, external ear: 3 and 4, auricular cartilage: 3, scapha; 4, concha; 5, annular cartilage; 6, external ear canal, vertical part; 6′, external ear canal, horizontal part; 7–12, middle ear: 7, tympanic bulla; 8, septum bullae; 9, tympanic membrane; 10–12, ear ossicles: 10, malleus; 10′, manubrium; 10″, head; 11, incus; 11′, long crus, 11″, short crus; 12, stapes; 12′, base; 13, auditory tube; 14, petrous temporal bone; 15–17, osseous labyrinth: 15, osseous semicircular canals; 16, vestibule; 17, cochlea; 18, external acoustic meatus; 19, tympano-occipital fissure; 20, vestibular window; 21, cervical sympathetic trunk; 22, cranial cervical ganglion; 23, sympathetic rami; 24, facial nerve; 25, musculus tensor tympani; 26, musculus stapedius.

normal variations in some cats (Beck *et al.* 2020). Simple squamous epithelium or simple cuboidal epithelium lines the tympanic cavity and some of the more ventral epithelial cells have cilia. A thin layer of connective tissue is located between the tympanic epithelium and osseous surface (Cole 2009). The tympanic cavity gas is nitrogen (83%), oxygen (12%), and carbon dioxide (5%) in air-ventilated dogs (Ostfeld *et al.* 1980).

The structures within the tympanic cavity on the medial wall of the bulla include the promontory (a bony prominence that sympathetic fibers traverse in the cat), the cochlear or round window, and the vestibular or oval window (Figure 69.5). The cochlear window is located at the caudolateral aspect of the promontory (in the dog) and the membrane covering the opening dissipates energy-produced vibrations of perilymph in the scala tympani. In the cat, the dorsolateral compartment walls have four openings (apertures) that include the tympanic membrane laterally, the tympanic ostium (which leads to the auditory tube) rostrally, and the vestibular and cochlear windows medially (Hudson & Hamilton 1993) (Figure 69.2). The auditory ossicles of the cat are in the dorsolateral compartment and the cochlear window is located in a gap within the septum that bisects the tympanic cavity (Tobias & Morris 2005). The vestibular window located at the dorsolateral region of the promontory and its membranous covering are attached to the base of the stapes (Figure 69.2). The rostral portion of the tympanic cavity proper is the location of the opening of the auditory tube that extends rostrally to the nasopharynx. The auditory tube is lined by ciliated columnar pseudostratified epithelium, which contains goblet cells and has the primary function of equalizing pressure on each side of the tympanic membrane. The portion of the auditory tube that connects with the nasopharynx is cartilaginous and connects with the junctional and osseous (distal) aspects of the tube. The osseous portions of the auditory tube remain patent; however, the cartilaginous portion only opens during swallowing and is closed at rest (Cole 2009). The auditory tube is opened by contraction of the levator and tensor palatini muscles (Njaa *et al.* 2012). Auditory (Eustachian) tube dysfunction associated with a palatine defect has been reported to be associated with unilateral otitis externa and otitis media in a dachshund (Koch *et al.* 2019). Measurement of the acoustic reflex and tympanometry may be used to evaluate the functional integrity of the middle ear components, including intracavitary pressure and compliance of the tympanum. These tests have been used diagnostically in dogs (Cole *et al.* 2002).

Bacterial content within the canine middle ear, in normal ears and ears with otitis media, is shown in Table 69.2.

Inner ear

Auditory and vestibular systems are the two functional units within the inner ear. The petrous portion of the temporal bone, the medial boundary of the middle ear,

Table 69.2 Most common flora of the middle ear in the dog.

Normal flora (low numbers)	Flora in otitis media
Escherichia coli	Yeast (common)
Staphylococcus sp.	*Staphylococcus (pseudo) intermedius*
Branhamella sp.	
Streptococcus sp.	*Pseudomonas aeruginosa*
Enterococcus sp.	*Proteus* sp.
Bacillus sp.	Beta-streptococcus
Bordetella bronchiseptica	*Corynebacterium* sp.
Clostridium perfringens	Enterococcus sp.
Yeast	

Source: Adapted from Cole 2009.

provides the location of the inner ear structures. It is very dense bone and contains no marrow structures (Njaa *et al.* 2012). This region includes an osseous perilymphatic labyrinth, a membranous endolymphatic labyrinth, and an otic capsule that surrounds them. Essentially, the otic capsule is a protective shell within the petrous portion of the temporal bone (Hudson & Hamilton 1993). Three semicircular canals with ampullae, an interposed utricle, macula, vestibule, and saccule, and a spiral cochlea are included (Figure 69.6). Sophisticated imaging equipment is required to visualize these structures (Njaa *et al.* 2012). These sensory organs control hearing and balance and function, either by hair cell (cellular mechanoreceptor) detection of rotational acceleration of endolymph, linear acceleration or deceleration of endolympa, or static position (Evans 1993b; Kumar 2005). In addition, the vestibular window transmits vibrations via perilymph in the scala tympani through the cochlear duct to receptors (hair cell stereocilia) in the organ of Corti, where depolarization of synaptic connections occurs (Figure 69.7). The result is transmission of information via the vestibulocochlear nerve, which innervates the entire membranous labyrinth. The inward movement of the vestibular window ultimately results in an outward movement of the membrane over the cochlear window (Cole 2009). Brainstem auditory evoked potentials (BAER), an indication of central auditory detection of sound, can be measured in dogs and are averaged recordings of brain activity. The BAER measurements may be stimulated by an auditory click or may be bone induced and are dependent on both mechanical and neuronal mechanisms of the ear (Sims 1988). Avoiding trauma to the dorsal and caudal regions near the promontory, and the dorsorostral location of the ossicles, is important during myringotomy or surgery to prevent iatrogenic neurological and/or auditory complications, respectively (Njaa *et al.* 2012).

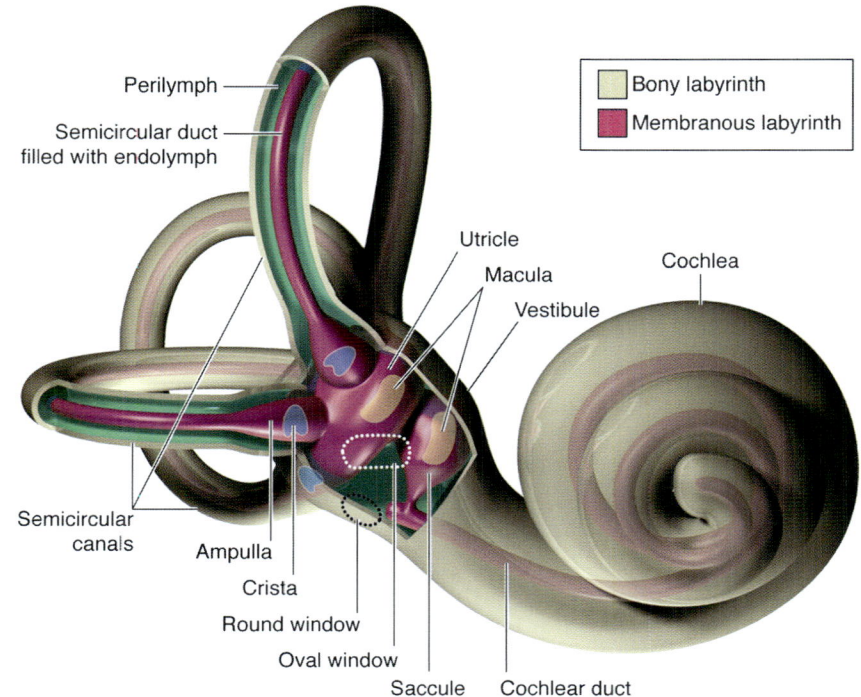

Figure 69.6 Schematic of the bony and membranous labyrinth of the inner ear. Source: Cole LK (2009) / with permission of The Ohio State University.

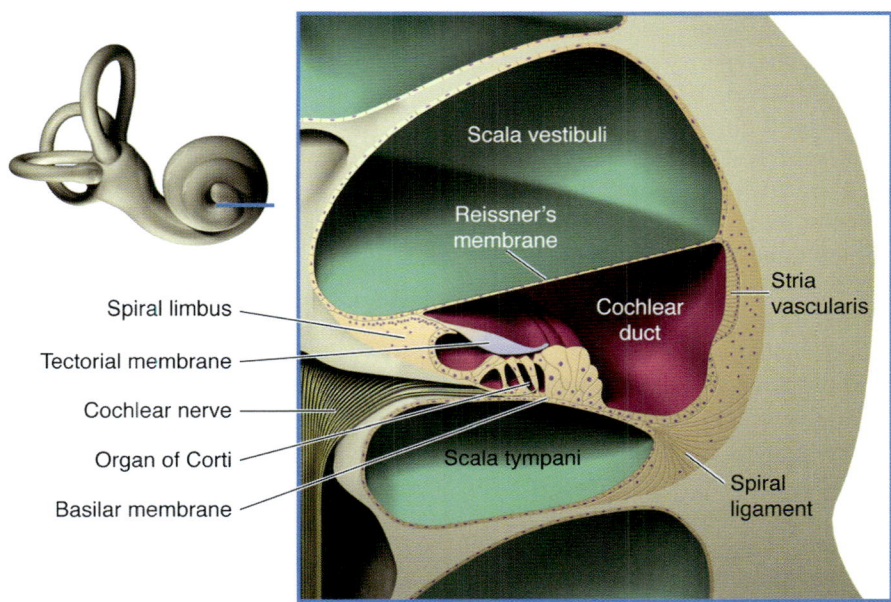

Figure 69.7 Cross-section of the cochlea. Source: Cole LK (2009) / with permission of The Ohio State University.

Innervation of the ear

In the dog, the facial nerve exits the skull from the stylomastoid foramen, which is located just ventral to the jugular process (a palpable prominence used for orientation in surgery) and caudal to the external acoustic meatus (Figure 69.8). The major portion of the nerve extends ventral to the horizontal ear canal and is directed rostrally to the face, where it splits into buccal, palpebral, and aural branches. Within the skull, the facial nerve is located within the facial canal of the petrous temporal

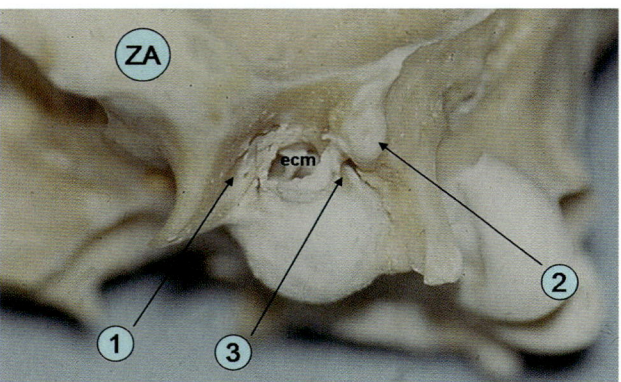

Figure 69.8 Photo of left lateral canine skull showing external acoustic meatus (ecm), retroarticular foramen (1), the mastoid process (2), and the stylomastoid canal (3). ZA, zygomatic arch.

bone after being accompanied by the vestibular and cochlear nerves through the internal acoustic meatus. In the middle ear, near the vestibular window, the stapedial nerve and the chorda tympani nerve leave the facial nerve. The facial nerve continues toward the stylomastoid foramen and just after exiting gives off muscular branches that supply auricular muscles, the caudal auricular nerve, and the caudal internal auricular nerve, which is sensory to the caudal aspect of the pinna. This small branch is transected during total ear canal ablation and is accompanied by a small vessel. Sensory innervation of the ear is from branches of the trigeminal, facial, vagus, and second cervical nerves (Evans 1993b).

The facial nerve is more exposed in the cat and is encountered in a more superficial location than in the dog. In the cat, nerves that traverse the middle ear to a distant location and nerves that have a primary function within the middle ear are subject to injury by disease or surgery within the cavity because they are more exposed than in dogs (Figure 69.2). Sympathetic postganglionic nerves lie under the mucous membrane and fan out as they pass over the promontory and extend under the rostrolateral septum bullae before exiting the bullae. Irritation of these fibers without transection can result in anisocoria (pupil dilatation in the ipsilateral eye) and retraction of the third eyelid. Damage to this innervation results in Horner's syndrome (characterized by ipsilateral miosis, protrusion of the third eyelid, and a narrow palpebral fissure; Hudson & Hamilton 1993). Nerves of the middle ear are listed in Table 69.3.

Blood supply to the ear

The external carotid artery that gives off the caudal auricular branch is followed by the superficial temporal artery that extends to the pinna to supply the majority of blood to the pinna. The caudal auricular artery gives off

Table 69.3 Nerves of the middle ear.

Postganglionic sympathetic nerve	Innervation of the eye and orbit
Chorda tympani nerve	Supply taste buds of the rostral tongue. Autonomic motor fibers innervate tongue glands that control vasodilatation and secretion
Tympanic nerve and plexus	Supply the mucous membrane that lines the tympanic bulla
Minor petrosal nerve	Supply the parotid and zygomatic salivary gland in part, and nerve injury can cause xerostomia
Tensor tympani nerve	Innervates the tensor tympani muscle
Stapedial nerve	Innervates the stapedius muscle
Facial nerve	In a location near the stapes, a short segment of the facial canal is not protected by a bony wall where the tendon of the stapedius muscle inserts on the stapes (Njaa et al. 2012)

the lateral, intermediate, deep, and medial auricular arteries, which supply the majority of blood to the caudal half of the pinna. There are many small foramina (channels) that allow blood vessels to course from the convex (outer) surface to the concave (inner) surface (Bacon 2012). The superficial temporal artery supplies the front half of the pinna. The vertebral artery provides arterial supply to the basilar artery and the bony labyrinth via the labyrinthine artery. The tympanum receives blood supply from the deep auricular and anterior tympanic branches of the maxillary artery, and from the stylomastoid branch of the posterior auricular artery (Cole 2009).

References

Bacon, N.J. (2012). Pinna and external ear canal. In: *Veterinary Surgery Small Animal*, vol. 2 (ed. K.M. Tobias and S.A. Johnston), 2059–2061. St. Louis, MO: Elsevier Saunders.

Beck, T., Bruhschwein, A., and Meyer-Lindenberg, A. (2020). Occurrence of tympanic bone spicules and bone crests in domestic cats. *Anatomia, Histologia, Embryologia* 49: 216–221.

Cole, L.K. (2009). Anatomy and physiology of the canine ear. *Veterinary Dermatology* 21: 221–231.

Cole, L.K., Kwochka, K.W., Podell, M. et al. (2002). Evaluation of radiography, otoscopy, pneumotoscopy, impedance audiometry and endoscopy for the diagnosis of otitis media. In: *Advances in Veterinary Dermatology*, vol. 4 (ed. K.L. Thoday, C.S. Foil and R. Bond), 49–55. Ames, IA: Iowa State Press.

Defalque, V.E., Rosenstein, D.S., and Rosser, E.J. (2005). Measurement of normal middle ear cavity volume in mesaticephalic dogs. *Veterinary Radiology & Ultrasound* 46: 490–493.

Evans, H.E. (1993a). The heart and arteries. In: *Miller's Anatomy of the Dog*, 3e (ed. H.E. Evans), 586–716. Philadelphia, PA: WB Saunders.

Evans, H.E. (1993b). The ear. In: *Miller's Anatomy of the Dog*, 3e (ed. H.E. Evans), 988–1008. Philadelphia, PA: WB Saunders.

Heine, P.A. (2004). Anatomy of the ear. In: *Veterinary Clinics of North America. Small Animal Practice*, vol. 34, 379–395.

Hudson, L.C. and Hamilton, W.P. (1993). Ear. In: *Atlas of Feline Anatomy for Veterinarians* (ed. L.C. Hudson and W.P. Hamilton), 228–237. Philadelphia, PA: WB Saunders.

Koch, S.N., Torres, S.M.F., and Kramek, B. (2019). Patulous Eustachian tube and palatine defect in a Dachshund with chronic unilateral otitis externa and otitis media. *Veterinary Dermatology* 31: 240–253.

Kumar, S. (2005). Anatomy of the canine and feline ear. In: *Small Animal Ear Diseases*, 2e (ed. L.N. Gotthelf), 1–21. St. Louis, MO: Elsevier Saunders.

Njaa, B.L., Cole, L.K., and Tabacca, N. (2012). Practical otic anatomy and physiology of the dog and cat. *Veterinary Clinics of North America. Small Animal Practice* 42: 1109–1126.

Ostfeld, E., Blonder, J., Crispin, M. et al. (1980). The middle ear gas composition in air-ventilated dogs. *Acta Oto-Laryngologica* 89: 105–108.

Radlinsky, M.G. (2016). Advances in otoscopy. *Veterinary Clinics of North America. Small Animal Practice* 46: 171–179.

Sims, M.H. (1988). Electrodiagnostic evaluation of auditory function. *Veterinary Clinics of North America. Small Animal Practice* 18: 913–944.

Steiss, J.E., Boosinger, T.R., Wright, J.C. et al. (1992). Healing of experimentally perforated tympanic membranes, demonstrated by electrodiagnostic testing and histopathology. *Journal of the American Animal Hospital Association* 28: 307–310.

Stern-Bertholtz, W., Sjostrom, L., and Hakanson, N.W. (2003). Primary secretory otitis media in the Cavalier King Charles spaniel: a review of 61 cases. *Journal of Small Animal Practice* 44: 253–256.

Stout-Graham, M., Kainer, R.A., Whalen, L.R. et al. (1990). Morphologic measurements of the external horizontal ear canal of dogs. *American Journal of Veterinary Research* 51: 990–994.

Tinling, S.P. and Chole, R.A. (2006). Gerbilline cholesteatoma development part I: epithelial migration pattern and rate on the gerbil tympanic memberane: comparisons with human and guinea pig. *Otolaryngology-Head and Neck Surgery* 134: 788–793.

Tobias, K.M. and Morris, D. (2005). The ear. In: *BSAVA Manual of Canine and Feline Head, Neck and Thoracic Surgery* (ed. D.J. Brockman and D.E. Holt), 56–72. Gloucester: British Small Animal Veterinary Association.

70

Surgery of the Pinna

Jamie R. Bellah

The pinna of dogs and cats is exposed and as a result is frequently injured by various types of trauma. Damage to the pinna may be self-inflicted by head shaking and ear scratching secondary to otitis externa, neoplasia, or inflammation. The extensive blood supply results in considerable hemorrhage when the pinna is lacerated or injured, and such a circumstance can be quite distressing to owners because of the apparent volume of blood loss and the mess that results from persistent head shaking and splattering of blood. Since the pinna of dogs and cats is an important part of the appearance of pets, a cosmetic result after surgery is always a goal.

Planning surgery involving the pinna is enhanced by recognizing the three zones of the pinna (horizontal zones dividing the length of the pinna into three equal areas), as has been described by Pavletic (2018). The skin of the lateral and lower aspects of the pinna of zone I is mobile, not fixed to the pinnal cartilage; the skin of the lateral aspect of zone II is less mobile; and the skin of the lateral aspect of zone III is thinner and is more fixed to the perichondrium, restricting its mobility. The skin lining the inner or concave surface of the pinna is fixed to the perichondrium in all three zones.

Lacerations

Managing lacerations of the pinna in dogs and cats depends on the nature and extent of the injury. Sharp laceration or crushing injury, partial or full thickness, and the presence of an architectural defect are examples (Figure 70.1). Lacerations that result from dog or cat fights may have ragged edges and require débridement.

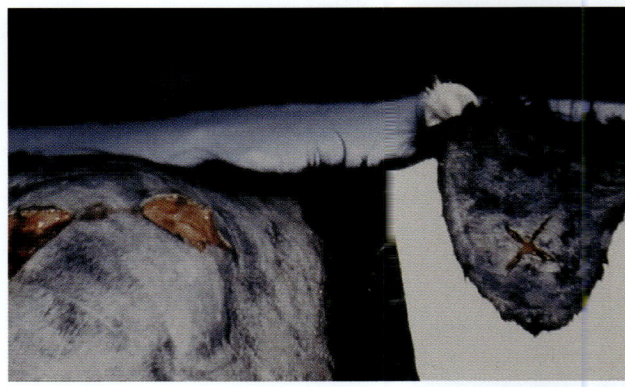

Figure 70.1 A cocker spaniel was hit by an arrow, creating a sharp laceration of the pinna and a shoulder laceration. The wound was sutured primarily and healed without complication.

Simple linear lacerations limited to the skin of the pinna usually require only hemostasis and measures to prevent self-trauma by the pet. The skin, particularly on the concave surface (rostrolateral), is securely fixed to the underlying cartilage and this tends to maintain some apposition of the skin margins. If undermining of the edges is evident or if the skin is flapped away from the cartilage, application of fine sutures to appose the skin margins is necessary. Dead space management, if necessary, can be accomplished by using a small-diameter closed-suction drain (Figure 70.2) or by using fine mattress sutures to limit space between the elevated skin and the perichondrium and cartilage.

Lacerations that involve the cartilage may require that the cartilage be apposed in addition to the skin for a

Small Animal Soft Tissue Surgery, Second Edition. Edited by Eric Monnet.
© 2023 John Wiley & Sons, Inc. Published 2023 by John Wiley & Sons, Inc.
Companion website: www.wiley.com/go/monnet/small

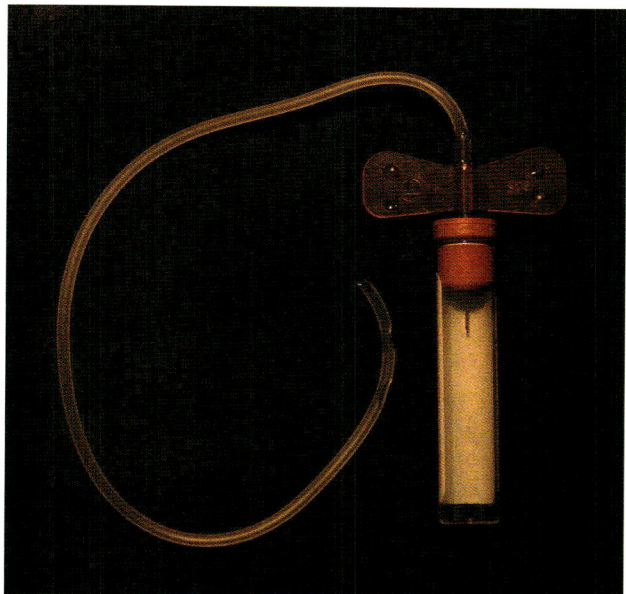

Figure 70.2 A simple closed-vacuum system. The luer lock tip of the butterfly catheter has been cut off and the tip of the catheter fenestrated about 1.5 cm. The tubing is placed through a small stab incision into a cavity and the needle tip is placed in a vacuum tube to create a closed-vacuum drainage system.

(a)

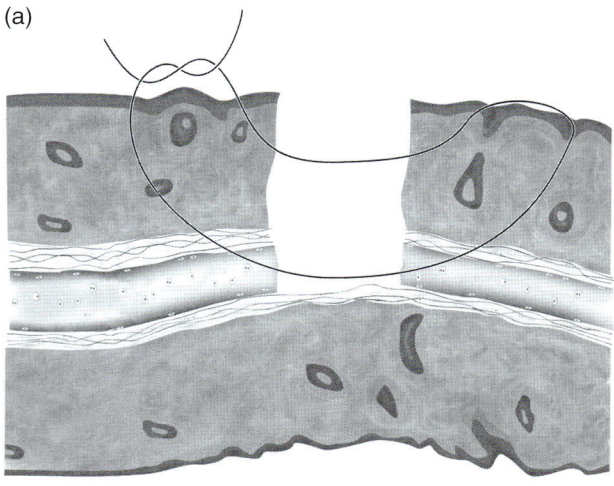

(b)

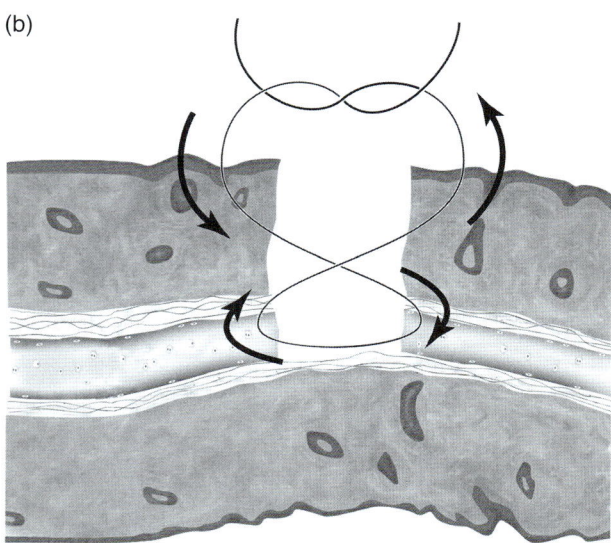

Figure 70.3 (a) A vertical mattress pattern used to appose a laceration on the concave surface of the ear; (b) A figure-of-eight pattern that apposes the cartilage and the skin of the concave surface.

satisfactory cosmetic result. The perichondrium and cartilage will hold sutures well, and incorporation of these layers can be done using suture patterns such as a vertical mattress pattern or a figure-of-eight pattern to appose both the cartilage and skin on one side of the pinna (Figure 70.3). Sometimes débridement of a portion of the cartilage is necessary.

If the laceration extends through both sides of the pinna (full thickness), both skin surfaces and the cartilage will need to be apposed. Lacerations may vary in direction from vertical to horizontal and often extend to the helical border of the pinna. The blood supply to the distal aspects of the pinna may be affected by some lacerations, particularly those that are horizontal, and tissue loss may complicate management. In addition, when cartilage lacerations occur, structural support of the pinna may be lost. Such structural support does not return until there is fibrous union between the cartilage surfaces and in some circumstances (i.e., erect ears that droop) cosmetic restoration is difficult or impossible. Wounds that involve cartilage, if allowed to heal by second intention, often disfigure the ear as a result of wound contraction.

Wounds of the pinna that completely perforate the ear should be sutured primarily if possible to limit wound contraction and subsequent deformation of the pinna. If allowed to occur, wound contraction widens the defect and creates permanent deformity (a gap), which may be

more difficult to correct. Suture patterns vary with the preference of the surgeon, but simple interrupted sutures and vertical mattress patterns have been used successfully (Henderson & Horne 2003).

Resection of portions of the pinna

There are many causes of architectural defects of the pinna, for example bite wounds causing fissures, neoplastic resections, inflammatory disease of the ear tips, thermal injury, fly strike injury and trauma, and avulsions. Correction of architectural defects is not always necessary nor possible without creating folds or exaggerated curvature of the pinna. Linear fissures may be débrided and sutured primarily. When the tips of the ears are involved, cosmetic amputation of the tips may be performed, as long as an attempt is made to keep them as symmetric as possible. Suturing the remaining margins may be done as previously described. It is critical to provide postoperative analgesia and protection from self-trauma, or head shaking and scratching will result in bleeding and untoward complications.

Wedge excision, partial amputation, and total pinnectomy

Fissures or small masses that extend to the helical border or are small and close to the edge of the pinna, respectively, may be managed by wedge excision. A long, triangular pattern allows the edges to be apposed (sometimes incompletely) in a cosmetic manner (Figure 70.4). It is important to pay attention to the vascular supply of the pinna so that loss of viability after resection is avoided. When partial amputations are performed, the excisions can be done with a scalpel or scissors while trying to retain the normal curvature of the ear. It is important to pay attention to achieving hemostasis and to avoid bulky ligatures. If ligatures are necessary, fine absorbable suture should be used. Electrocauterization is preferred and fine needlepoint tips work well. The skin edges are apposed over the cartilage carefully by a fine (5-0 or 4-0) simple continuous suture pattern.

Total pinnectomy is indicated when traumatic injury is severe and not repairable by reconstruction, to achieve adequate tissue margin when resecting neoplastic masses (i.e., squamous cell carcinoma in cats), and is sometimes done to provide tissue for reconstruction of head wounds (Bacon 2012). Closure of the wound varies depending on the depth of excision, with the skin of the convex surface of the incision being pulled over the concave surface of the auricular cartilage and sutured to the skin on the convex surface. Fine nonabsorbable suture in a continuous pattern is commonly used for apposition. Total pinnectomy is not done with the expectation of a cosmetic result.

Reconstruction of auricular margin defects

Larger defects of the pinna may be reconstructed with various techniques, depending on the location of the defect. The anterior and posterior edges of the base of the pinna may be reconstructed by using local transposition flaps (Figure 70.5) with the base of the flap anterior or posterior to the ear. Flaps may be oriented such that the base is adjacent to the base of the pinna and the peninsular portion of the flap extends ventrally (Pavletic 2010). The skin transposed to the pinna will have more hair and the direction of the hair may be different, but the flap allows reconstruction. In some situations a narrowed base of the pinna is acceptable and fairly cosmetic, so reconstruction is not always necessary. The reconstruction may prevent loss of the ear pinna, if there is exposed cartilage, and that is usually preferred by pet owners.

(a) (b) (c)

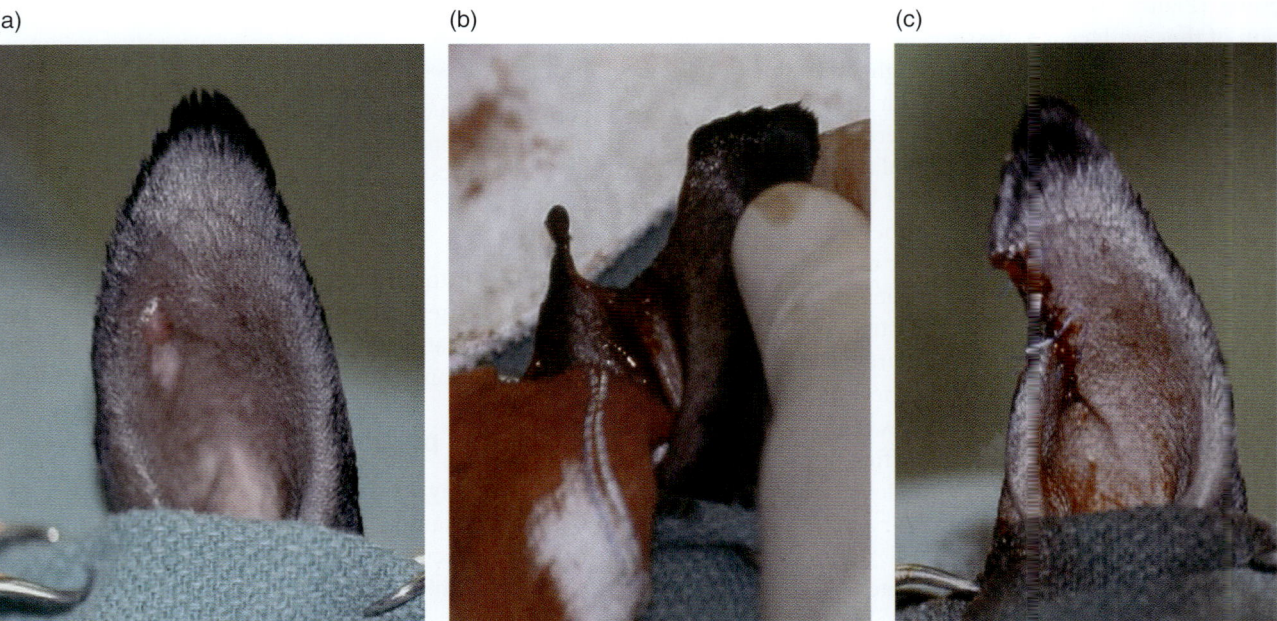

Figure 70.4 (a) The ear of a Boston terrier with a small nodular mast cell tumor near the caudal aspect of the pinna. (b) A triangular full-thickness wedge of the pinna is removed around the mast cell tumor. (c) The margins of the resection are apposed incompletely and the distal aspect of the incision is apposed over the exposed cartilage. The result was fairly cosmetic.

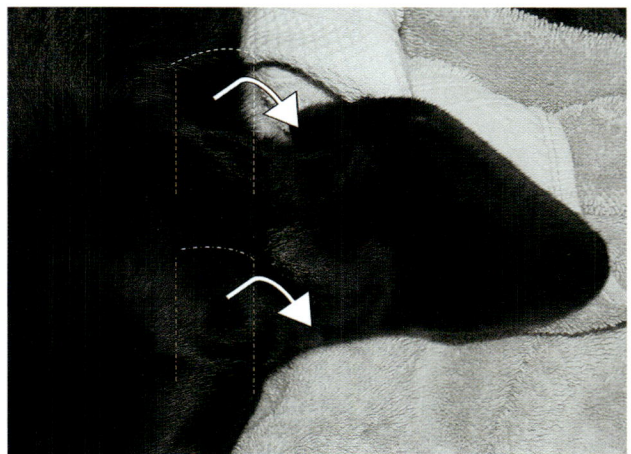

Figure 70.5 Two of the possible orientations for transposition flaps to repair defects near the base of the ear (arrows).

Distal and marginal defects of the pinna may be reconstructed by using skin of the head adjacent to the ear in the manner similar to a distant pedicle flap. The use of such flaps allows correction of architectural defects to salvage the shape of the pinna, but the amount and/or the direction of hair growth may vary and affect the final cosmetic result. Pendulous ears can be manipulated such that the donor site chosen will have hair growth in the same direction as the convex side of the pinna. In addition, the skin used for reconstruction will usually be thicker than that normally characteristic of the pinna (Pavletic 2010). The distant pedicle flap is left in place for 14 days so wound healing is complete, and the new collateral blood supply to the pedicle will be maintained after the pedicle is released. The flap is sutured to the remaining margins of the pinna. If two sides of the cartilage are exposed, it may require a two-stage technique to cover both concave and convex surfaces. Pedicles can be folded to cover both sides of the pinnal cartilage. Edema often occurs temporarily after apposition, but necrosis of the portion of the flap distal to the fold may also occur (Henderson & Horne 2003). If small defects remain after suturing the flap edges in place, they may be allowed to heal by second intention.

Aural hematoma

Pathogenesis

Aural hematoma is a very common abnormality affecting the pinna of dogs and less commonly cats (Figure 70.6) (Lanz & Wood 2004). It is hypothesized to be caused most commonly by trauma such as scratching the ear and head shaking (Lanz & Wood 2004; MacPhail 2016). The pathogenesis has been thought to involve separation of the skin of the inner pinna from the cartilage (Lanz &

Wood 2004). Others have suggested that the perichondrium separates from the cartilage, causing hemorrhage from the intrachondral vessels to accumulate within the subperiochondral space (Garbutt 1956), or as a result of separation of layers of cartilage with subperichondral hemorrhage (Stephenson 1941; Larson 1968; Dubielzig *et al.* 1984; Kuwahara 1986). Intrachondral clefts and intrachondral ruptures have been found in affected ears and have been suggested to result from head shaking that exceeds a critical velocity or a natural frequency that creates shear forces, which overstress the cartilage resulting in separation (Larson 1968; Dubielzig *et al.* 1984; MacPhail 2016; Lahiani & Niebauer 2020). Small intrachondral ruptures have been found histologically in normal dogs (Larson 1968), and have been shown to propagate widely, creating the fluid-filled cavity (Lahiani & Niebauer 2020). Histologic examination of cartilage samples has been done, and showed intrachondral separation in all dogs studied, with the presence of granulation tissue and no evidence of cartilage regeneration, and samples were without leucocyte infiltration (Lahiani & Niebauer 2020) (Figure 70.7). One attempt to induce aural hematoma in dogs by trauma was unsuccessful

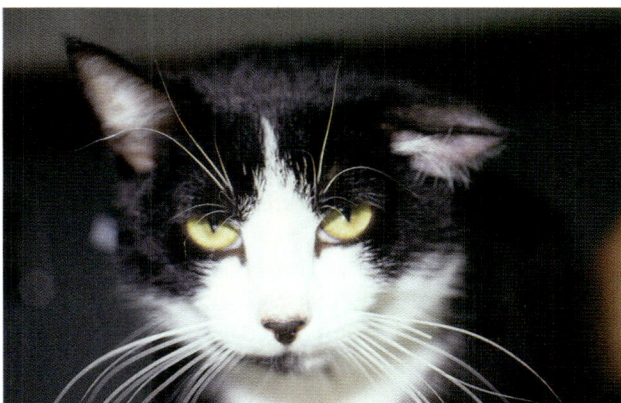

Figure 70.6 Domestic short-haired cat with an aural hematoma secondary to otocariasis.

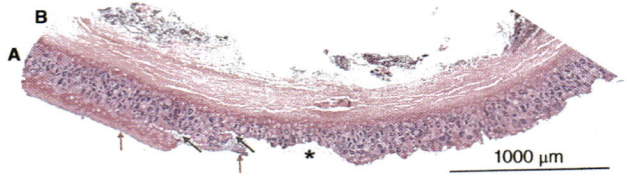

Figure 70.7 Histology of a cartilage sample stained with hematoxylin-eosin-saffron (x100). Intrachondral separation (black arrows) and erosion (asterisk) of the convex cartilage sheet (A) partially filled with granulation tissue (red arrows). No signs of cartilage regeneration or of leucocyte infiltration; no alteration of the subchondral tissue (B).

(Kuwahara 1986). Aural hematomas have been commonly associated with otitis externa (Stephenson 1941) and otocariasis (Kuwahara 1986), but others have noted that the condition commonly occurs without evidence of ear disease (Joyce 1994; Wilson 1983; Lahiani & Niebauer 2020). Treatment of coexisting otitis externa, if present, is a critical component of therapy contributing to the success of aural hematoma treatment (MacPhail 2016).

An autoimmune pathogenesis has been suggested to play a role in the development of aural hematoma (Kuwahara 1986). Serologic tests on blood and hematoma fluid from affected canine and feline ears that supported this conclusion included positive direct and indirect Coomb's tests in all affected animals, while 52.5% of antinuclear antibody (ANA) tests were positive (Kuwahara 1986; Joyce & Day 1997) and 19% of the ears had immunoglobulin (Ig)G deposition at the dermoepidermal junction, as seen by direct immunofluorescence (Kuwahara 1986). Corticosteroid therapy was successful in many of the affected animals and was considered supportive to the autoimmune hypothesis (Kuwahara 1986). A study of 15 dogs affected with aural hematoma showed none of the dogs to be Coomb's positive and no dog had a positive ANA titer. In this study, histopathologic evaluation of the cartilage showed minimal perichondral inflammation, erosion of auricular cartilage, and cartilage defects filled with fibrovascular granulation tissue (Joyce & Day 1997). Basement membrane zone deposition of IgG or IgM was seen in only two dogs. In this study 6 of 15 dogs had no evidence of otitis externa and an autoimmune pathogenesis was not supported (Joyce & Day 1997). Cytologic evaluation of the hematoma fluid revealed a low packed cell volume, low total protein, and low albumin compared with blood. Histopathologic examination of the dermis and the auricular cartilage revealed a predominance of mast cells and eosinophils, and may reflect an association with hypersensitivity disease. Joyce concluded that the pinnal skin was not the primary site of the hematoma formation and that an underlying primary immune event involving the auricular cartilage may play a role in the initiation of the condition (Joyce & Day 1997).

A more recent study of 10 dogs showed that the fluid-filled cavities of affected dogs had characteristics of a transudate with low hematocrits (median 3.9%), no blood clots, low total protein (median 4.8 g/dL), and low cellularity (median 3260 cells/mm³), and the comparisons to parameters in peripheral blood were significant. Cytologic examinations of fluid showed foamy erythrophagocytic macrophages, degenerating neutrophils, and cellular debris. Electrophoresis of the fluid within the aural cavities was quantitatively similar to peripheral blood (Lahiani & Niebauer 2020).

Treatment

Several objectives should be achieved in order to treat aural hematoma successfully in dogs and cats. If ear disease exists, identification of the cause and specific treatment will parallel treatment of the aural hematoma. Drainage of the aural hematoma and maintenance of apposition of the margins of the hematoma until healing occurs contribute to a successful outcome (Lanz & Wood 2004). Early drainage of the fluid from the aural cavity is important, as secondary fibrosis and contraction can result in permanent deformation of the pinna.

There are a number of treatment options that have been used successfully in dogs and cats (Brown 2010). Simple needle aspiration of the fluid from the aural cavity may be done, followed by bandaging to gently compress the internal margins of the pinna (Figure 70.8). Daily aspiration has been recommended (Lanz & Wood 2004). An anti-inflammatory dose of prednisone is used to lessen inflammation and subsequently decrease head shaking and scratching at the ear.

Various methods of long-term continuous drainage have been published previously and include teat cannula insertion, multiple variations of drain insertion (Lanz & Wood 2004), and multiple types of drains (Lanz & Wood 2004; MacPhail 2016; Chadzimisios et al. 2019). Chronic hematomas that have scarring or a lot of fibrin are not amenable to drainage techniques. All techniques are done by clipping and preparing the concave surface of the ear for surgery. Depending on the type of surgery, required anesthesia may vary from

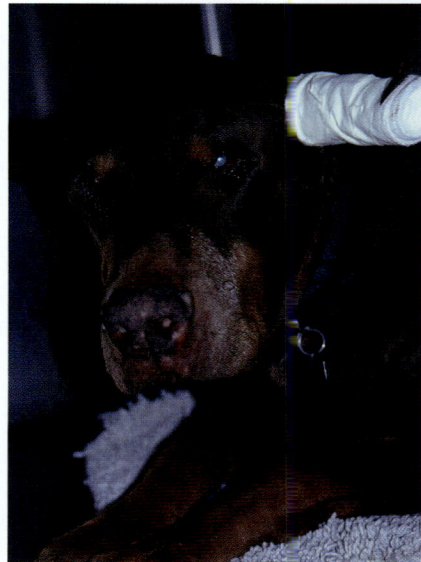

Figure 70.8 Gauze bandage rolling the ear and gently compressing the margins of aural hematoma together. Care must be taken with this technique, as if it is placed too tight loss of viability of the distal pinna can occur.

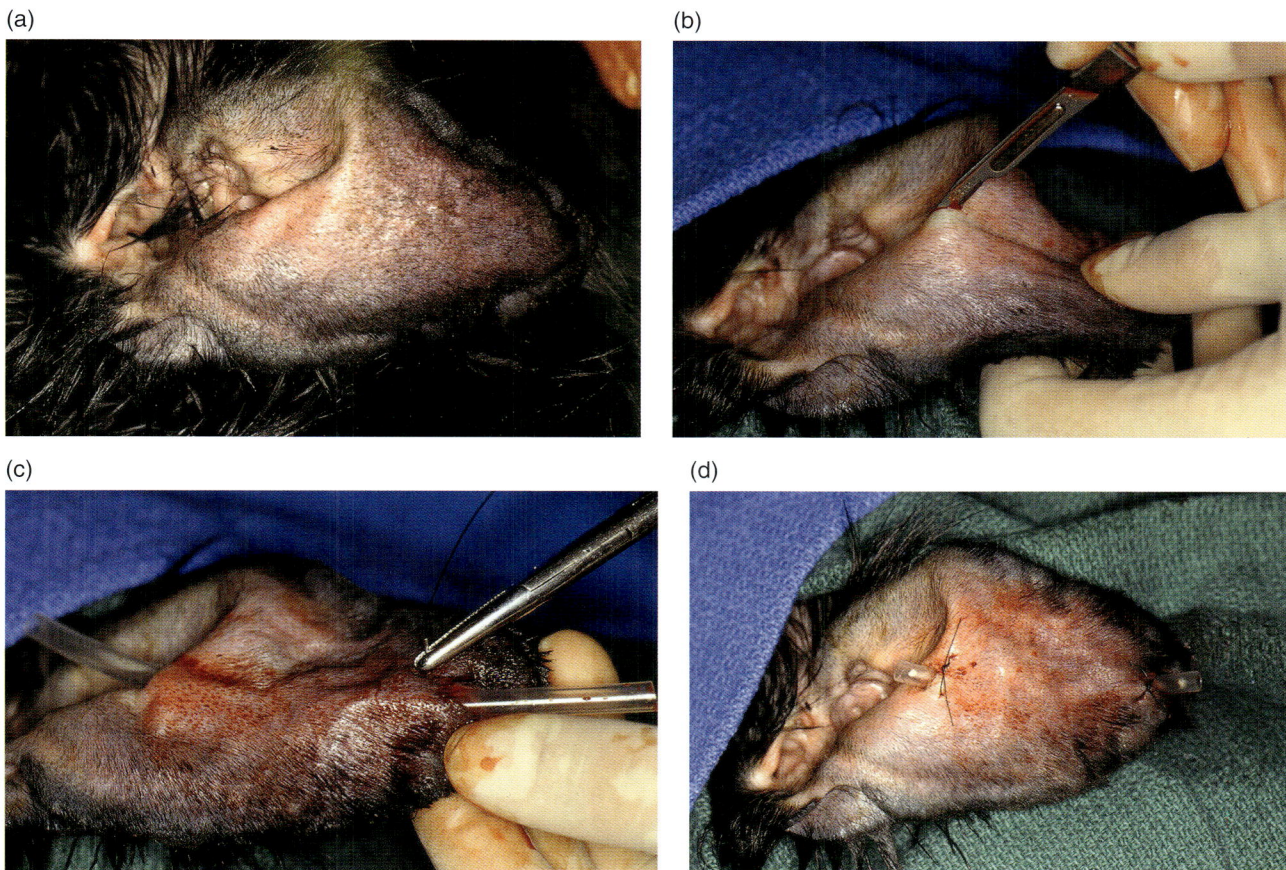

Figure 70.9 (a) Aural hematoma in a dog. (b) Small stab incisions are made after injection of a local anesthetic at the proximal and distal margins of the hematoma. The fluid is drained. (c) A small silastic tube is pulled through the hematoma using fine alligator forceps and the tubing is secured by placing two fine sutures. (d) The tubing is trimmed.

tranquilization and local infiltration of anesthetic to general anesthesia. Drainage can be accomplished by placing a silastic or Penrose drain through the hematoma (Figure 70.9). A small stab incision is made at both the apex and the base of the hematoma and the drain is pulled through. Fine sutures are placed through the skin and the drain to secure it in position. The drain orifices are periodically cleaned with saline and a cotton-tipped swab and pulled after 14 days. Alternatively, a teat cannula (Figure 70.10) is placed through a small incision at the apex of the hematoma (the dependent portion of the hematoma).

Closed-suction techniques are also simple to use by modifying a standard butterfly catheter (Swaim & Bradley 1996; Lanz & Wood 2004). The tubing near the injector port is fenestrated and the injector port is removed. After the hematoma is flushed with saline and the hematoma drained, the fenestrated portion of the butterfly tubing is inserted into the aural hematoma cavity at the base and a purse-string suture promotes an airtight seal. The butterfly catheter needle is inserted into a vacuum blood tube. The vacuum tube (container) is replaced periodically and the ear and tube are bandaged over the head to protect the system and ear. Incisional drainage is reserved for aural hematomas that have been of a more chronic duration or those that have recurred after less invasive techniques (Lanz & Wood 2004).

Laterally placed vacuum drains for successfully managing aural hematomas has been described (Pavletic 2015). Fenestrated silicon drains were used, placed in a minimally invasive technique, exited the base of the pinna adjacent to cervical skin, and were attached to a vacuum reservoir for continuous drainage (Figure 70.11). There is no need for open wound care or compressive dressings. A second report was similarly successful using a similar technique (9 of 10 dogs did not have recurrence at six months), but did report one dog that developed a persistent infection that was managed by drain removal, and two dogs where contamination was noted and resolved with the use of Blake drains and antimicrobials. The recommendation was made to use a 100 mL reservoir with and anti-reflux valve so that the reservoir is changed

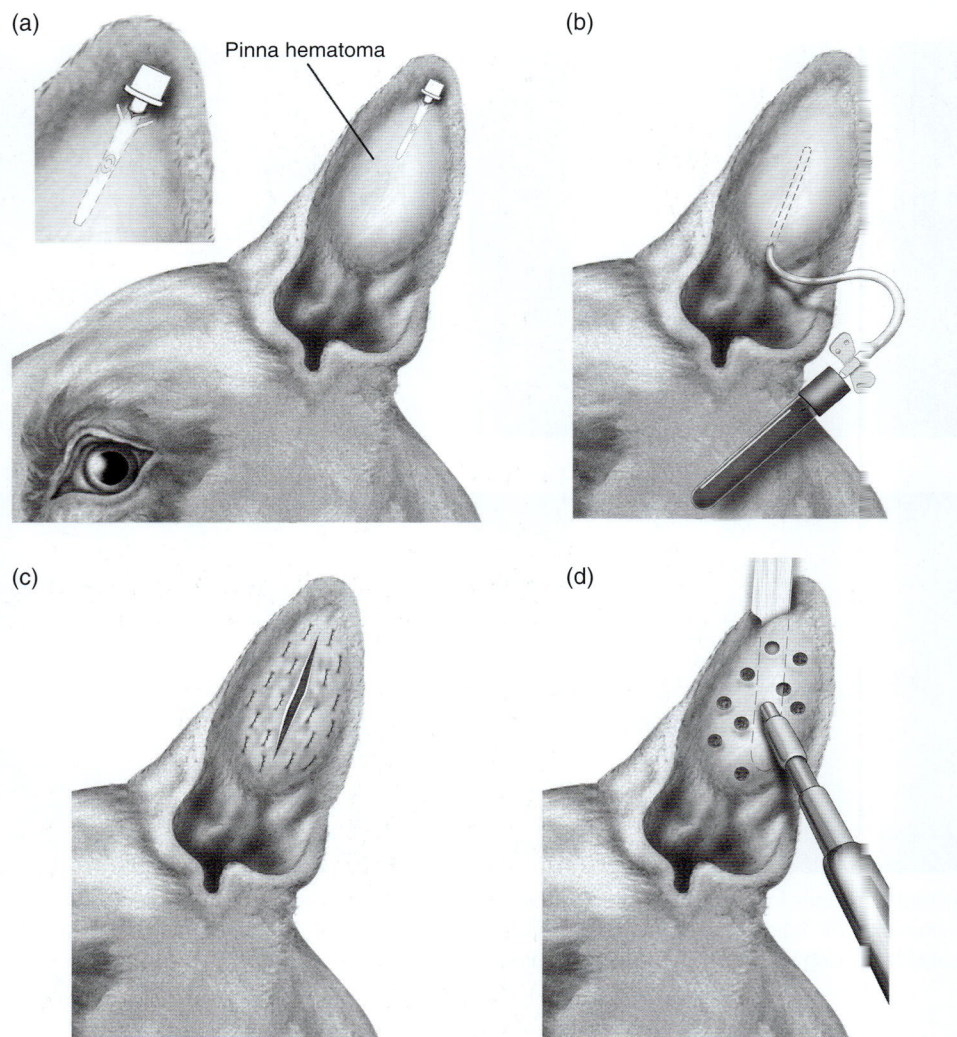

Figure 70.10 (a) A teat canula placed through a small incision into the cavity of the aural hematoma. The cannula may be placed in either the dorsal or ventral aspect of the hematoma. (b) A small vacuum drain has been placed in an aural hematoma and is secured by a fine purse-string suture. (c) Standard incision and suturing technique. Note that the sutures are placed parallel to the vasculature. (d) Aural hematoma treated by using a dermal punch to create small holes in the convex margin of the pinna. The tongue depressor prevents damage to the opposing margin of the hematoma.

once per week, and to attach the drain to a harness to lessen the tendency to rotate with the collar (Lahiani & Niebauer 2020).

A relatively new surgical technique, described in 23 dogs, places intradermal suture lines using absorbable sutures on each side of a linear incision, thus avoiding external sutures (Györffy & Szijártó 2014). There was no recurrence is the treated dogs and only one dog had an auricular deformity. The benefits of the technique included minimal aftercare, purportedly less irritation from external sutures, and no required suture removal. Use of a CO_2 laser has also been reported to be successful in eight dogs, as well as a sutureless surgical technique that utilizes a preshaped silicon pad that is

clipped to the pinna to apply compression to the aural hematoma post drainage. The device is left in place for a least three weeks and is examined daily for evidence of pressure necrosis (Hematoma Repair System, Pract vet, Phoenix, AZ, USA).

Surgical techniques remain a common method to treat aural hematomas and in a recent technique survey of veterinarians are perceived to be more likely to be successful with good cosmetic results (Hall *et al.* 2016). Surgical treatment includes an incision parallel to the long axis of the pinna, linear or S shaped, made on the concave surface of the ear, the hematoma cavity is lavaged with sterile saline, and all fibrin and clots are removed. Sutures are placed parallel to the vascular

(a)

(b)

(c)

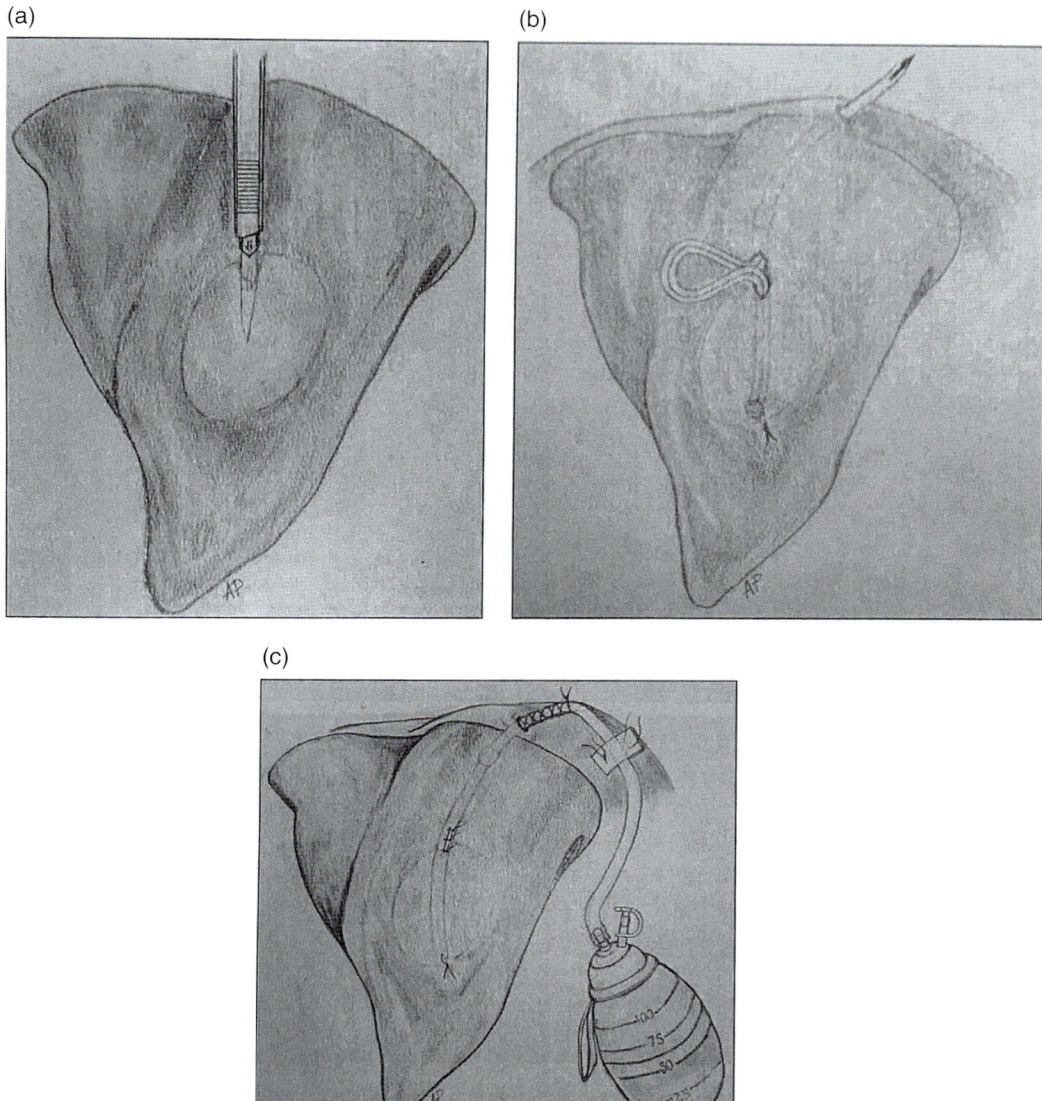

Figure 70.11 Placement of a vacuum drain in a dog with an aural hematoma. (a) A 1 cm skin incision is created at the base of the hematoma with a no. 15 scalpel blade, followed by insertion of a no. 11 blade to penetrate the hematoma cavity. (b) The fenestrated portion of the vacuum drain is shortened and advanced to traverse the length of the hematoma cavity. A suture is then placed through the skin at the apical end of the hematoma, capturing the tip of the drain. Once secured, a second 1 cm skin incision is created in the cervical skin located near the base of the ear. A hemostat is tunneled from the second skin incision to the first, and the end of the drain is drawn through the tunnel. Note that any excess portion of the nonfenestrated portion of the drain can be removed to facilitate this latter maneuver. (c) The initial incision is sutured with 3-0 nylon interrupted sutures. After ensuring sufficient laxity in the drain to allow normal ear movement, a purse-string suture is applied around the exit incision and incorporated into a finger-trap knot to secure the external drain; 2-0 nylon sutures are used to secure tabs created with surgical tape to the cervical skin as added security to prevent drain displacement. Finally, the external drain is shortened to connect to the vacuum reservoir, which will be secured to the dog's collar. © American Veterinary Medical Association.

supply and just tight enough to appose the surfaces of the ear. Knots are located on the convex surface of the pinna. Nonadherent bandaging technique allows absorption of fluid and protects the aural wound. When external sutures are used, it is recommended that suture removal is not done for 2–3 weeks (MacPhail 2016),

which allows time for remodeling of scar tissue and therefore achieving sufficient wound strength prior to removing ear protection.

A circular fenestration technique has also been used successfully on the concave surface of the ear. A dermal biopsy (4 mm) punch may be used and the holes are positioned about 1 cm apart. Bandaging is as for the suturing technique and restriction of ear position is done until the small circular wounds heal by second intention. A variation of the techniques utilizes a CO_2 laser to make the fenestrations. The laser was also used to make incisions that create focal adhesions subsequent to fibrosis from wound healing between the cartilage layers to aid in prevention of recurrence (Dye *et al.* 2002). Tissue welding was not used. Cyanoacrylates have been injected into aural hematomas to bond the edges together; however, granuloma formation has been reported and, given the success with other techniques that do not leave foreign material within the wound, it seems that using surgical glue is unnecessary.

Recurrence of aural hematoma may occur, particularly if proper care and bandaging are not long enough. The author feels that use of anti-inflammatory doses of prednisone over the period of bandaging is important in lessening inflammation and improving the comfort of the patient, so subjectively it seems that success has been improved with such use. Empirically, prednisone has been reported to be successfully used where surgical methods of treatment were not employed (Romatowski 1994). A human fibrin sealant has recently been reported as used in a dog with an aural hematoma; however, the hematoma recurred soon after ear protection was removed (Blätter *et al.* 2007).

Ear canal separation

Disruption of the ear canal may occur at the junction of the auricular and annular cartilage and at the junction of the horizontal ear canal and the external acoustic meatus. The injury occurs in both dogs and cats (Boothe *et al.* 1996; Connery *et al.* 2001; McCarthy *et al.* 1995; Kyles 2001; Smeak 1997; Tivers & Brockman 2009). It is suggested that the ligamentous connection between the auricular and annular cartilage is more susceptible to trauma and is therefore more commonly damaged (Boothe *et al.* 1996).

Treatment of acute ear canal separation is often by total ear canal ablation in both dogs and cats, and this procedure is typically done to resolve para-aural abscessation that may occur secondary to persisting discontinuity of the ear canal (McCarthy *et al.* 1995; Clarke 2004; Smeak 1997). The location of the tear dictates the possibility of repair: if the avulsion is from the external acoustic meatus, it is very difficult to appose the circumference of the horizontal ear canal. These injuries necessitate total ear canal ablation and lateral bulla osteotomy. Traumatic separation in more distal regions of the horizontal canal (such as the junction of the annular and auricular ligaments) may be resolved by vertical canal resection,

isolation of the opening of the horizontal canal, and apposition of the margins of this opening to the skin (Boothe *et al.* 1996). A caudal approach to the horizontal ear canal has been shown to allow repair of both acute and chronic separations between the annular and auricular cartilages when there is absence of middle ear disease in both dogs and cats (Tivers & Brockman 2009).

References

Bacon, N. (2012). Surgery of the pinna. In: *Veterinary Surgery Small Animal*, vol. 2 (ed. K.M. Tobias and S.A. Johnston), 2068–2070. St. Louis, MO: Elsevier.

Blätter, U.H., Mattison, O., and R.G. Rampelberg F. (2007). Short communication, "Fibrin sealant as a treatment of canine aural haematoma: a case history". *Veterinary Journal* 173: 697–700.

Boothe, H.W., Hobson, H.P., and McDonald, D.E. (1996). Treatment of traumatic separation of the auricular and annular cartilages without ablation: results in five dogs. *Veterinary Surgery* 25: 376–379.

Brown, C. (2010). Surgical management of canine aural hematoma. *Lab Animal* 39: 104–105.

Chadzimisios, K., Papazoplou, L.G. et al. (2019). Management of aural haematoma with Penrose drainage in dogs and cats: a retrospective study of 53 cases (1996–2016). *Hellenic Journal of Companion Animal Medicine* 8: 162–170.

Clarke, S.P. (2004). Surgical management of acute ear canal separation in a cat. *Journal of Feline Medicine and Surgery* 6: 283–286.

Connery, N.A., McCallister, H., and Hay, C.W. (2001). Para-aural abscessation following traumatic ear canal separation in a dog. *Journal of Small Animal Practice* 42: 253–256.

Dubielzig, R.R., Wilson, J.W., and Seireg, A.A. (1984). Pathogenesis of canine aural hematomas. *Journal of the American Veterinary Medical Association* 185: 873–875.

Dye, T.L., Teague, H.D., Ostwald, D.A., and Ferreira, S.D. (2002). Evaluation of a technique using the carbon dioxide laser for the treatment of aural hematomas. *Journal of the American Animal Hospital Association* 38: 385–390.

Garbutt, R.J. (1956). Surgical treatment of hematoma of the ear. *North American Veterinarian* 37: 1056–1059.

Györffy, A. and Szijártó, A. (2014). A new operative technique for aural haematoma in dogs: a retrospective clinical study. *Acta Veterinaria Hungarica* 62: 340–347.

Hall, J., Weir, S., and Ladlow, J. (2016). Treatment of canine aural haematoma by UK veterinarians. *Journal of Small Animal Practice* 57: 360–364.

Henderson, R.A. and Horne, R.D. (2003). The pinna. In: *Textbook of Small Animal Surgery*, 3e (ed. D. Slatter), 1737–1746. Philadelphia, PA: Saunders Elsevier Science.

Joyce, J.A. (1994). Treatment of canine aural haematoma using an indwelling drain and corticosteroids. *Journal of Small Animal Practice* 35: 341–344.

Joyce, J.A. and Day, M.J. (1997). Immunopathogenesis of canine aural haematoma. *Journal of Small Animal Practice* 38: 152–158.

Kuwahara, J. (1986). Canine and feline aural hematoma: clinical, experimental, and clinicopathologic observations. *American Journal of Veterinary Research* 47: 2300–2308.

Kyles, A.E. (2001). Traumatic separation of the auricular and annular cartilages in two cats. *Veterinary Surgery* 148: 696–697.

Lahiani, J. and Niebauer, G.W. (2020). On the nature of canine aural haematoma with continuous vacuum drainage. *Journal of Small Animal Practice* 61: 195–201.

Lanz, O.I. and Wood, B.C. (2004). Surgery of the ear and pinna. *Veterinary Clinics of North America* 34: 567–599.

Larson, S. (1968). Intrachondral rupture and hematoma formation in the external ear of dogs. *Pathologica Veterinaria* 5: 442–450.

MacPhail, C. (2016). Current treatment options for auricular hematomas. *Veterinary Clinics of North America. Small Animal Practice* 46: 635–641.

McCarthy, P.E., Hosgood, G., and Pechman, R.D. (1995). Traumatic ear canal separations and para-aural abscessation in three dogs. *Journal of the American Animal Hospital Association* 31: 419–424.

Pavletic, M.M. (2010). Atlas of small animal wound management and reconstructive surgery. In: *Closure Options for Select Pinnal Defects*, 3e, 666–667. Ames, IA: Wiley-Blackwell.

Pavletic, M.M. (2015). Use of laterally placed vacuum drains for management of aural hematomas in five dogs. *Journal of the American Veterinary Medical Association* 246: 112–117.

Pavletic, M.M. (2018). Atlas of small animal wound management and reconstructive surgery. In: *Pinnal Reconstructive Surgery*, 4e, 773–821. Ames, IA: Wiley-Blackwell.

Romatowski, J. (1994). Nonsurgical treatment of aural hematomas, Letters to the Editor. *Journal of the American Veterinary Medical Association* 204 (9): 1318.

Smeak, D.D. (1997). Traumatic separation of the annular cartilage from the external auditory meatus in a cat. *Journal of the American Medical Association* 4: 448–450.

Stephenson, H.C. (1941). Some diseases of the ear of dogs. *Journal of the American Veterinary Medical Association* 98: 138–142.

Swaim, S.F. and Bradley, D.M. (1996). Evaluation of closed-suction drainage for treating auricular hematomas. *Journal of the American Animal Hospital Association* 32: 36–43.

Tivers, M.S. and Brockman, D.J. (2009). Separation of the auricular and annular ear cartilages: surgical repair technique and clinical use in dogs and cats. *Veterinary Surgery* 38: 349–354.

Wilson, J.W. (1983). Treatment of auricular hematoma using a teat tube. *Journal of the American Veterinary Medical Association* 182: 1081–1083.

71

Aural Neoplasia

Brad M. Matz and Jamie R. Bellah

Neoplastic and nonneoplastic conditions frequently result in mass-forming lesions and can affect the pinna and ear canal. Most neoplasms of the ear are primary. Invasion of the structures of the ear canal can occur from neoplasia of the surrounding tissues. The incidence of aural neoplasia is generally low, particularly in comparison with the incidence of otic disease in general. However, neoplastic conditions can cause concurrent otitis. Neoplastic behavior in dogs is distributed nearly evenly between benign and malignant, although malignant behavior is more commonly observed in cats.

Origins, occurrence, and clinical signs

Neoplasia arises from histologic components of the surface and structural elements of all regions of the ear. Within the ear, neoplasia originates more commonly from tissue in the pinna and external ear canal than the middle or inner ear (Fan & de Lorimier 2004). Neoplasia such as parotid salivary gland adenocarcinoma may occur peripheral to the ear and subsequently involve or invade the ear canal (Figure 71.1). Cross-sectional imaging is helpful to evaluate regional anatomy. Neoplastic transformation of specific cell types leading to development of specific neoplasms involves epithelial cells (squamous and basal), glandular cells (ceruminous and sebaceous), mast cells, melanocytes, cutaneous plasma cells, and histiocytes, among others. Vascular endothelium, fibroblasts, chondrocytes, and other mesenchymal cells may also give rise to neoplasia within the supporting structures of the ear. Although common ear neoplasms in dogs and cats exist, most cutaneous tumors have been reported incidentally to involve the ear in both species (Vail & Withrow 2007). Inflammation resulting from chronic otitis externa with associated glandular dysplasia is thought to be a factor contributing to both benign and malignant tumor development, particularly in the cocker spaniel breed, which is overrepresented in aural neoplasia (Vail & Withrow 2007).

Clinical signs may not always be apparent, but observation or palpation of a mass are common indicators of aural neoplasia. Auricular discharge or odor may be noted, with other signs indicative of otitis externa or media. Aural neoplasia is usually unilateral, although three dogs with bilateral ear canal neoplasia have been reported (Zur 2005). Benign tumors tend to be less friable, nonulcerated, and pedunculated, whereas malignant masses can be ulcerated or broad based. These characteristics are tendencies and not always consistent with expected behavior. Neurologic signs such as facial paralysis, vestibular abnormalities, or Horner's syndrome may be seen and can be indicative of tumor invasion (Figure 71.2). Approximately 10% of dogs with malignant lesions will present with neurologic signs. Invasive tumors in both dogs and cats in the region of the tympanic bulla and within the bulla may result in neurologic signs such as facial nerve paralysis, Horner's syndrome, and temporomandibular joint pain from tumor interference (Yoshikawa et al. 2008). In cats, neurologic signs occur more commonly (25%) and may be associated with benign and malignant lesions (Vail & Withrow 2007). In cats and dogs, local invasion is common in most malignant tumors of the ear, but the frequency of distant metastasis is typically low (Hauck & Oblak 2020).

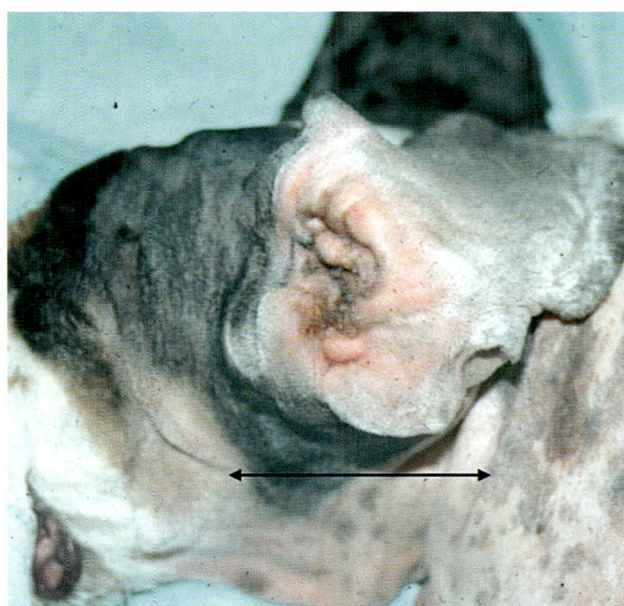

Figure 71.1 Parotid gland adenocarcinoma located ventral and encircling the left horizontal ear canal in a cocker spaniel dog. The arrow shows the diameter of the tumor. Pulmonary metastasis was noted at the time of diagnosis.

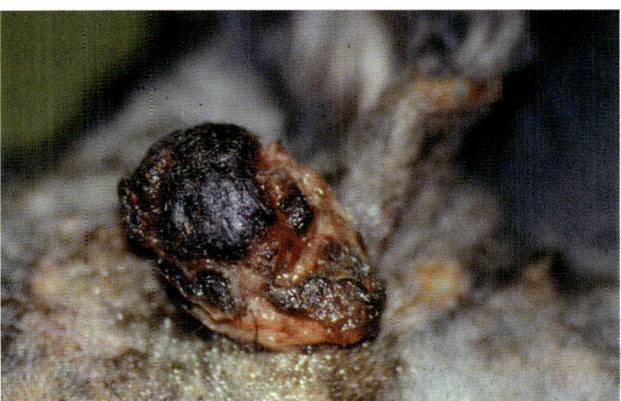

Figure 71.2 Basal cell tumor at the ventral aspect of the left ear canal in a chow.

Imaging modalities, reviewed in Chapter 75, are helpful in identifying the location and extent of neoplastic involvement (particularly cross-sectional imaging studies). Definitive diagnosis is by histopathologic examination of tissue. Fine-needle biopsy of external ear masses has been shown to accurately differentiate neoplastic processes from inflammatory polyps in cats; however, differentiation of malignant from benign neoplasms by fine-needle biopsy was not similarly precise (De Lorenzi *et al.* 2005). Median survival time following surgery for dogs and cats ranges from 4 to 180 months. Mitoses per high-powered field, degree of extension

beyond the ear canal, neurologic signs, and biopsy diagnosis all impact outcome (Hauck & Oblak 2020).

Tumors of the canine ear

Benign tumors

Benign tumors of the ear in dogs account for about 40% of ear neoplasms and include ceruminous gland adenoma, sebaceous gland adenoma, basal cell tumors (Figure 71.2), histiocytomas, papillomas, and fibromas (Berzon & Bunch 1980), inflammatory polyps (Pratschke 2003), and others (Fan & de Lorimier 2004; Vail & Withrow 2007) (Figure 71.3). Multiple follicular cysts were reported to obstruct the external ear canal in a dog, but are nonneoplastic (Gatineau *et al.* 2010). Ceruminous gland adenomas, which arise from modified apocrine glands termed ceruminous glands, are cured by complete excision.

In general, benign tumors may be treated by conservative surgical resection as long as adequate margins are attainable. Curative-intent resections, such as total ear canal

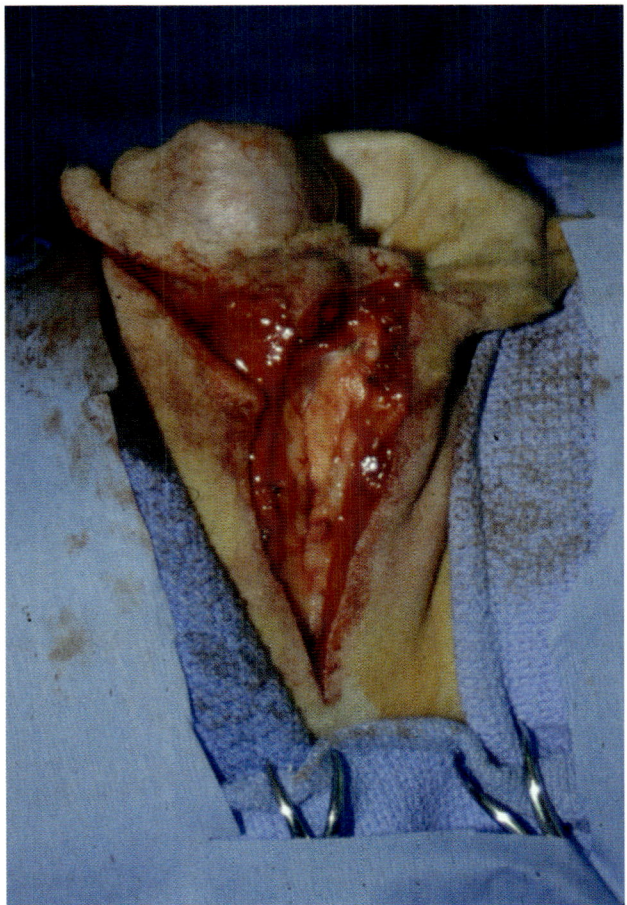

Figure 71.3 Hemangiopericytoma located on the rostral aspect of the pinna in a golden retriever.

ablation, are warranted when necessary to limit the possibility of regrowth and provide local control.

Histiocytomas, of epidermal Langerhans cell lineage, occur typically in young dogs as a solitary mass. These are rapidly growing tumors that usually regress spontaneously. The mechanism of regression is thought to be related to immunologic recognition (Kipar *et al.* 1998; Moore *et al.* 1996).

Three tumors that arise from sebaceous glands are benign: sebaceous hyperplasia, sebaceous epithelioma, and sebaceous adenoma. All tend to have a cauliflower appearance and can be greasy. Complete excision is curative (Scott & Anderson 1990).

Inflammatory polyps are not common in dogs but have been reported (Pollock 1971; Fingland *et al.* 1993; London *et al.* 1996; Pratschke 2003). It has been recommended that polypoid lesions in the canine nasopharynx or ear should not be considered as inflammatory polyps like in cats (Greci & Mortellaro 2016). Breeds that have been reported to be affected include shar-pei and cocker spaniel (Fan & de Lorimier 2004). The site of origin and management (traction or excision) of inflammatory polyps in dogs are similar to those in cats. Dogs with benign tumors of the middle ear may have long survival after surgery (Little *et al.* 1989). Other reports of benign tumors affecting the middle ear have included papilloma, basal cell tumor, and fibromyxoma (Bischel & Schärer 1985; Little *et al.* 1989).

Malignant neoplasms

Malignant neoplasms of the canine ear are slightly more common than benign tumors and ceruminous gland adenocarcinomas are overrepresented. In general, they tend to be locally invasive and associated with a suppurative to pyogranulomatous inflammatory response, but do not commonly metastasize (London *et al.* 1996; Moisan & Watson 1996).

Other malignant tumors include squamous cell carcinoma, carcinoma of undetermined origin, sebaceous cell carcinoma, and others such as melanoma and mesenchymal tumors (Figure 71.4). Most originate in the pinna or external ear canal. Ceruminous gland adenocarcinoma, sebaceous gland adenocarcinoma (Figure 71.5), a malignant jugulotympanic paraganglioma, and a malignant anaplastic neoplasm have been diagnosed in the middle ear (Little *et al.* 1989). Mast cell tumors may arise within the ear pinna and retrospective data suggest that their behavior at this location is aggressive, with greater than 40% being associated with regional lymph node metastasis (Higginbotham *et al.* 2000). Local recurrence is a risk if complete excision is not accomplished (Fan & de Lorimier 2004). A more recent article stated that margin status was not

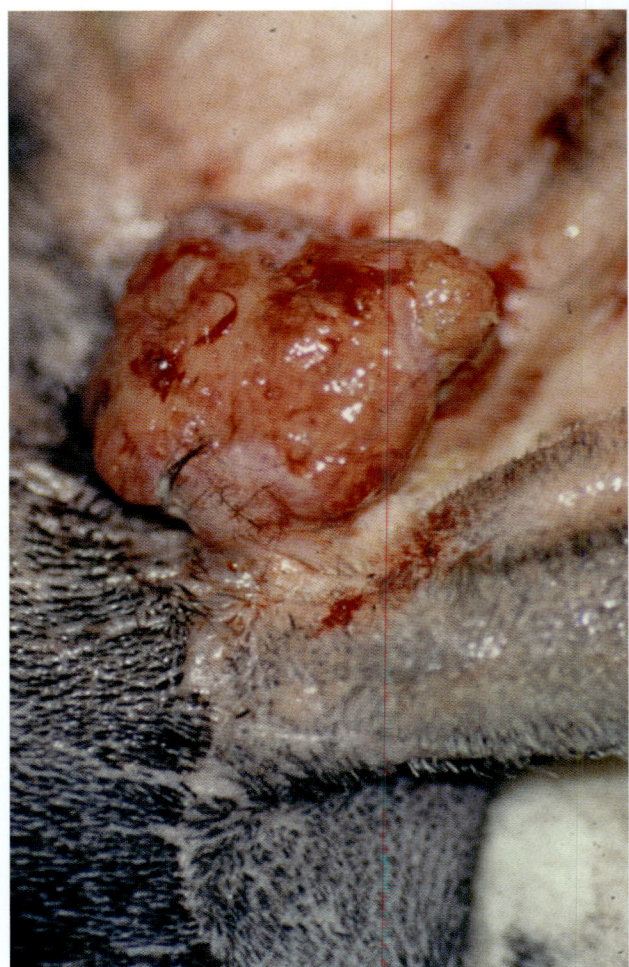

Figure 71.4 Recurrence of sebaceous gland adenocarcinoma after conservative excision in a cocker spaniel.

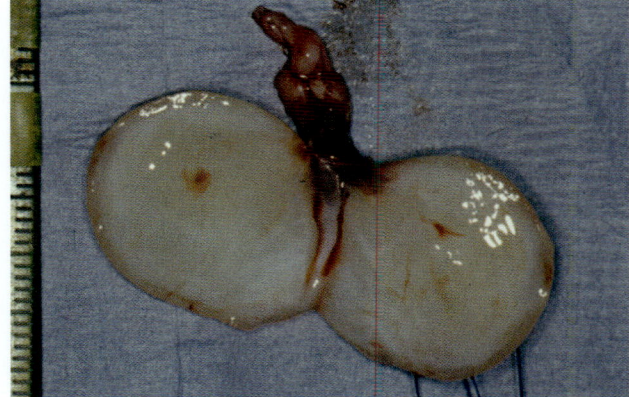

Figure 71.5 Feline inflammatory polyp showing typical fibrous appearance. This polyp extended down the eustachian tube to a nasopharyngeal location.

predictive of recurrence or survival time for pinnal mast cell tumors (Schwab *et al.* 2014) Aspirate cytology of the scar can be helpful in determining risk of regrowth or need for adjuvant therapy (Lee *et al.* 2021) Sebaceous gland adenocarcinomas are associated with local invasion and regional metastasis and may require adjunctive therapy in addition to curative intent surgical resection (Strafuss 1976). Neoplasia from structures that surround the ear canal, for example parotid salivary gland carcinoma, may encroach upon or invade neighboring aural tissues.

Curative-intent surgical resection is the best treatment for malignant neoplasms that involve the ear canal. Significant pinnal resection, vertical ear canal resection, and total ear canal ablation may be appropriate depending on the location, size, and depth of the mass. In one study in dogs with ceruminous gland adenocarcinoma, 3 of 4 dogs managed by less aggressive lateral ear resection showed recurrence, whereas in 11 dogs that underwent total ear canal ablation there was no recurrence 36 months after surgery (Marino *et al.* 1993). Deep masses that encroach upon or invade into the tympanum or external acoustic meatus or skull may not be amenable to complete excision. In situations where disease has been incompletely excised or metastasis to regional lymph nodes and beyond has occurred, consideration of adjunctive therapy such as regional radiation therapy and chemotherapy is appropriate. In general, poor prognostic factors relating to ear canal neoplasia in dogs include extensive tumor mass, invasion of the tympanic bulla, and conservative surgery (North & Banks 2009).

Tumors of the feline ear

Benign tumors

The most common benign aural neoplasms in cats are of ceruminous gland origin, while other tumor types are similar to those that occur in dogs. Benign tumors that originate in the cat's pinna include basal cell epithelioma, rhabdomyoma, and hemangioma (Miller *et al.* 1991; Fan & de Lorimier 2004). Other tumors like carcinoma, melanoma, and mast cell tumor may have a benign behavior. Cutaneous fibropapilloma (feline sarcoid) has been reported in a cat (Hanna & Dunn 2003).

Benign tumors are managed effectively by local excision, although rarely a basal cell tumor may invade neighboring and lymphatic and vascular structures (Day *et al.* 1994). Cryosurgical ablation is appropriate in select cases. Basal cell tumors and melanomas can be pigmented. Melanomas that involve the pinna are most commonly noninvasive; however, an aggressive phenotype with metastasis to regional lymph nodes can rarely

occur (Miller *et al.* 1991; Luna *et al.* 2000). Mast cell tumors are commonly found on the feline pinna and account for 59% of the tumors occurring in the region of the head. The incidence is highest in Siamese cats (Miller *et al.* 1991). Conservative local excision is sufficient to control mast cell tumors and local recurrence is uncommon in cats (Molander-McCrary *et al.* 1998; Johnson *et al.* 2002). Rhabdomyomas arise from striated skeletal muscle and are treated by local excision (Roth 1990). An unusual mass, a teratoma, involving the region of the ear canal has been reported and was successfully excised (Van Goethem *et al.* 2010).

Inflammatory polyps are the most common benign tumor of the feline ear (Fan & de Lorimier 2004). These masses are composed of a mixed inflammatory infiltrate amid loose fibrovascular tissue and covered by either stratified squamous or ciliated epithelium. Polyps usually project singularly into the external ear canal through the tympanum or into the nasopharynx from the eustachian tube (Figure 71.5). However, they have been reported to occur concurrently in the ear canal and the nasopharynx, and to develop in the contralateral ear (MacPhail *et al.* 2007). The origin of inflammatory polyps is the mucosa of the eustachian tube, pharynx, or middle ear, but the etiology remains undetermined. Ascending infection from the nasopharynx, chronic otitis media, long-standing inflammation of the upper respiratory tract, and a congenital origin are considered possible explanations (Fan & de Lorimier 2004). Attempts to detect feline herpesvirus 1 and calicivirus within inflammatory polyps by polymerase chain reaction (PCR) and reverse transcriptase PCR have produced variable results. It has been suggested that the lack of detection of these viruses may be secondary to immunologic clearance of the organisms prior to polyp diagnosis (Veir *et al.* 2002; MacPhail *et al.* 2007). Clinical signs include those typical of otitis externa and otitis media, with the additional stertorous respiration and nasal discharge that may accompany the nasopharyngeal polyp. Diagnosis is by visual or otoscopic inspection of the external ear canal and nasopharyngeal examination (polyps may be seen by retraction of the soft palate) and by imaging techniques (see Chapter 75). Histologic examination of biopsy specimens will confirm the diagnosis and is important, as some masses that appear as inflammatory polyps may be neoplastic (Tobias & Morris 2005). Surgical management of inflammatory polyps in cats is covered in Chapter 78.

Malignant neoplasms

In cats, over 80% of neoplasms originating in the ear are malignant (London *et al.* 1996). The most common malignant neoplasms involving the feline ear are squamous

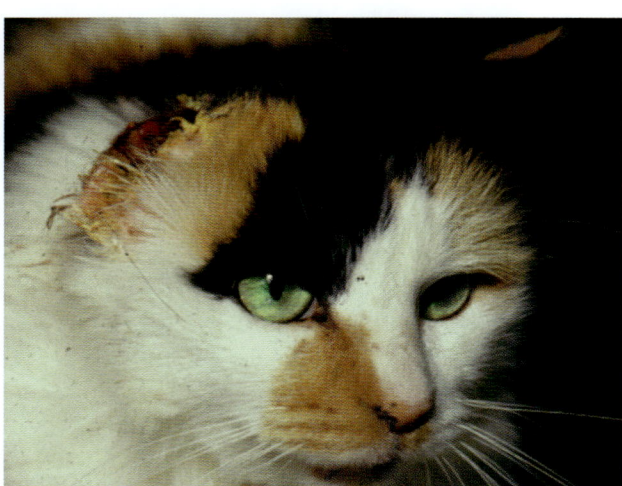

Figure 71.6 The right ear pinna and canal of this cat have been destroyed by a squamous cell carcinoma. The cat had facial paralysis and Horner's syndrome that were evident at presentation.

cell carcinoma (particularly involving the pinna) and ceruminous gland adenocarcinoma, with the mean age of diagnosis being 11 years (Vail & Withrow 2007). Ceruminous gland carcinoma is more common in the external ear canal (London *et al.* 1996). Sebaceous gland adenocarcinoma and carcinoma of undetermined origin also occur, and lymphoma has been reported (Carpenter *et al.* 1987; Trevor & Martin 1993; de Lorimier *et al.* 2003). One cat is reported to have had pulmonary metastasis in two investigations (Marino *et al.* 1994; London *et al.* 1996). Soft tissue infiltration is more commonly noted in cats (Fan & de Lorimier 2004). In cats with malignant aural tumors, 5–15% are reported to have regional lymph node or distant metastasis at the time of initial diagnosis, similar to 10% of dogs (Vail & Withrow 2007). Neoplastic infiltration of the external ear canal results in secondary otitis externa, but if primary neoplasia of the middle ear or invasion into middle ear structures occurs, otorrhea, a pain response on opening the mouth, vestibular signs, facial nerve paralysis, and Horner's syndrome (Figure 71.6) may be noted (Fiorito 1986; London *et al.* 1996). In some instances, dyspnea from tumor expansion or encroachment near respiratory structures may also occur (Fan & de Lorimier 2004). Ceruminous gland carcinoma has been shown to destroy the integrity of the ear canal (Miller & Lambrechts 2006).

Neurologic signs associated with aural neoplasia are often associated with deep neoplastic invasion. In one study, neurologic signs present at the time of tumor diagnosis were found in 9 of 13 cats with squamous cell carcinoma, and those that had squamous cell carcinoma or carcinoma of undetermined origin had shorter survival times (London *et al.* 1996). The incidence of neurologic signs in cats when aural neoplasia and benign polyps are combined is 25% (Vail & Withrow 2007). In a more recent investigation, only 5 of 59 cats with nonneoplastic middle ear disease noted at necropsy had associated clinical signs, namely peripheral vestibular disease and Horner's syndrome (Schlicksup *et al.* 2009). Meningeal carcinomatosis associated with aural squamous cell carcinoma, thought to occur by hematogenous spread, has been reported in two cats (Salvadori *et al.* 2004). Median survival times are affected by the presence of neurologic signs at the time of diagnosis: 15.5 months in cats without neurologic disease compared with 1.5 months when neurologic signs are noted (Vail & Withrow 2007). Similarly, cats that do not have lymphatic or vascular invasion at the time of diagnosis have a median survival time of 22 months, whereas those with invasion survive 4 months (Vail & Withrow 2007). Ceruminous gland carcinoma was reported to have a median survival time of 50.3 months after total ear canal ablation in 44 cats (Bacon *et al.* 2003). In the same report, the mitotic index (MI) could be used as a prognostic indicator, as cats with ceruminous gland carcinoma with an MI of 2 or less survived significantly longer that those that had an MI of 3 or more (Bacon *et al.* 2003). Incidentally, Horner's syndrome and facial nerve paralysis were present after surgery and thought to be secondary to hypothesized fragility of the feline tympanic plexus and facial nerve (Bacon *et al.* 2003). In another report of 16 cats with total ear canal ablation for ceruminous gland adenocarcinoma, the median disease-free interval was 42 months, with a recurrence rate of 25% (Marino *et al.* 1994).

In cats, squamous cell carcinomas are associated with anatomic regions exposed to sunlight, particularly those that lack skin pigmentation, where there is a 13.4 times greater risk of developing squamous cell carcinoma (Dorn *et al.* 1971). In addition, premalignant actinic keratosis and squamous cell carcinoma of the pinna have been shown to contain mutant p53, which is similar to the stepwise development of squamous cell carcinoma after chronic ultraviolet (UV) radiation exposure in humans (Albaric *et al.* 2001). Although the pinna is the most common region for squamous cell carcinoma to develop in the ear, all regions of the ear canal may be affected. Squamous cell carcinoma is locally aggressive and is multicentric in 15% of cats (Fan & de Lorimier 2004). Rarely, squamous cell carcinoma of the pinna that is more anaplastic or undifferentiated may undergo metastasis to regional lymph nodes or lung. Surgical management of squamous cell carcinoma in cats requires early resection regardless of the site. Pinnal amputation has been shown to cure squamous cell

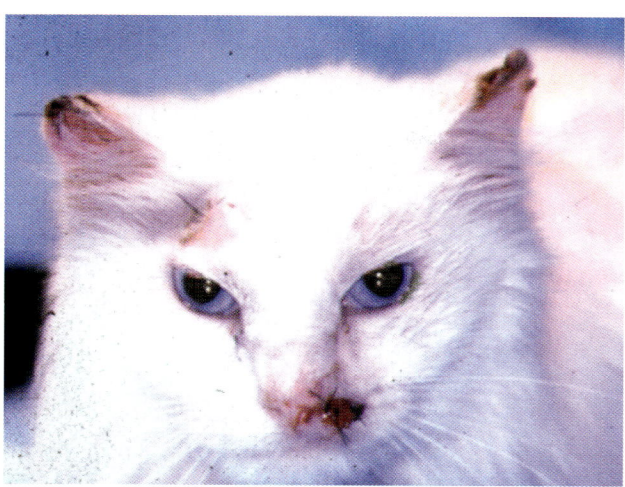

Figure 71.7 Bilateral hemangiosarcoma of the pinna with concomitant nasal and eyelid squamous cell carcinoma in a cat.

carcinoma in this location (Lana *et al.* 1997). Cryosurgery may be considered for superficial lesions of the pinna, and if done properly only one cycle of cryosurgery is required (Clarke 1991). Three freeze–thaw cycles are typically used. Photodynamic therapy has also been used as a local treatment modality for squamous cell carcinoma in cats and application to early lesions results in long-term responses, but lesion thickness is important (Stell *et al.* 2001; Vail & Withrow 2007). However, since damage from UV light has already occurred, future tumor development is likely unless the pinnae are removed. Regional hyperthermia, multiple forms of radiation therapy, and chemotherapy have been used adjunctively to treat squamous cell carcinoma in cats (Fan & de Lorimier 2004; Vail & Withrow 2007).

Malignant tumors of nonepithelial origin rarely occur in cats. Hemangiosarcomas have been reported in the pinna of cats (Figure 71.7) and behave aggressively, with local recurrence and a poor median disease-free survival of 9.5 months (Miller *et al.* 1992). In the aforementioned report, the hemangiosarcomas occurred in white cats and were consistent with the cutaneous vascular tumorigenesis associated with chronic exposure to sunlight in dogs (Nikula *et al.* 1992). Fibrosarcomas rarely involve the region of the ear in cats. The fibrosarcomas that are not associated with vaccination have low metastatic potential and are locally invasive (Hendrick *et al.* 1994). Lymphoma should also be considered as a differential diagnosis.

Poor prognostic indicators in cats with aural neoplasia include the presence of neurologic signs, invasion by squamous cell carcinoma or carcinoma of undetermined origin (undifferentiated carcinoma), or the presence of lymphatic or vascular invasion (North & Banks 2009).

Alternative or adjunctive therapy for ear neoplasia

Curative-intent surgical resection of aural neoplasia clearly provides the best chance for resolution of neoplastic disease. Other treatment modalities are useful in some circumstances, depending on the region of the tumor and the tumor behavior. Cryosurgery has been used with some success for neoplasia of the pinna, but does not allow margin assessment in comparison to sharp excision.

Radiation therapy can be used to support adjunctive treatment of aural neoplasia in two ways: (i) curative radiation therapy may be attempted and can be used as a primary mode of therapy or as an adjunct to incomplete excision; or (ii) it may be used in a palliative manner where the goal is to ameliorate pain rather than achieve cure. Such principles are applied in human patients and have been suggested to be applicable for use in small animals (Yoshikawa *et al.* 2008). Reports of the efficacy of radiation therapy of aural neoplasia are infrequent. Ceruminous gland adenocarcinoma was treated by external beam radiotherapy (48 Gy) in five dogs and six cats and resulted in a median progression-free interval of 40 months and a 1-year survival rate of 56% (Theon *et al.* 1994). Four animals had tumor recurrence and three had distant metastasis. The efficacy of radiation therapy has been more frequently reported for other regions of the head and neck, particularly nasal squamous cell carcinoma in cats (Fan & de Lorimier 2004).

Photodynamic therapy has been used for aural tumors (Lucroy 2007). A photosensitizing agent that is preferentially retained by the neoplasm is administered intravenously or topically. The subsequent interaction with a light-emitting diode source results in activation of the agent and, since it is concentrated within the tumor, a focused region of treatment occurs. Cytotoxic free radicals are produced within the tumor when oxygen interacts with the photosensitizing agent. Factors that affect the efficacy of this therapy include the type of photosensitizing agent used, the tumor to normal tissue photosensitizer ratio, and the energy dose received by the target tissue (Merkel & Biel 2001). Photodynamic therapy is used for superficial neoplasms because of the limitation of light penetration through tissue, and therefore photosensitizers that are too deep to be activated by light will have no tissue impact (Fan & de Lorimier 2004). Photosensitizing agents that have been used in cats include 5-aminolevulinic acid (topical) and aluminum phthalocyanine tetrasulfonate (intravenous). Cats treated by these agents have good initial responses to treatment, but regrowth within 18 months or only a partial response is indicative of poor long-term control (Peaston *et al.* 1993; Hahn *et al.* 1998; Stell *et al.* 2001).

Regional hyperthermia (>42 °C) has been shown to have direct cytotoxic effects and to potentiate the anticancer effects of chemotherapy, immunotherapy, and radiation therapy. Targeted tissues may be treated using electrodes positioned to direct radiofrequency current though tissue positioned between the electrodes (Fan & de Lorimier 2004). One disadvantage, as with cryosurgery, is that tumor margins cannot be adequately ascertained.

Topical immune response modification and stimulation with imiquimod, an immune system modifier that possesses antitumor and antiviral activity, is used to treat actinic keratoses in humans. Clinical resolution of actinic keratoses and squamous cell carcinoma in a cat was noted after 12 weeks of topical therapy (5% imiquimod, three times per week). No relapse of pinnal lesions was noted in 5 months, but biopsies were not done to confirm resolution of disease (Peters-Kennedy *et al.* 2008).

Attempts to provide local disease control using laser surgery (Nd:YAG), various types of radiation therapy, and radiation brachytherapy have been attempted in cats and dogs with variable success (Fan & de Lorimier 2004). Many reports are for nonaural uses, particularly nasal tumors, but the results may or may not be applicable to aural neoplasia. Systemic and intralesional chemotherapy has been used in cats with nonresectable squamous cell carcinoma. Intralesional chemotherapy for treatment of squamous cell carcinoma in cats has produced complete cure in 64–73.3% of cases reported (Fan & de Lorimier 2004). Most of the aforementioned therapies have been used for nasal planum squamous cell carcinoma in cats, but they may be applicable to aural neoplasms as well, depending on the location and extent of disease.

References

Albaric, O., Bret, L., Amardeihl, M., and Delverdier, M. (2001). Immunohistochemical expression of p53 in animal tumors: a methodological study using four anti-human p53 antibodies. *Histology and Histopathology* 16: 113–121.

Bacon, N.J., Gilbert, R.L., Bostock, D.E., and White, R.A. (2003). Total ear canal ablation in the cat: indications, morbidity and long-term survival. *Journal of Small Animal Practice* 44: 430–444.

Berzon, J.L. and Bunch, S.E. (1980). Recurrent otitis externa-media secondary to a fibroma in the middle ear. *Journal of the American Animal Hospital Association* 16: 73–77.

Bischel, P. and Schärer, V. (1985). Un néoplasme de l'oreille moyenne á l'orinine d'un syndrôme vestibularire chez le chien. *Schweizer Archiv für Tierheilkunde* 127: 717–722.

Carpenter, J.C., Andrews, L.K., and Holzworth, J. (1987). Tumors and tumorlike lesions. In: *Diseases of the Cat* (ed. J. Holzworth), 565–569. Philadelphia, PA: WB Saunders.

Clarke, R.E. (1991). Cryosurgical treatment of cutaneous squamous cell carcinoma. *Australian Veterinary Practice* 21: 148–153.

Day, D.G., Couto, C.G., Weisbrode, S.E. and Smeak, D.D. (1994). Basal cell carcinoma in two cats. *Journal of the American Animal Hospital Association* 30: 265–269.

De Lorenzi, D., Bonfanti, U., Masserdotti, C., and Tranquillo, M. (2005). Fine-needle biopsy of external ear canal masses in the cat: cytologic results and histologic correlations in 27 cases. *Veterinary Clinical Pathology* 34: 100–105.

Dorn, C.R., Taylor, D.O., and Schneider, R. (1971). Sunlight exposure and risk of developing cutaneous and oral squamous cell carcinoma in white cats. *Journal of the National Cancer Institute* 46: 1073–1078.

Fan, T.M. and de Lorimier, L.P. (2004). Inflammatory polyps and aural neoplasia. *Veterinary Clinics of North America: Small Animal Practice* 34: 489–509.

Fingland, R.B., Gratzek, A., Vorhies, M.W. and Kirpensteijn, J. (1993). Nasopharyngeal polyp in a dog. *Journal of the American Animal Hospital Association* 29: 311–314.

Fiorito, D.A. (1986). Oral and peripheral vestibular signs in a cat with squamous cell carcinoma. *Journal of the American Veterinary Medical Association* 188: 71–72.

Gatineau, M., Lussier, B., and Alexander, K. (2010). Multiple follicular cysts of the ear canal in a dog. *Journal of the American Animal Hospital Association* 46: 107–114.

Greci, V. and Mortellaro, C.M. (2016). Management of otic and nasopharyngeal, and nasal polyps in cats and dogs. *Veterinary Clinics of North America: Small Animal Practice* 46: 643–661.

Hahn, K.A., Panjehpour, M., and Legendre, A.M. (1998). Photodynamic therapy response in cats with cutaneous squamous cell carcinoma as a function of fluence. *Veterinary Dermatology* 9: 3–7.

Hanna, P.E. and Dunn, D. (2003). Cutaneous fibropapilloma in a cat (feline sarcoid). *Canadian Veterinary Journal* 44: 601–602.

Hauck, M.L. and Oblak, M.L. (2020). Tumors of the skin and subcutaneous tissues. In: *Withrow and MacEwen's Small Animal Clinical Oncology*, 6e (ed. D.M. Vail, D.H. Thamm and J.M. Liptak), 352–366. St. Louis, MO: Elsevier.

Hendrick, M.J., Sofer, F.S., and Goldschmidt, M.H. (1994). Comparison of fibrosarcomas that developed at vaccination sites and at nonvaccination sites in cats: 239 cases (1991–1992). *Journal of the American Veterinary Medical Association* 205: 1425–1429.

Higginbotham, M.L., Henry, C.J., Watson, Z. et al. (2000). Biological behavior of canine aural mast cell tumors. In: *Proceedings of the 20th Annual Meeting of the Veterinary Cancer Society*, vol. 52. Pacific Grove, CA: Veterinary Cancer Society.

Johnson, T.O., Schulman, F.Y., Lipscomb, T.P., and Yantis, L.D. (2002). Histopathology and biologic behavior of pleomorphic cutaneous mast cell tumors in fifteen cats. *Veterinary Pathology* 39: 452–457.

Kipar, A., Baumgartner, W., Kremmer, E. et al. (1998). Expression of major histocompatibility complex class II antigen in neoplastic cells of canine cutaneous histiocytoma. *Veterinary Immunology and Immunopathology* 62: 1–13.

Lana, S.E., Ogilvie, G.K., Withrow, S.J. et al. (1997). Feline cutaneous squamous cell carcinoma of the nasal planum and the pinnae: 61 cases. *Journal of the American Animal Hospital Association* 199: 329–332.

Lee, C.E., Lindley, S.S., Smith, A.N. et al. (2021). Predictive ability of fine-needle aspirate cytology for incompletely resected mast cell tumor surgical sites. *Canadian Veterinary Journal* 62: 141–144.

Little, C.J.L., Pearson, G.R., and Lane, J.G. (1989). Neoplasia involving the middle ear cavity of dogs. *Veterinary Surgery* 124: 54–57.

London, C.A., Dubilzeig, P.R., Vail, D.M. et al. (1996). Evaluation of dogs and cats with tumors of the ear canal: 145 cases (1978–1992).

Journal of the American Veterinary Medical Association 208: 1413–1418.

de Lorimier, L.P., Alexander, S.D., and Fan, T.M. (2003). T-cell lymphoma of the tympanic bulla in a feline leukemia virus-negative cat. *Canadian Veterinary Journal* 4: 987–999.

Lucroy, M.D. (2007). Photodynamic therapy. In: *Withrow and MacEwen's Small Animal Clinical Oncology*, 4e (ed. S.J. Withrow and D.M. Vail), 283–289. Philadelphia, PA: WB Saunders.

Luna, L.D., Higginbotham, M.L., Henry, C.L. et al. (2000). Feline non-ocular melanoma: a retrospective study of 23 cases (1991–1999). *Journal of Feline Medicine and Surgery* 2: 173–181.

MacPhail, C.M., Kudnig, S.T., and Lappin, M.R. (2007). Atypical manifestations of feline inflammatory polyps in three cats. *Journal of Feline Medicine and Surgery* 9: 219–225.

Marino, D.J., MacDonald, J.M., Matthiesen, D.T., and Patnaik, A.K. (1994). Results of surgery in cats with ceruminous gland adenocarcinoma. *Journal of the American Animal Hospital Association* 30: 54–58.

Marino, D.J., MacDonald, J.M., Matthiesen, D.T. et al. (1993). Results of surgery and long-term follow-up in dogs with ceruminous gland adenocarcinoma. *Journal of the American Animal Hospital Association* 29: 560–563.

Merkel, L.K. and Biel, M.A. (2001). Photodynamic therapy. In: *Withrow and MacEwen's Small Animal Clinical Oncology*, 3e (ed. S.J. Withrow and E.G. MacEwen), 86–91. Philadelphia, PA: WB Saunders.

Miller, J.M. and Lambrechts, N. (2006). What is your diagnosis. *Journal of the American Veterinary Medical Association* 229: 1245–1246.

Miller, M.A., Nelson, S.L., and Turk, J.R. (1991). Cutaneous neoplasia in 340 cats. *Veterinary Pathology* 28: 389–395.

Miller, M.A., Ramos, J.A., and Kreeger, J.M. (1992). Cutaneous vascular neoplasia in 15 cats: clinical, morphologic, and immunohistochemical studies. *Veterinary Pathology* 29: 329–336.

Moisan, P.G. and Watson, G.L. (1996). Ceruminous gland tumors in dogs and cats: a review of 124 cases. *Journal of the American Animal Hospital Association* 32: 449–443.

Molander-McCrary, H., Henry, C.J., Potter, K. et al. (1998). Cutaneous mast cell tumors in cats: 32 cases (1991–1994). *Journal of the American Animal Hospital Association* 34: 281–284.

Moore, P.F., Schrenzel, M.D., Affolter, V.K. et al. (1996). Canine cutaneous histiocytoma is an epidermotropic Langerhans cell histiocytosis that expresses CD1 and specific beta 2-integrin molecules. *American Journal of Pathology* 148: 1699–1708.

Nikula, K.J., Benjamin, S.A., Angleton, G.M. et al. (1992). Ultraviolet radiation, solar dermatosis, and cutaneous neoplasia in beagle dogs. *Radiation Research* 129: 11–18.

North, S. and Banks, T. (2009). *Small Animal Onology: An Introduction*. Philadelphia, PA: Elsevier.

Peaston, A.E., Leach, M.W., and Higgins, R.J. (1993). Photodynamic therapy for nasal and aural squamous cell carcinoma in cats. *Journal of the American Veterinary Medical Association* 202: 1261–1265.

Peters-Kennedy, J., Scott, D.W., and Miller, W.H. (2008). Apparent clinical resolution of pinnal actinic keratoses and squamous cell carcinoma in a cat using topical imiquimod 5% cream. *Journal of Feline Medicine and Surgery* 10: 593–599.

Pollock, S. (1971). Nasopharyngeal polyp in a dog. A case study. *Veterinary Medicine, Small Animal Clinician* 66: 705–706.

Pratschke, K.M. (2003). Inflammatory polyps of the middle ear in 5 dogs. *Veterinary Surgery* 32: 292.

Roth, L. (1990). Rhabdomyoma of the ear pinna in four cats. *Journal of Comparative Pathology* 103: 237–240.

Salvadori, C., Cantile, C., and Arispici, M. (2004). Meningeal carcinomatosis in two cats. *Journal of Comparative Pathology* 131: 246–251.

Schlicksup, M.D., Van Winkle, T.J., and Holt, D.E. (2009). Prevalence of clinical abnormalities in cats found to have nonneoplastic middle ear disease at necropsy: 59 cases (1991–2007). *Journal of the American Veterinary Medical Association* 235: 841–843.

Schwab, T.M., Popovitch, C., DeBiasio, J., and Goldschmidt, M. (2014). Clinical outcome for MCTs of canine pinnae treated with surgical excision (2004-2008). *Journal of the American Animal Hospital Association* 50: 187–191.

Scott, D.W. and Anderson, W.I. (1990). Canine sebaceous gland tumors: a retrospective analysis of 172 cases. *Canine Practice* 15: 19–21, 24–27.

Stell, A.J., Dobson, J.M., and Langmack, K. (2001). Photodynamic therapy of feline superficial squamous cell carcinoma using topical 5-aminolaevulinic acid. *Journal of Small Animal Practice* 42: 164–169.

Strafuss, A.C. (1976). Sebaceous gland adenocarcinoma in dogs. *Journal of the American Veterinary Medical Association* 169: 640–642.

Theoń, A.P., Barthez, P.Y., Madewell, B.R., and Griffey, S.M. (1994). Radiation therapy of ceruminous gland carcinoma in dogs and cats. *Journal of the American Veterinary Medical Association* 205: 566–569.

Tobias, K.M. and Morris, D. (2005). The ear. In: *BSAVA Manual of Canine and Feline Head, Neck and Thoracic Surgery* (ed. D.J. Brockman and D.E. Holt), 56–72. Gloucester: British Small Animal Veterinary Association.

Trevor, P.B. and Martin, R.A. (1993). Tympanic bulla osteotomy for treatment of middle-ear disease in cats: 19 cases (1984–1991). *Journal of the American Veterinary Medical Association* 202: 123–128.

Vail, D.M. and Withrow, S.J. (2007). Tumors of the skin and subcutaneous tissues. In: *Withrow and MacEwen's Small Animal Clinical Oncology*, 4e (ed. S.J. Withrow and D.M. Vail), 374–394. Philadelphia, PA: WB Saunders.

Van Goethem, B., Bosmanns, T., and Chiers, K. (2010). Surgical resection of a mature teratoma on the head of a young cat. *Journal of the American Animal Hospital Association* 46: 121–126.

Veir, J.K., Lappin, M.R., Foley, J.E., and Getzy, D.M. (2002). Feline inflammatory polyps: historical, clinical, and PCR findings for feline calici virus and feline herpes virus-1 in 28 cases. *Journal of Feline Medicine and Surgery* 4: 195–199.

Yoshikawa, H., Mayer, M.N., Linn, K.A. et al. (2008). A dog with squamous cell carcinoma in the middle ear. *Canadian Veterinary Journal* 49: 877–879.

Zur, G. (2005). Bilateral ear canal neoplasia in three dogs. *Veterinary Dermatology* 16: 276–280.

72

Otitis Externa

Robert Kennis

Canine otitis externa can be defined as an inflammatory process involving the external ear canal and or the pinnae. Involvement of the tympanic membrane(s) and middle ear would be considered otitis media and will be discussed in Chapter 73. Neoplastic, allergic, autoimmune, developmental, parasitic, and metabolic disorders will be included in this chapter as the clinical approach will be similar and may have an inflammatory component. The historical and clinical lesions will be reviewed in each section to assist in achieving an accurate diagnosis. There will be an emphasis on surgical intervention for various otitis disorders.

The signalment may be helpful in determining the cause of the otitis. Young dogs with otitis may point toward a parasitic or developmental cause. Juvenile cellulitis may present as a pustular otitis in dogs younger than 4 months of age (Hutchings 2003). Those breeds predisposed to allergy (food allergy or atopy) are likely to develop otitis. There does not appear to be a sex predisposition to the development of otitis; however, female dogs seem to be more likely to develop atopy than male dogs.

The history at time of presentation is of utmost importance (Rosser 2004). Age of onset, duration of the problem, and a thorough medical history should be evaluated. It is helpful to determine whether the otitis is recurrent or chronic. A recurrent problem may point toward an allergic or metabolic disorder. Those that are chronic may be due to neoplasia, autoimmune, and other systemic problems. Inadequate or inappropriate treatment may lead to chronic otitis. Pruritus may be the cause of or a consequence of otitis.

A physical evaluation of the ear canals and pinnae should be performed prior to otoscopic evaluation. The hair on the pinnae should be assessed for alopecia. It should be noted whether the alopecia is symmetric or not, whether the alopecia is traumatically induced, and whether the alopecia is associated with skin lesions. All primary and secondary skin lesions should be documented. The primary lesions will be targeted if a biopsy for histopathology is indicated. The ear pinnae should be palpated to determine skin thickness. Subtle aural hematomas may be discovered along with crusting or pustular lesions that may not be readily visible. Occasionally, a pinnal–pedal reflex may be initiated when the pinnae are rubbed. This is suggestive of but not diagnostic for parasitic otitis caused by *Sarcoptes scabiei var. canis*. The ear canals should also be palpated to determine the presence of dystrophic mineralization.

It should be noted whether the otitis is unilateral or bilateral. Unilateral disease is suggestive of foreign body or neoplasia, but there are exceptions (Zur 2005). Bilateral otitis would be suggestive of systemic disease. Perpetuating factors such as bacteria or yeast infections may be unilateral or bilateral and may be different in each ear.

It has been theorized that canine otitis externa is a multifactorial disorder (August 1988). Further, the possible components can be broken down into the following categories: predisposing, primary, and perpetuating factors. In order for successful resolution of otitis externa, all of these factors must be addressed. Not all cases will have each factor present. Conversely, some cases may present with multiple factors.

The predisposing factors are those that allow for an otitis externa to develop (see Table 72.1). Consider predisposing factors to be risk factors. Stenotic ear canals are an example. Some breeds such as the shar-pei are prone to stenotic ear canals and surgical intervention may be indicated. Inflammatory polyps may be considered either a predisposing or a perpetuating factor. Increases in moisture due to environmental humidity (Gray *et al.* 2005), bathing, or frequent swimming are considered risk factors for the development of otitis and are frequently a cause of recurrent otitis. The use of otic preparations containing astringents may be helpful in reducing excessive moisture. Iatrogenic trauma from the excessive use of cleaning agents or homemade preparations may lead to excessive moisture or irritation of the epithelium of the ear canal and/or pinnae. Some dogs have hair present within the ear canal. For some patients, it can be ignored. Some dogs may present with abundant hair that can function as a foreign body by trapping moisture and ceruminous debris. Gentle mechanical removal may be helpful. However, overzealous removal may lead to inflammation and secondary infection. Each case should be evaluated individually. The use of liquid depilatory agents developed for human beings should be avoided.

Primary factors are those disease processes that directly produce otitis externa. These are summarized in Table 72.1. The goal of therapy is to identify and treat the primary factor(s). An accurate assessment is essential prior to initiating surgical intervention.

The perpetuating factors of otitis externa are bacterial or fungal infections. Malassezia organisms are common pathogens (Morris 1999). Polyps may be considered in this category as they are typically a result of chronic inflammation. Surgical intervention is usually indicated to remove polyps, but medical management is sometimes helpful. Dystrophic mineralization may be considered both a perpetuating factor and progressive pathologic change (Roth 1988).

There is sparse information in the literature regarding feline otitis. Predisposing factors such as increased moisture are less of a concern. This may be due to the upright conformation of most cat breeds as well as the fastidious nature of the cat. Ear mites and the feline scabies mite, *Notoedres cati*, are easily identified with skin scrapings, ear exudate smears, and otoscopic evaluation. Atopy and adverse food reactions may be causes of recurrent otitis. Autoimmune disorders, especially pemphigus foliaceus, will often affect the feline pinna and ear canal. Bacterial and yeast infections occur, but less frequently than in the dog. Recurrent infections will frequently have an underlying allergic cause. Oropharyngeal polyps may be a cause or effect of recurrent infections. Surgical removal

Table 72.1 Predisposing, primary, and perpetuating factors of otitis externa.

Predisposing factors of otitis externa
Moisture
Stenosis
Foreign body
Trauma
Primary factors of otitis externa
Parasitic
    Sarcoptes scabiei
    Demodex canis
    Otodectes cynotis
    Ticks
    Fly bites
    Leishmaniasis
Allergic
    Atopy
    Food allergy
    Allergic contact dermatitis
Neoplasia
Vasculitis
Autoimmune diseases
    Pemphigus foliaceus
    Pemphigus erythematosus
    Pemphigus vulgaris
    Lupus-like disorders
Adverse cutaneous drug reaction
Irritant or caustic topical reaction
Metabolic disorders
    Hyperadrenocorticism
    Hypothyroidism
Nutritional disorders
Infectious causes
Dermatophytosis
Perpetuating factors of otitis externa
Bacteria
Yeast
Progressive pathologic changes
Polyp formation

is usually indicated. Otitis media may occur without overt clinical signs of otitis externa. The tympanic membrane may be intact in these cases. Surgical and diagnostic procedures are outlined in Chapter 73.

The diagnostic procedures indicated will be different for each patient and will depend upon the differential diagnoses. In general, skin scrapings, evaluation of direct impression skin samples, a fungal culture to evaluate for dermatophytosis, and evaluation of ear exudate cytology (Figure 72.1) should be considered to be a minimum data base. Additionally, a trichogram could be performed

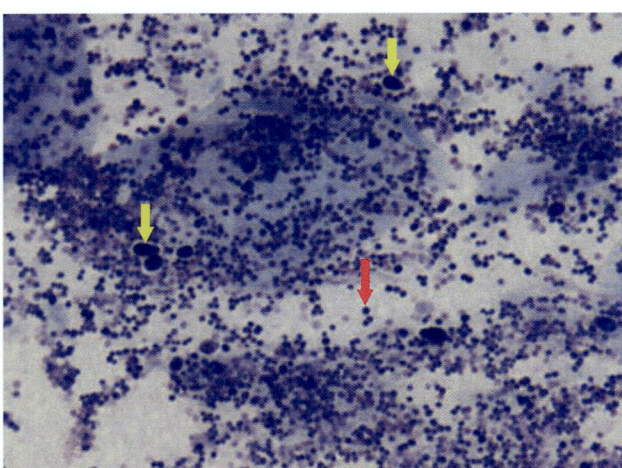

Figure 72.1 Photomicrograph of *Malassezia* organisms (yellow arrows) and cocci (red arrow) collected from ear exudation from the external ear canal of a dog. This was stained with a modified Wright's stain and viewed with an oil immersion objective.

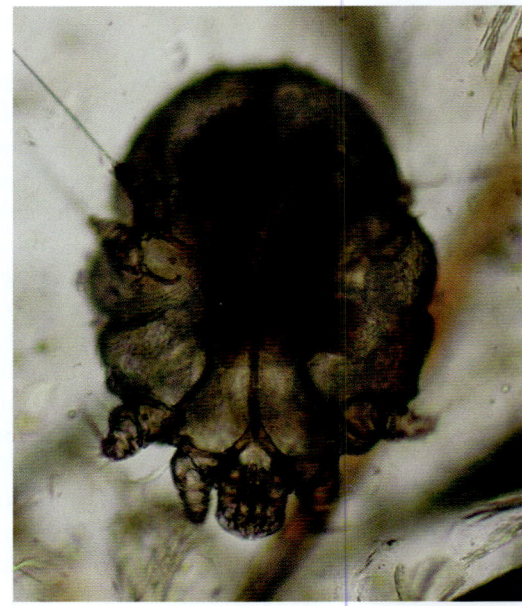

Figure 72.2 *Sarcoptes scabiei var. canis* collected from a superficial skin scraping of an ear margin.

to determine if the alopecia is traumatically induced. The same hairs will be evaluated for the presence of fungal spores suggestive of dermatophytosis. Deep skin scrapings should be performed on all alopecic pinnae to look for demodicosis. Superficial skin scrapings should be performed to look for *Sarcoptes scabiei var. canis* (Figure 72.2) if pinnal margin disease is present and if intense pruritus is present. Direct impression samples of pinnal lesions should be collected. Bacterial and/or yeast infections may be identified. Additionally, acantholytic cells suggestive of pemphigus complex disorders may be identified (Figure 72.3). Acetate tape-collected samples are an alternative to direct impression-collected samples and may be beneficial for dry and scaling lesions.

An otoscopic evaluation is always indicated. An otoscope will help to evaluate lesions present within the ear canal and assist with identifying foreign bodies or masses. It is the only way to assess the status of the tympanic membranes. Sedation and/or anesthesia may be indicated prior to an otoscopic evaluation. Ear cleaning may be necessary for a thorough evaluation. If severe stenosis prevents an otoscopic evaluation, the judicious use of oral and/or topical glucocorticoid medications may be indicated.

There are several indications for surgical intervention of canine otitis externa. Stenotic ear canals due to congenital causes can be corrected with lateral or vertical ear resection. A poor response to oral anti-inflammatory doses of glucocorticoids would be an indication to consider surgery of chronically inflamed ear canals. These procedures are rarely effective as a sole treatment for allergic causes of otitis externa. It is usually better to pursue medical management of chronically inflamed ears

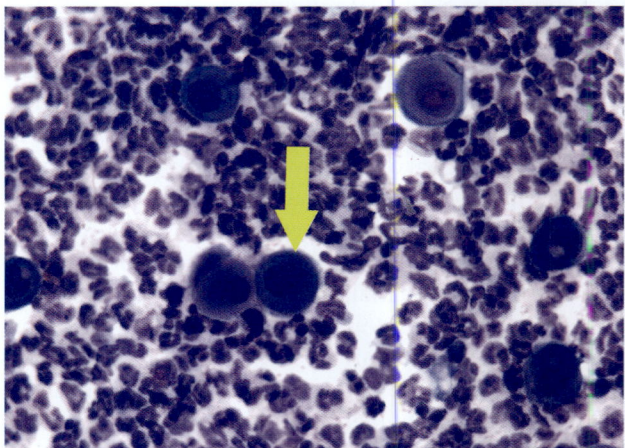

Figure 72.3 Photomicrograph of acantholytic cells (yellow arrow) collected by direct impression from a pinnal lesion, stained with a modified Wright's stain. Note myriad neutrophils in the background for size comparison.

due to allergic causes. Lateral ear resection may help with treatment of secondary infections, but will not resolve the pruritic stimulation. Ear masses due to neoplasia or polyps refractory to medical management must be excised by appropriate procedures (Figure 72.1). Dystrophic mineralization of the external ear canal will require surgical intervention. The extent of the procedure is dependent upon the severity and distribution of the mineralization within the ear. A total ear canal ablation is generally indicated. This is because dystrophic mineralization is a progressive pathologic change. Even with appropriate treatment of the primary cause of otitis, the mineralization is likely to continue. Dystrophic mineralization is often associated with clinical pain. Surgical intervention is likely to be associated with an improved quality of life.

Biopsy samples for histopathology are helpful to achieve a definitive diagnosis for pinnal disorders. The indications for performing a biopsy are without limits. Chronic lesions and those refractory to therapy would warrant a biopsy. Any odd-looking lesions or masses should be biopsied. The collected specimens can be submitted in neutral buffered formalin.

Biopsy samples can be performed with a myriad of techniques. Invariably, general anesthesia and/or regional ring block of the pinna are indicated. A recent publication reviewed regional anesthesia of the canine ear including techniques for blocking the two major sensory nerves to the ear (Layne 2019). Crusted, erythematous, papular, or pustular lesions can be sampled with a Baker biopsy punch. Care should be taken to attempt to maintain the integrity of the pustule if possible. A 3–4 mm punch can be used. The epithelium is gently cut without going into the cartilage of the pinna. The skin can be dissected with sharp scissors, scalpel blade, or syringe needle. Blood should be blotted from the sample before placing onto a piece of a wooden tongue blade, subcutaneous side down. This will help to maintain the integrity of small pieces of tissue within the formalin. A pencil can be used to label each tissue sample. Alternatively, tissue chambers can be used. These samples are small, so it is beneficial to collect several from affected areas. The hemorrhage should be minimal and can usually be managed with pressure. Cautery or tissue glue may also be considered. Those lesions with "interesting" margins are best sampled by scalpel excision. A surgical ellipse should be taken perpendicular to the leading margin (Figure 72.4). This will ensure that the biopsy samples will be cut along the long axis of the biopsy sample and will demonstrate the pathology of the transition from affected to nonaffected skin. This technique is preferred for ulcerated lesions and those lesions that are too large for a punch biopsy sample. Intact pustules and vesicles should be collected with surgical excision. Care should be taken to create as small an excision as possible. Suturing of these sample sites may lead to conformational defects of the pinnae.

Lesions of the ear margins due to vasculitis, autoimmunity, or seborrheic disorders may be more difficult to biopsy. It is sometimes beneficial to perform a cosmetic ear trim (Figure 72.5) of the affected pinna to provide an adequate sample for histopathology. The lesion can eas-

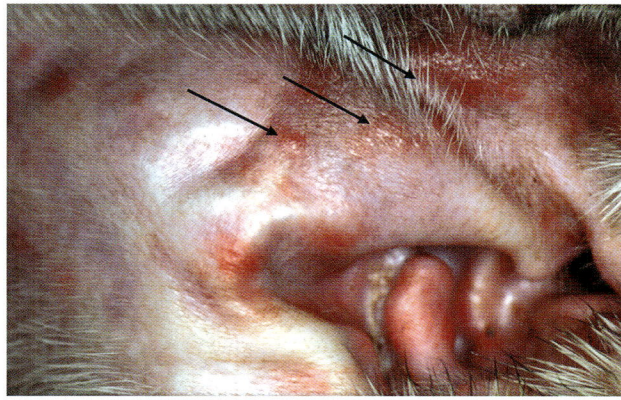

Figure 72.4 Suggested biopsy sites from a dog with vasculitis due to rickettsial infection.

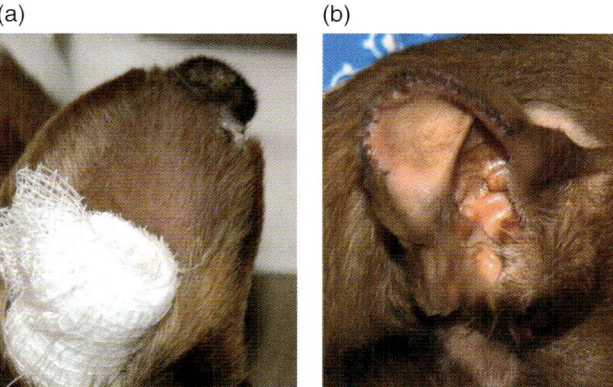

(a) (b)

Figure 72.5 Before (a) and after (b) cosmetic surgery to correct severe pinnal vasculitis, refractory to medical management.

ily be sutured with an interrupted or continuous pattern. Obviously there will be a permanent defect. Alternatively, a wedge resection through the cartilage can be performed (Angarano 1988). It is sometimes difficult to suture these lesions to control hemorrhage. Also, a permanent defect will be created. Care should be taken to extend the surgical site into the clinically normal ear pinna. Some cases of pinnal vasculitis are missed by conservative biopsy technique.

Masses are sometimes visible with otoscopic evaluation. A decision must be made regarding collecting a biopsy sample for histopathology or pursuing surgical excision. With appropriate sedation, anesthesia, and analgesia, fine-needle aspirates can be collected. A clamshell forceps or alligator forceps may be used to dislodge a portion of tissue for histopathology. Unfortunately, the tissue samples are usually crushed and not as good as surgically excised samples. Hemorrhage may be difficult to manage. Nonetheless, this may assist the surgeon with a plan and the owner with a prognosis prior to more extensive surgery.

Indications for surgical treatment

There are several indications for surgical intervention of canine otitis externa. Stenotic ear canals due to congenital causes can be corrected with later or vertical ear resection. A poor response to oral anti-inflammatory doses of glucocorticoids (prednisolone 1.5 mg/kg/day) or potent topical glucocorticoid medications would be an indication to consider surgery of chronically inflamed ear canals. These procedures are rarely effective as the sole treatment for allergic causes of otitis externa. It is usually better to pursue medical management of chronically inflamed ears due to allergic causes. Lateral ear resection may help with treatment of secondary infections, but will not resolve the pruritic stimulation.

Ear masses due to proliferative otitis, neoplasia, or polyps refractory to medical management must be excised by appropriate procedures (Figure 72.6). A recent publication reviewed the use of carbon dioxide laser surgery for chronic proliferative and obstructive otitis externa in 26 dogs (Aslan *et al.* 2021). Findings indicated that the carbon dioxide laser is an effective treatment for proliferative otitis externa causing obstruction,

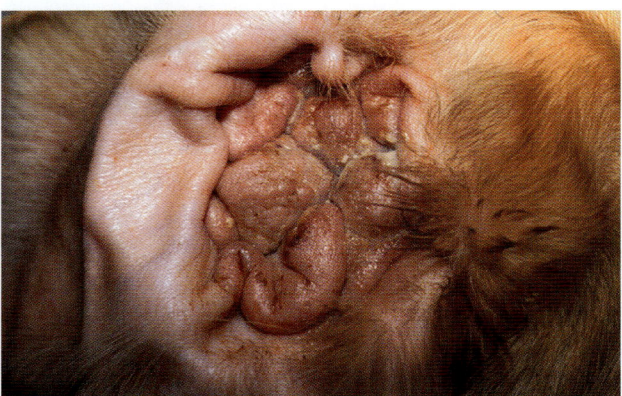

Figure 72.6 Proliferative otitis externa obstructing the horizontal ear canal.

and suggested that it should be considered an alternative to total ear canal ablation and bulla osteotomy (TECABO).

Dystrophic mineralization of the external ear canal will require surgical intervention. The extent of the procedure depends upon the severity and distribution of mineralization with the ear. A total ear canal ablation is generally indicated. This is because the dystrophic mineralization is a progressive pathologic change. Even with appropriate treatment of the primary cause of the otitis, the mineralization is likely to continue. Dystrophic mineralization is often associated with clinical pain that is commonly refractory to medical management. Surgical intervention is likely to be associated with an improved quality of life.

References

Angarano, D.W. (1988). Diseases of the pinna. *Veterinary Clinics of North America: Small Animal Practice* 18 (4): 869–884.

Aslan, J., Shipstone, M.A., and Mackie, J.T. (2021). Carbon dioxide laser surgery for chronic proliferative and obstructive otitis externa in 26 dogs. *Veterinary Dermatology* 32: 262–267.

August, J.R. (1988). Otitis externa. A disease of multifactorial etiology. *Veterinary Clinics of North America: Small Animal Practice* 18 (4): 731–742.

Gray, R.F., Sharma, A., and Vowler, S.L. (2005). Relative humidity of the external auditory canal in normal and abnormal ears, and its pathogenic effect. *Clinical Otolaryngology* 30 (2): 105–111.

Hutchings, S.M. (2003). Juvenile cellulitis in a puppy. *Canadian Veterinary Journal* 44 (5): 418–419.

Layne, E.A. (2019). Clinical techniques in veterinary dermatology; regional anesthesia of the canine ear. *Veterinary Dermatology* 30: 470–473.

Morris, D.O. (1999). Malassezia dermatitis and otitis. *Veterinary Clinics of North America: Small Animal Practice* 29 (6): 1303–1310.

Rosser, E.J. Jr. (2004). Causes of otitis externa. *Veterinary Clinics of North America: Small Animal Practice* 34 (2): 459–468.

Roth, L. (1988). Pathologic changes in otitis externa. *Veterinary Clinics of North America: Small Animal Practice* 18 (4): 755–764.

Zur, G. (2005). Bilateral ear canal neoplasia in three dogs. *Veterinary Dermatology* 16 (4): 276–280.

73

Feline and Canine Otitis Media

Dawn Logas

Otitis media is defined as inflammation of the middle ear cavity including the tympanum, tympanic bulla, and eustachian tube. The true incidence of canine and feline otitis media remains unknown because of the difficulty in accurately diagnosing the condition. Reported incidence ranges from 16% in acute otitis externa to 80% in chronic otitis externa (Little *et al.* 1991b; Cole *et al.* 1998).

Causes

Otitis media can arise from a variety of infectious and noninfectious causes. Infectious agents include bacteria, fungi, and viruses. Viruses are thought to be the least common cause of otitis media in dogs and cats. They enter the middle ear through the eustachian tube or via hematogenous spread. Bacteria, the most common infectious agent cultured, and fungi enter the middle ear from the external ear canal, eustachian tube, or less commonly the vascular system. Currently, the most common entry point is thought to be through a tympanum damaged by otitis externa. The most common bacteria cultured from the middle ears of dogs with chronic otitis externa include *Staphylococcus pseudintermedius*, *Pseudomonas aeruginosa*, β-hemolytic *Streptococcus*, and *Staphylococcus epidermidis* (Cole *et al.* 1998; Colombini *et al.* 2000).

The importance of the eustachian tube as an entry point for pathogenic bacteria in dogs and cats is unknown. In feline cases of otitis media not associated with otitis externa, bacteria normally associated with upper airway disease such as *Bordetella* and *Mycoplasma* were cultured (Trevor & Martin 1993). In cases of feline and canine otitis media associated with chronic sinusitis rather than otitis externa, the organisms cultured from the middle ear are often the same as those cultured from the sinuses. This is similar to what is seen in children with chronic otitis and sinusitis, where the microbiologic concordance between the middle ear and sinuses is 69% (Brook *et al.* 2000). Finally, the importance of bacterial biofilms in the development of feline or canine otitis media is unknown. Since biofilms play a pivotal role in the development of chronic hard-to-treat otitis media in children, it is probable they will be found to play a similar role in dogs and cats with otitis media (Hall-Stoodley *et al.* 2006). This is especially likely since *Pseudomonas* spp., which are often involved in canine and feline otitis media, very commonly form biofilms.

Malassezia pachydermatis is the most common fungal cause of otitis media in the dog and cat. It typically occurs as an extension of yeast otitis externa. *Aspergillus* spp., *Penicillium* spp., and other saprophytic fungi can also infrequently cause canine and feline otitis externa/media. They may appear as black or white fungal plaques on the walls of the external canal and tympanic bulla. They look similar to the plaques seen on moldy bread. It is important to note that these fungal infections can be seen in patients with competent immune systems as well as in those who are immunosuppressed.

Multiple noninfectious inflammatory processes can also lead to otitis media. Neoplastic growths in the middle ear, although rare, can initiate otitis media by directly causing inflammation or by inhibiting normal middle ear function, which can then lead to inflammatory changes. In cats, various carcinomas (including squamous cell carcinoma) and lymphoma have been reported (Trevor & Martin 1993; Fan & de Lorimier 2004). In

Small Animal Soft Tissue Surgery, Second Edition. Edited by Eric Monnet.
© 2023 John Wiley & Sons, Inc. Published 2023 by John Wiley & Sons, Inc.
Companion website: www.wiley.com/go/monnet/small

dogs, adenomas, adenocarcinomas, and squamous cell carcinomas have been described (Little *et al.* 1989; Yoshikawa *et al.* 2008).

Nonneoplastic causes of otitis media include lymphoid hyperplasia, inflammatory polyps, cholesteatomas, and primary secretory otitis media. Lymphoid hyperplasia can be seen in the tympanic bulla of both dogs and cats. It can appear as a yellowish firm plaque or lobulated nodule on the surface of the tympanic bulla. It is unknown at this time if the lymphoid hyperplasia initiates the otitis media or if it is a consequence of the otitis media.

Inflammatory polyps are of unknown etiology and arise from the mucosal lining of the middle ear, eustachian tube, or pharynx of dogs and cats (Fan & de Lorimier 2004). Many are thought to be congenital, although clinical signs may not be apparent for years (mean is about two years in cats). The polyps consist of fibrovascular tissue covered by an epithelial layer accompanied by a mixed inflammatory infiltrate. They can remain in the tympanic bulla cavity, extend through the eustachian tube into the pharynx, or extend into the external ear canal by rupturing or expanding the tympanic membrane. These polyps can cause stridor or dysphagia if they reside in the pharynx or otitis externa/media if they reside in the middle ear cavity or external ear canal.

Primary secretory otitis media is a well-documented syndrome in Cavalier King Charles spaniels, in which a plug of gelatinous mucus fills the tympanic bulla, causing pain and sometimes neurologic signs (Stern-Bertholtz *et al.* 2003). Although not documented in the literature, primary secretory otitis media has also been observed in other dog breeds and cats. Clinically, these patients may present with pain, manifested as unwillingness to chew hard food or open their mouth widely. They may also manifest with neurologic signs including vestibular signs, Horner's syndrome, and facial paralysis. Large gelatinous mucous plugs are removed from the affected tympanic bulla. These plugs are often found to be sterile on culture.

Cholesteatomas are congenital epithelial inclusion cysts arising from the stratified squamous epithelium of the tympanum. They can also be the result of an acquired involution of the tympanum into the middle ear cavity. Over time a cholesteatoma can fill the entire ventral cavity and cause destruction of the bony structures of the tympanic bulla (Little *et al.* 1991a; Fan & de Lorimier 2004). Congenital cholesteatomas are not uncommonly seen in children. They appear as small, white, pearl structures in the middle ear enclosed behind the tympanic membrane (Koltai *et al.* 2002). If left untreated they can continue to grow, with disastrous consequences. Unfortunately, the prevalence of congenital cholesteatomas in dogs is hard to estimate since they are usually associated with long-term otitis by the time of discovery. Most canine cholesteatomas are considered a consequence of chronic otitis externa and/or media, although a few are considered congenital. The exact mechanism of cholesteatoma formation in dogs is not known, but there are two possible mechanisms that have been demonstrated in various other species. The first involves a reversal of the normal outward epithelial migration in the external ear canal by experimental ligation or occlusion of the external ear canal. This leads to a rapid build-up of keratin debris, medial displacement of the tympanic membrane, and potential erosion of the bone of the tympanic bulla (McGinn *et al.* 1984). Theoretically, this could occur with severe otitis externa, which causes a functional occlusion of the external ear canal and reversal of epithelial migration. Another experimental mechanism suggests that once the epithelium in the middle ear has been disrupted and granulation tissue forms, the granulation tissue can form a bridge from the mucoperiosteum to the tympanic membrane. If there is perforation of the tympanic membrane, stratified squamous epithelium from the external ear canal can transmigrate into the middle ear through the perforation (Goycoolea *et al.* 1999). This squamous epithelium can then form a cholesteatoma, which can be open to the external canal or enclosed in the middle ear cavity if the tympanum heals.

Pathogenesis

The pathogenesis of otitis media appears to be similar no matter what the inciting cause (Little *et al.* 1991b). Before the pathogenesis of otitis media can be completely understood, it is important to have a working knowledge of the microanatomy and physiology of the middle ear.

The tympanum is composed of three distinct layers: the outer layer of stratified squamous epithelium, the middle layer of fibrous connective tissue, and the inner layer of simple mucosal epithelium. The mucoperiosteum that covers the majority of the tympanic bulla consists of a one-cell thick simple mucosal epithelium with a few ciliated cells. Close to the eustachian tube, the mucoperiosteum becomes a pseudostratified columnar epithelium with an abundance of ciliated cells and a few goblet cells. The eustachian tube itself is also lined by pseudostratified ciliated columnar epithelium containing a few goblet cells. The eustachian tube is normally collapsed and protects the middle ear from nasopharyngeal secretions. When patent, it allows ventilation of the middle ear and drainage of middle ear secretions.

Currently, it is thought that the eustachian tube evacuates the gas and mucus produced by the middle ear mucosa by peristaltic motion along with ciliary clearance (Cohen *et al.* 2009). Dysfunction of the eustachian tube is very important in the pathogenesis of otitis media in various species, including dogs and probably cats as well (Tojo *et al.* 1985; Vicente *et al.* 2007; Hueb & Goycoolea 2009). This dysfunction may be the result of primary anatomic abnormalities or be due to secondary causes such as inflammation or neoplasia.

Acute inflammation in the middle ear cavity initially induces a thickening of the middle ear mucosa due to vasodilatation, edema, and infiltration of inflammatory cells (Tojo *et al.* 1985). If left untreated, the thickening of the mucosa continues and can lead to a functional occlusion of the eustachian tube. In purulent otitis media this occlusion may be caused by a decrease in the surface tension-lowering substance normally present in the eustachian tube. Increased adherence of the tubal walls follows and leads to occlusion of the tube (Birken & Brookler 2009). After several months of eustachian tube occlusion and otitis media, there is degeneration and loss of the ciliated cells, which further impairs the normal clearance of fluid from the middle ear (Nell *et al.* 2000; Smirnova *et al.* 2004). At this time a significant increase in the number of goblet cells and formation of mucous glands are also noted. These glands form in areas where there is a break in the thickened epithelium, allowing invaginations that become lined with secretory cells (Goycoolea 2001). This hyperproliferation leads to increased mucus production and a mucoid effusion in the middle ear. The physical and histochemical qualities of the mucus also change at this time. The concentration of sulfated glycoproteins in the mucus is significantly increased, while the concentration of neutral glycoproteins is decreased (Jin *et al.* 1991). This leads to more gelatinous or viscous mucus that is much harder to clear. If this viscous mucus becomes organized and contacts the underlying fibrous tissue through breaks in the epithelial layer of the mucoperiosteum, it can act as a nidus for the formation of granulation tissue and cholesterol granulomas (Fliegner *et al.* 2007; Hueb & Goycoolea 2009). Over time this process can also lead to the formation of cholesteatomas in susceptible individuals (Goycoolea *et al.* 1999).

In addition to changes in the epithelial structures of the tympanic bulla, an increase in fibrous tissue and new bone formation has been demonstrated in many species (Vicente *et al.* 2007). When this occurs in the progression of the disease and to what extent vary, depending on the species. If left unchecked, the inflammation may also lead to osteomyelitis and bony destruction of the tympanic bulla.

Finally, there are changes in the permeability of the round window that occur with otitis media. In otitis media secondary to eustachian tube obstruction, the round window becomes thickened and its permeability decreases dramatically after just one week (Schachern *et al.* 1987). The opposite is seen in bacterial otitis media, in which the presence of potent cytolysins can lead to an increase in round window membrane permeability (Engel *et al.* 1995). It has been proposed that similar changes may be seen in the tympanic membrane in cases of otitis media, but these findings have not been confirmed.

Clinical signs

Clinical signs of otitis media are extremely variable. The clinical signs in many dogs and cats with both otitis media and otitis externa cannot be differentiated in any way from those with just otitis externa. Patients with both otitis externa and media can have general ear pain, a head tilt, and some hearing loss. Some cases of otitis media will have more evidence of pain on palpation of the bulla and may be reluctant to open their mouths or chew hard food. If the nerves that course around the base of the ear or through the tympanic bulla are mildly affected, keratoconjunctivitis sicca and dryness of the nasal planum on the ipsilateral side may occur.

In more severe cases the patient may show signs of Horner's syndrome and facial nerve palsy, with drooping of the facial muscles and skin along with drooling (Kern & Erb 1987). Complete deafness can result from otitis media, but otitis interna is necessary for there to be true vestibular disease (Kent *et al.* 2010). Although well documented, these neurologic signs are not seen in most cases of otitis media in the dog, but are seen more commonly in the cat. In one study of 43 dogs with confirmed otitis media, only one had facial nerve paralysis and one had keratoconjunctivitis sicca (Saridomichelakis *et al.* 2007). In a retrospective study of 16 cats with otitis media without nasopharyngeal polyps, 11/16 had neurologic signs (Swale *et al.* 2017).

Examination of the ear canal can be helpful in the diagnosis of otitis media if the tympanum can be visualized. In many cases with concurrent otitis externa, the external ear canal is swollen or fibrotic, making tympanic membrane visualization impossible. If the tympanum can be visualized it is often thickened or scarred, especially in patients with chronic otitis externa. A bulging or perforated membrane is indicative of otitis media. Perforations are less commonly seen since the tympanum heals quickly even in the face of infections. The tympanum is intact in up to 70% of confirmed cases of otitis media (Little *et al.* 1991b; Cole *et al.* 1998).

Diagnosis

If the tympanum is intact and not bulging, various other tests have been employed to help diagnose otitis media. Pneumotoscopy, tympanometry, and the acoustic reflex are all normally used in human medicine to help diagnose otitis media. When evaluated in dogs, all these tests had high false-negative results and were not considered very useful in the diagnosis of canine otitis media (Cole *et al.* 2000).

Diagnostic imaging that may be useful in the diagnosis of otitis media includes plain radiography, computed tomography (CT), magnetic resonance imaging (MRI), and ultrasound. Plain radiography, though easily accessible, has fairly high false-negative rates for diagnosing otitis media, particularly in less severe cases (Cole *et al.* 2000; Rohleder *et al.* 2006). CT is more accurate and reliable than radiography in diagnosing otitis media in moderate to severe cases, but also becomes less reliable in mild cases (Rohleder *et al.* 2006). Ultrasound examination of the bulla for fluid or air in both dogs and cats is more accurate than radiography, but still inferior to CT (Dickie *et al.* 2003; King *et al.* 2007). Ultrasound is also inferior to video otoscopy (Classen *et al.* 2016). MRI appears to be more useful in the diagnosis of vestibular disease and otitis interna than otitis media (Bischoff & Kneller 2004). It is accurate in detecting the soft tissue changes associated with otitis media, but bony changes in the bulla are more difficult to assess than with CT.

The most reliable and accurate way to diagnose otitis media is by video-otoscopic examination and myringotomy (Cole *et al.* 2000). Before a proper examination can occur the external ear canal must be cleared of wax and other debris. The increased magnification and illumination provided by video-otoscopes allow visualization of more subtle changes in the tympanum than can be detected with hand-held otoscopes. Small tears or perforations in the tympanum and/or fluid and debris behind the tympanum are more easily seen. If the tympanum is intact and otitis media is suspected, a myringotomy should be performed. This can be accomplished using a blunt tomcat catheter, video-otoscope biopsy forceps, or a 2–5 mm blunt buck curette. Myringotomy should always be performed in the caudoventral aspect of the tympanum to avoid the delicate structures protected by the round window and the germinal centers of the tympanum. In cases of otitis media, the tympanum usually ruptures easily with the application of very little pressure. If the tympanum is scarred and thickened, an endoscopic biopsy cup may be needed to penetrate the tympanum. This is particularly true when a cholesteatoma or thick-walled abscess is present in the middle ear. Fluid from the middle ear cavity should be examined cytologically for the presence of inflammatory cells and infectious agents. A sample of the fluid should also be submitted for bacterial culture and sensitivity testing. Once the tympanum is open, the middle ear cavity can be examined with the video-otoscope, a rigid cystoscope, or a small flexible endoscope. If necessary, a biopsy of the mucoperiosteum can be taken with an endoscopic biopsy cup.

Treatment

Medical treatment for otitis media can be attempted if the mucosa of the bulla is not invaded by neoplastic cells or by a thick layer of granulation tissue. The first step in the medical treatment of otitis media is the removal of any debris that has collected in the bulla cavity (Palmeiro *et al.* 2004). Cleaning of the middle ear cavity should be accomplished while the patient is under general anesthesia. The potential complications of lavaging the middle ear cavity include vestibular dysfunction, hearing loss, facial nerve paralysis, and Horner's syndrome. These complications are extremely rare in canine patients; Horner's syndrome and vestibular dysfunction occur more often in cats, since the nerves run more superficially through the feline tympanic bulla.

Topical and systemic antimicrobial therapy should be chosen based on cytology and culture/susceptibility results from specimens of the middle ear (Morris 2004). Reported treatment lengths range from 30 to 360 days, but the average case clears in 2–3 months. One of the greatest concerns with topical treatment for otitis media is the reported ototoxicity of most topical agents used, except the fluoroquinolones (Kavanagh *et al.* 2009). Unfortunately, the organisms cultured are frequently sensitive only to agents that are potentially ototoxic. In these cases the owners should be warned of both the potential side effects of the topical therapy and the damage that could occur to the middle ear if no topical therapy is used.

The use of glucocorticoids in the treatment of otitis media is controversial, but many veterinary dermatologists use both topical and systemic steroids to help reverse the inflammatory changes seen in the bulla. Glucocorticoids may potentially decrease middle ear effusion and maintain more normal function of the eustachian tube.

Canine and feline otitis media is more common than previously thought. It is most often associated with otitis externa, but as our ability to diagnose milder cases of this condition improves, more cases of primary otitis media may be found. If diagnosed early, otitis media is very amenable to medical treatment. Unfortunately, diagnosis often occurs after the bulla has been severely compromised. Surgical management with either a ventral bulla osteotomy or a total ear canal ablation then becomes the best option.

References

Birken, E.A. and Brookler, K.H. (2009). Surface tension lowering substance of the eustachian tube in non-suppurative otitis media: an experiment with dogs. *Laryngoscope* 83: 255–258.

Bischoff, M.G. and Kneller, S.K. (2004). Diagnostic imaging of the canine and feline ear. *Veterinary Clinics of North America: Small Animal Practice* 34: 437–458.

Brook, I., Yocum, P., and Shah, K. (2000). Aerobic and anaerobic bacteriology of concurrent chronic otitis media with effusion and chronic sinusitis in children. *Archives of Otolaryngology - Head and Neck Surgery* 126: 174–176.

Classen, J., Bruehschwein, A., Meyer-Lindenberg, A., and Mueller, R.S. (2016). Comparison of ultrasound imaging and video otoscopy with cross-sectional imaging for the diagnosis of canine otitis media. *Veterinary Journal* 217: 68–71.

Cohen, D., Raveh, D., Peleg, U. et al. (2009). Ventilation and clearance of the middle ear. *Journal of Laryngology and Otology* 123: 1314–1320.

Cole, L.K., Kwochka, K.W., Kowalski, J.J., and Hillier, A. (1998). Microbial flora and antimicrobial sensitivity patterns of isolated pathogens from the horizontal ear canal and middle ear in dogs with otitis media. *Journal of the American Veterinary Medical Association* 212: 534–538.

Cole, L.K., Kwochka, K.W., Podell, M. et al. (2000). Evaluation of radiography, otoscopy, pneumotoscopy, impedance audiometry and endoscopy for the diagnosis of otitis media in the dog. In: *Advances in Veterinary Dermatology*, vol. 4 (ed. K.L. Thoday, C.S. Foil and R. Bond), 49–56. Oxford: Blackwell Science.

Colombini, S., Merchant, S.R., and Hosgood, G. (2000). Microbial flora and antimicrobial susceptibility patterns from dogs with otitis media. *Veterinary Dermatology* 11: 235–239.

Dickie, A.M., Doust, R., and Cromarty, L. (2003). Comparison of ultrasonography, radiography and a single computed tomography slice for the identification of fluid within the canine tympanic bulla. *Research in Veterinary Science* 75: 209–211.

Engel, F., Blatz, R., Kellner, J. et al. (1995). Breakdown of the round window membrane permeability barrier evoked by Streptolysin O: possible etiologic role in development of sensorineural hearing loss in acute otitis media. *Infection and Immunity* 63: 1305–1310.

Fan, T.M. and de Lorimier, L. (2004). Inflammatory polyps and aural neoplasia. *Veterinary Clinics of North America: Small Animal Practice* 34: 489–509.

Fliegner, R.A., Jubb, K.V.F., and Lording, P.M. (2007). Cholesterol granuloma associated with otitis media and destruction of the tympanic bulla in a dog. *Veterinary Pathology* 44: 547–549.

Goycoolea, M.V. (2001). Gland formation in otitis media. An ultrastructural study in humans. *Acta Oto-Laryngologica* 121: 182–184.

Goycoolea, M.V., Hueb, M.M., Muchow, D., and Paparella, M.M. (1999). The theory of the trigger, the bridge and the transmigration in the pathogenesis of acquired cholesteatomas. *Acta Oto-Laryngologica* 119: 244–248.

Hall-Stoodley, L., Hu, F.Z., Gieseke, A. et al. (2006). Direct detection of bacterial biofilms on the middle-ear mucosa of children with chronic otitis media. *Journal of the American Medical Association* 296: 202–211.

Hueb, M.M. and Goycoolea, M.V. (2009). Experimental evidence suggestive of early intervention in mucoid otitis media. *Acta Oto-Laryngologica* 129: 444–448.

Jin, C.S., Majima, Y., Hamaguchi, Y. et al. (1991). Quantitative histochemical study of secretory cells after short term tubal obstruction in the cat. *Acta Oto-Laryngologica* 111: 515–523.

Kavanagh, K.R., Parham, K., and Schoem, S.R. (2009). Auditory function after a prolonged course of ciprofloxacin–dexamethasone otic suspension in a murine model. *Archives of Otolaryngology – Head and Neck Surgery* 135: 238–241.

Kent, M., Platt, S.R., and Schatzberg, S.J. (2010). The neurology of balance: function and dysfunction of the vestibular system in dogs and cats. *Veterinary Journal* 185: 247–258.

Kern, T.J. and Erb, H.N. (1987). Facial neuropathy in dogs and cats: 95 cases (1974–1985). *Journal of the American Veterinary Medical Association* 191: 1604–1609.

King, A.M., Weinrauch, S.A., Doust, G. et al. (2007). Comparison of ultrasonography, radiography and a single computed tomography slice for fluid identification within the feline tympanic bulla. *Veterinary Journal* 173: 638–644.

Koltai, P.J., Nelson, M., Castellon, R.J. et al. (2002). The natural history of congenital cholesteatoma. *Archives of Otolaryngology – Head and Neck Surgery* 128: 804–809.

Little, C.J.L., Pearson, G.R., and Lane, J.G. (1989). Neoplasia involving the middle ear cavity of dogs. *Veterinary Record* 124: 54–57.

Little, C.J.L., Lane, J.G., Gibbs, C., and Pearson, G.R. (1991a). Inflammatory middle ear disease of the dog: the clinical and pathological features of cholesteatomas, a complication of otitis media. *Veterinary Record* 128: 319–322.

Little, C.J.L., Lane, J.G., and Pearson, G.R. (1991b). Inflammatory middle ear disease of the dog: the pathology of otitis media. *Veterinary Record* 128: 293–296.

McGinn, M.D., Chole, R.A., and Henry, K.R. (1984). Cholesteatomas induction: consequences of external auditory canal ligation in gerbils, cats, hamsters, guinea pigs, mice and rats. *Acta Oto-Laryngologica* 97: 297–304.

Morris, D.O. (2004). Medical therapy of otitis externa and otitis media. *Veterinary Clinics of North America: Small Animal Practice* 34: 541–555.

Nell, M.J., Koerten, H.K., and Grote, J.J. (2000). Bactericidal/permeability-increasing protein prevents mucosal damage in an experimental rat model of chronic otitis media with effusion. *Infection and Immunity* 68: 2992–2994.

Palmeiro, B.S., Morris, D.O., Wiemelt, S.P., and Shofer, F.S. (2004). Evaluation of outcome of otitis media after lavage of the tympanic bulla and long-term antimicrobial drug treatment and long-term antimicrobial drug treatment in dogs: 44 cases (1998–2002). *Journal of the American Veterinary Medical Association* 225: 548–553.

Rohleder, J.J., Jones, J.C., Duncan, R.B. et al. (2006). Comparative performance of radiography and computed tomography in the diagnosis of middle ear disease in 31 dogs. *Veterinary Radiology and Ultrasound* 47: 45–52.

Saridomichelakis, M.N., Farmaki, R., Leontides, L.S., and Koutinas, A.F. (2007). Aetiology of canine otitis externa: a retrospective study of 100 cases. *Veterinary Dermatology* 18: 341–347.

Schachern, P.A., Paparella, M.M., Goycoolea, M.V. et al. (1987). The permeability of the round window membrane during otitis media. *Archives of Otolaryngology – Head and Neck Surgery* 113: 625–629.

Smirnova, M.G., Birchall, J.P., and Pearson, J.P. (2004). The immunoregulatory and allergy-associated cytokines in the aetiology of the otitis media with effusions. *Mediators of Inflammation* 13: 75–88.

Stern-Bertholtz, W., Sjostrom, L., and Hakanson, N.W. (2003). Primary secretory otitis media in the Cavalier King Charles spaniel: a review of 61 cases. *Journal of Small Animal Practice* 44: 253–256.

Swale, N., Foster, A., and Barnard, N. (2017). Retrospective study of presentation, diagnosis and management of 16 cats with otitis media not due to nasopharyngeal polyp. *Journal of Feline Medicine and Surgery* 20 (12): 1082–1086.

Tojo, M., Matsuda, H., Fukui, K. et al. (1985). Experimental induction of secretory and purulent otitis media by surgical obstruction of the eustachian tube in dogs. *Journal of Small Animal Practice* 26: 81–89.

Trevor, P.B. and Martin, R.A. (1993). Tympanic bulla osteotomy for the treatment of middle ear disease in cats. *Journal of the American Veterinary Medical Association* 202: 123–128.

Vicente, J., Trinidad, A., and Ramírez-Camacho, R. (2007). Evolution of middle ear changes after permanent eustachian tube blockage. *Archives of Otolaryngology – Head and Neck Surgery* 133: 587–592.

Yoshikawa, H., Mayer, M.N., Linn, K.A. et al. (2008). A dog with squamous cell carcinoma in the middle ear. *Canadian Veterinary Journal* 49: 877–879.

74

Surgery of the Vertical Ear Canal

Anne Sylvestre

Lateral wall resection

Resection of the lateral wall of the vertical ear canal was originally described by Lacroix and improved upon by Zepp with the addition of a ventral drain board or baffle. The drain board prevents growth of hair into the opening of the horizontal canal (Zepp 1949). There have been few changes to this procedure since the addition of the ventral drain board.

Indications

Lateral wall resection is mainly indicated to facilitate management of otitis externa that is controllable with topical therapy. The purpose of lateral wall resection, in the treatment of otitis externa, is to alter the microenvironment within the ear canal and improve drainage. Postoperatively, the improved drainage and aeration within the horizontal canal result in decreased temperature, humidity, and moisture within the canal, presumably creating an environment less conducive to the growth of microbial organisms (Fraser *et al.* 1969). It also helps in the delivery of medical treatment deeper in the ear canal. Numerous reports have shown that the success rate of lateral ear resection varies from 35% to 50% (Tufvesson 1955; Gregory & Vasseur 1983; Sylvestre 1998). One retrospective study found a failure rate of 86.5% in cocker spaniels, and a success rate of 80% in shar-peis (Sylvestre 1998). The procedure is not indicated in patients with hyperplasia of the ear canal, especially cocker spaniels. If the horizontal ear canal is stenotic, lateral ear resection is contraindicated because drainage of the middle ear will not be improved.

The procedure is also used to manage severe trauma to that portion of the ear and for the correction of a hypoplastic lateral ear canal, which is more commonly seen in the shar-pei.

Lateral wall resection is indicated for removal of benign masses of the vertical and horizontal ear canals. The procedure allows good exposure during local excision. A biopsy should be performed prior to lateral ear resection. If the mass is malignant, a total ear canal ablation with lateral bulla osteotomy is indicated to obtain wider margins.

It is imperative that owners be well informed of the potential postoperative outcomes and need for ongoing medical management so that their expectations are reasonable.

Surgical technique

The pinna and lateral aspect of the head are shaved and aseptically prepared for surgery. The ear canal can be cleaned before surgery with a saline flush to remove as much debris as possible. The patient is positioned in lateral recumbency with the head slightly elevated. Laser and electrocautery are useful instruments to control hemorrhage during this procedure.

A curved hemostat is placed within the ear canal to help identify the ventral-most extent of the vertical canal (Figure 74.1). Two parallel skin incisions are made, one starting from the pretragic and the other from the intertragic incisures; both are extended ventrally approximately 1.5 times the length of the vertical canal. The two incisions are then connected at their ventral-most point (Figure 74.2). The skin is elevated and reflected dorsally to its attachment on the tragus (Figure 74.3). An incision is

Small Animal Soft Tissue Surgery, Second Edition. Edited by Eric Monnet.
© 2023 John Wiley & Sons, Inc. Published 2023 by John Wiley & Sons, Inc.
Companion website: www.wiley.com/go/monnet/small

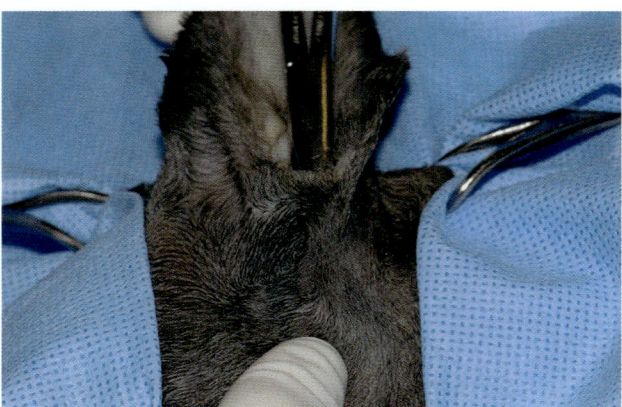

Figure 74.1 Left ear: probe inserted within the external ear canal, finger pointing to ventral-most aspect of the vertical canal. Cranial is to the left.

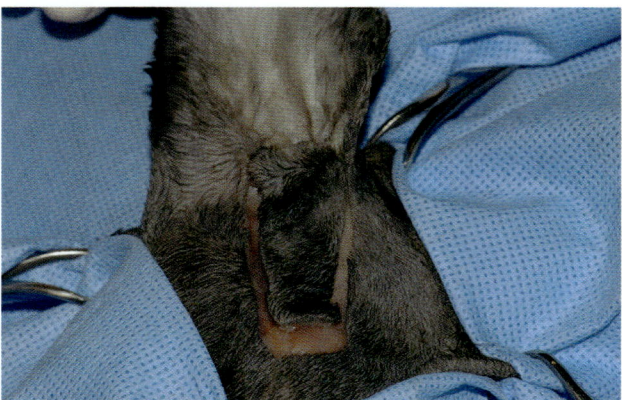

Figure 74.2 Two parallel skin incisions are made from the pre-tragic and intertragic incisures. The incisions extend ventrally approximately 1.5 times the length of the vertical canal. The two incisions are then connected at their ventral-most aspect.

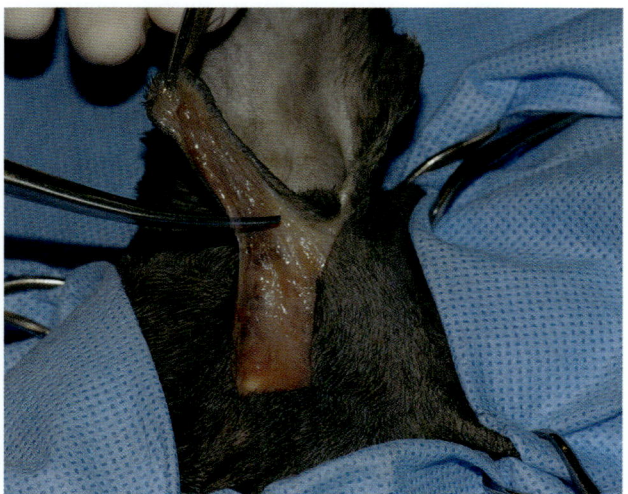

Figure 74.3 The connective tissues underneath the incised skin are cleared until the cartilage of the lateral wall of the vertical canal is evident.

made in the subcutaneous tissues directly over the lateral wall of the vertical canal. The tissues are elevated caudally and rostrally using sharp and blunt dissection techniques, until the cartilaginous lateral wall is clearly visible (Figure 74.4). The rostral auricular vein, located just ventral to the tragus, is cauterized or ligated before transection. The parotid gland must be reflected ventrally to allow full exposure of the lateral wall; gentle technique is necessary to avoid damaging the gland. The facial nerve is located deep (medial) to the surgical site, but one should exercise caution nonetheless, as aberrant anatomy or an overzealous dissection can lead to damage of this nerve.

The next part of the procedure is best accomplished with the surgeon positioned on the dorsal side of the patient. Looking into the lumen of the vertical canal, incisions are made along its rostral and caudal borders. These are best accomplished by making small advancing cuts with Mayo scissors, alternating frequently between the caudal and rostral incisions (Figure 74.5). It is important not to allow the two incisions to converge because the drain board will become too narrow. The incisions are continued ventrally to the junction of the vertical (auricular cartilage) and horizontal (annular cartilage) canals.

The lateral wall of the vertical canal can now be reflected ventrally to create the drain board (Figure 74.6). There should be minimal tension on the reflected lateral wall; if it does not lie flat, it may be because the incisions have not been extended to the level of the ligament between the horizontal and vertical canals. Otherwise, scoring the underside (ventral aspect) of the drain board may be helpful. A drain board of 1–2 cm in length is created by discarding a portion of the lateral wall of the vertical canal and attached skin flap (Figure 74.7).

The aural epithelium and cartilage are sutured to the skin. The first few sutures should focus on securing (i) the end of the drain board to the ventral-most skin incision and (ii) the horizontal canal, cranially and caudally (Figures 74.7 and 74.8). Sutures are then placed along the drain board and, finally, the two incisions dorsal to the level of the horizontal canal are closed. A 3-0 or 4-0 monofilament nonabsorbable suture is used to close the surgical site (Figure 74.9). Cartilage exposure and infection can increase the rate of dehiscence after surgery. Sedation of the patient may be necessary for suture removal.

Postoperative care and complications

Appropriate use of pain management is required after ear surgery. A bandage or Elizabethan collar may be necessary to prevent self-mutilation, which can increase the risk of dehiscence. The lateral ear resection is a contaminated surgery and therefore systemic antibiotics are

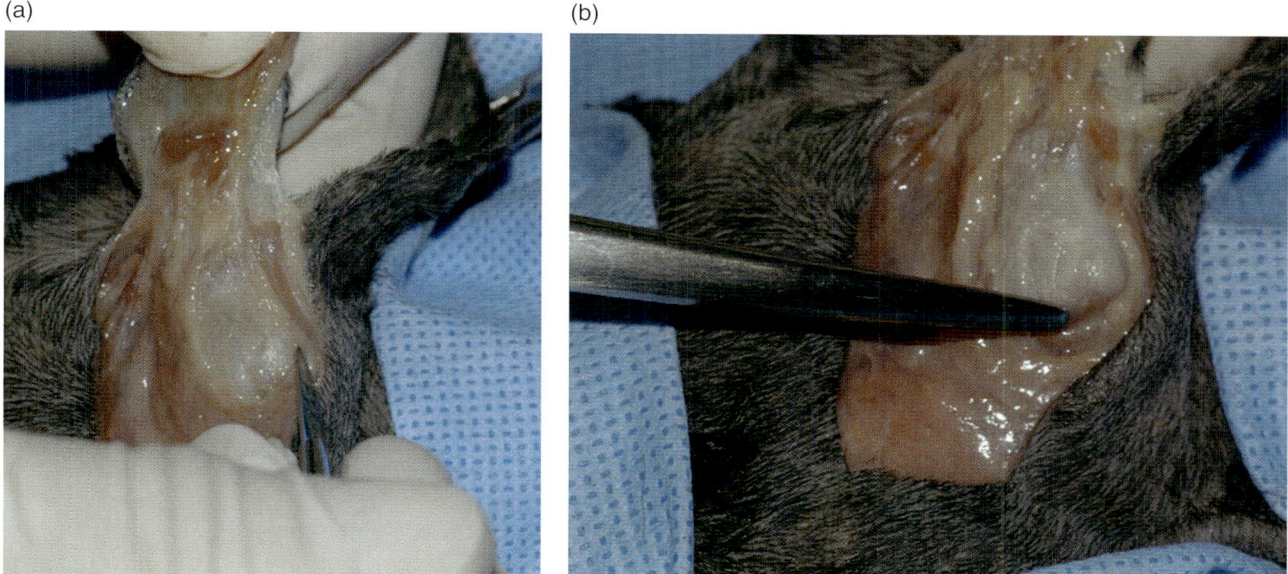

Figure 74.4 The connective tissues have been cleared (a) and the most ventral aspect of the lateral wall of the vertical canal is clearly visible (b).

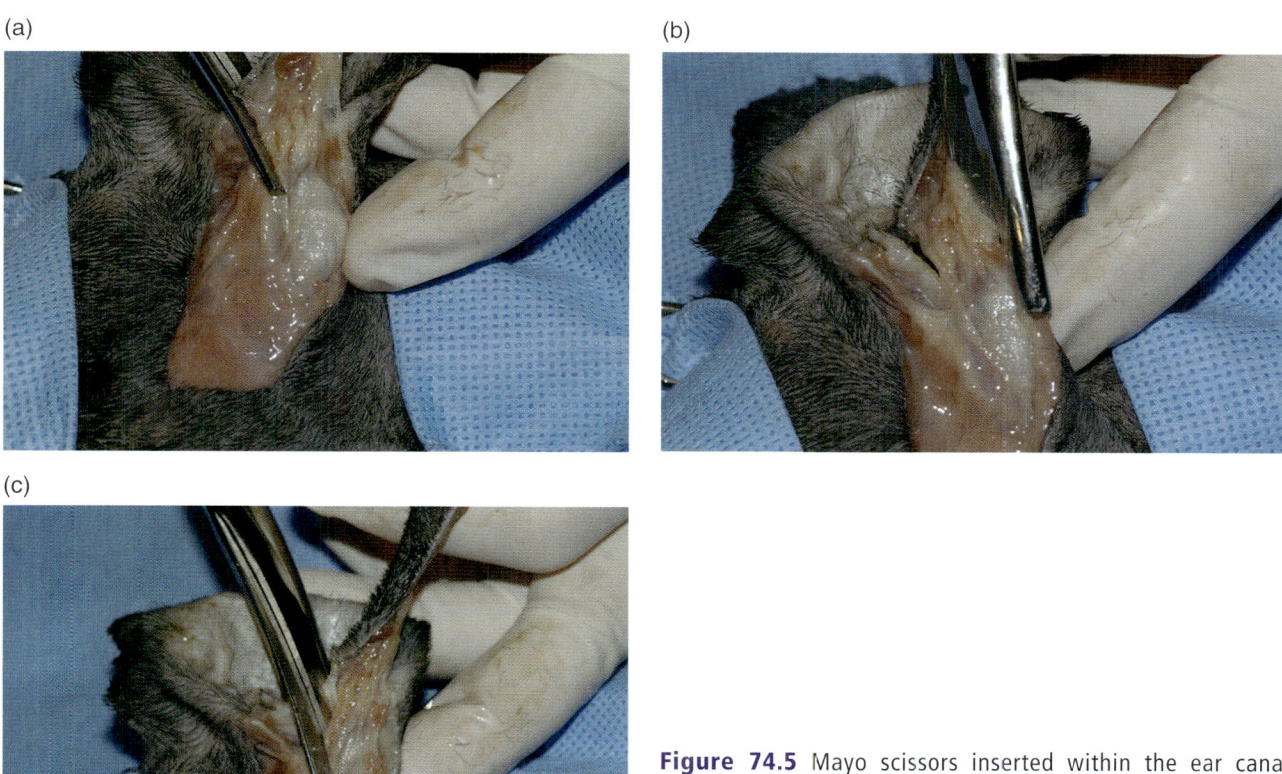

Figure 74.5 Mayo scissors inserted within the ear canal and cutting down the lateral wall of the vertical canal using short advancing cuts alternating along the cranial (a, c) and caudal (b) borders of the canal. It is important that the two incisions do not converge as they progress distally. The incisions extend to the level of the annular cartilage (horizontal canal).

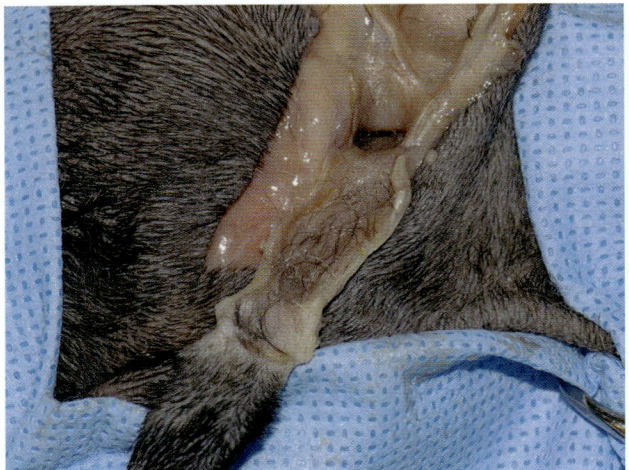

Figure 74.6 The incisions in the vertical canal are completed and the lateral wall has been opened ventrally, exposing the horizontal canal.

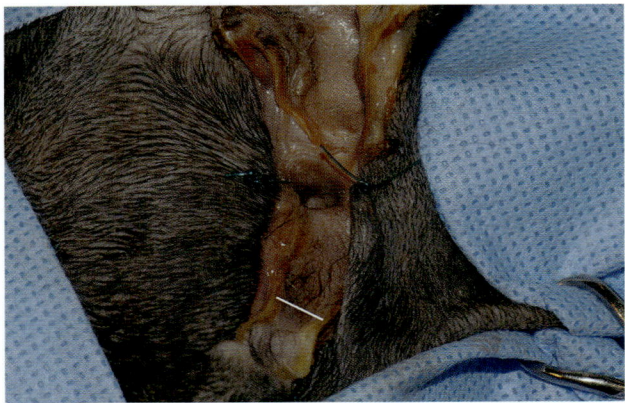

Figure 74.7 The skin is sutured to the aural epithelium starting at the level of the horizontal canal. The lateral wall of the vertical canal will then be cut at the level of the white line.

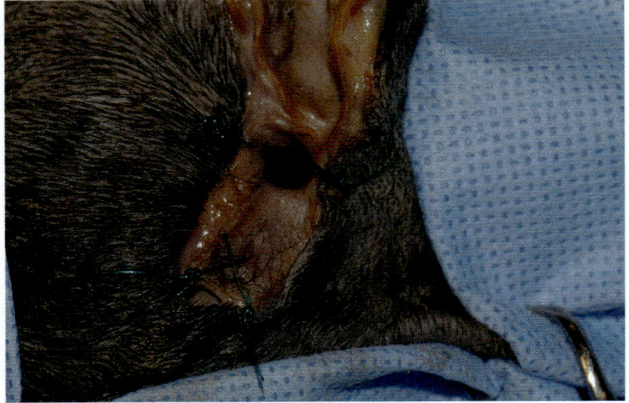

Figure 74.8 Next, the baffle or drain board is sutured to the ventral-most aspect of the skin incision.

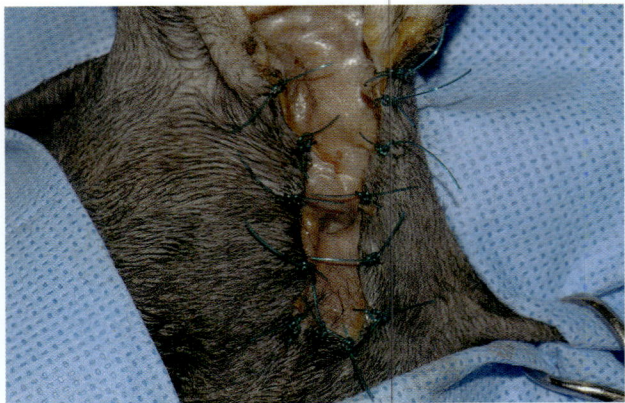

Figure 74.9 The final product: left ear lateral wall resection.

indicated. At the end of the surgery before closure of the surgical site, a swab should be performed to obtain a culture and sensitivity. Continued treatment of a preexisting condition such as otitis externa is also important.

The most common complication of this procedure is failure of the horizontal canal to remain patent. Reasons for failure include poorly identified and/or managed underlying disease, concurrent otitis media, and inappropriate case selection. Stricture of the horizontal canal by converging rather than diverging incisions in the vertical canal, as well as failure to completely open the lateral wall all the way to the annular ligament, will result in continued poor drainage and failure of the procedure (Lane & Little 1986). Partial wound dehiscence can also be a problem given that the tissues involved are often inflamed and infected. Second intention healing is frequently the treatment of choice in these cases.

Vertical ear canal ablation

Indications

Vertical ear canal ablation will accomplish the same objectives as lateral ear resection, with the advantage of removing more of the diseased tissue. The resultant effect is less postoperative pain and exudative discharge. This technique is used in cases such as neoplasia or hyperplasia of the epithelium of the vertical canal, with a relatively healthy horizontal ear canal. Although the surgical technique can be more challenging than lateral ear resection, some surgeons consider vertical ear resection to be more esthetically pleasing. Failure rates of 5–19% are reported for this technique (Siemering 1980; Tirgari 1988; McCarthy & Caywood 1992). Tirgari described a modified "pull-through" technique, the results of which were then published in a case series from which the failure rate of 19% was extrapolated.

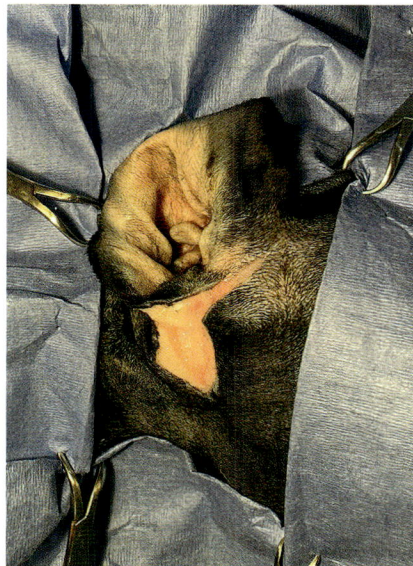

Figure 74.10 A T-shaped incision on the left ear: the horizontal incision is located at the base of the auditory meatus and the vertical incision is made along the vertical ear canal, ending just past its base.

A partial resection of the vertical ear canal has been reported (Pavletic 2019) in two cats with a benign growth at the junction of the auditory meatus and dorsal third of the vertical ear canal. The outcomes with the partial resections were successful for these patients.

Surgical technique

Preparation and positioning of the patient are the same as for the lateral wall resection procedure.

Place a probe in the vertical ear canal to help visualize its borders. A T-shaped skin incision is made at the ventral-most aspect of the auditory meatus and then along the vertical canal (Figure 74.10). Another incision is made around the auditory meatus, joining the ends of the horizontal part of the T-shaped incision. (Figure 74.11). Starting with the T-shaped incision, rather than only a circular incision around the meatus, will facilitate the closure.

Incise the subcutaneous tissues directly over the lateral wall of the vertical canal. The tissues are elevated caudally and rostrally using sharp and blunt dissection techniques, until the complete lateral cartilaginous wall of the vertical ear canal is clearly visible (Figure 74.12). Damage to the parotid gland can be minimized by working close to the ear canal itself. The rostral auricular vein, located just ventral to the tragus, is cauterized or ligated before transection.

The medial border of the vertical is dissected free from its muscular attachments. This is best accomplished scalpel blade and/or cautery (Figure 74.13).

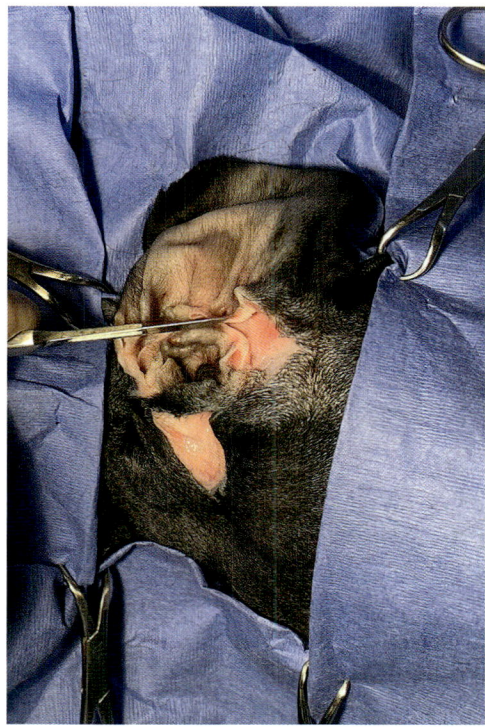

Figure 74.11 Another incision is made around the auditory meatus, joining the ends of the horizontal part of the T-shaped incision. Left ear.

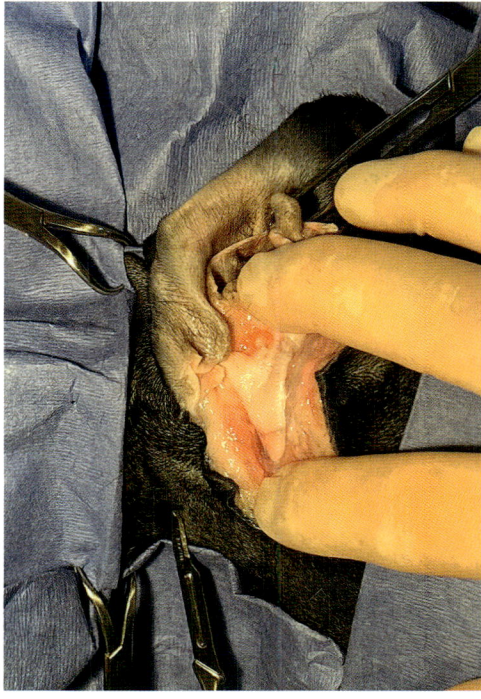

Figure 74.12 The connective tissues over the lateral wall of the vertical ear canal are elevated using sharp and blunt dissection techniques until the complete lateral cartilaginous wall of the vertical ear canal is clearly visible.

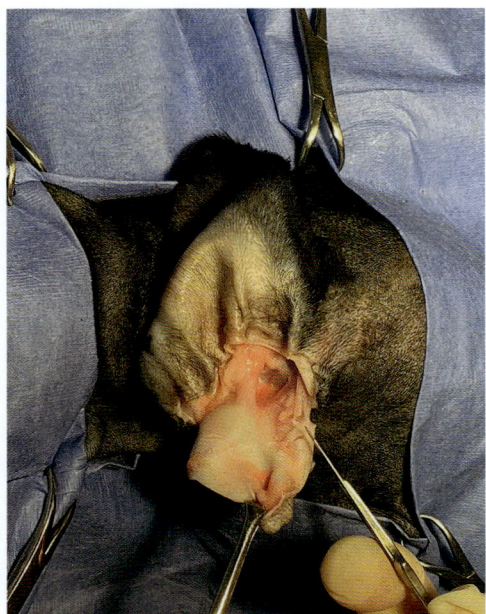

Figure 74.13 The medial border of the vertical canal is dissected free from its muscular attachments. This is best accomplished with a scalpel blade and/or cautery.

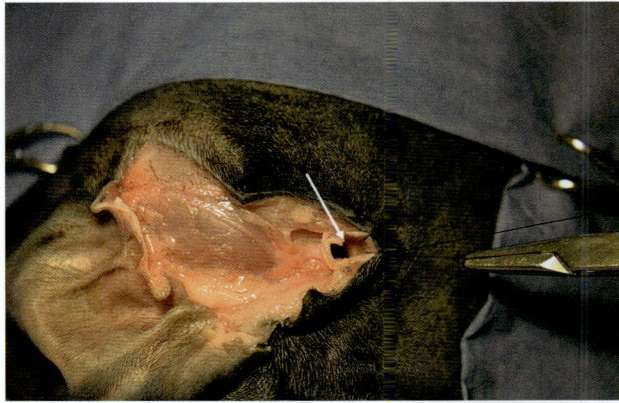

Figure 74.15 Small cuts are made in the rostral and caudal aspects of the horizontal canal (arrow; the caudal cut is not as visible due to the angle of the photo). The skin is sutured to the aural epithelium of the horizontal canal.

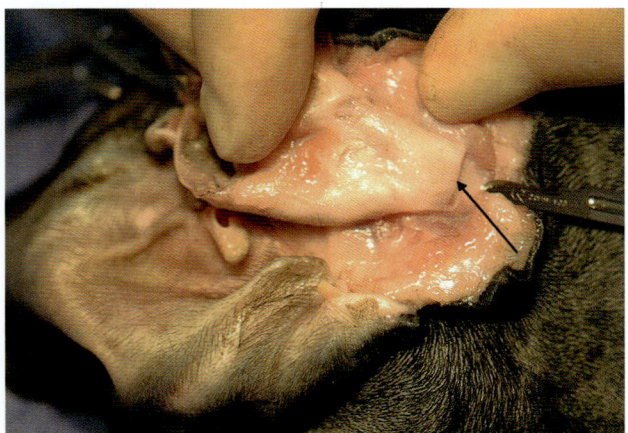

Figure 74.14 The junction of the vertical and horizontal canals is clearly visible (arrow). The vertical canal can be amputated at this junction.

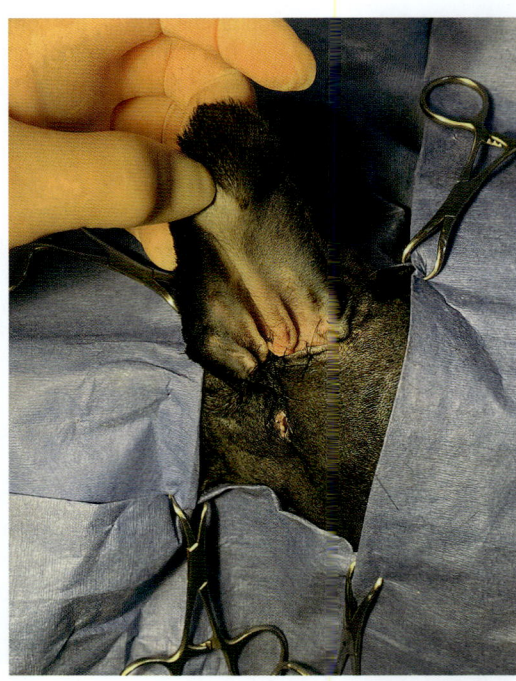

Figure 74.16 The vertical and horizontal portions of the skin incision are sutured closed. The natural curvature of the pinna should be maintained.

Once the vertical canal is completely freed from the surrounding tissues, it is amputated at the junction of the vertical and horizontal canal (Figure 74.14), or further distally, depending on the location of the lesion within the canal. A small cut is made in the rostral and caudal aspects of the horizontal canal to allow the edges to spatulate open. This will serve to create a slightly larger stoma and thereby help prevent stricture formation.

The skin is sutured to the aural epithelium of the horizontal canal (Figure 74.15). The vertical skin incision is then sutured closed. When closing the horizontal, or upper, portion of the surgical site, one should take the time to ensure that the natural curvature of the pinna is maintained (Figure 74.16). A monofilament, nonabsorbable, 3-0 or 4-0 suture material is appropriate for the closure.

Postoperative care and complications

The postoperative care for these patients is similar to that for the lateral wall resection procedure. Bandaging or an Elizabethan collar may be necessary to prevent self-mutilation. Pain management is required. Appropriate antibiotic therapy as well as continued management of the underlying condition is necessary.

Postoperative complications include stenosis of the horizontal canal as well as wound dehiscence. The use of the dorsal and ventral cartilage flaps may decrease the occurrence of stenosis. Owners should be forewarned that the ear carriage will be affected and may be especially notable in dogs with erect ears.

Lateral wall resection versus vertical canal ablation

It can sometimes be difficult to accurately assess the condition of the ear canal prior to surgery, making it difficult to confidently decide which procedure would be most beneficial to the patient. In these instances, it is best to start with the lateral wall resection procedure. This approach allows the surgeon to better assess the condition of the external canals. The surgeon may decide to continue with the lateral wall resection, proceed with the vertical ear canal resection, or alter the procedure to a total ear canal ablation. If converting to a vertical canal ablation and the disease in the vertical canal permits, a portion of the medial wall can be used to create a slightly longer dorsal baffle. This improvement to the technique aids in preventing hair from growing into the opening and minimizes stenosis (Lane & Little 1986).

References

Fraser, G., Gregor, W.W., Mackenzie, C.P. et al. (1969). Canine ear disease. *Journal of Small Animal Practice* 10: 725–754.

Gregory, C.R. and Vasseur, P.B. (1983). Clinical results of lateral ear resection in dogs. *Journal of the American Veterinary Medical Association* 182: 1087–1090.

Lane, J.G. and Little, C.J.L. (1986). Surgery of the canine external auditory meatus: a review of failures. *Journal of Small Animal Practice* 27: 247–254.

McCarthy, R.J. and Caywood, D.D. (1992). Vertical ear canal resection for end stage otitis externa in dogs. *Journal of the American Animal Hospital Association* 28: 545–552.

Pavletic, M.M. (2019). Partial vertical ear canal resection in two cats. *Journal of the American Veterinary Medical Association* 255: 1365–1368.

Siemering, G.H. (1980). Resection of the vertical ear canal for treatment of chronic otitis externa. *Journal of the American Animal Hospital Association* 16: 753–758.

Sylvestre, A.M. (1998). Potential factors affecting the outcome of dogs with a resection of the lateral wall of the vertical ear canal. *Canadian Veterinary Journal* 39: 157–160.

Tirgari, M. (1988). Long term evaluation of the pull-through techniques for vertical ear canal ablation for the treatment of otitis externa in dogs and cats. *Journal of Small Animal Practice* 29: 165–175.

Tufvesson, G. (1955). Operation for otitis externa in dogs according to Zepp's method. *American Journal of Veterinary Research* 16: 565–570.

Zepp, C.P. (1949). Surgical technique to establish drainage of the external ear canal and correction of hematoma of the dog and cat. *Journal of the American Veterinary Medical Association* 115: 91–92.

75

Imaging of the Ear for Surgical Evaluation

Robert Cole, Kaitlin Fiske, and John Hathcock

Choosing the best surgical therapy for ear disease may require evaluation of the middle and inner ear, as well as associated external ear soft tissue structures that cannot be evaluated by external examination alone. Conventional radiographic examination of the external ear and middle ear has been used routinely for such evaluations. This type of imaging examination can provide valuable information for the diagnosis of, and proper treatment planning for, many diseases of the ear. Radiographic contrast studies and ultrasonography have also been used occasionally to evaluate the ear. However, the cross-sectional imaging modalities of computed tomography (CT) and magnetic resonance imaging (MRI) extend the capabilities of diagnostic imaging of the external, middle, and inner ear beyond traditional radiographic examination. Studies have shown the cross-sectional modalities of CT and MRI to be more sensitive in the detection of changes in the middle and inner ear when compared with conventional radiology (Love *et al.* 1995; Garosi *et al.* 2003; Rohleder *et al.* 2006; Doust *et al.* 2007).

Radiology

Radiographic examination is the most readily available imaging technique for most practices. Some assessment of the external ear canals and tympanic bulla can be made with radiographic examination, but positioning of the skull for the radiographic views is critical for proper interpretation. Therefore the patient needs to be sedated or under general anesthesia to allow precise positioning for the multiple views needed. The ventrodorsal (or dorsoventral) view of the skull, which may be preferable to ensure more accurate positioning, allows good evaluation of the external ear canals bilaterally (Garosi *et al.* 2003; Benigni & Lamb 2006). The tympanic bullae are superimposed over the dense petrous temporal bone, making evaluation difficult, but they can be compared with each other for changes in opacity (Garosi *et al.* 2003). In the true lateral views of the skull, the tympanic bullae are superimposed over each other, so the oblique views of each tympanic bulla (lateroventral–laterodorsal) allow isolation and evaluation of each individual bulla (Hoskinson 1993; Garosi *et al.* 2003; Bischoff & Kneller 2004; Benigni & Lamb 2006). Additionally, the rostroventral–caudodorsal open-mouth view allows visualization of the bullae side by side without superimposition of the petrous portion of the temporal bones (Garosi *et al.* 2003; Bischoff & Kneller 2004). For feline patients, a rostro 10° ventro-caudodorsal oblique view may be easier to perform than the rostroventral-caudodorsal open-mouth view (Hammon *et al.* 2005).

Radiographic examination can evaluate for narrowing of the external ear canals and presence of mineralization of the external ear canal cartilages. In addition, it can evaluate for changes within the tympanic bullae, including increased soft tissue opacity, irregularities, thickening, or bony lysis (Figures 75.1 and 75.2). These findings may indicate chronic inflammation in the external ear canal and middle ear (Garosi *et al.* 2003; Forrest 2007; Benigni & Lamb 2006). Fluid accumulation, thickened inflammatory tissue, and polyps in the tympanic bulla cause increased radiopacity and may look similar. Lysis of the bulla may also be seen and could indicate severe

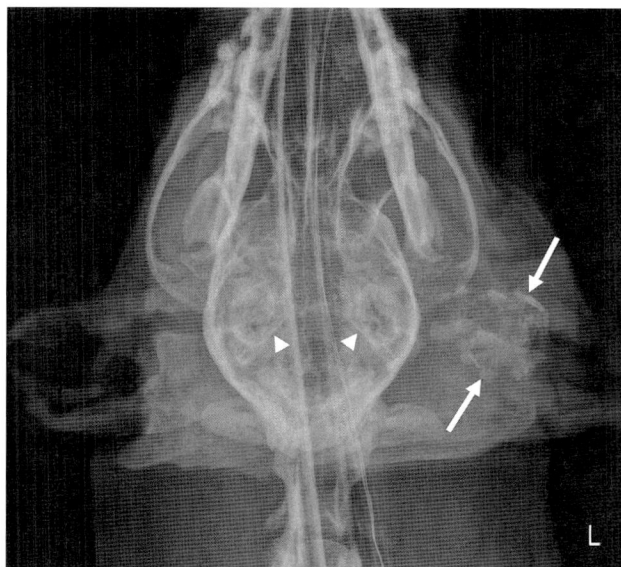

Figure 75.1 Ventrodorsal view of a skull of a dog with chronic otitis externa. Extensive mineralization around the left external ear canal is present (arrows). There is a normal-appearing external ear canal on the right side. Note the superimposition of the tympanic bullae over the skull (arrowheads), although they appear similar in opacity.

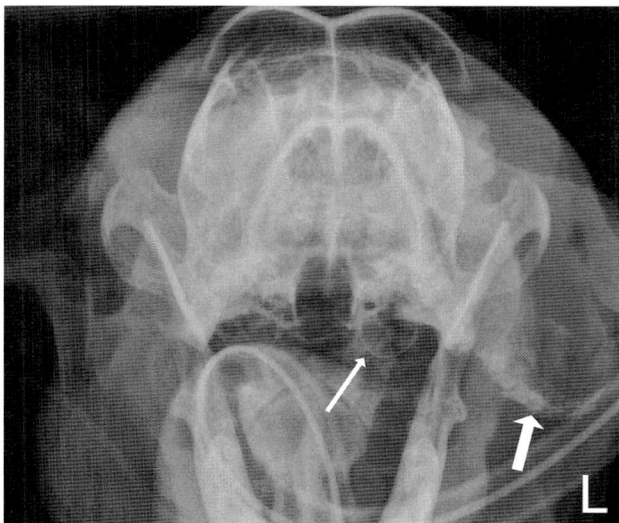

Figure 75.2 Rostrocaudal open-mouth view of the skull of the dog from Figure 75.1. The normal-appearing tympanic bullae can be seen as air-filled cavities surrounded by a uniform, thin bony wall (thin arrow). (The endotracheal tube is superimposed over the normal right tympanic bulla.) The mineralization of the left external ear canal can also be seen in this view (thick arrow).

infection or a neoplastic process involving the bulla (Garosi *et al.* 2003). Positive contrast studies (canalography) of the ear canal have also been used to evaluate for rupture of the tympanic membrane (Trower *et al.* 1998). In this procedure, positive contrast medium is instilled

into the external ear canal and post-contrast radiographs are compared with pre-installation images, looking for the presence of contrast medium in the tympanic bulla. This technique can also be used for evaluating external canal diameter (Eom *et al.* 2000).

Ultrasonography

Ultrasonography has been used to evaluate the external ear canal, tympanic bulla, and tympanic membrane and has been suggested as a noninvasive technique that does not require sedation or general anesthesia (Lee *et al.* 2006; Dickie *et al.* 2003a,b). Multiple different frequency ultrasound transducers have proven successful in imaging the external ear canal and tympanic bulla, and the best transducer may depend on the patient's size and the goals of the evaluation. A high-frequency (11–12 MHz) linear array transducer provides good image resolution and the superficial location of the tympanic bulla in cats proves favorable for this transducer type (King *et al.* 2007). This transducer type was also useful when imaging the external ear canal, tympanic membrane, and tympanic bulla in one plane due to its larger footprint (Lee *et al.* 2006). A microconvex array transducer with its smaller footprint can be easier to navigate the cutaneous surfaces of the base of the ear in dogs, but typically will have a lower frequency than the linear array transducer, reducing resolution (Dickie *et al.* 2003a). Regardless of the transducer type, the fur should be clipped ventral to the pinna and acoustic coupling gel should be used for image optimization. Although many cadaveric studies have described imaging patients in lateral recumbency, sternal recumbency may provide better visualization of fluid in a partially fluid-filled tympanic bulla due to the effects of gravity (Doust *et al.* 2007).

To view the tympanic bulla in a dog, both lateral and ventral windows have been described. The lateral window is achieved by angling the transducer perpendicular to the patient's head in between the zygomatic arch and wing of the atlas, ventral to the pinna. This view places the hypoechoic parotid salivary gland in the near field and the tympanic bulla deep to it, which is seen as a convex hyperechoic line with distal acoustic shadowing (Figure 75.3). The ventral approach involves angling the transducer dorsally along the ventral aspect of the skull at the level of the mandibular salivary gland, resulting in a hypoechoic mandibular salivary gland and hypoechoic digastricus muscle superficial to the tympanic bulla (Figure 75.4). If fluid is present in the tympanic bulla, then the far wall of the tympanic bulla is present as a concave hyperechoic line with distal acoustic shadowing (Dickie *et al.* 2003a).

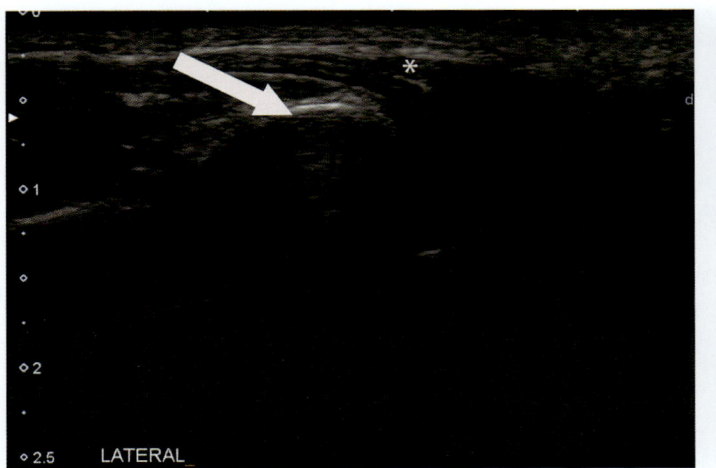
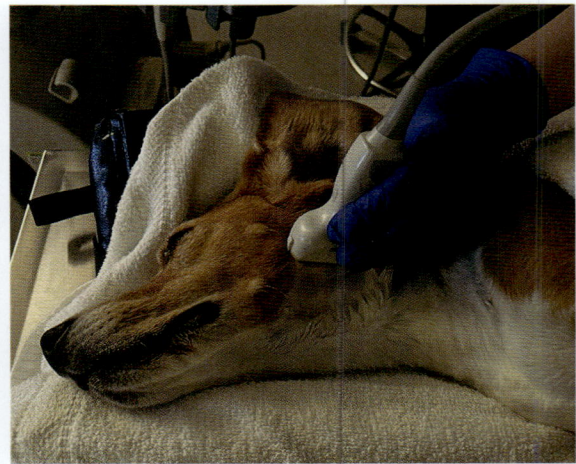

Figure 75.3 Sonographic appearance and accompanying photo of the tympanic bulla in a canine using the lateral transducer position. The image was acquired with a high-frequency (18 MHz) linear array probe. The wall of the tympanic bulla nearest the probe is a curvilinear hyperechoic line (white arrow) just deep to the parotid salivary gland (asterisk).

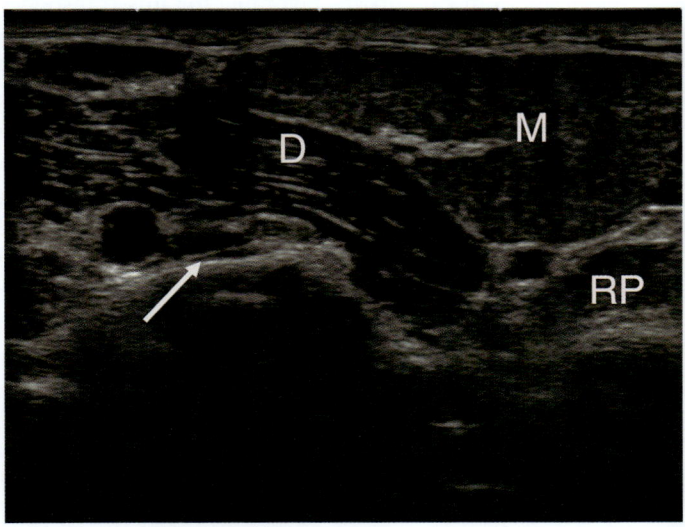
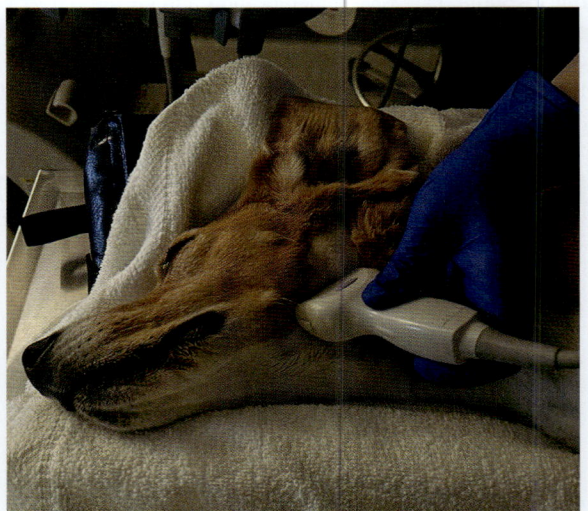

Figure 75.4 Sonographic appearance and accompanying photo of the normal tympanic bulla in a canine using the ventral transducer position. The image was acquired with a high-frequency (18 MHz) linear array probe. The wall of the tympanic bulla nearest the probe is a curvilinear hyperechoic line (white arrow) deep to the mandibular salivary gland (M) and digastricus muscle (D) and cranial to the retropharyngeal lymph node (RP).

In the cat, a ventral approach is preferred, since the gas-filled external ear canal obscures evaluation of the tympanic bulla. The tympanic bulla is easily palpated on the ventral aspect of the skull, caudal to the mandible. The tympanic bulla appears as a similar convex hyperechoic line with acoustic shadowing. Ventral to the tympanic bulla lie the digastricus muscle, subcutaneous fascia, and platysma muscle. Rostral and caudal landmarks include the styloglossus muscle and the mandibular salivary gland, respectively. In the transverse plane, the tympanic bulla is again present deep to the digastricus muscle, fascia, and platysma, and the sternomastoideus muscle,

longus capitus muscle, and basioccipital bone are present medial to the tympanic bulla (in superficial to deep order). Fluid within the tympanic bulla in a cat will result in anechoic material deep to the hyperechoic ventral aspect of the tympanic bulla and visualization of a convex hyperechoic line representing the osseous septum, which separates the larger ventral compartment from the dorsal compartment of the tympanic bulla. The dorsal compartment of the tympanic bulla cannot be visualized with ultrasound (King *et al.* 2007).

Infusing the external ear canal with sterile saline is a technique that may provide information on the status of the tympanic membrane and offer a better acoustic window to visualize the tympanic bulla (Lee *et al.* 2006).

Ultrasonography was 100% specific and sensitive in detecting fluid in the tympanic bulla of canine cadavers, in contrast to radiographs (sensitivity 80% and specificity 65%) according to one study (Griffiths *et al.* 2003). A study evaluating different imaging modalities in dogs clinically affected with otitis externa and otitis media concluded that ultrasound was better at detecting more severe changes associated with otitis media, since a tympanic bulla that is only partially filled with fluid or soft tissue material can be difficult to differentiate from a gas-filled bulla, as an acoustic shadow may still obscure the far wall of the tympanic bulla (Doust *et al.* 2007). Video otoscopy is considered a superior imaging technique to diagnose otitis media and externa when compared to ultrasound (Classen *et al.* 2016).

Computed tomography

CT has greatly enhanced the evaluation of all portions of the ear, especially the middle ear. Currently, many veterinarians rarely take radiographs to assess the ear or to evaluate other structures of the skull, instead opting for CT examination. The absence of superimposition of adjacent structures and the superior tissue contrast over conventional radiographic examination greatly aid in the evaluation of the structures of the ear. For proper positioning of the head, patients do require sedation or general anesthesia.

We place the patient in sternal recumbency with the head extended so that the hard palate is parallel with the table surface. The forelimbs should be pulled caudally out of the scanning field. The transverse scan plane is perpendicular to the hard palate. When evaluating just the tympanic bullae, thin slices (1 mm or thinner) are made through the tympanic bulla with a bone algorithm to enhance osseous detail.

One advantage of CT is the ability to manipulate the images to emphasize the bony structures or the soft tissue structures by selecting the range of CT numbers over which the gray scale (or shades of gray) can be assigned. To view the fine bony detail of the bullae, a bone window (a wide range of CT numbers with a high center CT number) is chosen to view these images. For our images, a bone window utilizing a window width (WW; i.e., the CT number range) of a minimum of 2000–2500 and a window level (WL; i.e., the center CT number) of 400–500 is chosen. Although the external ear canals can also be well visualized on these images, the primary purpose is to evaluate the tympanic bulla and petrous temporal bone. If a soft tissue mass associated with the ears needs to be evaluated, a scan using a soft tissue

algorithm through the entire area is obtained, and then the study is repeated after intravenous administration of iodine contrast. These images are viewed with a soft tissue window (a narrow range of CT numbers combined with a lower center CT number, such as WW 250–400, WL 30–50), which allows evaluation of the brain and calvarium to assess for extension of disease from the middle ear or for the presence of a primary lesion within the brain. Multiplanar reconstruction in the sagittal and dorsal planes may be made from the transverse images with image viewing software and may provide additional information.

The anatomy of the canine middle and inner ear on CT images has been described (Russo *et al.* 2002). The CT appearance of the feline middle and inner ear has also been described (Seifert *et al.* 2012). The thickness of the air-filled cavity of the bullae can be clearly seen on transverse images along with the air-filled external ear canals (Figure 75.5). Otitis media is indicated by increased soft tissue attenuation in the bulla (caused by fluid accumulation or proliferative soft tissue within the bulla) and alteration in the bulla contour caused by bony proliferation or lysis (Love *et al.* 1995; Garosi *et al.* 2003; Belmudes *et al.* 2018). Care must be taken when evaluating the thickness of the bulla, depending on whether the bulla is air-filled or fluid-filled. Air-filled bullae appear to have thinner walls compared with fluid-filled bullae (Barthez *et al.* 1996). Narrowing of the ear canals and

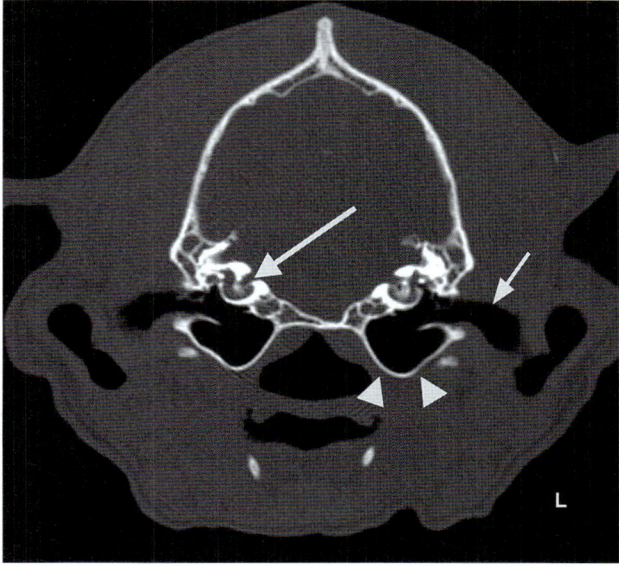

Figure 75.5 Transverse computed tomography image of the normal tympanic bullae of a dog (1 mm thick, bone algorithm, WW 2500 and WL 480). Note normal air-filled thin-walled bullae (arrowheads) and air-filled external ear canal (short arrow). Osseous detail of the temporal bone is evident, which includes the cochlea and semicircular canals (long arrow).

mineralization of the external ear canal cartilages due to otitis externa may also be seen (Figures 75.6–75.8). The changes may be unilateral or bilateral and the severity of the changes caused by otitis externa will vary.

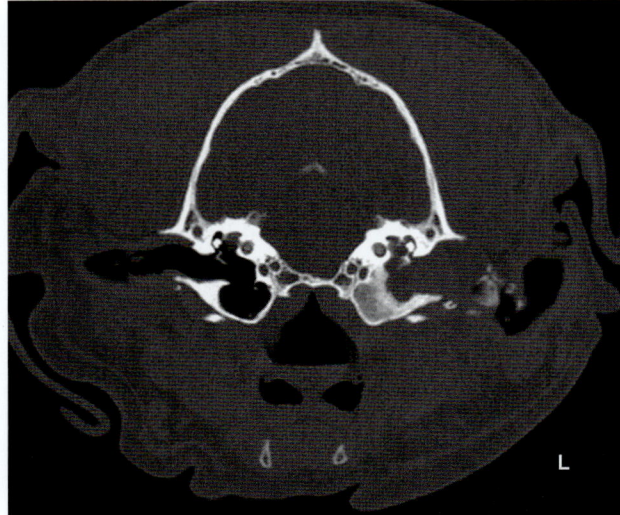

Figure 75.6 Transverse computed tomography image of a dog with chronic otitis externa and media (1 mm thick, bone algorithm, WW 2500, WL 480). There is proliferative bone in the left tympanic bulla as well as soft tissue opacity material in the bulla and distal external ear canal. Note the widened appearance of the opening into the bulla and mineralization in the external ear canal cartilages.

Polyps in the middle ear are thought to be due to chronic inflammation and appear as increased soft tissue attenuation (Seitz et al. 1996), often with a rim of contrast enhancement (Oliveira et al. 2012) (Figures 75.9 and 75.10). The polyps may extend into the external ear canal or into the nasopharynx through the auditory tube. Though most commonly thought of as occurring in cats, inflammatory polyps may also be found in dogs (Pratschke 2003; Blutke et al. 2010).

Chronic infection and neoplasia have to be considered when there is unilateral lysis of the bulla (Figures 75.11 and 75.12). Most neoplasias do not arise directly from the middle ear, but affect the middle ear by extension from surrounding structures (Forrest 2007). The lytic changes and adjacent soft tissue mass are often more extensive than that seen with chronic infection (Forrest 2007) (Figure 75.12). Cholesteatomas (epidermoid cysts containing keratin) have been described by CT and must also be differentiated from neoplasia (Figure 75.13). The change predominantly found with cholesteatomas is a nonenhancing, hyperattenuating mass causing expansile-type lysis of the tympanic bulla (Travetti et al. 2010; Greci et al. 2011; Risselada 2016). A cholesteatoma has also been reported in the cat and has a similar CT appearance (Alexander et al. 2019).

Club-shaped, well-defined hyperostotic tympanic bone spicules (HTBS) located on the tympanic bulla

(a)

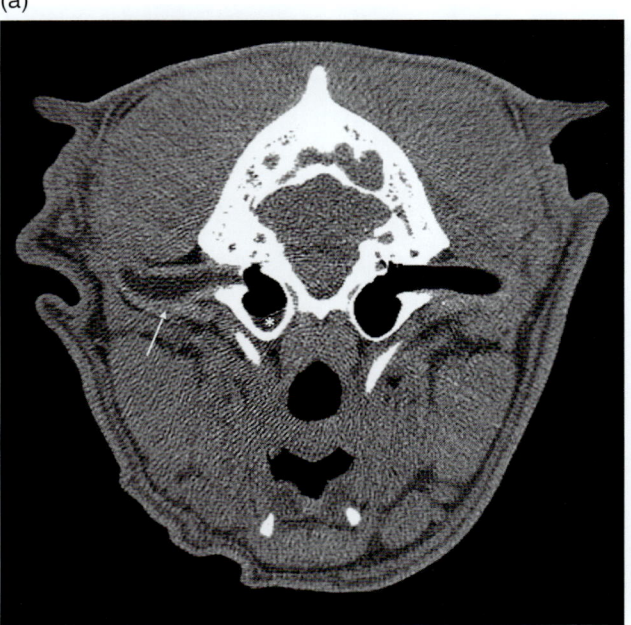

(b)

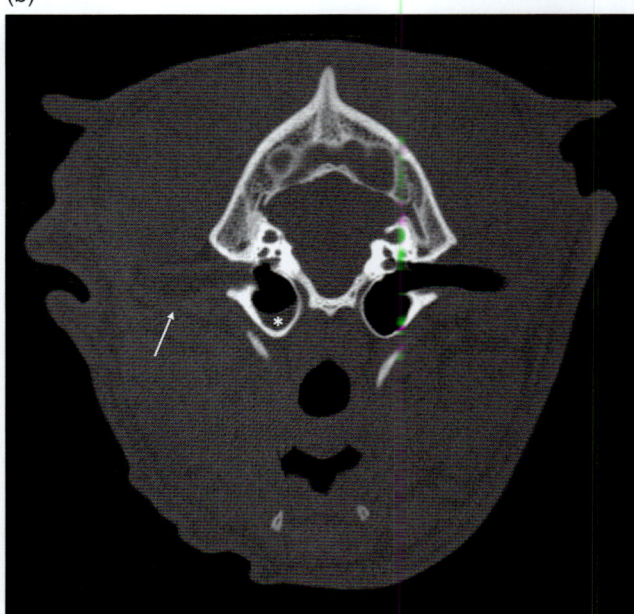

Figure 75.7 Transverse computed tomography images of a dog with chronic otitis external and externa (625 mm thick, bone algorithm): (a) a soft tissue window with WW 400, WL 40; (b) a bone window with WW 2500 and WL 400. There is thickening of the right external ear canal (white arrow) with fluid noted in the lumen of the external ear canal. There is fluid-attenuating material in the left tympanic bulla (asterisk) and mild thickening of the bulla wall compared to the thin bulla wall noted with the left ear.

septum can be seen on CT (Parzefall *et al.* 2014). Concretions (otoliths) within the tympanic bulla have also been reported and have been described as smooth, round, well-defined concretions that may be single or multiple (Ziemer *et al.* 2003). These may represent HTBS or true concretions (Parzefall *et al.* 2014). It is thought that otoliths and HTBS are associated with either active or previous otitis media (Ziemer *et al.* 2003; Parzefall *et al.* 2014).

Magnetic resonance imaging

MRI provides superior soft tissue contrast to both conventional radiographic examination and CT. However, the bone detail of the thin tympanic bulla may not be as well visualized as that seen with CT examination, especially if the bulla is air-filled. Bone and air are both low signal on MRI, which makes differentiating them difficult (Benigni & Lamb 2006; Lorek *et al.* 2020).

If the area of interest is the inner ear and/or the clinical suspicion is high for intracranial disease or extension of otitis media or interna, then MRI may be the choice for imaging evaluation (Sturges *et al.* 2006). The external ear canal, associated surrounding tissues, and middle ear can also be evaluated (Figure 75.14). The inner ear contains fluid in the membranous labyrinth of the cochlea and semicircular canals and is seen as high signal intensity on T2-weighted images (Figure 75.14). The inner ear may be best visualized by acquiring thin slices from T2-weighted volume-acquisition sequences specifically obtained to evaluate this area (Garosi *et al.* 2001; Lorek *et al.* 2020). The tympanic cavity and external ear canals have a signal void due to normally being air-filled. The adjacent brain and calvarium are also easily evaluated. Contrast can then be administered, and the T1-weighted images are reacquired to more thoroughly evaluate any soft tissue changes in the external ear, the

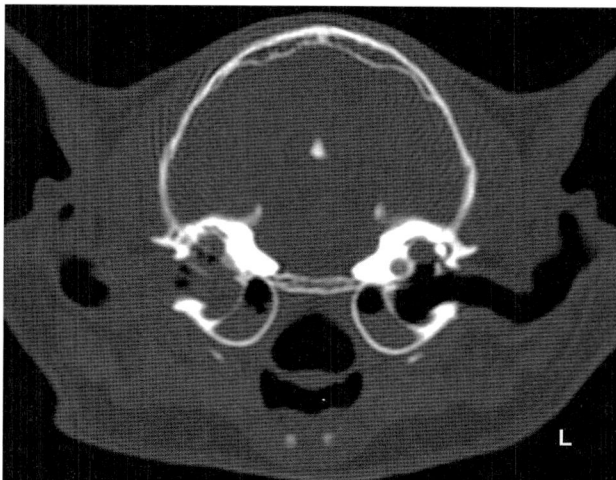

Figure 75.8 Transverse computed tomography image at the level of the tympanic bulla of the skull of a cat with otitis externa and media (1 mm thick, bone algorithm, WW 2500, WL 480). The medial and lateral compartments of the feline tympanic bulla can be seen. Both compartments of the right bulla and the medial compartment of the left bulla contain material of soft tissue opacity. The dependent location of the soft tissue and the presence of a meniscus in the medial compartments of both bullae suggest fluid accumulation. Soft tissue opacity material is also present in the distal right external ear canal. The thickness of the bullae appears normal. The left external ear canal is normal.

(a)

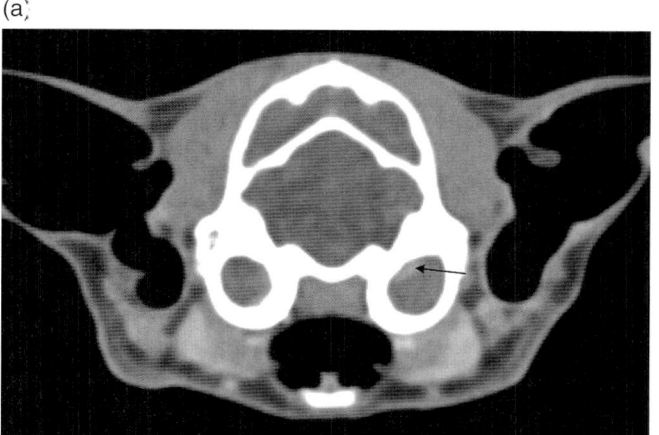

(b)

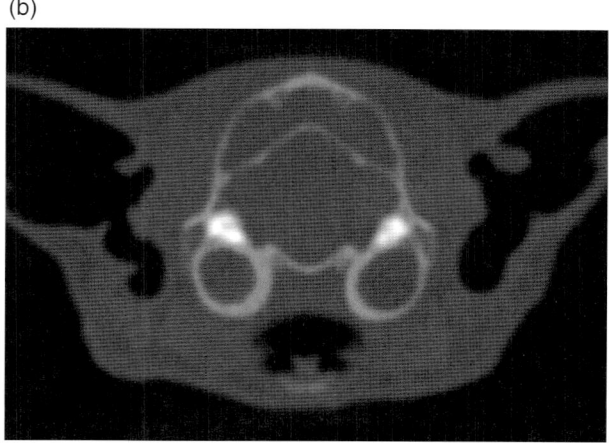

Figure 75.9 Transverse computed tomography image at the level of the tympanic bulla of the skull of a cat with inflammatory polyps and otitis media (0.625 mm thick, soft tissue algorithm): (a) post contrast in a soft tissue window (WW 400, WL 40); (b) post contrast in a bone window (WW 2500, WL 400). There is soft tissue attenuating material in the tympanic bullae of both ears with concurrent thickening of the bulla wall. There is contrast enhancement noted at the periphery of the left tympanic bulla denoted by the black arrow. Peripheral enhancement is often seen with polyps.

(a)

(b)

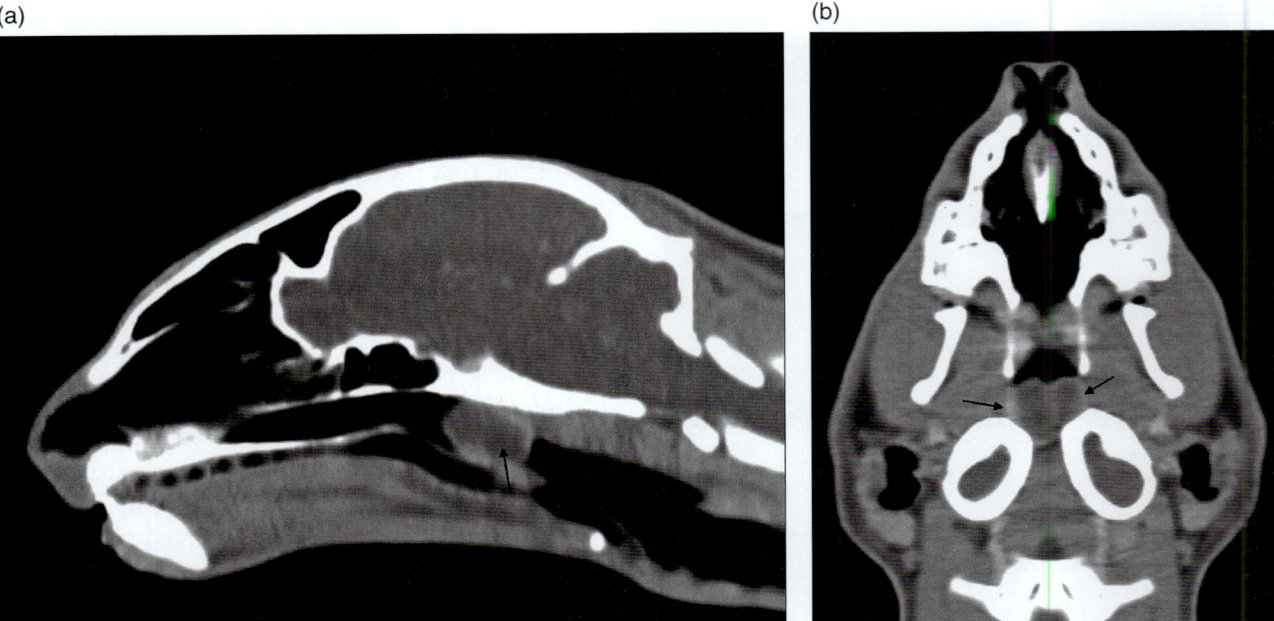

Figure 75.10 (a) Sagittal and (b) dorsal plane reformatted images from the same patient as Figure 75.9. The inflammatory polyps are denoted by the black arrows.

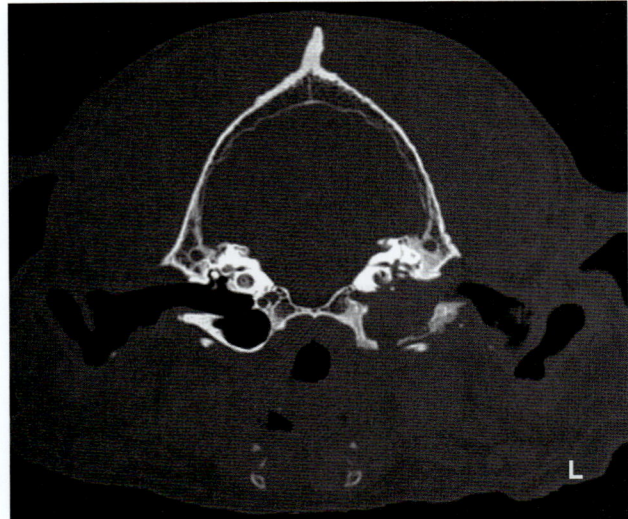

Figure 75.11 Transverse computed tomography image at the level of the tympanic bulla of the skull of a dog with chronic otitis media (1 mm thick, bone algorithm, WW 4800, WL 480). There is expansile-type enlargement of the left bulla with lysis and thickening. The bulla is also filled with soft tissue opacity material, and the petrous temporal bone appears more irregular than the opposite side.

middle ear, or within the calvarium. The absence of the normal high signal intensity of the inner ear has been reported to indicate inner ear abnormality (Garosi *et al.* 2000) (Figure 75.15).

Abnormalities in the tympanic bulla and external ear canal are indicated by replacement of the black appearance (normal signal void) by increased signal intensity material (relative to gray matter) on T1-weighted and T2-weighted images (Dvir *et al.* 2000; Garosi *et al.* 2000; Owen *et al.* 2004; Lorek *et al.* 2020) (Figure 75.16). Contrast media can also be used to assess enhancement characteristics of the auditory tissues (Allgoewer *et al.* 2000) and the mucosal lining of the tympanic bulla may contrast enhance with middle ear disease (Lorek *et al.* 2020). The character of the perilymph fluid within the inner ear can be evaluated with T2-weighted fluid-attenuated inversion recovery sequences (FLAIR). Normal perilymph would suppress on a T2-weighted FLAIR sequence (and would be hyperintense on a regular T2-weighted sequence), but in cases of otitis interna the perilymph may show decreased suppression when compared to the unaffected ear, indicating a proteinaceous and/or cellular perilymph (Castillo *et al.* 2020) (Figure 75.17). MRI also has the advantage of providing multiple planes to evaluate any abnormalities found (Allgoewer *et al.* 2000).

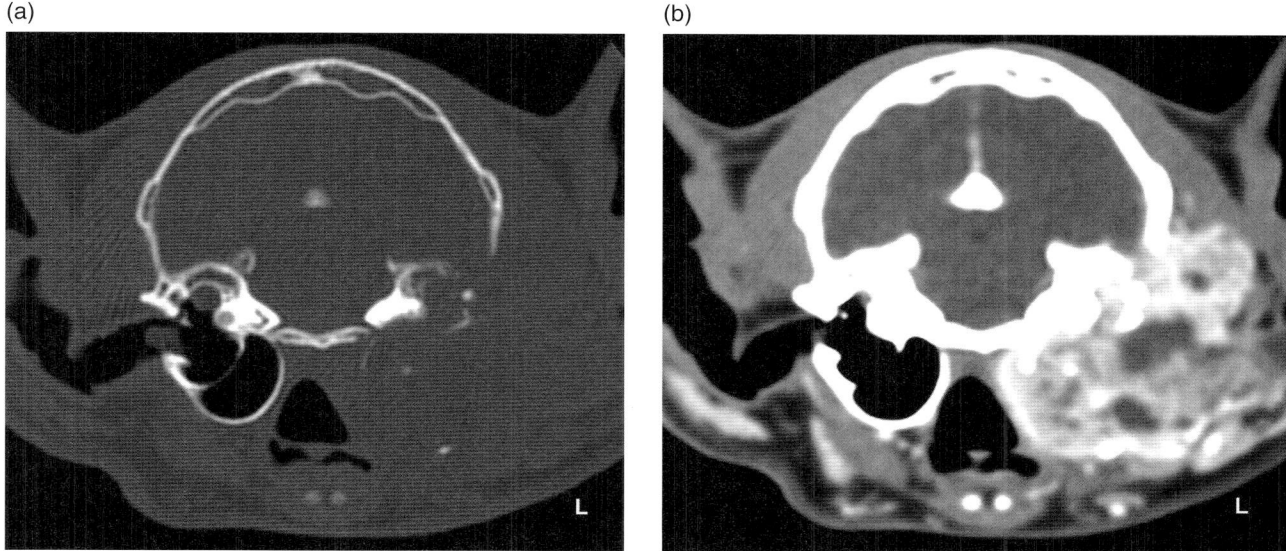

Figure 75.12 (a) Bone window and (b) soft tissue window post-contrast transverse computed tomography images of a cat with squamous cell carcinoma. (a) On the bone window image (1 mm thick, bone algorithm, WW 2500, WL 480) there is extensive lysis of the left tympanic bulla that extends to the adjacent petrous temporal. (b) A large contrast-enhancing soft tissue mass replacing the osseous bulla is present that extends into the calvarium through the lytic temporal bone (1 mm thick, soft tissue algorithm, WW 350, WL 90).

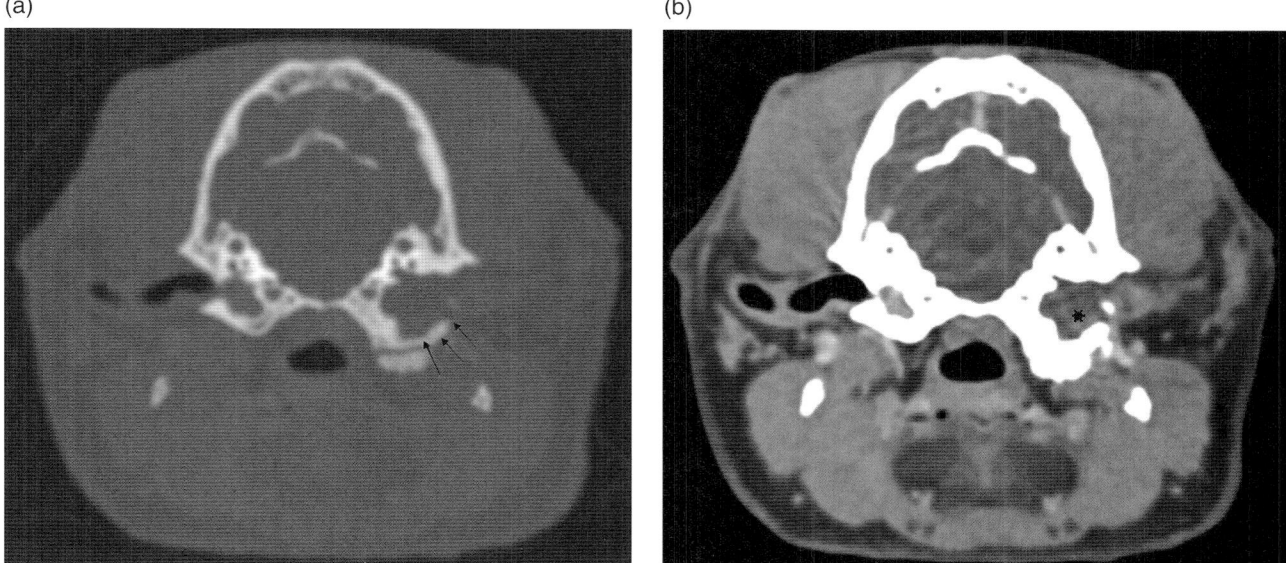

Figure 75.13 (a) Bone window and (b) soft tissue window transverse computed tomography images of a dog with a cholesteatoma in the left ear. There is expansile-type lysis of the left tympanic bulla (black arrows) with heterogeneous hyperattenuating material in the tympanic bulla (asterisk). This can be difficult to differentiate from more aggressive neoplasia and will require biopsy for confirmation. The right tympanic bulla also contains abnormal content and has concurrent otitis media and externa.

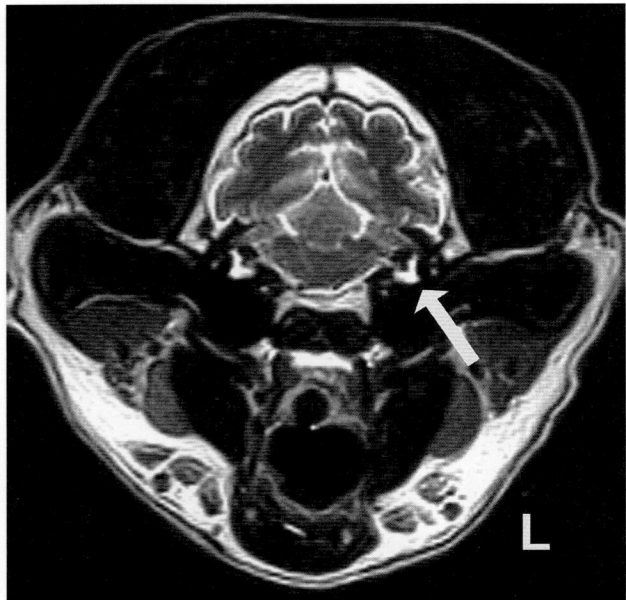

Figure 75.14 T2-weighted transverse spin echo magnetic resonance image (2.5 mm thick) at the level of the bullae of a normal dog. Note the normal-appearing high signal intensity in the membranous labyrinth of the inner ear (arrow). This has been described as being in the shape of a duck (Lamb & Garosi 2000). The normal signal void in the bullae and external ear canals can also be seen.

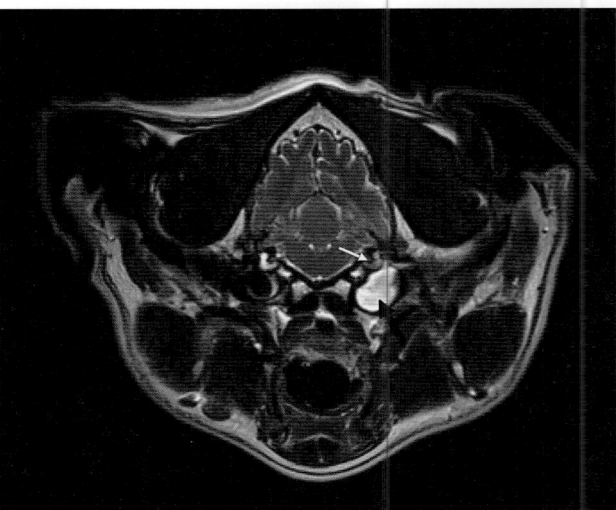

Figure 75.15 T2-weighted transverse spin echo magnetic resonance image at the level of the bullae of a dog with otitis media and interna of the left ear. Note the loss of the high signal intensity in the membranous labyrinth of the inner ear (white arrow) and the high signal fluid in the tympanic bulla (black arrow).

(a)

(b)

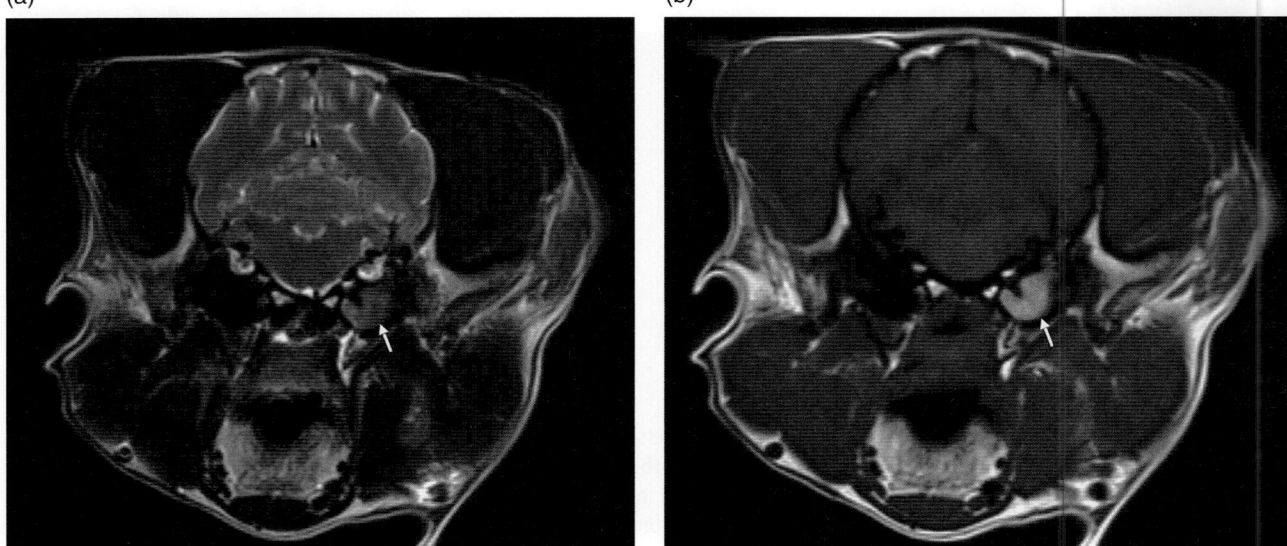

Figure 75.16 (a) T2-weighted and (b) T1-weighted transverse spin echo images at the level of the tympanic bullae of a canine patient. There is high signal material in the left tympanic bullae on both sequences. This is often seen with secretory otitis media.

(a)

(b)

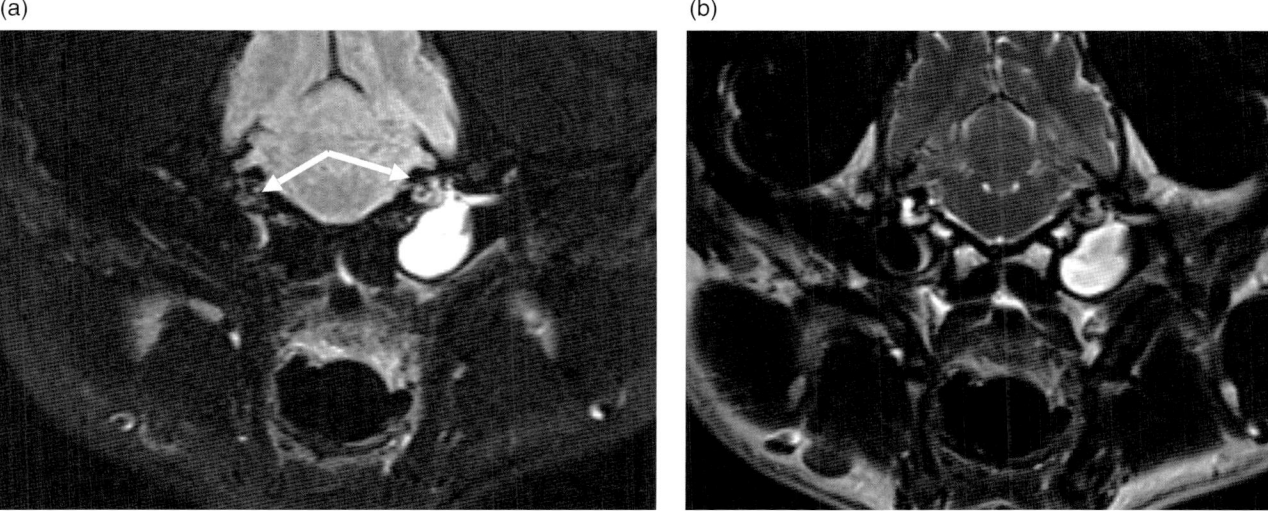

Figure 75.17 (a) T2-weighted fluid-attenuated inversion recovery sequences (FLAIR) and (b) T2-weighted transverse magnetic resonance images of a canine patient with otitis media and interna of the left ear. The normal high signal in the perilymph of the internal ear should suppress on the FLAIR sequence. In this case there is retention of the signal in the perilymph of the left internal ear canal relative to the right (white arrows). Note also the lower signal in the perilymph on the T2-weighted image of this same ear. These findings support proteinaceous or cellular fluid typical of otitis interna.

References

Alexander, A., Mahoney, P., Scurrell, E., and Baines, S. (2019). Cholesteatoma in a cat. *Journal of Feline Medicine and Surgery Open Reports* 5 (1): 2055116919848086.

Allgoewer, I., Lucas, S., and Schmitz, S.A. (2000). Magnetic resonance imaging of the normal and diseased feline middle ear. *Veterinary Radiology and Ultrasound* 41: 413–418.

Barthez, P.Y., Koblik, P.D., Hornof, W.J. et al. (1996). Apparent wall thickening in fluid filled versus air filled tympanic bulla in computed tomography. *Veterinary Radiology and Ultrasound* 37: 95–98.

Belmudes, A., Pressanti, C., Barthez, P. et al. (2018). Computed tomographic findings in 205 dogs with clinical signs compatible with middle ear disease: a retrospective study. *Veterinary Dermatology* 29: 45–50.

Benigni, L. and Lamb, C. (2006). Diagnostic imaging of ear disease in the dog and cat. *Companion Animal Practice* 28 (3): 122–130.

Bischoff, M.G. and Kneller, S.K. (2004). Diagnostic imaging of the canine and feline ear. *Veterinary Clinics of North America. Small Animal Practice* 34: 437–458.

Blutke, A., Parzefall, B., Steger, A. et al. (2010). Inflammatory polyp in the middle ear of a dog: a case report. *Veterinární Medicína* 55: 289–293.

Castillo, G., Parmentier, T., Monteith, G., and Gaitero, L. (2020). Inner ear fluid-attenuated inversion recovery MRI signal intensity in dogs with vestibular disease. *Veterinary Radiology and Ultrasound* 41: 531–539.

Classen, J., Bruehschwein, A., Meyer-Lindenberg, A., and Mueller, R. (2016). Comparison of ultrasound imaging and video otoscopy with cross-sectional imaging for diagnosis of canine otitis media. *Veterinary Journal* 217: 68–71.

Dickie, A.M., Doust, R., Cromarty, L. et al. (2003a). Ultrasound imaging of the canine tympanic bulla. *Research in Veterinary Science* 75: 121–126.

Dickie, A.M., Doust, R., Cromarty, L. et al. (2003b). Comparison of ultrasonography, radiography, and a single computed tomography slice for the identification of fluid within the canine tympanic bulla. *Research in Veterinary Science* 75: 209–216.

Doust, R., King, A., Hammond, G. et al. (2007). Assessment of middle ear disease in the dog: a comparison of diagnostic imaging modalities. *Journal of Small Animal Practice* 48: 188–192.

Dvir, E., Kirberger, R.M., and Terblanche, A.G. (2000). Magnetic resonance imaging of otitis media in a dog. *Veterinary Radiology & Ultrasound* 41: 46–49.

Eom, K.-D., Lee, H.-C., and Yoon, J.-H. (2000). Canalographic evaluation of the external ear canal in dogs. *Veterinary Radiology and Ultrasound* 41: 231–234.

Forrest, L.J. (2007). Cranial nasal cavities: canine and feline. In: *Textbook of Veterinary Diagnostic Radiology*, 5e (ed. D.E. Thrall), 119–141. St. Louis, MO: WB Saunders.

Garosi, L.S., Lamb, C.R., and Targett, M.P. (2000). MRI findings in a dog with otitis media and suspected otitis interna. *Veterinary Record* 146: 501–502.

Garosi, L.S., Dennis, R., Penderis, J. et al. (2001). Results of magnetic resonance imaging in dogs with vestibular disorders: 85 cases (1996–1999). *Journal of the American Veterinary Medical Association* 218: 385–391.

Garosi, L.S., Dennis, R., and Schwarz, T. (2003). Review of diagnostic imaging of ear diseases in the dog and cat. *Veterinary Radiology and Ultrasound* 44: 137–146.

Greci, V., Olga, T., Di Giancamillo, M. et al. (2011). Middle ear cholesteatoma in 11 dogs. *Canadian Veterinary Journal* 52: 631–636.

Griffiths, L., Sullivan, M., O'Neill, T., and Reid, S. (2003). Ultrasonogrpahy versus radiography for detection of fluid in the canine tympanic bulla. *Veterinary Radiology and Ultrasound* 44: 210–213.

Hammon, G., Sullivan, M., Weinrauch, S., and King, A. (2005). A comparison of the rostrocaudal open mouth and rostro 10° ventro-caudodorsal oblique radiographic views for imaging fluid in the feline tympanic bulla. *Veterinary Radiology and Ultrasound* 46: 205–209.

Hoskinson, J.J. (1993). Imaging techniques in the diagnosis of middle ear disease. *Seminars in Veterinary Medicine and Surgery (Small Animal)* 8: 10–16.

King, A., Weinrauch, S., Doust, R. et al. (2007). Comparison of ultrasonography, radiography and a single computed tomography slice for fluid identification within the feline tympanic bulla. *Veterinary Journal* 173: 638–634.

Lamb, C.R. and Garosi, L. (2000). Images in medicine. *Veterinary Radiology and Ultrasound* 41: 292.

Lee, J., Eom, K., Seong, Y. et al. (2006). Ultrasonographic evaluation of the external ear canal and tympanic membrane in dogs. *Veterinary Radiology and Ultrasound* 47: 94–98.

Lorek, A., Dennis, R., Van Dijk, J., and Bannoehr, J. (2020). Occult otitis media in dogs with chronic otitis externa-magnetic resonance imaging and association with otoscopic and cytological findings. *Veterinary Dermatology* 31: 146–e28.

Love, N.E., Kramer, R.W., Spodnick, G.J., and Thrall, D.E. (1995). Radiographic and computed tomographic evaluation of otitis media in the dog. *Veterinary Radiology and Ultrasound* 36: 375–379.

Oliveira, C., O'Brien, R., Matheson, J., and Carrera, I. (2012). Computed tomographic features of feline nasopharyngeal polyps. *Veterinary Radiology and Ultrasound* 53: 406–411.

Owen, M.C., Lamb, C.R., Lu, D., and Targett, M.P. (2004). Material in the middle ear of dogs having magnetic resonance imaging for investigation of neurologic signs. *Veterinary Radiology and Ultrasound* 45: 149–155.

Parzefall, B., Rieger, A., Volk, H. et al. (2014). Prevalence and characterization of small tympanic bone spicules and drumstick-like hyperostotic tympanic bone spicules in the middle ear cavity of dogs. *Veterinary Radiology and Ultrasound* 56: 25–32.

Pratschke, K.M. (2003). Inflammatory polyps of the middle ear in 5 dogs. *Veterinary Surgery* 32: 292–296.

Risselada, M. (2016). Diagnosis and management of cholesteatomas in dogs. *Veterinary Clinics of North America. Small Animal Practice* 46: 623–634.

Rohleder, J.J., Jones, J.C., Duncan, R.B. et al. (2006). Comparative performance of radiography and computed tomography in the diagnosis of middle ear disease in 31 dogs. *Veterinary Radiology and Ultrasound* 47: 45–52.

Russo, M., Covelli, E.M., Meomartino, L. et al. (2002). Computed tomographic anatomy of the canine inner and middle ear. *Veterinary Radiology and Ultrasound* 43: 22–26.

Seifert, H., Roher, U., Staszyk, C. et al. (2012). Optimising μCT imaging of the middle and inner cat ear. *Anatomia, Histologia, Embryologia* 41: 113–121.

Seitz, S.E., Losonski, J.M., and Marretta, S.M. (1996). Computed tomographic appearance of inflammatory polyps in three cats. *Veterinary Radiology and Ultrasound* 7: 99–104.

Sturges, B.K., Dickinson, P.J., Kortz, G.D. et al. (2006). Clinical signs, magnetic resonance imaging features and outcome after surgical and medical treatment of otogenic intracranial infection in 11 cats and 4 dogs. *Journal of Veterinary Internal Medicine* 20: 648–656.

Travetti, O., Guidice, C., Greci, V. et al. (2010). Computed tomography features of middle ear cholesteatoma in dogs. *Veterinary Radiology and Ultrasound* 51: 374–379.

Trower, N.D., Gregory, S.P., Renfrew, H., and Lamb, C.R. (1998). Evaluation of the canine tympanic membrane by positive contrast ear canalography. *Veterinary Record* 142: 78–81.

Ziemer, L.S., Schwarz, T., and Sullivan, M. (2003). Otolithiasis in three dogs. *Veterinary Radiology and Ultrasound* 44: 28–31.

76

Total Ear Canal Ablation and Lateral Bulla Osteotomy

Daniel D. Smeak

Total ear canal ablation (TECA) involves complete removal of the vertical and horizontal ear canals with associated secretory epithelium, including that within the osseous acoustic meatus. This salvage procedure is most often performed for irreversible inflammatory ear canal disease in dogs (Fraser *et al.* 1970; Spivack *et al.* 2013; Coleman & Smeak 2016) (Figure 76.1). Irreversible inflammatory disease is characterized by proliferative epithelial hyperplasia, causing concentric stenosis or collapse of the ear canal, which is often coupled with calcified peri-auricular tissue (Fraser *et al.* 1970; Little *et al.* 1991; Smeak & Kerpsack 1993) (Figure 76.2). Even when ear canal disease is not deemed irreversible, owners may elect this procedure if they are either unwilling or unable to provide appropriate medical therapy, especially when repeated attempts have failed (Smeak & Kerpsack 1993). Other less common indications for this procedure include severe ear canal trauma, invasive neoplasia, acquired aural cholesteatoma, certain congenital ear canal malformations or atresia, failed ear surgery, and ear canal avulsion (Smeak & Dehoff 1986; McCarthy *et al.* 1995; Hardie *et al.* 2008; Risselada 2016; Greci *et al.* 2011). In cats, TECA is most often performed for neoplastic invasion of the ear canal (ceruminous gland adenocarcinoma, squamous cell carcinoma) or global polypoid inflammatory disease, ceruminous cystomatosis, and more rarely for other indications as listed for dogs (Bacon *et al.* 2003; Soohoo *et al.* 2017). Without concurrent end-stage external ear disease, when surgery is indicated, primary middle ear infections and polyps in cats are treated via ventral bulla osteotomy alone; TECA is generally not indicated (Donnelly & Tillson 2004; Schlicksup *et al.* 2009).

A lateral bulla osteotomy (LBO) is nearly always performed with TECA, since otitis media is often associated with long-standing otitis externa in dogs, and the tympanic cavity can be explored through the same surgical approach (Cole *et al.* 1998; Smeak & Inpanbutr 2005). Debris and secretory epithelium may be found within the bulla in chronic inflammatory processes, and these have been implicated as causes for chronic deep infection after TECA (Holt *et al.* 1996; Smeak *et al.* 1996). When TECA was performed without bulla osteotomy in an original retrospective study, a high rate of infection-related complications was encountered (Smeak & Dehoff 1986). Later, the complication rate was decreased considerably when the procedure was combined with curettage of the tympanic bulla lining following an LBO (Mason *et al.* 1988; Beckman *et al.* 1990; Matthieson & Scavelli 1990; White & Pomeroy 1990). An aggressive bulla osteotomy involving the lateral bulla and floor, sometimes coined subtotal bulla osteotomy, has been advocated more recently, since wide exposure is necessary to ensure that any debris or epithelial remnants are completely removed, and it may allow more efficient drug delivery and immune defense, since there is better access for regional vascular tissue to reach the tympanic cavity (McAnulty *et al.* 1995; Smeak & Inpanbutr 2005). The ventral approach to the tympanic cavity provides better exposure and may allow exploration of the cavity with less risk of damage to neural structures (Boothe 1997). However, when the ventral approach was combined with TECA in a series of dogs with end-stage otitis externa and media, there was a high rate of complications, including facial nerve damage and recurrence of

Small Animal Soft Tissue Surgery, Second Edition. Edited by Eric Monnet.
© 2023 John Wiley & Sons, Inc. Published 2023 by John Wiley & Sons, Inc.
Companion website: www.wiley.com/go/monnet/small

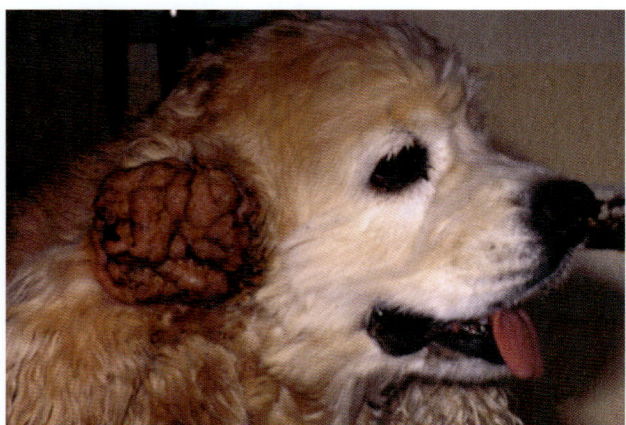

Figure 76.1 End-stage proliferative otitis externa in an adult cocker spaniel.

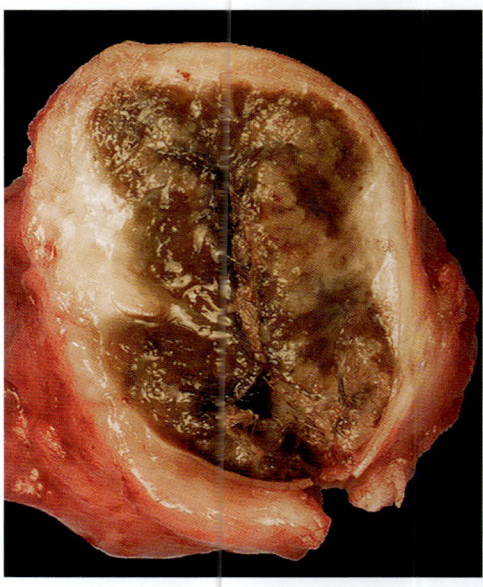

Figure 76.2 Cross-sectional view of excised ear canal after total ear canal ablation from dog shown in Figure 76.1. Note the concentric occlusion of the vertical ear canal with severe epithelial hyperplasia.

deep infection. This combined approach offers no advantage to the standard TECA/LBO technique (Sharp 1990). If the external ear disease process does not involve the middle ear, epithelium within the osseous external acoustic meatus and tympanic membrane should be carefully removed (McAnulty *et al.* 1995), but an extensive LBO may not be necessary, in the author's opinion.

For select patients with end-stage global ear disease, bilateral TECA/LBO procedures can be performed successfully during the same anesthetic episode. The findings of a retrospective study in dogs showed no significant difference in major anesthetic or overall surgical complication rates when TECA/LBO was performed bilaterally compared to dogs undergoing staggered procedures (Coleman & Smeak 2016). Some surgeons elect to stagger the procedures, choosing to perform the second side when the first procedure has completely healed, and any early complications have been resolved. This may be prudent in elderly and at-risk dogs to avoid the deleterious effects of prolonged anesthesia, especially if advanced imaging is elected during the same anesthetic episode. In the author's experience, risk of breathing difficulty from upper airway obstruction after surgery is increased, since more edema and swelling in the pharynx may be expected after aggressive bilateral TECA/LBO procedures (especially when there is preexisting upper airway obstruction, such as is seen in brachycephalic dogs).

If bilateral procedures are elected, the second side should be considered a completely separate procedure. Gowns and gloves are exchanged, the second side is prepped and draped, and additional sterile packs are used, since carryover of bacterial contamination may occur if the original instruments are used.

Owner education

Owners should be made thoroughly aware of the purpose and expectations after TECA/LBO, due to the risk of serious postoperative complications (see the section on complications). The major aim of the surgery is to make the pet more comfortable by completely removing the source of the chronic infection. Elimination of further ear cleaning duties and the malodorous discharge are added benefits (Beckman *et al.* 1990).

Before surgery, owners tend to be most concerned about the appearance of their pet and whether their animal will be deaf after surgery. The appearance in floppy-eared dogs, such as cocker spaniels, is unchanged after surgery, even if the ear canal excision is extended well up into the base of the pinna (Smeak & Kerpsack 1993) (Figure 76.3). The author prefers to remove all diseased ear tissue, despite the potential for poor ear carriage in erect-eared dogs and cats, since continued head shaking and scratching can be expected if proliferative ear tissue remains after TECA (Mason *et al.* 1988; Beckman *et al.* 1990; Matthieson & Scavelli 1990). A modified technique that preserves the distal vertical ear canal (hence maintains ear carriage in erect-eared dogs and cats), called a subtotal ear canal ablation, may be indicated when the disease process is limited to the horizontal ear canal (see Chapter 77) (Mathews *et al.* 2006). If this procedure is elected, owners should be warned that the portion of the vertical ear canal remaining after subtotal ear canal ablation may be a continued source of

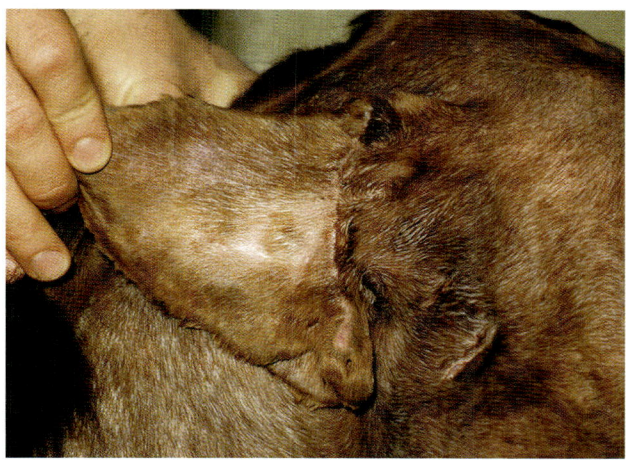

Figure 76.3 Appearance after total ear canal ablation in a dog that had proliferative tissue extension well into the medial pinna skin.

irritation and infection, particularly in dogs with progressive systemic skin conditions.

It is likely that most dogs with chronic external and middle ear infection have diminished hearing ability even *before* surgery (Smeak & Kerpsack 1993; Mason *et al.* 1988). Subjectively, if owners are made aware of their pet's auditory deficits in the preoperative evaluation, there is a low percentage of owners who believe that the auditory function decreased in the postoperative period (Smeak & Kerpsack 1993). Whether or not TECA/LBO contributes to hearing loss has been objectively examined. In one study, 100% of normal dogs were "deaf" after experimental TECA/LBO (when the tympanic membrane and ossicles were purposely removed), as determined by electronic measurements of air-conducted brainstem auditory evoked potentials (BSAEP) (McAnulty *et al.* 1995). Two dogs retained some hearing, but were subsequently found to have retained tympanic membranes and ossicles. In previous experimental studies, many dogs retained some hearing ability, but the tympanic membrane and ossicles were routinely not found or were removed during the surgery (Payne *et al.* 1989; Krahwinkel *et al.* 1993). Dogs retain bone-conducted BSAEP after TECA/LBO, and this would be expected because the surgery disrupts the sound conduction mechanisms but not the sensorineural components of the auditory pathway. Bone-conducted hearing alone is not likely to be practically relevant (McAnulty *et al.* 1995). In this study, retention of the tympanic membrane promoted reformation of the tympanic cavity, impedance of soft tissue ingrowth, and formation of epithelialized cavities and accumulated keratinized cellular debris, and this likely will increase the risk of late deep infection after TECA (McAnulty

et al. 1995). Therefore, it is recommended to remove the tympanic membrane with the epithelial lining of the external osseous meatus, despite the risk of diminished hearing (McAnulty *et al.* 1995; Smeak & Inpanbutr 2005).

In most cases, owners report high satisfaction after TECA/LBO is performed on their pets, in the experience of the author and others (Kim *et al.* 2003; Spivack *et al.* 2013). Owners should be reminded that this procedure is considered elective and rare, and that serious complications such as blood loss, upper airway obstruction, inner ear damage, recurrent deep infection, and death have been reported during and after surgery (Smeak & Dehoff 1986; Mason *et al.* 1988; Matthieson & Scavelli 1990; McAnulty *et al.* 1995).

Preoperative work-up

A complete preoperative blood and physical work-up, including a dermatologic examination, is essential to determine the extent and nature of the chronic ear disease process, and to help predict possible surgical or anesthetic complications.

Physical examination

During routine physical examination, the external ear, deeper ear canals, and regional lymph nodes are palpated and examined. In the examination, when the ear discharge appears mostly as blood, neoplasia should be highly suspected (Smeak & Dehoff 1986; Matthieson & Scavelli 1990). A complete cranial nerve examination should be performed to evaluate for facial nerve dysfunction (represented as either hemifacial spasm and/or poor palpebral reflex and lip droop), inner ear involvement, and Horner's syndrome. About 15% of dogs presenting for TECA consideration have either partial or complete facial nerve deficits (Matthieson & Scavelli 1990). Dogs with facial neuropathy are much more likely to have otitis media/interna, particularly cocker spaniels (Kern & Erb 1987). Concurrent middle ear disease increases the risk of infection complications after surgery (Smeak & Dehoff 1986). Significant pain elicited when opening the mouth of the patient generally signifies an aggressive middle ear condition (neoplasia, cholesteatoma, or severe infection) (Smeak 2016; Hardie *et al.* 2008).

In dogs, and much less likely in cats, chronic ear problems are manifestations of a systemic skin disorder, so a complete dermatologic examination should be performed. This is important since if the primary dermatologic disorder is not corrected after surgery, progression of the disease in the remaining ear tissue or in the opposite ear may occur (Mason *et al.* 1988; Beckman *et al.* 1990; Matthieson & Scavelli 1990). This progression may be seen as a failure of the surgical procedure from the owner's point of view (Smeak & Kerpsack 1993).

Appropriate staging is performed in animals with suspected neoplastic ear disease. Local lymph nodes are palpated, and fine-needle aspirate samples are examined cytologically when appropriate. Chest radiographs are evaluated for evidence of metastatic disease or other problems that may be found in older patients. If ear neoplasia is detected, it is important to determine if the disease has invaded structures of the skull or has extended past ear cartilage limits. In many cases, when neoplastic processes are confined within the external ear canal, cats and dogs can achieve long survival times (>42 months) following TECA and LBO alone (Marino *et al.* 1994; London *et al.* 1996; Bacon *et al.* 2003).

Otoscopic examination

A complete otoscopic examination is best performed while the patient is anesthetized. After thorough cleaning, the ear canal is examined and appropriate samples are collected for bacterial culture and susceptibility, and cytologic examination (Cole 2004). Particular attention is directed at locating tumors or growths and determining the amount of stenosis of the horizontal ear canal. Fine-needle aspirates of suspicious masses can be quite helpful in distinguishing benign versus malignant ear disease (Lorenzi *et al.* 2005). Otitis media can be assumed to be present if no tympanic membrane can be found and the tympanic bulla is filled with debris during otoscopic examination.

Imaging evaluation

Radiographic imaging of the external, middle, and internal ear is recommended to determine if there is evidence of otitis media or, when neoplasia is suspected, to look for evidence of tympanic bulla lysis or proliferation. Plain film, computed tomography (CT), or magnetic resonance imaging (MRI) can be used to examine the external ear canal, tympanic membrane, and tympanic bulla. Although plain film radiography continues to be used commonly to evaluate patients with chronic ear disease, it is not a modality that is sensitive to demonstrating changes in dogs with otitis media (Remedios *et al.* 1991). Positive-contrast ear canalography has also been used to determine if there is evidence of either a ruptured tympanic membrane or stenosis of the horizontal ear canal (Trower *et al.* 1998; Eom *et al.* 2000). In dogs with ear disease, canalography may be more sensitive for diagnosing otitis media than either otoscopic examination or plain film radiography (Trower *et al.* 1998).

In a comparison between CT evaluation and plain film radiographs for evaluation of otitis media, CT evaluation was found to be more sensitive for the diagnosis of otitis media and involvement of surrounding middle/inner ear structures (Rohleder *et al.* 2006). In cases with evidence of otitis with concurrent vestibular signs when it is not possible to differentiate between a central and peripheral vestibular syndrome, MRI has been advocated to evaluate possible caudal fossa parenchyma brain lesions and middle ear pathology (Dvir *et al.* 2000). In most cases, however, if the index of suspicion for otitis media is high based on the presence of chronic otitis externa or associated neurologic deficits, surgical exploration of the middle ear is indicated despite equivocal imaging results (Remedios *et al.* 1991). CT imaging is recommended before surgery particularly in those dogs with neurologic deficits, pain on opening the mouth during physical examination, or signs of upper airway obstruction, as these often indicate a more aggressive middle ear process (Hardie *et al.* 2008; Smeak 2016).

Aural cholesteatoma, an epidermoid cyst forming within the tympanic cavity, should be identified before considering surgery, because owners should be warned that recurrence of middle ear disease after TECA/LBO is common (Hardie *et al.* 2008; Risselada 2016; Greci *et al.* 2011). Most dogs have acquired forms of this condition, since most have a history of chronic ear disease, and epithelial migration is thought to occur through a perforated tympanic membrane into the tympanic cavity. CT radiographic changes consistent with this disease include osteoproliferation (particularly when *expansion* of the bulla is seen), bulla lysis, and bone lysis of the petrosal or squamous portion of the temporal bone (Hardie *et al.* 2008; Risselada 2016; Greci *et al.* 2011). It should be noted that cholesteatoma has been identified recently in a cat with clinical signs related to an oropharyngeal mass (Alexander *et al.* 2019).

Preoperative antibiotic and analgesia regimen choice

A proliferative and stenotic ear canal is difficult to prepare aseptically, so contamination is inevitable during surgery (Vogel *et al.* 1999). Bacterial contaminants are frequently isolated in the subcutaneous tissues during TECA/LBO. Cefazolin is not recommended as a perioperative antibiotic since many of these subcutaneous contaminants are not susceptible to this antibiotic (Vogel *et al.* 1999; Hettlich *et al.* 2005). Prophylactic intravenous antibiotic therapy should be initiated before the skin incision. In one report 90% of isolates from TECA procedures were susceptible to amoxicillin–clavulanate, aminoglycoside, or ticarcillin antibiotics (Vogel *et al.* 1999). If possible, the author prefers to use preoperative culture data of ear exudate, since this was found to be an accurate method to determine the choice for perioperative antibiotics during TECA in dogs (Cole *et al.* 2005). In addition to antibiotic use, gentle tissue handling, repeated wound irrigation, and complete removal of debris and infected epithelium are critical to reduce infection risk postoperatively (McAnulty *et al.* 1995; Smeak & Inpanbutr 2005). Ideally, medical treatment should be attempted before surgery for dogs presenting with draining tracts and severe infection in the region of the affected ear. Successful treatment of acute infection helps reduce surrounding inflammation and diminishes the risk of excessive hemorrhage and contamination during the procedure (Smeak & Kerpsack 1993).

TECA/LBO is known to be a very painful procedure in small animals (Buback *et al.* 1996). Preemptive analgesia should be considered, because it decreases the intensity and duration of postoperative pain and minimizes the likelihood of a chronic pain state being established (Tranquilli *et al.* 2004). In addition, it may help reduce the dosage and thus some of the deleterious effects of certain general anesthetics utilized during the procedure (Dyson 2008). Local nerve blockade before TECA/LBO is a technique used by some surgeons, but in one study it was not found to decrease observed and metabolic markers of postoperative pain and anxiety; however, subjectively these dogs were easier to manage anesthetically (Buback *et al.* 1996). Intraoperative analgesia can be attempted using a single splash block of bupivacaine, or a device can be placed that allows for continuous local infusion of bupivacaine in the postoperative period. However, in two reports neither single nor continuous nerve blockade was found to be clinically useful for decreasing observed or metabolic markers of pain in the postoperative period for TECA patients (Radlinsky *et al.* 2005; Buback *et al.* 1996). In the past the author preferred to utilize continuous incisional lidocaine delivery, since it was shown to be an equipotent and viable method of providing postoperative analgesia compared with intravenous morphine in a series of TECA procedures in dogs. Lidocaine delivery resulted in a trend toward lower pain scores, significantly lower sedation scores, and no dogs requiring analgesic rescue. Uncommon wound complications secondary to local infusion were minor and self-limiting (Wolfe *et al.* 2006). More recently, the author has utilized liposomal incapsulated bupivacaine (Nocita®, Aratana Therapeutics, Leawood, KS, USA) for general tissue infiltration at the time of surgery. Nocita is injected in superficial tissues and wound edges while the wound is still open after TECA/LBO (Grubb & Lobprise 2020). Subjectively, the author has observed that dogs have improved comfort and require less narcotic administration postoperatively. However, it is not uncommon to encounter facial nerve dysfunction lasting up to 48 hours after surgery following intraoperative tissue infiltration of Nocita.

Surgical anatomy

Detailed illustrations of the surgical anatomy related to TECA/LBO, are offered in a review article by Smeak and Inpanbutr (2005).

Surgical equipment

In addition to instruments included in a standard general surgery pack, several types of bone rongeurs and retractors are handy for TECA/LBO. The author prefers Cleveland or Zaufal rongeurs to remove the thicker bone of the lateral tympanic bulla and osseous external auditory meatus. In larger-breed dogs with extensive bulla bone proliferation, a double-action Ruskin rongeur may be used. A Kerrison down-bite laminectomy punch is very useful in the author's hands for safe bone removal of the caudal and ventral aspect of the external auditory meatus. Delicate Lempert or Beyer rongeurs help clean up rough edges of the osteotomy site. In lieu of rongeurs, some surgeons equipped with air-driven instruments prefer burrs to remove bone. When using burrs to remove bone, great care is required to avoid catching soft tissue and injuring neighboring neurovascular structures. Allow the burr to completely stop before adjusting the burr tip location. An ultrasonic bone curette (Sonopet®, Stryker Neurosurgical, Kalamazoo, MI, USA) proved useful when removing the osseous proliferation during TECA in several West Highland white terriers (Beever *et al.* 2019). Freer periosteal elevators are handy to reflect soft tissue attached around the ventrolateral bulla face. For deeper tissue retraction and exposure, delicate Senn or the larger Army-Navy or malleable retractors suffice. The author cautions using Gelpi retractors within the deeper aspects of the wound, because this may increase the risk of iatrogenic trauma to the facial nerve and nearby vascular structures (Smeak & Inpanbutr 2005). In the author's experience, Lone Star retractors (Cooper Surgical, Trumbull, CT, USA) are useful, particularly when performing this procedure with limited assistance. Angled 0° or 30° Daubenspeck bone curettes and malleable Halle bone curettes are handy for reaching the deep recesses of the tympanic cavity (Smeak & Inpanbutr 2005). The author finds it highly beneficial to utilize unipolar electrotomy during ear canal excision to reduce hemorrhage and maximize identification of important deeper structures.

Surgical technique

For more detailed descriptions and illustrations of the TECA and LBO procedure, refer to Smeak and Kerpsack (1993) and Smeak and Inpanbutr (2005).

Total ear canal ablation

After anesthesia is induced, clip and aseptically prepare the patient's entire pinna and lateral aspect of the head for surgery. Repeatedly lavage the ear canal with diluted antiseptic solution to remove as much debris and contamination as possible before aseptic preparation. Administer the appropriate intravenous antibiotic before the skin incision is made. Position the animal in lateral recumbency with the head obliqued and elevated with a towel to a level parallel to the chest wall, with the nose pointing slightly downward.

Begin the procedure by making a T-shaped incision; make the horizontal incision parallel and just below the tragus and create the vertical incision perpendicular from the midpoint of the horizontal incision to a point just ventral to the horizontal ear canal (Figure 76.4a). A circular incision is also possible. Undermine and retract the two resulting skin flaps and expose the lateral aspect of the vertical canal from surrounding connective tissue using electrotomy or blunt dissection (Figure 76.4b). Dissect around the proximal and medial portion of the vertical canal, staying as close as possible to the cartilage to avoid damaging the vascular supply to the pinna. Starting from the *caudal* aspect, cut through the medial aspect of the vertical canal with serrated Mayo scissors or a unipolar wand and continue the incision until the ear canal opening has been completely separated from the head (Figure 76.4c). Be sure to include all proliferative tissue in the region of the base of the pinna with the medial incision. Free the remaining soft tissue from the

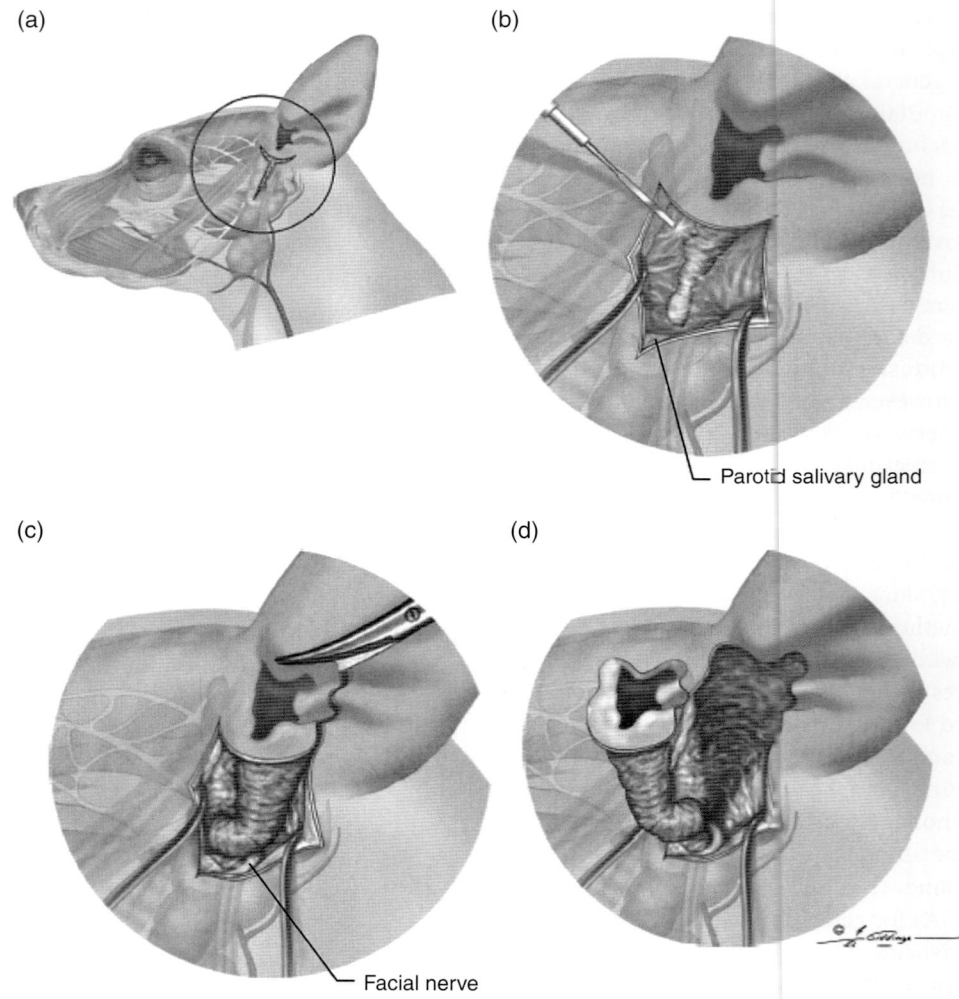

(a)

(b)

Parotid salivary gland

(c)

(d)

Facial nerve

Figure 76.4 (a) A T-shaped incision is made to expose the vertical ear canal. (b) Loose connective tissue is reflected from the vertical ear canal. Avoid damaging the parotid gland in the ventral aspect of the wound. (c) The vertical and horizontal ear canals are isolated from surrounding soft tissue by blunt and sharp dissection. The facial nerve is isolated and gently retracted. (d) The entire cartilaginous ear canal is isolated.

(a)

(b)

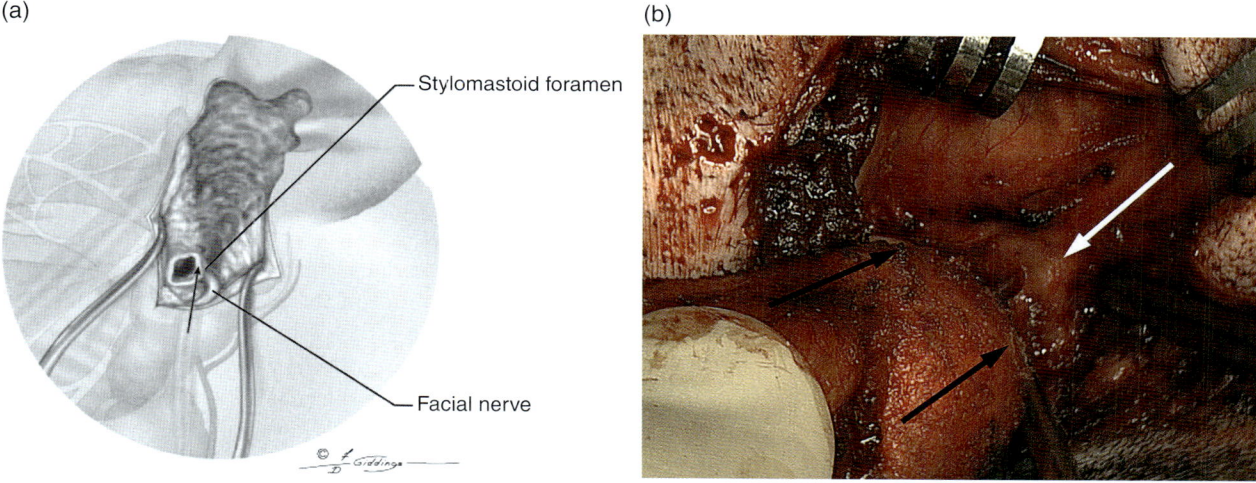

Stylomastoid foramen

Facial nerve

Figure 76.5 (a) Surgeon's lateral view of external auditory meatus after the cartilaginous ear canal has been excised. A thin rim of cartilage remains attached at the external auditory meatus. A prominent ridge (arrow – a consistent landmark) divides the stylomastoid foramen from the external auditory meatus. Note the location of the facial nerve and stylomastoid foramen. © D. Giddings. (b) The facial nerve (white arrow) is buried in adipose tissue close to the horizontal ear canal (black arrow) at the level of the external auditory meatus. Source: Smeak, D.D. and Inpanbutr, N. (2005). Lateral approach to subtotal bulla osteotomy in dogs. *Compendium*, May: 377–384.

vertical ear canal. An assistant can facilitate exposure of the surgical site by retracting the ear canal with a pair of Allis tissue forceps during dissection. Apply traction on the freed-up ear canal in a direction opposite the intended dissection plane. When the annular ligament is exposed, dissect soft tissue from the rostral and dorsal horizontal ear canal until the bony rim of the external auditory meatus is palpated. Dissection is first completed in this manner because this helps expose deeper tissue in the important area of the facial nerve. Irrigate the surgery site repeatedly during surgery. since this has been shown to decrease the number of bacterial contaminants in the wound by more the 33% (Hettlich *et al.* 2005).

Slowly and delicately begin dissection of the soft tissue from the ventral and caudal aspect of the proximal horizontal ear canal. The facial nerve may be found free from the canal (especially in cats), or in more chronic cases in dogs the nerve may be entrapped in the caudal aspect of the deep horizontal canal. Carefully free the nerve and note its location to keep it isolated and safe during the remaining part of the procedure. Dissect all soft tissue from the horizontal canal and excise the ear canal from the external auditory meatus (Figure 76.4d). If this attachment is thick and calcified, use rongeurs to disconnect the strong attachment to the external auditory meatus; otherwise a no. 15 blade will suffice (Figure 76.5). During this sharp dissection, be sure to direct the sharp-honed edge of the scalpel blade away from the course of the facial nerve (Figure 76.6). Submit the ear canal for histologic evaluation, and middle ear tissue samples for culture and susceptibility.

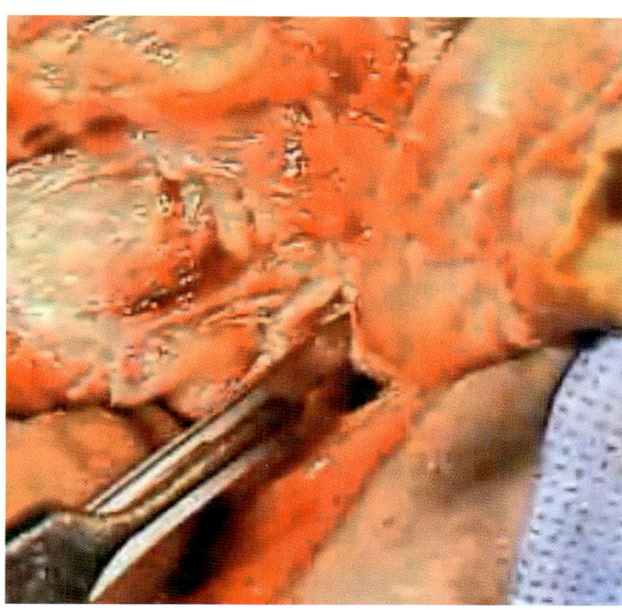

Figure 76.6 As the ear canal is retracted rostrally, a no. 15 BP blade shown being used to incise the proximal horizontal ear canal attachment to the external auditory meatus. Note that the blade is directed away from the course of the caudally located facial nerve, shown just to the left of the blade.

Subtotal bulla osteotomy

As the bulla is approached, take into account that the bulla may be extensively remodeled (expanded) from bulla osteitis or an expanding cholesteatoma (Smeak & Inpanbutr 2005; Hardie *et al.* 2008). Important neurovascular structures may be draped and tightly adhered to the ventral aspect of the tympanic bone. Always attempt to retract soft tissue for exposure of deeper structures surrounding the bulla without *directly* placing tension on the facial nerve. The author prefers to begin the bulla exposure by bluntly elevating soft tissue from the lateral face of the bulla using Freer elevators (Figure 76.7). Avoid sharp dissection or curettage in the region just rostral to the external auditory meatus to avoid damaging the retroarticular vein (Figure 76.8) (Smeak & Inpanbutr 2005). Remove the ventral aspect of the osseous ear canal first with rongeurs, and carefully strip out all epithelium and the tympanic membrane

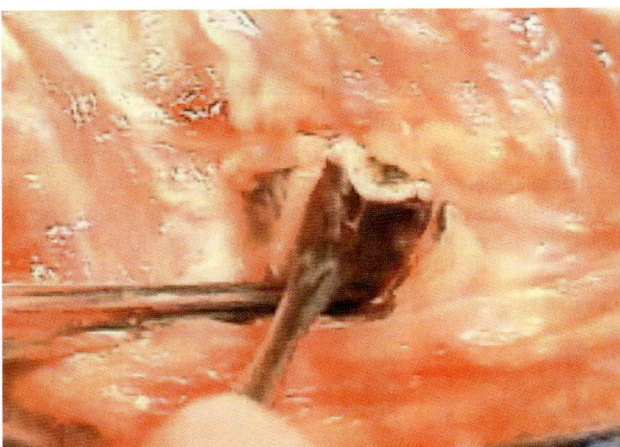

Figure 76.7 A Freer elevator is shown retracting the facial nerve (white vertical structure adjacent to the elevator) ventrally while freeing soft tissue from the deeper surface of the lateral bulla. A DeBakey forceps points to the nerve just caudal to the elevator.

(the malleus usually comes with the tympanic membrane as it is removed) within the external osseous meatus. Remove the remaining ventrolateral aspect of the bulla with rongeurs if there is any concern about debris or epithelium within the tympanic cavity. In subtotal bulla osteotomy, most of the lateral, caudal, and ventral bulla bone are removed (Figure 76.9) (Smeak & Inpanbutr 2005).

Occasionally in dogs, a greenish-brown epithelialized pouch will be found on the face of the bulla extending ventrally from the external auditory meatus. This pouch appears to be an outcropping of hyperplastic epithelium traveling between the external osseous meatus and ventral horizontal ear canal (Figure 76.10). Note that this pouch is often tightly adhered to structures under the floor of the bulla, and it must be carefully separated from these attachments (the external carotid artery typically is adhered to this pouch) to avoid profuse hemorrhage (Figure 76.11).

Carefully inspect the interior aspect of the tympanic bulla after irrigating with tepid sterile saline. Remove all debris and abnormal epithelium (seen as a greenish-brown thickened tissue) from the rostral, ventral, and caudal aspects of the tympanic cavity. There is no need to remove the remaining ossicles unless abnormal soft tissue is adhered to them in the epitympanic recess (Beckman *et al.* 1990; Smeak & Kerpsack 1993). The rostral tympanic cavity recess (opening of the auditory canal) and dorsal aspect of the tympanic bulla just medial to the external auditory meatus are carefully

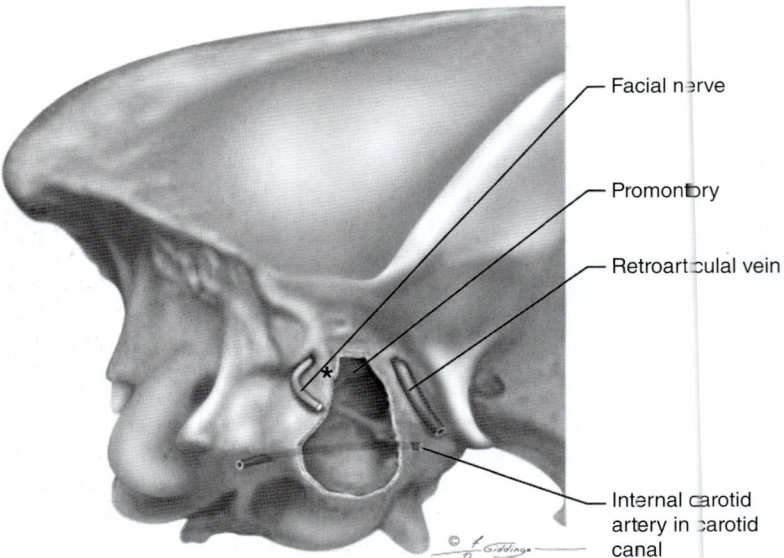

Figure 76.8 Close-up oblique ventrolateral view of important structures surrounding the tympanic bulla of the skull. The retroarticular vein is located just rostral to the entrance to the osseous ear canal and tympanic bulla. A distinct bony rim separates the osseous external auditory meatus from the stylomastoid foramen (i.e., exit site for the facial nerve). Source: Smeak, D.D. and Inpanbutr, N. 2005). Lateral approach to subtotal bulla osteotomy in dogs. *Compendium* May: 377–384.

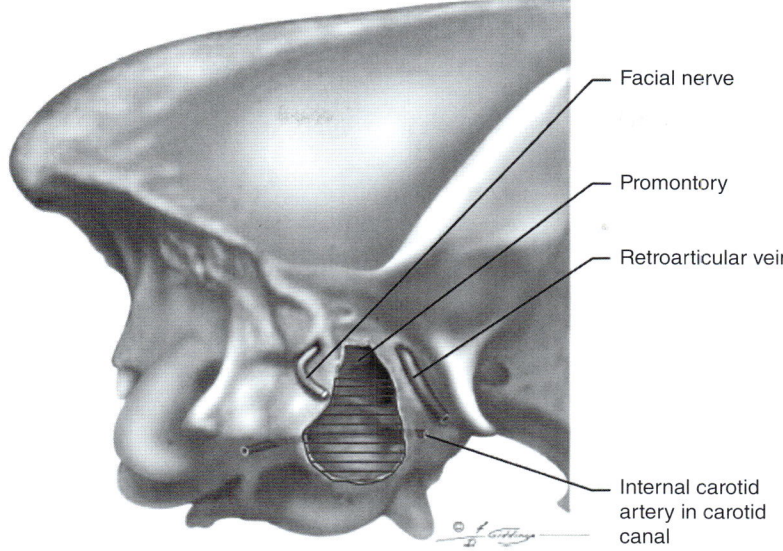

- Facial nerve
- Promontory
- Retroarticular vein
- Internal carotid artery in carotid canal

Figure 76.9 The ventral and lateral aspect of the tympanic bulla is removed with rongeurs (crosshatched area) to expose the bulla cavity.

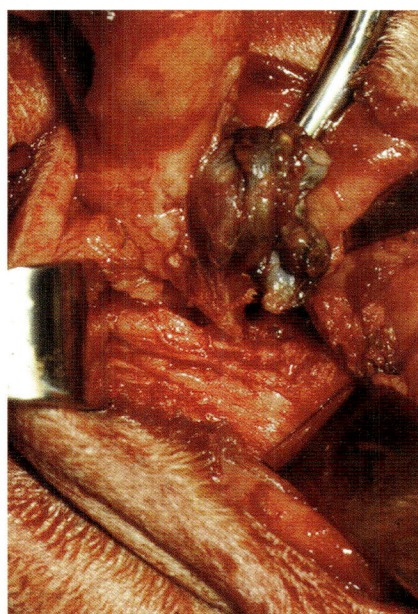

Figure 76.10 Partially isolated epithelial pouch found between ventral aspect of proximal horizontal ear canal (upper left of image) and tympanic bulla.

inspected for epithelial remnants (Watt *et al.* 2020). Remnants are submitted for biopsy, and culture and susceptibility. Complete removal of any epithelial remnants is critical to avoid recurrent deep infection after surgery (Smeak *et al.* 1996). The dorsal surface of the tympanic cavity is not curetted because damage to the promontory area and subsequent inner ear damage may occur. It is enough to simply tease any attached soft tissue from this area with hemostatic forceps.

Running within a canal on the medial aspect of the tympanic bone, the internal carotid artery may be damaged when freeing soft tissue in that area, especially when there is evidence that this bone has been eroded on CT imaging (Figure 76.12).

Provided that hemostasis is complete, the use of a video-otoscope during surgery provides excellent visualization of the inner tympanic cavity and may help identify debris and epithelial remnants (Haudequet *et al.* 2006; Rossello & Pelaez 2020). In one recent retrospective study of 51 TECA/LBO procedures, residual infected tissue was found with intraoperative endoscopy in 96% of cases after traditional bulla curettage (Rossello & Pelaez 2020). In another experimental study, intraoperative rigid endoscopy (1.9 mm) was used to help identify the most common locations of epithelial remnants after tympanic curettage. Epithelial remnants were consistently found after TECA/LBO, especially in the rostral compartment (Figure 76.13). Endoscopy should be considered during initial TECA/LBO or revision surgeries to help ensure complete removal of retained epithelium (Watt *et al.* 2020).

A Jackson–Pratt active suction drain may be placed in the depths of the wound if there is hemorrhage and gross contamination during surgery or when a para-aural abscess is discovered during dissection. Otherwise, the author does not routinely drain the wound (provided that the middle ear has been thoroughly evacuated and remaining wound surfaces are healthy). Rates of infection and wound complications were found to be similar whether or not TECA wounds were drained postoperatively in a previous retrospective study (Devitt *et al.* 1997).

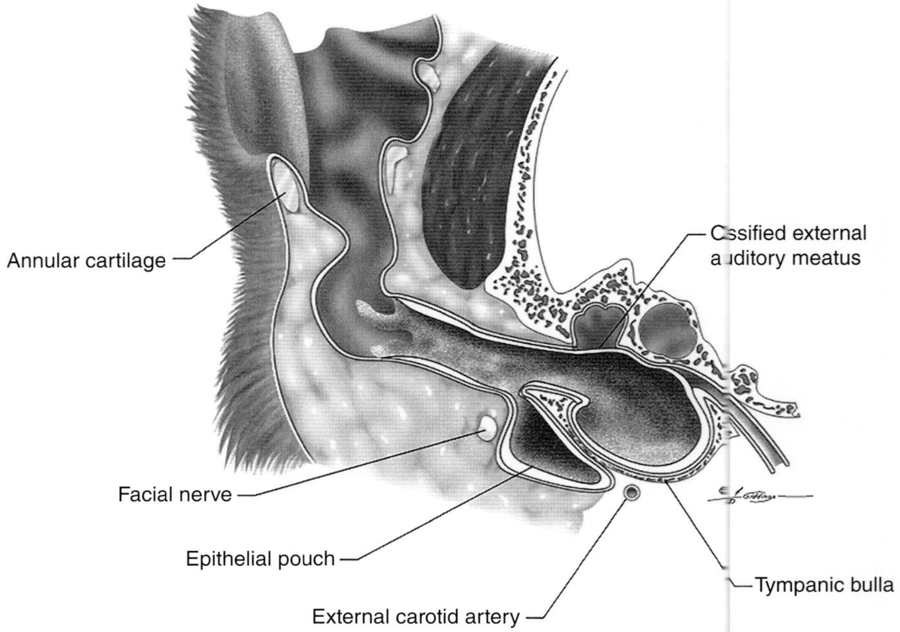

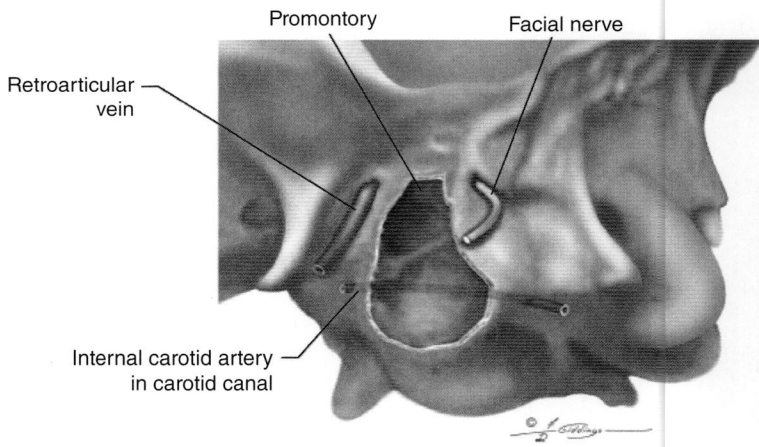

Figure 76.11 Transverse section through the head showing horizontal canal and tympanic bulla. A pouch of secretory epithelium often forms between the annular cartilage and the tympanic bulla extending into the external auditory meatus. Soft tissues are carefully dissected from the pouch and ventral aspect of the tympanic bulla. Source: Smeak, D.D. and Kerpsack, S.J. (1993). Total ear canal ablation and lateral bulla osteotomy for management of end stage otitis. *Seminars in Veterinary Medicine and Surgery (Small Animal)* 8:30–41.

Figure 76.12 Oblique ventrolateral view of skull after the lateral wall of the tympanic bulla has been removed. The internal carotid artery, a major blood supply to the brain, is illustrated. The internal carotid artery enters the caudal carotid foramen in the Petro occipital fissure and traverses the carotid canal. The medial wall of the tympanic bulla forms the lateral wall of the carotid canal.

While the wound remains open after TECA/LBO, a local anesthetic delivery system can be placed for postoperative analgesia (Figure 76.14) (Wolfe *et al.* 2006). Alternately, incised wound tissues can be infiltrated with liposomal encapsulated bupivacaine (Nocita). The dead space in the wound is closed by placing simple interrupted 4-0 absorbable monofilament suture material. It is important not to include the facial nerve within deeper suture bites intended to reduce dead space. The hypodermal layer of the T-shaped incision is apposed with interrupted 4-0 absorbable monofilament sutures. Attached soft tissues directly under the cut pinna cartilage are apposed to the hypodermis under the horizontal skin incision with interrupted suture (in buried knot fashion). The skin is routinely closed with 4-0 percutaneous monofilament nonabsorbable sutures, taking care to ensure that no pinna cartilage is exposed and that dermal edges are well apposed.

Variations in TECA/LBO in cats

A single pedicle advancement flap with a ventrally located base has been described to maintain normal ear carriage after TECA in cats (Figure 76.15) (McNabb & Flanders 2004). Generally, soft tissues are not strongly adhered to the ear canal in cats, so the horizontal and vertical ear canals can be readily freed from surrounding tissue. If neoplastic tissue extends past the ear canal cartilage, as much healthy soft tissue is removed as possible with the canal to help achieve a clean excision. The facial nerve is rarely incorporated in the ear canal (as typically observed in dogs) and often can be readily found loosely draped caudal and ventral to the horizontal ear canal.

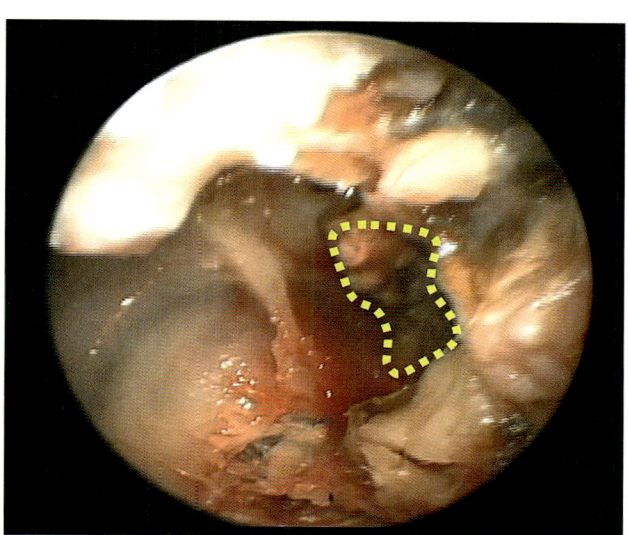

Figure 76.13 Endoscopic view of the tympanic cavity from a lateral bulla osteotomy. The yellow dotted line denotes retained greenish epithelium in the rostral compartment.

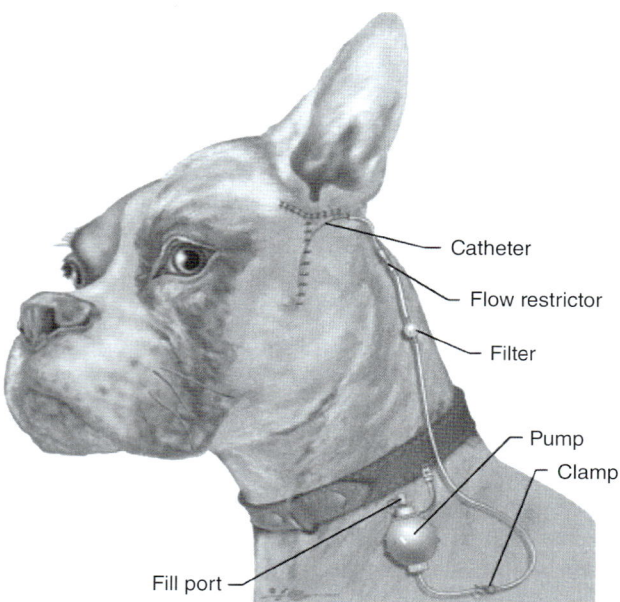

Figure 76.14 Application of the ON-Q local anesthetic infusion system in a total ear canal ablation.

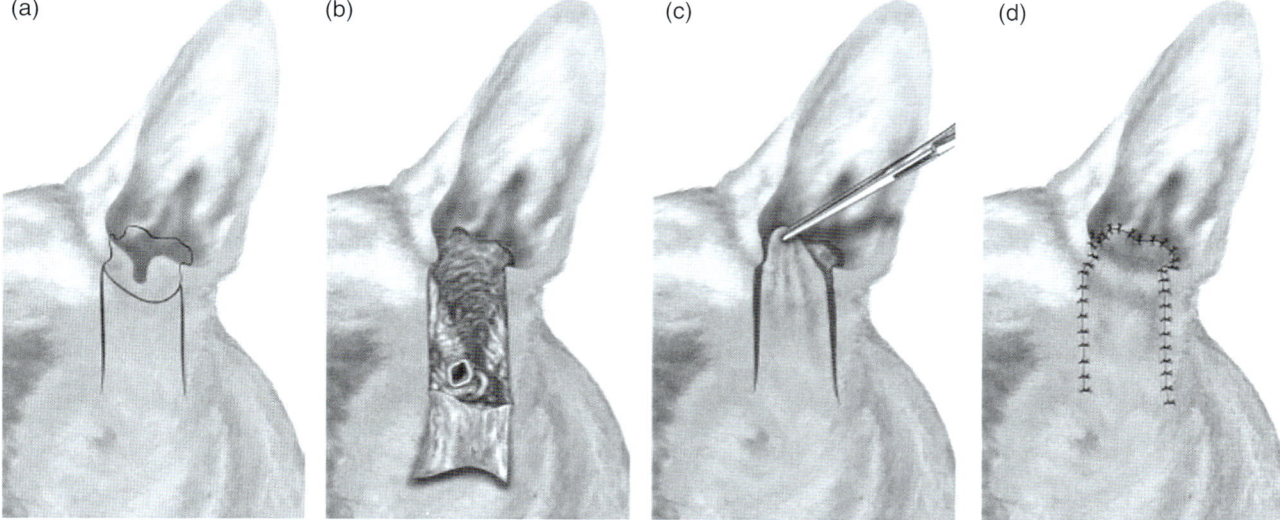

Figure 76.15 Technique for construction of single pedicle advancement flap at the base of the pinna in the modified ear canal ablation. (a) Vertical incisions are made at the rostral and caudal ends of the elliptical incision centered around the external auditory meatus. (b) The single pedicle advancement flap is dissected ventrally, allowing exposure of the subcutaneous tissue over the vertical ear canal. (c) After lateral bulla osteotomy and excision of the ear canal, the top of the advancement flap is pulled to the base of the pinna to determine if further release of the flap is necessary to reduce tension of the pinna. (d) The skin flap is sutured to the base of the pinna. Source: McNabb, A.H. and Flanders, J.A. (2004). Cosmetic results of a ventrally based advancement flap for closure of total ear canal ablations in 6 cats: 2002–2003. *Veterinary Surgery* 33:435–439.

Direct retraction of the nerve is avoided during canal and bulla dissection to reduce iatrogenic nerve damage. Routinely separate the attachment of the horizontal ear canal to the osseous auditory meatus with a no. 15 blade, directing the sharp edge away from the course of the facial nerve. In most cats undergoing TECA the tympanic bulla is not involved with the disease process, so a limited bulla osteotomy is performed to ensure that the tympanic cavity is clean and the epithelium and tympanic membrane in the osseous ear canal have been removed. When this is performed carefully, both chambers should be exposed from the lateral approach if full bulla exploration is indicated. In a recent study, larger bulla osteotomies help ensure adequate exposure to the hypotympanum (Mehrkens *et al.* 2019).

Postoperative care

Care immediately following surgery consists of routine monitoring for anesthetic recovery, analgesia, and antibiotic therapy. The author generally does not bandage the head following TECA/LBO. If excessive head shaking is observed, use a loosely applied stockinette to secure the pinna and to hold 4 × 4 sponges on the wound for the first 24 hours after surgery. If head-encircling bandages are used, be sure to avoid applying them too tightly, since respiratory difficulty from airway obstruction can be encountered (Lanz & Wood 2004).

Facial nerve dysfunction is evaluated when the animal is recovered from anesthesia and if deficits are seen, eye lubricants are applied to reduce corneal ulcers after surgery. Owners should continue using eye lubricants at home, particularly in patients with exophthalmos or diminished tear production, until the palpebral reflex has recovered.

Administration of the same antibiotic that was used intraoperatively is resumed until the culture and susceptibility results are complete. Antibiotic therapy is adjusted according to the culture and susceptibility results (Petersen *et al.* 2002). Treatment with enrofloxacin is not recommended for a bacterial organism intermediate or resistant in susceptibility to enrofloxacin, since appropriate levels will not be attained in the middle ear (Cole *et al.* 2009). The appropriate duration of antibiotic therapy has not been established; however, it would be prudent to continue antibiotics at least past the period when acute wound infection generally becomes apparent (usually within 7–10 days). If acute wound infection signs appear and progress despite hot-packing and appropriate antibiotic therapy, opening the wound for drainage and reculturing deep tissues to help guide further antibiotic management are required. Elizabethan collars are applied until sutures are removed in 10–14 days. Partial wound dehiscence is treated by local wound cleansing and second-intention healing.

Administration of injectable opiate medications by either intermittent or continuous-rate infusion (preferred) is recommended for the first 24–48 hours after surgery. The author prefers to combine narcotic administration with lidocaine and ketamine as a constant-rate infusion for the first 24 hours postoperatively, when a continuous local anesthetic wound infusion regimen is not elected. In the author's hand, tissue infiltration of liposomal encapsulated bupivacaine intraoperatively provides excellent analgesia for up to three days after surgery. It should be noted that in one randomized clinical trial in dogs, local infiltration of (nonliposomal encapsulated) bupivacaine after TECA did not appear to improve the control of pain after surgery in dogs receiving morphine (Radlinsky *et al.* 2005). Alternately, Lidoderm® patches (5% lidocaine patch, Endo Pharmaceuticals, Chadds Ford, PA, USA) shaped in a V pattern can be placed over the surgical incision site for the first 12 hours. After this time, administration of oral analgesics, either nonsteroidal anti-inflammatory drugs (NSAIDs) or opiate/NSAID combinations, is recommended for an additional 3–5 days after surgery (Tranquilli *et al.* 2004). The author has successfully used continuous nerve blockade (Wolfe *et al.* 2006) controlled by either an infusion pump or silastic bulb and an inline rate limiter (ON-Q® PainBuster® Post-Op Pain Relief System, i-Flow Corporation, Kimberly Clark, Lake Forest, CA, USA) for the first 24 hours postoperatively, and narcotics are reserved for any observable breakthrough pain. The patient is routinely transitioned over to NSAID/gabapentin on the second postoperative day as indicated. These drugs are continued at home for 3–5 additional days.

Complications and treatment

There are numerous complication risks associated with TECA/LBO. Severe hemorrhage during surgery is rare, but has been reported and may result in the death of the patient (Smeak & Dehoff 1986; Mason *et al.* 1988; McAnulty *et al.* 1995). Brisk hemorrhage from the retroarticular vein can usually be controlled with bone wax packed in the retroglenoid foramen (McAnulty *et al.* 1995; Smeak & Inpanbutr 2005). Hemorrhage deep within the tympanic cavity is suspected to come from damage to the internal carotid artery within the medial bulla wall. In the author's experience, this source of bleeding is difficult to control, but packing the bulla tightly with gauze stripping (1/4 in. umbilical tape) is usually successful. The gauze packing is slowly pulled, where it was exited adjacent to the sutured wound, the day following surgery. The author has also observed severe upper airway obstruction following recovery from anesthesia, presumably from an overtight head bandage coupled with pharyngeal edema. Therefore, constant monitoring of the patient after surgery is important, particularly during the first 12–24 hours.

Most complications related to surgery (wound infection/dehiscence, neurologic deficits) are short-lived and resolve within two weeks (Smeak & Dehoff 1986; Matthieson & Scavelli 1990). Extensive contamination during surgery to remove deep-seated chronically infected ears is expected despite proper wound preparation (Vogel *et al.* 1999). Acute wound complications are reported commonly in the literature (ranging from 8% to 41%) and include acute cellulitis/abscessation, incisional hematoma, incisional dehiscence, and extended wound drainage (Lane & Little 1986; Smeak & Dehoff 1986; Mason *et al.* 1988; Matthieson & Scavelli 1990; White & Pomeroy 1990). If wound complications develop, most are treated successfully with antibiotic therapy and local wound care until second-intention healing occurs. Pinna necrosis occurs from damage to the pinna vasculature during medial dissection of the vertical ear canal and is most often found along the proximal edge of the caudal pinna margin (Smeak & Kerpsack 1993). Therapy for this complication consists of débridement of the devitalized tissue and open wound management until second-intention healing occurs.

The most troubling long-term complication encountered after TECA/LBO involves recurrent otitis media (Smeak 2016). This can present itself as pain upon opening the mouth or diffuse swelling on the affected side, and when this infection becomes fulminate and chronic, draining tracts develop cranial and ventral to the initial incision. The most common underlying reason for recurrent infection is incomplete removal of the secretory epithelium lining the tympanic bulla or external osseous meatus, or incomplete removal of a portion of the horizontal ear canal (Beckman *et al.* 1990; White & Pomeroy 1990; Smeak *et al.* 1996; Hardie *et al.* 2008; Smeak 2016). Other factors purported in the literature that may be implicated in deep infection after TECA include osteomyelitis of the ossicles and the wall of the bulla, inadequate drainage of the middle ear through the eustachian tube, and parotid salivary gland damage (Smeak *et al.* 1996). Even when an LBO and proper curettage of the tympanic bulla are performed, the rate of recurrent deep infection is up to 14% (Smeak & Dehoff 1986; Mason *et al.* 1988; Beckman *et al.* 1990; Matthieson & Scavelli 1990; Smeak 2016). Clinical signs of deep infection may appear up to several years following TECA/LBO (Smeak 2016). When TECA/LBO is performed for aural cholesteatoma, recurrence of deep infection approaches 50%. Preoperative risk factors for recurrence identified in one case series included inability

to open the mouth or neurologic signs on admission, and lysis of any portion of the temporal bone on CT imaging (Hardie *et al.* 2008; Risselada 2016; Greci *et al.* 2011).

Long-term antibiotic therapy may be successful for *managing* signs of deep infection after TECA/LBO, but for those that do not respond or have recurrent signs after antibiotic withdrawal, surgical exploration of the region is recommended (Smeak *et al.* 1996; Hardie *et al.* 2008; Smeak 2016). Surgical approaches used for reexploration of the middle ear include the lateral approach and ventral bulla osteotomy (Smeak *et al.* 1996; Holt *et al.* 1996). Contrast CT imaging is very helpful to the author in determining the most useful surgical approach to remove the infected nidus (Smeak 2016). The infected nidus often is surrounded by a contrast-enhanced rim. The lateral approach is best used in the author's experience when it is believed that a portion of the nidus is identified lateral to and outside the bulla cavity (Figure 76.16) (Smeak 2016). The lateral approach may result in more complications associated with facial nerve deficits after surgery, since anatomic structures are obscured by scar tissue from the original surgery, although in most cases the deficits are temporary (Holt *et al.* 1996). The author prefers the ventral approach if the nidus of infection is isolated within the middle ear, since this approach offers excellent exposure and ventral drainage. Anatomy in this approach has not been altered by previous surgery, so identification of structures and dissection is easier in the author's hands (Smeak *et al.* 1996). When imaging shows that a portion of the

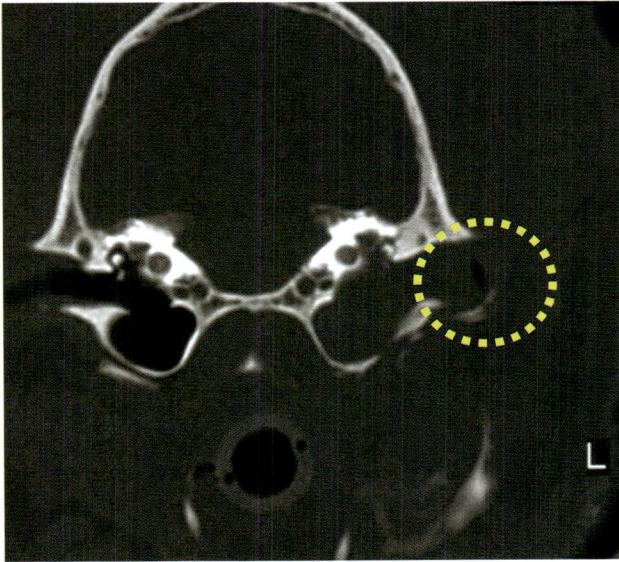

Figure 76.16 Computed tomography image of a dog after total ear canal ablation. Epithelial remnants of the proximal ear canal (yellow dashed circle) were found through a lateral approach.

horizontal ear canal remains after TECA/LBO, the lateral approach is chosen, because removal of retained ear canal tissue lateral to the bulla is very difficult if not impossible from the ventral approach (Smeak 2016).

Chronic dermatitis of the pinna is observed in up to 20% of dogs after TECA, and this complication results from either progression of an underlying dermatologic problem, and/or incomplete removal of proliferative tissue when making the medial incision around the vertical ear canal opening (Smeak & Kerpsack 1993).

Horner's syndrome, facial nerve paralysis, and vestibular syndrome are encountered after TECA and LBO. Facial nerve paralysis was present in 21–77% of cases after surgery in early retrospective case series (Smeak & Dehoff 1986; Matthiessen & Scavelli 1990; Spivack et al. 2013). Most of these neurologic signs regress within 3–4 weeks after surgery. If these signs persist for more than four weeks, they can be expected to be permanent (Smeak & Dehoff 1986; Matthiessen & Scavelli 1990). If the facial nerve has been transected during surgery, the deficit will be permanent. One clinical case has been reported of successful early microsurgical epineural repair of a severed facial nerve in a West Highland white terrier (Calvo et al. 2014).

A higher incidence of Horner's syndrome and facial nerve damage has been seen in cats following TECA and LBO. Horner's syndrome signs are expected to appear in 42% and facial nerve damage in 56–78% of cats after this procedure (Williams & White 1992; Bacon et al. 2003; Spivack et al. 2013). Increased risk of nerve damage after surgery is thought to be attributed to the greater fragility of the feline tympanic plexus and facial nerve compared to the dog (Bacon et al. 2003). In one more recent case series, the prevalence of facial nerve defects after TECA/LBO in dogs versus cats was not significantly different, although cats were more likely to have residual postoperative deficits at one year (Spivack et al. 2013). Most affected cats have temporary nerve damage; 14–27% have permanent Horner's syndrome, and 28–47% have permanent facial nerve dysfunction following TECA/LBO (Bacon et al. 2003; Williams & White 1992). Cats with otic neoplasia in one study were twice as likely to have facial nerve paralysis postoperatively compared to cats with other aural diseases, presumably due to the more extensive deep dissection and retraction necessary to help remove the neoplastic process (Bacon et al. 2003). Full recovery after facial nerve damage from traumatic ear canal avulsion appears to be variable following TECA (Smeak 1997; Clark 2004). Wound infections are less common in cats after TECA/LBO than in dogs, presumably since severely stenotic, deeply infected ear canals are more rarely encountered in cats (Williams & White 1992; Bacon et al. 2003; Spivack et al. 2013).

References

Alexander, A., Mahoney, P., and Scurrell, E. (2019). Cholesteatoma in a cat. *Journal of Feline Medicine and Surgery Open Reports* 5 (1): 2055116919848086.

Bacon, N.J., Gilbert, R.L., Bostock, D.E. et al. (2003). Total ear canal ablation in the cat: indications, morbidity and long-term survival. *Journal of Small Animal Practice* 44: 430–434.

Beckman, S.L., Henry, W.B., and Cechner, P. (1990). Total ear canal ablation. Combining bulla osteotomy and curettage in dogs with chronic otitis externa and media. *Journal of the American Veterinary Medical Association* 196: 84–90.

Beever, L., Swinbourne, F., Priestnall, S.L. et al. (2019). Surgical management of chronic otitis secondary to craniomandibular osteopathy in three West Highland white terriers. *Journal of Small Animal Practice* 60: 254–260.

Boothe, H.W. (1997). Ventral bulla osteotomy: dog and cat. In: *Current Techniques in Small Animal Surgery*, 4e (ed. M.J. Bojrab), 109–112. Baltimore, MD: Lippincott, Williams & Wilkens.

Buback, J.L., Boothe, H.W., Carroll, G.L. et al. (1996). Comparison of three methods for relief of pain after ear canal ablation in dogs. *Veterinary Surgery* 25: 380–385.

Calvo, I., Espadas, I., Hammond, G. et al. (2014). Epineural repair of an iatrogenic facial nerve neurotmesis after total ear canal ablation and lateral bulla osteotomy in a dog with concurrent craniomandibular osteopathy. *Journal of the South African Veterinary Association* 85: 1–4.

Clark, S.P. (2004). Surgical management of acute ear canal separation in a cat. *Journal of Feline Medicine and Surgery* 6: 283–286.

Cole, L.K. (2004). Otoscopic evaluation of the ear canal. *Veterinary Clinics of North America. Small Animal Practice* 34: 397–410.

Cole, L.K., Kwochka, K.W., Kowalski, J.J. et al. (1998). Microbial flora and antimicrobial susceptibility patterns of isolated pathogens from the horizontal ear canal and middle ear in dogs with otitis media. *Journal of the American Veterinary Medical Association* 212: 534–538.

Cole, L.K., Kwochka, K.W., Hillier, A. et al. (2005). Comparison of bacterial organisms and their susceptibility patterns from otic exudate and ear tissue from the vertical ear canal of dogs undergoing a total ear canal ablation. *Veterinary Therapeutics* 6: 252–259.

Cole, L.K., Papich, M.G., Kwochka, K.W. et al. (2009). Plasma and ear tissue concentrations of enrofloxacin and its metabolite ciprofloxacin in dogs with chronic end-stage otitis externa after intravenous administration of enrofloxacin. *Veterinary Dermatology* 20: 51–59.

Coleman, K.A. and Smeak, D.D. (2016). Complication rates after bilateral versus unilateral total ear canal ablation with lateral bulla osteotomy for end-stage inflammatory ear disease in dogs: 79 ears. *Veterinary Surgery* 45: 659–663.

Devitt, C.M., Seim, H.B. 3rd, Willer, R. et al. (1997). Passive drainage versus primary closure after total ear canal ablation-lateral bulla osteotomy in dogs: 59 dogs (1985–1995). *Veterinary Surgery*. 26: 210–216.

Donnelly, K.E. and Tillson, M.D. (2004). Feline inflammatory polyps and ventral bulla osteotomy. *Compendium*. June: 446–453.

Dvir, E., Kirberger, R.M., and Terblanche, A.G. (2000). Magnetic resonance imaging of otitis media in a dog. *Veterinary Radiology & Ultrasound* 41: 46–49.

Dyson, D.H. (2008). Analgesia and chemical restraint for the emergent veterinary patient. *Veterinary Clinics of North America. Small Animal Practice* 38: 1329–1352.

Eom, K., Lee, H., and Yoon, J. (2000). Canalographic evaluation of the external ear canal in dogs. *Veterinary Radiology & Ultrasound* 41: 231–234.

Fraser, G., Gregor, W.W., Mackenzie, C.P. et al. (1970). Canine ear disease. *Journal of Small Animal Practice* 10: 725–754.

Greci, V., Travetti, O., Di Giancamillo, M. et al. (2011). *Canadian Veterinary Journal* 52: 631–636.

Grubb, T. and Lobprise, H. (2020). Local and regional anaesthesia in dogs and cats: descriptions of specific local and regional techniques (Part 2). *Veterinary Medicine and Science* 6: 218–234.

Hardie, E.M., Linder, K.E., and Pease, A.P. (2008). Aural cholesteatoma in twenty dogs. *Veterinary Surgery* 37: 763–770.

Haudequet, P.H., Gauthier, O., and Renard, E. (2006). Total ear canal ablation associated with lateral bulla osteotomy with the help of otoscopy in dogs and cats: retrospective study of 47 cases. *Veterinary Surgery* 35: E1–E20.

Hettlich, B.E., Boothe, H.W., Simpson, R.B. et al. (2005). Effect of tympanic cavity evacuation and flushing on microbial isolates during total ear canal ablation with lateral bulla osteotomy in dogs. *Journal of the American Veterinary Medical Association* 227: 748–755.

Holt, D., Brockman, D.J., Sylvestre, A.M. et al. (1996). Lateral exploration of fistulas developing after total ear canal ablations: 10 cases (1989–1993). *Journal of the American Animal Hospital Association* 32: 527–530.

Kern, T.J. and Erb, H.N. (1987). Facial neuropathy in dogs and cats: 95 cases (1975–1985). *Journal of the American Veterinary Medical Association* 191: 1604–1609.

Kim, J.Y., Jeong, S.W., Jeong, M. et al. (2003). Total ear canal ablation and lateral bulla osteotomy for chronic otitis externa and media in dogs: postoperative recovery and long-term follow-up. *Journal of Veterinary Clinics* 1: 26–32.

Krahwinkel, D.J., Parco, A.D., Sims, M.H. et al. (1993). Effect of total ablation of the external auditory meatus and bulla osteotomy on auditory function in dogs. *Journal of the American Veterinary Medical Association* 202: 949–952.

Lane, J.G. and Little, C.J.L. (1986). Surgery of the canine external auditory meatus: a review of failures. *Journal of Small Animal Practice* 27: 247–254.

Lanz, O.I. and Wood, B.C. (2004). Surgery of the ear and pinna. *Veterinary Clinics of North America. Small Animal Practice* 34: 567–599.

Little, C.J.L., Lane, J.G., and Pearson, G.R. (1991). Inflammatory middle ear disease of the dog: the pathology of otitis media. *Veterinary Record* 128: 293–296.

London, C.A., Dubilzeig, R.R., Vail, D.M. et al. (1996). Evaluation of dogs and cats with tumors of the ear canal: 145 cases (1978–1992). *Journal of the American Veterinary Medical Association* 208: 1413–1418.

Lorenzi, D., Bonfanti, U., Masserdotti, C. et al. (2005). Fine-needle biopsy of external ear canal masses in the cat: cytologic results and histologic correlations in 27 cases. *Veterinary Clinical Pathology* 34: 100–105.

Marino, D.J., MacDonald, J.M., Matthieson, D.T. et al. (1994). Results of surgery in cats with ceruminous gland adenocarcinoma. *Journal of the American Animal Hospital Association* 30: 54–58.

Mason, L.K., Harvey, C.E., and Orsher, R.J. (1988). Total ear canal ablation combined with lateral bulla osteotomy for end-stage otitis in dogs – results in thirty dogs. *Veterinary Surgery* 17: 263–268.

Mathews, K.G., Hardie, E.M., and Murphy, K.M. (2006). Subtotal ear canal ablation in 18 dogs and one cat with minimal distal ear canal pathology. *Journal of the American Animal Hospital Association* 42: 371–380.

Matthieson, D.T. and Scavelli, T. (1990). Total ear canal ablation and lateral bulla osteotomy in 38 dogs. *Journal of the American Animal Hospital Association* 26: 257–267.

McAnulty, J.F., Hattel, A., and Harvey, C.E. (1995). Wound healing and brain stem auditory evoked potentials after experimental total ear canal ablation and lateral bulla osteotomy in dogs. *Veterinary Surgery* 24: 1–8.

McCarthy, P.E., Hosgood, G., and Pechman, R.D. (1995). Traumatic ear canal separations and para-aural abscessation in three dogs. *Journal of the American Animal Hospital Association* 31: 419–424.

McNabb, A.H. and Flanders, J.A. (2004). Cosmetic results of a ventrally based advancement flap for closure of total ear canal ablations in 6 cats: 2002–2003. *Veterinary Surgery* 33: 435–439.

Mehrkens, L., Townsend, K., Cooley, S. et al. (2019). Experience level as a predictor of entry into the hypotympanum during TECA-LBO in feline cadavers. Scientific Abstracts 2019 ACVS Surgery Summit. *Veterinary Surgery* 48: 1138.

Payne, J.T., Shell, L.G., Flora, R.M. et al. (1989). Hearing loss in dogs subjected to total ear canal ablation. *Veterinary Surgery* 18: 60.

Petersen, A.D., Walker, R.D., Bowman, M.M. et al. (2002). Frequency of isolation and antimicrobial susceptibility patterns of Staphylococcus intermedius and *Pseudomonas aeruginosa* isolates from canine skin and ear samples over a 6-year period (1992–1997). *Journal of the American Animal Hospital Association* 38: 407–413.

Radlinsky, M.G., Mason, D.E., Roush, J.K. et al. (2005). Use of a continuous, local infusion of bupivacaine for postoperative analgesia in dogs undergoing total ear canal ablation. *Journal of the American Veterinary Medical Association* 227: 414–419.

Remedios, A.M., Fowler, J.D., and Pharr, J.W. (1991). A comparison of radiographic versus surgical diagnosis of otitis media. *Journal of the American Animal Hospital Association* 27: 183–188.

Risselada, M. (2016). Diagnosis and management of cholesteatomas in dogs. *Veterinary Clinics of North America. Small Animal Practice* 46: 623–634.

Rohleder, J.J., Jones, J.C., Duncan, R.B. et al. (2006). Comparative performance of radiography and computed tomography in the diagnosis of middle ear disease in 31 dogs. *Veterinary Radiology & Ultrasound* 47: 45–52.

Rossello, C. and Pelaez, J. (2020). Endoscopic tympanic cavity lavage and debridement following total ear canal ablation and lateral bulla osteotomy. Scientific Abstracts 29th Annual Scientific Meeting of the ECVS. *Veterinary Surgery* 49: 212.

Schlicksup, M.D., Van Winkle, T.J., and Holt, D.E. (2009). Prevalence of clinical abnormalities in cats found to have nonneoplastic middle ear disease at necropsy: 59 cases (1991–2007). *Journal of the American Veterinary Medical Association* 235: 841–843.

Sharp, N.J.H. (1990). Chronic otitis externa and otitis media treated by total ear canal ablation and ventral bulla osteotomy in thirteen dogs. *Veterinary Surgery* 19: 162–166.

Smeak, D.D. (1997). Traumatic separation of the annular cartilage from the external auditory meatus in a cat. *Journal of the American Veterinary Medical Association* 211: 448–450.

Smeak, D.D. (2016). Treatment of persistent deep infection after total ear canal ablation and lateral bulla osteotomy. *Veterinary Clinics of North America. Small Animal Practice* 46: 609–621.

Smeak, D.D. and Dehoff, W.D. (1986). Total ear canal ablation clinical results in the dog and cat. *Veterinary Surgery* 17: 161–170.

Smeak, D.D. and Inpanbutr, N. (2005). Lateral approach to subtotal bulla osteotomy in dogs. *Compendium* May: 377–384.

Smeak, D.D. and Kerpsack, S.J. (1993). Total ear canal ablation and lateral bulla osteotomy for management of end stage otitis. *Seminars in Veterinary Medicine and Surgery (Small Animal)* 8: 30–41.

Smeak, D.D., Crocker, C.B., and Birchard, S.J. (1996). Treatment of recurrent otitis media that developed after total ear canal ablation and lateral bulla osteotomy in dogs. Nine cases (1996-1994). *Journal of the American Veterinary Medical Association* 209: 937–942.

Soohoo, J., Lange, C.E., and Loft, K.E. (2017). Feline ceruminous cystomatosis in the ears of 25 cats (2014–2016) [abstract]. In: *Veterinary Dermatology: Abstracts of the North American Veterinary Dermatology Forum*, 26–29 April. Orlando FL, USA.

Spivack, R.E., Elkins, D., Moore, G.E. et al. (2013). Postoperative complications following TECA-LBO in the dog and cat. *Journal of the American Animal Hospital Association* 49: 160–168.

Tranquilli, W.J., Grimm, K.A., and Lamont, L.A. (2004). *Pain Management for the Small Animal Practitioner*, 2e. Jackson, WY: Teton NewMedia.

Trower, N.D., Gregory, S.P., Renfrew, H. et al. (1998). Evaluation of the canine tympanic membrane by positive contrast ear canalography. *Veterinary Record* 142: 78–81.

Vogel, P.L., Komtebedde, J., Hirsch, D.C. et al. (1999). Wound contamination and antimicrobial susceptibility of bacteria cultured during total ear canal ablation and lateral bulla osteotomy in dogs. *Journal of the American Veterinary Medical Association* 214: 1641–1643.

Watt, M.M., Regier, P.J., Ferrigno, C.A. et al. (2020). Otoscopic evaluation of epithelial remnants in the tympanic cavity after total ear canal ablation and lateral bulla osteotomy. *Veterinary Surgery* 49 (7): 1406–1411.

White, R.A.S. and Pomeroy, C.J. (1990). Total ear canal ablation and lateral bulla osteotomy in the dog. *Journal of Small Animal Practice* 31: 547–553.

Williams, J.M. and White, R.A.S. (1992). Total ear canal ablation combined with lateral bulla osteotomy in the cat. *Journal of Small Animal Practice* 33: 225–227.

Wolfe, T.M., Bateman, S.W., Cole, L.K. et al. (2006). Evaluation of a local anesthetic delivery system for the postoperative analgesic management of canine total ear canal ablation: a randomized, controlled, double-blinded study. *Veterinary Anaesthesia and Analgesia* 33: 328–339.

77

Subtotal Ear Canal Ablation

Kyle G. Mathews

Total ear canal ablation (TECA) with lateral bulla osteotomy is a treatment option for dogs and cats with end-stage otitis externa, or masses confined to the ear canal. As described, the procedure involves a circumferential incision around the funnel-shaped auricular cavity and through the auricular cartilage (Beckman *et al.* 1990). A skin incision is then made over the vertical ear canal. The vertical and horizontal ear canals are dissected free of the soft tissues to the level of the tympanic bulla and a bulla osteotomy is performed.

A modification of this technique for dogs with erect ears has been described (Okamoto *et al.* 2001). The purpose of the modification was to avoid change in the ear carriage associated with excision of the medial portion of the auricular cartilage. An inverted L-shaped skin incision is made over the vertical canal just ventral to the auricular cavity to facilitate exposure. The annular cartilage of the vertical canal is transected at this point, followed by routine dissection and removal of the remaining vertical and horizontal canals. The horizontal portion of the L-shaped skin incision is sutured to the remaining cut end of the vertical canal. The distal portion of the vertical canal is thus preserved, resulting in a stoma just ventral to, and communicating with, the external orifice. This procedure was performed in three dogs with chronic otitis externa/media with no apparent problems reported at one-year follow-up (Okamoto *et al.* 2001).

Another report evaluated the cosmetic outcome of a modified TECA technique in six cats (McNabb & Flanders 2004). Erect ear carriage was maintained by creating a ventrally based advancement flap after circumferential incision around the external acoustic meatus and removal of the entire vertical and horizontal ear canals.

Indications

Many owners of animals with erect ears are not concerned about ear droop following standard TECA, yet methods to prevent its occurrence should be discussed prior to surgery. Subtotal ear canal ablation preserves erect ear carriage and eliminates dissection through and around the medial aspect of the auricular cartilage that is required for a standard TECA.

Subtotal ear canal ablation was expanded to include a subset of dogs with pendulous ears (Mathews *et al.* 2006). In each case, the medial surface of the pinna and the distal auricular cavity were free of, or minimally affected by, the underlying disease process. The technique is similar to a previously reported modification of lateral ear canal resection (Bardens 1962).

Animals with masses or gross changes to the vertical ear canal secondary to otitis externa are not candidates for subtotal ear canal ablation. This would include most pendulous-eared breeds, including cocker spaniels, which typically have significant involvement of the distal ear canal and auricular cavity by the time TECA is considered. The risk of recurrent disease in the remaining vertical canal would be too great to warrant these tissue-sparing techniques.

Surgical technique

A single vertical incision is made overlying the vertical ear canal from just ventral to the midpoint of the external orifice to ventral to the horizontal ear canal. With the aid of retractors, the central portion of the vertical ear canal is freed from its soft tissue attachments using blunt and sharp dissection and then transected (Figures 77.1 and 77.2). The proximal portion of the vertical canal and

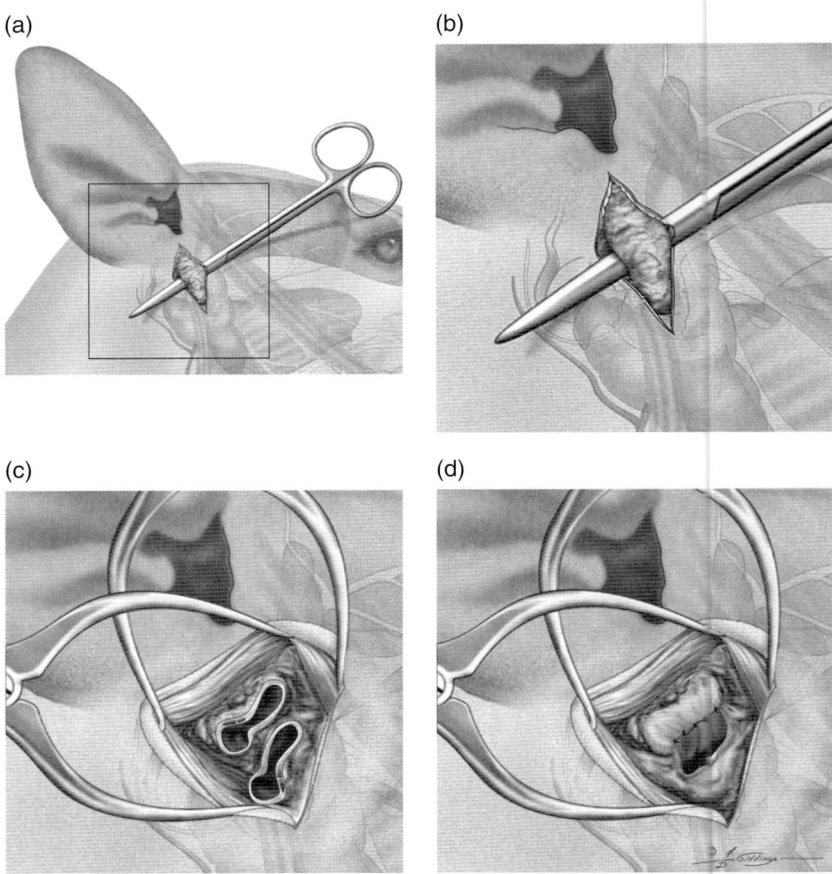

(a)

(b)

(c)

(d)

Figure 77.1 (a) The location of the skin incision parallel to, and directly over, the vertical ear canal (b) The vertical canal is dissected free of its attachments and elevated by passing an instrument (Metzenbaum scissors) behind the canal. (c) The canal is transected and the distal portion closed with cruciate sutures placed in the cut edges of the cartilage while avoiding the epithelium. (d) Following closure of the distal canal, the proximal vertical canal and horizontal canal are followed down to the tympanic bulla as with a standard total ear canal ablation. © D. Giddings.

the horizontal canal are then removed as for a standard TECA. Following lateral bulla osteotomy and curettage, the cut end of the distal vertical ear canal is grasped and elevated. The medial and lateral vertical ear canal cartilages are apposed with multiple simple interrupted or cruciate sutures using absorbable monofilament material (Figures 77.1 and 77.2). Care is taken to avoid penetrating the epithelium of the vertical canal with the sutures. Subcutaneous and skin closures are then performed in a routine manner. The result is a shallow, blind-ended auricular cavity with preservation of the entire circumference of annular cartilage surrounding the external orifice (Figure 77.3).

Outcome

Subtotal ear canal ablation was performed in 18 dogs and 1 cat (Mathews *et al.* 2006). One dog and the one cat had benign masses present within the horizontal ear canal. Animals with otitis had minimal or no involvement of the distal ear canal. Postoperative dermatologic problems associated with the remaining ear canal and pinnae were minor in four animals and protracted in four others. All complications resolved with medical management. Median time to follow-up was 12 months (mean 21 months, range 3–53 months). Normal ear carriage is maintained in animals with erect ears, and this technique results in an ear that appears surgically unaltered. Of 24 ears, 6 (25%) developed protracted auricular cavity skin infections that eventually resolved with medical management (Mathews *et al.* 2006). This compares with a similar presence of recurrent dermatologic problems associated with the pinna in 10 (26%) of 38 dogs following the standard TECA technique (Matthiesen & Scavelli 1990). Although all superficial infections were corrected with medical management, owners should be made aware of this possibility prior to the performance of subtotal ear canal ablation, even if

(a)

(b)

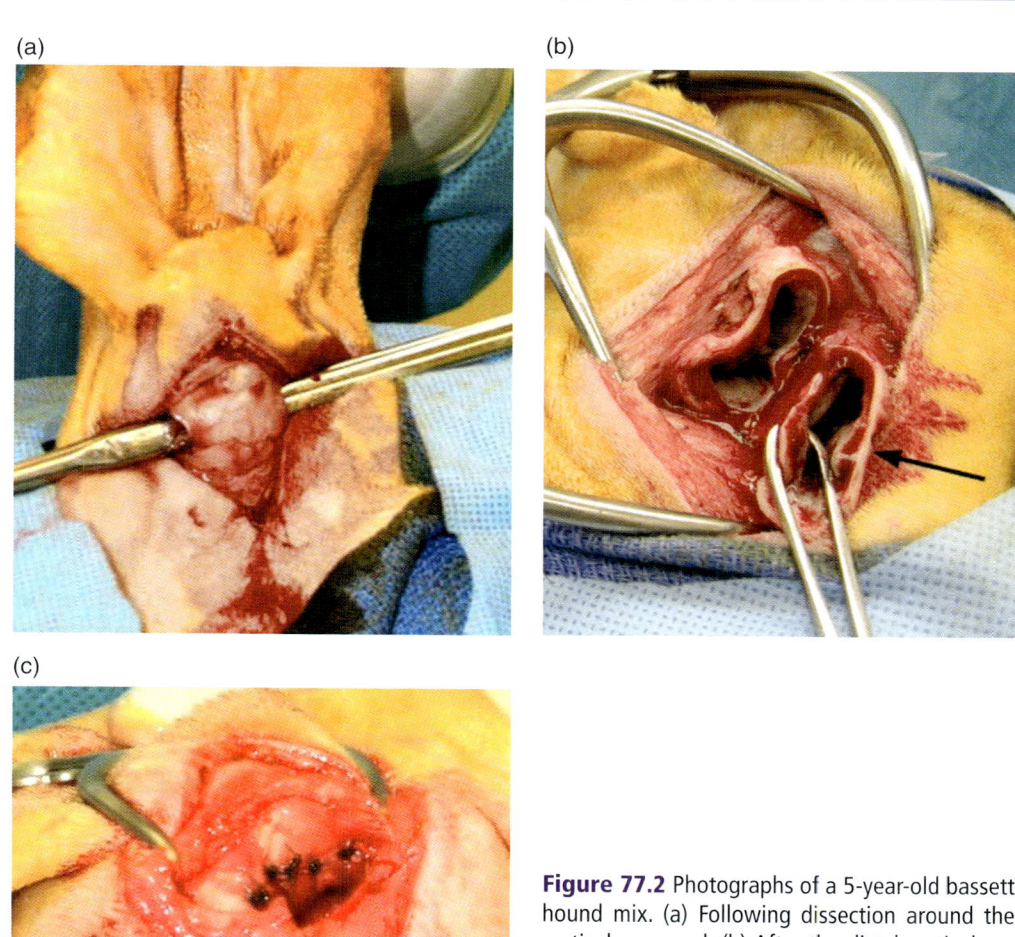

(c)

Figure 77.2 Photographs of a 5-year-old bassett hound mix. (a) Following dissection around the vertical ear canal. (b) After the distal vertical ear canal has been transected. The proximal portion of the vertical ear canal (arrow) and the entire horizontal ear canal will be removed as for a standard total ear canal ablation. (c) Following closure of the distal vertical ear canal with monofilament absorbable sutures that engage only the cartilage. Care is taken to make sure the sutures do not penetrate the epithelium of the ear canal.

(a)

(b)

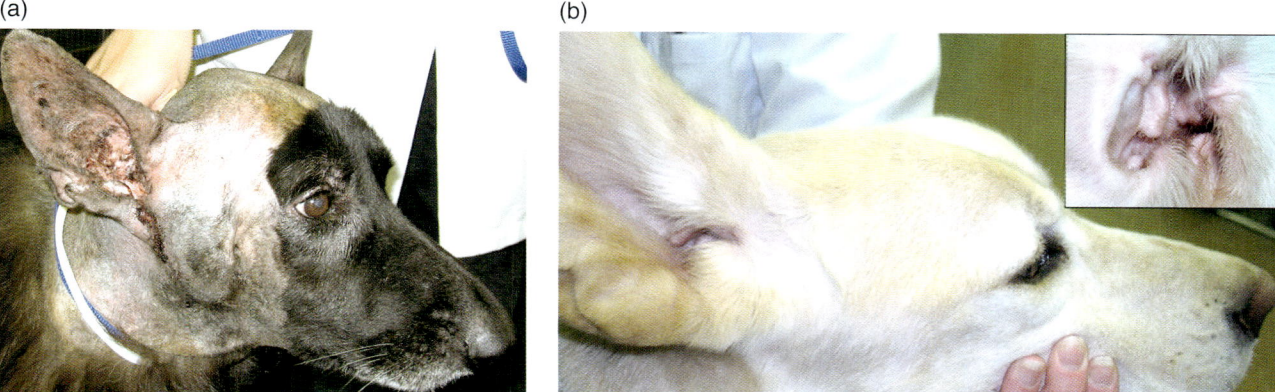

Figure 77.3 (a) Postoperative photograph of a German shepherd dog showing the location of the skin incision. (b) Follow-up photograph of the dog in Figure 77.2 showing a normal-appearing auricular cavity (inset).

there is no distal involvement at the time of surgery, and standard TECA with lateral bulla osteotomy should be discussed as an alternative.

Five animals (26%) without neurologic signs at presentation developed transient facial nerve paresis/paralysis (Mathews *et al.* 2006). While retraction could have contributed to facial nerve trauma in these cases, the frequency of this complication is similar to previous evaluations of the standard TECA technique (Smeak & Dehoff 1986; Beckman *et al.* 1990; Matthiesen & Scavelli 1990). The subjective impression of the surgeons who have performed this procedure is that facial nerve identification and retraction are no more difficult than with a standard TECA, although in the cat the skin incision was modified to improve exposure. As with the standard technique, owners should be made aware of the possibility of postoperative neurologic complications. My subjective impression is that subtotal ear canal ablation is easier to perform than a standard TECA, results in less hemorrhage, and may be less painful. Prospective studies are needed to address these issues. Because of these potential benefits, as observed following performance of subtotal ear canal ablation on several dogs with erect ears, it was subsequently performed on nine dogs with pendulous ears and minimal or no distal ear canal involvement.

References

Bardens, J.W. (1962). Relocation of the auditory canal in chronic otitis. *Small Animal Clinician* 2: 383–385.

Beckman, S.L., Henry, W.B. Jr., and Cechner, P. (1990). Total ear canal ablation combining bulla osteotomy and curettage in dogs with chronic otitis externa and media. *Journal of the American Veterinary Medical Association* 196: 84–90.

Mathews, K.G., Hardie, E.M., and Murphy, M. (2006). Subtotal ear canal ablation: results in 18 dogs and one cat with minimal distal ear canal pathology. *Journal of the American Animal Hospital Association* 42: 371–380.

Matthiesen, D.T. and Scavelli, T. (1990). Total ear canal ablation and lateral bulla osteotomy in 38 dogs. *Journal of the American Animal Hospital Association* 26: 257–267.

McNabb, A.H. and Flanders, J.A. (2004). Cosmetic results of a ventrally based advancement flap for closure of total ear canal ablations in 6 cats: 2002–2003. *Veterinary Surgery* 33: 435–439.

Okamoto, Y., Miyatake, K., Inoue, T. et al. (2001). Total ear-canal ablation preserving the auricular annular cartilage. *Journal of the Japanese Veterinary Medical Association* 54: 791–794.

Smeak, D.D. and Dehoff, W.D. (1986). Total ear canal ablation. Clinical results in the dog and cat. *Veterinary Surgery* 15: 161–170.

78

Surgical Diseases of the Middle Ear

Marije Risselada and Elizabeth M. Hardie

The middle ear ("tympanic bulla") is a complex structure. It has a one main bony cavity in dogs ("tympanic cavity"), and a smaller secondary cavity in cats, separated by an incomplete septum. The tympanic cavity is separated from the external ear canal by a tympanic membrane, with three ossicles transferring signals from the tympanic membrane to the inner ear. Sympathetic nerve fibers lie close to the surface at the promontory. Only a fibrous membrane covers the opening to the inner ear.

Surgical diseases of the middle ear include chronic otitis media (discussed in Chapter 74), fistulation or complications post-total ear canal ablation (TECA), polyps, cholesteatomas, and granulomas. Rarely, neoplasia may be present. Two main approaches to the bulla exist: lateral bulla osteotomy (LBO) and ventral bulla osteotomy (VBO). An LBO is typically performed in conjunction with TECA (discussed in Chapter 77), but can in rare instances be indicated if post-TECA complications arise. A VBO allows the surgeon visualization and exposure to remove masses and fluid accumulations within the middle ear cavity, while protecting these structures as much as possible.

Diseases of the middle ear

Polyps

Middle ear polyps are benign fibrous growths covered with epithelium. They usually originate at the junction of the auditory tube and the tympanic bulla, but can arise anywhere within the auditory tube and middle ear. They are found most commonly in young cats, but have been reported in older cats or dogs (Pratschke 2003;

Donnelly & Tillson 2004). The polyp may extend through the auditory tube into the nasopharynx or through the tympanic membrane into the external auditory canal (Figure 78.1). Polyps are routinely unilateral

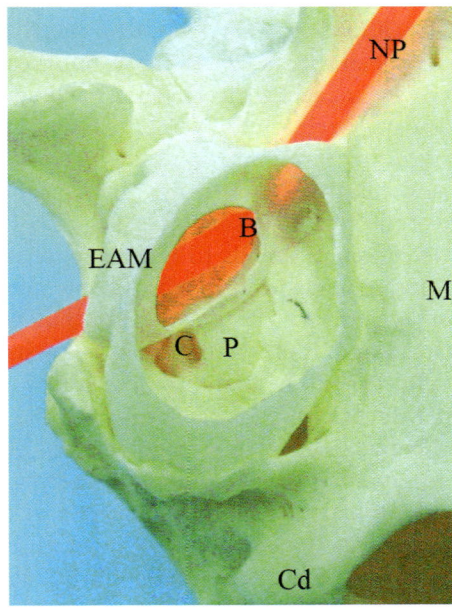

Figure 78.1 Feline skull: ventral view of the right bulla. The ventromedial and dorsolateral compartments have been opened. The orange string illustrates the two routes that polyps can take as they expand from the lateral compartment: (1) through the external acoustic meatus (EAM) into the external ear canal; or (2) through the auditory tube into the nasopharynx (NP). B, usual base of polyp; C, cochlear window; Cd, caudal; M, medial; P, promontory.

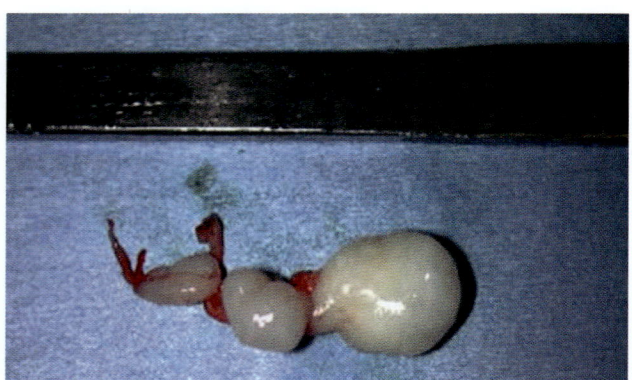

Figure 78.2 Ear polyp showing the stalk and the expanded bulb.

and solitary, but bilateral lesions and multiple polyps originating from the same ear have been reported (MacPhail *et al.* 2007).

The cause of polyp formation is not fully understood. Congenital and infectious causes have been postulated. Bacteria have been cultured from the middle ear of cats with polyps, but most polyps are not associated with otitis media (Kapatkin *et al.* 1990). Chronic viral infection has also been suggested as a cause, but no evidence for the presence of calicivirus or feline herpesvirus 1 in polyp tissue has been found (Veir *et al.* 2002). It possible, however, that viral infection may incite polyp formation and that polyp growth then occurs after clearance of the virus.

The polyp tissue expands to fill the space in which it is growing. Expansion through the tympanic membrane does occur, but the polyp tissue but does not invade or expand into surrounding bony structures (Kirpensteijn 1993). The shape of most polyps is that of a bulb on a stalk (Figure 78.2). The stalk is the portion contained in the auditory tube or dorsolateral compartment of the tympanic bulla, while the bulb represents the expanded portion in the nasopharynx or external ear canal. Clinical signs depend on the path of polyp growth (Kapatkin *et al.* 1990; Muilenburg & Fry 2002; Donnelly & Tillson 2004). Clinical signs associated with growth into the nasopharynx include increased respiratory noise, inappropriate respiratory effort, nasal discharge, sneezing, voice change, and dysphagia. Growth of the polyp into the external ear canal often results in otitis externa and clinical signs include aural discharge and head shaking. The polyp may be grossly visible within the external auditory canal. Rarely, signs associated with middle and inner ear disease (head tilt, nystagmus, ataxia, deafness) may be seen.

Polyps that are exerting pressure on the tympanic membrane or expanding into the external ear canal can be observed with a hand-held otoscope or by video-enhanced endoscopy. Polyps extending into the nasopharynx can be visualized by retracting the soft palate and viewing the caudal nasopharynx directly or with a retroflexed endoscope. Computed tomography (CT) is the preferred imaging modality, although magnetic resonance imaging (MRI) can be used as well and can provide more information about potential intracranial extension. CT provides detailed information on the bone of the bulla, the contents of the bulla, presence of a nasopharyngeal component, as well as potential extension in surrounding tissues. Nasopharyngeal polyps are visualized on MRI as a well-defined mass, hypo- to isointense (T1WI) and hyperintense (T2WI), compared to gray matter with strong rim enhancement post contrast (T1WI) (Tanaka *et al.* 2018). Radiography of the middle ear can be obtained using an open-mouth view, but some changes might not be visible (Love *et al.* 1995; Bischoff & Kneller 2004; Hammond *et al.* 2005; Lee *et al.* 2008).

Cholesteatoma

Aural cholesteatomas are epidermoid cysts forming within the middle ear (Little *et al.* 1991; Hardie *et al.* 2008). They are composed of keratin debris surrounded by keratinizing stratified squamous epithelium. They have been mostly reported in dogs, with only one case report in a cat (Alexander *et al.* 2019). They can be congenital or acquired. Congenital cholesteatoma is a developmental defect that occurs when a squamous epithelial cyst forms within the middle ear behind an intact tympanic membrane. Acquired cholesteatomas occur when retraction of the tympanic membrane into the middle ear or migration of squamous epithelium through a perforated tympanic membrane leads to cyst formation. Typically, formation of an acquired cholesteatoma requires both an inflammatory stimulus (chronic otitis media/externa) and a pathway for keratinizing stratified squamous epithelium to migrate into the middle ear (a ruptured tympanic membrane). Once the cyst is formed, it can expand slowly, with limited accumulation of keratin debris, or can expand rapidly because of massive production of sebaceous material. The inflammatory response associated with a cholesteatoma may be mild or severe, depending on cytokine production by the epithelium, exposure of tissues outside the cyst to sebaceous material, and the presence or absence of infection. Once present, infection is difficult to resolve because of poor blood supply to the infected material and because biofilms form (Gersdorff *et al.* 2006). In its most severe form, cholesteatoma causes expansion and destruction of the surrounding bone, pressure on surrounding structures, inflammation, and necrosis (Figure 78.3).

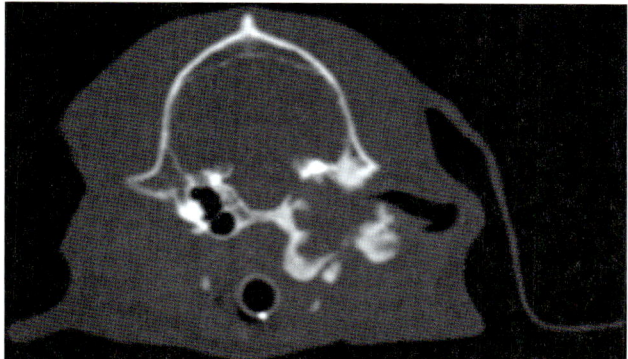

Figure 78.3 Computed tomographic image of a dog with cholesteatoma demonstrating bone lysis in the petrosal portion of the temporal bone. Source: Hardie *et al.* (2008). Reproduced with permission from John Wiley & Sons.

Clinical signs associated with cholesteatoma are those of chronic otitis externa (discharge, swelling, redness, and/or pain), pain on opening the mouth, inability to fully open the mouth, head tilt, unilateral facial palsy, ataxia, nystagmus, circling, and unilateral atrophy of the temporalis and masseter muscles (Little *et al.* 1991; Hardie *et al.* 2008). If bulla expansion into the nasopharynx and oropharynx occurs (Figure 78.4), increased respiratory noise and inappropriate respiratory effort may occur.

A presumptive diagnosis of cholesteatoma involves viewing typical imaging changes or direct observation of keratin debris within a cystic structure at surgery (Little *et al.* 1991; Hardie *et al.* 2008). Changes observed on CT include the presence of opacities within the bulla, osteoproliferation, lysis of the bulla, expansion of the bulla, bone lysis within the squamous or petrosal portions of the temporal bone, and enlargement of associated lymph nodes (Figure 78.3). Heterogeneous contrast medium enhancement of the tissue in the middle ear is common. Definitive diagnosis requires cooperation between the surgeon and the pathologist. The surgeon must carefully indicate that the origin of the tissue is the middle ear. The pathologist then looks for the presence of ciliated epithelium (to confirm that the origin of the tissue is middle ear), presence of metaplastic epithelium, presence of cornification, and accumulation of keratin-rich cornified material (ideally lamination is observed).

The prognosis for cholesteatoma depends on the size and invasiveness of the lesion at the time of diagnosis. In a study in which 19 dogs had TECA/LBO or VBO with the intent to cure, 9 dogs had no further signs of middle ear disease, but 10 had persistent or recurrent clinical signs (Hardie *et al.* 2008). Risk factors for recurrence after surgery were inability to open the mouth or neurologic signs on admission and lysis of any portion of the

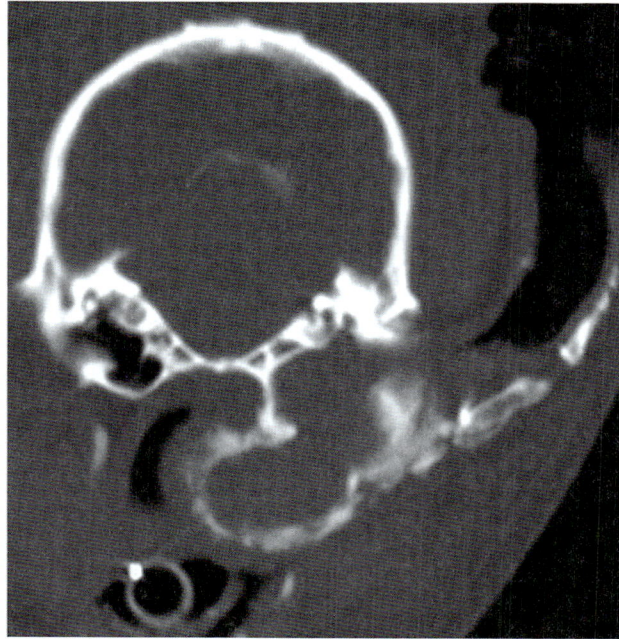

Figure 78.4 Computed tomographic image of a dog with cholesteatoma demonstrating expansion of the bulla into the oropharynx.

temporal bone on CT imaging. Dogs admitted with neurologic signs or inability to open the mouth had a median survival of 16 months.

Cholesterol granuloma

Chronic inflammation in the middle ear can result in granuloma formation. In particular, cholesterol granuloma, in which the granulomatous tissue contains cholesterol crystals, has been reported in dogs (Cox & Payne-Johnson 1995; Fliegner *et al.* 2007). These lesions may occur when hemorrhage, interference with drainage, and obstruction of air exchange occur within an aerated bony cavity. The source of the cholesterol may be erythrocyte membranes, mucosa, or transudate. The cholesterol precipitates, crystals are formed, and a secondary granulomatous reaction occurs. Clinical signs and imaging findings are similar to those associated with cholesteatoma. At surgery, the lesions may also appear similar, although copious accumulation of keratinaceous debris occurs only with cholesteatoma.

The diagnosis of cholesterol granuloma is based on observation of multiple acicular clefts surrounded by fibrous tissue and infiltrates of mononuclear inflammatory cells on histopathologic examination. It should be noted that because granuloma formation and cholesteatoma formation are both consequences of chronic infection, they can coexist in the same middle ear. In two reported cases of aural cholesterol granuloma formation in dogs, disease resolved following VBO (Cox & Payne-Johnson 1995; Fliegner *et al.* 2007).

Neoplasia

Reported cases of neoplasia originating in the middle ear are rare and typically affect cats over 10 years of age and dogs over 6 years of age (Little *et al.* 1989; Kirpensteijn 1993; Fan & de Lorimier 2004). Squamous cell carcinoma is the most commonly reported tumor of middle ear origin in the cat. Other reported feline tumors include papillary adenoma, ceruminous gland adenocarcinoma, adenocarcinoma possibly arising from the glandular epithelium of the auditory tube, anaplastic carcinoma, lymphoblastic lymphosarcoma, and lymphoma. Tumors originating in the middle ear of dogs are usually benign, but malignant tumors from surrounding structures may invade the middle ear. Reported tumors include basal cell tumor, papilloma, papillary adenoma, ceruminous gland adenocarcinoma, squamous cell carcinoma, sebaceous gland adenocarcinoma, and anaplastic neoplasia (Little *et al.* 1989; Yoshikawa *et al.* 2008).

Clinical signs of neoplasia include purulent otic discharge, nystagmus, head tilt, ataxia, pain on opening the mouth, ptosis (dropped eyelid), seizures, and Horner's syndrome. Imaging changes include the presence of opacities within the bulla, osteoproliferation, lysis of the bulla, bone lysis within the squamous or petrosal portions of the temporal bone, contrast-enhancing lesions within the cranium, and enlargement of associated lymph nodes. Surgical treatment of middle ear tumors is rarely reported, but mostly indicates a poor prognosis. One cat with papillary adenoma and one cat with adenocarcinoma treated with aggressive surgical debulking using VBO and craniectomy were alive at 840 days and 630 days after surgery, respectively (Lucroy *et al.* 2004). In a study of 11 dogs with middle ear tumors, 5 dogs with squamous papilloma, basal cell tumor, sebaceous adenocarcinoma, or papillary adenoma had survival times ranging from eight months to four years after undergoing surgical debulking (Little *et al.* 1989).

Fistulas post total ear canal ablation

Remnant epithelial tissue after a TECA-LBO might cause local abscessation due to recurrent otitis media with or without fistulating tracts. These might develop shortly after surgery, but can occur as long as several years postoperatively (Smeak 2016). Treatment typically includes excision of all fistulating tracts, and a lateral approach to the bulla, although a ventral approach could be considered (see Chapter 76).

Treatment and surgical recommendations

Presurgical treatment

Before recommending VBO, other less invasive treatment methods should be considered. Accumulations of fluid or pus may be removed using myringotomy, with flushing under video-enhanced endoscopic observation (Palmeiro *et al.* 2004). Polyps may be treated with traction and corticosteroids (Anderson *et al.* 2000; Muilenburg & Fry 2002). Per-endoscopic trans-tympanic excision has been used to remove ear polyps (Diel 2008).

Treatment of polyps may involve traction alone, traction and corticosteroid administration, or traction and VBO. Treatment with traction (with or without corticosteroids) is most likely to be successful for nasopharyngeal polyps that do not have evidence of middle ear disease (Muilenburg & Fry 2002; Veir *et al.* 2002). The higher recurrence rates for polyps with evidence of middle ear disease or those growing into the external auditory canal are likely due to the difficulty of completely removing polyp tissue that has expanded within the middle ear and through the tympanic membrane. Recurrence rates of feline polyps treated with traction (with or without corticosteroids) range from 11% for nasopharyngeal polyps to 50% for ear polyps (Anderson *et al.* 2000; Muilenburg & Fry 2002; Veir *et al.* 2002). Treatment of feline polyps with both traction and VBO is associated with recurrence rates of 0–4% (Faulkner & Budsberg 1990; Kapatkin *et al.* 1990), but is also associated with a risk of iatrogenic damage, usually temporary, to sympathetic nerve fibers or inner ear structures in up to 94% of cases (Faulkner & Budsberg 1990; Kapatkin *et al.* 1990; Anders *et al.* 2008). The prognosis for dogs affected with middle ear polyps appears to be similar to that of cats (Fingland *et al.* 1993; Pratschke 2003).

Small cholesteatomas may be treated with appropriate long-term antibiotic therapy with or without vitamin A (Rao *et al.* 2009). If the decision is made to enter the tympanic cavity using surgery, a choice must be made between LBO and VBO. LBO is indicated when TECA is also being performed to control otitis externa or to remove external ear canal masses (Smeak & Inpanbutr 2005). VBO is indicated when preservation of the external auditory canal is desired or when complete exposure of the tympanic cavity is needed in order to more fully remove mass lesions (McAnulty *et al.* 1995a,b; Smeak *et al.* 1996; Silva *et al.* 2003; Anders *et al.* 2008).

Perioperative care

VBO requires planning for adequate pain control. Local anesthesia can be administered before or during surgery by performing an auricular block. The efficacy of this treatment has not been demonstrated in dogs or cats.

Once the nerves and vessels surrounding the bulla have been identified during surgery, the soft tissues around the surgical site can be infused with bupivacaine. Injectable opioid-based analgesics are often needed for at least 12–24 hours after surgery, with the duration dependent on the amount of tissue dissection and bone removal that was performed. Nonsteroidal anti-inflammatory drugs (NSAIDs) can be added for a multi-modal approach, unless corticosteroids were required during recovery. If there are vestibular signs after surgery, the animal may need to be sedated, put on intravenous fluids, and placed in a padded cage to protect it from self-injury, depending on the severity. Centrally acting antiemetics may be administered to reduce nausea and disorientation.

Ventral bulla osteotomy

Surgical preparation and draping

The ventral head and neck are clipped from the mid-mandible to the mid-neck. If a polyp extending into the ear is present, it can be helpful also to clip the affected ear, so that it can be included in the sterile field. The animal is positioned in dorsal recumbency with a towel or positioning device under the junction of the head and neck. If the ear is to be included in the sterile field, the head is tilted to one side and the pinna suspended off the table using a towel clamp attached by tape to a hook above the table. After surgical preparation, the appropriate area is draped, the towel clamp removed, and the skull is leveled. If the ear is not included in the sterile field, the skull can be leveled and taped before surgical preparation and draping. Inclusion of the entire caudal skull in the sterile field allows the surgeon to use the contralateral side to confirm normal anatomy and allows bilateral VBO to be performed. If a bilateral VBO is intended, then the head is leveled, and the maxilla can be taped to avoid movement. Taping the maxilla through the oral cavity rather than a tape over the mandible will allow the anesthesia team access to the oral cavity throughout the procedure without having to undo the tape.

Approach

The horizontal ramus and angular process of the mandible, the larynx, and the wing of the atlas are palpated before incision. In the cat, the ventral aspect of the bulla can be palpated through the skin. A paramedian incision is made from the caudal aspect of the mandible to the middle of the wing of the atlas. This incision will be about 1–1.5 cm lateral to the midline in the cat and 2 cm in the dog. The platysma and sphincter colli muscles are incised and separated. The incision will be over the

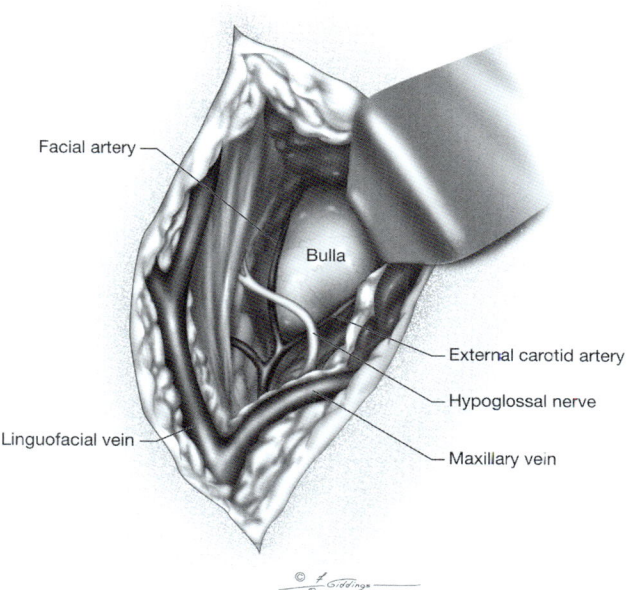

Figure 78.5 Ventral approach to the left canine bulla. The linguofacial vein and facial artery are medial. © D. Giddings.

jugular and linguofacial veins; these structures must be located and retracted. In the dog, the branch of the linguofacial vein draining the mandibular salivary gland must be severed and ligated or cauterized. In bilateral VBOs, making two separate incisions directly over the bulla is preferred over making a midline incision. The dissection is deepened between the mandibular salivary gland and the digastricus muscle. The external carotid artery, lingual artery, and hypoglossal nerve are located as the dissection proceeds between the digastricus and glossal muscles. The bulla will be in the triangle formed by the external carotid artery laterally and the lingual artery and the hypoglossal nerve medially (Figure 78.5). It is possible to palpate the stylohyoid bone on the caudolateral aspect of the bulla. The surgeon should also identify the origin of the digastricus muscle on the jugular process of the occiput (Figure 78.6). The bulla is just cranial and medial to this structure.

Surgery

Once the bulla is located, the periosteum is incised and elevated from the bone. On the medial aspect of the bulla, the ascending pharyngeal artery is immediately adjacent to the bulla and must be protected (especially important in the cat). The bulla is penetrated using a Steinmann pin in a Jacob's chuck. The opening is enlarged using Lempert or Kerrison rongeurs, being careful not to entrap any soft tissues as the bone is cut. The opening is enlarged until the majority of the ventral surface of the bulla has been removed. Fluid, mucus,

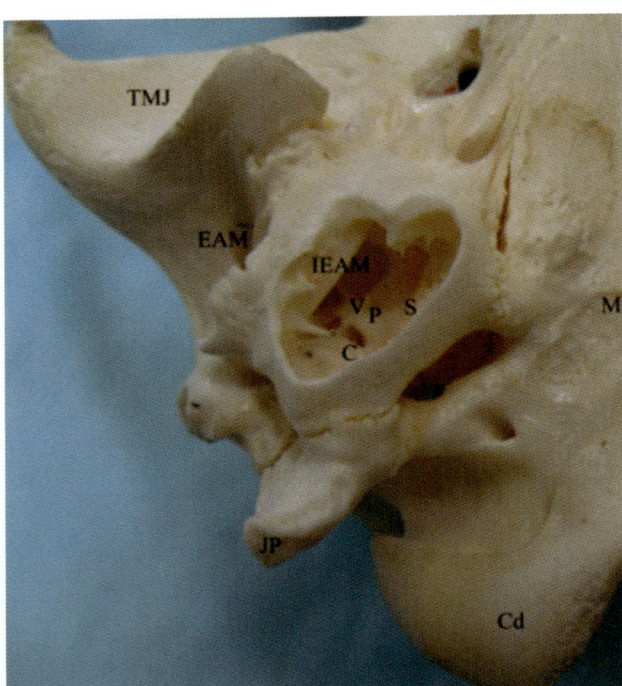

Figure 78.6 Ventral view of the right canine bulla. C, cochlear window; Cd, caudal; EAM, external acoustic meatus; IEAM, inner external acoustic meatus; JP, jugular process; M, medial; P, promontory; S, septum (incomplete in the dog, although some dogs may have an almost complete septum); TMJ, temporomandibular joint; V, vestibular window is dorsal (under a shelf of bone).

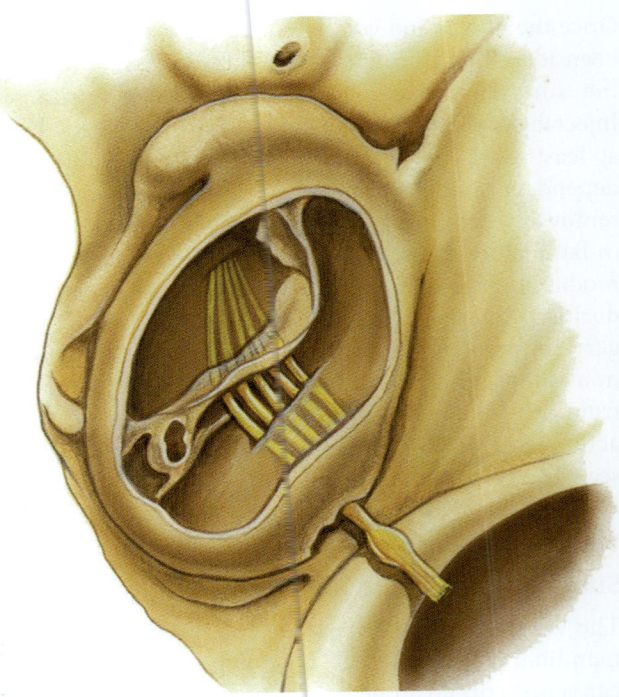

Figure 78.7 Ventral view of the right feline bulla with both compartments open showing the sympathetic nerves traversing the promontory. Source: Hudson, L.C and Hamilton, W.P. (2010). *Atlas of Feline Anatomy for Veterinarians*, 2e. Jackson, WY: Teton NewMedia.

pus, or keratin debris can be removed with a small curette and samples taken for culture. Care should be taken to avoid disturbing the cochlear window in both the dog and the cat. Additionally, care should be taken to protect the sympathetic fibers coursing over the promontory in the cat (Figure 78.7). In the cat, the ventral aspect of the lateral compartment is located. The bone is penetrated on the lateral aspect and the hole expanded using rongeurs until the lateral compartment can be clearly visualized.

Polyps usually originate in the cranial portion of the lateral compartment. A small curette and thumb forceps are used to remove the polypoid material, the epithelial attachments, and any accumulated debris. This is done carefully to avoid permanent damage to the sympathetic nerves in the cat. The surgeon should understand the location of the vestibular window and attempt to avoid penetrating this structure.

Once the attachments are severed within the bulla, traction can be used to remove the bulk of the polyp in the external auditory canal or the nasopharynx. If the ear has been included in the surgical field, the surgeon can provide traction on the ear polyp. Removal of nasopharyngeal polyps can be performed by the anesthetist

during surgery using traction. This is facilitated if an Allis tissue forceps or hemostat has been previously placed across the polyp. If this option is chosen, the surgeon can observe the base of the polyp as traction is applied to ensure that all attachments within the bulla are removed. If the nasopharyngeal polyp is too large to easily remove during surgery, it can be removed using traction after completion of the VBO. The cat will be repositioned in sternal recumbency with the maxilla suspended to provide better visualization. In cranial/rostral located polyps at the edge of hard palate to soft palate, an incision through the soft palate might be required to gain access to the polyp. Stay sutures are placed bilaterally and a midline incision is made in the soft palate, taking care to leave the free, caudal edge of the soft palate intact. After removal of the polyp, the palate is closed in two layers (nasopharyngeal mucosa and oral mucosa) using absorbable suture, and the stay sutures removed.

The removal of masses other than polyps (granulomas, small cholesteatomas, adenomas) is similar to the removal of polyps. The mass is removed along with any epithelial attachments. Small cholesteatomas may have a stalk that extends through the external acoustic meatus. If a cholesteatoma or cholesterol granuloma has resulted in expansion and distortion of the bulla, it can help to have the CT images present within the surgery suite. This allows the surgeon to repeatedly confirm the location of the bulla before penetration and to note the location of critical structures with the abnormal structure. If a large cholesteatoma is present, the surgeon will typically encounter copious amounts of keratin debris surrounded by inflamed thickened epithelium. If possible, the surgeon should attempt to elevate the epithelium from the surface of the bone, removing the debris and the epithelium together as one cystic structure. If the epithelium has expanded into the bony recesses of the bulla, this will not be possible. The keratin debris is removed. The abnormal epithelium is removed using a curette, a periosteal elevator, or a hemostat. The expanded ventral and lateral abnormal bone is removed to prevent impingement on normal structures and to allow safe access to the dorsal aspect of the middle ear. The anesthetist can repeatedly open the jaw during surgery to confirm the location of the temporomandibular joint and to ensure that the jaw can move freely at the conclusion of surgery.

Cholesteatomas and tumors can result in invasion into or through the petrous temporal bone, affecting the inner ear and brain. Lateral craniotomy has been used to access the inner surface of the petrous temporal bone to complete debulking of invasive middle ear masses after VBO. Approaching the brain through the inner ear is not recommended due to the risk of fatal hemorrhage and/or neurologic damage.

Masses and debris removed from the middle ear should be cultured for bacteria, as chronic infection is often present. Long-term antibiotic therapy may be needed after surgery to prevent recurrence of otitis media or cholesteatoma. When placing mass samples into formalin jars, the location of the mass should be carefully noted, as accurate diagnosis may require identifying that the location of the particular type of epithelium is abnormal (Little *et al.* 1991; Hardie *et al.* 2008).

Once debris, masses, and abnormal epithelium have been removed, the bulla is gently lavaged with warm saline to remove any remaining debris. The use of a video-otoscope during the surgery provides excellent visualization of the inner tympanic cavity during TECA and LBO, and may help identify debris and epithelial remnants (Haudiquet 2006).

A transoral approach to the ventral aspect of the bulla in dogs has been described in cadavers (Manou et al. 2017), but has not been described in cats nor clinically assessed in either species. The ventral aspect of the bulla was palpable in all dogs, but easier in mesati- and dolichocephalic than in brachycephalic dogs. Access was by drilling a k-wire, and increase in exposure using

Kerrison forceps. Further dissection revealed no damage to surrounding neurovascular structures.

Lateral Bulla Osteotomy

If performing an LBO for recurrent otitis media, positioning the patient in lateral recumbency and similar to positioning for a routine TECA is the most commonly used approach. If fistulating tracts are present, methylene blue can be injected to facilitate dissection around the tracts and down to the bulla. Advanced imaging such as CT will aid in finding landmarks in approaching the osseous meatus. The meatus might be scarred over with fibrous tissue, and the facial nerve and vessels might be more difficult to identify due to fibrous tissue, making the risks for complications higher. Care should be taken to remove all epithelial lining within the tympanic cavity. Given the abnormal tissue architecture laterally, some surgeons opt to approach the bulla ventrally through tissue that has not previously been incised. In a recent case report where cholesteatoma was found post LBO in two dogs, the elected approach for the one case that was surgically managed was a VBO, with no recurrence at five months postoperatively (Schuenemann & Oechtering 2012).

Postoperative care and complications

The use of Elizabethan collars after ear surgery is controversial. A soft Elizabethan collar can be used to prevent the patient from scratching the ear. Use of drains or soaker catheters in this location is not common. Bandages are typically avoided as they may slip, causing compression. Even a loosely placed bandage might put the patient at risk for upper airway obstruction if local tissue swelling or edema in conjunction with the bandage might create upper airway compression and obstruction.

Complications after VBO include respiratory distress (De Gennaro *et al.* 2017; Wainberg *et al.* 2019), Horner's syndrome (mainly in cats), vestibular disease, deafness, wound drainage, hemorrhage, facial or hypoglossal nerve damage, respiratory distress, and recurrence of disease (Faulkner & Budsberg 1990; Kapatkin *et al.* 1990; Sharp 1990; McAnulty *et al.* 1995b; Muilenburg & Fry 2002; Anders *et al.* 2008). Life-threatening respiratory distress can occur during recovery after VBO, especially after bilateral VBOs or if concurrent oral surgery for polyp extraction is needed. A significantly higher mortality rate (47% [30/64] vs. 9% [18/211]) has been described in single-stage bilateral versus unilateral VBO in cats (Wainberg *et al.* 2019).

Temporary Horner's syndrome has been reported in up to 94% of cats, resolving within weeks of the surgery (Kapatkin *et al.* 1990). Permanent Horner's syndrome occurs in up to 17% of feline patients (Faulkner & Budsberg 1990). In the same study, head tilt, nystagmus, and/or axatia were present in 5 of 12 cats (42%) after surgery and present long term in 2 of 12 cats (17%) (Faulkner & Budsberg 1990). In three different studies, *de novo* signs of vestibular disease were present after surgery in 0–17% of cats, but resolved with time (Kapatkin *et al*. 1990; Trevor & Martin 1993; Anders *et al*. 2008). In one study, deafness occurred after surgery in 1 of 12 cats (8%) that could hear before surgery, and hearing returned by the recheck at 668 days after surgery (Anders *et al*. 2008). In contrast, head tilt was permanent in 3 of 4 cats (75%) that had head tilt before surgery and hearing did not return in 7 cats that were deaf before surgery (Anders *et al*. 2008).

In normal dogs undergoing VBO, 1 of 12 dogs had markedly reduced hearing, as measured by brainstem auditory evoked potentials, approximately 5–6 weeks after surgery (McAnulty *et al*. 1995b). Four out of five dogs undergoing a VBO without TECA for otitis media had a satisfactory result, with one dog having continued purulent otic discharge (Holt & Walker 1997). No outcome data on a larger number of dogs undergoing VBO for clinical disease have been reported. Outcomes for dogs treated with VBO for cholesteatoma vary, and do not include large case numbers: four out of six dogs treated with VBO had no recurrence (Hardie *et al*. 2008) and one dog treated with VBO only had no recurrence at 12 months (Greci *et al*. 2011).

Healing and outcome after bulla osteotomy

In a study of 20 normal cats examined 8 or 16 weeks after VBO, there was reformation of the tympanic cavity in all cats. The defect in the bony septum between the lateral and medial compartments remained open in five cats. Connective tissue was found in the closed bone defects in most cats, but woven bone was present in four cats (da Silva *et al*. 2009). Cats undergoing VBO as treatment for middle ear polyps usually do not require long-term therapy (Donnelly & Tillson 2004).

In a study of VBO in normal dogs examined 1–6 weeks after surgery, 9 of 12 dogs reformed the tympanic bulla (McAnulty *et al*. 1995b). The defect was closed with fibrous connective tissue. Of the 12 dogs, 9 also had subperiosteal new bone formation from the inner surface of the bulla. In 3 dogs the bulla was filled with new bone. In a study in which 5 dogs with otitis media underwent ventral bulla osteotomy, partial or complete reformation of the bulla was found 60–78 months after surgery (Holt & Walker 1997). Close follow-up and monitoring of dogs after VBO are needed if there is any concern that all abnormal tissue was not removed. Many of the lesions associated with middle ear disease in dogs are the result of

chronic infection and the dogs will require ongoing antibiotic treatment. In a study of 19 dogs that underwent surgery with intent to cure cholesteatoma, 4 were managed long term (often years) with antibiotics to prevent recurrence of clinical signs (Hardie *et al*. 2008). Three dogs needed a second surgery to remove keratinaceous debris or abnormal bone, and one dog required removal of keratinaceous debris using a video-otoscope. Cats and dogs with neoplasia may require adjunctive therapy (Kirpensteijn 1993; Fan & de Lorimier 2004).

Summary

In summary, the major diseases of the middle ear in cats and dogs are otitis media, polyp, cholesteatoma, and cholesterol granuloma. Primary neoplasia is rare. VBO is used to gain access to the middle ear when preservation of the external ear canal is indicated or when better exposure of abnormal lesions can be achieved with a ventral approach. Mass removal from the middle ear requires detailed knowledge of middle ear anatomy, if iatrogenic damage to critical structures is to be avoided.

References

Alexander, A., Mahoney, P., Scarrell, E., and Baines, S. (2019). Cholesteatoma in a cat. *Journal of Feline Medicine and Surgery Open Reports* 5 (1): 2055116919848086.

Anders, B.B., Hoelzler, M.G., Scavelli, T.D. et al. (2008). Analysis of auditory and neurologic effects associated with ventral bulla osteotomy for removal of inflammatory polyps or nasopharyngeal masses in cats. *Journal of the American Veterinary Medical Association* 233: 580–585.

Anderson, D.M., Robinson, R.K., and White, R.A. (2000). Management of inflammatory polyps in 37 cats. *Veterinary Record* 147: 684–687.

Bischoff, M.G. and Kneller, S.K. (2004). Diagnostic imaging of the canine and feline ear. *Veterinary Clinics of North America. Small Animal Practice* 34: 437.

Cox, C.L. and Payne-Johnson, C.E. (1995). Aural cholesterol granuloma in a dog. *Journal of Small Animal Practice* 36: 25–28.

De Gennaro, C., Vettorato, E., and Corletto, F. (2017). Severe upper airway obstruction following bilateral ventral bulla osteotomy in a cat. *Canadian Veterinary Journal* 58: 1313–1316.

Diel, J.M. (2008). Removal of an ear polyp via perendoscopic transtympanic excision (PTTE) in two cats. *Der Praktische Tierarzt* 89: 94–98.

Donnelly, K.E. and Tillson, D.M. (2004). Feline inflammatory polyps and ventral bulla osteotomy. *Compendium on Continuing Education for the Practicing Veterinarian* 26: 446–454.

Fan, T.M. and de Lorimier, L.-P. (2004). Inflammatory polyps and aural neoplasia. *Veterinary Clinics of North America. Small Animal Practice* 34: 489–509.

Faulkner, J.E. and Budsberg, S.C. (1990). Results of ventral bulla osteotomy for treatment of middle ear polyps in cats. *Journal of the American Animal Hospital Association* 26: 496–499.

Fingland, R.B., Gratzek, A., Vorhies, M.W., and Kirpensteijn, J. (1993). Nasopharyngeal polyp in a dog. *Journal of the American Animal Hospital Association* 29: 311–314.

Fliegner, R.A., Jubb, K.V., and Lording, P.M. (2007). Cholesterol granuloma associated with otitis media and destruction of the tympanic bulla in a dog. *Veterinary Pathology* 44: 547–549.

Gersdorff, M.C.H., Debaty, M.E., and Tomasi, J.P. (2006). Pathophysiology of cholesteatoma. *Revue de Laryngologie Otologie Rhinologie* 127: 115–119.

Greci, V., Travetti, O., Di Giancamillo, M. et al. (2011). Middle ear cholesteatoma in 11 dogs. *Canadian Veterinary Journal* 52: 631–636.

Hammond, G.J., Sullivan, M., Weinrauch, S., and King, A.M. (2005). A comparison of the rostrocaudal open mouth and rostro 10° ventro-caudodorsal oblique radiographic views for imaging fluid in the feline tympanic bulla. *Veterinary Radiology and Ultrasound* 46: 205–209.

Hardie, E.M., Linder, K.E., and Pease, A.P. (2008). Aural cholesteatoma in twenty dogs. *Veterinary Surgery* 37: 763–770.

Haudiquet, P. (2006). Total ear canal ablation associated with lateral bulla ostectomy with the help of otoscopy in dogs and cats: retrospective study of 47 cases [abstract]. *Veterinary Surgery* 35: E3.

Holt, D.E. and Walker, L. (1997). Radiographic appearance of the middle ear after ventral bulla osteotomy in five dogs with otitis media. *Veterinary Radiology and Ultrasound* 38: 182–184.

Kapatkin, A.S., Matthiesen, D.T., Noone, K.E. et al. (1990). Results of surgery and long-term follow-up in 31 cats with nasopharyngeal polyps. *Journal of the American Animal Hospital Association* 26: 387–392.

Kirpensteijn, J. (1993). Aural neoplasms. *Seminars in Veterinary Medicine and Surgery (Small Animal)* 8: 17–23.

Lee, Y.-W., Kang, S.-K., and Choi, H.-J. (2008). Fluid accumulation in canine tympanic bulla: radiography, CT and MRI examinations. *Journal of Veterinary Clinics* 25: 176–181.

Little, C.J., Pearson, G.R., and Lane, J.G. (1989). Neoplasia involving the middle ear cavity of dogs. *Veterinary Record* 124: 54.

Little, C.J., Lane, J.G., Gibbs, C., and Pearson, G.R. (1991). Inflammatory middle ear disease of the dog: the clinical and pathological features of cholesteatoma, a complication of otitis media. *Veterinary Record* 128: 319–322.

Love, N.E., Kramer, R.W., Spodnick, G.J., and Thrall, D.E. (1995). Radiographic and computed tomographic evaluation of otitis media in the dog. *Veterinary Radiology and Ultrasound* 36: 375–379.

Lucroy, M.D., Vernau, K.M., Samii, V.F., and LeCouteur, R.A. (2004). Middle ear tumours with brainstem extension treated by ventral bulla osteotomy and craniectomy in two cats. *Veterinary and Comparative Oncology* 2: 234–242.

MacPhail, C.M., Innocenti, C.M., Kudnig, S.T. et al. (2007). Atypical manifestations of feline inflammatory polyps in three cats. *Journal of Feline Medicine and Surgery* 9: 219–225.

Manou, M., Moissonnier, P.H.M., Jardel, N. et al. (2017). Transoral approach for ventral tympanic bulla osteotomy in the dog: a descriptive cadaveric study. *Veterinary Surgery* 46: 773–779.

McAnulty, J.F., Hattel, A., and Harvey, C.E. (1995a). Wound healing and brain stem auditory evoked potentials after experimental total ear canal ablation with lateral tympanic bulla osteotomy in dogs. *Veterinary Surgery* 24: 1–8.

McAnulty, J.F., Hattel, A., and Harvey, C.E. (1995b). Wound healing and brain stem auditory evoked potentials after experimental ventral tympanic bulla osteotomy in dogs. *Veterinary Surgery* 24: 9–14.

Muilenburg, R.K. and Fry, T.R. (2002). Feline nasopharyngeal polyps. *Veterinary Clinics of North America. Small Animal Practice* 32: 839–849.

Palmeiro, B.S., Morris, D.O., Wiemelt, S.P., and Shofer, F.S. (2004). Evaluation of outcome of otitis media after lavage of the tympanic bulla and long-term antimicrobial drug treatment in dogs: 44 cases (1998–2002). *Journal of the American Veterinary Medical Association* 225: 548–553.

Pratschke, K.M. (2003). Inflammatory polyps of the middle ear in 5 dogs. *Veterinary Surgery* 32: 292–296.

Rao, U.S.V., Srinivas, D.R., Humbarwadi, R.S., and Malhotra, B.K. (2009). Role of vitamin A in the evolution of cholesteatoma. *Indian Journal of Otolaryngology and Head and Neck Surgery* 61: 150–152.

Schuenemann, R.M. and Oechtering, G. (2012). Cholesteatoma after lateral bulla osteotomy in two brachycephalic dogs. *Journal of the American Animal Hospital Association* 48: 261–268.

Sharp, N.J. (1990). Chronic otitis externa and otitis media treated by total ear canal ablation and ventral bulla osteotomy in thirteen dogs. *Veterinary Surgery* 19: 162–166.

da Silva, A.M., Padilha Filho, J.G., Monteiro, C.M.R., and Teixeira, A.J. (2003). Comparison between ventral and lateral approaches to tympanic bulla osteotomy in dogs. *A Hora Veterinária* 22 (132): 69–71.

da Silva, A.M., de Souza, W.M., de Carvalho, R.G. et al. (2009). Morphological aspects of tympanic bulla after ventral osteotomy in cats. *Acta cirurgica brasileira/Sociedade Brasileira para Desenvolvimento Pesquisa em Cirurgia* 24: 177–182.

Smeak, D.D. (2016). Treatment of persistent deep infection after total ear canal ablation and lateral bulla osteotomy. *Veterinary Clinics of North America. Small Animal Practice* 46: 609–621.

Smeak, D.D. and Inpanbutr, N. (2005). Lateral approach to subtotal bulla osteotomy in dogs: pertinent anatomy and procedural details. *Compendium on Continuing Education for the Practicing Veterinarian* 27: 377–384.

Smeak, D.D., Crocker, C.B., and Birchard, S.J. (1996). Treatment of recurrent otitis media that developed after total ear canal ablation and lateral bulla osteotomy in dogs: nine cases (1986–1994). *Journal of the American Veterinary Medical Association* 209: 937–942.

Tanaka, T., Akiyoski, H., Mie, K., and Nishida, H. (2018). MRI findings, including diffusion-weighted imaging and apparent diffusion coefficient value, in two cats with nasopharyngeal polyps and one cat with lymphoma. *Journal of Feline Medicine and Surgery Open Reports* 4 (2): 2055116918812254.

Trevor, P.B. and Martin, R.A. (1993). Tympanic bulla osteotomy for treatment of middle-ear disease in cats: 19 cases (1984–1991). *Journal of the American Veterinary Medical Association* 202: 123–128.

Veir, J.K., Lappin, M.R., Foley, J.E., and Getzy, D.M. (2002). Feline inflammatory polyps: historical, clinical, and PCR findings for feline calicivirus and feline herpes virus-1 in 28 cases. *Journal of Feline Medicine and Surgery* 4: 195–199.

Wainberg, S.H., Selmic, L.E., Haagsman, A.N. et al. (2019). Comparison of complications and outcome following unilateral, staged bilateral, and single-stage bilateral ventral bulla osteotomy in cats. *Journal of the American Veterinary Medical Association* 255: 828–836.

Yoshikawa, H., Mayer, M.N., Linn, K.A. et al. (2008). A dog with squamous cell carcinoma in the middle ear. *Canadian Veterinary Journal* 49: 877–879.

Section 11

Cardiac

79

Coagulation Disorders and Surgery

Sara Shropshire and Benjamin Brainard

Understanding hypocoagulability

Hypocoagulability refers to an inherited or acquired disorder of coagulation that could result in perioperative hemorrhage. An understanding of the underlying physiology of clot formation allows focused discussion of the causes of hypocoagulability and the options for therapy.

Primary hemostasis

Primary hemostasis refers to the activity of platelets in coagulation; platelets can be first responders to an area of vascular damage and become activated following exposure to subendothelial collagen or other soluble factors. Following activation, platelets undergo a shape change, release additional procoagulant factors, and experience a change in their membrane phospholipid structure that supports assembly of the plasma-based coagulation factor system and the ultimate formation of a fibrin clot (Smith 2009). Because platelets play such a key role in hemostasis, disorders of platelet number (thrombocytopenia) or function (thrombocytopathia) are risk factors for bleeding. Clinical signs of impaired primary hemostasis include mucosal hemorrhage (e.g., epistaxis, hematuria, gastrointestinal bleeding, oral mucosal bleeding), in addition to prolonged bleeding from cut skin surfaces in surgery. Petechiae are small, pinpoint hemorrhages that can be seen on glabrous skin such as ear pinnae and the inguinal area. Petechiae may also be seen on the gums and sclera in affected animals. Ecchymosis describes coalescing petechiae, which are more consistent with subcutaneous hemorrhage or bruising (but less severe than a hematoma), and may also be present in thrombocytopenic animals.

Macrothrombocytopenia is a heritable condition in Cavalier King Charles spaniels and English toy spaniels, characterized by a mean platelet volume that is much larger than normal (Tvedten *et al.* 2008). Dogs with macrothrombocytopenia do not have an increased tendency for bleeding, but the diagnosis of conditions such as consumptive coagulopathy can be difficult in these dogs. Thrombocytopenia secondary to consumption is a common condition in veterinary medicine, and is often a sequela to diverse diseases including hemorrhage, neoplasia, infections, or immune-mediated disease (where the thrombocytopenia is triggered by systemic inflammation). Thrombocytopenia can also be secondary to immune-mediated platelet destruction that can be idiopathic or triggered by medications (e.g., trimethoprim-sulfa drugs), infectious diseases, or neoplasia.

Iatrogenic impairment of platelet function occurs from the use of therapeutics designed to decrease platelet activity, such as clopidogrel. In addition, nonsteroidal anti-inflammatory drugs (NSAIDs; including aspirin) can interfere with platelet production of thromboxane and prevent activation and recruitment of other platelets to areas of hemorrhage (Brainard *et al.* 2007). Hetastarch and tetrastarches can cause a dose-related decrease in platelet function and should be used cautiously in patients at risk for hemorrhage (Epstein *et al.* 2014).

Spontaneous bleeding is unlikely in patients with platelet counts above 20×10^3 platelets/μL, and surgical bleeding is less likely in patients with platelet counts above 50×10^3 platelets/μL (Callan *et al.* 2009). Immune thrombocytopenia (ITP) frequently results in platelet counts below 20×10^3 platelets/μL (Callan *et al.* 2009). These animals are at high risk for spontaneous and surgical bleeding and may require platelet transfusion prior to invasive procedures (see later). Other heritable conditions that affect platelet function include von Willebrand disease (vWD), in which platelets are unable to localize to areas of vascular injury due to loss of the tethering von Willebrand molecule that is released from endothelial cells (Barr & McMichael 2012).

Secondary hemostasis

Secondary hemostasis is the process of formation of a fibrin clot from the activation of soluble plasma coagulation factors. Fibrin forms a meshwork over areas of vascular injury and is stabilized into a clot when it is cross-linked by coagulation factor XIII (Smith 2009).

Hemophilia is the most common heritable condition affecting coagulation function in veterinary species. Hemophilia describes decreased activity of one of the coagulation factors, specifically coagulation factor VIII (hemophilia A), IX (hemophilia B), or XI (hemophilia C) (Barr & McMichael 2012). Patients with hemophilia have variably severe bleeding phenotypes, but are highly likely to bleed from invasive procedures. Other heritable coagulation factor deficiencies have been reported in veterinary species (Barr & McMichael 2012). In general, transfusion with fresh frozen plasma (FFP, containing fully formed coagulation factors) will temporarily restore coagulation function and allow invasive procedures and perioperative hemodynamic stability.

Acquired coagulopathies that impact secondary hemostasis are common in veterinary medicine. Intoxications with anticoagulant rodenticide or iatrogenic use of anticoagulant medications such as heparin, warfarin, or other oral anticoagulants can result in significant coagulopathy. Because most coagulation factors are synthesized in the liver, significant hepatic disease can impair the production of factors (Webster 2017). Moderate to severe hemorrhage can result in consumption of coagulation factors, in the same manner as it can cause thrombocytopenia, and a transient impairment of coagulation function may occur. Clinical signs of secondary coagulopathies include cavity bleeding (hemarthrosis, hemothorax, hemoperitoneum, hemopericardium) and subcutaneous hematoma formation, and animals are more likely to present with hypovolemic or hemorrhagic shock, compared to those with primary hemostatic deficiencies.

Disseminated intravascular coagulation (DIC) is a syndrome associated with the activation of the coagulation system by systemic inflammation. Inflammation can activate platelets and secondary coagulation, leading to consumption of both. Triggers that are implicated for the initiation of DIC include circulating tissue factor-bearing cells or particles (monocytes, microparticles)

and thrombin produced during coagulation. Thrombin can also activate white blood cells, supporting continued inflammation (Brainard & Brown 2011). Initially, the body can compensate for DIC-associated consumption; this compensated state is characterized by a mild to moderate drop in platelet count, with normal to slightly prolonged coagulation times (see later). Compensated DIC is also termed "non-overt" (Levi et al. 2009). Eventually, with continued consumption, systemic coagulation competence can decrease, and the animal develops a hypocoagulable phenotype. Once DIC leads to hypocoagulability, platelet counts decrease further, and coagulation times become definitively prolonged; this is overt DIC. Other components of DIC can include thrombosis and hyperfibrinolysis. Fibrinolysis is triggered by the presence of an intravascular clot, as the endothelium releases tissue plasminogen activator, which activates plasminogen to plasmin and begins to break down formed clots. While fibrinolysis is necessary under normal conditions to restore blood flow following endothelial repair, the upregulation during DIC results in breakdown of clots before the endothelium has had a chance to completely heal and can contribute to the hypocoagulable phenotype.

Therapy for DIC is focused on resolution of the underlying cause of inflammation. In animals with hypocoagulability, FFP is indicated to resolve secondary coagulopathy if active bleeding is present (or prophylactically in the perioperative period to prevent intraoperative hemorrhage). Platelet counts do not usually drop below a threshold for spontaneous bleeding, and resolution of inflammation will allow rapid restoration of platelet count from the bone marrow. Because of the wide variety of conditions that have been associated with the initiation of DIC and subsequent coagulopathy, it is indicated to verify coagulation status and platelet count prior to surgery if there is a clinical suspicion for inflammatory disease, especially in cases of neoplasia and sepsis or septic shock.

The acute coagulopathy of trauma and shock (ACOTS) is a syndrome that is related to severe diffuse tissue trauma, resulting in a DIC-like phenotype but occurring acutely, as opposed to DIC, which usually has a longer time of onset (Gando et al. 2013). In addition to tissue damage causing activation of coagulation and disruption of blood flow, fibrinolysis is upregulated, and patients can present a similar appearance to patients with DIC.

As noted, fibrinolysis plays an important role in normal hemostasis, but if disordered can contribute to perioperative bleeding. Some dog breeds, notably sighthounds, have been hypothesized to have hyperactive fibrinolytic systems, resulting in delayed postoperative bleeding (Marín *et al.* 2012). It is unclear if this phenomenon is triggered by postoperative inflammation or if this is consistently present. Regardless, it is an important perioperative concern, and current recommendations include the administration of anti-fibrinolytic drugs to these patients in the perioperative period. Clinically, patients with hyperfibrinolysis may have persistent cavitary bleeding after procedures or may develop petechiae and bruising at diverse locations on the body. Diagnostic testing to evaluate primary and secondary hemostasis is usually normal, but laboratory markers of fibrinolysis (see later) may be increased.

Assessment of coagulation status

An evaluation of primary hemostasis starts with measurement of the platelet count. If evaluating a blood smear, each platelet observed on a 100× high-power field represents 15 000 circulating platelets/μL (Callan *et al.* 2009). Automated complete blood count machines are generally accurate, but low counts should be verified by evaluation of a blood smear, especially in cats, who have a tendency to develop platelet clumps that are not accurately counted by machines. Patients that have signs of primary hemostatic dysfunction but a normal platelet count may have heritable defects in platelet function, or may be animals with vWD. Circulating von Willebrand factor (vWF) can be measured at specialized laboratories (e.g., Cornell University Comparative Coagulation Laboratory) for the diagnosis of vWD Although vWD classically occurs in Doberman pinschers, it has been reported in many other breeds, and animals with compatible clinical signs should be tested. The buccal mucosal bleeding time (BMBT) is a simple test to evaluate the ability of an animal's platelets to form the initial platelet plug in areas of hemorrhage. The test is performed in dogs using the buccal mucosa by lifting a lip, and in cats by using the oral mucosa just above the canine teeth, due to their small lips. The test must be performed using a standardized tool (e.g., Simplate II, Organon Teknika, Durham, NC, USA) so that the length and depth of the incision are constant between animals. Sedation may be necessary in cats and some dogs to perform this test accurately. The platelet function analyzer (PFA) is a proprietary test that uses a cartridge to aspirate citrated whole blood through a small aperture coated with collagen and ADP to stimulate platelet activation. If platelet function is normal, the aperture will be occluded by platelets in a standard amount of time. Patients with vWD or other platelet dysfunction will have prolonged time to occlusion ("closure time"; Callan & Giger 2002). Both PFA and BMBT will be prolonged in patients with platelet counts below 100×10^3 platelets/μL (Jandrey 2012). Platelet aggregometry, either using

whole blood (impedance aggregometry) or platelet-rich plasma (optical aggregometry), is an advanced assay that evaluates the platelet aggregation response to specific agonists and is generally only available in specialized laboratories (Jandrey 2012).

Testing of secondary coagulation is generally performed on citrated plasma. The prothrombin time (PT) and activated partial thromboplastin time (aPTT) measure the extrinsic and intrinsic coagulation pathways, respectively, and reflect the activity of the plasma factors. Factor deficiencies are reflected in prolongations of PT (factor VII) or aPTT (factors VIII, IX, XI), or both (factors X, V, II). Mixed disturbances can occur with consumptive conditions, hepatic failure, vitamin K antagonist toxicity, and therapy with anticoagulants such as unfractionated heparin. As already noted, non-overt DIC is characterized by moderate prolongations in aPTT without changes in PT, with a moderate decrease in platelet count, while overt DIC is distinguished by moderate to severe prolongations in both aPTT and PT, with decreased platelet counts. In patients where specific factor deficiency is suspected, specialized laboratories (e.g., Cornell Comparative Coagulation Laboratory) can help to assess factor activities in plasma samples. Point-of-care coagulation monitors are also available, and generally use whole blood instead of citrated plasma (Dixon-Jimenez *et al.* 2013).

In addition to the other procoagulant factor activities, fibrinogen concentration can be measured. Fibrinogen is important not only as a procoagulant factor, but also as an acute-phase protein that can indicate the presence of systemic inflammation. In overt DIC, fibrinogen is consumed and low fibrinogen contributes to the hypocoagulable phenotype. In addition, DIC is characterized by increased fibrinolysis, and the breakdown of cross-linked clots into fibrin degradation products (FDPs), specifically d-dimers, provide an easily measurable biomarker of fibrinolysis. Circulating d-dimer concentration is increased in any situation with increased fibrinolysis, including DIC, as well as following thrombotic conditions, although it is not a reliable single diagnostic tool for the diagnosis of thromboembolism in veterinary species.

Global assessments of coagulation using whole blood analysis have become popular in veterinary medicine over the past 20 years. The most common tests are thromboelastography (TEG, Haemonetics Corp., Braintree, MA, USA) and rotational thromboelastometry (ROTEM). These tests graphically document the progression of clot formation as blood progresses from a liquid to a gelid solid (Kol & Borjesson 2010). The classic tracing resembles a tuning fork (Figure 79.1), with the initial time to initiation

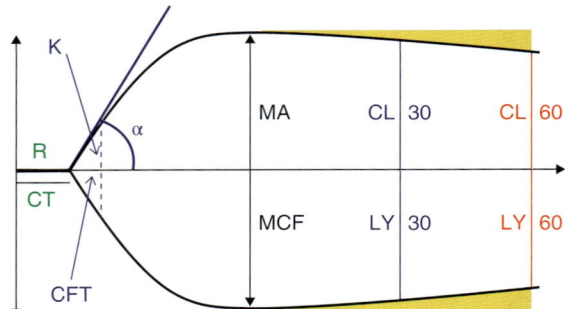

Figure 79.1 Representative thromboelastography (TEG)/thromboelastometry (ROTEM) tracing showing the TEG parameters above and ROTEM parameters below the center line. Reaction time (R) or clotting time (CT) represents the time until coagulation starts. The K-time or clot formation time represents the time for the tracing to achieve a specified width. The alpha angle represents the speed of clot formation. The maximum amplitude (MA) or maximum clot firmness (MCF) represents the final clot strength. The clot lysis (CL) and lysis index (LY) measured 30 and 60 minutes after MA or MCF are also depicted and represent clot breakdown due to fibrinolysis.

of coagulation (reaction time or clot formation time) corresponding roughly to the aPTT, the rate of split (angle) representing the speed of clot formation and the contribution of platelets, and the maximum width (maximum amplitude/maximum clot firmness) corresponding to the final clot strength and the contribution of platelets and fibrinogen. The decrease in the width of the tracing with time (measured usually at 30 and 60 minutes after the maximum amplitude) can indicate fibrinolysis, although the degree to which this occurs in dogs is minimal. To address the slow fibrinolysis, modified assays using added tissue plasminogen activator have been employed, but are not necessarily commonly used (Brown *et al.* 2016). It is important to have clearly defined protocols when using viscoelastic testing, as there can be significant variability between operators. It seems that the use of a strong activator such as 1 : 3400 dilution of tissue factor minimizes preanalytic variability in the assay (Smith *et al.* 2010).

Therapy for hypocoagulable patients

If patients are bleeding, consideration should be given to transfusions that include red blood cells, either as packed red blood cells, or as part of a transfusion of fresh or stored whole blood. The benefit of giving fresh whole blood is that both platelets and coagulation factors are transfused along with the red blood cells, and this addresses many diverse causes of coagulopathy. If animals are not anemic and the source of bleeding can be localized to a specific defect in primary or secondary hemostasis, more targeted therapies can be used.

Patients with vWD can be treated in the perioperative period with cryoprecipitate, which contains high concentrations of vWF, fibrinogen, and factor VIII (Prittie 2021). Cryoprecipitate is available as a frozen or lyophilized product, and appropriate dosages vary with product. In patients with vWD, cryoprecipitate transfusion should start during the presurgical preparation, continue through surgery as a slow infusion, and be completed in the postoperative period to ensure that adequate vWF is available for clot formation (Barr & McMichael 2012). Hypofibrinogenemia may also be treated with cryoprecipitate. Desmopressin (DDAVP) can cause a limited release of vWF from endothelial cells (depending on the type of vWD), and is indicated prior to emergent surgical conditions when cryoprecipitate is not available (Callan & Giger 2002). For patients with acquired platelet function deficits, guidance for the timing of surgery with regard to cessation of drug therapy has been reviewed (Brainard *et al.* 2019). In general, if the surgery is elective, cessation of therapy 3–5 days in advance for drugs that have an irreversible effect on platelets is prudent. Emergent surgery can continue with appropriate attention to hemostasis.

For conditions of platelet function defects, or in cases of thrombocytopenia, platelet transfusion may be considered. Platelets are part of a fresh whole blood transfusion, and also may be administered as platelet-rich plasma, obtained from a slow centrifugation of fresh whole blood (Callan *et al.* 2009). Platelet concentrate is frequently used in human medicine and is made either by sequential centrifugation of platelet-rich plasma, or through pheresis. Because these platelet concentrates have specific storage requirements (room temperature under continuous agitation, for five days), they are not widely available to the veterinary market except by special order. DMSO-stabilized frozen platelet concentrate is commercially available, and may provide some hemostatic capacity, although the function is decreased significantly from fresh platelet concentrate (Guillaumin *et al.* 2010). Lyophilized platelet concentrate may also provide hemostatic support for patients with thrombocytopenia and has the added benefit of room-temperature storage (Goggs *et al.* 2020).

FFP is obtained from fresh whole blood following centrifugation and contains all of the soluble coagulation factors in plasma. It can be used to treat inherited and acquired hemostatic disorders characterized by decreases in the function of one or multiple coagulation factors, including fibrinogen. In humans, FFP is considered to be adequate for complete factor replacement for one year following collection, after which the activity of factors V and VIII decreases (Culler *et al.* 2017). At this point, the plasma becomes stored plasma, and retains the activity of the more stable coagulation factors (e.g., factors II, VII, IX, X) for an additional four years. Thus acute coagulopathies are most effectively treated using FFP, although specific ones, such as anticoagulant rodenticide toxicosis, may be amenable to therapy with stored plasma, as it can replace all of the vitamin K-dependent coagulation factors.

DIC, as already noted, is a complex disorder that is characterized by concurrent hemorrhage and thrombosis. In patients with disturbances of secondary hemostasis and clinical bleeding due to DIC, it is indicated to replace active coagulation factors with FFP. Because FFP contains endogenous antithrombin, transfusion may also result in a decrease of circulating free thrombin and decrease coagulation or leukocyte activation. FFP administration in the absence of clinical hemorrhage in patients with DIC is controversial and should be considered in light of other aspects of disease, such as ease and duration of treatment and the overall inflammatory state of the patient.

In patients where the primary cause of hemorrhage is thought to be due to a hyperfibrinolytic state, as opposed to a factor or platelet deficiency, therapy should be directed toward strengthening formed clots to prevent premature lysis. Aminocaproic acid and tranexamic acid are both lysine analogs that act to decrease fibrinolysis. These drugs may be given orally or intravenously, and also may be used topically in certain circumstances. Dosing recommendations based on resolution of *in vitro* hyperfibrinolysis have been published in dogs (Brown *et al.* 2016; Osekavage *et al.* 2018), and the drugs are relatively well tolerated, with the exception of emesis that can result from rapid intravenous administration of tranexamic acid. There are not clear dosing recommendations for cats, but it is likely that doses may be lower than in dogs due to the more robust endogenous fibrinolysis in this species.

Hypercoagulability: a clinical conundrum

It is without a doubt that over the last 10 years, the topic of hypercoagulability has garnered a great deal of attention in veterinary medicine. Although more studies have been published and additional drug therapies have been investigated for use in dogs and cats with hypercoagulability or thrombosis, it is still challenging to know which patients should receive treatment, particularly in the surgical setting. Recently, consensus guidelines were published that reported on various known conditions that are associated with hypercoagulability or thrombosis in dogs and cats (deLaforcade *et al.* 2019). Conditions that were associated with a high risk of thrombosis in dogs included immune-mediated hemolytic anemia and protein-losing nephropathy, whereas in cats, cardiomyopathies

with concurrent risk factors (i.e., left atrial dilatation) were considered high risk. Conditions that surgeons would more commonly encounter in their canine patients that were described as having a risk factor for thrombosis include pancreatitis, neoplasia, and sepsis (deLaforcade *et al.* 2019), in addition to the hypercoagulable phase of DIC (Ralph & Brainard 2012). In cats, this does not seem to be as much of a clinical concern with surgical procedures even in the setting of a concurrent stable cardiomyopathy. Additionally, high-risk patients are dogs and cats that have more than one risk factor for thrombosis (deLaforcade *et al.* 2019) and prior surgery is associated with increased risk in human and veterinary medicine (Bates & Ginsberg 2004; Kim *et al.* 2013; Galanaud *et al.* 2016; Flynn *et al.* 2019; Respess *et al.* 2012). Consequently, many patients can appear hypercoagulable via different testing modalities simply because they have undergone a surgical procedure, since coagulation is intertwined with inflammation. In human patients, postoperative fibrinogen concentrations can remain elevated up to two weeks after surgery, and the magnitude of the increase is a function of the invasiveness of the surgery (Siemens *et al.* 1999). Increases in fibrinogen can also be seen in dogs postoperatively (Moldal *et al.* 2012). However, there are no surgical procedures where anticoagulation or thromboprophylactic therapy is routinely recommended and there are no universally accepted protocols. As a result, each patient is evaluated individually and therapy is tailored to that patient and clinical scenario.

Because of the direct relationships between coagulation and inflammation, it is important to critically assess surgical patients to determine their individual risk for thrombosis. This approach is recommended rather than labeling a patient as hypercoagulable and instituting therapy based on the results of a single test or diagnosis, because coagulation is dynamic and complex. Initially, patients should be assessed for the presence of the previously mentioned risk factors. Subsequent assessment for evidence of hypercoagulability or risk of thrombosis should be focused on what is known about the pathophysiology of thrombus formation. According to Virchow's triad, components that will lead to the formation of a thrombus include the absence of normal laminar blood flow, which includes endothelial damage and blood stasis. In addition to these factors, an imbalance between endogenous procoagulant and anticoagulant molecules can promote a procoagulant state (Kitrell & Berkwitt 2012; deLaforcade 2012).

Examples of situations where blood stasis may occur in surgical patients are vascular surgeries, vascular anomalies, abnormal blood flow or aneurysmal dilatations due to cardiovascular disease, or aberrant vasculature associated with neoplastic conditions. Additionally, perioperative occurrences such as hypovolemia related to procedural bleeding, preoperative hyperviscocity conditions, or recumbency of surgical patients postoperatively can contribute to hypercoagulability (deLaforcade 2012; Kaboli *et al.* 2003). Endothelial damage occurs in almost every surgical procedure and has the potential to activate the coagulation system through loss of the smooth endothelial surface and upregulation of endothelial adhesion molecules that can trigger coagulation (deLaforcade *et al.* 2019). Many factors can result in a systemic procoagulant state or hypercoagulability, including increased platelet activation and aggregation, increase in circulating procoagulants such as thrombin or fibrinogen, decrease in anticoagulants such as antithrombin, and decrease in fibrinolytic proteins such as tissue plasminogen activator or plasminogen (Kitrell & Berkwitt 2012; deLaforcade 2012). As previously stated, surgical procedures result in various levels of tissue trauma that range from very mild to more severe depending on the procedure. This tissue trauma not only leads to activation of coagulation, but also leads to inflammation that can become systemic. Systemic inflammation can result in platelet activation through a variety of mechanisms and results in increases in thrombin and fibrinogen in addition to decreases in antithrombin (Xu *et al.* 2016; Petäjä 2011; O'Brien 2012). Consequently, it can be reasonable to see why surgical patients have several factors aside from preexisting conditions (e.g., protein-losing nephropathy) that could put them at risk for clot formation. However, thousands of dogs and cats undergo surgical procedures every day and most patients do not suffer from clinically apparent thrombotic complications. Most patients can maintain a hemostatic balance, but if the balance is tipped into a procoagulant state, as might be caused by preexisting inflammation, then hypercoagulability and thrombus formation or a thromboembolic event can occur.

The diagnosis of hypercoagulability in veterinary medicine should be based on the individual patient assessment. The diagnosis of hypercoagulability can be challenging in both human and veterinary medicine. Additionally, even if evidence of a thrombus is found (e.g., incidental splenic vein thrombosis), it may not indicate that the patient is currently hypercoagulable, further complicating patient assessment and management. Serial coagulation assessment of patients is thus imperative for optimal patient care, as it provides a clearer view of a progression toward or away from hypercoagulability. Table 79.1 provides a list of various parameters or test assay results that can be consistent with hypercoagulability in veterinary patients.

More than one factor typically must be present to cause a patient to be more prone to clot formation or

Table 79.1 Parameters or test assays that can be consistent with hypercoagulability.

Parameter	Mechanism
Thrombocytosis	Inflammation, lack of removal by the spleen, hyperadrenocorticism
Hyperfibrinogenemia	Inflammation
Decreased antithrombin	Negative acute-phase protein, consumption, loss (urinary or gastrointestinal)
Increased D-dimers and FDPs[a]	Result of clot breakdown
Thromboelastography	Findings consistent with hypercoagulability; definitions vary depending on institution (e.g., increased maximum amplitude)
Thromboelastometry	Findings consistent with hypercoagulability; definitions vary depending on institution (e.g., maximum clot firmness)

[a] Fibrin (fibrinogen) degradation products (FDPs).

hypercoagulable, and tissue trauma or endothelial damage following surgery may be adequate in some animals to tip the balance. Additionally, in DIC, patients may be hypercoagulable or hypocoagulable, so if a patient has findings consistent with DIC (see the hypocoagulability section), they also may be at risk for clot formation depending on the clinical scenario.

Inflammation is common and expected following surgical procedures. Therefore, it is recommended that anticoagulant therapy or thromboprophylaxis should only be pursued in patients that have been fully assessed for risk factors, and when the pros and cons of therapeutic interventions have been considered. For example, it is the authors' opinion that it is not appropriate to start anticoagulant therapy in a patient that has no risk factors other than surgery, in whom the only testing results consistent with hypercoagulability are a mild hyperfibrinogenemia and a postoperative hypercoagulable TEG tracing, without clinical signs of thrombosis. However, it could be appropriate to initiate therapy in a patient that has high-risk factors for clot formation, testing consistent with hypercoagulability such as hyperfibrinogenemia or a hypercoagulable TEG tracing, and clinical signs concerning for hypercoagulability (e.g., acute respiratory distress due to suspect pulmonary thromboembolism postoperatively). Again, the decision to treat should be based on more than a single test result, and ideally serial assessment of the same animal. Treatment for hypercoagulability in surgical patients could include preoperative, perioperative, and postoperative medications, but there are few veterinary guidelines at this time (Blais *et al.* 2019). Options for therapy can include platelet inhibitors such as aspirin or clopidogrel, anticoagulants such as warfarin, unfractionated heparin, low molecular weight heparin, direct oral anticoagulants such as apixaban or rivaroxaban, and pro-fibrinolytic medications such as tissue plasminogen activator (Blais *et al.* 2019). Table 79.2 lists various treatment options, dosage guidelines, and considerations for treatment of surgical patients. These recommendations come from the recent consensus guidelines in addition to the authors' experience (Goggs *et al.* 2019; Sharp *et al.* 2019).

Another common consideration for therapy includes combination therapy. Although there are few established guidelines in veterinary medicine, combination therapy is reasonable when dealing with patients with overt thrombosis, that are considered extremely high risk for thrombosis formation, or in clinical scenarios where a thrombosis would be disastrous should one occur (e.g., thrombosis of a prosthetic heart valve in a cardiac patient) (Blais *et al.* 2019). It is the authors' opinion that when combination therapy is indicated in dogs and cats, that antiplatelet therapy (e.g., clopidogrel) is combined with an anticoagulant such as a direct oral anticoagulant (apixaban or rivaroxaban) due to the overall predictability, safety, and ease of administration of these medications.

Hypercoagulability in veterinary patients and particularly surgical patients can be challenging to diagnose and treatment protocols are not universally accepted or established. However, when patients are critically evaluated, the risk factors for thrombosis are understood, and diagnostics are viewed in light of the entire clinical picture rather than in isolation, the morbidity and mortality associated with aberrant clot formation can decrease so that surgical patients do not succumb to thromboembolic complications in the preoperative, perioperative, or postoperative period.

Table 79.2 Therapeutic options for hypercoagulability in surgical patients.

Medication	Indications	Dosage	Considerations
Platelet inhibition			
Aspirin	Dogs: prevention and treatment of aortic thromboembolism	Dogs: 1–3 mg/kg p.o. q24 h	Variable platelet inhibition, low dose inhibits platelet function in approximately one-third of healthy dogs
	Cats: none	Cats: not recommended	
Clopidogrel	Dogs: Prevention and treatment of aortic or venous thromboembolism or arterial thrombus/thromboembolism	Dogs: 2–4 mg/kg p.o. q24 h Loading dose 4–10 mg/kg once[a]	Response to clopidogrel therapy can be evaluated through platelet function assays, but future clinical studies need to be performed to determine how clinically beneficial monitoring is for an individual patient
	Cats: Same	Cats: 18.75 mg p.o. q24 h Loading dose 37.5 mg once[a]	
Anticoagulants			
Warfarin	Dogs: Not recommended, but could be considered for treatment of aortic thrombus/thromboembolism	Dogs: 0.05–0.2 mg/kg p.o. q24 h	Great deal of variability and absorption issues. Requires consistent and frequent monitoring. Dogs: monitor with PT_{INR} to achieve a target of 2–3, or 1.5–2.0 times the baseline PT
	Cats: Not recommended	Cats: Not recommended	
Unfractionated heparin	Dogs: Prevention and treatment of aortic or venous thromboembolism or arterial thrombus/thromboembolism	Dogs: 100 U/kg bolus i.v., then 20–35 U/kg/h c.r.i. 150–300 U/kg s.c. q6–8 h	Multiple issues with bioavailability, individual variation, and monitoring availability. May be less effective if antithrombin is very low. Dogs: monitor with anti-Xa target of 0.35–0.7 U/mL. Cats: unknown target for anti-Xa, but can use the same range as in dogs
	Cats: same	Cats: 200–250 U/kg s.c. q6–8 h	

(*Continued*)

Table 79.2 (Continued)

Medication	Indications	Dosage	Considerations
Low molecular weight heparin	Dogs: Prevention and treatment of aortic or venous thromboembolism or arterial thrombus/thromboembolism	Dalteparin: Dogs: 100–175 U/kg s.c. q8 h Cats: 75–100 U/kg s.c. q6 h	Safe and fewer bleeding complications than with unfractionated heparin. No established monitoring protocols currently
	Cats: Same	Enoxaparin: Dogs: 0.8 mg/kg s.c. q6 h Cats: 0.75–1 mg/kg s.c. q6–12 h	
Apixaban	Dogs: Prevention and treatment of aortic or venous thromboembolism or arterial thrombus/thromboembolism	Dogs: 0.25–1.0 mg/kg q8–12 h	Typically very well tolerated and safe to use in dogs and cats. No established monitoring protocols currently. For dogs, recommend q8 h dosing in known thrombosis or high-risk cases and q12 h for maintenance. Consider dose reduction if severe azotemia is present
	Cats: Same	Cats: <5 kg: 0.625 mg q12 h, >5 kg: 1.25 mg q12 h	
Rivaroxaban	Dogs: Prevention and treatment of aortic or venous thromboembolism or arterial thrombus/thromboembolism	Dogs: 0.5–2 mg/kg p.o. q24 h	Typically well tolerated and safe to use in dogs and cats. No established monitoring protocols currently
	Cats: Same	Cats: 0.5–1 mg/kg p.o. q24 h	
Thrombolytic Tissue plasminogen activator	Dogs: Only should be considered when rapid thrombolysis is required	Dogs: 0.2 mg/kg i.v. bolus, then 0.7 mg/kg i.v. over 30 min, then 0.5 mg/kg i.v. over 1 h for a total of 1.4 mg/kg	Assess patient after each dosage for signs of bleeding and stop if any are noted, but graduated protocol is typically well tolerated in dogs and cats where active thrombolysis is necessary
	Cats: Same	Cats: Dosages vary depending on the institution, but the dog protocol can also be followed. Alternatively, can give 0.1 mg/kg i.v. bolus followed by 0.9 mg/kg i.v. over 1 h with a total maximum dose of 8 mg	

c.r.i., continuous-rate infusion; INR, international normalized ratio; i.v., intravenous; p.o., orally; PT, prothrombin time; q, every; s.c., subcutaneous.

[a] Loading doses may be considered in patients where rapid plasma concentrations are desired such as during an acute thrombotic event.

References

Barr, J.W. and McMichael, M. (2012). Inherited disorders of hemostasis in dogs and cats. *Topics in Companion Animal Medicine* 27 (2): 53–58.

Bates, S.M. and Ginsberg, J.S. (2004). Clinical practice. Treatment of deep-vein thrombosis. *New England Journal of Medicine* 15: 268–277.

Blais, M.C., Bianco, D., Goggs, R. et al. (2019). Consensus on the rational use of antithrombotics in veterinary critical care (CURATIVE): domain 3-defining antithrombotic protocols. *Journal of Veterinary Emergency and Critical Care (San Antonio)*. 29 (1): 60–74.

Brainard, B.M. and Brown, A.J. (2011). Defects in coagulation encountered in small animal critical care. *Veterinary Clinics of North America: Small Animal Practice* 41 (4): 783–803.

Brainard, B.M., Meredith, C.P., Callan, M.B. et al. (2007). Changes in platelet function, hemostasis, and prostaglandin expression after treatment with nonsteroidal anti-inflammatory drugs with various cyclooxygenase selectivities in dogs. *American Journal of Veterinary Research* 68 (3): 251–257.

Brainard, B.M., Burikc, Y., Good, J. et al. (2019). Consensus on the rational use of antithrombotics in veterinary critical care (CURATIVE): domain 5-discontinuation of anticoagulant therapy in small animals. *Journal of Veterinary Emergency and Critical Care (San Antonio)*. 29 (1): 88–97.

Brown, J.C., Brainard, B.M., Fletcher, D.J. et al. (2016). Effect of aminocaproic acid on clot strength and clot lysis of canine blood determined by use of an in vitro model of hyperfibrinolysis. *American Journal of Veterinary Research* 77 (11): 1258–1265.

Callan, M.B. and Giger, U. (2002). Effect of desmopressin acetate administration on primary hemostasis in Doberman Pinschers with type-1 von Willebrand disease as assessed by a point-of-care instrument. *American Journal of Veterinary Research* 63 (12): 1700–1706.

Callan, M.B., Appleman, E.H., and Sachais, B.S. (2009). Canine platelet transfusions. *Journal of Veterinary Emergency and Critical Care (San Antonio)* 19 (5): 401–415.

Culler, C.A., Iazbik, C., and Guillaumin, J. (2017). Comparison of albumin, colloid osmotic pressure, von Willebrand factor, and coagulation factors in canine cryopoor plasma, cryoprecipitate, and fresh frozen plasma. *Journal of Veterinary Emergency and Critical Care (San Antonio)* 27 (6): 638–644.

deLaforcade, A., Bacek, L., Blais, M.C. et al. (2019). Consensus on the rational use of antithrombotics in veterinary critical care (CURATIVE): domain 1 – defining populations at risk. *Journal of Veterinary Emergency and Critical Care* 29: 37–48.

Dixon-Jimenez, A.C., Brainard, B.M., Cathcart, C.J., and Koenig, A. (2013). Evaluation of a point-of-care coagulation analyzer (Abaxis VSPro) for identification of coagulopathies in dogs. *Journal of Veterinary Emergency and Critical Care (San Antonio)* 23 (4): 402–407.

Epstein, K.L., Bergren, A., Giguère, S., and Brainard, B.M. (2014). Cardiovascular, colloid osmotic pressure, and hemostatic effects of 2 formulations of hydroxyethyl starch in healthy horses. *Journal of Veterinary Internal Medicine* 28 (1): 223–233.

Flynn, E., Huang, J.Y., Hardikar, W. et al. (2019). Antithrombotic management and thrombosis rates in children post-liver transplantation: a case series and literature review. *Pediatric Transplantation* 23: e13420.

Galanaud, J.P., Blanchet-Deverly, A., Pemod, G. et al. (2016). Management of pulmonary embolism: a 2–15 update. *Journal des Maladies Vasculaires* 41: 51–62.

Gando, S., Wada, H., and Thachil, J. (2013). Scientific and Standardization Committee on DIC of the International Society on Thrombosis and Haemostasis (ISTH). Differentiating disseminated intravascular coagulation (DIC) with the fibrinolytic phenotype from coagulopathy of trauma and acute coagulopathy of trauma-shock (COT/ACOTS). *Journal of Thrombosis and Haemostasis* 11 (5): 826–835.

Goggs, R., Bacek, L., Bianco, D. et al. (2019). Consensus on the rational use of antithrombotics in veterinary critical care (CURATIVE): domain 2 – defining rational therapeutic usage. *Journal of Veterinary Emergency and Critical Care (San Antonio)*. 29: 49–59.

Goggs, R., Brainard, B.M., LeVine, D.N. et al. (2020). Lyophilized platelets versus cryopreserved platelets for management of bleeding in thrombocytopenic dogs: a multicenter randomized clinical trial. *Journal of Veterinary Internal Medicine* 34 (6): 2384–2397.

Guillaumin, J., Jandrey, K.E., Norris, J.W., and Tablin, F. (2010). Analysis of a commercial dimethyl-sulfoxide-stabilized frozen

canine platelet concentrate by turbidimetric aggregometry. *Journal of Veterinary Emergency and Critical Care (San Antonio)*. 20 (6): 571–577.

Jandrey, K.E. (2012). Assessment of platelet function. *Journal of Veterinary Emergency and Critical Care (San Antonio)* 22 (1): 81–98.

Kaboli, P., Henderson, M.C., and White, R.H. (2003). DVT prophylaxis and anticoagulation in the surgical patient. *Medical Clinics of North America* 87: 77–110.

Kim, S.M., Park, J.M., Shin, S.H. et al. (2013). Risk factors for postoperative venous thromboembolism in patients with malignancy of the lower limb. *Bone & Joint Journal* 95: 558–562.

Kitrell, D. and Berkwitt, L. (2012). Hypercoagulability in dogs: pathophysiology. *Compendium of Continuing Education for Veterinarians* 34: E1–E5.

Kol, A. and Borjesson, D.L. (2010). Application of thrombelastography/thromboelastometry to veterinary medicine. *Veterinary Clinical Pathology* 39 (4): 405–416.

de Laforcade, A. (2012). Diseases associated with thrombosis. *Topics in Companion Animal Medicine* 27: 59–64.

Levi, M., Toh, C.H., Thachil, J., and Watson, H.G. (2009). Guidelines for the diagnosis and management of disseminated intravascular coagulation. British Committee for Standards in Haematology. *British Journal of Haematology* 145 (1): 24–33.

Marín, L.M., Iazbik, M.C., Zaldivar-Lopez, S. et al. (2012). Epsilon aminocaproic acid for the prevention of delayed postoperative bleeding in retired racing greyhounds undergoing gonadectomy. *Veterinary Surgery* 41 (5): 594–603.

Moldal, E.R., Kristensen, A.T., Peeters, M.E. et al. (2012). Hemostatic response to surgical neutering via ovariectomy and ovariohysterectomy in dogs. *American Journal of Veterinary Research* 73 (9): 1469–1476.

O'Brien, M. (2012). The reciprocal relationship between inflammation and coagulation. *Topics in Companion Animal Medicine* 27: 46–52.

Osekavage, K.E., Brainard, B.M., Lane, S.L. et al. (2018). Pharmacokinetics of tranexamic acid in healthy dogs and assessment of its antifibrinolytic properties in canine blood. *American Journal of Veterinary Research* 79 (10): 1057–1063.

Petäjä, J. (2011). Inflammation and coagulation. *Thrombosis Research* 127: S34–S37.

Prittie, J. (2021). The role of cryoprecipitate in human and canine transfusion medicine. *Journal of Veterinary Emergency and Critical Care (San Antonio)* 31: 204–214.

Ralph, A.G. and Brainard, B.M. (2012). Updated on disseminated intravascular coagulation: when to consider it, when to expect it, when to treat it. *Topics in Companion Animal Medicine* 27: 65–72.

Respess, M., O'Toole, T.E., Taeymans, O. et al. (2012). Portal vein thrombosis in 33 dogs: 1998–2011. *Journal of Veterinary Internal Medicine* 26: 230–237.

Sharp, C.R., deLaforcade, A.M., Koenig, A.M. et al. (2019). Consensus on the rational use of antithrombotics in veterinary critical care (CURATIVE): domain 4 – refining and monitoring antithrombotic therapies. *Journal of Veterinary Emergency and Critical Care (San Antonio)*. 29: 75–87.

Siemens, H.J., Brueckner, S., Hagelberg, S. et al. (1999). Course of molecular hemostatic markers during and after different surgical procedures. *Journal of Clinical Anesthesia* 11 (8): 622–629.

Smith, S.A. (2009). The cell-based model of coagulation. *Journal of Veterinary Emergency and Critical Care* 19: 3–10.

Smith, S.A., McMichael, M., Galligan, A. et al. (2010). Clot formation in canine whole blood as measured by rotational thromboelastometry is influenced by sample handling and coagulation activator. *Blood Coagulation & Fibrinolysis* 21 (7): 692–702.

Tvedten, H., Lilliehöök, I., Hillström, A., and Häggström, J. (2008). Plateletcrit is superior to platelet count for assessing platelet status in Cavalier King Charles Spaniels. *Veterinary Clinical Pathology* 37 (3): 266–271.

Webster, C.R. (2017). Hemostatic disorders associated with hepatobiliary disease. *Veterinar Clinics of North America. Small Animal Practice* 47 (3): 601–61.

Xu, X.R., Zhang, D., and Gwald, B.E. (2016). Platelets are versatile cells: new discoveries in hemostasis, thrombosis, immune responses, tumor metastasis and beyond. *Critical Reviews in Clinical Laboratory Sciences* 53: 409–430.

80

Heart Surgery Strategies

E. Christopher Orton

Beating heart surgery

Most cardiac surgeries in animals are performed on a beating heart without circulatory or cardiac arrest. These include surgery on structures outside the heart, such as patent ductus arteriosus ligation or pulmonary artery banding; surgery performed by passing instruments through small portals controlled by suture tourniquets, such as closed-valve dilatation; and surgery performed with the aid of tangential vascular clamps, such as systemic-to-pulmonary shunts. A central principle of all cardiac surgery is to plan the surgery so that control of bleeding is always maintained. This is especially true during beating heart surgery, where there are few fall-back options once significant bleeding occurs. It is important to have instrumentation available to control hemorrhage in the event that a cardiac structure is inadvertently opened or ruptured. Sutures should be buttressed with pledgets to prevent them from cutting through cardiac tissues. Vascular clamps should be deeply placed to prevent slippage and to ensure adequate margins for closure of cardiac incisions. Advanced planning and a deliberate approach are important in preventing crisis situations during cardiac surgery.

Motion is an intrinsic aspect of beating heart surgery. Cardiac motion adds to both the psychological and technical challenges of cardiac surgery. Gentle compression on the surface of the heart is useful in controlling cardiac motion during suture placement. Placement of fingers within the ring handles of a needle holder, as opposed to "palming" the instrument, provides greater instrument control that facilitates suturing on the beating heart. Pharmacologic manipulation of the heart rate during

beating heart surgery is not necessary and should be avoided given its inherent risks. As surgeons become familiar with operating on the beating heart, they soon realize that it is not fundamentally different from surgery on other tissues or organs.

Inflow occlusion

Inflow occlusion is a strategy for performing brief open cardiac repairs. It involves interruption of venous blood returning to the heart and a brief period of complete circulatory arrest. It is indicated for cardiac surgeries that require only a short period for open heart repair. Its principal advantages are simplicity, lack of need for specialized equipment, and associated minimal cardiopulmonary, metabolic, and hematologic derangement after surgery. The principal disadvantages of inflow occlusion are the restricted time it provides to perform cardiac surgery, motion of the surgical field, and limited availability of a rescue strategy should delays occur in the completion of surgery. As a result, cardiac surgery performed during inflow occlusion must be meticulously planned and executed.

Ideally, the duration of circulatory arrest in a normothermic patient should be 2 minutes or less to minimize the risk of cerebral injury and ventricular fibrillation. If necessary, inflow occlusion can be repeated to allow completion of a cardiac surgery. If repeated, adequate time for complete recovery of the myocardium should be allowed between inflow occlusions. Circulatory arrest time can be prolonged up to 4 minutes with mild whole-body hypothermia (32–34 °C). However, the risk of cardiac arrest increases as the circulatory arrest time

Small Animal Soft Tissue Surgery, Second Edition. Edited by Eric Monnet.
© 2023 John Wiley & Sons, Inc. Published 2023 by John Wiley & Sons, Inc.
Companion website: www.wiley.com/go/monnet/small

increases, regardless of whether deliberate hypothermia is employed. The temperature should not be allowed to fall below 32 °C because the risk of ventricular fibrillation increases significantly below this temperature. After surgery, surface warming with water blankets or beds is used to return the animal to normal temperature.

Inflow occlusion can be accomplished from a left or right thoracotomy, or a median sternotomy, depending on the cardiac procedure being performed. Tourniquets are placed on the venae cavae and azygous vein to accomplish inflow occlusion. The right phrenic nerve should be excluded during placement of tourniquets on the venae cavae to avoid injury to the nerve. Direct access to the venae cavae and azygous vein for inflow occlusion is readily achieved from a right thoracotomy or median sternotomy (Figure 80.1). Attaining access for inflow occlusion is more difficult from a left thoracotomy, particularly when the heart is enlarged. When approaching via a left thoracotomy, the venae cavae and azygous vein are accessed by dissecting through the mediastinum.

Drugs and equipment for full cardiac resuscitation should be immediately available during inflow occlusion. Ventilation should be discontinued during inflow occlusion to prevent pulmonary blood from being pushed into the surgical field during inspiration. De-airing the heart is a critical step at termination of venous inflow occlusion to avoid a fatal air embolus. This is accomplished by simultaneous release of one tourniquet and a large positive-pressure breath (i.e., Valsalva maneuver) just prior to closure of the cardiac incision. Gentle cardiac massage may be necessary after inflow occlusion to help reestablish cardiac function. Digital occlusion of the descending aorta during this period helps direct the available cardiac output to the heart and brain. Cardiac incisions are initially closed with vascular clamps to minimize the length of circulatory arrest times. After cessation of inflow occlusion and cardiac function is restored, the cardiac incisions are closed with suture. If ventricular fibrillation occurs, the heart should be defibrillated by direct electrical shock as soon as the incision is clamped.

Cardiopulmonary bypass

Cardiopulmonary bypass (CPB) is a procedure where an extracorporeal system provides a flow of oxygenated blood to the patient. CPB provides a motionless and bloodless operative field and permits time to perform more complex cardiac repairs. CPB can be successfully employed to treat a variety of cardiac conditions in dogs. Successful CPB requires a team approach. The primary bypass team consists of a surgeon, assistant surgeon, perfusionist, anesthesiologist, and scrub nurse.

(a) (b)

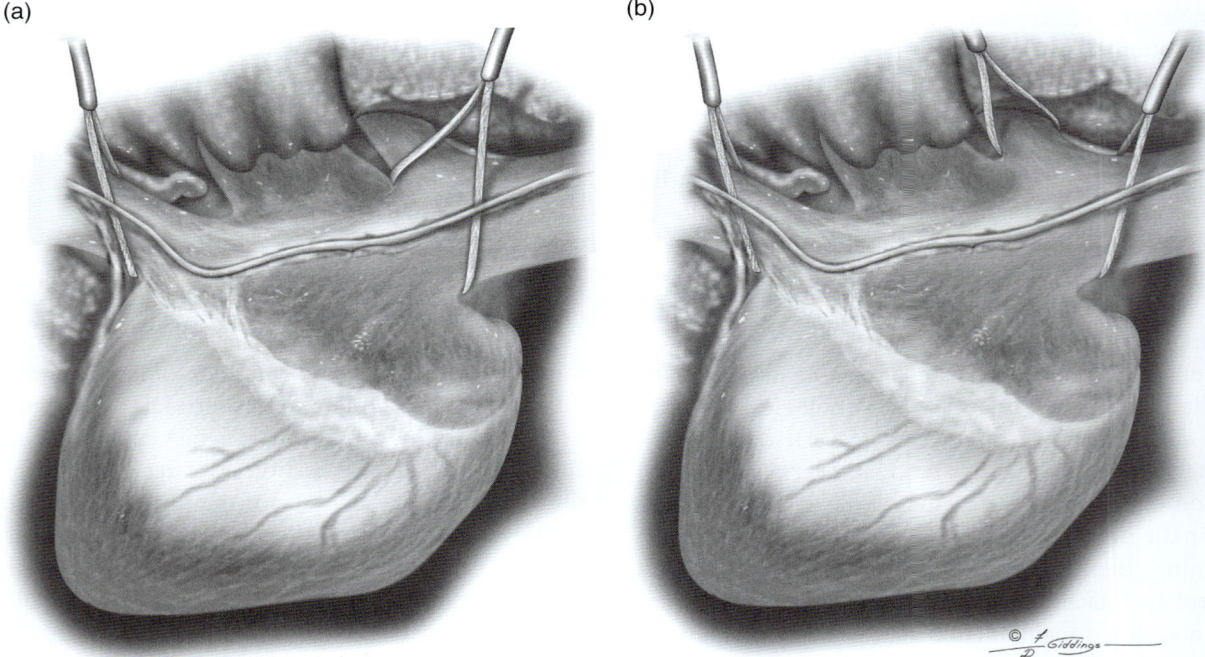

Figure 80.1 (a, b) Inflow occlusion, right thoracotomy. Venous inflow occlusion from a right thoracotomy is accomplished by passing tape or heavy-suture tourniquets around the cranial and caudal venae cavae and azygous vein. Tourniquets may be passed inside or outside of the pericardium. The phrenic nerve should be excluded if the tourniquets are passed outside the pericardium. Brief circulatory arrest by venous inflow occlusion is accomplished by tightening the tourniquets. © D. Giddings.

Initiation, maintenance, and discontinuation of CPB require a coordinated and practiced effort between these individuals. Consequently, there must be clear communication between team members.

CPB is accomplished with a heart–lung machine. The major components of a heart–lung machine include three to five pumps, a temperature-controlled circulating heater/cooler water bath, an oxygen blender, a gas flow meter, and an anesthetic vaporizer. The primary bypass circuit consists of a reservoir, pump, membrane oxygenator, heat exchanger, and circulating heater/cooler water bath. A membrane-type oxygenator should be used to minimize injury to the blood. A pediatric-size oxygenator is preferred in dogs under 40 kg to minimize the volume necessary to prime the circuit. During CPB, blood is drawn away from the patient to the reservoir by gravity flow. Blood is then pumped through the oxygenator under pressure and returned to the patient by means of a roller or centrifugal pump. The heater/cooler water bath is used to control body temperature by means of a heat exchanger built into the primary circuit. Blood in the operative field is collected and returned to the reservoir by one to three suction lines driven by additional roller pumps.

Prior to surgery, a catheter is placed into a jugular vein to provide central venous access and to monitor central venous pressure (CVP). An arterial catheter is placed to monitor direct arterial pressure and arterial blood-gas status. The electrocardiogram, arterial blood pressure, CVP, end-tidal CO_2, and esophageal and rectal temperatures are monitored continuously during surgery. The following parameters are measured throughout the procedure: arterial and venous blood gases, activated clotting time (ACT), electrolyte concentrations (Na^+, K^+, ionized Ca^{2+}), hematocrit, total protein, and lactate. Cannulation for CPB can be accomplished from a right or left thoracotomy, or median sternotomy, depending on the cardiac procedure being performed. Oxygenated blood is returned to the patient via the arterial cannula and line. Arterial cannulation is performed prior to cardiac manipulations and placement of other cannulas. If bleeding occurs before initiation of CPB, blood can be salvaged from the operative field and returned to the patient via the arterial cannula and line. Arterial cannulation of a femoral or carotid artery is preferred over direct aortic cannulation in dogs and should be performed before the thoracic cavity is opened (Figure 80.2). If a lateral thoracotomy approach is used, the femoral artery on the opposite-side (down) limb is chosen for cannulation. A straight arterial cannula, ranging in size from 8 to 14 F, is used.

Blood is diverted from the right heart to the CPB circuit by means of one or two venous cannulas and a venous line. Venous cannulation is accomplished using several configurations depending on the cardiac surgery undertaken. Bicaval venous cannulation is required for cardiac surgeries that require a right atrial cardiac approach such as septal defect repairs and tricuspid valve surgery (Figure 80.3). Alternatively, venous cannulation is accomplished by introducing a single two-stage

(a)   (b)

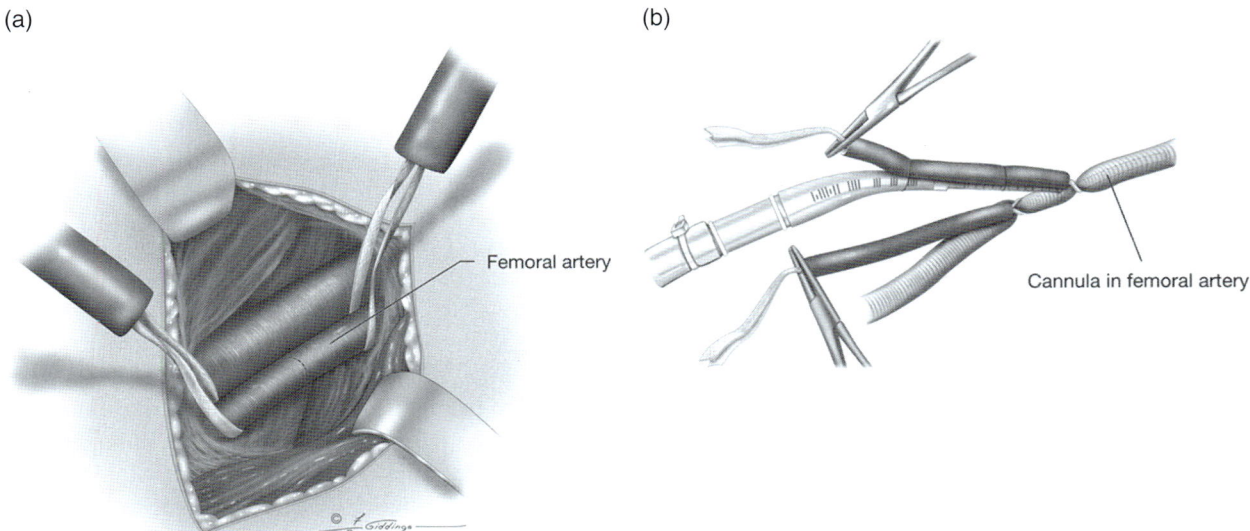

Figure 80.2 Femoral arterial cannulation for cardiopulmonary bypass. (a) The femoral artery is surgically exposed high in the femoral triangle. Two tape or silk suture tourniquets are passed around the artery. (b) An arterial cannula is passed into the artery to the level of the external iliac artery. The proximal tape tourniquet is tightened around the cannula and then tied to the cannula to secure it. © D. Giddings.

(a)

(b)

(c)

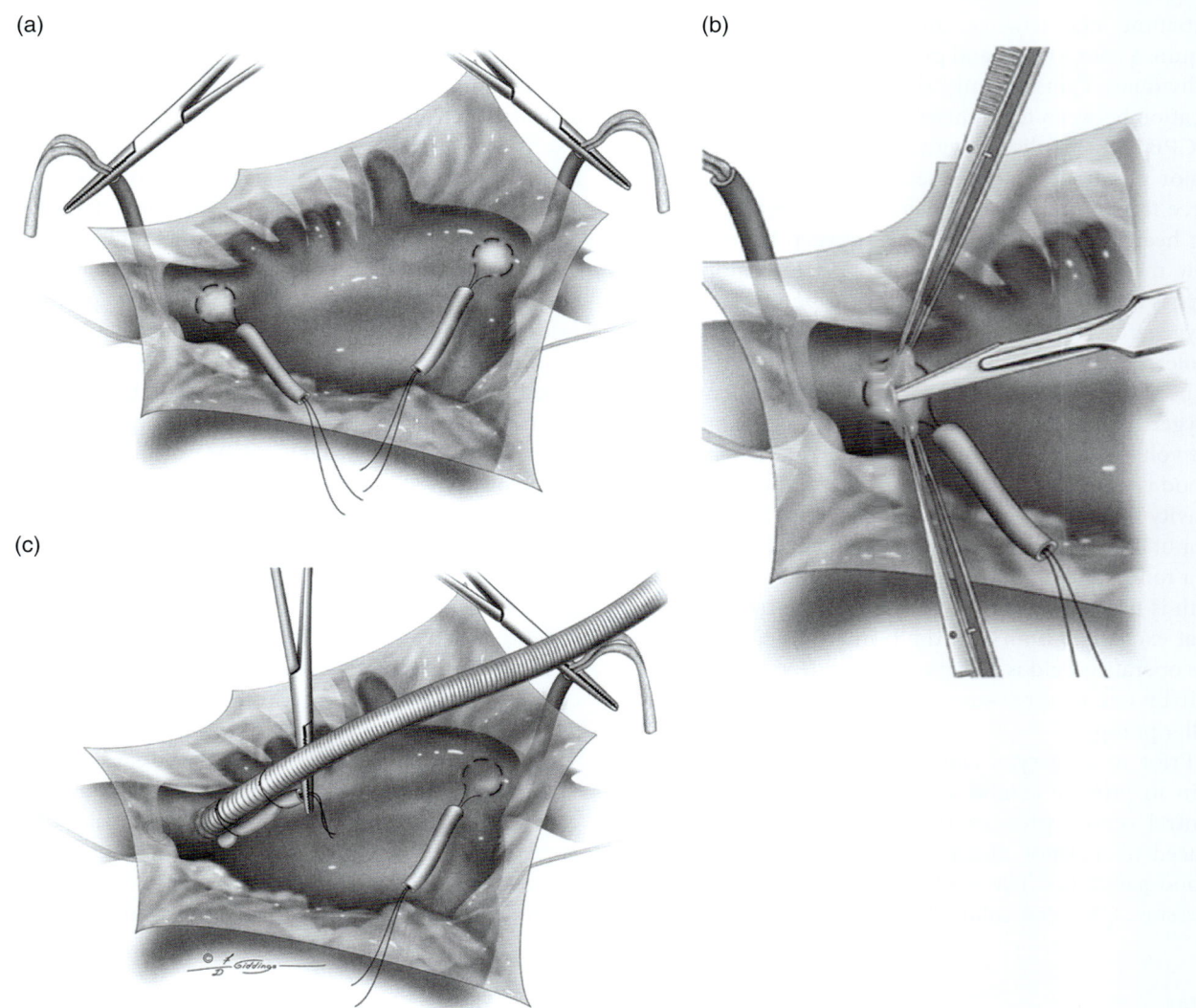

Figure 80.3 Bicaval venous cannulation for cardiopulmonary bypass. (a) Bicaval venous cannulation is accomplished through a right thoracotomy. Tape tourniquets are placed around the cranial and caudal venae cavae and azygos vein outside the pericardium. The pericardium is opened and sutured to the thoracotomy incision. Purse-string sutures are placed at each atrial–caval junction and passed through tourniquets. (b) The cannulation site is grasped with two forceps and incised with a no. 11 blade. (c) Bleeding is controlled during cannula insertion by bringing the forceps together to close the incision. A venous cannula is placed into the caudal vena cava, and the purse-string suture is tightened to control bleeding. The tourniquet is tied to the cannula to secure it. The process is repeated to place the cranial cannula. Complete diversion of venous return and isolation of the right atrium is accomplished by tightening the tape tourniquets around the venous cannulas. After cannula removal, the purse-string sutures are tied to close the cannulation incisions. © D. Giddings.

cavoatrial cannula through the right auricle (Figure 80.4). Cavoatrial cannulation is the only option for venous cannulation for CPB from a left thoracotomy.

Hemodilution is desirable during CPB to counter the effects of increased blood viscosity during hypothermia (Gravlee *et al.* 2008). The goal is to decrease the hematocrit to approximately 25–28%. Hemodilution is accomplished by priming the bypass circuit with a calculated volume of crystalloid solution. The hematocrit decreases when the patient's blood mixes with the circuit prime. A balanced pH-adjusted (7.4) crystalloid solution should be used to prime the circuit. Whole blood can be added to the prime solution if the volume of crystalloid is insufficient to adequately prime the circuit without causing excessive hemodilution. Other additives to the crystalloid prime include $NaHCO_3$ and heparin.

Prior to cannulation and initiation of CPB, the animal must undergo complete anticoagulation by administration of heparin (300 units/kg). The ACT is monitored every 30 minutes during bypass and maintained above

(a)

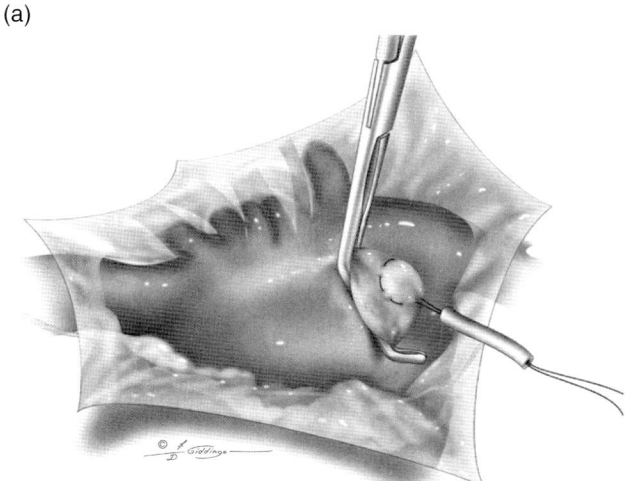

(b)

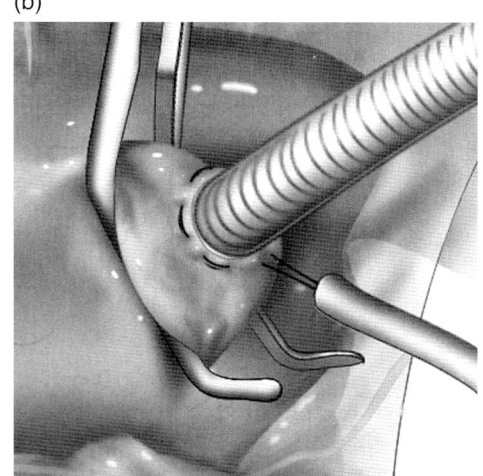

(c)

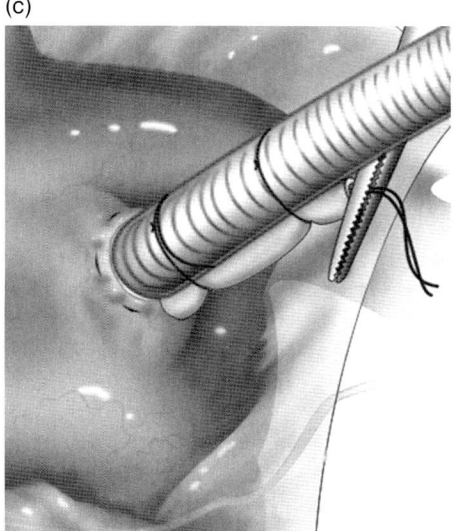

Figure 80.4 Cavoatrial venous cannulation for cardiopulmonary bypass. (a) Cavoatrial venous cannulation is accomplished by passing a straight two-stage venous cannula through the right auricle. A purse-string suture is placed around the circumference of the atrial appendage and passed through a tourniquet. (b) A vascular clamp is placed at the base of the auricle, and the end of the auricle is excised. A two-stage straight venous cannula is passed through the atriotomy as the vascular clamp is released. (c) The distal ports of the two-stage cannula are directed into the caudal vena, and the proximal ports are positioned in the right atrium. The purse-string tourniquet is tightened and tied to the cannula to secure it. The purse-string suture is tied after cannula removal, and a second ligature is tied around the appendage to close the incision. © D. Giddings.

480 seconds. Perfusion flow rates during bypass are dependent on several factors, including patient size, temperature, and hematocrit (50–80 mL/kg/min). Standard CPB perfusion strategies with mild to moderate hypothermia can be used for dogs weighing over 10 kg (Klement *et al.* 1987). Deep hypothermic (15–18 °C) low-flow (20 mL/kg/min) CPB may be a more appropriate strategy for small dogs (<10 kg) to decrease adverse effects associated with bypass (Lew *et al.* 1997). Ultimately, perfusion flow should be kept at the lowest level that meets the requirements of the patient with goals of maintaining a venous oxygen saturation of 70% or greater and normal lactate levels. Mean arterial pressure should be 50–70 mmHg during bypass. Phenylephrine (0.05–0.1 mg/kg intravenously [i.v.]) is administered as necessary to increase vascular resistance and maintain adequate mean arterial pressures. Arterial pressure usually falls dramatically for several minutes after initiation of bypass because of sudden hemodilution.

Esophageal and rectal temperatures are monitored continuously during CPB. Dogs are cooled to between 25 and 28 °C during cardiac surgery using the heater/cooler water bath and heat exchanger in the pump circuit. The requirement for inhalation and other anesthetic drugs decreases during hypothermia. During CPB, the oxygenator receives a continuous flow of a mixture of oxygen and nitrogen from the oxygen blender. The fraction of inspired oxygen should be adjusted to keep the PaO_2 above 120 mmHg during CPB. The $PaCO_2$ is adjusted during CPB by varying the total gas flow (L/min). Blood gases should be measured every 30 minutes during CPB. An alpha-stat strategy for acid–base management is most appropriate during CPB (Gravlee *et al.* 2008). Metabolic acidosis during CPB should be corrected by administration of $NaHCO_3$.

Complete CPB is accomplished by cross-clamping the ascending aorta (Figure 80.5). Protection of the

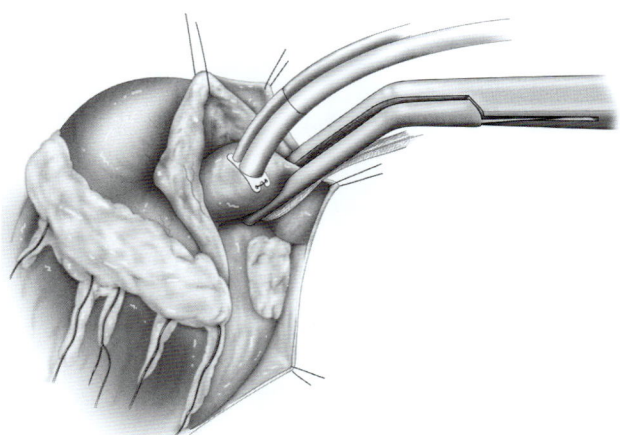

Figure 80.5 Antegrade cardioplegia and aortic cross-clamp. A tape is passed around the aorta. Antegrade administration of cardioplegia solution is accomplished through a cannula placed in the aortic root. The cannula is introduced through a pledget-buttressed mattress suture tourniquet. The aorta is cross-clamped just before administering cardioplegia solution. The mattress suture is tied after removal of the cannula. © D. Giddings.

myocardium from ischemic injury during aortic cross-clamping is accomplished by cessation of electromechanical activity and rapid cooling of the myocardium. This is achieved by administration of cold cardioplegia solution into the coronary circulation just after the aortic cross-clamp has been placed. The solution contains a high concentration of potassium that arrests the electrical and mechanical activities of the myocardium, thereby reducing its metabolic requirements. Cooling the myocardium to approximately 4–8 °C further decreases its metabolic requirement. Sanguineous–crystalloid cardioplegia solutions are superior to pure crystalloid cardioplegia solutions (Barner 1991). A sanguineous–crystalloid cardioplegia solution is made by blending a crystalloid cardioplegia solution with heparinized blood from the bypass circuit. Cardioplegia solution is delivered via a cannula placed in the ascending aorta prior to aortic cross-clamping. Electrical activity on the electrocardiogram should cease after cardioplegia administration. Cardioplegia is repeated every 20–40 minutes while the aorta is cross-clamped depending on the cardioplegia solution. Aortic cross-clamp time should ideally be kept >90 minutes.

Free air is evacuated from the heart before discontinuing bypass. This is accomplished by diverting venous blood back to the heart and allowing the cardiac incisions to overflow just prior to closure. The anesthesiologist assists by applying continuous positive pressure to the lungs to push pulmonary blood back toward the heart. After the aortic cross-clamp is removed, continuous low-pressure suction is applied to the cardioplegia cannula to scavenge air bubbles ejected from the left heart. The left ventricle, left atrium, and left auricle should be manipulated to release trapped air prior to reestablishing left ventricular ejection.

After closure of cardiac incisions, the aortic cross-clamp is removed, and coronary circulation is reestablished. If ventricular fibrillation occurs, the heart is electrically defibrillated with direct current and internal paddles (20–50 J). If initial attempts at defibrillation are unsuccessful, defibrillation is repeated every few minutes as the patient is rewarmed until a normal rhythm is restored. Rewarming begins as the cardiac surgery is being completed, while the cardiac incisions are being closed. After the patient is rewarmed to 37 °C and an effective cardiac rhythm established, a gradual process of weaning from CPB is begun. During this period, CaCl (10 mg/kg i.v.) and dobutamine (1–10 µg/kg/min i.v.) are usually required to support cardiovascular function. Once the animal has been fully weaned from CPB and is hemodynamically stable, the cannulas are removed in the reverse order in which they were introduced. Protamine sulfate (0.5–1 mg/100 units of heparin administered) is given to reverse the heparin anticoagulation. Protamine has a very potent hypotensive effect in dogs and must be administered slowly. The ACT should return to less than 150 seconds. Administration of fresh whole blood is indicated after CPB.

CPB initiates a systemic inflammatory response that has a profound effect on management after surgery (Gravlee *et al.* 2008). The first 12 hours after CPB are most critical. Major problems that can occur during this period include hemorrhage, hypoxemia, circulatory collapse, cardiac arrhythmias, low urine output, and electrolyte and acid–base abnormalities. Hemorrhage is a major postoperative concern after CPB. Hemorrhage can be surgical, biological, or both. Surgical hemorrhage results from bleeding from cardiotomy sites and is best prevented by careful inspection of cardiotomy sites prior to closure of the thoracotomy. Even with perfect closure of cardiotomy sites, significant bleeding can occur after CPB due to the biological effects of CPB. Dilutional and consumptive thrombocytopenia, acquired platelet dysfunction, consumptive and dilutional coagulopathy, and fibrinolysis all contribute to biological bleeding after surgery. In most cases, hemorrhage after CPB is biological and is best managed conservatively with supportive care. Administration of fresh whole blood to restore red blood cells, platelets, and clotting factors is indicated and should begin in the operating room. Additional stored blood or plasma may also be necessary in the postoperative period. Shed blood can be collected, washed with a cell washer, and returned to the patient as necessary.

Some degree of hypoxemia is usually present after CPB due to pulmonary injury and increased pulmonary vascular permeability (Gravlee *et al.* 2008). Ventilatory support is generally unnecessary after CPB in dogs. Circulatory support after CPB should include volume expansion to maintain CVP between 4 and 10 mmHg. Because of the generalized increase in vascular permeability after CPB, volume deficits should be restored primarily with plasma or blood. The hematocrit should be maintained above 30%. Administration of high volumes of crystalloid fluids should be avoided after CPB. Inotropic support may be necessary after surgery to maintain adequate cardiac output and mean systemic blood pressure. Ventricular tachycardia often occurs after CPB and should be controlled with intravenous lidocaine (50–80 µg/kg/min). Urine output should be monitored for 12 hours after surgery to ensure adequate renal function. Hypokalemia and hypocalcemia are frequently encountered after surgery and should be corrected.

References

Barner, H.B. (1991). Blood cardioplegia: a review and comparison with crystalloid cardioplegia. *Annals of Thoracic Surgery* 52: 1354–1367.

Gravlee, G.P., Davis, R.F., Stammers, A.H., and Ungerleider, R.M. (ed.) (2008). *Cardiopulmonary Bypass: Principles and Practice*, 3e. Baltimore, MD: Lippincott Williams & Wilkins.

Klement, P., del Nido, P.J., Mickleborough, L. et al. (1987). Technique and postoperative management for successful cardiopulmonary bypass and open-heart surgery in dogs. *Journal of the American Veterinary Medical Association* 190: 869–874.

Lew, L.J., Egger, C.M., Thomson, D.J. et al. (1997). Deep hypothermic low flow cardiopulmonary bypass in small dogs. *Veterinary Surgery* 26: 281–289.

81

Congenital Cardiac Shunts

E. Christopher Orton

Patent ductus arteriosus

The ductus arteriosus is a fetal vessel that connects the main pulmonary artery to the descending aorta and directs venous blood away from the collapsed fetal lungs. The ductus arteriosus closes soon after birth during the transition from fetal to extrauterine life. Continued patency of the ductus arteriosus for more than a few days after birth causes the condition of patent ductus arteriosus (PDA).

PDA is the most common congenital heart defect seen in dogs, accounting for 25–30% of congenital malformations (Buchanan 1999). The defect also occurs in cats, but with a lower prevalence. PDA is seen more commonly in purebred dogs, with a predilection for females. A heritable basis for PDA is established in poodles (Patterson 1965). PDA is caused by hypoplasia and segmental asymmetry of the ductus muscle mass that results in failure of ductus contraction (Buchanan 2001; Buchanan & Patterson 2003).

Pathophysiology

PDA allows left-to-right shunting of blood from the aorta to the pulmonary artery, resulting in severe volume overload of the left heart leading to left ventricular and atrial dilatation, progressive myocardial deterioration, and left-sided congestive heart failure. Progressive functional mitral regurgitation further overloads the left ventricle. Atrial fibrillation occurs as a late sequela. Most dogs and cats with untreated PDA die from progressive heart failure early in life. Some animals with PDA develop pulmonary hypertension that can reverse the direction of flow through the shunt, resulting in hypoxemia and cyanosis that are more intense in the caudal portions of the body.

Indication for surgery

Based on the poor long-term prognosis, PDA closure is indicated in dogs and cats with left-to-right PDA with few exceptions, preferably before 16 weeks of age. Older animals should undergo surgery as soon as possible after the diagnosis. Even animals with severe secondary myocardial failure and functional mitral regurgitation will benefit from PDA closure. Animals that present in congestive heart failure should be treated and undergo closure as soon as they are stable. Animals with pulmonary hypertension can undergo PDA closure so long as pulmonary artery pressures have not reached systemic levels. Surgical ligation of a fully right-to-left PDA is contraindicated. Treatment with a phosphodiesterase 5 inhibitor such as sildenafil can lower pulmonary artery pressures sufficiently to reestablish left-to-right shunt in some cases, especially cats.

Transcatheter ductal occlusion is now an established option for PDA closure in dogs. Given its decreased invasiveness and lower risk for ductal rupture, transcatheter ductal occlusion is generally preferred over surgical PDA ligation in most dogs (Goodrich et al. 2007; Gordon et al. 2010). Limitations of transcatheter ductal occlusion include small patient size and nontapering ductal anatomy that does not allow anchoring of an occluder. The cost of the device or lack of imaging equipment can sometimes also be limiting. Dogs that are not candidates for transcatheter ductal occlusion for whatever reason

Small Animal Soft Tissue Surgery, Second Edition. Edited by Eric Monnet.
© 2023 John Wiley & Sons, Inc. Published 2023 by John Wiley & Sons, Inc.
Companion website: www.wiley.com/go/monnet/small

become candidates for surgical PDA ligation. Surgical ligation is generally the only option for cats with PDA.

Patent ductus arteriosus ligation

Surgical PDA ligation is accomplished through a left fourth thoracotomy in dogs and a left fourth or fifth thoracotomy in cats. A lateral thoracic radiograph can be consulted to determine that appropriate intercostal space. The lungs are rotated caudally to expose the base of the heart. The vagus nerve courses over the ductus arteriosus and serves as an anatomic landmark for identification of the ductus arteriosus (Figure 81.1). The vagus nerve is isolated at the level of the ductus and gently retracted dorsally or ventrally with one or two sutures. Occasionally a persistent left cranial vena cava may overlie the ductus arteriosus. In this case, the vein should be isolated and retracted with the vagus nerve. The ductus arteriosus is isolated for ligation outside of the pericardium. Right-angled forceps are first passed transversely behind the ductus to establish a dissection plane. A dissection plane between the aorta and cranial ductus can also be established by angling the forceps 45° caudally. The forceps are passed medial to the ductus in a caudal to cranial direction. Blunt dissection medial to the ductus by opening and closing the forceps should be strictly avoided. Rather, the forceps should be allowed to find their way around the ductus by careful manipulation of the forceps

considering the three-dimensional shape of the ductus. Once the tip of the forceps can be visualized through the adventitial tissues between the aorta and cranial ductus, passage of the forceps can be safely completed. Heavy silk ligatures are grasped and passed around the ductus. The ductus arteriosus is closed by slowly tightening and tying the silk ligature.

Outcomes

Surgical mortality rates of 0–7% have been reported in retrospective studies involving 50 or more dogs (Eyster *et al.* 1976a; Birchard *et al.* 1990; Buchanan 1994; Hunt *et al.* 2001; Bureau *et al.* 2005; Goodrich *et al.* 2007). PDA ligation is curative in the majority of cases when it is performed at an early age (<6 months of age) (Van Israel *et al.* 2003; Bureau *et al.* 2005). Mitral regurgitation and secondary myocardial failure are generally reversible after surgery. Complete resolution of even severe mitral regurgitation is possible. Secondary changes may not be entirely reversible in older animals, particularly in large-breed dogs (Goodwin & Lombard 1992). PDA closure is still indicated in these animals as it will be associated with significant palliation.

Rupture of the ductus arteriosus or great vessels during dissection resulting in severe hemorrhage is the most serious complication associated with PDA ligation and the most common cause of operative mortality (Birchard *et al.* 1990; Buchanan 1994; Hunt *et al.* 2001). The risk of

(a)   (b)

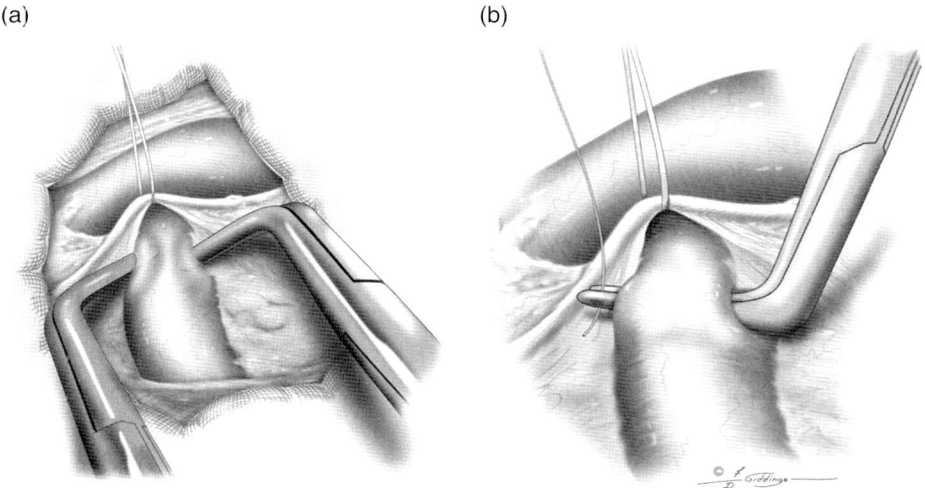

Figure 81.1 Patent ductus arteriosus (PDA) ligation. (a) PDA ligation is accomplished through a left thoracotomy. The vagus nerve courses over the ductus arteriosus and serves as an anatomic landmark for identification of the PDA. The vagus nerve is isolated by sharp dissection at the level of the ductus and gently retracted with a suture. (b) The PDA is isolated by blunt dissection without opening the pericardium. Dissection of the caudal ductus is accomplished by passing right-angled forceps behind the ductus parallel to the transverse plane. Dissection of the cranial aspect of the ductus is accomplished by angling the forceps caudally approximately 45°. Dissection is completed by passing the forceps medial to ductus in a caudal to cranial direction. Blunt dissection medial to the ductus by opening and closing the forceps should be avoided. Ligatures are passed around the ductus by grasping the ligature with right-angled forceps. The ductus arteriosus is closed by slowly tightening and tying the ligature. © D. Giddings.

this complication decreases with surgeon experience and increases in older animals. Small ruptures, especially those on the back side of the ductus, often will respond to gentle tamponade, but will enlarge and worsen if the dissection is continued. Large ruptures must be controlled immediately with vascular clamps. In most instances, simple ligation of the ductus arteriosus will not be feasible or safe after a rupture has occurred. Two surgical options can be considered. The PDA can be closed or at least attenuated with several wide buttressed mattress sutures across the ductus. This option not only attenuates ductal flow, but also provides a tamponade effect to control hemorrhage. The advantage of this method is that it is safer than dividing the ductus. The disadvantage is that the risk of significant residual shunt flow after surgery is high. Alternatively, the PDA can be divided between vascular clamps and oversewn. In this case the ductus is isolated between deeply placed tangential vascular clamps and divided. The open ends of the ductus are closed with pledget-reinforced interrupted mattress sutures oversewn with a simple continuous pattern. This method assures complete correction of shunt flow, but is more technically demanding.

Ventricular septal defect

Ventricular septal defect (VSD) is a congenital defect resulting from incomplete development of the membranous or muscular ventricular septum. Perimembranous defects are most common in companion animals and are bordered by the central fibrous body and the inlet, trabecular, or infundibular (outlet) portion of the muscular septum. These defects are medial to the septal leaflet of the tricuspid valve, inferior to the crista supraventricularis, and closely associated with the conduction tissues of the heart. Inlet perimembranous VSDs are associated with the spectrum of defects associated with atrioventricular septal defect (AVSD). Muscular defects are less common, bordered entirely by muscle, and occur within the inlet, trabecular, or infundibular muscular septum. Doubly committed subarterial VSDs occur high in the infundibular septum where the conjoined leaflets of the pulmonary and aortic valve form part of the rim of the defect. This defect, also known as juxta-arterial or conal septal VSD, is often associated with the aortic insufficiency due to prolapse of the right coronary cusp.

VSD accounts for about 10% of congenital heart defects in dogs and is among the most common congenital malformations in cats (Buchanan 1999). The etiology of VSD is incompletely understood, but is suspected to be heritable, particularly when it occurs in a breed with a high prevalence. VSD has been demonstrated to be a polygenic trait in keeshonds (Patterson et al. 1974).

Pathophysiology

The pathophysiologic consequences of VSD depend on its size and location. A large VSD allows left-to-right shunting of blood that overloads the left and possibly right ventricle, resulting in progressive heart failure. High-flow shunts can also trigger progressive pulmonary vascular remodeling, leading to pulmonary hypertension and reversal of shunt flow (Eisenmenger syndrome). Residence at altitude increases the likelihood and accelerates the development of pulmonary hypertension. Aortic insufficiency associated with doubly committed subarterial VSD is caused by prolapse of the right coronary aortic cusp into the defect and adds to left ventricular volume overload.

Indications

Surgical correction of VSD is indicated for high-flow shunts to prevent progressive heart failure or pulmonary hypertension. Progressive aortic insufficiency is also an indication to consider surgery (Shimizu et al. 2006). Several parameters suggest that a VSD is hemodynamically significant, including radiographic evidence of pulmonary vascular enlargement, radiographic or echocardiographic evidence of left ventricular chamber dilation, Doppler-measured pulmonary velocity >2.5 M, and $Q_P/Q_S > 1.5$.

Pulmonary artery banding

Pulmonary artery banding is an effective surgical option for palliation of VSD. The goal of pulmonary artery banding is to increase right ventricular systolic pressure and thereby decrease the pressure gradient driving the shunt flow. A method for placement of a dilatable pulmonary artery band has been described in cats (Sutherland et al. 2019). A dilatable pulmonary band allows the option of transcatheter balloon dilatation if the band becomes too tight as immature animals grow. Pulmonary artery banding is accomplished through a left fourth thoracotomy (Figure 81.2). The pericardium is opened and sutured to the thoracotomy incision. The pulmonary artery is separated from the aorta by a combination of sharp and blunt dissection. A polytetrafluoroethylene (PTFE) tape is passed around the pulmonary artery just dorsal to the pulmonary valve. A mattress suture in placed in the pulmonary artery distal to the band and a catheter is introduced for measurement of pulmonary arterial pressures during tightening of the band. The tape is progressively tightened by sequential placement of hemostatic clips on the band. Optimal

(a)

(b)

(c)

(d)

(e)

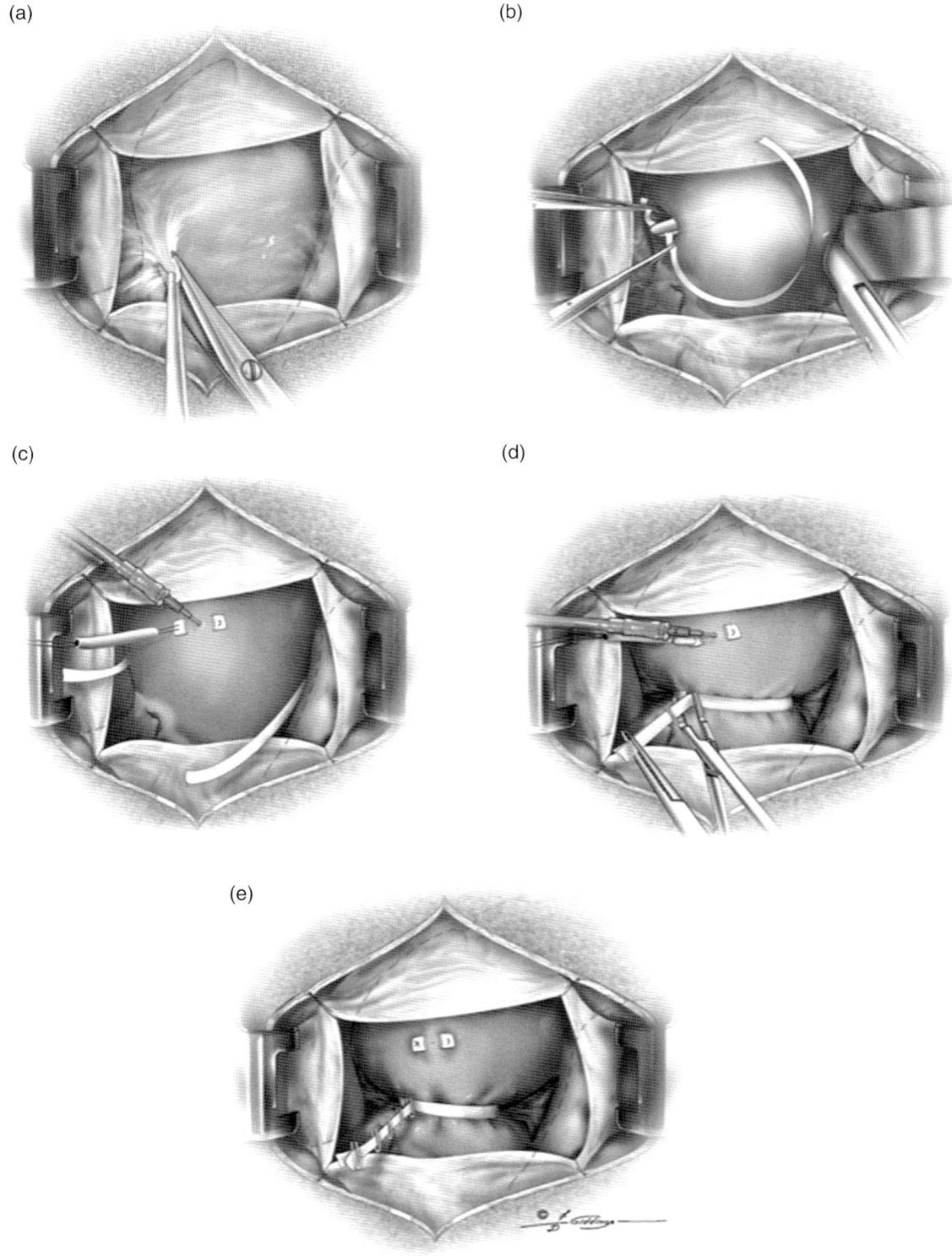

Figure 81.2 Pulmonary artery banding. (a) Pulmonary artery banding is accomplished through a left fourth thoracotomy. The pericardium is opened and sutured to the thoracotomy incision. The pulmonary artery is separated from the aorta by sharp and blunt dissection. (b) Tape is passed around the pulmonary artery just dorsal to the pulmonary valve. (c) A mattress suture is placed in the pulmonary artery distal to the band and a catheter is introduced for measurement of pulmonary arterial pressures during tightening of the band. (d) The tape is progressively tightened by sequential placement of hemostatic clips on the band. (e) After final tightening of the band, a 6-0 mattress suture is placed in the tape just behind the last clamp. © D. Giddings.

banding is judged when pulmonary systolic arterial pressure distal to the band is decreased, ideally to <30 mmHg, and the increase in systemic arterial pressures just begins to plateau. Intraoperative epicardial echocardiography evaluation of shunt flow can also be used to guide band tightening. After final tightening of the band, a 6-0 mattress suture is placed in the tape just behind the last clamp. The hemostatic clips should not protrude beyond the width of the tape to avoid later puncture of the pulmonary artery.

Open repair for ventricular septal defect

Open repair of VSD is accomplished under cardiopulmonary bypass. Perimembranous VSD is corrected through a right fifth thoracotomy. Arterial cannulation for cardiopulmonary bypass is in the left femoral artery. Venous cannulation is bicaval to allow complete isolation of the right atrium (Figure 81.3). The VSD is accessed through a right atriotomy. The septal leaflet of the tricuspid valve is retracted to expose the defect.

(a)

(b)

(c)

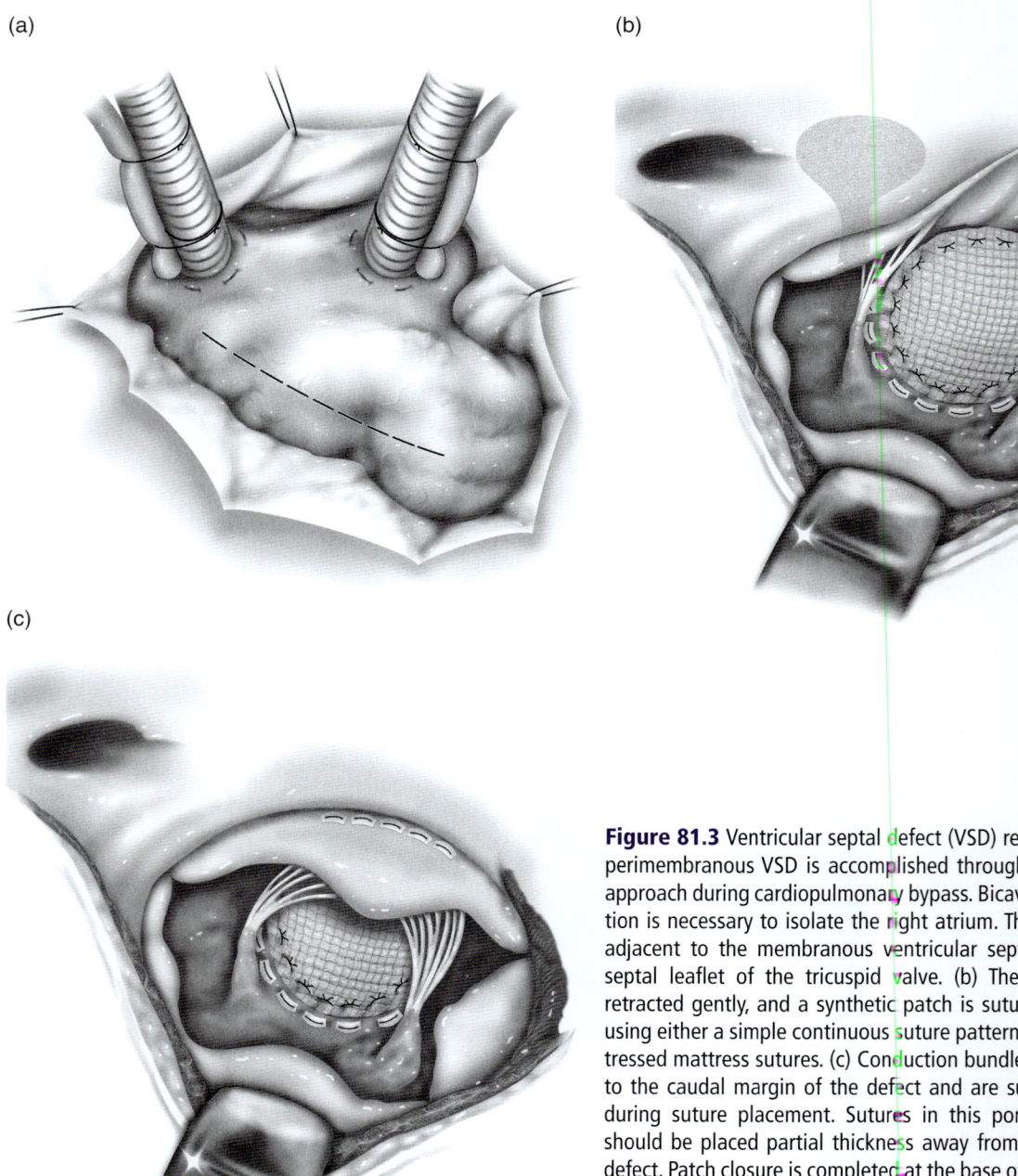

Figure 81.3 Ventricular septal defect (VSD) repair. (a) Repair of a perimembranous VSD is accomplished through a right atriotomy approach during cardiopulmonary bypass. Bicaval venous cannulation is necessary to isolate the right atrium. The defect is located adjacent to the membranous ventricular septum medial to the septal leaflet of the tricuspid valve. (b) The tricuspid valve is retracted gently, and a synthetic patch is sutured into the defect using either a simple continuous suture pattern or interrupted buttressed mattress sutures. (c) Conduction bundles are located close to the caudal margin of the defect and are susceptible to injury during suture placement. Sutures in this portion of the defect should be placed partial thickness away from the margin of the defect. Patch closure is completed at the base of the tricuspid valve by passing the sutures through the tricuspid valve annulus. The atriotomy incision is closed with a continuous mattress suture pattern oversewn with a simple continuous pattern. © D. Giddings.

Pledget-reinforced mattress sutures are placed around the circumference of the septal defect. The defect is closed with PTFE or Dacron cardiovascular graft. The major conduction bundles are located close to the caudal margin of the defect and are susceptible to injury during suture placement. Sutures in this portion of the defect should be placed partial thickness away from the caudal margin of the defect. Perimembranous defects typically are bordered by tricuspid valve annulus and do not have a dorsal margin. In this case, graft closure is completed by passing sutures through the tricuspid annulus into the atrial side of the valve. The atriotomy is closed with a continuous mattress suture pattern oversewn with a simple continuous pattern. Infundibular and doubly committed subarterial defects can be accessed through the outflow portion of the right ventricular wall via a median sternotomy. Cannulation for cardiopulmonary bypass and closure is similar to that for perimembranous defects. Closure of ventriculotomy is by pledget-reinforced mattress sutures.

Outcomes

Palliation of VSD has been reported in dogs and cats for up to seven years after surgery (Eyster *et al.* 1977). Long-term palliation of VSD can be achieved with pulmonary artery banding in small animals. The most serious early complication is overtightening of the band, leading to reversal of shunt flow and hypoxemia. This complication can be largely avoided by measurement of systemic and pulmonary arterial pressures and shunt flow during the procedure. Progressive obstruction and late reversal of shunt flow can result from growth of the animal, progressive fibrosis of the pulmonary artery band, progressive right ventricular hypertrophy, or any combination of these.

Definitive closure of VSD under cardiopulmonary bypass is considered curative in humans so long as it is undertaken prior to development of severe pulmonary hypertension or secondary myocardial failure (de Leval 1994a). Although reports in dogs are limited, a similar expectation after definitive closure of VSD in dogs is reasonable (Shimizu *et al.* 2006).

Atrial and atrioventricular septal defect

Atrial septal defects (ASDs) are classified as sinus venosus defects, coronary sinus ASD, ostium secundum (fossa ovalis type) ASD, or patent foramen ovale (Stark 1994). Sinus venosus defects are located dorsal in the atrial septum at the junction of the cranial or caudal vena cava and are usually associated with anomalous pulmonary venous return. Coronary sinus ASD or unroofed coronary sinus results from incomplete separation between the coronary sinus and the left atrium due to the persistence of a left cranial vena cava. Ostium secundum ASD (fossa ovalis type) occurs in the mid-dorsal portion of the atrial septum. Patent foramen ovale is usually a secondary defect caused by increased right atrial pressure associated with concurrent right heart defects.

AVSD represents a spectrum of malformations involving the septum primum, the inlet portion of the ventricular septum, and the AV valves (Pacifico 1994). AVSDs are classified as having communication at the atrial level, ventricular level, or both with a common AV valve. AVSD with communication at the atrial level consists of an ostium primum defect and a trifoliate left AV valve with bridging leaflets directed toward the inlet portion of the ventricular septum (Potter *et al.* 2022). The latter, formally known as a mitral cleft, can result in significant left AV valve regurgitation. Complete AVSD with atrioventricular communication, formally known as an endocardial cushion defect, consists of an ostium primum defect, inflow VSD, and a single AV valve with bridging leaflets that are common to the right and left ventricle.

Pathophysiology

ASD causes a predominantly left-to-right shunt that volume overloads the right ventricle. Progressive right heart dilatation and right-sided congestive heart failure can result if the shunt fraction is large. Bidirectional or right-to-left shunt with hypoxemia occurs when right atrial pressures are increased by congestive heart failure, pulmonary hypertension, or concurrent right-sided structural heart defects. AVSD can result in volume overload of the right and/or left ventricle, depending on the level of septal communication and the presence of AV valve regurgitation.

Indication for surgery

The decision to perform surgery to correct an ASD is based on clinical signs and the hemodynamic significance of the defect. The degree of cardiac chamber enlargement, pulmonary overcirculation on radiographs, and pulmonary flow velocity can be considered in evaluating hemodynamic significance. A septal shunt flow velocity above 0.45 m/s suggests a significant shunt flow (Marx *et al.* 1985).

Open repair for atrial and atrioventricular septal defects

Open repair of ASD is accomplished with the aid of cardiopulmonary bypass through a right fifth thoracotomy (Figure 81.4). Cannulation for cardiopulmonary bypass is as described for VSD. The defect is approached through a right atriotomy. The septal defect is closed

(a)

(b)

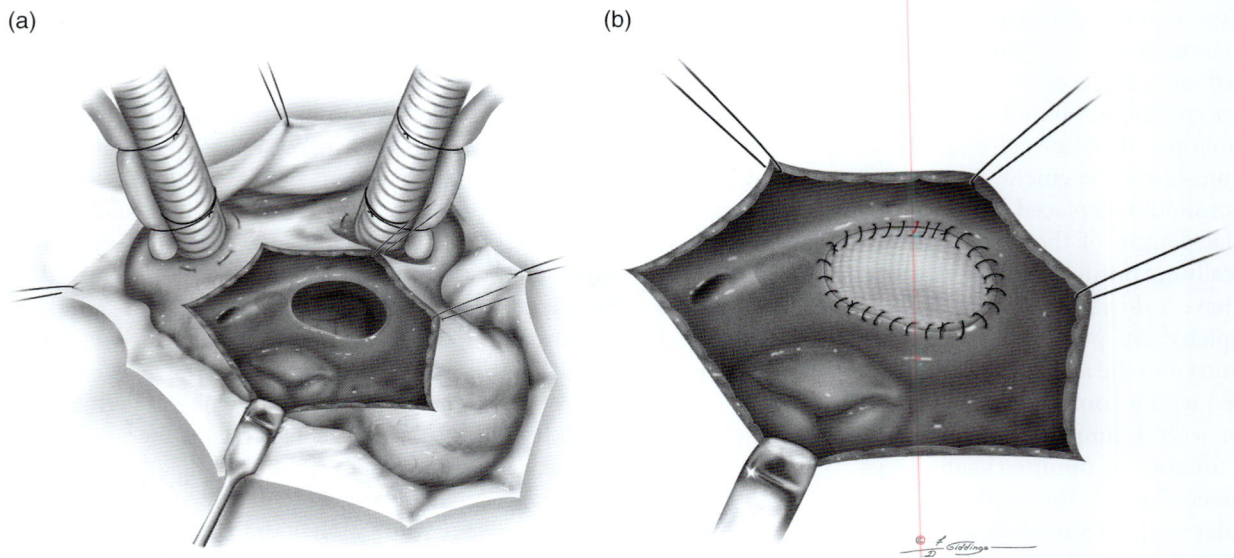

Figure 81.4 Atrial septal defect (ASD) repair. (a) Repair is accomplished through a right atriotomy approach during cardiopulmonary bypass. Bicaval venous cannulation is necessary to isolate the right atrium during bypass. (b) The septal defect is closed with an autogenous pericardium or polytetrafluoroethylene (PTFE) patch using a simple continuous suture pattern. The atriotomy incision is closed with a continuous mattress suture pattern oversewn with a simple continuous pattern. © D. Giddings.

with autogenous pericardium harvested before the pericardium or PTFE cardiovascular patch. Sinus venosus defects may require concurrent correction of anomalous pulmonary venous return. This is accomplished by extending the patch closure to the right of the ostia of the anomalous veins, functionally leaving their flow on the leftward side of the patch.

AVSD repair generally requires closure of the trifoliate left AV valve prior to closing the septal defect (Figure 81.5). This is accomplished by directly suturing the bridging leaflets together before closing the septal defect and performing an annuloplasty if necessary (see Chapter 82). The ostium primum defect is closed with autogenous pericardium or PTFE patch. In order to avoid injury to the atrioventricular conduction, the patch is extended around the coronary sinus, leaving coronary flow to the left side of the patch. The atriotomy is closed with a continuous horizontal mattress pattern and oversewn with a simple continuous pattern.

Outcomes

Successful surgical correction has been described for ASD and AVSD in dogs (Eyster *et al.* 1976b; Monnet *et al.* 1997; Akiyama *et al.* 2005; Seo *et al.* 2021). Open repair of ASD or AVSD can be considered curative, assuming that the magnitude of pulmonary hypertension or secondary myocardial failure present is not

severe at the time of surgery. For partial AVSD, long-term outcome also depends on the magnitude of residual AV valve regurgitation (Monnet *et al.* 1997). As with VSD, complete AV block is a possible operative complication of open repair.

Tetralogy of Fallot

Tetralogy of Fallot is a congenital heart defect that consists of pulmonary stenosis, an infundibular perimembranous VSD, a dextropositioned overriding aorta, and right ventricular hypertrophy. Tetralogy of Fallot is the most common cyanotic heart defect in companion animals, but accounts for only about 4% of cardiac malformations in dogs (Buchanan 1999). Tetralogy occurs in cats and a variety of canine breeds including keeshonds, poodles, schnauzers, terriers, collies, and shelties (Ringwald & Bonagura 1988). In keeshonds, tetralogy of Fallot is genetically transmitted as part of the spectrum of conotruncal defects (Patterson *et al.* 1974).

Pathophysiology

From a functional standpoint, tetralogy of Fallot can be simplified into the combined effects of the pulmonary stenosis and the VSD. The pathophysiologic consequences of tetralogy depend on the relative magnitude of these two defects. Animals with severe pulmonary stenosis and right-to-left shunt have moderate to severe cyanosis, exercise intolerance, and progressive

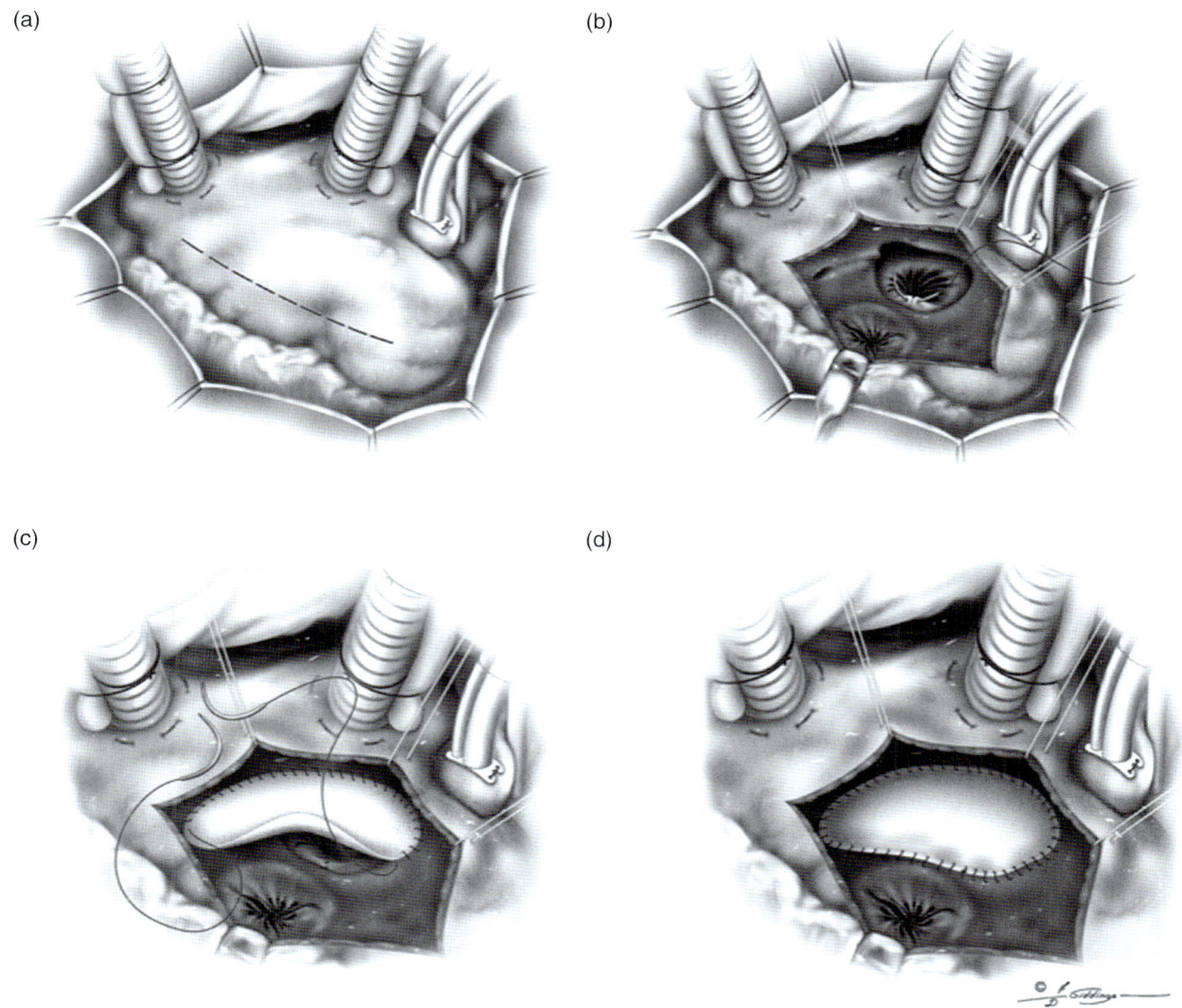

(a) (b) (c) (d)

Figure 81.5 Atrioventricular septal defect (AVSD) repair with communication at the atrial level and trifoliate left AV valve. (a) Repair is accomplished via a right atriotomy with bicaval venous cannulation for cardiopulmonary bypass. A cardioplegia cannula is placed in the ascending aorta and secured with a pledget-reinforced mattress suture. The ascending aorta is cross-clamped. (b) The right atrium is incised parallel and dorsal to the atrioventricular groove. The zone of apposition between the left AV valve bridging leaflets is closed with simple interrupted sutures of 6-0 suture through the ostium primum defect. (c and d) A polytetrafluoroethylene (PTFE) patch is sutured to the ventral, cranial, and dorsal rims of the ostium primum defect with continuous sutures of 5-0 suture. The patch is extended around the coronary sinus, leaving the coronary sinus on the leftward side of the patch to avoid injury to the atrioventricular node.

erythrocytosis. A shortened lifespan can be expected due to complications associated with chronic hypoxemia and erythrocytosis.

Indications

The long-term prognosis for tetralogy of Fallot depends on the ratio of pulmonary to systemic blood flow. Some animals may live for several years without surgical intervention, although they will be moderately to severely exercise intolerant. Animals with resting hypoxemia and

progressive polycythemia will likely succumb to the effects of the defect early in life. Surgery should be considered for animals with exertional cyanosis to lessen clinical signs and prolong life. Debilitating exercise intolerance, erythrocytosis (hematocrit >70%), and resting hypoxemia (arterial oxygen saturation <60%) are indications for surgery. Animals with predominantly left-to-right shunt, termed acyanotic tetralogy, may function reasonably well so long as the shunt flow remains low and does not cause heart failure, and so long as progressive infundibular hypertrophy of the right ventricle does not worsen the pulmonary stenosis and reverse the shunt.

Palliative interventions for tetralogy of Fallot include isolated correction of the pulmonary stenosis or creation of a systemic-to-pulmonary shunt (Sreeram *et al.* 1991; de Leval 1994b). The goal of both palliative approaches is to increase pulmonary blood flow without creating an overwhelming left-to-right shunt. Procedures aimed at relieving pulmonary stenosis alone risk overcorrection of the defect and creation of an overwhelming left-to-right shunt. From this standpoint, dilatation valvuloplasty is preferred over a more definitive surgery (Sreeram *et al.* 1991).

Systemic-to-pulmonary shunts increase pulmonary blood flow to a more predictable degree, and thereby improve arterial oxygen saturation while lessening the risk of excessive pulmonary overcirculation. Several systemic-to-pulmonic shunts have been devised for palliation of tetralogy of Fallot, including the Blalock–Taussig (BT; subclavian to pulmonary artery anastomosis), Potts (aorticopulmonary anastomosis), Waterston (aorta to right pulmonary artery anastomosis), and Glenn (vena cava to pulmonary arterial anastomosis) (de Leval 1994a,b). Modified BT consisting of a synthetic graft between the left subclavian artery and pulmonary artery has resulted in successful long-term palliation in dogs (Brockman *et al.* 2007). Definitive open correction for tetralogy of Fallot can be undertaken in dogs with curative intent.

Modified Blalock–Taussig shunt

The BT shunt is the preferred palliative procedure for tetralogy of Fallot in dogs. The magnitude of increase in pulmonary flow is determined by the diameter of the subclavian artery that is known to be appropriate. The original BT shunt consisted of dividing the left subclavian artery and performing an end-to-side anastomosis of the proximal end of the divided artery to the pulmonary artery. In animals, the left subclavian artery does not have sufficient length to reach the pulmonary without kinking at its origin on the aorta. A modification of the classic procedure consisting of a synthetic vascular graft between the left subclavian and pulmonary arteries is now preferred in dogs and humans (Figure 81.6). An additional advantage of the modified BT shunt is that the subclavian artery does not need to be sacrificed. Administration of clopidogrel for three months after surgery is recommended to decrease the likelihood of graft thrombosis.

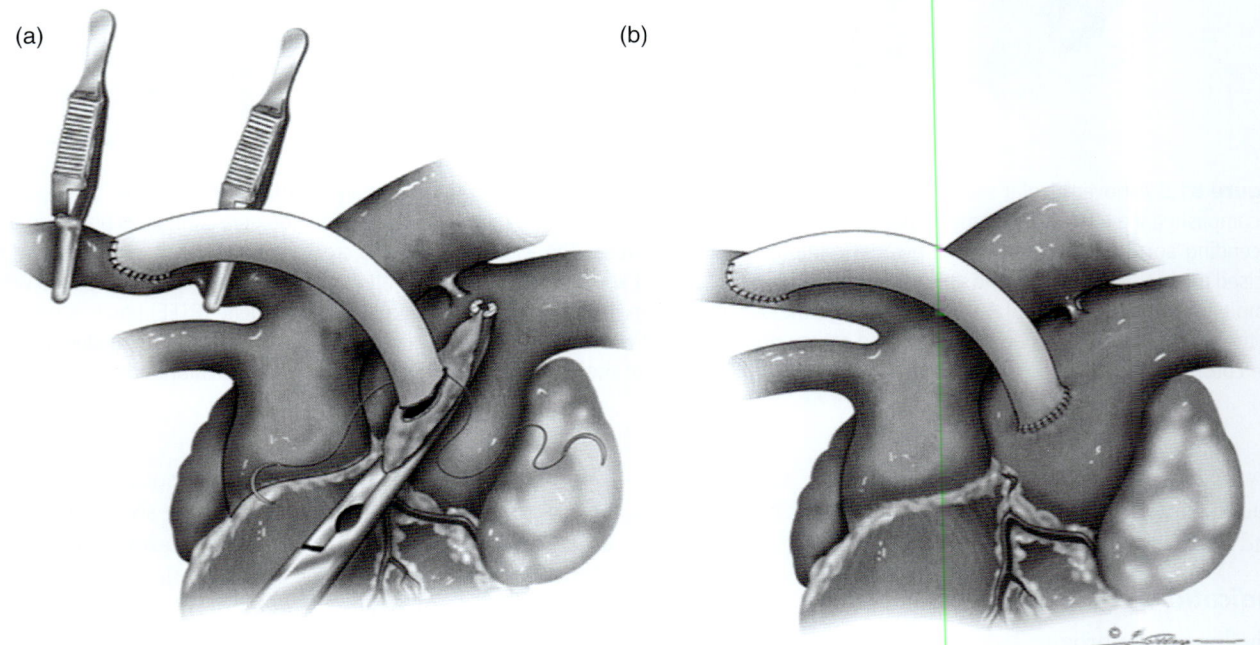

(a)   (b)

Figure 81.6 Modified Blalock–Taussig shunt. Surgery is performed via a left fourth intercostal thoracotomy. The left subclavian artery is isolated with vascular clamps or tourniquets. (a) A 5 or 6 mm PTFE vascular graft is anastomosed to the left subclavian artery. (b) A side-biting vascular clamp is placed on the pulmonary artery and the vascular graft is anastomosed to the pulmonary artery. © D. Giddings.

(a)

(b)

(c)

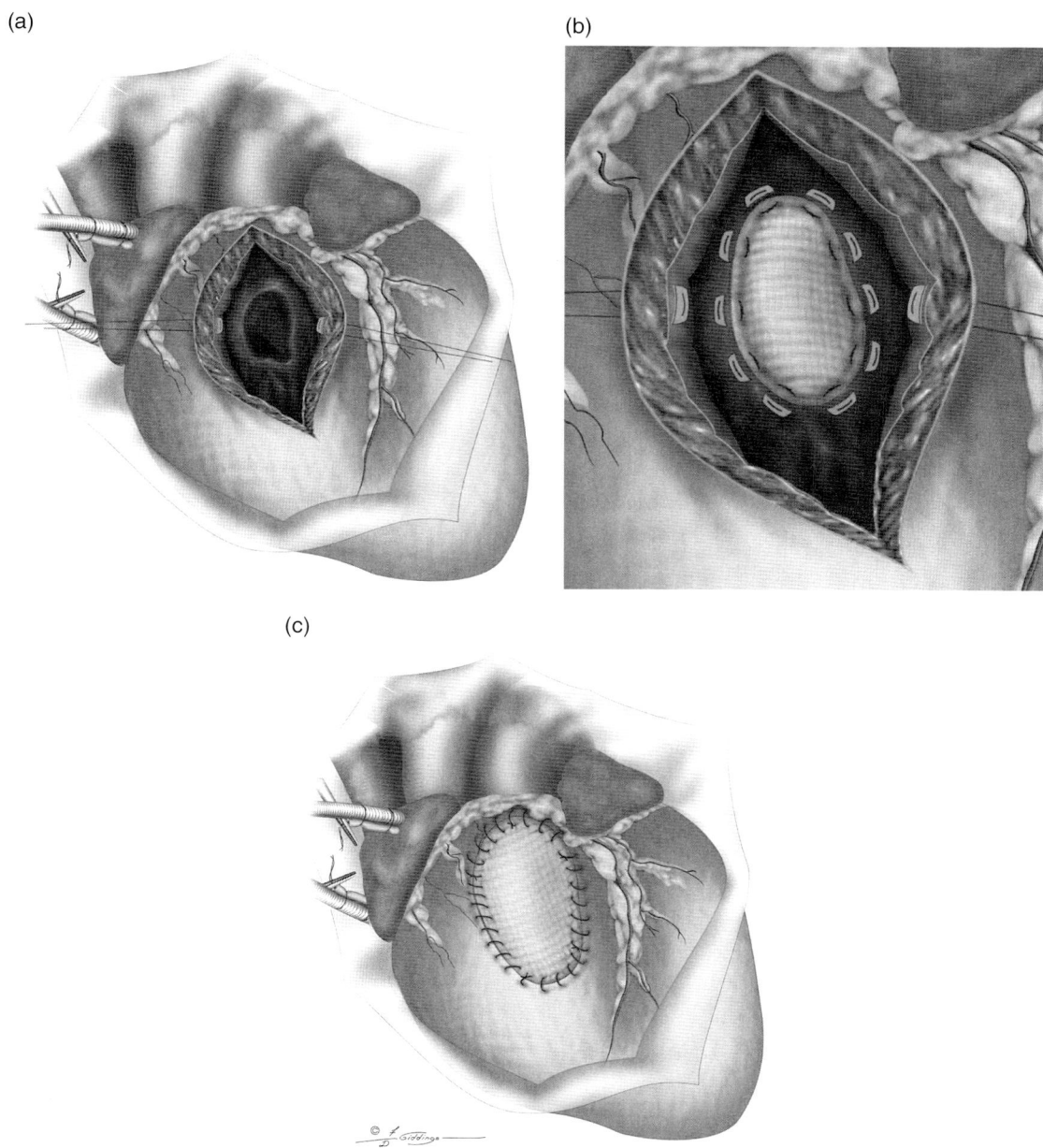

Figure 81.7 Tetralogy of Fallot repair. Open repair of tetralogy of Fallot is accomplished via median sternotomy during cardiopulmonary bypass. (a) After the pericardium is opened, a ventriculotomy is made in the right ventricular outflow tract (RVOT). The ventricular septal defect is visualized, typically below the crista supraventricularis. (b) The septal defect and overriding aorta are corrected with synthetic patch secured with interrupted buttressed mattress sutures. If the defect is in close proximity to the tricuspid annulus, some of the mattress sutures may be placed through the annulus from the atrial side. (c) The RVOT obstruction is corrected by placement of an oval synthetic patch within the ventriculotomy. The patch may or may not need to be extended across the pulmonary valve annulus. depending on whether valvular stenosis is contributing to the outflow obstruction. © D. Giddings.

Open repair of tetralogy of Fallot

Definitive repair of tetralogy of Fallot can be undertaken in dogs with the aid of cardiopulmonary bypass (Orton *et al.* 2001). The surgical approach is by median sternotomy (Figure 81.7). Arterial cannulation for cardiopulmonary bypass is in the left femoral artery. Venous cannulation should be bicaval, with direct cannulation of the cranial vena cava. The caudal vena cava cannula can be introduced via the right auricle. The aorta is cross-clamped and antegrade cardioplegia administered. The cardiac approach is via a longitudinal ventriculotomy in the right ventricular outflow tract. Patch closure of the VSD is performed, taking care to avoid injury to the tricuspid valve and conduction tissues. The pulmonary stenosis is corrected by excision of the subpulmonary muscular bands and imposition of an oval patch graft across the stenosis. In some dogs, the obstruction will consist entirely of a subpulmonary fibromuscular band. In this case, the band is excised and a patch graft is placed within the ventriculotomy approach, without extending the incision across the pulmonary valve annulus. In other cases, valvular pulmonary stenosis is present and a transannular pulmonary patch graft will be necessary. In both cases, preoperative planning must exclude the possibility of a prepulmonary coronary artery anomaly.

Outcomes

Successful short-term palliation of tetralogy of Fallot by systemic-to-pulmonary shunt has been described in dogs and cats (Miller *et al.* 1985; Ringwald & Bonagura 1988; Brockman *et al.* 2007). Long-term palliation of tetralogy of Fallot by modified BT shunt has been reported in dogs (Brockman *et al.* 2007). Successful definitive correction for tetralogy of Fallot has also been reported in dogs (Orton *et al.* 2001) and is associated with resolution of clinical signs and a normal life expectancy after surgery.

References

Akiyama, M., Tanaka, R., Maruo, K., and Yamane, Y. (2005). Surgical correction of a partial atrioventricular septal defect with a ventricular septal defect in a dog. *Journal of the American Animal Hospital Association* 41: 137–143.

Birchard, S.J., Bonagura, J.D., and Fingland, R.B. (1990). Results of ligation of patent ductus arteriosus in dogs: 201 cases (1969–1988). *Journal of the American Veterinary Medical Association* 196: 2011–2013.

Brockman, D.J., Holt, D.E., Gaynor, J.W., and Theman, T.E. (2007). Long-term palliation of tetralogy of Fallot in dogs by use of a modified Blalock–Taussig shunt. *Journal of the American Veterinary Medical Association* 231: 721–726.

Buchanan, J.W. (1994). Patent ductus arteriosus. *Seminars in Veterinary Medicine and Surgery (Small Animal)* 9: 168–176.

Buchanan, J.W. (1999). Prevalence of cardiovascular disorders. In: *Textbook of Canine and Feline Cardiology*, 2e (ed. P.R. Fox, D.D. Sisson and N.S. Moise), 457. Philadelphia, PA: WB Saunders.

Buchanan, J.W. (2001). Patent ductus arteriosus morphology, pathogenesis, types and treatment. *Journal of Veterinary Cardiology* 3 (1): 7–16.

Buchanan, J.W. and Patterson, D.F. (2003). Etiology of patent ductus arteriosus in dogs. *Journal of Veterinary Internal Medicine* 17: 167–171.

Bureau, S., Monnet, E., and Orton, E.C. (2005). Evaluation of survival rate and prognostic indicators for surgical treatment of left-to-right patent ductus arteriosus in dogs: 52 cases (1995–2003).

Journal of the American Veterinary Medical Association 227: 1794–1799.

Eyster, G.E., Eyster, J.T., Cords, G.B., and Johnston, J. (1976a). Patent ductus arteriosus in the dog: characteristics of occurrence and results of surgery in one hundred consecutive cases. *Journal of the American Veterinary Medical Association* 168: 435–438.

Eyster, G.E., Anderson, L.K., Krehbeil, J.D. et al. (1976b). Surgical repair of atrial septal defect in a dog. *Journal of the American Veterinary Medical Association* 169: 1081–1084.

Eyster, G.E., Whipple, R.D., Anderson, L.K. et al. (1977). Pulmonary artery banding for ventricular septal defect in dogs and cats. *Journal of the American Veterinary Medical Association* 170: 434–438.

Goodrich, K.R., Kyles, A.E., Kass, P.H., and Campbell, F. (2007). Retrospective comparison of surgical ligation and transarterial catheter occlusion of treatment of patent ductus arteriosus in two hundred and four dogs (1993–2003). *Veterinary Surgery* 36: 43–49.

Goodwin, J.K. and Lombard, C.W. (1992). Patent ductus arteriosus in adult dogs: clinical features of 14 cases. *Journal of the American Animal Hospital Association* 28: 349–354.

Gordon, S.G., Saunders, A.B., Achen, S.E. et al. (2010). Transarterial ductal occlusion using the Amplatz Canine Duct Occluder in 40 dogs. *Journal of Veterinary Cardiology* 12: 85–92.

Hunt, G.B., Simpson, D.J., Beck, J.A. et al. (2001). Intraoperative hemorrhage during patent ductus arteriosus ligation in dogs. *Veterinary Surgery* 30: 58–63.

de Leval, M. (1994a). Ventricular septal defects. In: *Surgery for Congenital Heart Defects*, 2e (ed. J. Stark and M. de Leval), 355. Philadelphia, PA: WB Saunders.

de Leval, M. (1994b). Systemic-to-pulmonary artery shunts. In: *Surgery for Congenital Heart Defects*, 2e (ed. J. Stark and M. de Leval), 247. Philadelphia, PA: WB Saunders.

Marx, G.R., Allen, H.D., Goldberg, S.J., and Finn, C.J. (1985). Transatrial septal velocity measurement by Doppler echocardiography in atrial septal defect: correlation with Qp:Qs ratio. *American Journal of Cardiology* 55: 1162–1167.

Miller, C.W., Holmberg, D.L., Bowen, V. et al. (1985). Microsurgical management of tetralogy of Fallot in a cat. *Journal of the American Veterinary Medical Association* 186: 708–709.

Monnet, E., Orton, E.C., Gaynor, J. et al. (1997). Partial atrioventricular septal defect: diagnosis and surgical repair in two dogs. *Journal of the American Veterinary Medical Association* 211: 569–572.

Orton, E.C., Mama, K., Hellyer, P., and Hackett, T.B. (2001). Open surgical repair of tetralogy of Fallot in two dogs. *Journal of the American Veterinary Medical Association* 219: 1089–1093.

Pacifico, A.D. (1994). Atrio-ventricular septal defects. In: *Surgery for Congenital Heart Defects*, 2e (ed. J. Stark and M. de Leval), 373. Philadelphia, PA: WB Saunders.

Patterson, D.F. (1965). Congenital heart disease in the dog. *Annals of the New York Academy of Sciences* 127: 541–569.

Patterson, D.F., Pyle, R.L., Van Mierop, L. et al. (1974). Hereditary defects in the conotruncal septum on Keeshond dogs: pathologic and genetic studies. *American Journal of Cardiology* 34: 187–205.

Potter, B.M., Scansen, B.A., Chi, I.J.B. et al. (2022). Trifoliate left atrioventricular valve with and without intact septal structures in four dogs: echocardiographic findings and surgical repair. *Journal of Veterinary Cardiology* 41: 70–78.

Ringwald, R.J. and Bonagura, J.D. (1988). Tetralogy of Fallot in the dog: clinical findings in 13 cases. *Journal of the American Animal Hospital Association* 24: 33–43.

Seo, J., Kurosawa, T.A., Luis Fuentes, V. et al. (2021). Surgical management of three dogs with an interatrial communication and atrioventricular valve abnormalities. *CASE* 5: 252–259.

Shimizu, M., Tanaka, R., Hoshi, K. et al. (2006). Surgical correction of ventricular septal defect with aortic regurgitation in a dog. *Australian Veterinary Journal* 84: 117–121.

Sreeram, N., Saleem, M., Jackson, M. et al. (1991). Results of balloon pulmonary valvuloplasty as a palliative procedure in tetralogy of Fallot. *Journal of the American College of Cardiology* 18: 159–165.

Stark, J. (1994). Secundum atrial septal defect and partial anomalous pulmonary venous return. In: *Surgery for Congenital Heart Defects*, 2e (ed. J. Stark and M. de Leval), 343. Philadelphia, PA: WB Saunders.

Sutherland, B.J., Pierce, K.V., Gagnon, A.L. et al. (2019). Dilatable pulmonary artery banding for ventricular septal defect: surgical technique and case report of three cats. *Journal of Veterinary Cardiology* 25: 32–40.

Van Israel, N., Dukes-McEwan, J., and French, A.T. (2003). Long-term follow up of dogs with patent ductus arteriosus. *Journal of Small Animal Practice* 44: 480–490.

82

Valvular Heart Disease

E. Christopher Orton

Mitral regurgitation

Mitral regurgitation is the most frequent cause of cardiac disability and death in dogs. Causes of mitral regurgitation in dogs are degenerative (myxomatous) mitral valve disease, congenital mitral valve dysplasia, and secondary functional mitral regurgitation.

Myxomatous degeneration is the most frequent cause of mitral regurgitation in dogs. The condition accounts for 40–75% of heart disease in dogs (Buchanan 1999; Atkins *et al.* 2009). It is characterized by varying degrees of nodular thickening and distortion of the valve leaflets, elongation and rupture of the chordae tendineae, and dilatation of the valve annulus. Mitral regurgitation results from the combination of leaflet prolapse/flail and annular dilatation.

Congenital mitral valve dysplasia occurs in cats and several large and giant breeds of dog. A genetic basis for the disease is suspected. A broad spectrum of lesions is possible, including shortening and thickening of the leaflets, cleft lesions of the leaflets, malformations (fusion, shortening, elongation, abnormal insertion, or absence) of the chordae tendineae, and malformation or mispositioning of papillary muscles. Mitral regurgitation typically results from restrictive leaflet motion (i.e., the valve does not completely close) and secondary annular dilatation. Mitral valve stenosis is a less common manifestation that accompanies mitral regurgitation in some cases.

Functional mitral regurgitation occurs secondary to left ventricular chamber dilatation associated with dilated cardiomyopathy, degenerative mitral valve disease, or congenital shunts. Mitral regurgitation is caused by a failure of leaflet coaptation due to dilatation of the mitral annulus.

Pathophysiology

Mitral regurgitation causes volume overload of the left heart. The left atrium and ventricle dilate in response to the overload. The response is initially adaptive, but becomes maladaptive as ventricular chamber dilatation becomes severe and the ventricular walls thin. Dilatation of the mitral valve annulus contributes to the progression by causing functional mitral regurgitation. Left-sided congestive heart failure develops in response to a neuroendocrine-mediated increase in left atrial pressure. Secondary myocardial failure contributes to the progression of heart failure. Atrial fibrillation may develop secondary to atrial dilatation, further compromising cardiac function.

Indications for surgery

Mitral valve surgery is an option for dogs with hemodynamically significant mitral regurgitation. Indications for considering mitral valve surgery are diuretic-dependent (stage C) congestive heart failure or significant left ventricular remodeling (stage B2) with activity intolerance. Dogs with secondary systolic dysfunction or atrial fibrillation can tolerate mitral valve surgery, but morbidity and mortality are higher in these patients.

Surgical options for correction of mitral regurgitation are valve repair or valve replacement. Mitral valve repair has the advantages of not requiring a prosthesis, being minimally thrombogenic, and not requiring

---

anticoagulation therapy after surgery. Valve repair preserves myocardial function better than valve replacement (Dalrymple-Hay *et al*. 1998). Disadvantages of valve repair include a more variable result and less certain durability. Valve repair is technically difficult, and results are dependent on surgeon experience.

Valve replacement has the advantage of being technically easier to perform than valve repair. Additionally, it provides more predictable complete correction of regurgitation. The disadvantage of valve replacement is the requirement for a valve prosthesis and the associated shortcomings. Valve prosthesis options are a mechanical prothesis or a glutaraldehyde-fixed bioprosthetic valve. Mechanical valves have excellent durability, but are thrombogenic and require lifetime anticoagulation therapy (Bonow *et al*. 2008). Mechanical protheses should not be used in dogs due to the high incidence of valve thrombosis despite anticoagulation (Orton *et al*. 2005). Bioprosthetic valves have the principal advantage of lower thrombogenicity. Anticoagulation therapy with warfarin is necessary for three months after surgery (Bonow *et al*. 2008). Warfarin therapy after valve replacement is guided by monitoring the international normalized ratio (INR) based on the prothrombin time (Triplett 1998; Winter *et al*. 2012). A target INR of 2.0–3.0 is recommended in humans after mitral valve replacement (Bonow *et al*. 2008). Because of size limitations in currently available valve prostheses, valve replacement is generally limited to dogs >10 kg.

Mitral valve repair

Mitral valve repair employs a variety of surgical techniques to address the functional causes of mitral regurgitation. These include annular dilatation (type I defect), excessive leaflet motion (type II defect), or restricted leaflet motion (type III defect) (Carpentier 1983). Annular dilatation is assumed to be a component of mitral regurgitation whenever substantial atrial and ventricular dilatation are present. Mitral valve leaflets are assessed for evidence of prolapse or restrictive motion before surgery by echocardiography. Color-flow patterns of regurgitant flow are also informative. Leaflet prolapse causes an eccentric regurgitant jet directed away from a prolapsing leaflet. Assessment of valve function during surgery is accomplished by infusing cold saline into the ventricle and observing regurgitant flow through the valve.

Mitral valve repair is accomplished through left thoracotomy. Standard femoral arterial cannulation for cardiopulmonary bypass is employed. Venous cannulation is accomplished with a two-stage cannula passed through the right atrial appendage. Approach to the mitral valve is via a left atriotomy. Annuloplasty corrects the annular dilatation component of mitral regurgitation and is necessary in virtually all mitral valve repairs regardless of original cause (Carpentier 1983; Griffiths *et al*. 2004; Uechi 2012). A fundamental principle of mitral valve annuloplasty is that the mural, but not the septal, portion of annulus stretches and dilates. Thus, it is the mural portion of the annulus that must be corrected by annuloplasty. The size of the annuloplasty ring is based on an approximation of the area of the septal leaflet measured with sizing obturators. Commercial annuloplasty bands are available, or a band is fashioned from cardiovascular graft material (Dacron® [INVISTA, Kennesaw, GA, USA] or polytetrafluoroethylene [PTFE]). Annuloplasty is achieved by preplacing double-armed sutures into the mural portion of the annulus (Figure 82.1). The ends of the suture are then passed through the band. The band is seated into position and the sutures are tied.

(a)   (b)

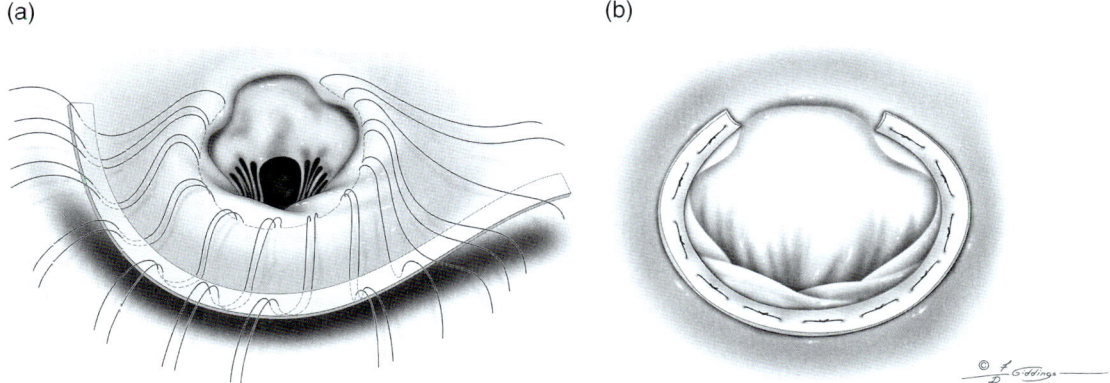

Figure 82.1 Mitral partial ring annuloplasty. The size of the annuloplasty ring is chosen or fashioned to match the circumference of the septal leaflet. (a) Double-armed 3-0 sutures are preplaced in the annulus from the atrial side. Sutures are placed with wide bites so the portion of the annulus within the suture will be imbricated when the ring is seated. Both ends of the sutures are passed through the ring. (b) The ring is seated and the sutures are tied. © D. Giddings.

(a)   (b)

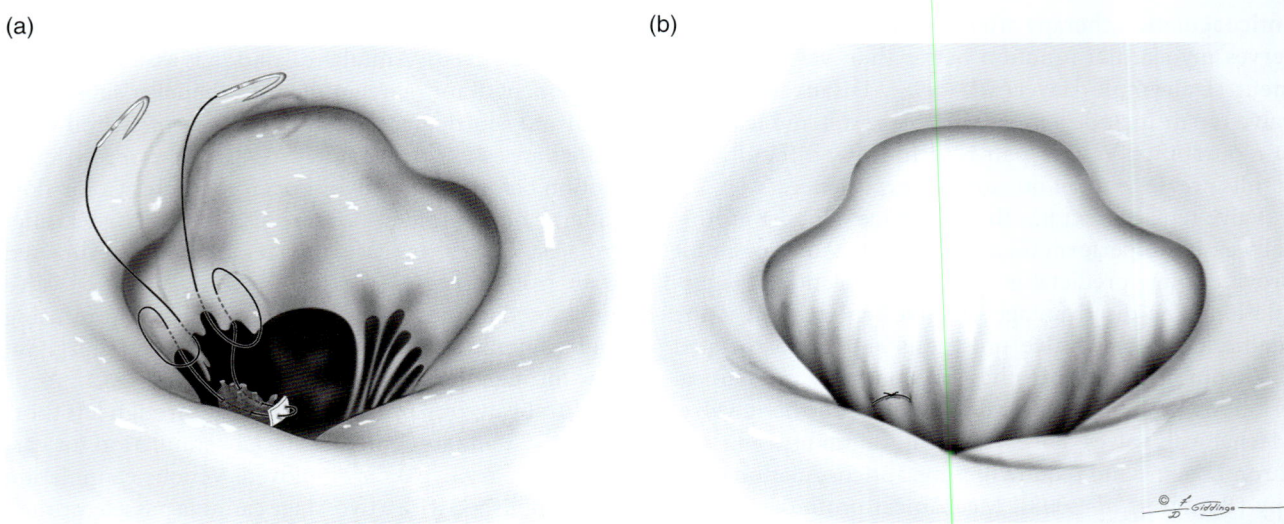

Figure 82.2 Artificial chordae tendineae repair is used to correct leaflet prolapse secondary to rupture or elongation of the chordae tendineae. (a) A pledget-buttressed double-armed polytetrafluoroethylene (PTFE) suture is passed through the appropriate papillary muscle and then twice through the margin of the leaflet. The length of the suture is determined by matching the leaflet margin with the margin of the opposing leaflet. (b) The suture is then tied. © D. Giddings.

Leaflet prolapse or flail is addressed by artificial chordae (Figure 82.2). PTFE monofilament sutures are placed in the papillary muscle and then brought through the leaflet margin (Griffiths *et al.* 2004; Uechi *et al.* 2012). Edge-to-edge repair for leaflet prolapse is accomplished by suturing the free edge of a prolapsing leaflet to the free edge of the facing leaflet (Maisano *et al.* 1998; Griffiths *et al.* 2004) (Figure 82.3). The correction results in a double-orifice valve.

A variety of repairs have been described for restrictive leaflet motion associated with mitral valve dysplasia. These include commissurotomy, resection of secondary chordae, papillary muscle splitting, or fenestration of fused thickened chordae (Carpentier 1994). Short chordae can be addressed dividing the chordal attachments from the tip of the papillary muscle and reattaching with a PTFE mattress suture, as described later in the chapter for repair of tricuspid valve dysplasia (TVD).

(a)   (b)

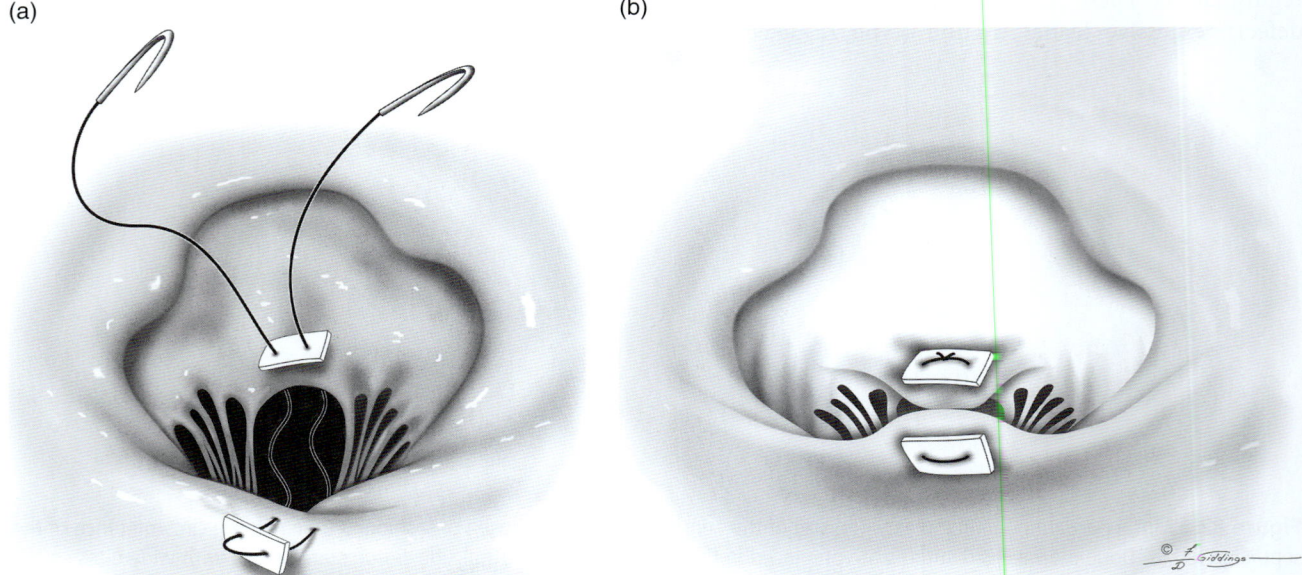

Figure 82.3 Edge-to-edge repair for leaflet prolapse. (a) A buttressed mattress suture is placed in the free edges of the septal and mural valve leaflets at the point of greatest leaflet prolapse. (b) The mattress suture is tied, resulting in a double-orifice valve. © D. Giddings.

Mitral valve replacement

Mitral valve replacement with a bioprosthetic valve is favored over replacement with a mechanical prosthesis in dogs with severe mitral regurgitation, because of the risk of valve prosthesis thrombosis and the limitations of long-term anticoagulation in dogs (Orton *et al.* 2005). The most common indication for mitral valve replacement is mitral valve dysplasia with severe leaflet anomaly, including mitral stenosis. Mitral valve replacement can be undertaken through left thoracotomy. Standard femoral arterial cannulation for cardiopulmonary bypass is employed. Venous cannulation is accomplished with a two-stage cannula passed through the right atrial appendage. Approach to the mitral valve is via a left lateral atriotomy. Surgery is performed under cardioplegic arrest with the aorta cross-clamped. Visualization of the mitral valve by the surgeon is enhanced by standing on the dorsal side of the animal.

The size of the mitral annulus is determined with an obturator and an appropriately sized prosthesis is chosen for implantation. The septal leaflet and associated chordae tendineae are excised, leaving a 3 mm margin of leaflet at the annulus (Figure 82.4). The mural leaflet is retained to preserve myocardial function (Heath *et al.* 1991). Between 12 and 15 buttressed mattress sutures are preplaced through the valve annulus. The mural leaflet is plicated into the mattress sutures to prevent it from interfering with the valve prosthesis. The mattress sutures are then passed through the sewing ring of the prosthesis. The prosthesis is seated into the valve annulus and the sutures are tied. A left ventricular vent cannula is temporary placed through the atriotomy and valve prostheses as the atriotomy is being closed. The left atrium is de-aired and closed with a continuous horizontal mattress pattern and oversewn with a simple continuous pattern. Dogs undergoing valve replacement with a bioprosthesis should be placed on anticoagulation therapy with warfarin (Winter *et al.* 2012), or a combination of an oral factor Xa inhibitor such as apixaban and clopidogrel (Gagnon *et al.* 2021) for three months after surgery to prevent thrombosis of the valve.

Outcomes

Based on both clinical and experimental results, the short- and long-term performance of bioprosthetic valves has been favorable in dogs (Behr *et al.* 2007; Takashima *et al.* 2007, 2008). In our clinical experience, bioprosthetic valves have performed well in dogs for periods of at least five years.

Successful mitral valve repair has been reported in dogs with degenerative mitral valve disease and congenital mitral dysplasia (Kamemoto *et al.* 1990; Boggs *et al.* 1996; Borenstein *et al.* 2004; Griffiths *et al.* 2004;

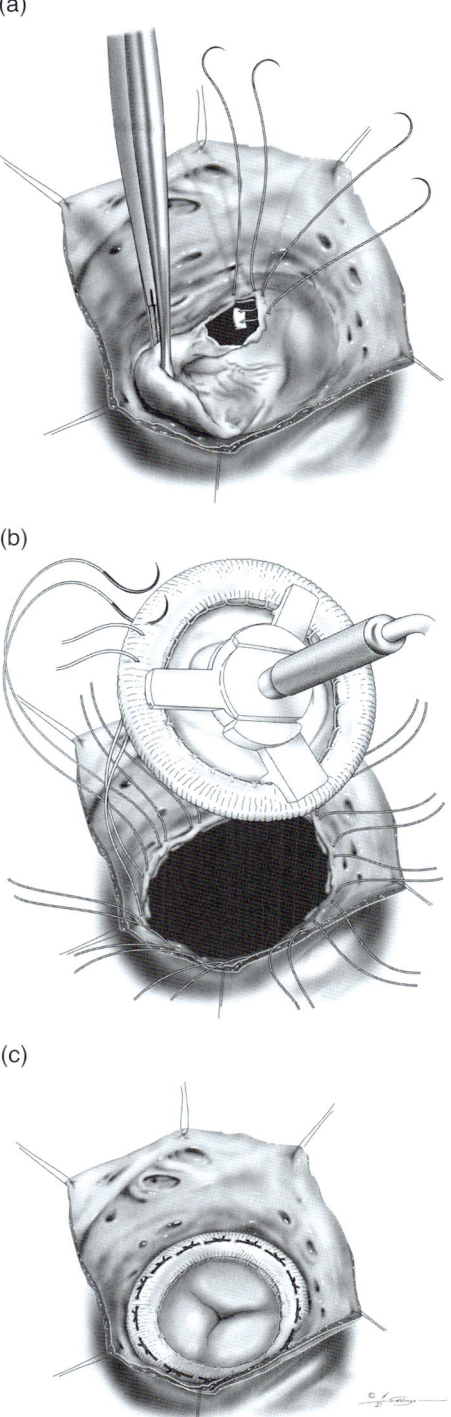

(a)

(b)

(c)

Figure 82.4 Heart valve replacement. (a) The septal valve leaflet and chordal apparatus are excised, leaving a 3 mm curtain of leaflet at the annulus. For mitral valve replacement, the mural leaflet is preserved and imbricated into the mattress sutures. (b) Buttressed mattress sutures are placed through the valve annulus using 2-0 or 3-0 double-armed polyester suture. The mattress sutures are passed through the sewing ring of the prosthesis. (c) The prosthesis is seated into the valve annulus and the sutures are tied. © D. Giddings.

Uechi *et al.* 2012). The expectation for mitral valve repair in dogs should be palliative rather than curative, because of the difficulty of achieving complete resolution of mitral regurgitation in dogs. However, dogs have survived for as long as seven years after mitral repair.

Tricuspid valve dysplasia

TVD is a congenital malformation of the tricuspid valve that occurs in dogs and cats. The reported prevalence for the defect is approximately 5% of cardiac malformations in dogs, although it may be emerging as a more important defect (Buchanan 1999). Labrador retrievers, golden retrievers, German shepherds, and other large-breed dogs are predisposed to the condition. A broad spectrum of pathologic lesions has been associated with tricuspid dysplasia. The most common manifestations are multiple direct attachments of large papillary muscles to the mural leaflet and an immobile septal leaflet that is "tethered" to the ventricular septum by multiple short fine chordae. The result is restrictive leaflet motion and torrential tricuspid regurgitation. Tricuspid stenosis results from failure of commissure separation of the mural and septal leaflets. Tricuspid regurgitation causes progressive right atrial and ventricular volume overload and dilatation, progressively worsening the tricuspid regurgitation. Most dogs with massive or torrential tricuspid regurgitation develop right-sided congestive heart failure within the first three years of life. Atrial fibrillation is a frequent late sequela that contributes to the progression of heart failure.

Indications for surgery

Tricuspid valve repair is the preferred surgical option for dogs with the typical TVD (Sutherland *et al.* 2021). Indications for tricuspid valve repair include torrential tricuspid regurgitation, severe right atrial and ventricular dilatation, and/or early evidence of hepatic venous congestion. Surgical intervention should be undertaken before congestive heart failure becomes established. Once right-sided congestive heart failure becomes medically refractory or atrial fibrillation is long-standing, dogs are poor candidates for surgery. Tricuspid valve replacement with a bioprosthesis can be undertaken for dogs with severe tricuspid regurgitation that are not amenable to surgical repair (Arai *et al.* 2011). Typically, dogs with malformation of the leaflets and/or tricuspid stenosis will not be amenable to valve repair.

Tricuspid valve repair

Tricuspid valve repair is performed via a right-sided thoracotomy through the fifth intercostal space. Cannulation for cardiopulmonary bypass is femoral arterial and bicaval venous. The surgery is performed under antegrade cardioplegia with the aorta cross-clamped. The tricuspid valve accessed is a right atriotomy. Surgical repair is directed at mobilization of the mural and septal leaflets and annuloplasty to restore the normal annular area (Sutherland *et al.* 2021). Mobilization of leaflets is accomplished by division of abnormal leaflet attachments and resuspension with artificial chordae (Figure 82.5).

Tricuspid valve replacement

Tricuspid valve replacement with a porcine bioprosthetic valve is accomplished through a right atriotomy with bicaval venous cannulation. The procedure is like that described for mitral valve replacement (Figure 82.4). Between 12 and 15 double-armed 3-0 or 2-0 buttressed mattress sutures are preplaced in the valve annulus. The leaflets are excised or imbricated within the mattress sutures to prevent them from interfering with the motion of the valve prosthesis. Dilatation of the tricuspid annulus is corrected by taking wide bites with each mattress suture. Mattress sutures are passed through the sewing ring of the valve prosthesis. The valve is seated into place and the sutures are tied. The atriotomy is closed with a continuous horizontal mattress pattern and oversewn with a simple continuous pattern. Dogs undergoing valve replacement with a bioprosthesis should be placed on anticoagulation therapy with warfarin (Winter *et al.* 2012) or a combination of an oral factor Xa inhibitor such as apixaban and clopidogrel (Gagnon *et al.* 2021) for three months after surgery to prevent thrombosis of the valve.

Outcomes

Tricuspid valve repair for tricuspid dysplasia generally does not abolish tricuspid regurgitation, but rather decreases torrential regurgitation to levels that can be tolerated for several years. Substantial reverse remodeling of the right heart can be expected, and this may further improve tricuspid regurgitation. Supraventricular tachyarrhythmias are sometimes observed as a late sequela. These are usually manageable with appropriate medical therapy and/or cardioversion. Results of dogs undergoing bioprosthesis valve replacement for TVD are reported (Arai *et al.* 2011). The surgery can be considered essentially curative provided that the valve prosthesis remains functional. Prosthesis-associated complications include thrombosis or late valve inflammatory pannus. Early valve thrombosis can usually be managed by more aggressive oral anticoagulation. Dogs undergoing bioprosthetic tricuspid valve replacement have remained free from clinical signs for periods of seven years or longer.

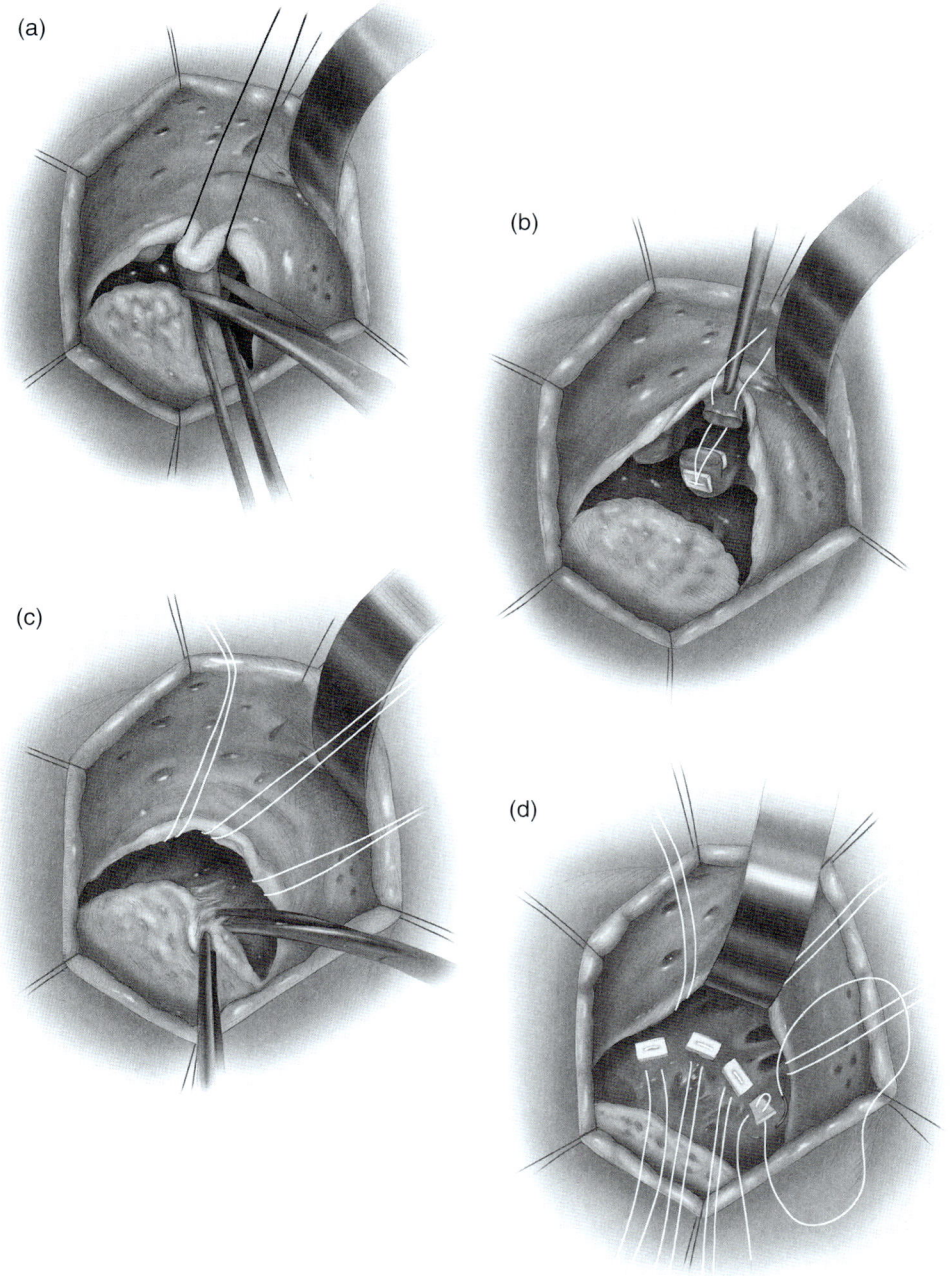

Figure 82.5 Tricuspid valve repair. (a) The direct papillary attachments to the mural leaflet are transected. (b) Polytetrafluoroethylene (PTFE) mattress sutures are placed between the cut end of the papillary and residual muscle on the leaflet. (c) The septal leaflet is then elevated from the septum by cutting shortened chordae and (d) resuspended with PTFE mattress sutures placed in the septum or right ventricular free wall. (e) Sutures are preplaced in the mural portion of the annulus and then through the annuloplasty band. (f) The annuloplasty band is tied down, the length of the neochords is adjusted, and they are tied. (g) A completed repair. © D. Giddings.

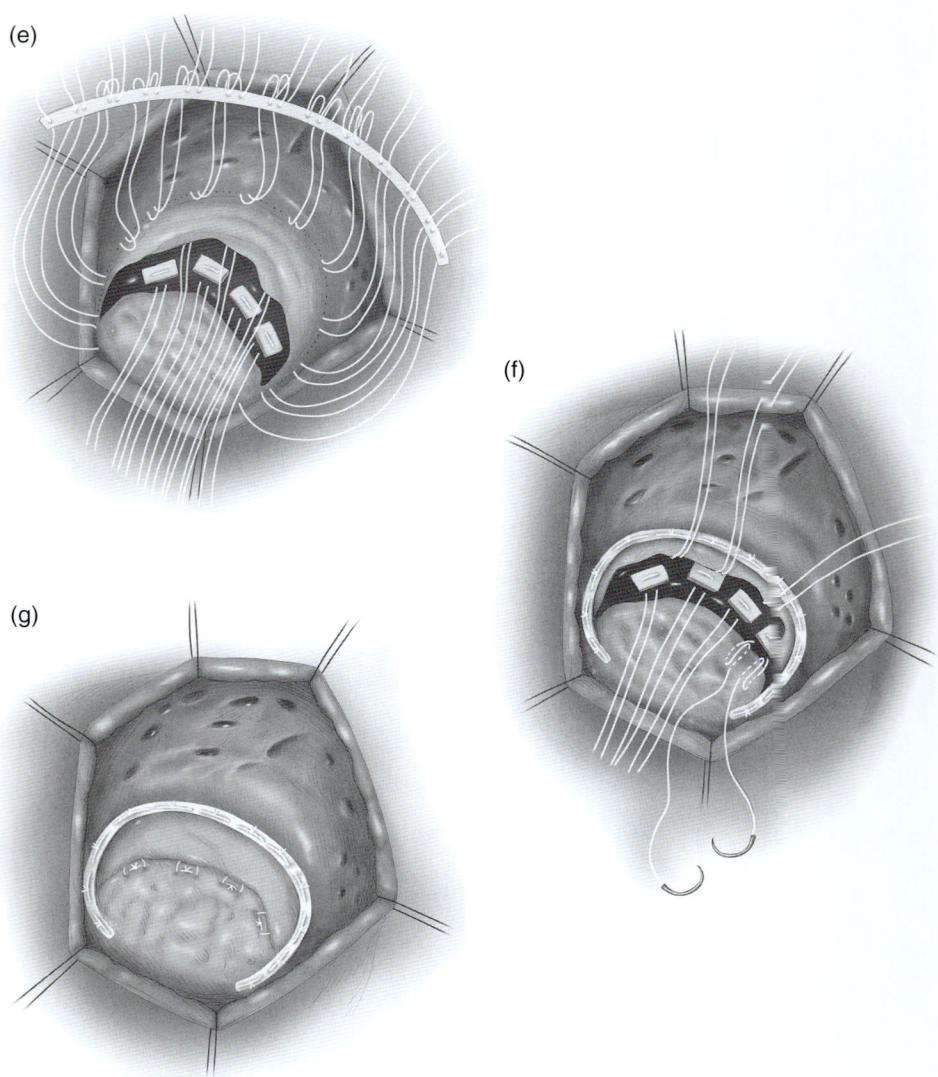

Figure 82.5 (Continued)

References

Arai, S., Griffiths, L.G., Mama, K. et al. (2011). Bioprosthesis valve replacement in dogs with congenital tricuspid valve dysplasia: technique and outcome. *Journal of Veterinary Cardiology* 13: 91–99.

Atkins, C., Bonagura, J., Ettinger, S. et al. (2009). Guidelines for the diagnosis and treatment of canine chronic valvular heart disease. *Journal of Veterinary Internal Medicine* 23: 1142–1150.

Behr, L., Chetboul, V., Sampedrano, C.C. et al. (2007). Beating heart mitral valve replacement with a bovine pericardial bioprosthesis for treatment of mitral valve dysplasia in a bull terrier. *Veterinary Surgery* 36: 190–198.

Boggs, L.S., Dewan, S.J., and Ballard, S.E. (1996). Mitral valve reconstruction in a toy-breed dog. *Journal of the American Veterinary Medical Association* 209: 1872–1876.

Bonow, R.O., Carabello, B.A., Chatterjee, K. et al. (2008). 2008 Focused update incorporated into the ACC/AHA 2006 guidelines for the management of patients with valvular heart disease: a report of the American College of Cardiology/American Heart Association Task Force on Practice Guidelines. *Circulation* 118: e523–e661.

Borenstein, N., Daniel, P., Behr, L. et al. (2004). Successful surgical treatment of mitral valve stenosis in a dog. *Veterinary Surgery* 33: 138–145.

Buchanan, J.W. (1999). Prevalence of cardiovascular disorders. In: *Textbook of Canine and Feline Cardiology*, 2e (ed. F.R. Fox, D.D. Sisson and N.S. Moise), 457. Philadelphia, PA: WB Saunders.

Carpentier, A. (1983). Cardiac valve surgery: the "French correction". *Journal of Thoracic and Cardiovascular Surgery* 86: 323–337.

Carpentier, A. (1994). Congenital malformations of the mitral valve. In: *Surgery for Congenital Heart Defects*, 2e (ed. J. Stark and M. de Leval), 599. Philadelphia, PA: WB Saunders.

Dalrymple-Hay, M.J.R., Bryant, M., Jones, R.A. et al. (1998). Degenerative mitral regurgitation: when should we operate. *Annals of Thoracic Surgery* 66: 579–1584.

Gagnon, A.L., Scansen, B.A., Olver, C. et al. (2021). Phase I clinical trial of an antithrombotic drug protocol combining apixaban and clopidogrel in dogs. *Journal of Veterinary Cardiology* 36: 105–114.

Griffiths, L.G., Boon, J., and Orton, E.C. (2004). Evaluation of techniques and outcomes of mitral valve repair in dogs. *Journal of the American Veterinary Medical Association* 224: 1941–1945.

Heath, B.J., Warren. E.T., and Nickels, B. (1991). Mitral valve replacement: techniques to eliminate myocardial rupture and prevent valvular disruption. *Annals of Thoracic Surgery* 52: 839–841.

Kamemoto, I., Shibata, S., Noguchi, H. et al. (1990). Successful mitral valvuloplasty for mitral regurgitation in a dog. *Japanese Journal of Veterinary Science* 52: 411–414.

Maisano, F., Torracca, L., Oppizzi, M. et al. (1998). The edge-to-edge technique: a simplified method to correct mitral insufficiency. *European Journal of Cardiothoracic Surgery* 13: 240–245.

Orton, E.C., Hackett, T.A., Mama, K., and Boon, J.A. (2005). Technique and outcome of mitral valve replacement in dogs. *Journal of the American Veterinary Medical Association* 226: 1508–1511.

Sutherland, B.J., Pierce, K.V., Heffner, G.G. et al. (2021). Surgical repair for canine tricuspid valve dysplasia: technique and case report. *Journal of Veterinary Cardiology* 33: 34–42.

Takashima, K., Soda, A., Tanaka, R., and Yamane, Y. (2007). Short-term performance of mitral valve replacement with porcine bioprosthetic valves in dogs. *Journal of Veterinary Medical Science* 69: 793–798.

Takashima, K., Soda, A., Tanaka, R., and Yamane, Y. (2008). Long-term clinical evaluation of mitral valve replacement with porcine bioprosthetic valves in dogs. *Journal of Veterinary Medical Science* 70: 279–283.

Triplett, D.A. (1998). Current recommendations for warfarin therapy. Use and monitoring. *Medical Clinics of North America* 82: 601–611.

Uechi, M. (2012). Mitral valve repair in dogs. *Journal of Veterinary Cardiology* 14: 185–192.

Uechi, M., Mizukoshi, T., Mizuno, T. et al. (2012). Mitral valve repair under cardiopulmonary bypass in small-breed dogs: 48 cases (2006–2009). *Journal for the American Veterinary Medical Association* 240: 1194–1201.

Winter, R.L., Sedacca, C.D., Adams, A., and Orton, E.C. (2012). Aortic thrombosis in dogs: presentation, therapy, and outcome in 26 cases. *Journal of Veterinary Cardiology* 14: 333–342.

83

Cardiac Neoplasia

E. Christopher Orton

A variety of primary intramural and intracavitary neoplasms have been reported in dogs, including hemangiosarcoma, fibrosarcoma, chondrosarcoma, rhabdomyosarcoma, ectopic thyroid carcinoma, fibroma, myxoma, and chemodectoma (Aronsohn 1985; Hayes & Sass 1988; Bright *et al.* 1990; Ware & Hopper 1999; Vicari *et al.* 2000). Lymphosarcoma and metastatic neoplasia are the most frequent cardiac neoplasms in cats (Tilley *et al.* 1981).

Hemangiosarcoma

Hemangiosarcoma is the most common cardiac neoplasm in dogs (Ware & Hopper 1999). The right auricle is the most frequent cardiac site for cardiac hemangiosarcoma. The most common clinical presentation for right atrial hemangiosarcoma is acute cardiac tamponade resulting from intrapericardial hemorrhage. Echocardiography confirms pericardial effusion and usually demonstrates a mass on the right auricle. Micrometastasis is present in virtually all cases at the time of diagnosis and hemangiosarcoma is regarded as universally fatal. Pericardiocentesis provides temporary relief of acute tamponade. Excision of the right atrial mass and subtotal pericardiectomy can be considered in some cases for palliative relief of recurrent cardiac tamponade (Figure 83.1). Median survival time after excision of right atrial hemangiosarcoma without adjuvant chemotherapy is approximately four months (Aronsohn 1985; Wykes *et al.* 1986). Survival times may be extended for dogs with adjuvant chemotherapy if

clean surgical margins at the primary surgery site can be achieved (Ogilvie *et al.* 1996; Weisse *et al.* 2005). Pericardiectomy without surgical excision of the primary tumor does not prolong survival (Dunning *et al.* 1998).

Aortic body tumors

Aortic body tumors account for approximately 80% of chemodectomas (Hayes & Sass 1988). Boxers, English bulldogs, and Boston terriers are affected most frequently. Residence at altitude and chronic hypoxia are thought to increase the risk for developing chemodectoma. Aortic body tumors are located at the base of the heart, between the outer wall of the ascending aorta and surrounding cardiac structures, including the pulmonary artery, right atrium, left atrium, or any combination of these. A strong presumptive diagnosis of aortic body tumor can be made based on this typical location. Aortic body tumors are highly vascular, slow growing, and moderately locally invasive. Initial growth of aortic body tumors displaces surrounding cardiac structures without causing adverse effects on cardiac function. Late in their course, aortic body tumors can grow into cardiac chambers, eventually resulting in obstruction to blood flow and heart failure. Aortic body tumors can also cause pericardial effusion, and this is the most likely reason for clinical signs early in their course. Aortic body tumors are often discovered incidentally on thoracic radiography or echocardiography performed for other reasons. Small heart base tumors can be surgically

(a)

(b)

(c)

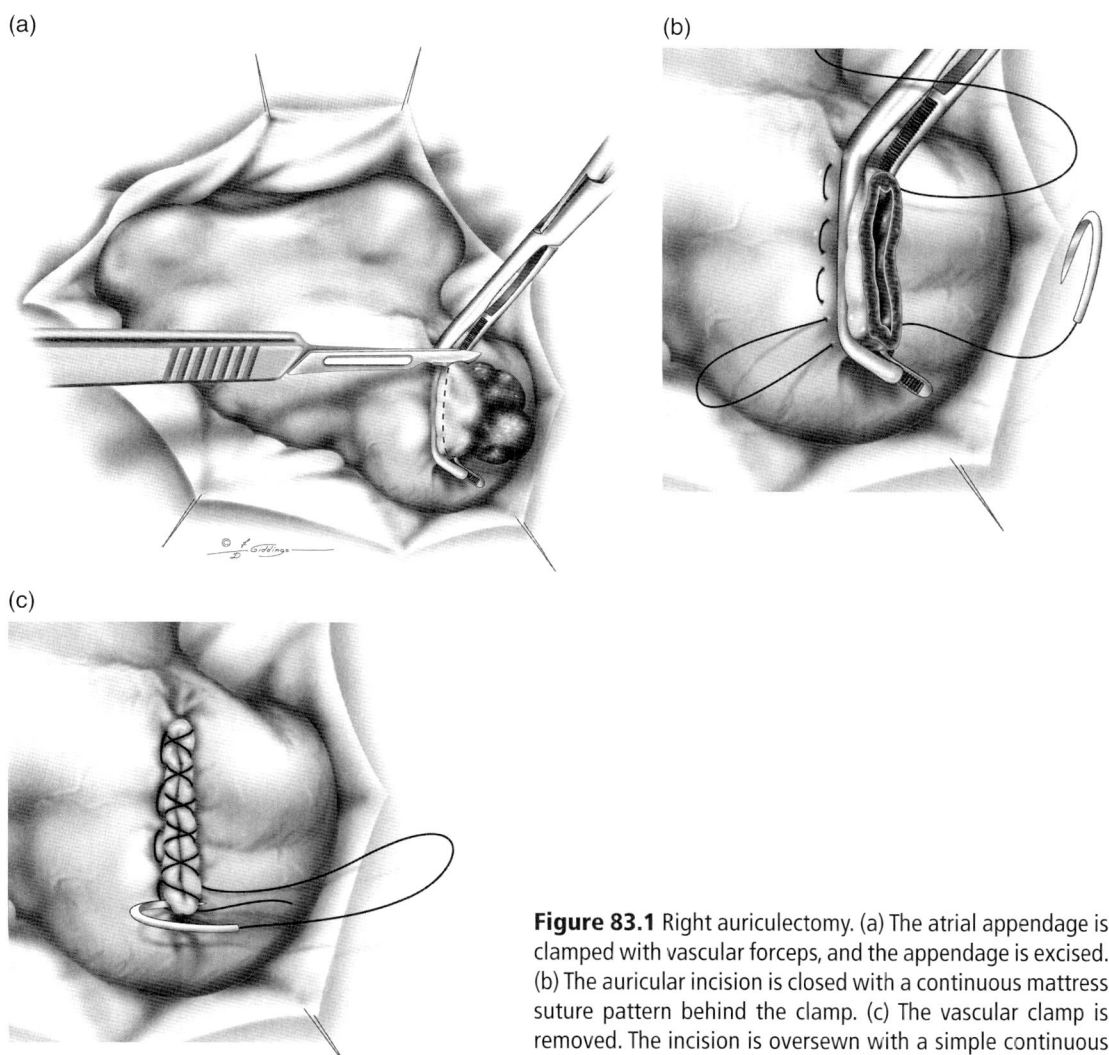

Figure 83.1 Right auriculectomy. (a) The atrial appendage is clamped with vascular forceps, and the appendage is excised. (b) The auricular incision is closed with a continuous mattress suture pattern behind the clamp. (c) The vascular clamp is removed. The incision is oversewn with a simple continuous pattern.

excised, but given their slow growth and the inherent risks associated with surgery (i.e., bleeding and vagal nerve injury), there is little evidence that surgical removal is beneficial. Large heart base tumors that have penetrated a cardiac chamber are not operable. Pericardectomy prolongs survival in dogs with aortic body tumors and should be considered as a palliative procedure regardless of whether pericardial effusion is present (Ehrhart *et al.* 2002).

Intraluminal tumors

Well-defined intraluminal tumors that obstruct blood flow through the right atrium or ventricle are occasionally seen in dogs. Most often these tumors are benign myxomas or thyroid carcinomas in the right heart (Bright *et al.* 1990; Bracha *et al.* 2009). Removal of these well-defined masses through the right atriotomy or ventriculotomy with inflow occlusion is possible in selected cases.

References

Aronsohn, M. (1985). Cardiac hemangiosarcoma in the dog: a review of 38 cases. *Journal of the American Veterinary Medical Association* 187: 922–926.

Bracha, S., Caron, I., Holberg, D.L. et al. (2009). Ectopic thyroid carcinoma causing right ventricular outflow tract obstruction in a dog. *Journal of the American Animal Hospital Association* 45: 138–141.

Bright, J.M., Toal, R.L., and Blackford, L.M. (1990). Right ventricular outflow obstruction caused by primary cardiac neoplasia: clinical features in two dogs. *Journal of Veterinary Internal Medicine* 4: 12–16.

Dunning, D., Monnet, E., Orton, E.C., and Salman, M.D. (1998). Analysis of prognosis indicators for dogs with pericardial effusion: 46 cases (1985–1996). *Journal of the American Veterinary Medical Association* 212: 1276–1280.

Ehrhart, N., Ehrhart, E.J., Willis, J. et al. (2002). Analysis of factors affecting survival in dogs with aortic body tumors. *Veterinary Surgery* 31: 44–48.

Hayes, H.M. and Sass, B. (1988). Chemoreceptor neoplasia: a study of the epidemiological features of 357 canine cases. *Journal of Veterinary Medicine Series A* 35: 401–408.

Ogilvie, G.K., Powers, B.E., Mallinckrodt, C.H., and Withrow, S.J. (1996). Surgery and doxorubicin in dogs with hemangiosarcoma. *Journal of Veterinary Internal Medicine* 10: 379–384.

Tilley, L.P., Bond, B., Patnaik, A.K., and Liu, S.K. (1981). Cardiovascular tumors in the cat. *Journal of the American Animal Hospital Association* 17: 1009–1021.

Vicari, E., Brown, D.C., Brockman, D.J. et al. (2000). Heart-base tumors in dogs: a retrospective study of 25 cases. *Veterinary Surgery* 29: 478.

Ware, W.A. and Hopper, D.L. (1999). Cardiac tumors in dogs: 1982–1995. *Journal of Veterinary Internal Medicine* 13: 95–103.

Weisse, W.C., Soares, N., Beal, M.W. et al. (2005). Survival times in dogs with right atrial hemangiosarcoma treated by means of surgical resection with or without adjuvant chemotherapy: 23 cases (1986–2000). *Journal of the American Veterinary Medical Association* 226: 575–579.

Wykes, P.M., Rouse, G.P., and Orton, E.C. (1986). Removal of five canine cardiac tumors using a stapling instrument. *Veterinary Surgery* 15: 103–106.

84

Congenital Pericardial Diseases

Eric Monnet

Congenital pericardial diseases or defects are rarely reported in small animals, probably because they do not induce a clinical condition. Most of the time, congenital pericardial diseases are diagnosed at the time of necropsy.

Absence of pericardium and pericardial defects

Absence of the pericardium is rare in dogs and cats (van den Ingh 1976; Bellah *et al*. 1989a). It does not precipitate clinical signs and is usually detected only at necropsy. Pericardial defects are typically associated with other congenital defects (Gaag & Luer 1976; Bellah *et al*. 1989a). Partial pericardial defects occur and represent a risk for cardiac herniation (Gaag & Luer 1976; van den Ingh 1976). Herniation of the right atrial appendage has been diagnosed in a young Labrador (Sisson & Thomas 1999).

Peritoneopericardial diaphragmatic hernia

Peritoneopericardial diaphragmatic hernia is the most common congenital pericardial defect in dogs and cats. As a result of the defect, abdominal contents can migrate into the pericardial sac (Figure 84.1). According to the Veterinary Medical Data Base at Purdue, from January 1993 to May 1994 peritoneopericardial diaphragmatic hernia was diagnosed in 0.015% of dogs and in 0.037% of cats presented at the Veterinary Medical Center (Sisson & Thomas 1999).

The condition results from faulty development of the septum transversum or from failure of the lateral pleuroperitoneal folds and the pars sternalis to unite (Evans & Biery 1980; Neiger 1996). It can occur as an isolated defect or very commonly with other midline defects such as umbilical hernia, cranial abdominal hernia, cardiac defect, or pectum excavatum (Figure 84.2) (Eyster *et al*. 1977; Bellah *et al*. 1989a,b). In cats, peritoneopericardial diaphragmatic hernia may be due to an autosomal recessive gene (Saperstein & Leipold 1976). Female cats may be more represented than male cats (Neiger 1996). For more information about peritoneopericardial diaphragmatic hernia, see Chapter 31.

Pericardial cysts

Pericardial cysts have been described mostly in companion animals aged under 3 years. Cysts are either unilocular or multilocular masses (Marion *et al*. 1970; Sisson *et al*. 1993; Less *et al*. 2000). On histologic analysis, some are thought to be cystic hematomas since they do not have an epithelial cell lining. Intrapericardial cysts have been associated with peritoneopericardial diaphragmatic hernia (Sisson *et al*. 1993). Cysts can be on a stalk at the apex of the pericardium. This suggests that pericardial cysts result from entrapment of omentum, falciform ligament, or liver in the pericardium during development (Bouvy & Bjorling 1991a,b; Sisson *et al*. 1993; Less *et al*. 2000).

Clinical findings

Dogs with pericardial cysts may show no clinical signs or may present with signs related to cardiac tamponade. Muffled heart sounds, distended jugular veins, a weak femoral pulse, ascites, and pleural effusion occur in dogs with pericardial cysts (Marion *et al*. 1970; Bouvy & Bjorling 1991b).

(a)

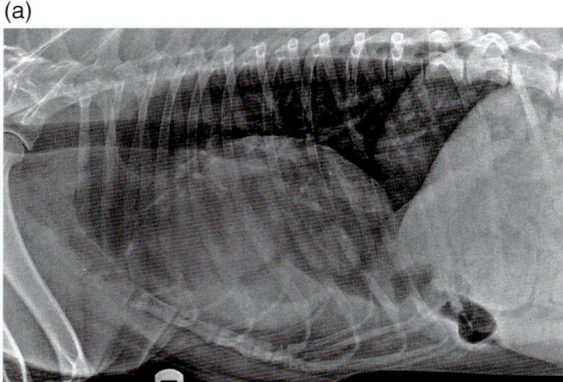

(b)

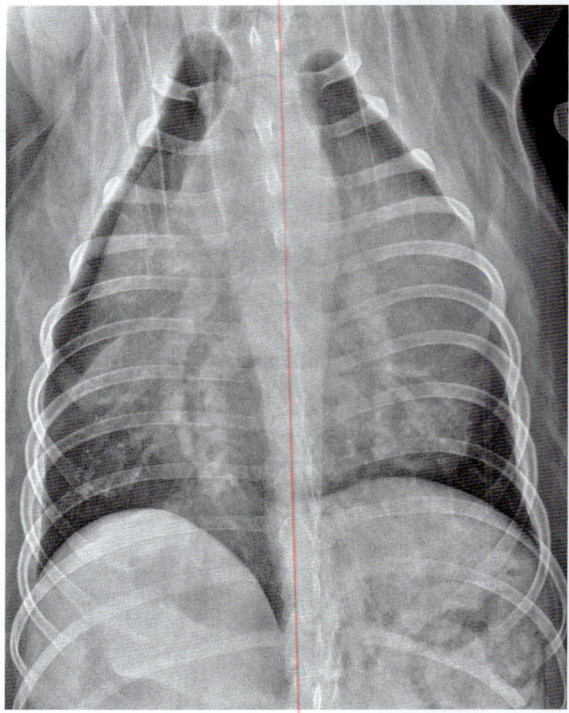

Figure 84.1 (a) Lateral thoracic radiograph of a dog with peritoneopericardial diaphragmatic hernia. Loops of bowel are present in the pericardial sac. The last two sternebrae have an abnormal conformation. (b) Ventrodorsal radiograph of the same dog. The pericardial sac is distended.

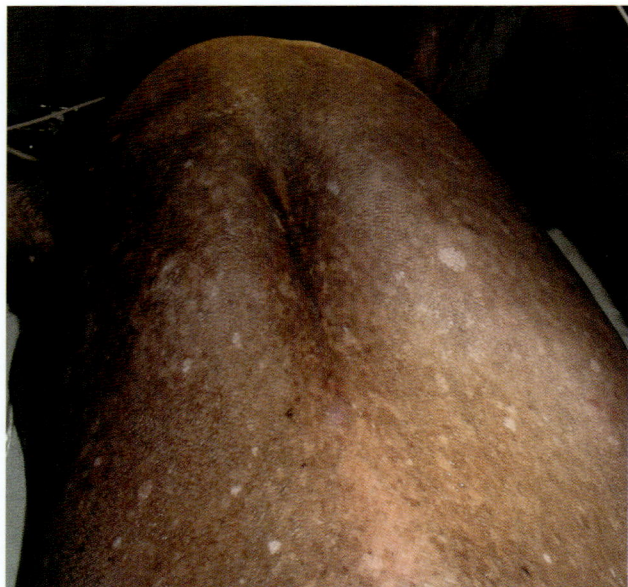

Figure 84.2 Cranial abdominal hernia in a dog with peritoneopericardial diaphragmatic hernia.

Direct impingement of the cyst on the left or right ventricle or fluid accumulation within the pericardium limits cardiac filling and reduces cardiac output (Less *et al.* 2000). Electrocardiography may show a decrease in the QRS amplitude with a modification of the mean electrical axis.

Thoracic radiography shows either a globoid or odd-shaped cardiac silhouette. Echocardiography allows visualization and definitive diagnosis of the pericardial cyst.

Treatment

If cardiac tamponade is due to excessive pericardial fluid, pericardiocentesis or cystocentesis is required before surgery. Median sternotomy facilitates exploration of the thoracic cavity, resection of the pericardial cyst, subtotal pericardiectomy, and repair of peritoneopericardial diaphragmatic hernia if needed. The prognosis is good if the cyst can be removed completely.

References

Bellah, J.R., Spencer, C.P., Brown, D.J., and Whitton, D.L. (1989a). Congenital cranioventral abdominal wall, caudal sternal, diaphragmatic, pericardial, and intracardiac defects in cocker spaniel littermates. *Journal of the American Veterinary Medical Association* 194: 1741–1746.

Bellah, J.R., Whitton, D.L., Ellison, G.W., and Phillips, L. (1989b). Surgical correction of concomitant cranioventral abdominal wall, caudal sternal, diaphragmatic, and pericardial defects in young dogs. *Journal of the American Veterinary Medical Association* 195: 1722–1726.

Bouvy, B.M. and Bjorling, D.E. (1991a). Pericardial effusion in dogs and cats. Part I. Normal pericardium and causes and pathophysiology of pericardial effusion. *Compendium on Continuing Education for the Practicing Veterinarian* 13: 417–424.

Bouvy, B.M. and Bjorling, D.E. (1991b). Pericardial effusion in dogs and cats. Part II. Diagnostic approach and treatment. *Compendium on Continuing Education for the Practicing Veterinarian* 13: 633–642.

Evans, S.M. and Biery, D.N. (1980). Congenital peritoneopericardial diaphragmatic hernia in the dog and cat: a literature review and 17 additional case histories. *Veterinary Radiology* 21: 108–116.

Eyster, G.E., Evans, A.T., Blanchard, G.L. et al. (1977). Congenital pericardial diaphragmatic hernia and multiple cardiac defects in a litter of collies. *Journal of the American Veterinary Medical Association* 170: 516–520.

Gaag, I.V. and Luer, J.T. (1976). Eight cases of pericardial defects in the dog. *Veterinary Pathology* 14: 14–18.

Less, R.D., Bright, J.M., and Orton, E.C. (2000). Intrapericardial cyst causing cardiac tamponade in a cat. *Journal of the American Animal Hospital Association* 36: 115–119.

Marion, J., Schwartz, A., Ettinger, S. et al. (1970). Pericardial effusion in a young dog. *Journal of the American Veterinary Medical Association* 157: 1055–1063.

Neiger, R. (1996). Peritoneopericardial diaphragmatic hernia in cats. *Compendium on Continuing Education for the Practicing Veterinarian* 18: 461–478.

Saperstein, G. and Leipold, H.W. (1976). Congenital defects in domestic cats. *Feline Practice* 6: 18–43.

Sisson, D. and Thomas, W.P. (1999). Pericardial disease and cardiac tumors. In: *Textbook of Canine and Feline Cardiology*, 2e (ed. P.R. Fox, D.D. Sisson and N.S. Moise), 679–699. Philadelphia, PA: WB Saunders.

Sisson, D., Thomas, W.P., Reed, J. et al. (1993). Intrapericardial cysts in the dog. *Journal of Veterinary Internal Medicine* 7: 364–369.

van den Ingh, T.S. (1976). Pericardial defect with incarceration of the heart in a dog. *Schweizer Archiv für Tierheilkunde* 119: 473–476.

85

Constrictive Pericarditis

Eric Monnet

Constrictive pericarditis compromises cardiac filling by causing a nondistensible, thickened, and fibrotic pericardium. This condition has been reported in dogs aged 3–10 years (Thomas *et al.* 1984; Campbell *et al.* 1995; Wright *et al.* 1996).

Etiology

Constrictive pericarditis is the end stage of an inflammatory process involving the pericardium. It can result from any chronic pericarditis (LeWinter & Kabbani 2005). Chronic idiopathic pericardial effusion, neoplasia, foreign material (e.g., bullets), and infection (coccidiomycosis) are most commonly reported in cases with constrictive pericarditis (Thomas *et al.* 1984; Wright *et al.* 1996; Sisson & Thomas 1999; Miller & Sisson 2000).

In most cases, the parietal pericardium is more severely affected than the visceral pericardium. The parietal pericardium can be up to 8 mm thick. In some cases, the visceral and parietal pericardium are both affected with severe adhesions between them. Pericardial fluid may be present and if so the condition is called effusive-constrictive pericarditis. Mesothelial proliferation, inflammation, and fibrous tissue are common findings on histology (Thomas *et al.* 1984; Wright *et al.* 1996; Sisson & Thomas 1999; Miller & Sisson 2000). The fibrosis and scarring are usually uniform and impede filling of all the cardiac chambers. Filling pressures in all the chambers rise and are equalized across the heart. Systemic and pulmonary vein pressures rise as the heart tries to compensate.

The resultant clinical signs are consistent with right-sided heart failure (LeWinter & Kabbani 2005).

Pathophysiology

Constrictive pericarditis affects late diastole. During early diastole the ventricles fill abnormally rapidly because of elevated atrial pressures. The filling is accentuated because of active early suction from the ventricles. The suction of the ventricles is increased because of small end-systolic volumes. During mid-diastole, ventricular filling is abruptly halted when the limit of pericardial distensibility is reached. Therefore, most ventricular filling occurs during early to mid-diastole. Systemic venous congestion induces congestion of the liver, resulting in rounding of the liver edges, distension of hepatic veins, and ascites. Peripheral edema can develop in very severe cases. Cardiac output is reduced as a consequence of reduced left ventricular filling. Myocardial contractile function is preserved, although ejection fraction may appear reduced because of reduced preload. If the inflammatory process reaches the myocardium and fibrosis occurs, true contractile dysfunction can result that will impair the efficacy of a pericardiectomy (LeWinter & Kabbani 2005) Fibrosis of the pericardium interferes with the transmission of intrathoracic pressure changes to the cardiac chambers during respiration. However, those changes are still transmitted to the pulmonary circulation. In inspiration the drop in intrathoracic pressure is transmitted to the pulmonary veins but not the left atrium. Therefore the pressure gradient between the pulmonary vein and the left atrium is reduced, creating a decreased flow of blood into the atrium and across the mitral valve. This reduction in left ventricular filling allows a septal shift to occur that results in an increase in right ventricular filling (Wolozin *et al.* 1988; Oh *et al.* 1994). Inhibition of atrial natriuretic peptide and reduction in cardiac output stimulate sodium retention, which will exacerbate systemic venous congestion (Wolozin *et al.* 1988). Fluid retention and signs of right-sided congestive heart failure can result from activation of the renin–angiotensin system.

The atrial and ventricular pressure tracings classically show a rapid *y* descent followed by an abrupt rise to an elevated diastolic plateau. This is referred to as the "square root sign" and is considered diagnostic for pericardial constriction. If a small amount of pericardial fluid is present, the rapid *y* descent is absent.

Pulmonary capillary wedge pressure and right ventricular, right atrial, and left ventricular diastolic pressures are all elevated and equal with constrictive pericarditis. If localized fibrosis is affecting one cardiac chamber more than the other, this hemodynamic finding may not hold. Also, if the patient is volume contracted (e.g., from diuretics), volume loading with crystalloid fluids may be required to demonstrate these classic hemodynamic changes. As the fibrosis worsens, cardiac output declines.

Central venous pressure does not decrease during inspiration because negative intrathoracic pressure during inspiration is not transmitted to the cardiac chambers. Augmentation or no change of systemic venous pressure during inspiration with constrictive pericarditis is referred to as the Kussmaul sign.

Diagnosis

History and physical examination

Dogs usually present with exercise intolerance, weakness, dyspnea, and collapse. Weight loss has been reported in chronic cases. Physical examination usually reveals signs of right-sided heart failure, including distended jugular veins and abdominal distension due to ascites. Heart sounds are decreased only if pericardial effusion is present (Thomas *et al.* 1984; Sisson & Thomas 1999; Miller & Sisson 2000).

Electrocardiography

Sinus tachycardia with prolonged P-wave duration and reduced QRS complex amplitude are common findings with constrictive pericarditis. Supraventricular tachycardia or atrial fibrillation is also common (Thomas *et al.* 1984; Sisson & Thomas 1999).

Radiography

On thoracic radiographs, the heart may appear globoid with loss of cardiac waist. Caudal vena cava enlargement and pleural effusion may be present. Reduction in the motion of the wall of the cardiac chambers is visible on fluoroscopy. Compression of the right ventricular outflow tract has been reported in dogs (Thomas *et al.* 1984; Sisson & Thomas 1999).

Echocardiography

It is difficult to definitely determine pericardial thickening on echocardiography except in extreme cases. If pericardial fluid is present, the thickness of the pericardium can be appreciated. M-mode often reveals flattening of the mid to late diastolic motion of the left ventricular free wall, which supports a finding of pericardial constriction. During ventricular filling, the left ventricular wall abruptly stops and becomes flat. A rapid early diastolic slope of the mitral valve may be present. Doppler flow–velocity measurements reveal exaggerated respiratory variation in both mitral inflow velocity and tricuspid–mitral inflow differences, with a pathologically elevated E/A ratio. Even in the face of concurrent cardiac tamponade, these inflow patterns have good sensitivity and specificity for constrictive pericarditis, and also help distinguish it from restrictive cardiomyopathy. Mitral E velocity is increased by at least 25% in expiration compared with inspiration. During inspiration the decrease in left ventricular filling results in a leftward septal shift, allowing flow in the right ventricle with an elevated tricuspid E velocity. Premature opening of the pulmonary valve may also be present because of elevated right ventricular pressures (Feigenbaum 1994; Armstrong 2005; LeWinter & Kabbani 2005).

Cardiac catheterization

After placement of an introducer in the jugular vein, a pulmonary artery catheter is introduced through the jugular vein and passed into the pulmonary artery. The pulmonary artery catheter is connected to a fluid-filled pressure transducer and pressure monitoring equipment. The pressure transducer is placed at the level of the right atrium. Pulmonary capillary wedge pressure is measured by inflation of the balloon at the tip of the pulmonary artery catheter. Pulmonary capillary wedge pressure is measured at the end of expiration. After recording the pulmonary capillary wedge pressure, the pulmonary artery catheter is withdrawn while the pressure monitor records the pressure wave at the tip of the pulmonary artery catheter. Pulmonary artery, right ventricular, and right atrial pressures will be successively traced. Diastolic pressures in the right ventricle and right atrium and the pulmonary capillary wedge pressures are then compared to establish the diagnosis of constrictive pericarditis.

Differentiating constrictive pericarditis from restrictive cardiomyopathy

The most important differential diagnosis is with restrictive cardiomyopathy. Usually patients with restrictive cardiomyopathy have thick-walled ventricles due to the infiltrative process occurring in the cardiac muscle, in contrast to those with constrictive pericarditis who have thickening of the pericardium on echocardiography. Doppler echocardiography shows an enhanced respiratory variation in mitral inflow velocity (>25%). During cardiac catheterization the diastolic pressure in the left ventricle is higher than that in the right ventricle with restrictive cardiomyopathy, while these pressures are equal with constrictive pericarditis. Marked elevation of right ventricular systolic pressure is present with restrictive cardiomyopathy associated with pulmonary hypertension (LeWinter & Kabbani 2005).

Treatment

Subtotal or complete pericardiectomy is the treatment of choice for constrictive pericarditis when the parietal pericardium is involved (Figure 85.1). A median sternotomy is recommended to visualize both sides of the heart during the dissection. The clinical outcome of the procedure is expected to be favorable. However, if the epicardium is involved, decortication of the affected tissue is required and the prognosis is more guarded (Figure 85.2). Laceration of a coronary artery, pulmonary thromboembolism, and arrhythmias are possible complications of cardiac decortication (Orton 1995; Sisson & Thomas 1999; LeWinter & Kabbani 2005).

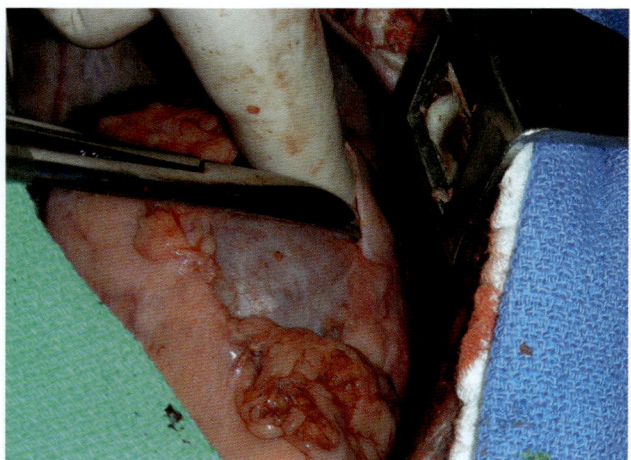

Figure 85.1 Constrictive pericarditis: the pericardium is very fibrotic and is dissected.

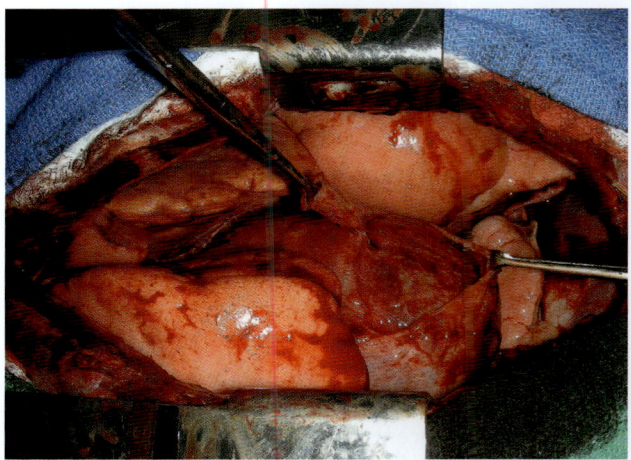

Figure 85.2 Constrictive pericarditis and epicarditis requiring decortication.

References

Armstrong, W.F. (2005). Echocardiography. In: *Braunwald's Heart Disease: A Textbook of Cardiovascular Medicine*, 7e (ed. D.P. Zipes, P. Libby, R.O. Bonow and E. Braunvald), 187–270. Philadelphia, PA: Elsevier Saunders.

Campbell, S.L., Forrester, S.D., Johnston, S.A. et al. (1995). Chylothorax associated with constrictive pericarditis in a dog. *Journal of the American Veterinary Medical Association* 206: 1561–1564.

Feigenbaum, H. (1994). Pericardial disease. In: *Echocardiography*, 656–676. Philadelphia, PA: Lea & Febiger.

LeWinter, M.M. and Kabbani, S. (2005). Pericardial disease. In: *Braunwald's Heart Disease. A Textbook of Cardiovascular Medicine*, 7e (ed. D.P. Zipes, P. Libby, R.O. Bonow and E. Braunwald), 1757–1780. Philadelphia, PA: Elsevier Saunders.

Miller, M.W. and Sisson, D.D. (2000). Pericardial disorders. In: *Textbook of Veterinary Internal Medicine* (ed. S J. Ettinger and E.C. Feldman), 923–936. Philadelphia, PA: WB Saunders.

Oh, J.K., Hatle, L.K., Seward, J.B. et al. (1994). Diagnostic role of Doppler echocardiography in constrictive pericarditis. *Journal of the American College of Cardiology* 23: 154–162.

Orton, E.C. (1995). Pericardium. In: *Small Animal Thoracic Surgery* (ed. E.C. Orton, T.O. McCracken and C.C. Cann), 177–185. Baltimore, MD: Williams & Wilkins.

Sisson, D. and Thomas, W.P. (1999). Pericardial disease and cardiac tumors. In: *Textbook of Canine and Feline Cardiology*, 2e (ed. P.R. Fox, D.D. Sisson and N.S. Moise), 679–699. Philadelphia, PA: WB Saunders.

Thomas, W.P., Reed, J.R., Bauer, T.G., and Breznock, E.M. (1984). Constrictive pericardial disease in the dog. *Journal of the American Veterinary Medical Association* 184: 546–553.

Wolozin, M.W., Ortola, F.V., Spodick, D.H., and Seifter, J.L. (1988). Release of atrial natriuretic factor after pericardiectomy for chronic constrictive pericarditis. *American Journal of Cardiology* 62: 1323–1325.

Wright, K.N., DeNovo, R.C. Jr., Patton, C.S. et al. (1996). Effusive-constrictive pericardial disease secondary to osseous metaplasia of the pericardium in a dog. *Journal of the American Veterinary Medical Association* 209: 2091–2095.

86

Pericardial Effusion

Eric Monnet

The pericardium is composed of two layers. The visceral pericardium is a serous membrane of a single layer of mesothelial cells firmly adhered to the epicardium. The parietal pericardium is fibrous, with a thickness of 2 mm in a normal patient. It is acellular and contains mostly collagen and elastin fibers. The fibers of collagen are organized in wavy bundles that can stretch. When they align, the stiffness of the pericardium is increased. The parietal pericardium is attached to the great vessels. The visceral pericardium reflects back at the level of the great vessels to become the inner layer of the parietal pericardium. The parietal pericardium is covered by the visceral pleura on the outside (LeWinter & Kabbani 2005). Between the two layers of pericardium a small amount of pericardial fluid is present. The fluid is mostly present at the level of the atrioventricular groove (Santamore et al. 1990).

Etiology

Any infection, autoimmune disease, or inflammatory process that can trigger a pericarditis can cause pleural effusion (Brownlie & Clayton-Jones 1985; de Madron 1990; Bouvy & Bjorling 1991a; Berg 1994; Dunning et al. 1998; Sisson & Thomas 1999; Covey & Connolly 2018; Lakhdhir et al. 2020). Neoplasia of the heart can also cause pericardial effusion. Noninflammatory disease, including hypothyroidism and amyloidosis, has been reported to cause pericardial effusion in human patients (Cacoub et al. 2000; LeWinter & Kabbani 2005). Pericardial effusion is most commonly idiopathic in origin in dogs (Dunning et al. 1998; Aronsohn & Carpenter 1999).

Pericardial effusions are categorized by the clinicopathologic characteristics of the fluid that accumulates. A transudate occurs secondary to congestive heart failure, peritoneopericardial diaphragmatic hernia, hypoalbuminemia, or increased vascular permeability (Lombard 1983; Berg & Wingfield 1984; Berg et al. 1984; Brownlie & Clayton-Jones 1985; de Madron et al. 1987; de Madron 1990; Bouvy & Bjorling 1991b; Berg 1994; Dunning et al. 1998; Sisson & Thomas 1999). Hemorrhagic pericardial effusion results from trauma, rupture of the left atrium secondary to mitral valve disease, intoxication with anticoagulants, or neoplasia, or it may be idiopathic (Price & Mullen 1966; Buchanan 1972; Kagan 1980; Berry et al. 1988a; Vogtli et al. 1997; Petrus & Henik 1999). An exudate results from infectious on noninfectious pericarditis (Bouvy & Bjorling 1991a; de Laforcade et al. 2005).

Pericarditis

Pericarditis has been associated with feline cardiomyopathy and feline infectious peritonitis (Owens 1977; Fossum et al. 1994). Fungal pericarditis is unusual, with the exception of that caused by *Coccidioides immitis* in dogs living in the southwestern USA (Miller & Sisson 2000; Heinritz et al. 2005). Infectious pericardial effusion has been reported in dogs (Aronson & Gregory 1995).

Idiopathic pericardial effusion

Idiopathic pericardial effusion is the most common cause of acute or chronic nonneoplastic hemorrhagic pericardial effusion in the dog (Berg et al. 1984; Dunning

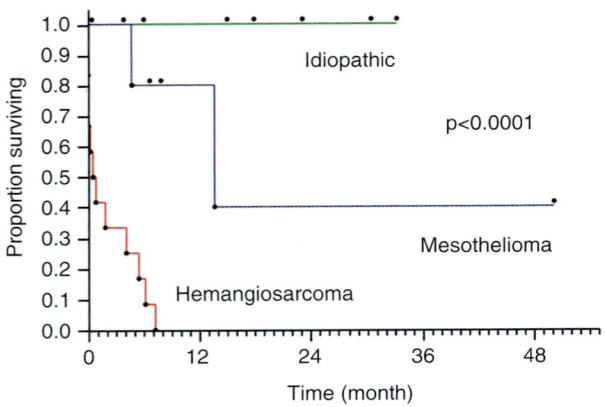

Figure 86.1 Kaplan–Meier actuarial survival curve of dogs presented with pericardial effusion. Dogs with an idiopathic pericardial effusion have an excellent prognosis. Source: From Dunning et al. (1998).

et al. 1998; Aronsohn & Carpenter 1999; Miller & Sisson 2000). The prognosis of dogs with idiopathic pericardial effusion is excellent (Figure 86.1) (Dunning et al. 1998).

Neoplastic pericardial effusion

Neoplasia of the heart, heart base, or pericardium is the second most common cause of hemorrhagic pericardial effusion in dogs.

Hemangiosarcoma of the right atrium

Hemangiosarcoma of the right atrium is the most common cardiac neoplasm (Berg & Wingfield 1984; Aronsohn 1985; Rush et al. 1990; de Madron 1991; Bradley et al. 1992; Gonin-Jmaa et al. 1996; Dunning et al. 1998; Closa et al. 1999; Miller & Sisson 2000). This tumor is often multicentric, involving the spleen or liver at the time of pericardial effusion. Echocardiography is the most sensitive test for the diagnosis of a right atrial tumor. Hemangiosarcoma of the right atrium carries a poor prognosis because by the time of diagnosis the tumor has already metastasized (Dunning et al. 1998; Weisse et al. 2005). In a study on 46 dogs with pericardial effusion, Dunning et al. (1998) showed that the median survival of the 11 dogs with hemangiosarcoma was 16 days. Pericardiectomy did not improve long-term survival of the dogs with a right atrial appendage. In a study on 23 dogs with pericardial effusion and hemangiosarcoma of the right atrium, Weisse et al. (2005) showed that atrial appendage resection was associated with a low complication rate. The median survival of dogs in that study was 46 days after pericardiectomy and right atrial appendage resection and 164 days after pericardiectomy, right atrial appendage resection, and chemotherapy.

Chemodectoma or heart base tumor

The term "heart base tumor" has been used to describe any kind of tumor situated at the base of the heart. Chemodectoma is the most common tumor at the base of the heart and the second most common cardiac tumor (Berg & Wingfield 1984; Aronsohn 1985; Rush et al. 1990; de Madron 1991; Bradley et al. 1992; Gonin-Jmaa et al. 1996; Dunning et al. 1998; Closa et al. 1999; Miller & Sisson 2000; Macdonald et al. 2009; Hansen et al. 2021). Ectopic thyroid mass, mesothelioma, lymphosarcoma, and sarcomas have been diagnosed at the base of the heart (Macdonald et al. 2009). A heart base tumor is most commonly seen in brachycephalic dogs, which is thought to be related to hypoxemia (Patnaik et al. 1975). It is usually undiagnosed until the dog has a pericardial effusion severe enough to induce clinical signs or cardiac tamponade with collapse. Pericardiectomy alone significantly improves survival. Median survival of dogs with a heart base tumor was 730 days after pericardiectomy alone and 42 days without surgery (Ehrhart et al. 2002).

Mesothelioma

Mesothelioma of the pericardium is another cause of a hemorrhagic pericardial effusion (Berg & Wingfield 1984; Aronsohn 1985; Rush et al. 1990; de Madron 1991; Bradley et al. 1992; Gonin-Jmaa et al. 1996; Dunning et al. 1998; Closa et al. 1999; Miller & Sisson 2000). Cytology is not diagnostic for mesothelioma. The diagnosis requires histologic evaluation of the pericardium and mediastinal lymph nodes draining the pericardium and pleural surface (McDonough et al. 1992; Sisson & Thomas 1999). Pericardiectomy palliates the clinical signs and is associated with a 15-month median survival (Dunning et al. 1998). A severe pleural effusion usually develops after pericardiectomy (Sisson & Thomas 1999).

Pathophysiology of cardiac tamponade

Cardiac tamponade is a life-threatening, slow, or rapid compression of the heart due to the pericardial accumulation of fluids, blood, or pus (Spodick 2003). The pericardium is fairly noncompliant. The stress–strain curve of the normal pericardium is J-shaped. Pericardial pressure begins to rise after 5–60 mL of fluid accumulates within the pericardium. The capacitance of the pericardium is influenced by the rate of fluid accumulation. Hypertrophy of the pericardium by slow stretching allows augmentation of pericardial volume and rightward shift of the pressure–volume curve of the pericardium. As a result, the pericardium can accumulate a larger volume of fluid before pressure begins to rise. However, beyond a certain point the volume of the pericardium is fixed and pressure increases quickly with a small additional increase in volume. When the pericardium is thickened, as is the case with constrictive pericardial disease, a minor increase in volume causes a significant increase in pericardial pressure (Reddy & Curtiss 1990; Ameli & Shah 1991; Kirkland & Taylor 1992; Fowler 1994; Hancock 1994; Spodick 1998, 2003).

Elevation in pericardial pressure decreases myocardial compliance, which increases diastolic pressure within the heart. In the normal condition, right atrial pressure and pericardial pressure are equal. Therefore a slight increase in pericardial pressure will affect the right atrium first. Raised pericardial pressure first collapses the thin right atrium, then the right ventricle. The left ventricle is barely, if at all, directly compressed. As fluid accumulation increases, the right and left atrial pressures and ventricular diastolic pressures gradually rise and equilibrate with pericardial pressure. Pericardial pressure dictates intracavitary filling pressure. Since transmural filling pressures of the cardiac chambers are very low, cardiac volume decreases until they are very small, inducing a small stroke volume and cardiac output (Reddy & Curtiss 1990; Ameli & Shah 1991; Kirkland & Taylor 1992; Fowler 1994; Hancock 1994; Spodick 1998, 2003; LeWinter & Kabbani 2005; Shabetai 2007).

Cardiac tamponade increases ventricular interaction, resulting in pulsus paradoxus, a greater than normal reduction of systolic pressure during inspiration. A decrease in systolic blood pressure exceeding 10 mmHg on inspiration is a common finding in mild to severe cardiac tamponade (Shabetai 2007). Cardiac volume is not changed but redistributed during inspiration. Pulsus paradoxus affects both the pulmonary and systemic circulations, but the effects are almost 180° out of phase, with the peak systolic pressure of one ventricle highest when that of the other ventricle is lowest (LeWinter & Kabbani 2005; Shabetai 2005, 2007). During inspiration, pericardial pressure and right ventricular pressure decrease. Venous return to the right atrium and ventricle is increased. However, because the volume is limited by the pericardium, there is a leftward shift of the septum. Left ventricular end-diastolic volume is decreased, resulting in a reduction in cardiac output and arterial pressure during inspiration. Venous return is confined to the ejection phase, instead of taking place during the ejection period and after opening of the atrioventricular valves during the diastolic phase. Therefore, the jugular pulse shows a prominent x descent but not a y descent. Pulsus paradoxus is not pathognomonic for cardiac tamponade, but can occur with constrictive pericarditis, pulmonary embolism, hypovolemic shock, and pulmonary disease (asthma, emphysema) with large variations in intrathoracic pressure (LeWinter & Kabbani 2005).

Decreased cardiac output results in activation of the renin–angiotensin–aldosterone system, causing retention of sodium and water. Activation of the sympathetic nervous system results in inotropic and chronotropic effects, and vasoconstriction (Friedman *et al.* 1977). Patients on β-blockers may not exhibit a normal sympathetic response to cardiac tamponade and may show clinical signs earlier (Friedman *et al.* 1977; LeWinter & Kabbani 2005). Atrial natriuretic factor is not increased during cardiac tamponade to counteract these effects, because the atrium is still supported by the pericardium, which limits its dilatation. As a result, cardiac tamponade is associated with increases in systemic venous and portal pressures causing jugular distension, fluid transudation from systemic capillary beds to produce peripheral edema, and liver congestion and ascites (Reddy & Curtiss 1990; Ameli & Shah 1991; Kirkland & Taylor 1992; Fowler 1994; Hancock 1994; Spodick 1998, 2003).

Diagnosis

The manifestations of pericardial effusion depend on the rate of effusion formation and rise in intrapericardial pressure. Animals present with signs of chronic pericardial effusion more often than they do with acute pericardial effusion. Animals with chronic pericardial effusion due to idiopathic causes or right atrial tumor may present with apparent acute manifestation because of the acute onset of bleeding. Clinical signs of the underlying disease such as disseminated neoplasia or infection might predominate at presentation. A left apical systolic murmur suggests the possibility of a left atrial tear due to chronic mitral regurgitation (Berg & Wingfield 1984; Berg *et al.* 1984, 1985; Rush *et al.* 1990; Dunning *et al.* 1998; Aronsohn & Carpenter 1999).

Signalment and history

Acute pericardial effusion causes acute hypotension, rapidly progressing weakness, dyspnea, collapse, and cardiogenic shock. Death may occur. This is the most common presentation for animals with left atrial tears, acute neoplastic hemorrhage, or traumatic laceration of a coronary artery (Berg & Wingfield 1984; Berg *et al.* 1984, 1985; de Madron *et al.* 1987; Rush *et al.* 1990; Bouvy & Bjorling 1991b; Dunning *et al.* 1998; Aronsohn & Carpenter 1999).

Animals with chronic pericardial effusions present with a history of exercise intolerance, lethargy, anorexia, dyspnea, and weakness. Occasionally, owners report

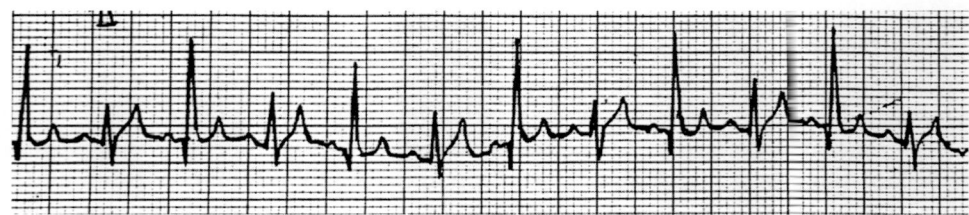

Figure 86.2 Electrocardiogram of a dog with severe pericardial effusion. The amplitude of the QRS complexes alternates between tall and short.

collapsing episodes, and they often report gradual onset of abdominal distension.

Physical examination

The classic signs for chronic pericardial effusion consist of muffled heart sounds, weak femoral pulse, and distended systemic veins. Chronic pericardial effusion commonly induces signs of right-sided congestive heart failure such as pleural effusion or ascites (Berg & Wingfield 1984; Berg *et al.* 1984, 1985; de Madron *et al.* 1987; Rush *et al.* 1990; Bouvy & Bjorling 1991b; Dunning *et al.* 1998; Aronsohn & Carpenter 1999; Miller & Sisson 2000).

Cardiac tamponade is associated with jugular venous distension, weak femoral pulse, and tachycardia. Central venous pressure frequently exceeds 10–12 mmHg. The lateral saphenous veins are usually distended. With the animal in lateral recumbency, the saphenous vein does not collapse when a pelvic limb is raised above the level of the heart. Heart sounds are diminished on auscultation. Abdominal distension with abdominal fluid and an enlarged liver are frequent findings. Pulsus paradoxus can be present in severe cases. Weight loss is common in dogs with chronic pericardial effusion (Berg & Wingfield 1984; Berg *et al.* 1984, 1985; de Madron *et al.* 1987; Rush *et al.* 1990; Bouvy & Bjorling 1991b; Dunning *et al.* 1998; Aronsohn & Carpenter 1999; Miller & Sisson 2000).

Laboratory evaluation

While bloodwork will not provide a specific diagnosis for pericardial effusion, the importance of performing a complete blood count and chemistry profile relates to the assessment of anesthetic eligibility and the evaluation of concurrent diseases that might be present. Liver enzymes may be elevated because of liver congestion resulting from decreased venous return.

Cytology and analysis of pericardial effusion are important for differentiating between a transudate, exudate, or hemorrhage (Berg & Wingfield 1984; Berg *et al.* 1984, 1985; de Madron *et al.* 1987; Rush *et al.* 1990; Bouvy & Bjorling 1991b; Dunning *et al.* 1998; Aronsohn & Carpenter 1999; Miller & Sisson 2000). Usually

pericardial fluid does not clot unless active hemorrhage is present. The packed cell volume of the fluid is less than the packed cell volume of the peripheral blood, unless there is active hemorrhage. The presence of an exudate would indicate active pericarditis. A transudate would be present with congestive heart failure.

Cytology of the pericardial fluid is not reliable for determining the presence of neoplasia (Sisson *et al.* 1984; Edwards 1996; de Laforcade *et al.* 2005). Reactive mesothelial cells are often present and do not correlate with a diagnosis of mesothelioma. The pH of freshly sampled effusate has been suggested to determine the origin of the pericardial effusion (Edwards 1996). An effusion of neoplastic origin is reputed to have a pH greater than 7.5 (Edwards 1996). In a study on 41 dogs with pericardial effusion, pH, bicarbonate and chloride were significantly lower in dogs with neoplasia, whereas lactate, hematocrit, and urea nitrogen were significantly higher in the pericardial fluid of dogs with neoplasia (de Laforcade *et al.* 2005). However, these differences were not clinically significant enough to differentiate a benign from a malignant pericardial effusion (de Laforcade *et al.* 2005). If cytology is suggestive of infection, a sample should be submitted for bacterial and fungal culture.

Electrocardiography

A reduction in QRS amplitude may be present on several or all leads when pericardial fluid is present. Electrical alternans, due to motion or swinging of the beating heart, may be present on the electrocardiogram (Figure 86.2) (Bonagura 1981).

Radiography

Thoracic radiography usually demonstrates abnormalities. When there is significant accumulation of pericardial fluid, the cardiac silhouette loses its angles and waists (Figure 86.3). If the effusion is chronic, the cardiac silhouette becomes globoid in shape. Pulmonary vasculature is often reduced as a result of low perfusion. Heart base tumors may deviate the trachea dorsally or laterally (Berg *et al.* 1984; Farrow 1984; Aronsohn 1985; Gores *et al.* 1994). Computed tomography and magnetic

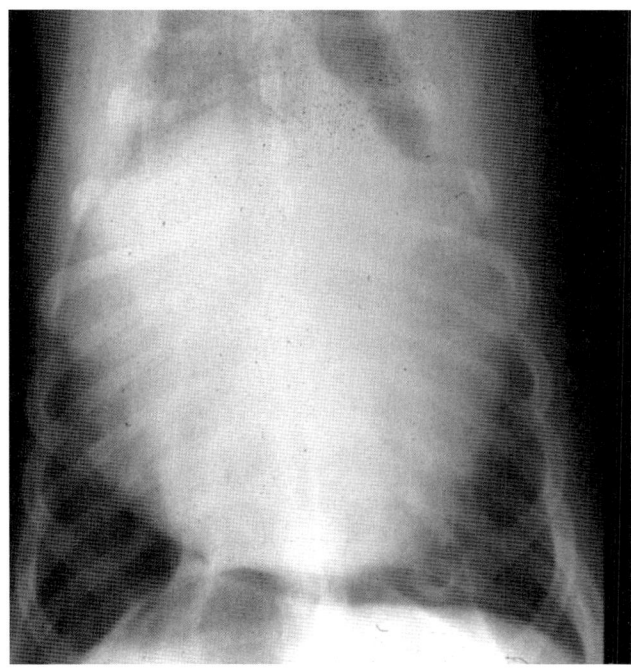

Figure 86.3 Thoracic radiograph of a dog with severe pericardial effusion. The pericardium/heart has a globoid shape.

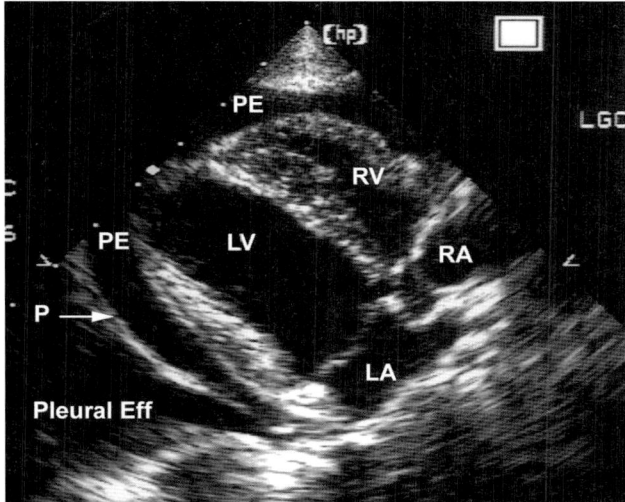

Figure 86.4 Echocardiography of a dog with pericardial effusion. A space is present between the epicardium and the pericardium. LA, left atrium; LV, left ventricle; P, pericardium; PE, pericardial effusion; RA, right atrium; RV, right ventricle. Source: Courtesy of June Boon, Colorado State University.

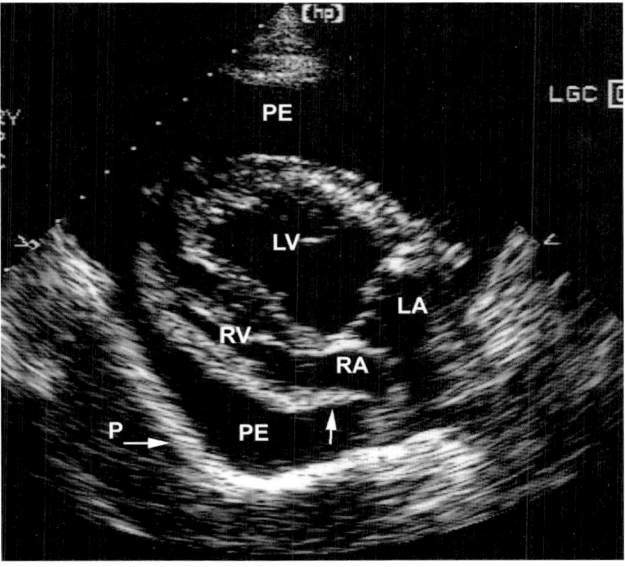

Figure 86.5 Echocardiography of a dog with severe pericardial effusion inducing cardiac tamponade. The right atrium is collapsing. LA, left atrium; LV, left ventricle; P, pericardium; PE, pericardial effusion; RA, right atrium; RV, right ventricle. Source: Courtesy of June Boon, Colorado State University.

resonance imaging are useful for the diagnosis of cardiac neoplasia, constrictive pericarditis, and pericardial cyst (Gouliamos *et al.* 1984; Soulen 1991).

Echocardiography

Echocardiography is a very sensitive technique for demonstrating pericardial effusion. It is capable of detecting as little as 15 mL of pericardial fluid (Bonagura & Herring 1985; Berry *et al.* 1988b). An anechoic space between the epicardium and the pericardial sac is the classic echocardiographic finding in pericardial effusion (Figure 86.4). Right and left ventricular dimensions are often diminished and the ventricular walls appear thicker than normal when pericardial effusion is severe and cardiac filling is impaired. Collapse of the right atrium or ventricle during diastole suggests significant elevation of intrapericardial pressure and cardiac tamponade (Figure 86.5). However, the absence of these findings does not exclude significant impairment of cardiac function (Bonagura & Herring 1985; Berry *et al.* 1988b).

Echocardiography allows visualization of cardiac masses or myocardial infiltration. Even though it does not provide histologic diagnosis, a right atrial mass is suggestive of hemangiosarcoma (Figure 86.6) while a mass adjacent to the ascending aorta is most likely a chemodectoma (Figure 86.7). Myocardial infiltration, visible as diffuse hyperechogenicity in a cat, is suggestive of lymphosarcoma (Brummer & Moise 1989).

Two-dimensional echocardiography has been reported to be 80–90% sensitive for the detection of cardiac masses in dogs (Thomas *et al.* 1984; Sisson & Thomas 1999). However, false negatives are possible. In a study on 107 dogs with pericardial effusion, sensitivity and specificity of echocardiography were 82% and 100% respectively for detection of a cardiac mass, 82% and

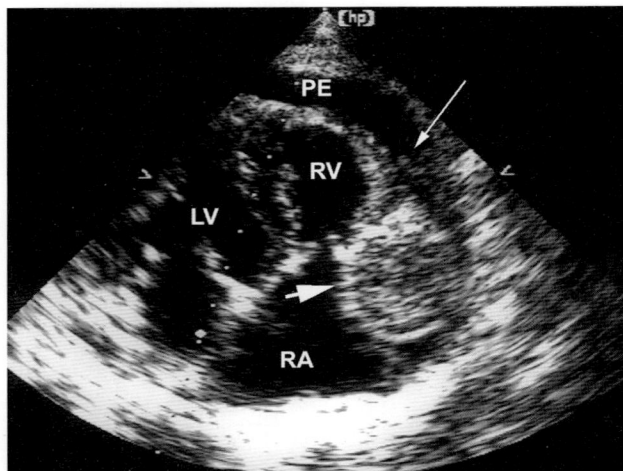

Figure 86.6 Echocardiography of a dog with a right atrial tumor (large arrow). LV, left ventricle; PE, pericardial effusion; RA, right atrium; RV, right ventricle. Source: Courtesy of June Boon, Colorado State University.

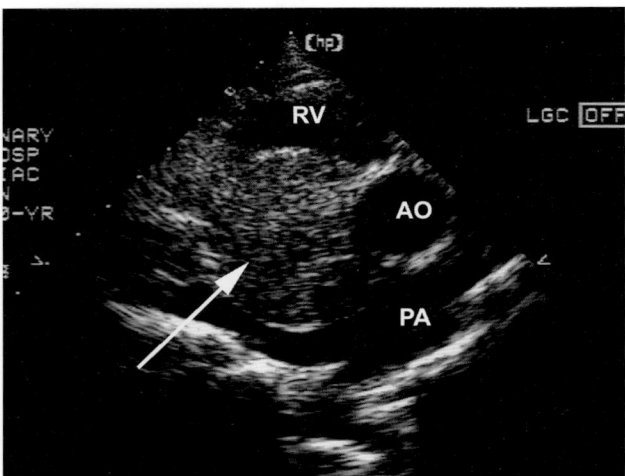

Figure 86.7 Echocardiography of a dog with a mass around the ascending aorta (arrow). AO, aorta; PA, pulmonary artery; RV, right ventricle. Source: Courtesy of June Boon, Colorado State University.

99% respectively for detection of a right atrial mass, and 74% and 98% respectively for detection of a heart base mass (Macdonald *et al.* 2009).

Treatment

Pericardiocentesis

Pericardiocentesis with a needle or catheter is the most appropriate emergency treatment for cardiac tamponade (Ettinger 1974). It is associated with minimal complications if performed properly. Local anesthesia can be used to block the intercostal space. The puncture is most often performed between the fourth and sixth intercostal spaces

on the right side to avoid major coronary arteries. A 20-gauge needle or catheter attached to an extension set, three-way stopcock, and syringe are used. The needle or catheter is advanced in the intercostal space while observing the electrocardiogram. If the needle or catheter touches the myocardium, a premature complex will occur and the needle or catheter should be withdrawn slightly. Negative pressure should be applied to the needle or catheter while it is advanced into the pericardial space. Fluid in the pericardial sac is often hemorrhagic and must be distinguished from blood arising from inadvertent cardiac puncture. The fluid should not clot and the packed cell volume should be significantly lower than that of peripheral blood. Fluid should be saved for cytology and culture (Ettinger 1974; Sisson & Thomas 1999). If cardiac tamponade is present, drainage of pericardial fluid causes decreased heart rate, augmentation of amplitude of QRS complexes, decreased central venous pressure, and improvement in arterial pulse quality.

Pericardial catheter has been placed for the treatment of acute pericardial effusion and maintained for 18 hours while the dogs were stabilized in the critical care unit (Cook *et al.* 2019). It has been associated with the induction of arrhythmias.

Pericardiectomy

Pericardiectomy is curative for idiopathic pericardial effusion and mostly palliative for neoplastic pericardial effusion by preventing recurrence of cardiac tamponade (Berg & Wingfield 1984; Berg *et al.* 1984; Dunning *et al.* 1998). Pericardiectomy decreases the surface area of pericardium producing the fluid, and increases the surface area for absorption of the fluid by allowing fluid into the pleural cavity. If an infection is suspected, a portion of the pericardium should be submitted for culture and sensitivity.

Complete or subtotal pericardiectomy can be performed through a median sternotomy or right thoracotomy. Median sternotomy has the advantage of allowing direct visualization of both phrenic nerves. A subtotal pericardiectomy is the technique most commonly used. After identification of both phrenic nerves (Figure 86.8), the pericardium is resected ventral to the phrenic nerves (Figure 86.9). Visualization of the phrenic nerves can be difficult for cases with severe pericarditis. Complete pericardiectomy requires dissection of both phrenic nerves from the pericardium prior to complete resection of the pericardium at the base of the heart. Complete pericardiectomy is not thought to have significant benefit over subtotal pericardiectomy in most cases. However, for the treatment of a chylous effusion, the author recommends a pericardiectomy as dorsal as possible to completely liberate the left and right atrium.

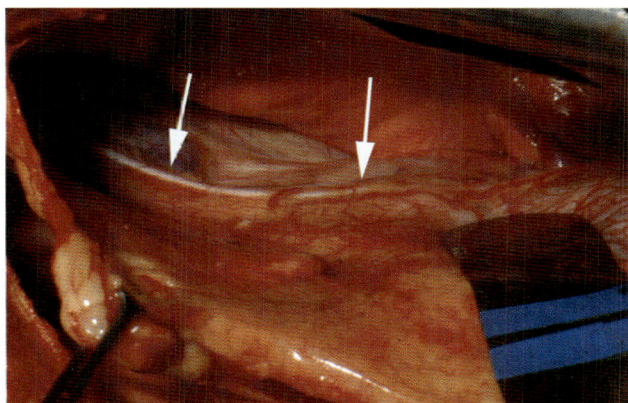

Figure 86.8 Visualization of the phrenic nerve (arrows) on the pericardium at the level of the atrioventricular groove.

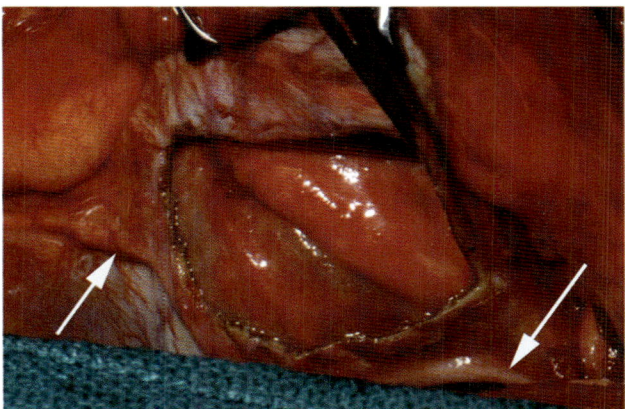

Figure 86.9 The incision in the pericardium is performed ventral to the phrenic nerve (arrow) to complete a subtotal pericardiectomy.

After completing the median sternotomy, the mediastinum is dissected from the sternum. The mediastinum and pericardium can be manipulated during the surgery with Allis tissue forceps (Figure 86.10) and the pericardial sac is opened with Metzenbaum scissors. The pericardial fluid is aspirated. It is recommended that electrocautery be used to perform the pericardiectomy because of the rich vascular supply present on the pericardium that can result in significant blood loss during and after surgery (Orton 1995; Aronsohn & Carpenter 1999). When using electrocautery it is important to lift the pericardium away from the heart to avoid contacting the myocardium with the electrocautery device.

Subtotal pericardiectomy can also be performed via thoracoscopy (Dupré *et al.* 2001; Michelotti *et al.* 2019). It will require a transdiaphragmatic subxiphoid approach or right intercostal approach. The mediastinum is dissected, the phrenic nerves on the right and left sides

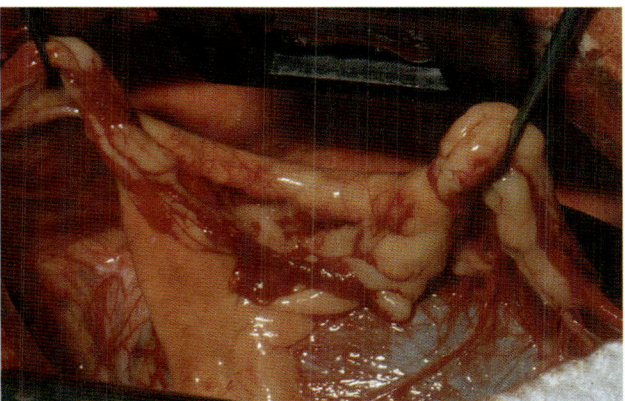

Figure 86.10 The pericardium is manipulated with Allis tissue forceps.

visualized, and a subtotal pericardiectomy is performed. It does not require one-lung ventilation (Dupré *et al.* 2001).

Pericardial window

A pericardial window can be performed with thoracoscopy (Jackson *et al.* 1999; Walsh *et al.* 1999; Monnet 2009). This is a minimally invasive procedure that prevents recurrence of cardiac tamponade. It is a viable option for dogs with neoplastic effusion and is a palliative procedure (Dunning *et al.* 1998). Minimally invasive surgery to palliate cardiac tamponade is an appealing option for these cases. Thoracoscopy can be performed using an intercostal or transdiaphragmatic approach. The intercostal approach gives better visualization of the right atrial appendage and aortic root.

For a transdiaphragmatic approach, the patient is placed in dorsal recumbency (Website Chapter 86: Heart/pericardium/thoracoscopy pericardial window). Three ports are required. One port is placed transdiaphragmatically from a subxiphoid position. Two additional ports are placed in either the fourth and seventh intercostal spaces ventrally on the right side or in the seventh intercostal in the right and the left side. If cannulas are placed in the left and right sides, the mediastinum has to be detached from the sternum with electrocautery (Figure 86.11). The transdiaphragmatic port is used to place the thoracoscope, while the other two ports are used to introduce Metzenbaum scissors and graspers. Electrocautery is connected to insulated Metzenbaum scissors designed for minimally invasive surgery. Bipolar sealing technology can also be used to perform the pericardial window. The ventral mediastinum is opened to allow complete exploration of the thoracic cavity with the thoracoscope. Exploration is performed before the pericardium is opened. Fluid within the thoracic cavity may interfere with good

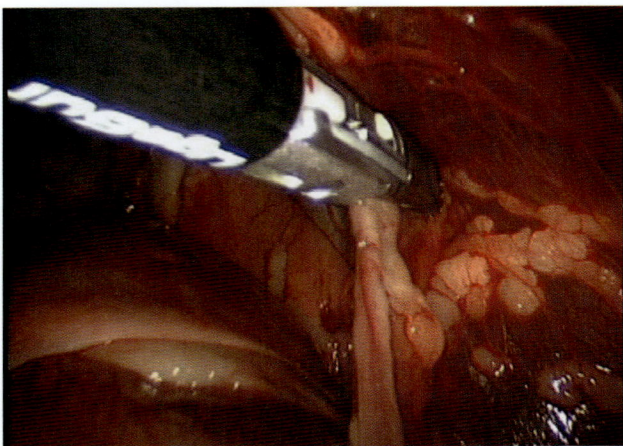

Figure 86.11 Dissection of the mediastinum during a transdiaphragmatic approach with thoracoscopy.

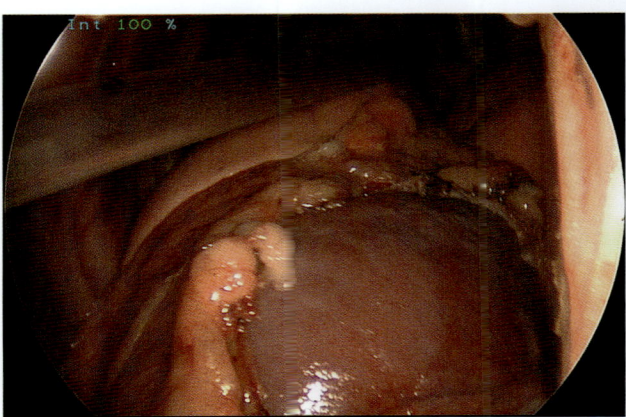

Figure 86.13 A pericardial window (3 × 3 cm) is then completed with electrocautery and scissors.

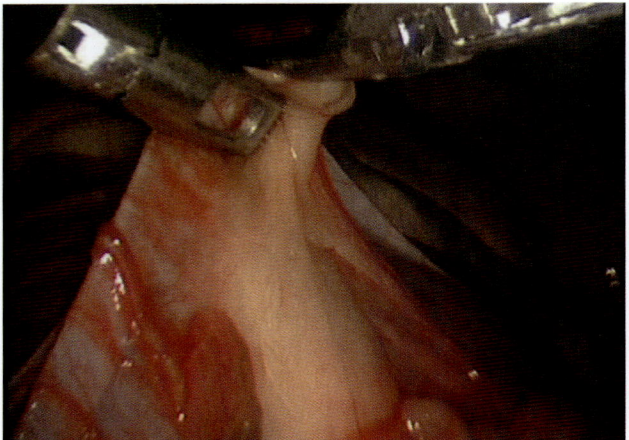

Figure 86.12 The pericardium is being held with grasping forceps at the level of the apex to avoid traumatizing a right atrial tumor.

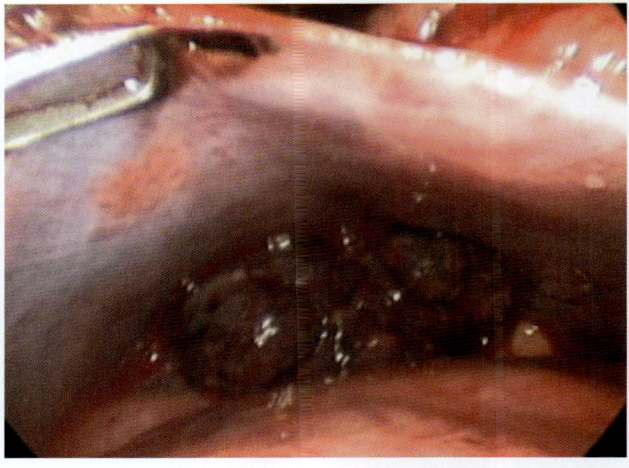

Figure 86.14 Visualization of a right atrial tumor during thoracoscopy.

visualization of the thoracic cavity and should be removed. After exploration of the thoracic cavity, the pericardium is mobilized with graspers and tented at the level of the ventricles to avoid inadvertent grasping and cutting of the right atrial appendage (Figure 86.12). A small hole is made in the pericardium with Metzenbaum scissors and pericardial fluid is aspirated with a surgical aspirator. Using a combination of electrocautery and cutting, the Metzenbaum scissors are used to complete the pericardial window (Figure 86.13). A window of 3 × 3 cm is sufficient to drain the pericardial sac without risking herniation of the heart through the window in a larger-breed dog. The right atrium can be visualized after the window has been made and the thoracoscope introduced into the pericardial sac (Figure 86.14). The aortic root can also be inspected to visualize a heart base tumor. The transdiaphragmatic approach allows

visualization and biopsy of the sternal lymph nodes if necessary.

After creating a pericardial window, a pericardioscopy can be performed, especially if an idiopathic pericardial effusion is suspected. During pericardioscopy, the inside of the pericardium, the epicardium, and the heart base can be visualized and biopsied if needed. This technique increases the chance of diagnosis of mesothelioma and other tumors (Skinner et al. 2014; Carvajal et al. 2019).

Percutaneous balloon pericardiotomy

Pericardiotomy has been performed in human and dogs as a palliative treatment for cardiac tamponade. A balloon catheter is introduced into the pericardial space under fluoroscopy. The balloon is inflated and retrieved to tear the pericardium (Busadori et al. 1998).

Right trial tumor resection and heart base tumor resection

A right atrial tumor can be resected after performing a subphrenic pericardiectomy because it will improve exposure. The right atrial appendage is isolated with a Satinsky clamp at its base (Figure 86.15). The right atrial appendage is resected, leaving enough tissue to be able to place two simple continuous suture lines to seal the atriectomy (Figures 86.16 and 86.17). Nonabsorbable monofilament suture size 4-0 is used to complete the closure.

A right atrial tumor can be resected with a thoracoscopy if the tumor is small and located toward the tip of the right atrial appendage (Ployart *et al.* 2013). A thoracoscopy can also be used to evaluate the size and

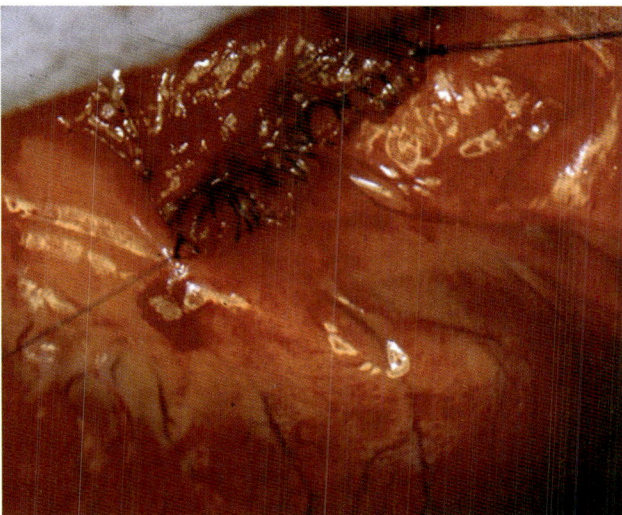

Figure 86.17 Two simple continuous sutures have been placed to close the right atrial appendage; 3-0 polypropylene suture is used.

location of the tumor and decide if it is resected with a thoracoscopy, with an open approach, or is not resectable.

Heart base tumors are rarely resected because they are very firmly attached to the major vessels (aorta and pulmonary artery). They are highly vascular and have a tendency to be associated with severe hemorrhage during dissection. Heart base tumors are treated with radiation therapy with improved survival (Ehrhart *et al.* 2002; Hansen *et al.* 2021).

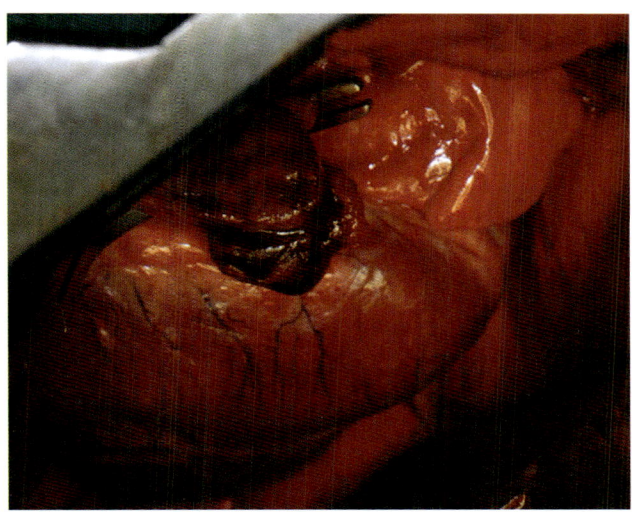

Figure 86.15 A tangential clamp has been placed at the base of the right atrium.

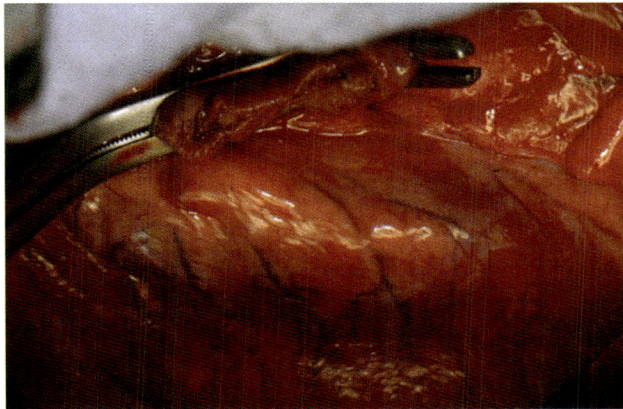

Figure 86.16 The right atrial appendage has been resected, making sure enough tissue is left to suture the right atrial appendage.

References

Ameli, S. and Shah, P.K. (1991). Cardiac tamponade. Pathophysiology, diagnosis, and management. *Cardiology Clinics* 9: 665–674.

Aronsohn, M.G. (1985). Cardiac hemangiosarcoma in the dog: a review of 38 cases. *Journal of the American Veterinary Medical Association* 187: 922–926.

Aronsohn, M.G. and Carpenter, J.L. (1999). Surgical treatment of idiopathic pericardial effusion in the dog: 25 cases (1985–1993). *Journal of the American Animal Hospital Association* 35: 521–525.

Aronson, L.R. and Gregory, C.R. (1995). Infectious pericardial effusion in five dogs. *Veterinary Surgery* 24: 402–407.

Berg, J. (1994). Pericardial disease and cardiac neoplasia. *Seminars in Veterinary Medicine and Surgery (Small Animal)* 9: 185–191.

Berg, R.J. and Wingfield, W. (1984). Pericardial effusion in the dog: a review of 42 cases. *Journal of the American Animal Hospital Association* 20: 721–730.

Berg, R.J., Wingfield, W.E., and Hoopes, P.J. (1984). Idiopathic hemorrhagic pericardial effusion in eight dogs. *Journal of the American Veterinary Medical Association* 185: 988–992.

Berg, R.J., Wingfield, W.E., and Hoopes, P.J. (1985). Idiopathic hemorrhagic pericardial effusion in 8 dogs. *Veterinary Surgery* 14: 46–47.

Berry, C.R., Lombard, C.W., Hager, D.A., and Ackerman, N. (1988a). Pericardial effusion secondary to chronic endocardiosis and left atrial rupture in a dog. *Compendium on Continuing Education for the Practicing Veterinarian* 10: 800–805.

Berry, C.R., Lombard, C.W., Hager, D.A. et al. (1988b). Echocardiographic evaluation of cardiac tamponade in dogs before and after pericardiocentesis: four cases (1984–1986). *Journal of the American Veterinary Medical Association* 192: 1597–1603.

Bonagura, J.D. (1981). Electrical alternans associated with pericardial effusion in the dog. *Journal of the American Veterinary Medical Association* 178: 574–579.

Bonagura, J.D. and Herring, D.S. (1985). Echocardiography. Acquired heart disease. *Veterinary Clinics of North America: Small Animal Practice* 15: 1209–1224.

Bouvy, B.M. and Bjorling, D.E. (1991a). Pericardial effusion in dogs and cats. Part I. Normal pericardium and causes and pathophysiology of pericardial effusion. *Compendium on Continuing Education for the Practicing Veterinarian* 13: 417–424.

Bouvy, B.M. and Bjorling, D.E. (1991b). Pericardial effusion in dogs and cats. Part II. Diagnostic approach and treatment. *Compendium on Continuing Education for the Practicing Veterinarian* 13: 633–642.

Bradley, G.A., Tye, J., Lozano-Alarcon, F. et al. (1992). Hemopericardium in a dog due to hemorrhage originating in a heart base thymic remnant. *Journal of Veterinary Diagnostic Investigation* 4: 211–212.

Brownlie, S.E. and Clayton-Jones, D.G. (1985). Successful removal of a heartbase tumour in a dog with pericardial haemorrhagic effusion. *Journal of Small Animal Practice* 26: 191–197.

Brummer, D.G. and Moise, N.S. (1989). Infiltrative cardiomyopathy responsive to combination chemotherapy in a cat with lymphoma. *Journal of the American Veterinary Medical Association* 195: 1116–1119.

Buchanan, J.W. (1972). Spontaneous left atrial rupture in dogs. *Advances in Experimental Medicine and Biology* 22: 315–334.

Bussadori, C., Grasso, A., and Santilli, R.A. (1998) []. Percutaneous pericardiotomy with balloon catheter in the treatment of malignant pericardial effusion in dogs]. *Radiologia Medica* 96: 503–506.

Cacoub, P., Axler, O., De Zuttere, D. et al. (2000). Amyloidosis and cardiac involvement. *Annales de Médecine Interne* 151: 611–617.

Carvajal, J.L., Case, J.B., Mayhew, P.D. et al. (2019). Outcome in dogs with presumptive idiopathic pericardial effusion after thoracoscopic pericardectomy and pericardioscopy. *Veterinary Surgery* 48: O105–O111.

Closa, J.M., Font, A., and Mascort, J. (1999). Pericardial mesothelioma in a dog: long-term survival after pericardiectomy in combination with chemotherapy. *Journal of Small Animal Practice* 40: 383–386.

Cook, S., Cortellini, S., and Humm, K. (2019). Retrospective evaluation of pericardial catheter placement in the management of pericardial effusion in dogs (2007-2015): 18 cases. *Journal of Veterinary Emergency and Critical Care (San Antonio, Tex.)* 29: 413–417.

Covey, H.L. and Connolly, D.J. (2018). Pericardial effusion associated with systemic inflammatory disease in seven dogs (January 2006–January 2012). *Journal of Veterinary Cardiology* 20: 123–128.

Dunning, D., Monnet, E., Orton, E.C., and Salman, M.D. (1998). Analysis of prognostic indicators for dogs with pericardial effusion: 46 cases (1985–1996). *Journal of the American Veterinary Medical Association* 212: 1276–1280.

Dupré, G.P., Corlouer, J.P., and Bouvy, B.M. (2001). Thoracoscopic pericardectomy performed without pulmonary exclusion in 9 dogs. *Veterinary Surgery* 30: 21–27.

Edwards, N.J. (1996). The diagnostic value of pericardial fluid pH determination. *Journal of the American Animal Hospital Association* 32: 63–67.

Ehrhart, N., Ehrhart, E.J., Willis, J. et al. (2002). Analysis of factors affecting survival in dogs with aortic body tumors. *Veterinary Surgery* 31: 44–48.

Ettinger, S.J. (1974). Pericardiocentesis. *Veterinary Clinics of North America: Small Animal Practice* 4: 403–412.

Farrow, C.S. (1984). Exercise in radiology [globose cardiomegaly compatible with pericardial effusion; dog]. *Canadian Veterinary Journal* 25: 302–303.

Fossum, T.W., Miller, M.W., Rogers, K.S. et al. (1994). Chylothorax associated with right-sided heart failure in five cats. *Journal of the American Veterinary Medical Association* 204: 84–89.

Fowler, N.O. (1994). Pulsus paradoxus. *Heart Disease and Stroke* 3: 68–69.

Friedman, H.S., Lajam, F., Zaman, Q. et al. (1977). Effect of autonomic blockade on the hemodynamic findings in acute cardiac tamponade. *American Journal of Physiology* 232: H5–H11.

Gonin-Jmaa, D., Paulsen, D.B., and Taboada, J. (1996). Pericardial effusion in a dog with rhabdomyosarcoma in the right ventricular wall. *Journal of Small Animal Practice* 37: 193–196.

Gores, B.R., Berg, J., Carpenter, J.L., and Aronsohn, M.G. (1994). Surgical treatment of thymoma in cats: 12 cases (1987–1992). *Journal of the American Veterinary Medical Association* 204: 1782–1785.

Gouliamos, A., Andreou, J., Sterotis, J. et al. (1984). Detection of pericardial heart disease by computed tomography. *Clinical Radiology* 35: 397–400.

Hancock, E.W. (1994). Cardiac tamponade. *Heart Disease and Stroke* 3: 155–158.

Hansen, K.S., Theon, A.P., Willcox, J.L. et al. (2021). Long-term outcomes with conventional fractionated and stereotactic radiotherapy for suspected heart-base tumours in dogs. *Veterinary and Comparative Oncology* 19: 191–200.

Heinritz, C.K., Gilson, S.D., Soderstrom, M.J. et al. (2005). Subtotal pericardectomy and epicardial excision for treatment of coccidioidomycosis-induced effusive-constrictive pericarditis in dogs: 17 cases (1999–2003). *Journal of the American Veterinary Medical Association* 227: 435–440.

Jackson, J., Richter, K.P., and Launer, D.P. (1999). Thoracoscopic partial pericardiectomy in 13 dogs. *Journal of Veterinary Internal Medicine* 13: 529–533.

Kagan, K.G. (1980). Thoracic trauma. *Veterinary Clinics of North America: Small Animal Practice* 10: 641–653.

Kirkland, L.L. and Taylor, R.W. (1992). Pericardiocentesis. *Critical Care Clinics* 8: 699–712.

de Laforcade, A.M., Freeman, L.M., Rozanski, E.A., and Rush, J.E. (2005). Biochemical analysis of pericardial fluid and whole blood in dogs with pericardial effusion. *Journal of Veterinary Internal Medicine* 19: 833–836.

Lakhdhir, S., Viall, A., Alloway, E. et al. (2020). Clinical presentation, cardiovascular findings, etiology, and outcome of myocarditis in dogs: 64 cases with presumptive antemortem diagnosis (26 confirmed postmortem) and 137 cases with postmortem diagnosis only (2004–2017). *Journal of Veterinary Cardiology* 30: 44–56.

LeWinter, M.M. and Kabbani, S. (2005). Pericardial disease. In: *Braunwald's Heart Disease. A Textbook of Cardiovascular Medicine*, 7e (ed. D.P. Zipes, P. Libby, R.O. Bonow and E. Braunwald), 1757–1780. Philadelphia, PA: Elsevier Saunders.

Lombard, C.W. (1983). Pericardial disease. *Veterinary Clinics of North America: Small Animal Practice* 13: 337–353.

Macdonald, K.A., Cagney, O., and Magne, M.L. (2009). Echocardiographic and clinicopathologic characterization of pericardial effusion in dogs: 107 cases (1985–2006). *Journal of the American Veterinary Medical Association* 235: 1456–1461.

de Madron, E. (1990). Seven cases of pericardial effusion of cancerous origin in dogs. Clinical, electrocardiographic, radiographic and echocardiographic aspects. *Pratique Médicale et Chirurgicale de l'Animal de Compagnie* 25: 59–69.

de Madron, E. (1991). Malignant pericardial effusion in dogs: seven cases clinical, electrocardiographic, radiographic, and echocardiographic aspects. *European Journal of Companion Animal Practice* 1: 52–62.

de Madron, E., Prymak, C., and Hendricks, J. (1987). Idiopathic hemorrhagic pericardial effusion with organized thrombi in a dog. *Journal of the American Veterinary Medical Association* 191: 324–326.

McDonough, S.P., MacLachlan, N.J., and Tobias, A.H. (1992). Canine pericardial mesothelioma. *Veterinary Pathology* 29: 256–260.

Michelotti, K.P., Youk, A., Payne, J.T., and Anderson, J. (2019). Outcomes of dogs with recurrent idiopathic pericardial effusion treated with a 3-port right-sided thoracoscopic subtotal pericardiectomy. *Veterinary Surgery* 48: 1032–1041.

Miller, M.W. and Sisson, D.D. (2000). Pericardial disorders. In: *Textbook of Veterinary Internal Medicine* (ed. S.J. Ettinger and E.C. Feldman), 923–936. Philadelphia, PA: WB Saunders.

Monnet, E. (2009). Interventional thoracoscopy in small animals. *Veterinary Clinics of North America: Small Animal Practice* 39: 965–975.

Orton, E.C. (1995). Pericardium. In: *Small Animal Thoracic Surgery* (ed. E.C. Orton, T.O. McCracken and C.C. Cann), 177–185. Baltimore, MD: Williams & Wilkins.

Owens, J.M. (1977). Pericardial effusion in the cat. *Veterinary Clinics of North America: Small Animal Practice* 7: 373–383.

Patnaik, A.K., Liu, S.K., Hurvitz, A.I., and McClelland, A.J. (1975). Canine chemodectoma (extra-adrenal paragangliomas): a comparative study. *Journal of Small Animal Practice* 16: 785–801.

Petrus, D.J. and Henik, R.A. (1999). Pericardial effusion and cardiac tamponade secondary to brodifacoum toxicosis in a dog. *Journal of the American Veterinary Medical Association* 215: 647–648.

Ployart, S., Libermann, S., Doran, I. et al. (2013). Thoracoscopic resection of right auricular masses in dogs: 9 cases (2003–2011). *Journal of the American Veterinary Medical Association* 242: 237–241.

Price, E.K. and Mullen, P.A. (1966). A case of haemopericardium in the dog. *Veterinary Record* 78: 480–485.

Reddy, P.S. and Curtiss, E.I. (1990). Cardiac tamponade. *Cardiology Clinics* 8: 627–637.

Rush, J.E., Keene, B.W., and Fox, P.R. (1990). Pericardial disease in the cat: a retrospective evaluation of 66 cases. *Journal of the American Animal Hospital Association* 26: 39–46.

Santamore, W.P., Constantinescu, M.S., Bogen, D., and Johnston, W.E. (1990). Nonuniform distribution of normal pericardial fluid. *Basic Research in Cardiology* 85: 541–549.

Shabetai, R. (2005). Cardiac tamponade, myocardial stress, and reverse remodeling. *Journal of Cardiac Failure* 11: 134–136.

Shabetai, R. (2007). Heart failure in cardiac tamponade, contrictive pericarditis, and restrictive cardiomyopathy. In: *Congestive Heart Failure* (ed. J.D. Hosenpud and B.H. Greenberg), 395–413. Philadelphia, PA: Lippincott Williams & Wilkins.

Sisson, D. and Thomas, W.P. (1999). Pericardial disease and cardiac tumors. In: *Textbook of Canine and Feline Cardiology*, 2e (ed. P.R. Fox, D.D. Sisson and N.S. Moise), 685–699. Philadelphia, PA: WB Saunders.

Sisson, D., Thomas, W.P., Ruehl, W.W., and Zinkl, J.G. (1984). Diagnostic value of pericardial fluid analysis in the dog. *Journal of the American Veterinary Medical Association* 184: 51–55.

Skinner, O.T., Case, J.B., Ellison, G.W., and Monnet, E. (2014). Pericardioscopic imaging findings in cadaveric dogs: comparison of an apical pericardial window and sub-phrenic pericardectomy. *Veterinary Surgery* 43: 45–51.

Soulen, R.L. (1991). Magnetic resonance imaging of great vessel, myocardial, and pericardial disease. *Circulation* 84 (Suppl 3): I311–I321.

Spodick, D.H. (1998). Pathophysiology of cardiac tamponade. *Chest* 113: 1372–1378. [Erratum appears in *Chest* 1998; 114: 662.].

Spodick, D.H. (2003). Acute cardiac tamponade. *New England Journal of Medicine* 349: 684–690.

Thomas, W.P., Reed, J.R., Bauer, T.G., and Breznock, E.M. (1984). Constrictive pericardial disease in the dog. *Journal of the American Veterinary Medical Association* 184: 546–553.

Vogtli, T., Gaschen, F., Vogtli-Burger, R., and Lombard, C. (1997) []. Hemorrhagic pericardial effusion in dogs. A retrospective study of 10 cases (1989–1994) with a review of the literature]. *Schweizer Archiv für Tierheilkunde* 139: 217–224.

Walsh, P.J., Remedios, A.M., Ferguson, J.F. et al. (1999). Thoracoscopic versus open partial pericardectomy in dogs: comparison of postoperative pain and morbidity. *Veterinary Surgery* 28: 472–479.

Weisse, C., Soares, N., Beal, M.W. et al. (2005). Survival times in dogs with right atrial hemangiosarcoma treated by means of surgical resection with or without adjuvant chemotherapy: 23 cases (1986–2000). *Journal of the American Veterinary Medical Association* 226: 575–579.

87

Pacemaker Therapy

Eric Monnet

Pacemaker therapy is indicated in veterinary medicine for symptomatic bradyarrhythmias including atrioventricular (AV) block, sick sinus syndrome, and persistent atrial standstill (Bigler *et al.* 1981; Buchanan *et al.* 1968; Fingeroth 1994; Hackett *et al.* 1995; Musselman *et al.* 1976; Pibarot *et al.* 1993; Sykes 1979; Zymet 1981; Wess *et al.* 2006; Santilli *et al.* 2019; Moise 1999; Ward *et al.* 2015, 2016; Cervenec *et al.* 2017; Noszczyk-Nowak *et al.* 2019).

Pacemaker therapy improves cardiac output and decreases the risk of sudden cardiac death associated with these arrhythmias by maintaining the heart rate above a predetermined rate.

A complete diagnostic work-up including physical examination, laboratory blood work, thoracic radiographs, echocardiography, and electrocardiogram should be performed prior to implantation of a permanent pacemaker.

Indications

Atrioventricular block

Pathophysiology and pathology

AV block is characterized by varying degrees of conduction delay or block through the AV node. AV block is graded according to its degree of severity. First-degree AV block is a delay in impulse conduction through the AV node. Second-degree is an intermittent failure of impulse conduction through the AV node. Second-degree AV block can be low grade (i.e., impulses conducted > impulses blocked) or high grade (i.e., impulses conducted < impulses blocked). Third-degree AV block

is a complete and persistent failure of impulse conduction through the AV node. The result is complete AV dissociation and establishment of a ventricular origin escape rhythm.

Whereas first-degree and low-grade second-degree AV block are generally the result of exaggerated parasympathetic influence on the AV node, high-grade second-degree and third-degree AV block are generally the result of an intrinsic pathologic process within the AV node. Pathologic causes of AV block include degeneration of conduction tissues, invasion of conduction tissues by endocarditis or neoplasia, or traumatic or iatrogenic surgical injury to conduction pathways.

High grade second-degree and third-degree AV block effectively limit ventricular systole to a slow rate and thereby decrease the output capacity of the heart. The pathophysiologic consequences of this restricted cardiac output include exercise intolerance, collapse, syncope, and sudden cardiac death. Bradycardia-mediated low cardiac output initiates the same neuroendocrine mechanisms induced by other chronic causes of low cardiac output. Initially this response is adaptive, resulting in blood volume expansion, ventricular chamber dilatation, and enhanced stroke volume that counter the effects of bradycardia. Over time, however, the neuroendocrine response becomes maladaptive, causing the syndrome of congestive heart failure.

Clinical presentation

Clinical signs associated with AV block depend upon several factors, including the ventricular rate, the presence or absence of concurrent cardiac disease, and

---

whether the bradycardia is persistent or intermittent. Severe lethargy, exercise intolerance, collapse, and syncope are possible complaints at presentation. The heart rate is slow and fixed. The femoral pulse is usually strong because of the increased stroke volume. Intermittent jugular pulsation may be present with third-degree AV block due to AV dissociation (cannon a waves). Systemic venous congestion, ascites, or pulmonary edema may occur as a result of congestive heart failure.

Diagnosis

Diagnosis of AV block is based on electrocardiogram. First-degree AV block is recognized as a prolongation of the P-R interval. Second-degree heart block is characterized by intermittent P waves that are not followed by a QRS complex. The condition may be low or high grade. Third-degree AV block is characterized by complete AV dissociation and a slow escape rhythm. The escape rhythm is classically recognized as a wide-complex QRS consistent with ventricular origin (Figure 87.1). Sometimes the escape rhythm is a narrow-complex QRS that presumably originates below the site of AV block, but still high in the His-Purkinge conduction system.

First-degree and low-grade second-degree AV block generally are not associated with clinical signs and are abolished by the administration of atropine. These rhythms generally do not warrant further diagnostics. High-grade second-degree and third-degree AV block often cause clinical signs and are not responsive to the administration of atropine. Echocardiography should be performed on animals with high-grade second-degree or third-degree AV block to assess myocardial function and to rule out possible underlying causes of AV block such as endocarditis or neoplasia.

Indication for pacemaker

Pacemaker implantation is indicated in companion animals with high-grade second-degree or third-degree AV block when clinical signs such as exercise intolerance, syncope, or congestive heart failure are present (Hackett *et al.* 1995; Moise 1999; Ward *et al.* 2015; Weder *et al.* 2015; Noszczyk-Nowak *et al.* 2019). Some animals do not show overt clinical signs related to bradycardia at the time of clinical presentation. The likelihood of degeneration of the rhythm, the risk for sudden cardiac death, and the ventricular escape rate are also taken into consideration. Cats with third-degree AV block that have a escape heart rate above 100 bpm are often not symptomatic and may not need a pacemaker. If the escape rate in a cat drops below 90 bpm, a pacemaker is recommended. Dogs with third-degree AV block usually exhibit lethargy, syncope, or congestive heart failure when the heart rate is below 50 bpm.

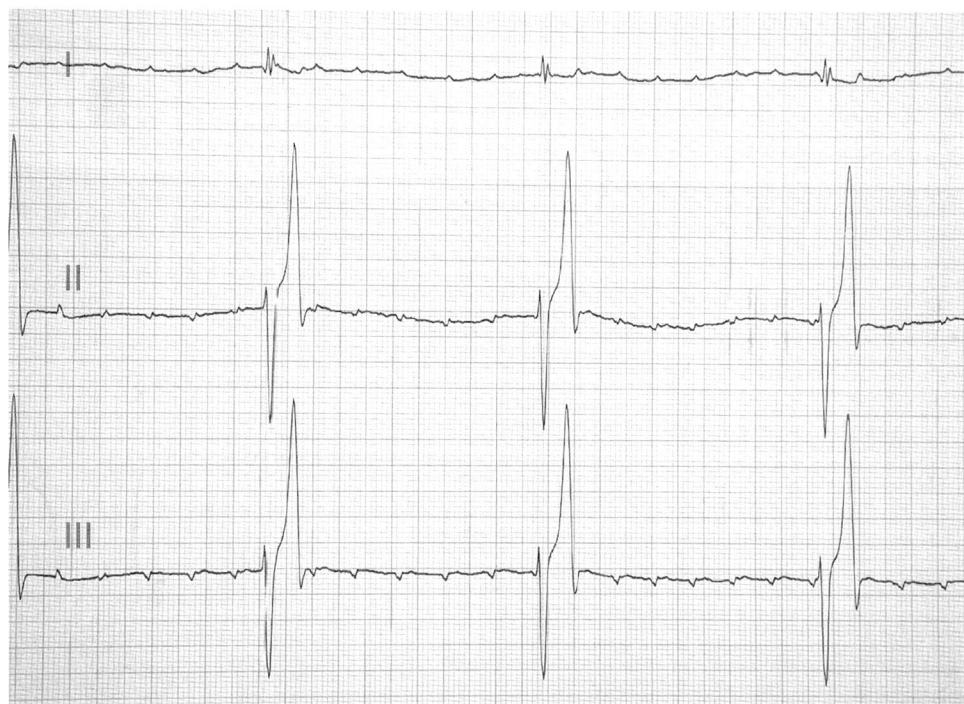

Figure 87.1 Electrocardiogram from a dog with a third-degree atrioventricular (AV) block (leads I, II, and III). Complete AV dissociation with a wide-complex (ventricular) escape rhythm is present.

Sick sinus syndrome

Pathophysiology and pathology

Sick sinus syndrome is a collective term given to a number of electrophysiologic abnormalities of the sinoatrial (SA) node that result in bradycardia or long periods of sinus pause, or both. When episodes of supraventricular tachycardia are also present, the condition is termed bradycardia-tachycardia syndrome. Sick sinus syndrome is an affliction of the SA node that either disrupts SA impulse generation or blocks the conduction of SA impulses into the atrium. This condition may be due to pathologic changes in or around the SA node, or it may be associated with abnormal autonomic nervous system function. Pathologic lesions of the SA node include a decrease in the number of impulse-generating P cells and fibrosis of the SA node. Extrinsic influences from the autonomic nervous system may exacerbate the condition. Sick sinus syndrome occurs most commonly in middle-aged miniature schnauzers, cocker spaniels, and West Highland white terriers (Ward *et al.* 2016). The condition also occurs in other breeds of dog.

Clinical presentation

Animals with sick sinus syndrome present with progressive lethargy, exercise intolerance, and frequent syncope. Physical examination is fairly unremarkable except for prolonged pauses in the heart rhythm. Clinical signs related to congestive heart failure are uncommon.

Diagnosis

Diagnosis of sick sinus syndrome is based on the presence of clinical signs, usually frequent syncope, and characteristic findings on the electrocardiogram. The most characteristic electrocardiographic finding is long periods of sinus pause lasting up to 10 seconds (Figure 87.2). The sinus pauses may be terminated by a junctional escape complex or by paroxysmal supraventricular tachycardia. The sinus pauses may or may not be abolished by administration of atropine (0.002–0.004 mg/kg intramuscularly or intravenously).

Indication for pacemaker

Implantation of a pacemaker is indicated for dogs with sick sinus syndrome who are symptomatic and whose sinus pauses are not abolished by atropine (Burrage 2012; Ward *et al.* 2016). Long sinus pauses are often observed in dogs during sleep that disappear when the animal is awake or during exercise. Pacemaker implantation is not indicated for asymptomatic dogs whose sinus pauses disappear with exercise or administration of atropine.

Atrial standstill

Pathophysiology and pathology

Atrial standstill occurs when the atrial muscle is not capable of conducting a wave of depolarization. The cardiac impulse may originate in the SA node and be conducted by internodal pathways to the AV node, or may originate from a junctional escape rhythm. Temporary atrial standstill is caused by hyperkalemia. Persistent atrial standstill is associated with a heritable form of cardiomyopathy known as atrioventricular muscular dystrophy and is most commonly seen in English springer spaniels.

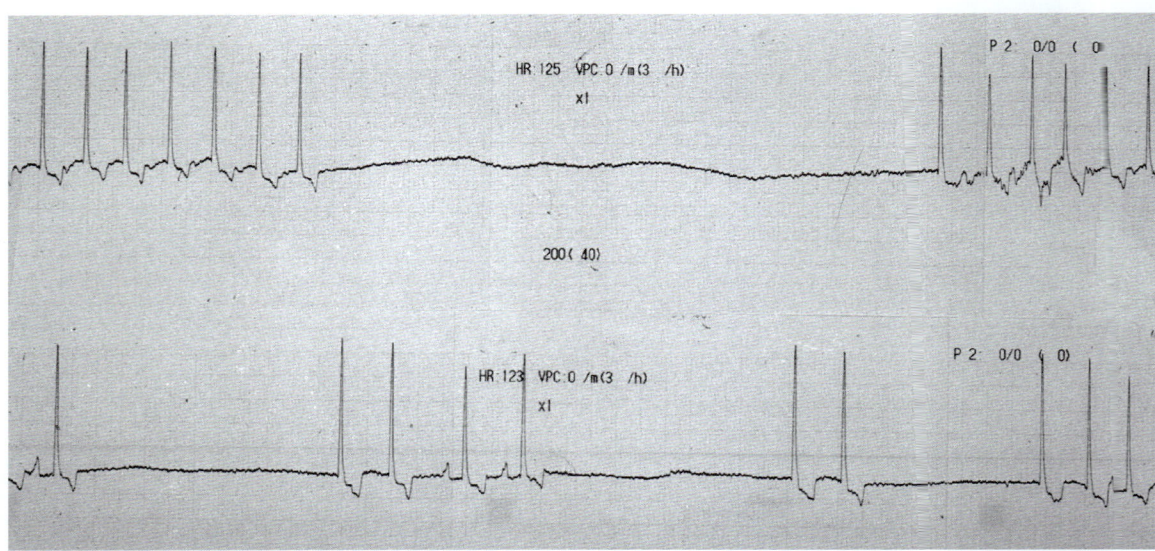

Figure 87.2 Electrocardiogram from a schnauzer with sick sinus syndrome. The electrocardiogram shows long periods of sinus pause terminated by junctional escape complexes.

Clinical presentation

Animals with persistent atrial standstill present with a history of progressive lethargy, exercise intolerance, and syncope. Physical examination is unremarkable except for bradycardia. Signs of congestive heart failure may occur. Animals with temporary atrial standstill present with clinical signs referable to the underlying cause of hyperkalemia. Causes of acute hyperkalemia include hypoadrenalcorticism, obstructive uropathy, acute oliguric renal failure, diabetic ketoacidosis, reperfusion injury, and drug toxicities.

Diagnosis

Electrocardiographic diagnosis of atrial standstill is based on an absence of P waves in all leads including unipolar thoracic leads (Figure 87.3). A slow narrow- or wide-complex escape rhythm will be present. Laboratory analysis should be performed urgently to rule out hyperkalemia. If hyperkalemia is not present, then persistent atrial standstill should be suspected. Echocardiographic evaluation of ventricular diastolic filling confirms absence of an atrial filling phase. Evidence of ventricular systolic dysfunction may also be present.

Indication for pacemaker

Pacemaker implantation is indicated for dogs with persistent atrial standstill who have a slow escape rhythm and signs referable to bradycardia (Cervenec *et al.* 2017). Pacemaker implantation in these animals may only be palliative because of progressive systolic dysfunction of the ventricles. Animals with temporary atrial standstill should undergo urgent medical therapy for hyperkalemia and its underlying cause.

Theories of artificial cardiac stimulation

For an electrical stimulus to trigger a self-propagating wave of depolarization within the myocardium, an electrical field of sufficient intensity must be applied between the two stimulating electrodes. The total energy (E) of a pacing stimulus is determined by the voltage (V), the current amplitude (I), and the duration of the stimulus (t):

$$E = VIt$$

Total energy can also be defined by the total impedance (R), V, and t:

$$E = V2t/R$$

The stimulation threshold is the minimum stimulus energy required to consistently achieve myocardial depolarization outside the refractory period of the heart. Stimulation thresholds have been expressed by varying different parameters that effect stimulus energy, including current (mA), voltage potential (V), total energy (micro-Joules), charge (Coulombs), pulse width (ms), and voltage quantity (V-sec).

Chronaxie and rheobase

The intensity of electrical stimulus required to capture the myocardium is dependent on the amount of time for which the stimulus is applied (i.e., pulse width or duration). This interaction of stimulus amplitude and pulse duration defines the strength duration curve (Figure 87.4). The total energy required for myocardial stimulation has an exponential relation with pulse duration, with a relatively flat curve at pulse durations greater than 1 ms and a rapidly rising curve at pulse durations less than 0.25 ms. Because of this relationship, pulses of

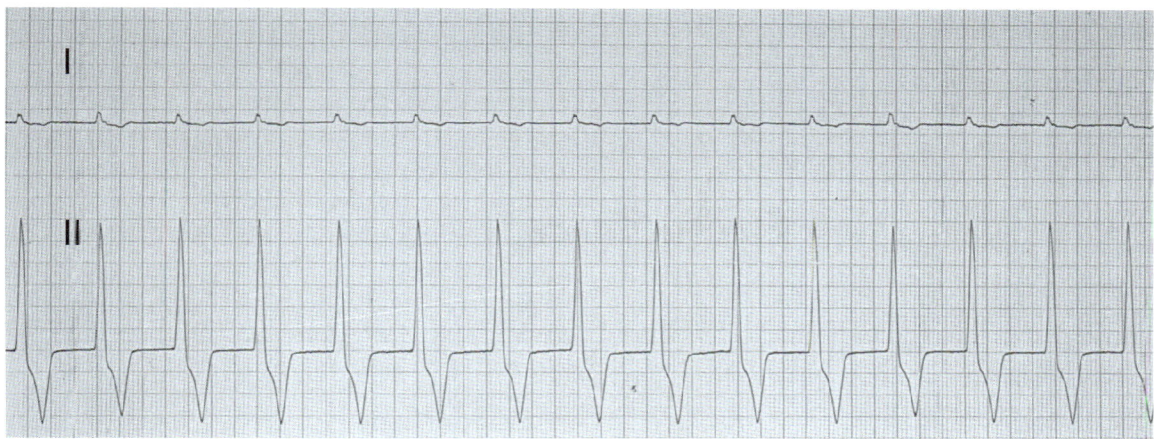

Figure 87.3 Electrocardiogram from a springer spaniel with a persistent atrial standstill (leads I and II). P waves were not present in any lead. A wide-complex (ventricular) escape rhythm is present.

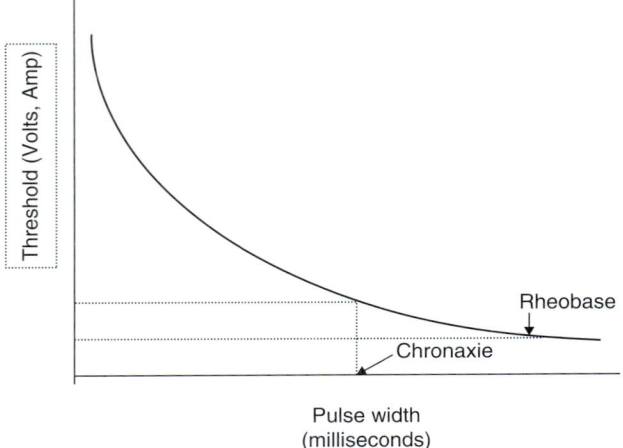

Figure 87.4 Strength–duration stimulation threshold curve. Rheobase is the current (amp) or voltage threshold that is independent of the pulse width. Chronaxie is the pulse width at twice the rheobase.

very short duration must have a higher intensity than pulses of longer duration to capture the myocardium. Conversely, increasing the pulse width over 1 ms has little influence on the intensity of the stimulus that is required to capture the heart.

The rheobase is defined as the lowest stimulus current (or voltage) that results in capture of the heart at an infinitely long pulse duration (Figure 87.4). A stimulus with a voltage below the rheobase does not capture the myocardium. Chronaxie is then defined as the threshold pulse width at twice rheobase stimulus current (or voltage). In most cases, chronaxie represents the best compromise between adequate pacing reliability and generator longevity.

A strength–duration curve can be determined for each patient if a pacemaker system analyzer (PSA) is available (Figure 87.5). For several pulse durations, the amplitude of the electrical stimulus can be decreased until the heart is not captured. Chronaxie and rheobase are then determined. Another, simpler technique is to determine the rheobase first by applying a pulse with a duration longer than 1 ms and determining the lowest amplitude required to capture the myocardium. The current intensity can be set to twice the rheobase and the chronaxie can be determined by varying the pulse width or duration. The pulse generator is then set at twice the stimulus threshold near the chronaxie pulse width to achieve the best pacing stimulus.

Pacing equipment

Pulse generator

A pulse generator must perform many functions. It must provide pacing therapy by generating appropriately

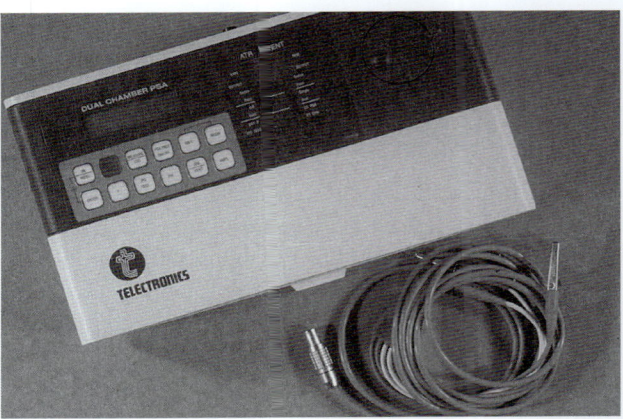

Figure 87.5 Pacemaker system analyzer. This device is used to determine the pacing and sensing thresholds of the electrodes and to measure electrode impedance.

timed stimulation pulses that are synchronized to the intrinsic cardiac rhythm. To do this, it needs an output and a sensing amplifier. For a rate-adaptive generator, the device must interpret physiologic or biophysical parameters that indicate changes in metabolic demand. The pulse generator must allow its parameters to be modified by a programmer (telemetry interface). Finally, the pulse generator needs a battery of either zinc-mercury or lithium.

Rate-responsive generators

Among the most important functions of the cardiovascular system is the appropriate adjustment of cardiac output during rest, exercise, and metabolic stress. Modulation of cardiac output is achieved by a change in both heart rate or stroke volume. When greater cardiac output is needed, an increase in heart rate is the dominant contributor, providing approximately 66–80% of the total increase in cardiac output for the normal heart. Initially, cardiac pacemakers were incapable of providing any increase in heart rate during periods of physiologic stress. More recent designs are able to change the pacing rate in response to physiologic stress and are called rate-adaptive pacemakers (Benditt & Duncan 1995). The most commonly used technology to detect body activity is a piezoelectric device inside the generator that is activated by vibration or movement of the body. Newer-generation pacemakers use sensors for right ventricular dP/dt, body temperature, minute ventilation, or mixed venous saturation as sources of information about physiologic activity (Benditt & Duncan 1995).

Five-letter code

The Mode Code Committee of the North American Society of Pacing and Electrophysiology introduced the

Table 87.1 Five-letter system to identify pacemaker function.

1st letter	2nd letter	3rd letter	4th letter	5th letter
Chamber paced	Chamber sensed	Response to sensing	Programmability/rate modulation	Anti-tachyarrhythmia functions
O: None	O: None	O: None	O: None	O: None
A: Atrium	A: Atrium	I: Inhibited	P: Simple programmable	P: Pacing (anti-tachyarrhythmia)
V: Ventricle	V: Ventricle	T: Triggered	M: Multiprogrammable	S: Shock
D: Dual (A&V)	D: Dual (I&T)	C: Communicating	D: Dual (P&S)	R: Rate modulation

pacing code in most common use at present (Table 87.1). The first three letters of the code describe the anti-bradycardia pacing functions. The fourth letter describes the degree of programmability of the device, or the presence or absence of rate modulation. By definition, a pacemaker is rate responsive if it is programmable. The fifth letter indicates the presence of one or more active anti-tachycardia functions and is only present for pacemakers that have these functions.

In veterinary medicine the most common pacing modes used are VVI, or VVIR when the pacemaker is implanted with an open surgical approach. The ventricle is the site of both pacing and sensing, and the pacing impulse is inhibited when a naturally occurring heartbeat is sensed. Different configurations can be used with a transvenous approach when both the atrium and the ventricle can be paced or sensed (DDDR). Dual-chamber pacing is the most desirable method to avoid the pacemaker syndrome. It requires placing of multiple transvenous leads and is associated with a longer surgical time (Genovese *et al.* 2013). Dual-chamber pacing can also be performed with epicardial implantation but requires an intercostal thoracotomy (Weder *et al.* 2015)

Leads

Leads conduct current from the pulse generator to the myocardium. They consist of one or two electrodes in contact with myocardium, a conductor surrounded by insulation, and a connector to the generator.

Electrodes

In an electrical circuit, electrons flow from the cathode to the anode to complete the circuit. By strict definition, all electrical circuits are bipolar. When applied to a pacemaker lead, the terms unipolar and bipolar simply indicate the number of electrodes in contact with the heart (Figure 87.6). Unipolar leads have only one electrode (the cathode) in contact with the heart. The current flows from the negatively charged cathode to the heart and returns to the pulse generator (anode) to complete the circuit. In a bipolar lead, both electrodes are a

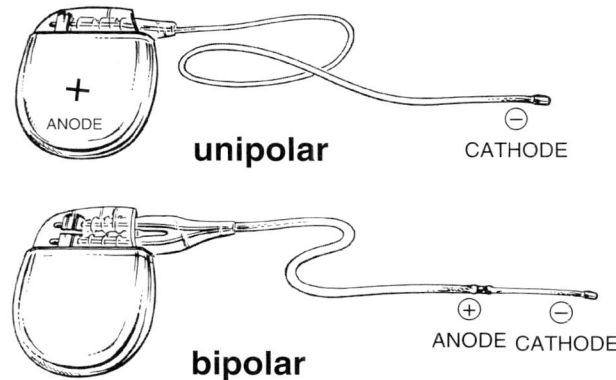

Figure 87.6 Differences between unipolar and bipolar lead systems. Source: Mond, H.G. and Helland, J.R. Engineering and clinical aspect of pacing leads. In Ellenbogen, K.A., Kay, G.N., and Wilkoff, B.L. eds. (1995). *Clinical Cardiac Pacing*, 69. Philadelphia, PA: W.B. Saunders.

short distance from each other at the distal end of the lead and both are in contact with the heart. The tip electrode is usually the cathode, and a ring electrode proximal to this serves as the anode. Bipolar leads were originally thicker and stiffer than unipolar leads. Today, bipolar leads have become almost as thin as unipolar leads, with less risk of obstructing veins or perforating the right ventricle. Stimulation thresholds are low and equivalent in both lead systems because the lead impedance is similar (Mond & Helland 1995).

Bipolar and unipolar electrodes are equally sensitive for detecting the intracardiac electrocardiogram. Bipolar atrial electrodes seem to be less sensitive to ventricular activity (known as far-field sensing) compared to unipolar atrial electrodes. Unipolar electrodes are also more susceptible to oversensing of skeletal myopotentials adjacent to the implanted pulse generator (Gialafos *et al.* 1985; Kay & Ellenbogen 1995; Lau *et al.* 1989; Levine & Klein 1983). Skeletal muscle twitching resulting from anodal stimulation of the muscle is also more common with unipolar electrodes than with bipolar electrodes. One advantage of a unipolar electrode is that the stimulus artifact can be recorded more easily on an electrocardiogram than can a bipolar artifact. Because of this difference, bipolar pacemakers can be more difficult to evaluate by external electrocardiogram alone.

The performance of the pacing electrodes is a major determinant of the stimulus intensity required to produce a self-propagating wavefront in the myocardium (Mond & Helland 1995).

The electrodes also affect lead impedance, a major factor that influences pulse generator longevity. Lastly, electrodes determine the sensing characteristics of the pacing system. The size, surface structure, and biological response to electrodes are critical factors in the design of pacing electrodes (Mond & Helland 1995).

The stimulation threshold varies as an inverse function of the size or geometric surface area of the stimulating electrode. By reducing the surface area of the electrodes, high current density and lower stimulation levels are obtained. A surface area of $8 \, mm^2$ seems to provide the optimum compromise between a small surface area that allows a low stimulus threshold and an acceptably high surface area for sensing (Mond & Helland 1995). Experimental studies have shown that electrodes with a porous surface that allows tissue ingrowth have a thinner fibrous capsule and a lower chronic threshold than electrodes with a solid or polished surface. Porosity of the electrodes allows a reduction of the polarization, the electrochemical impedance due to the accumulation of charge occurring at the electrode–myocardium interface. Polarization represents 30–40% of the total impedance. Electrode pores create areas of low polarization and zones of high current density (Mond & Helland 1995; Bobyn et al. 1981; Karpawich et al. 1988; Ormerod et al. 1988; Ripart & Mugica 1983).

Electrode size, pore size, and material influence the biological response of the myocardium to the foreign material. After implantation of the electrode, edema and fibrinolysis appear. Macrophages infiltrate the field and granulation tissue develops. Fibroblasts are attracted by chemotaxis. Macrophages also produce free radicals that induce cell death. A collagen capsule develops and impedance increases. The collagen capsule is conductive but not excitable. The thickness of the capsule is added to the size of the electrode to know the virtual diameter of the electrode. The collagen capsule is not a response to the electrical stimulus but rather a foreign-body reaction (Stokes & Kay 1995). Porous steroid-eluting electrodes induce the least amount of fibrous tissue production, whereas polished platinum electrodes induce the most amount of fibrous tissue (Bobyn et al. 1981; Hua et al. 1997; Karpawich et al. 1988; Radovsky et al. 1988; Schuchert et al. 1990).

The composition of the electrode is an important determinant of long-term function. Electrodes can corrode and degrade over time. Platinum is relatively nonreactive. Platinum powder creates a porous electrode with low polarization potential. Alloying platinum with 10% iridium increases its mechanical strength without altering its mechanical performances (Karpawich et al. 1988; Kertes et al. 1983; Mond & Helland 1995; Ripart & Mugica 1983).

Lead fixation

Lead fixation to the myocardium can be passive or active. Most common passive fixation designs are tines positioned immediately behind the electrode (Figure 87.7). Tines and other devices are extensions of the insulation material that are designed to become entrapped in the trabeculae of the right atrial appendage or right ventricle. Tined leads are the most popular method of endocardial lead fixation (Kertes et al. 1983; Mond & Sloman 1980).

Active lead fixation consists of an electrically active electrode screw at the distal end of the lead (Figures 87.8a and 87.9). Bipolar epicardial lead can be secure over the epicardium with mattress sutures (Figures 87.8b and 87.10). In the case of a transvenous lead, the screw is retractable or covered with a dissolving mannitol plug that prevents premature fixation during lead implantation. Active-fixation leads cause more tissue trauma and are more likely to result in significant elevations of the stimulation thresholds after implantation.

Lead connector

The connector is the portion of the lead used to connect the lead to the pulse generator. The standard lead connector is a low-profile 3.2 mm unipolar or bipolar

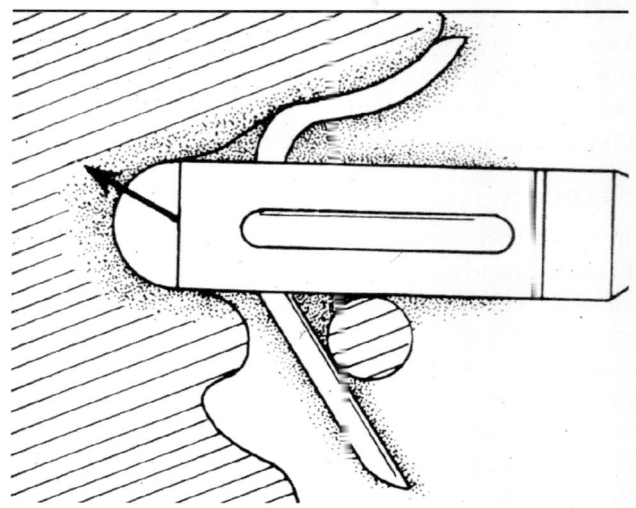

Figure 87.7 Passive lead fixation with tines.

(a)

(b)

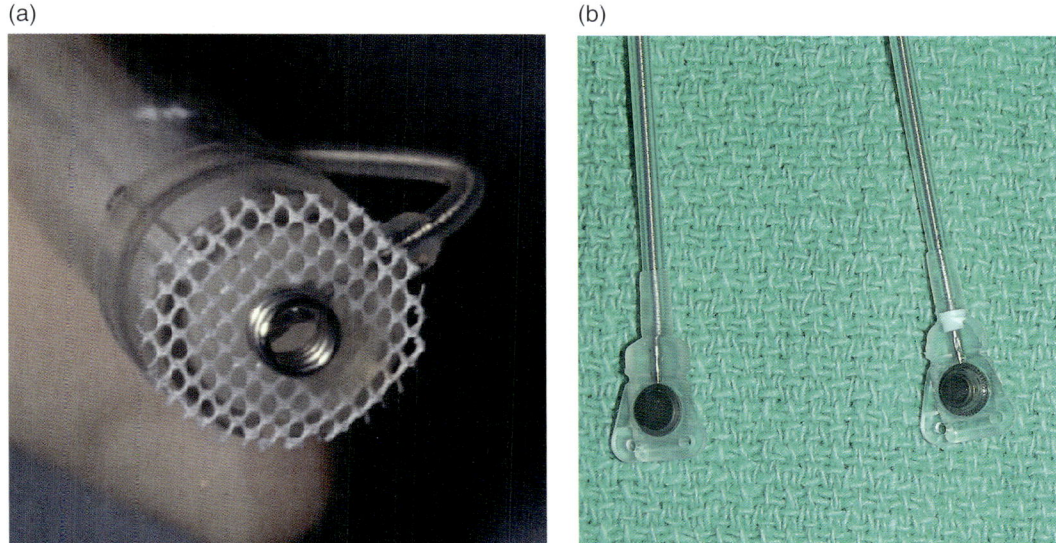

Figure 87.8 (a) Epicardial screw-in lead for active lead fixation. The electrode is implanted by turning the lead a specified number of turns. (b) Bipolar epicardial leads. They are secured on the epicardium with mattress sutures placed in the holes of the leads.

(a)

(b)

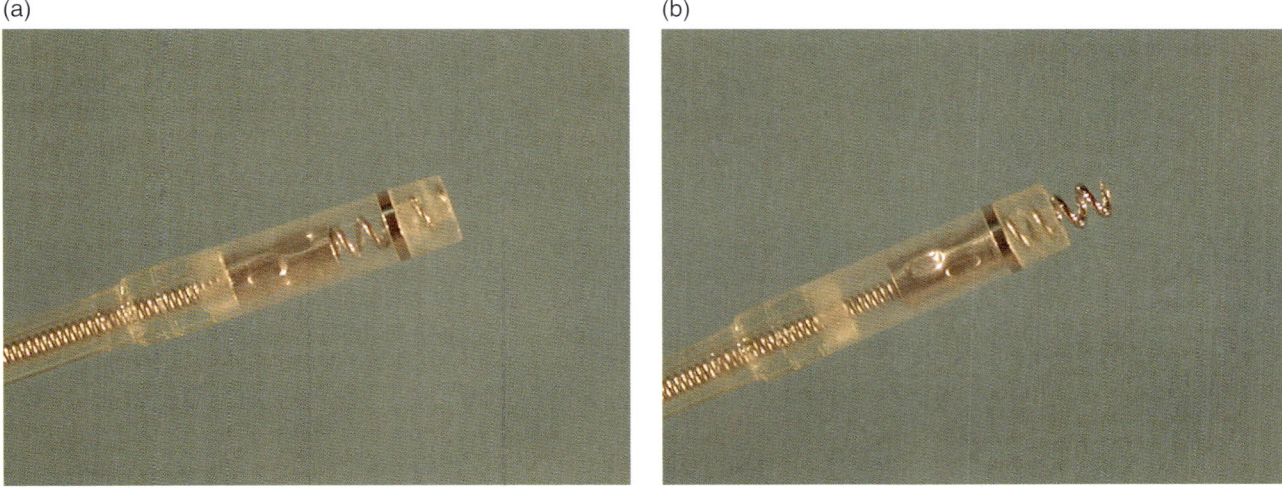

Figure 87.9 Endocardial screw-in lead. (a) The screw-in mechanism is retracted during introduction of the lead in the right ventricle. (b) The screw-in mechanism is exposed for active fixation in the myocardium of the right ventricle.

connector designated Voluntary Standard 1 (VS-1). Sealing rings are placed on the connectors between the anode and the cathode ring (Mond & Helland 1995).

Lead conductor and insulation

The lead conductor is usually made of an alloy of nickel, chromium, cobalt, and molybdenum that is very resistant to corrosion. Bipolar leads require two conductors. The coaxial design allows the creation of a bipolar lead that is as small as a unipolar lead. Lead insulation is made from different types of polyurethane (Kertes *et al.* 1983; Woscoboinik *et al.* 1992).

Surgical technique

Pacemakers can be implanted using either a transdiaphragmatic epicardial or a transvenous endocardial approach (Fox *et al.* 1986; Orton 2019). The transdiaphragmatic approach is more invasive because it requires a midline celiotomy and opening of the thoracic cavity. A mini-thoracotomy technique has also been described (Orton 2019). A transvenous approach can be used for either temporary or permanent pacemaker implantation, or both (Bellenger *et al.* 1990; Bigler *et al.* 1981; Flanders *et al.* 1999; Musselman *et al.* 1976; Reef *et al.* 1986; Sisson *et al.* 1991). The transvenous approach is the standard approach for placement of a permanent pacemaker in dogs because of its less invasive nature and reliability. A transdiaphragmatic epicardial approach can still be considered for small dogs and dogs with coagulation disorders and risk of thrombosis of the jugular vein and cranial vena cava (Wess *et al.* 2006; Van de Wiele *et al.* 2008; Cunningham *et al.* 2009; Mulz *et al.* 2010; Ward *et al.* 2016; Orton 2019).

Prior to implantation of a permanent pacemaker, it is usually necessary to increase the heart rate either with a temporary external pacemaker or pharmacologically. If a temporary external pacemaker is available, a flow-directed balloon-tip bipolar electrode is introduced into the jugular vein through a venous introducer and wedged in the trabeculae of the right ventricle under local anesthesia and light sedation. Prior to introduction, the transvenous electrode is connected to an external pacer set at 5 V and a rate of 100 bpm. The transvenous electrode is advanced into the right atrium where the balloon at the tip is inflated. The electrode is carried by the blood flow into the right ventricle. The electrocardiogram documents capture of the ventricle when the electrode is properly wedged into the trabeculae. Fluoroscopy may be used to assist with placement of the electrode and confirm its position. For sick sinus syndrome, the right atrium can be paced instead of the right ventricle. Percutaneous temporary pacing is also possible by placing two electrodes, one on each side of the thoracic cavity (Lee *et al.* 2010; Noomanova *et al.* 2010). If a temporary external pacemaker is not available, constant intravenous infusion of a β-adrenergic agonist such as isoproterenol (0.01 µg/kg/min) can be used during anesthesia to increase the rate of the escape rhythm, but this method is less reliable. Intraoperative antibiotic therapy is recommended during pacemaker implantation to reduce the risk of implant infection.

Transdiaphragmatic approach

Permanent transdiaphragmatic pacemaker implantation is accomplished through a ventral midline celiotomy. Balfour retractors are placed, the liver is gently retracted caudally, and the phrenicohepatic ligament is incised. A midline incision is made in the diaphragm to expose the pericardium and the apex of the heart. Stay sutures or tissue forceps are placed on the edge of the diaphragm for retraction (Figure 87.10). The pericardium is opened and retracted to expose the apex of the left ventricle. A screw-in unipolar epicardial electrode is implanted in the myocardium at the apex of the left ventricle, avoiding coronary arteries. The screw-in electrode is turned clockwise into the myocardium with a number of turns specified by the manufacturer. Epicardial electrodes can also be sutured to the epicardium at the apex of the left ventricle (Figures 87.11 and 87.12a).

Ideally, electrical impedance of the electrode should be measured to confirm appropriate implantation of the electrode.

A PSA allows measurement of total lead impedance and stimulation threshold after lead implantation. Lead impedance at implantation should be between 250 and 1000 Ω. A broken lead will have an impedance over 1000 Ω, whereas a leaking lead due to damage to the insulation will have an impedance below 250 Ω. The capture voltage (i.e., the lowest voltage at which the heart is paced) also can be determined. The PSA unit is set for a pulse width of 11 ms. The lowest voltage required to capture the myocardium is then determined by decreasing the pacing voltage from the PSA unit. The voltage for capture at this pulse width is equivalent to the rheobase.

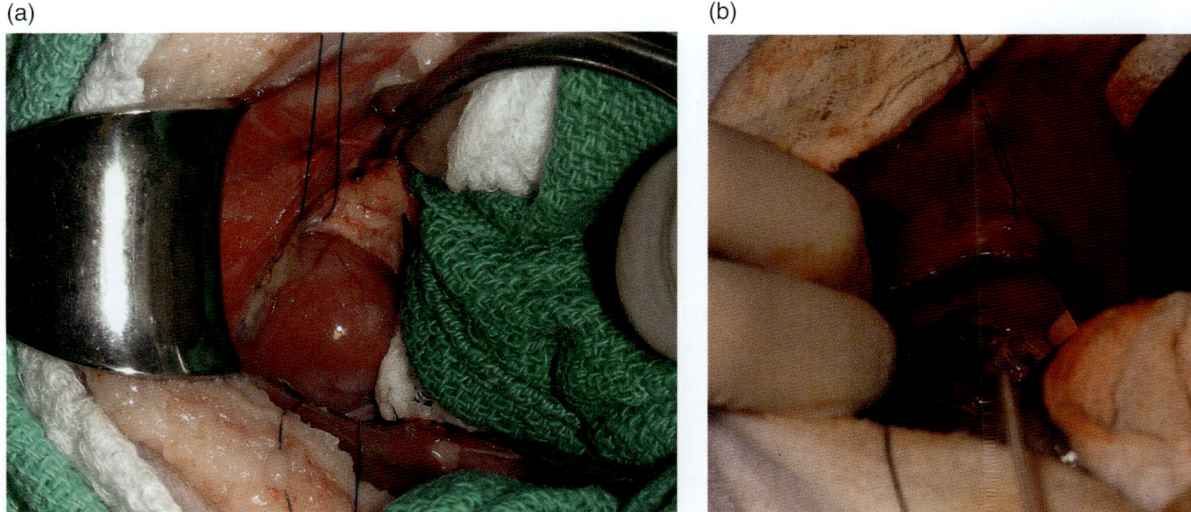

(a)   (b)

Figure 87.10 Transdiaphragmatic epicardial lead placement. (a) The apex of the left ventricle is exposed through the diaphragm and the pericardium. (b) The epicardial lead is screwed into the apex of the left ventricle after opening of the diaphragm and the pericardium. The tip of the electrode is turned a specific number of turns.

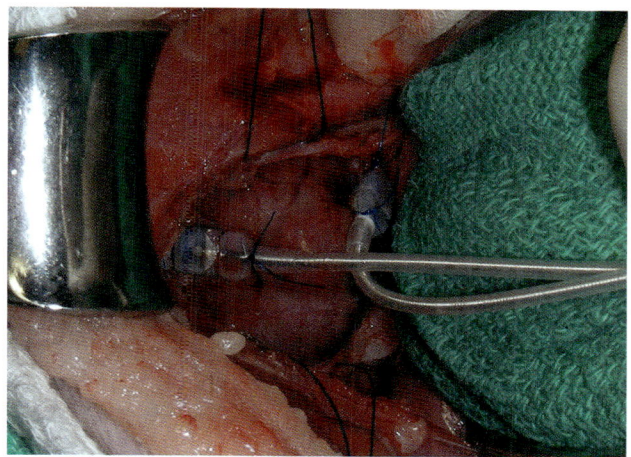

Figure 87.11 A bipolar epicardial lead has been sutured to the apex of the left ventricle with a transdiaphragmatic approach.

The chronaxie is then determined by doubling the rheobase and decreasing the pulse width until the myocardium is not captured. The lowest value for the pulse width is the chronaxie. Then the pacemaker should be set at twice the chronaxie voltage for safety. If pulse width is over 0.2 ms or the voltage over 3 V, the lead should be repositioned. Setting the pacemaker parameters with this technique allows for optimization of the longevity of the battery of the pulse generator without compromising the safety of the patient.

After the lead is tested and stimulation parameters are determined, the other end of the unipolar lead is connected and tightly secured with the pulse generator. The generator then is placed in a pouch between the transverse abdominalis muscle and the internal oblique (Figures 87.12a and 87.13). As soon as the pulse

(a)

(b)

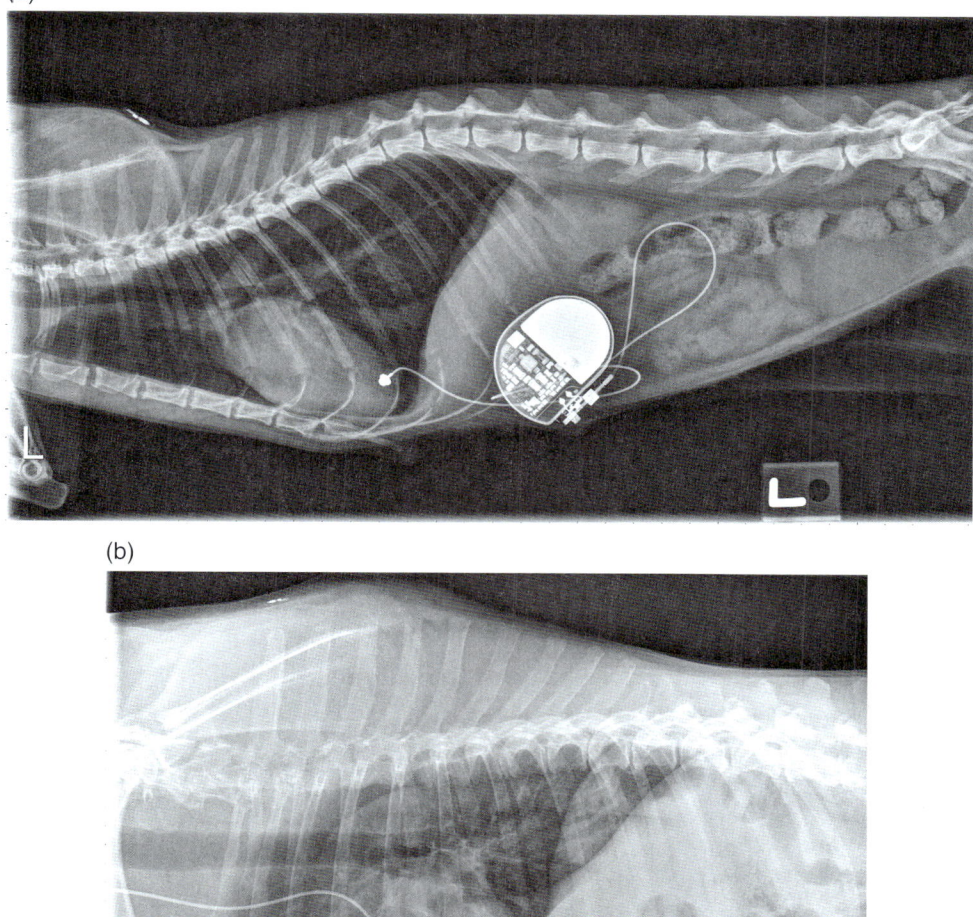

Figure 87.12 (a) Lateral radiograph after implantation of a screw-in epicardial lead in a cat. (b) Lateral radiograph after implantation of a transvenous endocardial lead in a dog.

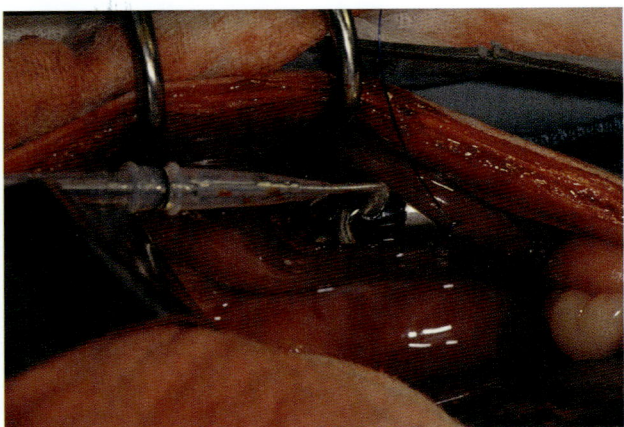

Figure 87.13 Transdiaphragmatic generator implantation. A pouch is developed in the abdominal wall between the transverse abdominalis muscle and the internal oblique muscle.

generator is placed in contact with the patient, temporary pacing is stopped and the permanent pacemaker paces the heart. A subcostal thoracostomy tube is implanted. The diaphragmatic incision, muscular pouch, and celiotomy are closed in a routine fashion. Care is taken not to damage the lead during suturing.

Mini-thoracotomy approach

A mini-thoracotomy on the left side can be performed to expose the apex of the left ventricle (Orton 2019). A skin incision is made caudal to the last rib and a pocket is created in the abdominal wall between the external and internal oblique muscles. After implantation of the epicardial electrodes, the leads are tunneled caudally in the subcutaneous space toward the pocket made in the abdominal wall. The generator is connected to the leads and then buried in the pocket, as described in the transdiaphragmatic approach.

Transvenous approach

The animal is placed in lateral recumbency with neck and space between the scapulae surgically prepared (Figure 87.14). The jugular vein is surgically exposed and retracted between two silk sutures. The sutures are pulled up to stop blood flow through the jugular vein. A no. 11 blade is used to make a transverse incision in the jugular vein between the two stay sutures. A vessel dilator is used to increase the opening of the jugular vein. The transvenous endocardial bipolar lead is advanced under fluoroscopy into the right ventricle (Figure 87.12b). The lead is either wedged in the trabeculae or screwed in the endocardium, according to the lead design. The total lead impedance is measured as for the transdiaphragmatic epicardial implantation. Bipolar leads should have an impedance between 250

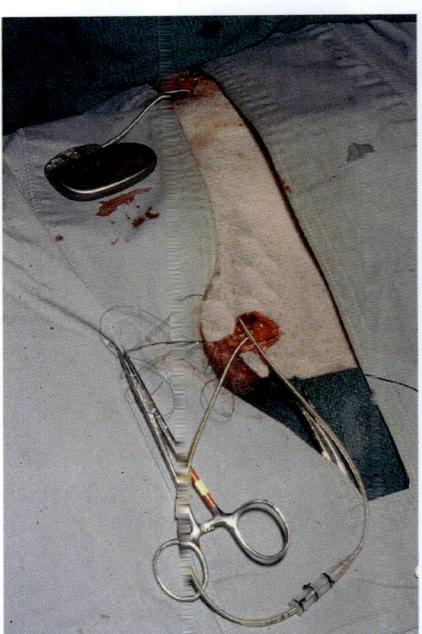

Figure 87.14 Transvenous endocardial lead placement. The jugular vein is exposed and the lead introduced into the vein. The lead is advanced into the right heart under fluoroscopic guidance. A loop of lead is left outside of the jugular vein to prevent dislodgment. The connector and the lead are tunneled between the scapulae. The pulse generator is implanted between the scapulae.

and 500 Ω. Some extra length of lead is left in the right ventricle to avoid traction on the lead during each cardiac cycle that could cause lead dislodgment. The silk sutures are tied around the lead. A 5 cm incision is made between the scapulae and a pocket is created in the subcutaneous tissues for the pulse generator. The lead is tunneled through the subcutaneous tissues of the neck to the subcutaneous pocket. A loop of lead is left next to the jugular vein to avoid excessive traction on the lead during lateral motion of the neck. The lead is connected to the pulse generator. The pulse generator is then placed in the subcutaneous pocket. The subcutaneous tissues and skin are closed.

Postoperative evaluation

After surgery, animals should undergo continuous electrocardiographic monitoring for 24 hours to confirm proper function of the pacemaker (Figure 87.15). The heart rate should not drop below the preset rate of the pacemaker. Pacemakers are usually set at an impulse rate between 80 and 100 bpm, according to the size of the animal and its projected activity level. Ventricular premature contractions often are seen after surgery due to myocardial injury associated with lead implantation. Lidocaine can be used to suppress ventricular premature contractions, but

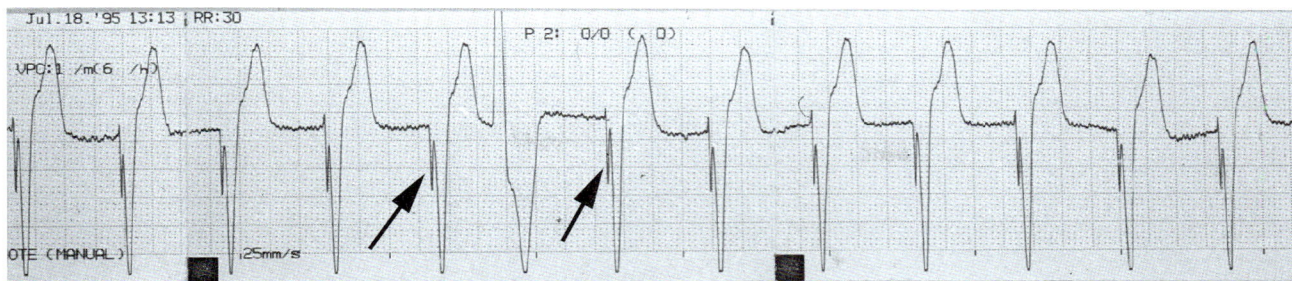

Figure 87.15 Electrocardiogram of a dog with normal VVI pacing. Electrical impulses from the pacemaker are seen as a negative spike on the electrocardiogram just before the QRS complex (arrows). Each pacing artifact is immediately followed by a wide-complex QRS-T indicating normal capture of the ventricle by the pacemaker. The pacemaker sensing function is normal because a single ventricular premature contraction was detected and pacing was briefly paused to avoid a competitive rhythm.

usually this is not necessary. The temporary transvenous lead may be left in place for 24 hours as a back-up in case of problems with the permanent pacemaker.

Pacing complications are due either to failure to capture, failure to sense, failure to capture and sense, or battery failure (Bonagura *et al.* 1983; Fingeroth 1994; Fox *et al.* 1991; Love & Hayes 1995; Sisson *et al.* 1991; Tilley *et al.* 1986; Wess *et al.* 2006; Johnson *et al.* 2007; Ward *et al.* 2015).

Failure to capture

Failure to capture is characterized on an electrocardiogram by pacemaker spikes that are not followed by a QRS-T complex (Figure 87.16). Recognition is more of a challenge with bipolar leads because pacing spikes are not always readily visible on a surface electrocardiogram. Augmentation of total lead impedance after implantation is the most common cause of failure to capture. Total lead impedance is due to resistance of the conducting lead, resistance between the electrode and the myocardium, and the resistance caused by polarization. Increased lead impedance from fibrous tissue deposition around the lead is the most common cause of the augmentation of total lead impedance after implantation. It takes approximately 4–6 weeks for sufficient fibrous tissue to develop and create an increase in impedance. Increasing the output voltage of the pulse generator by telemetry usually corrects this problem. Other causes of failure to capture are lead fracture, lead insulation failure, or lead dislodgment (Figure 87.17). A thoracic radiograph can help identify a lead fracture.

Measurement of lead impedance differentiates between a lead fracture or a lead insulation failure. Lead impedance should be less than 1000 Ω and more than 250 Ω. The impedance is higher than 2000 Ω with a lead fracture, while it is less than 250 Ω with an insulation leakage. Lead replacement will then be needed. Kits from the manufacturer are available to repair a broken

lead or an insulation failure. Lead dislodgment was common with early-style passive endocardial leads. Newer designs for passive fixation have substantially decreased this problem.

Failure to sense

Failure to sense intrinsic cardiac activity is classified as oversensing or undersensing. Failure to properly sense places the animal at risk for competitive tachycardia and ventricular fibrillation (i.e., undersensing) or to failure of appropriate pacing (i.e., oversensing) (Love & Hayes 1995; Kay & Ellenbogen 1995). Sensing of electrical activities other than QRS complexes is known as oversensing. Oversensing can be due to extracardiac or intracardiac signals. Oversensing causes inappropriate cessation of pacing by the pacemaker, which is programmed to sense and not compete with QRS complexes. Extracardiac signals are electromagnetic interference due to radio, television, radar, arc welding equipment, or medical equipment (electrocautery, magnetic resonance imaging) and skeletal myopotentials. Skeletal myopotential inhibition is the most common extracardiac cause of oversensing. Intracardiac oversensing occurs from far-field sensing (i.e., sensing P wave by ventricular electrode or sensing T wave by an atrial electrode), T wave sensing by a ventricular lead, afterpotential sensing (electrical activity due to polarization at the electrode–myocardium interface), or interaction with a temporary pacemaker (Figure 87.18). Variation of lead impedance from lead fracture, insulation failure, and loose connection to the generator can also contribute to oversensing (Kay & Ellenbogen 1995; Hauser & Susmano 1981). A blanking period prevents sensing of activity immediately after firing an impulse. This blanking period avoids T wave or afterpotential sensing. Changing the sensing threshold usually corrects oversensing, except when it is due to a lead problem. Turning *off* the sensing function of the pacemaker might be required in some cases.

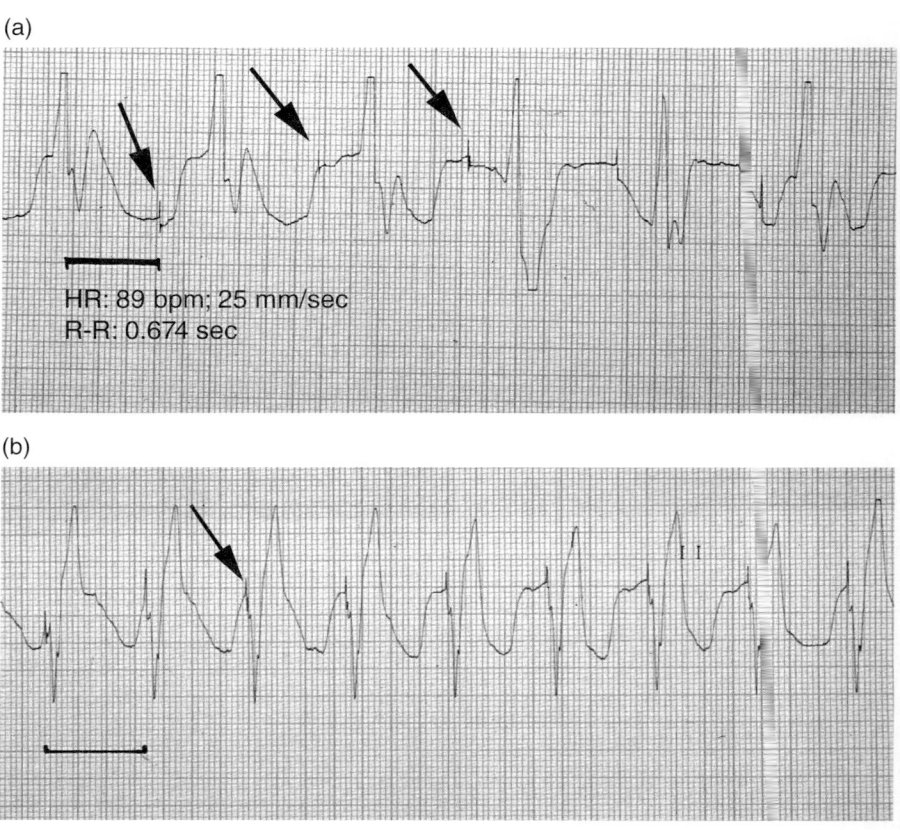

Figure 87.16 (a) Electrocardiogram from a dog with failure to capture. Pacing artifacts (arrows) are present that are not followed by a QRS-T complex. (b) Electrocardiogram for the same dog after adjustment of the output voltage. Pacing has been restored because pacing artifacts (arrow) are now followed by a QRS-T complex.

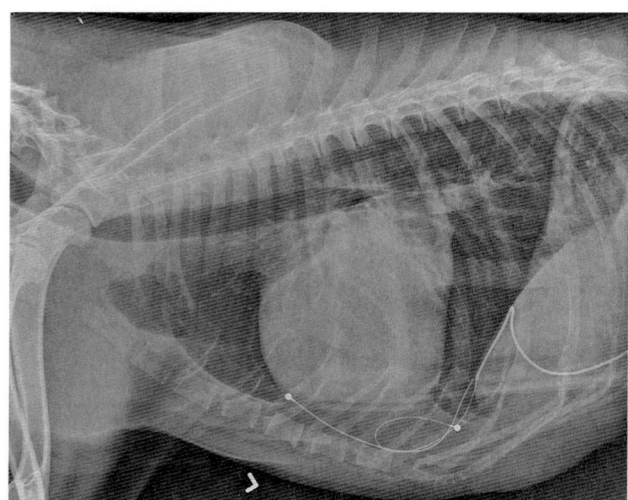

Figure 87.17 Lateral radiograph showing epicardial lead being detached from the epicardium.

Failure to sense an intrinsic QRS complex may result from lead fracture, lead insulation failure, lead dislodgment, improper fixation of the lead connector in the pulse generator, cross-talk in a dual-chamber device, or increased impedance at the lead–myocardium interface. Failure to sense is recognized on an electrocardiogram by the presence of a nonpaced QRS complex between two normally timed paced QRS complexes. Adjusting the sensitivity threshold generally corrects the problem (Kay & Ellenbogen 1995).

Fusion is defined as depolarization of the ventricle resulting from electrical activation occurring at two or more sites (Figure 87.19). Ventricular fusion usually results when ventricular activation occurs over the AV node–Purkinje conduction system as well as from a pacing stimulus. Fusion is manifested by a QRS complex wider than that seen during normal intrinsic ventricular activation. Pseudofusion refers to the electrocardiographic appearance of a pacemaker spike that fails to capture the ventricle that is superimposed on a QRS complex originating from normal atrioventricular conduction. Even if the pacing amplitude is sufficient to capture the myocardium, it is delivered after most of the myocardium has been depolarized (Figure 87.20).

(a)

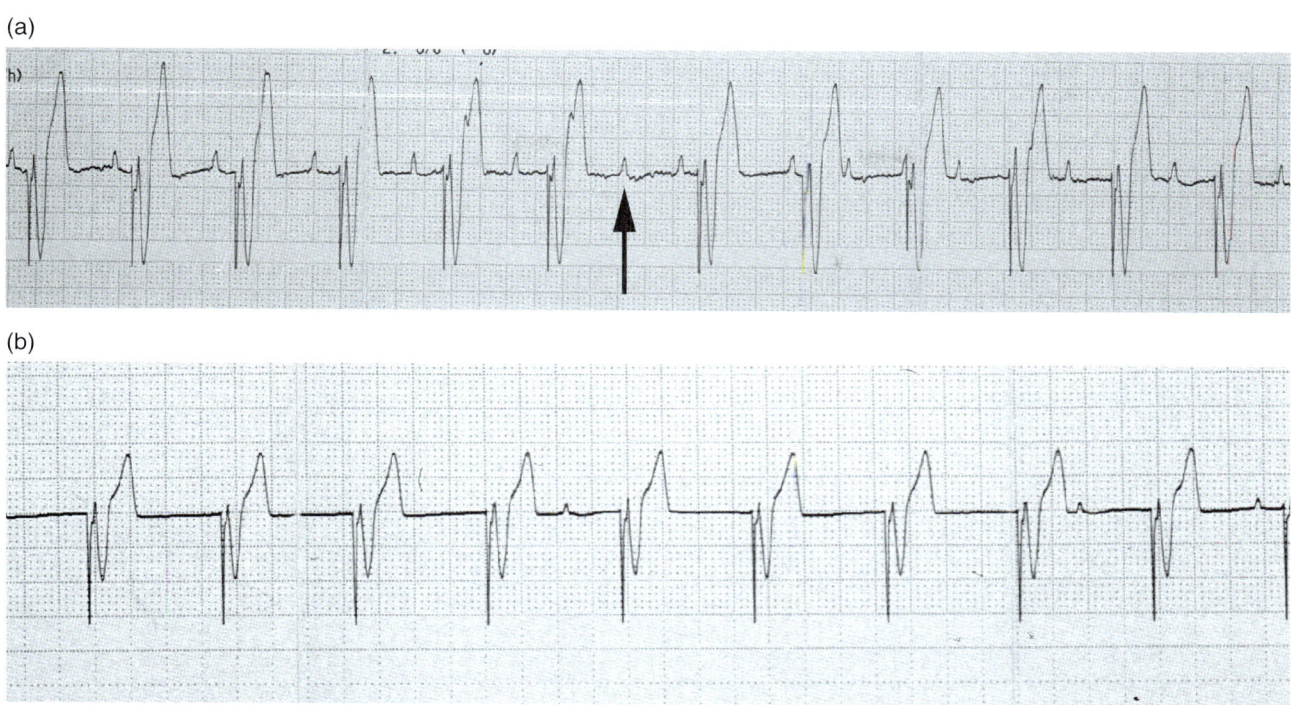

(b)

Figure 87.18 (a) Electrocardiogram of a dog with oversensing of the P wave (arrow) during VVI pacing. (b) Electrocardiogram of the same dog after turning off the sensing function of the pacemaker.

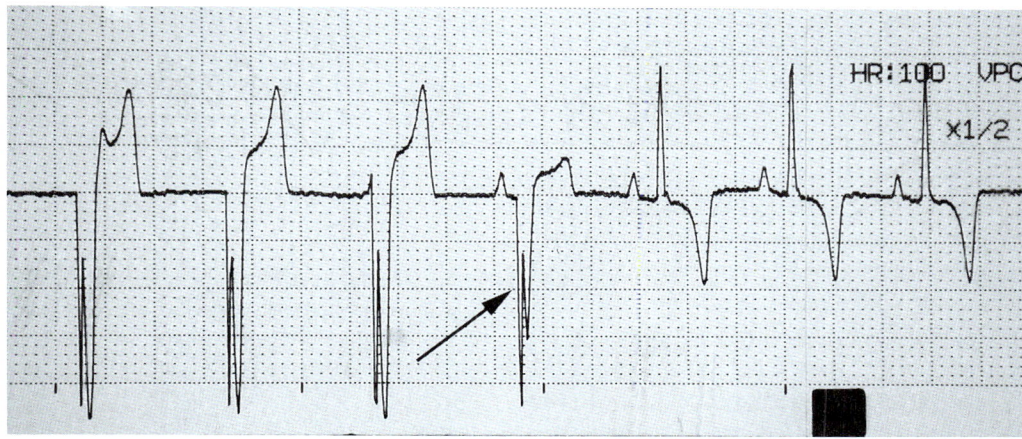

Figure 87.19 Electrocardiogram demonstrating a fusion complex (arrow) during VVI pacing in a dog. The was caused by nearly simultaneous activation of the ventricle by the pacemaker and an intrinsic complex.

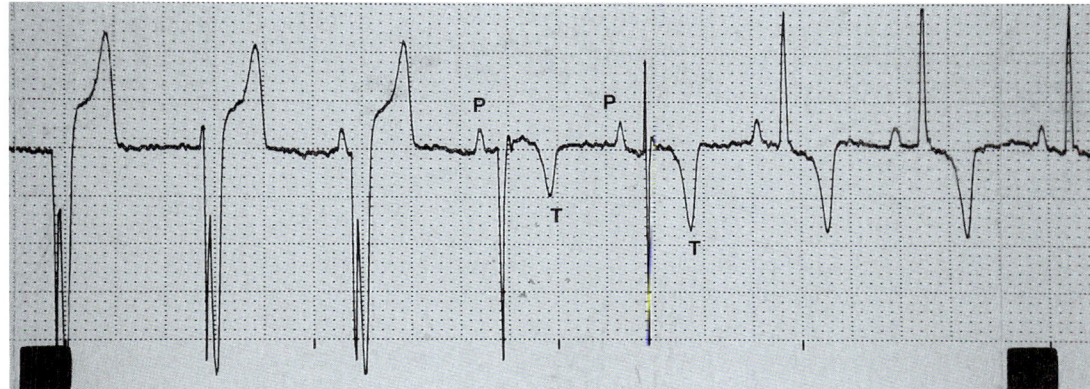

Figure 87.20 Electrocardiogram demonstrating a pseudofusion complex (fifth complex) during VVI pacing in a dog. The pacemaker delivered an impulse of adequate intensity, but did not capture because it occurred during the refractory period of an intrinsic beat.

Battery failure

A gradual decrease in the pacing rate indicates impending battery failure. Battery failure can also cause erratic behavior of the pacemaker (e.g., failure to capture, or to sense, or both). Confirmation of a battery failure is usually made after elimination of the other problems. The battery level of the newer generation of pacemakers can be measured by telemetry. A failing battery requires replacement of the pacemaker generator.

Seroma

A seroma can sometimes develop around the pacemaker. It has mostly been reported for pulse generators implanted in the neck, because of the motion of the neck area in companion animals. Implantation of the pacemaker between the shoulders seems to prevent this problem and keeps the pacemaker in a location easily accessible for interrogation and programming by telemetry.

A seroma is usually treated conservatively with hot packing. If the seroma does not resolve, the generator could be implanted in a different site (i.e., between the shoulders).

Hemodynamic effect of pacing: pacemaker syndrome

Pacemaker syndrome can result from the selection of a suboptimal pacing mode in animals with concurrent severe cardiac dysfunction. It is characterized by a reduction of arterial pressure and cardiac output, and the progression of congestive heart failure (Ellenbogen & Stambler 1995; Furman 1994; Levine et al. 1983; Travill & Sutton 1992). It is most commonly due to a loss of AV synchronization during single-chamber ventricular pacing. Atrial contraction contributes up to 30% of ventricular filling and cardiac output (Ogawa et al. 1978; Levine 1992; Janosik & Labovitz 1995). Loss of AV synchronization occurs with VVI pacing for third-degree AV block or atrial standstill. Further, atrial contraction against closed AV valves can contribute to atrial dilation and exacerbate signs of pulmonary congestion (Ogawa et al. 1978).

Pacemaker syndrome can be recognized at the time of implantation when arterial pressure drops by more than 20 mmHg after implanting the pacemaker. Pacemaker syndrome is corrected by dual-chamber AV synchronous pacing (DDI).

References

Bellenger, C.R. et al. (1990). Transvenous pacemaker leads in the dog: an experimental study. *Research in Veterinary Science* 49: 211.

Benditt, D.G. and Duncan, J.L. (1995). Activity-sensing rate-adaptive pacemakers. In: *Clinical Cardiac Pacing*, 1e (ed. K.A. Ellenbogen, G.N. Kay and B.L. Wilkoff), 167–186. Philadelphia, PA: WB Saunders.

Bigler, B., Gertsch, M., Schübach, P., and Häusermann, L. (1981). Implantation of an intravenous pacemaker system in a dachshund with a 3d grade AV-block and Margagni-Adams-Stokes crises. *Schweizer Archiv für Tierheilkunde* 123: 545.

Bobyn, J.D., Wilson, G.J., Mycyk, T.R. et al. (1981). Comparison of the porous-surfaced with a totally porous ventricular endocardial pacing electrode. *Pacing and Clinical Electrophysiology* 4: 405.

Bonagura, J.D., Helphrey, M.L., and Muir, W.W. (1983). Complications associated with permanent pacemaker implantation in the dog. *Journal of the American Veterinary Medical Association* 182: 149.

Buchanan, J.W., Dear, M.G., Pyle, R.L., and Berg, P. (1968). Medical and pacemaker therapy of complete heart block and congestive heart failure in a dog. *Journal of the American Veterinary Medical Association* 152: 1099.

Burrage, H. (2012). Sick sinus syndrome in a dog: treatment with dual-chambered pacemaker implantation. *Canadian Veterinary Journal* 53: 565–568.

Cervenec, R.M., Stauthammer, C.D., Fine, D.M. et al. (2017). Survival time with pacemaker implantation for dogs diagnosed with persistent atrial standstill. *Journal of Veterinary Cardiology* 19: 240–246.

Cunningham, S.M., Ames, M.K., Rush, J.E., and Rozanski, E.A. (2009). Successful treatment of pacemaker-induced stricture and thrombosis of the cranial vena cava in two dogs by use of anticoagulants and balloon venoplasty. *Journal of the American Veterinary Medical Association* 235: 1467–1473.

Ellenbogen, K.A. and Stambler, B.S. (1995). Pacemaker syndrome. In: *Clinical Cardiac Pacing* (ed. K.A. Ellenbogen, G.N. Kay and B.L. Wilkoff), 419. Philadelphia, PA: WB Saunders.

Fingeroth, J.M. (1994). Pacemaker therapy for bradycardias. *Seminars in Veterinary Medicine and Surgery (Small Animal)* 9: 192.

Flanders, J.A., Moïse, N.S., Gelzer, A.R. et al. (1999). Introduction of an endocardial pacing lead through the costocervical vein in six dogs. *Journal of the American Veterinary Medical Association* 215: 46.

Fox, P.R., Matthiesen, D.T., Purse, D., and Brown, N.O. (1986). Ventral abdominal, transdiaphragmatic approach for implantation of cardiac pacemakers in the dog. *Journal of the American Veterinary Medical Association* 189: 1303

Fox, P.R., Moise, N.S., Woodfield, J.A., and Darke, P.G. (1991). Techniques and complications of pacemaker implantation in four cats. *Journal of the American Veterinary Medical Association* 199: 1742.

Furman, S. (1994). Pacemaker syndrome. *Pacing and Clinical Electrophysiology* 17: 1.

Genovese, D.W., Estrada, A.H., Maisenbacher, H.W. et al. (2013). Procedure times, complication rates, and survival times associated with single-chamber versus dual-chamber pacemaker implantation in dogs with clinical signs of bradyarrhythmia: 54 cases (2004–2009). *Journal of the American Veterinary Medical Association* 242: 230–236.

Gialafos, J., Maillis, A., Kalogeropoulos, C. et al. (1985). Inhibition of demand pacemakers by myopotentials. *American Heart Journal* 109: 984.

Hackett, T.B., Van Pelt, D.R., Willard, M.D. et al. (1995). Third degree atrioventricular block and acquired myasthenia gravis in four dogs. *Journal of the American Veterinary Medical Association* 206: 1173.

Hauser, R.G. and Susmano, A. (1981). After-potential oversensing by a programmable pulse generator. *Pacing and Clinical Electrophysiology* 4: 391.

Hua, W., Mond, H.G., and Strathmore, N. (1997). Chronic steroid-eluting lead performance: a comparison of atrial and ventricular pacing. *Pacing and Clinical Electrophysiology* 20: 17.

Janosik, D.L. and Labovitz, A.J. (1995). Basic physiology of cardiac pacing. In: *Clinical Cardiac Pacing* (ed. K.A. Ellenbogen et al.), 367–398. Philadelphia, PA: WB Saunders.

Johnson, M.S., Martin, M.W., and Henley, W. (2007). Results of pacemaker implantation in 104 dogs. *Journal of Small Animal Practice* 48: 4–11.

Karpawich, P.P., Stokes, K.B., Helland, J.R. et al. (1988). A new low threshold platinized epicardial pacing electrode: comparative evaluation in immature canines. *Pacing and Clinical Electrophysiology* 11: 1139.

Kay, G.N. and Ellenbogen, K.A. (1995). Sensing. In: *Clinical Cardiac Pacing* (ed. K.A. Ellenbogen et al.), 36–68. Philadelphia, PA: WB Saunders.

Kertes, P., Mond, H., Sloman, G. et al. (1983). Comparison of lead complications with polyurethane tined, silicone rubber tined, and wedge tip leads: clinical experience with 822 ventricular endocardial lads. *Pacing and Clinical Electrophysiology* 6: 957.

Lau, C.P., Linker, N.J., Butrous, G.S. et al. (1989). Myopotential interference in unipolar rate responsive pacemakers. *Pacing and Clinical Electrophysiology* 12: 1324.

Lee, S., Nam, S.J., and Hyun, C. (2010). The optimal size and placement of transdermal electrodes are critical for the efficacy of a transcutaneous pacemaker in dogs. *Veterinary Journal* 183: 196–200.

Levine, P.A. (1992). Benefits of dual-chamber pacemakers. *Western Journal of Medicine* 156: 70.

Levine, P.A. and Klein, M.D. (1983). Myopotential inhibition of unipolar pacemakers: a disease of technologic progress. *Annals of Internal Medicine* 98: 101.

Levine, P.A., Seltzer, J.P., and Pirzada, F.A. (1983). The "pacemaker syndrome" in a properly functioning physiologic pacing system. *Pacing and Clinical Electrophysiology* 6: 279.

Love, C.J. and Hayes, D.L. (1995). Evaluation of pacemaker malfunction. In: *Clinical Cardiac Pacing* (ed. K.A. Ellenbogen et al.), 656–683. Philadelphia, PA: WB Saunders.

Moise, N.S. (1999). Pacemaker therapy. In: *Textbook of Canine and Feline Cardiology* (ed. P.R. Fox, D. Sisson and N.S. Moise), 400–425. Philadelphia, PA: WB Saunders. pp. 400–425

Mond, H.G. and Helland, J.R. (1995). Engineering and clinical aspects of pacing leads. In: *Clinical Cardiac Pacing* (ed. K.A. Ellenbogen et al.), 69–90. Philadelphia, PA: WB Saunders.

Mond, H. and Sloman, G. (1980). The small-tined pacemaker lead – absence of dislodgement. *Pacing and Clinical Electrophysiology* 3: 171.

Mulz, J.M., Kraus, M.S., Thompson, M., and Flanders, J.A. (2010). Cranial vena caval syndrome secondary to central venous obstruction associated with a pacemaker lead in a dog. *Journal of Veterinary Cardiology* 12: 217–223.

Musselman, E.E., Rouse, G.P., and Parker, A.J. (1976). Permanent pacemaker implantation with transvenous electrode placement in a dog with complete atrioventricular heart block, congestive heart failure and Stokes–Adams syndrome. *Journal of Small Animal Practice* 17: 149.

Noomanova, N., Perego, M., Perini, A., and Santilli, R.A. (2010). Use of transcutaneous external pacing during transvenous pacemaker implantation in dogs. *Veterinary Record* 167: 241–244.

Noszczyk-Nowak, A., Michalek, M., Kapturska, K. et al. (2019). Retrospective analysis of indications and complications related to implantation of permanent pacemaker: 25 years of experience in 31 dogs. *Journal of Veterinary Research* 63: 133–140.

Ogawa, S., Dreifus, L.S., Shenoy, P.N. et al. (1978). Hemodynamic consequences of atrioventricular and ventriculoatrial pacing. *Pacing and Clinical Electrophysiology* 1: 8.

Ormerod, D., Walgren, S., Berglund, J., and Heil, R. Jr. (1988). Design and evaluation of a low threshold, porous tip lead with a mannitol coated screw-in tip ("Sweet Tip"). *Pacing and Clinical Electrophysiology* 11: 1784.

Orton, E.C. (2019). Epicardial pacemaker implantation in small animals. *Journal of Veterinary Cardiology* 22: 65–71.

Pibarot, P., Vrins, A., Salmon, Y., and Difruscia, R. (1993). Implantation of a programmable atrioventricular pacemaker in a donkey with complete atrioventricular block and syncope. *Equine Veterinary Journal* 25: 248.

Radovsky, A.S., Van Vleet, J.F., Stokes, K.B., and Tacker, W.A. Jr. (1988). Paired comparisons of steroid-eluting and nonsteroid endocardial pacemaker leads in dogs: electrical performance and morphologic alterations. *Pacing and Clinical Electrophysiology* 11: 1085.

Reef, V.B., Clark, E.S., Oliver, J.A., and Donawick, W.J. (1986). Implantation of a permanent transvenous pacing catheter in a horse with complete heart block and syncope. *Journal of the American Veterinary Medical Association* 189: 449.

Ripart, A. and Mugica, J. (1983). Electrode-heart interface: definition of the ideal electrode. *Pacing and Clinical Electrophysiology* 6: 410.

Santilli, R.A., Giacomazzi, F., Porteiro Vazquez, D.M., and Perego, M. (2019). Indications for permanent pacing in dogs and cats. *Journal of Veterinary Cardiology* 22: 20–39.

Schuchert, A., Hopf, M., Kuck, J.H., and Bleifeld, W. (1990). Chronic ventricular electrograms: do steroid-eluting leads differ from conventional leads? *Pacing and Clinical Electrophysiology* 13: 1879.

Sisson, D., Thomas, W.P., Woodfield, J. et al. (1991). Permanent transvenous pacemaker implantation in forty dogs. *Journal of Veterinary Internal Medicine* 5: 322.

Stokes, K.B. and Kay, G.N. (1995). Artificial electric cardiac stimulation. In: *Clinical Cardiac Pacing* (ed. K.A. Ellenbogen, G.N. Kay and B.L. Wilkoff), 3–37. Philadelphia, PA: WB Saunders.

Sykes, G.P. (1979). Pacemaker and sutureless lead implantation in a dog with third-degree heart block. *Veterinary Medicine* 74: 1463.

Tilley, L.P., Miller, M.S., and Owens, J.M. (1986). Radiographic aspects of cardiac pacemakers. *Seminars in Veterinary Medicine and Surgery (Small Animal)* 1: 165.

Travill, C.M. and Sutton, R. (1992). Pacemaker syndrome: an iatrogenic condition. *British Heart Journal* 68: 163.

Van De Wiele, C.M., Hogan, D.F., Green, H.W. 3rd, and Parnell, N.K. (2008). Cranial vena caval syndrome secondary to transvenous pacemaker implantation in two dogs. *Journal of Veterinary Cardiology* 10: 155–161.

Ward, J.L., DeFrancesco, T.C., Tou, S.P. et al. (2015). Complication rates associated with transvenous pacemaker implantation in dogs with high-grade atrioventricular block performed during versus after normal business hours. *Journal of Veterinary Internal Medicine* 29: 157–163.

Ward, J.L., DeFrancesco, T.C., Tou, S.P. et al. (2016). Outcome and survival in canine sick sinus syndrome and sinus node dysfunction: 93 cases (2002–2014). *Journal of Veterinary Cardiology* 18: 199–212.

Weder, C., Monnet, E., Ames, M., and Bright, J. (2015). Permanent dual chamber epicardial pacemaker implantation in two dogs with complete atrioventricular block. *Journal of Veterinary Cardiology* 17: 154–160.

Wess, G., Thomas, W.P., Berger, D.M., and Kittleson, M.D. (2006). Applications, complications, and outcomes of transvenous pacemaker implantation in 105 dogs (1997–2002). *Journal of Veterinary Internal Medicine* 20: 877–884.

Woscoboinik, J.R. et al. (1992). Pacing lead survival: performance of different models. *Pacing and Clinical Electrophysiology* 15: 1991.

Zymet, C.L. (1981). Use of a pacemaker to correct sinus bradycardia in a dog. *Veterinary Medicine* 76: 65.

Section 12

Hematopoietic

88

Surgical Treatment of Splenic Disease

Kyla Walter and William T.N. Culp

The spleen performs many important functions in companion animals; however, removal of part or all of the spleen can be performed and generally results in no untoward consequences. Despite this, surgery should not be taken lightly, as complications associated with splenic disease and spleen-related surgical procedures can be severe. Pathologic conditions of the spleen are relatively common in dogs and cats and understanding the preoperative, intraoperative, and postoperative scenarios that can be encountered is important for reaching a successful outcome.

Splenic diseases

Neoplasia

Hemangiosarcoma

Hemangiosarcoma represents 45–51% of canine splenic malignancies (Brown *et al.* 1985; Eberle *et al.* 2012; Prymak *et al.* 1988; Spangler & Culbertson 1992b; Spangler & Kass 1997). Some authors have suggested that hemangiosarcoma is the most common splenic pathology diagnosed in dogs (Day *et al.* 1995); however, results of a large retrospective evaluation of splenic diseases revealed that hyperplastic splenic nodules were diagnosed over twice as often as hemangiosarcoma (Spangler & Culbertson 1992b). Hemangiosarcoma is the third most common tumor affecting feline spleens (Spangler & Culbertson 1992a).

Hemangiosarcoma is diagnosed more often in the spleen of dogs than in any other organ (Brown *et al.* 1985; Clifford *et al.* 2000). When evaluating visceral hemangiosarcoma in cats, both the spleen and the liver have been shown to be the most common location for heman-

giosarcoma, depending on the study (Culp *et al.* 2008; Scavelli *et al.* 1985). In dogs with splenic hemangiosarcoma, just over half are classified as grade III (metastatic disease noted at the time of diagnosis) (Brown *et al.* 1985), and dogs with multiple-lesion splenic hemangiosarcoma have been shown to have a worse prognosis than dogs with single-lesion splenic hemangiosarcoma (Spangler & Kass 1997). The typical sites of metastasis include the liver, omentum, mesentery, and lungs. The presence of concurrent splenic and cardiac hemangiosarcoma is reported in ~9% of cases (Boston *et al.* 2011).

Dogs are often diagnosed with splenic hemangiosarcoma as a result of clinical signs associated with ruptured tumors (Eberle *et al.* 2012; Hammond & Pesillo-Crosby 2008; Pintar *et al.* 2003). The cause of nontraumatic hemoperitoneum is most likely to be splenic in origin (~60–75%); however, in small dogs (<20 kg) the prevalence is lower (~43% splenic origin) (Aronsohn *et al.* 2009; Fleming *et al.* 2018; Story *et al.* 2020; Pintar *et al.* 2003). In dogs with hemorrhage resulting from splenic lesions, hemangiosarcoma was diagnosed in 56–70%, as opposed to nonmalignant splenic pathology (Aronsohn *et al.* 2009; Eberle *et al.* 2012; Hammond & Pesillo-Crosby 2008; Pintar *et al.* 2003). The prevalence of hemangiosarcoma in dogs with incidentally identified splenic masses is lower (30–50%) (Cleveland & Casale 2016; Day *et al.* 1995; Spangler & Culbertson 1992b).

Overall, the prognosis for dogs with splenic hemangiosarcoma is poor, with median survival times in the 2–3-month range (Batschinski *et al.* 2018; Brown *et al.* 1985; Hammond & Pesillo-Crosby 2008; Kim *et al.* 2007; Wood *et al.* 1998). However, the administration of chemotherapy significantly improves median survival times to approximately 4.5–6.5 months, with a doxorubicin-based protocol generally being the chemotherapy regimen of choice (Clifford *et al.* 2000; Story *et al.* 2020; Ogilvie *et al.* 1996). Several other protocols have been attempted and often involve the addition of other chemotherapeutic drugs such as vincristine and cyclophosphamide to a protocol incorporating doxorubicin (Hammer *et al.* 1991; Sorenmo *et al.* 1993). Another anthracycline drug called epirubicin was evaluated in dogs with splenic hemangiosarcoma and similar survival times were noted in these dogs when compared to historical survival times in dogs receiving doxorubicin-based protocols (Kim *et al.* 2007). That same study also noted a significantly longer median survival time (345 days) in stage I dogs undergoing splenectomy and receiving epirubicin compared to stage II (93 days) and III (68 days) dogs with similar treatment protocols (Kim *et al.* 2007). A prospective evaluation of adjuvant doxorubicin and dacarbazine (ADTIC) with traditional doxorubicin and cyclophosphamide (AC) demonstrated longer survival times in dogs treated with ADTIC compared with those receiving AC (>550 days vs. 142 days mean survival time) (Finotello *et al.* 2017). Alvarez *et al.* (2013) suggested that a vincristine, doxorubicin, and cyclophosphamide chemotherapy protocol may provide some survival benefit for dogs with stage III hemangiosarcoma; however, this protocol may be associated with high toxicities.

Many researchers are targeting other treatment modalities in an effort to improve outcome in dogs diagnosed with hemangiosarcoma (Clifford *et al.* 2000; Lana *et al.* 2007; U'Ren *et al.* 2007; Sorenmo *et al.* 1993). Dogs with splenic hemangiosarcoma have been treated with a daily low-dose oral chemotherapy drug protocol (etoposide, cyclophosphamide, piroxicam), and outcome in those dogs was at least as good as outcomes in dogs receiving doxorubicin (Lana *et al.* 2007). The administration of intracavitary pegylated liposomal encapsulated doxorubicin was shown to decrease the serosal, mesenteric, and omental metastases in dogs with splenic hemangiosarcoma; however, this treatment did not prevent intra-abdominal recurrence of hemangiosarcoma (Sorenmo *et al.* 1993). Adding an immune stimulant to chemotherapy has shown a survival advantage over the administration of chemotherapy alone, and that study provided an impetus for evaluation of a tumor vaccine in dogs with hemangiosarcoma (U'Ren *et al.* 2007). The vaccine was shown to be safe in dogs and induced an immune response in dogs receiving doxorubicin (U'Ren *et al.* 2007). Further study into this potential treatment option is needed.

Hemangioma

Splenic hemangiomas are exceedingly rare. In dogs, splenic hemangiomas have been diagnosed in <1–3% of cases of pathologic splenic samples (Spangler & Culbertson 1992b; Spangler & Kass 1997). No cases of splenic hemangioma were diagnosed in 455 feline splenic disease samples in one study (Spangler & Culbertson 1992a). In a group of four dogs diagnosed with splenic hemangioma, survival data was available for two; one dog was still alive 17 months post splenectomy, and one dog died four years after splenectomy from heart failure (Day *et al.* 1995).

Lymphoma

Splenectomy is often recommended in dogs and cats diagnosed with lymphoma that is isolated to the spleen. When canine splenic lymphoma is diagnosed, the spleen is generally the only site affected (Valli *et al.* 2006). Canine splenic lymphoma more often forms a mass lesion that extends outward from the splenic capsule in a localized region (Valli *et al.* 2006). Dogs with splenic lymphoma treated by splenectomy had a one-year survival rate of 58.8% (van Stee *et al.* 2015) and B-cell lymphoma held a better prognosis for survival than other variants. Confinement of disease to the spleen was a positive prognostic indicator and adjuvant chemotherapy did not provide a survival benefit. Marginal zone lymphoma, a form of indolent B-cell lymphoma, was associated with a prolonged survival time following splenectomy in patients with no clinical signs (1153 days compared to 309 days in dogs with clinic signs) (O'Brien *et al.* 2013).

Nonlymphomatous/nonangiogenic sarcomas

Histiocytic disease affecting the spleen is still being characterized, but veterinary literature discussing this disease process is increasing (Affolter & Moore 2002; Hendrick *et al.* 1992; Morris *et al.* 2002; Latifi *et al.* 2020; Spangler & Kass 1998). In a previous retrospective case series of dogs with splenic fibrohistiocytic nodules (SFHN), the lymphoid : fibrohistiocytic proportion and mitotic index of the cells composing the nodule were shown to influence survival (Spangler & Kass 1998). Dogs with a higher proportion of lymphoid to fibrohistiocytic-type cells had longer survival times compared to dogs with lower proportions (Spangler & Kass 1998). More recent work has confirmed that this group of dogs with SFHN included a heterogeneous group of disease that did not correspond with SFHN grade or percentage of lymphocytes (Moore *et al.* 2012). The large number of diagnoses makes it difficult to evaluate prognosis.

Histiocytic sarcoma can be diagnosed in either a local or systemic form, and the spleen is often the primary location (Affolter & Moore 2002). Metastasis from splenic histiocytic sarcoma is commonly diagnosed in the lymph nodes and liver (Affolter & Moore 2002). Localized splenic histiocytic sarcoma is poorly understood, but may have a longer survival time than disseminated histiocytic sarcoma. Dogs undergoing splenectomy with adjuvant lomustine-based chemotherapy had a median survival time of 427 days (Latifi *et al.* 2020).

Other nonlymphomatous/nonangiogenic sarcomas have been identified in the spleen and include fibrosarcoma, undifferentiated sarcoma, leiomyosarcoma, osteosarcoma, chondrosarcoma, rhabdomyosarcoma, mesenchymoma, myxosarcoma, leiomyoma, plasma cell myeloma, lipoma-myelolipoma, and liposarcoma (Knapp *et al.* 1993; Langenbach *et al.* 1998; Smolowitz & Carpenter 1988; Spangler & Culbertson 1992a,b; Spangler *et al.* 1994; Spangler & Kass 1997; Zimmer & Stair 1983). Of these tumors, the malignant forms have demonstrated poor median survival times (2.5–4 months), with mortality rates of 80–100% at one year after diagnosis (Langenbach *et al.* 1998; Spangler *et al.* 1994). The mitotic index of this group of tumors affects prognosis, as tumors with a mitotic index >9 have significantly shorter survival times than those with a lower mitotic index (Spangler *et al.* 1994). Additionally, cases with metastatic disease noted at the time of splenectomy have a median survival time of one month, which is significantly worse than cases without metastatic disease (Weinstein *et al.* 1989).

Mast cell tumors

Mast cell tumors are the most common malignant tumor affecting the spleen in cats (Figure 88.1) (Spangler & Culbertson 1992a); however, splenic mast cell disease is uncommon in dogs, accounting for less than 1% of all

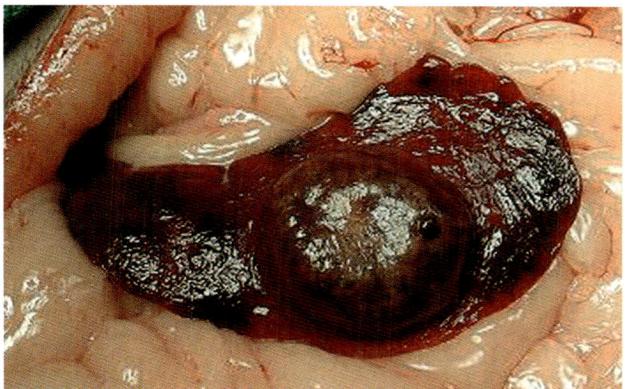

Figure 88.1 Mast cell tumors are the most common malignant tumor affecting the spleen in cats.

splenic lesions (Spangler & Culbertson 1992b). The occurrence of mast cell disease in the spleen of dogs with cutaneous mast cell disease negatively affects prognosis (Stefanello *et al.* 2009). In dogs with mast cell infiltration of the spleen and/or liver, a median survival time of 34 days was noted; this is in contrast to dogs without splenic and liver infiltration that demonstrated a median survival time of 733 days (Stefanello *et al.* 2009).

Hematoma

Hematomas, while accounting for 11–33% of pathologic splenic samples in dogs, are uncommonly diagnosed in cats (~2%) (Aronsohn *et al.* 2009; Spangler & Culbertson 1992a,b; Spangler & Kass 1997; Wrigley *et al.* 1989). Similar to splenic hemangiosarcoma, hemoperitoneum and cardiac arrhythmias are regularly diagnosed in association with splenic hematomas (Aronsohn *et al.* 2009; Knapp *et al.* 1993; Marino *et al.* 1994; Pintar *et al.* 2003). Between 7% and 27% of nontraumatic hemoperitoneum cases are secondary to splenic hematoma rupture, and cardiac arrhythmias are noted in approximately 33% of cases diagnosed with splenic hematoma (Aronsohn *et al.* 2009; Knapp *et al.* 1993; Marino *et al.* 1994; Pintar *et al.* 2003).

Distinction between splenic hemangiosarcoma and splenic hematomas generally cannot be made based on physical examination, radiographic or ultrasonographic findings, or gross intraoperative appearance (Aronsohn *et al.* 2009; Wrigley *et al.* 1989). For this reason, it is always recommended to perform a complete splenectomy with submission of the entire spleen for histopathologic evaluation. Authors evaluating canine anatomic evidence have suggested that splenic hyperplastic nodules and splenic hematomas are closely associated (Spangler & Culbertson 1992b).

Postsplenectomy prognosis is significantly better for dogs diagnosed with splenic hematoma as compared to splenic hemangiosarcoma (Spangler & Kass 1998). Of dogs diagnosed with splenic hematoma, 83% were alive at two months in one study, compared to 31% of dogs with splenic hemangiosarcoma (Spangler & Kass 1998). In that same study, 64% of dogs diagnosed with splenic hematomas were alive at one year (Spangler & Kass 1998).

Splenic trauma

Injuries to the spleen that occur secondary to trauma are uncommon in companion animals. In a large retrospective case series of dogs being struck by a vehicle, only 31 of 600 dogs experienced abdominal trauma (Kolata & Johnston 1975). In the group of 31 dogs, 3 had splenic trauma, which included contusions, ruptures of the parenchyma, and development of hematomas (Kolata & Johnston 1975). In a separate study, 7/12 dogs that developed hemoperitoneum secondary to trauma were hemorrhaging from the spleen (Mongil *et al.* 1995). Recently, in a study evaluating major abdominal evisceration after trauma or postoperative dehiscence, 2 of the 12 dogs and cats included experienced a splenic evisceration. Of those cases, 1 required a splenectomy (Gower *et al.* 2009).

Recommendations for surgical intervention in a dog or cat with splenic trauma are variable. Many cases do not require surgery, and medical management can be effective at controlling a bleed secondary to trauma. When abdominal exploration is pursued, repair of a splenic laceration can be difficult due to splenic friability, and partial or complete splenectomy may need to be considered.

Splenitis/splenic abscessation

Splenic inflammation is a very uncommon diagnosis, being found in 2% of feline splenic submissions and <1–1% of canine splenic submissions (Gower *et al.* 2009; Spangler & Culbertson 1992a,b; Spangler & Kass 1997). Infectious agents associated with splenitis in the dog have included *Monocillium indicum* (Mackie *et al.* 2004), *Mycobacterium avium* (Spangler & Kass 1997; O'Toole *et al.* 2005), coagulase-positive *Staphylococcus aureus* (Spangler & Kass 1997; O'Toole *et al.* 2005), and leishmania (Ferri *et al.* 2017). A foreign body resulted in splenitis and intra-abdominal infection with *b-Streptococcus*, *Clostridium perfringens*, and *Prevotella bivia* in a cat (Culp & Aronson 2008). The true cause of splenitis/splenic abscessation is usually unknown in dogs and cats, and complete splenectomy is often recommended in companion animals when these diseases are diagnosed.

Splenic torsion

Splenic torsion is most likely to occur secondary to other diseases such as neoplasia or gastric dilatation and volvulus (Weber 2000). German Shepherd dogs and Great Danes have demonstrated a predisposition toward splenic torsion, and some authors suggest that dogs with splenic torsion may be more likely to develop gastric dilatation and volvulus (Neath *et al.* 1997; Weber 2000). Thus, prophylactic gastropexy may be warranted in dogs undergoing splenectomy to treat a splenic torsion. Complications that have been recorded in association with splenic torsion include hemoperitoneum, cardiac arrhythmias, and a compromised cardiovascular state (Robinson *et al.* 1993; Neath *et al.* 1997; Weber 2000; Aronsohn *et al.* 2009).

Torsion of the splenic pedicle can result in life-threatening consequences (Weber 2000). Surgery involves complete splenectomy, and the spleen should not be returned to normal position prior to removal to decrease the chance of reperfusion injury (Neath *et al.* 1997; Weber 2000). The outcome with surgery can be favorable in dogs, as survival rates of 74–100% have been reported (Neath *et al.* 1997; Weber 2000).

Splenic infarction

Splenic infarction is often associated with other disease processes in the dog (Hardie *et al.* 1995). Common diseases implicated in the development of splenic infarction include coagulopathies, splenomegaly, cardiac disease, liver disease, renal disease, neoplasia, and immune-mediated diseases (Hardie *et al.* 1995; Kim *et al.* 2020). Some authors have advocated medical management over splenectomy, as concurrent disease processes may predispose these cases to other medical problems when surgery is pursued (Hardie *et al.* 1995).

Immune-mediated hemolytic anemia/ immune-mediated thrombocytopenia

Generally, immune-mediated hemolytic anemia (IMHA) is managed medically (Weinkle *et al.* 2005; Piek *et al.* 2008); however, some success has been seen in dogs when splenectomy is combined with immunosuppressive medications in refractory IMHA cases, as is commonly performed in humans with IMHA (Horgan *et al.* 2009). One study evaluated 10 dogs that underwent splenectomy in conjunction with the administration of immunosuppressive medications (Horgan *et al.* 2009). Positive findings in that study included a significant increase in postsplenectomy packed cell volume and a significant decrease in postsplenectomy blood transfusions (Horgan *et al.* 2009). In addition, 9/10 dogs survived to 30 days, and immunosuppressive medications were discontinued in 4 dogs (Horgan *et al.* 2009).

Similar to IMHA, medical management is pursued initially in the treatment of immune-mediated thrombocytopenia (IMT), and many dogs will respond favorably to this alone (Jans *et al.* 1990). Surgery is not considered as a first-line therapy, as many dogs will experience only a single episode and not require long-term medical therapy (Jans *et al.* 1990). One study found that splenectomy may aid in discontinuing corticosteroid therapy while still maintaining a platelet count of >200 000 in dogs with multiple episodes of IMT relapse (Jans *et al.* 1990). Lastly, a study evaluating IMHA, IMT, and Evan's syndrome found that 8/9 dogs evaluated were able to cease corticosteroid intake and demonstrated clinical improvement over the 12 months following splenectomy (Feldman *et al.* 1985).

Diagnostics

Clinical signs/physical examination

The clinical signs of dogs and cats with splenic pathology are variable. Splenic disease is often noted incidentally during geriatric evaluations of patients with no outward clinical signs or when a patient with another disease process is being evaluated. Dogs and cats with splenic pathology can be presented to a veterinary clinic for nondescript clinical signs such as lethargy, anorexia, vomiting, or diarrhea, or with life-threatening signs secondary to hemorrhage and hemodynamic collapse (Prymak *et al.* 1988; Pintar *et al.* 2003; Culp *et al.* 2008). Some owners will report that their pet has exhibited waxing and waning decreased activity levels, which ultimately are likely due to slow or intermittent intraperitoneal bleeds (Wood *et al.* 1998).

In animals with splenic disease, general physical examination may be unrewarding from a diagnostic standpoint. Dogs and cats with hemoperitoneum may have signs such as prolonged capillary refill time, poor pulse quality, anemia-related heart murmurs, abdominal distension, a palpable abdominal mass, abdominal pain, and/or an abdominal fluid wave (Prymak *et al.* 1988; Wood *et al.* 1998; Hanson *et al.* 2001; Pintar *et al.* 2003). In one study, the presence of hemoperitoneum associated with a splenic mass was strongly associated with a diagnosis of splenic hemangiosarcoma (Hammond & Pesillo-Crosby 2008).

Bloodwork

Bloodwork is important in the staging of splenic disease, both as a preanesthetic test and in judging the severity of disease secondary to splenic pathology. Veterinary patients with hemoperitoneum often have decreased packed cell volumes and total solid concentrations (Hanson *et al.* 2001; Pintar *et al.* 2003; Wood *et al.* 1998). Coagulation profiles may demonstrate decreased platelet counts or prolongation of prothrombin time and partial thromboplastin time, depending on the length of time the hemoperitoneum has occurred as well as the severity (Pintar *et al.* 2003).

A recent study evaluating dogs with hemoperitoneum noted that dogs diagnosed with splenic hemangiosarcoma had significantly lower total solid concentrations and platelet counts than dogs with other splenic lesions (Hammond & Pesillo-Crosby 2008). Further, a cutoff value of <5.8 mg/dL for total solid concentration had a positive predictive value of 87% (negative predictive value 43%) for hemangiosarcoma, and a cutoff value of <90 000 platelets had a positive predictive value of 92% (negative predictive value 42%) for hemangiosarcoma (Hammond & Pesillo-Crosby 2008). An association between splenic hemangiosarcoma and acanthocytosis has also been suggested (Gelberg & Stackhouse 1977; Hirsch *et al.* 1981). Lastly, dogs with splenic hemangiosarcoma were shown to be significantly more likely to

have a neutrophilic leukocytosis in comparison to dogs with splenic hematoma (Marino *et al.* 1994).

Radiographs

The most common findings associated with splenic disease on abdominal radiographs include loss of serosal detail (secondary to hemoperitoneum), splenomegaly, and abdominal mass effect (displacement of other abdominal organs) (Figure 88.2) (Neath *et al.* 1997; Pintar *et al.* 2003; Stickle 1989; Weinstein *et al.* 1989; Wood *et al.* 1998). When considering abdominal surgery to treat splenic disease, the performance of thoracic radiographs prior to anesthesia is highly recommended. Splenic neoplasia is often malignant and metastasis to the pulmonary parenchyma occurs regularly.

Ultrasound

Ultrasonography is the most commonly described tool in the diagnosis of splenic disease in veterinary medicine (Ballegeer *et al.* 2007; Cruz-Arámbulo *et al.* 2004; Cuccovillo & Lamb 2002; Hanson *et al.* 2001; Ivancić *et al.* 2009; Ohlerth *et al.* 2008; Ramirez *et al.* 2002; Sato & Solano 2004; Stefanello *et al.* 2009; Wrigley *et al.* 1988a, 1988b). Significant factors in the diagnosis of specific splenic diseases may be noted during ultrasonographic examination. In dogs noted to have splenic and hepatic target lesions (typically a mass or nodule with a hypoechoic outer zone and a hyperechoic inner zone compared to the outer zone) during an ultrasound examination, the positive predictive value for a malignant diagnosis is 81% for multiple target lesions and 74% for a single target lesion (Cuccovillo & Lamb 2002). Single discrete masses are significantly more likely to be

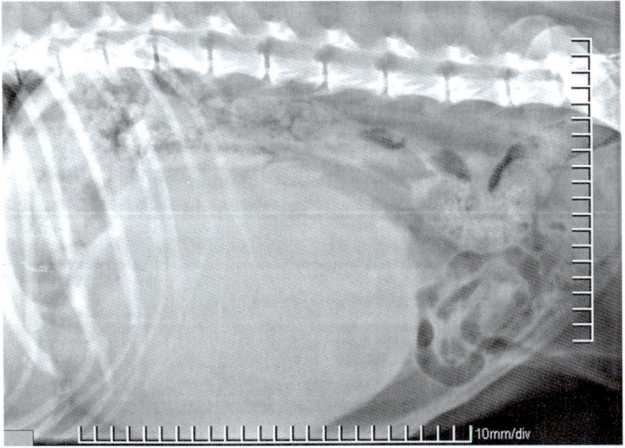

Figure 88.2 The most common findings associated with splenic disease on abdominal radiographs include loss of serosal detail (secondary to hemoperitoneum), splenomegaly, and abdominal mass effect (displacement of other abdominal organs).

benign, and multiple, similar-appearing masses are more likely to be malignant (Ballegeer *et al.* 2007).

Several studies have described the ultrasonographic findings of specific neoplastic diseases affecting the spleen. The spleen is the abdominal organ most often affected by histiocytic neoplasia, accounting for 80–83% of documented cases (Ramirez *et al.* 2002; Cruz-Arámbulo *et al.* 2004). The most common ultrasonographic finding associated with histiocytic neoplasia is the presence of hypoechoic nodules dispersed throughout the splenic parenchyma (Ramirez *et al.* 2002; Cruz-Arámbulo *et al.* 2004). Malignant histiocytosis predominates (73% of cases) over other forms of histiocytic disease such as histiocytic sarcoma and malignant fibrous histiocytoma; however, these diseases cannot be differentiated based on ultrasound alone (Cruz-Arámbulo *et al.* 2004).

For dogs with splenic hemangiosarcoma, a mass is often identified within the splenic parenchyma or extending outward from the spleen (Wrigley *et al.* 1988b). Differing from histiocytic neoplasia, a study has reported that splenic hemangiosarcoma tends to have a mixed echogenicity, with the majority of lesions having anechoic and hyperechoic regions (Wrigley *et al.* 1988b). Another study, however, found that 61% of splenic hemangiosarcoma cases were extensively or moderately hypoechoic (Ohlerth *et al.* 2008). The sensitivity of abdominal ultrasound to detect masses of the spleen, liver, and mesentery is reported to be 87.4%, 37.3%, and 31.3%, respectively (Cudney *et al.* 2021); several dogs in that study had diffuse peritoneal nodular metastasis that was not detected on abdominal ultrasound.

The ultrasonographic interpretations of both dogs and cats with splenic lymphosarcoma have also been reported (Wrigley *et al.* 1988b). The vast majority (83%) of cats with splenic lymphosarcoma demonstrate splenomegaly on ultrasound examination (Hanson *et al.* 2001). Dogs with splenic lymphosarcoma are noted to have a nonhomogeneous echoic pattern, with hypoechoic to anechoic nodules being diagnosed regularly (Wrigley *et al.* 1988a). Focal splenic masses are less commonly noted, being diagnosed in only 3/12 cases in one canine study (Wrigley *et al.* 1988a). The ultrasonographic honeycomb pattern commonly associated (Bertal *et al.* 2018) with splenic lymphoma in dogs can be associated with either benign or malignant disorders in the cat.

Variability exists in the echogenic appearance of splenic mast cell tumors, precluding a diagnosis based on ultrasound alone (Sato & Solano 2004; Stefanello *et al.* 2009). Of cats with splenic mast cell disease, 93% have splenomegaly (Kim *et al.* 2007). Dogs may also have a subjective increase in splenic size on ultrasound evaluation (Sato & Solano 2004; Stefanello *et al.* 2009).

Recently, the use of contrast harmonic ultrasonography has gained popularity for evaluating splenic masses (Ohlerth *et al.* 2007, 2008; Ivancić *et al.* 2009). Contrast harmonic ultrasonography utilizes a microbubble contrast medium that enhances ultrasound signals and improves an ultrasonographer's ability to evaluate tissue perfusion (Ohlerth *et al.* 2007, 2008). In one study evaluating the use of contrast harmonic imaging, malignant splenic lesions were significantly more likely to have extensive to moderate hypoechogenicity in comparison to adjacent spleen, as opposed to benign lesions (Ohlerth *et al.* 2008). In a separate study, splenic hemangiosarcoma was indistinguishable from splenic hematomas when contrast harmonic ultrasonography was used (Ivancić *et al.* 2009). However, contrast harmonic ultrasonography demonstrated 100% accuracy in determining metastatic disease to the liver from splenic hemangiosarcoma (Ivancić *et al.* 2009).

Computed tomography

Computed tomography (CT) has been shown to be highly accurate in the evaluation of canine spleen volumes (Moss *et al.* 1981). Recent evidence suggests that CT is also useful in distinguishing malignant from non-malignant splenic lesions (Fife *et al.* 2004). Malignant masses have significantly lower mean Hounsfield units and are more likely to hypoattenuate in comparison to their nonmalignant counterparts (hematoma, hyperplasia) (Fife *et al.* 2004). CT has also been used successfully to identify splenic torsion (Patsikas *et al.* 2001).

Magnetic resonance imaging

Magnetic resonance imaging (MRI) is not a useful technique for differentiating between specific types of benign lesions affecting the spleen such as lymphoid hyperplasia and extramedullary hematopoiesis; however, MRI has a sensitivity and specificity of 100% in the delineation of benign versus malignant lesions (Clifford *et al.* 2004). It remains uncommon to perform MRI evaluations of the abdomen to assess splenic disease in veterinary medicine, as most cases present on an emergency basis, precluding the practical use of MRI (Clifford *et al.* 2004).

Splenic aspiration and biopsy

The decision to perform splenic aspiration is clinician dependent. The knowledge gained from the cytology of a splenic aspirate is likely related to the exfoliative nature of the aspirated lesions. In general hematopoietic cells exfoliate more readily than mesenchymal cells (Christopher 2003). A few studies have correlated findings of cytology to histopathologic diagnosis, and these studies have varied in results (Ballegeer *et al.* 2007; O'Keefe & Couto 1987). In one study, 100% of cytologic diagnoses correlated with histopathologic diagnoses; however, over half of the cases in that study did not have histopathology performed, resulting in low case numbers for comparison (O'Keefe & Couto 1987). In a more recent study, the correlation between cytologic diagnosis and histopathologic diagnosis was 61.3% (Ballegeer *et al.* 2007). Of the 19 cases in that study that had a correlation between cytology and histopathology, 11 were benign conditions, 8 were malignant diseases, and 1 was an infectious disease (Ballegeer *et al.* 2007). In 16.1% of cases, the cytologic diagnosis was incorrect when compared with the histopathologic diagnosis. Yankin *et al.* (2020) found that aspiration of splenic nodules and parenchyma identified a clinically relevant diagnosis in 20% of dogs.

If incisional biopsies utilizing tissue-core biopsy instruments are performed preoperatively, ultrasound guidance is recommended (de Rycke *et al.* 1999). The accuracy of these instruments to obtain splenic tissue was shown to be as high as 90% in one study (de Rycke *et al.* 1999). However, the diagnostic value can be low due to poor sample quality and small size of the specimens (de Rycke *et al.* 1999).

Performing an incisional splenic biopsy intraoperatively is unusual and the indications are few. Obtaining splenic samples laparoscopically has been described, though, with some success (Barnes *et al.* 2006). Organs that are biopsied with the use of an endoscopic stapling device experience less bleeding, fibrin deposition, fibrosis, and coagulation necrosis versus those obtained by use of a harmonic scalpel (Barnes *et al.* 2006). Despite this, both techniques result in similarly sized samples that typically allow for diagnosis (Barnes *et al.* 2006).

When splenic pathology is suspected during abdominal exploratory surgery, excisional biopsies of the entire spleen are recommended. If a histopathologic diagnosis is not consistent with a clinician's clinical suspicion of the splenic disease process, further sectioning of the sample or reevaluation of the microscopic characteristics of the lesion should be requested. A description of the procedures used for splenic biopsy follows later.

Biomarkers

Proteins such as vascular endothelial growth factor, basic fibroblast growth factor, bcl-2, and survivin have been shown to be more commonly expressed in malignant neoplasia (hemangiosarcoma) when compared to benign neoplasia (hemangioma) (Murakami *et al.* 2008; Yonemaru *et al.* 2006). Plasma vascular endothelial growth factor was more likely to be detectable in dogs

with hemangiosarcoma than in healthy dogs (Clifford *et al.* 2001). Signal transducer and activator of transcription 3 (STAT3) protein is expressed in hemangiosarcoma significantly more than in hemangioma (Petterino *et al.* 2006). In addition, serum big endothelin-1 (big ET-1) levels in dogs with splenic hemangiosarcoma were significantly higher than in dogs with other splenic malignancies or benign splenic pathology (Fukumoto *et al.* 2015). These findings may provide targets for diagnostics or therapeutics in the future; further investigation is necessary before the clinical utility of these markers is known.

Management of splenic disease

Preoperative management

As stated previously, dogs with splenic pathology may be asymptomatic and the preoperative planning may be limited to the evaluation of laboratory work (complete blood count, serum chemistry profile, and urinalysis) for anesthetic planning, as well as thoracic radiographs and abdominal ultrasound. In patients with hemoperitoneum and associated hypovolemic shock, a more intensive work-up and stabilization period are essential. At a minimum, bloodwork should include a complete blood count, serum chemistry profile, coagulation profile, blood typing, and blood cross-matching; lactate measurements can be used to assess appropriate resuscitation. Thoracic radiographs should also be performed to rule out metastatic neoplasia and other underlying disease. Close anesthetic monitoring is critical in these cases, as these dogs are often cardiovascularly unstable. Access to blood pressure monitoring, pulse oximetry, electrocardiography, and blood bank facilities is recommended. If the dog is stable, an echocardiogram may be indicated to evaluate the patient for the presence of a right atrial mass.

When planning splenic surgery, it is necessary to have a thorough understanding of the specific disease processes that may affect the spleen, so that proactive measures can be taken in order to try to limit serious perioperative complications that can arise. Mast cell disease, which can infiltrate the spleen, can cause systemic anaphylaxis and hemorrhage secondary to release of histamine and heparin from within the granules of the neoplastic mast cells (Marconato *et al.* 2008). Gastrointestinal ulceration and perforation can occur secondary to an increased release of hydrochloric acid that is induced by mast cell-released histamine (Misdorp 2004). In addition, it is important to recognize that splenectomy may not be recommended in some cases of splenic lymphoma. In cases of multiorgan involvement, chemotherapy is often recommended as an alternative treatment (Brooks *et al.* 1987).

Patients with splenic pathology can be diagnosed with irregular heart rhythms, with the most likely manifestation being ventricular tachyarrhythmias (Knapp *et al.* 1993; Marino *et al.* 1994). The pathogenesis for the development of ventricular tachyarrhythmias with splenic disease is not fully known; however, hypoxemia secondary to abdominal bleeding, reperfusion injury, release of myocardial depressant factors associated with pancreatic ischemia, and sympathetic stimulation have been proposed (Knapp *et al.* 1993; Marino *et al.* 1994). General guidelines exist for the treatment of ventricular tachyarrhythmias in dogs, and current recommendations for initiating treatment include the development of polymorphic ventricular tachycardia, heart rates greater than 180–200 bpm with ventricular tachycardia, pulse deficits, and potentially the development of the R on T phenomenon. Current treatment recommendations include the administration of anti-arrhythmic medications such as lidocaine, procainamide, sotalol, and β- blockers (Pariaut 2009).

Intraoperative management

Splenic biopsy

Incisional splenic biopsies can be performed similarly to biopsies performed elsewhere in the body. In general, a biopsy instrument such as a Tru-Cut® biopsy needle (Travenol Laboratories, Deerfield, IL, USA) or a BioPince™ full-core biopsy instrument (Angiotech Pharmaceuticals, Vancouver, BC, Canada) is utilized with ultrasound guidance or during a laparoscopic or open procedure. Alternatively, a skin biopsy punch can also be used. To perform the biopsy punch technique, the region that is to be biopsied should be isolated from other abdominal organs and draped with sterile laparotomy sponges. The size of the biopsy punch is based on the size of the lesion, but a 4–6 mm punch is often sufficient. A twisting motion should be utilized while the biopsy punch is held in a perpendicular plane to the spleen; the punch biopsy instrument should be gently buried into the spleen until the blade is completely seated in splenic parenchyma. After this has been accomplished, the biopsy punch should be gently retracted from the splenic parenchyma. In some cases, the biopsy sample will be drawn out of the spleen with the biopsy punch. If the biopsy sample remains within the splenic parenchyma, forceps should be used to gently grasp a small section of the splenic capsule overlying the biopsy sample. When the sample has been pulled free from the spleen by the forceps, it may need to be freed from the spleen by incising the deep margin with scissors. A piece of a hemostatic agent such as a gelatin sponge (Gelfoam®, Pharmacia & Upjohn, Kalamazoo,

MI, USA) may be inserted into the defect made by the biopsy punch. Alternatively, a simple interrupted horizontal mattress suture may be placed across the biopsy site, closing one side of splenic capsule to its opposite counterpart.

Splenectomy

For all splenectomies (regardless of the technique utilized), the patient should be placed in dorsal recumbency, and a liberal clip of the fur on the patient's ventral surface should be performed. The skin incision for a splenectomy should extend from the xyphoid to a few centimeters cranial to the cranial aspect of the pubis. After incising through the linea alba, a complete abdominal exploratory should be performed. When a persistently bleeding vessel is noted, it should be ligated prior to completion of a full abdominal exploratory so that further cardiovascular compromise does not occur; if this is necessary, it is imperative to complete a thorough exploratory before closing the abdomen. A liver biopsy is recommended in all cases of suspected splenic malignant pathology.

After performing an abdominal exploratory, the spleen should be mobilized out of the abdomen and isolated from the other abdominal organs by laparotomy sponges. The spleen should be oriented properly, and the location of the splenic vessels should be determined. In some cases of splenic pathology, the omentum will be adhered to the splenic lesion. This will need to be separated from the spleen before pursuing splenectomy. The omentum should be retracted away from the spleen, and sections of the omentum that are closely approximated to the spleen should be isolated. Hemostasis can be achieved by ligation, application of staples (using a Ligate-Divide stapler, United States Surgical, a division of Tyco Healthcare Group LP, Norwalk, CT, USA; or Ligaclips®, Ethicon, Somerville, NJ, USA), application of electrocautery, or utilization of a vessel-sealing unit (LigaSure®, Valleylab, a division of Tyco Healthcare Group, Boulder, CO, USA; or EnSeal®, Ethicon).

Partial splenectomy

A partial splenectomy may be performed for cases of localized splenic trauma or for obtaining a biopsy. However, the indications for partial splenectomy are few, and the risks may outweigh the benefits. Risks include postoperative hemorrhage, as well as leaving malignant cells in the remaining spleen, if malignant pathology is present. Performing a partial splenectomy will likely entail longer operating times compared to complete splenectomy (Waldron & Robertson 1995). After a partial splenectomy, the remaining spleen does not regenerate (Bar-Maor *et al.* 1988).

Partial splenectomies can be performed by either ligation or stapling techniques (Furneaux 1975; Bellah 1994; Waldron & Robertson 1995). To perform a partial splenectomy by ligation, the blood vessels closest to the hilus that are supplying the portion of spleen to be removed should be ligated first. This will result in a line of demarcation denoting the portion of spleen where the vascular supply has been compromised. Next, the splenic pulp is milked into the area that is to be removed, two Carmalt clamps are placed along the line of demarcation, and the spleen is incised between these two clamps. The cut surface of the spleen that is remaining in the patient is then oversewn with a 3-0 absorbable suture, and the clamp is removed. The cut end should be monitored closely for bleeding (Bellah 1994; Waldron & Robertson 1995).

To perform a partial splenectomy with stapling equipment, the area to be removed is again devascularized with ligation of the splenic hilar vessels supplying that section (Bellah 1994; Waldron & Robertson 1995). A surgical stapling device (generally a thoracoabdominal stapling device, United States Surgical) is placed on the line of demarcation and the staples are applied. A Carmalt forceps is placed on the section of spleen to be removed, to prevent bleeding from the cut edge. The surgical stapling device is removed, and the cut edge of the spleen that is remaining within the patient is evaluated for bleeding. If bleeding is noted, ligatures may need to be placed.

Complete splenectomy

Several techniques have been utilized to perform a complete splenectomy. Ligation of the main splenic artery and vein is considered by many the technique of choice (Hosgood et al. 1989). For this procedure, the splenic artery (distal to the left pancreatic lobe branches and proximal to the continuation as the left gastroepiploic artery), the short gastric arteries, the left gastroepiploic artery, and all associated veins are ligated (Hosgood et al. 1989). The vessels are gently isolated by blunt dissection in a direction parallel to the vessels. The vessels are then tied individually with two ligatures on the proximal end of the vessel that remains in the patient. The splenic artery should be transfixed to prevent suture migration. The distal end of each vessel is ligated with a single ligature, and the vessel is sectioned between the second and third ligatures from proximal to distal. The separation of the main splenic artery and vein prevents the formation of an arterio-venous fistula. Alternatively, the splenic hilar vessels can be ligated individually, but this technique may result in longer operative times (Hosgood et al. 1989).

The use of vessel-sealant devices is becoming more popular in veterinary medicine, and most laparoscopic splenectomies in humans are performed with such devices (Romano et al. 2002; Barbaros et al. 2007). These devices have been used successfully in canine and feline patients to perform a myriad of cases (Mayhew 2009; Monnet 2009), and as their availability increases, their use for both open and laparoscopic splenectomies will also likely increase. These devices can be used on the splenic hilar vessels and some are capable of sealing vessels that are up to 7 mm in diameter (Soon et al. 2006). The use of a bipolar vessel-sealant device has not been associated with differences in short-term mortality (Sirochman et al. 2020).

Laparoscopic and laparoscopic-assisted splenectomy

In human medicine, laparoscopic splenectomy (LS) has become the standard of care for surgical disease of the spleen (Gamme et al. 2013). Despite the longer reported surgical times, multiple studies have shown a reduction in postoperative complications as well as shorter hospitalization times when compared to open splenectomy (Farah et al. 1997; Winslow & Brunt 2003; Kucuk et al. 2005). With the increasing utilization of minimally invasive surgery (MIS) in veterinary patients, a variety of techniques for laparoscopic splenectomy have been reported in both healthy dogs (Stedile et al. 2009; Khalaj et al. 2012) and in dogs and cats with naturally occurring splenic disease (Collard et al. 2010; O'Donnell et al. 2013; Shaver et al. 2015; Wright et al. 2016). Laparoscopic splenectomy in veterinary patients presents specific challenges and the need for careful case selection is critical for successful outcomes. The most common indication for splenectomy in veterinary patients is the presence of a mass (whereas splenectomy is typically performed for hematologic disease in humans), and the spleen is a relatively larger organ in dogs than humans when compared to body size. In addition, many patients requiring splenectomy have active hemoperitoneum or significant omental adhesions at the time of surgery, which limits laparoscopic visualization. Intracorporeal manipulation of a large spleen containing a mass lesion can also be technically challenging and may result in significant hemorrhage. Therefore, total laparoscopic or laparoscopic-assisted splenectomy (LAS) is generally only considered in dogs without hemoperitoneum and in those with modest-sized splenic masses less than 5–6 cm in diameter (Collard et al. 2010; Mayhew et al. 2018; Shaver et al. 2015) or 55.2 cm^3/kg volume (McGaffey et al. 2022).

In patients who are appropriate candidates, LS has the proposed benefits of decreased postoperative pain, shorter hospitalization time, decreased incisional infection rates, and decreased blood loss (Stedile et al. 2009;

Khalaj *et al.* 2012; Shaver *et al.* 2015; Wright *et al.* 2016; Maurin *et al.* 2020). Techniques for laparoscopic-assisted and full laparoscopic, single- and multi-port, splenectomy have been described. When LAS is performed, the abdomen is initially explored and staged using single -or multi-port laparoscopy prior to splenectomy. Then the subumbilical incision is extended into a mini-laparotomy and a wound retraction device is inserted. The tail of the spleen is then partially exteriorized and the splenic hilus and omental adhesions sealed and transected with a vessel-sealant device (Collard *et al.* 2010; Wright *et al.* 2016). Total LS has been described using a variety of multi-port techniques, with port placement dependent on surgeon preference and concurrent procedures being performed (Shaver *et al.* 2015). The spleen is excised using a laparoscopic vessel-sealant device, with simultaneous retraction with a blunt probe to perform a hilar splenectomy. Ultimately, the spleen is exteriorized through an extended midline port or paracostal incision, with incision size depending on the size of the spleen. Single-port LS has also been reported in dogs with naturally occurring splenic disease using either a single-incision laparoscopic surgery (SILS) port or a GelPOINT® access system (Applied Medical, Rancho Santa Margarita, CA, USA) and laparoscopic vessel-sealant device (Mayhew *et al.* 2018). Following splenectomy, the spleen is exteriorized through the SILS port incision or using a specimen retrieval device.

Generally, the outcomes of all reported techniques for LAS and LS are excellent, with minimal complications. Among the six studies reported and a total of 204 canine splenectomies, 99% (202/204) survived to the time of discharge. One dog died from progressive respiratory distress, presumed to be secondary to pulmonary thromboembolism (Mayhew *et al.* 2018), and one died from a suspected portal vein thrombus (McGaffey *et al.* 2022). No additional life-threatening complications were reported. The overall incidence of conversion to open celiotomy was 5% (10/204). Reasons for conversion included large splenic dimensions, adhesion formation, and poor visualization from abundant falciform fat or hemorrhage (Mayhew *et al.* 2018; McGaffey *et al.* 2022; Shaver *et al.* 2015). Mayhew *et al.* (2018) reported that heavier body weight was significantly associated with conversion from single-port LS to LAS, and suggested that single-port LS may be best suited for smaller dogs with smaller masses, whereas larger dogs or those with larger masses may be better candidates for LAS. Minor complications were inconsistently reported between studies.

Postoperative management

Some veterinary patients have a quick recovery after undergoing splenectomy, and are therefore able to be discharged within the first few postoperative days. Other patients, such as those with significant compromise preoperatively, may require more intensive monitoring and treatment, thereby necessitating longer hospital stays. Additionally, complications associated with splenic pathology, such as ventricular tachyarrhythmias, may manifest after splenic surgery and can require therapy with anti-arrhythmics. Blood products such as packed red blood cells may be necessary postoperatively in cases that are significantly anemic, and plasma may be indicated to address prolongations in coagulation times.

Certain factors have been identified that impact post-splenectomy complications and prognosis. Dogs with ruptured splenic masses are more likely than those without to develop rapid ventricular tachycardia postoperatively, and likewise, dogs with splenic hemangiosarcoma are more likely to develop rapid ventricular tachycardia compared to other splenectomized dogs, because it is commonly associated with a hemoabdomen and hypovolemic shock (Marino *et al.* 1994). Dogs with malignant lesions of the spleen generally have a poorer prognosis than dogs with benign splenic disease (Spangler & Kass 1997). In one study, 6?% of dogs were accurately diagnosed with splenic neoplasia when anemia and splenic rupture were noted in concordance with splenomegaly (Spangler & Kass 1997). Among malignant splenic tumors, dogs with single lesions tend to have an improved prognosis versus those with multiple lesions (Spangler & Kass 1997).

References

Affolter, V.K. and Moore, P.F. (2002). Localized and disseminated histiocytic sarcoma of dendritic cell origin in dogs. *Veterinary Pathology* 39 (1): 74–83.

Alvarez, F.J., Hosoya, K., Lara-Garcia, A. et al. (2013). VAC protocol for treatment of dogs with stage III hemangiosarcoma. *Journal of the American Animal Hospital Association* 49 (6): 370–377.

Aronsohn, M.G., Dubiel, B., Roberts, B., and Powers, B.E. (2009). Prognosis for acute nontraumatic hemoperitoneum in the dog: a retrospective analysis of 60 cases (2003–2006). *Journal of the American Animal Hospital Association* 45 (2): 72–77.

Ballegeer, E.A., Forrest, L.J., Dickinson, R.M. et al. (2007). Correlation of ultrasonographic appearance of lesions and cytologic and histologic diagnoses in splenic aspirates from dogs and cats: 32 cases (2002–2005). *Journal of the American Veterinary Medical Association* 230 (5): 690–696.

Barbaros, U., Dinccag, A., Deveci, U. et al. (2007). Use of electrothermal vessel sealing with LigaSure device during laparoscopic splenectomy. *Acta Chirurgica Belgica* 107 (2): 162–165.

Bar-Maor, J.A., Sweed, Y., and Shoshany, G. (1988). Does the spleen regenerate after partial splenectomy in the dog? *Journal of Pediatric Surgery* 23 (2): 128–129.

Barnes, R.F., Greenfield, C.L., Schaeffer, D.J. et al. (2006). Comparison of biopsy samples obtained using standard endoscopic instruments and the harmonic scalpel during laparoscopic and laparoscopic-assisted surgery in normal dogs. *Veterinary Surgery* 35 (3): 243–251.

Batschinski, K., Nobre, A., Vargas-Mendez, E. et al. (2018). Canine visceral hemangiosarcoma treated with surgery alone or surgery and doxorubicin: 37 cases (2005–2014). *Canadian Veterinary Journal* 59 (9): 967–972.

Bellah, J.R. (1994). Surgical stapling of the spleen, pancreas, liver, and urogenital tract. *Veterinary Clinics of North America: Small Animal Practice* 24 (2): 375–394.

Bertal, M., Norman Carmel, E., Diana, A. et al. (2018). Association between ultrasonographic appearance of splenic parenchyma and cytology in cats. *Journal of Feline Medicine and Surgery* 20 (1): 23–29.

Boston, S.E., Higginson, G., and Monteith, G. (2011). Concurrent splenic and right atrial mass at presentation in dogs with HSA: a retrospective study. *Journal of the American Animal Hospital Association* 47 (5): 336–341.

Brooks, M.B., Matus, R.E., Leifer, C.E., and Patnaik, A.K. (1987). Use of splenectomy in the management of lymphoma in dogs: 16 cases (1976–1985). *Journal of the American Veterinary Medical Association* 191 (8): 1008–1010.

Brown, N.O., Patnaik, A.K., and MacEwen, E.G. (1985). Canine hemangiosarcoma: retrospective analysis of 104 cases. *Journal of the American Veterinary Medical Association* 186 (1): 56–58.

Christopher, M.M. (2003). Cytology of the spleen. *Veterinary Clinics of North America: Small Animal Practice* 33 (1): 135–152.

Cleveland, M.J. and Casale, S. (2016). Incidence of malignancy and outcomes for dogs undergoing splenectomy for incidentally detected nonruptured splenic nodules or masses: 105 cases (2009-2013). *Journal of the American Veterinary Medical Association* 248 (11): 1267–1273.

Clifford, C.A., Mackin, A.J., and Henry, C.J. (2000). Treatment of canine hemangiosarcoma: 2000 and beyond. *Journal of Veterinary Internal Medicine* 14 (5): 479–485.

Clifford, C.A., Hughes, D., Beal, M.W. et al. (2001). Plasma vascular endothelial growth factor concentrations in healthy dogs and dogs with hemangiosarcoma. *Journal of Veterinary Internal Medicine* 15 (2): 131–135.

Clifford, C.A., Pretorius, E.S., Weisse, C. et al. (2004). Magnetic resonance imaging of focal splenic and hepatic lesions in the dog. *Journal of Veterinary Internal Medicine* 18 (3): 330–338.

Collard, F., Nadeau, M.E., and Carmel, E.N. (2010). Laparoscopic splenectomy for treatment of splenic hemangiosarcoma in a dog *Veterinary Surgery* 39 (7): 870–872.

Cruz-Arámbulo, R., Wrigley, R., and Powers, B. (2004). Sonographic features of histiocytic neoplasms in the canine abdomen. *Veterinary Radiology & Ultrasound* 45 (6): 554–558.

Cuccovillo, A. and Lamb, C.R. (2002). Cellular features of sonographic target lesions of the liver and spleen in 21 dogs and a cat. *Veterinary Radiology & Ultrasound* 43 (3): 275–278.

Cudney, S.E., Wayne, A.S., and Rozanski, E.A. (2021). Diagnostic utility of abdominal ultrasonography for evaluation of dogs with nontraumatic hemoabdomen: 94 cases (2014–2017). *Journal of the American Veterinary Medical Association* 258 (3): 290–294.

Culp, W.T. and Aronson, L.R. (2008). Splenic foreign body in a cat. *Journal of Feline Medicine and Surgery* 10 (4): 380–383.

Culp, W.T., Drobatz, K.J., Glassman, M.M. et al. (2008). Feline visceral hemangiosarcoma. *Journal of Veterinary Internal Medicine* 22 (1): 148–152.

Day, M.J., Lucke, V.M., and Pearson, H. (1995). A review of pathological diagnoses made from 87 canine splenic biopsies. *Journal of Small Animal Practice* 36 (10): 426–433.

Eberle, N., von Babo, V., Nolte, I. et al. (2012). Splenic masses in dogs. Part 1: epidemiologic, clinical characteristics as well as histopathologic diagnosis in 249 cases (2000–2011). *Tierärztliche Praxis. Ausgabe K, Kleintiere/Heimtiere* 40 (4): 250–260.

Farah, R.A., Rogers, Z.R., Thompson, W.R. et al. (1997). Comparison of laparoscopic and open splenectomy in children with hematologic disorders. *Journal of Pediatrics* 131 (1 Pt 1): 41–46.

Feldman, B.F., Handagama, P., and Lubberink, A.A. (1985). Splenectomy as adjunctive therapy for immune-mediated thrombocytopenia and hemolytic anemia in the dog. *Journal of the American Veterinary Medical Association* 187 (6): 617–619.

Ferri, F., Zini, E., Auriemma, E. et al. (2017). Splenitis in 33 dogs. *Veterinary Pathology* 54 (1): 147–154.

Fife, W.D., Samii, V.F., Drost, W.T. et al. (2004). Comparison between malignant and nonmalignant splenic masses in dogs using contrast-enhanced computed tomography. *Veterinary Radiology & Ultrasound* 45 (4): 289–297.

Finotello, R., Stefanello, D., Zini, E., and Marconato, L. (2017). Comparison of doxorubicin-cyclophosphamide with doxorubicin-dacarbazine for the adjuvant treatment of canine hemangiosarcoma. *Veterinary and Comparative Oncology* 15 (1): 25–35.

Fleming, J., Giuffrida, M.A., Runge, J.J. et al. (2018). Anatomic site and etiology of hemorrhage in small versus large dogs with spontaneous hemoperitoneum. *Veterinary Surgery* 47 (8): 1031–1038.

Fukumoto, S., Miyasho, T., Hanazono, K. et al. (2015). Big endothelin-1 as a tumour marker for canine haemangiosarcoma. *Veterinary Journal* 204 (3): 269–274.

Furneaux, R.W. (1975). Symposium on surgical techniques in small animal practice. Surgical techniques for the spleen and liver. *Veterinary Clinics of North America* 5 (3): 363–381.

Gamme, G., Birch, D.W., and Karmali, S. (2013). Minimally invasive splenectomy: an update and review. *Canadian Journal of Surgery* 56 (4): 280–285.

Gelberg, H. and Stackhouse, L.L. (1977). Three cases of canine acanthocytosis associated with splenic neoplasia. *Veterinary Medicine, Small Animal Clinician* 72 (7): 1183–1184.

Gower, S.B., Weisse, C.W., and Brown, D.C. (2009). Major abdominal evisceration injuries in dogs and cats: 12 cases (1998–2008). *Journal of the American Veterinary Medical Association* 234 (12): 1566–1572.

Hammer, A.S., Couto, C.G., Filppi, J. et al. (1991). Efficacy and toxicity of VAC chemotherapy (vincristine, doxorubicin, and cyclophosphamide) in dogs with hemangiosarcoma. *Journal of Veterinary Internal Medicine* 5 (3): 160–166.

Hammond, T.N. and Pesillo-Crosby, S.A. (2008). Prevalence of hemangiosarcoma in anemic dogs with a splenic mass and hemoperitoneum requiring a transfusion: 71 cases (2003–2005). *Journal of the American Veterinary Medical Association* 232 (4): 553–558.

Hanson, J.A., Papageorges, M., Girard, E. et al. (2001). Ultrasonographic appearance of splenic disease in 101 cats. *Veterinary Radiology & Ultrasound* 42 (5): 441–445.

Hardie, E.M., Vaden, S.L., Spaulding, K., and Malarkey, D.E. (1995). Splenic infarction in 16 dogs: a retrospective study. *Journal of Veterinary Internal Medicine* 9 (3): 141–148.

Hendrick, M.J., Brooks, J.J., and Bruce, E.H. (1992). Six cases of malignant fibrous histiocytoma of the canine spleen. *Veterinary Pathology* 29 (4): 351–354.

Hirsch, V.M., Jacobsen, J., and Mills, J.H. (1981). A retrospective study of canine hemangiosarcoma and its association with acanthocytosis. *Canadian Veterinary Journal* 22 (5): 152–155.

Horgan, J.E., Roberts, B.K., and Schermerhorn, T. (2009). Splenectomy as an adjunctive treatment for dogs with immune-mediated hemolytic anemia: ten cases (2003–2006). *Journal of Veterinary Emergency and Critical Care* 19 (3): 254–261.

Hosgood, G., Bone, D.L., Vorhees, W.D. 3rd, and Reed, W.M. (1989). Splenectomy in the dog by ligation of the splenic and short gastric arteries. *Veterinary Surgery* 18 (2): 110–113.

Ivančić, M., Long, F., and Seiler, G.S. (2009). Contrast harmonic ultrasonography of splenic masses and associated liver nodules in dogs. *Journal of the American Veterinary Medical Association* 234 (1): 88–94.

Jans, H.E., Armstrong, P.J., and Price, G.S. (1990). Therapy of immune mediated thrombocytopenia. A retrospective study of 15 dogs. *Journal of Veterinary Internal Medicine* 4 (1): 4–7.

Khalaj, A., Bakhtiari, J., and Niasari-Naslaji, A. (2012). Comparison between single and three portal laparoscopic splenectomy in dogs. *BMC Veterinary Research* 8: 161.

Kim, S.E., Liptak, J.M., Gall, T.T. et al. (2007). Epirubicin in the adjuvant treatment of splenic hemangiosarcoma in dogs: 59 cases (1997–2004). *Journal of the American Veterinary Medical Association* 231 (10): 1550–1557.

Kim, S.M., Kim, G.N., Jeong, S.W., and Kim, J.H. (2020). Multiple splenic infarctions in a dog with immune-mediated hemolytic anemia: therapeutic implications. *Iranian Journal of Veterinary Research* 21 (1): 65–69.

Knapp, D., Aronsohn, M., and Harpster, N.J.J. (1993). Cardiac arrhythmias associated with mass lesions of the canine spleen. *Journal of the American Animal Hospital Association* 29 (2): 122.

Kolata, R.J. and Johnston, D.E. (1975). Motor vehicle accidents in urban dogs: a study of 600 cases. *Journal of the American Veterinary Medical Association* 167 (10): 938–941.

Kucuk, C., Sozuer, E., Ok, E. et al. (2005). Laparoscopic versus open splenectomy in the management of benign and malign hematologic diseases: a ten-year single-center experience. *Journal of Laparoendoscopic & Advanced Surgical Techniques. Part A* 15 (2): 135–139.

Lana, S., U'Ren, L., Plaza, S. et al. (2007). Continuous low-dose oral chemotherapy for adjuvant therapy of splenic hemangiosarcoma in dogs. *Journal of Veterinary Internal Medicine* 21 (4): 764–769.

Langenbach, A., Anderson, M.A., Dambach, D.M. et al. (1998). Extraskeletal osteosarcomas in dogs: a retrospective study of 169 cases (1986–1996). *Journal of the American Animal Hospital Association* 34 (2): 113–120.

Latifi, M., Tuohy, J.L., Coutermarsh-Ott, S.L. et al. (2020). Clinical outcomes in dogs with localized splenic histiocytic sarcoma treated with splenectomy with or without adjuvant chemotherapy. *Journal of Veterinary Internal Medicine* 34 (6): 2645–2650.

Mackie, J.T., Padhye, A.A., Sutherland, R.J. et al. (2004). Granulomatous lymphadenitis and splenitis associated with *Monocillium indicum* infection in a dog. *Journal of Veterinary Diagnostic Investigation* 16 (3): 248–250.

Marconato, L., Bettini, G., Giacoboni, C. et al. (2008). Clinicopathological features and outcome for dogs with mast cell tumors and bone marrow involvement. *Journal of Veterinary Internal Medicine* 22 (4): 1001–1007.

Marino, D.J., Matthiesen, D.T., Fox, P.R. et al. (1994). Ventricular arrhythmias in dogs undergoing splenectomy: a prospective study. *Veterinary Surgery* 23 (2): 101–106.

Maurin, M.P., Mullins, R.A., Singh, A., and Mayhew, P.D. (2020). A systematic review of complications related to laparoscopic and laparoscopic-assisted procedures in dogs. *Veterinary Surgery* 49 (Suppl 1): O5–O14.

Mayhew, P.D. (2009). Advanced laparoscopic procedures (hepatobiliary, endocrine) in dogs and cats. *Veterinary Clinics of North America: Small Animal Practice* 39 (5): 925–939.

Mayhew, P.D., Sutton, J.S., Singh, A. et al. (2018). Complications and short-term outcomes associated with single-port laparoscopic splenectomy in dogs. *Veterinary Surgery* 47 (S1): O67–O74.

McGaffey, M.E.S., Singh, A., Buote, N.J. et al. (2022). Complications and outcomes associated with laparoscopic-assisted splenectomy in dogs. *Journal of the American Veterinary Medical Association* 260 (11): 1309–1315.

Misdorp, W. (2004). Mast cell and canine mast cell tumours. A review. *Veterinary Quarterly* 26 (4): 156–169.

Mongil, C.M., Drobatz, K.J., and Hendricks, J.C. (1995). Traumatic hemoperitoneum in 28 cases: a retrospective review. *Journal of the American Animal Hospital Association* 31 (3): 217–222.

Monnet, E. (2009). Interventional thoracoscopy in small animals. *Veterinary Clinics of North America: Small Animal Practice* 39 (5): 965–975.

Moore, A.S., Frimberger, A.E., Sullivan, N., and Moore, P.F. (2012). Histologic and immunohistochemical review of splenic fibrohistiocytic nodules in dogs. *Journal of Veterinary Internal Medicine* 26 (5): 1164–1168.

Morris, J.S., McInnes, E.F., Bostock, D.E. et al. (2002). Immunohistochemical and histopathologic features of 14 malignant fibrous histiocytomas from flat-coated retrievers. *Veterinary Pathology* 39 (4): 473–479.

Moss, A.A., Friedman, M.A., and Brito, A.C. (1981). Determination of liver, kidney, and spleen volumes by computed tomography: an experimental study in dogs. *Journal of Computer Assisted Tomography* 5 (1): 12–14.

Murakami, M., Sakai, H., Kodama, A. et al. (2008). Expression of the anti-apoptotic factors Bcl-2 and survivin in canine vascular tumours. *Journal of Comparative Pathology* 139 (1): 1–7

Neath, P.J., Brockman, D.J., and Saunders, H.M. (1997). Retrospective analysis of 19 cases of isolated torsion of the splenic pedicle in dogs. *Journal of Small Animal Practice* 38 (9): 387–392.

O'Brien, D., Moore, P.F., Vernau, W. et al. (2013). Clinical characteristics and outcome in dogs with splenic marginal zone lymphoma. *Journal of Veterinary Internal Medicine* 27 (4): 949–954.

O'Donnell, E., Mayhew, P., Culp, W., and Mayhew, K. (2013). Laparoscopic splenectomy: operative technique and outcome in three cats. *Journal of Feline Medicine and Surgery* 15 (1): 43–52.

Ogilvie, G.K., Powers, B.E., Mallinckrodt, C.H., and Withrow, S.J. (1996). Surgery and doxorubicin in dogs with hemangiosarcoma. *Journal of Veterinary Internal Medicine* 10 (6): 379–384.

Ohlerth, S., Rüefli, E., Poirier, V. et al. (2007). Contrast harmonic imaging of the normal canine spleen. *Veterinary Radiology & Ultrasound* 48 (5): 451–456.

Ohlerth, S., Dennler, M., Rüefli, E. et al. (2008). Contrast harmonic imaging characterization of canine splenic lesions. *Journal of Veterinary Internal Medicine* 22 (5): 1095–1102.

O'Keefe, D.A. and Couto, C.G. (1987). Fine-needle aspiration of the spleen as an aid in the diagnosis of splenomegaly. *Journal of Veterinary Internal Medicine* 1 (3): 102–109.

O'Toole, D., Tharp, S., Thomsen, B.V. et al. (2005). Fatal mycobacteriosis with hepatosplenomegaly in a young dog due to Mycobacterium avium. *Journal of Veterinary Diagnostic Investigation* 17 (2): 200–204.

Pariaut, R. (2009). Ventricular tachyarrhythmias. In: *Small Animal Critical Care Medicine* (ed. D. Silverstein and K. Hopper), 202–210. St. Louis, MO: WB Saunders.

Patsikas, M.N., Rallis, T., Kladakis, S.E., and Dessiris, A.K. (2001). Computed tomography diagnosis of isolated splenic torsion in a dog. *Veterinary Radiology & Ultrasound* 42 (3): 235–237.

Petterino, C., Rossetti, E., and Drigo, M. (2006). Immunodetection of the signal transducer and activator of transcription-3 in canine haemangioma and haemangiosarcoma. *Research in Veterinary Science* 80 (2): 186–188.

Piek, C.J., Junius, G., Dekker, A. et al. (2008). Idiopathic immune-mediated hemolytic anemia: treatment outcome and prognostic factors in 149 dogs. *Journal of Veterinary Internal Medicine* 22 (2): 366–373.

Pintar, J., Breitschwerdt, E.B., Hardie, E.M., and Spaulding, K.A. (2003). Acute nontraumatic hemoabdomen in the dog: a retrospective analysis of 39 cases (1987–2001). *Journal of the American Animal Hospital Association* 39 (6): 518–522.

Prymak, C., McKee, L.J., Goldschmidt, M.H., and Glickman, L.T. (1988). Epidemiologic, clinical, pathologic, and prognostic characteristics of splenic hemangiosarcoma and splenic hematoma in dogs: 217 cases (1985). *Journal of the American Veterinary Medical Association* 193 (6): 706–712.

Ramirez, S., Douglass, J.P., and Robertson, I.D. (2002). Ultrasonographic features of canine abdominal malignant histiocytosis. *Veterinary Radiology & Ultrasound* 43 (2): 167–170.

Robinson, T.C., Sarchet, R.W., and Van Dongen, P.L. (1993). Splenic torsion in dogs. *Veterinary Record* 133 (2): 48.

Romano, F., Caprotti, R., Franciosi, C. et al. (2002). Laparoscopic splenectomy using Ligasure. *Surgical Endoscopy* 16 (11): 1608–1611.

de Rycke, L.M., van Bree, H.J., and Simoens, P.J. (1999). Ultrasound-guided tissue-core biopsy of liver, spleen and kidney in normal dogs. *Veterinary Radiology & Ultrasound* 40 (3): 294–299.

Sato, A.F. and Solano, M. (2004). Ultrasonographic findings in abdominal mast cell disease: a retrospective study of 19 patients. *Veterinary Radiology & Ultrasound* 45 (1): 51–57.

Scavelli, T.D., Patnaik, A.K., Mehlhaff, C.J., and Hayes, A.A. (1985). Hemangiosarcoma in the cat: retrospective evaluation of 31 surgical cases. *Journal of the American Veterinary Medical Association* 187 (8): 817–819.

Shaver, S.L., Mayhew, P.D., Steffey, M.A. et al. (2015). Short-term outcome of multiple port laparoscopic splenectomy in 10 dogs. *Veterinary Surgery* 44 (Suppl 1): 71–75.

Sirochman, A.L., Milovancev, M., Townsend, K., and Grimes, J.A. (2020). Influence of use of a bipolar vessel sealing device on short-term postoperative mortality after splenectomy: 203 dogs (2005–2018). *Veterinary Surgery* 49 (2): 291–303.

Smolowitz, R.M. and Carpenter, J.L. (1988). Canine splenic sarcomas with an osteosarcomatous component. *Veterinary Pathology* 25 (3): 246–248.

Soon, P.S., Yeh, M.W., Sywak, M.S., and Sidhu, S.B. (2006). Use of the ligaSure vessel sealing system in laparoscopic adrenalectomy. *ANZ Journal of Surgery* 76 (9): 850–852.

Sorenmo, K.U., Jeglum, K.A., and Helfand, S.C. (1993). Chemotherapy of canine hemangiosarcoma with doxorubicin and cyclophosphamide. *Journal of Veterinary Internal Medicine* 7 (6): 370–376.

Spangler, W.L. and Culbertson, M.R. (1992a). Prevalence and type of splenic diseases in cats: 455 cases (1985–1991). *Journal of the American Veterinary Medical Association* 201 (5): 773–776.

Spangler, W.L. and Culbertson, M.R. (1992b). Prevalence, type, and importance of splenic diseases in dogs: 1,480 cases (1985–1989). *Journal of the American Veterinary Medical Association* 200 (6): 829–834.

Spangler, W.L. and Kass, P.H. (1997). Pathologic factors affecting postsplenectomy survival in dogs. *Journal of Veterinary Internal Medicine* 11 (3): 166–171.

Spangler, W.L. and Kass, P.H. (1998). Pathologic and prognostic characteristics of splenomegaly in dogs due to fibrohistiocytic nodules: 98 cases. *Veterinary Pathology* 35 (6): 488–498.

Spangler, W.L., Culbertson, M.R., and Kass, P.H. (1994). Primary mesenchymal (nonangiomatous/nonlymphomatous) neoplasms occurring in the canine spleen: anatomic classification, immunohistochemistry, and mitotic activity correlated with patient survival. *Veterinary Pathology* 31 (1): 37–47.

Stedile, R., Beck, C.A., Schiochet, F. et al. (2009). Laparoscopic versus open splenectomy in dogs. *Pesquisa Veterinaria Brasileira* 29: 653–660.

van Stee, L.L., Boston, S.E., Singh, A. et al. (2015). Outcome and prognostic factors for canine splenic lymphoma treated by splenectomy (1995–2011). *Veterinary Surgery* 44 (8): 976–982.

Stefanello, D., Valenti, P., Faverzani, S. et al. (2009). Ultrasound-guided cytology of spleen and liver: a prognostic tool in canine cutaneous mast cell tumor. *Journal of Veterinary Internal Medicine* 23 (5): 1051–1057.

Stickle, R.L. (1989). Radiographic signs of isolated splenic torsion in dogs: eight cases (1980–1987). *Journal of the American Veterinary Medical Association* 194 (1): 103–106.

Story, A.L., Wavreille, V., Abrams, B. et al. (2020). Outcomes of 43 small breed dogs treated for splenic hemangiosarcoma. *Veterinary Surgery* 49 (6): 1154–1163.

U'Ren, L.W., Biller, B.J., Elmslie, R.E. et al. (2007). Evaluation of a novel tumor vaccine in dogs with hemangiosarcoma. *Journal of Veterinary Internal Medicine* 21 (1): 113–120.

Valli, V.E., Vernau, W., de Lorimier, L.P. et al. (2006). Canine indolent nodular lymphoma. *Veterinary Pathology* 43 (3): 241–256.

Waldron, D.R. and Robertson, J. (1995). Partial splenectomy in the dog: a comparison of stapling and ligation techniques. *Journal of the American Animal Hospital Association* 31 (4): 343–348.

Weber, N.A. (2000). Chronic primary splenic torsion with peritoneal adhesions in a dog: case report and literature review. *Journal of the American Animal Hospital Association* 36 (5): 390–394.

Weinkle, T.K., Center, S.A., Randolph, J.F. et al. (2005). Evaluation of prognostic factors, survival rates, and treatment protocols for immune-mediated hemolytic anemia in dogs: 151 cases (1993–2002). *Journal of the American Veterinary Medical Association* 226 (11): 1869–1880.

Weinstein, M.J., Carpenter, J.L., and Schunk, C.J. (1989). Nonangiogenic and nonlymphomatous sarcomas of the canine spleen: 57 cases (1975–1987). *Journal of the American Veterinary Medical Association* 195 (6): 784–788.

Winslow, E.R. and Brunt, L.M. (2003). Perioperative outcomes of laparoscopic versus open splenectomy: a meta-analysis with an emphasis on complications. *Surgery* 134 (4): 647–653.

Wood, C.A., Moore, A.S., Gliatto, J.M. et al. (1998). Prognosis for dogs with stage I or II splenic hemangiosarcoma treated by splenectomy alone: 32 cases (1991–1993). *Journal of the American Animal Hospital Association* 34 (5): 417–421.

Wright, T., Singh, A., Mayhew, P.D. et al. (2016). Laparoscopic-assisted splenectomy in dogs: 18 cases (2012–2014). *Journal of the American Veterinary Medical Association* 248 (8): 916–922.

Wrigley, R.H., Konde, L.J., Park, R.D., and Lebel, J.L. (1988a). Ultrasonographic features of splenic lymphosarcoma in dogs: 12 cases (1980–1986). *Journal of the American Veterinary Medical Association* 193 (12): 1565–1568.

Wrigley, R.H., Park, R.D., Konde, L.J., and Lebel, J.L. (1988b). Ultrasonographic features of splenic hemangiosarcoma in dogs: 18 cases (1980–1986). *Journal of the American Veterinary Medical Association* 192 (8): 1113–1117.

Wrigley, R.H., Konde, L.J., Park, R.D., and Lebel, J.L. (1989). Clinical features and diagnosis of splenic hematomas in dogs: 10 cases (1980 to 1987). *Journal of the American Animal Hospital Association* 25 (4): 371–375.

Yankin, I., Nemanic, S., Funes, S. et al. (2020). Clinical relevance of splenic nodules or heterogeneous splenic parenchyma assessed by cytologic evaluation of fine-needle samples in 125 dogs (2011–2015). *Journal of Veterinary Internal Medicine* 34 (1): 125–131.

Yonemaru, K., Sakai, H., Murakami, M. et al. (2006). Expression of vascular endothelial growth factor, basic fibroblast growth factor, and their receptors (flt-1, flk-1, and flg-1) in canine vascular tumors. *Veterinary Pathology* 43 (6): 971–980.

Zimmer, M.A. and Stair, E.L. (1983). Splenic myelolipomas in two dogs. *Veterinary Pathology* 20 (5): 637–638.

89

Surgical Treatment of Thymic Disease

Erin A. Gibson and William T.N. Culp

The thymus has been an organ of interest to anatomists for many centuries. Descriptions of the human thymus can be found dating back as far as 1659, and similar descriptions in dogs and cats were reported in the early to mid-nineteenth century (Latimer 1954). The roles of the thymus in providing immune functions are well documented (Levin & Snyder 1969; Chapman & Bopp 1970; Aronsohn 1985; Monroe & Roth 1986; Aspinall & Andrew 2000; Taub & Longo 2005), but the thymus also has an important function as an endocrine gland (Monroe & Roth 1986). Thymic disease is uncommon, but when it is encountered, surgery is most often the treatment of choice. The surgeon choosing to pursue thymic surgery should have a full understanding of thymic anatomy and intraoperative/postoperative potentialities, as well as a grasp of the paraneoplastic syndromes that can manifest in association with thymic pathology.

Thymic anatomy

The thymus is a bilobed organ with clearly defined cortical and medullary regions (Taub & Longo 2005; Bezuidenhout 1993; Dyce *et al.* 1996b). Immature thymocytes are found within the lobes and are intertwined within a thymic epithelial stroma (Taub & Longo 2005; Hollander 2005). Thymopoiesis (developing and outputting T cells) takes place within the thymic epithelial space, which is the area encompassing both the cortex and the medulla (Aspinall & Andrew 2000; Taub & Longo 2005; Gorgollón & Ottone-Anaya 1978). Surrounding the thymic epithelial space is a perivascular space, which is separated from the thymic epithelial space by a basement membrane (Taub & Longo 2005). No thymocytes are located in the perivascular space.

It is imperative to have a thorough understanding of the various regions of the thymus, and of the changes that occur in the thymus throughout the mammalian lifespan, so that thymic disease can be understood. As development occurs, the thymic epithelial space decreases in size as the perivascular space increases (Taub & Longo 2005). As mammals age, the perivascular space begins to fill with adipocytes, fibroblasts, and lymphoid cells (Taub & Longo 2005). The alteration of the perivascular space to these other cell types is the essential process that leads to thymic atrophy (involution). As thymic atrophy progresses, thymopoiesis decreases, and this results in a reduced capacity for T-cell differentiation within the thymus, which can potentially lead to an increased risk of infection (Taub & Longo 2005; Day 1997; Zlamy & Prelog 2009).

In the dog, the thymus continues to increase in weight until 6 months of age; however, the organ to body weight ratio increases until 2 months and then begins to decrease (Yang & Gawlak 1989). This correlates with the current understanding that the thymus grows in young animals during the first few months of life and then progressively decreases in size during adulthood as atrophy occurs (Bezuidenhout 1993).

The thymus is located in the cranial mediastinum in a cranioventral location (Bezuidenhout 1993; Dyce *et al.* 1996a). When it has reached maximum size it can extend from the sternum ventrally to the trachea dorsally (Aronsohn 1985; Bezuidenhout 1993). The thymus extends more prominently along the left side of the pericardium than along the right (Dyce *et al.* 1996a). The

Small Animal Soft Tissue Surgery, Second Edition. Edited by Eric Monnet.
© 2023 John Wiley & Sons, Inc. Published 2023 by John Wiley & Sons, Inc.
Companion website: www.wiley.com/go/monnet/small

primary thymic blood supply comes from the internal thoracic arteries, which give off the thymic arterial branches that supply both lobes of the thymus (Bezuidenhout 1993; Dyce *et al.* 1996a). Other arterial supply may also originate from the left subclavian artery and the brachiocephalic trunk (Dyce *et al.* 1996a). Venous drainage occurs by thymic veins that are satellites of the thymic arteries. The thymus is innervated by both sympathetic and parasympathetic nerves (Bezuidenhout 1993).

Diagnostics

Clinical signs/physical examination

Thymic pathology is often noted incidentally in dogs and cats during routine geriatric thoracic radiographic screening. When this is the case, owners do not typically report any associated clinical signs (Bellah *et al.* 1983). Despite this, there are certain key physical examination and historical findings that can lead toward a diagnosis of thymic pathology.

Due to the thymic location in the cranial mediastinum and its relative proximity to the respiratory tract, clinical signs seen with thymic disease include dyspnea, coughing, and dysphonia (Day 1997; Bellah *et al.* 1983; Atwater *et al.* 1994; Gores *et al.* 1994; Zitz *et al.* 2008). Other less specific signs include anorexia, lethargy, and weight loss (Aronsohn 1985; Day 1997; Atwater *et al.* 1994; Gores *et al.* 1994; Zitz *et al.* 2008). Megaesophagus may develop secondary to mechanical obstruction from a thymic mass or due to the presence of the paraneoplastic syndrome myasthenia gravis, and clinical signs such as regurgitation and gagging may also be encountered (Aronsohn 1985; Day 1997; Klebanow 1992; Rusbridge *et al.* 1996; Smith *et al.* 2001).

When a diagnosis of vena caval syndrome is made, it is imperative to evaluate for the presence of thymic disease (Peaston *et al.* 1990; Hunt *et al.* 1997; Holsworth *et al.* 2004). Vena caval syndrome is a manifestation of cranial vena caval obstruction, and this can be caused by a mediastinal mass, such as a thymic mass (Hunt *et al.* 1997). Signs associated with this syndrome include distension of the jugular veins (due to increased hydrostatic pressure) and edema, which is most commonly present in the sternal or cervical region or the forelimbs (Hunt *et al.* 1997; Holsworth *et al.* 2004).

Bloodwork

While bloodwork will not provide a specific diagnosis of the thymic pathology that is present, the importance of performing a complete blood count and chemistry profile is in the assessment of anesthetic eligibility, as well as for evaluation of concurrent diseases that might be present. In addition, hypercalcemia is a paraneoplastic syndrome that may be associated with thymomas (Atwater *et al.* 1994; Klebanow 1992; Harris *et al.* 1991). In one study, a dog diagnosed with a thymoma demonstrated resolution of hypercalcemia after removal of the tumor (Harris *et al.* 1991). Additionally, dogs that develop aspiration pneumonia secondary to megaesophagus may have a leukocytosis with left shift (Aronsohn 1985). Elevated troponin levels have been associated with the reported paraneoplastic syndromes of giant cell-like myocarditis, suspected to be secondary to anti-striational antibodies. Myocarditis may be clinically silent unless significant arrhythmias develop, which may be identified on physical examination or during anesthesia. In one dog, myasthenia gravis and polymyositis were also identified consistent with deranged autoimmune activation (Perillo *et al.* 2021).

Radiographs

Due to the location of the thymus in the cranial mediastinum and the involution that occurs during maturity, the normal thymus is generally not seen in adult animals when thoracic radiographs are performed. Radiographs can be very useful in identifying a cranial mediastinal mass, as 86–100% will be noted on thoracic radiographs (Figure 89.1) (Aronsohn 1985; Atwater *et al.* 1994; Gores *et al.* 1994; Zitz *et al.* 2008). For thymomas, regular findings on thoracic radiographs include identification of a soft tissue opacity in the cranial mediastinum, dorsal displacement of the trachea on lateral projections, and widening of the mediastinum in the ventrodorsal projection (Aronsohn 1985; Atwater *et al.* 1994; Gores *et al.* 1994; Zitz *et al.* 2008). Some reports state that a thymoma is likely to exhibit more growth on the left

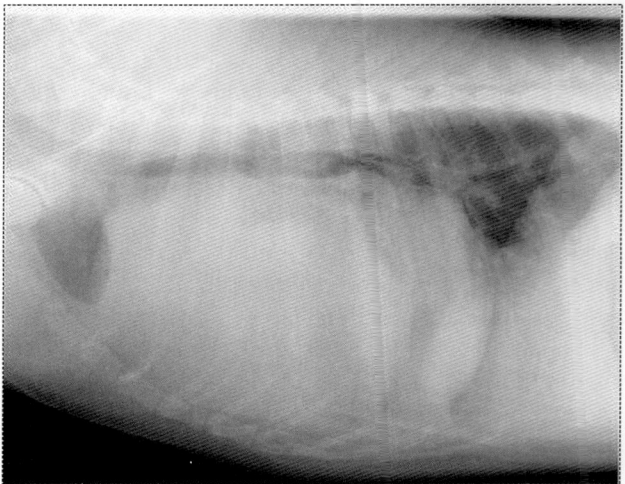

Figure 89.1 Lateral thoracic radiograph of dog with a large thymoma in the cranial mediastinum.

side, which can be detected radiographically (Bellah *et al.* 1983; Hunt *et al.* 1997). Pleural effusion is noted in 25–67% of cases (Atwater *et al.* 1994; Gores *et al.* 1994; Zitz *et al.* 2008). Other potential radiographic findings can include megaesophagus and aspiration pneumonia (Aronsohn 1985; Klebanow 1992). The presence of pulmonary metastatic disease is rare with thymomas, as this tumor is locally invasive but has low metastatic potential (Yang & Gawlak 1989; Gores *et al.* 1994; Robat *et al.* 2013; Martano *et al.* 2021; Turek 2003).

Ultrasound

Ultrasound is useful in the diagnosis of cranial mediastinal masses. Additionally, ultrasound is an excellent tool to aid in fine-needle aspiration and biopsy collection (Gores *et al.* 1994). Thymomas can have variable ultrasonographic appearances. In one study, two dogs and one cat had thymomas that appeared solid with ultrasound evaluation, whereas two dogs and one cat had thymomas that were composed of fluid-filled cavities (Zitz *et al.* 2008). In a study comparing ultrasound characteristics of mediastinal lymphoma to thymoma, cystic and heterogenous appearance was significantly associated with thymoma and may aid in differentiating the two entities (Patterson & Marolf 2014). Pleural effusion is often noted on ultrasonographic examination as well (Zitz *et al.* 2008).

Computed tomography

Computed tomography (CT) is superior to both radiographs and ultrasound in characterizing the extent of thymic disease (Yoon *et al.* 2004; Hylands 2006). One recent study reported on the use of CT in the evaluation of cranial mediastinal masses in dogs and cats (Yoon *et al.* 2004). That study evaluated 9 patients with thymomas, and 7 of 9 demonstrated a maximum tumor width to thoracic width of 70% or greater (Patterson & Marolf 2014). That study further categorized the relationship between the thymoma and regional anatomic structures based on CT (Yoon *et al.* 2004). Findings included that in 83% (dogs) and 67% (cats) thymomas were immediately adjacent to the aortic root; in 50% (dogs) and 100% (cats) thymomas were immediately adjacent to the cranial vena cava; in 11% (dogs) and 33% (cats) compression of the cranial vena cava was noted; 11% of dogs had displacement and compression of the cranial vena cava; 33% of dogs had tumor invasion into the cranial vena cava; 83% (dogs) and 67% (cats) had displacement of the subclavian vessels; 33% of dogs had esophageal displacement; and 50% (dogs) and 33% (cats) had tracheal displacement. CT was found to provide accurate local staging information (Yoon *et al.* 2004). In a large retrospective study of canine CT

scans comparing mediastinal lymphoma to thymic epithelial neoplasia, findings of homogeneity and envelopment of the vena cava were more commonly associated with mediastinal lymphoma, while thymic epithelial neoplasms tended to be more heterogenous (Reeve *et al.* 2020). The injection of intravenous contrast material in concordance with CT imaging is recommended to evaluate the patient for vascular invasion from the thymoma (Rosado-de-Christenson *et al.* 2008).

Magnetic resonance imaging/positron emission tomography

Magnetic resonance imaging (MRI) is not routinely utilized in veterinary or human patients for the evaluation of thymic pathology (Rosado-de-Christenson *et al.* 2008). In one human study, MRI was found to be significantly better at the identification of tumor capsule, intratumoral septa, and intrinsic lesion hemorrhage (Sadohara *et al.* 2006); however, the main utility of MRI would be in assessing the extent of vascular invasion or vascular patency (Rosado-de-Christenson *et al.* 2008).

Positron emission tomography (PET) is not currently readily available in veterinary clinics, but is increasing in use in human medical facilities (Rosado-de-Christenson *et al.* 2008). Advantages of PET for evaluation of thymic disease include improved anatomic localization and improved assessment of lymph nodes for metastatic disease (Rosado-de-Christenson *et al.* 2008). In the future, PET will likely be utilized for staging and restaging of neoplastic disease in veterinary medicine (Rosado-de-Christenson *et al.* 2008).

Cytology/histopathology

The two most common cranial mediastinal masses found in dogs and cats are lymphoma and thymoma (Lana *et al.* 2006). As chemotherapy, and not surgery, is the first-line treatment option for cranial mediastinal lymphoma, determining the diagnosis of a cranial mediastinal mass is of the utmost importance (Zitz *et al.* 2008). Fine-needle aspiration of the cranial mediastinal mass combined with cytologic evaluation is the least invasive means of obtaining a diagnosis. The predominant cells contained within a thymoma are thymic epithelial cells and lymphocytes, but other cell types (mast cells, eosinophils, neutrophils) are often found as well (Atwater *et al.* 1994; Zitz *et al.* 2008; Burkhard & Meyer 1996). A diagnosis has been reported to be obtained by cytologic evaluation in 25–78% of cases (Atwater *et al.* 1994; Gores *et al.* 1994; Zitz *et al.* 2008; Rae *et al.* 1989).

Due to the inconsistent results obtained with cytology of cranial mediastinal masses alone, a recent study evaluated the use of flow cytometry to aid in the diagnosis of these masses (Lana *et al.* 2006). More than 80% of thymocytes express the cell surface markers CD4 and CD8, a trait unique to thymocytes in contrast to lymphocytes (Lana *et al.* 2006). This study found that aspirates producing ≥10% CD4+ CD8+ small lymphocytes were 100% specific for the diagnosis of thymoma. Consequently, if <10% of the small lymphocytes were CD4+ CD8+, thymoma could be eliminated as a differential diagnosis (Lana *et al.* 2006). Fine-needle aspiration with subsequent cytologic evaluation and flow cytometry is recommended when confronted with a mediastinal mass.

In cases where fine-needle aspiration does not reveal a definitive diagnosis, a core biopsy can be considered. Potential complications associated with core biopsy of the thymus include hemorrhage and pneumothorax, and owners should be educated prior to pursuing this diagnostic test. Thymomas often have cystic regions, and biopsies taken in these cystic regions have an increased chance of being nondiagnostic (Aronsohn 1985). Additionally, due to the close association with many of the intrathoracic great vessels and heart, iatrogenic bleeding is possible. It is recommended to utilized ultrasound or CT guidance when performing a core biopsy of thymic pathology. Success rates of preoperatively determining a diagnosis with a core biopsy of a thymoma vary between 50% and 100%; in the study with 100% success, CT guidance was utilized (Atwater *et al.* 1994; Zitz *et al.* 2008). Thoracoscopic-guided thoracic exploratory surgery is progressively becoming more utilized in veterinary medicine, and a biopsy can be performed during this procedure as well.

Staging

Staging of thymic epithelial neoplasia remains a controversial topic in human medicine (Kondo *et al.* 2004; Rena *et al.* 2005; Weydert *et al.* 2009). Thymomas can be either benign or malignant, but histologic differentiation is difficult (Rae *et al.* 1989; Masaoka *et al.* 1981). For this reason, some authors have proposed a staging system for thymomas based on certain characteristics other than histopathologic findings (Masaoka *et al.* 1981). Historically, thymic epithelial neoplasia was divided into four stages, with location of tumor growth, invasiveness, and metastasis being the major considerations (Weydert *et al.* 2009). Other components that assist in staging include the development of a paraneoplastic syndrome or nonthymic malignant tumors (Masaoka *et al.* 1981). Five-year survival rates are different in humans based on the stage: stage I = 92.6%, stage II = 85.7%, stage III = 69.6%, and stage IV = 50%.

The veterinary literature has often adopted the human staging system, and this has been reported in a few

studies (Aronsohn 1985; Bellah *et al.* 1983). In general, the surgeon resecting a thymic epithelial neoplasm should consider the status of the thymic capsule (intact or penetrated by tumor), invasiveness into surrounding organs/blood vessels, and the presence or absence of metastatic disease.

Thymic diseases

Thymoma

A thymoma is a tumor of the thymic epithelial cells; however, variable amounts of lymphocytes are generally found in a thymoma and may predominate (Aronsohn 1985; Zitz *et al.* 2008). Thymomas are uncommon tumors, but when a mass is noted in the cranial mediastinum, the level of suspicion is heightened (Figure 89.2). Several histopathologic subtypes are recognized, including epithelial, lymphocyte rich, and clear cell. Lymphocyte-rich tumors have been associated with a better prognosis in some studies (Zitz *et al.* 2008), although this is not consistently corroborated (Robat *et al.* 2013). Thymic carcinoma, a more histopathologically malignant manifestation of thymic epithelial tumor, has been described in dogs and may have decreased overall survival compared to thymomas (Martano *et al.* 2021; MacIver *et al.* 2017). Other tumors that are commonly noted in the cranial mediastinum include lymphoma, chemodectoma, and ectopic thyroid/parathyroid tumors (Zitz *et al.* 2008). As mentioned previously, diagnosis of a thymoma can be achieved in some cases by cytology; however, the

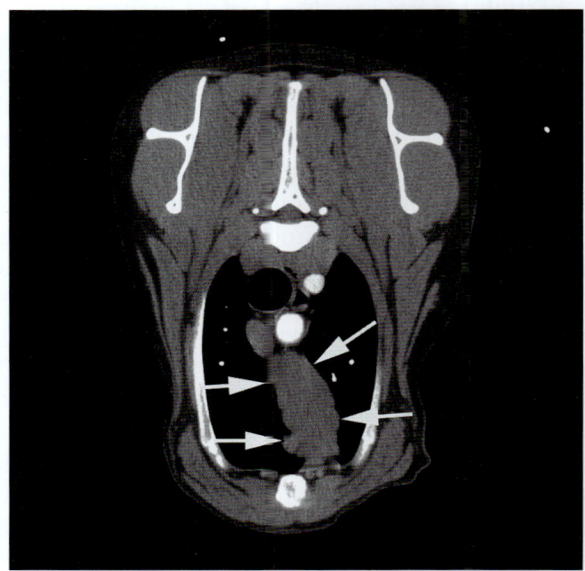

Figure 89.2 Computed tomography angiogram of a dog with a thymoma (white arrows). It is not invading the cranial vena cava or the brachiocephalic trunk.

addition of flow cytometry increases the chance of obtaining a definitive diagnosis (Lana *et al.* 2006).

Several paraneoplastic syndromes have been described in concordance with thymomas. When these syndromes occur, evaluation for a mediastinal mass should be pursued (Aronsohn 1985). The most commonly described paraneoplastic syndrome to occur in conjunction with thymomas is myasthenia gravis (Day 1997; Atwater *et al.* 1994; Gores *et al.* 1994; Zitz *et al.* 2008; Klebanow 1992; Robat *et al.* 2013; Martano *et al.* 2021; Hall *et al.* 1972; Darke 1975; Lainesse *et al.* 1996; Shelton *et al.* 2001; Wood *et al.* 2001; Uchida *et al.* 2002). Myasthenia gravis occurs when acetylcholine receptors are targeted by autoantibodies (Klebanow 1992; Robat *et al.* 2013; Martano *et al.* 2021; Shelton *et al.* 2001; Wood *et al.* 2001; Uchida *et al.* 2002). When the autoantibodies bind to the receptors, neuromuscular transmission at the muscular endplate is halted (Klebanow 1992; Shelton *et al.* 2001; Wood *et al.* 2001). Clinically, this is manifested as muscle weakness and fatigue that can be exacerbated with exercise (Klebanow 1992; Lainesse *et al.* 1996; Shelton *et al.* 2001). Myasthenia gravis also can result in megaesophagus, which can cause regurgitation; this likely occurs due to dysfunction of the striated muscle composition of the canine esophagus (Klebanow 1992; Lainesse *et al.* 1996). Megaesophagus can lead to life-threatening aspiration pneumonia, which may need to be treated before surgical removal of the thymoma can be considered (Klebanow 1992; Lainesse *et al.* 1996). Diagnosis of myasthenia gravis is made by detecting circulating antibodies against the acetylcholine receptors (Lainesse *et al.* 1996; Shelton *et al.* 2001).

The prognosis for improvement of signs associated with myasthenia gravis after removal of a thymoma is variable. Some studies have reported complete resolution of clinical signs associated with myasthenia gravis, and a decrease in acetylcholine receptor antibody after tumor removal (Zitz *et al.* 2008; Darke 1975); however, these findings are not universal (Klebanow 1992; Rusbridge *et al.* 1996). In a recent survey of dogs diagnosed and treated for myasthenia gravis, 11% were diagnosed with concurrent thymomas; a clinical remission rate up to 31% was reported, regardless of whether medical or surgical treatment was pursued (Forgash *et al.* 2021). Dogs and cats should be monitored post thymectomy for continued megaesophagus and owners should be made aware of this possibility, as well as the potential need for use of immunosuppressive medications if myasthenia gravis persists.

Other documented paraneoplastic syndromes that occur in conjunction with thymomas include polymyositis (Perillo *et al.* 2021; Darke 1975), myocarditis (Perillo *et al.* 2021), hypercalcemia (Atwater *et al.* 1994;

Smith *et al.* 2001; Harris *et al.* 1991), neutropenia (O'Connell *et al.* 2018), and exfoliative dermatitis (Scott *et al.* 1995; Forster-van Hijfte *et al.* 1997; Rottenberg *et al.* 2004). The cause of polymyositis is unknown, and the association between thymomas and hypercalcemia is speculative. In one study, a single dog was reported to experience normalization of plasma calcium after thymectomy (Harris *et al.* 1991). Authors have suggested that hypercalcemia associated with thymoma is secondary to the release of a humoral factor from tumor cells that increases systemic bone resorption (Harris *et al.* 1991; Barthez *et al.* 1995). Exfoliative dermatitis, or erythroderma, results in generalized scaling and erythema in cats, and it has been suggested that there is an association with thymomas (Perillo *et al.* 2021; Scott *et al.* 1995; Forster-van Hijfte *et al.* 1997; Rottenberg *et al.* 2004; Singh *et al.* 2010). The condition is generally nonpruritic, and long-term effects can include alopecia and loss of hair coat pigment (Scott *et al.* 1995; Rottenberg *et al.* 2004). The reason for the association between thymoma and exfoliative dermatitis is currently unknown (Scott *et al.* 1995; Rottenberg *et al.* 2004). Regression of exfoliative dermatitis has been noted in two cats that underwent thymectomy, further suggesting a connection between these diseases (Forster-van Hijfte *et al.* 1997; Rottenberg *et al.* 2004).

Surgical resection is the most well-documented treatment modality for thymomas (Atwater *et al.* 1994; Gores *et al.* 1994; Zitz *et al.* 2008). In two retrospective canine case series, outcomes post thymectomy were variable (Atwater *et al.* 1994; Zitz *et al.* 2008). The presence of megaesophagus significantly decreased survival time in one of the studies, likely resulting in the poorer outcomes in that group of dogs (Atwater *et al.* 1994). In dogs without megaesophagus, one-year survival rates range from 64% to 83% (Atwater *et al.* 1994; Zitz *et al.* 2008). Other studies have documented overall median survival time in dogs post thymectomy of 635–1340 days (Zitz *et al.* 2008; Robat *et al.* 2013; Martano *et al.* 2021). In two dogs treated with thoracoscopic resection of thymomas, one died 5 days postoperatively from aspiration pneumonia, and one was alive 18 months postoperatively (Mayhew & Friedberg 2008). A larger retrospective study evaluating dogs undergoing minimally invasive treatment of cranial mediastinal masses identified an intraoperative survival rate of 94%, and 76% of operated dogs were discharged. Importantly, all dogs who died within the perioperative period were diagnosed with myasthenia gravis and megaesophagus (MacIver *et al.* 2017). Orthostatic hypotension secondary to compression of great vessels and possible paraneoplastic derangement of the autonomic nervous system secondary to thymoma during anesthesia has also been reported in one dog (Hansford & Henao-Guerrero 2020). This highlights the importance of cautious and thorough monitoring during anesthesia in companion animals with cranial mediastinal masses. Rates of recurrence following surgical treatment range from 15% to 25% (Zitz *et al.* 2008; Robat *et al.* 2013; Martano *et al.* 2021), with a reported median time to recurrence of 518 days (Robat *et al.* 2013).

In one study, 2 of 12 cats did not survive the immediate postoperative period; in the nonsurviving cats, one cat died secondary to postoperative hemorrhage and the other cat developed a pleural fungal infection (Gores *et al.* 1994). However, none of the other cats in that study developed local tumor recurrence or metastasis for a median follow-up period of 21 months (Gores *et al.* 1994). The median survival time post thymectomy for 9 cats with thymoma in a separate study was 1825 days, and the one-year survival rate was 89% (Zitz *et al.* 2008).

Preoperative planning with a thoracic CT scan can assist the surgeon in being prepared for the degree of tumor invasion that will be encountered intraoperatively. However, in some cases thymectomy is attempted based on CT findings, and complete surgical removal is not possible. Radiation therapy should be considered in those cases (Meleo 1997). Radiation therapy has been evaluated as both a primary treatment and an adjunctive treatment postoperatively (Klebanow 1992; Hitt *et al.* 1987; Kaser-Hotz *et al.* 2001). In a cohort of 20 cases (17 dogs, 3 cats), an overall response rate of 75% was achieved, including two complete responses attributable to radiation therapy alone (Smith *et al.* 2001). The median survival time of the dogs and cats in that study was 248 days and 720 days, respectively (Smith *et al.* 2001). Stereotactic body radiotherapy (SBRT) is a regionally tissue-sparing modality that has been compared to non-modulated radiotherapy in the treatment of thymomas in dogs; median survival time was 250 and 169 days, respectively, in those two groups. The only significant difference between the cohorts was incidence of radiation side effects in the heart and lung, occurring at a much higher rate in the nonmodulated group (71%) compared to the SBRT group (25%) (Trageser *et al.* 2022). Further research evaluating the efficacy and safety of SBRT-based protocols is necessary, but early reports are promising. Presurgical low-dose intensity-modulated radiotherapy of a thymoma combined with intratumoral fluid aspiration led to tumor shrinkage of 80% in one cat, allowing successful surgical removal (Kutara *et al.* 2020).

Thymic lymphoma

In a review of thymic pathology in 66 dogs and cats, 31 (47%) of the cases were diagnosed with thymic lymphoma (Day 1997). However, very little literature has been dedicated to this disease. In a group of 12 dogs, 8 thymic lymphomas were diagnosed ante mortem, but respiratory signs had been previously noted in only 3 of those cases. The majority of dogs experienced nonspecific clinical signs such as vomiting, diarrhea, anorexia, weight loss, and depression (Day 1997). Hypercalcemia was noted in 3 of 5 cases that were evaluated (Day 1997). Cats are more likely to present with respiratory signs related to thymic lymphoma, as 12 of 18 cats in one study presented with dyspnea (Day 1997). Case reports of two dogs with thymic lymphoma with leukemia have also been published (Cheetham & Murphy 1982; Finlay 1982), as has a case report of a puppy that developed hypercalcemia and bone lesions secondary to a thymic lymphoma (Barthez *et al.* 1995).

Other thymic disease

Thymic branchial cysts represent remnants of the branchial arch system of the fetus (Liu *et al.* 1983). The components of the branchial arch system should disappear during normal development, but this does not always occur and can lead to the development of a cystic structure in the thymus (Day 1997; Liu *et al.* 1983). One study in beagles showed that the incidence of branchial arch cysts actually increased with age in that group (Newman 1971). The most common clinical sign in dogs and cats with thymic branchial cysts is dyspnea, being noted in 76% of cases (Liu *et al.* 1983). The presence of pleural effusion is also a regular finding, and the cysts will often rupture, leading to severe chronic inflammatory reactions, hemorrhage, and edema (Liu *et al.* 1983). In a group of seven dogs undergoing resection of thymic branchial cysts, two died intraoperatively, two died from surgical complications postoperatively, and three survived for at least 18 months (Liu *et al.* 1983). A cystic thymus has been reported in two other feline cases: one case in conjunction with myasthenia gravis and one case associated with thymic hyperplasia (Day 1997; O'Dair *et al.* 1991).

Thymic hemorrhage has been reported in several case reports and case series, and the causes in these cases were variable (Day 1997; Klopfer *et al.* 1985; van der Linde-Sipman & van Dijk 1987; Bradley *et al.* 1992; Glaus *et al.* 1993; Coolman *et al.* 1994; Liggett *et al.* 2002). An idiopathic etiology was given to the earliest group of described cases, of which the first 70 reported cases died (Coolman *et al.* 1994). Some have suggested that an increased blood pressure in a thymus that is involuting may cause vessel rupture (van der Linde-Sipman & van Dijk 1987; Bradley *et al.* 1992; Coolman *et al.* 1994). Others have stated that the bleeding encountered within the thymus is secondary to a known trauma or repeated microtrauma (van der Linde-Sipman & van Dijk 1987;

Bradley *et al.* 1992). It is likely that thymic hemorrhage is due to a combination of these events, which ultimately results in the development of idiopathic thymic hemorrhage. A series of dogs that developed thymic hemorrhage secondary to anticoagulant rodenticide intoxication has also been described (Liggett *et al.* 2002).

Surgical management of thymic disease

Most thymic pathology is surgically treated in a similar manner. The discussion of the surgical management here will focus on the removal of thymomas, as this is the most common thymic disease that is encountered.

Surgical approach

The thymus can be approached surgically in three ways: median sternotomy, lateral thoracotomy, and thoracoscopically. The approach chosen is based on the size of the thymic pathology, suspected invasiveness, and clinician preference/experience.

Median sternotomy

For a median sternotomy, the patient is placed in dorsal recumbency and the fur is clipped from the ventral and lateral thorax, extending from the mid-cervical region cranially to the last rib caudally, and dorsally to the dorsal third of the ribs. A skin incision is made extending from a few centimeters cranial to the manubrium to a few centimeters caudal to the xyphoid. The subcutaneous tissues are bluntly and sharply dissected to expose the midline of the sternum. The muscular attachments on the ventral aspect of the sternum are elevated laterally by use of a periosteal elevator and/or electrocautery. An oscillating saw or sternal saw is then used to transect the sternum. When transecting the sternum, a few key principles should be adhered to. First, an attempt should be made to leave the caudal (xyphoid) aspect of the sternum intact. This provides stability to the sternal repair and allows for better reduction of the sternum upon closure. Transecting the manubrium may allow better visualization and assist the surgeon during the dissection process. Second, the saw cut should be oriented in the mid-sternum to avoid accidental transaction of the ribs.

Once the sternum has been split, the thoracic cavity is exposed, and further retraction is performed by placing Finochietto retractors to retract the sternum laterally (Figure 89.3). Connective tissue is often adhered to the sternum, and this will need to be transected to allow for complete visualization of the thymus. The use of electrocautery or vessel-sealant devices for the transection of this tissue is recommended. Care should be taken to avoid causing trauma to the internal thoracic vessels that traverse the region of the sternum.

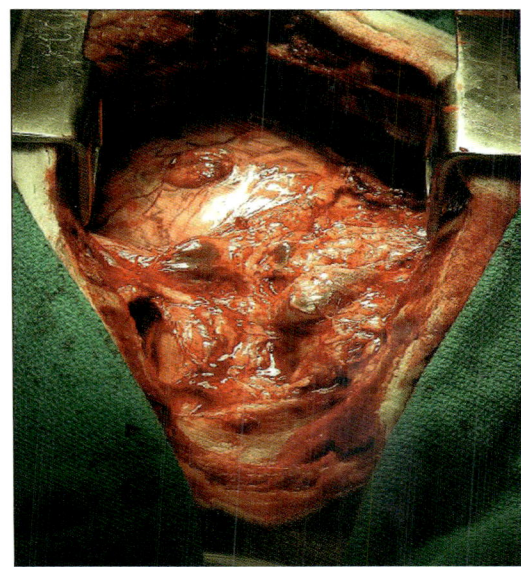

Figure 89.3 Median sternotomy in a dog with a large thymoma.

Lateral thoracotomy

For a lateral thoracotomy, the patient is placed in lateral recumbency, with the side that appears to be more affected (based on auscultation, radiographs, or CT scan) away from the table. If neither side demonstrates a larger proportion of the mass, a left lateral approach should be performed. The lateral thorax is clipped free of fur from the first rib cranially to the thirteenth rib caudally and from the dorsal spinous processes of the vertebrae dorsally to the sternum ventrally. In general, an approach through the fifth or sixth intercostal space is recommended. A skin incision is made extending from the dorsal third of the ribs to the ventral third of the ribs. The subcutaneous tissues are bluntly and sharply dissected to expose the underlying muscles. The panniculus muscle is transected and the latissimus dorsi and scalenus muscles are exposed. The scalenus muscle attaches to the fifth rib caudally and will allow for orientation when this muscle is visualized. The latissimus dorsi and scalenus muscles (or external abdominal oblique muscle if performing a sixth intercostal approach) are transected. Next, the serratus ventralis muscle is separated to expose the intercostal space. The external intercostal muscles will be visualized and are transected, followed by transection of the internal intercostal muscles. The parietal pleura is then visualized and gently transected with scissors. The ribs are spread by use of Finochietto retractors.

Thoracoscopy

To perform a thoracoscopic approach to the thymus, the patient is placed in dorsal recumbency and prepared in the same manner as used for a median sternotomy; this is done so that conversion to an open procedure can be performed if necessary. The patient is tilted slightly to the right side to allow for better access to the left side. A three-port technique is utilized for thoracoscopic thymectomy: (i) paraxyphoid; (ii) right side, eighth intercostal space; and (iii) left side, fourth intercostal space (Mayhew & Friedberg 2008). The paraxyphoid trocar is placed first, and the thoracoscope is introduced through this trocar to perform a thoracic cavity exploration. The left-sided trocar is then placed using thoracoscopic guidance in the fourth intercostal space, followed by placement of the right-sided trocar in the eighth intercostal space (Mayhew & Friedberg 2008).

Procedures

Thymectomy (open approach)

When visualization of the thoracic cavity is achieved, a complete exploration of the thoracic cavity is recommended. For lateral thoracotomy and thoracoscopic approaches, exploration of only the side that has been entered is possible unless the mediastinum is opened. Upon completion of the exploration, the surgeon should gently palpate the extent of the thymic pathology. Due to the location of the thymus within the cranial mediastinum, adherence of tumor to the surrounding vasculature and pericardium is frequently noted (Figure 89.3). Vascular invasion can be evaluated preoperatively with the use of ultrasound and CT; however, the extent is not always appreciated until palpation and visual inspection are performed at the time of surgery.

As thymomas are often very vascular, the use of electrocautery or vessel-sealant units is recommended during dissection. When possible, the goal during initiation of thymoma removal is to isolate a single side of the mass. If the cranial or caudal aspects of the mass can be freed from the surrounding tissue, the thymoma can be mobilized more easily, thereby allowing for better visualization of the great vessels and the heart. If the cranial border of the thymoma can be dissected from the cranial vena cava, then a good plane of dissection can be created from cranial to caudal, preventing accidental penetration of the vena cava. Dissection should continue along the lateral aspect of the thymoma to allow for dissection of the area closest to the great vessels (dorsal); this should not be performed until maximal visualization has been achieved. It is also important to locate the phrenic nerves (dorsolateral), as they are often intertwined within the tumor and/or surrounding tissues. Occasionally, a pericardial resection will need to be performed to obtain a clean margin.

Thoracoscopic thymectomy

Thoracoscopic thymectomy has been reported in dogs, and careful case selection is essential (MacIver et al. 2017; Mayhew & Friedberg 2008). It is not recommended to perform a thoracoscopic thymectomy without advanced imaging (CT), as thoracoscopic techniques should not be pursued if significant vascular invasion exists (MacIver et al. 2017; Mayhew & Friedberg 2008). After placing the trocars as already described, a thoracic exploration is performed. The mediastinal attachments to the thymus are broken down with a blunt probe, vessel-sealant unit (ENSEAL®, Ethicon Endo-Surgery, Cincinnati, OH, USA; or LigaSure™, Valleylab, a division of Tyco Healthcare Group, Boulder, CO, USA), or harmonic scalpel (Harmonic ACE™, Ethicon Endo-Surgery) to allow for exposure to both hemithoraces. The mass is then manipulated with forceps or a grasping instrument to allow for blunt and sharp dissection or exposure to a vessel-sealant unit or harmonic scalpel. Once fully dissected free from the surrounding tissue, the thymoma should be placed in a specimen retrieval bag for removal from the thorax (Mayhew & Friedberg 2008). A chest tube should be placed prior to closure, and closure should proceed with suture placement in the muscle layer, subcutaneous layer, and skin.

Venotomy associated with thymectomy

Tumor invasion into the great vessels is occasionally encountered (Hunt et al. 1997; Holsworth et al. 2004). Partial amputation of the ventral aspect of the tumor should be avoided, but is sometimes necessary to allow for visualization of the invading vessel(s). Prior to undertaking the removal of tumor from within a vessel, the surgeon should consider the length of the venotomy that is needed, as well as the ability to close the incision/defect that is created. A full complement of cardiovascular instruments should be readily available.

To proceed with tumor removal from within a vessel, laparotomy sponges should be used to isolate the vessel from surrounding structures as thoroughly as possible. Rommel tourniquets are then placed proximal and distal to the invaded section of vessel to control bleeding. The pericardium may need to be removed from the vena cava to be able to place a tourniquet between the mass and the right atrium. After the thymoma has been isolated on a pedicle entering the cranial vena cava, the tourniquets are closed to interrupt blood flow. This will likely not affect cardiac function, as the blood flow in the cranial vena cava is already compromised by the presence of the mass.

A stay suture with 5-0 monofilament nonabsorbable polypropylene can be placed on each side of the venotomy to control the wall of the vein. The venotomy is performed by using a no. 11 blade to make an incision on each side of the pedicle. The incision can be extended with scissors. The tumor is gently massaged out of the vessel while an attempt is made to remove the tumor in a single piece (avoiding breakage). The two stay sutures are then grabbed and pulled together to facilitate the placement of a vascular clamp. The vascular clamp is placed along the venotomy incision (with the jaws parallel to the incision), with a goal of not completely occluding the vena cava, and the Rommel tourniquets are gently loosened. A 5-0 monofilament nonabsorbable polypropylene suture line is placed in a simple continuous pattern along the exposed portion of the incision. Alternatively, an interrupted horizontal mattress pattern can be utilized to close the venotomy incision. It is recommended to place pledgets on the sutures to prevent vessel tearing. After suturing is completed, the vascular clamp is gently removed, and the vessel is checked for hemorrhage. If leakage is encountered, the vascular clamp is replaced, and additional sutures are placed where needed.

References

Aronsohn, M. (1985). Canine thymoma. *Veterinary Clinics of North America* 15: 755–767.

Aspinall, R. and Andrew, D. (2000). Thymic involution with aging. *Journal of Clinical Immunology* 20: 250–256.

Atwater, S.W., Powers, B.E., Park, R.D. et al. (1994). Thymoma in dogs: 23 cases (1980–1991). *Journal of the American Veterinary Medical Association* 205: 1007–1013.

Barthez, P.Y., Davis, R., Pool, R.R. et al. (1995). Multiple metaphyseal involvement of a thymic lymphoma associated with hypercalcemia in a puppy. *Journal of the American Animal Hospital Association* 31: 82–85.

Bellah, J.R., Stiff, M.E., and Russell, R.G. (1983). Thymoma in the dog: two case reports and review of 20 additional cases. *Journal of the American Veterinary Medical Association* 183: 306–311.

Bezuidenhout, A.J. (1993). The lymphatic system. In: *Miller's Anatomy of the Dog*, 3e (ed. H.E. Evans), 753–755. Philadelphia, PA: WB Saunders.

Bradley, G.A., Tye, J., Lozano-Alarcon, F. et al. (1992). Hemopericardium in a dog due to hemorrhage originating in a heart base thymic remnant. *Journal of Veterinary Diagnostic Investigation* 4: 211–212.

Burkhard, M.J. and Meyer, D.J. (1996). Invasive cytology of internal organs. *Veterinary Clinics of North America* 26: 1203–1222.

Chapman, A.L. and Bopp, W.J. (1970). Electron microscopy of vascular barrier in thymus, tonsil, and lymph node of beagle pups. *American Journal of Veterinary Research* 31: 1255–1268.

Cheetham, C.J. and Murphy, S.K.B. (1982). Thymic lymphosarcoma cell leukaemia. *Veterinary Record* 110: 457.

Coolman, B.R., Brewer, W.G., D'Andrea, G.H. et al. (1994). Severe idiopathic thymic hemorrhage in two littermate dogs. *Journal of the American Veterinary Medical Association* 205: 1152–1153.

Darke, P.G.G. (1975). Myasthenia gravis, thymoma and myositis in a dog. *Veterinary Record* 97: 392–394.

Day, M.J. (1997). Review of thymic pathology in 30 cats and 36 dogs. *Journal of Small Animal Practice* 38: 393–403.

Dyce, K.M., Sack, W.O., and Wensing, C.J.G. (1996a). The thorax of the carnivores. In: *Textbook of Veterinary Anatomy*, 2e (ed. K.M. Dyce). 412. Philadelphia, PA: WB Saunders.

Dyce, K.M., Sack, W.O., and Wensing, C.J.G. (1996b). The cardiovascular system. In: *Textbook of Veterinary Anatomy*, 2e (ed. K.M. Dyce), 257–258. Philadelphia, PA: WB Saunders.

Finlay, D.E. (1982). Thymic lymphosarcoma-cell leukaemia in a crossbred bitch. *Veterinary Record* 110: 337–338.

Forgash, J.T., Chang, Y.M., Mittelman, N.S. et al. (2021). Clinical features and outcome of acquired myasthenia gravis in 94 dogs. *Journal of Veterinary Internal Medicine* 35 (5): 2315–2326.

Forster-van Hijfte, M.A., Curtis, C.F., and White, R.N. (1997). Resolution of exfoliative dermatitis and *Malassezia pachydermatis* overgrowth in a cat after surgical thymoma resection. *Journal of Small Animal Practice* 38: 451–454.

Glaus, T.M., Rawlings, C.A., Mahaffey, E.A. et al. (1993). Acute thymic hemorrhage and hemothorax in a dog. *Journal of the American Animal Hospital Association* 29: 489–491.

Gores, B.R., Berg, J., Carpenter, J.L. et al. (1994). Surgical treatment of thymoma in cats: 12 cases (1987–1992). *Journal of the American Veterinary Medical Association* 204: 1782–1785.

Gorgollón, P. and Ottone-Anaya, M. (1978). Fine structure of canine thymus. *Acta Anatomica* 100: 136–152.

Hall, G.A., Howell, J.M., and Lewis, D.G. (1972). Thymoma with myasthenia gravis in a dog. *Journal of Pathology* 108: 177–180.

Hansford, J. and Henao-Guerrero, N. (2020). Orthostatic hypotension secondary to a suspected thymoma in a dog: a case report. *BMC Veterinary Research* 16 (1): 388.

Harris, C.L., Klausner, J.S., Caywood, D.D. et al. (1991). Hypercalcemia in a dog with thymoma. *Journal of the American Animal Hospital Association* 27: 281–284.

Hitt, M.E., Shaw, D.P., Hogan, P.M. et al. (1987). Radiation treatment for thymoma in a dog. *Journal of the American Veterinary Medical Association* 190: 1187–1190.

Hollander, G. (2005). Thymic functions related to the pathogenesis of IBD. *Journal of Pediatric Gastroenterology and Nutrition* 40: S10–S12.

Holsworth, I.G., Kyles, A.E., Bailiff, N.L. et al. (2004). Use of a jugular vein autograft for reconstruction of the cranial vena cava in a dog with invasive thymoma and cranial vena cava syndrome. *Journal of the American Veterinary Medical Association* 225: 1205–1210.

Hunt, G.B., Churcher, R.K., Church, D.B. et al. (1997). Excision of a locally invasive thymoma causing cranial vena caval syndrome in a dog. *Journal of the American Veterinary Medical Association* 210: 1628–1630.

Hylands, R. (2006). Veterinary diagnostic imaging: thymoma. *Canadian Veterinary Journal* 47: 593–596.

Kaser-Hotz, B., Rohrer, C.R., Fidel, J.L. et al. (2001). Radiotherapy in three suspect cases of feline thymoma. *Journal of the American Animal Hospital Association* 37: 483–488.

Klebanow, E.R. (1992). Thymoma and acquired myasthenia gravis in the dog: a case report and review of 13 additional cases. *Journal of the American Animal Hospital Association* 28: 63–69.

Klopfer, U., Perl, S., Yakobson, B. et al. (1985). Spontaneous fatal hemorrhage in the involuting thymus of dogs. *Journal of the American Animal Hospital Association* 21: 261–264.

Kondo, K., Yoshizawa, K., Tsuyuguchi, M. et al. (2004). WHO histologic classification is a prognostic indicator in thymoma. *Annals of Thoracic Surgery* 77: 1183–1188.

Kutara, K., Mochizuki, Y., Ohnishi, A. et al. (2020). The outcome and CT findings of low-dose intensity modulated radiation therapy with SQAP in a cat with thymoma. *Veterinary Sciences* 7 (4): 203.

Lainesse, M.F.C., Taylor, S.M., Myers, S.L. et al. (1996). Focal myasthenia gravis as a paraneoplastic syndrome of canine thymoma: improvement following thymectomy. *Journal of the American Animal Hospital Association* 32: 111–117.

Lana, S., Plaza, S., Hampe, K. et al. (2006). Diagnosis of mediastinal masses in dogs by flow cytometry. *Journal of Veterinary Internal Medicine* 20: 1161–1165.

Latimer, H.B. (1954). The prenatal growth of the thymus in the dog. *Growth* 18: 71–77.

Levin, J.M. and Snyder, C.C. (1969). The thymus gland and immunity. *American Surgeon* 35: 321.

Liggett, A.D., Thompson, L.J., Frazier, K.S. et al. (2002). Thymic hematoma in juvenile dogs associated with anticoagulant rodenticide toxicosis. *Journal of Veterinary Diagnostic Investigation* 14: 416–419.

van der Linde-Sipman, J.S. and van Dijk, J.E. (1987). Hematomas in the thymus in dogs. *Veterinary Pathology* 24: 59–61.

Liu, S., Patnaik, A.K., and Burk, R.L. (1983). Thymic branchial cysts in the dog and cat. *Journal of the American Veterinary Medical Association* 182: 1095–1098.

MacIver, M.A., Case, J.B., Monnet, E.L. et al. (2017). Video-assisted extirpation of cranial mediastinal masses in dogs: 18 cases (2009–2014). *Journal of the American Veterinary Medical Association* 250 (11): 1283–1290.

Martano, M., Buracco, P., and Morello, E.M. (2021). Canine epithelial thymic tumors: outcome in 28 dogs treated by surgery. *Animals (Basel)* 11 (12): 3444.

Masaoka, A., Monden, Y., Nakahara, K. et al. (1981). Follow-up study of thymomas with special reference to their clinical stages. *Cancer* 48: 2485–2492.

Mayhew, P.D. and Friedberg, J.S. (2008). Video-assisted thoracoscopic resection of noninvasive thymomas using one-lung ventilation. *Veterinary Surgery* 37: 756–762.

Meleo, K.A. (1997). The role of radiotherapy in the treatment of lymphoma and thymoma. *Veterinary Clinics of North America* 27: 115–129.

Monroe, W.E. and Roth, J.A. (1986). The thymus as part of the endocrine system. *Compendium on Continuing Education for the Practicing Veterinarian* 8: 24–32.

Newman, A.J. (1971). Cysts of branchial arch origin in the thymus of the beagle. *Journal of Small Animal Practice* 12: 681–685.

O'Connell, E., Harper, A., Blundell, R., and Batchelor, D. (2018). Paraneoplastic immune-mediated neutropenia in a dog following thymoma excision with later development of metastatic thymic carcinoma treated with toceranib phosphate. *Veterinary Record Case Reports* 6: e000548.

O'Dair, H.A., Holt, P.E., Pearson, G.R. et al. (1991). Acquired immune-mediated myasthenia gravis in a cat associated with a cystic thymus. *Journal of Small Animal Practice* 32: 198–202.

Patterson, M.M. and Marolf, A.J. (2014). Sonographic characteristics of thymoma compared with mediastinal lymphoma. *Journal of the American Animal Hospital Association* 50 (6): 409–413.

Peaston, A.I., Church, D.B., Allsen, G.S. et al. (1990). Combined chylothorax, chylopericardium, and cranial vena cava syndrome in a dog with thymoma. *Journal of the American Veterinary Medical Association* 197: 1354–1356.

Perillo, R., Menchetti, M., Giannuzzi, P.A. et al. (2021). Acquired myasthenia gravis with concurrent polymyositis and myocarditis secondary to a thymoma in a dog. *Open Veterinary Journal* 11 (3): 436–440.

Rae, C.A., Jacombs, R.M., and Couto, C.G. (1989). A comparison between the cytological and histological characteristics in thirteen canine and feline thymomas. *Canadian Veterinary Journal* 30: 497–500.

Reeve, E.J., Mapletoft, E.K., Schiborra, F. et al. (2020). Mediastinal lymphoma in dogs is homogeneous compared to thymic epithelial neoplasia and is more likely to envelop the cranial vena cava in CT images. *Veterinary Radiology & Ultrasound* 61 (1): 25–32.

Rena, O., Papalia, E., Maggi, G. et al. (2005). World Health Organization histologic classification: an independent prognostic factor in resected thymomas. *Lung Cancer* 50: 59–66.

Robat, C.S., Cesario, L., Gaeta, R. et al. (2013). Clinical features, treatment options, and outcome in dogs with thymoma: 116 cases (1999–2010). *Journal of the American Veterinary Medical Association* 243 (10): 1448–1454.

Rosado-de-Christenson, M.L., Strollo, D.C., and Marom, E.M. (2008). Imaging of thymic epithelial neoplasms. *Hematology/Oncology Clinics of North America* 22: 409–431.

Rottenberg, S., vonTscharner, C., and Roosje, P.J. (2004). Thymoma-associated exfoliative dermatitis in cats. *Veterinary Pathology* 41: 429–433.

Rusbridge, C., White, R.N., Elwood, C.M. et al. (1996). Treatment of acquired myasthenia gravis associated with thymoma in two dogs. *Journal of Small Animal Practice* 36: 376–380.

Sadohara, J., Fujimoto, K., Müller, N.L. et al. (2006). Thymic epithelial tumors: comparison of CT and MR imaging findings of low-risk thymomas, high-risk thymomas, and thymic carcinomas. *European Journal of Radiology* 60: 70–79.

Scott, D.W., Yager, J.A., and Johnson, K.M. (1995). Exfoliative dermatitis in association with thymoma in three cats. *Feline Practice* 23: 8–13.

Shelton, G.D., Skeie, G.O., Kass, P.H. et al. (2001). Titin and ryanodine receptor autoantibodies in dogs with thymoma and late-onset myasthenia gravis. *Veterinary Immunology and Immunopathology* 78: 97–105.

Singh, A., Boston, S.E., and Poma, R. (2010). Thymoma-associated exfoliative dermatitis with post-thymectomy myasthenia gravis in a cat. *Canadian Veterinary Journal* 51: 757–760.

Smith, A.N., Wright, J.C., Brawner, W.R. et al. (2001). Radiation therapy in the treatment of canine and feline thymomas: a retrospective study (1985–1999). *Journal of the American Animal Hospital Association* 37: 489–496.

Taub, D.D. and Longo, D.L. (2005). Insights into thymic aging and regeneration. *Immunological Reviews* 205: 72–93.

Trageser, E., Martin, T., Hoaglund, E. et al. (2022). Outcomes of dogs with thymoma treated with intensity modulated stereotactic body radiation therapy or non-modulated hypofractionated radiation therapy. *Veterinary and Comparative Oncology* 20: 491–501.

Turek, M.M. (2003). Cutaneous paraneoplastic syndromes in dogs and cats: a review of the literature. *Veterinary Dermatology* 14: 279–296.

Uchida, K., Awamura, Y., Nakamura, T. et al. (2002). Thymoma and multiple thymic cysts in a dog with acquired myasthenia gravis. *Journal of Veterinary Medical Science* 64: 637–640.

Weydert, J.A., DeYoung, B.R., and Leslie, K.O. (2009). Recommendations for the reporting of surgically resected thymic epithelial tumors. *American Journal of Clinical Pathology* 132: 10–15.

Wood, S.L., Rosenstein, D.S., and Bebchuk, T. (2001). Myasthenia gravis and thymoma in a dog. *Veterinary Record* 148: 573–574.

Yang, T.J. and Gawlak, S.L. (1989). Lymphoid organ weights and organ:body weight ratios of growing beagles. *Lab Animal* 23: 143–146.

Yoon, J., Feeney, D.A., Cronk, D.E. et al. (2004). Computed tomographic evaluation of canine and feline mediastinal masses in 14 patients. *Veterinary Radiology & Ultrasound* 45: 542–546.

Zitz, J.C., Birchard, S.J., Couto, G.C. et al. (2008). Results of excision of thymoma in cats and dogs: 20 cases (1984–2005). *Journal of the American Veterinary Medical Association* 232: 1186–1192.

Zlamy, M. and Prelog, M. (2009). Thymectomy in early childhood: a model for premature T cell immunosenescence? *Rejuvenation Research* 12: 249–258.

Index

Note: Page references in *italics* refer to Figures; those in **bold** refer to Tables.

Small Animal Soft Tissue Surgery, Second Edition. Edited by Eric Monnet.
© 2023 John Wiley & Sons, Inc. Published 2023 by John Wiley & Sons, Inc.
Companion website: www.wiley.com/go/monnet/small